NEURAL BLOCKADE

IN CLINICAL ANESTHESIA AND MANAGEMENT OF PAIN

edited by

MICHAEL J. COUSINS, M.B.,B.S., M.D. (SYD.), F.F.A.R.A.C.S., F.F.A.R.C.S.
Professor and Chairman
Department of Anaesthesia and Intensive Care and
Chairman, Pain Management Unit
Flinders Medical Centre
The Flinders University of South Australia
Adelaide, Australia

PHILLIP O. BRIDENBAUGH, M.D.

Professor and Chairman
Department of Anesthesia
University of Cincinnati Medical Center College of Medicine
Cincinnati, Ohio

Cover illustration and color illustrations by Alan Bentley
Department of Medical Illustration and Media
Flinders Medical Centre
Adelaide, Australia

With 41 Contributors

NEURAL BLOCKADE

IN CLINICAL ANESTHESIA AND MANAGEMENT OF PAIN

Second Edition

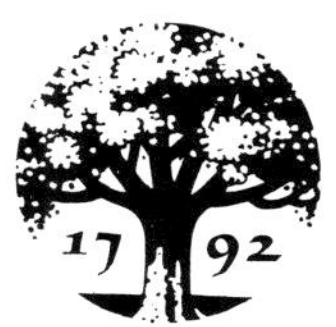

J. B. LIPPINCOTT COMPANY
PHILADELPHIA
LONDON NEW YORK SÃO PAULO
MEXICO CITY ST. LOUIS SYDNEY

Acquisitions Editor: Susan M. Gay
Sponsoring Editor: Sanford Robinson
Manuscript Editor: Leslie E. Hoeltzel
Indexer: Ruth Elwell
Design Director: Tracy Baldwin
Design Coordinator: Don Shenkle
Designer: Maria S. Karkucinski
Production Manager: Kathleen P. Dunn
Production Coordinator: Caren Erlichman
Compositor: Digitype, Inc.
Printer/Binder: Kingsport Press
Insert Printer: Princeton Polychrome Press

2nd Edition

6 5 4 3 2

Library of Congress Cataloging in Publication Data

Neural blockade in clinical anesthesia and management of pain.

Includes bibliographies and index.
1. Nerve block. 2. Nerves—Effect of drugs on. 3. Pain—Physiological aspects. I. Cousins, Michael J. II. Bridenbaugh, Phillip O., 1932– . [DNLM: 1. Nerve Block. 2. Pain—therapy. WO 300 N494]
RD84.N48 1987 617'.96 86-21443
ISBN 0-397-50562-0

The authors and publisher have exerted every effort to ensure that drug selection and dosage set forth in this text are in accord with current recommendations and practice at the time of publication. However, in view of ongoing research, changes in government regulations, and the constant flow of information relating to drug therapy and drug reactions, the reader is urged to check the package insert for each drug for any change in indications and dosage and for added warnings and precautions. This is particularly important when the recommended agent is a new or infrequently employed drug.

To patients with acute or chronic pain

The theoretical and practical information in this text is dedicated to more enlightened and effective use of neural blockade for the management of all types of pain and for prevention of the harmful sequelae of severe unrelieved pain.

CONTRIBUTORS

C. Richard Bennett, D.D.S., Ph.D., F.A.C.D.
Professor and Chairman, Department of Anesthesia, University of Pittsburgh School of Dental Medicine; Staff Anesthesiologist, Presbyterian–University Hospital, Pittsburgh, Pennsylvania

Robert A. Boas, M.B., B.S., F.F.A.R.A.C.S.
Associate Professor, Department of Pharmacology and Clinical Pharmacology, University of Auckland School of Medicine, Auckland, New Zealand

Nikolai Bogduk, M.B., Ph.D., Dip. Anat.
Senior Lecturer in Anatomy, Visiting Medical Officer to the Pain Clinic, Princess Alexandra Hospital, University of Queensland, Brisbane, Queensland, Australia

John J. Bonica, M.D., D.Sc.
Emeritus Professor, Department of Anesthesiology, University of Washington, Seattle, Washington

L. Donald Bridenbaugh, M.D.
Professor, Department of Anesthesiology, The Mason Clinic, Seattle, Washington

Phillip O. Bridenbaugh, M.D.
Professor and Chairman, Department of Anesthesia, University of Cincinnati College of Medicine, Cincinnati, Ohio

Philip R. Bromage, M.B., B.S., F.F.A.R.A.C.S.
Formerly Professor and Chairman, Department of Anesthesiology, University of Colorado Health Sciences Center, Denver, Colorado
Currently Professor of Anaesthesia, King Khalid University Hospital, Riyadh, Saudi Arabia

T. C. Kester Brown, M.D., F.F.A.R.A.C.S.
Director, Department of Anaesthesia, Royal Childrens' Hospital, Parkville, Victoria, Australia

Peter Brownridge, M.B., Ch.B., D.R.C.O.G., F.F.A.R.C.S.
Senior Lecturer and Director of Obstetric Anaesthesia, Department of Anaesthesia and Intensive Care, Flinders Medical Centre, The Flinders University of South Australia, Adelaide, South Australia, Australia

Robert Chase, M.D.
Emile Holman Professor of Surgery, Stanford University Medical Center, Stanford, California

David A. Cherry, M.B., B.S., F.F.A.R.A.C.S.
Director, Pain Management Unit, Department of Anaesthesia and Intensive Care, Flinders Medical Centre, Adelaide, South Australia, Australia

Sheila E. Cohen, M.B., B.S., F.F.A.R.C.S.
Associate Professor of Anesthesia (Clinical), Co-Director of Obstetric Anesthesia, Department of Anesthesia, Stanford University School of Medicine, Stanford, California

Michael J. Cousins, M.B., B.S., M.D., (Syd.), F.F.A.R.A.C.S., F.F.A.R.C.S.
Professor and Chairman, Department of Anaesthesia and Intensive Care, Flinders Medical Centre, The Flinders University of South Australia, Adelaide, South Australia, Australia

Benjamin G. Covino, Ph.D., M.D.
Professor and Chairman, Department of Anesthesia, Brigham and Women's Hospital, Harvard Medical School, Boston, Massachusetts

Brian Dwyer, M.B., B.S. (Sydney), F.F.A.R.C.S., F.F.A.R.A.C.S.
Formerly Director of Anaesthesia and Director of Pain Clinic, Department of Anaesthesia, St. Vincent's Hospital, Sydney, New South Wales, Australia

Lorne Eltherington, M.D.
Associate Professor of Anesthesia (Clinical), Director, Stanford Pain Service, Stanford University Medical Center, Stanford, California

Marianne E. Feitl, M.D.
Department of Ophthalmology, Washington University School of Medicine, St. Louis, Missouri

B. Raymond Fink, M.D.
Professor Emeritus, Department of Anesthesiology, University of Washington, Seattle, Washington

David Gibb, M.B., B.S. (Sydney), M.Sc. (Med), F.F.A.R.C.S., F.F.A.R.A.C.S.
Chairman, Department of Anaesthetics, St. Vincent's Hospital, Darlinghurst, New South Wales, Australia

Geoffrey K. Gourlay, Ph.D.
Principal Hospital Scientist and Lecturer, Pain Management Unit, Department of Anaesthesia and Intensive Care, Flinders Medical Centre, The Flinders University of South Australia, Adelaide, South Australia, Australia

Nicholas M. Greene, M.D.
Professor, Department of Anesthesiology, Yale University School of Medicine, New Haven, Connecticut

C. McK. Holmes, M.B., B.Ch., F.F.A.R.C.S., F.F.A.R.A.C.S.
Consultant Anaesthetist, Department of Anaesthesia and Intensive Care, University of Otago Medical School, Dunedin Hospital, Dunedin, New Zealand

Jordan Katz, M.D.
Professor of Anesthesiology, University of California, San Diego, La Jolla, California

Henrik Kehlet, M.D., Ph.D.
Professor, Department of Surgical Gastroenterology, Hvidovre Hospital, Hvidovre, Denmark

Theodore Krupin, M.D.
Chief of Glaucoma Service, Department of Ophthalmology, Scheie Eye Institute, Presbyterian–University of Pennsylvania Medical Center, Philadelphia, Pennsylvania

J. Bertil Löfström, M.D., Ph.D.
Professor, Department of Anesthesiology, Linkoping University, Linkoping, Sweden

Laurence E. Mather, Ph.D., F.F.A.R.A.C.S.
Reader, Department of Anaesthesia and Intensive Care, Flinders Medical Centre, The Flinders University of South Australia, Adelaide, South Australia, Australia

Ronald Melzack, Ph.D.
Professor, Department of Psychology, McGill University, Montreal, Quebec, Canada

Daniel C. Moore, M.D.
Professor, Department of Anesthesiology, University of Washington, Seattle, Washington

Terence M. Murphy, M.B., Ch.B., F.F.A.R.C.S.
Professor, Department of Anesthesiology, University of Washington School of Medicine, Seattle, Washington

Robert R. Myers, Ph.D.
Associate Professor of Anesthesiology and Neurosciences, University of California, San Diego, School of Medicine, La Jolla, California

P. Prithvi Raj, M.D.
Professor, Department of Anesthesiology, University of Texas Medical Center, Houston, Texas

Otto Schulte-Steinberg, M.D.D.A. (McGill)
Formerly Chief, Department of Anaesthesia, Keiskrankenhaus, Starnberg, Germany

D. Bruce Scott, M.D., F.R.C.P.E., F.F.A.R.C.S.
Consultant Anaesthetist, Department of Anaesthetics, Royal Infirmary, Edinburgh, Scotland

Gary R. Strichartz, Ph.D.
Associate Professor of Pharmacology in Anesthesia, Department of Anesthesia, Brigham and Women's Hospital, Harvard Medical School, Boston, Massachusetts

Mark Swerdlow, M.D., M.Sc., F.F.A.R.C.S., D.A.
Formerly Director, North West Regional Pain Relief Centre, Hope Hospital, University of Manchester School of Medicine, Salford, England

Ronald R. Tasker, M.D.
Professor, Department of Surgery, University of Toronto; Head, Division of Neurosurgery, Toronto General Hospital, Toronto, Ontario, Canada

Gale E. Thompson, M.D.
Director, Department of Anesthesiology, The Mason Clinic, Seattle, Washington

Geoffrey T. Tucker, B.Pharm., Ph.D.
Reader in Clinical Pharmacology and Therapeutics, Department of Therapeutics, University of Sheffield Medical School, Royal Hallamshire Hospital, Sheffield, England

Richard J. Willis, M.B., B.S., F.F.A.R.A.C.S.
Senior Specialist Anaesthetist, Department of Anaesthesia and Intensive Care, Flinders Medical Centre, Adelaide, South Australia, Australia

Tony L. Yaksh, Ph.D.
Professor, Section of Neurosurgical Research, Mayo Clinic, Rochester, Minnesota

FOREWORD

Neural Blockade in Clinical Anesthesia and Management of Pain must be the most ambitious project of its kind ever undertaken. This book ranges from a consideration of the physiology, pharmacology, and toxicology of the local analgesic agents in common use to a number of the less orthodox methods of relieving suffering of various origins. The book is indeed encyclopedic in its coverage, and, like encyclopedias in other sciences, each section has been entrusted to a recognized world authority in his own special field. No book on local analgesia could have a sounder pedigree.

There are situations in which, manifestly, local anesthesia is preferable to general. Apart from these, improved sedation and longer-acting analgesic drugs have improved patient acceptance, but the practitioner still has to acquire the necessary "know-how" to deposit the solution with reasonable accuracy for it to be effective. Both editors are renowned for their practical teaching, which should be a sound guarantee that both the expert and the tyro can turn to this book for guidance and profit.

Neural blockade offers far more to the patient than merely analgesia during surgery. Rapid growth in application of neural blockade to postoperative, post-traumatic, and obstetric pain management is extensively covered in this textbook. Even more extensive is the breadth and depth of scientific information and clinical application of neural blockade in chronic pain; this is presented as completely and concisely as possible.

Sir Robert Macintosh,
D.M., F.R.C.S. (EDIN), HON F.F.A.R.C.S.,
England, Ireland, Australasia
Emeritus Nuffield Professor of Anaesthetics, University of Oxford

PREFACE

The Second Edition of *Neural Blockade in Clinical Anesthesia and Management of Pain* is substantially larger and more comprehensive than the textbook that first appeared in 1980 under this name. This is a reflection of some very considerable advances in the knowledge of anatomy, physiology, and pharmacology of neural blockade and in the techniques of neural blockade. To a greater extent, it reflects a very rapid rate of development of knowledge and of improved treatment for all forms of severe pain. We, the editors, have chosen authors for the 36 chapters on the basis of their preeminence; thus the book retains an international flavor, with authors drawn from ten countries: Australia, Canada, Denmark, England, Germany, New Zealand, Scotland, Sweden, Saudi Arabia, and the United States of America. In this Second Edition are 24 new contributors, all of whom have played a key role in the field that is the subject of their chapter.

In the field of *acute pain* substantial advances in basic and clinical research have been very rapidly applied to the treatment of surgical and postoperative pain, obstetric pain, and, to a lesser extent, pain in patients with acute medical conditions and in the critical care setting. Advances in physiology and pharmacology have been so great that every chapter in Part One has been completely rewritten by the acknowledged authorities. A new chapter has been added that discusses the effects of neural blockade on the response to surgical trauma. The chapters of Part Two detail the techniques of neural blockade, and each chapter has been very substantially rewritten as a result of developments in basic knowledge, refinement of existing methods, and description of new techniques. Such advances reflect a continuation of the increased scientific and clinical activity that convinced us of the need for this book.

Interest in the causes and treatment of *chronic pain* has been more intense than in any other field of medicine. Part Three of *Neural Blockade* is greatly expanded and begins with an overview of acute and chronic pain, including a summary of the new international classification of chronic pain syndromes and descriptions of pain terms. This is followed by 11 new chapters and 1 chapter from the First Edition that has been greatly expanded. The extensive literature on neurologic mechanisms of pain is distilled into easily readable form. Psychological aspects of pain are summarized and implications for neural blockade highlighted. The wide range of techniques now available for *acute* pain management is placed in a very practical context. Diagnostic, prognostic, and therapeutic local anesthetic blocks are critically examined, and guidance is given on the role they play in comparison to other options now available. Back pain is accorded its own chapter, with some original information that challenges traditional ideas. The intense scientific and clinical interest in spinal opioids indicated the need for a new major chapter that discusses the scientific basis and use of the techniques in acute and chronic pain. Another new chapter provides very recent information on the neuropathology of neurolytic agents and other drugs, including local anesthetics. Neurolytic and neurodestructive techniques have been refined and greatly expanded since the First Edition, and these sections have been revised and expanded accordingly. Neurostimulation by both transcutaneous and dorsal column (epidural) techniques has also been refined, and its place in the treatment of acute and chronic pain is discussed. The use of neural blockade in the multidisciplinary pain clinic is presented by the founding father of this important concept of pain management.

Since the First Edition, there has been a further increase in the use of neural blockade for surgery and for acute pain relief, in part because of a better understanding of the pharmacology, physiology, and anatomy of neural blockade. Emphasis on practical teaching of neural blockade techniques in anesthesiology training programs has also played a major role in this resurgence of use of neural blockade. Professional organizations such as the American and European Societies of Regional Anesthesia have played an important part. Patients have begun to perceive that there is often an alternative to general anesthesia. This is in part a "spin off" of a large increase in the successful use of epidural blockade for cesarean section and in the performance of much "day surgery" under local and regional anesthesia.

The huge costs of chronic pain in terms of human suffering, and the financial burden, have reached prominence in the eyes of the public and governments. The high annual costs in the United States (more than $50 billion) have been confirmed in other countries. This has stimulated the formation of special governmental advisory groups with the aim of defining research and treatment strategies to improve treatment of chronic pain. Cancer pain has been identified as a major world health problem, as has noncancer pain. The World Health Organization (WHO) and the International Association for the Study of Pain (IASP) are collaborating in programs to improve education about the treatment of chronic pain and to implement effective treatment throughout the world. Techniques of neural blockade play a part in diagnosis and treatment of chronic pain. Properly applied, they may relieve the suffering of many patients; however, it is emphasized in many places in this book that neural blockade must be used in the context of a full range of physical and psychological assessments and as only one of the options for treatment of pain. The aim of those treating pain should always be to use the simplest and least invasive options that will relieve pain before progressing to more invasive approaches. *Neural Blockade in Clinical Anesthesia and Management of Pain* aims to give a balanced view of the safe and effective use of neural blockade and to provide a critical review of those situations in which it may be helpful to patients in pain.

MICHAEL J. COUSINS, M.B., B.S., M.D.
PHILLIP O. BRIDENBAUGH, M.D.

ACKNOWLEDGMENTS

The Second Edition of *Neural Blockade in Clinical Anesthesia and Management of Pain* has been an even larger undertaking than the First Edition. As indicated in the Preface extraordinary growth in this exciting field over the past 7 years has made it necessary to add 24 new authors out of a total of 41 contributors from ten different countries. The administrative and logistical exercise of developing the book and bringing it to the final stage has placed great demands on the two editors, on their staff, their families, and the publisher. The editors wish to thank their professional colleagues in the Department of Anaesthesia and Intensive Care, Flinders Medical Centre, Flinders University of South Australia, and the Department of Anesthesia, University of Cincinnati, for their support, interest, and understanding. In Adelaide, particular thanks are due to Josephine O'Grady, secretary to Professor Cousins, and in Cincinnati to Marianne Cost, secretary to Professor Bridenbaugh.

The love and support of the editors' families made it possible for the editors to cope with the demands of the Second Edition; it helped greatly to know that the families believed their work was worthwhile.

To their teachers and peers, the editors owe their early interest in the scientific basis and clinical aspects of neural blockade and pain management. Professor Cousins developed his interest in neural blockade while working with Professor Philip Bromage at McGill University, Montreal; while at McGill his interest in pain was kindled by the lectures of Professor Ronald Melzack on the new Melzack–Wall "Gate Theory of Pain." He subsequently developed a commitment to the multidisciplinary approach to pain management as a result of working closely with Professor John Bonica on the Council of the International Association for the Study of Pain. Editorial skills can, to a degree, be learned "on the job"; however, a term on the editorial board of *Anesthesia and Analgesia* provided superb experience under the masterly leadership of Nicholas M. Greene. At Stanford University a keen appreciation was gained of scientific method and critical appraisal of the scientific literature from Professors Richard Mazze, John P. Bunker, Ellis Cohen, and C. Philip Larson, Jr.

Professor Bridenbaugh began his clinical and academic involvement in neural blockade at the very start of his specialist career while at the Virginia Mason Clinic in Seattle (Drs. L. D. Bridenbaugh and Daniel C. Moore). He subsequently began a commitment to scientific work in this field while at Stanford University, then at Oxford University (Sir Robert Macintosh) and also in association with Professor Ben Covino (Harvard University). His knowledge and his perspective of neural blockade have been greatly influenced by his colleagues in the American Society of Regional Anesthesia and by his experience as an editor and then as Editor-in-Chief of *Regional Anesthesia.*

The editors have been fortunate to have the services of a medical illustrator of extraordinary talent. Alan Bentley of the Department of Medical Illustration and Media, Flinders Medical Centre, prepared the artwork for the cover and drew all of the color illustrations and many of the anatomic illustrations in black and white. Each one of these figures resulted from observation of actual block procedures and anatomic dissections, careful study of many original source materials, and long hours of discussion. The editors thank Alan Bentley for his artistic skill while preserving anatomic integrity and his willingness to persevere with the editors' and authors' attempts to explain the practical points they wished to illustrate.

Particular thanks are due to Sir Robert Macintosh and E & S Livingstone, Edinburgh, for granting permission to redraw and adapt a number of illustrations from Sir Robert's classic monographs: *Local Analgesia, Abdominal Surgery* (1962); *Local Analgesia, Head and Neck,* Second Edition (1955); and *Lumbar Puncture and Spinal Analgesia* (edited by J. A. Lee and R. S. Atkinson, 1978). Many other authors and publishers gave permission for their works to be quoted or reproduced, and due acknowledgment has been given in the text.

Color illustrations are very expensive but are believed to be essential in a textbook relying on anatomic clarity. The use of color was supported by Astra Chemicals, Australia and the United States; Ciba-Geigy, Australia; Roche, Australia; Glaxo Company, Australia; and Spembly Ltd, England.

The First Edition of *Neural Blockade in Clinical Anesthesia and Management of Pain* was begun by Professor Michael Cousins and the then Editor-in-Chief of Medical Books, The J. B. Lippincott Company, Mr. Lewis Reines. Soon afterward Professor Phillip Bridenbaugh began working on the book, and both editors rapidly appreciated the benefits of a running partner. The Second Edition has been the result of a very close and rewarding collaboration between the two editors. The staff of J. B. Lippincott, acknowledged on page iv, have been of great assistance. Particular thanks are due to J. Stuart Freeman, Jr., Sanford Robinson, and Leslie E. Hoeltzel.

In Adelaide, Michele Cousins, B.A., provided editorial assistance to Professor Cousins, proofread a substantial portion of the manuscript, and checked the extensive bibliography.

CONTENTS

INTRODUCTION

part one

PHARMACOLOGY AND PHYSIOLOGY OF NEURAL BLOCKADE

part two

TECHNIQUES OF NEURAL BLOCKADE

NEURAL BLOCKADE

IN CLINICAL ANESTHESIA AND MANAGEMENT OF PAIN

INTRODUCTION

1 HISTORY OF NEURAL BLOCKADE

B. RAYMOND FINK

PHYSIOLOGY OF PAIN

Fundamental to modern neural blockade is the concept that pain is a sensory warning conveyed by specific nerve fibers, amenable, in principle, to modulation or interruption anywhere in the nerve's pathway. This outlook may be traced back to developments in the study of physiology that finally supplanted the view, first expressed by Plato and Aristotle, that pain, like pleasure, is a passion of the soul, that is, an emotion and not one of the senses. Philosophical changes ensuing on the great revolutions of the 18th century and the birth of biology gradually, although not entirely, effaced the religious connotations of pain in Western civilization.[19]

The doctrine of specific energies of the senses was first promulgated by Johannes P. Mueller (1801–1858) in 1826.[73] This doctrine, although it did not posit specificity for the conduction of pain, initiated the movement of scientific thought toward analysis and classification of the specific characters of different nerves. The theory that pain was a separate and distinct sense was first definitely formulated by Moritz S. Schiff (1823–1896) in 1858, following experiments on animals.[25] Its rival, the intensity theory, was stated explicitly by Erb in 1874 but had been anticipated by Erasmus Darwin (1731–1802), who said that pain results "whenever the sensorial motions are stronger than usual."[25] Attempts to influence neuralgic pain by applying a drug to the transmitting nerve appear first to have been published by Francis Rynd (1801–1861).[75] Rynd's idea may be said to have foreshadowed both nerve block and, at a remoter stretch, opioid regional analgesia.

According to some accounts of the 1850s, Pravaz in Lyon and Wood in Edinburgh respectively invented the syringe and hypodermic hollow needle. A thorough sifting of the historical evidence[47] and independent reexamination of the sources support the following outline of the facts. Rynd in 1845 described the idea of introducing a solution of morphine hypodermically in the neighborhood of a peripheral nerve,[75] with the intention of allaying neuralgic pain in that nerve. However, he introduced the solution not by syringe but by means of gravity, allowing it to enter passively through a cannula after removal of the trocar. The moment of invention of the syringe is lost in the mists of several centuries preceding Alexander Wood (1817–1884). Wood's contribution was his procedure of subcutaneous injection, which he performed in 1855 with a graduated glass syringe and hollow needle supplied by Ferguson.[91] This equipment had been manufactured by Ferguson for a different purpose, namely the injection of ferric perchloride into an aneurysm to produce a coagulum, as proposed by Charles-Gabriel Pravaz (1791–1853) in 1853 following experiments in animals;[69] Pravaz himself had used a syringe and trocar ("trois-carre"). Wood thus originated the practice of percutaneous subcutaneous injection to medicate locally a peripheral nerve. His technique was adopted by C. Hunter and renamed hypodermic injection, ostensibly because Hunter had in view a different purpose, to wit, systemic absorption of the drug.

Carl Koller (1857–1944; Fig. 1-1) searched for a surgical local surface anesthetic and hit upon cocaine in 1884, and immediately demonstrated its startling

This account is based on dates of first publication and generally omits anecdotal priorities.

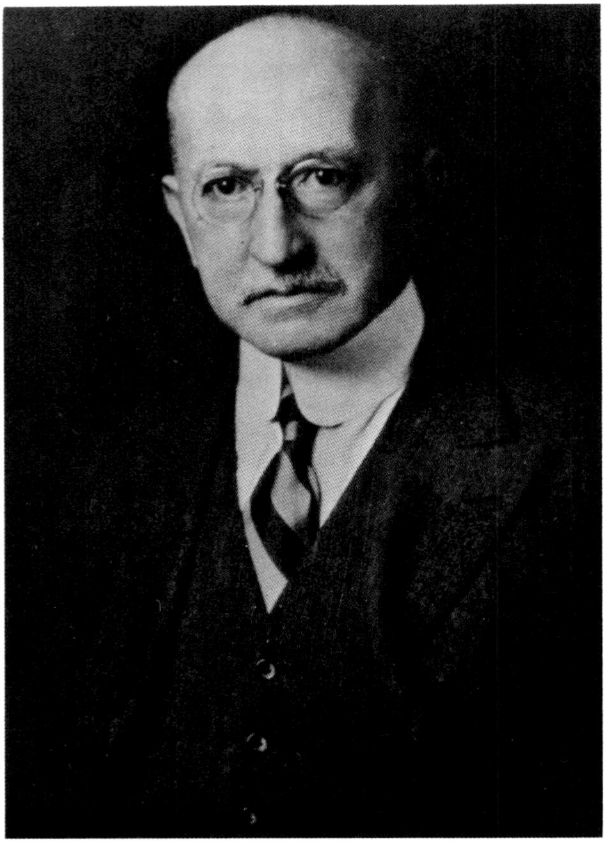

FIG. 1-1. Carl Koller, M.D. (1857–1944)

effectiveness on the cornea.[50] This opened the vast new world of local and regional analgesic therapy. James Leonard Corning (1855–1923)[22] conceived and attempted the direct application of an analgesic to the spinal cord, but a defective rationale and unserviceable technique stultified his approach to the management of chronic pain. A deeper knowledge of the underlying mechanisms was requisite. Understanding of these mechanisms remained relatively superficial until the era of electrophysiologic and neuropharmacologic microexploration following World War II.

Melzack and Wall's hypothesis that a spinal gate controls the cephalad transmission of nociception[64] was based on evidence suggesting that the intensity and quality of pain perceived do not bear a push-button, straight-through, one-to-one relationship to the intensity of the stimulus, but are instead determined by a multiplicity of physiologic and psychologic variables. This led directly to the reintroduction of electrical stimulation as a method of treating chronic pain. The search for the mechanism of opiate analgesia and opiate addiction resulted in Reynolds' spectacular demonstration in 1969 of the analgesic effect of electrical stimulation of the periaqueductal gray matter.[72] This seminal discovery gave enormous impetus to pain research and led to the uncovering of a system of descending neurons that inhibit pain and are activated by opiate drugs acting at endorphinergic synapses. Brilliant experimental work in rats enabled Yaksh and Rudy[93] to produce analgesia mediated by a direct spinal action of narcotics, a landmark advance from which important clinical developments have sprung. The progression of clinical applications sharply illustrates the process and value of basic medical research (see Appendix A at the end of this chapter).

COCAINE ANESTHESIA

The mid-nineteenth century was a period of growing ferment in Western science and technology. In 1865, six years after the publication of Charles Darwin's epochal book, Lister opened a new era in surgery by applying Pasteur's proof of nonspontaneous generation to the elimination of sepsis. Pflüger showed that the seat of respiration was in the tissues and not in the blood, and in 1882, the same year that produced the world's first electrical power station (in New York), Ringer demonstrated the need for calcium and potassium salts to maintain the excitability of the heart. The establishment of the coal tar industry in Germany led to large-scale production of pharmaceuticals, of which the marketing of cocaine by Merck was one result. The year 1886 saw the introduction of steam sterilization of dressings by von Bergmann, and the year 1890, the use of surgical rubber gloves, initially for the purpose of protecting the hands of Halsted's instrument nurse from disinfectant.

Koller's demonstration of ocular surface anesthesia with cocaine[50] had antecedents almost as numerous as those of general anesthesia 40 years earlier. Albert Niemann (1834–1861) was successful in isolating and naming the alkaloid from the leaves of *Erythroxylon coca,* as first recorded in 1860 in a report signed W. (for H. Wöhler), which also related the passionate chewing of the leaves by the *coqueros* of Peru and the deleterious mental effects this had on them.[65] A thorough pharmacologic investigation of the properties of the alkaloid in frogs was presented by von Anrep in 1880 in a 35-page report, which ended as follows:

"the animal experiments have no practical application; nevertheless I would recommend trying cocaine as a local anesthetic in persons of melancholy disposition."[87] Plainly, von Anrep was most impressed by the stimulating properties of cocaine, and these seem also to have been uppermost in the mind of Sigmund Freud (1856 – 1939) when he suggested a study of the drug to Koller.[6]

Freud wanted to know more about the analeptic action of cocaine, which, he hoped, because of reports from the United States, might be useful in curing one of his great friends of addiction to morphine. This friend was a pathologist and had developed an unbearably painful thenar neuroma after accidentally cutting himself while performing an autopsy. Freud obtained a supply of cocaine from the manufacturing firm of Merck and shared it with Koller, who was to help him investigate its effects on the nervous system. Koller was a junior intern in the Ophthalmological Clinic at the University of Vienna and longed to obtain the coveted appointment of assistant in the clinic, on the strength of a worthy piece of research. The research proved worthy enough, but animosities intervened, and it did not secure him the appointment. Deeply disappointed, he moved to the Netherlands and, 2 years later, emigrated to the United States of America.

Koller's discovery was no accident for he was keenly aware of the limitations of general anesthesia in ophthalmologic surgery. He had delved into the literature and presumably read von Anrep's suggestion about local anesthesia, and had taken it seriously enough to try it experimentally. After making some dramatic tests on animals, Koller tried it on himself and then performed an operation for glaucoma with cocaine topical anesthesia on September 11, 1884, 4 days before the Congress of Ophthalmology was due to meet in Heidelberg. Koller immediately wrote a paper for the Congress, but, being an impecunious intern, he could not afford the train fare to Heidelberg so he gave the paper to a visiting ophthalmologist from Trieste, Dr. Brettauer, who had stopped in Vienna on his way to the Congress. Brettauer's news from Heidelberg reached New York in a letter from H.D. Noyes, an American ophthalmologist who had attended the Heidelberg Congress.[66]

Noyes's letter to the New York Medical Record excited numerous readers to test the new wonder drug and many of them rushed into print with astounding experiences. One of the most striking, published within 5 weeks of Noyes's communication, was that of N.J. Hepburn, a New York ophthalmologist.[44] There were no standards for drug trials in those days, and the tradition of self-experimentation was inviolate. If a researcher or physician wanted to know whether a drug was safe, he tried it on himself. Hepburn describes how on October 16, 1884, he experimented with a 2% solution of cocaine, giving himself a series of subcutaneous injections of 0.4 ml (8 mg) at intervals of 5 minutes. He noted that by the time of the eighth injection, the agreeable stimulating effects of the drug — rapid respiration and pulse, a feeling of warmth, pleasant hallucinations — had reached such a point that he felt it best to stop. For reasons that Hepburn does not state, he repeated the performance 2 days later, and then found it possible to carry the number of 0.4-ml injections to 16 before the general disturbance persuaded him to cease. He records that four days later he was at it again, and this time he tried a larger unit volume and amount (10 mg), and was able to tolerate 16 of these doses. It seems likely that Hepburn was already in the grip of addiction. Otherwise, why would he have increased the size of the injections?

By November 29, 1884, the ophthalmologist Bull was able to report that he had used the drug to produce anesthesia of the cornea and conjunctiva in more than 150 cases.[16] He gave sound reasons for his enthusiasm: he saved the time required for complete etherization and avoided the enormous engorgement of the ocular blood vessels produced by the ether, the danger of vomiting, and the disadvantage that almost any apparatus for producing anesthesia by inhalation was a physical interference for the operator.

CONDUCTION ANESTHESIA

After the publication of Noyes's letter, the idea of injecting cocaine directly into tissues in order to render them insensible occurred simultaneously to several American surgeons. W.B. Burke injected five minims (drops) of 2% solution close to a metacarpal branch of the ulnar nerve and painlessly extracted a bullet from the base of his patient's little finger.[17] But it was William Stewart Halsted (1852 – 1922) and his associates who most clearly saw the great possibilities of conduction block.[41–43] The term was introduced by François-Franck 7 years later,[35] though he may well have borrowed part of it from Corning, for in 1886 Corning was writing that "the thought of producing anaesthesia by abolishing conduction in sensory nerves, by suitable means, should have been rife in the minds of progressive physicians." Corning himself quite possibly got the idea from Halsted, for Halsted later attested that Corning was a frequent observer at the Roosevelt Hospital in New York, where Halsted, assisted by Hall, performed his teaching. In 1884 Hall described how he blocked a cutaneous branch of the ulnar nerve in his own forearm.[40] He and Halsted made injections into the musculocutaneous nerve of the leg and the ulnar nerve. Hall noted the appearance of marked constitutional symptoms, giddiness, severe nausea, cold perspiration, and dilated pupils, but this did not daunt these bold pioneers, and the same evening Halsted blocked Hall's supratrochlear nerve and removed an adjoining congenital cystic tumor. He also induced Nash, a dental surgeon, to tend to Hall's own upper incisor tooth after injection of cocaine into the infraorbital nerve at the infraorbital foramen, and Halsted thereafter performed an inferior dental nerve block on a medical student volunteer and later did the same to Hall. Hall's report was quite explicit in predicting that, once the limits of safety had been determined, this mode of administration would find very wide application in the outpatient department.

The daring experimenters at the Roosevelt Hospital unfortunately became addicted to the new drug, and no more was heard from them about its use in surgery. But that Hall and Halsted were the true progenitors of conduction anesthesia can scarcely be doubted.[40,62]

The great advantage of local anesthesia with cocaine was, of course, that it anesthetized only the part of the body on which the operation was to be performed. However, a price was paid in toxicity and time. Rapid absorption limited the safe quantity of cocaine to 30 mg and the useful duration of anesthesia to 10 to 15 minutes. In 1885 Corning sought a means of prolonging the local anesthetic effects for surgical and other purposes, although he was primarily interested in the application of the drug to the therapeutics of neurologic disease.[21] His notion of pharmacokinetics was that after the introduction of cocaine beneath the skin, a certain period of time elapsed during which the anesthetic agent was diffused throughout the surrounding tissue, the capillary circulation having a dual effect, first as a distributor and afterward as a dilutor and rapid remover of the anesthetic substance. In his first article of 1885, Corning described how he experimentally injected 0.3 ml of a 4% solution of cocaine into the lateral antebrachial nerve and obtained immediate anesthesia of the skin supplied by this nerve as far as the wrist. He found that simple arrest of the circulation in the involved part by compression or constriction proximal to the point of injection intensified the anesthesia and prolonged it indefinitely. He used an Esmarch bandage for this purpose and pointed out that the method was readily applicable to surgery of all the extremities. The Riva-Rocci cuff tourniquet had not yet been invented. Esmarch had introduced his elastic bandage in 1874 for the purpose of producing a bloodless field in major amputations.[32]

As has briefly been mentioned, François-Franck was the first to apply the term *blocking* to the infiltration of a nerve trunk in any part.[35] He found that the effect of the blocking drug was not limited to the purely sensory fibers because it paralyzed all nerves, whether motor or sensory, and that the sensory anesthesia was manifested much more promptly than was the motor paralysis, a confirmation of von Anrep's observations of 1879 to 1880. François-Franck spoke of the action of cocaine as a "physiological section," transitory and noninjurious.

Corning's principle of prolonging the local anesthetic action of cocaine by arresting the circulation in the anesthetized area inspired Heinrich F.W. Braun (1862–1934) to dispense with the elastic tourniquet and substitute epinephrine, a "chemical tourniquet" as he called it.[13] Epinephrine had become available in pure form after Abel isolated it from the suprarenal medulla in 1897.[1]

The suggestion for this use of epinephrine came from ophthalmologic practice, in which it had been introduced to limit hemorrhage and to render the conjunctiva bloodless, as well as to treat certain diseases, notably glaucoma, in which it was found to prolong the local effect of other drugs in general and of cocaine in particular. This observation had been confirmed by rhinologists and had enabled them to reduce the concentration and dose of cocaine and correspondingly to limit the hazard of toxicity.[63] Initially, in Braun's solution, the epinephrine was present in concentrations from 1:10,000 to 1:100,000. The first experiments to determine the dosage to be injected subcutaneously were made by Braun on himself. He found his limit of tolerance was 0.5 mg (0.5 ml of 1:1000 solution), after which general symptoms occurred and he had to lie down.

Braun introduced the term *conduction anesthesia,* and he felt that the use of epinephrine rendered conduction anesthesia in other parts of the body as effective as that in an extremity. In 1905 Braun published a textbook on local anesthesia, giving detailed descriptions of the technique for every region.[14]

INFILTRATION ANESTHESIA

Some 10 years earlier, a different approach, termed *infiltration anesthesia,* had been advocated by Karl Ludwig Schleich (1859–1922).[77] Schleich applied the principle that pure water has a weak anesthetic effect but is painful on injection, whereas physiologic saline is not.

The observation that subcutaneous injection of water produced local anesthesia was apparently first made by Potain in 1869. Halsted, in a short letter to the editor of the New York Medical Journal, dated September 19, 1885,[41] baldly asserted that "the skin can be completely anesthetized to any extent by cutaneous injections of water"; he had of late used water instead of cocaine in skin incisions, and the anesthesia did not always vanish just as soon as hyperemia supervened.

Schleich believed that there must be a solution of such a concentration between "normal" (0.6% salt solution) and pure water that would not provoke pain on injection and yet be usefully anesthetic, and he thought a 0.2% solution of sodium chloride was ideal. To this, he added cocaine to a concentration of 0.02% and employed the mixture to produce a field of cutaneous anesthesia in the surgery of hydrocele, sebaceous cyst, hemorrhoids, and small abscesses.

The reason why Schleich's hypotonic solutions containing a miniscule amount of cocaine produced impairment of sensation does not appear to have been explained. In the light of later work, it seems possible that loss of electrolyte from nerve fibers may have been involved.

Braun dismissed Schleich's solutions as nonphysiologic and insisted that injections into the tissues for whatever purpose must be composed of fluids of the same osmotic tension as the body fluids. Inasmuch as most local anesthetic solutions are hypotonic, a corresponding amount of an indifferent salt, such as sodium chloride, must be added to prevent any injurious action upon the tissue.

Nevertheless, Schleich's infiltration technique was an important advance in that it extended the field of usefulness of a small quantity of anesthetic. Schleich was probably indebted to Paul Reclus for the idea of using a weak solution of cocaine to avoid toxic reactions and fatalities. Enthusiasm for local anesthesia had diminished owing to casualties, but Reclus clearly understood that the basic cause of accidental deaths was overdose from the use of unnecessarily high concentrations.[71] He realized that undue absorption was avoidable by using lower concentrations, and he eventually reduced the strength of his cocaine solutions to 0.5%.

The toxicity of cocaine, coupled with its vast potential for usefulness in surgery, led to an intensive search for less toxic substitutes. However, decreased toxicity without increased irritancy—or impractically brief effectiveness—proved elusive until the synthesis of procaine (Novocaine) by Einhorn in 1904.[12] Additional crucial properties, chemical stability and absence of sensitization, were achieved with lidocaine, synthesized by Löfgren and announced in 1948.[57]

INTRAVENOUS REGIONAL ANESTHESIA

In 1908, August K.G. Bier (1851–1949) devised a very effective method of bringing about complete anesthesia and motor paralysis of a limb.[9] He injected a solution of procaine into one of the subcutaneous veins that were exposed between two constricting bands in a space that had previously been rendered bloodless by an elastic rubber bandage extending from fingers or toes. The injected solution permeated the entire section of the limb very quickly, producing what Bier called *direct vein anesthesia* in 5 to 15 minutes. The anesthesia lasted as long as the upper constricting band was kept in place. After it was removed, sensation returned in a few minutes.

SPINAL ANESTHESIA

Somewhat paradoxically, the first spinal anesthesia occurred 5 years before the first lumbar puncture. The term *spinal anesthesia* was introduced by Corning in his famous second paper of 1885.[22] It was the fruit of a brilliant yet erroneous idea, because what he had in mind was neither spinal nor epidural anesthesia as presently understood. Corning was under the mistaken impression that the interspinal blood vessels communicated with those of the spinal cord, and his intention was to inject cocaine into the minute interspinal vessels and have it carried by communicating vessels into the spinal cord. He made no mention of the cerebrospinal fluid, nor of how far he introduced the needle into the spinal space.

Corning's objective was clearly expressed by the title of his article, "Spinal Anaesthesia and Local Medication of the Cord with Cocaine."[22] There is no doubt that Corning was quite literally aiming directly at the spinal cord, as he introduced a hypodermic needle—he does not say of what size—between the spinous processes of the T11 and T12 vertebrae. He wrote, "I reasoned that it was highly probable that, if the anesthetic was placed between the spinous processes of the vertebrae, it would be rapidly transported by the blood to the substance of the cord and would give rise to anaesthesia of the sensory and perhaps also of the motor tracts of the same. To be more explicit, I hoped to produce artificially a temporary condition of things analogous in its physiological consequences to the effects observed in transverse myelitis or after total section of the cord." Corning's report was based on a series of two: one dog and one man. In the case of the man, he injected a total of 120 mg of cocaine, about four times the potentially lethal dose, in a period of 8 minutes. Corning implies that he was using the procedure partly as a treatment of masturbation. What he achieved in the man was probably what is now called *epidural* or *extradural anesthesia,* and, in the dog, which received 13 mg, *spinal anesthesia,* as judged by the rates of onset. Corning certainly did have an original idea, as he was at no small pains to indicate, but the results were a lucky accident because the experiment could easily have been fatal and was conceived on the basis of an entirely erroneous notion of the local circulation.

There is, of course, no direct communication between the extradural capillaries and those of the spinal cord so it is rather difficult to understand on what Corning based his expectations. At least as early as 1870, *Gray's Anatomy* had a section on the meninges, including the subarachnoid space and cerebrospinal fluid,[37] but Corning apparently was unaware of its existence. He kept the syringe connected to the needle with rubber tubing and thus would not have seen cerebrospinal fluid drip from the needle. Although English language anatomy books clearly delineated the spinal meninges and cerebrospinal fluid, the contemporary German and French language textbooks did not. Corning had a long line of New England ancestors, but he received his medical education in Europe at the University of Wurtzburg,[10] and so possibly never learned the basic facts of meningeal anatomy. In any case, how he got the idea that there were vascular channels between the spinous processes of the vertebrae which were a direct avenue into the spinal cord remains unclear.

LUMBAR PUNCTURE

Corning was a neurologist, not a surgeon, and he thought of his spinal use of cocaine as a new means of managing neurologic disorders. He did foresee that it would probably find application as a substitute for etherization in genitourinary or other branches of surgery. However, nothing came of his suggestion until 14 years later, perhaps because conceptual errors flawed his technique at a time when the procedure of lumbar puncture had not yet been invented, let alone standardized. It fell to Heinrich Irenaeus Quincke (1842–1922) to do this, by basing his approach on the anatomical ground that the subarachnoid spaces of the brain and spinal cord were continuous and ended in the adult at the level of S2, whereas the spinal cord extended only to L2.[70] Thus, a puncture effected in the third or fourth lumbar intervertebral space would not damage the spinal cord.

Lumbar puncture, as the title of Quincke's article indicated,[70] was invented as a treatment for hydrocephalus. Quincke acknowledged in his communication that he followed in the steps of Essex Wynter, who 6 months earlier had described the use of a Southey's tube and trocar for a similar purpose.[92] This device was originally designed to drain edema fluid in cases of dropsy. Wynter introduced the tube between the lumbar vertebrae, after making a small incision in the skin, for the purpose of instituting drainage of the fluid in two cases of tuberculous meningitis. Quincke's method was a vast improvement and became the standard technique, thanks to a detailed description that is still up to date. Quincke prescribed bed rest for the 24 hours following the puncture. Quincke's needles had an internal diameter of from 0.5 to 1.2 mm, and only the larger ones were equipped with a stylet. It is interesting to note that he entered the skin 5 to 10 mm from the midline. Thus, the paramedian approach is and has always been the classic one, and not the median approach as is sometimes taught.

It took 8 years for Quincke's technique to be applied to the production of what is now called *spinal anesthesia.* No doubt, great courage was required to introduce a drug as toxic as cocaine directly into the nervous system, as Corning had attempted in 1885. Unfortunately, Corning's audacity had no direct sequel unless the title of Bier's paper is taken as an implied tribute to Corning. (Bier does not mention him by name.) August Bier published his celebrated paper on spinal anesthesia in 1899, under the title "Versuche über Cocainisirung des Rückenmarkes" ("Researches on Cocainisation of the Spinal Cord").[8] Apparently Bier also assumed that intrathecal injection of cocaine produced anesthesia by a direct action on the spinal cord. Bier had a certain amount of luck on his side; he worked at the same institution as Quincke and would have been familiar with his technique and might even have borrowed his needles.

Bier, of course, was a surgeon, and it is noticeable that for many years virtually all the extensions of technique in the use of local anesthetics were developed by surgeons. They first performed the block and then performed the operation. This makes Corning's interest in cocaine all the more remarkable because he was genuinely an outsider in the field and may well have been viewed as such. He seems to have eluded the hazard to which several of the American surgical pioneers of regional anesthesia fell victim when their conscientious zeal led them to experiment on themselves before trying their ideas on patients.

Bier wanted to apply cocaine anesthesia for major operations and saw spinal anesthesia as a way to safely produce a maximum area of anesthesia with a minimum amount of drug. It was his opinion that the spectacular insensitivity to pain evoked by small amounts of cocaine injected into the dural sac resulted from its spread in the cerebrospinal fluid and that it acted not only on the surface of the spinal cord but especially on the unsheathed nerves that traverse the intramembranous space. However, this understanding was not conclusive. The extent of the anesthesia produced was somewhat unpredictable, so Bier decided to obtain an improved insight by experimenting on himself. His assistant, Hildebrandt, performed the lumbar puncture on Bier, but when the time came to attach the syringe to the needle, a crisis developed; the needle did not fit. A considerable amount of cerebrospinal fluid and most of the cocaine dripped onto the floor. To salvage the experiment, Hildebrandt volunteered his own body. This time there was a good fit and complete success.

However, the success was not without sequel. The experimenters celebrated with wine and cigars, and the next day Bier suffered an oppressive headache that lasted for 9 days. Hildebrandt's "hangover" developed even before the night ended. Moreover, while he was anesthetized, Hildebrandt had been scientifically kicked in the shins to demonstrate the depth of the analgesia, and in the aftermath he duly developed painful bruises in places where no pain had been.

As Bier emphasized in his paper, his experiences proved that by the injection of extraordinarily small amounts of cocaine (5 mg) into the dural sac, about two thirds of the entire body could be made insensible enough for the painless performance of major operations. Complete loss of sensation lasted about 45 minutes. Bier decided that the escape of a considerable amount of cerebrospinal fluid was probably responsible for the after-effects. He believed that in his own case some type of circulatory disturbance was present, because he felt absolutely well in a supine position but had a sensation of very strong pressure in the head and felt dizzy only if he sat up. Bier concluded that the escape of cerebrospinal fluid should be avoided if possible, and strict rest in bed should be observed. Bier said that the size of the needle should be very fine and that, after the dural sac had been entered, the stylet should be withdrawn and the opening immediately closed with a finger so that as little cerebrospinal fluid as possible escaped.

Halsted had introduced the use of rubber gloves at operations in the winter of 1889 to 1890, as noted earlier in this chapter, but not with the intention of avoiding wound infection. That consequence was actually serendipitous. His motive was to spare the hands of his operating room nurse (whom he later married), who had developed a dermatitis from mercurous chloride. Soon the operators took to wearing them as well, but only out of convenience. It was not until 1894 that the wearing of gloves was recommended as part of aseptic technique.[43] It surely is a fortunate coincidence that Bier did not start his work on spinal anesthesia until after this important prophylactic measure had become generally available.

The news of Bier's work, published in April 1899, spread quickly, and, although he abandoned it himself, his method of subarachnoid spinal anesthesia was soon brought into prominence by Théodore Tuffier (1857–1929).[84] In the Spring of 1900, in a report on 63 operations, Tuffier enunciated the rule "never inject the cocaine solution until the cerebrospinal fluid is distinctly recognized."[85] The sensation caused by Tuffier's demonstrations is well conveyed by Hopkins, who wrote: "To be able to converse with a patient during the performance of a hysterectomy, the patient all the while evincing not the slightest indication of pain (and even being unable to tell where the knife was being applied) was certainly a marvel, and was well worth crossing the Atlantic to see."[46]

In the United States, spinal anesthesia was adopted for obstetrics by Marx (see under Obstetric and Epidural Anesthesia, later in this chapter) and for general surgery by a number of surgeons, most prominently Rudolph Matas (1860–1957).[61] Matas's article begins with a critical historical review of older methods of local and regional anesthesia. In his description of spinal anesthesia, cocaine hydrochloride, in the amount of 10 to 20 mg, was dissolved in distilled water. The solution instilled was therefore clearly hypotonic. Fowler preferred to have his patients in the sitting position for the injection and not surprisingly was often astonished by the rapidity and completeness of the anesthesia.[34] Gravity methods were not yet understood.

Aseptic precautions were strictly observed, and E.W. Lee mentions that the injection he used consisted of 12 to 20 minims of a 2% sterilized solution prepared in hermetically sealed tubes by Truax, Green and Company of Chicago.[55] This appears to be the earliest published reference to this method of packaging, an important advance because previously it was necessary for the surgeon to prepare his own solution from tablets and sterilize it.

In 1912, Gray and Parsons of Birmingham, England, undertook an extensive study of variations in blood pressure associated with the induction of spinal anesthesia.[38] They concluded that the bulk of the fall in arterial blood pressure during high spinal anesthesia is attributable to the diminished negative intrathoracic pressure during inspiration, which is dependent on abdominal and lower thoracic paralysis. They noted that when the negative pressure in the thorax is increased, the arterial blood pressure rises.

It was by then quite clear that one of the principal dangers of spinal anesthesia is the lowering of the blood pressure. Believing this to be the primary hindrance to its more universal adoption among urologists, Smith, working with Porter, reported in 1915 the results of 50 experiments on cats.[81] They found that the quantity of anesthetic solution was more important for diffusion than its concentration, dilute solutions usually spreading farther than concentrated ones. The introduction of procaine beneath the dura in the region in which the splanchnic nerves arise caused as profound a fall in blood pressure as was caused by complete resection of the cord in the upper thoracic region. This, they thought, proved that the fall in blood pressure was not due to toxicity of the drug or to paralysis of the bulbar vasomotor center but to paralysis of the vasomotor fibers that regulate the tonus of the blood vessels in the splanchnic area. Since these nerve roots originate between T2 and T7, Smith and Porter believed that the main clinical objective was to prevent cephalad diffusion of the drug from reaching this height and paralyzing these nerve roots.

Gaston Labat (1877–1934)[52] emphasized that the danger of spinal anesthesia was not the fall in blood pressure as such but rather the associated cerebral anemia, both being attributable to the increased volume of blood in the viscera caused by splanchnic vascular paralysis and vasomotor collapse. He expressed the belief that this cerebral anemia could be avoided by placing the patient in the Trendelenburg position immediately following the intraspinal injection and that, by this procedure, the brain would be kept amply supplied with blood, and irremediable respiratory failure would be avoided. To ensure that the blood pressure would not drop during spinal anesthesia, the practice of administering ephedrine subcutaneously was introduced.

The idea of making the injected solution hyperbaric with glucose, in order to obtain control over the intrathecal spread of the solution, originated with Arthur E. Barker.[5] Barker employed stovaine, euphoniously so called from the English translation of its inventor's name, Fourneau.[27] Stovaine was less toxic than cocaine but was very slightly irritating and was eventually superseded by procaine. Barker's stovaine came directly from the laboratory of Billon in Paris, where it was made up in 5% glucose especially for Barker and packaged in sterile ampules. Barker was a professor of surgery at the University of London, and his article is exceedingly thoughtful, based on some 80 cases. He describes experiments with a glass model of the spinal canal, conforming to the shape seen in a mesial section of a cadaver and bearing a T-junction in the lumbar region to simulate the injection site.

Years later, Pitkin, in 1928, and Etherington-Wilson, in 1934, experimented with a similar apparatus but without acknowledging any debt to Barker.[33,68] Their goal was the opposite of Barker's, to obtain control over the rate of ascent of the drug by making the injected solution hypobaric. Control was achieved by varying the time the patient was kept sitting upright after the injection. Pitkin did this by mixing alcohol with the procaine solutions, a mixture he called *spinocaine,* but he categorically warned against having the patient in the sitting position during injection. He controlled level of blockade by tilting the table and illustrated this with a figure showing an "altimeter" attachment.

Barker stressed such points of technique as raising the head on pillows: whenever he injected a heavy fluid intradurally, he kept the level of analgesia below the transverse nipple line. At times, he seated the patient on the edge of the table with the feet on a low chair to make the fluid run into the sacral end of the dural sac, where it quickly affected the roots of the nerves supplying the anus and the perineum.

Barker advocated puncture in the midline as being easier and allowing more even spread of the injected fluid than the paramedian approach. He, too, emphasized that in no case should the analgesic solution be injected unless the cerebrospinal fluid ran satisfactorily. Above all else, perfect asepsis throughout the entire procedure was absolutely necessary. Moreover, no trace of germicides should be left on the skin, because they could be conveyed by the needle into the spinal canal, where their irritating qualities were particularly undesirable. Barker enjoined that all needles, syringes, and other instruments for the procedure were to be kept apart for this sole use, including the little sterilizer in which they were boiled. Billon's sterilized, sealed ampules were to be opened only a moment before use.

Barker's rational approach to the use of a hyperbaric solution for spinal anesthesia was apparently forgotten when stovaine was replaced by improved drugs and had to be rediscovered after trials of quasi-isobaric solutions of several new drugs led to unsatisfactory control of level. The lessons of the past were ignored or forgotten by surgeons and not yet learned by anesthesiologists. Indeed, at that time there were few anesthesiologists to learn. In 1920, W.G. Hepburn[45] revived Barker's technique with stovaine, and Sise, an anesthesiologist at the Lahey Clinic, applied it to procaine in 1928 and to tetracaine in 1935.[79,80]

Tetracaine's great advantage as a spinal anesthetic was its relatively prolonged duration of action without undue toxic effects, but this advantage was partially negated by the vagaries of its segmental spread, which resulted from its being used in an approximately isobaric solution. Therefore, Sise mixed the solution with an equal or greater volume of 10% glucose and injected it while the patient lay on his side on a table tilted head down 10°. The patient was then turned on his back and a good-sized pillow inserted under his head and shoulders to flex the cervical spine forward as much as possible; the slope of the table was adjusted during the next few minutes as dictated by the level of analgesia needed.

A refinement of this technique was the saddle-block method described in detail by Adriani and Roman-Vega.[3] Anesthesia deliberately confined to the perineal area was obtained by performing the lumbar puncture and injection of hyperbaric solution with the patient sitting on the operating table and remaining so for 35 to 40 seconds after the injection.

An article that announced a hypobaric solution and the associated modifications in the technique of spinal anesthesia was published by W.W. Babcock in 1912.[4] He dissolved 80 mg of stovaine in 2 ml of 10% alcohol, thus obtaining a solution whose specific gravity was less than 1.000, well below that of the cerebral spinal fluid, which he took to be 1.0065. He believed that the anesthesia that resulted was chiefly a nerve root anesthesia and not the "true spinal cord anesthesia" obtained with the standard solutions. Babcock said that the lightness of this particular anesthetic solution caused it to rise rapidly within the cavity of the arachnoid. He stressed that the patient should promptly have the head and shoulders lowered after the injection, but he rather perversely insisted that during the injection the patient should be sitting on the operating table, the legs hanging over the side of the table. He further remarked that "in most cases spinal anesthesia enables me to operate entirely free from the worry and watchfulness associated with etherization by an untrained assistant. . . . I have thus been able to operate successfully upon the neck, face, and even the cranium. . . ." But let us not fail to note that Babcock also promulgated the following dictum: *"Death from spinal anesthesia usually indicates inefficient or insufficiently prolonged methods of resuscitation."* The emphasis is his.

A method for continuous spinal anesthesia was described by W.T. Lemmon in 1940.[56] It was performed with the aid of a special mattress, a malleable needle, and special tubing, and was proposed for long operations that required abdominal relaxation. The equipment was original but not the main idea. In 1907, H.P. Dean wrote of having so arranged the exploring needle that it could be left *in situ* during the operation and another dose injected without moving the patient beyond a slight degree.[26] He proposed that additional injections be made postoperatively to treat pain or abdominal distention. Whether anything ever came of his proposal, he did not say. Lemmon's ponderous technique was quickly simplified by E.B. Tuohy.[86] He performed continuous spinal anesthesia by means of a ureteral catheter introduced in the subarachnoid space through a needle with a Huber point.

OBSTETRIC AND EPIDURAL ANESTHESIA

Tuffier's favorable experience with spinal anesthesia for operative interventions on the lower limbs and urogenital organs led O. Kreis of Basel to give the method a trial in childbirth.[51] He injected 10 mg of cocaine at the L4-5 level, in five parturients, and claimed that this alleviated pain with little impairment of muscular power or uterine motility; however, he recommended the method particularly for forceps delivery. S. Marx[60] in the United States quickly followed with several reports praising the ability of lumbar cocainization to still "the agonizing and maniacal shrieks of these poor women" for 1 to 5 hours, without cessation of uterine contractions; spontaneous bearing down was eliminated, although when told to do so the patient was capable of bringing her abdominal muscles into play as powerfully as under normal conditions. All of this occurred in the year 1900, but the enthusiasm soon waned.

Interest in obstetrical regional anesthesia was revived when W. Stoeckel[82] developed what he termed *sacral anesthesia* with procaine. The feasibility of injecting a local anesthetic by the caudal route was demonstrated by Fernand Cathelin (1873–1945) in 1901. Cathelin based his approach on a thorough anatomical study of the sacral canal and its contents.[18] He found that fluids injected into the extradural space through the sacral hiatus rose to a height proportional to the amount and speed of injection. His objective was to develop a method that would be less dangerous but just as effective as subarachnoid lumbar anesthesia. He was successful in reducing the danger, but his efforts to demonstrate the efficiency of the caudal injection for surgical operations were disappointing, and indeed Cathelin himself thought its principal sphere of usefulness lay in the treatment of bladder incontinence and of enuresis in children.

Reflecting on the similarities in the innervation of the bladder and uterus, the gynecologist W. Stoeckel thought that if the pain of childbirth was largely uterine in origin, as seemed probable, the caudal epidural method of the urologist Cathelin offered an ideal approach to painless obstetrics. Cathelin himself had considered pregnancy a contraindication to epidural injection because of the hazard of toxic absorption of cocaine. Stoeckel, however, had begun to use procaine and considered the reduced toxicity of the new drug acceptable. Stoeckel gave the method careful study. He injected colored fluid into the sacral canal of cadavers and noted its extensive spread upward and, contrary to Cathelin's observations, also through the sacral foramina. In 1909 Stoeckel described his experience with caudal anesthesia in the management of labor. He wrote that various concentrations of procaine and epinephrine produced predictably varying degrees of success after a single injection. Pain relief averaged 1 to 1½ hours in duration, but, warned Stoeckel, the greater the analgesic effect, the greater the hazard of impairing the forces of labor. These reservations, of course, would not apply to the use of caudal anesthesia for surgical operations, and Läwen, in 1910, described how he used Stoeckel's experience and Cathelin's ideas to perform a variety of interventions in the vicinity of the perineum.[53]

Läwen had tested the effectiveness of various concentrations and volumes of procaine–sodium chloride solutions with indifferent success, until he took to preparing and using the bicarbonate salt, as recommended by O. Gros.[39] Gros, in the pharmacology laboratory, had established that bicarbonate salts penetrated the nerve sheaths more rapidly than the hydrochloride salts. Läwen exploited this discovery by using increased volumes and stronger concentrations (20 to 25 ml of a 1.5% to 2% solution) to produce anesthesia in the gluteal region, rectum, anus, skin of the scrotum, penis, upper and inner parts of the thigh, and the vulva and vagina. The anesthesia developed after a delay of 20 minutes and lasted for 1½ to 2 hours. He performed all the common operations on these parts and, hence, was the first to employ sacral anesthesia for operative work, reporting 47 cases with an incidence of failure of 15%.

Pauchet, in 1914, was credited with overcoming this incidence of failure by injecting the sacral nerves individually through the posterior sacral foramina, a method that has become known as *transsacral anesthesia*.

The duration of satisfactory anesthesia from a single peridural injection was limited to a few hours. After Lemmon's demonstration of continuous spinal anesthesia in 1940,[56] it was not long before the "continuous" technique (actually replenishments at half-hour intervals) was transferred by Edwards and Hingson to obstetrical delivery, in which it had an important sphere of usefulness.[31] This was a rational development, following on the seminal work of Cleland, which identified the pathways of uterine pain and clarified the sources of failure and success of regional obstetric block.[20] Cleland had determined that all the sensory fibers that supply the fallopian tubes and uterus enter the spinal cord through T11 and T12, and he blocked them paravertebrally, while those from the cervix and perineum were interrupted by caudal block.[20] Edwards and Hingson realized that the continuous method enabled them to start the anesthesia early and to continue it for as long as necessary, 5 or 6 hours on the average, to the completion of labor and repair of an episiotomy or laceration. An initial dose of 30 ml of 1.5% metycaine in physiologic saline produced freedom from pain within 5 minutes.

Caudal block by catheter in obstetrics was announced by Manalan in 1942,[58] independently of Hingson's group, but his described technique of injection was not "continuous." He introduced a No. 4 ureteral silk catheter through the lumen of a 14-gauge needle, advanced the catheter until stopped by the dura, and then withdrew the needle, leaving the catheter in place. The injection, 30 ml of 1% procaine with epinephrine, was withheld until required. Later, he substituted a nylon catheter for the silk catheter because the nylon one could be more easily sterilized. Block and Rochberg devised a continuous gravity drip of procaine and instituted it from the outset, so as to detect any untoward symptoms before a large amount of the drug had been introduced.[11]

However, the earliest intimation of continuous regional anesthesia in the practice of obstetrics came from Eugene Aburel of Rumania.[2] For the first stage of labor he used a specially made combination of catheter and needle: he introduced the needle paravertebrally into the lumbosacral plexus, injected 30 ml of 0.05% dibucaine solution, and then introduced an elastic silk catheter similar to a ureteral catheter through the needle, before withdrawing the needle and fixing the catheter with adhesive tape. Repeated paravertebral injections were given through the catheter, which was "tolerated well, during a rather long period of time." For the second stage he administered a single (caudal) injection of 30 to 35 ml or infiltrated the perineum. He declared that continuous local anesthesia for obstetrics was henceforth a proven practical procedure but this claim apparently failed to persuade contemporary obstetricians.

PARAVERTEBRAL CONDUCTION ANESTHESIA

Matas, the eminent American pioneer and historian of regional anesthesia, recorded that Sellheim, injecting close to the posterior roots of T8 to T12, in addition to the ilioinguinal and iliohypogastric nerves, was able to perform abdominal operations successfully.[62] Sellheim was, therefore, credited by Matas as being the originator of the paravertebral method of anesthesia.

It was 6 years later, Kappis having in the meantime greatly improved on Sellheim's technique, that the method was first used in urologic surgery. According to Kappis, success with conduction anesthesia of the trigeminal nerve led him to seek an anatomically reliable approach to conduction anesthesia of the spinal nerves at their exit from between the vertebrae.[48] In his paper, he described posterior approaches to the lower seven cervical nerves for the purposes of cervical and brachial plexus block. He cautioned against blocking C4 bilaterally at the same time. He made up his own solution of procaine–epinephrine and let it stand for an hour because he believed this improved its effectiveness. The method for paravertebral block of the thoracic nerves and the first four lumbar nerves was given in this same paper, and was used in a great many upper abdominal operations. Finally, Kappis pointed out that these techniques could also be used to treat acute and chronic pain with procaine, or even with alcohol if motor function could be disregarded. Two years later, Kappis described his posterior approach to the splanchnic plexus.[49]

In 1922, Läwen found unilateral paravertebral block of selected spinal nerves useful in the differential diagnosis of intra-abdominal disease.[54] For example, he observed that a 10-ml injection of 2% procaine at T10 could completely relieve the pain of a severe biliary colic for 3 hours. The use of segmental paravertebral block for the differential diagnosis of painful conditions was an original idea of Läwen's. At the suggestion of Pal, it was then tried by Brunn and Mandl in 1924[15] as a therapeutic measure in the hopes of obtaining pain relief in acute cholecystitis, but without significant success. Kappis had treated a case of angina pectoris in this manner in 1923, and von Gaza used 0.5% procaine diagnostically prior to resection of the affected paravertebral nerves.[88]

In 1925 Mandl reported 16 cases of angina pectoris in which he injected procaine, 0.5%, paravertebrally with excellent results.[59] The next year Swetlow attempted to destroy the afferent sensory fibers altogether by substituting 85% alcohol for the procaine and for the most part obtained satisfactory relief of pain for several months.[83]

The pioneer of alcohol injection for the purpose of producing a long-lasting interruption of neural conduction was Schloesser.[78] Schloesser presented the method as a means of managing convulsive facial tic; he obtained paralysis that lasted from days to months, according to the quantity of alcohol injected. He suggested that the method would also be useful for supraorbital neuralgia and tic douloureux. Like many a pioneer, he was too far ahead of his time to gain an immediate following.

Segmental peridural anesthesia, under the name of *metameric anesthesia,* was used for the first time in 1921 by Fidel Pagés, a Spanish military surgeon.[67] To Dogliotti, however, belongs the credit for systematizing and popularizing the peridural principle to produce what he termed *segmental peridural spinal anesthesia.*[28,30] In the light of later theory, which requires that three consecutive internodes be blocked to prevent saltatory conduction, it is interesting to note Dogliotti's iteration of the need to bathe a sufficient length of the spinal nerves. He emphasized that if the anesthetic solution is injected in sufficient quantity (50–60 ml) and under adequate pressure, it will be quite easy to subject the spinal nerves to the action of the injected fluid throughout their length in the spinal canal and the intervertebral foramina, and even beyond. Dogliotti's method was easier and, without question, simpler than paravertebral regional block, since only one puncture was needed. He stressed the sudden loss of resistance when the point of the needle, having pierced the ligamentum flavum, entered the epidural space. The usefulness of this technique was extended further when Curbelo decided to apply the Tuohy armamentarium for continuous spinal anesthesia to continuous segmental peridural anesthesia.[23] In one case, he left the catheter in place for as long as 4 days and administered a total of 10 injections of 15 ml each of 2% procaine solution for the production of a continuous sympathetic lumbar block.

DIAGNOSTIC PROCAINE BLOCK

The pioneer in the use of procaine for determining the pathways of obscure pain was von Gaza.[88] But it was left to White to discover and demonstrate the wide diagnostic usefulness of procaine block of sensory or sympathetic nerves, as the case may be, in determining the pathways of peripheral pain.[90] White emphasized the advantage to the surgeon and the patient of knowing exactly how much relief of suffering or improvement of circulation might be expected from an operation.

Conceptually, it was but a short step from diagnostic block to therapeutic block, and indeed the step was taken by von Gaza and by Brunn and Mandl in 1924 in the management of visceral pain. In the same year, Royle in Australia demonstrated that relief of deforming contractions and spastic paralyses (Little's disease) could be obtained by interrupting the sympathetic nerve supply to the musculature of the affected parts.[74] Long-term pain relief by neurolytic injection of alcohol was developed by Swetlow for the interruption of cardiac afferent inflow and subsequently applied to paravertebral sympathetic block in the treatment of severe intractable pain, particularly the pain of malignant disease.[83]

Dogliotti, in 1930, took the bold step of injecting absolute alcohol into the subarachnoid space, hoping to produce by simple chemical means a posterior rhizotomy equivalent to that previously attainable only by surgery.[29] At the opposite end of the local anesthetic concentration spectrum, Sarnoff and Arrowood exploited the continuous subarachnoid injection of dilute procaine (0.2%) to obtain a differential block limited to efferent sympathetic fibers and afferent fibers subserving pain.[76]

Wertheim and Rovenstine, anesthesiologists at the New York University College of Medicine, devised and described a technique of suprascapular nerve block in the treatment of intractable shoulder pain, such as subacromial bursitis.[89] They reported that the analgesic effect of a 2% procaine injection may continue for 4 to 6 weeks.

ANESTHESIOLOGY AS A SPECIALTY PRACTICE

One of the more noticeable and surprising features in the history of the first 50 years of neural blockade is the almost total uninvolvement of anesthesiologists. Virtually all the developments were devised by surgeons and basic scientists. Also surprising is the miniscule nature of the contribution from Britain, the country of Snow and Lister and pioneering investigation in general. This was not a case of noncommunication, since the very first notice of Koller's discovery in the foreign press had appeared in the London *Lancet.* There is no easy explanation. In most of the medical world, the practice of anesthesia was considered a poor relation, comparatively unhonored and unskilled, seemingly offering little opportunity or incentive for innovative work. In the British quarter of the globe, general anesthesia was administered by physicians and perhaps generated a certain sense of security and a tendency to leave well enough alone. Everywhere, if local anesthesia was the choice, the surgeon did both the choosing and the injecting. It was not until nerve block began to be perceived as an independent diagnostic and therapeutic tool that a demand arose for regional anesthetic skill independent of surgical operation. In the United States, this period saw the beginnings of anesthesiology as an individual specialty, welcomed by forward-looking surgeons such as William Mayo, who established Labat, one of the first regional anesthesiologists, as a lecturer at the renowned Mayo Clinic in Minnesota.

Not least of the services rendered by the development of regional anesthesia was the stimulation of a higher level of vigilance and physiologic awareness in anesthetic practice as a whole. No better proof of this trend could be desired than that provided by anesthesia records. Charted records of the vital signs during an operation were apparently being kept by Dr. Codman at the Massachusetts General Hospital at the close of the 19th century, stimulated by the recommendations of Cushing.[7] It must be remembered that a convenient method of measuring the blood pressure of a patient was not available until Riva-Rocci invented the arm cuff in 1896, and that 10 years were to elapse before Korotkoff, a Russian army surgeon, discovered the auscultatory method. Thus, the analgesia charts of Codman at first showed only the pulse rate, and when blood pressure was added, only the systolic pressure. Cushing's insistence on charted records was of a piece with other aspects of his greatness as a medical scientist and surgeon. Following the lead of Crile, he sought to combat shock in major amputations by cocainizing the large nerve trunks before dividing them and he kept graphic track of the patient's condition by having the vital signs measured every 5 minutes.[24]

The first publication, however, of a chart for recording the progress of a patient during anesthesia should be credited to Sydney Ormond Goldan (1869–1944), who presented a facsimile of one in the *Philadelphia Medical Journal,* November 3, 1900.[36] It was designed specifically for registering the course of "intraspinal cocainization" and provided for the recording of three vital signs, pupil, pulse, and respiration, every 10 minutes (Fig. 1-2).* Goldan's paper has a further title to scholarly distinction; it seems to have been the earliest article in the literature of local anesthesia to include a list of bibliographic citations. Historically, Goldan's contribution is also of interest for his concluding remark: ". . . a remedy for the headache may be found not in simple analgesics, but drugs exerting their influences upon the circulation. . . . Increasing the blood-pressure favors an increased tension in the veins retarding absorption."

*R.A. Gordon (Can. Anaesth. Soc. J., *25*:75–80, 1978) has drawn attention to an anesthetic chart for use in hospital practice, arranged by C. O'Reilly and published in Canada (Lancet, *34*:636, 1901).

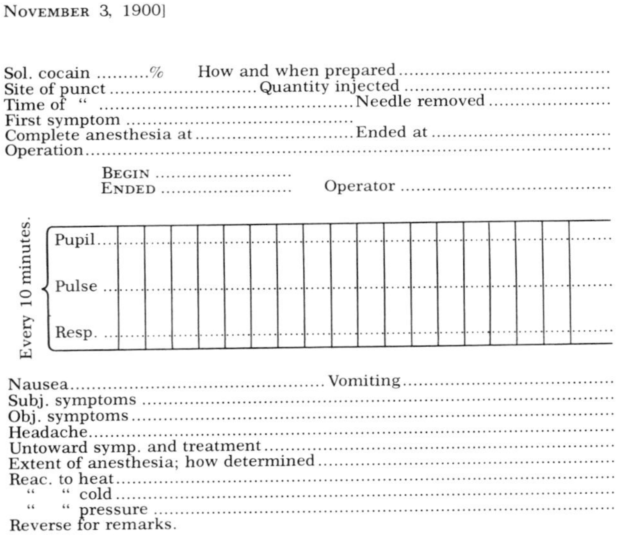

NOVEMBER 3, 1900]

Sol. cocain ....% How and when prepared ....
Site of punct .... Quantity injected ....
Time of " .... Needle removed ....
First symptom ....
Complete anesthesia at .... Ended at ....
Operation ....
BEGIN ....
ENDED .... Operator ....

Every 10 minutes. { Pupil ... / Pulse ... / Resp. ...

Nausea .... Vomiting ....
Subj. symptoms ....
Obj. symptoms ....
Headache ....
Untoward symp. and treatment ....
Extent of anesthesia; how determined ....
Reac. to heat ....
" " cold ....
" " pressure ....
Reverse for remarks.

FIG. 1-2. Facsimile of Goldan's chart, the earliest published anesthesia chart. (Goldan, S.O.: Intraspinal cocanization for surgical anesthesia. Philadelphia Med. J., *6*:850, 1900.)

Goldan gave full details of 16 cases of spinal anesthesia, a large series for that time, and explicitly described himself as an anesthetist. Thus, the practice of careful record keeping in the operating room, an indispensable foundation to the progress of anesthesiology, was initiated publicly by the first physician to describe himself as an anesthetist in the United States of America. It is worth noting that Goldan, a much forgotten trailblazer, was also incontrovertibly the first anesthetist to practice regional block anywhere in the world.

REFERENCES

1. Abel, J.J.: On the blood-pressure-raising constituent of the suprarenal capsule. Johns Hopkins Hosp. Bull., *8*:151, 1897.
2. Aburel, E.: L'anesthésie locale continue (prolongée) en obstétrique. Bull. Soc. Obstét. Gynecol., *20*:35, 1931.
3. Adriani, J., and Roman-Vega, D.: Saddle block anesthesia. Am. J. Surg., *71*:12, 1946.
4. Babcock, W.W.: Spinal anesthesia; with report of surgical clinics. Surg. Gynecol. Obstet., *15*:606, 1912.
5. Barker, A.E.: Clinical experiences with spinal analgesia in 100 cases and some reflections on the procedure. Br. Med. J., *1*:665, 1907.
6. Becker, H.K.: Carl Koller and cocaine. Psychoanal. Q., *32*:309, 1963.
7. Beecher, H.K.: The first anesthesia records (Codman, Cushing). Surg. Gynecol. Obstet., *71*:789, 1940.
8. Bier, A.: Versuche über Cocainisirung des Rückenmarkes. Dtsch. Z. Chir., *51*:361, 1899.
9. Bier, A.: Ueber einen neuen Weg Localanästhesie an den Gliedmassen zu erzeugen. Arch. Klin. Chir., *86*:1007, 1908.
10. Biographical sketch of Doctor James Leonard Corning of New York City, and his recent remarkable discoveries in local anesthesia. Va. Med. Mon., *12*:713, 1886.
11. Block, N., and Rochberg, S.: Continuous caudal anesthesia in obstetrics. Am. J. Obstet. Gynecol., *45*:645, 1943.
12. Braun, H.: Ueber einige neuer örtliche Anaesthetica (Stovain, Alypin, Novocain). Dtsch. Klin. Wochenschr., *31*:1667, 1905.
13. Braun, H.: Ueber den Einfluss der Vitalität der Gewebe auf die örtlichen und allgemeinen Giftwirkungen localanästhesirender Mittel und über die Bedeutung des Adrenalins für die Localanästhesie. Arch. Klin. Chir., *69*:541, 1903.
14. Braun, H.: Local Anesthesia: Its Scientific Basis and Practical Use, ed. 3. Philadelphia, Lea & Febiger, 1914.
15. Brunn, F., and Mandl, F.: Die paravertebrale Injektion zur Bekämpfung visceraler Schmerzen. Wien. Klin. Wochenschr., *37*:511, 1924.
16. Bull, C.S.: The hydrochlorate of cocaine as a local anaesthetic in ophthalmic surgery. N.Y. Med. J., *40*:609, 1884.
17. Burke, W.C., Jr.: Hydrochlorate of cocaine in minor surgery. N.Y. Med. J., *40*:616, 1884.
18. Cathelin, F.: Une nouvelle voie d'injection rachidienne. Méthodes des injections épidurales par le procédé du canal sacré.

Applications à l'homme. C.R. Soc. Biol. (Paris), *53*:452, 1901.
19. Caton, D.: The secularization of pain. Anesthesiology, *62*:493, 1985.
20. Cleland, J.G.: Paravertebral anesthesia in obstetrics. Surg. Gynecol. Obstet., *57*:57, 1938.
21. Corning, J.L.: On the prolongation of the anaesthetic effect of the hydrochlorate of cocaine, when subcutaneously injected. An experimental study. N.Y. Med. J., *42*:317, 1885.
22. Corning, J.L.: Spinal anaesthesia and local medication of the cord. N.Y. Med. J., *42*:483, 1885.
23. Curbelo, M.M.: Continuous peridural segmental anesthesia by means of a ureteral catheter. Anesth. Analg. (Cleve.), *28*:13, 1949.
24. Cushing, H.: On the avoidance of shock in major amputations by cocainization of large nerve-trunks preliminary to their division. Ann. Surg., *36*:321, 1902.
25. Dallenbach, K.M.: Pain: History and present status. Am. J. Psychol., *52*:331, 1939.
26. Dean, H.P.: Relative value of inhalation and injection methods of inducing anaesthesia. Br. Med. J., *2*:869, 1907.
27. De Lapersonne, F.: Un nouvel anesthésique local, la stovaïne. Presse Med., *12*:233, 1904.
28. Dogliotti, A.M.: Eine neue Methode der regionaren Anästhesie: "Die peridurale segmentäre Anästhesie." Zentralbl. Chir., *58*:3141, 1931.
29. Dogliotti, A.M.: Proposta di un nuovo metodo di cura delle algie periferiche. L'alcoolizzazione sottomeningea delle radici posteriori. Considerazioni sulle prime 30 osservazione cliniche. Minerva Med., *1*:536, 1931.
30. Dogliotti, A.M.: A new method of block anesthesia. Segmental peridural spinal anesthesia. Am. J. Surg., *20*:107, 1933.
31. Edwards, W.B., and Hingson, R.A.: Continuous caudal anesthesia in obstetrics. Am. J. Surg., *57*:459, 1942.
32. Esmarch, F.: Ueber künstliche Blutleere. Arch. Klin. Chir., *17*:292, 1874.
33. Etherington-Wilson, E.: Intrathecal nerve root block. Some contributions and a new technique. Proc. R. Soc. Med., *27*:325, 1934.
34. Fowler, R.G.: Cocaine analgesia from subarachnoid injection, with a report of forty-four cases together with a report of a case in which antipyrin was used. Philadelphia Med. J., *6*:843, 1900.
35. François-Franck, C.A.: Action paralysante locale de la cocaïne sur les nerfs et les centres nerveux. Applications à la technique expérimentale. Arch. Physiol. Norm. Pathol., *24*:562, 1892.
36. Goldan, S.O.: Intraspinal cocainization for surgical anesthesia. Philadelphia Med. J., *6*:850, 1900.
37. Gray, H.: Anatomy: Descriptive and Surgical, ed. 5, pp. 572–574. Philadelphia, Henry C. Lea, 1870.
38. Gray, H.T., and Parsons, L.: Blood pressure variations associated with lumbar puncture and the induction of spinal anesthesia. Q. J. Med., *5*:339, 1912.
39. Gros, O.: Ueber die Narkotika und Localanästhetika. Arch. exp. Pathol. Pharmakol., *63*:80, 1910.
40. Hall, R.J.: Hydrochlorate of cocaine. N.Y. Med. J., *40*:643, 1884.
41. Halsted, W.S.: Water as a local anesthetic. N.Y. Med. J., *42*:327, 1885.
42. Halsted, W.S.: Practical comments on the use and abuse of cocaine; suggested by its invariably successful employment in more than a thousand minor surgical operations. N.Y. Med.J., *42*:294, 1885.
43. Halsted, W.S.: Surgical Papers by William Steward Halsted, vol. 1, pp. 37–39. Baltimore, Johns Hopkins Press, 1924.
44. Hepburn, N.J.: Some notes on hydrochlorate of cocaine. Medical Record, *26*:534, 1884.
45. Hepburn, W.G.: Stovain spinal analgesia. Am. J. Surg., *34*:87, 1920.
46. Hopkins, G.S.: Anesthesia by cocainization of the spinal cord. Philadelphia Med. J., *6*:864, 1900.
47. Howard-Jones, N.: A critical study of the origins and early development of hypodermic medication. J. Hist. Med. *2*:201, 1947.
48. Kappis, M.: Ueber Leitungsanästhesie an Bauch, Burst, Arm und Hals durch Injektion ans Foramen intervertebrale. Munch. Med. Wochenschr., *1*:794, 1912.
49. Kappis, M.: Erfahrungen mit Lokalanästhesie bei Bauchoperationen. Verh. Dtsch. Ges. Chir., *43*:87, 1914.
50. Koller, C.: On the use of cocaine for producing anaesthesia on the eye. Lancet, *2*:990, 1884.
51. Kreis, O.: Ueber Medullarnarkose bei Gebärenden. Zentralbl. Gynakol., *24*:724, 1900.
52. Labat, G.: Circulatory disturbances associated with subarachnoid nerve block. Long Island Med. J., *21*:573, 1927.
53. Läwen, A.: Uber die Verwertung der Sakralanästhesie fur chirurgische Operationen. Zentralbl. Chir., *37*:708, 1910.
54. Läwen, A.: Ueber segmentäre Schmerzaufhebung durch paravertebrale Novokaininjektionen zur Differentialdiagnose intra-abdominaler Erkrankungen. Med. Wochenschr., *69*:1423, 1922.
55. Lee, E.W.: Subarachnoidean injections of cocaine as a substitute for general anesthesia in operations below the diaphragm, with report of seven cases. Philadelphia Med. J., *6*:865, 1900.
56. Lemmon, W.T.: A method for continuous spinal anesthesia. Ann. Surg., *111*:141, 1940.
57. Löfgren, N.: Studies on Local Anesthetics. Xylocaine: A New Synthetic Drug. Inaugural dissertation. Stockholm, Hoeggstroms, 1948.
58. Manalan, S.A.: Caudal block anesthesia in obstetrics. J. Indiana State Med. Assoc., *35*:564, 1942.
59. Mandl, F.: Die Wirkung der paravertebralen Injektion bei "Angina pectoris." Arch. Klin. Chir., *136*:495, 1925.
60. Marx, S.: Analgesia in obstetrics produced by medullary injections of cocain. Philadelphia Med. J., *6*:857, 1900.
61. Matas, R.: Local and regional anesthesia with cocain and other analgesic drugs, including the subarachnoid method, as applied in general surgical practice. Philadelphia Med. J., *6*:820, 1900.
62. Matas, R.: Local and regional anesthesia: A retrospect and prospect. Am. J. Surg., *25*:189, 1934.
63. Mayer, E.: Clinical experience with adrenaline. Philadelphia Med. J., *7*:819, 1901.
64. Melzack, R., and Wall, P.D.: Pain mechanisms: A new theory. Science, *150*:971–975, 1965.
65. Niemann, A.: Ueber eine organische Base in der Coca. Annalen Chemie, *114*:213, 1860.
66. Noyes, H.D.: The ophthalmological congress in Heidelberg. Medical Record, *26*:417, 1884.

67. Pagés, F.: Anestesia metamerica. Rev. Sanid. Milit. Argent., *11*:351–365.
68. Pitkin, G.: Controllable spinal anesthesia. Am. J. Surg., *5*:537, 1928.
69. Pravaz, C.G.: Sur un nouveau moyen d'opérer la coagulation du sang dans les artères, applicable à la guérison des anéurismes. C.R. Acad. Sci. (Paris), *36*:88, 1853.
70. Quincke, H.: Die Lumbalpunction des Hydrocephalus. Ber. Klin. Wochenschr., *28*:929, 1891.
71. Reclus, P.: Analgésie locale par la cocaïne. Rev. Chir., *9*:913, 1889.
72. Reynolds, D.V.: Surgery in the rat during electrical analgesia induced by focal brain stimulation. Science, *164*:444–445, 1969.
73. Riese, W., and Arrington, G.E., Jr.: The history of Johannes Müller's doctrine of the specific energies of the senses: Original and later versions. Bull. Hist. Med., *37*:179–183, 1963.
74. Royle, N.D.: A new operative procedure in the treatment of spastic paralysis and its experimental basis. Med. J. Aust., *1*:77, 1924.
75. Rynd F.: Neuralgia–Introduction of fluid to the nerve. Dublin Medical Press, *13*:167, 1845.
76. Sarnoff, S.J., and Arrowood, J.G.: Differential spinal block. Surgery, *20*:150, 1946.
77. Schleich, C.L.: Zur Infiltrationsanästhesie. Therapeutisch Monathefte, *8*:429, 1894.
78. Schloesser: Heilung peripharer Reizzustände sensibler und motorischer Nerven. Klin. Monatsbl. Augenheilkd., *41*:244, 1903.
79. Sise, L.F.: Spinal anesthesia for upper and lower abdominal operations. N. Engl. J. Med., *199*:61, 1928.
80. Sise, L.F.: Pontocain-glucose for spinal anesthesia. Surg. Clin. North Am., *15*:1501, 1935.
81. Smith, G.S., and Porter, W.T.: Spinal anesthesia in the cat. Am. J. Physiol., *38*:108, 1915.
82. Stoeckel, W.: Ueber sakrale Anästhesie. Zentralbl. Gynaekol., *33*:1, 1909.
83. Swetlow, G.I.: Paravertebral alcohol block in cardiac pain. Am. Heart J., *1*:393, 1926..
84. Tuffier, T.: Analgésie chirurgicale par l'injection sous-arachnoidienne lombaire de cocaine. C.R. Soc. Biol., 11th Series, *1*:882, 1899.
85. Tuffier, T.: Anesthésie medullaire chirurgicale par injection sous-arachnoidienne lombaire de cocaine; technique et resultats. Semaine medicale, *20*:167, 1900.
86. Tuohy, E.B.: Continuous spinal anesthesia: Its usefulness and technic involved. Anesthesiology, *5*:142, 1944.
87. von Anrep, B.: Ueber die physiologische Wirkung des Cocain. Pflugers Arch., *21*:38, 1880.
88. von Gaza, W.: Die Resektion der paravertebralen Nerven und die isolierte Durchschneidung des Ramus communicans. Arch. Klin. Chir., *133*:479, 1924.
89. Wertheim, H.M., and Rovenstine, E.A.: Suprascapular nerve block. Anesthesiology, *2*:541, 1941.
90. White, J.C.: Diagnostic novocaine block of the sensory and sympathetic nerves. A method of estimating the results which can be obtained by their permanent interruption. Am. J. Surg., *9*:264, 1930.
91. Wood, A.: New method of treating neuralgia by the direct application of opiates to the painful points. Edinburgh Med. Surg. J., *82*:265, 1855.
92. Wynter, W.E.: Four cases of tuberculosus meningitis in which paracentesis of the theca vertebralis was performed for the relief of fluid pressure. Lancet, *1*:981, 1891.
93. Yaksh, T.L., and Rudy, T.A.: Analgesia mediated by a direct spinal action of narcotics. Science, *192*:1357–1358, 1976.

APPENDIX A: CHRONOLOGY OF IDEAS CONCERNING PAIN AND NEURAL BLOCKADE

ca. 500 B.C. **Alcmaeon (Croton)**
The brain is associated with the organs of sense

ca. 375 B.C. **Plato (Athens)**
Pain is an emotion that dwells in the brain

ca. 200 **Galen (Pergamon)**
Recognized the functional unity of the brain, spinal cord, and peripheral nerves

1752 **Haller (Germany)**
Only certain specific parts of the body react to pain, disclosing sensibility

1826 **Mueller (Germany)**
Asserted the doctrine of specific sensory energies, that there is no direct correlation between the external stimulation and the impression received. It is the nerves that determine the kind of ideas contained in the mind

1855 **Wood (UK)**
Neuralgic pain can be treated by circumneural injection of pain-relieving drug

1885 **Corning (USA)**

Pain can be treated by "medication of the spinal cord"

1900 Cushing (USA)
Nerve block to prevent pain and "shock" of amputation

1908 Crile (USA)
"Anociassociation"—neural blockade to prevent noxious stimulation

1933 Brouwer (Netherlands)
Proposed centrifugal influence on centripetal systems in the brain

1934 O'Shaughnessy and Slome (UK)
Spinal anesthesia decreased mortality in dogs with limb trauma

1953 Bonica (USA)
Publication of an encyclopedic treatise on the management of acute pain and chronic pain

1957 Hagbarth and Kerr (Australia)
Evidence of descending control of sensory input

1958 Bromage (Canada)
Epidural block restored respiratory function after abdominal surgery

1963 Hume and Egdahl
Spinal lesions or spinal anesthesia modified the stress response to surgery in man

1965 Melzack and Wall (Canada and UK)
A spinal gate in the dorsal horn controls the transmission of nociceptive messages

1969 Reynolds (USA)
Pain-inhibitory impulses descend from the midbrain to the spinal cord. The pathway is activatable by electrical stimulation and morphine

1971 Bromage (Canada)
Epidural block in humans modifies stress response during and after surgery

1976 Yaksh and Rudy (USA)
Spinal application of morphine inhibits nociceptive transmission

1979 Cousins and colleagues (Australia)
Epidural administration of opioids in humans results in "selective spinal analgesia" on the basis of studies of pharmacokinetics and neural effects

1981 Duggan (Australia)
More than one population of opioid receptors in spinal cord

1983 Yaksh (USA)
Several different spinal receptor systems mediating antinociception

APPENDIX B: CHRONOLOGY OF LOCAL ANESTHESIA

1564 Paré (France)
Local anesthesia by nerve compression

1600 Valverdi (Italy)
Regional anesthesia by compression of nerves and blood vessels supplying operative area

1646 Severino (Italy)
Refrigeration anesthesia by use of freezing mixtures of snow and ice

1656 Wren (England)
First experiments with intravenous injection

1784 Moore (England)
Local anesthesia of extremity by compression of nerve trunks

1839 Taylor and Washington (USA)
Hypodermic injection

1843 Wood (Scotland)
Morphine injection (published 1855)

1845 Rynd (Dublin)
Hypodermic Needle

1853 Pravaz (France)
Hypodermic Syringe

1855 Gaedcke (Germany)
Isolation of alkaloid from leaves of cocoa plant

1860 Niemann (Germany)
Purification and naming of cocaine

1873 Bennett (Scotland)
Anesthetic properties of cocaine

1878 von Anrep (Germany)
Pharmacologic effects of cocaine (published 1879–1880)

1884 Koller (Austria)
First topical use of cocaine (eye surgery)

Halsted and Hall (USA)

Neural blockade with cocaine (in each other)
Burke (USA)
Removal of bullet from finger under nerve block with cocaine

1885 **Corning (USA)**
"Spinal anesthesia" (actually injected epidurally)

1890 **Reclus (France)**
Early use of infiltration anesthesia

1891 **Quincke (Germany)**
Lumbar puncture technique

1892 **Schleich (Germany)**
Introduced infiltration anesthesia
François-Franck
Coined term nerve *blocking*

1897 **Braun (Germany)**
Cocaine toxicity related to absorption; advocated use of epinephrine

1898 **Bier (Germany)**
First planned spinal anesthetic

1899 **Tuffier (France)**
Report of 125 spinal anesthetics
Tait and Caglieri (USA)
First use of spinal anesthesia in USA (". . . never inject . . . until CSF . . . recognized")

1900 **Tait and Caglieri (USA)**
Detailed studies of subarachnoid space and spinal anesthesia in animals and humans

1901 **Cathelin and Sicard (France)**
Independently discovered caudal epidural block using cocaine

1902 **Braun (Germany)**
Use of epinephrine in nerve blocking—term *conduction anesthesia*

1904 **Einhorn (Germany)**
Synthesis of procaine (Novocaine)

1905 **Braun (Germany)**
Text *Local Anesthesia*

1907 **Barker (UK)**
Introduction of hyperbaric spinal anesthetic solutions

1908 **Crile (USA)**
Anociassociation: regional block plus light general anesthesia

1912 **Gray and Parsons (UK)**

1915 **Smith and Porter (USA)**
Blood pressure changes during spinal anesthesia

1922 **Labat (USA)**
Text *Regional Anesthesia: Its Technique and Clinical Application*
Founded American Society of Regional Anesthesia (1923)

1942 **Allen (USA)**
Refrigeration anesthesia for amputation
Edwards and Hingson (USA)
Continuous caudal anesthesia in obstetrics

APPENDIX C: CHRONOLOGY OF LOCAL ANESTHETIC AGENTS

Cocaine
1860 Purification and naming by Niemann (Germany)
1884 First clinical use, topical, by Koller (Germany)
First clinical use, nerve block, by Halsted (USA)

Procaine
1904 Synthesis by Einhorn (Germany)
1905 Clinical introduction by Braun (Germany)

Stovaine*
1904 Synthesis by Fourneau (France)

Cinchocaine (Nupercaine, dibucaine)
1925 Synthesis by Meischer
1930 Clinical introduction by Uhlmann

Amethocaine (Pontocaine, Tetracaine)
1928 Synthesis by Eisleb
1932 Clinical introduction

Lignocaine (Lidocaine)
1943 Synthesis by Löfgren and Lundqvist
1947 Clinical introduction (Gordh)

Mepivacaine
1956 Synthesis by Ekstam and Egner
1957 Clinical introduction (Dhunér)

Prilocaine
1959 Synthesis by Lofgren and Tegner
1960 Clinical introduction by Wielding

Bupivacaine
1957 Synthesis by Ekstam
1963 Clinical introduction by Widman

Etidocaine
1971 Synthesis by Takman
1972 Clinical introduction by Lund

*Discarded, too toxic.

APPENDIX D: CHRONOLOGY OF INDIVIDUAL NEURAL BLOCKADE TECHNIQUES

Spinal analgesia
1898 Bier (Germany)
First use for surgery in humans
1940 Lemmon (USA)
Continuous spinal anesthesia
1946 Adriani and Roman-Vega (USA)
Saddle block spinal

Lumbar epidural analgesia
1921 Pagés (Spain)
First use for surgery
1931 Dogliotti (Italy)
Popularized surgical use
1949 Curbelo
Used Tuohy equipment for continuous blockade

Caudal epidural analgesia
1901 Sicard, Cathelin (France)
First use for surgery
1909 Stoeckel
Use in obstetrical pain
1910 Läwen (Germany)
Popularized surgical use
1913 Danis (Belgium)
Transsacral approach
1942 Edwards and Hingson (USA), Manalan
Continuous caudal

"Continuous" regional techniques
1931 Aburel (Rumania)
Continuous paravertebral lumbosacral plexus block

Paravertebral somatic block
1906 Sellheim
Thoracic paravertebral block
1912 Kappis
Paravertebral block for surgery and also for pain relief
1922 Läwen
Use in diagnosis of abdominal disease

Celiac block
1906 Braun
Anterior surgical approach
1914 Kappis
Posterior approach

Paravertebral lumbar sympathetic block
1926 Mandl

Stellate ganglion (cervicothoracic sympathetic) **block**
1930 Labat
Posterior approach
1934 Leriche and Fontaine
Anterior approach (used for cerebrovascular accidents)
1948 Apgar
Anterior approach
1954 Moore
Paratracheal approach

Brachial plexus block
1884 Halsted
Injection under direct vision
1897 Crile
1911 Hirschel
"Blind" axillary injection
Kulenkampff
Supraclavicular technique
1940 Patrick
Basis of current supraclavicular technique
1958 Burnham
Axillary perivascular technique
1964 Winnie and Collins
Subclavian
1970 Winnie
Interscalene

Cervical plexus block
1939 Rovenstine and Wertheim

Intravenous regional analgesia
1908 Bier
Injection between two cuffs
1963 Holmes
Injection below a single cuff after exsanguination

Intra-arterial regional anesthesia
1912 Goyanes (Spain)
Arterial injection below a cuff

Diagnostic blockade in pain management
1924 von Gaza
Procaine blockade in investigation of pain pathways
1930 Mandl
Paravertebral procaine block in diagnosis of angina pectoris
1930 White
Blockade of sensory and sympathetic nerves in pain diagnosis

Therapeutic nerve block in pain management
1899 Tuffier
Spinal cocaine for pain of sarcoma of leg
1901 Cushing

Regional anesthesia used to describe pain relief by nerve block
1903 Schloesser
Trigeminal alcohol block
1924 von Gaza, Braun, Mandl
Local anesthetic neural blockade for management of visceral pain
1924 Royle
Surgical sympathectomy for pain of spastic paralysis
1926 Swetlow
Neurolytic sympathetic block with alcohol for angina pectoris and abdominal pain
1930 Dogliotti
Neurolytic subarachnoid alcohol block
1941 Wertheim and Rovenstine
Suprascapular local anesthetic nerve block for shoulder pain

APPENDIX E: CHRONOLOGY OF THE STUDY OF COMPLICATIONS OF NEURAL BLOCKADE

1884 Halsted and associates (USA)
Cocaine addiction
1889 Reclus (France)
Toxicity due to systemic absorption defined
Bier and colleagues (Germany)
Severe postlumbar puncture headache
1900 Goldan (USA)
Development of anesthetic record of "intraspinal" cocainization
1901 Dandois (Belgium)
Paraplegia after subarachnoid cocaine
1906 Koenig (USA)
Permanent neurologic sequelae in several patients following spinal cocaine
1907 Barker (UK)
Recognition of need to control level of block
1912 Gray and Parsons (UK)
Recognition of vascular pooling due to sympathetic blockade
1927–1928 Labat (USA)
Emphasis on maintenance of cerebral perfusion
1952 Sancetta and colleagues
Cardiovascular effects of "low and high" spinal anesthesia
1953 Gillies (UK)
Studies of cardiovascular effects
1953– Green (USA)
Studies of physiologic effects of spinal anesthesia
1954 Dripps and Vandam (USA)
Long-term follow-up of 10,098 spinal anesthetics; failure to discover major neurologic sequelae
Importance of meticulous technique and safe handling of drugs stressed
1960– Bromage and colleagues (Canada)
Studies of physiology and pharmacology of epidural blockade
1965– Braid and Scott (UK); Tucker and Mather (USA); Boyes and Covino (USA); Harrison and colleagues (USA); De Jong and colleagues (USA)
Studies of pharmacokinetics and toxicity of local anesthetics
1970– Bonica and colleagues (USA)
Studies of cardiovascular effects of central neural blockade

part one

PHARMACOLOGY AND PHYSIOLOGY OF NEURAL BLOCKADE

2 NEURAL PHYSIOLOGY AND LOCAL ANESTHETIC ACTION

GARY R. STRICHARTZ

OVERVIEW OF THE NEURON

Local anesthetic drugs have in common the ability to reversibly block conduction of nerve impulses at the level of the axonal membrane. Thus it is pertinent to review briefly the structure and function of neurons, the impulse generating and conducting units of the nervous system. As shown in Figure 2-1, a typical neuron comprises a cell body (perikaryon), dendrites, with multiple small branches close to cell bodies, and a single axon for each neuron.

Sensory neurons have their cell bodies in dorsal root ganglia and are *unipolar,* that is, they have only one "process," an axon with a long branch extending to the periphery and a shorter branch to the spinal cord. Impulses are generated in the small peripheral branches (arborizations) at specialized sensory endings that serve as the "receptor" component of the neuron (see also Chap. 24, Table 24-1); axons then *conduct* these impulses to the spinal cord. Of note, sensory neurons subserving internal organs (visceral) are essentially the same and have their cell bodies in the dorsal root ganglion (see Chap. 24a). *Sympathetic (efferent) neurons* are described in Chapter 13 in detail, and an outline is shown in Figure 2-1.

Motor neurons have their cell bodies in the ventral horn of the spinal cord gray matter. They are *multipolar* in that they have many dendrites in addition to one axon that follows a long course to the periphery (Fig. 2-1). The dendrites and cell body of the motoneuron are specially developed for integrating postsynaptic currents to determine the output activity, as impulse generation, and the axon *conducts* these impulses to its branched terminal enlargements, which contain neurotransmitters to activate effector organs. *Interneurons* comprise a vast intermediate network with synapses between afferent (sensory) neurons and efferent (motor and sympathetic) neurons and other interneurons. Indeed, the overwhelming majority of all nerve cells are interneurons.

AXONS AND PERIPHERAL NERVES

Axons are cylinders of axoplasm encased in the axonal membrane, which is similar to other plasma membranes (Fig. 2-2). Axons are always enveloped by a Schwann cell. Many unmyelinated axons lie within invaginations of a single Schwann cell (Fig. 2-2C). In contrast, the thick myelin sheath of a myelinated axon is formed by a single Schwann cell wrapped many times round the axon (Fig. 2-2B). This myelin sheath is interrupted periodically at the so-called nodes of Ranvier, where the extracellular medium has access to the axolemma.

Nerve impulses travel along nonmyelinated axons as a uniform wave, in a manner similar to the way a flame progressively ignites the fuse of a firecracker. The nerve impulse, or *action potential,* is a change in the electrical voltage across the membrane that is due to changes in the permeability of ionic channels in the axon membrane (see below). In nonmyelinated axons

Parts of this chapter are based on the chapter by R. H. de Jong that appeared in the first edition of *Neural Blockade in Clinical Anesthesia and Management of Pain.*

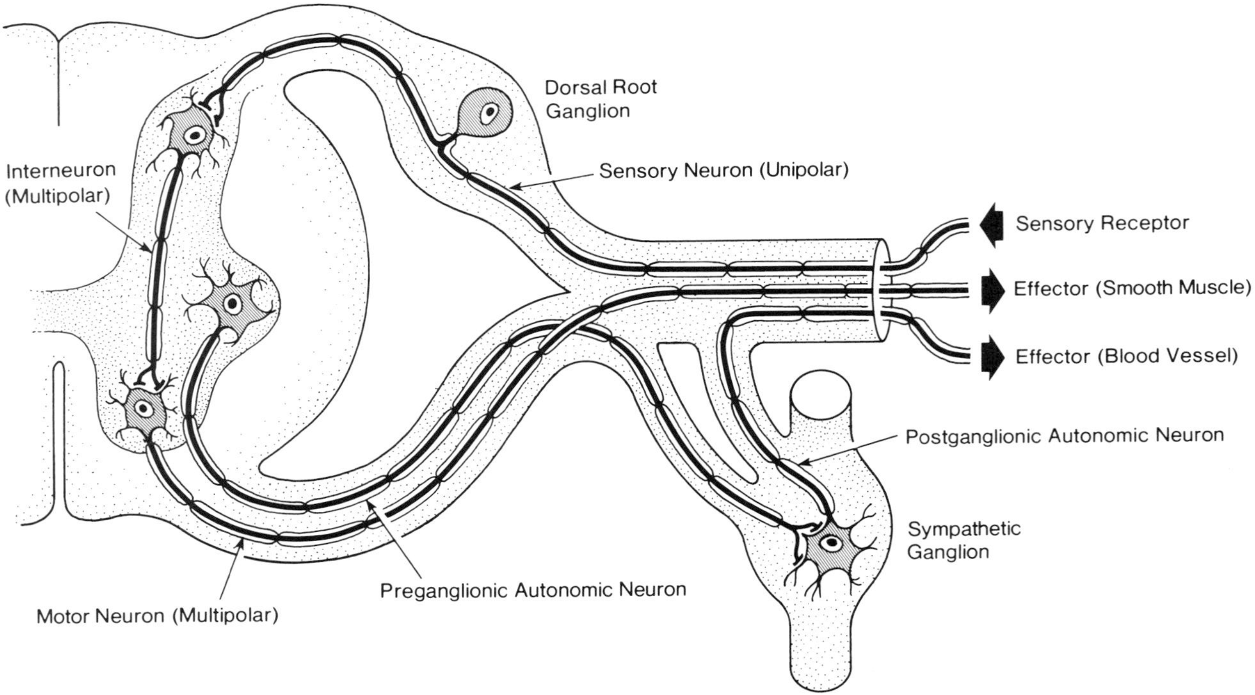

FIG. 2-1. The neuron. *Sensory neuron*, with a cell body (perikaryon) and an axon with long peripheral and short central branches ("unipolar" neuron). *Interneuron* with numerous dendrites, a cell body and one short axon ("multipolar" neuron). *Motor neuron* with a great many dendrites, a cell body, and a long peripheral axon ("multipolar" neuron). Two *sympathetic neurons*, one with a cell body in the spinal cord and the other with its cell body in the sympathetic chain, are also shown. Each has several dendrites and a medium length axon.

these permeability changes occur uniformly along the axon, supporting a wave of inward ionic current that underlies the depolarization of the nerve impulse. In myelinated axons, however, the membrane permeability changes, and associated inward currents occur only at the nodes of Ranvier; the myelinated *internode* of the axon is depolarized by the passive spread of current from the nodes. Thus impulse conduction in these axons is continuous but not homogeneous (see Fig. 2-8).

Axonal Membrane

The fluid mosaic model depicts the axonal membrane as a bilayer of phospholipid molecules with their fatty acyl chains facing each other, thus making the inner portion of the membrane hydrophobic. The surfaces of the membrane facing the cytoplasm and extracellular fluid are formed by the charged and polar hydrophilic groups of the phospholipid molecules. Globular proteins are also present, and some of these penetrate the entire thickness of the membrane. Ionic channels are composed of such transmembrane proteins (Fig. 2-3). The presence of globular proteins was confirmed by the technique of freeze-fracture electron microscopy. These globular proteins are the subject of intense investigation, with final details of structure and function as yet unknown (see below). It now seems likely, however, that the following functions are important: acting as ionic channels, pumping ions and transporting metabolites, acting as enzymes, receptors for hormones and transmitters, and as structural proteins.

Organization of a Peripheral Nerve. In clinical practice, local anesthetics must diffuse across a number of structures before reaching their site of action in the axonal membrane. Peripheral nerves contain both afferent and efferent axons (Fig. 2-4). These axons and their Schwann cells are surrounded by a delicate layer of fine connective tissue (endoneurium), which allows easy diffusion of local anesthetics.

Bundles of axons are enclosed in a squamous cellular sheath, the *perineurium,* which comprises several layers of cells and acts as a semipermeable barrier to local anesthetics. One or more perineurial bundles are covered by an outermost, easily permeable connective tissue layer, *epineurium.* This layer also carries the nutritional blood vessels of larger nerves (see also Figs. 29-1–29-3). Factors with an important influence on local anesthetic diffusion will thus include (see also Chap. 3) the perineurium, the presence or absence of myelin, and the size and position of the axons, either in the outermost or innermost aspects of the nerve (see Fig. 2-12).

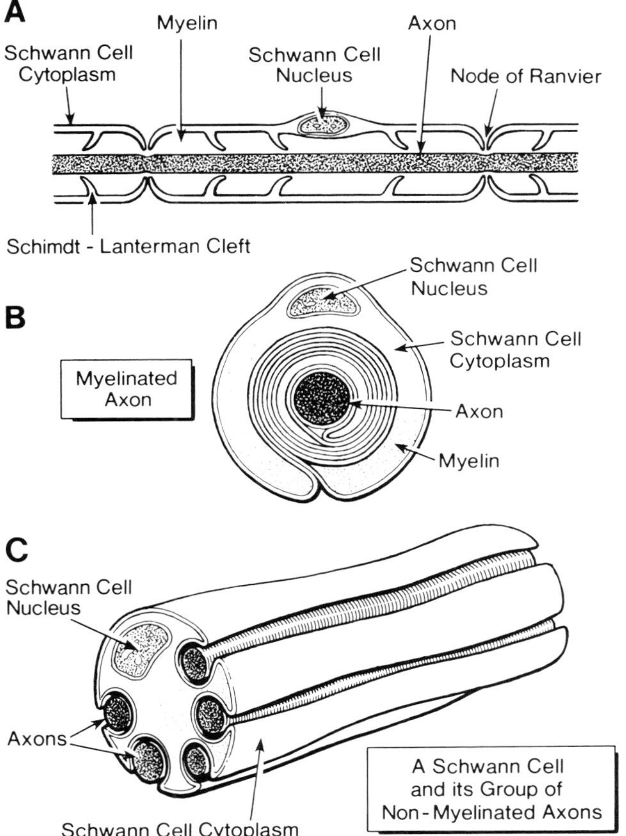

FIG. 2-2. Diagram of axon. *Myelinated axon.* **A.** Longitudinal section shows the relation of the myelin sheath to the nodes of Ranvier where myelin is absent, but one overlying Schwann cell and a thin layer of "gap substance" are present. The extranodal area is highly specialized and, because of anionic charges bound within it, tends to attract cationic substances such as local anesthetics. **B.** Transverse section of a myelinated fiber shows how the Schwann cell wraps around one axon many times to form the multiple layers of the myelin sheath. **C.** In transverse section many nonmyelinated axons can be seen embedded in the folds of a single Schwann cell. The Schwann cell surrounds the axon loosely, thus allowing uniform spread of depolarization directly along the axon (see below).

NERVE MEMBRANES AND IMPULSES

The generation and the propagation of impulses in excitable nerve and muscle cells are dependent on the flow of specific ionic currents through channels that span the plasma membrane. These channels open and close in response to the electrical potential of the cell membrane and are the targets for local anesthetics as they block impulse propagation. A major purpose of this chapter is to describe the role of ion channels in impulse behavior and thereby explain many of the physiologic effects of local anesthetics. Most ion channels appear to be very similar in the peripheral and central nervous systems, in cell bodies, and in axons. Thus a single description will serve to characterize the actions of local anesthetics associated with blockade of axonal conduction in peripheral nerve or those actions associated with cardiac and central nervous system toxicity.

This knowledge provides a basis for increasing the efficacy of neural blockade and for helping to prevent and treat the complications from local anesthesia.

IONIC BASIS OF THE IMPULSE

The important elements for impulse generation are contained in the plasma membrane of excitable cells. Two factors contribute to electric potentials in cells: concentration gradients of ions across membranes, and selective permeation of ions through membranes. The gradients, in conjunction with existing electric potentials, produce forces that tend to move the ions; the selective changes in permeability permit that tendency to be manifested as ionic current. Energy from the cell's metabolism is used to create and maintain the gradients.

The concentration of potassium ions inside a cell is about ten times greater than the extracellular K^+ concentration, and *vice versa* for sodium ions. A special protein in the membrane (the Na–K pump) actively transports K^+ into the cell and Na^+ out of the cell,

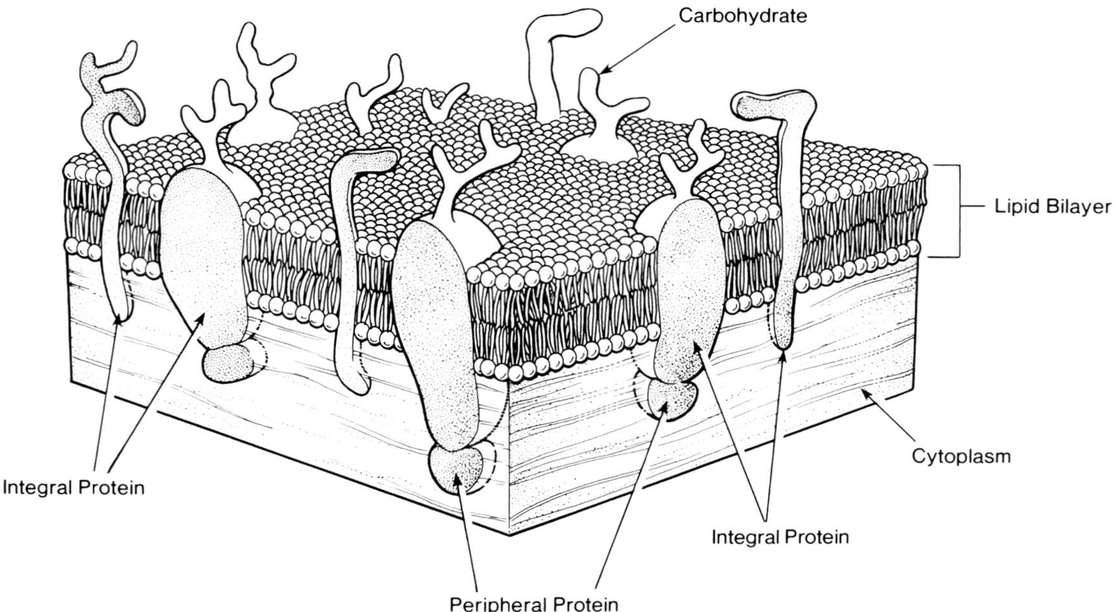

FIG. 2-3. Axonal membrane. The axonal membrane is similar to the plasma membrane of other cells. This diagram is modified from the classic Singer–Nicholson fluid-mosaic model (Singer and Nicholson, 1972). Carbohydrate molecules attached to proteins and lipids on the extracellular surface of the membrane form a "cell coat." The lipid bilayer comprises densely packed phospholipids which, nevertheless, freely diffuse laterally in the plane of the membrane. Integral proteins of varying shapes and peripheral protein only on the cytoplasmic surface are associated with enzymatic and receptor functions.

using ATP as the source of energy (see below in Fig. 2-8).[41] In the resting axon membrane there is a selective permeability to K^+ ions, allowing the net efflux of a small number of K^+ ions and leaving the axoplasm electrically negative (polarized) while making the outside electrically positive. This accounts, for the most part, for the cell's "resting potential," which typically equals −70 to −80 millivolts (Fig. 2-5).

Sodium ions tend to flow into the axon because it is now electrically negative inside and the Na^+ ions are more concentrated outside. A selective permeability to Na^+ arises when specific "sodium channels" in the axon membrane are opened.[28] Figure 2-5 shows the contributions of ionic currents during a propagated nerve impulse. Note that the initial depolarization of the membrane precedes the increase in ionic current; this early depolarization is a result of "local circuit" current flowing down the axon from an adjacent excited region of axon. The large inward Na current (I_{Na^+}) dominates the total ionic current (I_i) and accounts for the *rising phase* of the impulse. Opening of Na^+ channels occurs as the membrane is "depolarized" from the resting potential, that is, as it becomes less negative. Such opening is an intrinsic behavior of Na^+ channels, arising from their molecular structure. As the membrane potential becomes less negative, more Na^+ channels open, and they open more rapidly; as more channels open, more Na^+ ions enter the cell, and depolarization is accelerated (Fig. 2-6). This cycle accounts for the regenerative behavior of nerve impulses.[29]

Impulse depolarizations are transient events. Repolarization of the membrane to the negative resting value occurs because of three factors: The force moving Na^+ into the cell diminishes as the axoplasmic potential becomes less negative; the sodium channels eventually close during a depolarization; new potassium channels open and allow a large, outward K^+-current that returns the axoplasmic potential toward its resting value, or beyond (see Fig. 2-5). In simple terms, impulses have a depolarization phase and a repolarization phase. Inward currents, carried by Na^+ ions, depolarize the cell whereas outward currents, carried by K^+ ions, repolarize the cell. It must be

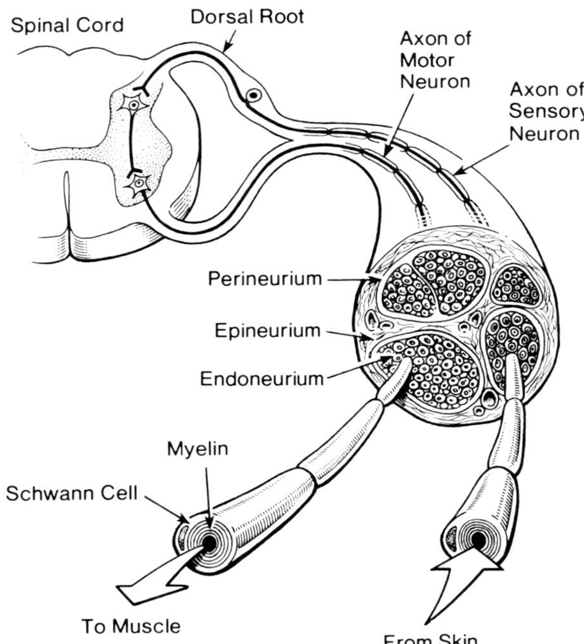

FIG. 2-4. Diagram of a peripheral nerve. The *epineurium*, with its easily permeable collagen fibers, is oriented along the long axis of the nerve. The *perineurium* is a discrete layer of cells, whereas the *endoneurium* is a delicate matrix of connective tissue embedding bundles of axons. Both afferent (sensory) and efferent (motor) axons are shown. Sympathetic efferent axons (not shown) are also present in mixed peripheral nerves.

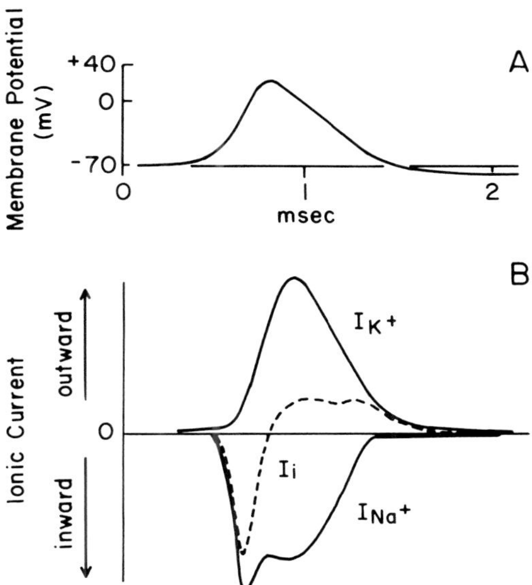

FIG. 2-5. A propagating action potential and the membrane currents that produce it. **A.** The membrane potential rises from its resting value, about −70 mV in this squid axon, to reverse its sign, becoming positive inside, and then repolarizes. A hyperpolarization actually follows the impulse in this, but not in all, axons. **B.** Inward sodium current ($I_{Na}+$) and outward potassium current ($I_K +$) together yield the net ionic current across the membrane (I_i). The maximum rate of depolarization corresponds to the peak of net inward current, that of repolarization to the largest net outward current.

emphasized that the total number of ions moving across the membrane is small and that the most modest concentration changes occur, even during a tetanic train of impulses.[30] These changes stimulate the Na^+-K^+ transport pump, which then restores the original gradient over a period of seconds to minutes. Because the pump moves unequal numbers of Na^+ and K^+ ions, it creates a net current and can mildly hyperpolarize the axon through this action. In this way, and in other ways, such as ion accumulation, the preceding activity in a nerve will influence the conduction properties of subsequent impulses, for times considerably longer than the traditional refractory period.

THRESHOLD

In order to initiate an impulse, conditions must exist wherein a *net* inward current occurs. This requires

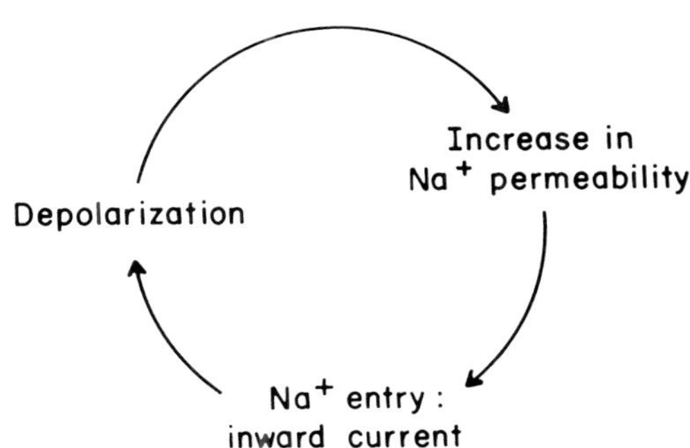

FIG. 2-6. The positive feedback cycle that underlies the depolarization phase of regenerative action potentials. Each of the three components in the cycle is increased by the preceding one and, in turn, increases the subsequent one. The cycle is initiated by a source of current "external" to the membrane area being studied, for example, an adjacent excited region, a sensory ending depolarized by a physiologic stimulus, or a dendritic arbor that collects postsynaptic currents.

that a sufficient number of sodium channels be opened in order to overcome the actions of the outward current pathways; outward current is carried by the "leak" channels, which are open at rest, plus the voltage-dependent K^+ channels. Small depolarizations, of 15 to 20 mV, are usually sufficient to initiate an impulse in a resting axon, but larger stimulating depolarizations are needed shortly after a preceding impulse, that is, threshold is greater during such a "refractory" period.[42] Other circumstances that elevate threshold are pathologic, such as demyelination of myelinated axons, and pharmacologic, such as the presence of local anesthetics.[55] Often threshold rises because there are fewer available Na^+ channels. Then additional reductions in the impulse amplitude, rate of depolarization, and conduction speed also occur. Partial blockade of impulses occurs in regions of individual axons where some, but not all, of the sodium channels are blocked. These reduced impulses still exhibit threshold behavior and are characterized as all-or-nothing phenomena.

IMPULSE PROPAGATION

Inward current entering the axon during the depolarizing phase of an impulse flows within the conducting medium of the axoplasm and spreads to adjacent, inactive regions. These adjacent regions are thus rapidly depolarized by the "local circuit" current, usually to levels far in excess of those for threshold conditions, and the regenerative impulse "invades" this region, generating its own inward current. Figure 2-7 shows how the propagating impulse potential is spread over axons during one instant. The spatial spread of the potential change is large compared to the nerve diameter. If we assume that the impulse lasts for a duration of 1 msec, and is conducted at a velocity of 1 m/sec in the small, nonmyelinated C fibers (of less than 1 μm diameter), then the potential change extends over 1 mm, 1000 times the axon diameter. For large myelinated axons, of 20 μm diameter, impulses travel at 60 to 100 m/sec and thus extend over distances of 60 to 100 mm. In these fibers

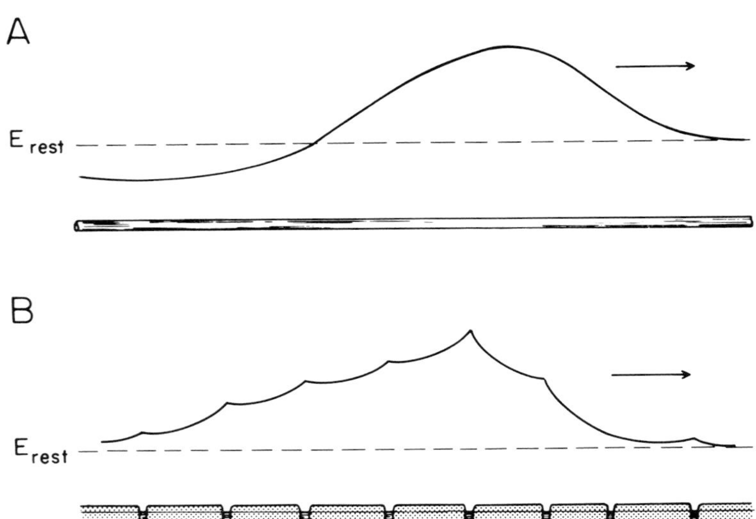

FIG. 2-7. Instantaneous spatial distribution of the membrane potential change during the propagation of an action potential conducted to the right, as shown by the arrows. **A.** In the smaller, nonmyelinated axon (*e.g.*, a mammalian C-fiber) the potential changes in the same smooth, continuous shape that it has when measured in time at one narrow region of the axon. This occurs because the axon is a cable with uniform properties along its length and the impulse propagates at a constant velocity. **B.** Conduction in a myelinated axon is also characterized by continuous potential changes along the axon. Regions in which large inward currents flow into the axon, the nodes of Ranvier, depolarize the adjacent internodes, which have no sodium channels and generate no active inward ionic current. (The lengths of nodes and internodes are not drawn to scale.) Note that during an impulse many nodes of Ranvier are simultaneously at some level of depolarization; thus the impulse travels much further in the same time in a myelinated axon (see text).

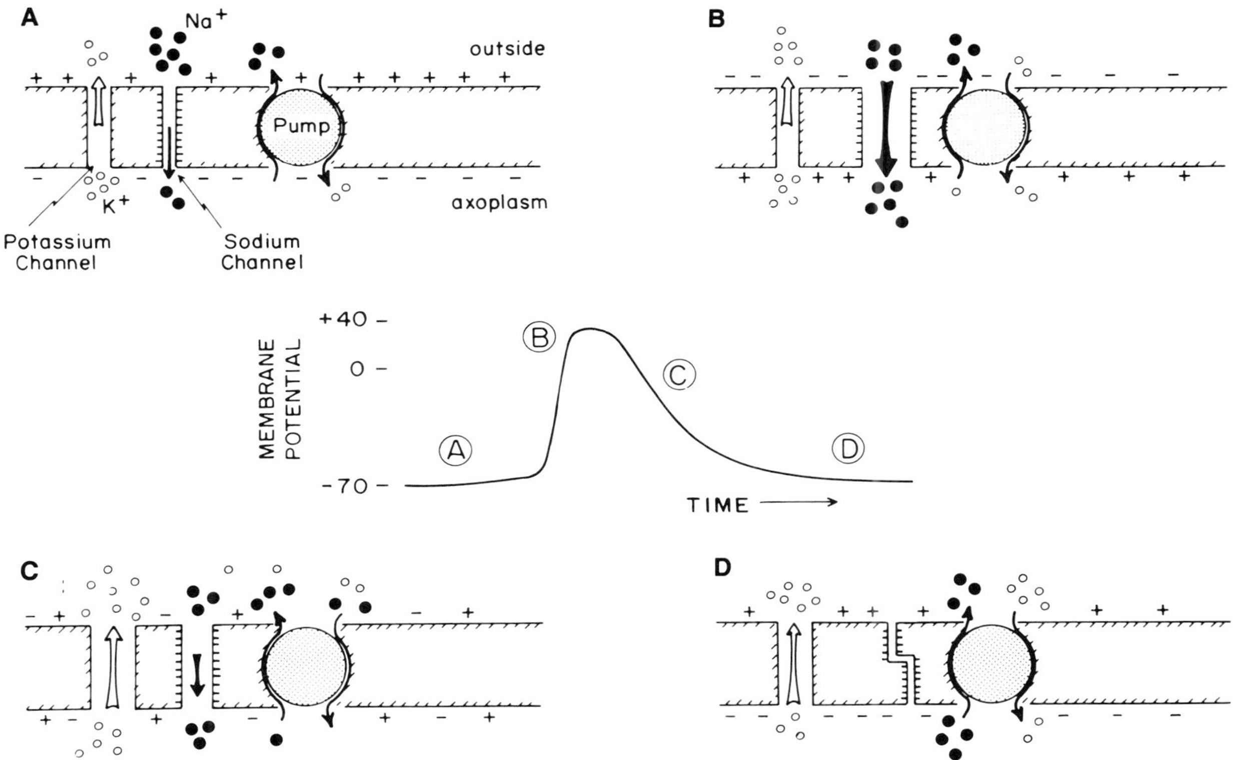

FIG. 2-8. Diagram of the states of membrane activities at different phases of the action potential. Potassium channels *(open arrows)*, sodium channels *(filled arrows)*, and the (Na^+-K^+) pump are shown. The size of the arrows indicates the magnitude of the current through the specific channel; the "width" of the channels is proportional to the relative permeability of that channel, or to the fractions of channels that are open. **A.** In the resting membrane a small efflux of K^+ and influx of Na^+ are balanced by basal activity of the pump, which always transports $^3Na^+$ out for each $^2K^+$ it brings in. **B.** At the rising phase, the rapid depolarization is driven by a large Na^+ current. **C.** During repolarization more K^+ channels are opened and the Na^+ channels begin to close, by inactivation, resulting in a net outward current. **D.** Directly after the impulse many Na^+ channels are inactivated and cannot open in response to a depolarizing stimulus. The impulse-related increase in intracellular Na^+ accelerates the pump, which also removes some of the K^+ that may have accumulated in the extra-axonal space. The combination of ion accumulation and depletion, electrogenic pump activity, and slow recovery of channel conformational changes accounts for the multiphasic changes in firing threshold that follow nerve impulses.

the active Na^+ currents are entering the axon at the nonmyelinated nodes of Ranvier, which are separated from one another by several millimeters of insulated myelin.[31] Obviously, many nodes are being depolarized simultaneously, although to differing degrees, as an impulse propagates along these axons. Inward currents from all the active nodes integrate as they spread toward inactive regions, ensuring that impulse propagation will continue. Therefore, complete block of impulses in about three to five nodes in sequence is necessary for the total prevention of impulse propagation.[44]

A visualization of the molecular events around a nerve impulse helps to summarize the forgoing (Fig. 2-8). In the resting axon the membrane is selectively permeable to K^+ ions; basal activity of the Na^+-K^+ pump maintains the ion gradients against a background "leak" through the resting membrane. Local depolarizations rapidly increase the permeability to Na^+ ions and, if sufficient, trigger an increase in Na^+ current large enough to produce the full impulse depolarization. The K^+ permeability also increases, although more slowly, and in conjunction with inactivation of the Na^+ permeability results in a net outward current. This repolarizes the membrane. The small changes in ion concentrations, particularly the increase in intracellular Na^+, stimulate the Na^+-K^+ pump to act more rapidly, thus restoring the original conditions.

MECHANISMS OF ANESTHETIC ACTION

Local anesthetics block impulses by interfering with the function of sodium channels.[24,59] In the presence of local anesthetics, sodium channels are less likely to open in response to a stimulating depolarization,[10] the resulting Na^+ current is decreased, and at sufficiently high anesthetic concentrations enough channels are blocked to prevent impulse generation. Because they lessen the probability that channels will open, local anesthetics have an effect similar to that of a preceding depolarization. They shift channels toward an "inactivated" state that cannot be directly opened by stimulation but must first be converted to the "resting" state from which opening normally occurs.[14]

A detailed analysis of the mechanism of local anesthetic action encounters three salient questions: Which species of the drug, neutral or protonated, is the active form? Where does the anesthetic molecule act? What is the molecular mechanism of channel interference? These interrelated questions are addressed next.

ACTIVE SPECIES

Being tertiary amines (see Table 3-1, Chap. 3), local anesthetics under physiologic conditions exist in rapid equilibrium between the neutral and protonated, charged species:

$$\overset{|}{\underset{/\ \backslash}{\mathrm{N}:}} \quad + \quad \mathrm{H}^+ \rightleftharpoons \overset{|}{\underset{/\ \backslash}{\mathrm{NH}^+}}$$

Nonionized + proton base (neutral) — Ionized (charged) "protonated" conjugate acid

The pKa values of the tertiary amines range from about 7.5 to 9.5; thus in solution all these drugs are charged more of the time than they are uncharged (see Chap. 3, Tables 3-1, 3-2). Evidence suggests that both species can inhibit Na^+ channels. Quaternary derivatives that are permanently charged, such as QX-314, when directed into the axoplasmic space are potent blockers of impulses and of Na^+ currents.[21,53] Interestingly, these drugs are without effect when placed outside the axon; their charge and low hydrophobicity greatly restrict their passage into and through the membrane. Perpetually uncharged, benzocaine also effectively blocks impulses and sodium channels.[26,46] The potency of tertiary amine local anesthetics in blocking sodium channels in single cells is faster and larger when the drug is applied externally at alkaline external *p*H[25] or by direct internal perfusion at neutral or slightly acidic internal *p*H.[37] Both of these observations are consistent with a model where the neutral form of the anesthetic dissolves in and passes through the axon membrane and, having reached its site of action, becomes protonated (see Chap. 3, Table 3-2). Thus, *p*H effects anesthetic potency on single fibers by two, conflicting means. An extracellular alkaline *p*H favors the neutral membrane-permeant form of the drug, but an acidic cytoplasmic *p*H favors the more potent blocking species at the site of action. Thus both neutral and charged forms of anesthetics participate in impulse blockade. (Of course, during most clinical procedures, the functional potency of local anesthetics is determined largely by the fraction of injected drug that passes through tissue barriers into the nerve bundle, and alkaline conditions that favor the penetrating, neutral species are desirable.)[12,47]

LOCUS OF ACTION

In principle, local anesthetics could act at any of three phases in nerve membranes: at the membrane : solution interface, in the membrane's hydrocarbon interior, or at the sodium channel itself. The last possibility is probably the case for traditional local anesthetic agents (Fig. 2-9). The quaternary derivatives, mentioned above, are known to bind at the interface of lipid bilayer membranes and thus to alter the local membrane properties,[36,52] but they act on nerves only from the axoplasmic surface. Thus the general perturbation of the interface cannot be a mechanism for nerve block.

Many compounds can dissolve in the hydrocarbon

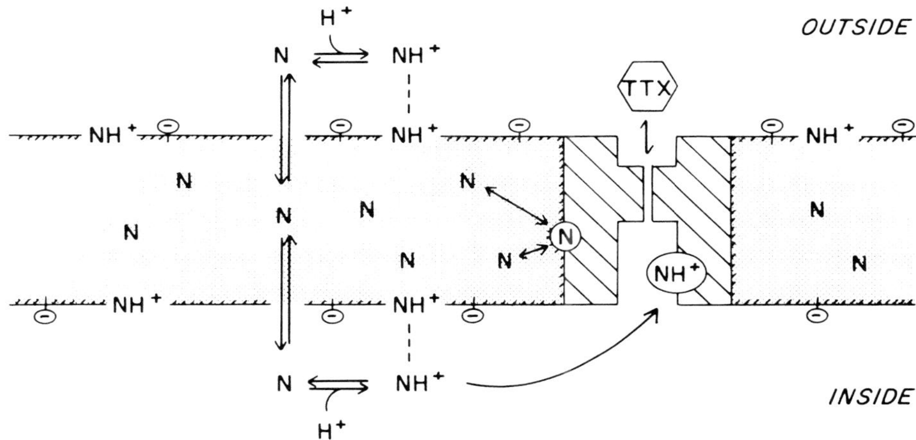

FIG. 2-9. Tertiary amine local anesthetics exist as neutral base *(N)* and protonated *(NH^+)* species in physiologic solution. These forms interact in various modes with phospholipids and proteins in nerve membranes: *N* preferentially partitions into the hydrophobic membrane interior, whereas NH^+ adsorbs at the negatively charged membrane surface, through hydrophobic and electrostatic interactions. Two primary reactions with Na^+ channel proteins are shown: rapid binding of the neutral form at the lipid:protein interface and slower binding of the charged form by means of the inner mouth of the channel; the latter depends on the conversion of the channel to open or activated conformations (see text). The natural "local anesthetics" tetrodotoxin (TTX) and saxitoxin bind at the external surface of the channel and have no obvious interactions with local anesthetics.

interior of cell membranes, but few of these block impulse conduction at concentrations as low as those that perturb the membrane interior.[51]

In contrast, there is ever-increasing evidence that local anesthetics specifically associate with the sodium channel itself. For example, the inhibition of channels is enhanced by the application of patterns of membrane potential that favor the opening of sodium channels.[14,53] This potentiation of anesthetic block by repetitive depolarizations is called "use-dependent" or "phasic" block. The degree of inhibition of single impulses, measured without recently preceding stimulation, is called resting or "tonic" block. Local anesthetics also are more potent, tonically, on channels in depolarized membranes than on those in normally polarized membranes.[14,26] Other features of tonic and phasic blocks will be described in the following section.

Another observation supporting the notion of the sodium channel as anesthetic receptor is the stereoselective block by anesthetic enantiomers. The presence of asymmetric carbons in the aromatic moiety, or in the cyclic amine of molecules like bupivacaine, results in a potency difference of two to five between isomers[2]; however, isomers around asymmetric carbons in the intermediate linkage show no stereoselective potency.[18]

Finally, the effects of local anesthetics are modified by other drugs and treatments that specifically affect Na^+ channels. Activator compounds, which allow channels to open at the resting potential and thus produce spontaneous depolarizations of the cell, are antagonized by local anesthetics, competitively.[33,34] Enzymatic digestion of a portion of the channel facing the axoplasm greatly reduces the phasic blocking action of anesthetics, although tonic block is little affected.[8] These observations all point to the sodium channel itself as a *specific receptor* for local anesthetic molecules.

MOLECULAR MECHANISMS OF ACTION

How exactly do local anesthetics interfere with the operation of Na^+ channels? The answer must be framed by our limited knowledge of channel structure and function. Sodium channels have been isolated and purified from eel electric organ and mammalian brain and muscle. The channels are composed of at least one, very large protein (200,000 daltons) and perhaps one or two smaller proteins (each about 40,000 daltons).[1,4,22] The protein is bound to many sugar residues that probably extend into the extracellular interface. An unusually high percentage of these sugars are negatively charged sialic acid groups (see Fig. 2-3). The channel is unstable and denatures irreversibly when removed from the membrane by solubilization with nonionic detergents, but stability is gained by addition of phospholipids to the detergent.[1] Such solubilized channels can be inserted into artificial lipid bilayer membranes and will perform similarly to native sodium channels.[48] Apparently the structural integrity and functional capacity of channels is dependent on an intimate association with phospholipids. The primary sequence of amino acids is now known for the large protein from the electric eel's sodium channel, and speculations about its three-dimensional structure are inevitable.[39] Despite these structural details, the functional roles of identified regions of the channel protein remain unknown.

All the information about mechanisms of local anesthetics comes from physiologic studies. Some of these have been reviewed above. Anesthetics inhibit stimulated channels (phasic block) more than resting channels (tonic block). Phasic block is much more stereospecific than tonic block.[64] Quaternary anesthetic derivatives, active only from the axoplasm, seem to bind selectively to channels in the open conformation and to dissociate very slowly from these channels once they have closed, leading researchers to identify an anesthetic binding site in the channel's pore.[9,53] In contrast, neutral anesthetics like benzocaine provide almost no phasic block.[26] If they also bind in the pore, they can dissociate rapidly from closed channels, perhaps by leaving through a hydrophobic pathway into the hydrophobic core of the membrane. By comparison, tertiary amine anesthetics produce a phasic block that is dependent on the extracellular *p*H.[49] At high *p*H, when they are less charged, they behave like benzocaine, and at low *p*H, when they are more charged, they behave like the quaternary compounds.

A single explanation for tonic and phasic block has been formalized as the modulated receptor hypothesis (MRH) (see Fig. 2-10). The hypothesis rests on the accepted notion that sodium channels normally respond to membrane depolarizations by passing through defined conformational "states," beginning at rest (R), activating through closed intermediate

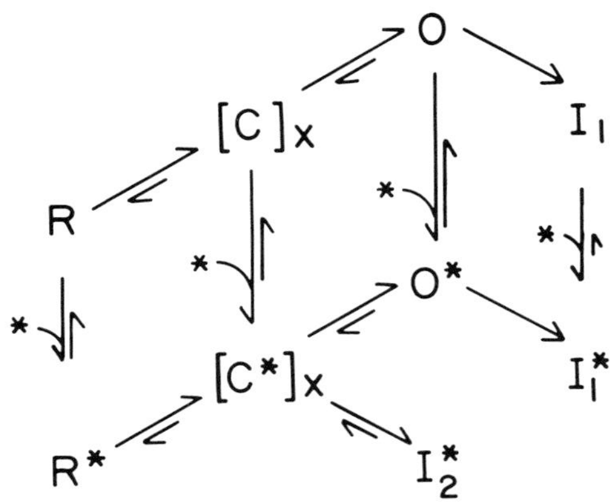

FIG. 2-10. The revised modulated receptor model. Each letter represents a state of the sodium channel: *R*, resting; C_x, any one of several intermediate states between *R* and *O*, which is the open, ion conducting state; I_1, an inactivated (nonopenable) state that is formed from *O;* and I_2, a different inactivated state that is formed from the anesthetic-bound *C** states, without going through *O*. The vertical arrows indicate binding reactions of a local anesthetic molecule, indicated by the asterisk (*). States *C* and *O* and *I* have higher affinities for anesthetics than does *R*. The $[C^*]_x \leftrightarrows I_2^*$ reaction may account for much of the resting, tonic blocking activity of local anesthetics, and thus favor the neutral, more hydrophobic drugs. Anesthetic binding reactions of *O* and *I* conformations are activated by rapid depolarizations (*e.g.*, action potentials), with the fomer being faster than the latter. Charged drugs bound to *O** and I_1 and I_2^* dissociate slowly, accounting for much of the phasic blocking behavior.

forms (C) to reach an open (O) form, and then closing to an inactivated (I) state. According to the MRH, local anesthetics have a higher affinity for open and, especially, inactivated Na^+ channels than for resting channels.[27] During stimulation, channels that are opened and inactivated bind local anesthetics more tightly. This binding thus stabilizes the channels in a nonconducting state, and increasingly so with each stimulating pulse. Eventually some anesthetic-bound channels will return to the resting equilibrium, and a steady-state level of phasic block will be reached wherein increased inhibition during a depolarization is exactly reversed by drug dissociation in the time between pulses.

The original MRH has been modified on the basis of recent experiments showing that channels that have been modified chemically to prevent inactivation still can be blocked by local anesthetics, both phasically and tonically. Therefore, the normal inactivated state is not essential for block.[56] It appears that open and activated channels react most rapidly with anesthetic molecules and that inactivated channels react more slowly but still have a greater equilibrium drug affinity than resting channels. During one relatively brief nerve impulse the formation of inactivated channels is limited, and drug binding to this state probably contributes little to the observed phasic block. In contrast, during a cardiac (ventricular) action potential (see Fig. 2-13) the long depolarized plateau populates the inactivated state for a sufficiently long time to allow significant anesthetic binding to that conformation. Therefore, this reaction pathway is probably important for the antiarrhythmic action of local anesthetics, as described later in this chapter. Regardless of the kinetic details, the concept of selective, state-dependent binding of anesthetics lies at the core of the modulated receptor concept.

Does an anesthetic molecule that inhibits the channel act by "plugging" the pore, preventing ions from passing, or does it interfere with the conformational changes that underlie channel opening? Both possibilities are supported by experimental evidence, and indeed both may be occurring during the blockade of impulses by tertiary amine drugs. My own view is that tertiary amine drugs have two binding sites on the channel (see Fig. 2-9). One site is near enough to the pore to allow the anesthetic molecule to become protonated directly from the solution; this site favors the charged anesthetic species. Binding and unbinding of drug molecules from this site are slow reactions, with rates that approximate those of the channel gating processes. The other site is in a hydrophobic milieu where the probability of encountering a proton donor is low. This second site is bound during tonic block, and local anesthetics can bind to, and dissociate from it into the membrane relatively rapidly and easily. During phasic block, anesthetic molecules bind to the first site, from which dissociation is much slower. Interestingly, the stereoisomers that show the greater potency for phasic block are all relatively long, planar molecules compared to their less potent enantiomers, which show an acutely angled conformation.[18] The planar isomer probably slides easily into the phasic blocking site, whereas the angled one is sterically restricted from that locus. Our knowledge about molecular mechanisms of anesthetic action will expand greatly with the detailed structural analysis of purified sodium channels.

CLINICAL ASPECTS OF NERVE BLOCK

Consideration of factors beyond the molecular mechanism of action is necessary to describe the effects of local anesthetics as they are used clinically. Both anatomic and chemical factors determine the susceptibility of fibers to block by local anesthetics, the rate of onset, maximum degree, and duration of nerve block, and the differential actions of local anesthetics on different kinds of excitable tissues. All these aspects are discussed in this section.

Fiber Size and Function. The diameter and myelinization of a nerve fiber determine (to a degree) its sensitivity to local anesthetics as well as its message-carrying function. To simplify description, nerve fibers have been categorized into three major classes: Myelinated somatic nerves are called A fibers; myelinated preganglionic autonomic nerves, B fibers; and nonmyelinated axons, C fibers. The B and C fibers are small, ranging in diameter from about 2 μm to less than 1 μm, respectively, whereas the A fibers vary in diameter from about 4 to 20 μm (Table 2-1).

Accordingly, A fibers are further divided into four groups according to decreasing impulse conduction velocity and size: alpha, beta, gamma, and delta. Largest are the alpha fibers, related to motor function, proprioception, and reflex activity. Beta fibers also innervate muscle and transmit touch and pressure sensations, while gamma fibers control muscle spindle tone. The thinnest A fibers — the delta group — subserve pain and temperature functions and signal tissue damage.

The thinly myelinated B fibers are preganglionic autonomic axons that innervate vascular smooth muscle, among others; B fibers thus assume cardinal importance during spinal or peridural anesthesia. The nonmyelinated C fibers, like the myelinated A-delta fibers, subserve pain and temperature transmission, as well as postganglionic autonomic functions. C fibers are thinner than myelinated fibers (less than 1 μm diameter) and have a much lower conduction velocity than even A-delta fibers, less than 1 m/sec.

It is evident from this summary that humans are equipped with two separate impulse conducting systems that convey pain-related messages: One system relays signals rapidly and comprises myelinated A-delta fibers; the other comprises slowly conducting nonmyelinated C fibers.

TABLE 2-1. CLASSIFICATION AND PHYSIOLOGIC CHARACTERISTICS OF NERVE FIBERS

Class	A-alpha	A-beta	A-gamma	A-delta	B	C
Function	Motor	Touch/pressure	Proprioception	Pain/temperature	Preganglionic autonomic (sympathetic)	Pain/temperature
Myelin	+++	++	++	++	+	−
Diameter (μm)	12–20	5–12	5–12	1–4	1–3	0.5–1
Conduction speed (m/sec)	70–120	30–70	30–70	12–30	14.8*	1.2
Onset time	0 ←	0 ←	0 ←	0 ←	0 →	0
Regression	Reverse of onset time (note some exceptions with long-acting agents, *e.g.*, etidocaine sympathetic block offset before sensory)†					
C_m (parallels onset time)		Highest			Lowest	

Key: +++: heavily myelinated; ++: moderately myelinated; +: lightly myelinated; −: nonmyelinated.

*Faster onset than smaller C fibers because C fibers are grouped together in less accessible "Remak bundles."

†Data from Bromage P.R.: Physiology and pharmacology of epidural analgesia. Anesthesiology *28*:592, 1967.

(Data from de Jong, R.H., and Nace, R.A.: Nerve impulse conduction during intravenous lidocaine injection. Anesthesiology, *29*:22, 1968; Heavner, J.E., and de Jong, R.H.: Lidocaine blocking concentrations for B- and C-nerve fibers. Anesthesiology, *40*:228, 1974; Scurlock, J.E., Heavner, J.E., de Jong R.H.: Differential B and C fibre block by an amide- and an ester-linked local anesthetic. Br. J. Anaesth., *47*:1135 1975)

MINIMUM BLOCKING CONCENTRATION (C_m)

The minimum blocking concentration (C_m) is defined as the lowest concentration of local anesthetic *in vitro* that will block a given nerve within a reasonable time (commonly 10 min). The C_m of a local anesthetic is thus similar to the minimum alveolar anesthetic concentration (MAC) of a general anesthetic. Another similarity with inhalation agents is the need to administer initially a higher concentration of drug to achieve an effective concentration, rapidly, at the site of action in the nervous system; that is, MAC in the brain for inhalation agents, or C_m in the axon for local anesthetics. (It should be understood that C_m has been determined *in vitro;* thus for blockade of mixed somatic nerve function an administered concentration of 1% lidocaine *in vivo* appears to be necessary to achieve the measured C_m of approximately 0.07% [2–3 mM] lidocaine at the axons.) The concept is important clinically, for only drug concentrations greater than C_m will reliably anesthetize a nerve. As the pharmacologic potency of local anesthetics varies greatly, each agent has a C_m that must be further defined by the prevailing solution conditions, for example, *p*H, temperature, and Na^+ and Ca^{2+} concentrations.

The C_m of an axon with given diameter is the same whether it runs in a peripheral nerve or in a spinal rootlet. The local anesthetic pool, however, is subject to numerous influences that act to reduce the final anesthetic concentration reaching the nerve membrane. Dilution by tissue fluid, fibrous tissue barriers, absorption, metabolism, elimination, and distribution are examples. The final concentration of drug eventually arriving at the axon depends on the magnitude of these factors and on the length of exposure to them (see also Chap. 3). For instance, much less local anesthetic is needed for subarachnoid than for peridural block, not because the C_m changes when an axon transverses the vertebral canal, but because spinal roots are flimsily protected in the subarachnoid space. Additionally, the drug is absorbed faster into the bloodstream from the vascular extradural space than from the marginally perfused intradural space (see Chaps. 3, 4).

DIFFERENTIAL NERVE BLOCK

It is often noted when anesthetizing a peripheral nerve that pain is obtunded completely (A-delta and C fibers are blocked) but that motor function and touch (A-alpha and A-beta fibers) are unaffected.[43] Without forewarning, the patient's retention of muscle control might be disconcerting to a surgeon accustomed to equating anesthesia with limp muscles. Further, as large fibers convey touch and light pressure sensations, an anxious patient might misinterpret the perception of incision and tissue manipulation as pain. This situation is called a differential block.

If motor block is to accompany sensory blockade —desirable when setting a fracture, for instance—a more concentrated local anesthetic solution is used, which ensures that the C_m of even the larger motor fibers is reached. Further, during the block's induction phase the intraneural anesthetic concentration rises with time. Thus, merely waiting a few minutes may raise the anesthetic concentration above the C_m for motor nerves, and thus build up toward full motor blockade after all.

Differential blockade, observed clinically, has its basis in several possible sources. First, it may be a temporal rather than an equilibrium phenomenon, impulses in small fibers being blocked faster than those in large ones because of the time-course of drug diffusion into, as well as along the length of, nerve sufficient to block propagation through the anesthetized region. Second, some fibers may be more subject to impulse blockade by anesthetics than others because of anatomic features, such as the presence of myelin, which can effectively pool anesthetic molecules near the axon membrane, at steady-state, but draw them away from the axon during the onset of drug diffusion and block. Third, axons *per se* may be differentially sensitive to block because, for example, some have potassium channels and some do not,[13,45] the resting potentials differ, or the nature of the membrane lipids differs, and thus also the membrane concentration of anesthetics.[54]

These categories to explain differential block are speculations about a complex behavior observed clinically. The situation is not much clarified by experimental studies. The relation between C_m and fiber diameter is far more complex than is usually appreciated. Despite widespread belief, C_m does not increase simply as a function of fiber diameter.[43] This is especially true when comparing myelinated and nonmyelinated fibers. In separate experiments, it has been shown that both B-fibers and A-delta fibers are blocked at concentrations of local anesthetics lower than those required to block the smaller C fibers.[23,57] Among the myelinated fibers, however, a block of larger fibers does seem to require a higher C_m. In almost all such studies the amplitude of compound action potentials is measured; this signal represents the summed response of thousands of similar but nonidentical individual axons. Reduction of the maximum amplitude occurs because impulses in some fibers are slowed more than in others, in addition to the total blockade present in yet other fibers. In other words, the signal is spread out, or dispersed, as well as inhibited owing to complete block. The consequences of this dispersion for synaptic integration of afferent information in the spinal cord are unknown. Therefore, it would be fortuitous if a 50% reduction of the compound action potentials from A-delta and C-fibers results in a patient's perceiving only half as much pain.

PHASIC BLOCK *IN VIVO*

As described previously, differential block refers to complete blockade of one nerve modality (*e.g.*, sympathetic) with partial blockade of other modalities (*e.g.*, sensory and motor). Within one modality, it is possible to produce a blockade that may be ineffective under the following circumstances. When the C_m for a particular nerve and local anesthetic combination has just been reached, the nerve (by definition) no longer conducts a single impulse. A seeming inconsistency of the resultant threshold state of the nerve is that every second or third member of a train of impulses may breach the block. Such a threshold block effectively divides the frequency of a train of impulses by one half or one third.

This so-called Wedensky block has traditionally been explained on the basis that the nonconducted impulse (which precedes the conducted impulse) briefly lowers the firing threshold of the nerve; another impulse arriving during this period of facilitation was thought to induce just sufficiently more depolarization to trigger the membrane. An alternative explanation of frequency-dependent blockade, however, implies that each new impulse intensifies local anesthetic block. Thus, after the passage of an action potential, a nerve with a low concentration of local anesthetic remains super-refractory to further stimulation for a period of time, which results in the dropping out of every second or third impulse from a train of stimuli.[17] The mechanisms for phasic block, described in experimental situations, also can describe the threshold block observed clinically.

Whatever the underlying mechanism, the reduced ability of a marginally blocked axon to transmit fast trains of impulses becomes more pronounced in thinner axons.[20,57] As impulses generated by noxious stimuli generally occur in high-frequency barrages and are conducted along thin axons, the perception of pain is particularly vulnerable to threshold block phenomena.

When the anesthetic concentration at the nerve membrane rises beyond C_m, blockade becomes increasingly more profound, and progressively fewer impulses in a train are conducted. Because the local anesthetic concentrations that are used clinically far exceed the C_m, the threshold phase ordinarily is traversed swiftly. This phase is most easily demonstrated during recovery from a block when the concentration gradients are shallower and diffusion of drug from nerve occurs more slowly.

Even so, threshold block is encountered clinically. For instance, a patient may be insensitive to a pinprick stimulus when it is tested after nerve block, yet may still discern a high-intensity stimulus such as a surgical incision. To be sure, the incisional pain is much less intense than it would have been without the block; the burning component of pain, in particular, seems to be attenuated.

Factors Affecting the Time-Course of Neural Block*. At this point, the experimental evidence for local anesthetic action, based on knowledge of events in single axons, must be applied to the nerve, the complex structure with which anesthesiologists deal.

Intraneural injection is prone to damage axons and their blood vessels by compression because the nerve's tough outer sheath acts as a physical barrier that traps intraneural fluid. At the very least, intraneural injection is uncomfortable to the patient. For this reason alone, local anesthetic is always placed near, rather than inside, a nerve. How much drug eventually reaches the nerve (and how much is "wasted") largely depends on the location of the needle, and therefore on the anesthetist's knowledge of anatomy, his clinical skill, and on the various factors that affect the immediate distribution of local anesthetics (see Chap. 3).

Delivery Phase. Because the local anesthetic is generally injected into the fluid medium surrounding a nerve, the drug molecules must diffuse through many layers of fibrous and other tissue barriers before they reach individual axons. The density of non-neural tissue components in a peripheral nerve varies. Much fibrous tissue and even some fat are found in the sciatic nerve; considerably lesser amounts are found in other peripheral nerves. An exception to this is the spinal rootlets, floating nearly naked in the cerebral spinal fluid of the subarachnoid space; drug diffusion and penetration of these nerves accordingly is rapid, so that just a small amount of local anesthetic produces swift and solid blockade.

The first step in moving the anesthetic to its neural target site is mass movement (spread) of the injected solution. A large volume spreads farther and exposes more nerves to the anesthetic (but, of course, also increases the vascular absorption surface). Mass movement is particularly important in subarachnoid (spinal) anesthesia, with the drug spreading upward and downward in the spinal fluid, according to the specific gravity of the fluid that contains the local anesthetic (see Chap. 7).

*Reproduced substantially from the chapter by R. H. de Jong that appeared in the first edition of *Neural Blockade in Clinical Anesthesia and Management of Pain.*

Diffusion, the movement of drug molecules away from the site of injection, is governed by concentration gradients. Molecules move from an area of dense population (high concentration) to one of low concentration, the rate of diffusion being greater the steeper the concentration gradient. Because diffusion is a relatively slow process, the local anesthetic solution is continually being diluted with tissue fluid. At the same time, drug is continuously absorbed by vascular and lymphatic channels. In addition, a substantial portion of the supply of available anesthetic is bound to non-neural tissue elements encountered along the diffusion path; because this uptake is largely due to hydrophobic absorption, generally the more lipophilic the agent, the slower is the onset of block (see Chap. 3). Clearly, to produce anesthesia confidently, the blocking solution should be deposited as near to the nerve as possible.

Although proximity to the nerve is important, blockade can be enhanced further by limiting local vascular drug absorption. Absorption is most successfully slowed and the block correspondingly prolonged, by incorporating a vasoconstrictor into the local anesthetic solution. The vasoconstrictor (with epinephrine still considered most efficacious) restricts the local circulation so that the rate of local anesthetic vascular absorption is reduced.[5] Similarly, drug injected into highly perfused tissue (*e.g.*, peridural space) is absorbed much faster than is drug injected into a marginally perfused region, such as the lumbar subarachnoid space.[7] Highly fat-soluble local anesthetics, such as etidocaine and bupivacaine, are extensively bound to local tissue depots as well as to plasma proteins. Vascular uptake appears to be relatively less affected by the addition of epinephrine to solutions of these local anesthetics, and thus is less of an influence on the amount of drug available for action on the nerve.

Concentration Effect. Early reports implied that the more concentrated the anesthetic solution, the faster is the vascular absorption and the higher the blood level. Recent clinical studies, however, fail to demonstrate an important rise in blood level when the same net dose of local anesthetic is injected in more concentrated form (mepivacaine being one exception; see Chap. 3). This intuitively makes sense; while drug is absorbed more slowly from a dilute than from a concentrated solution, a greater volume of the weaker solution must be injected to reach the same total drug mass, thereby spreading absorption over a larger capillary surface area. The net rate of drug absorption, accordingly, remains nearly constant.[50]

The limiting factor controlling anesthetic uptake probably is tissue-binding capacity. If unoccupied tissue-binding sites remain, the ratio of free to bound drug is independent of concentration. If, however, tissue-binding sites become saturated, then proportionately more free (unbound) drug becomes available, the diffusion gradient steepens, and more drug is absorbed into the circulation. Saturation of tissue-binding sites probably explains why mepivacaine blood levels tend to rise with increasing concentration.[60]

It has been said that topical application of a high concentration of local anesthetic produces even higher blood concentrations. This seems to be the case with cocaine but certainly does not apply for topically used lidocaine.[32,61]

Induction Phase. After the local anesthetic has been deposited near a nerve trunk, it diffuses from the nerve's outer surface toward the nerve's center.[18a] Accordingly, axons that reside in the outer layers of the nerve (mantle fibers) are anesthetized well before axons that course through the nerve's inner layers (core fibers). Topographically, the fibers in a nerve trunk are arrayed in concentric layers. Fibers that innervate a limb's distal parts assume a central position in the nerve's core, whereas those that innervate the limb's proximal parts lie in the nerve's mantle.

As the local anesthetic diffuses through a nerve trunk from mantle to core, anesthesia tends to spread along the limb in a proximal to distal direction. This can easily be observed during axillary block; the subject first notes that the upper arm becomes numb, analgesia spreading from there down the arm to reach the fingers last (Fig. 2-11).

An excellent demonstration of concentric somatotopic innervation within a nerve derives from clinical experiments with intravenous regional anesthesia. (Local anesthetic solution is injected into an extremity vein, while inflow and outflow of blood are halted by an occlusive tourniquet applied proximally.) On cross-section, the nerve's core is more densely vascularized than the mantle region (see Chap. 12). Engorged with a backflow of local anesthetic, these veins then act as an anesthetic source centered in the core. Under these conditions, blockade progresses in a distal-to-proximal direction, as the drug now diffuses from core to mantle.[40] By the same principle, when the trunks of the brachial plexus are blocked as a result of the supraclavicular approach, paresis precedes analgesia because axons that innervate the

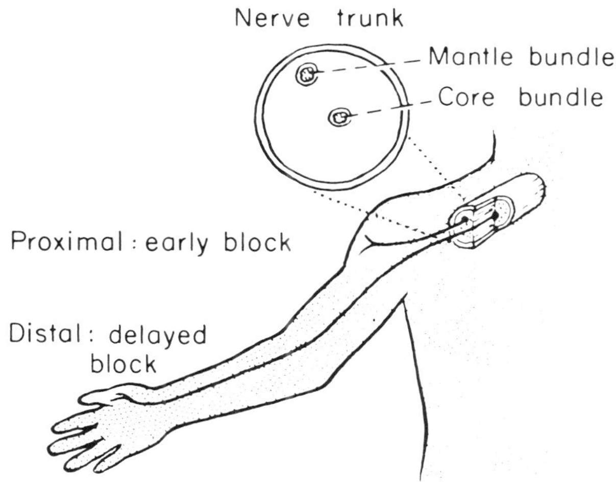

FIG. 2-11. Somatotopic distribution in peripheral nerve. Axons in large nerve trunks (*e.g.*, axillary terminus of brachial plexus) are arranged so that the outer (mantle) fibers innervate the more proximal structures, and the inner (core) fibers, the more distal parts of a limb. With the local anesthetic diffusing inward down the mantle-to-core gradient, the analgesia salient sweeps down the limb in proximal-to-distal fashion. (de Jong, R.H.: Physiology and Pharmacology of Local Anesthesia. Springfield, Ill., Charles C Thomas, 1970.)

shoulder-girdle muscles inhabit the mantle position high in the neck (Fig. 2-11).

The rapidity of onset of nerve block is (roughly) proportional to the logarithm of the concentration of the drug. This means that doubling the drug concentration will hasten the onset of block only modestly, although, of course, the more concentrated solution also will block the larger nerve fibers more effectively. Thus, concentrated anesthetic solutions increase the maximum extent of nerve penetration and the size of the fiber that can be blocked but have a lesser effect on the speed of onset of block. It must be remembered, however, that increasing the concentration also increases the total dose of the drug being given, and therefore the risk of systemic toxicity.

Recovery Phase. During recovery from nerve block, the diffusion gradient is reversed.[18a] The nerve core retains a higher anesthetic concentration than the exposed mantle, which, bathed in extracellular fluid, loses drug more readily than the well-shielded core. Accordingly, regression of analgesia takes place initially in territory innervated by mantle fibers and lastly in that supplied by core fibers, so that normal sensation returns initially to the proximal and lastly to the distal parts of the limb. Of course, to the extent that a vascular element lies in the nerve core, more centrally located fibers will also be freed of anesthetic early in the recovery phase. For example, recovery patterns after supraclavicular block suggest that at the origin of the brachial plexus drug absorption occurs faster from the core than from the mantle.[62]

Diffusion from the nerve and absorption into the vascular bed mainly account for termination of blockade. It has been found empirically that the duration of the block is related linearly to the logarithm of the anesthetic concentration. Thus, repeated doubling of the anesthetic concentration will have progressively less effect on duration, probably because with repeated injections, steady-state distributions of drug are achieved from which the duration of block is completely dependent on the saturation of local tissue depots. More important is the lipophilic solubility of the individual local anesthetic agents; for example, agents with high lipid solubility, such as bupivacaine and etidocaine, are highly concentrated in local tissue, such as cells around the nerve trunk and myelin sheaths around individual axons, and dislodge slowly from neural tissue. Blockade therefore persists for a long time (see Chap. 3). Lipophilic uptake by local tissues is also slow, accounting for the fact that maintenance of block by repeated drug injections does increase the time for recovery, albeit to a limited extent.

PERIODIC ("CONTINUOUS") NERVE BLOCK

A lengthy operation or prolonged labor might easily outlast the duration of a single anesthetic blockade and thus would require repeated administration to keep the patient pain-free. To facilitate reinjection, a catheter often is placed in the vicinity of the nerves to be blocked. Local anesthetic solution thereby can be replenished on an as-needed basis, a technique widely (although imprecisely) known as continuous nerve block.

Events during initial injection through the catheter are no different from those discussed above, progressing through induction, steady-state, and regression.[18a] They deviate, however, when the block starts to wear off and the patient begins to sense some vague discomfort. At this moment, the mantle fibers (being closest to the external environment) have suffered the greatest anesthetic loss through outward diffusion and have dropped their anesthetic content below C_m. It is this restoration of neural traffic in mantle fibers that the patient senses, and it is at this moment that anesthetic replenishment normally is instituted.

At this time, however, the core's anesthetic concentration still is comfortably above C_m, by virtue of its remoteness from the external environment. Thus, freshly injected anesthetic has to travel a much shorter distance because only the outer shell's anesthetic supply must be replenished throughout the nerve's entire innervation territory; accordingly, solid conduction blockade is quickly restored (Fig. 2-12).

Further setting the second (and subsequent) injections apart from the original injection is that a considerable amount of residual anesthetic remains lodged in the mantle fibers and in the accessory tissues because anesthetic concentrations below C_m, although falling short of supplying a sufficient mass of molecules to inhibit all impulses, nevertheless leave some sodium channels occupied. Hence, to block all impulses again, fewer free local anesthetic molecules are needed the next time. The local accessory tissues also have a reduced uptake capacity, being partially occupied by previously injected anesthetic. Conduc-

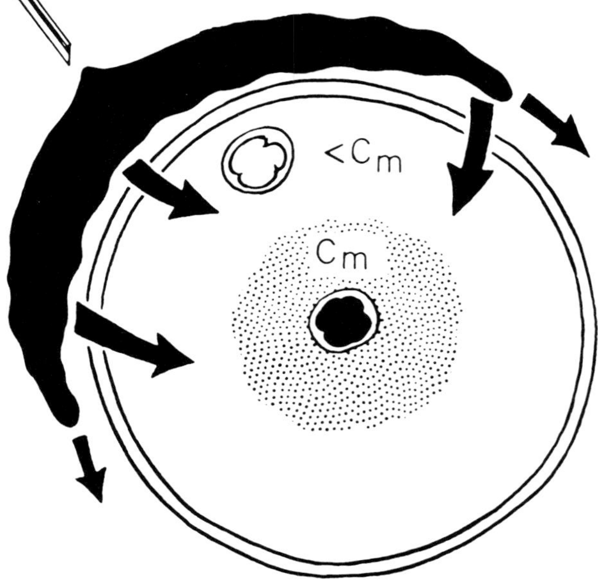

FIG. 2-12. Reinjection sequence for regional anesthesia. Fresh anesthetic solution is injected when sensory blockade just begins to wane. As the mantle fibers lie closest to the newly injected anesthetic puddle, their C_m is rapidly restored; the entire innervated territory is quickly reanesthetized owing to the preexposure of the nerve from previously injected anesthetic. (de Jong, R.H.: Physiology and Pharmacology of Local Anesthesia. Springfield, Ill., Charles C Thomas, 1970.)

tion block thus is reestablished not only sooner but also with less anesthetic than originally required.

By the same token, since the non-neural components also retain absorbed anesthetic, less drug is taken up for nonblocking purposes, leaving more anesthetic molecules free to attach to neural receptors. Hence, the quality ("depth") of the block, especially of the thicker, more resistant motor fibers, seems to improve during a continuous nerve block—a phenomenon called *augmentation*. Augmentation can also be observed clinically in epidural block if a small, repeated dose (3–4 ml) of local anesthetic is injected approximately 20 minutes after the first dose. There is no increase in the spatial extent of blockade; however, within the segments blocked, there is a more solid blockade of the entire range of fiber sizes. Presumably, the fibers with only partial blockade take up additional local anesthetic and thereby achieve the C_m.

Tachyphylaxis, a drug's declining effectiveness when it is given repeatedly, is often observed when a continuous nerve block is used over a long time. It is less likely to occur if a blocking agent is reinjected soon after the first signs of returning sensation; in fact, the aforementioned augmentation of blockade is more likely to occur than not under these conditions. When the block is allowed to lapse, however (as when attempting to provide postoperative pain relief), tachyphylaxis frequently occurs. Hallmarks of tachyphylaxis are even shorter duration of action, fading anesthetic potency, and shrinking analgesic field. Timing, evidently, is a prime consideration that determines whether augmentation or tachyphylaxis follows reinjection.[6]

Tachyphylaxis may well prove to be the result of several unrelated clinical factors. (In the laboratory, for instance, nerve block does not seem to lessen with time.) Important in this regard are anatomic causes such as perineural edema, microhemorrhage, or miniclots that may result from irritation by the catheter or from the anesthetic solution. Each, singly or combined, tends physically to shield the nerve from total contact with the anesthetic. In addition, the nerve's epineurium itself may become swollen. Other plausible causes are hypernatremia (from the anesthetic solution's saline carrier) and acidosis from anesthetic solutions at *p*Hs well below 7.

Although the mechanism may not be known exactly, the effects seem to be clear. To take advantage of augmentation, the local anesthetic solution should be reinjected soon after the patient senses discomfort, topping-up with a dose that is from one-fourth to one-third less than the original "priming" dose. If a delay of 10 or more minutes is unavoidable, more drug must be given to offset tachyphylaxis, on the order of one-fourth to one-third more than the priming dose.[6] Also, commercial solutions that contain epinephrine and acidic antioxidants, such as sodium metabisulfite (which lowers the *p*H of the solution and thus increases the likelihood of tachyphylaxis), should be avoided. Recent experiments demonstrate that bisulfite ions, combined with a low *p*H, may have deleterious effects on nerve conduction (see Chap. 4).

CARDIAC VERSUS NEURONAL ACTIONS OF LOCAL ANESTHETICS

The same drug is often used regionally as a local anesthetic and systemically as an antiarrhythmic. In what ways are the actions of these agents on nerve and heart similar? And to what extent do they differ?

Action potentials differ among the myocardial tissues. In atrial and ventricular musculature and in the fast conducting system of the His bundle and Purkinje fibers, there is a rapid phase of depolarization, primarily due to, as in nerve, inward current through sodium channels; a plateau phase due to the near balance of inward calcium and calcium currents and outward potassium currents; and a repolarization phase due to the eventual dominance of outward potassium currents (Fig. 2-13).[38] By comparison, action potentials in the SA and AV nodes have slower rising depolarizations primarily due to inward currents through calcium channels alone.[11]

At the doses of local anesthetic drugs administered systemically as antiarrhythmics (10–50 μm in blood), the primary target is the sodium channel. The other channels are affected by local anesthetics but at considerably higher (toxic) concentrations.[3,58,59] Inhibition of the sodium channel in heart under these conditions acts primarily to limit the rate of firing in ventricular tissue by raising the action potential threshold in a phasic manner. As in nerve, threshold is controlled by several factors, the availability of Na^+ channels being one important contributor. But two salient differences occur in heart: At the ventricular resting potential, or the mean diastolic potential, few of the channels are inactivated, whereas in nerve near 30% may be in that state; and the cardiac action potential produces a depolarization that endures for several hundred milliseconds, whereas the neuronal impulse is over in 1 msec.[16] Therefore, in the absence of impulses, myocardial channels are neither activated nor inactivated and thus have a lower anesthetic affinity than do the partially inactivated channels in nerve. In the presence of impulses, myocardial channels stay opened or inactivated for relatively long times, and thereby greatly enhance the effective channel affinity of local anesthetics. After a cardiac action potential, the anesthetics dissociate from the channels, eventually returning the membrane threshold to near the normal value. A drug that dissociates in only tens of milliseconds does not elevate threshold long enough to be an effective antiarrhythmic. One that dissociates in several seconds will be bradycardiogenic. Lidocaine, fortuitously, has just the right kinetics to be an effective antiarrhythmic.[15]

Cardiotoxicity from systemic local anesthetics has two forms: One is the bradycardia just mentioned; the other is an arrhythmogenic action, particularly evident with bupivacaine and leading to rare but potentially lethal episodes of cardiac collapse (see Chap. 4). The origins of this arrhythmogenic action are unknown, but several recent reports suggest that bupivacaine may have more of an effect on calcium release in heart than do other local anesthetics.[35,63]

The increase in sarcoplasmic Ca^{2+} that is essential for tension development occurs through a Ca^{2+}-dependent Ca^{2+} release process; a relatively small amount of Ca^{2+} that enters the muscle through the plasma membrane triggers the release of a far greater amount of Ca^{2+} from sarcoplasmic reticular stores (Fig. 2-13).[19] An inward Ca^{2+} current through the plasma membrane, which can be selectively expressed by a combination of elevated external K^+ and isoproterenol, was not altered by bupivacaine, although contractile tension was significantly reduced.[35,63] Apparently bupivacaine effects the storage or release of cytoplasmic Ca^{2+}. It is known that divalent cations, particularly in the cytoplasm, can strongly modulate membrane excitability.[41] Perhaps bupivacaine's arrhythmogenic toxicity derives from its ability to interfere with Ca^{2+} storage inside the heart, and thereby to influence indirectly membrane excitability (see also Chap. 4).

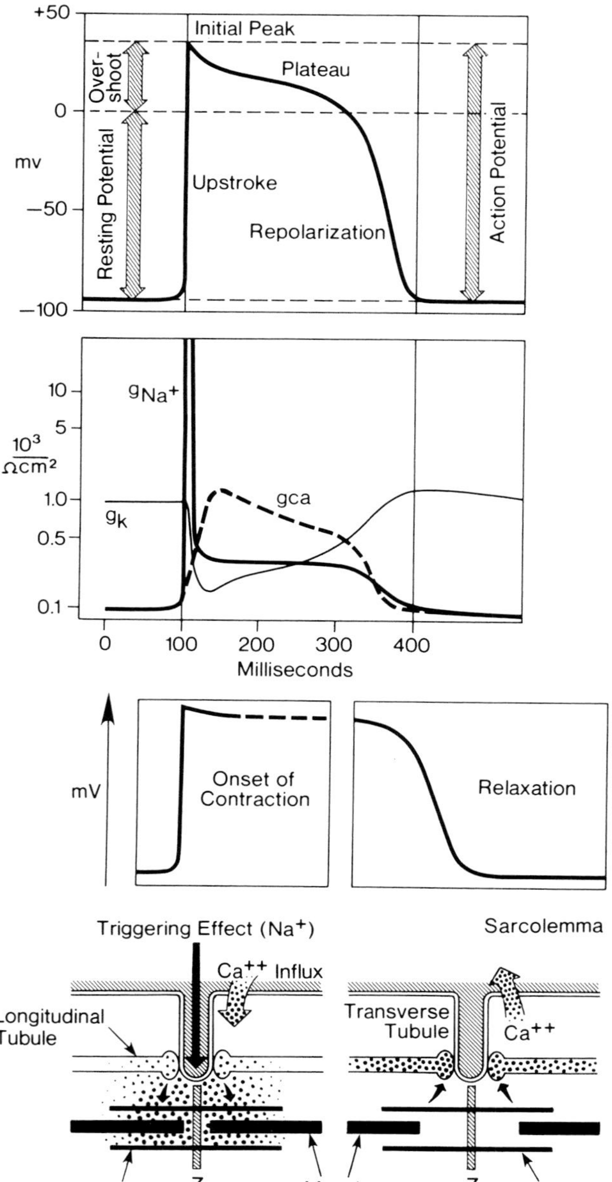

FIG. 2-13. Electrical and ionic events in myocardial muscle action potential (AP) leading to contraction. **Upper Panel.** The AP of cardiac ventricular muscle cells begins with a very rapid depolarization of membrane potential to the "initial peak." This is followed by a characteristic feature of cardiac muscle (and also Bundle of His and Purkinje tissue), a prolonged "plateau" responsible for the AP lasting more than 100 times longer than that of a peripheral nerve fiber. **Middle Panel.** Changes in Na^+, Ca^{++}, and K^+ conductance *(g)* that are responsible for the various phases of the AP: resting potential (G_K); initial peak ($G_{Na} + G_{Ca}$); plateau ($G_{Ca} + G_K$); and repolarization (gradual decrease in G_{Ca} and increase in G_K). Local anesthetics block the "fast Na^+ channel" except at very high concentrations where they may also block the "slow Ca^{++} channel" (see text). **Lower Two Panels:** Diagram of relationship of excitation, rapid triggering (Na^+), Ca^{++} movement, and action of contractile apparatus of cardiac muscle. During the AP there is an influx of Ca^{++}, which not only prolongs the AP, but also triggers the release of internal Ca^{++} from sarcoplasmic reticulum. Release of Ca^{++} leads to activation of the actin/myosin contractile apparatus.

SUMMARY

The impulse-blocking action of local anesthetics rests on their ability to interfere with the opening of voltage-gated sodium channels of excitable membranes. When enough channels cannot open, insufficient inward current (Na^+) flows into the cell to elicit or sustain a regenerative action potential. If this situation occurs along a sufficient length of axon, impulse propagation will terminate within the anesthetized region of that axon.

Although the final details remain to be specified, the molecular mechanism of anesthetic block has many known features. Both neutral and protonated versions of the tertiary amine anesthetics can block Na^+ channels, although not necessarily by identical mechanisms. Anesthetic molecules appear to bind to, and act directly on, the Na^+ channels themselves. Changes of channel conformation, such as appear during an impulse, often potentiate anesthetic block in a "use-dependent" manner.

The potency of anesthetics in clinical situations depends as much on their ability to reach the nerve fibers as it does on their intrinsic blocking activities. Factors such as sheath penetration, vascular absorption, and local tissue binding are all important determinants of functional potency. Volume, *p*H, and buffering capacity of the injected anesthetic solution are also important. Differential block of specific fiber types does occur but usually not in the order that it has been classically described. Smaller fibers subserving pain transmission are often blocked faster after regional injection or at a lower dose of anesthetic, but in several experimental cases larger myelinated A-delta or B fibers were blocked before the smallest, nonmyelinated C fibers.

Antiarrhythmic actions of local anesthetics can be explained by the same schemes that describe impulse-blocking actions; however, Na^+ channels in heart differ from those in nerve such that low concentrations of lidocaine will slow rapid, repetitive ventricular action potentials, through a use-dependent block, while having almost no effect on cardiac impulse firing at normal frequencies. Part of this action is a result of the long period of depolarization during a cardiac action potential, providing time for the extended binding of anesthetic molecules to inactivated Na^+ channels. The arrhythmogenic action of certain local anesthetics, such as bupivacaine, seems to concern the cytoplasmic metabolism of Ca^{2+} rather than any direct effect on channels in the myocardial plasma membrane.

Although local anesthetics are usually reliable drugs, they can be improved in several respects. Fast reversibility, to produce block of rapidly controlled duration, is desirable. Drugs of very long, but reversible, action would be useful for nerve block, such as intercostal block for postoperative pain. Selective block of functionally defined fiber types also would be a desirable clinical feature, allowing a differential titration of sensory and motor activities. In addition, reduced toxicity, both from accidental intravascular injection and from systemic accumulation after repeated injections, is a highly sought objective. As our knowledge about the relation between molecular properties of local anesthetics and their pharmacologic actions increases, we come closer to the reality of designing drugs and procedures to fulfill these criteria.

REFERENCES

1. Agnew, W.S., Levinson, S.R., Brabson, J.S., and Raftery, M.A.: Purification of the tetrodotoxin-binding component associated with the voltage-sensitive sodium channel from *Electrophorus electroplax* membranes. Proc. Natl. Acad. Sci. U.S.A., *75*:2606–2610, 1978.
2. Akerman, S.B., Camougis, G., and Sandberg, R.V.: Stereoisomerism and differential activity in excitation block by local anesthetics. Eur. J. Pharmacol., *8*:337–347, 1969.
3. Arhem, P., and Frankenhaeuser, B.: Local anesthetics: Effects on permeability properties of nodal membrane in myelinated nerve fibres from *Xenopus*. Potential clamp experiments. Acta Physiol. Scand., *91*:11–21, 1974.
4. Barchi, R.L., Cohen, S.A., and Murphy, L.E.: Purification from rat sarcolemma of the saxitoxin-binding component of the excitable membrane sodium channel. Proc. Natl. Acad. Sci. U.S.A., *77*:1306–1310, 1980.
5. Bonica, J.J., Akamatsu, T.J., Berges, P.U., Morikawa, K.I., *et. al.*: Circulatory effects of epidural block: II. Effects of epinephrine. Anesthesiology, *34*:514, 1971.
6. Bromage, P.R., Pettigrew, R.T., and Crowell, D.E.: Tachyphylaxis in epidural analgesia: I. Augmentation and decay of local anesthesia. J. Clin. Pharmacol., *9*:30, 1969.
7. Burfoot, M.F., and Bromage, P.R.: The effects of epinephrine on mepivacaine absorption from the spinal epidural space. Anesthesiology, *35*:488, 1971.
8. Cahalan, M.: Local anesthetic block of sodium channels in normal and pronase-treated squid giant axons. Biophys. J., *23*:285–311, 1978.
9. Cahalan, M.D., and Almers, W.: Interactions between quaternary lidocaine, the sodium channel gates and tetrodotoxin. Biophys. J., *27*:39–56, 1979.
10. Cahalan, M., Shapiro, B.I., and Almers, W.: Relationship between inactivation of sodium channels and block by quaternary derivatives of local anesthetics and other compounds. *In* Fink, B.R. (ed.): Molecular Mechanisms of Anesthesia (Progress in Anesthesiology, Vol. 2). New York, Raven Press, 1980.

11. Carmeliat, E., and Vereecke, J.: Electrogenesis of the action potential and automaticity. *In* Berne, R.M., Sperelakis, N., and Geiger, S., (eds.): Handbook of Physiology, Section 2: The Cardiovascular System, Vol. 1, The Heart, pp. 269–334. Bethesda, Md., American Physiological Society, 1979.
12. Catchlove, R.F.H.: The influence of CO_2 and pH on local anesthetic action. J. Pharmacol. Exp. Ther. *181*:298–309, 1972.
13. Chiu, S.Y., Ritchie, J.M., Rogart, R.B., and Stagg, D.: A quantitative description of membrane currents in rabbit myelinated nerve. J. Physiol., *292*:149–166, 1979.
14. Courtney, K.R.: Mechanism of frequency-dependent inhibition of sodium currents in frog myelinated nerve by the lidocaine derivative GEA-968. J. Pharmacol. Exp. Ther., *195*:225–236, 1975.
15. Courtney, K.R.: Structure-activity relations for frequency-dependent sodium channel block in nerve by local anesthetics. J. Pharmacol. Exp. Ther., *213*:114–119, 1980a.
16. Courtney, K.R.: Antiarrhythmic drug design: Frequency-dependent block in myocardium. *In* Fink, B.R. (ed.): Molecular Mechanisms of Anesthesia, pp. 111–118. New York, Raven Press, 1980b.
17. Courtney, K.R., Kendig, J.J., and Cohen, E.N.: Frequency-dependent conduction block: The role of nerve impulse pattern in local anesthetic potency. Anesthesiology *48*:111–117, 1978.
18. Courtney, K.R., and Strichartz, G.R.: Structural elements which determine local anesthetic activity. *In* Strichartz, G.R. (ed.): Handbook of Experimental Pharmacology: Local Anesthetics. New York, Springer-Verlag, 1986.
19. Fabiato, A., and Fabiato, F.: Contractions induced by a calcium-triggered release of calcium from the sarcoplasmic reticulum of single skinned cardiac cells. J. Physiol. (Lond.), *249*:469–495, 1975.
20. Franz, D.N., and Perry, R.S.: Mechanisms for differential block among single myelinated and non-myelinated axons by procaine. J. Physiol., *236*:193–210, 1974.
21. Frazier, D.T., Narahashi, T., and Yamada, M.: The site of action and active form of local anesthetics: II. Experiments with quaternary compounds. J. Pharamacol. Exp. Ther., *171*:45–51, 1970.
22. Hartshorne, R.P., and Catterall, W.A.: Purification of the saxitoxin receptor of the sodium channel from rat brain. Proc. Natl. Acad. Sci. U.S.A., *78*:4620–4624, 1981.
23. Heavner, J.E., de Jong, R.: Lidocaine blocking concentration for B- and C-nerve fibers. Anesthesiology, *40*:228, 1974.
24. Hille, B.: The common mode of action of three agents that decrease the transient change in sodium permeability in nerves. Nature, *210*:1220–1222, 1966.
25. Hille, B.: The pH-dependent rate of action of local anesthetics on the node of Ranvier. J. Gen. Physiol., *69*:475–496, 1977a.
26. Hille, B.: Local anesthetics: Hydrophilic and hydrophobic pathways for the drug-receptor reaction. J. Gen. Physiol., *69*:497–515, 1977b.
27. Hille, B.: Local anesthetic action on inactivation of the Na channel in nerve and skeletal muscle: Possible mechanisms for antiarrhythmic agents. *In* Morad, M. (ed.): Biophysical Aspects of Cardiac Muscle, pp. 55–74. New York, Academic Press, 1978.
28. Hille, B.: Ionic channels of excitable membranes. Sunderland, Ma., Sinauer Associates, 1984.
29. Hodgkin, A.L., and Huxley, A.F.: A quantitative description of membrane current and its application to conduction and excitation in nerve. J. Physiol., *117*:500–544, 1952b.
30. Hodgkin, A.L., and Keynes, R.D.: The potassium permeability of a giant nerve fibre. J. Physiol., *128*:61–88, 1955.
31. Huxley, A.F., and Stampfli, R.: Evidence for saltatory conduction in peripheral myelinated nerve fibers. J. Physiol., *108*:315–339, 1949.
32. Karvonen S., et. al.: Blood lidocaine concentration after arterial and venous local anesthesia of the respiratory tract using an ultrasonic nebulizer. Acta Anaesthesiol. Scand., *20*:156, 1976.
33. Khodorov, B.I.: Chemicals as tools to study nerve fiber sodium channels: Effects of batrachotoxin and some local anesthetics. *In* Tosteson, D.C., Ovchinnikov, Y.A., and Latorre, R. (eds.): Membrane Transport Processes, Vol. 2. New York, Raven Press, 1978.
34. Khodorov, B.I., Peganov, E., Revenko, S., and Shishkova, L.: Sodium currents in voltage clamped nerve fiber of frog under the combined action of batrachotoxin and procaine. Brain Res., *84*:541–546, 1975.
35. Lynch, C.: Local anesthetic effects upon myocardial excitation-contraction (E-C) coupling. Reg. Anaesth., *10*:38–39, 1985.
36. McLaughlin, S.: Local anesthetics and the electrical properties of phospholipid bilayer membranes. *In* Fink, B.R. (ed.): Molecular Mechanisms of Anesthesia, pp. 193–220. New York, Raven Press, 1975.
37. Narahashi, T., Frazier, D., and Yamada, M.: The site of action and active form of local anesthetics: I. Theory and pH experiments with tertiary compounds. J. Pharmacol. Exp. Ther., *171*:32–44, 1970.
38. Noble, D.: The Initiation of the Heartbeat. Oxford, Oxford University Press, 1975.
39. Noda, M., Shimizu, S., Tanabe, T., Takai, T., *et al.*: Primary structure of *Electrophorus electricus* sodium channel deduced from cDNA sequence. Nature, *312*:121–127, 1984.
40. Raj, P.P., Garcia, C.E., Burleson, J.W., and Jenkins, M.T.: The site of action of intravenous regional anesthesia. Anesth. Analg. (Cleve.), *51*:776, 1972.
41. Rang, H.P., and Ritchie, J.M.: On the electrogenic sodium pump in mammalian non-myelinated nerve fibers and its activation by various cations. J. Physiol., *196*:183–211, 1968.
42. Raymond, S.A.: Effects of nerve impulses on threshold of frog sciatic nerve fibers. J. Physiol., *290*:273–303, 1979.
43. Raymond, S.A., and Gissen, A.J.: Differential Nerve Block. *In* Strichartz, G.R. (ed.): Handbook of Experimental Pharmacology, Vol. 81, Local Anesthetics. New York, Springer-Verlag, 1986.
44. Ritchie, J.M.: Physiological basis for conduction in myelinated nerve fibers. *In* Morell, P. (ed.): Myelin, 2nd ed., pp. 117–145. New York, Plenum Press, 1984.
45. Ritchie, J.M., Rang, H.P., and Pellegrino, R.: Sodium and potassium channels in demyelinated and remyelinated mammalian nerve. Nature, *294*:257–259, 1981.
46. Ritchie, J.M., and Ritchie, B.R.: Local anaesthetics: Effect of pH on activity. Science, *162*:1394–1395, 1968.
47. Ritchie, J.M., Ritchie, B., and Greengard, P.: The effect of the nerve sheath on the action of local anesthetics. J. Pharmacol. Exp. Ther., *150*:160–164, 1965b.

48. Rosenberg, R.L., Tomiko, S.A., and Agnew, W.S.: Single-channel properties of the reconstituted voltage-regulated Na channel isolated from the electroplax of *Electrophorus electricus.* Proc. Natl. Acad. Sci., U.S.A., *81*:5594–5598, 1984.
49. Schwarz, W., Palade, P.T., and Hille, B.: Local anesthetics: Effect of pH on use-dependent block of sodium channels in frog muscle. Biophys. J., *20*:343–368, 1977.
50. Scott, D.B.: Evaluation of the toxicity of local anaesthesia agents in man. Br. J. Anaesth., *47*:56, 1975.
51. Seeman, P.: The membrane expansion theory of anesthesia. *In* Fink, B.R. (ed.): Molecular Mechanisms of Anesthesia, Progress in Anesthesiology, Vol. 1. New York, Raven Press, 1975.
52. Skou, J.C.: Local anesthetics: VI. Relation between blocking potency and penetration of a monomolecular layer of lipoids from nerves. Acta Pharmacol. Toxicol., *10*:325–337, 1954.
53. Strichartz, G.R.: The inhibition of sodium currents in myelinated nerve by quanternary derivatives of lidocaine. J. Gen. Physiol., *62*:37–57, 1973.
54. Strichartz, G.R.: The composition and structure of excitable nerve membrane. *In* Jamieson, G.A., Robinson, D.M. (eds.): Mammalian Cell Membranes, Vol. 3, pp. 173–205. London, Butterworths, 1977.
55. Strichartz, G., Hahin, R., and Cahalan, M.: Pharmacological models for sodium channels producing abnormal impulse activity. *In* Culp, W.J., Ochoa, J. (eds.): Abnormal Nerves and Muscles as Impulse Generations, pp. 98–129. New York, Oxford University Press, 1982.
56. Strichartz, G., and Wang, W.K.: The kinetic basis for phasic local anesthetic blockade of neuronal sodium channels. *In* Miller, K.W., Roth, S. (eds.): Molecular and Cellular Mechanisms of Anesthetics, pp. 217–226. New York, Plenum Publishing Corp., 1986.
57. Strichartz, G., and Zimmermann, M.: Selective conduction blockade among different fiber types in mammalian nerves by lidocaine combined with low temperature. Society for Neuroscience, Annual Meeting Abstracts, p. 675, 1983.
58. Tan, K.-N.: Receptor-mediated actions of thyrotropin-releasing hormone on calcium fluxes and prolactin release in pituitary cells in culture. Dissertation, Harvard Medical School, pp. 5.1–5.12. Ann Arbor, MI, University Microfilms, 1983.
59. Taylor, R.E.: Effect of procaine on electrical properties of squid axon membrane. Am. J. Physiol., *196*:1071–1078, 1959.
60. Tucker, G.T., Moore, D.C., Bridenbaugh, P.O., Bridenbaugh, L.D.: Systemic absorption of mepivacaine in commonly used regional block procedures. Anesthesiology *37*:277, 1972.
61. Van Dyke, C., Barash, P.G., Jatlow, P., and Byck, R.: Cocaine: Plasma concentrations after intranasal application in man. Science, *191*:859, 1976.
62. Winnie, A.P., LaVallee, D.A., Pesosa, B., and Masud, Z.K.: Clinical pharmacokinetics of local anaesthetics. Can. Anaesth. Soc. J., *24*:252, 1977.
63. Wojtczak, J.A., and Kaplan, J.A.: Bupivacaine cardiotoxicity: "Power failure" and its mechanisms. Reg. Anaesth. *10*:43, 1985.
64. Yeh, J.Z.: Blockage of sodium channels by stereoisomers of local anesthetics. Prog. Anesthesiol., *2*:35–44, 1980.

3 PROPERTIES, ABSORPTION, AND DISPOSITION OF LOCAL ANESTHETIC AGENTS

GEOFFREY T. TUCKER
LAURENCE E. MATHER

The use of regional anesthesia requires administration of sufficient local anesthetic to be effective but not so much that toxicity develops. Just as the anesthesiologist must have a thorough knowledge of the anatomic and physical landmarks, the anesthesiologist must also appreciate local anesthetic action through knowledge of the individual characteristics of each drug to be injected. This necessitates thorough familiarization with the kinetics of absorption and disposition of local anesthetics in the body.

In reviewing this aspect of the pharmacology of local anesthetics, it is important to examine relationships between the physicochemical properties of the agents and their fate in the body and to delineate the role of pharmacokinetics in the overall response to regional anesthesia. This response is a complex function of pharmacokinetics, pharmacodynamics, the physiologic consequences of neural blockade, and the pathophysiologic status of the patient. Each of these factors can influence the others.

STRUCTURE AND PHYSICOCHEMICAL PROPERTIES OF LOCAL ANESTHETICS

"Ester Caines". The grandfather of all local anesthetics was, of course, cocaine (Fig. 3-1). This naturally occurring compound was discovered in South America by German scientists during the 1850s and was first introduced into clinical medicine in the latter part of the 19th century. Notice the aromatic "hydrophobic head," the ester linkages at his "neck" and "hand," and the amino group dangling down in front.

The essential features of this "noble savage" were subsequently handed down to his more sophisticated son, procaine (Fig. 3-2), who was born just in time to take part in the First World War. After the war procaine, in turn, became the father of a large family of ester caines: Of these, chloroprocaine and tetracaine (Fig. 3-3) still remain popular with some anesthesiologists.

"Amide Caines". The early 1930s saw the introduction of dibucaine (Fig. 3-4), a "two-headed" compound with the ester linkage replaced by a carbamoyl group. This agent is rather toxic, and its use has been confined essentially to spinal anesthesia.

The next development occurred in Sweden, where some significant mutations resulted in a new, hardier breed of amide caines (Fig. 3-5). Thus, the labile ester linkage was again replaced, this time by the chemically sturdier amide grouping, the reverse of the carbamoyl link. Lidocaine was the first of these "Viking maidens," followed by mepivacaine, prilocaine, bupivacaine, and, more recently, their American cousin, etidocaine. Notice that prilocaine looks a little sad. This is because she has only one pigtail. The o-tolui-

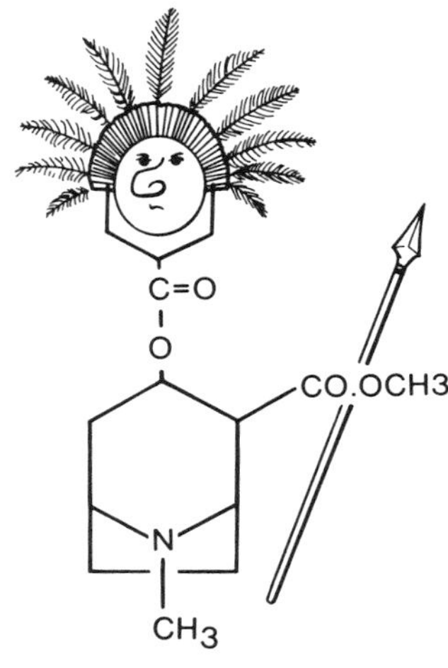

'Co' Sth. America (1850)

FIG. 3-1. Cocaine. (Tucker, G.T.: Transformation and toxicity of local anaesthetics. Acta Anaesthesiol. Belg., *26 [Suppl.]*:123, 1975.)

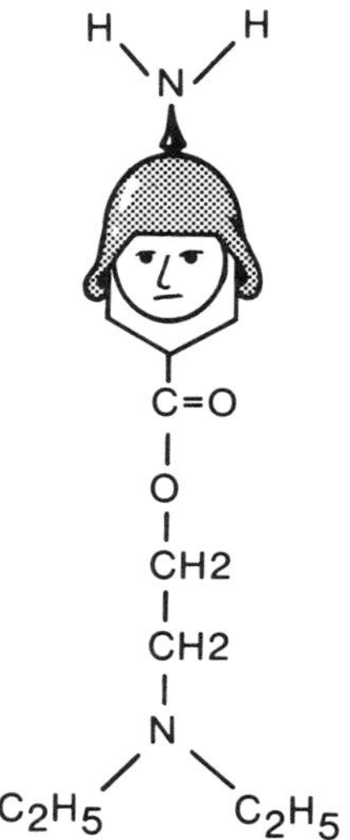

'Pro' Germany (1905)

FIG. 3-2. Procaine. (Tucker, G.T.: Biotransformation and toxicity of local anaesthetics. Acta Anaesthesiol. Belg., *26[Suppl.]*:123, 1975.)

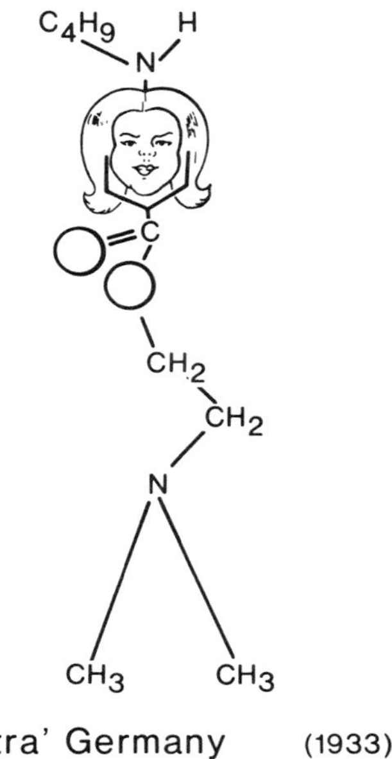

'Tetra' Germany (1933)

FIG. 3-3. Tetracaine. (Tucker, G.T.: Biotransformation and toxicity of local anaesthetics. Acta Anaesthesiol. Belg., *26[Suppl.]*:123, 1975.)

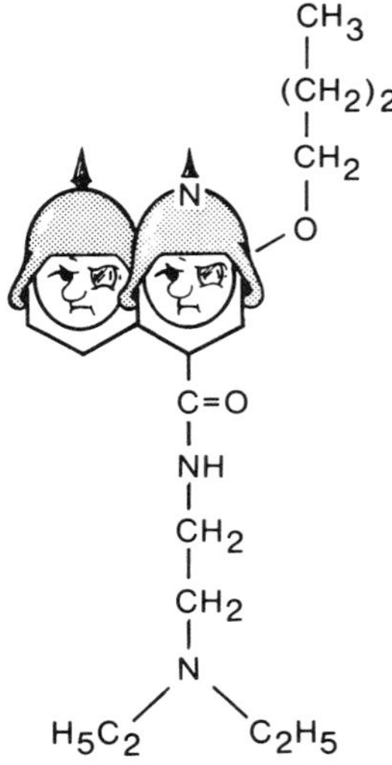

'Dibu' Germany (1932)

FIG. 3-4. Dibucaine.

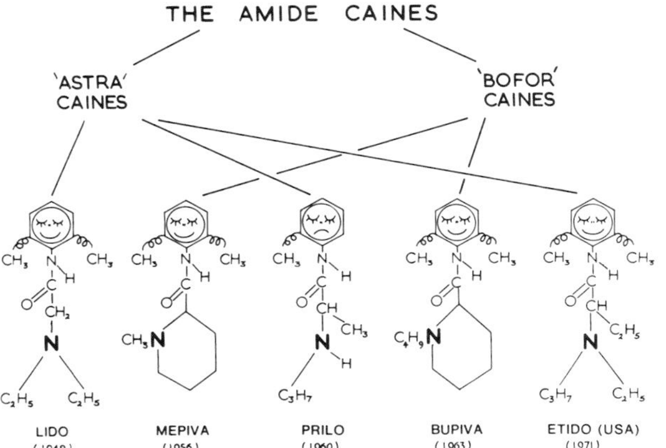

FIG. 3-5. The "amide caines." **Left to Right.** Lidocaine, mepivacaine, prilocaine, bupivacaine, and etidocaine. (Tucker, G.T.: Biotransformation and toxicity of local anaesthetics. Acta Anaesthesiol. Begl., *26[Suppl.]:* 123, 1975.)

dine moiety, unlike the 2,6-xylidine ring found in the other amides, is associated with methemoglobinemia at high doses. Prilocaine differs also in having one leg—the amino group is secondary rather than tertiary as in her near-relatives.

Mepivacaine, prilocaine, bupivacaine, and etidocaine, but not lidocaine, all have an asymmetric carbon atom (asymmetric because it has bonded to it four different functional groups). Consequently, although the racemates are used clinically, these agents can exist in two stereoisomeric forms having different physicochemical and pharmacologic properties.

PHYSICOCHEMICAL PROPERTIES

Basically three mechanisms are involved in the movement of local anesthetic molecules within the body: *bulk flow* of the injected solution at the site of administration; *diffusion* into and through aqueous and lipoprotein barriers; and *vascular transport*. Of these, diffusion is most directly dependent on the physicochemical properties of the agent.

According to Fick's Law, the rate of passive diffusion (dQ/dt) of a drug through a biologic membrane at steady-state may be approximated by equation 1, in which D is the diffusion coefficient of the drug in the membrane; A and δ are, respectively, the area and the thickness of the membrane; K is the partition coefficient of drug between the aqueous and membrane phases; and ΔC is the concentration gradient.

$$\frac{dQ}{dt} = -\frac{D.A.K.\Delta C}{\delta} \quad 1$$

Inasmuch as they determine D, K, and C, physicochemical properties will influence the rate of transport of local anesthetic at the membrane level, and potentially, therefore, the time-course of anesthetic and pharmacologic effects. By influencing the equilibrium distribution of the drugs between fluids and tissues, physicochemical properties also modulate activity and overall drug movement in the bloodstream.

Some physicochemical properties and features of the clinically used local anesthetics are given in Tables 3-1 and 3-2. As Table 3-1 shows, structural changes in the aromatic portion of the esters and in the amine group of the amides markedly alter physical properties such as lipid/aqueous partition coefficients and protein binding. These, in turn, have significant effects on potency, onset time, and duration of anesthesia. For example, addition of a four-carbon butyl group to the lipophilic aromatic amino end with subtraction of two carbons from the hydrophilic amino end of the ester procaine gives tetracaine and results in a 200-fold increase in partition coefficient, a 10-fold increase in protein binding, and a marked increase in potency. With the amide mepivacaine, substitution of a four-carbon butyl group for the one-carbon methyl group on the amine function gives bupivacaine with a 35-fold increase in partition coefficient, increased protein binding, and increased potency. Similarly, substitution in the lidocaine molecule of a propyl for an ethyl group at the amine end and addition of an ethyl group at the alpha carbon in the intermediate chain yield etidocaine. This results in a 50-fold increase in partition coefficient, increased protein binding and potency, and a duration of local anesthetic action at least twice that of lidocaine (see Chap. 4 for details of comparative clinical effects).

Molecular Weight. Molecular weights of the clinically useful agents vary from 220 to 288 (see Table 3-1); this feature is an important determinant of their diffusion coefficients. Because diffusion coefficient is inversely proportional to the square root of the molecular weight, however, differences in molecular weight among the agents might not be expected to contribute significantly to differences in rates of diffusion. Dural permeability is claimed to be more dependent on molecular weight than lipid solubility, but the relationship is unconvincing within a series of opioids having similar physicochemical properties to the amide local anesthetics.[288] There is evidence to

TABLE 3–1. PHYSICOCHEMICAL PROPERTIES OF LOCAL ANESTHETICS

	Chemical Configuration			Physicochemical Properties					Biologic Properties		
Agent	**Aromatic Lipophilic**	**Intermediate Chain**	**Amine Hydrophilic**	**Molecular Weight (Base)**	***pK′$_a$* (25°C)**	**Partition Coefficient†**	**Aqueous Solubility‡**	**Percent Protein Binding**	**Equieffective§ Anesthetic Concentration**	**Approximate Anesthetic Duration (min)§**	**Site of Metabolism**
Esters											
Procaine	H—N(H)—C_6H_4—	$COOCH_2CH_2$	—N(C_2H_5)(C_2H_5)	236	9.05	0.02	?	5.8‖	2	50	Plasma
Chloroprocaine	H_2N—C_6H_3(Cl)—	$COOCH_2CH_2$	N(C_2H_5)(C_2H_5)	271	8.97	0.14	?	?	2	45	Plasma
Tetracaine	H_9C_4N(H)—C_6H_4—	$COOCH_2CH_2$	—N(CH_3)(CH_3)	264	8.46	4.1	1.4	75.6‖	0.25	175	Plasma
Amides											
Prilocaine	C_6H_4(CH_3)—	NHCOCH(CH_3)	—N(H)(C_3H_7)	220	7.9	0.9	?	55 approx.	1	100	Liver, extra-hepatic tissues

Mepivacaine		NHCO	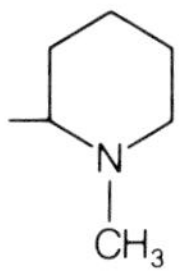 N–CH_3 (ring)	246	7.76	0.8	15	77.5¶	1	100	Liver
Lidocaine	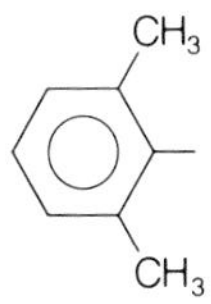 CH_3, CH_3 (ring)	$NHCOCH_2$	$-N(C_2H_5)(C_2H_5)$	234	7.91	2.9	24	64.3¶	1	100	Liver
Bupivacaine		NHCO	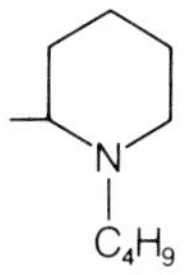 N–C_4H_9 (ring)	288	8.16	27.5	0.83	95.6¶	0.25	175	Liver
Etidocaine		$NHCOCH(C_2H_5)$	$-N(C_2H_5)(C_3H_7)$	276	7.7	141	?	94¶	0.25	200	Liver

* *p*H corresponds to 50% ionization.
‖ n-heptane/*p*H 7.4 buffer.
‡ Aqueous solubility (mg HCl Salt/ml at *p*H 7.37 and 37°C).
§ Data derived from rat sciatic nerve blocking procedure.
‖ Nerve homogenate binding.
¶ Plasma protein binding—2 μg/ml.

(Data from Ekenstam, B.: The effect of the structural variation on the local analgetic properties of the most commonly used groups of substances. Acta Anaesthesiol. Scand., *25* [*Suppl.*]: 10, 1966; Truant, A. P., and Takman, B.: Differential physical—chemical and neuropharmacologic properties of local anesthetic agents. Anesth. Analg. (Cleve.), *38*:478, 1959; Tucker, G. T.: Biotransformation and toxicity of local anaesthetics. Int. Anesthesiol. Clin., *13*:33, 1975; Mather, L.E.: Unpublished data; Kamaya, H., Hayes, J.J., and Ueda, I.: Dissociation constants of local anesthetics and their temperature dependence. Anesth. Analg. (Cleve.), *62*:1025, 1983; Dudziak, R., and Uihlein, M.: Loslichkeit von Lokalanaesthetika in Liquor cerebrospinalis und ihre Abhangigkeit von der Wasserstoffionenkonzentration. Anaesthesist, *27*:32, 1978.)

TABLE 3-2. FEATURES COMMON TO MOST LOCAL ANESTHETICS

Weak Bases with $pK_a > 7.4$. (Free base poorly water-soluble)
Thus dispensed as acidic solution, hydrochloride salts, (*p*H 4–7), which are more highly ionized and thus water-soluble
Exist in solution as equilibrium mixture of nonionized, lipid-soluble (free base) and ionized, water-soluble (cationic) forms
Body buffers raise *p*H and therefore increase amount of free base present
Lipid-soluble (free base) form crosses axonal membrane
Water-soluble (cationic) form is active blocker for most agents

suggest that molecular weight might be relevant to the diffusion of local anesthetics in the sodium channel of the nerve membrane.[103]

Lipid Solubility. The partition coefficients of drugs measured in aqueous/organic solvent systems *in vitro* are used to indicate their relative *in vivo* partition characteristics or degree of lipid solubility.[402] The values obtained may differ quantitatively between systems[203,417] such that their best use is in making comparisons between drugs within the same system. For example, Rosenberg and colleagues[342] have shown good rank order correlation between the n-heptane/buffer partition coefficients of bupivacaine, etidocaine, and lidocaine and their *in vitro* partition into rat sciatic nerve and human epidural and subcutaneous fat. Net lipid solubility, as reflected by heptane/buffer partition coefficients, is independent of ester or amide grouping. Tetracaine (ester) is highly lipid soluble, as are bupivacaine and etidocaine (amides) (see Table 3-1).

A high lipid solubility would be expected to promote drug entry into membranes by increasing diffusion rate. The net effect on onset of maximum anesthetic action is difficult to predict, however, because a faster rate of diffusion is offset by a greater capacity for uptake by a membrane. By promoting interaction with hydrophobic components of receptors, a high lipid solubility will increase potency and duration of effect.

Ionization. The inclusion of an amino group in the structure of most local anesthetics confers upon them the "split personality" of a weak base, meaning that they exist in solution partly as the nonionized free base and partly as the ionized cation (conjugate acid) (Equation 2):

$$\underset{\text{nonionized base}}{>\!\text{N}:} + \text{H}^+ \underset{\text{Ka}}{\rightleftharpoons} \underset{\text{ionized cation (conjugate acid)}}{>\!\text{N}:^+\text{H}} \qquad 2$$

The position of equilibrium depends on the dissociation constant (Ka) of the conjugate acid and on the local hydrogen ion concentration (Equation 3). Thus,

$$\text{Ka} = \frac{[\text{H}^+]\,[\text{base}]}{[\text{conjugate acid}]} \qquad 3$$

where the square brackets indicate concentration or, more properly, activity. By rearranging Equation 3 and taking logarithms, the familiar Henderson–Hasselbalch equation (Equation 4) is obtained:

$$\text{pKa} = p\text{H} - \log\frac{[\text{base}]}{[\text{conjugate acid}]} \qquad 4$$

where pKa is defined, by analogy to *p*H, as the negative logarithm of the dissociation constant of the conjugate acid under particular conditions of solvent and temperature.[417] Equation 4 shows that the pKa is equal to the *p*H at which the local anesthetic is 50% ionized, that is, when

$$\frac{[\text{base}]}{[\text{conjugate acid}]} = 1 \text{ and } \log 1 = 0.$$

The greater the pKa, the smaller is the proportion of nonionized form at any *p*H. Ester-type agents have relatively high pKa values (8.5–9.1) compared to the amides (7.6–8.2) (see Table 3-1), which accounts, in part, for relatively poor penetrance and the need to inject these agents close to neural tissue.

Ionization is relevant to the solubility and activity of local anesthetics (see Table 3-2) and their equilibrium distribution in various body compartments. Because the ionized forms are more water soluble than the free bases, the drugs are dispensed as their hydrochloride salts in acidic solutions, which also helps to stabilize the esters that readily hydrolyze in alkaline conditions. The *p*H of plain solutions of the ester-type agents may be as low as 2.8 compared to 4.4 to 6.4 for those of the amides.[279] The drugs are more lipid soluble in their free-base forms. Thus, the nonionized fraction becomes essential for passage through lipoprotein diffusion barriers to the site of action on the nerve membrane. Decreasing ionization by alkalinization will effectively raise the initial concentration gradient of diffusible drug, thereby increasing the rate of drug transfer and decreasing the latent period of a nerve block. Once at the nerve membrane, ionization is again necessary for complete anesthetic activity.[393]

The aqueous phases on either side of many body membranes differ in their *p*H values. Consequently, although nonionized drug concentrations in these phases will be at the same at equilibrium, different concentrations of ionized, and therefore of total, drug will exist on either side of the membrane depending on the *p*H gradient. For a weak base, the equilibrium ratio (R) of total drug concentration across the membrane is given by Equation 5. Thus,

$$R = \frac{1 + 10^{pKa\text{-}pH_1}}{1 + 10^{pKa\text{-}pH_2}} \qquad 5$$

where the subscripts 1 and 2 refer to the two aqueous compartments. Total drug concentration will be greater in the compartment having the lower *p*H because a greater proportion will be in the ionized form. Thus, for example, lowered *p*H owing to infection in tissues surrounding a nerve results in less nonionized drug, which is the form that can cross the axonal membrane (see also Chap. 2).

Aqueous Solubility. The aqueous solubility of a local anesthetic is directly related to its extent of ionization and inversely related to its lipid solubility (Table 3-1). Despite quite large differences in lipid solubility of the amide local anesthetic bases, the differences in aqueous solubility are smaller when compared between 50% and 90% ionized (Fig. 3-6).

Benzocaine, which lacks an amino group attached to the carbon chain, is almost insoluble in water. For this reason its use is essentially confined to topical anesthesia, although it has been injected for prolonged intercostal nerve block after solubilization with dextran (see Chap. 4).

A low aqueous solubility may be a limiting factor when selecting an agent for subarachnoid block. Thus, there has been concern over the possible neurotoxicity of 1% solutions of bupivacaine HCl since they become opalescent on mixing with CSF *in vitro*.[137] Although precipitation of the compound may occur *in vivo*,[117,276,384] animal studies indicate that morphologic effects of the less water-soluble agents on the spinal cord are apparent only after intrathecal injection of concentrations greater than 2%.[7,8]

Protein Binding. Besides being more lipid soluble, the longer-acting local anesthetics also exhibit higher

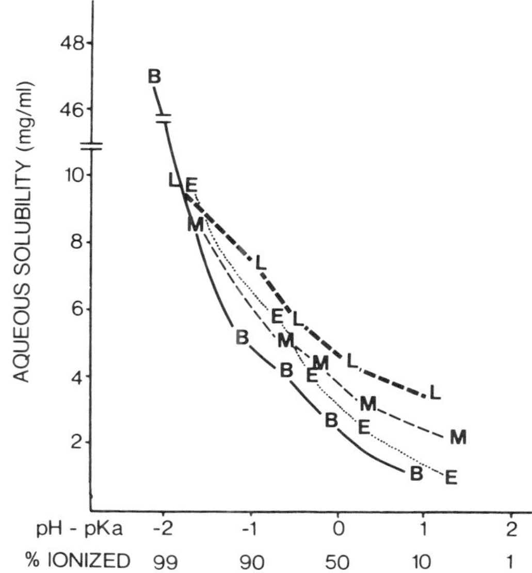

FIG. 3-6. Solubilities of lidocaine (*L*), mepivacaine (*M*), etidocaine (*E*), and bupivacaine (*B*) in aqueous buffer in relation to their pKa and degree of ionization. (Mather: Unpublished data.)

degrees of binding to plasma and tissue proteins (Table 3-1). This suggests that the binding forces are predominantly hydrophobic, which is also consistent with greater plasma binding at higher *p*H values.[83]

Adsorption of local anesthetics to binding sites within membranes or tissues, while producing relatively high apparent partition coefficients, may result in slower penetration rates. This may be considered either as a lowering of diffusion coefficient or as a decrease in ΔC, the effective concentration gradient of diffusible drug. Binding of the drugs to proteins associated with the aqueous phases on either side of a membrane will affect the transfer and equilibrium distribution of total drug, analogously to ionization. Only the unbound drug will diffuse readily, and, again, this will modify net drug transfer rate by an influence on ΔC.

At equilibrium, the concentration of unbound, nonionized drug will be the same on either side of the membrane, but total drug concentrations will differ depending on the relative capacities of the binding sites associated with the two aqueous phases and the *p*H values of these phases.[404]

On the basis of an appreciation of the different structures and physicochemical properties of local anesthetics and the expected consequences of these differences,[69] it is possible to inquire more specifically into their absorption and disposition in various parts of the body. In doing so, the fate of the agents is best divided into consideration of their local disposition, systemic absorption, and systemic disposition (Fig. 3-7).[256]

The term *disposition* has a special meaning; it refers collectively to the processes of drug distribution into and out of tissues and drug elimination by excretion and metabolism, while specifically excluding the process of absorption into the bloodstream.

LOCAL DISPOSITION

In contrast to many drugs, the primary effects of local anesthetics at both a pharmacologic level (neural blockade) and at the clinical level (analgesia and anesthesia) can be measured fairly objectively. The anesthesiologist is concerned particularly with the onset, spread, quality, and duration of nerve block. Ultimately, however, these variables depend on the distribution and dissipation of the drugs at the site of injection. Therefore, it would be valuable to have chemical measurements of the agents at these sites as a function of time in order to establish pharmacodynamic relationships. Regrettably, such data are sparse, even from animals. Therefore, knowledge of the local disposition, or neurokinetics, of local anesthetics remain largely theoretical and on the basis of spatiotemporal changes in anesthetic effect rather than direct measurements of intraneural and perineural drug concentrations.

Factors that affect local disposition of local anesthetics include dispersion by bulk flow of the injected solution, diffusion, and binding of the agent. Metabolic breakdown seems less important. Local blood supply is critical, but this will be discussed primarily in the context of systemic absorption.

BULK FLOW

The extent of spread of the injected solution might be expected to depend upon its volume, the force (speed) with which it is injected, the size of the injected space, the physical resistance offered by tissues and fluids, gravity, and the position of the pa-

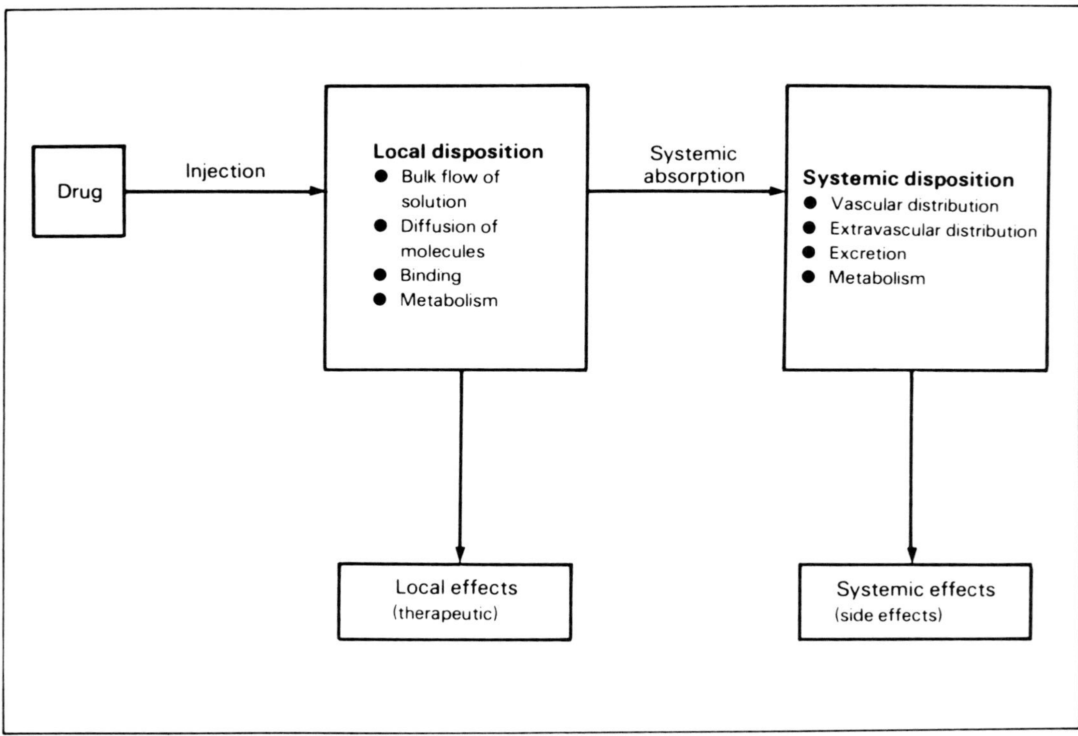

FIG. 3-7. Fate of local anesthetic agents. (Mather, L.E., and Cousins, M.J.: Local anaesthetics and their current clinical use. Drugs, *18:*185, 1979.)

tient during and after injection. Bulk flow of local anesthetic solutions has been assessed by the use of marker dyes, radiocontrast media, and external counting techniques.[65,80,285,306] Although the spread of analgesia may also indicate the extent of bulk flow, these two terms are not necessarily synonymous because spread of effect also depends on diffusion and local perfusion.

Subarachnoid Block. Hydrodynamic considerations are more important after subarachnoid injection than after any other regional anesthetic procedure. Using ^{131}I as a marker, Kitahara and colleagues[216] documented the spread of isobaric and hyperbaric local anesthetic solutions in relation to the level of analgesia and with patients in various positions. Hyperbaric solutions spread more cephalad than did isobaric ones; however, there is no difference in the spread of analgesia between isobaric and hypobaric solutions.[71] A head-down position does not cause extra cephalad spread in most patients.[374] Unilateral block can be obtained by maintaining the lateral position, but the block rapidly becomes bilateral when the patient is turned supine.[432]

Comparison of the same dose of local anesthetic in different volumes indicated no difference in the spread of analgesia in the supine position produced by 15 mg of bupivacaine given as 0.5% and 0.75% hyperbaric solutions but less cephalad spread when 10 mg was given as the 0.75% compared to the 0.5% solution.[90] Spread of analgesia may or may not be influenced when concentration is constant and volume is varied, depending on the concentration of hyperbaric bupivacaine and the posture of the patient (see Chap. 7 for further details).[28,90,391]

Epidural Block. Studies using radiopaque markers indicate that increasing the volume of injectate causes a disproportionately smaller increase in cephalad spread.[80,281] This may reflect greater spillage into the paravertebral spaces with larger volumes and is consistent with volume-spread of analgesia relationships.[65,178] Thus, below a limiting volume (constant dose), the spread and intensity of block become independent of volume, indicating that factors other than bulk flow are more important for the ultimate dispersion of the local anesthetic.

Neither Burn and associates nor Nishimura and associates could demonstrate any effect of the rate of injection on spread of solutions in the epidural space.[80,306] The results of studies on the spread of analgesia vary but, in general, indicate a minor influence of injection speed.[98,146,198,343] Confounding factors include the drug used, the age of the patient, the range of injection pressures, and the direction of the needle bevel.

Posture has a minimal influence on the spread of analgesia. No significant differences in cephalad spread occur in the sitting and lateral positions.[275,306,314] An exception is the obese patient who achieves a lower block when seated.[190] Caudad spread may be marginally less when the patient is sitting.[275] The lateral position favors spread of analgesia to the dependent side in both nonpregnant and pregnant patients, but this does not appear to be of great clinical significance.[17,112,179,198,275,369]

Increases in the duration and longitudinal spread of epidural anesthesia with increasing age have been assigned to reduced lateral leakage of solution, owing to progressive sclerotic closure of the paravertebral foramina.[65] This is supported by the finding of increased residual epidural pressure after injection in older people, evidence from epidurograms, and more extensive cephalad spread shown by an external counting method.[65,306] In contrast, although Burn and associates[80] found evidence of reduced lateral spread of solution with age using 20 ml lumbar injections, this was not seen with 40 ml solutions and, when there was less lateral spread, it was not accompanied by greater longitudinal flow. Further, while verifying a decline in dose requirements with age, recent studies have shown that the relationship is more complex than originally proposed.[179,312,313,370]

Intercostal Block. The distribution of marker substances after injection into the costal grooves of cadavers has been investigated. Whereas Nunn and Slavin[308] concluded that spread occurs to the nerves above and below the target one, Moore[280,284,285] found that spread was exclusive to the injected intercostal groove.

Brachial Plexus Block. Winnie and co-workers[439] used a mixture of bupivacaine and radiopaque dye to document the spread of solution following injection into the brachial plexus sheath and have made specific recommendations on technical and mechanical factors designed to improve the flow in the desired direction. These are based on the concept of a continuous, single fascial compartment surrounding the brachial plexus from its origins and extending peripherally as far as the axilla. Recently, Thompson and Rowe[400] have challenged this concept with evidence of individual fascial compartments around each of the major branches of the plexus (see Chap. 10).

DIFFUSION

Once the local anesthetic has been deposited and spread physically in the extraneural fluids, it finds its way to sites of action in and on the nerve membrane largely by the process of diffusion.

Subarachnoid Block. After subarachnoid injection, the relatively high lipid solubility of local anesthetics will promote local cord uptake rather than extensive cephalad spread via CSF flow. Thus drug concentrations in the CSF decline rapidly in both directions from the point of injection and exponentially at the site of injection as uptake proceeds.[220,276,327] Direct diffusion along the concentration gradient from CSF through the pia mater directly into the cord delivers drug only to the superficial parts of the structure. Access to deeper areas is effected by diffusion in the CSF contained in the spaces of Virchow–Robin which connect with perineural clefts surrounding the bodies of nerve cells within the cord.[175] Deeper penetration of drug into the cord may also occur by means of uptake into spinal radicular arteries (see Chap. 7).

The pattern of drug distribution within the cord is a complex function of accessibility by diffusion from the CSF, the relative myelin (lipid) content of various tracts, and the rate of drug removal by local perfusion. Studies in animals using radiolabeled lidocaine have shown that it accumulates along the posterior and lateral aspects of the spinal cord as well as in the spinal nerve roots, but not to such a degree in the dorsal root ganglion or in the more central parts of the cord. Uptake of drug was higher in the gray matter than in the white matter of the cord, and posterior nerve roots had higher concentrations than anterior roots.[66,96,194] The model proposed for subarachnoid injection of opioids[104] may be viewed as a reasonable representation of the fate of local anesthetics since, in general, these agents have similar physicochemical properties (see Fig. 28-6).

Epidural Block. Local anesthetics appear rapidly in the CSF after epidural injection.[433] Thus, peak drug concentrations in the CSF occur within 10 to 20 minutes and are sufficient to produce blockade of spinal nerve roots. By 30 minutes high drug concentrations are also achieved in the peripheral cord and in the spinal nerves in the paravertebral space.[66]

Apart from direct diffusion of drug across the dura, access to the cord, particularly the dorsal horn region, may be mediated by diffusion and bulk flow through the arachnoid villi at the dural root sleeves, by uptake into the posterior radicular branch of spinal segmental arteries, and by centripetal subneural and subpial spread from the remote paravertebral nerve trunks.[63,65] These suggestions are consistent with clinical observations of the distribution of analgesia during induction and regression of epidural block. A segmental pattern of analgesia during onset may be related to the initial drug diffusion into spinal nerves and roots, with subsequent nonsegmental regression resulting from ultimate diffusion to structures within the cord.[419] Again, the model proposed for epidural administration of opioids[104] (Fig. 28-17) may also represent the fate of local anesthetic agents.

Electrophysiologic studies in monkeys indicate that the depth of penetration of the cord varies considerably with the agent used, chloroprocaine being limited to dorsal horn gray matter, bupivacaine reaching both the dorsal horn and white matter, and etidocaine concentrating predominantly in the white matter.[109] These differences are, however, concentration-dependent. Thus, increased concentration of bupivacaine was shown to influence penetration at the dorsal root entry zone and, to a lesser degree, at the white tracts of the spinal cord.[110] A marked effect of etidocaine on lower limb reflexes after thoracic epidurals in humans is consistent with blockade of relatively deep motor tracts within the cord using this agent.[64]

Much of an epidural dose of local anesthetic may be sequestered temporarily in extraneural tissues at the site of injection. This nonspecific "binding" may have two effects: By lowering the amount of agent free to diffuse onto the nerves, it effectively lowers clinical potency; on the other hand, by providing a depot from which drug is slowly dissociated to maintain anesthetic concentrations in the nerve, it could prolong duration of block. Prolonged sequestration of local anesthetic drugs in epidural fat, particularly those that are more lipid soluble, has been demonstrated in the sheep (Fig. 3-8).

Brachial Plexus Block. Progression of blockade from upper arm to hand and then to fingers is explained by more rapid diffusion of local anesthetic into mantle fibers that innervate more proximal regions than do the core fibers.[116] To explain why the onset of motor block often precedes that of sensory loss, Winnie and colleagues[437] have suggested that the effect of the larger diameter of the motor fibers is offset by their more peripheral location in the median nerve compared to sensory fibers. According to the classic view, the sequence of recovery should be the same as that of onset: arm first, then hand and

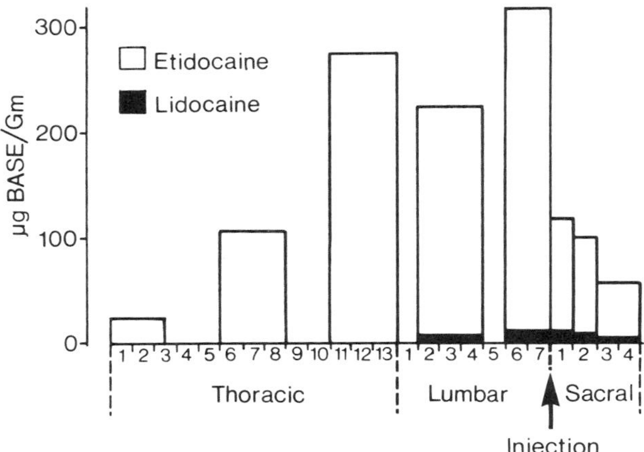

FIG. 3-8. Mean local anesthetic concentrations in peridural fat of sheep 12 hours after peridural injection. Dose is 80 mg of etidocaine hydrochloride, 50 mg of lidocaine hydrochloride, and 50 μg of epinephrine; n is 6. (Lebeaux, M., and Tucker, G.T.: Unpublished data.)

fingers.[116] This follows if the concentration gradient within the nerve now becomes reversed, decreasing from core to mantle. However, this has been challenged by Winnie and colleagues,[438] who observed the reverse order of recovery with significant motor block that outlasted analgesia. To account for these findings it was proposed that a more rapid vascular uptake of agent occurs near the more distally innervating sensory fibers located in the core of the nerve. As intraneural blood vessels pass from mantle to core they become increasingly branched and thus offer a larger surface area for drug absorption.

Differential Block. The propensity to produce a marked differential blockade is a characteristic of some local anesthetic agents, particularly tetracaine and etidocaine, which produce profound motor blockade, and bupivacaine, which provides good analgesia with a minimum of motor loss. In the case of epidural block, Bromage[64] has suggested that this phenomenon may be due to deeper penetration of the spinal cord by more lipid-soluble agents causing interference with long descending motor pathways. Bupivacaine, however, is more lipid soluble than tetracaine and lidocaine, which produce less differential sensory loss, and the differences in sensory–motor dissociation seen with the various agents are also apparent after peripheral nerve block procedures, in which penetration of the cord is not a factor.[240,330] To accommodate the latter, differences in the ability of the agents to diffuse into individual sensory and motor fibers have been postulated. Thus, from electrophysiologic studies with isolated rabbit vagus nerve, Gissen and co-workers[169] concluded that, compared to etidocaine, less lipid-soluble bupivacaine diffuses relatively slowly into fast-conducting A (motor) fibers at low concentrations. This is supported by other electrophysiologic studies,[161,310,341] although Fink and Cairns[158] discount diffusion within a nerve as a contributory factor to differential block.

The contribution of frequency-dependent block to differential nerve block is discussed in Chapter 2.

***p*H Effects.** Any factor that creates local extracellular acidosis should retard net diffusion of local anesthetic to the nerve by increasing drug ionization (see Equation 4). A low *p*H may be preexisting, for example, as a result of infection or may be induced by injection of the anesthetic solution. Likely effects of the injection on local *p*H have been reviewed by Rowland,[355] and the mechanisms suggested are summarized in Table 3-3. Of these, movement of carbon dioxide is probably fleeting; dilution of local bicarbonate stores is readily avoided; acidic solutions are rapidly counteracted by the buffer capacity of most tissues; and stabilizers may be circumvented by adding concentrated epinephrine before the injection rather than using a premixed acidic solution. The importance of vasoconstrictor and metabolic effects of epinephrine is indicated by the observation that whereas injection of a plain lidocaine solution lowers tissue *p*H for 30 minutes, solutions containing epinephrine (5 μg/ml) maintain tissue acidosis for 90 minutes or more. This effect of epinephrine was the same, however, whether the *p*H was 3.5 or 6.5.[428]

TABLE 3-3. MECHANISMS FOR LOWERING LOCAL EXTRACELLULAR *p*H BY LOCAL ANESTHETIC SOLUTIONS

Movement of intracellular carbon dioxide into solutions deficient in carbon dioxide
Dilution of local bicarbonate stores by large volumes of solution
Use of acidic solutions
To dissolve agents as their salts (*p*H 5–7)
To stabilize ester-type agents
To stabilize added epinephrine with addition of sodium bisulfite (*p*H 3–4)
Effect of added epinephrine, causing local ischemia and increased cellular metabolism

(Data from Rowland, M: Local anesthetic absorption, distribution and elimination. *In* Eger, E [ed.]: Anesthetic Uptake and Action, pp. 332–366. Baltimore, Williams & Wilkins, 1974.)

Despite these considerations, it has been shown that the addition of epinephrine to local anesthetic solutions at the time of injection does not prolong the onset of clinical epidural or subarachnoid nerve block with lidocaine or bupivacaine.[78] In fact, with etidocaine, the opposite has been found.[62,297]

Cohen and colleagues have suggested that acidosis could explain the development of tachyphylaxis to local anesthetics during multidose subarachnoid and epidural block.[97] They showed that repeated spinal injections of local anesthetic solutions in dogs resulted in a progressive fall in the *p*H of poorly buffered CSF from 7.4 to 6.8. This has been confirmed by others after single doses and would be accompanied by a reduction in the fraction of nonionized agent, and hence should decrease access of drug to the site of action (Table 3-4). Tachyphylaxis is not, however, explained adequately by *p*H effects alone.[255] In sheep, for example, duration of motor block after subarachnoid injections of local anesthetics was either longer or similar and showed a greater frequency when the *p*H of the solution was decreased from 6.5–7 to 4–4.5, although sensory blockade showed the expected opposite trend.[6,9]

Replacement of the hydrochloride salt solution of local anesthetic by carbonated solutions should obviate the movement of carbon dioxide out of the nerve. In contrast, rapid penetration of carbon dioxide into the nerve to cause a lowering of intraneural *p*H could promote a more rapid production of active ionized drug at the point where it is needed.[88] Open clinical studies have shown that carbonation of lidocaine significantly decreases onset time after epidural,[67] caudal,[104] and brachial plexus blocks. However, recent double-blind investigations, while showing that carbonation improves the quality of epidural analgesia, have not confirmed an effect on the onset of action of lidocaine.[254,295] Similarly, this process does not appear to hasten the effects of bupivacaine after epidural injection,[72] although it does so when this agent is used for brachial plexus block using the interscalene approach.[269]

METABOLISM

The evidence suggests that local metabolism has a negligible influence on the neurokinetics of local anesthetics and the time-course of conduction blockade. Thus when procaine is incubated with nerve tissue, it is hydrolyzed only to the extent of 2% to 4% per hour, which can be accounted for largely by nonenzymatic breakdown.[307,376] Hydrolysis of ester-type agents in the vicinity of the nerve also seems to be slow, since addition of a cholinesterase inhibitor to chloroprocaine solution did not prolong blockade.[242] On the other hand, subarachnoid injection of exogenous cholinesterase has been shown to reverse a tetracaine block in rabbits.[425]

Significant local metabolic alteration of the amide-type agents is most unlikely.

SYSTEMIC ABSORPTION

INTERPRETATION OF "BLOOD LEVELS"

The value of measurements of blood concentrations of local anesthetics after various routes of administration rests on the assumption that there is a closer relationship between drug concentrations in the circulation and systemic drug effects than between dose and effect.

Estimates have been made of threshold plasma concentrations of various local anesthetics associated with the onset of significant CNS toxicity in humans (Table 3-5). These range from 5 to 10 μg/ml for lidocaine and mepivacaine and from 2 to 4 μg/ml for bupivacaine and etidocaine. Although these values are useful guidelines, they refer to the mythical

TABLE 3-4. *p*H OF CEREBROSPINAL FLUID IN DOGS AFTER SUBARACHNOID INJECTION OF LOCAL ANESTHETIC SOLUTIONS

Time After Injection (min)	10% Dextrose in Saline Control (*p*H 5.5)	5% Lidocaine Hydrochloride + 7.5% Dextrose (*p*H 4.5)	0.75% Etidocaine Hydrochloride + 5% Dextrose (*p*H 4.2)	2% Procaine Hydrochloride (*p*H 4.2)	4% Tetracaine Hydrochloride (*p*H 4.2)
0	7.41	7.34	7.40	7.36	7.37
2	7.26	6.10	6.20	6.40	6.80
5	7.36	6.40	6.89	6.74	6.93
15		6.90	7.24	7.23	7.10
30		7.10	7.27	7.32	7.21

(Based on unpublished data from Mather, L. E., Pavlin, E., and Middaugh, M., 1975.)

"average subject" and must be interpreted in the light of a number of considerations. Other considerations are mentioned here briefly and amplified in the section on "Systemic Disposition." It is particularly important to differentiate between concentrations obtained under slowly equilibrating conditions (*i.e.*, under quasi-equilibrium between blood and target tissue) such as may occur after successful perineural injection and those obtained under rapidly changing conditions (*i.e.*, without equilibration between blood and target tissue) such as may occur after accidental intravascular injection.

1. *Plasma versus blood.* Plasma and whole blood concentrations of local anesthetics are not the same, and the ratio of the two varies with the agent.[413] Thus, bupivacaine is about 2.5 times as toxic to the CNS as lidocaine based on plasma concentrations but about 3.5 times as toxic based on blood concentrations. The estimate of relative toxicity based on dosage is generally considered to be about 4.
2. *Total versus free.* It is generally believed, but rather more difficult to prove, that non-protein-bound (free) concentrations of drugs in plasma relate to pharmacologic and toxic effects more closely than do total (bound plus free) concentrations. Some data suggest that this is so for lidocaine[322] and bupivacaine.[127]

   As discussed later, there is significant variation in the plasma binding of local anesthetics such that the same unbound plasma drug concentration can be associated with very different total concentrations in different subjects. Ideally, therefore, "minimal toxic levels" of the drugs should be quoted in terms of free drug. On this basis, bupivacaine is probably about 15 times as toxic as lidocaine.
3. *Ionized versus un-ionized.* The degree of ionization of local anesthetics will be sensitive to small changes in plasma *p*H because their pKa values are close to 7.4. Therefore, if the local anesthetic cation is responsible for effects in the brain, as it is at the nerve membrane, then brain tissue *p*H may be a significant determinant of toxicity. Englesson[144,145] has shown in cats that the CNS toxicity of local anesthetics is very sensitive to changes in acid–base balance. Therefore, in the absence of knowledge of brain *p*H, at least it may be important to specify the *p*H and $Paco_2$ of the plasma sample when relating the circulating concentration of local anesthetic to toxicity.
4. *(+)-Isomer versus (−)-isomer.* With the exception of lidocaine, the main amide-type local anesthetics are optically active and are administered as racemic mixtures. Methods are not yet available for routinely measuring the concentrations of the individual enantiomers in biological fluids. There is good reason to believe that the enantiomers differ in their pharmacokinetics and toxicity.[3,243,360] Thus precise interpretation of blood concentration-response data, or even blood concentration-time data, may be more complex than is commonly appreciated.
5. *Drug versus metabolite.* Some of the metabolic products of local anesthetics may contribute to the toxicity of the parent drug, and it may be important to measure their plasma concentrations also (see later).
6. *Artery versus vein.* Blood can never be considered as a homogenous drug-containing compartment if drug administration or elimination is taking place. Because drug concentrations in peripheral blood may be homogeneous only under steady-state conditions, caution should be used when interpreting absolute drug concentrations in arterial or venous blood vessels. Thus, large arteriovenous differences in the concentrations of local anesthetics have been observed (Figs. 3-9, 3-10). Under these dynamic conditions, the time profile of drug concentration in arterial blood will peak earlier than that at targets for toxicity in vital organs. (Fig. 3-11).[299] This probably explains why arterial plasma concentrations of etidocaine and bupivacaine in monkeys associated with the onset of convulsions were higher when the agents were injected at a faster rate, reflecting disequilibrium between drug in plasma and at sites of toxicity.[253] Drug concentrations in peripheral venous blood peak later than those in the brain, particularly if samples are taken from vessels draining a poorly perfused region without significant shunt flow. The significance of arteriovenous drug concentration differences will depend on the rate of change of drug concentration.

With due regard to the above considerations, a knowledge of the rates of systemic absorption of local anesthetics helps to set confidence limits on the likelihood of systemic toxic reactions after the various block procedures. Indirectly, these rates also suggest the relationship between blockade and the amount of drug remaining at the site of injection.

In humans, measurement of drug concentration–time profiles in the peripheral circulation has been used widely to assess systemic uptake of the different agents. Because these profiles are the net result of

TABLE 3-5. RELATIONSHIP BETWEEN PLASMA CONCENTRATIONS OF LOCAL ANESTHETICS AFTER INTRAVENOUS ADMINISTRATION AND CNS TOXICITY*

Agent	Author	Reference	Number of Subjects	Infusion Rate (mg/min)	Infusion Time (min)
Procaine	Usubiaga *et al.* (1966)	420	5	3-9/kg	To convulsions
Lidocaine	Foldes *et al.* (1960)	160	10	0.50/kg	12.8
	Jorfeldt *et al.* (1968)	205a	4	0.25/kg	20
	Scott (1975)	362a	5	20	12.5
Mepivacaine	Jorfeldt *et al.* (1968)	205a	11	0.25/kg	20
Bupivacaine	Jorfeldt *et al.* (1968)	205a	5	0.06/kg	20
	Mather *et al.* (1971b)	258	3	Avg. 5.6	14-18
	Scott (1975)	362a	5	10	8-12.5
	Wiklund and Berlin-Wahlen (1977)	429	7	2	150
	Mather *et al.* (1979)	264	8	7.5	10
Etidocaine	Scott (1975)	362a	5	10	12.5
			5	20	6.8-11
	Wiklund and Berlin-Wahlen (1977)	429	8	2	150
	Mather *et al.* (1979)	264	8	7.5	10

*For example, light headedness, circumoral numbness, disorientation.
†For example, muscular twitching, nystagmus, slurred speech.
‡M = maximum; T = threshold.
§V = peripheral venous; A = arterial.
||C = colorimetric; GC = gas chromatography.
¶Venous levels about 50% lower.
**Fatigue only.
(Tucker, G.T., and Mather, L.E.: Clinical pharmacokinetics of local anaesthetic agents. Clin. Pharmacokinet., *4*:241, 1979.)

both systemic absorption and disposition processes, they are of value mainly to determine relative changes in systemic drug uptake, for example, as a result of variation in dose, route of injection, concentration and volume of solution, and concentration of added vasoconstrictor. These variables are assumed not to influence systemic disposition kinetics.

If blood drug concentration-time profiles are also available after intravenous administration, it becomes possible to calculate absolute drug absorption rates with the aid of more sophisticated techniques of pharmacokintic analysis.[406,411] Measurement of the drug content of venous blood draining from the site of injection has also been used to provide estimates of absolute absorption rates.[77,148]

Because local anesthetics are relatively lipid-soluble compounds, their diffusion across the capillary endothelium is not likely to be rate limiting. Hence their absorption rates will primarily be related directly to local blood flow and inversely to local tissue binding.

Important determinants of systemic absorption include the physicochemical and vasoactive properties of the agent, the site of injection, dosage factors, the presence of additives such as vasoconstrictors in the injected solution, factors related to nerve block, and pathophysiologic features of the patient.

AGENT

Tucker and Mather[413] have tabulated the extensive data on peak blood and plasma concentrations of the amide-type agents and the times of their occurrence after various routes of injection in humans. These data are updated in Tables 3-6 to 3-10. For example, after epidural injection of plain solutions, the increment in peak whole blood drug concentration per 100 mg of dose is about 0.9 to 1.0 μg/ml for lidocaine and mepivacaine, slightly less for prilocaine, and about half as much for bupivacaine and etidocaine. Although differences in disposition kinetics contribute to this order (see later), it appears that despite similar peak times net absorption of the long-acting, more lipid-soluble agents is slower. This is consistent with data on residual concentrations of the agents in epidural fat after injection into sheep (see Fig. 3-8) and is confirmed by pharmacokinetic calculations of the time-course of unabsorbed drug in humans.[78,262,382,383,413] The latter show that systemic up-

TABLE 3-5. RELATIONSHIP BETWEEN PLASMA CONCENTRATIONS OF LOCAL ANESTHETICS AFTER INTRAVENOUS ADMINISTRATION AND CNS TOXICITY* ***(continued)***

Number of Subjects with Symptoms			Plasma Drug Concentration (mean—range or SD μg/ml)‡	Sampling Site§	Assay‖
Subjective*	**Objective†**	**Convulsions**			
5	5	5	38 (21–81) M	V	C
10	10	1	5.29 ± 0.55 M	V	C
Most	Most	1	4.9 M	A	C
5	2	0	~2.2 M	V	GC
Most	Most	0	6.0 M	A	C
Some	0	0	2.1 M	A	C
3	0	0	2.6–4.5 M	V	GC
5	4	0	2.24 ± 0.48 M	V	GC
6	2	0	~2.3 T	A	GC
7	0	0	2.2–4.2¶ T	A	GC
4	0	0	2.27 ± 0.24 M	V	GC
5	5	0	~2.2 M	V	GC
2**	0	0	1.96 ± 0.25 M	A	GC
6	0	0	2.1–5.3¶ T	A	GC

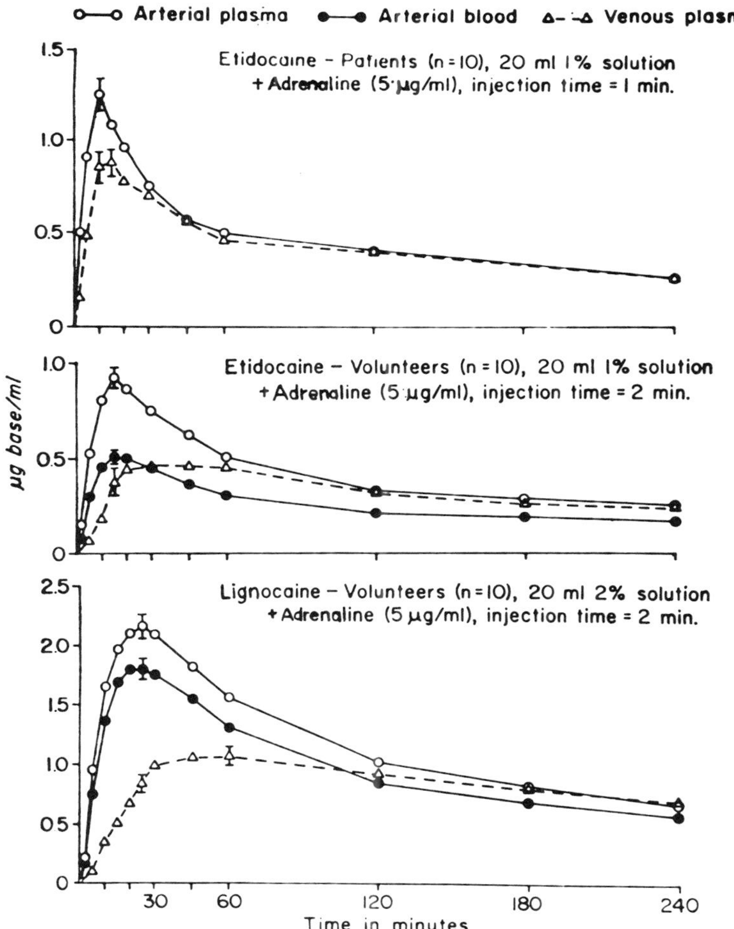

FIG. 3-9. Mean concentrations of etidocaine and lidocaine (lignocaine) after epidural injection in patients (female, 21 to 52 years, 110 to 178 lb, undergoing abdominal hysterectomy, started after 30 min) and healthy volunteers (male, 21 to 32 years, 159 to 200 lb.) (Tucker, G.T., and Mather, L.E.: Pharmacokinetics of local anaesthetic agents. Br. J. Anaesth., *47*:213, 1975.)

TABLE 3-6. LIDOCAINE: SYSTEMIC UPTAKE AFTER ADMINISTRATION FOR REGIONAL ANESTHESIA*

Author	Reference	Route	Dose (mg)	Concentration (%)	Epinephrine	Number of Subjects	Assay	Sampling Site	Maximum[1] Concentration (μm/ml)	Peak Time (min)	Maximum Concentration (μg/100 mg of dose)
Thomas *et al.* (1969)	395	TS (V)	400	-	–	9	GC	VP	0.55 (0.16–1.00)	50 (30–120)	0.14
		TS (P)	400	-	–	6			0.47 (0.24–0.82)	77 (30–150)	0.12
		TS (E)	1000	-	–	5			0.46 (0.20–0.65)	24 (10–45)	0.05
Bromage and Robson (1961)	70	Endo	280–520	4	–	12	C	VB	0.7–10.0	5–25	
Pelton *et al.* (1970)	316	Endo	3/kg	10	–	13	GC	VB	2.2	~5	1.05
								AB	2.5	~2	1.19
Chu *et al.* (1975)	95	Endo	200	4	–	6[d]	GC	VP	3.54 ± 0.76[b]	20[c]	1.77
Patterson *et al.* (1975)	315	Endo	180–380[e]	1	–	21	GC	VB	1.90 (0.58–18.20)	26 (5–75)	0.62
Viegas and Stoelting (1975)	423	Endo	2/kg	4	–	6[d]	GC	AB	1.7 ± 0.25[b]	9–15	1.21
			2/kg[e]	4	–	4[d]			2.4 ± 0.3[b]	4–15	1.71
Curran *et al.* (1975)	107	Endo	300	10	–	5[d,f]	GC	VB	5.1 (1.9–8.2)	10–15	1.70
			300	10	–	5[d,g]			1.1 (0.4–2.5)	10–20	0.37
Smith (1976)	378	Endo	2/kg	4	–	30	GC	B	0.1–2.0[h]		
Karvonen *et al.* (1976)	211	Endo	400	4	–	15	GC	AB	1.39 ± 0.66	20[c]	0.35
								VB	1.07 ± 0.54	20[c]	0.27
Scott *et al.* (1976)	364	Endo	100	5 or 10	–	5[d]	GC	VP	1.46 ± 0.43	10	1.46
		Endo	100		–	6			0.96 ± 0.25	20	0.96
		Endo	50		–	5			0.48 ± 0.25	5	0.96
Chinn *et al.* (1977)	92	Endo	280	4	–	5[i]	GC	VP	0.6	20	0.21
		Endo	400	4	–	5[i]			0.44	10	0.11
Cannell *et al.* (1975)	87	Perioral	40–160	2	–	9	GC	VB	0.4–2.0	~10	
			40–160	2	+	11		VP	0.4–1.5	30–60	
Schwartz *et al.* (1974)	362	SC[a,f]	200	2	–	8	GC	VB	0.49 ± 0.16	120	0.25
Scott *et al.* (1972)	363	SCA	400	2	–	10	C	VP	1.95 ± 0.23	~30	0.49
			400	2	+	10			1.02 ± 0.15	~15	0.26
		SCV	400	2	–	9			4.91 ± 0.43	~15	1.23
			400	2	+	9			2.50 ± 0.36	~15	0.62
Petrie *et al.* (1974)	318a	PCB	200	1	–	10	GC	VP	2.08 ± 0.09[b]	10	1.04
Mazze and Dunbar (1966)	267	BP	6.2/kg	1.5	+	7	GC	VP	2.5 ± 0.5	30 (20–60)	0.50
Raj *et al.* (1977)	331	BP	400[k]	2	–	5	GC	VP	~3.4	25	0.85
			400[k]	2	+	5			~2.4	25	0.60
Wildsmith *et al.* (1977)	431	BP[p]	450	2	–	5	GC	VP	4.51	15	1.00
			450	2	+	5			3.62	20	0.80
Scott *et al.* (1972)	363	IC	400	1	–	8	C	VP	6.8 ± 0.32	~15	1.70
			400	1	+[l]	12			5.28 ± 0.36	~20	1.32
			400	1	+[m]	10			4.87 ± 0.24	~10	1.22
			400	2	–	11			6.48 ± 0.38	~15	1.62
Braid and Scott (1965)	55	IC	400	4	–	13	C	VP	8.42 ± 0.26	~15	2.10
Bromage and Robson (1961)	70	Epid	300–500	2	–	15	C	VB	1.7–9.4	5–35	
			300–680	2	+	12			1.0–4.4	12–40	

Mazze and Dunbar (1966)	267	Epid	5.5/kg	1.5	+	4	GC	VP	3.1 ± 0.7	20–30	0.79
Lund and Cwik (1966)	247	Epid	600	2	+	?	C	VB	2.72 ± 1.26	30[c]	0.45
Scott *et al.* (1972)	363	Epid	200	2	–	11	C	VP	3.30 ± 0.07	~15	1.65
			400	2	–	23			4.27 ± 0.24	~20	1.07
			400	2	+[l]	15			2.95 ± 0.29	~15	0.74
			400	2	+[m]	13			3.09 ± 0.38	~30	0.77
			600	2	–	10			7.34 ± 0.37	~15	1.22
			600	3	–	8			6.31 ± 0.26	~15	1.05
Braid and Scott (1966)	56	Epid	700	2	–	9	C	VP	7.43 ± 0.23	~15	1.06
Raj *et al.* (1977)	331	Epid	300[k]	2	–	6	GC	VP	3.5	25	1.17
			300[k]	2	+	8			~2.6	25	0.75
Mather *et al.* (1976)	262	Epid	400	2	–	5	GC	AP	3.7 ± 0.5	12 ± 3	0.93
			400	2	+	5			2.1 ± 0.4	25 ± 4	0.53
Mazze and Dunbar (1966)	267	Caud	6.6/kg	1.5	+	4	GC	VP	1.8 ± 0.5	40 (10–60)	0.42
Spielman *et al.* (1983)	380	TS (F)	240	2	–	9	GC	VB	1.70 ± 0.34	30	0.71
Labedzki *et al.* (1983)	229	Endo	480–720	2–10	–	10	GC	VP	(1.9–7.4)	20–90	0.64
Jones *et al.* (1982)	205	Endo[j]	230–364	2–4	–	19	GC	VP	(0.95–3.34)	30–90	0.55
LeLorier *et al.* (1979)	234	Endo[s]	400–1000	2	–	12	GC	VP	(0.56–3.70)		0.40
		Endo[t]	40–320	2	–	8	GC	VP	(0.06–0.98)		0.42
Morrell *et al.* (1982)	296	Endo	160	4	–	24[d]	GC	AP	3.10 ± 0.29[b]	5–40	1.94
		Endo	160	4	–	22	GC	AP	2.50 ± 0.26[b]	10–40	1.56
Gomez *et al.* (1983)	172	Endo[s]	180–400	4	–	29	EMIT	VS	1.21 ± 0.64	30	-
McBurney *et al.* (1984)	268	Endo[j]	104–148[u]	4	–	10	GC	VP	0.66 ± 0.18	15–60	0.56
		Endo	200[v]	4	–	10	GC	VP	1.53 ± 1.20	20–60	0.76
Kanto *et al.* (1980)	209	SCC	0.8–3.7/kg	0.5	+	12	GC	VP	(0.6–1.0)	5–10	-
Blanco *et al.* (1982)	49	PCB	90–100	1	–	24	GC	P	1.32 ± 0.42	10	1.32
		PCB[r]	90–100	1	–	25	GC	P	1.72 ± 0.64	10	1.72
Giasi *et al.* (1979)	167	Epid	75	2	–	10	GC	VP	0.41 ± 0.07	15	0.55
Mayumi *et al.* (1983)	266	Epid	200	2	–	10	EMIT	AP	3.26 ± 0.97	10	1.63
		Epid (C)	200	2	–	10	EMIT	AP	3.84 ± 1.40	10	1.92
		Epid (T)	200	2	–	10	EMIT	AP	4.11 ± 0.79	10	2.05
Boster *et al.* (1982)	52	Endo[w]	5.7 ± 1.3[a] mg/kg	10	–	7	GC	VS	1.7–5.0	11–30	0.54[x]
Burm (1985)	78	Epid	400	2	–	10	GC	CeP	2.2 ± 0.2[a]	27 ± 12[a]	0.55
Burm (1985)	78	Epid	400	2	+	12	GC	CeP	1.7 ± 0.3[a]	32 ± 11[a]	0.43
Giasi *et al.* (1979)	167	SAB	75	5	–	10	GC	VP	0.32 ± 0.07[b]	15	0.43
Axelsson and Widman (1981)	27	SAB	100	5	–	16	GC	VB	0.28 ± 0.02[b]	120	0.28
		SAB	100	5	+	16	GC	VB	0.14 ± 0.03[b]	60	0.14
Burm *et al.* (1983)	79	SAB	75	5	–	7	GC	CeP	0.44 ± 0.20[a]	25–120	0.59
Burm (1985)	78	SAB	100	5	–	10	GC	CeP	0.53 ± 0.14[a]	71 ± 29[a]	0.53
		SAB	100	5	+	10	GC	CeP	0.38 ± 0.11[a]	58 ± 24[a]	0.38
Philipson *et al.* (1984)	319	Infiltr (P)	30–160	1–2	–	15	GC	KP	0.06 ± 2.4	3–12	

*For explanation of symbols and abbreviations used in this table, see glossary on p. 97.

(Tucker, G.T., and Mather, L.E.: Clinical pharmacokinetics of local anaesthetic agents. Clin. Pharmacokinet., *4*:241, 1979.)

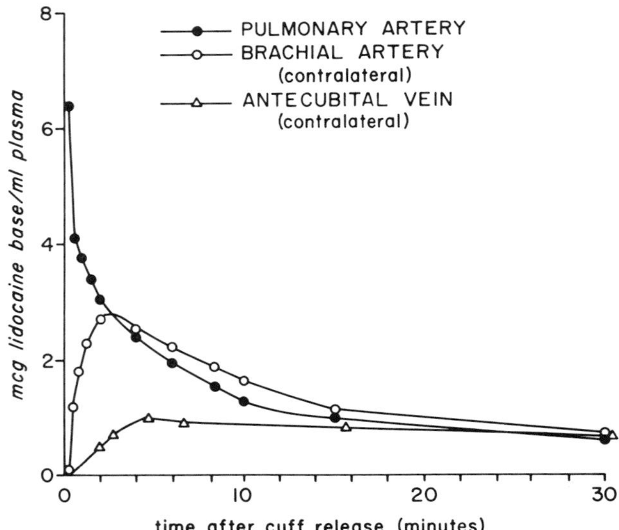

FIG. 3-10. Plasma lidocaine levels in a subject following cuff release after intravenous regional anesthesia with 3 mg/kg^{-1} lidocaine hydrochloride (0.5% solution; 45 minutes cuff time.) (Tucker, G.T., and Boas, R.A.: Pharmacokinetic aspects of intravenous regional anesthesia. Anesthesiology, *34*:538, 1971.)

take after epidural injection is a biphasic process (Fig. 3-12), the contribution of the initial rapid phase being greater for lidocaine than for the long-acting analogues. The slower net absorption of the latter provides them with a greater systemic safety margin despite their greater intrinsic toxicity (Fig. 3-13).

Differences in the absorption rates of the different agents have implications for the accumulation of the drugs during multiple-dose and continuous procedures. Whereas systemic accumulation is most marked with the short-acting amides, extensive local accumulation is predicted for bupivacaine and etidocaine, despite their longer dosage intervals.[410,411] Good agreement between predicted and observed plasma concentrations of etidocaine and lidocaine during short-term multiple dosage (Fig. 3-14) supports the indirect estimates of local accumulation of these agents (Fig. 3-15).

Observation of relatively low blood concentrations of prilocaine with respect to the toxic threshold, particularly after brachial plexus block (Fig. 3-16) and intravenous regional anesthesia, supports the claim that this compound should be the agent of choice for many medium duration single-dose procedures (except for obstetrics). In this case, however, a high systemic clearance, rather than slow absorption, is mainly responsible for the low blood drug concentrations. This also applies with respect to the ester-type agents.[226,282]

Although the rate of systemic absorption of local anesthetics is controlled largely by the extent of local binding, vasoactive properties of these drugs may also be a factor. Thus, studies involving local infiltration and intra-arterial injection of the agents and their application to isolated blood vessels have shown them to have direct effects on vascular smooth muscle. Therefore, by modifying local perfusion, they could influence their own systemic absorption and hence duration of anesthetic action. These effects vary with the agent, its concentration and stereoisomeric form, the site of injection, and the preexisting vascular tone.[19,20,47,111,113,152,204] Of the amides, bupivacaine and etiodocaine are most likely to produce vasodilatation, and prilocaine and mepivacaine are most likely to produce vasoconstriction. Increasing the concentration of the agents increases the frequency of vasodilatation. However, the contribution of these phenomena to the relative absorption of drugs after peripheral and central nerve block is difficult to evaluate. Spinal cord blood flow in animals was unaffected by subarachnoid injection of lidocaine or mepivacaine[134,340,379]; tetracaine increased flow in one study[221] but had no effect in another.[379]

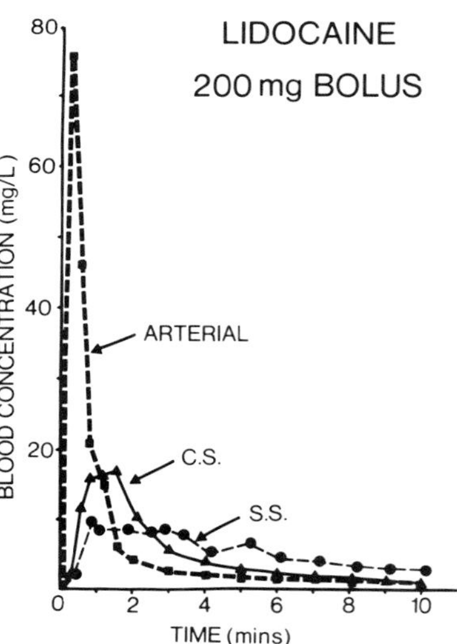

FIG. 3-11. Blood concentrations of lidocaine after an intravenous bolus dose of 200 mg in a 50-kg sheep. C.S., coronary sinus; S.S., sagittal sinus.

SITE OF INJECTION

Vascularity and the presence of tissue and fat that can bind local anesthetics are primary influences on their rate of removal from specific sites of injection. In general, and independent of the agent used, absorption rate decreases in the following order: intercostal block > caudal block > epidural block > brachial plexus block > sciatic and femoral nerve block (Fig. 3-17; Tables 3-6 to 3-10).

Intercostal Block. Circulating concentrations of the agents after intercostal blocks using plain solutions are often higher than those associated with CNS toxicity following short intravenous infusion; however, patients are often sedated by light general anesthesia and premedication during this procedure.

Epidural Block. Although the epidural space is more vascular than the intercostal site, most of the blood vessels contained within it transverse rather than drain it, while large quantities of fat are able to sequester local anesthetics and delay their uptake. Vascular uptake will take place into the epidural veins and thence to the azygos vein. In the presence of raised intrathoracic pressure, however, absorbed drug could also be redirected up the internal venous system to cerebral sinuses (see Chap. 28, Fig. 28-12). Vascular absorption from different regions of the epidural space appears to be similar, since Mayumi and co-workers.[266] found similar plasma concentration–time profiles of lidocaine after cervical, thoracic, and lumbar injections.

Brachial Plexus Block. Peak plasma drug concentrations are similar after brachial plexus block using the interscalene and axillary approaches, although the latter is associated with a slower rise to peak concentrations.[421]

Subarachnoid Block. Initial drug absorption after subarachnoid injections is relatively slow compared to the epidural route,[27,78,79] and, dose for dose, peak plasma drug concentrations are slightly lower.[78,167] Systemic uptake after spinal injection is believed to occur predominantly after dural diffusion into the more vascular epidural space,[96] as well as from blood vessels within the subarachnoid space, particularly those in the pia mater, and the cord itself.[175] Extensive diffusion into the epidural space might be expected to result in sequestration in epidural fat, thus, retarding the absorption of the longer-acting agents to a greater extent than the shorter-acting agents. The time-courses of plasma concentrations of lidocaine and bupivacaine after subarachnoid injection in humans confirm that there is net slower absorption of bupivacaine than lidocaine (Table 3-11) and the pattern differs from that after epidural injection. In contrast to the pattern of faster initial, slower secondary phases of absorption as seen after epidural injection of these agents, absorption of bupivacaine after subarachnoid injection was six-fold slower in the initial phase; for lidocaine, only the slower phase was observed.[78] The similarity of the slower absorption phases for subarachnoid and epidural routes for either drug also suggests that a distribution-equilibrium occurs with a common tissue structure—most probably epidural fat. There may be differences, however, in the pathways of systemic drug absorption for lumbar subarachnoid and epidural injections. Lumbar subarachnoid deposition of local anesthetic solution would lead to systemic absorption by means of the lumbar azygos veins into the inferior vena cava. Spread of local anesthetic solution in the epidural space would lead to more diffuse absorption by means of the lumbar azygos and thoracic hemiazygos veins into the inferior and superior vena cavae, respectively. Thus the time-courses of local anesthetic concentrations in blood from the inferior or superior vena cava or from an artery may differ. Accordingly, Denson and associates[118] observed that lidocaine concentrations in blood from the inferior vena cava markedly exceeded those in arterial blood, but Burm[78] observed only small differences between "central" and arterial concentrations without significant differences to the area under the curve.

Intravenous Regional Anesthesia. A pharmacokinetic analysis of plasma lidocaine concentrations measured after intravenous regional anesthesia has shown that if the cuff is correctly inflated for at least 10 minutes after injection, only about 20% to 30% of a 200 mg dose enters the systemic circulation during the first minute after cuff release. The rest emerges rather slowly, with about half of the dose still remaining in the arm after 30 minutes.[406] Direct experimental support for this prediction comes from observations of sustained high concentrations of local anesthetic in the venous drainage from the blocked arm compared to levels in the contralateral limb.[148] Longer application of the cuff has also been shown to result in a slower drug washout after release (see Chap. 12 for further details).

Endotracheal Administration. Endotracheal administration of lidocaine in doses up to 400 mg

TABLE 3-7. PRILOCAINE: SYSTEMIC UPTAKE AFTER ADMINISTRATION FOR REGIONAL ANESTHESIA*

Author	Reference	Route	Dose (mg)	Concentration (%)	Epinephrine
Wildsmith *et al.* (1977)	431	BP[p]	450	1.5	−
			450	1.5	+
Scott *et al.* (1972)	363	IC	400	1	−
			400	2	−
			400	2	+[l]
			400	2	+[m]
Lund and Cwik (1965)	246	Epid	600	2	−
			600	2	+
			900	3	−
			900	3	+
Scott *et al.* (1972)	363	Epid	200	2	−
			400	2	−
			400	2	+[l]
			400	2	+[m]
			600	2	−
			600	3	−

*For explanation of symbols and abbreviations used in this table, see glossary on p. 97.

TABLE 3-8. MEPIVACAINE: SYSTEMIC UPTAKE AFTER ADMINISTRATION FOR REGIONAL ANESTHESIA*

Author	Reference	Route	Dose (mg)	Concentration (%)	Epinephrine
Teramo and Rajamaki (1971)	394	PCB	200	1	−
			400	2	−
Matthes and Schabert (1966)	265	Periton	2/kg	0.5	+
Matthes and Schabert (1966)	265	BP	6/kg	2	−
			6/kg	2	+
Dhuner *et al.* (1965)	131	BP	5/kg	2	−
			5/kg	2	+
Tucker *et al.* (1972)	414	BP	500	1	−
			500	1	+
Tucker *et al.* (1972)	414	SF	500	1	−
			500	1	+
Tucker *et al.* (1972)	414	IC	500	2	−
			500	2	+
			500	1	−
			500	1	+
Lund and Cwik (1966)	247	Epid	600	2	−
			600	2	+
Matthes and Schabert (1966)	265	Epid	6/kg	2	−
			6/kg	2	+
Tucker *et al.* (1972)	414	Epid	500	2	−
			500	2	+
Tucker *et al.* (1972)	414	Caudal	500	2	−
			500	2	+
			500	1	−
			500	1	+
Vester-Andersen *et al.* (1981)	421	BP[p]	400	1	+
		BP[q]	400	1	+
Vester-Andersen *et al.* (1984)	422	BP[q]	400	1	+
			500	1	+
			600	1	+

*For explanation of symbols and abbreviations used in this table, see glossary on p. 97.

TABLE 3–7. PRILOCAINE: SYSTEMIC UPTAKE AFTER ADMINISTRATION FOR REGIONAL ANESTHESIA* ***(continued)***

Number of Subjects	Assay	Sampling Site	Maximum[a] Concentration (μg/ml)	Peak[a] Time (min)	Maximum Concentration (μg/100 mg of dose)
5	GC	VP	2.3	30	0.51
5			1.2	30	0.27
9	C	VP	5.09 ± 0.25	~15	1.27
13			4.46 ± 0.27	~15	1.11
16			3.63 ± 0.21	~20	0.91
10			2.79 ± 0.22	~15	0.70
?	C	VB	3.68 ± 2.05	20[c]	0.61
?			1.75 ± 0.84	20[c]	0.29
?			5.23 ± 2.57	20[c]	0.58
?			3.25 ± 1.40	20[c]	0.36
8	C	VP	1.69 ± 0.21	~15	0.84
31			2.67 ± 0.15	~15	0.67
27			2.21 ± 0.10	~20	0.55
36			2.23 ± 0.13	~20	0.56
9			4.47 ± 0.15	~20	0.74
12			4.90 ± 0.25	~20	0.82

TABLE 3–8. MEPIVACAINE: SYSTEMIC UPTAKE AFTER ADMINISTRATION FOR REGIONAL ANESTHESIA* ***(continued)***

Number of Subjects	Assay	Sampling Site	Maximum[a] Concentration (μg/ml)	Peak[a] Time (min)	Maximum Concentration (μg/100 mg of dose)
5	C	VP	1.86 (1.4–2.4)	30[c]	0.93
6			4.47 (2.1–5.6)	30[c]	1.12
7	C	VB	1.09 ± 0.30	10[c]	0.78
10	C	VB	2.07 ± 0.73	15[c]	0.49
10			1.49 ± 0.37	30[c]	0.35
15	C	VB	1.99 ± 0.18[b]	45	0.57
16			1.61 ± 0.13[b]	45	0.46
5	GC	AP	3.68 ± 0.83	24 (15–30)	0.74
5			2.96 ± 0.77	47 (15–120)	0.59
5	GC	AP	3.59 ± 1.25	31 (25–45)	0.72
5			3.06 ± 1.34	55 (20–110)	0.61
5	GC	AP	8.06 ± 1.62	9 (5–15)	1.61
5			3.94 ± 0.69	19 (5–45)	0.79
5			5.91 ± 1.58	11 (5–15)	1.18
5			3.69 ± 0.68	37 (10–60)	0.74
?	C	VB	5.56	20[c]	0.93
?			4.00	20[c]	0.67
6	C	VB	1.31 ± 0.39	30[c]	0.31
4			1.27 ± 0.20	60[c]	0.30
5	GC	AP	4.95 ± 0.86	16 (10–20)	0.99
5			3.19 ± 0.60	26 (15–45)	0.64
5	GC	AP	5.49 ± 1.52	13 (10–15)	1.10
5			4.60 ± 1.48	40 (25–60)	0.92
5			4.57 ± 1.65	25 (10–60)	0.91
5			2.38 ± 0.45	72 (30–120)	0.48
10	GC	VB	2.15 ± 0.90	30	0.54
10	GC	VB	1.91 ± 0.42	50	0.48
7	GC	VB	~1.4	40–70	0.35
8	GC	VB	~2.1	40–70	0.42
10	GC	VB	~2.5	40–70	0.42

TABLE 3–9. BUPIVACAINE: SYSTEMIC UPTAKE AFTER ADMINISTRATION FOR REGIONAL ANESTHESIA*

Author	Reference	Route	Dose (mg)	Concentration (%)	Epinephrine
Hollmen *et al.* (1969)	192	PCB	100	0.5	+
Hollmen *et al.* (1969)	193	PCB	100	0.5	−
Beazley *et al.* (1972)	35	PCB	50	0.25	−
			50	0.25	+
Belfrage *et al.* (1973)	37	Pudend	25	0.25	+
Moore *et al.* (1976a)	287	BP	300	0.5	+
Raj *et al.* (1977)	331	BP	150[n]	0.75	−
			150[n]	0.75	+
			150[k]	0.75	−
			150[k]	0.75	+
Wildsmith *et al.* (1977)	431	BP[p]	150	0.5	−
			150	0.5	+
Moore *et al.* (1976)	287	SF	400	0.5	+
Moore *et al.* (1976)	283	IC	400	0.5	+
Willdeck–Lund and Edstrom (1975)	434	IC	70	0.5	+
Fujimori *et al.* (1967)	165a	Epid	100	0.5	+
Wilkinson and Lund (1970)	433	Epid	150	0.5	+
			150	0.5	−
			225	0.75	+
Reynolds (1971)	337	Epid	70–100	0.5	+
Appleyard *et al.* (1974)	18	Epid	1.5/kg	0.5	−
			1.5/kg	0.5	+
			1.5/kg	0.5	−[o]
Lund *et al.* (1975)	244	Epid	150	0.5	+
			225	0.75	+
Belfrage *et al.* (1975)	38	Epid	1.58/kg	0.5	+
Belfrage *et al.* (1975)	39	Epid	25	0.25	+
Abdel-Salam *et al.* (1975)	2a	Epid	100	0.5	−
			100	0.5	+
Moore *et al.* (1976)	283	Epid	150	0.75	+
			225	0.75	+
Stanton–Hicks *et al.* (1976)	383	Epid	150	0.75	+
Raj *et al.* (1977)	331	Epid	112.5[n]	0.75	−
			112.5[n]	0.75	+
			112.5[k]	0.75	−
			112.5[k]	0.75	+
Spielman *et al.* (1983)	380	TS(F)	100	0.5	−
McBurney *et al.* (1984)	268	Endo[j]	8–25[u]	0.5	−
		Endo[j]	25	0.5	−
Tuominen *et al.* (1983)	416	BP[q]	3/kg	0.5	−
Biscoping *et al.* (1984)	46	Epid	112–150	0.75	−
Burm *et al.* (1983)	79	SAB	15	0.5	−
Neill and Watson (1984)	302	CPB	150–270	0.375–0.5	−
					+
Colley and Heavner (1981)	99	Infiltr (S)	1.03/kg	0.125	+
			1.25/kg	0.125	−
			2.02/kg	0.25	+
			2.00/kg	0.25	−
Burm (1985)	78	SAB	15	0.5	−
		SAB	15	0.5	+
Burm (1985)	78	Epid	100	0.5	−
		Epid	100	0.5	+

*For explanation of symbols and abbreviations used in this table, see glossary on p. 97.

TABLE 3–9. BUPIVACAINE: SYSTEMIC UPTAKE AFTER ADMINISTRATION FOR REGIONAL ANESTHESIA* ***(continued)***

Number of Subjects	Assay	Sampling Site	Maximum[a] Concentration (μg/ml)	Peak[a] Time (min)	Maximum Concentration (μg/100 mg of dose)
10	GC	VP	0.2 (0.16–1.25)	25 (10–60)	0.2
11	GC	VP	0.8 (0.30–1.87)	15 (5–30)	0.8
8	GC	VP	1.07 ± 0.14[b]	~15	2.14
8			0.53 ± 0.05[b]	~10	1.06
11	GC	VP	0.31 (0.11–0.54)	~20	1.24
10	GC	AP	1.71 (1.05–2.40)	30–35	0.57
		VP	1.55 (0.94–2.25)	30–35	0.52
5	GC	VP	~1.0	~25	0.67
5			~0.5	~30	0.33
4			~0.7	~30	0.47
5			~0.5	~30	0.33
5	GC	VP	2.16	15	1.44
5			1.19	20	0.79
10	GC	AP	1.89 (1.0–3.16)	15	0.47
		VP	1.60 (0.84–2.73)	15	0.40
10	GC	AP	3.29 (1.72–4.0)	10–20	0.82
		VP	2.52 (1.4–3.45)	10–20	0.63
19	GC	AB	0.38	5–10	0.54
		VB	0.26	5–10	0.37
21	C	AP	0.77 ± 0.32	30[c]	0.77
		VP	0.92 ± 0.23	30[c]	0.92
12	GC	VP	1.14	20	0.76
5			1.26	20	0.84
6			2.33	20	1.03
10	GC	VB	0.33 ± 0.04[b]	~30	0.38
8	GC	VB	~0.5	16[c]	0.48
8			~0.4	28[c]	0.38
8			~0.58	16[c]	0.55
?	GC	VP	1.14 ± 0.17[b]	~20	0.76
?			2.33 ± 0.41[b]	~20	1.03
8	GC	AP	1.01 ± 0.33[b]	20[c]	0.91
		VP	0.82 ± 0.36[b]	30[c]	0.74
27	GC	VP	0.16 ± 0.08	20[c]	0.64
9	GC	VP	0.79 ± 0.10[b]	5[c]	0.79
8			0.74 ± 0.09[b]	15[c]	0.74
10	GC	AP	1.46 (1.13–2.32)	15–20	0.97
		VP	1.19 (0.71–1.73)	15–20	0.79
10		AP	1.49 (1.12–2.15)	15–30	0.66
		VP	1.25 (0.78–1.70)	15–30	0.55
5	GC	AP	1.35 ± 0.63	20 ± 4	0.90
6	GC	VP	1.0	25	0.89
8			0.8	25	0.71
8			1.0	25	0.89
7			0.5	25	0.44
12	GC	VB	0.44 ± 0.15	60	0.44
9	GC	VP	0.27 ± 0.18	15–60	1.55
9	GC	VP	0.27 ± 0.06	15–45	1.09
7	GC	VB	(0.68–3.33)	30	0.70
10	GC	CeP	(0.89–2.76)	3–30	1.25
15	GC	CeP	0.06 ± 0.02	40–120	0.42
5	GC	P	4.95 ± 0.96	10–20	–
3	GC	P	3.56 ± 0.83	10–20	–
6	GC	AB	0.12 ± 0.06	5–10	0.2
5			0.77 ± 0.15	5–10	0.8
5			1.01 ± 0.67	5–10	0.7
5			1.23 ± 0.49	5–10	0.9
10	GC	CeP	0.070 ± 0.032	62 ± 33	0.41
10	GC	CeP	0.056 ± 0.015	59 ± 27	0.37
10	GC	CeP	0.73 ± 0.30	19 ± 8	0.73
10	GC	CeP	0.53 ± 0.13	21 ± 8	0.53

TABLE 3-10. ETIDOCAINE: SYSTEMIC UPTAKE AFTER ADMINISTRATION FOR REGIONAL ANESTHESIA*

Author	Reference	Route	Dose (mg)	Concentration (%)	Epinephrine
Lund *et al.* (1975)	244	BP	150	0.5	+
Wildsmith *et al.* (1977)	431	BP^{p}	150	0.5	−
			150	0.5	+
Bridenbaugh *et al.* (1974)	60, 61	IC	150	0.25	+
			150	0.5	+
			200	1	−
			200	1	+
			300	0.5	+
Willdeck-Lund and Edstrom (1975)	434	IC	140	1	+
Dhuner and Lund (1975)	132	IC	100	0.5	−
			100	0.5	+
Engberg *et al.* (1974)	143	Epid	300	1.5	+
Bridenbaugh *et al.* (1974)	60,61	Epid	50	0.25	+
			100	0.5	+
			150	0.75	+
			200	1	+
			300	1.5	−
			300	1.5	+
Lund *et al.* (1973, 1975)	244, 249	Epid	100	0.5	+
			150	0.5	+
			150	0.75	+
			300	1	−
			300	1	+
			300	1.5	+
			450	1.5	+
Abdel-Salam *et al.* (1975)	2a	Epid	100	0.5	−
			200	1	−
			200	1	+
Mather *et al.* (1976)	262	Epid	200	1	−
			200	1	+
Stanton-Hicks *et al.* (1976)	283	Epid	300	1.5	+
Lund *et al.* (1977)	250	Epid	250	1	−
			250	1	+
Lund *et al.* (1975)	244	Caudal	150	0.5	+

*For explanation of symbols and abbreviations used in this table, see glossary on p. 97.

usually produces peak plasma drug concentrations within 10 to 15 minutes well below the toxic threshold. The concentrations are significantly lower in spontaneously breathing patients than in those paralyzed with succinylcholine since the former are more likely to swallow a large proportion of the dose, which then undergoes considerable first-pass hepatic metabolism following absorption from the gut.[364] Application only to areas below the vocal cords may result in excessive plasma drug concentrations because of less transfer to the intestine and first-pass loss.[107]

DOSAGE FACTORS

Concentration and Volume. There is some evidence that the absorption rate of local anesthetic after central and peripheral nerve block and after intravenous regional anesthesia is faster from concentrated solutions than from more dilute solutions containing the same dose (Fig. 3-17).[54,406,414] These differences presumably reflect saturation of local binding sites or greater vasodilator effects produced by more concentrated solutions. Both of these mechanisms should result in disproportionate increases in plasma drug

TABLE 3-10. ETIDOCAINE: SYSTEMIC UPTAKE AFTER ADMINISTRATION FOR REGIONAL ANESTHESIA* *(continued)*

Number of Subjects	Assay	Sampling Site	Maximum[a] Concentration (μg/ml)	Peak[a] Time (min)	Maximum Concentration (μg/100 mg of dose)
13	GC	VP	0.64 ± 0.12[b]	~20	0.43
5	GC	VP	1.31	15	0.87
5			0.86	10	0.57
10	GC	AP	1.15 ± 0.23[b]	10-15	0.77
10			1.30 ± 0.23[b]	5-10	0.87
8			1.53 ± 0.11[b]	5-20	0.76
10			1.27 ± 0.09[b]	10-15	0.63
10			2.39 ± 0.26[b]	5-15	0.80
20	GC	AB	0.52	5-10	0.37
		VB	0.46	5-10	0.33
5	?	P	0.8	15	0.80
5			0.6	30	0.60
19	GC	VP	1.51	16	0.50
5	GC	AP	0.30 ± 0.04[b]	2-20	0.60
8			0.53 ± 0.02[b]	2-15	0.53
10			0.68 ± 0.03[b]	5-20	0.45
10			1.27 ± 0.09[b]	10-15	0.63
5			2.70 ± 0.31[b]	5-15	0.90
5			1.56 ± 0.22[b]	5-20	0.52
?	GC	VP	0.58 ± 0.10	20	0.58
6			0.60 ± 0.11[b]	20	0.40
?			0.66 ± 0.05[b]	20	0.44
?			1.31 ± 0.09[b]	20	0.44
?			1.18 ± 0.09[b]	20	0.39
?			1.69 ± 0.21[b]	20	0.56
?			2.44 ± 0.37[b]	20	0.54
9	GC	VP	0.86 ± 0.12[b]	15[c]	0.86
9			0.97 ± 0.10[b]	20[c]	0.43
9			0.69 ± 0.06[b]	10[c]	0.34
5	GC	AP	1.07 ± 0.16	15 ± 5	0.53
5			0.92 ± 0.19	16 ± 9	0.46
5	GC	AP	1.52 ± 0.64	14 ± 2	0.51
?	GC	VP	1.33 ± 0.36		0.53
?			1.26 ± 0.26		0.50
6	GC	VP	1.33 ± 0.3[b]	~10	0.89

concentrations when concentration and mass of drug are increased but volume is held constant. Up to a 300 mg epidural dose (constant volume) of etidocaine, plasma concentrations increase linearly with dose, but beyond this they become disproportionately higher.[60,244]

The rate of systemic absorption of lidocaine (30 mg) after subarachnoid injection in monkeys was found to be independent of concentration/volume (2% versus 5%).[121]

Speed of Injection. Compared to epidural injections given over 1 minute, those injected in 15 seconds resulted in 16% higher maximum plasma concentrations of lidocaine.[363] Plasma bupivacaine concentrations were not influenced by varying epidural injection speed from 20 to 100 seconds.[341]

Perivascular axillary injection of mepivacaine as a divided dose with an interval of 20 minutes resulted in slightly lower plasma drug concentrations up to 90 minutes than those after a single bolus dose, with no difference in sensory or motor blockade.[422]

The effects of speed of injection on the systemic absorption of local anesthetics are not clinically significant; however, a slow administration is advisable to allow early detection of an inadvertent i.v. injection before all of the dose has been given and to minimize the blood concentrations of drug.

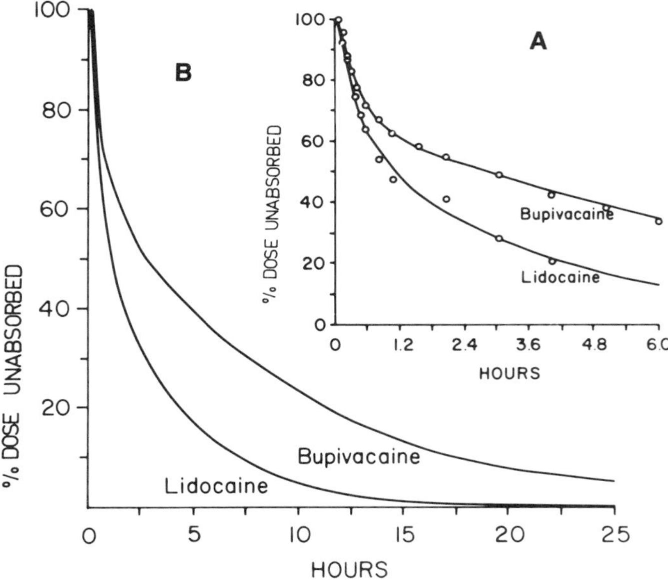

FIG. 3-12. Relation between fraction of dose unabsorbed after epidural injection and time, for bupivacaine and lidocaine. **Graph (A).** Mean experimental data from 20 ml 0.75% bupivacaine HCl or 2% lidocaine HCl, both with 5 μg/ml epinephrine. **Graph (B).** Computer predicted curves for extended time period based on data in **(A).** (Tucker, G.T., and Mather, L.T.: Clinical pharmacokinetics of local anaesthetic agents. Clin. Pharmacokinet., *4*:241, 1979.)

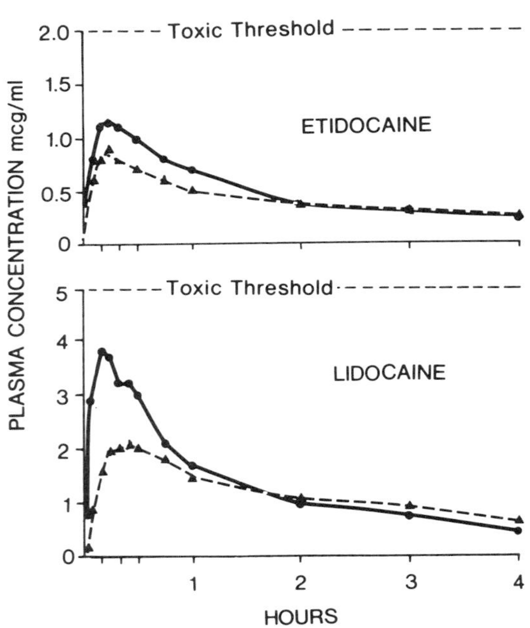

FIG. 3-13. Plasma concentrations following epidural injections of 20 ml of 1% etidocaine HCl or 2% lidocaine HCl in volunteer subjects. Plain solutions ●— —●; with epinephrine 5μg/ml (1:200,000) ▲— —▲. (Mather, L.E., and Cousins, M.J.: Local anaesthetics and their current clinical use. Drugs, *18*:185, 1979.)

ADDITIVES

Vasoconstrictors. To counteract increases in local blood flow resulting from vasomotor blockade and the direct vasodilator action of local anesthetics, vasoconstrictor agents are often added to local anesthetic solutions. The degree to which the desired effects of a decrease in systemic absorption rate of local anesthetic and a prolongation of anesthesia are achieved is a complex function of the type, dose, and concentration of both local anesthetic and vasoconstrictor and of the characteristics of the site of injection.

Although epinephrine is the vasoconstrictor most commonly used, it does have a dual action on blood vessels.[51] Skin and cutaneous vessels are always constricted, but muscle vessels may be constricted or dilated, which may explain why the addition of epinephrine decreases the absorption rate of mepivacaine to a greater extent after subcutaneous than after intramuscular injection. The action of epinephrine on blood vessels of mucous membranes is profound. Epinephrine significantly reduces blood cocaine concentrations after topical intranasal application of aqueous cocaine solutions and reduces blood loss after similar applications of paraffin paste solution.[236] Epinephrine (5 μg/ml) added to mepivacaine solutions for various block procedures prolongs the time

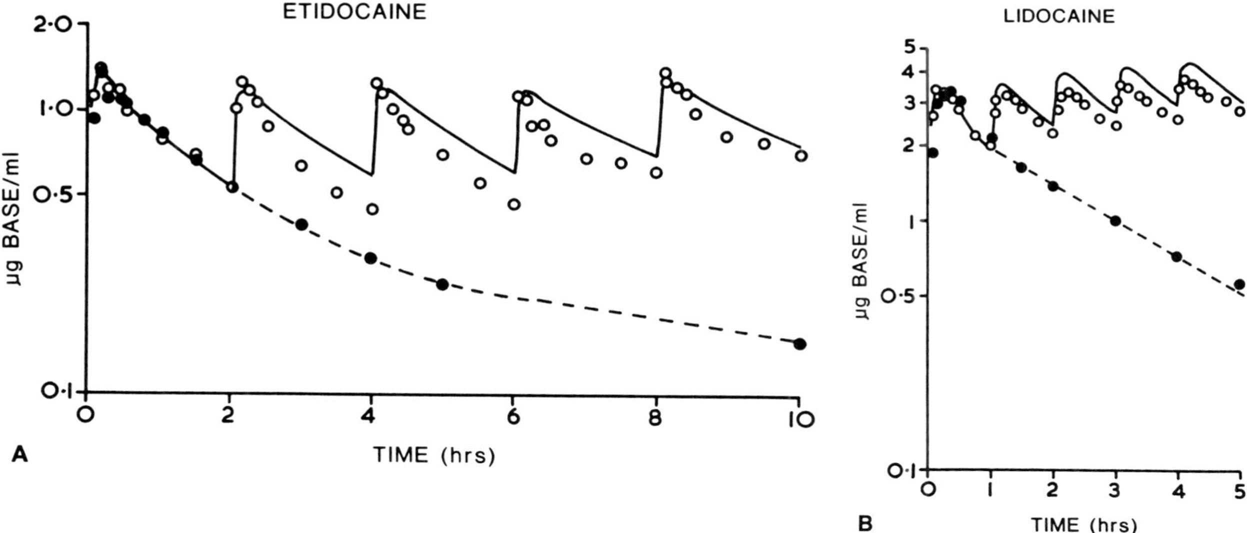

FIG. 3-14. Observed (○) and predicted (—) plasma concentrations following repeated epidural administration of **(A)** etidocaine and **(B)** lidocaine. (Data from Tucker, G.T., and Mather, L.E.: Pharmacokinetics of local anaesthetic agents. Br. J. Anaesth., *47*:213, 1975.) Observed (●) plasma concentrations following single epidural injection. (Data from Tucker, G.T., *et al.*,: Observed and predicted accumulation of local anaesthetic agent during continuous extradural analgesia. Br. J. Anaesth., *49*:237, 1977.)

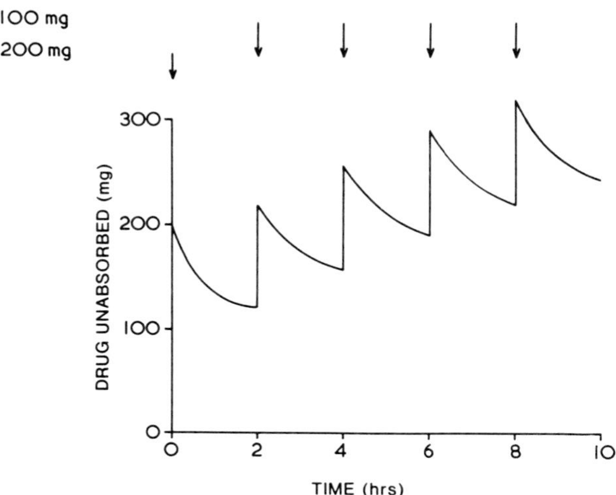

FIG. 3-15. Predicted local accumulation of etidocaine during repeated epidural injections. Two-hundred milliters given initially followed by 100 ml at 2-hour intervals. (Tucker, G.T., *et al.*: Observed and predicted accumulation of local anaesthetic agent during continuous extradural analgesia. Br. J. Anaesth., *49*:237, 1977.)

until maximum arterial plasma drug concentrations occur. Maximum plasma drug concentrations are also lowered, but the greatest effect, a 50% decrease, was seen with intercostal block with a 2% solution (Fig. 3-17). Tables 3-6 to 3-10 contain additional data on the effect of epinephrine on maximum plasma and blood concentrations of local anesthetics.

Results with lidocaine and prilocaine suggest that the use of epinephrine concentrations greater than 5 μg/ml produces only marginally greater decreases in maximum plasma local anesthetic concentration and should, therefore, be avoided in view of side-effects associated with excessive systemic levels of epinephrine.[130]

The importance of the dose of local anesthetic is also illustrated by results of studies with prilocaine. While epinephrine had little influence on a 400 mg epidural dose, the effect was significantly greater at 600 and 900 mg.[55,56]

Systemic absorption of local anesthetics after paracervical injection appear to be particularly sensitive to the effects of epinephrine, as indicated by the results of studies with bupivacaine.[35,192,193] For other

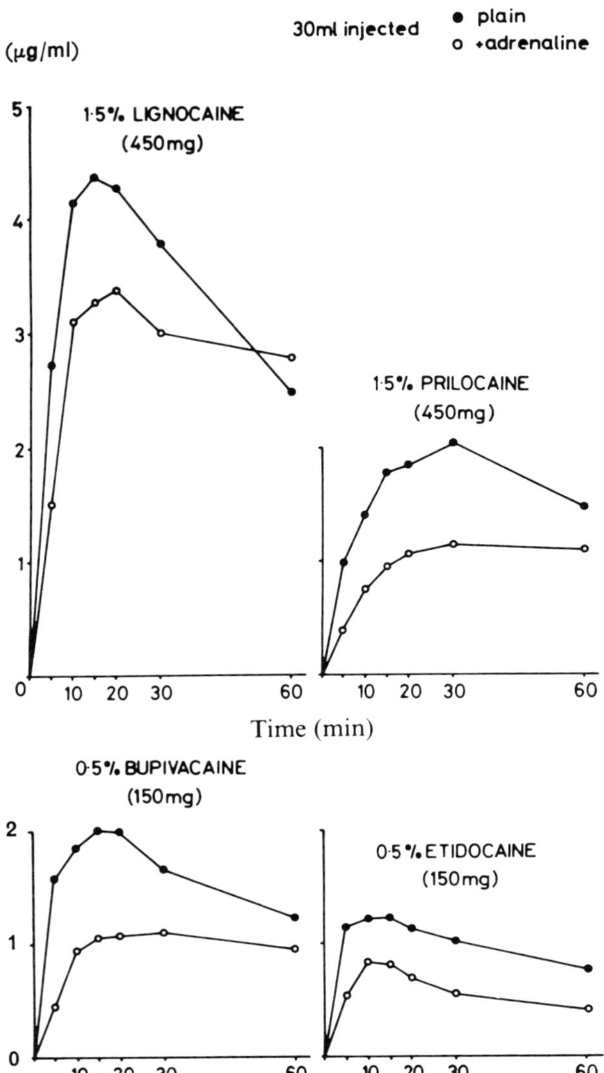

FIG. 3-16. Plasma concentrations of local anesthetic agents after interscalene brachial plexus injection of 30 ml with or without added epinephrine. (Wildsmith, et al., 1977: ref 431.)

routes, however, the data suggest that addition of epinephrine lowers the absorption rates of the long-acting agents somewhat less effectively than those of the short-acting analogues.[283,286] This is also seen in calculated absorption time profiles[411] and is presumably due to greater competition for available drug by tissue-binding sites.

Conflicting data are available on the effect of epinephrine on the systemic absorption of local anesthetics after subarachnoid injection. In monkeys[119] and dogs,[334] no effect on the absorption of lidocaine was found, whereas the addition of epinephrine was associated with lower plasma concentrations of lidocaine in humans[28,78] and of lidocaine and mepivacaine in cats.[379]

The clinical data on the effect of epinephrine on the time-course of subarachnoid block also are conflicting. Clinically insignificant prolongation of block by epinephrine may be due to a direct spinal analgesic action of the vasoconstrictor.[100] Whereas Chambers and colleagues[89] found a lack of a clinically significant prolongation of subarachnoid block in humans after the addition of epinephrine to lidocaine,[78] Burm[78] reported that the time to regression of two segments and the time to total recovery of sensory and motor responses were prolonged. In contrast, Burm[78] found no prolongation by epinephrine of subarachnoid block with bupivacaine but Chambers[91] did. The findings of Burm[78] in this regard were consistent with a lack of effect of epinephrine on bupivacaine plasma concentrations. Thus the effects of epinephrine mixed with the amide agents appear to be equivocal. In contrast to these agents, tetracaine block is prolonged to a clinically significant degree by epinephrine.[21,102] This difference may be explained, in part, by the observation that whereas epinephrine attenuates a hyperemic effect of tetracaine on cord blood flow,[221] neither lidocaine nor epinephrine appears to alter cord blood flow.[133,340,379] A more recent study,[222] however, suggests that epinephrine does prevent a late decrease in lumbosacral cord blood flow caused by lidocaine.

Vasopressor agents advocated as alternatives to epinephrine include octapressin[217] and the pure alpha-adrenoceptor agonist phenylephrine. Addition of the latter, at a concentration of 50 μg/ml, to lidocaine for epidural block was found to be less effective than epinephrine (5 μg/ml) in lowering blood concentrations of the local anesthetic.[381] Phenylephrine had no effect on lidocaine absorption after subarachnoid injection in monkeys, yet it prolonged neural blockade.[128] Like epinephrine, phenylephrine prolongs useful clinical blockade after spinal tetracaine[21,102] possibly because of α-agonist activity at spinal regions involved in antinociception (see Chap. 28).

Carbonation. The vasodilating effect of carbon dioxide and a greater availability of free drug base probably account for the faster systemic absorption

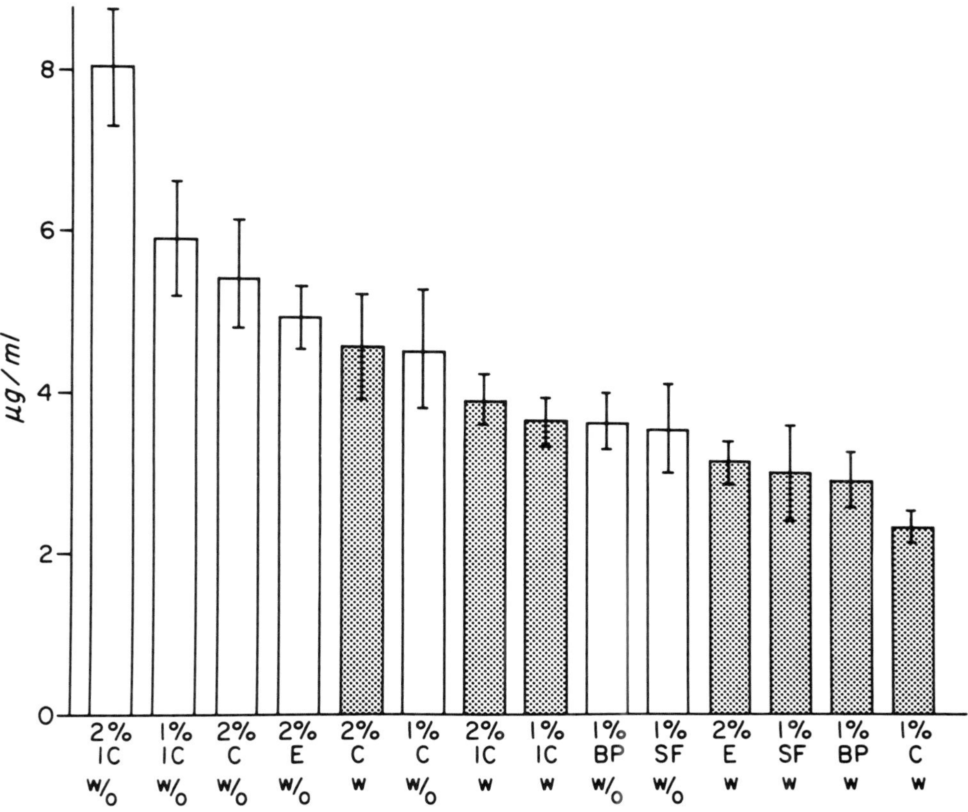

FIG. 3-17. Systemic absorption of mepivacaine in humans after various regional block procdures and the mean maximum plasma drug concentrations. (± SEM) IC, intercostal block; C, caudal block; E, epidural block; BP, brachial plexus block; SF, sciatic/femoral block; w/o, solution without epinephrine; w, plus epinephrine, 1 : 200,000 *(stippled blocks)*. (Tucker, G.T., Moore, D.C., Bridenbaugh, P.O., Bridenbaugh, L.D., *et al.*: Systemic absorption of mepivacaine in commonly used regional block procedures. Anesthesiology, *37*:277, 1972.)

TABLE 3-11. MEAN FRACTIONS AND HALF-LIVES, CHARACTERIZING THE ABSORPTION OF LIDOCAINE AND BUPIVACAINE AFTER SUBARACHNOID AND EPIDURAL ADMINISTRATION

	Lidocaine		Bupivacaine	
	Subarachnoid	Epidural	Subarachnoid	Epidural
F_1	–	0.38	0.35	0.29
$T_{1/2}$ fast (min)	–	9.3	50	8
F_2	–	0.58	0.61	0.64
$T_{1/2}$ slow (min)	71	82	408	371

*F_1 and F_2 are fractions of the doses absorbed in initial faster and subsequent slower phases proceeding with respective half-lives $T_{1/2}$ fast and $T_{1/2}$ slow.

(Burm, A.G.: Pharmacokinetics and clinical effects of lidocaine and bupivacaine following epidural and subarachnoid administration in man. Ph.D. Thesis, University of Leiden, 1985.)

of bupivacaine and lidocaine seen after epidural injection of the carbonated solution compared to plain and epinephrine-containing solutions.[18,254]

Dextran. A number of clinical reports have indicated that the addition of dextran (10%) to solutions of local anesthetics provides extended duration of intercostal block sufficient to reduce the need for repeat injections for postoperative pain relief after major surgery.[210,238] However, other controlled animal studies[365] and a clinical study[58] have failed to substantiate these findings. Rosenblatt and Fung[345] examined the underlying rationale for the use of dextran and pointed out that the alkalinity (*p*H 8.0) of some dextran solutions was the unifying factor in the apparent success or failure of the various studies. In addition, as pointed out by Loder,[239] other investigators used different dextrans in a lower concentration than those used in the original studies. Dextran (10%) has been shown to attenuate the systemic absorption rate of epinephrine after injection of lidocaine solutions into the scalp.[418]

Dextrose. In monkeys, the addition of dextrose (7.5%) to lidocaine solutions for subarachnoid block was found to decrease the systemic absorption rate of the local anesthetic.[121]

Sodium Bicarbonate. Studies of intravenous regional anesthesia in dogs have shown that the release of bupivacaine into the circulation after deflation of the tourniquet is slowed significantly by prior i.v. injection of sodium bicarbonate into the occluded limb.[134] The effect of the latter is to correct the acidosis caused by ischemia, thereby facilitating tissue uptake of the local anesthetic.

FACTORS RELATED TO NERVE BLOCK

The hypotension that often results from epidural anesthesia may prolong the duration of blockade owing to decreased perfusion of the epidural space and a slower systemic uptake of local anesthetic. This is supported by the observation that prophylactic subcutaneous or intravenous injection of ephedrine results in shorter durations of anesthesia and elevated blood concentrations of some local anesthetic agents.[143,263]

PHYSICAL AND PATHOPHYSIOLOGIC FACTORS

Age and Weight. In adults, plasma concentrations of local anesthetics after epidural and other nerve blocks are poorly correlated with age and weight.[283,287,363,414] Studies designed specifically to compare groups of young and elderly patients indicate a trend to more rapid absorption in the latter after epidural and caudal injections.[159,162,343]

Although plasma concentrations of local anesthetics are broadly comparable in children and adults on a mg/kg dosage basis, uptake appears to be particularly rapid from the respiratory tract in children younger than 3 years, and peak plasma drug concentrations are relatively low after caudal block in children (Table 3-12) (see also Chap. 21).

Pregnancy. Although engorgement of vertebral veins and a hyperkinetic circulation might be expected to enhance absorption of local anesthetic drugs after epidural block in pregnant women, plasma drug concentration–time profiles appear to be similar to those in nonpregnant women.[290]

Higher plasma concentrations of lidocaine after epidural injection were observed in preeclamptic compared to normal patients, but this was probably the result of a lower systemic drug clearance rather than enhanced absorption.[333]

Disease and Surgery. Changes in local perfusion associated with altered hemodynamics in certain disease-states or as a result of operative conditions may modify absorption of local anesthetics and hence duration of anesthesia. For example, acute hypovolemia slows lidocaine absorption after epidural injection in dogs[293] and prolongs anesthesia in patients undergoing thoracotomy with regional block.[329] Conversely, the hyperkinetic circulation that may accompany kidney disease could account partially for a decreased duration of brachial plexus block in patients with chronic renal failure, owing to enhanced systemic uptake of local anesthetic.[68,388]

SYSTEMIC DISPOSITION

After absorption from the site of administration, local anesthetic drugs are distributed by the bloodstream to the organs and tissues of the body and cleared,

TABLE 3-12. SYSTEMIC UPTAKE OF LOCAL ANESTHETICS AFTER ADMINISTRATION FOR REGIONAL ANESTHESIA IN CHILDREN

Author	Reference	Agent	Route	Dose (mg/kg)	Concentration (%)	Epinephrine
Eyers *et al.* (1978)	149	Lido	Caudal	4	1	–
			SC	4	1	–
			Endo	4	4	–
		Bupiv	Caudal	2	0.5	–
			SC	2	0.5	–
Eyres *et al.* (1983a)	150	Lido	Endo	4	4	–
Eyres *et al.* (1983b)	151	Bupiv	Caudal	3	0.25	–
Rothstein *et al.* (1981)	349	Bupiv	IC	2	0.5	+
			IC	3	0.5	+
			IC	4	0.5	+
Takasaki (1984)	392	Lido	Caudal	11	1.5	–
		Mepiv	Caudal	11	1.5	–
		Bupiv	Caudal	3.7	0.5	–
Ecoffey *et al.* (1984)	139	Lido	Caudal	5	1	–

Key: LC = high-pressure liquid chromatography; GC = gas chromatography; * more rapid in younger patients but peaks are similar; some patients had concentrations greater than 8 μg/ml without evidence of toxicity; + higher peaks in patients < 3 years of age; faster absorption in patients < 1 year of age.

mostly by metabolism and to a small extent by renal excretion. In pregnant women, a proportion of the dose also crosses the placenta into the baby.

A physiologic model useful in describing the time-course of these processes has been elaborated by Benowitz and associates.[42] This perfusion model (it assumes no diffusion limitations) is based upon an extrapolation of equilibrium tissue/blood partition coefficients of lidocaine from monkeys to humans and estimates of normal cardiac output, regional blood flows, and hepatic extraction. It simulates the duration of the agent in various tissues, and its validity is supported by a close prediction of the arterial blood concentration–time profile of lidocaine after intravenous injection (Fig. 3-18).[406] Similar curves are obtained experimentally with the other amide-type agents, and it may be presumed that the model is general for these compounds (Fig. 3-19). Ester-type agents are probably distributed in the same way, but they are set apart from the amides by the site and rate of their metabolism.

DISTRIBUTION

Role of the Lung

The first organ to be exposed to local anesthetic once it has entered the systemic circulation is the lung. This structure has the potential to provide an important buffer function by delaying the first-pass transmission of drug enroute to the arterial circulation. Hence the peak arterial blood drug concentration that hits the target organs for toxicity, the brain and the heart (via the coronary circulation), after rapid i.v. input may be attenuated considerably compared to the drug concentration in the pulmonary artery (see Fig. 3-10).[206,241,406] Arthur[22] has shown that lung uptake of prilocaine in humans exceeds that of lidocaine and contributes to its greater systemic safety margin. The rank order of uptake in rat lung slices at a fixed cation/base ratio was found to be bupivacaine > etidocaine > lidocaine.[325] The extravascular *p*H of the lung is low relative to plasma *p*H, and this will encourage ion-trapping of local anesthetics. Accordingly, lung uptake of lidocaine in pigs was found to increase with the value of arterial blood *p*H.[326] It should be emphasized that first-pass lung uptake consists of drug distribution, not drug clearance. Although lung tissue has the potential to metabolize drugs (including prilocaine), available evidence indicates that there is no pulmonary clearance of amide local anesthetics *in vivo*.[200,259]

Inadvertent injection of local anesthetic into the carotid or vertebral artery during attempted stellate ganglion or interscalene block will bypass the lung completely, resulting in a high probability of CNS toxicity. Further, Aldrete and associates[13,14] have shown that the introduction of local anesthetics under pressure into the lingual, brachial, or femoral

TABLE 3-12. SYSTEMIC UPTAKE OF LOCAL ANESTHETICS AFTER ADMINISTRATION FOR REGIONAL ANESTHESIA IN CHILDREN *(continued)*

Number of Subjects	Age	Assay	Sampling Site	Maximum Concentration (μg/ml)	Peak Time (min)	Maximum Concentration (μg/100 mg of dose)
7	5d-15y	GC	VP	~2	10-20	
13	5d-15y	GC	VP	1-2	~15	
27	5d-15y	GC	VP	3-7*	<10	
14	5d-15y	GC	VP	~0.6	~15	
12	5d-15y	GC	VP	~0.5	15-20	
96	2w-12y	LC	VP	5.1 ± 2.0⁺	8⁺	1.28
45	4m-12y	GC	AP	1.57 ± 0.45	15	0.52
7	55 ± 11m	GC	AB	0.77 ± 0.09	10	0.38
5	55 ± 11m	GC	AB	1.39 ± 0.12	10	0.46
11	55 ± 11m	GC	AB	1.99 ± 0.16	5	0.50
10	7m-7y	GC	VB	2.20 ± 0.26	45	0.20
10	7m-7y	GC	VB	2.53 ± 0.31	45	0.23
10	7m-7y	GC	VB	0.67 ± 0.08	45	0.18
11	3.5-9y	EMIT	VP	2.05 ± 0.08	28 ± 3	0.41

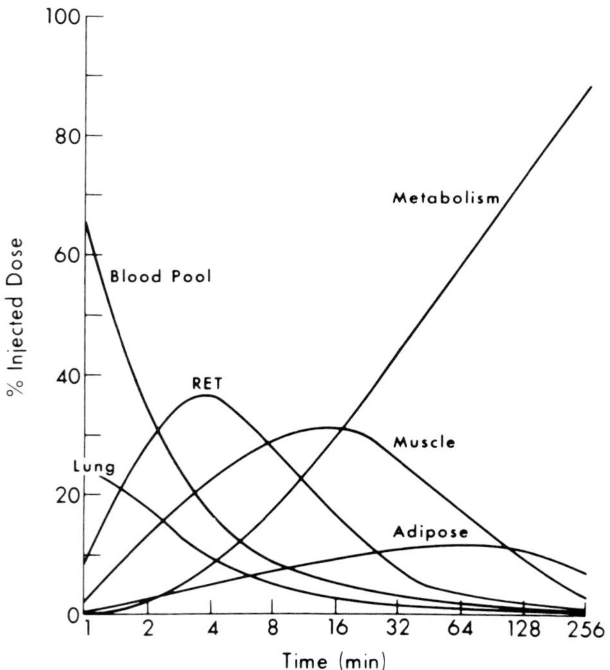

FIG. 3-18. Perfusion model of the distribution of lidocaine in various tissues and its elimination from humans after an intravenous infusion for 1 minute (RET = rapidly equilibrating tissues). Note the use of a logarithmic time scale to show more clearly the rapid changes immediately following injection. (Data from Benowitz, N., Forsyth, R.P., and Melmon, K.L.: Lidocaine disposition kinetics in monkey and man: I. Prediction by a perfusion model. Clin. Pharmacol. Ther., *16*:99, 1974.)

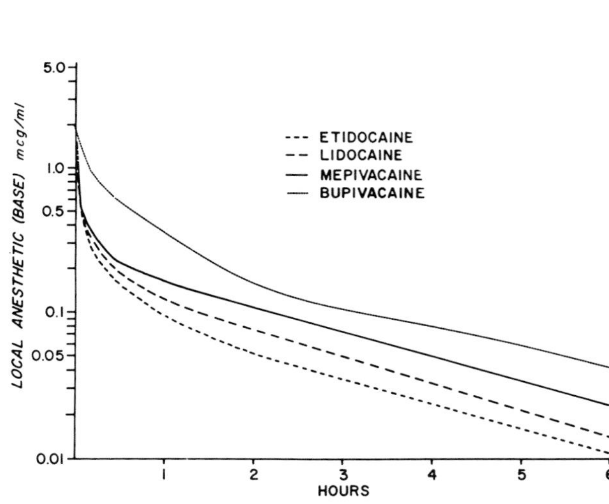

FIG. 3-19. Mean arterial whole blood concentrations of local anesthetics after intravenous infusion of 44.16 base equivalent of each drug at a constant rate over 10 minutes. (Tucker, G.T., and Mather, L.E.: Pharmacokinetics of local anaesthetic agents. Br. J. Anaesth., *47*:213, 1975)

artery of baboons and the facial artery of dogs can produce a retrograde flow permitting direct access of high concentrations of drug to the cerebral circulation.

Blood and Tissue Binding

After leaving the lung, local anesthetic is distributed to other organs according to the proportion of the cardiac output that they receive. The time taken to achieve distribution equilibrium in each organ (*i.e.*, when incoming arterial drug concentration equals outgoing venous concentration) is directly proportional to its capacity for drug uptake (mass × tissue/blood partition coefficient) and inversely proportional to its blood flow. Thus, drug equilibrates successively in, and redistributes from, the small vessel-rich organs, the muscles, and finally the fat, where it is relatively highly soluble (see Fig. 3-18). This progression, together with the process of drug elimination, accounts for the shape of the blood drug concentration–time profile, which is readily simulated by an empirical multiexponential function (see Fig. 3-19).[405,413]

Tissue/blood partition coefficients are determined by drug binding to plasma, erythrocytes, and tissue components and by the *p*H gradient between plasma and extravascular water spaces. Experimental determination of tissue/blood partition coefficients is complex. Such determinations are usually made postmortem and under non-steady-state conditions. It is not known what changes in tissue/blood equilibrium occur at, or after, death. Figure 3-20 shows *in vivo* data for lidocaine and bupivacaine brain/blood and heart muscle/blood partition coefficients at steady-state in the sheep before and during tonic skeletal muscle contraction and resulting acidemia.[299]

Blood Binding

The long-acting amides are bound in plasma to a greater extent than the short-acting ones (see Table 3-1). A feature of this binding is that it approaches saturation, that is, the unbound fraction increases at high total plasma drug concentrations (Fig. 3-21).[261,408]

Attachment of the agents to binding sites in or on the erythrocyte is of similar order to plasma binding.[411,413] In the presence of plasma proteins, however, plasma binding competes with binding to the red cells.[231] Hence blood/plasma drug concentration

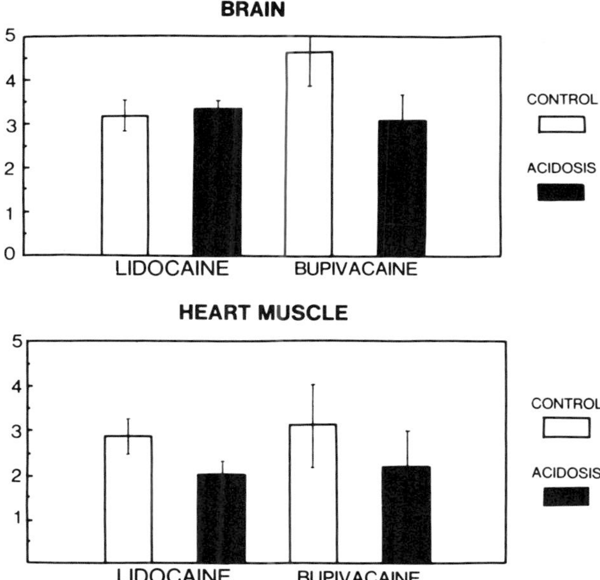

FIG. 3-20. Tissue:blood partition coefficients of lidocaine and bupivacaine in the sheep at steady-state at normal blood *p*H 7.48 and during combined metabolic and respiratory acidosis *p*H 7.05. (Nancarrow, 1986: ref 299.)

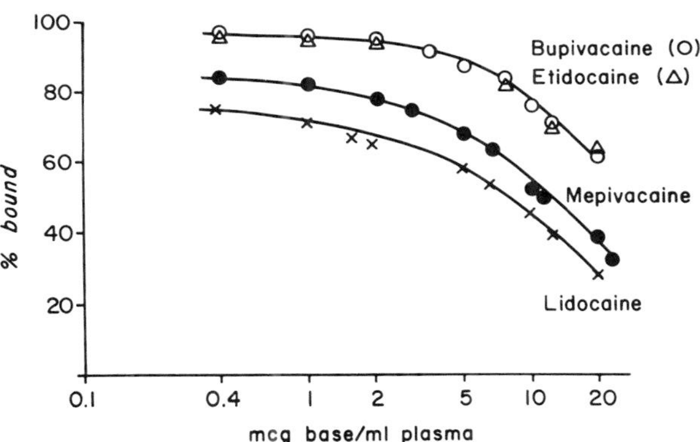

FIG. 3-21. Plasma binding of amide-type local anesthetics. (Tucker, G.T., and Mather, L.E.: Pharmacokinetics of local anaesthetic agents. Br. J. Anaesth., *47*:213, 1975.)

ratios are inversely related to plasma binding (Table 3-13).

There are two principal classes of plasma binding sites: a high-affinity, low-capacity site on alpha$_1$-acid glycoprotein and a quantitatively less important low-affinity, high-capacity site on albumin.[124,257,261,322,350]

The extent of binding varies with the plasma concentration of alpha$_1$-acid glycoprotein, and both are elevated considerably in patients with cancer,[201] chronic pain,[165] trauma,[140] and uremia,[177] in those receiving renal transplants,[177] and in postoperative[187] and postmyocardial infarction patients (Fig. 3-22).[30,351] Increased plasma binding is also anticipated in patients with inflammatory disease, in which plasma alpha$_1$-acid glycoprotein concentrations also rise as part of the stress response. There is a slight increase in the plasma binding of lidocaine with age.[114] One study suggests an increase in smokers,[270] but this was not confirmed by others.[114] Low plasma concentrations of alpha$_1$-acid glycoprotein in neonates are associated with much lower binding of local anesthetics compared to that in adult plasma.[292,318,321,440] Slightly lower concentrations of the main binding protein and higher free fractions of lidocaine were found in women taking oral contraceptives.[350,352] One study[440] showed less binding of lidocaine in pregnant compared to nonpregnant women, but another study[292] found equal binding of etidocaine in the two groups. In both of these studies, delivery was not associated with a significant change in the plasma concentration of alpha$_1$-acid glycoprotein.

A major difficulty in assessing the degree of binding pertains to differences in methodology used by

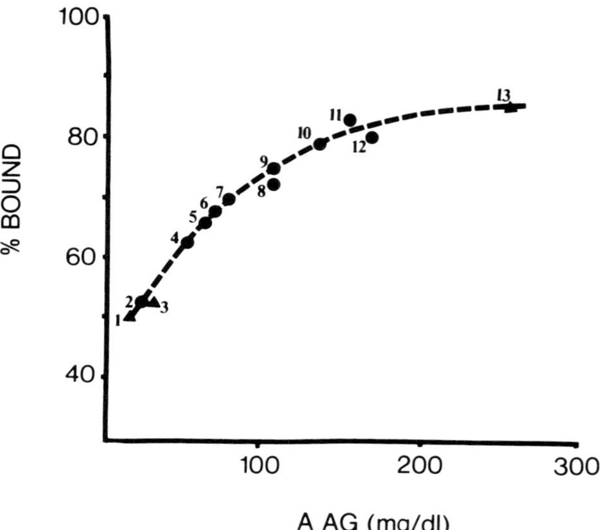

FIG. 3-22. Relation between the mean percentage of lidocaine bound and the concentration of α_1-acid glycoprotein in plasma in various clinical conditions. ●, patient group data; ▲, individual patient data; 1, patient with nephrotic syndrome; 2, neonates; 3, patient with carcinoma of prostate receiving high-dose estrogens; 4, females on oral contraceptives; 5, women under 40 years; 6, men under 40 years; 7, adults > 70 years; 8, epileptic subjects; 9, renal transplantation patients; 10, chronic renal failure patients; 11, cancer patients; 12, myocardial infarction patients; 13, patient with myocardial infarction. (Data from Jackson, et al., 1982: ref 201; and Routledge, et al., 1982: ref 354.)

TABLE 3-13. PHARMACOKINETIC VARIABLES DESCRIBING THE DISPOSITION KINETICS OF AMIDE-TYPE LOCAL ANESTHETICS IN ADULT MALES

	Prilocaine	Lidocaine	Mepivacaine	Bupivacaine	Etidocaine
λ	1.1	0.8	0.9	0.6	0.6
V_{ss}* (liters)	191	91	84	73	134
Vu_{ss} (liters)	?	253	382	1028	1478
CL* (liters/min)	2.37	0.95	0.78	0.58	1.11
E_H	?	0.65	0.52	0.38	0.74
$t_{1/2,z}$(h)	1.6	1.6	1.9	2.7	2.7
MBRT(h)	1.3	1.6	1.8	2.1	2.0

*Specified with respect to arterial total blood drug concentrations, with the exception of prilocaine data, which are specified with respect to peripheral venous blood drug concentration.

Key: λ = blood/plasma concentration ratio; V_{ss} = volume of distribution at steady-state; Vu_{ss} = volume of distribution at steady-state based on unbound drug concentrations in plasma water; CL = mean total body clearance; E_H = estimated hepatic extraction ratio; $t_{1/2,z}$ = terminal "elimination" half-life; MBRT = mean body retention time.

(Tucker, G.T.: Pharmacokinetics of local anaesthetics: Role in toxicity. *In* Scott, D.B., McClure, J., and Wildsmith, J.A.W. (eds.): Regional Anaesthesia 1884–1984, pp. 61–71. Sodertalje, ICM AB, 1984.)

various investigators — in particular the blood collection techniques and the choice of experimental conditions. The use of heparin in patients or blood sample containers may decrease the degree of binding in plasma and alter the equilibrium ratio between plasma and whole blood concentrations. There is evidence that this action is mediated through the action of heparin in activating lipoprotein lipase *in vivo* and in blood samples *in vitro* and it is not completely abolished by protamine.[136]

The binding of local anesthetics to alpha$_1$-acid glycoprotein is very sensitive to changes in plasma *p*H, which creates considerable difficulties in its measurement. It is known that binding decreases as *p*H decreases[16,83,106,180,271,323] so that failure of investigators to adjust *p*H of samples before determination of binding may be a source of error. There is also evidence in the rat for a circadian variation in the plasma binding and erythrocyte uptake of lidocaine.[75,76]

Plasma Binding and Toxicity

The role of plasma drug binding in the toxicity of local anesthetics is widely misunderstood. The issue resolves into two quite separate questions:

1. Does it influence the interpretation of plasma or blood drug concentration?
2. Does it influence the actual kinetics of a drug, thereby controlling its access to sites of action?

A third question that follows from these is, do changes in plasma binding ever necessitate changes in drug dosage?

The importance of allowing for plasma binding when comparing plasma or blood concentrations of local anesthetics in a particular patient with the "minimum toxic level" has been mentioned already. This is illustrated by data on total plasma concentrations of bupivacaine in postoperative patients receiving long-term infusions for neural blockade. Thus, Ross and associates[346] observed continuously rising plasma bupivacaine concentrations over 2 days during epidural infusions, and in four of their cases the concentrations exceeded 4 μg/ml. Despite these high levels, there were no signs of serious toxicity. Similarly, Richter and co-workers[338] found that plasma bupivacaine concentrations during prolonged epidural infusions were grossly underestimated by predictions from initial dose data. Others have also noted marked accumulation of plasma bupivacaine in postoperative patients.[336,344] The most likely explanation for this is the marked rise in plasma α_1-acid glycoprotein after surgery, which is not attenuated by sympathetic block and which is associated with increased plasma drug binding. Therefore, although total drug concentrations may exceed the minimum toxic level, free drug concentrations stay within acceptable limits. This is confirmed by a study in cholecystectomy patients receiving i.v. infusions of bupivacaine before and after surgery. Although total plasma drug concentrations were doubled postoperatively, the unbound (active) concentrations were similar to those measured preoperatively (Fig. 3-23).[187] Prolonged accumulation of total plasma drug concentrations is not seen during long-term perineural infusions in patients with chronic pain presumably because these patients have stable plasma protein concentrations.[122]

The kinetic implications of the plasma binding of local anesthetics have been discussed by Tucker.[405] When systemic drug input is gradual, as it would be after successful perineural injection, distribution of the dose is spread over time and a large extravascular distribution space, and extensive tissue binding (see below) ensures that only a small percentage remains in the blood at any time. Under these conditions any changes in plasma binding are likely to have little influence on free (active) drug concentrations, since these are effectively buffered by a high volume of distribution. Plasma binding does not limit the full extent of distribution significantly. Also, for drugs with relatively low hepatic extraction ratios such as bupivacaine (see Table 3-13), any increase in free drug concentration will be compensated by a faster elimination. Etidocaine may be an exception because it has a relatively high hepatic extraction ratio and theory predicts that, in this case, a decrease in plasma binding will be associated with a sustained increase in free drug concentration during continuous administration.

There is a theoretical possibility that plasma binding may limit the initial uptake of local anesthetics into the brain and myocardium following rapid, inadvertent i.v. injection, thereby modulating toxicity; however, it is probable that a toxic dose would produce sufficiently high blood drug concentrations to overwhelm the blood binding capacity so that most circulating drug would be free to diffuse into tissues. Indeed, similar fractions of doses of lidocaine and bupivacaine have been found in the hearts or brains of sheep killed by bolus doses of either local anesthetic.[299]

In vivo experiments in rats suggest that binding of lidocaine to human α_1-acid glycoprotein is rapidly reversible and does not rate-limit uptake of drug by

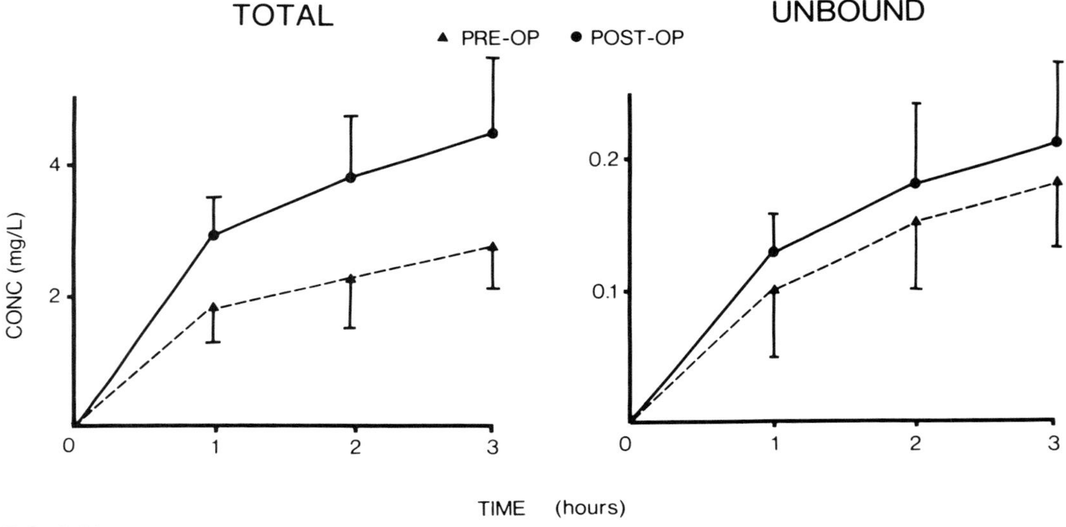

FIG. 3-23. Mean total and unbound plasma concentrations of bupivacaine during intravenous infusions of 2 mg/min of bupivacaine HCl in seven cholecystectomy patients studied 3 hours before surgery and 72 hours postoperatively.

the brain.[311] In contrast, binding to albumin does appear to inhibit brain uptake of lidocaine. However, this protein contributes much less to the net plasma binding of local anesthetics, and its influence on brain uptake appears to be attenuated in human plasma (Table 3-14). The observation that lumbar CSF concentrations of lidocaine may exceed the unbound concentration in plasma supports the notion that plasma binding alone does not control CNS penetration by local anesthetic agents.[232]

Tissue Distribution

In the amide series of local anesthetics, a greater extent of plasma binding is accompanied by a parallel increase in affinity for tissue components. These factors tend to balance out in producing mean volumes of distribution at steady-state (V_{ss}), based on whole blood drug concentrations, which vary only over a twofold range. Volumes based on unbound drug (V_{uss}) vary over a fivefold range, being greatest for

TABLE 3-14. EFFECTS OF NORMAL HUMAN SERUM, HUMAN ALPHA$_1$-ACID GLYCOPROTEIN (AAG), AND BOVINE SERUM ALBUMIN (BSA) ON RAT BRAIN EXTRACTION AND FREE PERCENTAGE OF LIDOCAINE

	Lidocaine	
Injectate*	**Brain Extraction**	**(%) Free Percentage**
Control	101 ± 5	100
AAG (1 mg/ml)	107 ± 2	73 ± 6
AAG (5 mg/ml)	93 ± 3	35 ± 3
BSA (5 g/dl)	40 ± 3	~80
Normal human serum (80%)	91 ± 4	43 ± 6

*A 200 μl bolus of Ringer's solution, pH 7.4, containing 1 μg/ml lidocaine with and without protein or serum was injected in less than 1 sec into the carotid artery and the rats were killed 15 sec later. Data are mean ± SE; n = 3–6.

(Data from Pardridge, W.M., Sakiyama, R., and Fierer, G.: Transport of propranolol and lidocaine through the rat blood-brain barrier. Primary role of globulin-bound drug. J. Clin. Invest., *71*:900, 1983.)

bupivacaine and etidocaine (see Table 3-13). The latter are more relevant than V_{ss} because they relate to the "active" drug concentration. A larger V_{uss} for etidocaine compared to bupivacaine encourages more rapid distribution away from vital organs. The large volumes of distribution of all of the agents militate against their effective removal from the body by hemodialysis after overdosage.

Toxicity, Acidosis, Hypercarbia, and Tissue Binding

The CNS toxicity of local anesthetics is increased significantly by acidosis and hypercarbia, particularly when respiratory acidosis is accompanied by an underlying metabolic acidosis.[144,145] Respiratory acidosis does not appear to be associated with altered tissue/blood ratios of local anesthetics, which would be consistent with proportional changes in intracellular and extracellular *p*H causing no increase in ion-trapping.[182] In contrast, local metabolic acidosis should have a more dramatic effect on local tissue drug uptake. Thus, Simon and associates[372,373] have shown that drug-induced status epilepticus in rats markedly elevates both brain and blood concentrations of lidocaine and its partition between brain and blood (Fig. 3-24). They suggested that this was the result of cerebral lactic acidosis causing increased ion-trapping of the drug, an increased brain–blood flow, and peripheral vasoconstriction delaying redistribution to muscle and fat.

Perfusion of heart and brain with blood rendered acidotic by perfusing tonic skeletal muscle (analogous to local anesthetic-induced seizure) does not result in increased uptake of either lidocaine or bupivacaine. The partition coefficients of both of these agents into heart, and that of bupivacaine into brain, are decreased despite decreased plasma binding. In fact, this is what would be expected as the metabolic component of the acidosis is not generated in these tissues (see Fig. 3-20).[299] Prompt treatment of convulsions from local anesthetic toxicity is important; the longer the delay, the more difficult it becomes for

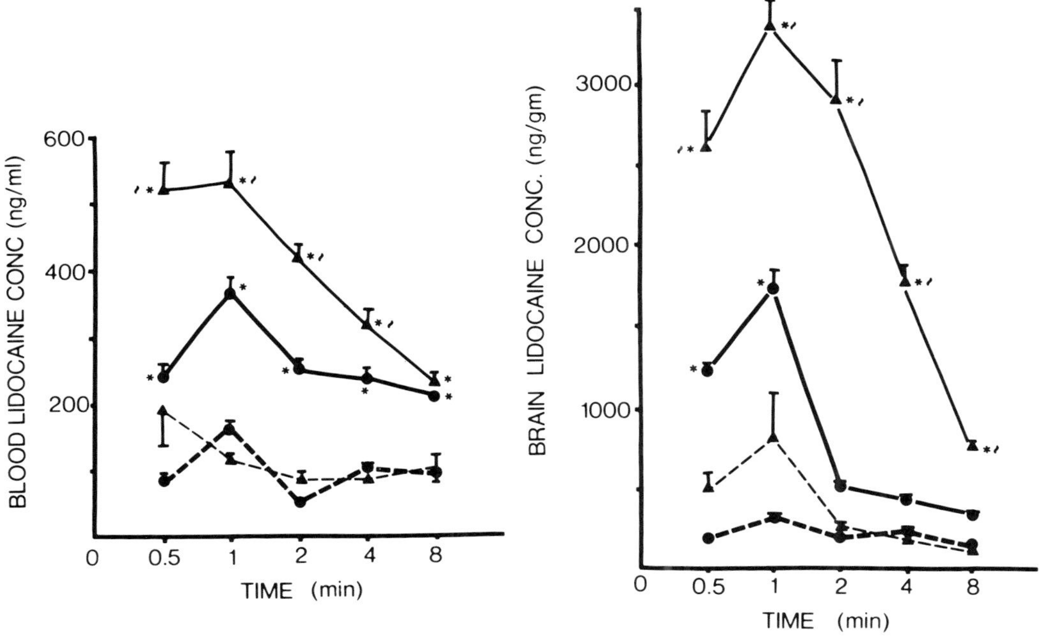

FIG. 3-24. Lidocaine concentrations in femoral artery and brain tissue of the rat after bolus injection at time 0. Solid lines, animals convulsing from intravenous injection of pentylenetetrazol; broken lines, nonconvulsing animals; ▲, animals paralyzed with gallamine and ventilated with 30:70 nitrous oxide: oxygen; ●, unrestrained animals; *p < 0.001 convulsing versus nonconvulsing animals; p < 0.001 paralyzed versus nonparalyzed animals. (Simon, et al., 1984: ref 373.)

the drug to leave the brain. Treatment by paralysis and artificial ventilation, however, exacerbates the entry into brain, since prevention of the systemic acidosis, but not the cerebral acidosis, increases the effect of *p*H partition of drug. Ventilation with oxygen is necessary to meet metabolic oxygen demand during acidosis. Anticonvulsants may be required for continuation of ventilation until the drug is cleared from the brain. However, local anesthetic-induced myocardial depression is antagonized by autonomic responses during convulsions. Thus, abolition of convulsions may unmask the drug-induced myocardial depression and produce even more profound hemodynamic disturbances.

Although it might be argued that systemic acidosis could retard the elimination of local anesthetics from the body, available evidence indicates that nonsystematic changes in hepatic blood flow occur accompanied by a small decrease in hepatic extraction ratio but no overall decrease in the rate of removal of either lidocaine or bupivacaine by the liver of the sheep made acidotic.[299]

Excretion

Renal excretion of unchanged local anesthetics is a minor route of elimination, accounting for less than 1% to 6% of the dose under normal conditions.[11,36,163,213,260,337,415] Acidification of the urine to about *p*H 5 increases this proportion to 5% to 20%, depending on the agent, which is consistent with less tubular reabsorption of drug as a result of greater ionization. This increase in net excretion is clearly insufficient, however, to warrant acidification of the urine as a means of speeding the elimination of local anesthetics in patients with toxic symptoms. Estimates of the renal clearances of the amide-type agents indicate that they enter the tubular fluid by both glomerular filtration and tubular secretion.[147]

Secretion of unchanged local anesthetics down the *p*H gradient between blood and gastric juice is also a potential route of excretion; however, most of the drug that appears in the stomach contents is subsequently reabsorbed from the intestine and undergoes first-pass metabolism in the liver. Although the use of a stomach pump has been advocated for treatment of local anesthetic toxicity, especially in neonates,[111] it is unlikely that this is of any value. Gastric juice/blood drug concentration ratios may be high, but the proportion of the dose recycled by way of the stomach is unlikely to be significant.

Metabolism

Local anesthetics are eliminated largely by metabolic conversion to more polar compounds that are more easily removed by the kidney. Although this is generally considered to be a detoxification process, the possibility that metabolic products may retain some of the activity of the parent drug or have quite different pharmacologic or toxic effects should not be ignored. A knowledge of both the nature of the metabolic products and of the rate of metabolic clearance of the parent drug is important.[403]

ESTERS

Cocaine. The main routes of breakdown of cocaine in humans are ester hydrolysis and N-demethylation. The former involves nonenzymatic loss of the methyl group to give benzoylecgonine, enzymatic loss of the benzoyl group in plasma and liver yielding ecgonine methyl ester, and further hydrolysis of both of these compounds to ecgonine. Norcocaine, the product of N-demethylation, undergoes an analogous series of hydrolysis steps.[386,387] Of these metabolites, only norcocaine is believed to have significant pharmacologic activity, but it is not a major product.[188,301] Norcocaine nitroxide has been suggested as a potential hepatotoxic metabolite of cocaine.[218]

Values of the mean intravenous plasma half-life of cocaine in humans vary from 40 to 150 minutes; 1% to 20% of the dose is excreted unchanged in the urine, with about 40% as benzylecgonine.[31,157,202 219]

Procaine and Its Congeners. The procaine derivatives are also detoxified by ester hydrolysis, partly in blood by plasma pseudocholinesterase and red cell esterases and partly in the liver.[18,62,85,86,174,208] Procaine itself is cleaved to diethylamino ethanol and para-amino benzoic acid (Fig. 3-25). The most striking feature of the hydrolysis of these compounds by plasma pseudocholinesterase is its speed, *in vitro* half-lives in plasma from normal adults being less than 1 minute for chloroprocaine and procaine and a little longer for tetracaine (Fig. 3-26).[160]

As a consequence of rapid hydrolysis in blood, circulating concentrations of the esters after normal doses for regional anesthesia are extremely low compared to those of the amides.[226,282,309,427] After high-dose i.v. infusions (1-1.5 mg/min/kg) dose-dependent plasma clearances of procaine between 0.04 and 0.08 liters/min/kg and elimination half-lives of 7 to 8 minutes have been observed.[367]

The clinical implication of these rapid clearance

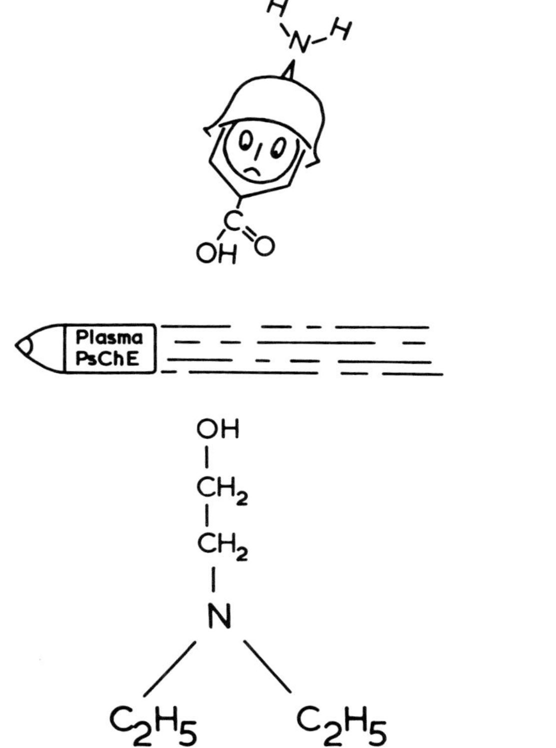

FIG. 3-25. Hydrolysis of procaine. (Tucker, G.T.: Biotransformation and toxicity of local anaesthetics. Acta Anaesthesiol. Belg., *26[Suppl.]*:123, 1975)

values is that if a toxic concentration is attained, the ensuing reaction should be relatively short-lived. If, however, the esterase becomes saturated or substrate inhibited[208] because of a very high concentration of drug, or if the enzyme is genetically atypical,[160] then toxicity may be prolonged. Nevertheless, apparent inadvertent i.v. injection of an epidural dose of 2-chloroprocaine was not accompanied by any adverse effects despite a plasma drug concentration of 17 μg/ml at 10 minutes.[176]

The hydrolysis products of procaine and 2-chloroprocaine have been measured in human plasma and are claimed to be pharmacologically inactive,[62,226,309] although the aminobenzoic acids may contribute to the rare allergic reaction. Krogh and Jellum[223] found that most of the chlorobenzoic acid (CABA) formed from 2-chloroprocaine is metabolized further and excreted as the N-acetyl product. The latter may be the CABA conjugate observed in urine by Kuhnert and associates[227] and Krogh and Jellum.[224] Small amounts of the N-oxide of tetracaine have been found in animal urine,[164,278] but no data are available on this metabolite in humans.

Amides. Clearance of these agents can be equated almost entirely with metabolic clearance because renal excretion of unchanged forms is so low. Total clearances in humans vary in the order: bupivacaine < mepivacaine < lidocaine < etidocaine < prilocaine (see Table 3-13), showing no relationship to anes-

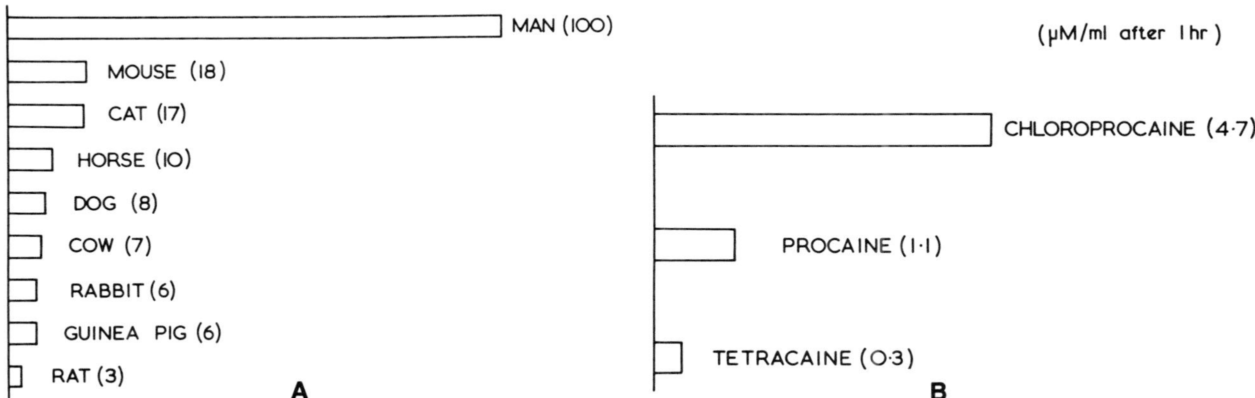

FIG. 3-26. **A.** Relative rates of procaine hydrolysis in plasma of different mammalian species. (Aven, M.H., Light, A., and Foldes, F.F.: Hydrolysis of procaine in various mammalian plasmas. Fed. Proc., *12*(Abstr. 986):299, 1953.) **B.** Hydrolysis rates of esters in pooled human plasma. (Data from Foldes, F.F., Davidson, G.N., Duncalf, D., and Kuwabarra, S.: The intravenous toxicity of local anesthetic agents in man. Clin. Pharmacol. Ther., *6*:328, 1965.)

thetic potency or to lipid solubility/protein binding. Terminal elimination half-lives after rapid i.v. injection are between 2 and 3 hours for all of the agents. With the exception of prilocaine (which has a clearance value in excess of liver blood flow, suggesting some metabolism outside the liver), metabolic clearance is virtually synonymous with hepatic clearance.[415] Etidocaine clearance is dependent mostly on liver perfusion, whereas that of bupivacaine should be more sensitive to changes in intrinsic hepatic enzyme function.[405] Although clearance of the former compound is double that of the latter, and they are intrinsically equitoxic, any advantage that this might offer for etidocaine is offset by the fact that twice the dose is required to establish the same quality of sensory blockade as that produced by bupivacaine.

During short i.v. infusions, the agents appear to increase their own clearance by stimulating liver blood flow.[415] On the other hand, a significant decrease in the clearance of lidocaine and extension of its half-life have been observed during prolonged i.v. infusions for the control of cardiac arrhythmias in postmyocardial infarction patients.[33,233,328,354] Reasons for this include a progressive increase in plasma binding as α_1-acid glycoprotein levels rise[351] and, possibly, product-inhibition by lidocaine metabolites.[235]

Identification of the biotransformation products of the amides indicates three main sites of metabolic attack: aromatic hydroxylation, N-dealkylation, and amide hydrolysis. The relative importance of these routes varies considerably among the different compounds (Table 3-15) and between different species.

Lidocaine. About 80% of a dose of lidocaine has been accounted for as metabolites (Fig. 3-27). In humans, 3′-hydroxylation is a minor pathway, the primary route of metabolism being N-deethylation to monoglycinexylidide (MEGX) followed by further N-deethylation to glycinexylidide (GX) and 3′-hydroxylation, but mostly amide hydrolysis to give 2,6-xylidine. The latter is then converted to 4-hydroxy-2,6-xylidine, the major urinary product of lidocaine in humans.[54,213] Original studies suggested that amide hydrolysis took place only after N-deethylation, but more recent work[304] has demonstrated at least 35% of a dose of lidocaine in urine as N,N-diethylglycine, a product of direct hydrolysis of the parent drug.

Other metabolites of lidocaine have been proposed, but their existence is more controversial. A cyclic metabolite, claimed initially to be excreted in human urine, was subsequently shown largely to be an artifact arising from the reaction of MEGX with trace amounts of acetaldehyde in solvents used in isolation procedures.[57,303] Nevertheless, experiments in monkeys suggested that it may be formed *in vivo* if a patient receiving lidocaine has also ingested alcohol and has an elevated body burden of acetaldehyde.[303] Mather and Thomas[260] presented indirect evidence for the urinary excretion of the amide N-hydroxy derivatives of lidocaine and MEGX; however, the presence of these compounds in urine could not be verified by others, although this does not preclude their existence as intermediates in the formation of subsequent metabolites.[305]

MEGX, GX, and the 4-hydroxy product formed from lidocaine have all been measured in human plasma.[29,33,48,181,225,300,328,390] Of these, there is evidence that only MEGX contributes to the effects of the parent drug. Thus, steady-state unbound plasma concentrations of MEGX in humans are about 70% those of lidocaine,[135] and this metabolite has been shown to have comparable antiarrhythmic and convulsant activity in animals.[25,50,82,377] Plasma GX concentrations are much lower than those of lidocaine in humans; it is much less antiarrhythmic and is devoid of convulsant effect in animals.[50,82,389] Direct intravenous injection of GX into two subjects did not reproduce any of the major toxic effects associated with lidocaine, although there was some impairment of mental concentration.[389] MEGX has a relatively short elimination half-life, slightly longer than that of lidocaine itself.[181,300] It is eliminated primarily by further metabolism; only about 12% of the dose is excreted unchanged in the urine. GX has a much longer half-life (about 10 hours), and 50% of a dose is excreted unchanged[389]; consequently, it may accumulate during long-term administration of lidocaine, especially in patients with renal disease.[101]

Prilocaine. Prilocaine is split at the amide linkage to yield o-toluidine which, in turn, is converted to 4- and 6-hydroxytoluidine, probably by rearrangement of an amide N-hydroxy intermediate (Fig. 3-28). These hydroxylation steps are responsible for the methemoglobinemia seen when the dose of prilocaine exceeds about 600 mg.[189] They cannot occur with the 2,6-xylidine ring of other amide-type local anesthetics. Therefore, methemoglobinemia is not a complication of the administration of these compounds.[251]

Mepivacaine. The structures of various mepivacaine metabolites found in human urine are shown in Figure 3-29.[273,274,397] About 1% of an oral dose is re-

TABLE 3-15. RENAL EXCRETION OF AMIDE-TYPE LOCAL ANESTHETICS AND THEIR METABOLITES (% DOSE)

			Aromatic Hydroxylation		N-Dealkylation		Amide Hydrolysis		
Agent	**Subject**	**Unchanged**	**3-Hydroxy***	**4-Hydroxy***	**Mono-**	**Di-**	**2,6-Xylidine***	**40H-Xylidine***	**Total**
Lidocaine	Adult	1.9[a] (0.6–4.7)	<1[b,c]	<1[b,c]	2.6[a] (0.9–4.8)	2.3	2.2[a] (1.6–2.4)	65.1[a] (53.1–74.4)	~74
	Neonate	19.7[a]	ND	ND	19.7[a] (4.2–48.9)	ND	2.7[a] (1.2–4.3)	8.9[a] (0–22.2)	~51 ~34
Mepivacaine	Adult	4.0[a] (2.8–5.2)	15.9[d] (11.9–20.3)	11.5[d] (8.5–14.3)	2.5[d] (1.8–3.1)	Not possible	ND	ND	~34
	Neonate	43.3[e] (21.8–64.9)	<2[e]	<2[e]	11.4[e] (6.5–17.2)	Not possible	ND	ND	~55
Bupivacaine	Adult	2.6[f] ± 0.3	~2[g]	~2[g]	0.2[f] ± 0.3 (5–20[g])	Not possible	~0[g]	~0[g]	~10
Etidocaine	Adult	0.3[h] ± 0.3	~5[h]	~5[h]	2.6[h] ± 4.3	13.1[h] ± 4.0*	0.9[h] ± 0.7	3.2[h] ± 2.3	~30

*Free and conjugated.
[a]Mihaly et al. (1978): 4 adults, i.v.; normal *p*H; 8 neonates, s.c.[277]
[b]Keenaghan and Boyes (1972): 2 adults, p.o.; normal *p*H.[213]
[c]Nelson et al. (1977): 3 adults, p.o.; normal *p*H.[304]
[d]Meffin et al. (1973): 3 adults, i.v.; normal *p*H.[272]
ND = not determined.
[e]Moore et al. (1978); 5 neonates, s.c.[289a]
[f]Reynolds (1971a): 4 adults, i.v.; acid urine.[337]
[g]Mather et al. (1971b) and unpublished data: 3 adults, i.v.; acid urine.[258]
[h]Morgan et al. (1977) and unpublished data: 9 adults, epidural, i.v.; normal *p*H.[291]
(Tucker, G.T., and Mather, L.E.: Clinical pharmacokinetics of local anaesthetic agents. Clin. Pharmacokinet., *4*:241, 1979.)

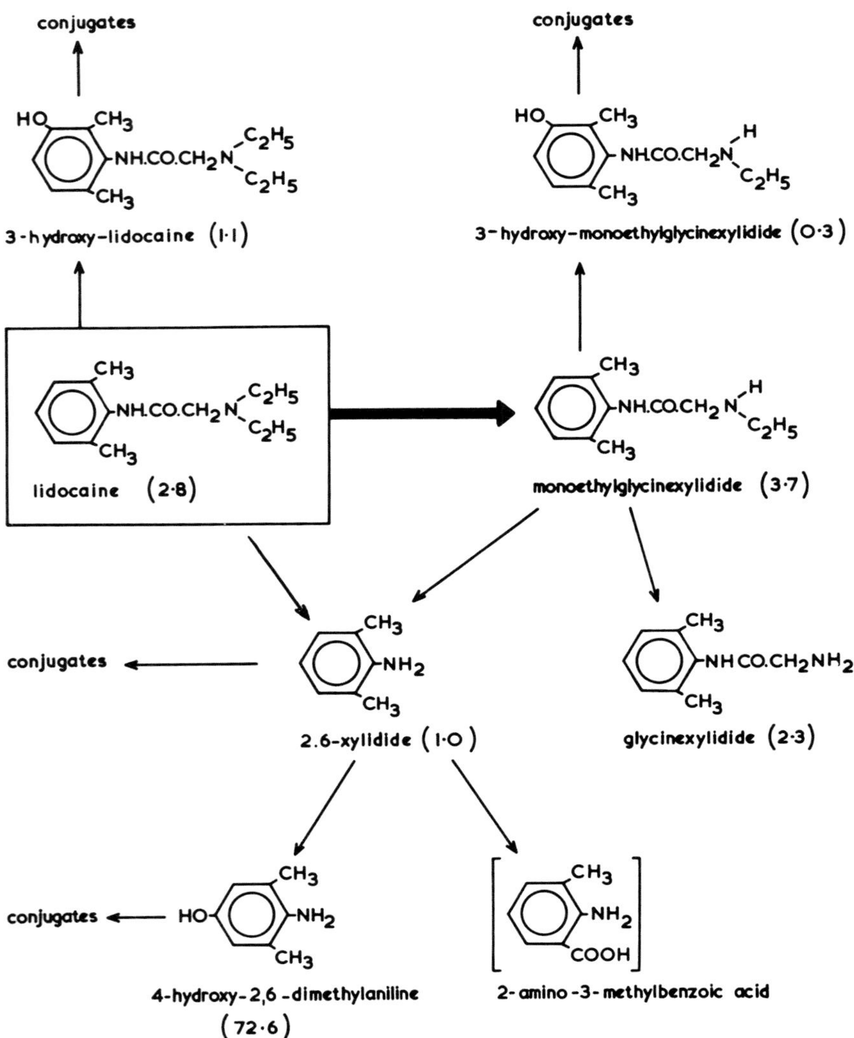

FIG. 3-27. Pathways for the biotransformation of lidocaine in humans. Values in parentheses indicate percentages of dose found in urine. (Boyes, R.N., A review of the metabolism of amide local anaesthetic agents. Br. J. Anaesth., *47*:225, 1975; and Keenaghan, J.B., and Boyes, R.N.: The tissue distribution, metabolism and excretion of lidocaine in rats, guinea pigs, dogs, and man. J. Pharmacol. Exp. Ther. *180*:454, 1972.)

covered as the N-demethylated derivative, 2,6-pipecolylxylidide (PPX). A further 15% to 20% appears as conjugates of the 3′-hydroxy compound, probably formed from an epoxide intermediate; 10% to 14% as conjugates of the 4′-hydroxy compound, possibly formed by means of an amide N-hydroxy intermediate; and 10% as various neutral lactams. Animal data indicate that PPX and the 4′-hydroxy metabolite are 68% and 36%, respectively, as toxic as mepivacaine.[184] Plasma concentrations of PPX in humans, however, are less than 0.1% those of the parent compound.[272] Direct administration of PPX in humans resulted in a 50% urinary recovery of the unchanged compound.[337]

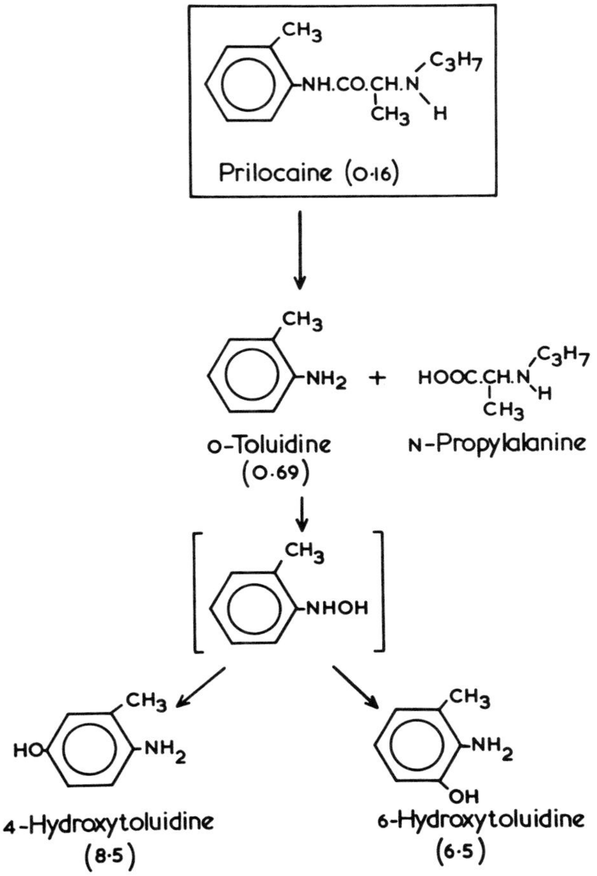

FIG. 3-28. Pathways for the biotransformation of prilocaine in humans. Values in parentheses indicate percentages of dose found in urine. (Akerman, B., Astrom, A., Ross, S., and Telc, A.: Studies on the absorption, distribution and metabolism of labelled prilocaine and lidocaine in some animal species. Acta Pharmacol. Toxicol. (Kbh.), *24*:389, 1966.)

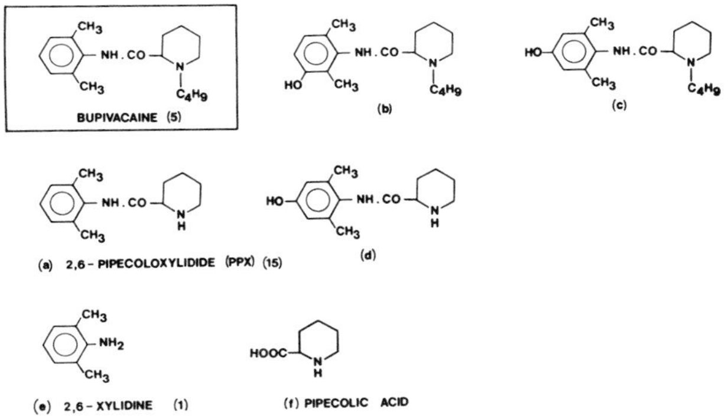

Bupivacaine. Products of the biotransformation of bupivacaine in humans are poorly characterized. This drug shares a common N-dealkylation metabolite, PPX, with mepivacaine. Urinary recovery of PPX after giving both drugs is very low. In rats, a large proportion of a dose of bupivacaine is excreted as conjugates of the 3′- and 4′-hydroxy derivatives, whereas the monkey excretes over 50% as the hydrolysis product pipecolic acid.[84,170] Some of the known metabolites of bupivacaine are shown in Figure 3-30. Peak plasma concentrations of PPX after epidural injection of bupivacaine are only one tenth those of parent drug, but PPX has a longer elimination half-life.[228]

Etidocaine. Although 20 metabolites of etidocaine have been found in the urine of patients treated with etidocaine (some of which are shown in Figure 3-31), only 30% of the dose has been recovered.[290,398,424] The two mono-N-dealkylated products of etidocaine have been measured in plasma,[291] but the clinical significance of this is unknown.

Dibucaine. Studies of the metabolism of dibucaine in rats, rabbits, and humans have led to the identification in urine of ten basic metabolites, representing 10% of the dose.[199] These include products of O-dealkylation, N-dealkylation, and N-oxidation, as well as diols and alcohols formed by ω-1 hydroxylation of the alkoxy side-chain.

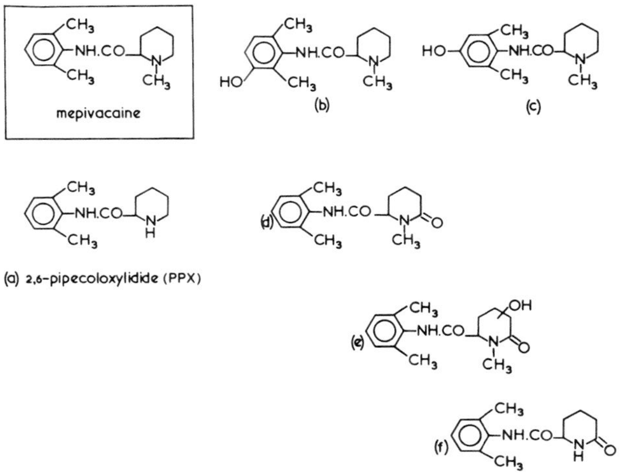

FIG. 3-29. Biotransformation products of bupivacaine.

FIG. 3-30. Biotransformation products of mepivacaine in humans.

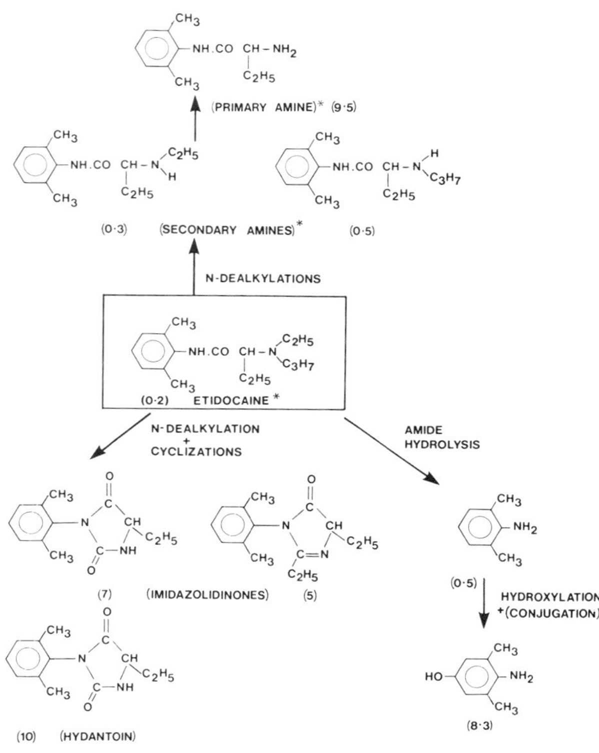

FIG. 3-31. Biotransformation products of etidocaine in humans. Values in parentheses indicate percentages of dose found in urine.

Physical and Pathophysiologic Factors

Weight. Limited data on amide-type agents indicate a poor correlation among body weight, surface area or lean body mass, and drug disposition kinetics in young male volunteers with normal height: weight ratios.[356,411] In obese subjects of either sex, with no evidence of cardiac or renal dysfunction, a 50% increase in the terminal elimination half-life of lidocaine was noted. This was explained by a change in volume of distribution rather than clearance.[4]

Age. No differences in the disposition kinetics of lidocaine were found between young (24–34 years) and older (52–57 years) normal subjects.[356] In contrast, Abernethy and Greenblatt[5] observed that elderly men (65–75 years), but not women (64–88 years), had lower clearances of lidocaine (35%) than did young controls, resulting in a 60% increase in half-life. Earlier studies had found no change in clearance in geriatric patients but longer half-lives associated with increased volumes of distribution (see also Chap. 21).[108,300]

Gender. There are suggestions that women may have up to 50% longer half-lives of lidocaine than men. One study assigns this to a significant (64%) difference in volume of distribution,[436] whereas another found small (15%) differences in clearance.[4]

Race. No differences in the disposition kinetics and plasma binding of lidocaine have been found in white, Oriental, and black subjects.[171]

Posture. Prolonged bed rest is associated with decreases in plasma and extracellular fluid volumes, and hepatic blood flow is less when standing. Thus, posture might be expected to alter drug disposition. However, although Bennett and colleagues[40] showed that the clearance of lidocaine was lowered on standing, others found no influence of prolonged recumbency on the disposition and plasma binding of this drug.[212]

Factors Related to Nerve Block

High epidural block in healthy humans may be associated with a 20% lowering of hepatic blood flow.[215] It is not known whether this decreases significantly the systemic clearance of local anesthetic used in patients since other factors, for example, maintenance of correct fluid balance, may offset the hemodynamic effect. Blockade to T6–7 with epidural tetracaine did not influence the disposition kinetics of intravenous etidocaine in healthy humans.[411] Similarly, Runciman[357] did not observe alterations in total body clearance, hepatic or renal extraction ratio, and hepatic or renal clearance of lidocaine in sheep having T6 subarachnoid blockade with tetracaine. In monkeys, Sivarajan and associates[375] observed significant falls in coronary, hepatic, renal, and cerebral blood flows during T1 epidural anesthesia. These changes might be expected to have a profound influence on local anesthetic kinetics.

Apart from effects on central hemodynamics, epidural block also causes changes in peripheral blood flows. Thus, lumbar sympathetic block results in vasodilatation in the legs with compensatory vasoconstriction in the arms and a lowering of arm blood flow. This is reflected in considerable arteriovenous concentration difference in plasma concentrations of local anesthetics (see Fig. 3-9), that across the arm being much greater than that across the leg.[262,411] Presumably, these differences mirror those in the rate of tissue uptake of drug and the extent of cutaneous shunting of both blood and drug.

Cardiovascular Disease. Plasma concentrations of lidocaine after intravenous injection in patients with congestive heart failure were found to be about twice as high as those in control subjects receiving the same dose.[41,401] Concentrations of MEGX, formed from lidocaine, may also be elevated.[181] These findings reflect significant decreases in the volume of distribution and clearance of the compounds (Table 3-16). Changes in the rate of drug distribution are a consequence of autoregulatory redistribution of blood away from the periphery to the vital organs. An increase in the extent of distribution, however, as measured by V_{ss}, presumably reflects altered tissue/blood partition coefficients or vascular shunting. The impaired clearance appears to be associated with diminished hepatic blood flow secondary to a low cardiac output or impaired hepatic extraction secondary to hepatocellular dysfunction or intrahepatic shunting.[43,401] Hypovolemia,[26] hypotension,[153] and cardiopulmonary resuscitation[91,94] are associated with changes in the disposition of lidocaine similar to those seen in heart failure.

After the use of local anesthetics for regional anesthesia in patients with circulatory depression or diminished cardiac output, abnormally elevated blood drug concentrations may not be achieved owing to impaired peripheral perfusion and slower uptake of drug from the site of injection.[293] Also, autoregulatory vasoconstriction may be impaired by extensive sympathetic blockade with concomitant effects on the volume of distribution of the drug.

Surprisingly, only minor decreases in the clearance and volume of distribution of lidocaine were observed in patients studied immediately after cardiopulmonary bypass surgery.[191] More marked changes seen on the third and seventh postoperative days were explained, in part, by an increase in plasma drug binding accompanying a rise in alpha$_1$-acid glycoprotein levels.

TABLE 3-16. LIDOCAINE DISPOSITION IN VARIOUS GROUPS OF PATIENTS

	$t_{1/2,z}$ (h)	V_{ss} (liters/kg)	CL (ml/min/kg)
Normal	1.8	1.32	10.0
Heart failure	1.9	0.88	6.3
Liver cirrhosis	4.9	2.31	6.0
Renal disease	1.3	1.2	13.7

(Data from Thompson, P., *et al.*: Lidocaine pharmacokinetics in advanced heart failure, liver disease, and renal failure in humans. Ann. Intern. Med., *78*:499, 1973.) See glossary to Tables 3-6 to 3-10 for definitions (p. 97). Underlined values differ significantly in comparison to normal subjects.

Liver Disease. Although plasma half-life values of procaine are longer in patients with liver disease (Table 3-16), presumably owing to decreased synthesis of pseudocholinesterase, normal esterase activity is preserved in their erythrocytes.[85] This, and the fact that the absolute rate of plasma hydrolysis remains high, suggests that these patients may not be much more susceptible to toxicity.

The clinical significance of altered disposition of the amides in liver disease is greater than that of the esters and depends upon the type of liver disease. In severe cirrhosis there are considerable increases in the half-life and volume of distribution and a decrease in the clearance of lidocaine (Table 3-16). The mechanism of the change in distribution may be related to altered plasma or tissue binding, or both. The lowered clearance reflects decreased enzyme activity plus extrahepatic shunting.[196] Clearly, systemic accumulation of the amides will be more extensive and prolonged in patients with cirrhosis and the regression of systemic effects will be slower.[10] In contrast, chronic hepatitis appears to be associated with a higher lidocaine clearance than normal,[195] although V_{ss} is also increased secondary to a decreased plasma drug binding.[197] The acute phase of viral hepatitis is accompanied by increases in lidocaine half-life and volume of distribution and a trend toward a lower clearance. No differences in the plasma binding of the drug were seen in the acute and recovery phases of the disease.[435]

Renal Disease. Procaine hydrolysis in sera from patients with impaired renal function is slowed in proportion to the blood urea nitrogen value (Table 3-17).[335] A decreased synthesis of pseudocholinesterase, rather than inhibition or inactivation of the enzyme by other components of uremic serum, appears to be responsible for this effect.[86] As in patients with liver disease, red cell esterase activity is preserved in renal disease,[85] and the change in plasma hydrolysis rate may be of little clinical significance.

As might be expected of drugs that are eliminated almost entirely by the liver, the disposition kinetics of the amides are unaffected by renal disease (see Table 3-15).[401] In contrast to the parent drugs, however,

TABLE 3-17. *IN VITRO* PLASMA $t_{1/2\beta}$ OF CHLOROPROCAINE AND PROCAINE (SEC ± SD)

	Author	Reference	Normals*	Pregnant	Liver Disease	Renal Disease	Pulmonary Disease	Heart Failure	Neonates
Chloroprocaine	Finster *et al.* (1973)	156a	21 ± 2 (M) 25 ± 1 (F)	21 ± 1					43 ± 2
Procaine	Reidenberg *et al.* (1972)	335	39 ± 8		138 ± 54	84 ± 50			84 ± 30
	duSouich and Erill (1977)	138	43 ± 6				83 ± 16	92 ± 11	

*M = male; F = female.
(Tucker, G.T., and Mather, L.E.: Clinical pharmacokinetic of local anaesthetic agents. Clin. Pharmacokinet., *4*:241, 1979.)

polar metabolites will tend to accumulate in patients with renal insufficiency. This is true of GX, formed from lidocaine, although the evidence suggests that the plasma concentrations reached are not likely to cause major toxicity.[101]

Pulmonary Disease. Despite the fact that compromised pulmonary function is one of the indications for regional anesthesia, relationships between the disposition and toxicity of local anesthetics and lung pathology and hypoxia are poorly defined.

A compromise in pulmonary perfusion, especially if shunting occurs, or alteration in the integrity of lung tissue might allow local anesthetic to escape early lung uptake with delivery of excessive drug concentrations to the heart and brain[406]; however, studies in ventilated intensive care patients have indicated that pulmonary uptake of lidocaine is not lowered markedly by severe respiratory insufficiency.[207] In animals, acute hypoxia is associated with a substantial lowering of hepatic blood flow; this may have consequences for the clearance of some local anesthetics,[347] although capillary recruitment may increase the hepatic extraction in order to compensate.[359]

Ingestion of Food

Through its influence on splanchnic hemodynamics and elevation of plasma concentrations of lipids, ingestion of food has the potential to alter the disposition of drugs. The consumption of a high protein meal was shown to increase the clearance of intravenously administered lidocaine, without alteration of plasma binding, in a manner consistent with its high hepatic clearance and the known effects of splanchnic blood flow.[142]

Drug-Drug Interactions

Ideally, interpretation of pharmacokinetic data on drug-drug interactions should be based on measurements of unbound plasma drug concentrations because these are believed to relate more closely to drug effects than total concentrations. It becomes especially important in this context to stress the following point: Although the unbound *fraction* of local anesthetic in plasma may be increased by a second drug, this does not necessarily mean that its unbound plasma *concentration* will be significantly greater *in vivo,* and therefore that the risk of toxicity will be increased. Failure to appreciate this point has led to a confused literature.

An increasing number of drugs have been shown to alter the disposition kinetics of local anesthetics, but the clinical significance of the changes is largely unknown.

Local Anesthetics. There is *in vitro* evidence that plasma concentrations of etidocaine and bupivacaine in the clinical range can inhibit the hydrolysis of chloroprocaine by 10% to 40%.[230,332] Clinically relevant concentrations of bupivacaine may also increase the free *fractions* of lidocaine[173,270] and mepivacaine[185] in plasma; however, the suggestion that a toxic reaction to a combined block with bupivacaine and mepivacaine was due to such a displacement reaction increasing the free concentration of mepivacaine is unlikely.[186]

No differences in plasma concentration-time profiles of etidocaine were observed when intercostal block was performed with etidocaine alone and when it was given with bupivacaine for bilateral block.[59,60] Similarly, the plasma concentration-time profiles of lidocaine and bupivacaine were independent of whether they were used alone or in combinations for epidural block.[368]

General Anesthetics. The rate of elimination of lidocaine in dogs was lower under halothane anesthesia than while breathing nitrous oxide[81] or air.[53] Similarly, a 34% lower clearance of lidocaine and a trend toward a smaller V_{ss} were found in patients receiving maintenance anesthesia with halothane and nitrous oxide-oxygen compared with a control group administered fentanyl, thiopentone, and nitrous oxide-oxygen. Pharmacokinetic parameters for the latter were similar to those for unanesthetised subjects.[44] All of these results are consistent with the effects of halothane in decreasing hepatic and renal blood flow,[361] renal tubular secretory activity, and mixed function oxidase activity.[120,358] Studies specifically designed to examine the effects of halothane on lidocaine clearance, however, did not observe consistent effects on lidocaine hepatic extraction so that lidocaine hepatic clearance varied principally in proportion to hepatic blood flow.[259] In view of the profound effects of general anesthetics on drug clearance,[358] it is surprising that DeRick and colleagues[129] did not note any alteration in lidocaine blood concentrations in dogs anesthetized with methoxyflurane-nitrous oxide.

Addition of sodium thiopental to human serum did not alter the protein binding of bupivacaine.[23] General anesthesia lowers the pulmonary extraction of lidocaine in humans to a small extent.[206,207]

Premedicants. Arteriovenous concentration differences of amide local anesthetics measured in the arm were found to be less in premedicated patients than in volunteers receiving similar epidural injections. It was suggested that the administration of premedicants, such as meperidine, to patients caused a generalized vasodilation and opening of cutaneous shunts, which antagonized the compensatory vasoconstriction in the upper limbs produced by lumbar sympathetic block.[298,411]

At clinically relevant plasma concentrations, meperidine does not influence the free fractions of lidocaine or bupivacaine in plasma.[123,173,412] Although it has been suggested that diazepam may influence plasma concentrations of etidocaine and bupivacaine through alterations in plasma binding,[168] recent reports have not found a plasma binding interaction between these drugs.[126] As diazepam binds to albumin and the local anesthetics preferentially bind to α_1-acid glycoprotein, an interaction would not have been expected.

Sympathomimetics. Benowitz and colleagues[43] have documented the effects of norepinephrine (alpha-adrenoceptor stimulation) and of isoproterenol (beta-adrenoceptor stimulation) on the disposition kinetics of lidocaine in monkeys. The former decreased initial volume of distribution, decreased clearance by lowering hepatic blood flow, and increased half-life; the latter had the opposite effects.

Inclusion of epinephrine in solutions for epidural block often results in a significant increase in cardiac output and falls in peripheral resistance and arterial blood pressure over a period of about an hour.[51] These effects, together with an increase in liver blood flow (mediated partly through the increase in cardiac output and also by direct action on intrahepatic β_2-receptors), could influence the systemic disposition of local anesthetics. Studies in monkeys[15] and in healthy humans[215] showed that epinephrine absorbed from the epidural space offsets temporarily the lowering of hepatic blood flow caused by sympathetic blockade.

Intravenous injection of 20 mg of ephedrine was found to increase the clearance of lidocaine by stimulating hepatic blood flow.[430] Whether this also happens in the presence of sympathetic blockade is not known.

Beta-Adrenoceptor Antagonists. In therapeutic doses, propranolol lowers the clearance of lidocaine in humans by about 40%, mainly by direct inhibition of mixed-function oxidase activity and partly by decreasing liver blood flow, through its effects on cardiac output and by intrahepatic β_2-blockade. Other beta-adrenoceptor antagonists have less marked effects, depending upon their lipid-solubility, cardioselectivity, and intrinsic sympathomimetic activity.[34,407] Propranolol does not impair the plasma binding of lidocaine at clinically relevant concentrations.[173,271]

Patients receiving therapy with a variety of beta-blockers were reported to have higher mean plasma concentrations of bupivacaine after intercostal block, compared to a group in whom the drugs had been withdrawn. The differences, however, were not significant statistically.[324]

Propranolol has been shown to decrease first-pass pulmonary extraction of bupivacaine by about 10% in rabbits, presumably by competing for tissue binding sites.[348]

H2-Antagonists. Therapeutic doses of cimetidine lower the clearance of lidocaine in humans by 20% to

30%, mainly by direct inhibition of metabolism rather than through any influence on liver blood flow.[32,154,426,436] Some studies also indicate that cimetidine decreases the V_{ss} of lidocaine, presumably by altering plasma and tissue binding, and prolongs its terminal half-life. In contrast to cimetidine, ranitidine has little[339] or no[155] effect on the disposition of lidocaine.

Data in rats and monkeys suggest that cimetidine also inhibits the metabolism of bupivacaine.[399]

Enzyme-Inducing Agents. The systemic clearance of free (unbound) lidocaine was found to be about 25% greater in epileptic patients receiving phenytoin than in a group of age-matched control subjects.[317,353] This is a consequence of the enzyme-inducing properties of the anticonvulsant. Long-term therapy with phenytoin also leads to the induction of α_1-acid glycoprotein synthesis, enhanced plasma binding of lidocaine and a lowering of its red blood cell/plasma concentration ratio.[353] This effect is not common to all enzyme-inducing agents, however, because rifampicin has no influence on α_1-acid glycoprotein levels and the plasma binding of lidocaine.[156]

Other Therapeutic Agents. Administration of inhibitors of plasma pseudocholinesterase, for example, neostigmine and ecothiophate, should be avoided in patients receiving ester-type local anesthetics, as should acetazolamide, which blocks hydrolysis by the red cell esterase.[85] Nitroprusside in hypotensive doses was shown to have no effect on lidocaine clearance in dogs.[371]

Many basic drugs have been shown to displace lidocaine from plasma binding sites but only when added at supratherapeutic concentrations.[166,173,271,412]

PLACENTAL TRANSFER

Esters. After maternal injection, 2-chloroprocaine appears in both maternal and cord plasma in very low concentrations.[1,2,226] Thus, even though elimination half-lives of chloroprocaine and procaine are twice as long in cord plasma as in maternal plasma and pregnancy is associated with a decrease in pseudocholinesterase activity (see Table 3-17),[226,309,335] the absolute rate of hydrolysis in the mother remains fast and helps to reduce placental transfer and intoxication of the fetus. Also, the enzyme activity still seems adequate despite the fact that administration of these drugs in itself lowers cholinesterase activity in maternal and cord plasma by 70% to 80%.[226]

Amides. At delivery, mean values of cord/maternal plasma concentration ratios of the amides decrease in the following order: prilocaine (1.0 – 1.1), lidocaine (0.5 – 0.7), mepivacaine (0.7), bupivacaine (0.2 – 0.4), and etidocaine (0.2 – 0.3),[413] although individuals may differ markedly. These differences reflect differential maternal and fetal plasma binding of the drugs owing to relatively low fetal concentrations of α_1-acid glycoprotein (Fig. 3-32).[257,261,318,321,408,440] As such, however, these ratios are not direct predictors of relative fetal toxicity because they are based on measurements of *total* plasma drug concentrations. Concentration ratios of unbound (active) drug across the placenta are probably close to unity for all of the agents[396] or somewhat greater owing to ion-trapping as a result of fetal acidosis.[45,74,214,319,394,409] The important calculation is the ratio of free drug concentration associated with toxicity to the free drug concentration in fetal blood after normal maternal dosage. This may be significantly greater for bupivacaine and etidocaine than for lidocaine and mepivacaine, indicating their higher safety margin.

Kuhnert and colleagues[228] have suggested that relatively low cord/maternal ratios of bupivacaine, based on total plasma drug concentrations are not due to relatively high maternal plasma binding but to extensive fetal tissue uptake. Such an explanation is kinetically unsound and certainly cannot explain low umbilical venous to maternal ratios.

In theory, a high maternal/fetal plasma binding ratio should delay equilibration of drug in the fetal tissues.[115] However, observations that the placental transfer of the agents is perfusion limited[183] and that fetal scalp capillary/maternal blood concentration ratios of both lidocaine and bupivacaine are relatively stable after 20 minutes indicate that this may be of importance only when delivery occurs soon after injection.[38,441] Similar umbilical artery/umbilical vein concentration ratios observed for the various agents also suggest that their equilibration rates in the fetus are similar.[409]

Some studies have reported much higher fetal blood concentrations of mepivacaine than those in the maternal circulation after paracervical block. Thus, it was proposed that direct diffusion of drug into the uterine artery occurs close to the site of injection, resulting in the delivery of high drug concentrations directly to the placenta, and hence fetal toxicity.[24,385] In contrast, others have found an association

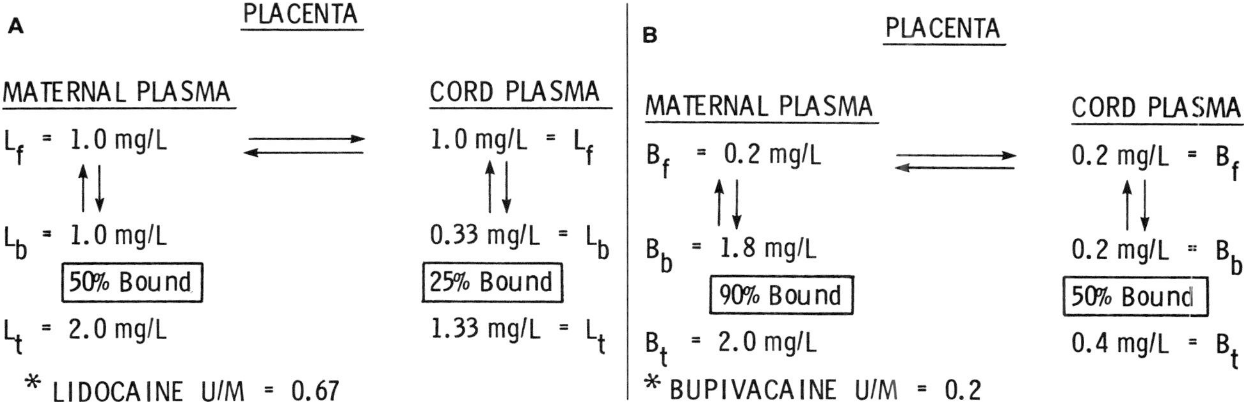

FIG. 3-32. Schematic showing how transplacentral distribution of local anesthetics may be predicted from differences in binding of the drugs in maternal and cord plasma. **A.** Lidocaine. **B.** Bupivacaine, f, b, t, represent free, bound, and total drug concentrations, respectively.

between fetal bradycardia after paracervical block and fetal/maternal drug concentration ratios of less than one, and lower than those seen when the heart rate was unchanged.[237,394] Thus, Liston and associates proposed that the problem of fetal bradycardia is not related to a direct toxic effect of the local anesthetic in the fetus but to some factor that causes impaired placental perfusion, thereby reducing both fetal oxygen supply and the extent of drug transfer.[237]

Metabolites of local anesthetics have been measured in fetal blood after maternal injection of the parent drugs.[48,225,228] The significance of this in relation to fetal toxicity is not known.

NEONATAL DRUG DISPOSITION

Having left the womb, the newborn can no longer rely on the placenta as a means of returning local anesthetic from whence it came. Clearance of the drugs now depends on the ability of immature hepatic and renal systems to deal with them.

Any investigation of the kinetics of local anesthetics in the newborn following neural blockade in the mother is handicapped by the difficulty of knowing how much of a dose the patient received. Further, when drug metabolites are detected, it is difficult to separate the quantity manufactured by the infant from the contribution donated *in utero* by the mother. Despite these problems, studies have indicated that fetal liver is able to metabolize local anesthetics.

Measurement of plasma concentrations and urinary excretion rates of lidocaine and mepivacaine given subcutaneously to facilitate arterial catheterization in neonates has indicated rapid absorption followed by monoexponential elimination over at least 24 hours.[277,289] Comparison with data from adults showed a twofold to threefold prolongation of the terminal half-life of both agents, related in part to a twofold increase in weight-corrected volume of distribution (Table 3-18). Lower plasma binding in the infants probably contributes to these findings. Mean plasma and blood clearance (based on body weight) of mepivacaine were more than halved in neonates, whereas those of lidocaine were similar to adult values; renal excretion of both drugs was eightfold to ninefold greater in neonates than in adults. When clearances were divided into renal and hepatic components, renal clearance of both drugs was found to be elevated significantly in neonates, whereas the hepatic clearance of mepivacaine, but not of lidocaine, was considerably reduced. The first observation may be due to decreased protein binding in neonatal blood and decreased tubular reabsorption owing to higher urine flow rates and lower urine *p*H in newborns. Less impairment of the hepatic clearance of lidocaine might be explained by a greater dependence on hepatic perfusion compared to mepivacaine, the elimination of which should be affected more by the function of immature liver enzymes.

Compared to adults, the capacity of the newborn to carry out direct aromatic hydroxylation of amide-

TABLE 3-18. COMPARISON OF THE DISPOSITION KINETICS OF AMIDE-TYPE LOCAL ANESTHETICS IN ADULTS AND NEONATES

	Lidocaine		Mepivacaine		Bupivacaine		Etidocaine	
Parameter	Adult	Neonate	Adult	Neonate	Adult	Neonate	Adult	Neonate
$t_{1/2,z}$ (h)	1.8[a] (1.2–2.2)	3.2[b] (3.0–3.3) 3[c]	3.2[d] (1.7–7.9)	8.7[d] (6.2–12.2) 9[c]	2.7 ± 1.3[e]	8.1 ± 2.5[f] 18 ± 6[g]	2.6 ± 1.1[e]	6.42 ± 2.73[h]
V_{ss}* (liters/kg)	1.11[a] (0.58–1.91)		1.02[d] (0.68–1.52)					
V* (liters/kg)		2.75[b] (1.44–4.99)		1.71[d] (1.14–2.77)				
CL* (ml/min/kg)	9.2[a] (5.3–12.1)	10.2[b] (5.1–19.0)	5.5[d] (2.9–8.9)	2.3[d] (1.7–3.1)				
f_e**	0.019[b] (0.006–0.047)	0.160[b] (0.015–0.313)	0.038[d] (0.021–0.057)	0.357[d] (0.197–0.527)				

**Fraction of dose excreted unchanged in urine.
*Specified with respect to venous plasma concentrations.
[a]Rowland *et al.* (1971).[356] [b]Mihaly *et al.* (1978).[277] [c]Brown *et al.* (1975).[73] [d]Moore *et al.* (1978).[289] [e]Tucker *et al.* (1977a).[415] [f]Magno *et al.* (1976).[252] [g]Caldwell *et al.* (1976).[84] [h]Morgan *et al.* (1978)—urine data.[291]
(Tucker, G.T., and Mather, L.E.: Clinical pharmacokinetics of local anaesthetic agents. Clin. Pharmacokinet., *4*:241, 1979.)

type local anesthetics is negligible, N-dealkylation is viable, but further metabolism of the products of this reaction may be impaired; amide hydrolysis to form 2,6-xylidine seems similar, but further hydroxylation of this compound may be deficient, although conjugation of the 4-hydroxy product is as extensive as in adults (Table 3-18).

Estimates of the terminal elimination half-lives of lidocaine and mepivacaine in neonates after epidural administration to their mothers agree closely with those derived from direct injection. Half-lives of bupivacaine and etidocaine in the neonate after maternal epidural injection also indicate prolonged elimination in the newborn, although mean estimates vary widely (8–18 hours) (Table 3-18).

Hypothermia associated with acidosis and hypertension have been shown to slow the clearance of lidocaine in puppies,[294] and acidosis in human neonates is accompanied by a significant increase in the elimination half-life of bupivacaine.[113]

Clinical implications of the data accumulated on placental transfer and neonatal disposition of local anesthetics are thought to favor the use of either rapidly metabolized 2-chloroprocaine or bupivacaine. Mepivacaine appears less safe than lidocaine because of its longer elimination half-life in the newborn (Fig. 3-33), whereas prilocaine is avoided because of the possibility of inducing methemoglobinemia, especially in an already hypoxic fetus.

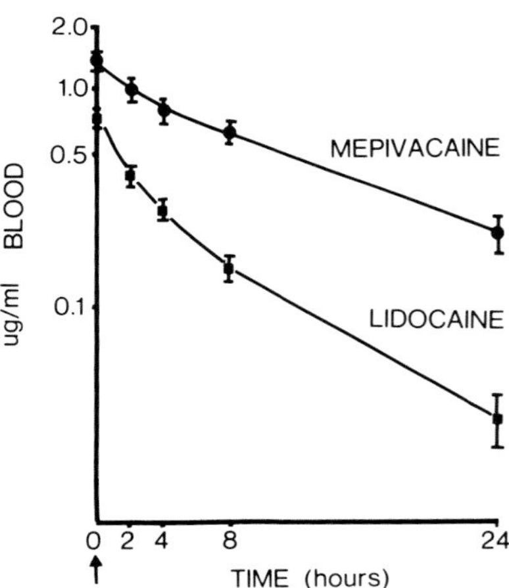

FIG. 3-33. Postnatal, neonatal blood concentrations of local anesthetic after peridural injection into their mothers. (Brown, W.U., *et al.*: Newborn blood levels of lidocaine and mepivacaine in the first postnatal day following epidural anesthesia. Anesthesiology, *42*:698, 1975.)

GLOSSARY OF SYMBOLS FOR TABLES

a	Mean ± SD	TS (V)	Topical spray (vaginal)
b	SE	TS (P)	Topical spray (perineal)
c	Time of mean maximum concentration	TS (E)	Topical spray (episiotomy repair)
d	Paralyzed	Endo	Endotracheal
e	With lidocaine lubricant	SAB	Subarachnoid block
f	Sprayed below vocal cords only	SCA	Subcutaneous abdominal
g	Sprayed above and below vocal cords	SCV	Subcutaneous vaginal
h	High concentrations of glycinexylidide observed	PCB	Paracervical block
i	Endotracheal intermittent positive pressure breathing	BP	Brachial plexus block
j	Endotracheal nebulizer	SF	Sciatic/femoral block
k	With bupivacaine	IC	Intercostal block
l	1:200,000	Epid	Lumbar epidural block
m	1:80,000	Caudal	Caudal block
n	With chloroprocaine	Periton	Peritonsillar block
o	Carbonated solution	Pudend	Pudendal block
p	Interscalene approach	GC	Gas chromatography
q	Axillary approach	C	Colorimetry
r	With laminaria tents	A	Arterial
s	For bronchoscopy	V	Venous
t	For gastroscopy	Epid (C)	Cervical epidural block
u	Upper respiratory tract	Epid (T)	Thoracic epidural block
v	Lower respiratory tract	TS (F)	Topical spray (fallopian tubes)
w	Percutaneous transcricothyroid injection	SCC	Subcutaneous cranial
x	Per mg/kg injected	CPB	Cervical plexus block
P	Plasma	Infiltr (S)	Scalp infiltration
B	Whole blood	Infiltr (P)	Perineal infiltration
CeP	Central Plasma	EMIT	Enzyme immunoassay
kg	Kg body weight	Ce	Central venous

REFERENCES

1. Abboud, T.K., Kim, K.C., Noueihed, R., Kuhnert, B.R., *et al.*: Epidural bupivacaine, chloroprocaine, or lidocaine for Cesarian section—Maternal and neonatal effects. Anesth. Analg. (Cleve.), *62*:914, 1983.
2. Abboud, T.K., Afrasiabi, A., Sarkis, F., Daftarian, F., *et al.*: Continuous infusion epidural analgesia in parturients receiving bupivacaine, chloroprocaine, or lidocaine—Maternal, fetal, and neonatal effects. Anesth. Analg. (Cleve.), *63*:421, 1984.

2a. Abdel-Salam, A.R., Vonwiller, J.B., and Scott, D.B.: Evaluation of etidocaine in extradural block. Br. J. Anaesth., *47*:1081, 1975.

3. Aberg, G.: Toxicological and local anaesthetic effects of optically active isomers of two local anaesthetic compounds. Acta Pharmacol. Toxicol. (Kbh.), *31*:273, 1972.
4. Abernethy, D.R., and Greenblatt, D.J.: Lidocaine disposition in obesity. Am. J. Cardiol., *53*:1183, 1984a.
5. Abernethy, D.R., and Greenblatt, D.J.: Impairment of lidocaine clearance in elderly male subjects. J. Cardiovasc. Pharmacol., *5*:1093, 1984b.
6. Adams, H.J.: Effect of pH on spinal anaesthesia with lidocaine in sheep. Pharmacol. Res. Commun. *7*:551, 1975.
7. Adams, H.J., Mastri, A.R., Eicholzer, A.W., and Kilpatrick, G.: Morphological effects of intrathecal etidocaine and tetracaine on the rabbit spinal cord. Anesthesiology, *53*:904, 1974.
8. Adams, H.J., Mastri, A.R., and Doherty, J.: Bupivacaine: Morphological effects on spinal cords of cats and durations of spinal anesthesia in sheep. Pharmacol. Res. Commun., *9*:847, 1977.
9. Adams, H.J., Charron, D.M., and Takman, B.H.: Spinal anesthesia in sheep with local anesthetic solutions at pH 4 and pH 7. Acta Anaesthesiol. Scand., *28*:270, 1984.
10. Adjepon-Yamoah, K.K., Nimmo, J., and Prescott, L.F.: Gross impairment on hepatic drug metabolism in a patient with chronic liver disease. Br. Med. J., *4*:387, 1974.
11. Adjepon-Yamoah K.K., and Prescott, L.F.: Lignocaine metabolism in man. Br. J. Pharmacol., *47*:672, 1974.
12. Akerman B., Astrom, A., Ross, S., and Telc, A.: Studies on the absorption, distribution and metabolism of labelled prilocaine and lidocaine in some animal species. Acta Pharmacol. Toxicol. (Kbh.), *24*:389, 1966.
13. Aldrete, J.A., Nicholson, J., Sada, T., Davidson, W., *et al.*: Cephalic kinetics of intra-arterially injected lidocaine. Oral Surg., *44*:167, 1977.
14. Aldrete, J.A., Romo-Salas, F., Arora, S., Wilson, R., *et al.*:

Reverse arterial blood flow as a pathway for central nervous systemic toxic responses following injection of local anesthetics. Anesth. Analg. (Cleve.), *57*:428, 1978.

15. Amory, D.W., Sivarajan, M., and Lindbloom, L.E.: Systemic and regional blood flow during epidural anesthesia with epinephrine in the rhesus monkey. Acta Anaesthesiol. Scand., *21*:423, 1977.
16. Apfelbaum, J.L., Gross, J.B., Shaw, L.M., Spaulding, B.C., *et al.*: Changes in lidocaine protein binding may explain its increased CNS toxicity at elevated CO_2 tensions. Anesthesiology, *61*:A213, 1984.
17. Apostolou, G.A., Zarmakoupis, P.K., and Mastrokostopoulos, G.T.: Spread of epidural anesthesia and the lateral position. Anesth. Analg. (Cleve.)., *60*:584, 1981.
18. Appleyard, T.N., Witt, A., Atkinson, R.E., and Nicholas, R.D.G.: Bupivacaine carbonate and bupivacaine hydrochloride: A comparison of blood concentrations during epidural blockade for vaginal surgery. Br. J. Anaesth., *46*:530, 1974.
19. Aps, C., and Reynolds, F.: The effect of concentration in vasoactivity of bupivacaine and lignocaine. Br. J. Anaesth., *48*:1171, 1976.
20. Aps, C., and Reynolds, F.: An intradermal study of the local anaesthetic and vascular effects of the isomers of bupivacaine. Br. J. Clin. Pharmacol., *6*:63, 1978.
21. Armstrong, I.R., Littlewood, D.G., and Chambers, W.A.: Spinal anesthesia with tetracaine—Effect of added vasoconstrictors. Anesth. Analg. (Cleve.), *62*:793, 1983.
22. Arthur, G.R.: Distribution and elimination of local anaesthetic agents: The role of lung, liver and kidney. Ph.D. Thesis, University of Edinburgh, 1981.
23. Arthur, G.R., Denson, D.D., and Coyle, D.E.: Effect of sodium thiopental on the serum protein binding of bupivacaine. Reg. Anesth., *9*:171, 1984.
24. Asling J.H., Shnider, S.M., Margolis, A.J., Wilkinson, G.R., *et al.*: Paracervical block in obstetrics: II. Etiology of fetal bradycardia following paracervical block anesthesia. Am. J. Obstet. Gynecol., *107*:626, 1970.
25. Astrom, A.: General pharmacology and toxicology of lidocaine. In Scott, D.B., and Julian, D.V. (eds.): Lidocaine in the Treatment of Ventricular Arrhythmias, pp. 128–138. Baltimore, Williams & Wilkins, 1971.
26. Aven, M.H., Light, A., Foldes, F.F.: Hydrolysis of procaine in various mammalian plasmas. Fed. Proc., *12*:986, 1953.
27. Axelsson, K.H., and Widman, B.: Blood concentration of lidocaine after spinal anaesthesia using lidocaine and lidocaine with adrenaline. Acta Anaesthesiol. Scand., *25*:240, 1981.
28. Axelsson, K.H., Edstrom, H.H., Sundberg, A.E.A., and Widman, G.B.: Spinal anaesthesia with hyperbaric 0.5% bupivacaine: Effects of volume. Acta Anaesthesiol. Scand., *26*:439, 1982.
29. Barchowsky, A., Stargel, W.W., Shand, D.G., and Routledge, P.A.: Saliva concentrations of lidocaine and its metabolites in man. Ther. Drug Monit., *4*:335, 1982.
30. Barchowsky, A., Shand, D.G., Stargel, W.W., Wagner, G.S., *et al.*: On the role of alpha-1-acid glycoprotein in lignocaine accumulation following myocardial infarction. Br. J. Clin. Pharmacol., *13*:411, 1981.
31. Barnett, G., Hawks, R., and Resnick, R.: Cocaine pharmacokinetics in humans. J. Ethnopharamacol., *3*:353, 1981.
32. Bauer, L.A., Edwards, W.A.D., Randolph, F.P., and Blouin, R.A.: Cimetidine-induced decrease in lidocaine metabolism. Am. Heart J., *108*:413, 1984.
33. Bax, N.D.S., Tucker, G.T., and Woods, H.F.: Lignocaine and indocyanine green kinetics in patients following myocardial infarction. Br. J. Clin. Pharmacol., *10*:353, 1980.
34. Bax, N.D.S., Tucker, G.T., Lennard, M.S., and Woods, H.F.: The impairment of lignocaine clearance by propranolol—Major contribution from enzyme inhibition. Br. J. Clin. Pharmacol. *19*:597, 1985.
35. Beazley, J.M., Taylor, G., and Reynolds, F.: Placental transfer of bupivacaine after paracervical block. Obstet. Gynecol., *39*:2, 1972.
36. Beckett, A.H., Boyes, R.N., and Appleton, P.J.: The metabolism and excretion of lignocaine in man. J. Pharm. Pharmacol., *18*:76S, 1966.
37. Belfrage, P., Berlin, A., Linstedt, M., and Raabe, N.: Plasma levels of bupivacaine following pudendal block in labour. Br. J. Anaesth., *45*:1067, 1973.
38. Belfrage, P., Raabe, N., and Berlin, A.: Lumbar epidural analgesia with bupivacaine in labour. Am. J. Obstet. Gynecol., *121*:360, 1975.
39. Belfrage, P., Irestedt, L., and Berlin, A.: Concentration of bupivacaine in arterial and venous plasma after epidural anaesthesia in man and after intramuscular administration in dog. Acta Anaesthesiol. Scand., *19*:85, 1975.
40. Bennett, P.N., Aarons, L.J., Bending, M.R., Steiner, J.A., *et al.*: Pharmacokinetics of lidocaine and its deethylated metabolite: Dose and time dependency studies in man. J. Pharmacokinet. Biopharm., *10*:265, 1982.
41. Benowitz, N.L., and Meister, W.: Clinical pharmacokinetics of lignocaine. Clin. Pharmacokinet., *3*:177, 1978.
42. Benowitz N., Forsyth, R.P., and Melmon, K.L.: Lidocaine disposition kinetics in monkey and man: I. Prediction by a perfusion model. Clin. Pharmacol. Ther., *16*:87, 1974.
43. Benowitz, N., Forsyth, R.P., Melmon, K.L., and Rowland, M.: Lidocaine disposition kinetics in monkey and man: II. Effects of hemorrhage and sympathomimetic drug administration. Clin. Pharmacol. Ther., *16*:99, 1974.
44. Bentley, J.B., Glass, S., and Gandolfi, A.J.: The influence of halothane on lidocaine pharmacokinetics in man. Anesthesiology, *59*:A246, 1983.
45. Biehl, D., Shnider, S.M., Levinson, G., and Callender, K.: Placental transfer of lidocaine: Effects of acidosis. Anesthesiology, *48*:409, 1978.
46. Biscoping, J., Salomon, F., and Hempelmann, G.: Plasmaspiegel nach lumbaler Periduralanaesthesie mit Bupivacain 0.75%. Reg. Anaesth., *7*:48, 1984.
47. Blair, M.R.: Cardiovascular pharmacology of local anaesthetics. Br. J. Anaesth., *47*[*Suppl.*]:247, 1975.
48. Blankenbaker, W.L., DiFazio, C.A., and Berry, F.A.: Lidocaine and its metabolites in the newborn. Anesthesiology, *42*:325, 1975.
49. Blanco, L.J., Reid, P.R., and King, T.M.: Plasma lidocaine levels following paracervical infiltration for aspiration abortion. Obstet. Gynecol., *60*:506, 1982.

50. Blumer, J., Strong, J.M., and Atkinson, A.J.: The convulsant potency of lidocaine and its N-dealkylated metabolites. J. Pharmacol. Exp. Ther., *186*:31, 1973.
51. Bonica, J.J., Akamatsu, T.J., Berges, P.U., Morikawa, K., *et al.*: Circulatory effects of peridural block: II. Effects of epinephrine. Anesthesiology, *34*:514, 1971.
52. Boster, S.R., Danzl, D.F., Madden, R.J., and Jarboe, C.H.: Translaryngeal absorption of lidocaine. Ann. Emerg. Med., *11*:461, 1982.
53. Boyce, J.R., Cervenko, F.W., and Wright, F.J. Effects of halothane on the pharmacokinetics of lidocaine in digatalis-toxic dogs. Can. Anaesth. Soc. J., *25*:323, 1978.
54. Boyes, R.N.: A review of the metabolism of amide local anaesthetic agents. Br. J. Anaesth., *47*:225 ,1975.
55. Braid, D.P., and Scott, D.B.: The systemic absorption of local analgesic drugs. Br. J. Anaesth., *37*:394, 1965.
56. Braid, D.P., and Scott, D.B.: The effect of adrenaline on the systemic absorption of local anaesthetic drugs. Acta Anaesthesiol. Scand., *23*[*Suppl.*]:334, 1966.
57. Breck, G.D, and Trager, W.F.: Oxidative N-dealkylation: A Mannich intermediate in the formation of a new metabolite of lidocaine in man. Science, *173*:544, 1971.
58. Bridenbaugh, L.D.: Does the addition of low molecular weight dextran prolong the duration of action of bupivacaine? Reg. Anaesth., *3*:6, 1978.
59. Bridenbaugh, P.O.: Intercostal nerve blockade for evaluation of local anaesthetic agents. Br. J. Anaesth., *47*:306, 1975.
60. Bridenbaugh, P.O., Tucker, G.T., Moore, D.C., Bridenbaugh, L.D., *et al.*: Preliminary clinical evaluation of etidocaine (Duranest): A new long-acting local anesthetic agent. Acta Anaesthesiol. Scand., *18*:165, 1974.
61. Bridenbaugh, P.O., Tucker, G.T., Moore, D.C., Bridenbaugh, L.E., *et al.*: Role of epinephrine in the regional block anesthesia with etidocaine: A double-blind study. Anesth. Analg. (Cleve.), *53*:430, 1974.
62. Brodie, B.B., Lief, P.A., and Poet, R.: The fate of procaine in man following its intravenous administration and methods for the estimation of procaine and diethylaminoethanol. J. Pharmacol. Exp. Ther., *94*:359, 1948.
63. Bromage, P.R.: Physiology and pharmacology of epidural analgesia. Anesthesiology, *28*:592, 1967.
64. Bromage, P.R.: Lower limb reflex changes in segmental epidural analgesia. Br. J. Anaesth., *46*:504, 1974.
65. Bromage, P.R.: Mechanisms of action of extradural analgesia. Br. J. Anaesth., *47*[*Suppl.*]:199, 1975.
66. Bromage, P.R., Joyal, A.C., and Binney, J.C.: Local anesthetic drugs: Penetration from the spinal extradural space into the neuraxis. Science, *140*:392, 1963.
67. Bromage, P.R., Burfoot, M.E., Crowell, D.E., and Truant, A.P.: Quality of epidural blockade: III. Carbonated local anaesthetic solutions. Br. J. Anaesth., *39*:197, 1967.
68. Bromage, P.R., and Gertel, M.: Brachial plexus anesthesia in chronic renal failure. Anesthesiology, *36*:488, 1972a.
69. Bromage, P.R., and Gertel, M.: Improved brachial plexus blockade with bupivacaine hydrochloride and carbonated lidocaine. Anesthesiology, *36*:479, 1972.
70. Bromage, P.R., and Robson, J.G.: Concentrations of lignocaine in the blood after intravenous, intramuscular, epidural and endotracheal administration. Br. J. Anaesth., *16*:461, 1961.
71. Brown, D.T., Wildsmith, J.A.W., Covino, B.G., and Scott, D.B.: Effect of baricity on spinal anaesthesia with amethocaine. Br. J. Anaesth., *52*:589, 1980a.
72. Brown, D.T., Morison, D.H., Covino, B.G., and Scott, D.B.: Comparison of carbonated bupivacaine and bupivacaine hydrochloride for extradural anaesthesia. Br. J. Anaesth., *52*:419, 1980b.
73. Brown, W.U., Bell, G.C., Lurie, A.O., Weiss, J.B., *et al.*: Newborn blood levels of lidocaine and mepivacaine in the first postnatal day following maternal epidural anesthesia. Anesthesiology, *42*:698, 1975.
74. Brown, W.U., Bell, G.C., and Alper, M.H.: Acidosis, local anesthetics and the newborn. Obstet. Gynecol., *48*:27, 1976.
75. Bruguerolle, B., Valli, M., Bouyard, L., Jadot, G., *et al.*: Effect of the hour of administration on the pharmacokinetics of lidocaine in the rat. Eur. J. Drug Metab. Pharmacokinet., *8*:233, 1983a.
76. Bruguerolle, B., Valli, M., Jardot, G., Bouyard, L., *et al.*: Variations circadiennes du passage intraerthrocytaire de la lidocaine. J. Pharmacol. (Paris), *14*:189, 1983b.
77. Burfoot, M.F., and Bromage, P.R.: The effects of epinephrine on mepivacaine absorption from the spinal epidural space. Anesthesiology, *35*:488, 1971.
78. Burm, A.G.: Pharmacokinetics and clinical effects of lidocaine and bupivacaine following epidural and subarachnoid administration in man. Ph.D. Thesis, University of Leiden, 1985.
79. Burm, A.G., van Kleef, J.W., Gladines, M.P., Spierdijk, J., *et al.*: Plasma concentrations of lidocaine and bupivacaine after subarachnoid administration. Anesthesiology, *59*:191, 1983.
80. Burn, J.M., Guyer, P.B., and Langdond, L.: The spread of solutions injected into the epidural space. A study using epidurograms in patients with the lumbosciatic syndrome. Br. J. Anaesth., *45*:338, 1973.
81. Burney, R.G., and DiFazio, C.A.: Hepatic clearance of lidocaine during N_2O anesthesia in dogs. Anesth. Analg. (Cleve.), *55*:322, 1976.
82. Burney, R.G., DiFazio, C.A., Peach, M.J., Petrie, K.A., *et al.*: Anti-arrhythmic effects of lidocaine metabolites. Am. Heart. J., *88*:65, 1974.
83. Burney, R.G., DiFazio, C.A., and Foster, J.H.: Effects of pH on protein binding of lidocaine. Anesth. Analg. (Cleve.), *57*:478, 1978.
84. Caldwell, J., Moffatt, J.R., Smith, R.L., Lieberman, A.B., *et al.*: Determination of bupivacaine in human fetal and neonatal blood samples by gas liquid chromatography mass spectrometry. Biomed. Mass Spectrom., *4*:322, 1977.
85. Calvo, R., Carlos, R., and Erill, S.: Effects of disease and acetazolamide on procaine hydrolysis by red cell enzymes. Clin. Pharmacol. Ther., *27*:175, 1980.
86. Calvo, R., Carlos, R., and Erill, S.: Procaine hydrolysis defect in uraemia does not appear to be due to carbamylation of plasma esterases. Eur. J. Clin. Pharmacol., *24*:533, 1983.
87. Cannell, H., Walters, H., Beckett, A.H., and Saunders, A.:

Circulating levels of lignocaine after per-oral injections. Br. Dent. J., *138*:87, 1975.

88. Catchlove, R.F.H.: The influence of CO_2 and pH on local anesthetic action. J. Pharmacol. Exp. Ther., *181*:298, 1972.
89. Chambers, W.A., Littlewood, D.G., Logan, M.R., and Scott, D.B.: Effect of added epinephrine on spinal anesthesia with lidocaine. Anesth. Analg. (Cleve.), *60*:417, 1981.
90. Chambers, W.A., Littlewood, D.G., Edstrom, H.H., and Scott, D.B.: Spinal anaesthesia with hyperbaric bupivacaine: Effects of concentration and volume administered. Br. J. Anaesth., *54*:75, 1982.
91. Chambers, W.A., Littlewood, G.D., and Scott, D.B.: Spinal anesthesia with hyperbaric bupivacaine: Effect of added vasoconstrictors. Anesth. Analg. (Cleve.), *62*:793, 1983.
92. Chinn, W.M., Zavala, D.C., and Ambre, J.: Plasma levels of lidocaine following nebulized aerosol administration. Chest, *71*:346, 1977.
93. Chow, M.S.S., Ronfeld, R.A., Ruffett, D., and Fieldman, A.: Lidocaine pharmacokinetics during cardiac arrest and external cardiopulmonary resuscitation. Am. Heart J., *102*:799, 1981.
94. Chow, M.S.S., Ronfeld, R.A., Hamilton, R.A., Helmink, R., *et al.*: Effect of external cardiopulmonary resuscitation on lidocaine pharmacokinetics in dogs. J. Pharmacol. Exp. Ther., *224*:531, 1983.
95. Chu, S.S., Rah, K.H., Brannan, M.D., and Cohen, J.L.: Plasma concentrations of lidocaine after endotracheal spray. Anesth. Analg. (Cleve.), *54*:438, 1975.
96. Cohen, E.N.: Distribution of local anesthetic agents in the neuraxis of the dog. Anesthesiology, *29*:1002, 1968.
97. Cohen, E.N., Levine, D.A., Colliss, J.E., and Gunther, R.E.: The role of pH in the development of tachyphylaxis to local anesthetic agents. Anesthesiology, *29*:994, 1968.
98. Cohen, S., Luykx, W.M., and Marx, G.F.: High versus low flow rates during lumbar epidural block. Reg. Anaesth., *9*:8, 1984.
99. Colley, P.S., and Heavner, J.E.: Blood levels of bupivacaine after injection into the scalp with and without epinephrine. Anesthesiology, *54*:81, 1981.
100. Collins, J.G., Matsumoto, M., and Kitahara, L.M.: Suppression by spinally administered epinephrine of noxiously evoked dorsal horn neuron activity in cats: Evidence for spinal epinephrine analgesia. Anesth. Analg. (Cleve.), *62*:253, 1983.
101. Collinsworth, K.A., Strong, J.M., Atkinson, A.J., Winkle, R.A., *et al.*: Pharmacokinetics and metabolism of lidocaine in patients with renal failure. Clin. Pharmacol. Ther., *18*:59, 1975.
102. Concepcion, M., Maddi, R., Francis, D., Rocco, A.G., *et al.*: Vasoconstrictors in spinal anesthesia with tetracaine—A comparison of epinephrine and phenylephrine. Anesth. Analg. (Cleve.), *63*:134, 1984.
103. Courtney, K.R.: Structure-activity relations for frequency-dependent sodium channel block in nerve by local anesthetics. J. Pharmacol. Exp. Ther., *213*:114, 1980.
104. Cousins, M.J., and Bromage, P.R.: A comparison of the hydrochloride and carbonated salts of lignocaine for caudal analgesia in outpatients. Br. J. Anaesth., *43*:1149, 1971.
105. Cousins, M.J., and Mather, L.E.: Intrathecal and epidural administration of opioids. Anesthesiology, *61*:276, 1984.
106. Coyle, D.E., Denson, D.D., Thompson, G.A., Myers, J.A., *et al.*: The influence of lactic acid on the serum protein binding of bupivacaine: Species differences. Anesthesiology, *61*:127, 1984.
107. Curran, J., Hamilton, C., and Taylor, T.: Topical analgesia before tracheal intubation. Anaesthesia, *30*:765, 1975.
108. Cusack, B., Kelly, J.G., Lavan, J., Noel, J., *et al.*: Pharmacokinetics of lignocaine in the elderly. Br. J. Clin. Pharmacol., *9*:293P, 1980.
109. Cusick, J.F., Myklebust, J.B., and Abram, S.E.: Differential neural effects of epidural anesthetics. Anesthesiology, *53*:299, 1980.
110. Cusick, J.F., Myklebust, J.B., Abram, S.E., and Davidson, A.: Altered neural conduction with epidural bupivacaine. Anesthesiology, *57*:31, 1982.
111. Datta, S., Houle, G.L., and Fox, G.S.: Concentration of lidocaine hydrochloride in newborn gastric fluid after elective caesarian section and vaginal delivery with epidural analgesia. Can. Anaesth. Soc. J., *22*:79, 1975.
112. Datta, S., Alper, M.H., Ostheimer, G.W., Brown, W.U., *et al.*: Effects of maternal position on epidural anesthesia for Cesarian section, acid-base status, and bupivacaine concentrations at delivery. Anesthesiology, *50*:205, 1979.
113. Datta, S., Brown, W.U., Ostheimer, G.W., Weiss, J.B., *et al.*: Epidural anesthesia for Cesarian section in diabetic parturients: Maternal and neonatal acid-base status and bupivacaine concentration. Anesthesiology, *60*:574, 1981.
114. Davis, D., Grossman, S.H., Kitchell, B.B., Shand, D.G., *et al.*: The effects of age and smoking on the plasma protein binding of lignocaine and diazepam. Br. J. Clin. Pharmacol., *19*:261, 1985.
115. Dawes, G.S.: A theoretical analysis of fetal drug equilibration. *In* Boreus, L. (ed.): Fetal Pharmacology, pp. 381–399. New York, Raven Press, 1973.
116. DeJong, R.H.: Local Anesthetics, pp. 63–83. Springfield, Ill., Charles C Thomas, 1977.
117. Dennhardt, R., and Ammon, K.: Untersuchungen zur Loslichkeit von Bupivacain im Liquor cerebrospinalis. Anaesthesist, *29*:10, 1980.
118. Denson, D.D., Ritschel, W.A., Turner, P.A., Ohlweiler, D.F., *et al.*: A comparison of intravenous and subarachnoid lidocaine pharmacokinetics in the Rhesus monkey. Biopharm. Drug Dispos., *2*:367, 1981.
119. Denson, D.D., Bridenbaugh, P.O., Turner, P.A., Phero, J.C., *et al.*: Neural blockade and pharmacokinetics following subarachnoid lidocaine in the rhesus monkey: I. Effects of epinephrine. Anesth. Analg. (Cleve.), *61*:746, 1982.
120. Denson, D.D., Myers, J.A., Watters, C., and Raj, P.P.: Selective inhibition of the aromatic hydroxylation of bupivacaine by halothane. Anesthesiology, *57*:A242, 1982.
121. Denson, D.D., Bridenbaugh, P.O., Turner, P.A., and Phero, J.C.: Comparison of neural blockade and pharmacokinetics after subarachnoid lidocaine in the rhesus monkey: II. Effects of volume, osmolality, and baricity. Anesth. Analg. (Cleve.), *62*:995, 1983.
122. Denson, D.D., Raj, P.P., Saldahna, F., Finnsson, R.A., *et al.*:

Continuous perineural infusion of bupivacaine for prolonged analgesia: Pharmacokinetic considerations. Int. J. Clin. Pharmacol. Ther. Toxicol., *21*:591, 1983.

123. Denson, D.D., Myers, J.A., and Coyle, D.E.: The clinical relevance of the drug displacement interaction between meperidine and bupivacaine. Res. Commun. Chem. Pathol. Pharmacol., *45*:323, 1984.

124. Denson, D.D., Coyle, D.E., Thompson, G., and Myers, J.A.: Alpha$_1$-acid glycoprotein and albumin in human serum bupivacaine binding. Clin. Pharmacol. Ther., *35*:409, 1984.

125. Denson, D.D., Coyle, D.E., Thompson, G.A., Santos, D., *et al.*: Bupivacaine protein binding in the term parturient: Effects of lactic acidosis. Clin. Pharmacol. Ther., *35*:702, 1984.

126. Denson, D.D., Myers, J.A., Thompson, G.A., and Coyle, D.E.: The influence of diazepam on the serum protein binding of bupivacaine at normal and acidic pH. Anesth. Analg. (Cleve.), *63*:980, 1984.

127. Denson, D.D., Myers, J.A., Hartrick, C.T., Pither, C.P., *et al.*: The relationship between free bupivacaine concentration and central nervous system toxicity. Anesthesiology, *63*:A211, 1984.

128. Denson, D.D., Turner, P.A., Bridenbaugh, P.O., and Thompson, G.A.: Pharmacokinetics and neural blockade after subarachnoid lidocaine in the rhesus monkey: III. Effects of phenylephrine. Anesth. Analg. (Cleve.), *63*:129, 1984.

129. DeRick, A., Rossel, M.T., Belpaire, F., and Bogaert, M.: Lidocaine plasma concentrations obtained with a standardized infusion in the awake and anaesthetized dog. J. Vet. Pharmacol. Ther., *4*:129, 1981.

130. Dhuner, K.G., Frequency of general side reactions after regional anaesthesia with mepivacaine with and without vasoconstrictors. Acta Anaesthesiol. Scand., *48*[*Suppl.*]:23, 1972.

131. Dhuner, K.G., Harthon, J.G.L., Herbring, B.G., and Lie, T.: Blood levels of mepivacaine after regional anaesthesia. Br. J. Anaesth., *37*:746, 1965.

132. Dhuner, K.G., and Lund, N.: Intercostal blocks with etidocaine. Acta Anaesthesiol. Scand., *60*[*Suppl.*]:39, 1975.

133. Dohi, S., Matsumiya, N., Takeshima, R., and Naito, H.: The effects of subarachnoid lidocaine and phenylephrine on spinal cord and cerebral blood flow in dogs. Anesthesiology, *61*:238, 1984.

134. Donchin, Y., Ramu, A., Olshwang, D., Neiman, Z., *et al.*: Effect of sodium bicarbonate on the kinetics of bupivacaine in i.v. regional anaesthesia in dogs. Br. J. Anaesth., *52*:969, 1980.

135. Drayer, D.E., Lorenzo, B., Werns, S., and Reidenberg, M.M.: Plasma levels, protein binding, and elimination data of lidocaine and active metabolites in cardiac patients of various ages. Clin. Pharmacol. Ther., *34*:14, 1983.

136. Dubé, L.M., Ngoc, A.H., Davies, R.F., Beanlands, D.S., *et al.*: Influence of protamine on heparin-induced increases of lidocaine free fraction. Res. Commun. Chem. Pathol. Pharmacol., *42*:401, 1983.

137. Dudziak, R., and Uihlein, M.: Loslichkeit von Lokalanaesthetika im Liquor cerebrospinalis und ihre Abhangigkeit von der Wasserstoffion-enkonzentration. Anaesthesist, *27*:32, 1978.

138. DuSouich, P., and Erill, S.: Altered metabolism of procainamide and procaine in patients with pulmonary and cardiac diseases. Clin. Pharmacol. Ther., *21*:101, 1977.

139. Ecoffey, C., Desparmet, J., Berdeaux, A., Maury, M., *et al.*: Pharmacokinetics of lignocaine in children following caudal anaesthesia. Br. J. Anaesth., *56*:1399, 1984.

140. Edwards, D.J., Lalka, D., Cerra, F., and Slaughter, R.L.: Alpha$_1$-acid glycoprotein concentration and protein binding in trauma. Clin. Pharmacol. Ther., *31*:62, 1982.

141. Ekenstam, B.: The effect of the structural variation on the local analgetic properties of the most commonly used groups of substances. Acta Anaesthesiol. Scand., *25*[*Suppl.*]:10, 1966.

142. Elvin, A.T., Cole, A.F.D., Pieper, J.A., Rolbin, S.H., *et al.*: Effects of food on lidocaine kinetics: Mechanisms of food-related alteration in high intrinsic clearance drug elimination. Clin. Pharmacol. Ther., *30*:455, 1981.

143. Engberg, G., Holmdahl, M.H., and Edstrom, H.H.: A comparison of the local anesthetic properties of bupivacaine and two new long-acting agents, HS-37 and etidocaine, in epidural analgesia. Acta Anaesthesiol. Scand., *18*:277, 1974.

144. Englesson, S.: The influence of acid-base changes on central nervous system toxicity of local anaesthetic agents: I. An experimental study in cats. Acta Anaesthesiol. Scand., *18*:79, 1974.

145. Englesson, S., and Grevsten, S.: The influence of acid-base changes on central nervous system toxicity of local anaesthetic agents: II. Acta Anaesthesiol. Scand., *18*:88, 1974.

146. Erdemir, H.A., Soper, L.E., and Sweet, R.E.: Studies of the factors affecting peridural anesthesia. Anesth. Analg. (Cleve.), *44*:400, 1966.

147. Eriksson, E.: Prilocaine, an experimental study in man of a new local anaesthetic with special regards to efficacy, toxicity and excretion. Acta Chir. Scand., *358*[*Suppl.*]:55, 1966.

148. Evans, C.J., Dewar, J.A., Boyes, R.N., and Scott, D.B.: Residual nerve block following intravenous regional anaesthesia. Br. J. Anaesth., *46*:668, 1974.

149. Eyres, R.L., Kidd, J., Oppenheim, R., and Brown, T.C.K.: Local anaesthetic plasma levels in children. Anaesth. Intens. Care, *6*:243, 1978.

150. Eyres, R.L., Bishop, W., Oppenheim, R.C., and Brown, T.C.K.: Plasma lignocaine concentrations following topical laryngeal application. Anaesth. Intensive Care, *11*:23, 1983.

151. Eyres, R.L., Bishop, W., Oppenheim, R.C., and Brown, T.C.K.: Plasma bupivacaine concentrations in children during caudal epidural analgesia. Anaesth. Intensive Care, *11*:20, 1983.

152. Fairley, J.W., and Reynolds, F.: An intradermal study of the local anaesthetic and vascular effects of the isomers of mepivacaine. Br. J. Anaesth., *53*:1211, 1981.

153. Feely, J., Wade, D., McAllister, C.B., Wilkinson, G.R., *et al.*: Effect of hypotension on liver blood flow and lidocaine disposition. N. Engl. J. Med., *307*:866, 1982.

154. Feely, J., Wilkinson, G.R., McAllister, C.B., and Wood, A.J.J.: Increased toxicity and reduced clearance of lidocaine by cimetidine. Ann. Intern. Med., *96*:592, 1982.

155. Feely, J., and Guy, E.: Lack of effect of ranitidine on the disposition of lignocaine. Br. J. Clin. Pharmacol., *15*:378, 1983.
156. Feely, J., Clee, M., Pereira, L., and Guy, E.: Enzyme inhibition with rifampicin; lipoproteins and drug binding to alpha$_1$-acid glycoprotein. Br. J. Clin. Pharmacol., *16*:195, 1983.
156a. Finster, M., Perel, J.M., Hinsvark, O.N., and O'Brien, J.E.: Reassessment of the metabolism of 2-chloroprocaine hydrochloride (Nesacaine). *In* Abstracts of Scientific Papers—Annual Meeting, San Francisco. Chicago, American Society of Anesthesiologists, 1973.
157. Fish, F., and Wilson, W.D.C.: Excretion of cocaine and its metabolites in man. J. Pharm. Pharmacol., *21*:153s, 1969.
158. Fink, B.R., and Cairns, A.M.: Diffusional delay in local anesthetic block in vitro. Anesthesiology, *61*:555, 1984.
159. Finucane, B.T., and Hammonds, W.D.: Influence of age on vascular absorption of lidocaine injected epidurally in man. Reg. Anaesth., *9*:36, 1984.
160. Foldes, F.F., Davidson, G.N., Duncalf, D., and Kuwabarra, S.: The intravenous toxicity of local anesthetic agents in man. Clin. Pharmacol. Ther., *6*:328, 1965.
161. Ford, D.J., Raj, P.P., Regan, K.M., and Ohlweiler, D.: Differential peripheral nerve block by local anesthetics in the cat. Anesthesiology, *60*:28, 1984.
162. Freund, P.R., Bowdle, T.A., Slattery, J.T., and Bell, L.E.: Caudal anesthesia with lidocaine or bupivacaine: Plasma local anesthetic concentration and extent of sensory spread in old and young patients. Anesth. Analg. (Cleve.), *63*:1017, 1984.
163. Friedman, G.A., Rowlingson, J.C., DiFazio, C.A., and Donegan, M.F.: Evaluation of the analgesic effect and urinary excretion of systemic bupivacaine in man. Anesth. Analg. (Cleve.), *61*:23, 1982.
164. Fukuda, J., and Momose, A.: Determination of tetracaine N-oxide in urine by gas chromatography. Yakugaku Zasshi, *95*:480, 1975.
165. Fukui, T., Hameroff, S.R., and Gandolfi, A.J.: Alpha-1-acid glycoprotein and beta-endorphin alterations in chronic pain patients. Anesthesiology, *60*:494, 1984.
165a. Fijimori, M., Kato, M., Nishimura, K., and Kataoka, T.: LAC-43 (Marcain) in epidural anesthesia and its blood concentrations. Jpn. J. Anesthesiol., *16*:307, 1967.
166. Ghoneim, M.M., and Pandya, H.: Plasma protein binding of bupivacaine and its interaction with other drugs in man. Br. J. Anaesth., *46*:435, 1974.
167. Giasi, R.M., D'Agostino, E., and Covino, B.G.: Absorption of lidocaine following subarachnoid and epidural administration. Anesth. Analg. (Cleve.), *58*:360, 1979.
168. Giasi, R.M., D'Agostino, E., and Covino, B.G.: Interaction of diazepam and epidurally administered local anesthetic agents. Reg. Anaesth., *3*:8, 1980.
169. Gissen, A.J., Covino, B.G., and Gregus, J.: Differential sensitivity of fast and slow fibers in mammalian nerve: III. Effect of etidocaine and bupivacaine on fast/slow fibers. Anesth. Analg. (Cleve.), *61*:570, 1982.
170. Goehl, T.J., Davenport, J.B., and Stanley, M.J.: Distribution, biotransformation and excretion of bupivacaine in the rat and the monkey. Xenobiotica, *3*:761, 1973.
171. Goldberg, M.J., Spector, R., and Johnson, G.F.: Racial background and lidocaine pharmacokinetics. J. Clin. Pharmacol., *22*:391, 1982.
172. Gomez, F., Barrueco, M., Lanao, J.M., Vicente, M.T., *et al.*: Serum lidocaine levels in patients undergoing fibrobronchoscopy. Ther. Drug Monit., *5*:201, 1983.
173. Goolkasian, D.L., Slaughter, R.L., Edwards, D.J., and Lalka, D.: Displacement of lidocaine from serum alpha$_1$-acid glycoprotein binding sites by basic drugs. Eur. J. Clin. Pharmacol., *25*:413, 1983.
174. Greene, N.M.: The metabolism of drugs employed in anesthesia. Anesthesiology, *29*:327, 1968.
175. Greene, N.M.: Uptake and elimination of local anesthetics during spinal anesthesia. Anesth. Analg. (Cleve.), *62*:1013, 1983.
176. Gross, T.L., Kuhnert, P.M., and Kuhnert, B.R.: Plasma levels of 2-chloroprocaine and lack of sequelae following an apparent inadvertent intravenous injection. Anesthesiology, *54*:173, 1981.
177. Grossman, S.H., Davis, D., Kitchell, B.B., Shand, D.G., *et al.*: Diazepam and lidocaine plasma protein binding in renal disease. Clin. Pharmacol. Ther., *31*:350, 1982.
178. Grundy, E.M., Ramamurthy, S., Patel, K.P., Mani, M., *et al.*: Extradural analgesia revisited. Br. J. Anaesth., *50*:805, 1978.
179. Grundy, E.M., Rao, L.N., and Winnie, A.P.: Epidural anesthesia and the lateral position. Anesth. Analg. (Cleve.), *57*:95, 1978.
180. Ha, H.R., Vozeh, S., and Follath, F.: Measurement of free lidocaine serum concentration by equilibrium dialysis and ultrafiltration techniques. The influence of pH and heparin. Clin. Pharmacokinet., *9*[*Suppl.*]:96, 1984.
181. Halkin, H., Meffin, P., Melmon, K.L., and Rowland, M.: Influence of congestive heart failure on blood levels of lidocaine and its active monodeethylated metabolite. Clin. Pharmacol. Ther., *17*:669, 1975.
182. Halpern, S.H., Eisler, E.A., Shnider, S.M., Shapiro, D.A., *et al.*: Myocardial tissue uptake of bupivacaine and lidocaine after intravenous injection in normal and acidotic rabbits. Anesthesiology, *61*:A208, 1984.
183. Hamshaw-Thomas, A., Rogerson, N., and Reynolds, F.: Transfer of bupivacaine, lignocaine and pethidine across the rabbit placenta: Influence of maternal protein binding and fetal flow. Placenta, *5*:61, 1984.
184. Hansson, E., Hoffmann, P., and Kristerson, L.: Fate of mepivacaine in the body: II. Excretion and biotransformation. Acta Pharmacol. Toxicol. (Kbh.), *22*:213, 1965.
185. Hartrick, C.T., Dirkes, W.E., Coyle, D.E., Raj, P.P., *et al.*: Influence of bupivacaine on mepivacaine protein binding. Clin. Pharmacol. Ther., *36*:546, 1984.
186. Hartrick, C.T., Raj, P.P., Dirkes, W.E., and Denson, D.D.: Compounding of bupivacaine and mepivacaine for regional anesthesia. A safe practice? Reg. Anaesth., *9*:94, 1984.
187. Hasselstrom, L., Nortved–Sorensen, J., Kehlet, H., Juel–Christensen, N., *et al.*: Influence of systemically administered bupivacaine on cardiovascular function in cholecystectomised patients. Acta Anaesthesiol. Scand. (in press).
188. Hawks, R.L., Kopin, I.J., Colburn, R.W., and Thoa, N.B.: Norcocaine: A pharmacologically active metabolite of cocaine found in brain. Life Sci., *15*:2189, 1974.

189. Hjelm, M., and Holmdahl, M.H.: Biochemical effects of aromatic amines: II. Cyanosis, methaemoglobinaemia and Heinz-body formation induced by a local anaesthetic agent (prilocaine). Acta Anaesthesiol. Scand., *9*:99, 1965.
190. Hodgkinson, R., and Husain, F.J.: Obesity, gravity and spread of epidural anesthesia. Anesth. Analg. (Cleve.), *60*:421, 1981.
191. Holley, F.O., Ponganis, K.V., and Stanski, D.R.: Effects of cardiac surgery with cardiopulmonary bypass on lidocaine disposition. Clin. Pharmacol. Ther., *35*:617, 1984.
192. Hollmen, A., Korhonen, M., and Ojala, A.: Bupivacaine in paracervical block: Plasma levels and changes in maternal and foetal acid–base balance. Br. J. Anaesth., *41*:603, 1969.
193. Hollmen, A., Ojala, A., and Korhonen, M.: Paracervical block with marcaine/adrenaline. Acta Anaesthesiol. Scand., *13*:1, 1969.
194. Howarth, F.: Studies with a radioactive spinal anaesthetic. Br. J. Pharmacol., *4*:333, 1949.
195. Huet, P-M., and LeLorier, J.: Effects of smoking and chronic hepatitis B on lidocaine and indocyanine green kinetics. Clin. Pharmacol. Ther., *28*:208, 1980.
196. Huet, P-M., and Villeneuve, J–P.: Determinants of drug disposition in patients with cirrhosis. Hepatology, *3*:913, 1983.
197. Huet, P-M., Arsene, D., and Richer, D.: The volume of distribution of lidocaine in chronic hepatitis: Relationship with serum alpha$_1$-acid glycoprotein and serum protein binding. Clin. Pharmacol. Ther., *29*:252, 1981.
198. Husemeyer, R.P., and White, D.C.: Lumbar extradural injection pressures in pregnant women. An investigation of relationships between rate of injection, injection pressures and extent of analgesia. Br. J. Anaesth., *52*:55, 1980.
199. Igarishi, K., Kasuya, F., and Fukui, M.: Metabolism of dibucaine: Isolation and identification of urinary basic metabolites in the rat, rabbit and man. J. Pharmacobiodyn. *6*:538, 1983.
200. Irestedt, L., Andreen, M., Belfrage, P., and Fagerstrom, T.: The elimination of bupivacaine (Marcain) after short intravenous infusion in the dog with special reference to the role played by the liver and lung. Acta Anaesthesiol. Scand., *22*:413, 1978.
201. Jackson, P.R., Tucker, G.T., and Woods, H.F.: Altered plasma binding in cancer: Role of alpha$_1$-acid glycoprotein and albumin. Clin. Pharmacol. Ther., *32*:295, 1982.
202. Javaid, J.I., Musa, M.N., Fischman, M., Schuster, C.R., *et al.*: Kinetics of cocaine in humans after intravenous and intranasal administration. Biopharm. Drug Dispos., *4*:9, 1983.
203. Johansson, P–A.: Liquid–liquid distribution of lidocaine and some structurally related antiarrhythmic drugs and some local anaesthetics. Acta Pharm. Suec., *19*:137, 1982.
204. Johns, R.A., DiFazio, C.A., and Longnecker, D.E.: Lidocaine constricts or dilates rat arterioles in a dose-dependent manner. Anesthesiology, *62*:141, 1985.
205. Jones, D.A., McBurney, A., Stanley, P.J., Tovey, C., *et al.*: Plasma concentrations of lignocaine and its metabolites during fibreoptic bronchoscopy. Br. J. Anaesth., *54*:853, 1982.
205a. Jorfeldt, L., Lofstrom, B., Pernow, B., Persson, B., *et al.*: The effect of local anaesthetics on the central circulation and respiration in man and dog. Acta Anaesthesiol. Scand., *12*:153, 1968.
206. Jorfeldt, L., Lewis, D.H., Lofstrom, B., and Post, C.: Lung uptake of lidocaine in healthy volunteers. Acta Anaesthesiol. Scand., *23*:567, 1979.
207. Jorfeldt, L., Lewis, D.H., Lofstrom, B., and Post, C.: Lung uptake of lidocaine in man as influenced by anaesthesia, mepivacaine infusion or lung insufficiency. Acta Anaesthesiol. Scand., *27*:5, 1983.
208. Kalow, W.: Hydrolysis of local anesthetics by human serum cholinesterase. J. Pharmacol. Exp. Ther., *104*:122, 1952.
209. Kanto, J., Jalonen, J., Laurikainen, E., Nieminen, V., *et al.*: Plasma concentrations of lidocaine (lignocaine) after cranial subcutaneous injection during neurosurgical operations. Acta Anaesthesiol. Scand., *24*:178, 1980.
210. Kaplan, J.A., Miller, E.D., and Gallagher, E.G.: Postoperative analgesia for thoracotomy patients. Anesth. Analg. (Cleve.), *54*:773, 1975.
211. Karvonen, S., Jokinen, K., Karvonen, P., and Hollmen, A.: Arterial and venous blood lidocaine concentrations after local anaesthesia of the respiratory tract using an ultrasonic nebulizer. Acta Anaesthesiol. Scand., *20*:156, 1976.
212. Kates, R.E., Harapat, S.R., Keefe, D.L.D., Goldwater, D., *et al.*: Influence of prolonged recumbency on drug disposition. Clin. Pharmacol. Ther., *27*:624, 1980.
213. Keenaghan, J.B., and Boyes, R.N.: The tissue distribution, metabolism and excretion of lidocaine in rats, guinea pigs, dogs and man. J. Pharmacol. Exp. Ther., *180*:454, 1972.
214. Kennedy, R.L., Erenberg, A., Robilliard, J.E., Merkow, A., *et al.*: Effects of the changes in maternal–fetal pH on the transplacental equilibrium of bupivacaine. Anesthesiology, *51*:50, 1979.
215. Kennedy, W.F., Everett, G.B., Cobb, L.A., and Allen, G.D.: Simultaneous systemic and hepatic hemodynamic measurements during high peridural anesthesia in normal men. Anesth. Analg. (Cleve.), *50*:1069, 1971.
216. Kitahara, T., Juri, S., and Yoshida, J.: The spread of drugs used for spinal anesthesia. Anesthesiology, *17*:295, 1956.
217. Klingenstrom, P., Nylen, B., and Westermark, L.: A clinical comparison between adrenaline and octapressin as vasoconstrictors in local anaesthesia. Acta Anaesthesiol. Scand., *11*:35, 1967.
218. Kloss, M.W., Rosen, G.M., and Rauckman, E.J.: Cocaine-mediated hepatotoxicity. Biochem. Pharmacol., *33*:169, 1984.
219. Kogan, M.J., Verebey, K.G., Depace, A.C., Resnick, R.B., *et al.*: Quantitative determination of benzoylecgonine and cocaine in human biofluids by gas-liquid chromatography. Anal. Chem., *49*:1965, 1977.
220. Koster, H., Shapiro, A., and Leikensohn, A.: Procaine concentration changes at the site of injection in subarachnoid anesthesia. Am. J. Surg., *33*:245, 1936.
221. Kozody, R., Palahniuk, R.J., and Cumming, M.O.: Spinal cord blood flow following subarachnoid tetracaine. Can. Anaesth. Soc. J., *32*:23, 1985.
222. Kozody, R., Swartz, J., Palahniuk, R.J., Biehl, D., *et al.*: Spinal cord blood flow following subarachnoid lidocaine. Anesth. Analg. (Cleve.), *64*:185, 1985.
223. Krogh, K., and Jellum, E.: Urinary metabolites of chloropro-

caine studied by combined gas chromatography-mass spectrometry. Anesthesiology, *54*:329, 1981.

224. Krogh, K., and Jellum, E.: Urinary metabolites of chloroprocaine. Anesthesiology, *56*:483, 1982.

225. Kuhnert, B.R., Knapp, D.R., Kuhnert, P.M., and Prochaska, A.L.: Maternal, fetal, and neonatal metabolism of lidocaine. Clin. Pharmacol. Ther., *26*:213, 1979.

226. Kuhnert, B.R., Kuhnert, P.M., Prochaska, A.L., and Gross, T.L.: Plasma levels of 2-chloroprocaine in obstetric patients and their neonates after epidural anesthesia. Anesthesiology, *53*:21, 1980.

227. Kuhnert, B.R., Kuhnert, P.M., Reese, A.L.P., Philipson, E.H., *et al.*: Maternal and neonatal elimination of CABA after epidural anesthesia with 2-chloroprocaine during parturition. Anesth. Analg. (Cleve.), *62*:1089, 1983.

228. Kuhnert, P.M., Kuhnert, B.R., Stitts, J.M., and Gross, T.L.: The use of a selected ion monitoring technique to study the disposition of bupivacaine in mother, fetus, and neonate following epidural anesthesia for Cesarian section. Anesthesiology, *55*:611, 1981.

229. Labedzki, L., Ochs, H.R., Abernethy, D.R., and Greenblatt, D.J.: Potentially toxic serum lidocaine concentrations following spray anesthesia for bronchoscopy. Klin. Wochenschr., *61*:379, 1983.

230. Lalka, D., Vicuna, N., Burrow, S.R., Jones, D.J., *et al.*: Bupivacaine and other amide local anesthetics inhibit hydrolysis of chloroprocaine by human serum. Anesth. Analg. (Cleve.), *57*:534, 1978.

231. LaRosa, C., Morgan, D.J., and Mather, L.E.: Pethidine binding in whole blood: Methodology and clinical significance. Br. J. Clin. Pharmacol. *7*:405, 1984.

232. Laurikainen, E., Marttila, R., Lindberg, R., and Kanto, J.: Penetration of lidocaine and its active desethylated metabolite into cerebrospinal fluid in man. Eur. J. Clin. Pharmacol., *25*:639, 1983.

233. LeLorier, J., Grenon, D., Latour, Y., Caille, G., *et al.*: Pharmacokinetics of lidocaine after prolonged intravenous infusions in uncomplicated myocardial infarction. Ann. Intern. Med., *87*:700, 1977.

234. LeLorier, J., Larochelle, P., Bolduc, P., Clermont, R., *et al.*: Lidocaine plasma concentrations during and after endoscopic procedures. Int. J. Clin. Pharmacol. Biopharm., *17*:53, 1979.

235. Lennard, M.S., Tucker, G.T., and Woods, H.F.: Time-dependent kinetics of lignocaine in the isolated perfused rat liver. J. Pharmacokinet. Biopharm., *11*:165, 1983.

236. Lips, F.J., O'Reilly, J., Close, D., Beaumont, G.D., *et al.*: The effects of formulation and addition of adrenaline to cocaine for haemostasis in intranasal surgery. Anaesth. Intensive Care (in press).

237. Liston, W.A., Adjepon-Yamoah, K.K., and Scott, D.B.: Foetal and maternal lignocaine levels after paracervical block. Br. J. Anaesth., *45*:750, 1973.

238. Loder, R.E.: A local anaesthetic solution with longer action. Lancet, *2*:346, 1960.

239. Loder, R.E.: Lidocaine-dextran solutions. Anesthesiology, *53*:522, 1980.

240. Lofstrom, B.: Blocking characteristics of etidocaine (Duranest). Acta Anaesthesiol. Scand., *60*[*Suppl.*]:21, 1975.

241. Lofstrom, B.: Tissue distribution of local anesthetics with special reference to the lung. Int. Anesthesiol. Clin., *16*:53, 1978.

242. Luduena, F.P.: Duration of local anesthesia. Annu. Rev. Pharmacol., *9*:503, 1969.

243. Luduena, F.P., Bogado, E.F., and Tullar, B.F.: Optical isomers of mepivacaine and bupivacaine. Arch. Int. Pharmacodyn. Ther., *200*:359, 1972.

244. Lund, P.C., Bush, D.F., and Covino, B.G.: Determinants of etidocaine concentration in the blood. Anesthesiology, *42*:497, 1975.

245. Lund, P.C., and Covino, B.G.: Distribution of local anesthetics in man following peridural anesthesia. J. Clin. Pharmacol., *7*:324, 1967.

246. Lund, P.C., and Cwik, J.C.: Citanest: A clinical and laboratory study. Anesth. Analg. (Cleve.), *44*:623, 1965.

247. Lund, P.C., and Cwik, J.C.: A correlation of the differential penetration and the systemic toxicity of lidocaine, mepivacaine and prilocaine in man. Acta Anaesthesiol. Scand., *23*[*Suppl.*]:475, 1966.

248. Lund, P.C., and Cwik, J.C., and Gannon, R.T.: Etidocaine (Duranest): A clinical and laboratory evaluation. Acta Anaesthesiol. Scand., *18*:176, 1974.

249. Lund, P.C., and Cwik, J.C., and Pagdanganan, R.T.: Etidocaine: A new long-acting local anesthetic agent. Anesth. Analg. (Cleve.), *52*:482, 1973.

250. Lund, P.C., Cwik, J.C., Gannon, R.T., and Vassallo, H.G.: Etidocaine for Caesarian section—Effects on mother and baby. Br. J. Anaesth., *49*:457, 1977.

251. McLean, S., Starmer, G.A., and Thomas, J.: Methaemoglobin formation by aromatic amines. J. Pharm. Pharmacol., *21*:441, 1969.

252. Magno, R., Berlin, A., Karlsson, K., and Kjellmer, I.: Anesthesia for Cesarian section IV: Placental transfer and neonatal elimination of bupivacaine following epidural analgesia for elective Cesarian section. Acta Anaesthesiol. Scand., *20*:141, 1976.

253. Malagodi, M.H., Munson, E.S., and Embro, M.J.: Relation of etidocaine and bupivacaine toxicity to rate of infusion in rhesus monkeys. Br. J. Anaesth., *49*:121, 1977.

254. Martin, R., Lamarche, Y., and Tetreault, L.: Comparison of the clinical effectiveness of lidocaine hydrocarbonate and lidocaine hydrocloride with and without epinephrine in epidural anaesthesia. Can. Anaesth. Soc. J., *28*:217, 1981.

255. Mather, L.E.: Tachyphylaxis in regional anaesthesia: Can we reconcile clinical observation and laboratory measurements? Anaesth. Intenzivemed. *176*:3, 1986.

256. Mather, L.E., and Cousins, M.J.: Local anaesthetics and their current clinical use. Drugs, *18*:185, 1979.

257. Mather, L.E., Long, G.J., and Thomas, J.: The binding of bupivacaine to maternal and foetal plasma proteins. J. Pharm. Pharmacol., *23*:359, 1971.

258. Mather, L.E., Long, G.J., and Thomas, J.: The intravenous toxicity and clearance of bupivacaine in man. Clin. Pharmacol. Ther., *12*:935, 1971.

259. Mather, L.E., Runciman, W.B., Carapetis, R.J., Ilsley, A.H., *et al.*: Hepatic and renal clearances of lidocaine in conscious and anesthetized sheep. Anesth. Analg. (Cleve.), *65*:943, 1986.

260. Mather, L.E., and Thomas, J.: Metabolism of lidocaine in man. Life Sci., *11*:915, 1972.
261. Mather, L.E., and Thomas, J.: Bupivacaine binding to plasma protein fractions. J. Pharm. Pharmacol., *30*:653, 1978.
262. Mather, L.E., Tucker, G.T., Murphy, T.M., Stanton-Hicks, M., *et al.*: Effect of adding adrenaline to etidocaine and lignocaine in extradural anaesthesia. II: Pharmacokinetics. Br. J. Anaesth., *48*:989, 1976.
263. Mather, L.E., Tucker, G.T., Murphy, T.M., Stanton-Hicks, M., *et al.*: Haemodynamic drug interactions: Peridural lignocaine and intravenous ephedrine. Acta Anaesthesiol. Scand., *20*:207, 1976.
264. Mather, L.E., Tucker, G.T., Murphy, T.M., Stanton-Hicks, M., *et al.*: Cardiovascular and subjective central nervous system effects of long-acting local anaesthetics in man. Anaesth. Intensive Care, *7*:215, 1979.
265. Matthes, H., and Schabert, P.: Vergleichende Undersuchungen uber Blutspiegel von mepivacain nach Resorption aus verscheidenen geweben. Acta Anaesthesiol. Scand., *23*[*Suppl.*]:371, 1966.
266. Mayumi, T., Dohi, S., and Takahashi, T.: Plasma concentrations of lidocaine associated with cervical, thoracic, and lumbar epidural anesthesia. Anesth. Analg. (Cleve.), *62*:578, 1983.
267. Mazze, R.I., and Dunbar, R.W.: Plasma lidocaine concentrations after caudal, lumbar epidural, axillary block and intravenous regional anesthesia. Anesthesiology, *27*:574, 1966.
268. McBurney, A., Jones, D.A., Stanley, P.J., and Ward, J.W.: Absorption of lignocaine and bupivacaine from the respiratory tract during fibreoptic bronchoscopy. Br. J. Clin. Pharmacol., *17*:61, 1984.
269. McClure, J.H., and Scott, D.B.: Comparison of bupivacaine hydrochloride and carbonated bupivacaine in brachial plexus block interscalene technique. Br. J. Anaesth., *53*:523, 1981.
270. McNamara, P.J., Slaughter, R.L., Visco, J.P., Elwood, C.M., *et al.*: Effect of smoking on binding of lidocaine to human serum proteins. J. Pharm. Sci., *69*:749, 1980.
271. McNamara, P.J., Slaughter, R.L., Pieper, J.A., Wyman, W.G., *et al.*: Factors influencing serum protein binding of lidocaine in humans. Anesth. Analg. (Cleve.), *60*:395, 1981.
272. Meffin, P., Long, G.J., and Thomas, J.: Clearance and metabolism of mepivacaine in the human neonate. Clin. Pharmacol. Ther., *14*:219, 1973.
273. Meffin, P., Robertson, A.V., Thomas, J., and Winkler, J.: Neutral metabolites of mepivacaine in humans. Xenobiotica, 3:191, 1973.
274. Meffin, P., and Thomas, J.: The relative rates of formation of the phenolic metabolites of mepivacaine in man. Xenobiotica, *3*:625, 1973.
275. Merry, A.F., Cross, J.A., Mayadeo, S.V., and Wild, C.J.: Posture and spread of extradural analgesia in labour. Br. J. Anaesth., *55*:303, 1983.
276. Meyer, J., and Nolte, H.: Liquorkonzentrationen zur bupivacain nach subduraler applikation. Anaesthesist, *29*:38, 1978.
277. Mihaly, G.W., Moore, R.G., Thomas, J., Triggs, E.G., *et al.*: The pharmacokinetics of the anilide local anaesthetic in neonates. I: Lignocaine. Eur. J. Clin. Pharmacol., *13*:143, 1978.
278. Momose, A., and Fukuda, J.: A new metabolite of tetracaine. Chem. Pharm. Bull., *24*:1637, 1976.
279. Moore, D.C.: The pH of local anesthetic solutions. Anesth. Analg. (Cleve.), *60*:833, 1981.
280. Moore, D.C.: Intercostal nerve block: Spread of India ink injected to the rib's costal groove. Br. J. Anaesth., *53*:325, 1981.
281. Moore, D.C., Bridenbaugh, L.D., Van Ackeren, E.G., Belda, F.B., *et al.*: Spread of radio-opaque solutions in the epidural space of the human adult corpse. Anesthesiology, *19*:377, 1957.
282. Moore, D.C., Bridenbaugh, L.D., Bridenbaugh, P.O., Thompson, G.E., *et al.*: Does compounding of local anesthetic agents increase their toxicity in humans? Anesth. Analg. (Cleve.), *51*:579, 1972.
283. Moore, D.C., Mather, L.E., Bridenbaugh, L.D., Balfour, R.I., *et al.*: Arterial and venous plasma levels of bupivacaine (Marcaine) following epidural and intercostal nerve blocks. Anesthesiology, *45*:39, 1976.
284. Moore, D.C., Bush, W.H., and Scurlock, J.E.: Intercostal nerve block: A roentgenographic anatomic study of technique and absorption in humans. Anesth. Analg. (Cleve.), *59*:815, 1980.
285. Moore, D.C., Bush, W.H., and Burnett, L.L.: Celiac plexus block: A roentgenographic, anatomic study of technique and spread of solution in patients and corpses. Anesth. Analg. (Cleve.), *60*:369, 1981.
286. Moore, D.C., Mather, L.E., Bridenbaugh, P.O., Balfour, R.I., *et al.*: Arterial and venous plasma levels of bupivacaine following peripheral nerve blocks. Anesth. Analg. (Cleve.), *55*:763, 1976.
287. Moore, D.C., Mather, L.E., Bridenbaugh, L.D., Thompson, G.E., *et al.*: Bupivacaine (Marcaine): An evaluation of its tissue and systemic toxicity in humans. Acta Anaesthesiol. Scand., *21*:109, 1977.
288. Moore, R.A., Bullingham, R.E.S., McQuay, H.J., Hand, C.W., *et al.*: Dural permeability to narcotics: In vitro determination and application to extradural administration. Br. J. Anaesth., *54*:1117, 1982.
289. Moore, R.G., Thomas, J., Triggs, E.J., Thomas, B.D., *et al.*: The pharmacokinetics and metabolism of the anilide local anaesthetics in neonates. III: Mepivacaine. Eur. J. Clin. Pharmacol., *14*:203, 1978.
290. Morgan, D.J., Smyth, M.P., Thomas, J., and Vine, J.: Cyclic metabolites of etidocaine in humans. Xenobiotica, *7*:365, 1977.
291. Morgan, D.J., Cousins, M.J., McQuillan, D., and Thomas, J.: Pharmacokinetics and metabolism of the anilide local anaesthetics in neonates. II: Etidocaine. Eur. J. Clin. Pharmacol., *13*:365, 1978.
292. Morgan, D.J., Koay, B.B., and Paull, J.D.: Plasma protein binding of etidocaine during pregnancy and labour. Eur. J. Clin. Pharmacol., *22*:451, 1982.
293. Morikawa, K.I., Bonica, J.J., Tucker, G.T., and Murphy, T.M.: Effect of acute hypovolaemia on lignocaine absorption and cardiovascular response following epidural block in dogs. Br. J. Anaesth., *46*:631, 1974.

294. Morishima, H.O., Mueller-Heubach, E., and Shnider, S.M.: Body temperature and disappearance of lidocaine in newborn puppies. Anesth. Analg. (Cleve.), *50*:938, 1971.

295. Morison, D.H.: A double blind comparison of carbonated lidocaine and lidocaine hydrochloride in epidural anaesthesia. Can. Anaesth. Soc. J., *28*:387, 1981.

296. Morrell, D.F., Chappell, W.A., and White, I.W.C.: Topical analgesia of the upper airway with lignocaine. Absorption and its relationship to toxic and anti-arrhythmic levels. S. Afr. Med. J., 551, April 10, 1982.

297. Murphy, T.M., Mather, L.E., Stanton-Hicks, M.d'A., Bonica, J.J., *et al.*: Effects of adding adrenaline to etidocaine and lignocaine in extradural anaesthesia. I: Block characteristics and cardiovascular effects. Br. J. Anaesth., *48*:893, 1976.

298. Murphy, T.M., Mather, L.E., Zachariah, P., Butler, S.H., *et al.*: Effects of premedication on the blood concentrations and cardiovascular effects of lidocaine used in epidural block. Anesth. Analg. (Cleve.) (submitted).

299. Nancarrow, C.: Acute Toxicity of Lignocaine and Bupivacaine. Ph.D. Thesis, Flinders University of South Australia, 1986.

300. Nation, R.L., Triggs, E.J., and Selig, M.: Lignocaine kinetics in cardiac patients and aged subjects. Br. J. Clin. Pharmacol., *4*:439, 1977.

301. Nayak, P.K., Misra, A.Z., and Mule, S.J.: Physiological disposition and biotransformation of ^{3}H-cocaine in acutely and chronically treated rats. J. Pharmacol. Exp. Ther., *196*:556, 1976.

302. Neill, R.S., and Watson, R.: Plasma bupivacaine concentrations during combined regional and general anaesthesia for resection and reconstruction of head and neck carcinomata. Br. J. Anaesth., *56*:485, 1984.

303. Nelson, S.D., Breck, G.D., and Trager, W.F.: *In vivo* metabolite condensations. Formation of N1-ethyl-2-methyl-N3-(2,6-dimethylphenyl)-4-imidazolinone from the reaction of a metabolite of alcohol with a metabolite of lidocaine. J. Med. Chem., *16*:1106, 1973.

304. Nelson, S.D., Garland, W.A., Breck, G.D., and Trager, W.F.: Quantification of lidocaine and several metabolites utilizing chemical-ionization mass spectrometry and stable isotope labelling. J. Pharm. Sci., *66*:1180, 1977.

305. Nelson, S.D., Garland, W.A., and Trager, W.F.: Lack of evidence for the formation of N-hydroxyamide metabolites of lidocaine in man. Res. Commun. Chem. Pathol. Pharmacol., *8*:45, 1974.

306. Nishimura, N., Kitahara, T., and Kusakabo, T.: The spread of lidocaine and I-131 solution in the epidural space. Anesthesiology, *20*:785, 1959.

307. Nordqvist, P.: The occurrence of procaine esterase in peripheral nerve and its influence on procaine block. Acta Pharmacol. Toxicol. (Kbh.), *8*:217, 1952.

308. Nunn, J.E., and Slavin, G.: Posterior intercostal nerve block for pain relief after cholecystectomy. Br. J. Anaesth., *52*:253, 1980.

309. O'Brien, J.E., Abbey, V., Hinsvark, O., Perel, J., *et al.*: Metabolism and measurement of chloroprocaine, an ester-type local anesthetic. J. Pharm. Sci., *68*:75, 1979.

310. Palmer, S.K., Bosnjak, Z.J., Hopp, F., von Colditz, J.H., *et al.*: Lidocaine and bupivacaine differential blockade of isolated canine nerves. Anesth. Analg. (Cleve.), *62*:754, 1983.

311. Pardridge, W.M., Sakiyama, R., and Fierer, G.: Transport of propranolol and lidocaine through the rat blood-brain barrier. Primary role of globulin-bound drug. J. Clin. Invest., *71*:900, 1983.

312. Park, W.Y., Massengale, M., Kin, S-I., Poon, K.C., *et al.*: Age and the spread of local anesthetic solutions in the epidural space. Anesth. Analg. (Cleve.), *59*:768, 1980.

313. Park, W.Y., Hagins, F.M., Rivat, E.L., and MacNamara, T.E.: Age and epidural dose response in adult men. Anesthesiology, *56*:318, 1982.

314. Park, W.Y., Hagins, F.M., Massengale, M.D., and MacNamara, T.E.: The sitting position and anesthetic spread in the epidural space. Anesth. Analg. (Cleve.), *63*:863, 1984.

315. Patterson, J.R., Blaschke, T.F., Hunt, K.K., and Meffin, P.J.: Lidocaine blood concentrations during fiberoptic bronchoscopy. Am. Rev. Respir. Dis., *112*:53, 1975.

316. Pelton, D.A., Daly, M., Cooper, P.D., and Conn, A.W.: Plasma lidocaine concentrations following topical aerosol application to the trachea and bronchi. Can. Anaesth. Soc. J., *17*:250, 1970.

317. Perucca, E., and Richens, A.: Reduction of oral bioavailability of lignocaine by induction of first-pass metabolism in epileptic patients. Br. J. Clin. Pharmacol., *8*:21, 1979.

318. Petersen, M.C., Moore, R.G., Nation, R.L., and McMeniman, W.: Relationship between the transplacental gradients of bupivacaine and alpha$_1$-acid glycoprotein. Br. J. Clin. Pharmacol., *12*:859, 1981.

318a. Petrie, R.H., Paul, W.L., Miller, F.C., Arca, J.J., *et al.*: Placental transfer of lidocaine following paracervical block. Am. J. Obstet. Gynecol., *120*:791, 1974.

319. Philipson, E.H., Kuhnert, B.R., and Syracuse, C.D.: Maternal, fetal, and neonatal lidocaine levels following local perineal infiltration. Am. J. Obstet. Gynecol., *149*:403, 1984.

320. Piafsky, K.M., and Knoppert, D.: Binding of local anesthetics to alpha$_1$-acid glycoprotein. Clin. Res., *26*:836A, 1979.

321. Piafsky, K.M., and Woolner, E.A.: The binding of basic drugs to alpha$_1$-acid glycoprotein in cord serum. J. Pediatr., *5*:820, 1982.

322. Pieper, J.A., Wyman, M.G., Goldreyer, B.N., Cannom, D.S., *et al.*: Lidocaine toxicity: Effects of total versus free lidocaine concentrations. Circulation, *62*(III):181, 1980.

323. Ponganis, K.V., and Stanski, D.R.: Factors affecting the measurement of lidocaine protein binding by equilibrium dialysis in human serum. J. Pharm. Sci., *74*:57, 1985.

324. Ponten, J., Biber, B., Henriksson, B-A., and Jonsteg, C.: Bupivacaine for intercostal nerve blockade in patients on long-term beta-receptor blocking therapy. Acta Anaesthesiol. Scand., *76*[*Suppl.*]:70, 1982.

325. Post, C., Andersson, R.G.G., Ryrfeldt, A., and Nilsson, E.: Physicochemical modification of lidocaine uptake in rat lung tissue. Acta Pharmacol. Toxicol., *44*:103, 1979.

326. Post, C., and Eriksdotter-Behm, K.: Dependence of lung uptake of lidocaine in vivo on blood pH. Acta Pharmacol. Toxicol., *51*:136, 1982.

327. Post, C., and Freedman, J.: A new method for studying the

distribution of drugs in spinal cord after intrathecal injection. Acta Pharmacol. Toxicol., *54*:253, 1984.

328. Prescott, L.F., Adjepon-Yamoah, K.K., and Talbot, R.G.: Impaired lignocaine metabolism in patients with myocardial infarction and cardiac failure. Br. Med. J., *1*:939, 1976.

329. Quimby, C.W.: Influence of blood loss on the duration of regional anesthesia. Anesth. Analg. (Cleve.), *44*:387, 1965.

330. Radtke, H., Nolte, H., Fruhstorfer, H., and Zenz, M.: A comparative study between etidocaine and bupivacaine in ulner nerve block. Acta Anaesthesiol. Scand., *60*[*Suppl.*]:17, 1975.

331. Raj, P.P., Rosenblatt, R., Miller, J., Katz, R.L., *et al.*: Dynamics of local anesthetic compounds in regional anesthesia. Anesth. Analg. (Cleve.), *56*:110, 1977.

332. Raj, P.P., Ohlweiler, D., Hitt, B.A., and Denson, D.D.: Kinetics of local anesthetic esters and effects of adjuvant drugs on 2-chloroprocaine hydrolysis. Anesthesiology, *53*:307, 1980.

333. Ramanathan, J., Bottorff, M., and Sibai, B.M.: Maternal and neonatal effects of epidural lidocaine in preeclamptic women undergoing Cesarian section. Anesth. Analg. (Cleve.), *64*:268, 1985.

334. Ravindran, R.S., Viegas, O.J., Pantazis, K.L., and Baldwin, S.J.: Serum lidocaine levels following spinal anesthesia with lidocaine and epinephrine in dogs. Reg. Anaesth., *8*:6, 1983.

335. Reidenberg, M.M., James, M., and Dring, L.G.: The rate of procaine hydrolysis in serum of normal subjects and diseased patients. Clin. Pharmacol. Ther., *13*:279, 1972.

336. Renck, H., Edstrom, H., Kinnberger, B., and Brandt, G.: Thoracic epidural analgesia: II. Prolongation in the early postoperative period by continuous injection of 1.0% bupivacaine. Acta Anaesthesiol. Scand., *20*:47, 1976.

337. Reynolds, F.: Metabolism and excretion of bupivacaine in man: A comparison with mepivacaine. Br. J. Anaesth., *43*:33, 1971.

338. Richter, O., Klein, K., Abel, J., Ohnesorge, F.K., *et al.*: The kinetics of bupivacaine (Carbostesin) plasma concentrations during epidural anesthesia following intraoperative bolus injection and subsequent continuous infusion. Int. J. Clin. Pharmacol. Ther. Toxicol., *22*:611, 1984.

339. Robson, R.A., Wing, L.M.H., Miners, J.O., Lillywhite, K.J., *et al.*: The effect of ranitidine on the disposition of lignocaine. Br. J. Clin. Pharmacol., *20*:170, 1985.

340. Rosayro, A.M., Tait, A.R., LaBond, V., Ketcham, T.R., *et al.*: The effect of subarachnoid lidocaine and epinephrine on spinal cord blood flow. Anesthesiology, *59*:A208, 1983.

341. Rosenberg, P.H., and Heinonen, E.: Differential sensitivity of A and C nerve fibres to long-acting amide local anaesthetics. Br. J. Anaesth., *55*:143, 1983.

342. Rosenberg, P.H., Kytta, J., and Alila, A.: Uptake of bupivacaine, etidocaine, lignocaine and ropivacaine in n-hepatane, rat sciatic nerve and human epidural and subcutaneous fat. Br. J. Anaesth., *58*:310, 1986.

343. Rosenberg, P.H., Saramies, L., and Alila, A.: Lumbar epidural anaesthesia with bupivacaine in old patients: Effect of speed and direction of injection. Acta Anaesthesiol. Scand., *25*:270, 1981.

344. Rosenblatt, R., Pepitone-Rockwell, F., and McKillop, M.J.: Continuous axillary analgesia for traumatic hand injury. Anesthesiology, *51*:565, 1979.

345. Rosenblatt, R., and Fung, D.L.: Mechanism of action for dextran prolonging regional anesthesia. Reg. Anesth., *5*:3, 1980.

346. Ross, R.A., Clarke, J.E., and Armitage, E.N.: Postoperative pain prevention by continuous epidural infusion. Anaesthesia, *35*:663, 1980.

347. Roth, R.A., and Rubin, R.J.: Role of blood flow in carbon monoxide and hypoxic hypoxia-induced alterations in hexobarbital metabolism in rats. Drug. Metab. Dispos., *5*:460, 1976.

348. Rothstein, P., and Pitt, B.R.: Pulmonary extraction of bupivacaine and its modification by propranolol. Anesthesiology, *59*:A189, 1983.

349. Rothstein, P., Arthur, G.R., Feldman, H., Barash, P.G., *et al.*: Pharmacokinetics of bupivacaine in children following intercostal block. Anesthesiology, *57*:A426, 1981.

350. Routledge, P.A., Barchowsky, A., Bjornsson, T.D., Kitchell, B.B., *et al.*: Lidocaine plasma protein binding. Clin. Pharmacol. Ther., *27*:347, 1980a.

351. Routledge, P.A., Stargel, W.W., Wagner, G.S., and Shand, D.G.: Increased alpha$_1$-acid glycoprotein and lidocaine disposition in myocardial infarction. Ann. Intern. Med., *93*:701, 1980b.

352. Routledge, P.A., Stargel, W.W., Kitchell, B.B., Barchowsky, A., *et al.*: Sex-related differences in the plasma protein binding of lignocaine and diazepam. Br. J. Clin. Pharmacol., *11*:245, 1981a.

353. Routledge, P.A., Stargel, W.W., Finn, A.L., Barchowsky, A., *et al.*: Lignocaine disposition in blood in epilepsy. Br. J. Clin. Pharmacol., *12*:663, 1981b.

354. Routledge, P.A., Stargel, W.W., Barchowsky, A., Wagner, G.S., *et al.*: Control of lidocaine therapy: New perspectives. Ther. Drug Monit., *4*:265, 1982.

355. Rowland, M.: Local anesthetic absorption, distribution and elimination. *In* Eger, E., II.(ed.): Anesthetic Uptake and Action, Pp. 332–366. Baltimore, Williams & Wilkins, 1974.

356. Rowland, M., Thomson, P., Guichard, A., and Melmon, K.L.: Disposition kinetics of lidocaine in normal subjects. Ann. N.Y. Acad. Sci., *179*:383, 1971.

357. Runciman, W.B.: The Effects of General and Spinal Anaesthesia on Regional Blood Flow and Drug Disposition in the Sheep. Ph.D. Thesis, Flinders University of South Australia, 1982.

358. Runciman, W.B., Mather, L.E.: Effects of anaesthesia on drug disposition. *In:* Feldman, S.A., Scurr, C.F., and Paton, W. Mechanisms of action of drugs in anaesthetic practice (in press).

359. Runciman, W.B., Mather, L.E., Upton, R.N., Shepherd, T.M., *et al.*: The effects of hypoxia and haemodilution on chlormethiazole kinetics. Clin. Exp. Pharmacol. Physiol. [*Suppl.*], *9*: 49, 1985.

360. Runciman, W.B., Mather, L.E., Ilsley, A.H., Carapetis, R.J., *et al.*: A sheep preparation for studying interactions between blood flow and drug disposition: II. Experimental applications. Br. J. Anaesth., *56*:1117, 1984.

361. Runciman, W.B., Mather, L.E., Ilsley, A.H., Carapetis, R.J., *et al.*: A sheep preparation for studying interactions between blood flow and drug disposition. III: Effects of general and spinal anaesthesia on regional blood flow and oxygen tensions. Br. J. Anaesth., *56*:247, 1984.

362. Schwartz, M.L., Covino, B.G., Narang, R.M., Sethi, V., *et al.*: Blood levels of lidocaine following subcutaneous administration prior to cardiac catheterization. Am. Heart J., *88*:721, 1975.

362a. Scott, D.B.: Evaluation of the toxicity of local anaesthetic agents in man. Br. J. Anaesth., *47*:56, 1975.

363. Scott, D.B., Jebson, P.J.R., Braid, D.P., Ortengren, B., *et al.*: Factors affecting plasma levels of lignocaine and prilocaine. Br. J. Anaesth., *44*:1040, 1972.

364. Scott, D.B., Littlewood, D.G., Covino, B.G., and Drummond, G.B.: Plasma lignocaine concentrations following endotracheal spraying with an aerosol. Br. J. Anaesth., *48*:899, 1976.

365. Scurlock, J.E., and Curtis, B.M.: Dextran-local anesthetic interactions. Anesth. Analg. (Cleve.), *59*:335, 1980.

366. Schulte-Steinberg, O., Hartmuth, L., and Schutt, L.: Carbon dioxide salts of lignocaine in brachial plexus block. Anaesthesia, *25*:191, 1970.

367. Seifen, A.B., Ferrari, A.A., Seifen, A.A., Thompson, D.S., *et al.*: Pharmacokinetics of intravenous procaine infusion in humans. Anesth. Analg. (Cleve.), *58*:382, 1979.

368. Seow, L.T., Lips, F.J., Cousins, M.J., and Mather, L.E.: Lidocaine and bupivacaine mixtures for epidural blockade. Anesthesiology, *56*:177, 1982.

369. Seow, L.T., Lips, F.J., and Cousins, M.J.: Effect of lateral posture on epidural blockade for surgery. Anaesth. Intensive Care, *11*:97, 1983.

370. Sharrock, N.E.: Epidural anesthetic dose responses in patients 20 to 80 years old. Anesthesiology, *49*:425, 1978.

371. Shiroff, R.A., Schneck, D.W., Pritchard, J.F., Luderer, J., *et al.*: Effects of acute blood pressure reduction by sodium nitroprusside on serum lidocaine levels. Fed. Proc., *36*:958, 1977.

372. Simon, R.P., Benowitz, N.L., Bronstein, J., and Jacob, P.: Increased brain uptake of lidocaine during bicuculline-induced status epilepticus in rats. Neurology, *32*:196, 1982.

373. Simon, R.P., Benowitz, N.L., and Culala, S.: Motor paralysis increases brain uptake of lidocaine during status epilepticus. Neurology, *34*:384, 1984.

374. Sinclair, C.J., Scott, D.B., and Edstrom, H.H.: Effect of the Trendelenberg position on spinal anaesthesia with hyperbaric bupivacaine. Br. J. Anaesth., *54*:497, 1982.

375. Sivarajan, M., Amory, D.W., Lindboom, L.E.: Systemic and regional blood flow during epidural anesthesia without epinephrine in the rhesus monkey. Anesthesiology, *45*:300, 1976.

376. Skou, J.C.: Local anaesthetics: III. Distribution of local anaesthetics between the solid phase/aqueous phase of peripheral nerves. Acta Pharmacol. Toxicol. (Kbh.), *10*:297, 1954.

377. Smith, E.R., and Duce, B.R.: The acute antiarrhythmic and toxic effects in mice and dogs of 2-ethylamino-2′, 6′-acetoxylidine (L-86), a metabolite of lidocaine. J. Pharmacol. Exp. Ther., *179*:580, 1971.

378. Smith, R.B.: Uptake of lidocaine from the trachea. Anesthesiology, *44*:269, 1976.

379. Smith, S.L., Albin, M.S., Watson, W.A., Pantoja, G., *et al.*: Spinal cord and cerebral blood flow responses to intrathecal local anesthetics with and without epinephrine. Anesthesiology, *59*:A312, 1983.

380. Spielman, F.J., Hulka, J.F., Ostheimer, G.W., and Mueller, R.A.: Pharmacokinetics and pharmacodynamics of local analgesia for laparoscopic tubal ligations. Am. J. Obstet. Gynecol., *146*:821, 1983.

381. Stanton-Hicks, M.D'A., Berges, P.U., and Bonica, J.J.: Circulatory effects of peridural block: IV. Comparison of the effects of epinephrine and phenylephrine. Anesthesiology, *39*:308, 1973.

382. Stanton-Hicks, M., Murphy, T.M., Bonica, J.J., Mather, L.E., *et al.*: Effects of peridural block: V. Properties, circulatory effects and blood levels of etidocaine and lidocaine. Anesthesiology, *42*:398, 1975.

383. Stanton-Hicks, M., Murphy, T.M., Bonica, J.J., Mather, L.E., *et al.*: Effects of extradural block: Comparison of the properties, circulatory effects and pharmacokinetics of etidocaine and bupivacaine. Br. J. Anaesth., *48*:575, 1976.

384. Starke, P., and Nolte, H.: pH des liquor spinalis wahrend subduraler blockade. Anaesthesist, *27*:41, 1978.

385. Steffenson, J.L., Shnider, S.M., and de Lorimer, A.A.: Transarterial diffusion of mepivacaine. Anesthesiology, *32*:459, 1970.

386. Stewart, D.J., Inaba, T., Lucassen, M., and Kalow, W.: Cocaine metabolism: Cocaine and norcocaine hydrolysis by liver and serum esterases. Clin. Pharmacol. Ther., *25*:464, 1979.

387. Stewart, D.J., Inaba, T., Tang, B.K., and Kalow, W.: Hydrolysis of cocaine in human plasma by cholinesterase. Life Sci., *20*:1557, 1977.

388. Strasser, K., Abel, J., Breulmann, M., Schumacher, I., *et al.*: Plasmakonzentration von etidocain in der ersten zwei Stunden nach axillarer blockade bei gesunden und bei Patienten mit Niereninsuffizienz. Reg. Anaesth., *4*:14, 1981.

389. Strong, J.M., Mayfield, D.E., Atkinson, A.J., Burris, B.C., *et al.*: Pharmacological activity, metabolism, and pharmacokinetics of glycinexylidide. Clin. Pharmacol. Ther., *17*:184, 1975.

390. Strong, J.M., Parker, M., and Atkinson, A.J.: Identification of glycinexylidide in patients treated with intravenous lidocaine. Clin. Pharmacol. Ther., *14*:67, 1973.

391. Sundnes, K.O., Vaagenes, P., Skretting, P., Lind, B., *et al.*: Spinal analgesia with hyperbaric bupivacaine: Effects of volume of solution. Br. J. Anaesth., *54*:69, 1982.

392. Takasaki, M.: Blood concentrations of lidocaine, mepivacaine and bupivacaine during caudal analgesia in children. Acta Anaesthesiol. Scand., *28*:211, 1984.

393. Takman, B.: The chemistry of local anaesthetic agents. Br. J. Anaesth., *47*:183, 1975.

394. Teramo, K., and Rajamaki, A.: Foetal and maternal plasma levels of mepivacaine and foetal acid-base balance and heart rate after paracervical block during labour. Br. J. Anaesth., *43*:300, 1971.

395. Thomas, J., Long, G., and Mather, L.E.: Plasma lignocaine concentrations following topical aerosol application. Br. J. Anaesth., *41*:442, 1969.

396. Thomas, J., Long, G., Moore, G., and Morgan, D.: Plasma protein binding and placental transfer of bupivacaine. Clin. Pharmacol. Ther., *19*:426, 1976.

397. Thomas, J., and Meffin, P.: Aromatic hydroxylation of lidocaine and mepivacaine in rats and humans. J. Med. Chem. *15*:1046, 1972.

398. Thomas, J., Morgan, D., and Vine, J.: Metabolism of etidocaine in man. Xenobiotica, *6*:39, 1986.

399. Thompson, G.A., Myers, J.A., Turner, P.A., Denson, D.D., *et al.*: Influence of cimetidine on bupivacaine disposition in rat and monkey. Drug Metab. Dispos., *12*:625, 1984.

400. Thompson, G.E., and Rowe, D.H.: Functional anatomy of the brachial plexus sheaths. Anesthesiology, *59*:117, 1983.

401. Thompson, P., Melmon, K.L., Richardson, J.A., and Rowland, M.: Lidocaine pharmacokinetics in advanced heart failure, liver disease and renal failure in humans. Ann. Intern. Med., *78*:499, 1973.

402. Truant, A.P., and Takman, B.: Differential physical-chemical and neuropharmacologic properties of local anesthetic agents. Anesth. Analg. (Cleve.), *38*:478, 1959.

403. Tucker, G.T.: Biotransformation and toxicity of local anaesthetics. Acta Anaesthesiol. Belg., *26*[*Suppl.*]:123, 1975.

404. Tucker, G.T.: Plasma binding and disposition of local anesthetics. Int. Anesthesiol. Clin., *13*:33, 1975.

405. Tucker, G.T.: Pharmacokinetics of local anaesthetics: Role in toxicity. *In* Scott, D.B., McClure, J., and Wildsmith, J.A.W. (eds.): Regional Anaesthesia 1884–1984, pp. 61–71. Sodertalje, Sweden, ICM AB, 1984.

406. Tucker, G.T., and Boas, R.A.: Pharmacokinetic aspects of intravenous regional anesthesia. Anesthesiology, *34*:538, 1971.

407. Tucker, G.T., Bax, N.D.S., Lennard, M.S., Al-Asady, S., *et al.*: Effects of beta-adrenoceptor antagonists on the pharmacokinetics of lignocaine. Br. J. Clin. Pharmacol., *17*[*Suppl.* 1]:21S, 1984.

408. Tucker, G.T., Boyes, R.N., Bridenbaugh, P.O., and Moore, D.C.: Binding of anilide-type local anesthetics in human plasma. I: Relationships between binding, physicochemical properties and anesthetic activity. Anesthesiology, *33*:287, 1970.

409. Tucker, G.T., Boyes, R.N., Bridenbaugh, P.O., and Moore, D.C.: Binding of anilide-type local anesthetics in human plasma. II: Implications *in vivo* with special reference to transplacental distribution. Anesthesiology, *33*:304, 1970.

410. Tucker, G.T., Cooper, S., Littlewood, D., Buckley, S.P., *et al.*: Observed and predicted accumulation of local anaesthetic agent during continuous extradural analgesia. Br. J. Anaesth., *49*:237, 1977.

411. Tucker, G.T., and Mather, L.E.: Pharmacokinetics of local anaesthetic agents. Br. J. Anaesth., *47*:213, 1975.

412. Tucker, G.T., and Mather, L.E.: Plasma protein binding of bupivacaine and its interaction with other drugs in man. Br. J. Anaesth., *47*:1029, 1975.

413. Tucker, G.T., and Mather, L.E.: Clinical pharmacokinetics of local anaesthetic agents. Clin. Pharmacokinet., *4*:241, 1979.

414. Tucker, G.T., Moore, D.C., Bridenbaugh, P.O., Bridenbaugh, L.D., *et al.*: Systemic absorption of mepivacaine in commonly used regional block procedures. Anesthesiology, *37*:277, 1972.

415. Tucker, G.T., Wiklund, L., Berlin, A., and Mather, L.E.: Hepatic clearance of local anesthetics in man. J. Pharmacokinet. Biopharm., *5*:111, 1977.

416. Tuominen, M., Rosenberg, P.H., and Kalso, E.: Blood levels of bupivacaine after single dose, supplementary dose and during continuous infusion in axillary plexus block. Acta Anaesthesiol. Scand., *27*:303, 1983.

417. Ueda, I., Katsuji, O., and Arakawa, K.: True oil/water partition coefficients of procaine and lidocaine and estimation of their dissociation constants in organic solvents. Anesth. Analg. (Cleve.), *61*:56, 1982.

418. Ueda, W., Hirakawa, M., and Mori, K.: Inhibition of epinephrine absorption by dextran. Anesthesiology, *62*:72, 1985.

419. Urban, B.J.: Clinical observations suggesting a changing site of action during induction and recession of spinal and epidural anesthesia. Anesthesiology, *39*:496, 1973.

420. Usubiaga, J.E., Wikinski, F.A., Ferrero, R., Usubiaga, L.E., *et al.*: Local anesthetic induced convulsions. An electroencephalographic study. Anesth. Analg. (Cleve.), *45*:611, 1966.

421. Vester-Andersen, T., Christiansen, C., Hansen, A., Sorensen, M., *et al.*: Interscalene brachial plexus block: Area of analgesia, complications and blood concentrations of local anesthetics. Acta Anaesthesiol. Scand., *25*:81, 1981.

422. Vester-Andersen, T., Husum, B., Lindeburg, T., Borrits, L., *et al.*: Perivascular axillary block. V: Blockade following 60ml of mepivacaine 1% injected as a bolus or as 30 + 30ml with a 20-min interval. Acta Anaesthesiol. Scand., *28*:612, 1984.

423. Viegas, O., and Stoelting, R.K.: Lignocaine in arterial blood after laryngotracheal administration. Anesthesiology, *43*:491, 1975.

424. Vine, J., Morgan, D., and Thomas, J.: The identification of eight hydroxylated metabolites of etidocaine by chemical ionization mass spectrometry. Xenobiotica, *8*:509, 1978.

425. Wang, B.C., Spielholz, N.I., Hillman, D.E., and Turndorf, H.: Reversal of tetracaine spinal block by exogenous subarachnoid cholinesterase. Anesthesiology, *59*:A209, 1983.

426. Webb, T.D., and Ward, D.S.: Elimination of lidocaine following regional block is inhibited by cimetidine. Anesthesiology, *59*:A213, 1983.

427. Weiss, R.R., Halevy, S., Almonte, R.O., Gundersen, K., *et al.*: Comparison of lidocaine and 2-chloroprocaine in paracervical block: Clinical effects and drug concentrations in mother and child. Anesth. Analg. (Cleve.), *62*:168, 1983.

428. Wennberg, E., Haljamae, H., Edwall, G., and Dhuner, K-G.: Effects of commercial (pH 3.5) and freshly prepared (pH 6.5) lidocaine-adrenaline solutions on tissue pH. Acta Anaesthesiol. Scand., *26*:524, 1982.

429. Wiklund, L., and Berlin-Wahlen, A.: Splanchnic elimination and systemic toxicity of bupivacaine and etidocaine in man. Acta Anaesthesiol. Scand., *21*:521, 1977.

430. Wiklund, L., Tucker, G.T., and Engberg, G.: Influence of intravenously administered epinephrine on splanchnic haemodynamics and clearance of lidocaine. Acta Anaesthesiol. Scand., *21*:275, 1977.

431. Wildsmith, J.A.W., Tucker, G.T., Cooper, S., Scott, D.B., *et al.*: Plasma concentrations of local anaesthetics after interscalene brachial plexus block. Br. J. Anaesth., *49*:461, 1977.

432. Wildsmith, J.A.W., McClure, J.H., Brown, D.T., and Scott, D.B.: Effects of posture on the spread of isobaric and hyperbaric amethocaine. Br. J. Anaesth., *53*:273, 1981.

433. Wilkinson, G.R., and Lund, P.C.: Bupivacaine levels in plasma and cerebrospinal fluid following peridural administration. Anesthesiology, *33*:482, 1970.

434. Willdeck-Lund, G., and Edstrom, H.: Etidocaine in intercostal nerve block for pain relief after thoracotomy: A comparison with bupivacaine. Acta Anaesthesiol. Scand., *60*[*Suppl.*]:33, 1975.

435. Williams, R., Blaschke, T.F., Meffin, P.J., Melmon, K.L., *et al.*: Influence of viral hepatitis on the disposition of two compounds with high hepatic clearance: Lidocaine and indocyanine green. Clin. Pharmacol. Ther., *20*:290, 1976.

436. Wing, L.M.H., Miners, J.O., Birkett, D.J., Foenander, T., *et al.*: Lidocaine disposition—Sex differences and effects of cimetidine. Clin. Pharmacol. Ther., *35*:695, 1984.

437. Winnie, A.P., Lavallee, D.A., Sosa, B.P., and Masud, K.Z.: Clinical pharmacokinetics of local anaesthetics. Can. Anaesth. Soc. J., *24*:252, 1977.

438. Winnie, A.P., Tay, C-H., Patel, K.P., Ramamurthy, S., *et al.*: Pharmacokinetics of local anesthetics during plexus blocks. Anesth. Analg., (Cleve.), *56*:852, 1977.

439. Winnie, A.P., Radonjic, R., Akkineni, S.R., and Durrani, Z.: Factors influencing distribution of local anesthetic injected into the brachial plexus sheath. Anesth. Analg. (Cleve.), *58*:225, 1979.

440. Wood, M., and Wood, A.J.J.: Changes in plasma drug binding and alpha$_1$-acid glycoprotein in mother and newborn infant. Clin. Pharmacol. Ther., *29*:522, 1981.

441. Zador, G., Engelsson, S., and Nilsson, B.A.: Low dose intermittent epidural anaesthesia in labour. I: Clinical efficacy and idocaine concentrations in maternal and foetal blood. Acta Obstet. Gynecol. Scand. *34*[*Suppl.*]:3, 1974.

4 CLINICAL PHARMACOLOGY OF LOCAL ANESTHETIC AGENTS

BENJAMIN G. COVINO

A description of the clinical pharmacology of any drug should include a review of factors that influence the usefulness and potential toxicity of that specific agent or class of agents. With local anesthetic drugs, the properties that determine their clinical usefulness are the inherent anesthetic potency of the agent and the onset and duration of anesthesia. The toxicity of local anesthetic agents includes adverse systemic effects involving the central nervous system and the cardiovascular system, local irritant actions, allergy and miscellaneous reactions such as methemoglobinemia, and addiction. A large number of local anesthetic agents are commercially available for clinical use. These agents differ markedly in terms of their clinical profiles and their potential for producing toxic reactions. A knowledge of the clinical pharmacology of the various drugs is important in terms of selecting the appropriate agent for a specific clinical situation.

Clinically useful local anesthetic agents essentially fall into one of two chemically distinct groups: Agents that possess an ester link between the aromatic portion and the intermediate chain are referred to as amino esters and include procaine, chloroprocaine, and tetracaine; local anesthetics with an amide link between the aromatic portion and the intermediate chain are referred to as amino amides and include lidocaine, mepivacaine, prilocaine, bupivacaine, and etidocaine. The chemical structure of the various local anesthetic agents and the basic pharmacologic differences between the ester and amide compounds have been presented in Table 3-1. The clinical profile, available commercial solutions, maximum dosage, and primary area of clinical use of the different agents are summarized in Table 4-1.

PHARMACOLOGIC FACTORS AFFECTING ANESTHETIC ACTIVITY

In humans, the potency, onset, and duration of anesthesia are primarily determined by the physicochemical properties of the various agents and their inherent vasodilator activity. In addition, onset, duration, and depth of anesthesia may be altered by such factors as dosage administered, addition of vasoconstrictors to the local anesthetic solution, and the site of injection. Attempts have been made to alter the onset and duration of anesthesia by such factors as using mixtures of various agents, carbonation of local anesthetic solutions, and adding potassium and dextran to local anesthetic solutions.

Physicochemical Properties. The physicochemical properties that influence local anesthetic activity are primarily lipid solubility, protein binding, and pKa. The relative values for lipid solubility, protein binding, and pKa of the various local anesthetic agents are shown in Table 3-1.

Lipid solubility appears to be the primary determinant of intrinsic anesthetic potency (Fig. 4-1). Procaine and chloroprocaine, for example, represent agents of low lipid solubility, the partition coefficient values of which are less than 1. These drugs must be administered in relatively high concentrations, that

TABLE 4–1. CLINICAL PROFILE OF LOCAL ANESTHETIC AGENTS

Agent	Concentration (%)	Clinical Use	Onset	Usual Duration (h)	Recommended Maximum Single Dose (mg)	Comments	*pH* of Plain Solutions*
Amides							
Lidocaine	0.5–1.0	Infiltration	Fast	1.0–2.0	300	Most versatile agent	6.5
	0.25–0.5	i.v. Regional			500 + epinephrine		
	1.0–1.5	Peripheral nerve blocks	Fast	1.0–3.0	500 + epinephrine		
	1.5–2.0	Epidural	Fast	1.0–2.0	500 + epinephrine		
	4	Topical	Moderate	0.5–1.0	500 + epinephrine		
	5	Spinal	Fast	0.5–1.5	100		
Prilocaine	0.5–1.0	Infiltration	Fast	1.0–2.0	600	Least toxic amide agent	4.5
	0.25–0.5	i.v. Regional			600		
	1.5–2.0	Peripheral nerve blocks	Fast	1.5–3.0	600	Methemoglobnemia occurs usually above 600 mg	
	2.0–3.0	Epidural	Fast	1.0–3.0			
Mepivacaine	0.5–1.0	Infiltration	Fast	1.5–3.0	400 500 + epinephrine	Duration of plain solutions longer than lidocaine without epinephrine. Useful when epinephrine is contraindicated.	4.5
	1.0–1.5	Peripheral nerve blocks	Fast	2.0–3.0			
	1.5–2.0	Epidural	Fast	1.5–3.0			
	4.0	Spinal	Fast	1.0–1.5	100		
Bupivacaine	0.25	Infiltration	Fast	2.0–4.0	175 225 + epinephrine	Lower concentrations provide differential sensory/motor block. Ventricular arrhythmias and sudden cardiovascular collapse reported following rapid i.v. injection.	4.5–6
	0.25–0.5	Peripheral nerve blocks	Slow	4.0–12.0	225 + epinephrine		
	0.25–0.5	Obstetrical epidural	Moderate	2.0–4.0	225 + epinephrine		
	0.5–0.75	Surgical epidural	Moderate	2.0–5.0	225 + epinephrine		
	0.5–0.75	Spinal	Fast	2.0–4.0	20		
Etidocaine	0.5	Infiltration	Fast	2.0–4.0	300 400 + epinephrine	Profound motor block useful for surgical anesthesia but not for obstetrical analgesia.	4.5
	0.5–1.0	Peripheral	Fast	3.0–12.0	400 + epinephrine		
	1.0–1.5	Surgical epidural	Fast	2.0–4.0	400 + epinephrine		
Dibucaine	0.25–0.5 hyperbaric	Spinal	Fast	2.0–4.0	10	Recommended only for spinal and topical use	
	0.00067 hypobarbic	Spinal	Fast	2.0–4.0	10		
	1.0	Topical	Slow	30–60	50		
Esters							
Procaine	1.0	Infiltration	Fast	30–60	1000	Used mainly for infiltration and differential spinal blocks. Allergic	5–6.5
	1.0–2.0	Peripheral nerve blocks	Slow	30–60	1000		
	2.0	Epidural	Slow	30–60	1000		

(continued)

TABLE 4-1. CLINICAL PROFILE OF LOCAL ANESTHETIC AGENTS *(continued)*

Agent	Concentration (%)	Clinical Use	Onset	Usual Duration (h)	Recommended Maximum Single Dose (mg)	Comments	*p*H of Plain Solutions*
	10.0	Spinal	Moderate	30–60	200	potential after repeated use	
Chloroprocaine	1.0	Infiltration	Fast	30–60	800 1000 + epinephrine	Lowest systemic toxicity of all local anesthetics	2.7–4
	2.0	Peripheral nerve block	Fast	30–60	1000 + epinephrine	Intrathecal injection may be associated with sensory/motor deficits.	
	2.0–3.0	Epidural	Fast	30–60	1000 + epinephrine		
Tetracaine	0.5	Spinal	Fast	2.0–4.0	20	Use is primarily limited to spinal and topical anesthesia.	4.5–6.5
	2.0	Topical	Slow	30–60	20		
Cocaine	4.0–10.0	Topical	Slow	30–60	150	Topical use only. Addictive, causes vasoconstriction. CNS toxicity initially features marked excitation ("Fight and Flight" Response). May cause cardiac arrhythmias owing to sympathetic stimulation.	
Benzocaine	Up to 20	Topical	Slow	30–60	200	Useful only for topical anesthesia.	

**Note:* Epinephrine-containing solutions have a *p*H 1 to 1.5 units lower than plain solutions.

is, 2% to 3%, to attain effective conduction blockade in humans. On the other hand, tetracaine, bupivacaine, and etidocaine are compounds of high lipid solubility with partition coefficients varying from 4 to 140. These agents produce effective anesthesia at relatively low concentrations of 0.25% to 0.5%. Lidocaine, mepivacaine, and prilocaine are intermediate both in terms of lipid solubility (partition coefficients of about 1–3) and of their anesthetic potency *in vivo* (effective anesthetic concentration of 1–2%). A rather precise correlation exists between lipid solubility and anesthetic potency as determined on an isolated nerve; however, in humans the correlation between lipid solubility and anesthetic effectiveness is less precise owing to other biological considerations that exist *in vivo* but not in an *in vitro* preparation. In general, potency increases as a function of lipid solubility until a partition coefficient of about 4 is achieved. Further increases in lipid solubility do not appear to cause a further enhancement of anesthetic potency (Fig. 4-1).

The pKa of a chemical compound, which is essentially the *p*H at which the ionized and nonionized forms are present in equal amounts, will influence the onset of anesthesia because the uncharged form of the local anesthetic agent is primarily responsible for diffusion across the nerve sheath and nerve membrane.[95] The onset of action will be directly related to the amount of drug that exists in the base form. The percentage of a specific local anesthetic that is present in the base form when injected into tissue, the *p*H of which is 7.4, is inversely proportional to the pKa of that agent. Mepivacaine, lidocaine, prilocaine, and etidocaine, for example, possess a pKa of about 7.7. When these agents are injected into tissue at a *p*H of 7.4, about 65% of these

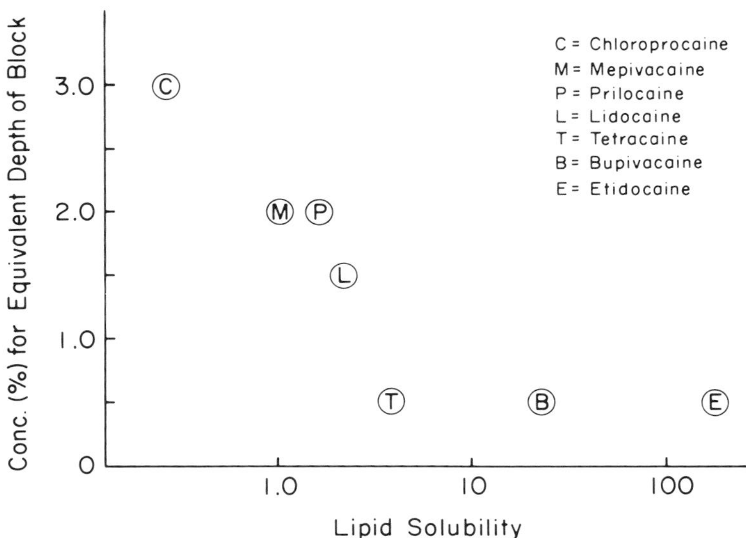

FIG. 4-1. Relation between lipid solubility and inherent potency of local anesthetic agents.

drugs exist in the ionized form and 35% in the nonionized base form. On the other hand, tetracaine possesses a pKa of 8.6, which means that only 5% is present in the nonionized form at a tissue *p*H of 7.4, whereas 95% exists in the charged cationic form. In humans, a correlation does exist between onset of conduction blockade and the pKa of the various local anesthetic agents (Fig. 4-2).[13,75] For example, the agents with relatively low pKa's, namely, lidocaine, mepivacaine, prilocaine, and etidocaine, have a fairly rapid onset of action. On the other hand, tetracaine and procaine, which have high pKa's, have a rather slow onset of action. Bupivacaine is intermediate, both in terms of pKa and onset of action. One exception to this rule appears to be chloroprocaine, which has a *high pKa* and a rapid onset of action in humans; however, if one considers that chloroprocaine generally is used at higher concentrations and larger dosages than other local anesthetics, the more rapid onset of action may be related simply to the larger number of molecules of this agent that are administered in order to achieve effective anesthesia.

Finally, the relative protein binding of various local anesthetics will influence the duration of anesthesia of the various agents (Fig. 4-2). If, indeed, a local anesthetic receptor site exists in the protein sodium channel in nerve membrane, then agents that possess a greater affinity for protein should remain at the receptor site for a longer time and therefore cause a longer duration of action. Thus, bupivacaine and etidocaine, which are about 95% protein bound, do demonstrate long durations of anesthesia. On the other hand, procaine, which is only 6% protein bound, has a relatively short duration of action. Prilocaine, mepivacaine, and lidocaine, which are intermediate in terms of protein binding (55–75%), are also intermediate in terms of anesthetic duration.

Vasodilator Properties. The clinical activity of the various local anesthetics is also modified by factors not related to the physicochemical properties of the different drugs. In particular, the effect of local anesthetics on vascular smooth muscle will indirectly influence the apparent potency and duration of action of these agents. Local anesthetics are absorbed into the vascular compartment from the region of their injection. The rate of vascular absorption will determine the number of molecules of local anesthetic available for diffusion to the receptor site of the nerve membrane, which in turn will influence their *in vivo* potency and duration of action. All local anesthetics except cocaine exhibit a biphasic effect on vascular smooth muscle.[9,61] At extremely low concentrations they cause enhanced activity of vascular smooth muscle, leading to vasoconstriction. At concentrations commonly used for regional anesthesia, however, local anesthetics tend to be vasodilators. Differences in the relative degree of vasodilation produced by local anesthetics will influence their anesthetic profile. For example, *in vitro* studies have shown that lidocaine is significantly more potent than mepivacaine on an isolated nerve, whereas duration of con-

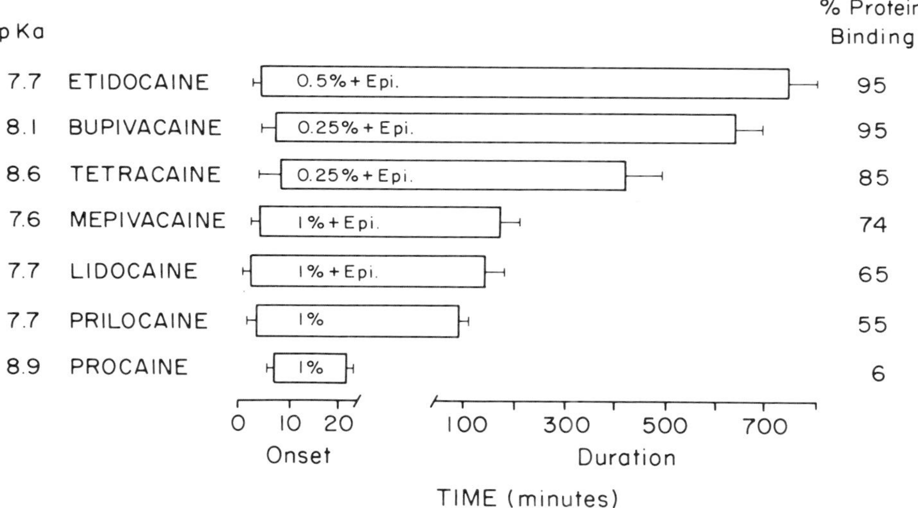

FIG. 4-2. Relation between pKa and onset of anesthesia (*left side* of figure) and relation between protein binding and duration of anesthsia (*right side* of figure).

duction block is similar.[30] Studies in humans, however, have indicated that little difference exists in the relative anesthetic potency between these two agents and the duration of action of mepivacaine is somewhat longer than that of lidocaine.[75] These differences are probably related to the greater degree of vasodilation induced by lidocaine. The addition of epinephrine to solutions of lidocaine and mepivacaine will essentially eliminate the difference in vasodilator activity produced by the two compounds. Under such conditions little difference in the duration of action is observed in humans when epinephrine-containing solutions of lidocaine and mepivacaine are used.[75]

In summary, the clinically important properties of local anesthetic agents include potency, onset, and duration of action. The clinical profile of the various agents is related primarily to their physicochemical properties. *In vivo,* however, the clinical activity of these drugs may be altered by other actions, such as their relative effects on vascular smooth muscle. On the basis of their anesthetic profile in humans, the various local anesthetics may be classified as follows:

1. Agents of low anesthetic potency and short duration of action, that is, procaine and chloroprocaine.
2. Agents of intermediate anesthetic potency and duration of action, that is, lidocaine, mepivacaine, and prilocaine.
3. Agents of high anesthetic potency and prolonged duration of action, that is, tetracaine, bupivacaine, and etidocaine.

In terms of onset, chloroprocaine, lidocaine, mepivacaine, prilocaine, and etidocaine possess a relatively rapid onset of action. Procaine and tetracaine have a long latency period except when used for spinal anesthesia, and bupivacaine is intermediate in terms of onset of anesthesia.

In addition to the anesthetic properties described above, one other important clinical consideration is the ability of local anesthetic agents to cause a differential blockade of sensory and motor fibers (Fig. 4-3). Although differential conduction blockade has been used for many years by altering the concentration of procaine administered intrathecally, this technique is useful primarily for the diagnosis of certain pain states. The introduction of bupivacaine into clinical practice provided anesthesiologists with the first agent that showed a relative specificity for sensory fibers such that adequate sensory analgesia without profound inhibition of motor fibers could be achieved for surgical, obstetric, and acute and chronic pain therapy.[17] Bupivacaine and etidocaine,

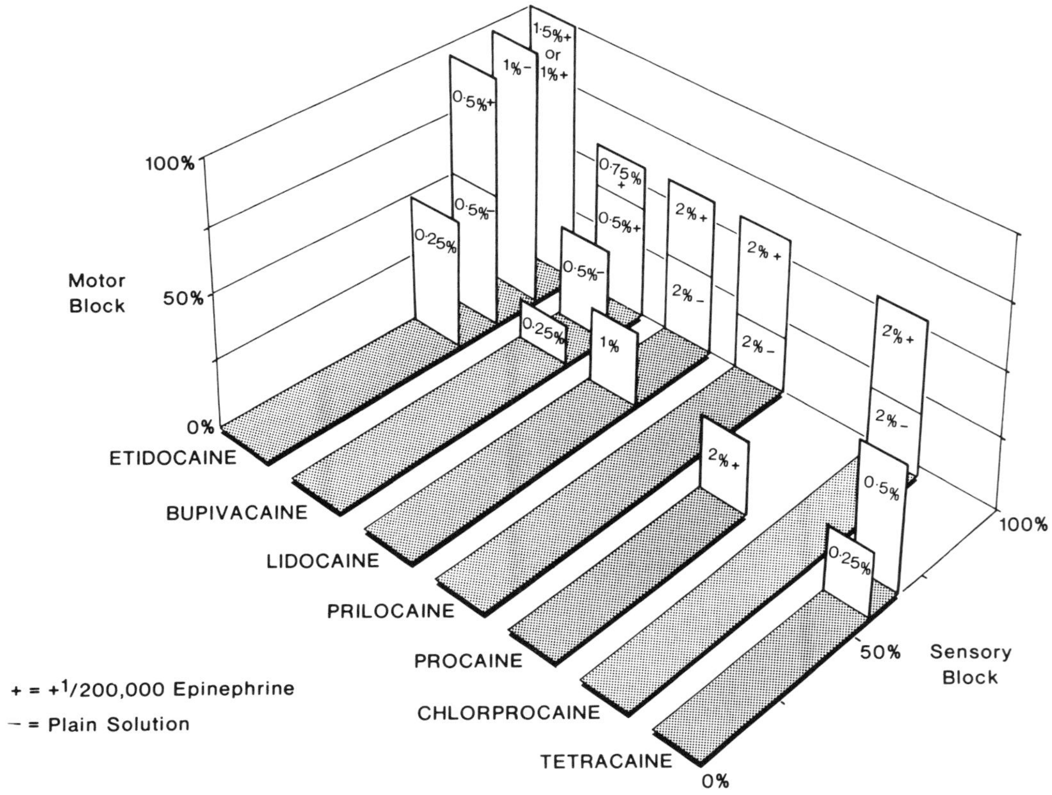

FIG. 4-3. Comparison of agents in epidural block. The percentage of motor blockade and the percentage of success of sensory blockade are illustrated for each agent. This illustration is based on subjective clinical data, and thus only approximate comparisons can be drawn.

the two most recent local anesthetic agents introduced into clinical practice, provide an interesting contrast in terms of their differential sensory/motor blocking activity, although they are both potent long-acting anesthetic agents. Bupivacaine, for example, is widely used epidurally for surgical and obstetric procedures and relief of pain postoperatively because of its ability to provide adequate sensory analgesia with minimal blockade of motor fibers, particularly when used as an 0.25% or 0.5% solution. Thus, the woman in labor can be rendered painfree and still be able to move her legs, which is one of the primary reasons why this agent has enjoyed popularity for continuous epidural blockade during labor. Increasing the concentration of bupivacaine to 0.75% will increase the depth of both sensory and motor blockade while also shortening latency and producing a more prolonged duration of anesthesia.[105] Etidocaine, on the other hand, shows little separation between sensory and motor blockade. To achieve adequate epidural sensory anesthesia, 1.5% concentrations of etidocaine are usually required. At these concentrations, etidocaine has an extremely rapid onset of action and a prolonged duration of anesthesia; however, sensory anesthesia is associated with a profound degree of motor blockade. Thus etidocaine is a valuable agent, particularly for epidural blockade in surgical situations in which optimum muscle relaxation is desirable, because it combines a rapid onset, prolonged duration, and satisfactory quality of anesthesia with profound motor blockade. This marked effect on motor function renders etidocaine of limited value, however, for obstetric analgesia and postoperative pain relief.

NONPHARMACOLOGIC FACTORS INFLUENCING ANESTHETIC ACTIVITY

Although the inherent pharmacologic properties of the various local anesthetic agents will basically determine their anesthetic profile, other factors may influence the quality of regional anesthesia, including [a] dosage of local anesthetic administered; [b] addition of a vasoconstrictor to the local anesthetic solution; [c] site of administration; [d] use of additives; and [e] mixtures of local anesthetic solutions.

Dosage of Local Anesthetic Solutions. The mass of drug administered will influence the onset, potency, and duration of anesthesia (Table 4-2).[17] As the dose of local anesthetic is increased, the frequency of satisfactory anesthesia and the duration of anesthesia will increase and the time for onset of anesthesia will decrease. In general, the dosage of local anesthetic administered can be increased by administering a larger volume of a less concentrated solution or a smaller volume of a more concentrated solution. In clinical practice, however, an increase in dosage is usually achieved by using a more concentrated solution of the specific agent. For example, a dose-response study involving the use of bupivacaine for epidural analgesia in women in labor showed that increasing the concentration from 0.125% to 0.5% while maintaining the same volume of injectate (10 ml) resulted in a decreased latency, improved incidence of satisfactory analgesia, and an increased duration of sensory analgesia.[70] A similar study involving the use of bupivacaine for surgical anesthesia also demonstrated that increasing the concentration from 0.5% to 0.75% with a concomitant increase in dosage from about 100 mg to 150 mg produced a more rapid onset and prolonged duration of sensory anesthesia.[105] In addition, the frequency of satisfactory sensory anesthesia was increased and the depth of motor blockade enhanced. The relative influence of volume, concentration, and dosage was demonstrated in a study in which prilocaine (600 mg) administered epidurally either as 30 ml of a 2% solution or 20 ml of 3% solution was evaluated.[32] No difference in onset, adequacy, or duration of anesthesia and onset, depth, and duration of motor blockade was observed despite differences in volume and concentration of anesthetic solution used, since the dosage was maintained constant. The volume of anesthetic solution administered may influence the spread of anesthesia; for example, 30 ml of 1% lidocaine administered into the epidural space was shown to produce a level of anesthesia that was 4.3 dermatomes higher than that achieved when 10 ml of 3% lidocaine was used.[42] Thus, except for the possible effect on the spread of anesthesia, the primary qualities of regional anesthesia, namely, onset, depth, and duration of blockade, are related to the mass of drug injected, that is, the product of volume times concentration.

TABLE 4-2. EFFECTS OF DOSE AND EPINEPHRINE ON LOCAL ANESTHETIC PROPERTIES

	Increased Dose (Concentration or Volume)	Addition of Epinephrine
Onset time	↓	↓ (Minimal effect for etidocaine)
Degree of motor blockade	↑	↑
Degree of sensory blockade	↑	↑
Duration of blockade	↑	↑
Area of blockade	↑	↑
Peak plasma concentration	↑	↓

Addition of a Vasoconstrictor to Local Anesthetic Solutions. Vasoconstrictors, particularly epinephrine, are frequently added to local anesthetic solutions. The decrease in the rate of vascular absorption that results from adding epinephrine will allow more anesthetic molecules to reach the nerve membrane, thereby improving the depth and duration of anesthesia (Table 4-2). Local anesthetic solutions usually contain a 1 : 200,000 (5 μg/ml) concentration of epinephrine, a concentration that has been reported to provide an optimal degree of vasoconstriction when used with lidocaine for epidural or intercostal use.[11] Little information is available on the optimum concentration of epinephrine when used with other local anesthetic agents. Other vasoconstrictor agents such as norepinephrine and phenylephrine have been used as additives to solutions of local anesthetics. Regional blood flow studies indicate that epinephrine is more effective as a vasoconstrictor than norepinephrine when combined with local anesthetic agents.[36] Phenylephrine has been reported to produce the greatest prolongation of spinal anesthesia when combined with tetracaine[78]; however, more recent studies conducted under double-blind conditions indicated that at equipotent doses no differences existed between the ability of epinephrine and phenylephrine to prolong the duration of spinal anesthesia produced by tetracaine (Fig. 4-4).[31]

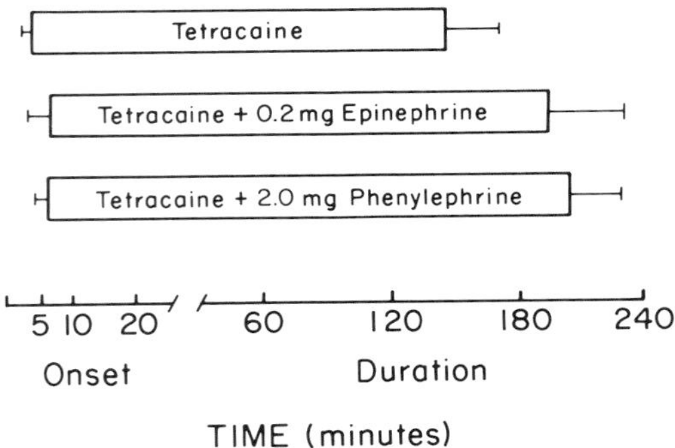

FIG. 4-4. Comparative effect of epinephrine and phenylephrine on the duration of spinal anesthesia produced by tetracaine. (Data derived from Concepcion, *et al.*: ref 31)

Differences exist in terms of the effect of epinephrine in prolonging the duration of action of various local anesthetic agents. Procaine, lidocaine, and mepivacaine, for example, benefit greatly from the addition of epinephrine in terms of prolonging the duration of infiltration anesthesia, peripheral nerve blocks, and epidural blockade.[1,15,54,111] The duration of action of prilocaine, bupivacaine, and etidocaine is also prolonged by adding epinephrine when these agents are used for infiltration and peripheral nerve blocks.[1,75,111] The duration of action of these agents is not, however, markedly affected by epinephrine following epidural blockade.[15,22,65] The decreased vasodilator action of prilocaine compared to that of lidocaine is believed responsible for the reduced effect of added epinephrine to solutions of prilocaine. With bupivacaine and etidocaine, the high lipid solubility of these agents may be responsible for the diminished effect of epinephrine. These agents are taken up substantially by epidural fat and then slowly released, which contributes to their prolonged duration of action; however, the interaction of epinephrine and the long-acting agents, such as bupivacaine, is dependent on the concentration of drug used. In epidural blockade for labor, for example, the frequency and the duration of adequate analgesia were improved when epinephrine 1 : 200,000 was added to 0.125% and 0.25% bupivacaine[70]; however, the addition of epinephrine to 0.5% and 0.75% bupivacaine was not associated with a significant improvement in the frequency of satisfactory epidural blockade in obstetric or surgical patients.[70,108] The degree of motor blockade is enhanced following the epidural administration of epinephrine-containing solutions of bupivacaine and etidocaine.[108] The differential effect of epinephrine in terms of prolonging the duration of action of local anesthetic agents is most apparent in the subarachnoid space. Epinephrine significantly extends the duration of spinal anesthesia when combined with tetracaine.[6,31] The duration of effective surgical anesthesia is not, however, markedly enhanced when solutions of lidocaine or bupivacaine with epinephrine are administered intrathecally.[24,25]

Site of Injection. The site of administration of local anesthetic agents will influence their anesthetic profile. Although local anesthetics are frequently classified as agents of short, moderate, or long duration with a slow or rapid onset of action, these general properties are influenced by the type of anesthetic procedure performed. Tetracaine, for example, is usually considered an agent of slow onset and long duration, but its onset of action is quite rapid (about 3 minutes) when administered intrathecally, whereas the duration of spinal anesthesia with tetracaine is only 2 to 3 hours.[31] In terms of latency, the most rapid onset of action occurs after the intrathecal or subcutaneous administration of local anesthetics, whereas the slowest onset times are observed during the performance of brachial plexus blocks.[29] With regard to the duration of anesthesia, an agent such as bupivacaine possesses a duration of surgical anesthesia of about 4 hours when administered into the epidural space (Fig. 4-5). When bupivacaine is administered for brachial plexus blockade, however, the duration of anesthesia averages 10 hours. Differences in the onset and the duration of anesthesia depending on the site of injection are partly due to the particular anatomy of the area of injection, the variation in the rate of vascular absorption, and the amount of drug used for various types of regional anesthesia. In the case of spinal anesthesia, the lack of a nerve sheath around the spinal cord and the deposition of the local anesthetic solution in the immediate vicinity of the spinal cord are responsible for the rapid onset of action. On the other hand, the relatively small amount of drug used for spinal anesthesia probably accounts for the relatively short duration of action associated with this particular technique. With brachial plexus blockade, the onset of anesthesia is slow due to the anesthetic agent usually being deposited at some distance from the nerve roots, and therefore time for diffusion to the nerve membrane is required before signs of anesthesia are apparent. The long duration of brachial plexus blockade observed with most local anesthetics but, in particular, with the longer-acting agents is probably related to the decreased rate of

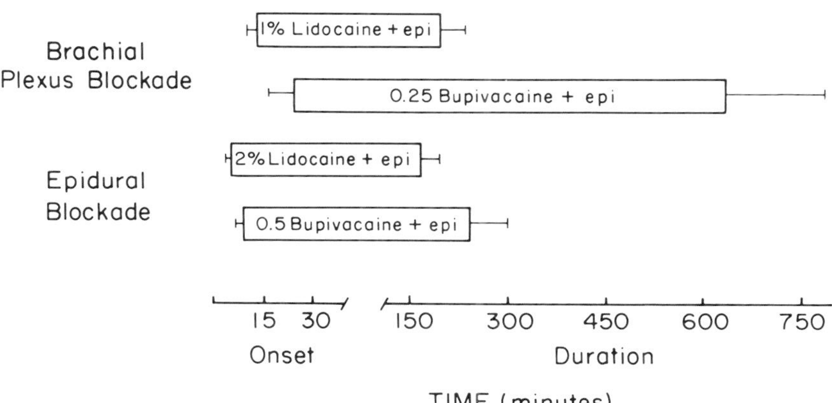

FIG. 4-5. Comparative onset and duration of anesthesia of lidocaine and bupivacaine following epidural and brachial plexus blockade.

vascular absorption from that site, and also the larger doses of drug commonly used for this regional anesthetic technique.

Use of Additives with Local Anesthetic Solutions. Attempts have been made to modify local anesthetic solutions in a number of ways in order to improve the onset of action or prolong the duration of anesthesia. Carbonation of local anesthetic solutions has been attempted to reduce the onset of action of various local anesthetics (Fig. 4-6). It has been clearly shown in isolated nerve preparations that carbon dioxide will enhance the diffusion of local anesthetics through nerve sheaths and produce a more rapid onset of conduction block.[23,52] The mechanism is believed related to the diffusion of carbon dioxide through the nerve membrane resulting in a decrease in intracellular *p*H. The lower *p*H will increase the intracellular concentration of the cationic form of the local anesthetic, which represents the active form that binds to a receptor in the sodium channel. In addition, the local anesthetic cation does not readily diffuse through membranes such that the drug remains entrapped within the axoplasm, a situation referred to as ion trapping. The enhanced formation of the local anesthetic cation and the process of ion trapping are believed responsible for the more rapid onset and more profound degree of conduction block. A number of clinical studies have been carried out with carbonated solutions of lidocaine. Initial investigations in humans found that lidocaine carbonate solutions had a more rapid onset of brachial plexus and epidural blockade compared to lidocaine hydrochloride solutions.[14,16] More recent double-blind studies, however, have failed to demonstrate a significantly more rapid onset of action when lidocaine carbonate was compared with lidocaine hydrochloride for epidural blockade.[84] In theory an agent such as bupivacaine that has a relatively slow onset of action should benefit greatly from the use of a carbonated solution, and it has been reported that bupivacaine–carbon dioxide is associated with a more rapid onset of action in humans[37]; however, double-blind studies in which bupivacaine carbonate was compared with bupivacaine hydrochloride for brachial plexus or epidural blockade have failed to confirm these earlier reports of a significantly shorter onset of action of the carbonated solution.[20,77] Thus, at present, it is not certain whether carbonation of local anesthetic solutions imparts any advantage to the various local anesthetic agents in terms of onset of block when used under clinical conditions, although the depth of anesthesia may be improved.

The discrepancy between *in vitro* and *in vivo* studies suggests that the injected carbon dioxide is rapidly buffered *in vivo* such that the intracellular *p*H is not sufficiently altered and significantly increased levels of the cationic form of the local anesthetic are not achieved to produce a more rapid onset of anesthesia.

Attempts have been made to improve the onset of conduction blockade by adding sodium bicarbonate to local anesthetic solutions immediately before injection.[50,59] Theoretically, sodium bicarbonate will increase the *p*H of the local anesthetic solution, which in turn will increase the amount of drug in the uncharged base form. Thus the rate of diffusion across the nerve sheath and nerve membrane should be enhanced, resulting in a more rapid onset of anesthesia. Several clinical studies have been performed in which the addition of sodium bicarbonate to solu-

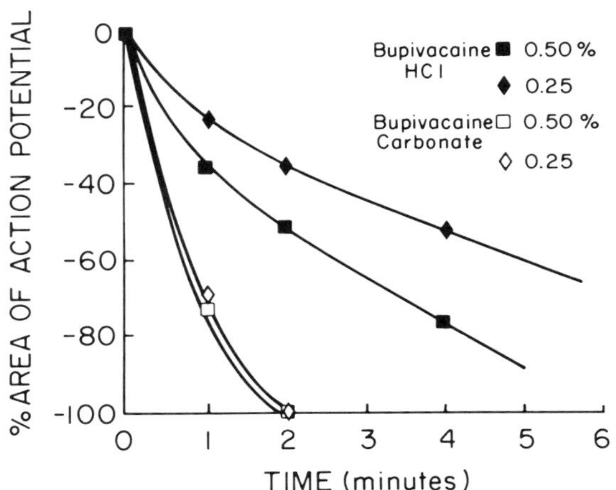

FIG. 4-6. Effect of CO_2 on the onset of conduction block in the isolated frog sciatic nerve.

tions of bupivacaine did appear to produce a significant decrease in the latency of brachial plexus blockade.[50,59] Moreover, it has been reported that the duration of anesthesia was prolonged by increasing the *p*H of the local anesthetic solution (Fig. 4-7).[59]

Potassium has also been added to local anesthetic solutions in an attempt to improve the quality of anesthesia. Addition of 1% KCl to lidocaine was found to shorten the latency of spread and intensify the quality of sensory block in the epidural space.[18] In a subsequent study, the duration of digital and ulnar blocks with lidocaine was prolonged by the addition of KCl, but the onset of anesthesia was unaffected.[4]

Various attempts have been made to prolong the duration of anesthesia by incorporating dextran into local anesthetic solutions.[74,99] Discrepancies exist in studies of the effectiveness of dextran in prolonging the duration of regional anesthesia. In one controlled clinical study, prolonged durations of anesthesia were observed in some patients, but the mean duration of intercostal nerve blockade was not significantly altered when solutions of bupivacaine with and without dextran were compared.[12]

Rosenblatt and Fung have suggested that the difference in results obtained by various investigators may be related to the *p*H of the dextran solution used.[98] These authors have reported that dextran solutions with a *p*H of 8.0 significantly prolong the duration of bupivacaine-induced coccygeal nerve blocks in rats, whereas the duration of block is not altered when dextran with a *p*H of 4.5 to 5.5 is added to bupivacaine.[98] These results indicate that alkalinization of the anesthetic solution may be responsible for prolonged conduction blockade rather than the dextran itself.

Mixtures of Local Anesthetics. The use of mixtures of local anesthetics for regional anesthesia has become relatively popular in recent years. The basis for this practice is to compensate for the short duration of action of certain agents such as chloroprocaine or lidocaine and the long latency of other agents such as tetracaine and bupivacaine. The combination of lidocaine or mepivacaine and tetracaine was commonly used in some centers before the advent of bupivacaine and etidocaine as long duration anesthetics. Because the slow onset of tetracaine for peripheral nerve blocks and epidural anesthesia was clinically unacceptable, the addition of lidocaine or mepivacaine provided a local anesthetic solution that afforded a relatively rapid onset of action and prolonged duration of anesthesia. Recently, mixtures of chloroprocaine and bupivacaine have been used to produce a local anesthetic solution with a rapid onset and long duration of action. The low systemic toxicity of chloroprocaine afforded an additional advantage to such a mixture; however, the use of a chloroprocaine–bupivacaine mixture has produced contradictory results. Cunningham and Kaplan originally reported that a mixture of chloroprocaine and bupivacaine did result in a short latency and prolonged duration of brachial plexus blockade.[33] On the other hand, Cohen and Thurlow found that the duration of epidural anesthesia produced by a mixture

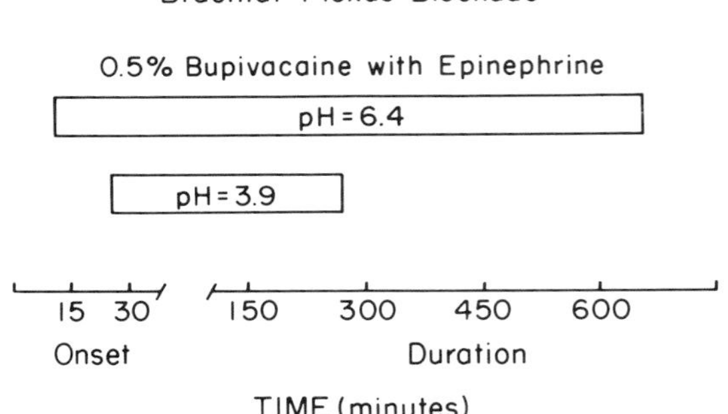

FIG. 4-7. Effect of *p*H on the onset and duration of brachial plexus blockade. (Data derived from Hilgier: ref 59)

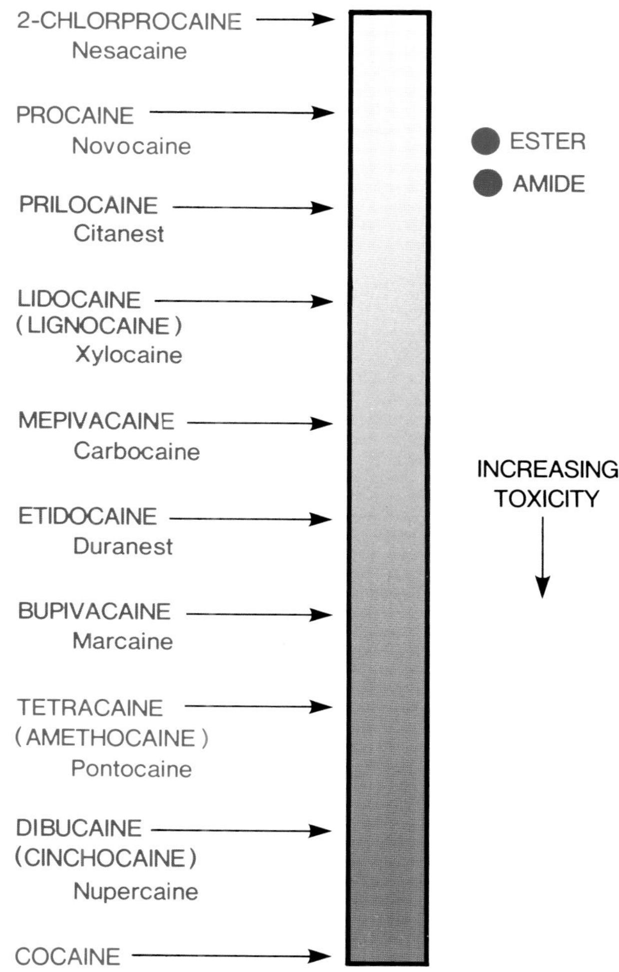

FIG. 4-8. Spectrum of local anesthetic agents. Agents are arranged in approximate order of increasing toxicity; it should be noted, however, that comparisons of all of the agents at "equi-effect" concentration, under the same conditions, have not yet been made in humans.

of chloroprocaine–bupivacaine was significantly shorter than that obtained with solutions of bupivacaine alone.[27] This reduced duration has been attributed in part to a decrease in *p*H, since chloroprocaine solutions have a *p*H of about 3.0.[49] Reduction in *p*H will decrease the amount of bupivacaine available in the uncharged base form, which may reduce the number of molecules able to penetrate the nerve sheath. In addition, data from isolated nerve studies suggest that a metabolite of chloroprocaine may inhibit the binding of bupivacaine to membrane receptor sites.[28] In a randomized prospective study of mixtures of various concentrations of lidocaine and bupivacaine, no difference in onset of blockade was observed among the solutions tested. Duration of blockade with a 50 : 50 mixture of lidocaine/bupivacaine was only marginally greater than that for lidocaine alone.[106] At present there do not appear to be any clinically significant advantages to using mixtures of local anesthetic agents. Etidocaine and bupivacaine provide clinically acceptable onsets of action and prolonged durations of anesthesia. In addition, the use of catheter techniques for epidural anesthesia and for brachial plexus blockade makes it possible to administer repeated injections of rapidly acting agents such as chloroprocaine or lidocaine, which will provide an anesthetic duration of indefinite length.

TOXICITY OF LOCAL ANESTHETICS

Various types of toxic reactions have been reported in humans in association with the use of local anesthetic agents. The adverse reactions observed include systemic toxicity involving primarily the central nervous system and the cardiovascular system, localized neural and skeletal muscle irritation, and specific side-effects such as methemoglobinemia, allergy, and addiction. CNS and cardiovascular toxicity and skeletal muscle irritation are toxicologic properties of all local anesthetic agents. The remaining adverse effects are associated with the use of certain specific drugs. If one considers the large number of local anesthetic administrations, the frequency of toxic reactions is extremely low. Moreover, most untoward effects are due to the inappropriate use of this class of drugs, such as accidental intravascular or intrathecal injections or administration of an excessive dosage.

SYSTEMIC TOXICITY

Most toxic reactions to local anesthetics in humans involve the CNS. Local anesthetic-induced cardiovascular depression occurs less frequently but tends to be more serious and more difficult to manage.

Local anesthetics vary considerably in terms of their potential for causing systemic toxic reactions. The relative toxicity of the commonly used agents is depicted in Figure 4-8.

Central Nervous System Toxicity

The signs and symptoms of local-anesthetic-induced CNS toxicity are shown in Figure 4-9. Human volunteers receiving intravenous infusions of local anesthetics describe feelings of lightheadedness and dizziness followed frequently by visual and auditory disturbances such as difficulty in focusing and tinnitus. Other subjective CNS symptoms include disorientation and occasional feelings of drowsiness. Objective signs of CNS toxicity are usually excitatory in nature and include shivering, muscular twitching, and tremors initially involving muscles of the face and distal parts of the extremities. Ultimately, generalized convulsions of a tonic–clonic nature occur. If a sufficiently large dose of a local anesthetic agent is administered systemically, the initial signs of CNS excitation are followed rapidly by a state of generalized CNS depression. Seizure activity ceases and respiratory depression and ultimately respiratory arrest occur. Occasionally in some patients CNS depression may occur without a preceding excitatory phase, particularly if other CNS depressant drugs have been used concomitantly.

The mechanism by which local anesthetic agents produce an initial state of CNS excitation involves the selective blockade of inhibitory pathways in the cerebral cortex.[34,60,112] The initial inhibition of inhibitory pathways by local anesthetic agents would allow facilitatory neurons to function in an unopposed fashion, which would result in an increase in excitatory activity, leading to convulsions. After an increase in the dose of local anesthetic administered, these agents would tend to inhibit both inhibitory and facilitatory pathways, resulting in a generalized state of CNS depression.

The potential CNS toxicity of various local anesthetic agents appears to be primarily related to their intrinsic anesthetic potency. In cats, for example, a dose of about 35 mg/kg of procaine was required to cause convulsions compared to a mean convulsive dose of 5 mg/kg of bupivacaine.[40] Lidocaine, mepivacaine, and prilocaine were intermediate with regard to the dose required to induce convulsions. A comparison of the intrinsic anesthetic potency and

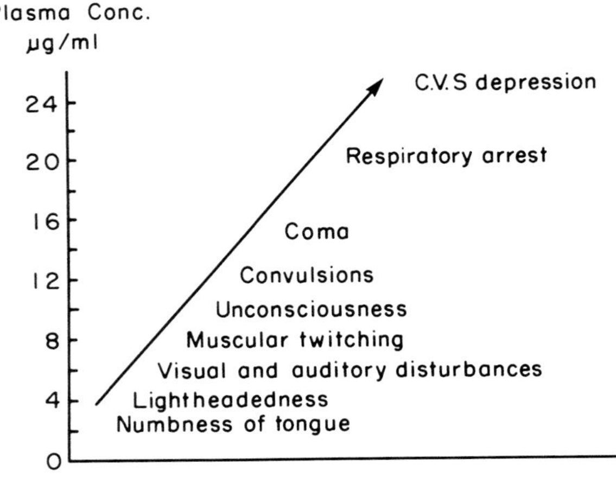

FIG. 4-9. Relationship of signs and symptoms of local anesthetic toxicity to plasma concentrations of lidocaine.

toxicity of these local anesthetics indicates that bupivacaine is about eight times more potent than procaine when used for production of regional anesthesia and about seven times more toxic than procaine with regard to the dose required to produce convulsive activity in cats. In a similar study in dogs a dose of about 20 mg/kg of lidocaine was required to produce convulsions compared to doses of 8 mg/kg for etidocaine and 5 mg/kg of bupivacaine.[73] Thus the relative CNS toxicity of bupivacaine, etidocaine, and lidocaine is about 4:2:1, which is similar to the relative anesthetic potency of these agents in humans. Intravenous infusion studies in human volunteers have also demonstrated a relationship between the intrinsic anesthetic potency of various local anesthetics and the dosage required to induce signs of CNS toxicity.[47,103,104]

A correlation also exists between the convulsive blood level of various local anesthetic agents and their relative anesthetic potencies. In monkeys, bupivacaine produced convulsions at a blood level of about 4.5 µg/ml, whereas lidocaine-induced convulsions were observed at a mean blood level of 25 µg/ml.[85] In humans, convulsions have been reported at venous blood levels of approximately 2 to 4 µg/ml of bupivacaine and etidocaine, whereas concentrations in excess of 10 µg/ml are usually required for production of convulsive activity when a less potent agent such as lidocaine is administered.

Although a general relationship exists between anesthetic potency and CNS toxicity, the rate of injection and rapidity with which a particular blood level is achieved will influence the toxicity of local anesthetic agents (Fig. 4-10). Scott, for example, has shown that human volunteers could tolerate an average dose of 236 mg of etidocaine and a venous blood level of 3.0 µg/ml before the onset of CNS symptoms when etidocaine was infused at the rate of 10 mg/min.[102] When the infusion rate was increased to 20 mg/min, however, the volunteers could only tolerate an average of 161 mg of etidocaine, which produced a venous plasma level of about 2 µg/ml.

The acid–base status of animals and patients can markedly effect the CNS activity of local anesthetic agents.[40] Studies in cats have shown that the convulsive threshold of various local anesthetics is inversely related to the arterial P_{CO_2} level (Table 4-3). The convulsive threshold dose of various local anesthetics was decreased by about 50% when the P_{CO_2} was elevated from 25–40 mm Hg to 65–81 mm Hg. A decrease in arterial *p*H is also associated with a decrease in the convulsive threshold of these agents. The relationship between P_{CO_2}, *p*H, and the CNS activity of local anesthetic agents has been evaluated by Englesson and Grevsten.[41] Respiratory acidosis with a resultant increase in P_{CO_2} and a decrease in arterial *p*H will consistently decrease the convulsant threshold of local anesthetic agents; however, an elevated P_{CO_2} and *p*H, as may occur during metabolic alkalosis, exert less of an effect on the convulsive threshold of local anesthetic agents, suggesting that *p*H is primarily responsible for the changes in CNS toxicity. Acidosis may alter the convulsive threshold

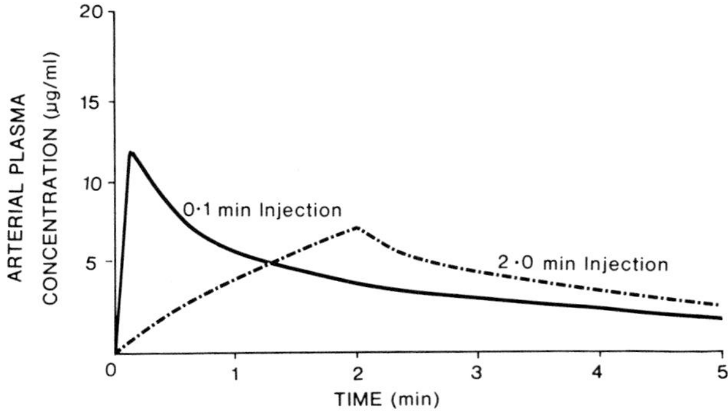

FIG. 4-10. Arterial plasma concentrations, following intravenous injection of 100 mg of lidocaine hydrochloride over 0.1 and 2 minutes, to simulate concentrations of an inadvertent intravenous injection during a block procedure. Note the reduction in peak concentrations brought about by prolonging injection time. (Data from Tucker, G.T., and Boas. R.A.: Pharmacokinetic aspects of intravenous regional anesthesia. Anesthesiology, *34*:538, 1971.)

TABLE 4-3. EFFECT OF P_{CO_2} ON THE CONVULSIVE THRESHOLD (CD_{100}) OF VARIOUS LOCAL ANESTHETICS IN CATS

Agent	CD (mg/kg) P_{CO_2} $25-40_{mm\ Hg}$	P_{CO_2} $65-81_{mm\ Hg}$	Change in CD_{100}
Procaine	35	17	51
Mepivacaine	18	10	44
Prilocaine	22	12	45
Lidocaine	15	7	53
Bupivacaine	5	2.5	50

Data derived from Englesson.[40]

in several ways. An elevation of P_{CO_2} will enhance cerebral blood flow so that more anesthetic agent is delivered to the brain. A decrease in intracellular *p*H will enhance the conversion of the base form of local anesthetic agents to the cationic form, which is responsible for the effect of these drugs on nerve membranes. The cationic form does not diffuse well, which will increase the intracellular concentration. Hypercarbia or acidosis, or both, will also decrease the plasma protein binding of local anesthetic agents.[5,21] Therefore, an elevation in P_{CO_2} or decrease in *p*H will increase the portion of free drug available for diffusion into the brain. On the other hand, acidosis will increase the cationic form of the local anesthetic, which will decrease the rate of diffusion.

In summary, local anesthetic agents can produce marked effects on the central nervous system. In general, signs of CNS excitation leading to frank convulsions are the most common manifestation of systemic local anesthetic toxicity. Excessive doses of these drugs may also lead to CNS depression and respiratory arrest. In general the potential CNS toxicity of local anesthetics correlates with the inherent anesthetic potency of the various agents.

Cardiovascular System Toxicity

Local anesthetic agents can exert a direct action both on cardiac muscle and on peripheral vascular smooth muscle.

Cardiac Effects. Detailed electrophysiologic studies on cardiac muscle have been carried out with various local anesthetics but particularly with lidocaine, because this agent is used for treating ventricular arrhythmias. Lidocaine decreases the maximum rate of depolarization without altering the resting membrane potential of cardiac muscle.[51] Action potential duration and the effective refractory period are decreased by lidocaine; however, the ratio of effective refractory period to action potential duration is increased both in Purkinje fibers and in ventricular muscle (see Fig. 2-13).

Considerable interest exists in the cardiac electrophysiologic effects of bupivacaine because of the observation that this agent may precipitate cardiac arrhythmias in various animal species, including man. Bupivacaine markedly depresses the rapid phase of depolarization (V max) in isolated guinea pig papillary muscle preparations.[26] In addition, the rate of recovery from a steady-state block was much slower in bupivacaine-treated papillary muscles as compared to lidocaine. This slow rate of recovery resulted in an incomplete restoration of V max between action potentials when heart rate exceeded 100 beats/min. In contrast, recovery from lidocaine was complete, even at rapid heart rates. A decrease in rate of depolarization and action potential duration leading to conduction block and electrical inexcitability was also observed in canine Purkinje fibers.[117] These results suggest that bupivacaine may produce unidirectional block and a reentrant type of cardiac arrhythmia.

Electrophysiologic studies in intact dogs and in humans essentially reflect the findings observed in isolated cardiac tissue.[69,110] As the dose and blood levels of lidocaine are increased, a prolongation of conduction time through various parts of the heart occurs that is reflected in the electrocardiogram as an increase in the PR interval and QRS duration. Extremely high concentrations of local anesthetics will depress spontaneous pacemaker activity in the sinus node, resulting in sinus bradycardia and sinus arrest. A similar depression at the AV node also occurs, resulting in prolonged PR intervals and partial and complete AV dissociation.

Because depolarization in the heart and nerve is related to the influx of sodium ions, local anesthetics are believed to act primarily at the sodium channels to inhibit sodium conductance (see Fig. 2-13). In cardiac tissue the depolarization phase of the action potential is related to the influx of sodium ions through so-called fast channels and to the influx of calcium ions through slow channels (see Fig. 2-13). The slow calcium channels are responsible for the spontaneous depolarization observed in the region of the SA node. Most investigators believe that local anesthetics have little effect on the slow inward calcium currents. Josephson and Sperelakis have reported, however, that high concentrations of lidocaine, procaine, and tetracaine can block slow calcium channels in the myocardial sarcolemma.[63]

Local anesthetic agents also exert profound effects on the mechanical activity of cardiac muscle. Studies on isolated guinea pig atria and isolated whole rabbit hearts have shown that all local anesthetics exert a dose-dependent negative inotropic action.[10,45] The more potent local anesthetic agents tend to depress cardiac contractility at lower doses and concentrations than do the less potent local anesthetic agents (Table 4-4).

Studies in dogs in which a strain gauge arch was sutured to the right ventricle revealed that a relationship exists between the local anesthetic potency of various agents and their ability to decrease myocardial contractility (Fig. 4-11).[109] Tetracaine, for example, which is about eight to ten times more potent than procaine as a local anesthetic, was found to be about eight times more depressant than procaine in intact dogs. The hemodynamic effects of the various clinically useful ester and amide local anesthetics were compared in closed-chest anesthetized dogs.[71,77] Again, a relationship existed between the anesthetic potency of the various agents and their depressant effect on heart rate, blood pressure, and cardiac output. The direct effect of lidocaine on myocardial contractility in patients under general anesthesia was evaluated by Harrison and colleagues during thoracic surgical procedures.[57] A strain gauge sutured to the right ventricle revealed that the intravenous administration of 2 to 4 mg/kg of lidocaine

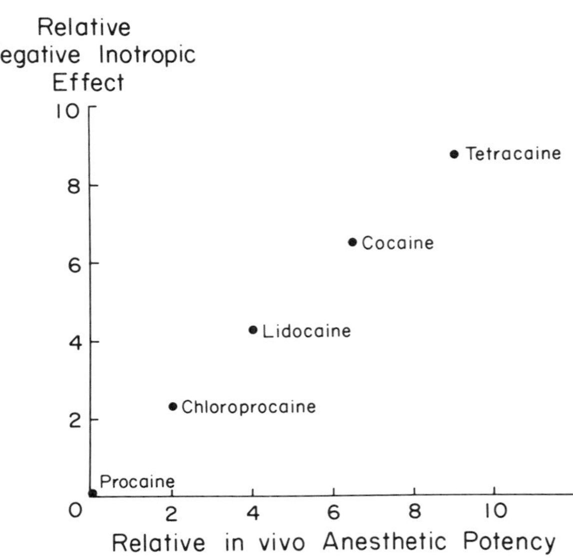

FIG. 4-11. Relation between anesthetic potency and negative inotropic effect of various local anesthetics. (Data derived from Stewart, *et al.*: ref 109)

TABLE 4-4. COMPARATIVE EFFECT OF VARIOUS LOCAL ANESTHETIC AGENTS ON CARDIAC CONTRACTILITY

		Local Anesthetic Concentrations (μg/ml) to Produce 25–50% Decrease in Cardiac Contractility	
Agent	**Relative Anesthetic Potency**	**Isolated Rabbit Heart* (25% ↓)**	**Isolated Guinea Pig Atria† (50% ↓)**
Procaine	1	–	277
Chloroprocaine	1	–	102
Cocaine	2	–	56
Lidocaine	2	16.4	67
Prilocaine	2	11.7	42
Mepivacaine	2	9.9	55
Etidocaine	6	1.3	–
Bupivacaine	8	1.4	6
Tetracaine	8	0.9	6

*Data derived from Block and Covino.[10]
†Data derived from Feldman et al.[45]

caused minimal changes in right ventricular contractile force.

The mechanism by which local anesthetics depress myocardial contractility is not precisely known. Both procaine and tetracaine can increase the release of calcium from isolated skeletal muscle preparations.[67] A similar displacement of calcium from cardiac muscle would result in a decrease in myocardial contractility; however, studies in the isolated guinea pig heart have shown that an increase in the extracellular concentration of calcium failed to reverse the negative inotropic action of bupivacaine or lidocaine.[113]

In recent years several case reports have appeared in the literature in which bupivacaine and etidocaine were associated with rapid and profound cardiovascular depression.[2,38,89] These cases differed from the usual cardiovascular depression seen with local anesthetics. The onset of cardiovascular depression occurred relatively early. In some cases, severe cardiac arrhythmias were observed, and the cardiac depression appeared resistant to various therapeutic modalities.

Insight into these clinical problems has been obtained in nonanesthetized sheep preparation with chronic vascular catheters.[83] After non-convulsion-producing graded bolus doses of both lidocaine and bupivacaine, dose-dependent reductions in left ventricular dp/dt max occurred (as an index of myocardial contractility), as did increases in left ventricular end diastolic pressure (LVEDP) (Fig. 4-12A). Both of these parameters returned to control values within 3 minutes in keeping with negative inotropic drug effects. In addition, within seconds of drug administration into the inferior vena cava, dose-dependent increases in pulmonary artery pressure were noted, suggesting a direct pulmonary vasoconstrictive effect (Fig. 4-12B). These effects were of similar magnitude when lidocaine and bupivacaine were administered in doses considered to be of equal potency, that is, lidocaine : bupivacaine = 4 : 1.

With convulsion-producing doses ($CD_{100} = 3.3$ mg/kg for lidocaine, 1.5 mg/kg for bupivacaine), the initial transient depression in the indices of myocardial contractility was rapidly reversed, presumably by autonomic responses to the convulsion. During convulsions, elevations in LVEDP were marked for both drugs, but without significant changes in intrathoracic pressure, suggesting decreased myocardial compliance as a possible causative factor.

The cardiotoxicity of the more potent agents such as bupivacaine appears to differ from that of lidocaine in the following manner: [1] The ratio of the dosage required for irreversible cardiovascular collapse and the dosage that will produce CNS toxicity (convulsions), that is, the CC/CNS ratio, is lower for bupivacaine and etidocaine than for lidocaine; [2] ventricular arrhythmias and fatal ventricular fibrillation may occur after the rapid intravenous administration of a large dose of bupivacaine (Fig. 4-12C) but not lidocaine; [3] the pregnant animal or patient may be more sensitive to the cardiotoxic effects of bupivacaine than the nonpregnant animal or patient; [4] cardiac resuscitation is more difficult after bupivacaine-induced cardiovascular collapse; and [5] acidosis and hypoxia markedly potentiate the cardiotoxicity of bupivacaine.

CC/CNS Ratio. Studies in adult sheep in which a continuous intravenous infusion of local anesthetics was administered have shown that a CC/CNS dose ratio of 7.1 ± 1.1 existed for lidocaine, indicating that seven times as much drug was required to induce irreversible cardiovascular collapse as was needed for the production of convulsions.[82,83] In comparison, the CC/CNS ratio for bupivacaine was 3.7 ± 0.5 and for etidocaine 4.4 ± 0.9. In terms of blood levels associated with CNS and cardiovascular collapse, lidocaine showed a CC/CNS blood level ratio of 3.6 ± 0.3 compared to values of 1.6 to 1.7 for bupivacaine and etidocaine (Fig. 4-12). Tissue levels of the various local anesthetics that were determined at the time of cardiovascular collapse indicate a greater uptake of bupivacaine and etidocaine by the myocardium compared to lidocaine (Fig. 4-13).

Ventricular Arrhythmias. deJong and colleagues initially reported that bupivacaine caused cardiac arrhythmias in awake but paralyzed cats, whereas no such changes were observed with lidocaine.[35] Studies in unanesthetized sheep confirmed that severe cardiac arrhythmias occur after the rapid intravenous administration of bupivacaine, whereas no cardiac irregularities were observed when lidocaine was injected intravenously.[66] Although no cardiac arrhythmias were observed in the canine toxicity studies conducted by Liu and co-workers, these dogs were anesthetized with pentobarbital.[71,77] Subsequent studies in unanesthetized dogs demonstrated the occurrence of ventricular tachycardia and ventricular fibrillation in some animals receiving intravenous bupivacaine.[100] No arrhythmias occurred when the same dogs were given intravenous lidocaine. The incidence of ventricular fibrillation has been ascertained in preliminary studies in awake dogs in which convulsant and supraconvulsant doses of lidocaine, mepivacaine, bupivacaine, and etidocaine were ad-

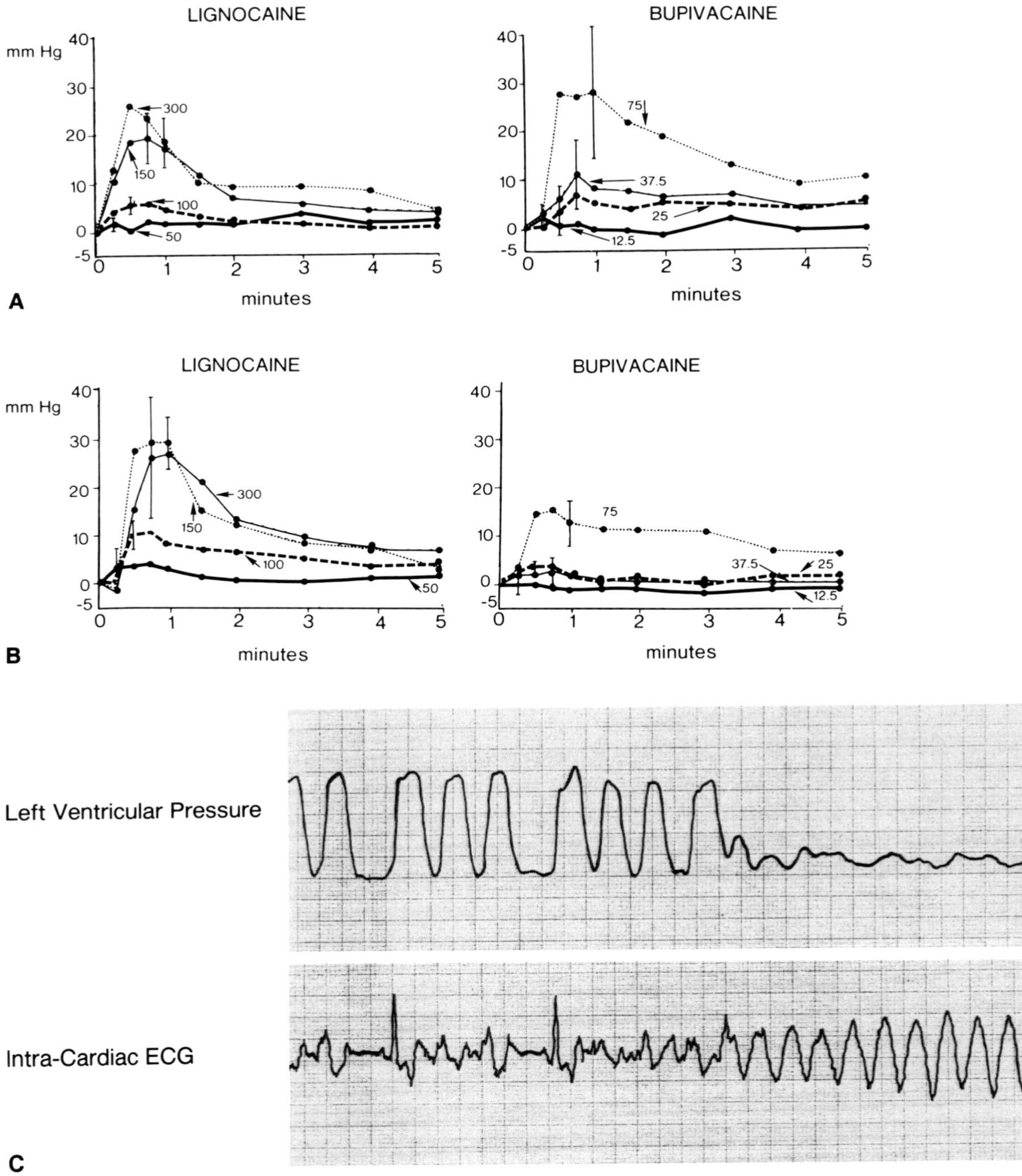

FIG. 4-12. Cardiovascular effects of local anesthetics in nonanesthetized sheep. **A.** Change in left ventricular end diastolic pressure (LVEDP) at increasing doses of lidocaine (lignocaine) and bupivacaine. **B.** Change in pulmonary artery pressure at the same doses of both drugs. The four doses (mg) were chosen for each drug to approximate equivalent clinical doses (lidocaine: bupivacaine = 4 : 1) (see text). **C.** Cardiac toxicity of bupivacaine. A rapid intravenous bolus of 150 mg of bupivacaine resulted in a fatal rapid decrease in left ventricular pressure (catheter tip transducer). Also ECG changed from a normal intracardiac quadripolar ECG pattern to that of ventricular tachycardia and subsequent ventricular fibrillation. (Reproduced with permission from Dr. C. Nancarrow: Acute Toxicity of Lignocaine and Bupivacaine. Ph.D. Thesis, Flinders University of Southern Australia, 1986.)[86]

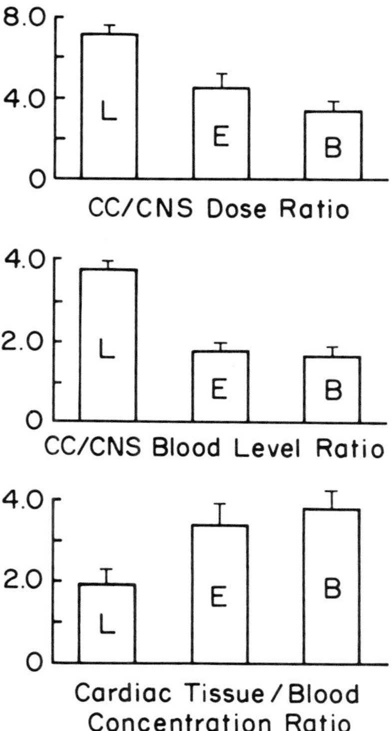

FIG. 4-13. Comparative CC/CNS toxicity dose ratio, CC/CNS toxicity blood level ratio, and myocardial tissue levels at time of cardiovascular collapse of lidocaine (*L*), bupivacaine (*B*), and etidocaine (*E*). (Data derived from Morishima, *et al.*: refs 82, 83)

ministered intravenously (Table 4-5).[44] Although the number of animals studied is relatively small in each group, it appears that ventricular fibrillation may occur in about 50% of dogs after the rapid intravenous injection of a convulsant or supraconvulsant dose of bupivacaine. Ventricular fibrillation was not observed in the lidocaine, etidocaine, or mepivacaine treated dogs. Ventricular arrhythmias were observed in awake paralyzed cats following the administration of etidocaine, although the frequency was less than that associated with the use of bupivacaine.[35] In addition, ventricular fibrillation was also observed in one of three dogs in which supraconvulsant doses of etidocaine were injected.[39] The results suggest that the occurrence of ventricular fibrillation is not related to the basic piperidine ring structure of bupivacaine because mepivacaine, which contains the piperidine moiety, failed to cause these cardiac abnormalities. Thus it appears that it is the bupivacaine molecule *per se* that is responsible for the actions on the heart.

The theory that ventricular arrhythmias are related to the degree of lipid solubility and protein binding may not be valid because etidocaine, which is more highly lipid soluble than bupivacaine and equally protein bound, appears to be associated with a lower incidence of ventricular fibrillation than is bupivacaine. In sheep, Nancarrow and colleagues found that mean values of maximum arterial drug concentrations during fatal experiments were 165 mg/liter (SD 22) for lidocaine-treated animals and 20.9 mg/liter (SD 7.9) after bupivacaine.[86] For both drugs, similar percentages of the initial dose (3% for lidocaine, 3.7% for bupivacaine) were found in the heart after analysis of tissue homogenate obtained postmortem.

Cardiac arrhythmias associated with bupivacaine do not appear related to the intensity of convulsive activity, although pentobarbital-treated dogs that did not convulse did not demonstrate these electrocardiographic abnormalities. Isolated guinea pig hearts perfused with a bupivacaine solution revealed evidence of conduction block and bigemeny and trigemeny, but did not when perfused with lidocaine.[113] In addition, Reiz has observed the development of ventricular fibrillation in intact pigs in which bupivacaine was injected directly into the left anterior descending coronary artery (Reiz, S.: Personal communication). Thus these ventricular arrhythmias apparently are not related to the occurrence of convulsive activity.

The etiology of bupivacaine-associated ventricular arrhythmias is not known. As mentioned previously, electrophysiologic studies have shown that bupivacaine can markedly depress the rapid phase of depolarization (V max) of the cardiac action potential and prolong the recovery phase, leading to conduction block and electrical inexcitability. These data suggest possible unidirectional blockade of conducting pathways, which may cause a reentrant type of arrhythmia.[26,117]

TABLE 4-5. FREQUENCY OF VENTRICULAR FIBRILLATION (VF) FOLLOWING THE I.V. ADMINISTRATION OF CONVULSANT OR SUPRACONVULSANT DOSES OF VARIOUS LOCAL ANESTHETICS IN UNANESTHETIZED DOGS

Drug	Number of Dogs	Dose (mg/kg)	Frequency of VF
Lidocaine	10	11-33	0
Mepivacaine	5	13-26	0
Etidocaine	8	4.6-9.2	13
Bupivacaine	16	3.4-13.6	44

Data derived from Eicholzer et al,[39] Feldman et al,[44] and Sage et al.[100]

Enhanced Cardiotoxicity in Pregnancy. Many of the cardiotoxic reactions reported after the use of bupivacaine have occurred in pregnant patients. As a result, the 0.75% solution is no longer recommended for use in obstetric anesthesia in the United States. It is not certain whether the pregnant patient is more susceptible to the toxic effects of local anesthetics. Studies in sheep have shown that the CC/CNS dosage ratio of bupivacaine decreased from 3.7 ± 0.5 in nonpregnant sheep to 2.7 ± 0.4 in pregnant sheep.[81] Little difference was observed, however, in the CC/CNS blood level ratio, which varied from 1.6 ± 0.1 in nonpregnant sheep to 1.4 ± 0.1 in pregnant ones. The myocardial uptake of bupivacaine in pregnant sheep at the time of cardiovascular collapse did not differ from that in nonpregnant sheep. Additional studies are clearly warranted to determine the relative cardiotoxicity of bupivacaine and other local anesthetics in pregnant and nonpregnant animals.

Cardiac Resuscitation. Cardiopulmonary resuscitation is apparently extremely difficult in patients in whom cardiotoxicity has occurred following the administration of a toxic dose of bupivacaine. Studies in acidotic and hypoxic sheep have also indicated that cardiac resuscitation following bupivacaine-induced toxicity is difficult.[114] Recent studies in hypoxic dogs rendered toxic with bupivacaine indicate that resuscitation is possible if massive doses of epinephrine and atropine are used.[64] It is not known whether the observed difficulty with cardiac resuscitation is unique to bupivacaine. Little information is available on resuscitation of animals in which similar degrees of cardiac depression have been produced by other local anesthetics.

Effect of Acidosis and Hypoxia. Changes in acid–base status will alter the potential cardiovascular toxicity of local anesthetic agents. Studies on isolated atrial tissues have shown that hypercarbia, acidosis, and hypoxia will tend to potentiate the negative chronotropic and inotropic action of lidocaine and bupivacaine.[101] In particular, the combination of hypoxia and acidosis appears to markedly potentiate the cardiodepressant effects of bupivacaine. Studies in intact sheep have also demonstrated that hypoxia and acidosis markedly increase the cardiotoxicity of bupivacaine.[114] This enhanced toxicity is not related to a greater myocardial tissue uptake of local anesthetic, since investigations in rabbits demonstrated a decreased cardiac concentration of bupivacaine in the presence of acidosis.[56] Marked hypercarbia, acidosis, and hypoxia occur very rapidly in some patients after seizure activity caused by the rapid accidental intravascular injection of local anesthetic agents.[79] Thus it has been postulated that the cardiovascular depression observed with the more potent agents such as bupivacaine may in part be related to the severe acid–base changes that occur following the administration of toxic doses of these agents (see also Chap. 3).

PERIPHERAL VASCULAR EFFECTS

Local anesthetics exert a biphasic action on smooth muscle of peripheral blood vessels.[9] For example, exposure of arterioles in the cremaster muscle of rats to concentrations of lidocaine of 10 to 10^3 μg/ml produced a dose-related state of vasoconstriction varying from 88% to 60% of the control vascular diameter.[61] An increase in the concentration of lidocaine to 10^4 μg/ml produced approximately a 27% increase in arteriolar diameter, indicating a significant degree of vasodilation. Other studies using an isolated rat portal vein preparation have also demonstrated that local anesthetic drugs stimulate spontaneous myogenic contractions and augment basal tone at low concentrations and inhibit myogenic activity at higher concentrations.[9]

In vivo studies have also confirmed the biphasic effect of local anesthetic on the peripheral vasculature. The intra-arterial administration of mepivacaine in human volunteers resulted in a decrease in forearm blood flow without any change in arterial pressure, which suggests that mepivacaine caused vasoconstriction, which increases peripheral vascular resistance.[62] Similar studies with lidocaine also showed an increased tone in capacitance vessels, with less consistent effect on resistance vessels. As the dose of local anesthetic agent is increased, the stimulatory or vasoconstrictor action of these agents changes to one of inhibition and vasodilation.

Cocaine is the only agent that produces a state of vasoconstriction at most doses. Direct blood flow studies in dogs have shown that the initial effect of cocaine is one of vasodilation, but this is followed by a long period of vasoconstriction regardless of the dose of cocaine administered.[87] This unique property of cocaine is not related to a direct effect of cocaine itself on vascular smooth muscle but is basically an indirect action of this agent. Cocaine has been shown to inhibit the uptake of norepinephrine by tissue binding sites. Thus, after the release of norepinephrine from postganglionic sympathetic fibers, the decrease in the reuptake of norepinephrine by tissue binding sites will result in an excess amount of free norepinephrine, which will lead to a prolonged, profound state of vasoconstriction. This property of cocaine to inhibit the reuptake of norepinephrine has not been demonstrated to occur with other local anesthetics.

In summary, the sequence of cardiovascular events that usually occurs after the systemic administration of local anesthetic agents is as follows: At relatively nontoxic blood levels of these agents, either no change in blood pressure or a slight increase in blood pressure may be observed. Concentrations of local anesthetics that produce CNS toxicity will result in a marked increase in heart rate, blood pressure, and cardiac output that is directly related to the degree and duration of convulsive activity.[100] A further increase in dosage and blood level of local anesthetic leads to cardiovascular depression. The initial fall in blood pressure is primarily related to a decrease in cardiac output that is transient in nature and spontaneously reversible in most patients. If the amount of local anesthetic administered is excessive, however, a profound state of cardiovascular depression occurs that is related to the negative inotropic and peripheral vasodilator action of these agents. Ultimately, the combined peripheral vasodilation, decreased myocardial contractility, and depressant effect on cardiac rate and conductivity will lead to cardiac arrest and circulatory collapse. In addition, certain agents such as bupivacaine may precipitate potentially fatal ventricular fibrillation.

Miscellaneous Systemic Effects

Other systemic actions have been ascribed to local anesthetic drugs, most of which are related to the generalized membrane stabilizing property of this class of drugs. For example, local anesthetics have been reported to possess neuromuscular blocking, ganglionic blocking, and anticholinergic activity. There is little evidence to suggest that any of these miscellaneous effects is clinically significant under normal conditions.

A unique systemic side-effect is the formation of methemoglobinemia following the administration of large doses of prilocaine.[58,76] A dose-response relationship exists between the amount of prilocaine administered and the degree of methemoglobinemia. In general, doses of prilocaine of approximately 600 mg are required before the development of clinically significant levels of methemoglobinemia. The formation of methemoglobinemia is believed to be related to the degradation of prilocaine in the liver to O-toluidine, which is actually responsible for the oxidation of hemoglobin to methemoglobin.[58] Although methemoglobinemia is of little clinical significance in most patients with normal oxygen carrying capacity, it has limited the use of this potentially valuable drug, since prilocaine is the least toxic of the amide local anesthetics in terms of CNS toxicity. The methemoglobinemia associated with the use of prilocaine is spontaneously reversible or may be treated by the intravenous administration of methylene blue.

ALLERGIC EFFECTS

Reports of allergic reactions, hypersensitivity, or anaphylactic responses to local anesthetic agents appear periodically.[19,58,94] Unfortunately, systemic toxic reactions to local anesthetic agents are frequently misdiagnosed as representing allergic- or hypersensitivity-type reactions.[46] The amino-ester agents such as procaine have been shown to produce allergic-type reactions. Because these agents are derivatives of para-aminobenzoic acid, which is known to be allergenic in nature, it is not unusual that a certain percentage of the population will demonstrate allergic reactions to this class of local anesthetics. The advent of the amino amide local anesthetics, that are not derivatives of para-aminobenzoic acid, markedly changed the incidence of allergic-type reactions to local anesthetic drugs. Reactions of an allergic type to the amino amides are extremely rare, although several cases have been reported in the literature in recent years which suggest that this class of agents can on rare occasions produce an allergic-type phenomenon.[19,46,94] It should be remembered that solutions of amino amide agents from multiple-dose containers may contain a preservative, methylparaben, whose chemical structure is similar to that of para-aminobenzoic acid. It has been shown that patients in whom methylparaben was administered intradermally demonstrated a positive skin reaction.[3] Also some patients are allergic to metabisulfite, which is present in epinephrine-containing local anesthetic solutions. Cross-sensitivity reactions are possible because many other drugs, foods, and beverages contain preservatives such as metabisulphite and hydroxybenzoate. Two patients suspected of having allergic reactions to local anesthetics were confirmed by challenge testing to have allergies to benzoate and metabisulphite.

Progressive challenge with dilute (1 : 1000) and then undiluted intradermal injection of local anesthetics has been successfully used to diagnose adverse responses to local anesthetics. It is important to use local anesthetic solutions without additives in such testing, and also for neural blockade in patients with a history of allergy to preservatives in foods and drugs.[46]

LOCAL TISSUE TOXICITY

Local anesthetic agents used clinically rarely produce localized nerve damage.[107] Recently, however, some concern has been expressed regarding the potential neurotoxicity of chloroprocaine. Prolonged sensory motor deficits were reported in four patients after the epidural or subarachnoid injection of large doses of this particular drug.[91,93] Subsequently, Moore reported signs of neural damage in five additional patients in whom chloroprocaine had been used.[80] Studies in animals have proved somewhat contradictory regarding the potential neurotoxicity of chloroprocaine (Table 4-6). Barsa and associates, using an isolated rabbit vagus nerve preparation, reported that chloroprocaine was associated with signs of neural irritation, whereas the use of lidocaine under similar conditions failed to cause local toxic effects.[7] Histologic examination of rabbit sciatic nerves exposed to chloroprocaine for 6 hours did not, however, reveal any signs of nerve damage.[88] Doses of chloroprocaine sufficient to cause total spinal anesthesia in dogs produced paralysis in about 30% of the animals, whereas dogs treated with bupivacaine did not show evidence of permanent neurologic sequelae.[92] Studies of a similar nature in sheep and monkeys failed to show any difference in neurotoxicity between chloroprocaine and other local anesthetics or control solutions.[97] Paralysis observed in rabbits in which chloroprocaine solutions were administered intrathecally was believed related to sodium bisulfite, which is used as an antioxidant in chloroprocaine solutions.[116] The use of pure solutions of chloroprocaine without sodium bisulfite did not cause paralysis, whereas sodium bisulfite alone was associated with paralysis. A detailed series of studies has been conducted on the isolated rabbit vagus nerve to investigate the neurotoxicity of the various components of commercial chloroprocaine solutions (Table 4-7).[53] Commercial solutions of 3% chloroprocaine contain the local anesthetic agent itself, 0.2% sodium bisulfite, and hydrogen ions, which yield a *p*H of approximately 3.0. Application of commercial 3% chloroprocaine to isolated vagus nerves for 30 minutes resulted in irreversible conduction blockade. The use of 3% chloroprocaine with sodium bisulfite solution buffered to a *p*H of 7.0 caused reversible conduction block. A 3% chloroprocaine solution with a *p*H of 3.0 but without sodium bisulfite also resulted in reversible blockade. Application of an 0.2% sodium bisulfite solution at a *p*H of 3.0 resulted in irreversible conduction block, whereas the use of a 0.2% sodium bisulfite solution with a *p*H of 7.0 caused no conduction block. The results of these studies suggest that the combination of a low *p*H and the presence of sodium bisulfite may be responsible for the neurotoxic reactions observed following the use of large amounts of chloroprocaine solution. Chloroprocaine, itself, does not appear to be neurotoxic. The tolerance of peripheral nerves to bisulfite seems to be much higher than that of spinal nerve roots. Ford and colleagues (personal communication) injected 10% bisulfite at *p*H 4.8 near the saphenous nerve of the cat, and no damage was detected; however, at *p*H 2.8 moderate damage occurred.

Skeletal muscle appears to be more sensitive to the local irritant properties of local anesthetic agents than other tissues. Skeletal muscle changes have been observed with most of the clinically used local anesthetic agents.[68,80] In general, the more potent longer-

TABLE 4-6. SUMMARY OF NEUROTOXICITY STUDIES INVOLVING CHLOROPROCAINE

		Signs of Neurotoxicity			
Reference	**Type of Study**	**2-CP**	**Lidocaine**	**Bupivacaine**	**$NaHSO_3$**
7	Isolated rabbit vagus nerve	+++	0	—	—
53	Isolated rabbit vagus nerve	+++	—	0	+++
88	Intact rabbit sciatic nerve	0	0	—	—
92	Dog—total spinal	+++	—	0	—
116	Rabbit—spinal	+++	—	—	+++
97	Sheep—total spinal	+	+	0	—
97	Monkey—total spinal	+	—	+	—

0 = no effect; + = mild toxicity; +++ = severe toxicity; — = not studied; 2-CP = commercial 2-chloroprocaine solution; $NaHSO_3$ = sodium bisulfite.

TABLE 4-7. EFFECT OF CHLOROPROCAINE, *pH*, AND BISULFITE ON A AND C FIBER CONDUCTION IN THE ISOLATED RABBIT VAGUS NERVE

Local Anesthetic	*pH*	Bisulfite (%)	Recovery Time (min) A	Recovery Time (min) C
3% chloroprocaine	3.0	0.2	α	α
3% chloroprocaine	7.2	–	60	120
3% chloroprocaine	3.2	–	60	120
3% chloroprocaine	7.3	0.2	60	120
–	7.0	0.2	–	–
–	3.3	0.2	α	α

– = no block; α = irreversible block.

acting agents such as bupivacaine and etidocaine appear to cause a greater degree of localized skeletal muscle damage than the less potent, shorter-acting agents such as lidocaine and prilocaine. This effect on skeletal muscle is reversible, and muscle regeneration occurs rapidly and is complete within 2 weeks after injection of local anesthetic agents. These changes in skeletal muscle have not been correlated with any overt clinical signs of local irritation.

FACTORS INFLUENCING SYSTEMIC LOCAL ANESTHETIC ACTIVITY

The CNS and cardiovascular toxicity of local anesthetics is clearly related to the blood level of these agents, which in turn will influence the concentration in the brain and heart. The blood levels of local anesthetics that are achieved following the use of appropriate dosages and appropriate regional anesthetic techniques rarely cause adverse systemic reactions; however, toxic blood levels can occur, usually caused by an accidental intravascular injection or the extravascular administration of an excessive dose.

Extremely high blood levels of local anesthetics are achieved following rapid intravascular injection. Under these conditions toxicity is primarily related to the intrinsic anesthetic potency of the specific agents. The concentration of a drug in blood following an extravascular injection is determined by the rate of absorption, tissue redistribution, and metabolism and excretion. Thus, following an extravascular injection, the blood level and the toxicity of local anesthetics are in part related to the intrinsic potency of the agent, but also to the pharmacokinetic profile of the drug. The pharmacokinetics of the various local anesthetic agents have been described in Chapter 3.

Absorption of local anesthetics is related to site of injection, choice of drug, dosage, and addition of vasoconstrictors.

Site of Injection. Absorption from any site depends on the blood supply to that site, with richly supplied areas favoring rapid absorption.[11] Figure 4-14 shows mean plasma concentration curves following the injection of 400 mg of lidocaine at four different sites. The highest concentrations occurred after intercostal block and the lowest after subcutaneous abdominal infiltration. These results agree with the relative blood supplies of the four anatomic areas.

Choice of Drug. Figure 4-15 shows the plasma concentrations after epidural block, using the same dose of lidocaine or prilocaine. As can be seen, prilocaine yields lower plasma concentrations than does lidocaine. These differences may indicate a slower absorption for prilocaine, but it is more likely that they result from more rapid metabolism and a larger volume of distribution than for lidocaine. They explain the fact that intravenous prilocaine causes less toxicity, and for a shorter time, than does the same dose of lidocaine.[43] Similarly, etidocaine blood levels are lower than those of bupivacaine when equal doses are administered. This difference in blood levels allows the use of higher concentrations and dosages

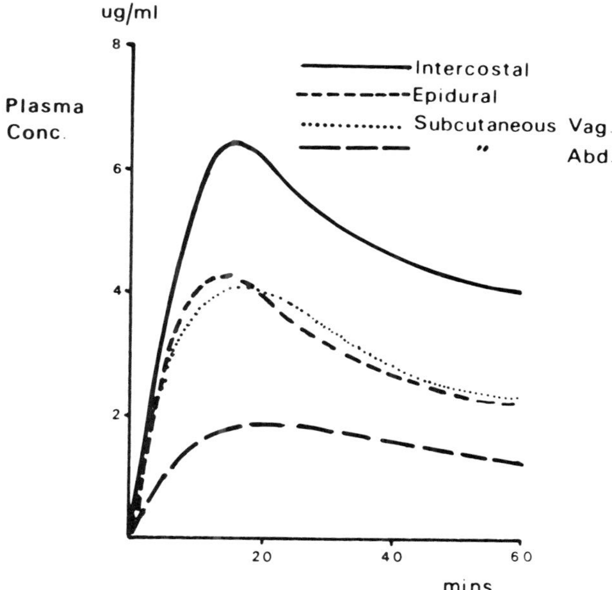

FIG. 4-14. Plasma concentrations of lidocaine following injection of 400 mg at four different sites.

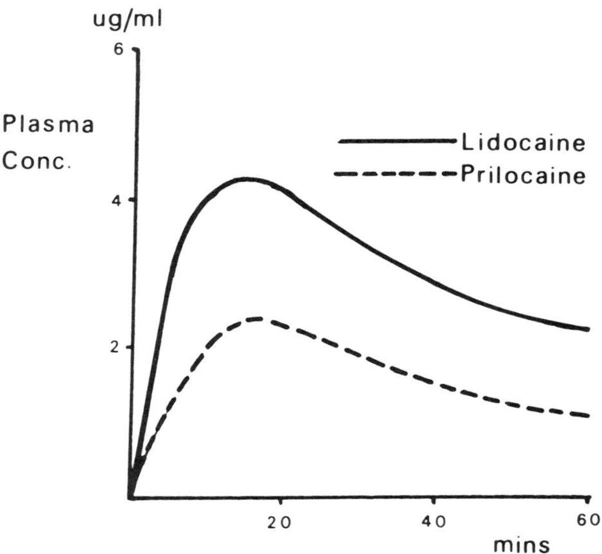

FIG. 4-15. Plasma concentrations of lidocaine and prilocaine following the epidural injection of 400 mg of each agent.

of etidocaine needed to achieve the same depth of anesthesia as buipvacaine. The epidural administration of 300 mg of etidocaine (20 ml of 1.5%) and 150 mg of bupivacaine (20 ml of 0.75%) produces similar depths and duration of anesthesia and similar blood levels.

Dosage. Within the clinical range of dosages for most local anesthetics, the relation between dosage and maximum plasma concentration appears reasonably linear (Fig. 4-16).

Addition of Epinephrine. The efficacy of epinephrine in reducing the absorption of local anesthetics depends on the sensitivity of the vasculature at the site of injection and the local anesthetic drug itself (Figs. 4-17, 4-18; see also Tables 3-6 to 3-10).

The rate of tissue redistribution, metabolism, and excretion varies considerably among different local anesthetics. Among the amino amides prilocaine has the shortest distribution half-life ($T_{1/2}\ \alpha$), whereas the rates of tissue redistribution of the other amide agents are similar. The elimination half-life ($T_{1/2}\,\beta$) is also lower for prilocaine than for the other amide drugs because of its rapid rate of hepatic metabolism and possible metabolism by extrahepatic organs. The elimination half-lives of lidocaine, mepivacaine, and etidocaine are similar, whereas bupivacaine pos-

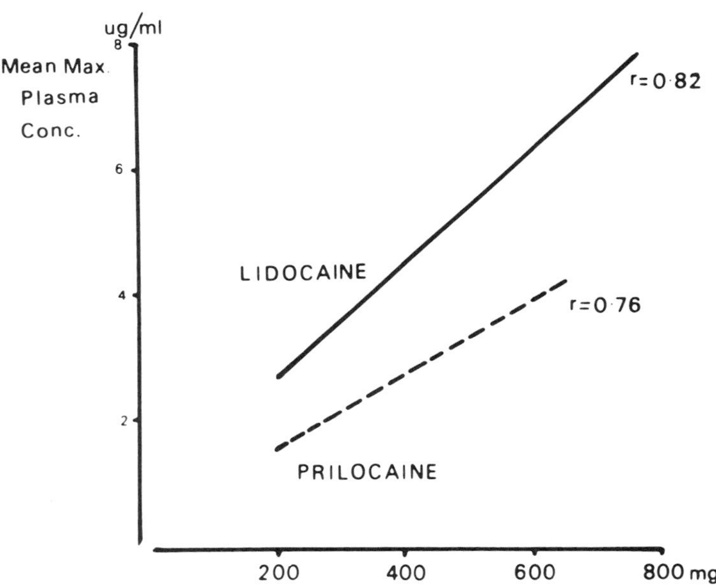

FIG. 4-16. Regression lines of mean maximum plasma concentration for lidocaine and prilocaine following epidural injection.

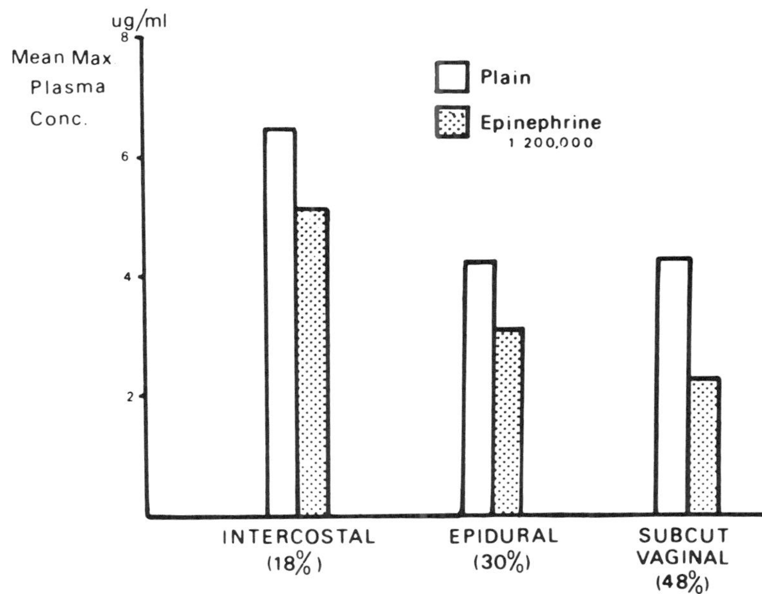

FIG. 4-17. Mean maximum concentrations of lidocaine with and without epinephrine, 1 : 200,000 given at three different sites. The most marked reduction caused by epinephrine occurs with the subcutaneous injection (48%), compared to 30% for epidural and 18% for intercostal (see also Fig. 3-13).

sesses the longest $T_{1/2}\beta$ value, which is indicative of a relatively slow rate of hepatic degradation. These differences in the pharmacokinetic and metabolic properties are responsible for the relatively low potential for systemic toxicity of prilocaine and the relatively high potential of bupivacaine.

Among the amino ester agents, chloroprocaine is hydrolyzed most rapidly, followed in order by procaine and tetracaine. The rate of hydrolysis of the ester agents is correlated with their relative potential for producing systemic toxicity; thus chloroprocaine tends to be least toxic, whereas tetracaine is the most toxic and procaine is intermediate in terms of its toxic potential.

The clinical status of the patient will influence the pharmacokinetic properties and toxic potential of the various local anesthetics. The half-life of amide local anesthetics is prolonged in patients with a low cardiac output.[115] In such cases, an intravenous bolus injection results in a much higher blood concentration that persists for a longer period of time such that the proportion of drug reaching the brain and myocardium will be higher (Fig. 4-19).

Low cardiac output states are, in addition, often

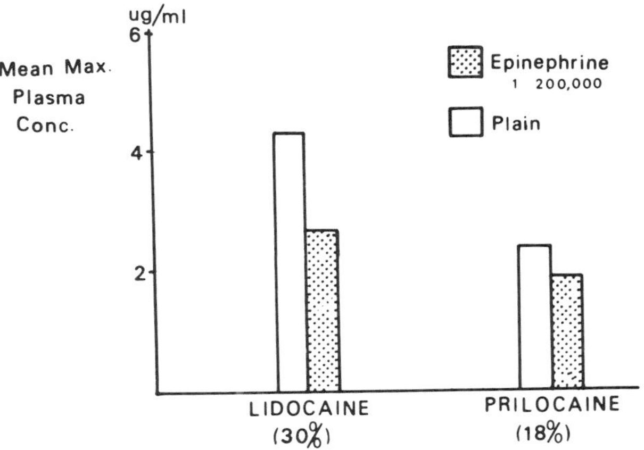

FIG. 4-18. Mean maximum concentration of lidocaine and prilocaine with and without epinephrine. 1 : 200,000, given epidurally. Epinephrine gives a larger reduction in plasma concentrations with lidocaine than with prilocaine (30% and 18%, respectively).

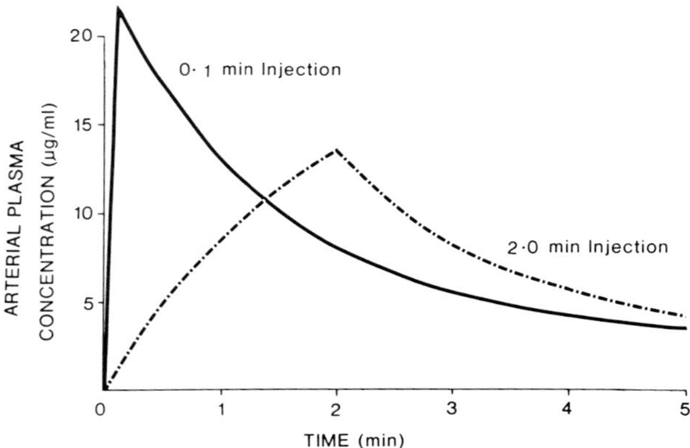

FIG. 4-19. Simulated arterial plasma concentrations of lidocaine, as described in Figure 4-10, show the likely outcome in patients with cardiac output reduced to about 50% of normal. (Data from Thomson, S.P. *et al.*: Lidocaine pharmacokinetics in advanced heart failure, liver disease, and renal failure in humans. Ann. Intern. Med., *78*:499, 1973.)

associated with a considerable reduction in liver blood flow.[55] Because the liver is responsible for detoxifying amide local anesthetics, reducing the liver blood flow will reduce the amount of drug available for degradation. This may produce very high blood concentrations during continuous intravenous infusion.[90] Hepatocellular disease could likewise reduce the speed of degradation and must be considered if high or repeated doses of local anesthetic are contemplated.

DIAGNOSIS, PREVENTION, AND TREATMENT OF TOXIC REACTIONS

The differential diagnosis of systemic local anesthetic reactions is described in Table 4-8. Most toxic effects are preventable by the careful performance of regional anesthetic procedures, selection of the appropriate agent and dose, and a knowledge of the factors that affect absorption, distribution, and elimination of local anesthetics.

Prevention. As indicated previously, most toxic reactions are due to an accidental intravascular injection. This can often be avoided by careful technique and by allowing sufficient time for reflux of the blood down the needle or catheter used for injection (see also Table 4-9). Very gentle syringe aspiration before and during injection is also useful, although a negative result may be due to collapse of the vessel wall against the needle orifice rather than correct placement extravascularly. The use of a short bevel needle with a clear plastic hub allows easier recognition of vascular entry when performing nerve blocks such as brachial plexus blockade. Injections should be made slowly or by use of a fractionated dose technique. For

TABLE 4-8. DIFFERENTIAL DIAGNOSIS OF LOCAL ANESTHETIC REACTIONS

Etiology	Major Clinical Features	Comments
Local anesthetic toxicity		
Intravascular injection	Immediate convulsion and/or cardiac toxicity	Injection into vertebral or a carotid artery may cause convulsion after administration of small dose
Relative overdose	Onset in 5 to 15 minutes of irritability, progressing to convulsions	
Reaction to vasoconstrictor	Tachycardia, hypertension, headache, apprehension	May vary with vasopressor used
Vasovagal reaction	Rapid onset Bradycardia Hypotension Pallor, faintness	Rapidly reversible with elevation of legs
Allergy		
Immediate	Anaphylaxis (↓ BP, bronchospasm, edema)	Allergy to amides extremely rare
Delayed	Urticaria	Cross-allergy possible, for example, with preservatives in local anesthetics and food
High spinal or epidural block	Gradual onset Bradycardia* Hypotension Possible respiratory arrest	May lose consciousness with total spinal block and onset of cardiorespiratory effects more rapid than with high epidural or with subdural block.
Concurrent medical episode (*e.g.*, asthma attack, myocardial infarct)	May mimic local anesthetic reaction	Medical history important

*Sympathetic block above T4 adds cardioaccelerator nerve blockade to the vasodilatation seen with blockade below T4; total spinal block may have rapid onset.

TABLE 4-9. MEASURES TO PREVENT TOXICITY FROM NEURAL BLOCKADE*

Patient evaluation
Identification of significant systemic disease, age, and other factors, to permit individualization of local anesthetic dose
Premedication
Diazepam or other appropriate CNS depressant in moderate dosage
Preparation
Resuscitative drugs
  Diazepam or thiopentone, succinylcholine, atropine, vasopressor
Equipment
  Oxygen administration and suction equipment
  Airway (oropharyngeal airway, laryngoscope, endotracheal tube)
Ensure adequate i.v. available
Discard any cloudy solutions or those containing crystals
Physically separate neural blockade tray from any other drugs
Prevention
Personally check dose of local anesthetic and vasoconstrictor
Use test dose, 5–10% of total dose
Aspirate frequently and discard solution colored by blood
Monitor cardiovascular signs (rapid ↑ heart rate if epinephrine injected i.v.)
Constant verbal contact with patient past time of peak plasma concentration

*Local anesthetic toxicity may result in convulsions; however, with rapid and appropriate treatment, these should never be fatal in themselves. See also cardiac effects of bupivacaine in text.

example, during the performance of an epidural block, 3 to 4 ml of the anesthetic may be administered through the needle, followed by an additional 3 to 4 ml of solution after insertion of an epidural catheter. Once the catheter is taped in place and the patient properly positioned, additional increments of 3 to 4 ml of solution can be injected at 3- to 5-minute intervals as needed for attainment of a satisfactory level of anesthesia. The patient should be questioned during the injection of the local anesthetic to determine the presence of early numbness or any warning signs of toxicity such as circumoral numbness and tinnitus. In addition, monitoring of heart rate, blood pressure, and ECG should be performed before, during, and after the administration of any local anesthetic.

The use of a test dose is frequently helpful to detect an accidental intravascular or intrathecal injection. Three milliliters to 5 ml of anesthetic solution usually is required for an appropriate test dose. If there is no medical contraindication to the use of epinephrine, an epinephrine-containing solution is of value because a sudden increase in heart rate and blood pressure is usually diagnostic of an intravascular injection unless the patient has been taking β-adrenergic blockers. A period of 3 to 5 minutes is usually required after an epidural test dose in order to elicit signs of subarachnoid block.

Treatment. Other than cessation of injection, it is seldom necessary to treat the minor signs and symptoms of toxicity (see Table 4-10) provided adequate respiration and cardiovascular function are maintained. Nevertheless, early signs of toxicity warrant constant verbal contact, cardiovascular monitoring, administration of oxygen, and encouragement to breathe at a normal minute volume.

Convulsions. If convulsions occur, the aim of treatment is to stop them and treat any respiratory or cardiovascular depression before cerebral hypoxia occurs. Currently, three pharmacologic approaches to controlling convulsions are available (see below). The simple nonpharmacologic measures should be carried out *before* any drug treatment is begun. The prevention of hypoxia and acidosis is the single most important feature of treatment.

Intravenous Barbiturates: Thiopental (50–100 mg) can rapidly abort a convulsive episode. This agent has the great advantage of being familiar and usually readily available to the anesthesiologist. The possibility of enhanced respiratory and cardiovascular depression should be minimal and transient considering the small dosage required. Respiration must be carefully observed and a clear airway obtained, if

TABLE 4-10. TREATMENT OF ACUTE LOCAL ANESTHETIC TOXICITY

Airway
Establish clear airway; suction, if required
Breathing
Oxygen with face mask
Encourage adequate ventilation (prevent cycle of acidosis, increased uptake of local anesthetic into CNS, and lowered seizure threshold)
Artificial ventilation, if required
Circulation
Elevate legs
Increase i.v. fluids if ↓ blood pressure
CVS support drug if ↓ blood pressure persists (see below) or ↓ heart rate
Cardioversion if ventricular arrhythmias occur
Drugs
CNS depressant
  Diazepam 5–10 mg, i.v.
  Thiopental 50 mg, i.v., incremental doses until seizures cease
Muscle relaxant
  Succinylcholine 1 mg/kg, if inadequate control of ventilation with above measures (requires artificial ventilation and may necessitate intubation)
CVS support
  Atropine 0.6 mg, i.v., if ↓ heart rate
  Ephedrine, 12.5–25 mg, i.v., to restore adequate blood pressure
  Epinephrine for profound cardiovascular collapse

necessary, by endotracheal intubation. If respiratory depression or apnea occurs, artificial ventilation with oxygen is required.

Diazepam: Diazepam may be administered intravenously in doses of 5 to 10 mg to control convulsions. Its onset may be somewhat slower than that of thiopental and its duration of action is longer. Respiration must be maintained and supported in the same fashion as described above. Although both thiopental and diazepam should abort the convulsions, they will not prevent the possibility of respiratory and cardiovascular depression.

Succinylcholine: Succinylcholine, a neuromuscular blocking agent, will also stop convulsions when administered intravenously. A dose of 50 mg is usually adequate, but administration is accompanied by paralysis and cessation of respiration. The patient should be immediately intubated and ventilated with oxygen. This agent should be used only by persons skilled in the art of endotracheal intubation. Of note, succinylcholine will inhibit muscular convulsive activity but not the convulsive process in the brain which might increase the oxygen demand of the brain; however, if respiration is controlled with oxygen and cardiovascular function is adequate, no deleterious CNS sequelae are likely.

Cardiovascular Depression. Hypotension should be treated by correction of hypoxia, elevation of legs, increased rate of infusion of intravenous fluids, and, if necessary, intravenous administration of a vasopressor agent. Because hypotension usually is due to a combination of myocardial depression and vasodilation, it is preferable to use an agent that stimulates both alpha- and beta-adrenergic receptors such as ephedrine (15–30 mg or incremental doses of 5 mg until a positive response is obtained). Atropine (0.4 mg) can also be used to reverse a state of bradycardia.

Profound cardiovascular depression requires the immediate institution of cardiopulmonary resuscitation. Ventricular tachycardia or fibrillation should be treated by electrical cardioversion, which may require the use of higher than normal electrical energy. It has been reported that the use of large doses of epinephrine and atropine can reverse the cardiovascular collapse produced by bupivacaine in dogs. It may be necessary to continue cardiopulmonary resuscitative efforts for an hour or longer in situations of profound circulatory collapse. All other treatment modalities should be carried out, such as controlled ventilation with oxygen and administration of sodium bicarbonate to treat acidosis.

Respiratory and cardiovascular depression caused by a total spinal block should be treated in the same manner as described above. Assisted or controlled ventilation with oxygen and endotracheal intubation, if deemed necessary, should be instituted promptly to prevent hypoxia and acidosis. Rapid infusion of intravenous fluids, vasopressors, and anticholinergic agents should be given to treat hypotension and bradycardia (see also Chapter 8). Aspiration of 10 to 20 ml of cerebrospinal fluid and replacement with saline may be useful for prevention of possible neural damage, particularly if solutions of chloroprocaine have been administered intrathecally.

Proper monitoring and immediate availability of resuscitative equipment are equally important when performing a regional or general anesthetic technique (see Chap. 6).

CLINICAL USE OF LOCAL ANESTHETICS

AMINO ESTER AGENTS

Procaine

Procaine is rarely used at present for peripheral nerve or extradural blocks because of its low potency, slow onset, and relatively short duration of action. Although the potential for systemic toxic reactions is quite small with procaine, this agent can cause allergic-type reactions. Currently, procaine is used mainly for infiltration anesthesia and differential spinal blocks in chronic pain patients.

Chloroprocaine

Chloroprocaine has enjoyed an increased use in recent years in the United States because of its rapid onset of action and low systemic toxicity. Although the potency of this agent is relatively low, it can be used for epidural anesthesia in a concentration of 3% because of its systemic safety. The duration of action of chloroprocaine is about 30 to 60 minutes. This agent has enjoyed its greatest popularity for epidural analgesia and anesthesia in obstetrics because of its rapid onset and low systemic toxicity in mother and fetus. Frequent injections are needed in order to provide adequate pain relief during labor. Often epidural analgesia is established in the pregnant woman with chloroprocaine, after which a longer-acting agent such as bupivacaine is used. As discussed previously, the epidural use of chloroprocaine may have declined somewhat because of reports of prolonged sensory/motor deficits following the accidental subarachnoid injection of this agent.

Chloroprocaine has also proved of value for peripheral nerve blocks and epidural anesthesia when the duration of surgery is not expected to exceed 30 to 60 minutes. Thus this drug is useful for ambulatory surgical procedures performed under regional anesthesia. Chloroprocaine has also been mixed with other agents such as bupivacaine or tetracaine in order to provide a rapid onset and prolonged duration of anesthesia; however, as discussed previously, such mixtures may not result in the long duration of anesthesia usually associated with bupivacaine.

Tetracaine

Tetracaine remains the most popular drug for spinal anesthesia in the United States. Tetracaine may be used as an isobaric, hypobaric, or hyperbaric solution for spinal blockade, although hyperbaric solutions of tetracaine are probably used most commonly. Tetracaine provides a relatively rapid onset of spinal anesthesia—about 3 to 5 minutes—a profound depth of anesthesia, and a duration of 2 to 3 hours. The addition of epinephrine can extend the duration of anesthesia to 4 to 6 hours.

Tetracaine is rarely used for other forms of regional anesthesia because of its extremely slow onset of action and the potential for systemic toxic reactions when the larger doses required for other types of regional blockade are used. Before the introduction of bupivacaine and etidocaine, mixtures of tetracaine and other local anesthetics with a more rapid onset such as lidocaine or mepivacaine were used for various regional anesthetic procedures.

Tetracaine does possess excellent topical anesthetic properties, and solutions of this agent were commonly used for endotracheal surface anesthesia. The absorption of tetracaine from the tracheobronchial area is, however, extremely rapid, and several fatalities have been reported following the use of an endotracheal aerosol of tetracaine.

Cocaine

The original local anesthetic, cocaine, is still used clinically for its topical anesthetic and vasoconstrictor properties. Cocaine solutions are frequently used to anesthetize the nasal mucosa before nasotracheal intubation.

AMINO AMIDE AGENTS

Lidocaine

Lidocaine was the first drug of the amino amide type to be introduced into clinical practice. This agent remains the most versatile and most commonly used local anesthetic because of its inherent potency, rapid onset, moderate duration of action, and topical anesthetic activity. Solutions of 0.5%, 1.0%, 1.5%, and 2.0% lidocaine are available for infiltration, peripheral nerve blocks, and epidural anesthesia. In addition, 5% lidocaine with 7.5% glucose is widely used for spinal anesthesia of 30 to 60 minutes' duration. Lidocaine is also used in ointment, jelly, and viscous and aerosol preparations for a variety of topical anesthetic procedures.

Although the duration of action of lidocaine is about 1 to 3 hours for various regional anesthetic procedures, the addition of epinephrine will significantly prolong the duration of this agent. Moreover, epinephrine will decrease the rate of absorption of lidocaine, which will significantly decrease its blood levels and potential for producing systemic toxic reactions (see Table 3-6).

Lidocaine also possesses a number of nonanesthetic uses. It is widely used as an intravenous antiarrhythmic agent in patients with ventricular arrhythmias. In addition, it has proved useful as an antiepileptic and intravenous analgesic agent. The systemic analgesic properties of lidocaine have proved to be of value in the treatment of certain chronic pain syndromes (see Chap. 27.2). In addition, the combination of intravenous lidocaine and CNS depressants such as barbiturates and general anesthetics has been used to provide a state of balanced analgesia and anesthesia. This systemic analgesic activity of lidocaine is apparently due to an action in the central nervous system and is not related to its effect on peripheral nerves.

Mepivacaine

Mepivacaine is similar to lidocaine in terms of its anesthetic profile. Mepivacaine can produce a profound depth of anesthesia with a relatively rapid onset and a moderate duration of action. This agent may be used for infiltration, peripheral nerve blocks, and epidural anesthesia in concentrations varying from 0.5% to 2.0%. In some countries 4% hyperbaric solutions of mepivacaine are also available for spinal anesthesia.

Differences do exist between mepivacaine and lidocaine. Mepivacaine is not effective as a topical anesthetic agent and thus is less versatile than lidocaine. In addition, the metabolism of mepivacaine is markedly prolonged in the fetus and newborn such that this agent is not usually used for obstetric anesthesia. In adults, however, mepivacaine appears to be somewhat less toxic than lidocaine. Moreover, the vasodilator activity of mepivacaine is less than that of lidocaine. Thus mepivacaine provides a somewhat longer duration of anesthesia than lidocaine when the two agents are used without epinephrine. The duration of action of mepivacaine can be significantly prolonged by the addition of a vasoconstrictor such as epinephrine (see Table 3-8).

A 3% solution of mepivacaine is available specifically for dental anesthesia. A 2% solution of mepivacaine with the vasoconstrictor levonordefrin (Neo-Cobefrin) is also prepared specifically for the dental field.

Prilocaine

The clinical profile of prilocaine is also similar to that of lidocaine. Prilocaine has a relatively rapid onset of action while providing a moderate duration of anesthesia and a profound depth of conduction blockade. This agent causes significantly less vasodilation than lidocaine and thus can be used without epinephrine. In general, the duration of prilocaine without epinephrine is similar to that of lidocaine with epinephrine (see Table 3-7). Thus prilocaine is particularly useful in patients in whom epinephrine may be contraindicated. Prilocaine is useful for infiltration, peripheral nerve blockade, and epidural anesthesia. Although prilocaine possesses topical anesthetic activity and can induce spinal anesthesia of short duration, no specific formulations of this agent are available for topical or spinal anesthesia.

The primary advantage of prilocaine compared to lidocaine is its significantly decreased potential for producing systemic toxic reactions. Studies in animals and human volunteers indicate that prilocaine is approximately 40% less toxic than lidocaine. Prilocaine is the least toxic of the amino amide local anesthetics. Thus this agent is particularly useful for intravenous regional anesthesia because CNS toxic effects are rarely seen after tourniquet deflation, even when early accidental release of the tourniquet may occur. Forty milliliters of 0.5% prilocaine (200 mg) provides effective anesthesia for hand surgery using the intravenous regional anesthetic technique (see Chap. 12).

The major deterrent to the use of prilocaine is related to the formation of methemoglobinemia with this drug. This unusual side-effect of prilocaine has essentially eliminated the use of this drug in obstetrics, although prilocaine has not been reported to cause any significant adverse effects in mother, fetus, or newborn; however, the cyanotic appearance of newborns delivered of mothers who have received prilocaine for epidural anesthesia during labor results in sufficient confusion concerning the etiology of the cyanosis such that the obstetric use of this potentially valuable drug has been virtually abandoned.

Bupivacaine

Bupivacaine has probably had the greatest influence on the practice of regional anesthesia since the introduction of lidocaine. Bupivacaine was the first local anesthetic that combined the properties of an acceptable onset, long duration of action, profound conduction blockade, and significant separation of sensory anesthesia and motor blockade. This agent is used in concentrations of 0.125%, 0.25%, 0.5%, and 0.75% for various regional anesthetic procedures, including infiltration, peripheral nerve blocks, and epidural and spinal anesthesia. Bupivacaine has not been used for topical anesthesia. The average duration of surgical anesthesia of bupivacaine varies from about 3 to 10 hours. Its longest duration of action occurs when major peripheral nerve blocks such as brachial plexus blockade are performed. In these situations, average durations of effective surgical anesthesia of 10 to 12 hours have been reported. In some patients, durations of brachial plexus block of 24 hours or more have been observed with complete recovery of sensation. The vascular absorption of bupivacaine is influenced to a variable extent by epinephrine, but less so than for lidocaine (see Table 3-9).

The major advantage of bupivacaine appears to be in the area of obstetric analgesia for labor. In this situation, bupivacaine administered epidurally in concentrations varying from 0.125% to 0.5% provides satisfactory pain relief for 2 to 3 hours, which significantly decreases the need for repeated injections in the pregnant woman. More importantly, adequate analgesia is usually achieved without significant motor blockade such that the woman in labor is able to move her legs. This differential blockade of sensory and motor fibers is also the basis for the widespread use of bupivacaine for postoperative epidural analgesia and for certain chronic pain states.

Unfortunately the obstetric use of bupivacaine has been tempered somewhat in recent years because of reports of sudden cardiovascular collapse following the accidental rapid intravenous administration of this agent. The cardiotoxicity of bupivacaine, which has been discussed previously, has occurred primarily in the United States in obstetric patients. As a result, the 0.75% solution of bupivacaine is no longer recommended for obstetric anesthesia in the United States.

Bupivacaine had become relatively popular for intravenous regional anesthesia. The advantage of bupivacaine for i.v. regional anesthesia is related to the suggestion that there was an extended duration of anesthesia that occurred after tourniquet deflation. Several reports of sudden cardiovascular collapse after accidental early cuff deflation have resulted, however, in a recommendation in the United States that bupivacaine not be used for i.v. regional anesthesia.

In recent years, bupivacaine has been used extensively for spinal anesthesia. Isobaric and hyperbaric solutions of 0.5% to 0.75% bupivacaine have been investigated for various surgical procedures performed under subarachnoid blockade. Onset of spinal anesthesia with bupivacaine usually occurs within 5 minutes, whereas the duration of surgical anesthesia persists for 3 to 4 hours. Comparative studies of bupivacaine and tetracaine suggest little difference between the two agents in terms of onset, spread, and duration of spinal blockade. Several investigations have suggested that the frequency of satisfactory anesthesia may be greater with bupivacaine than with tetracaine. In addition, less hypotension is apparent after the intrathecal administration of bupivacaine, even in patients with an exaggerated spread of sensory anesthesia. The degree of motor blockade is greater when isobaric solutions of bupivacaine are used as opposed to hyperbaric formulations (see Chap. 7).

Etidocaine

Etidocaine, which is chemically related to lidocaine, is the latest local anesthetic introduced for clinical use. This agent is characterized by very rapid onset, prolonged duration of action, and profound sensory and motor blockade. Etidocaine may be used for infiltration, peripheral nerve blockade, and epidural anesthesia. Although etidocaine and bupivacaine provide prolonged durations of anesthesia, significant differences exist with regard to the anesthetic profile of these two local anesthetics. Etidocaine has a significantly more rapid onset of action than bupivacaine. In addition, the concentrations of etidocaine required for adequate sensory anesthesia produce profound motor blockade. As a result, etidocaine is primarily useful as an anesthetic for surgical procedures in which muscle relaxation is required. Thus this agent is of limited use for obstetric epidural analgesia and for postoperative pain relief because it does not provide a differential blockade of sensory and motor fibers. It is possible to take advantage of the different pharmacologic profiles of etidocaine and bupivacaine in certain clinical situations. For example, it is possible to initiate epidural blockade with 1.5% etidocaine for lower limb orthopedic procedures, such as total hip replacements, and for abdominal surgical procedures. Under these conditions etidocaine will provide a rapid onset of action and a profound depth of anesthesia and muscle relaxation. Supplemental intraoperative and postoperative anesthesia is then provided by 0.5% bupivacaine, which produces excellent sensory anesthesia with minimal motor blockade. Effects of epinephrine on vascular absorption of etidocaine are summarized in Table 3-10.

MISCELLANEOUS

Dibucaine

Dibucaine is essentially used for spinal anesthesia. Interestingly, it is probably the most widely used spinal anesthetic drug outside the United States, but its use is rather limited in the United States. Comparative studies of dibucaine and tetracaine indicate that dibucaine is more potent than tetracaine, that is, 0.25% dibucaine provides a depth of anesthesia similar to that produced by 0.5% tetracaine.[96] The onset of action of the two agents is similar, whereas the duration of anesthesia is slightly longer with dibucaine. In addition, the degree of hypotension and the profoundness of motor blockade were less in patients receiving intrathecal dibucaine than in subjects in whom tetracaine was administered into the subarachnoid space, although the spread of sensory anesthesia was similar in the two groups (see Chap. 7).

Hyperbaric solutions of 0.25% and 0.5% dibucaine with 5% glucose are commonly available in most countries. A preformulated hypobaric solution of 0.667 mg/ml (1:1500) dibucaine is also available.

Benzocaine

Benzocaine, a local anesthetic used exclusively for topical anesthesia, is available in a variety of proprietary and nonproprietary preparations. The most common forms used in the operating room setting are aerosol solutions for endotracheal administration and an ointment for lubrication of endotracheal tubes.

Dyclonine

Dyclonine is also used exclusively for topical anesthesia because it is highly irritating if administered by injection. A comparative study of several topical anesthetic preparations suggested that dyclonine provides the greatest depth and longest duration of anesthesia following topical application to the gingival mucosa.

DRUGS USED WITH LOCAL ANESTHETICS

VASOCONSTRICTORS

Epinephrine is, of course, the active principal of the adrenal medulla. It is a powerful vasoconstrictor and has effects on both alpha- and beta-adrenergic receptors.

On exposure to air or light, epinephrine may rapidly lose potency as a result of degradation. For this reason, stabilizing agents, such as sodium metabisulphite, are used. They slow the breakdown of the drug to as little as 2% per year. These agents also allow epinephrine-containing solutions to be autoclaved once without appreciable loss of activity. Epinephrine-containing solutions cannot, however, be reautoclaved. Epinephrine-containing solutions have a lower *p*H (3–4.5) than do untreated solutions because of the added antioxidant.

When epinephrine is used with local anesthetic solutions, it must be in a concentration and dose to produce the desired vasoconstriction without leading to epinephrine overdose. Although the optimal concentration has been controversial, most authorities now agree on 1 : 200,000. More dilute solutions are of doubtful value; increasing the concentration does not achieve a correspondingly more effective vasoconstriction and increases the likelihood of toxicity. Even with 1 : 200,000, a total dose of 200 μg should not be exceeded.

The principal side-effects of epinephrine are hypertension, bradycardia or tachycardia, and cardiac arrhythmias. Such reactions are likely to occur if the local anesthetic solution is accidentally injected intravenously. Animal experiments have shown that epinephrine increases the toxicity of local anesthetics when given directly into the circulation. The favorable cardiovascular effects of slowly absorbed 1 : 200,000 epinephrine are similar to those observed during recently developed "low-dose" constant infusion of epinephrine in intensive therapy; this differs markedly from the adverse effects of a relatively large bolus dose rapidly injected directly into the circulation. It is wise to avoid the use of epinephrine in patients sensitive to catecholamines (*e.g.*, patients with hypertension, thyrotoxicosis).

Epinephrine also has local side-effects, the most important being vasoconstriction of terminal arteries, leading to gangrene, for example, in the digits if the drug is used in a local anesthetic for ring blocks.

Phenylephrine (Neosynephrine) is a sympathomimetic drug with predominately alpha-receptor activity. It has been extensively used in spinal anesthesia.

Felypressin (Octapressin) is a synthetic drug similar to the naturally occurring vasopressin but without the antidiuretic and coronary vasoconstrictor effects of vasopressin. It has been shown to increase the intensity and duration of dental nerve blocks, and it is used in local anesthesia for this purpose in a concentration of 0.03 U/ml. It is a useful alternative in patients who are sensitive to catecholamines.

Ornipressin (POR-8) is another octapeptide related to vasopressin. It is supplied in ampules of 5 IU in 1 ml. A dose of 5 IU in 50 ml of 2% lidocaine has been used for plastic surgery. It is claimed to have a direct effect on the peripheral vasculature with minimal or no direct cardiac effects. Animal studies have revealed teratogenicity in high, subcutaneous doses considerably in excess of the maximum clinical level.

Levonordefrin (Neo-cobefrin) is an alpha-receptor stimulator used with mepivacaine in dental blocks in a 1 : 20,000 concentration.

ANTIOXIDANTS

Most of the commonly used local anesthetics, especially of the amide type, are extremely stable compounds and will remain unchanged in solution indefinitely. Thus solutions do not require additives if they are stored in ampules. If epinephrine is included in the preparation, however, antioxidants must be added to prevent breakdown of the vasoconstrictor.

The agent used for this purpose is sodium metabisulphite in a concentration of 0.1%. Epinephrine-containing solutions will retain their potency for 2 years with this agent and will withstand single autoclaving.

Studies discussed above indicate that bisulphite in the presence of low *p*H (below 3) may cause neurotoxicity. Thus spinal and epidural local anesthetic solutions should contain only low concentrations of bisulphite (0.1%) and *p*H should be buffered to be above 4.5 (see above).

ANTIMICROBIALS

Except for minor infiltration, local anesthetic solutions should not contain antimicrobials. Thus the ideal presentation is in a single-use rubber-capped vial or ampule. Vials are preferred because their caps are easily removed, whereas glass fragments may contaminate solutions when ampules are opened.

In multiple-dose vials, methylparaben (1%) is often the antimicrobial included in the solution. Methylparaben is effective against gram-positive organisms and fungi but less so against gram-negative bacteria. It may be responsible for some of the allergic reactions attributed to local anesthetics — in theory, it should be considerably more antigenic than the local anesthetics. Chlorocresol has been used as an antibacterial agent and is more effective than methylparaben, but, like phenol, it is neurotoxic and should not be used in spinal, i.v., or plexus blocks or extradural injections.

SUMMARY

The clinical pharmacologic properties of local anesthetic agents affect both the anesthetic profile and potential toxicity of the various drugs in current clinical use. The most important anesthetic properties are potency, onset, duration of action, and relative blockade of sensory and motor fibers. These qualities are related to the physicochemical properties of the various compounds. The toxicity of local anesthetics involves the central nervous system and the cardiovascular system. The toxicity of the different drugs is generally correlated with their inherent anesthetic potency but can be modified by the pharmacokinetic and metabolic properties of the specific agents. In general, the local anesthetics for infiltration, peripheral nerve blockade, and epidural anesthesia can be divided into three groups: [1] agents of short duration, that is, procaine and chloroprocaine; [2] agents of moderate duration, that is, lidocaine, mepivacaine, and prilocaine; and [3] agents of long duration, that is, tetracaine, bupivacaine, and etidocaine. These local anesthetics also vary in terms of onset: Chloroprocaine, lidocaine, mepivacaine, prilocaine, and etidocaine have a rapid onset, whereas procaine, tetracaine, and bupivacaine are characterized by a longer latency period.

The agents specifically formulated for intrathecal use include lidocaine, mepivacaine, and procaine, which have a short duration of action, and tetracaine, dibucaine, and bupivacaine, which provide a prolonged duration of spinal anesthesia.

Agents used in topical anesthetic preparations include lidocaine, tetracaine, benzocaine, and dyclonine. Cocaine solutions are also used for topical anesthesia of the nasal mucosa.

With regard to the relative systemic toxicity of the various agents, chloroprocaine is the least toxic of the amino esters, whereas tetracaine is most toxic. Among the amino amides, prilocaine is least toxic, followed in order of increasing toxicity by mepivacaine, lidocaine, etidocaine, and bupivacaine.

An appreciation of the pharmacologic and toxicologic profile of the various local anesthetics should make it possible to match a specific agent to a particular clinical situation.

REFERENCES

1. Albert, J., and Lofstrom, B.: Bilateral ulnar nerve blocks for the evaluation of local anaesthetic agents. Acta Anaesthesiol. Scand., *9*:203, 1965.
2. Albright, G.A.: Cardiac arrest following regional anesthesia with etidocaine or bupivacaine. Anesthesiology, *51*:285, 1979.
3. Aldrete, J.A., and Johnson, D.A.: Evaluation of intracutaneous testing for investigation of allergy to local anesthetic agents. Anesth. Analg., *49*:173, 1970.
4. Aldrete, J.A., Barnes, D.R., Sidon, M.A., McMullen, R.B.: Studies on effects of addition of potassium chloride to lidocaine. Anesth. Analg., *48*:269, 1969.
5. Apfelbaum, J.L., Gross, J.B., Shaw, L.M., Spaulding, B.C., *et al.*: Changes in lidocaine protein binding may explain its increased CNS toxicity at elevated CO_2 tensions. Anesthesiology, *61*:A213, 1984.
6. Armstrong, I.R., Littlewood, D.G., and Chambers, W.A.: Spinal anesthesia with tetracaine — Effect of added vasoconstrictor. Anesth. Analg., *62*:793, 1983.
7. Barsa, J.E., Batra, M., Fink, B.R., Sumi, S.M.: Prolonged neural blockade following regional analgesia with 2-chloroprocaine. Anesth. Analg., *61*:961, 1982.
8. Benoit, P.W., and Belt, W.D.: Some effects of local anesthetic agents on skeletal muscle. Exp. Neurol., *34*:264, 1972.

9. Blair, M.R.: Cardiovascular pharmacology of local anaesthetics. Br. J. Anaesth., *47*:247, 1975.
10. Block, A., and Covino, B.G.: Effect of local anesthetic agents on cardiac conduction and contractility. Reg. Anaesth., *6*:55, 1982.
11. Braid, D.P., and Scott, D.B.: The systemic absorption of local analgesic drugs. Br. J. Anaesth., *37*:394, 1965.
12. Bridenbaugh, L.D.: Does the addition of low molecular weight dextran prolong the duration of action of bupivacaine? Reg. Anaesth., *3*:6, 1978.
13. Bridenbaugh, P.O.: Intercostal nerve blockade for the evaluation of local anaesthetic agents. Br. J. Anaesth., *47*:306, 1975.
14. Bromage, P.R.: A comparison of the hydrochloride and carbon dioxide salts of lidocaine and prilocaine in epidural analgesia. Acta Anaesthesiol. Scand. Suppl., *16*:55, 1965.
15. Bromage, P.R.: A comparison of the hydrochloride salts of lignocaine and prilocaine for epidural analgesia. Br. J. Anaesth., *37*:753, 1965.
16. Bromage, P.R.: An evaluation of two new local anesthetics for major conduction blockade. Can. Anaesth. Soc. J., *17*:557, 1970.
17. Bromage, P.R.: Mechanism of action of extradural analgesia. Br. J. Anaesth., *47*:199, 1975.
18. Bromage, P.R., and Burfort, M.D.: Quality of epidural blockade. II. Influence of physico-chemical factors: Hyaluronidase and potassium. Br. J. Anaesth., *38*:857, 1966.
19. Brown, D.T., Beamish, D., Wildsmith, J.A.W.: Allergic reaction to an amide local anaesthetic. Br. J. Anaesth., *53*:435, 1981.
20. Brown, D.T., Morrison, D.H., Covino, B.G., and Scott, D.B.: Comparison of carbonated bupivacaine and bupivacaine hydrochloride for extradural anaesthesia. Br. J. Anaesth., *52*:419, 1980.
21. Burney, R.G., DiFazio, C.A., and Foster, J.A.: Effects of pH on protein binding of lidocaine. Anesth. Analg., *57*:478, 1978.
22. Buckley, F.P., Littlewood, D.G., Covino, B.G., and Scott, D.B.: Effects of adrenaline and the concentration of solution on extradural block with etidocaine. Br. J. Anaesth., *50*:171, 1978.
23. Catchlove, R.F.H.: The influence of CO_2 and pH on local anesthetic action. J. Pharmacol. Exp. Ther., *181*:291, 1972.
24. Chambers, W.A., Littlewood, D.G., and Scott, D.B.: Spinal anesthesia with hyperbaric bupivacaine: Effect of added vasoconstrictors. Anesth. Analg., *61*:49, 1982.
25. Chambers, W.A., Littlewood, D.G., Logan, M.R., and Scott, D.B.: Effect of added epinephrine on spinal anesthesia with lidocaine. Anesth. Analg., *60*:417, 1981.
26. Clarkson, C.W., Hondeghem, L., Matsubara, T., and Levinson, G.: Possible mechanism of bupivacaine toxicity: Fast inactivation block with slow diastolic recovery. IARS Abstracts, A21, 1984.
27. Cohen, S.E., and Thurlow, A.: Comparison of a chloroprocaine-bupivacaine mixture with chloroprocaine and bupivacaine used individually for obstetric epidural analgesia. Anesthesiology, *51*:288, 1979.
28. Corke, B.G., Carlson, C.G., and Dettbarn, W.D.: The influence of 2-chloroprocaine on the subsequent analgesic potency of bupivacaine. Anesthesiology, *60*:25, 1984.
29. Covino, B.G., and Bush, D.F.: Clinical evaluation of local anesthetic agents. Br. J. Anaesth., *47*:289, 1975.
30. Covino, B.G., and Vassallo, H.G.: Local Anesthetics. Mechanisms of Action and Clinical Use. New York Grune & Stratton, 1976.
31. Concepcion, M., Maddi, R., Francis, D., Rocco, A.G., *et al.*: Vasoconstrictors in spinal anesthesia with tetracaine. A comparison of epinephrine and phenylephrine. Anesth. Analg., *63*:134, 1984.
32. Crawford, O.B.: Comparative evaluation in peridural anesthesia of lidocaine, mepivacaine, and L-67, a new local anesthetic agent. Anesthesiology, *25*:321, 1964.
33. Cunningham, N.L., and Kaplan, J.A.: A rapid onset long acting regional anesthetic technique. Anesthesiology, *41*:509, 1974.
34. DeJong, R.H., Robles, R., and Corbin, R.W.: Central actions of lidocaine—Synaptic transmission. Anesthesiology, *30*:19, 1969.
35. DeJong, R.H., Ronfeld, R.A., and DeRosa, R.A.: Cardiovascular effects of convulsant and supraconvulsant doses of amide local anesthetics. Anesth. Analg., *61*:3, 1982.
36. Dhuner, K.G., and Lewis, D.: Effect of local anaesthetics and vasoconstrictors upon regional blood flow. Acta Anaesthesiol. Scand., *23*:347, 1966.
37. Eckstein, K.L., Vincente-Eckstein, A., Steiner, R., and Missler, V.: Klinische erprobung von bupivacaine CO_2. Anaesthesist, *27*:1, 1978.
38. Edde, R.R., and Deutsch, S.: Cardiac arrest after interscalene brachial plexus block. Anesth. Analg., *55*:446, 1977.
39. Eicholzer, A.W., Feldman, H.S.: Acute toxicity of etidocaine following various routes of administration in the dog. Toxicol. Appl. Pharmacol., *37:13, 1976.*
40. Englesson, S.: The influence of acid-base changes on central nervous system toxicity of local anesthetic agents. I. An experimental study in cats. Acta Anaesthesiol. Scand., *18*:79, 1974.
41. Englesson, S., and Grevsten, S.: The influence of acid-base changes on central nervous system toxicity of local anaesthetic agents: II. Acta Anaesthesiol. Scand., *18*:88, 1974.
42. Erdimir, H.A., Soper, L.E., and Sweet, R.B.: Studies of factors affecting peridural anesthesia. Anesth. Analg., *44*:400, 1965.
43. Eriksson, E., Engelsson, S., Wahlquist, S., and Ortengren, B.: Study of the intravenous toxicity in man and some in vitro studies on the distribution and absorbability. Acta Chir. Scand., *358[Suppl]*:25, 1966.
44. Feldman, H.S., Arthur, G.R., Norway, S.B., Doucette, A.M., *et al.*: Cardiovascular effects of mepivacaine and etidocaine in the awake dog. Anesthesiology, *61*:A229, 1984.
45. Feldman, H.S., Covino, B.M., and Sage, D.J.: Direct chronotropic and inotropic effects of local anesthetic agents in isolated guinea pig atria. Reg. Anaesth., *7*:149, 1982.
46. Fisher, M. Mc.D., and Graham, R.: Adverse responses to local anaesthetics. Anaesth. Intensive Care *12*:325, 1984.
47. Foldes, F.F., Davidson, G.M., Duncalf, D., and Kuwabara, J.: The intravenous toxicity of local anesthetic agents in man. Clin. Pharmacol. Ther., *6*:328, 1965.
48. Ford, D.J., and Raj, P.R.: Personal communication.

49. Galindo, A., and Witcher, T.: Mixtures of local anesthetics: Bupivacaine-chloroprocaine. Anesth. Analg., *59*:683, 1980.

50. Galindo, A., Schou, M., Witcher, T.: pH adjusted local anesthetics. Proceedings of the American Society of Regional Anesthesia, p 50, 1981.

51. Gettes, L.S.: Physiology and pharmacology of antiarrhythmic drugs. Hosp. Pract., *16*:89, 1981.

52. Gissen, A.J., Covino, B.G., and Gregus, J.: Differential sensitivity of fast and slow fibers in mammalian nerve. IV. Effect of carbonation of local anesthetics. Reg. Anaesth., *10*:68, 1985.

53. Gissen, A.J., Datta, S., and Lambert, D.: The chloroprocaine controversy II. Is chloroprocaine neurotoxic? Reg. Anaesth., *9*:135, 1984.

54. Grambling, Z.W., Ellis, R.G., and Valpitto, P.P.: Clinical experiences with mepivacaine (Carbocaine). J.M.A. Georgia, *53*:16, 1964.

55. Harrison, D.C., and Alderman, E.L.: Relation of blood levels to clinical effectiveness of lidocaine. *In* Scott, D.B. and Julian, D.C. (eds): Lidocaine in the Treatment of Ventricular Arrhythmias, pp. 178–188. Edinburgh, E & S Livingston, 1971.

56. Halpern, S.H., Eisler, E.A., Shnider, S.M., *et al.*: Myocardial tissue uptake of bupivacaine and lidocaine after intravenous injection in normal and acidotic rabbits. Anesthesiology, *61*:A208, 1984.

57. Harrison, D.C., Sprouse, J.H., and Morrow, A.G.: The antiarrhythmic properties of lidocaine and procaine amide; clinical and physiologic studies of their cardiovascular effects in man. Circulation, *28*:486, 1963.

58. Hjelm, M., and Holmdahl, M.H.: Biochemical effects of aromatic amines II. Cyanosis, methemoglobinemia and Heinz-body formation induced by a local anaesthetic agent (prilocaine). Acta Anaesthesiol. Scand., *2*:99, 1965.

59. Hilgier, M.: Alkalinization of bupivacaine for brachial plexus block. Reg. Anaesth., *10*:59, 1985.

60. Huffman, R.D., and Yim, G.K.W.: Effects of diphenylaminoethanol and lidocaine on central inhibition. Int. J. Neuropharmacol., *8*:217, 1969.

61. Johns, R.A., DiFazio, C.A., and Longnecker, D.E.: Lidocaine constricts or dilates rat arterioles in a dose dependent manner. Anesthesiology, *61*:A204, 1984.

62. Jorfeldt, L., Lofstrom, B., Pernow, B., and Wahren, J.: The effect of mepivacaine and lidocaine on forearm resistance and capacitance vessels in man. Acta Anaesthesiol. Scand., *14*:183, 1970.

63. Josephson, I., and Sperelakis, N.: Local anesthetic blockade of Ca^{2+}-mediated action potentials in cardiac muscle. Eur. J. Pharmacol., *40*:201, 1976.

64. Kasten, G.W., and Martin, S.T.: Successful resuscitation after massive intravenous bupivacaine overdose in the hypoxic dog. Anesthesiology, *61*:A206, 1984.

65. Keir, L.: Continuous epidural analgesia in prostatectomy: comparison of bupivacaine with and without adrenaline. Acta Anaesthesiol. Scand., *18*:1, 1974.

66. Kotelko, D.M., Shnider, S.M., Dailey, P.A., *et al.*: Bupivacaine-induced cardiac arrhythmias in sheep. Anesthesiology, *60*:10, 1984.

67. Kuperman, A.S., Altura, B.T., and Chezar, J.A.: Action of procaine on calcium efflux from frog nerve and muscle. Nature, *217*:673, 1968.

68. Libelius, R., Sonesson, B., Stamenovic, B.A., Thesleff, S.: Denervation-like changes in skeletal muscle after treatment with a local anesthetic (Marcaine). J. Anat., *106*:297, 1970.

69. Lieberman, N.A., Harris, R.S., Katz, R.I., Lipschutz, H.M., *et al.*: The effects of lidocaine on the electrical and mechanical activity of the heart. Am. J. Cardiol., *22*:375, 1968.

70. Littlewood, D.G., Buckley, P., Covino, B.G., Scott, D.B., *et al.*: Comparative study of various local anesthetic solutions in extradural block in labour. Br. J. Anaesth., *51*:47, 1979.

71. Liu, P.L., Feldman, H.S., Covino, B.M., Giasi, R., *et al.*: Acute cardiovascular toxicity of procaine, chloroprocaine and tetracaine in anesthetized ventilated dogs. Reg. Anaesth., *7*:14, 1982.

72. Liu, P.L., Feldman, H.S., Covino, B.M., Giasi, R., *et al.*: Acute cardiovascular toxicity of intravenous amide local anesthetics in anesthetized ventilated dogs. Anesth. Analg., *61*:317, 1982.

73. Liu, P.L., Feldman, H.S., Giasi, R., Patterson, M.K., *et al.*: Comparative CNS toxicity of lidocaine, etidocaine, bupivacaine and tetracaine in awake dogs following rapid IV administration. Anesth. Analg., *62*:375, 1983.

74. Loder, R.E.: A local anesthetic solution with longer action. Lancet, *2*:346, 1960.

75. Lofstrom, J.B.: Ulnar nerve blockade for the evaluation of local anaesthetic agents. Br. J. Anaesth., *47*:297, 1975.

76. Lund, P.C., and Cwik, J.C.: Propitocaine (Citanest) and methemoglobinemia. Anesthesiology, *26*:569–571, 1965.

77. McClure, J.H., and Scott, D.B.: Comparison of bupivicaine hydrochloride and carbonated bupivacaine in brachial plexus block by the inter-scalene technique. Br. J. Anaesth., *53*:523, 1981.

78. Meagher, R.P., Moore, D.C., and DeVries, J.C.: The most effective potentiator of tetracaine spinal anesthesia. Anesth. Analg., *45*:134, 1966.

79. Moore, D.C., Crawford, R.D., and Scurlock, J.E.: Severe hypoxia and acidosis following local anesthetic-induced convulsions. Anesthesiology, *53*:259, 1980.

80. Moore, D.C., Spierdijk, J., VanKleef, J.D., Coleman, R.L., *et al.*: Chloroprocaine neurotoxicity: Four additional cases. Anesth. Analg., *61*:155, 1982.

81. Morishima, H.O., Pederson, H., Finster, M., Hiraoka, H., *et al.*: Bupivacaine toxicity in pregnant and nonpregnant ewes. Anesthesiology, *63*:134, 1985.

82. Morishima, H.O., Peterson, H., Finster, M., *et al.*: Is bupivacaine more cardiotoxic than lidocaine? Anesthesiology, *59*:A409, 1983.

83. Morishima, H.O., Pedersen, H., Finster, M., Feldman, H.S., *et al.*: Etidocaine toxicity in the adult, newborn and fetal sheep. Anesthesiology, *58*:342, 1983.

84. Morrison, D.H.: A double-blind comparison of carbonated lidocaine and lidocaine hydrochloride in epidural anaesthesia. Can. Anaesth. Soc., J., *28*:387, 1981.

85. Munson, E.S., Tucker, W.K., Ausinsch, B., and Malagodi, H.: Etidocaine, bupivacaine, and lidocaine seizure thresholds in monkey. Anesthesiology, *42*:471, 1975.

86. Nancarrow, C.: Acute Toxicity of Lignocaine and Bupivacaine. Ph.D. Thesis, Flinders University of South Australia, 1986.
87. Nishimura, N., Morioka, T., Sato, S., and Kuba, T.: Effects of local anesthetic agents on the peripheral vascular system. Anesth. Analg., *44*:135, 1965.
88. Pizzalato, D., and Reneger, O.J.: Histopathologic effects of long exposure to local anesthetics on peripheral nerves. Anesth. Analg., *38*:138, 1959.
89. Prentiss, J.E.: Cardiac arrest following caudal anesthesia. Anesthesiology, *50*:51, 1979.
90. Prescott, L.F., and Nimmo, J.: Plasma lidocaine concentrations during and after prolonged infusions in patients with myocardial infarction. *In* Scott, D.B. and Julian, D.C. (eds): Lidocaine in the Treatment of Ventricular +rrhythmias, pp. 178–188. Edinburgh, E & S Livingston, 1971.
91. Ravindran, R.S., Bond, V.K., Tasch, M.D., Gupta, C.D., *et al.*: Prolonged neural blockade following regional analgesia with 2-chloroprocaine. Anesth. Analg., *58*:447, 1980.
92. Ravindran, R.S., Turner, M.S., and Muller, T.: Neurological effects of subarachnoid administration of 2-chloroprocaine-CE, bupivacaine and low pH normal saline in dogs. Anesth. Analg., *61*:279, 1982.
93. Reisner, L.S., Hochman, B.N., and Plumer, M.H.: Persistent neuralgia deficit and adhesive arachnoiditis following intrathecal 2-chloroprocaine injection. Anesth. Analg., *58*:452, 1980.
94. Reynolds, F.: Allergy reaction to an amide local anaesthetic. Br. J. Anaesth., *53*:901, 1981.
95. Ritchie, J.M., Ritchie, B., and Greengard, P.: The active structure of local anesthetics. J. Pharmacol. Exp. Ther., *150*:152, 1965.
96. Rocco, A.G., Francis, D.M., Wark, J.A., Concepcion, M.A., *et al.*: A clinical double-blind study of dibucaine and tetracaine in spinal anesthesia. Anesth. Analg., *61*:133, 1982.
97. Rosen, M.A., Baysinger, C.L., Shnider, S.M., *et al.*: Evaluation of neurotoxicity of local anesthetics following subarachnoid injection. Anesthesiology, *57*:A196, 1982.
98. Rosenblatt, R.M., and Fung, D.L.: Mechanism of action of dextran prolonging regional anesthesia. Reg. Anaesth., *5*:3, 1980.
99. Rosenblatt, R.M., and Fung, D.L.: Optional ratio of bupivacaine and dextran for regional anaesthesia. Reg. Anaesth., *4*:2, 1979.
100. Sage, D., Feldman, H., Arthur, G.R., Covino, B.G.: Cardiovascular effects of lidocaine and bupivacaine in the awake dog. Anesthesiology, *59*:A210, 1983.
101. Sage, D.J., Feldman, H.S., Arthur, G.R., *et al.*: Influence of lidocaine and bupivacaine on isolated guinea pig atria in the presence of acidosis and hypoxia. Anesth., Analg., *63*:1, 1983.
102. Scott, D.B.: Evaluation of clinical tolerance of local anesthetic agents. Br. J. Anaesth., *47*:328, 1975.
103. Scott, D.B.: Evaluation of the toxicity of local anaesthetic agents in man. Br. J. Anaesth., *47*:56, 1975.
104. Scott, D.B.: Toxicity caused by local anaesthetic drugs., Br. J., Anaesth., *53:553, 1981.*
105. Scott, D.B., McClure, J.H., Giasi, R.M., Seo, J., *et al.*: Effects of concentration of local anaesthetic drugs in extradural block. Br. J. Anaesth., *52*:1033, 1980.
106. Seow, L.T., Lips, F.J., Cousins, M.J., and Mather, L.E.: Lidocaine and bupivacaine mixtures for epidural blockade. Anesthesiology, *56*:177, 1982.
107. Skou, J.C.: Local anaesthetics. II. The toxic potencies of some local anesthetics and of butyl alcohol, determined on peripheral nerve. Acta Pharmacol. Toxicol., *10*:292, 1954.
108. Sinclair, C.J., and Scott, D.B.: Comparison of bupivacaine and etidocaine in extradural blockade. Br. J. Anaesth., *56*:147, 1984.
109. Stewart, D.M., Rogers, W.P., Mahaffrey, J.E., and Witherspoon, S., *et al.*: Effect of local anesthetics on the cardiovascular system in the dog. Anesthesiology, *24*:620, 1963.
110. Sugimoto, T., Schaal, S.F., Dunn, N.M., and Wallace, A.G.: Electrophysiological effects of lidocaine in awake dogs. J. Pharmacol. Exp. Ther., *166*:146, 1969.
111. Swerdlow, M., and Jones, R.: The duration of action of bupivacaine, prilocaine, and lignocaine. Br. J. Anaesth., *42*:335, 1970.
112. Tanaka, K., and Yamasaki, M.: Blocking of cortical inhibitory synapses by intravenous lidocaine. Nature, *209*:207, 1966.
113. Tanz, R.D., Heskett, T., Loehning, R.W., and Fairfax, C.A.: Comparative cardiotoxicity of bupivacaine and lidocaine in the isolated perfused mammalian heart. Anesth. Analg., *63*:549, 1984.
114. Thigpen, J.W., Kotelko, D.M., Shnider, S.M., *et al.*: Bupivacaine cardiotoxicity in hypoxic-acidotic sheep. Anesthesiology, *59*:A204, 1983.
115. Thomson, S.P.: Lidocaine pharmacokinetics in advanced heart failure, liver disease, and renal failure in humans. Ann. Intern. Med., *78*:499, 1973.
116. Wang, B.C., Hillman, D.E., Spiedholz, N.I., and Turndorf, H.: Chronic neurological deficits and Nesacaine-CE—An effect of the anesthetic, 2-Chloroprocaine, or the antioxidant, sodium bisulfite? Anesth. Analg., *63*:445, 1984.
117. Wojtczak, J.A., Pratilas, V., Griffin, R.M., and Kaplan, J.A.: Cellular mechanisms of cardiac arrhythmias induced by bupivacaine. Anesthesiology, *61*:A37, 1984.

5 MODIFICATION OF RESPONSES TO SURGERY BY NEURAL BLOCKADE: CLINICAL IMPLICATIONS

HENRIK KEHLET

Surgical trauma is an injury that may range from minor elective procedures to a massive insult following major procedures complicated by sepsis. The body reacts to the noxious stimulus both locally and generally. The inflammatory reaction constitutes the local response and is considered to be important for healing and defense against infection. The general response is in the form of an endocrine metabolic activation leading to hypermetabolism with an acceleration of most biochemical reactions, including substrate mobilization. The general response is highly dependent on the severity of the injury and represents a stereotyped neurophysiologic reflex response. From a teleological viewpoint the stress response probably has evolved to provide a maximum chance of survival because of the resulting fluid preservation and supply of the increased demands for energy-generating substrates. If prolonged, however, the stress response may have a detrimental effect because of the resulting devastating nutritional consequences leading to depletion of several essential components of the body.

During the past few decades there has been a tremendous increase of knowledge within anesthesia and surgery, allowing even major procedures to be performed in patients with severe complicating disease, previously contraindicating surgery. A key factor in the development of safe convalescence has been the development of surgical biology, because the proper treatment of surgical trauma requires knowledge of its biochemical effects. Thus a favorable postoperative outcome will most probably occur through a collaboration between anesthesiologists and surgeons taking advantage of the knowledge of precipitating factors of the stress response and applying modulatory therapeutic methods, thereby minimizing profound changes in fluid and electrolyte balances, nutritional metabolism, and host defense mechanisms.

This chapter updates the developments in our understanding of the release mechanisms involved in the stress response to surgical procedures and in the techniques that can modulate these responses. A review of the literature will be presented on the modulating effect of neural blockade on the stress response to surgical procedures, and the implications for anesthetic practice will be delineated based on a review of controlled studies on the effect of neural blockade on postoperative morbidity.

GENERAL STRESS RESPONSE TO SURGERY

The response to surgical trauma may be divided into two phases: The initial acute "ebb" or "shock" phase is characterized by a hypodynamic state, a reduction in metabolic rate, and depression of most physiologic processes. With surgical trauma this phase is either absent or very transient during the operative period.

The second phase is the hyperdynamic "flow"

phase, which may last for a few days or weeks depending on the magnitude of the surgical insult or occurrence of complications. Characteristically, metabolic rate and cardiac output are elevated. A summary of the endocrine and metabolic changes to surgical trauma is given in Table 5-1. There is a change in the endocrine milieu whereby plasma concentrations of the catabolic active hormones are elevated while those of the anabolic active hormones are lowered. Post-traumatic changes in the biological activity of thyroid hormone have not been clarified but are not reflected by changes in circulating levels of T_3 and T_4. The influence of surgery on insulin secretion is biphasic, with an impaired insulin response to glucose during the initial phase followed by an increased insulin response but with a concomitant increased peripheral insulin resistance (postreceptor defect). Hepatic glucose production is stepped up due to an increased gluconeogenesis and an initially increased glycogenolysis, and total body glucose utilization is elevated. Lipid turnover and oxidation are enhanced and protein turnover is increased, probably with a reduction in protein synthesis and a slight increase in breakdown during elective surgery. During major trauma, however, the increased protein breakdown exceeds synthesis. Synthesis of some specific proteins, that is, acute-phase proteins, is increased. Concomitantly, fluid and electrolyte balance shows a shift toward water and sodium retention, while urinary potassium excretion is increased. Vascular permeability to albumin is increased. Peripheral blood neutrophils increase whereas lymphocytes decrease, and most parameters of specific as well as nonspecific immunofunction show a deterioration. Coagulation is activated and fibrinolysis inhibited except for an initial transient activation.

Although the metabolic response to surgery is a net effect of responses to injury and (semi-) starvation, the changes in energy metabolism and substrate flow are predominantly determined by the injury response. The intensity of the stress response to surgery is directly related to the degree of tissue trauma, that is, diagnostic procedures of short duration, procedures on the body surface, ear surgery, and superficial eye surgery evoke only a very slight, transient response, whereas procedures involving the thorax and abdominal cavity elicit a more pronounced response in which the flow phase may last up to several days or weeks if complications eventuate. Intracranial procedures lead to an intermediate, rather small, and short-lived response. A detailed description of the endocrine metabolic response to surgery and trauma has been given in recent reviews.[52,70,116,117,126,223]

TABLE 5-1. NEUROENDOCRINE AND METABOLIC RESPONSES TO SURGERY

Endocrine	
Catabolic	
Due to increase in:	ACTH, cortisol, ADH, GH, catecholamines, renin, angiotensin-II, aldosterone, glucagon, interleukin-1
Anabolic	
Due to decrease in:	Insulin, testosterone
Metabolic	
Carbohydrate	Hyperglycemia, glucose intolerance, insulin resistance
Due to increase in:	Hepatic glycogenolysis (epinephrine, glucagon)—gluconeogenesis (cortisol, glucagon, growth hormone epinephrine, free fatty acids)
Due to decrease in:	Insulin secretion/action
Protein	Muscle protein catabolism, increased synthesis of acute-phase proteins
Due to increase in:	Cortisol, epinephrine, glucagon, interleukin-1
Fat	Increased lipolysis and oxydation
Due to increase in:	Catecholamines, cortisol, glucagon, growth hormone
Water and Electrolyte Flux	Retention of H_2O and Na^+, increased excretion of K^+, decreased functional extracellular fluid with shifts to intracellular compartments
Due to increase in:	Catecholamines, aldosterone, ADH, cortisol, angiotensin-II, prostaglandins, and other factors

RELEASE MECHANISMS OF THE STRESS RESPONSE

In contrast to our detailed knowledge of the changes in various hormonal and metabolic compartments of the stress response, information on the exact nature and relative role of the various signals that may initiate and potentiate the response is limited and not fully understood (Fig. 5-1).

AFFERENT NEURAL STIMULI

Much evidence has accumulated to demonstrate that the peripheral and central nervous systems represent a major common pathway mediating the stress response.[222] The nociceptive signals to the central nervous system are transmitted primarily by small myelinated (A δ) and unmyelinated (C) sensory afferent fibers to the substantia gelatinosa in the dorsal horn, with further rostrad spread to the ventral-posterior nucleus of the thalamus.[225] Modulation of pain may occur at many levels, including midbrain, medulla, and spinal cord, by means of powerful descending inhibitory systems, as shown in Figure 5-2 (see also Chaps. 24 and 25). The relative role of the various nociceptive stimuli (pressure, vibration, chemical, thermal, intense mechanical) in arousing the stress response remains to be ascertained, as do the peripheral substrates (transmitters) involved; however, local synthesis in the traumatized area of histamine, serotonin, kinins, prostaglandins, and substance-P has been shown to facilitate the initiation of afferent neural stimuli. Afferent stimuli conducted through somatosensory and sympathetic pathways play a predominant role in precipitating the response to abdominal surgery compared to the vagal afferent pathway. The role of the afferent parasympathetic pathways through the pelvic nerves has not been evaluated. The influence of efferent neural stimuli in raising the stress response is discussed below. The importance of afferent neural stimuli versus other stimuli (see Fig. 5-1) in mediating the trauma response has been evaluated in clinical studies using different techniques of neural blockade (see below). These studies have demonstrated that during relatively minor, clean surgery the neural pathway is the main release mechanism of most of the classic endocrine metabolic responses (see Table 5-1), but not of postoperative changes in various protein systems (acute-phase proteins) and the coagulation and fibrinolytic systems. During major procedures, however, other stimuli (see Fig. 5-1) may potentiate the response.

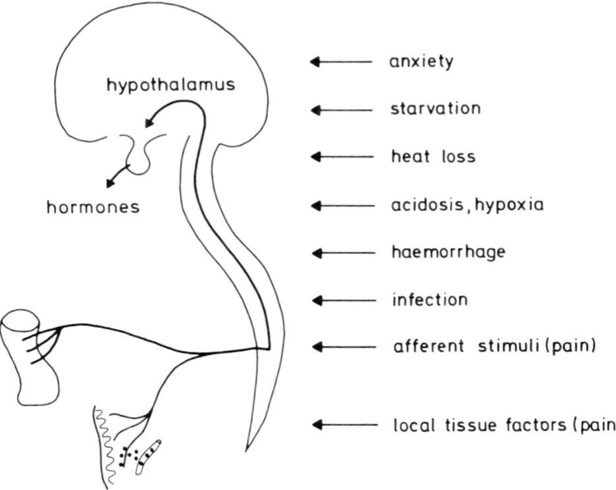

FIG. 5-1. Release mechanisms of the endocrine metabolic response to surgery. The principal mechanisms are afferent neural stimuli from the surgical area, local tissue factors released at the trauma site, and interleukin-1 from circulating macrophages. Psychological factors, starvation, heat loss, acidosis and hypoxia, hemorrhage, and infection all act as amplifiers of the response.

LOCAL TISSUE FACTORS

The observation that severe injury to a denervated limb elicited an adrenocortical response during various experimental settings has emphasized that factors other than afferent neural stimuli may initiate the response during a major insult. The nature of such substances, presumably released at the trauma site, has been studied extensively during recent years,[39,124,134] but a clear picture has not emerged. An initial reaction, leading to the inflammatory response, activation of the complement pathways, and coagulation and fibrinolysis, is activation of the plasma contact activation system;[39] the initial biochemical event initiating this surface-mediated defense reaction is unknown. Further, most nociceptive stimuli lead to a local release of histamine, serotonin, prostaglandins, substance-P, and the like,[225] but the exact role of these substrates in mediating the stress response apart from facilitating the afferent neural stimuli remains to be determined (Fig. 5-3). Recently, interleukin-1, which is synthesized by activated macrophages, has been demonstrated to be a key mediator of host responses to microbial invasion.[56] Al-

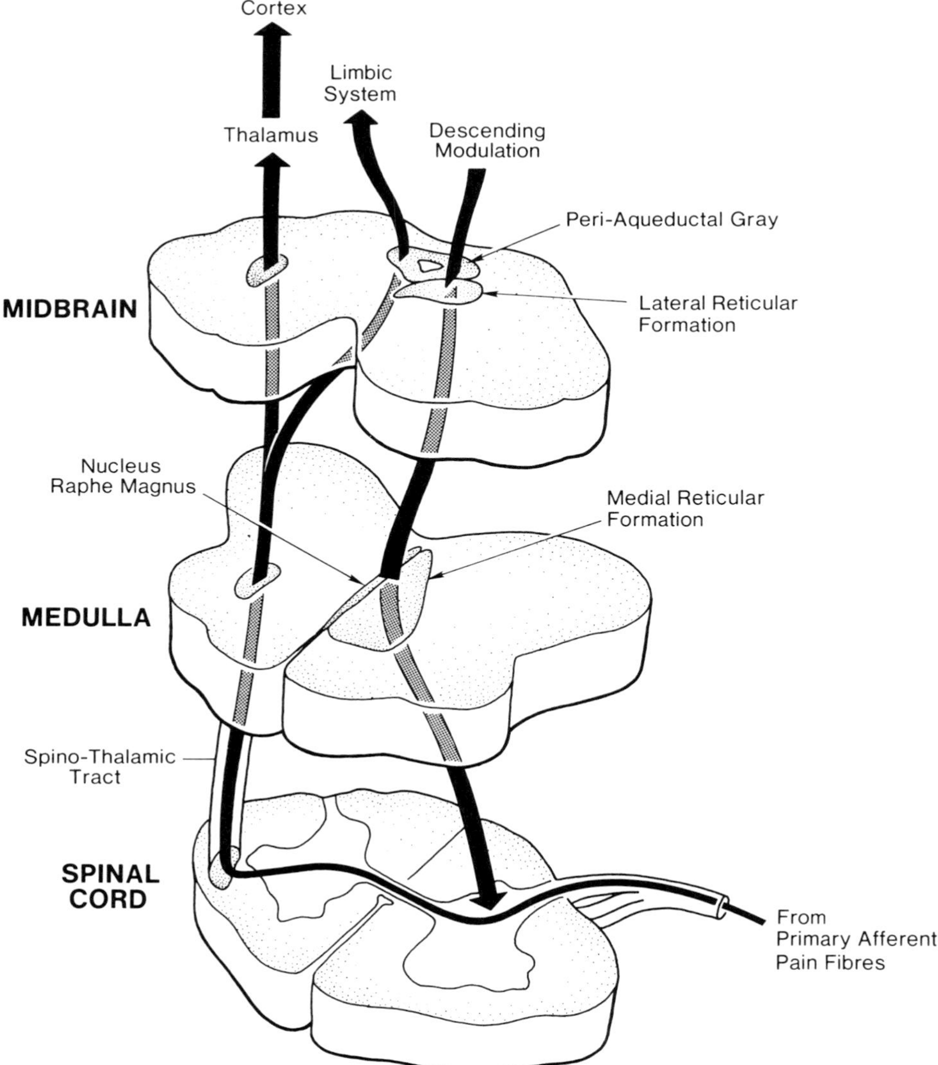

FIG. 5-2. Pain transmission and modulation. Primary afferent fibers are shown entering dorsal horn of spinal cord and crossing over to spinothalamic tract. Note descending modulation initiated in midbrain and medulla, impinging on primary afferernt pathway in dorsal horn. Modulation also occurs more centrally (see Chaps. 24 and 25), probably partly involving limbic system. (Reproduced with permission from Phillips, G.D., and Cousins, M.J.: Neurological mechanisms of pain and the relationship of pain, anxiety, and sleep. In Cousins, M.J. and Phillips, G.D. [eds.]: Acute Pain Management. London, Churchill Livingstone, 1986.)

though the amino acid sequence of interleukin-1 is still unknown, this circulating peptide has potent biologic activities, such as activation of various immunofunctions and a potentiating role in muscle proteolysis, hyperthermia, and acute-phase protein synthesis in the liver. The precise role of interleukin-1 in releasing various aspects of the stress response to surgical procedures remains to be ascertained but may be important, since combined hormonal infusions with epinephrine, norepinephrine, cortisol, and

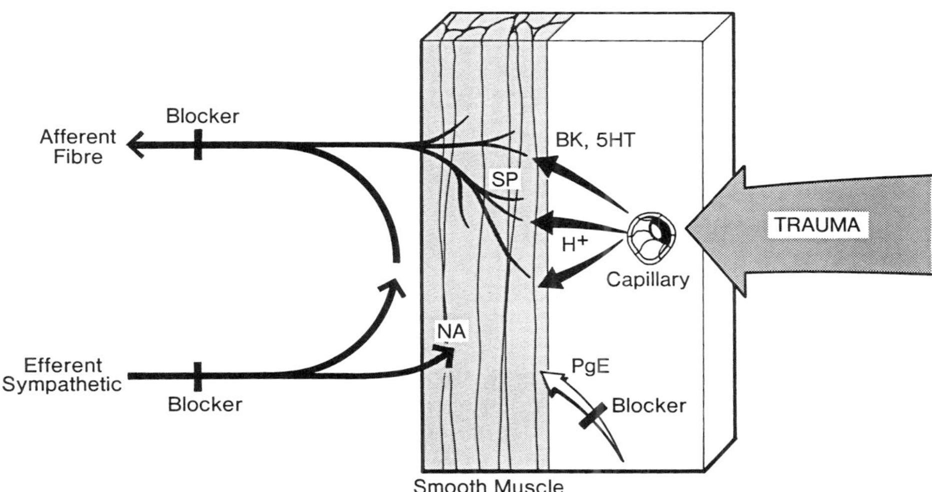

FIG. 5-3. Local tissue factors and peripheral pain receptors. The physical stimuli of "trauma," the chemical environment (*e.g.*, *H^+*), algesic substances (*e.g.*, serotonin [5-HT], bradykinin [BK]), and microcirculatory changes may all modify peripheral receptor activity. Efferent sympathetic activity may increase the sensitivity of receptors by means of noradrenaline *(NA)* (norepinephrine) release. Substance P may be the peripheral pain transmitter. Points of potential blockade of nociception are shown as "blocker." Other potential sites involve BK, 5-HT, NA, and SP. (Reproduced with permission from Phillips, G.D., and Cousins, M.J.: Neurological mechanisms of pain and the relationship of pain, anxiety, and sleep. In Cousins, M.J., and Phillips, G.D., [eds.]: Acute Pain Management. London, Churchill Livingstone, 1986.)

glucagon may only simulate some of the metabolic responses observed after surgery. Hyperthermia, the acute-phase protein response, and the magnitude of metabolic changes observed during major surgery are not, however, attained with these hormone infusions.[11,71]

ALTERED SET POINT OF ENDOCRINE METABOLIC FEEDBACK SYSTEMS

In our effort to find a rational explanation for the necessity of the stress response, we hypothesized that trauma leads to a change in the set point of various endocrine and substrate feedback systems because of an extra need for substrates during the hypermetabolic state and in healing tissues. In several studies, however, the administration of hormones (cortisol), substrates (glucose, fat, various proteins), and fluids could not be demonstrated to prevent the trauma-induced increase in cortisol secretion, gluconeogenesis, various protein systems, antidiuretic hormone, or aldosterone.[111,113] These findings may suggest that the stress response be considered as a reflex response rather than as a response elicited because of a primarily increased need for hormones or substrates, or both.

OTHER FACTORS

It is well documented that hemorrhage, even of small magnitude and not accompanied by hypotension, may activate atrial receptors and lead to an endocrine metabolic response. Similarly, acidosis and hypoxia may activate the response, and, if infection is superimposed on the surgical trauma, an exaggerated stress response will eventuate. All these factors, however, may not be considered as basic release mechanisms of the response but rather as amplifying factors.[111] Correspondingly, psychological factors *per se* may precipitate endocrine metabolic changes, but from a quantitative viewpoint these are negligible compared to the trauma-induced changes.

Heat loss, caused by the semi-nude condition of the patient and low ambient temperature of the operating room, may be an additional stimulus for increased metabolism in surgical patients. Heat loss is not, however, the causative factor of the stress response to surgery but may act as an amplifying factor, since prevention of heat loss by various methods has not been demonstrated to prevent the responses.[111,113]

MODIFYING FACTORS OF THE STRESS RESPONSE

The stress response to surgery and other injuries has usually been considered to be a homeostatic defense mechanism important for healing of tissue and adaptation to the noxious insult of injury. It has also been believed to enhance resistance to stress. In modern anesthesia and surgery, however, the biochemical changes after injury need not necessarily be considered as a homeostatic response important for survival and restitution, since physiologic disturbances may be prevented or repeatedly treated and substrates, blood, and other fluids are readily available. Concern about detrimental effects of surgery such as increased demands on various organs, myocardial infarction, pulmonary complications, thromboembolism, pain and convalescence with fatigue, and inability to work—all of which may not be considered as results of imperfections in surgical technique but rather as sequelae to the stress responses—has therefore led to studies of an eventual modulation of the trauma response. Thus, with the availability of current therapy, the stress responses may have become maladaptive, and instead the hypothesis has been proposed that the above-mentioned morbidity in high-risk surgical patients may be reduced by inhibiting the surgically induced endocrine response, hypermetabolism, and resulting increased demands on body mass and physiologic reserve.[111,113]

At present a variety of methods are available to modify the stress response to surgery (Fig. 5-4).[111,113]

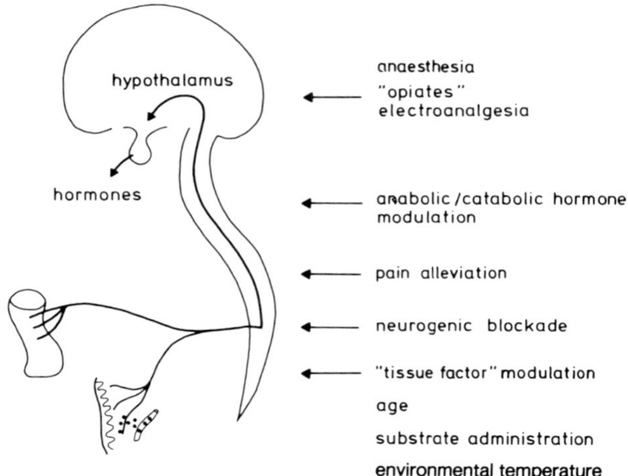

FIG. 5-4. Methods available to modify the endocrine metabolic response to surgery.

GENERAL ANESTHESIA

Although the use of general anesthesia may limit the perception of the injury, a vast amount of data have indicated that this may not necessarily be followed by a concomitant interference with the processing of the noxious stimuli to the hypothalamus and thereby an altered stress response. Generally it may be stated that almost all intravenous agents and volatile anesthetics in normal "low" doses have only a quantitatively minor influence on endocrine metabolic function *per se* and on endocrine metabolic changes induced by surgical trauma (see reviews in References 22, 109, 111, 161). In circumstances in which a slight inhibitory or stimulatory effect of an anesthetic has been demonstrated intraoperatively, the endocrine metabolic changes in the recovery period and late convalescence were *not* different from the usual pattern.

Exceptions to the general rule that general anesthetics are relatively inert as modifiers of the trauma response are ether and cyclopropane, both of which exert a stimulatory effect of the sympathetic nervous system and the adrenal cortex, and etomidate and high-dose opiate anesthesia, which have an inhibitory effect. Several studies have demonstrated that the hypnomimetic agent etomidate selectively inhibits the adrenocortical response to surgery through an inhibition of two enzymes in cortisol synthesis[68,213] but without influence on other responses. Much concern has arisen about the use of etomidate for anesthesia or intensive care,[128] since uncontrolled observations have suggested an increased mortality among intensive care patients receiving long-term sedation with etomidate. Further data are needed, however, before implications can be settled for the use of etomidate in low doses as an adjuvant to anesthesia for surgical procedures. No severe side-effects have been observed to the transient, selective inhibition of the cortisol response to surgical procedures by etomidate.

The use of "high"-dose (MAC* dose above 1.5) halothane and enflurane may suppress the initial surgically induced increase in plasma catecholamines due to skin incision,[179] but further data are needed during the intraoperative and postoperative period.

The use of "high"-dose opiate anesthesia has become popular especially during cardiovascular procedures, and it is well documented that this anesthetic principle may lead to a complete suppression of most endocrine and metabolic responses.[22,109,111] Most studies have been performed in patients undergoing open heart surgery, and the results have been rather uniform in demonstrating that morphine (2–4 mg/kg), fentanyl (50–200 μg/kg), and other synthetic opiates may either prevent or inhibit the initial endocrine metabolic response. This applies to the usual increase in plasma concentrations of cortisol, aldosterone, renin, vasopressin, growth hormone, epinephrine, and norepinephrine, glucose, and lactate. In most of these studies, however, the modifying effect disappeared during the cardiopulmonary bypass procedure, and no influence on flow-phase responses in the later postoperative period has been demonstrated. Similarly, studies performed during abdominal procedures with "high"-dose opiate anesthesia also failed to show any influence on postoperative metabolism.[153] No differences have been demonstrated among the various synthetic opiates with regard to their inhibitory effect on the surgical stress response.

In summary, "high"-dose opiate anesthesia has only a transient inhibitory effect on the stress response as long as high concentrations are maintained in the blood and tissues, but prolonged postoperative metabolic effects do not eventuate. The use of this technique for a sustained reduction of the stress response is therefore limited because of the concomitant depression of the respiratory system. Further, fentanyl (50 μg/kg) could not reverse the established metabolic and cortisol response to pelvic surgery when administered 60 minutes after skin incision.[10a] The use of "high"-dose opiate administration in the postoperative period needs further evaluation as a continuous intravenous infusion to prolong rewarming time and minimize shivering, heat loss, and metabolic demands and heart work.

*Minimum alveolar concentration of anesthetic that prevents movement in response to surgical stimulus in 50% of patients.

ANABOLIC/CATABOLIC HORMONE MODULATION

Because the endocrine response to surgery is characterized by increased secretion of catabolic active hormones (catecholamines, cortisol, glucagon) and impaired secretion or effect of anabolic active hormones (insulin, testosterone), the catabolic postoperative state may be transformed to anabolism either by antagonizing the action of catecholamines by adrenergic blockade or by administration of anabolic hormones.[111,113]

It is well documented that some aspects of the metabolic response to surgery may be modified by adrenergic blockade, and in this context β-adrenergic blockade is more effective than α-adrenergic blockade.[111,113] No information is available, however, on eventual modulation of postoperative metabolism by adrenergic blockade. Administration of insulin has also been demonstrated to reduce post-traumatic protein breakdown, but data from surgical patients in the postoperative period are not available. Administration of growth hormone may improve nitrogen balance in traumatized patients, and several studies have shown anabolic steroids to be effective to improve postoperative nitrogen balance.[111,113]

Thus endocrine manipulations may partly attenuate different metabolic responses after surgical trauma. A major reduction of the stress response will probably not be achieved, however, unless a multicomponent regimen is used, and this may still be without effect on certain hormones (thyroid), various neural transmitters, and interleukin-1, among others. Furthermore, additional treatment of pain is necessary.

PAIN ALLEVIATION

During recent years, basic research on the mechanisms by which nociceptive stimuli are processed in the central nervous system has led to an improved understanding of pain and treatment of pain (see Chaps. 24 and 25). The influence of pain relief on the stress response to surgery by the methods available (Fig. 5-5) will be reviewed in detail as concerns neural blockade by spinal and epidural analgesia with local anesthetic agents and epidural/intrathecal administration of opiates. The influence of other methods has been reviewed elsewhere[112] and will only be summarized below.

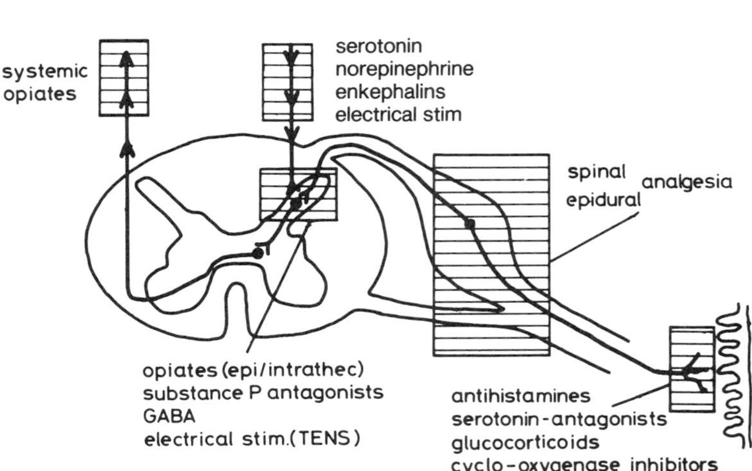

FIG. 5-5. Various techniques that may provide pain relief in surgical patients and thereby eventually modify the endocrine metabolic response. At present no information is available from antagonism of peripheral mediators of pain, while neural blockade with local anesthetics inhibits a major part of the stress response. Pain relief with epidural/intrathecal opiates is less efficient in reducing the stress response despite sufficient pain relief. The effect of stimulation of descending inhibitory pathways on the stress response is unknown. Administration of systemic opiates in usual low doses has no consistent influence on the stress response.

Influence of Pain Relief by Antagonizing Peripheral Mediators of Pain. As mentioned above several endogenous algesic substances may be released following a noxious stimulus. Agents that either prevent the release or antagonize these mediators may therefore be expected to provide pain relief and subsequently alter the stress response. Although several of the pharmacologic modulators as shown in Figure 5-5 may lead to pain relief, no information is available on a concomitant reduction in the stress responses following surgery.[112]

Pain Relief by Stimulation of Inhibitory Descending Pathways. Despite well-documented pain alleviation during experimental settings by stimulation of the descending inhibitory pathways (see Fig. 5-2) from the brain stem, using serotonin, norepinephrine and enkephalins as transmitters, no data are available on an eventual reduction in the stress response from experimental or from clinical studies.

Transcutaneous Electrical Stimulation (TENS). Several controlled studies have demonstrated the efficacy of TENS in relieving pain following different operative procedures,[205] but no information exists on subsequent modulation of the stress response.

Systemic Opiate Administration. Despite the widespread use of intermittent or continuous administration of various opiates for pain alleviation in surgical patients, very little information is available on subsequent mitigation of endocrine metabolic changes. The data suggest, however, that either none or only minor reductions will be obtained unless very high doses are used.[112] The recent use of systemic infusion of opiates by a demand technique has been shown to be an effective technique for postoperative pain relief, but the influence on the trauma response is unknown.

AGE

It has been suggested that elderly patients might undergo surgical procedures at an increased risk because of abnormal endocrine and metabolic responses, but few studies have focused on this problem with appropriate matched control groups. The limited data suggest that elderly patients elicit an increased cortisol response, whereas other responses may be similar to those of younger patients.[100a,111]

SUBSTRATE ADMINISTRATION

It may be hypothesized that if trauma leads to increased requirements for certain substrates, then administration of such substrates should attenuate or prevent the stress response. As a general conclusion, however, provision of substrates may to some degree improve single aspects of postoperative catabolism, but the fundamental characteristics of the trauma response are not prevented. This also applies to administration of various specific substrates such as branched chain amino acids and ketones. Such considerations, however, obviously should not be an argument against nutritional support *per se,* but rather serve to emphasize that the basic mechanism of the stress response is not a lack or an increased need of substrates.

REDUCTION OF HEAT LOSS

Because injury leads to increased heat production and a rise in body temperature, it has been suggested that the stimulus to the stress response is a change in the set point of thermal neutrality at the hypothalamic level caused by the need for a higher core temperature. A logical approach to attenuate the responses would therefore be to raise environmental temperature. This principle is further argued by the usual increased heat loss in surgical patients owing to the semi-nude state and relatively low temperature in the operating rooms and wards. As mentioned above, recent observations suggest that the increased heat production and rise in body temperature are mediated by a synergistic effect of cortisol, catecholamines, and glucagon with a superimposed influence of interleukin-1. There is no evidence, however, that an increase in environmental temperature or prevention of heat loss may result in a major reduction in the stress response, although avoidance of additional heat loss may mitigate some responses and demands on the cardiovascular system.[111,113]

MODIFICATION OF ENDOCRINE METABOLIC FUNCTION BY NEURAL BLOCKADE WITH LOCAL ANESTHETICS

The central role of the peripheral and central nervous system in mediating the response to surgical injury has stimulated research on the effects of blockade of nociceptive stimuli by peripheral or central nerve blocks on the injury response. Thus in 1910 George Crile launched the hypothesis of anociassociation,[50] suggesting that disruption of nociceptive stimuli by neural blockade might favorably affect post-traumatic outcome. Indeed the drawing on the cover of this book depicts this concept, with neural blockade "protecting" the nervous system from noxious input and preventing adverse neurohumoral responses. In contrast, Walter Cannon demonstrated the importance of the sympathetic nervous system in maintaining homeostasis in response to a variety of stresses, such as fluid deprivation, hemorrhage, and cold[31]; however, the theory of anociassociation was supported in experimental studies, demonstrating that spinal anesthesia effective before injury reduced mortality to blunt hind limb trauma.[160] Following the classic studies of Hume and Egdahl[100] demonstrating the importance of the peripheral and central nervous system in mediating the adrenocortical response to trauma, a vast amount of data have appeared during the last decades on the influence of neural blockade on various aspects of the responses to surgical injury. In the following sections these data are reviewed and the strength and limitations of these findings are discussed, aiming to identify issues relevant to future progress in our understanding of the surgical stress response. Finally, directions for future research are suggested.

INFLUENCE OF NEURAL BLOCKADE *PER SE* ON ENDOCRINE METABOLIC FUNCTION

The effects of neural blockade by spinal or epidural analgesia with local anesthetic agents have predominantly been studied within the 20- to 30-minute interval between initiation of anesthesia and start of surgery. It appears that neural blockade *per se* has only a limited influence of endocrine metabolic function, except for the effect on catecholamines and pancreatic islet function. The data suggest that epidural analgesia has no important effect on resting plasma cortisol and growth hormone levels,[74,77,162,171] whereas minor decreases in plasma prolactin LH and FSH have been observed.[77] In metabolic parameters, no significant changes have been noted in blood glucose, lactate, alanine, free fatty acids, glycerol, and ketones during 20 to 30 minutes of epidural analgesia (T4–S5).[108]

In contrast, plasma epinephrine and norepinephrine decreased in relation to a higher rostrad spread of sensory analgesia during spinal anesthesia with tetracaine (Fig. 5-6).[165] Other studies have found the same relation between changes in plasma catecholamines and sensory level of analgesia during spinal anesthesia with hyperbaric tetracaine and bupivacaine, although less significant.[14]

On average, no significant changes in plasma catecholamines are to be expected during blockade, in-

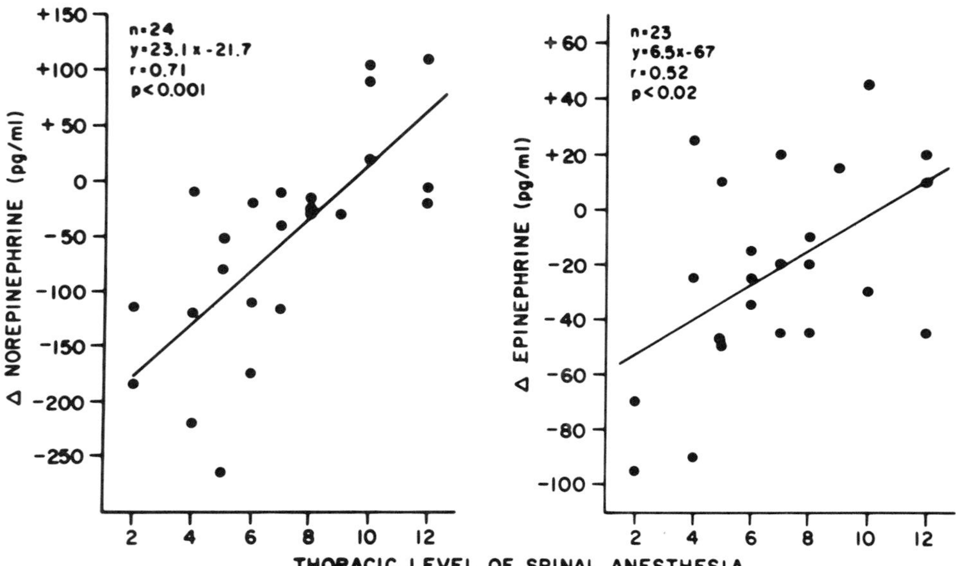

FIG. 5-6. Effect of spinal local anesthetic block *per se* on plasma catecholamines. Changes in plasma norepinephrine and epinephrine from preanesthesia to 30 minutes after subarachnoid injection of tetracaine. Regression analysis shows a significant correlation between thoracic level of anesthesia with both norepinephrine and epinephrine. (Reproduced with permission from Pflug, A.E., and Halter, J.B.: Effect of spinal anesthesia on adrenergic tone and the neuroendocrine responses to surgical stress in humans. Anesthesiology, *55*:120, 1981.)

cluding lower (T9 – T10) thoracic levels,[81,165] whereas decreased concentrations are seen during higher (T2 – T6) dermatome blockade.[64,81,165] Plasma norepinephrine, but not epinephrine, decreased during epidural analgesia extending to between T4 – T10, whereas plasma renin activity and vasopressin were unchanged.[59] During subsequent tilt, epidural analgesia did not modulate plasma catecholamines and renin, whereas vasopressin increased compared to tilt without epidural analgesia.[59]

The acute insulin response to hyperglycemia is inhibited by a high thoracic (T2 – T6) dermatome blockade, whereas a low (T9 – T10) blockade has no influence on insulin secretion, suggesting that a baseline adrenergic input is important for maintenance of normal pancreatic islet function.[81] Plasma glucagon responses to a glucose load may be augmented by a high dermatome blockade.[81]

No systematic studies have been published on a possible differential effect of spinal versus epidural analgesia or by different local anesthetic agents on endocrine metabolic function.

The influence of circulating levels of local anesthetics on endocrine metabolic function is debatable; initial studies with intravenous infusion of lidocaine, bupivacaine, and etidocaine, in amounts resulting in plasma concentrations at the same levels observed during administration in epidural analgesia, showed epinephrine-like responses such as increased splanchnic uptake of glycerol and lactate and release of 3-hydroxybuturate.[220] Recent controlled studies, however, did not observe any change in plasma catecholamines and various metabolites during infusion of bupivacaine unless plasma bupivacaine levels exceeded 3 to 4 μg/liter.[82]

INFLUENCE OF NEURAL BLOCKADE ON THE RESPONSE TO SURGICAL PROCEDURES

LOWER ABDOMINAL (GYNECOLOGIC) PROCEDURES AND OPERATIONS ON THE LOWER EXTREMITIES

The modifying effects of neural blockade on intraoperative and postoperative endocrine and metabolic responses are summarized in Tables 5-2 and 5-3.

TABLE 5-2. INFLUENCE OF NEURAL BLOCKADE (SPINAL/EPIDURAL) ON THE ENDOCRINE RESPONSE TO LOWER ABDOMINAL (GYNECOLOGIC) SURGERY OR TO PROCEDURES ON THE LOWER EXTREMITIES

Hormone (and Supporting References)	Intraoperative Response	Postoperative Response*
P-prolactin (9, 23, 77)	↓	↓
P-growth hormone (15, 23, 77, 155, 165)	↓	↓
P-ACTH (155)	↓	?
P-ADH (17, 166)	↓	↓
P-TSH	?	?
P-FSH (77)	→	↘
P-LH (77)	→	↘
P-beta-endorphin (66)	↓	?
P-cortisol (6, 23, 30, 43, 63, 74, 77, 94, 105, 108, 129, 152, 165, 171, 177)	↓	↓
P-aldosterone (28, 76)	↓	↓
P-renin (28, 76)	↓	↓
P-epinephrine (64, 165)	↓	↓
P-norepinephrine (64, 165)	↓	↓
P-insulin (6, 26, 30, 105)	↘	↘
P-C-peptide (6, 26)	↘	↘
P-glucagon (6, 23)	→	→
P-T_3 (24, 25)	→	→
P-T_4 (24, 25)	→	→
P-testosterone	?	?
P-estradiol	?	?
P-gastrointestinal hormones	?	?
P-neurotransmitters	?	?

*Continuous epidural analgesia only.
? = No data; ↓ = inhibition of response; → = no effect on response; ↘ = slight inhibition; P = plasma.

Most studies have been performed during hysterectomy,[9,15,17,23,25,26,30,43,63,129,152] vaginal surgery,[166] inguinal herniotomy and minor orthopedic procedures,[6,81,105,155,165] prostatectomy,[66] and hip replacement.[37,94,177,193]

Pituitary Hormones. The normal increase in plasma prolactin during surgery is prevented by neural blockade,[9,23,77] but this effect is caused both by afferent neural blockade and by the omission of general anesthesia, since many general anesthetics in themselves exert a stimulatory effect on prolactin secretion. Thus during surgery performed under combined general anesthesia and epidural analgesia, plasma prolactin levels may be elevated already before skin incision.[23]

Neural blockade also inhibits the growth hormone and ACTH response to surgery.[15,23,77,155,165] Similarly the usual increase in ADH is reduced by neural blockade.[17,166] Neural blockade accelerates the minor postoperative decrease in plasma FSH and LH in female patients[77]; no data are available on TSH changes. In one study the usual increase in beta-endorphin was prevented by spinal anesthesia during prostatectomy.[66]

Cortisol. Several studies have demonstrated that neural blockade with spinal or epidural analgesia may abolish or inhibit the cortisol response to surgery (Fig. 5-7).[6,23,30,36,43,63,74,77,94,105,108,129,165,171,177] In some of these studies, however, the influence was only marginal despite evidence that these patients had sufficient alleviation of pain. The variable success in inhibiting the cortisol response to surgery in these studies may be explained by insufficient afferent neural blockade (see below).

Aldosterone and Renin. The limited data on the influence of neural blockade on plasma aldosterone and renin changes suggest that these responses are reduced both intraoperatively and postoperatively during hysterectomy and hip surgery.[28,76]

Catecholamines. Neural blockade leads to an abolished epinephrine response to surgery,[64,165] in ac-

TABLE 5-3. INFLUENCE OF NEURAL BLOCKADE (SPINAL/EPIDURAL) ON THE METABOLIC RESPONSE TO LOWER ABDOMINAL (GYNECOLOGIC) SURGERY OR TO PROCEDURES ON THE LOWER EXTREMITIES

Metabolic Response (and Supporting References)	Intraoperative Response	Postoperative Response*
P-glucose (6, 23, 26, 30, 63, 108, 152, 171, 177)	↓	↓
Glucose tolerance (6, 30, 99, 105)	↑	→
Free fatty acids and glycerol (41, 78, 108)	↓	→
P-ketones (6, 108)	↓	↗
P-cAMP (157)	↓	↓
P-lactate (108, 193)	↓	→
Liver glycogen (7)	↓	?
Muscle amino acids (37)	?	↓
Nitrogen balance (27)	?	↑
P-creatinine phosphokinase (173)	?	↘
P-amino acids (37, 108)	→	→ ↘
P-acute-phase proteins (172)	→	→
Oxygen consumption (67, 175)	?	↘

*Continuous epidural analgesia only.
? = No data; ↑ = improvement or normalization (nitrogen balance, glucose tolerance); ↘ = slight inhibition of response; ↓ = inhibition of response; → = no effect on response; ↗ = slight increase; P = plasma.

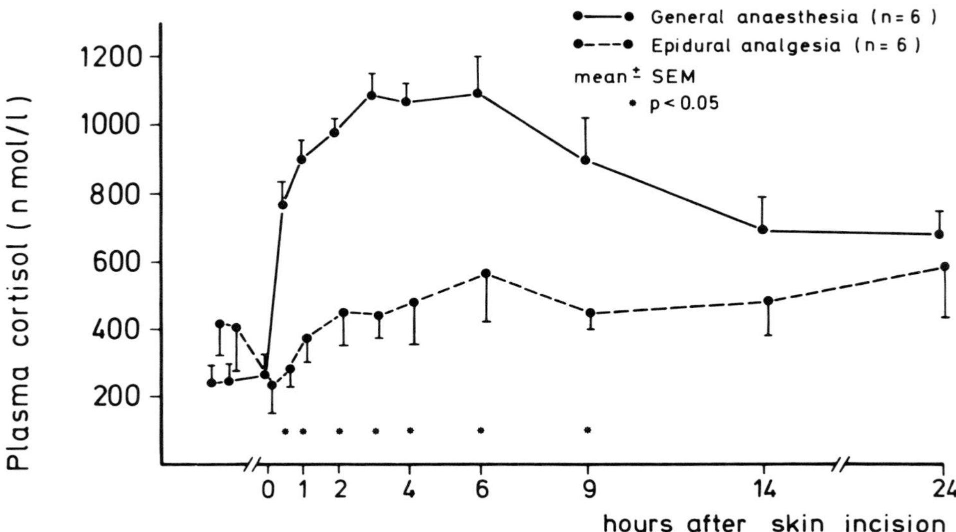

FIG. 5-7. Plasma cortisol: Comparison of intraoperative and postoperative changes in patients undergoing abdominal hysterectomy during general anesthesia (halothane) or continuous epidural analgesia with intermittent injections of plain bupivacaine 0.5%. Sensory level of analgesia was maintained from T_4 to S_5 during the 24-hour postoperative period. Plasma cortisol increased at all times after skin incision in patients operated on under general anesthesia, whereas no changes were observed in patients receiving continuous epidural analgesia. (Reproduced with permission from Brandt, M.R., Fernandes, A., Mordhorst, R., and Kehlet, H.: Epidural analgesia improves postoperative nitrogen balance. Br. Med. J., *1*:1106, 1978.)

cordance with the inhibited cyclic AMP response.[157] The data on intraoperative and postoperative changes in plasma norepinephrine are contradictory[64,165]; looking at the data from major (upper) abdominal procedures, however, an abolished norepinephrine response is most likely (see below).

Thyroid Hormones. Neural blockade has no major influence on plasma thyroxine (T_4),[24,25] but during combined general anesthesia and neural blockade an intraoperative and early postoperative increase in T_4 may be observed because several general anesthetic agents lead to hepatic release of T_4. Neural blockade alone or in combination with general anesthesia has no influence on the normal rapid decrease in plasma triiodothyronine (T_3) during hysterectomy or on the usual postoperative decrease in binding of thyroid hormones to plasma proteins.[24,25]

Insulin and Glucagon. Plasma insulin (and C-peptide) levels are unchanged during surgery under general anesthesia but may decrease during neural blockade (Fig. 5-8).[6,26] This is probably caused by blockade of resting adrenergic tone to the pancreatic islets, since baseline adrenergic input is important for normal islet function.[81] Plasma glucagon did not change during abdominal hysterectomy[23] or knee surgery[6] performed during general anesthesia or during combined general anesthesia and epidural analgesia[23] or epidural analgesia alone.[6]

Sex Hormones. No information is available on the influence of neural blockade on changes in plasma testosterone and estradiol.

Gastrointestinal Hormones and Neurotransmitters. No data are available.

Glucose Metabolism. The usual hyperglycemic response to surgery is reduced or blocked by neural blockade (Fig. 5-8).[23,26,30,63,108,152,171,177] This effect is not mediated through an increased insulin secre-

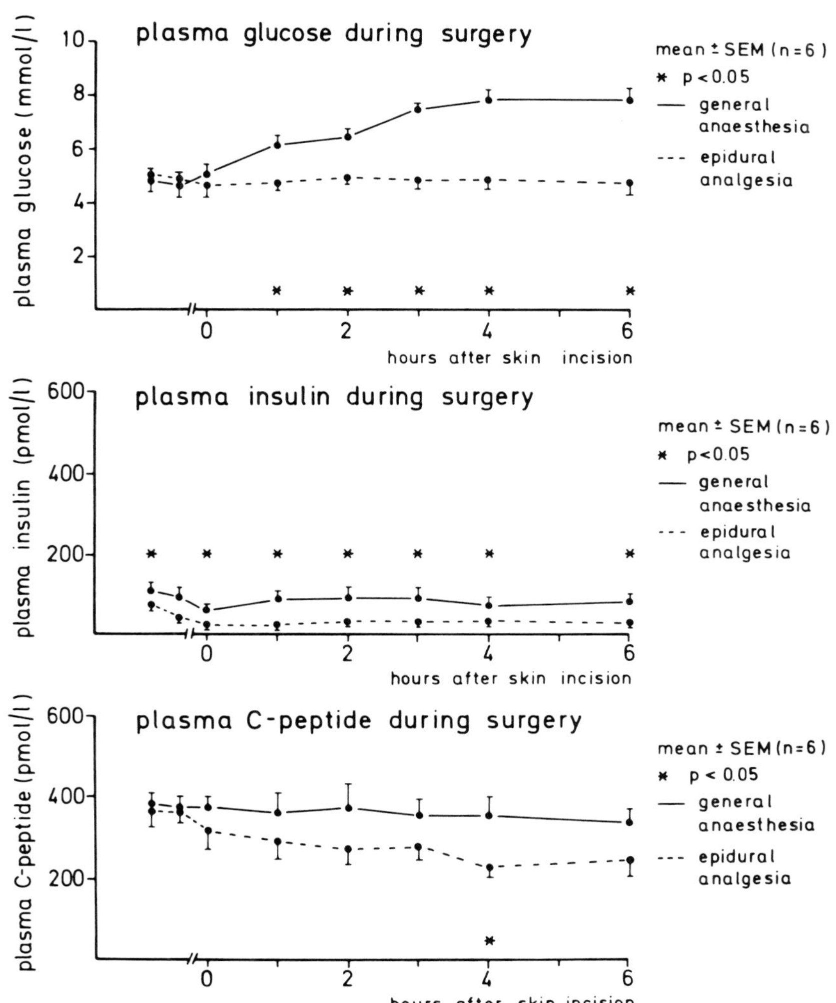

FIG. 5-8. Plasma glucose, insulin and C-peptide: Comparison of changes in patients undergoing abdominal hysterectomy during general anesthesia with halothane or enflurane or continuous epidural analgesia with intermittent injections of plain bupivacaine 0.5%. Sensory level of analgesia extended from T_4 to S_5 throughout the study. During general anesthesia plasma glucose increased after skin incision despite unchanged levels in insulin and C-peptide. In contrast, patients receiving epidural analgesia showed no changes in plasma glucose, probably because of concomitant inhibition of plasma catecholamines and cortisol. Insulin and C-peptide decreased after epidural analgesia because of blockade of adrenergic tone to pancreatic islets. (Reproduced with permission from Brandt, M.R., Kehlet, H. Faber, O., and Binder, C.: C-peptide and insulin during blockade on the hyperglycemic response to surgery by epidural analgesia. Clin. Endocrinol., 6:167, 1977.)

tion[6,26] but probably by inhibition of hepatic glycogenolytic response to surgery.[7] The inhibitory effect of neural blockade on the glycogenolytic response to surgery is caused by the abolished epinephrine responses[64,185] or blockade of efferent sympathetic neural pathways to the liver,[102,123] or both. Probably both efferent sympathetic nerves to the liver and the adrenals must be deactivated to block the glucose response to surgery.[123]

Lower glucose concentrations in patients operated on during neural blockade have also been demonstrated in skeletal muscle biopsies.[193] No differences, however, in muscle content of creatinine phosphate, adenosine triphosphate, lactate, or glucose-6-phosphate were found between patients operated on under epidural analgesia or neuroleptanesthesia.[193] An intravenous glucose tolerance test carried out during inguinal herniotomy[105] or hysterectomy[99] performed under neural blockade was normal, in contrast to the impaired glucose tolerance observed during surgery under general anesthesia. This effect of neural blockade on intraoperative glucose tolerance is probably caused by several factors. First, inhibition of hepatic glucose output may be important. Second, inhibition of the cortisol and epinephrine response to surgery may be of importance because both hormones inhibit peripheral glucose clearance.[11] Third, preservation of normal insulin response to glucose during neural blockade[79,80,99] may be a causative factor, although this could not be demonstrated in one study.[105] Also, omission of general anesthesia may be important because halothane has been shown to inhibit the acute insulin response to glucose independent of adrenergic mechanisms.[79,80] In two studies in which tests were performed 8 and 24 hours after surgery, glucose tolerance was found to be abnormal and similar to that of patients operated on under general anesthesia,[6,30] but in one of these the cortisol response was incompletely inhibited, suggesting insufficient afferent neural blockade.[30]

Altogether, the mechanisms involved in the modifying effect of neural blockade on glucose homeostasis, glucose tolerance, and insulin response to a glucose load are very complex. This is further emphasized by the demonstration that a high thoracic block (T2 – T6) inhibits resting efferent sympathetic tonic activity to the pancreatic islets, thereby leading to an impaired insulin response to glucose.[81] This may be a contributing mechanism to the impaired glucose tolerance and insulin response to glucose during the late postoperative period in patients having continuous epidural analgesia who are normoglycemic prior to glucose "challenge."[30] Further investigations using either a glucose clamp technique or labeled glucose for glucose clearance studies are needed to clarify the underlying mechanisms to the modifying effect of neural blockade on perioperative glucose homeostasis (see Tables 5-2 and 5-3).

Fat Metabolism. Neural blockade probably inhibits intraoperative lipolysis as indicated by reduced levels of plasma free fatty acids and glycerol during lower abdominal surgery.[41,108] Postoperatively, levels return to control values despite continuous epidural analgesia (see Table 5-3).[108]

Spinal anesthesia (T10 – L1) did not inhibit the increase in free fatty acids and glycerol during inguinal herniotomy unless the extent of analgesia was increased to high thoracic levels (T1 – T3).[78]

Although a reduction of postoperative lipolysis by neural blockade is to be expected because of the concomitant sympathetic blockade, further studies are needed using radioactive techniques to assess lipid turnover and oxidation.

Lactate and Ketones. The normal perioperative increase in blood lactate, which is partly caused by the general anesthetics, may be reduced by neural blockade.[108,193] The intraoperative increase in 3-hydroxybutyrate is reduced by neural blockade during hysterectomy,[108] whereas late postoperative levels tend to increase compared to those in patients undergoing hysterectomy or knee surgery under general anesthesia.[6,108]

Amino Acids and Nitrogen Balance. No influence of neural blockade could be demonstrated in the first 24-hour postoperative blood alanine profile,[108] but the 5-day cumulative postoperative nitrogen balance was significantly less negative (about 50%) in patients undergoing abdominal hysterectomy during epidural analgesia for 24 hours compared to general anesthesia (Fig. 5-9).[27] Correspondingly, continuous 24-hour postoperative epidural analgesia following hip replacement prevented the usual postoperative shifts in amino acid composition in muscle.[37] There are no data on 3-methylhistidine excretion.

Renal Function, Water, and Electrolyte Balance. Renal function and urinary excretion of water and electrolytes may be profoundly altered in connection with anesthesia and surgery,[46] and neural blockade may influence this response by several mechanisms: [1] changes in glomerular filtration rate (GFR), secondary to universal hemodynamic effects of sympathetic blockade; [2] effects mediated through an altered endocrine response to surgery by neural blockade; [3] direct renal effects owing to blockade of efferent neural pathways or interruption of neural renal reflexes (afferent/efferent), or both. Renal innervation originates from T10 – L1.[16] The influence of neural blockade on central and peripheral hemodynamics (see Chaps. 7 and 8) may also affect renal hemodynamics and decrease effective renal blood flow.[212] GFR has been found to decrease during epidural analgesia parallel to the decrease in systemic blood pressure.[104] The influence of neural blockade on the endocrine response to surgery has been described (Table 5-2). Since most of the hormones (cortisol, catecholamines, aldosterone, renin, ADH) that may affect kidney function[58] are modified by neural blockade, a major influence should be expected on kidney function. Further, experimental studies have shown efferent sympathetic nervous activity to be important for kidney function, since denervation led to an increase in sodium excretion and urine flow.[75,150] Also, neural blockade may interfere with reflexes recognized to influence efferent renal nerve activity and thereby tubular transport rates, although conclusive evidence has yet to be demonstrated.[150]

Despite the increased knowledge from both experimental and clinical studies on various mechanisms whereby neural blockade may influence kidney function in the perioperative period, no final conclu-

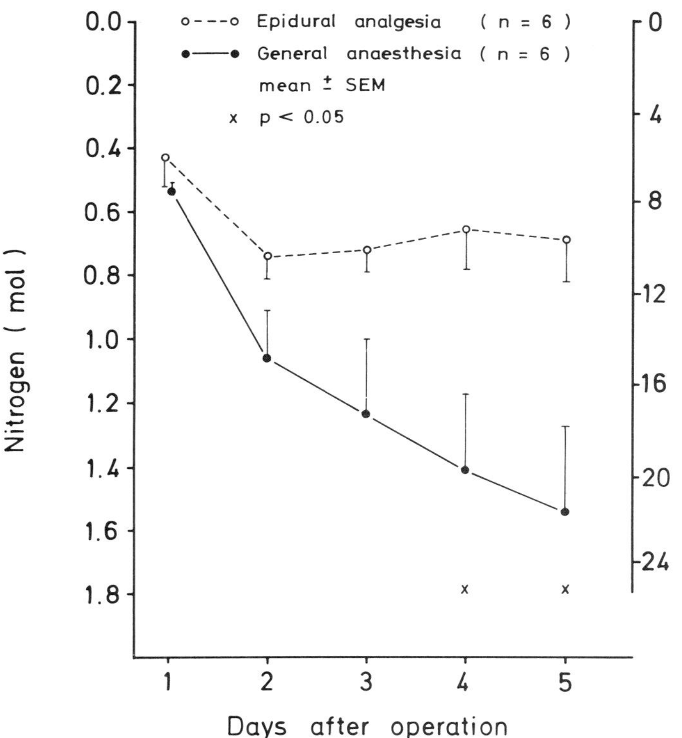

FIG. 5-9. Nitrogen balance: Comparison of urinary nitrogen excretion during the initial 5 days after abdominal hysterectomy in patients under general anesthesia with halothane or continuous epidural analgesia for 24 hours with intermittent injections of plain bupivacaine 0.5%. Sensory level of analgesia was held from T_4 to S_5. During the 5-day postoperative period, both groups received a hypocaloric oral intake amounting to 20 g of nitrogen and about 2900 calories. Patients receiving epidural analgesia had no intraoperative and postoperative increase in plasma cortisol and glucose, and concomitantly urinary nitrogen excretion was significantly reduced. (Reproduced with permission from Brandt, M.R., Fernandes, A., Mordhorst, R., and Kehlet, H.: Epidural analgesia improves postoperative nitrogen balance. Br. Med. J., *1*:1106, 1978.)

sion has emerged on the modifying effect of neural blockade on fluid and electrolyte balance in surgical patients. Thus the available data are very discordant (Table 5-4), and unfortunately the explanation hereto is not clear. A major problem hindering interpretation of these studies is that surgical procedures, extent and duration of neural blockade, fluid administration, and duration of the studies are not similar. The observation in experimental studies that neural blockade may reverse post-traumatic anuria[42] has not been elucidated in clinical settings.

Further studies on this important aspect of the injury response and its eventual modulation by neural blockade are needed.

Hepatic Function and Serum Enzymes. It is well documented that surgical trauma may lead to changes in various serum enzymes considered to be of hepatic origin and to increases in hepatic microsomal enzyme activity.[127] This may contribute to accelerated drug pharmacokinetics in the postoperative period.[61] These changes are predominantly observed within the first postoperative week and differ from results obtained intraoperatively where changes may be absent.[159] Although changes in hepatic functions and various serum enzymes probably are correlated to the intensity of the surgical trauma, the role of the general anesthetic agents in modifying hepatic function should not be overlooked. Thus, in experimental studies thiopentone anesthesia *per se* without surgery consistently decreased hepatic flow and extraction of test drugs, whereas these changes in hepatic function were not observed after high spinal anesthesia.[133] The effects of general anesthesia could be demonstrated up to 24 hours after application[133] and therefore should be reinvestigated in clinical settings.

TABLE 5-4. INFLUENCE OF NEURAL BLOCKADE ON PERIOPERATIVE FLUID AND ELECTROLYTE BALANCE

Surgery	Reference	Urinary H_2O Excretion	Urinary Na^+ Excretion	Urinary K^+ Excretion
Hysterectomy	28	→	→	↓
Herniotomy	21	↑	↑	→
Hip replacement	17	→		
Cholecystectomy	141		→	
Vagotomy/ pyloroplasty	11a	→	↑	↓
Abdominal/thoracic	187	→	→	→

→ = No influence; ↑ = increased excretion; ↓ = decreased excretion.

The effect of neural blockade on the surgically induced changes in hepatic function has not been fully evaluated. Studies performed during spinal anesthesia with assessments either during surgery[159] or within the initial postoperative 3 weeks[127] have shown no difference in hepatic microsomal enzyme activity measured by the aminopyrine breath test or by antipyrine clearance, compared to changes in patients operated on under general anesthesia. That a single dose spinal anesthesia has no effect on late postoperative hepative function is not, however, unexpected because studies on endocrine metabolic changes have shown only a transient (2–5 hours) inhibition (see below). In studies from patients operated on during continuous epidural analgesia no influence could be demonstrated on the normal postoperative changes in serum bilirubin, alkaline phosphatase, amino transferase, or aspartate amino transferase,[87,173] whereas the postoperative increase in serum lactate dehydrogenase and creatinine kinase was reduced.[173]

Oxygen Consumption, Thermoregulation, and Shivering. Epidural analgesia has been reported to reduce, although not normalize, the usual postoperative increase in oxygen consumption following prostatectomy[175] and major vascular surgery.[67] No effect could be demonstrated, however, following cholecystectomy.[101] Some reduction by neural blockade of the postoperative increases in oxygen consumption would be expected because the postoperative elevation in catabolic hormones (see Table 5-2) is reduced, thereby minimizing general metabolism.[11] Neural blockade may, however, have a dual effect on oxygen consumption because the vasodilatation of extensive neural blockade may predispose to hypothermia if vasodilated areas of the patient are left exposed in a cold environment. Most studies have shown a more pronounced decrease in central temperature following neural blockade and a prolonged rewarming period.[86,92,103,210] When changes in mean skin temperature were combined with changes in core temperature to provide an estimate for changes in total body heat, however, no differences were observed between epidural analgesia and general anesthesia.[92] A single dose epidural analgesia has no effect on the later hyperthermic response to surgery.[117a]

Another factor that may tend to eliminate the reducing effect of neural blockade on postoperative oxygen consumption is shivering, which may represent an inappropriately programmed thermal response to raise the body temperature by increasing metabolism. Observations on the occurrence of postoperative shivering in patients receiving neural blockade are not uniform, although most studies have found an increased incidence[86,92,210]; however, occurrence of postoperative shivering was not correlated to changes in central core temperature.[86] Efforts to minimize shivering by using warmed solutions of the local anesthetics have been negative,[214] but a combination of warmed local anesthetics and parenteral fluids did reduce shivering following epidural anesthesia in obstetrics.[139]

Further studies are needed on the effect of neural blockade on post-traumatic oxygen consumption and thermoregulation in order to reduce postoperative demands. Prevention of heat loss during anesthesia and postoperative recovery is important, as these measures have been demonstrated to reduce nitrogen excretion following abdominal surgery.[32]

Coagulation and Fibrinolysis. Surgical trauma initiates profound changes in both the coagulatory and fibrinolytic system. Thus the ability to coagulate is increased; changes in fibrinolysis are characterized by an initial, intraoperative enhanced fibrinolytic function and decreased fibrinolysis in the postoperative period. As representing one of the factors of the triad of Virchow, these postoperative changes in coagulation and fibrinolysis may contribute to development of thromboembolic complications.

Modulation of the surgically induced changes in coagulation and fibrinolysis by neural blockade may be due to effects of the neural afferent/efferent blockade or effects of the local anesthetics *per se* (Table 5-5). Most studies have considered the effect of continuous epidural analgesia on coagulation and fibrinolysis, since a single dose regional anesthesia probably will lead to prolonged effects in the postoperative period, in accordance with data on other stress responses (see above).

TABLE 5-5. INFLUENCE OF NEURAL BLOCKADE ON PERIOPERATIVE CHANGES IN COAGULATION AND FIBRINOLYSIS

	Parameter	Change (Reference)
Coagulation		
	Platelet count	No effect (83, 174)
	P-fibrinogen	No effect (83, 174)
	Prothrombin time	No effect (83, 174)
	Partial thromboplastin time	No effect (83)
	P-antithrombin III	No effect (174, 224)
	P-factor VIII antigen	Inhibition of response (174)
	Factor VIII capacity	Inhibition of response (148)
Fibrinolysis		
	Clot lysis time	No major effect (62, 174, 190)
	S-fibrinogen degradation products	No effect (174, 190)
	P-plasminogen, α_1-antitrypsin, α_2-macroglobin	No effect (174, 224)
	S-fibrinolysis inhibition activity	Inhibition of response (148)
	P-plasminogen activators and release after venous occlusion	Increased (148)
Effects of Local Anesthetics per se		
	Platelet aggregation	Inhibition (18)
	Prothrombin time, partial thromboplastin time, antithrombin-III platelets and aggregation, clot lysis time	No effect (40)
	Endothelial structure and leukocyte adherence	Preserving/inhibition (194)

P = Plasma; S = serum.

Neural blockade has no effect on postoperative blood platelet count[83,174]; no data are available on platelet aggregation. Similarly, neural blockade neither modulates postoperative changes in plasma fibrinogen,[83,174] prothrombin time,[83,174] partial thromboplastin time,[83] or plasma antithrombin III levels.[174,224] In contrast, epidural analgesia inhibits postoperative increase in plasma factor VIII antigen[174] and the capacity for activation of factor VIII.[148]

The influence of neural blockade on the fibrinolytic response to surgery is debatable. No major effects have been observed in intraoperative and postoperative clot lysis time,[62,174,190] fibrin degradation products,[174,190] or changes in plasma plasminogen, alpha-1 antitrypsin, and alpha-2 macroglobulin.[174,224] Continuous epidural anesthesia was found, however, to inhibit fibrinolysis inhibition activity in serum in patients undergoing hip surgery (Fig. 5-10).[148] Further, resting plasma concentrations of plasminogen activators and capacity for release of plasminogen activators after venous occlusion were increased.[148]

The explanation for the discordant results in the various investigations is not clear but may be due to different techniques to assess fibrinolytic function and to differences in amount of blood transfused between patients operated on under general anesthesia and neural blockade.

Besides the effects mediated through the afferent/efferent neural blockade on the trauma response, neural blockade *per se* or the local anesthetics themselves may influence coagulation and fibrinolysis. No data have been published on the effect of spinal or epidural analgesia *per se* on fibrinolysis and coagulation, but during eye surgery no changes or differences in factor II and X, antithrombin III, plasminogen, or alpha-2 antiplasmin were found between patients operated on under general and those under regional anesthesia.[176]

In *in vitro* studies lidocaine, bupivacaine, and tocainide caused an inhibition of ADP-induced platelet aggregation, but only at high and probably unphysiologic plasma levels.[18] Intravenous infusion of lidocaine (2 mg/min) for 6 days after hip surgery did not modulate various tests of coagulation and fibrinolytic function.[40] Local anesthetics may exert an antithrombotic effect by blocking leukocyte locomotion and by preventing these cells from adhering to and invading venous walls, thus preserving endothelial structure. (Fig. 5-11).[194]

The clinical effect of neural blockade on thrombo-

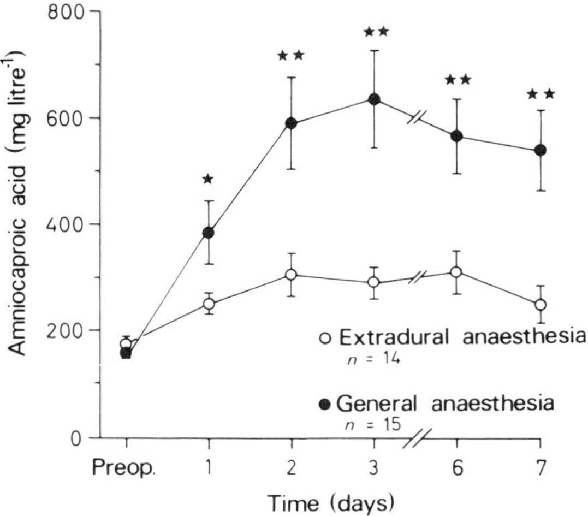

FIG. 5-10. Fibrinolysis inhibition activity expressed in dilution of aminocaproic acid in patients undergoing hip replacement under general anesthesia with nitrous oxide/oxygen and fentanyl or continuous epidural analgesia with intermittent injections of 0.5% bupivacaine with adrenaline for 24 hours. The results show that the increase in fibrinolysis inhibition activity in serum was avoided by epidural analgesia. At the same time the patients receiving epidural analgesia also showed higher concentrations of plasminogen activators and increased capacity for release of plasminogen activators; the capacity for activation of factor VIII was significantly reduced. Thus fibrinolytic function was improved by epidural analgesia. (Reproduced with permission from Modig, J., Borg, T., Bagge, L., and Saldeen, T.: Role of extradural and of general anaesthesia in fibrinolysis and coagulation after total hip replacement. Br. J. Anaesth., *55*:625, 1983.)

embolic complications is discussed later in this chapter.

Immunocompetence and Acute-Phase Proteins. Infectious complications continue to be one of the major factors leading to postoperative morbidity. Determinants of infection are host defense mechanisms, the environment where the infection takes place, and the microorganisms producing the infection. Studies performed during different degrees of surgical trauma combined with general anesthesia have concluded that changes in immunocompetence are predominantly correlated to the magnitude of trauma and that the general anesthesia *per se* has only a minor role in this context.[110] Immunocompetence is a multicomponent mechanism by which the body protects itself against foreign organisms or substances and involves either nonspecific or specific immune mechanisms. In the following sections the influence of neural blockade and local anesthetic agents on nonspecific and specific immune mechanisms is reviewed; the review of the influence of general anesthesia and different surgical procedures on immunocompetence has been discussed elsewhere.[110]

The influence of neural blockade *per se* on immunocompetence is probably negligible. Thus no influence on peripheral blood neutrophils and lymphocytes was found,[171,192] and the chemotactic response of neutrophils was not altered by epidural analgesia or spinal anesthesia, except for a slight depression when epinephrine was added to epidural analgesia.[192]

Neural blockade may alter some aspects of the surgically induced changes in nonspecific immunity. Thus postoperative granulocytosis may be reduced by continuous epidural analgesia[171] but not following single dose spinal or epidural anesthesia.[60,215] Late postoperative changes in leukocyte migration are not modified by a single dose epidural analgesia.[60] Complement[224] or acute-phase protein responses[172] (Fig. 5-12) are not modulated by continuous epidural anesthesia. In contrast, epidural analgesia has led to an improved monocyte function (spreading and lysis) during hip surgery.[94] This effect was not due to omission of general anesthesia because the same observations were made during combined epidural and general anesthesia.[97]

Neural blockade may also influence perioperative changes in specific immunity because the normal lymphopenic response may be obtunded.[171,215] Continuous epidural analgesia has no influence on postoperative changes in immunoglobulins.[172] A slight decrease in the number of T-cells following hip surgery was not modulated by epidural analgesia, and the ratio between T-suppressor (T8) cells and T-helper (T4) cells was unaffected.[98] A number of studies have considered the influence of neural blockade on the lymphoproliferative response of circulating lymphocytes to various immune stimuli, "mitogens," in the perioperative period. In several of these studies, however, interpretation of the results is impeded by the lack of appropriate control groups.[51,115,183] In other studies neural blockade by epidural analgesia[95] or spinal anesthesia[215] improved the normal decrease in blastogenic response of circulating lymphocytes to nonspecific and specific mitogens during hip surgery[95] during prostatectomy.[215] In contrast, the usual intraoperative increase and postoperative decrease in natural killer (NK) cell activity were not modified by epidural analgesia effective during major upper ab-

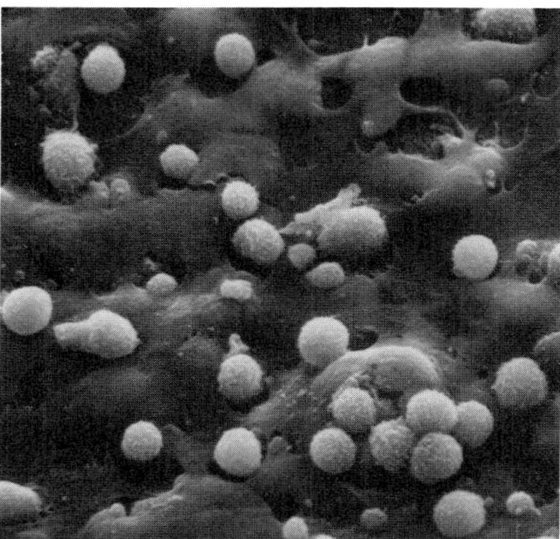

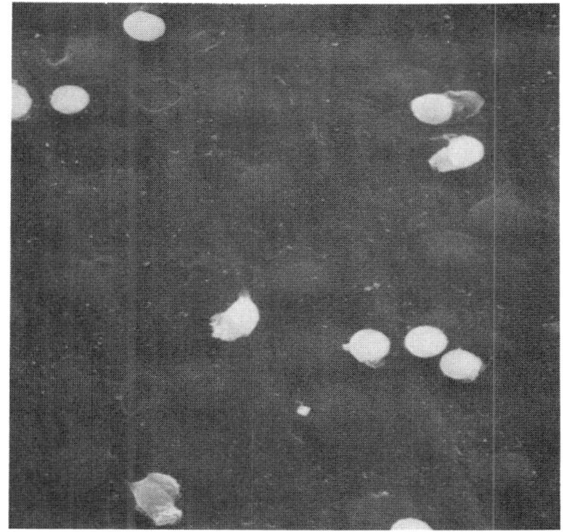

FIG. 5-11. Luminal surface of jugular vein taken for bypass grafting from canine model: (Scanning electron micrograph × 1,000). Vein was exposed and occluded briefly before local perfusion and fixation. **Left.** Control: Endothelium is extensively damaged by leukocytes that had adhered and forced their way across junctions between endothelium and basement membrane. **Right.** Lidocaine (load dose 1.25 mg/kg, then 0.125 mg/kg/min), 15 to 30 minutes before and during vein dissection and removal. Endothelial damage is greatly reduced, and leukocyte adherence and migration are essentially eliminated. (Reproduced with permission from Stewart, G.J.: Antithrombotic activity of local anesthetics in several canine models. Reg. Anaesth. 7:S89, 1982.)

dominal surgery despite inhibition of some aspects of the endocrine response.[206] A single dose epidural analgesia has no effect on late postoperative changes in lymphocyte response to phytohemagglutinin and pokeweed mitogen stimulation.[60] Epidural analgesia with combined administration of local anesthetics and morphine did not modify postoperative impairment in delayed hypersensitivity in patients undergoing major abdominal surgery,[89] but this regimen also failed to significantly alter the endocrine metabolic stress response.

Local anesthetic agents *per se* stabilize cell membrane function and may therefore influence neutrophil and lymphocyte function. Thus *in vitro* studies have demonstrated that lidocaine and bupivacaine reduce the blastogenic lymphocyte response to PHA stimulation[168] and lidocaine[211] and procaine[195] reduce NK-cell activity. In these studies, however, pharmacologic doses of local anesthetics were used, and extrapolation to the clinical situation is difficult. In other *in vitro* studies using local anesthetics in concentrations observed during epidural analgesia, no effect of lidocaine was observed on microbicidal oxidative function (neutrophil chemiluminescence)[217] or of bupivacaine on monocyte function (spreading and lysis) and lymphocyte blastogenic response to mitogens.[96] In experimental studies in rabbits, intravenous infusion of lidocaine (0.3 mg/kg/min) inhibited granulocyte adherence and suppressed delivery to inflammatory sites.[130a]

In summary, neural blockade may influence some aspects of the surgically induced impairment in various aspects of immunocompetence. The mechanism hereto has not been completely elucidated but may partly be explained by the concomitant inhibition of various endocrine metabolic responses.[96] The clinical relevance and implications for anesthetic practice have not, however, been settled. Nevertheless, the data on neural blockade and perioperative immunocompetence are extremely interesting and of potential value because post-traumatic immunodepression has been impossible to modulate by other therapeutic measures.

MAJOR (UPPER) ABDOMINAL AND THORACIC SURGERY

The influence of neural blockade with local anesthetics on the endocrine metabolic response to major

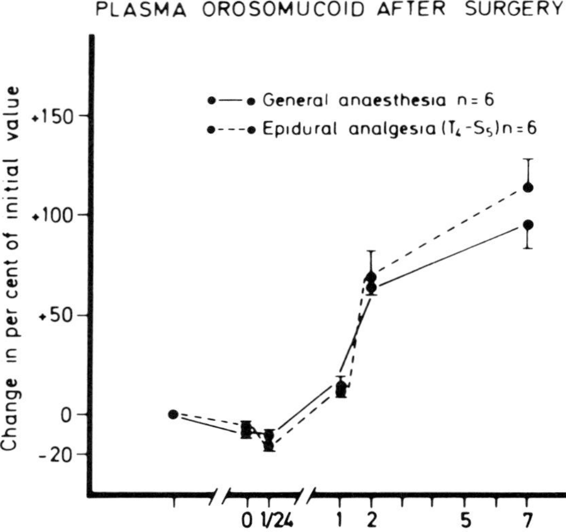

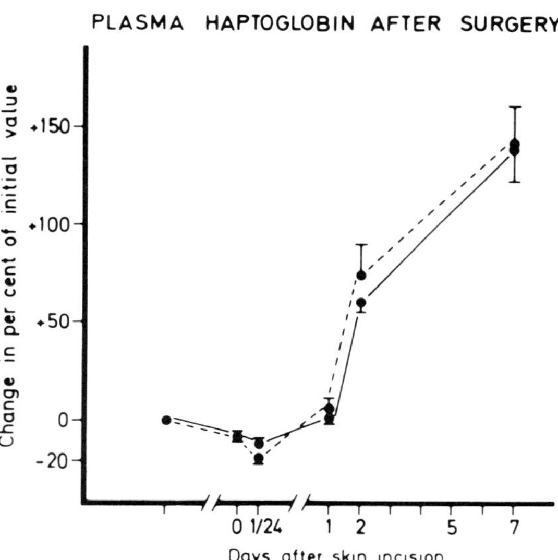

FIG. 5-12. Comparison of postoperative changes in plasma acute-phase proteins (orosomucoid and haptoglobin) in patients undergoing abdominal hysterectomy under general anesthesia (halothane) or continuous epidural analgesia with intermittent injections of bupivacaine 0.5% for 24 hours. The results show that acute-phase protein responses are not modified by epidural analgesia despite sufficient pain relief and concomitant reduction in other endocrine metabolic responses (cortisol and glucose). (Reproduced with permission from Rem, J., Saxtrup Nielsen, O., Brandt, M.R., Kehlet, H.: Release mechanisms of postoperative changes in various acute phase protein and immunoglobulins. Acta Chir. Scand., *502*:51, 1980.)

abdominal and thoracic procedures is summarized in Table 5-6. In most studies plain 0.5% bupivacaine has been used intraoperatively and a continuous technique with intermittent injections or continuous infusion of lower concentrations of bupivacaine postoperatively. The results of these studies are reasonably consistent in that pronounced inhibitory effects on several endocrine or metabolic responses were not obtained in any study, in contrast to changes observed during epidural analgesia in procedures on the lower part of the abdomen (see Tables 5-2 and 5-3); however, the influence of neural blockade on specific endocrine or metabolic changes varied among the different studies (see Table 5-6). This discrepancy may be due to several factors: [1] the extent of sensory analgesia varied, and in some studies had not been defined. Further, duration of neural blockade differed; [2] the technique of epidural analgesia and administration of local anesthetics varied, and in no study were data presented to document that the claimed area of analgesia was maintained throughout the study period. In most studies sufficient pain relief was reported, but only two studies[90,180] substantiated this by pain score assessments; [3] the surgical procedures differed, and especially the combination of thoracic and abdominal operations in some studies impeded interpretation[19,29,187]; and [4] in some studies perioperative administration of fluids, glucose, or other substrates was not defined and therefore impeded interpretation.[8,202–204] Despite these flaws in methodology, the conclusion seems valid that neural blockade with local anesthetics is less efficient in reducing the surgical stress response to thoracic and upper abdominal procedures than to operations performed in the lower part of the body. Nevertheless, some responses may be more reduced than others, as most studies have found a pronounced inhibition of the glucose, epinephrine, and norepinephrine response (see Table 5-6). In accordance with studies in the lower part of the body, epidural analgesia has no influence on changes in thyroid hormones and various proteins.

Several explanations may be given for the less pronounced effect of neural blockade in reducing the stress response to major abdominal and thoracic procedures compared to other operations (Fig. 5-13). Thus the unblocked *vagal afferent pathway* has been hypothesized to be of importance in this context,[29] but experimental studies in dogs with vagotomy, ventrolateral cordotomy, or combined vagotomy plus cordotomy failed to demonstrate an importance of the vagal pathway in the antidiuretic hormone response to surgery[207]; however, a concomitant

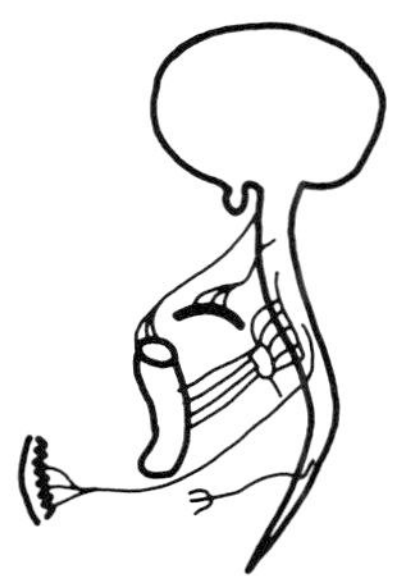

FIG. 5-13. Factors that may explain the demonstrated reduced inhibition of the surgical stress response by epidural analgesia during major (upper) abdominal procedures compared to procedures in the lower abdomen and lower extremities. Existent data suggest that the main cause is an insufficient afferent somatic and sympathetic block, whereas unblocked parasympathetic afferents probably are of minor importance. The role of potentiating humoral release mechanisms (local tissue factors and interleukin-1) and increased metabolism by shivering due to heat loss have not been fully evaluated.

neural blockade of sympathetic and somatic afferents was not performed. Correspondingly, clinical studies using infiltration of the vagal nerve with local anesthetics immediately after opening the abdomen[200] or preliminary surgical vagotomy or vagal blockade[203] failed to modify the stress response. The role of unblocked *phrenic afferents* is unknown. An insufficient *afferent sympathetic block* may be of importance because an additional coeliac plexus block was found to further reduce the stress response when combined with epidural analgesia.[204] According to previous observations neural blockade as assessed by sensory level of analgesia and extending to T_4 may also lead to an autonomic blockade of the sympathetic plexuses in the abdomen,[16] but recent studies assessing sympathetic blockade by skin conductance and skin blood flow and temperature suggest that the level of sympathetic blockade in spinal anesthesia may be lower than that of sensory blockade.[10,130] Thus the relative inefficiency of epidural analgesia in reducing the stress response to upper abdominal procedures may be due to inadequate inhibition of sympathetic afferent activity. The role of an insufficient *afferent somatic block* is difficult to assess because no consistent evaluation of the sensory blockade was reported in the various studies (see Table 5-6). Nevertheless, an insufficient afferent somatic block is probably an important factor contributing to the reduced inhibitory effect of neural blockade on the stress response to major (upper) abdominal procedures. Thus a pronounced variation in both proximal/distal and contralateral extent of analgesia has been demonstrated during continuous epidural analgesia with intermittent injections of identical doses of bupivacaine.[13] Also, epidural analgesia did not result in blockade of centrally recorded evoked potentials during electrical stimulation within an area of sensory analgesia.[185] The role of potentially unblocked *pelvic parasympathetic* afferents is unknown but may be of importance because, in most studies, blocks extending from T4 to L1-2 were used (see Table 5-6). Finally, potentiating *humoral release mechanisms* (see above) may also be more effective during major procedures than during minor procedures. *Heat loss and shivering,* which are more pronounced after major than minor procedures, are additional factors that may reduce the inhibitory effect of neural blockade on the surgical stress response, but quantitative assessments have not been performed.

In conclusion, the available data have clearly demonstrated neural blockade to be less efficient in reducing the surgical stress response to upper abdominal and thoracic procedures than to operations in the lower part of the body. The data suggest that this is due to both insufficient afferent sympathetic and somatic neural blockade, although other factors may also contribute.

MECHANISM OF MODIFYING EFFECTS OF NEURAL BLOCKADE ON THE STRESS RESPONSE

The basic mechanism of the blocking effect of neural blockade on the stress response to surgery is by attempting to prevent the nociceptive signal from the surgical area from reaching the central nervous system (see cover of this book). Although small myelinated (A delta) and unmyelinated (C) sensory fibers are primarily involved in the transmission of these stimuli, the ascending pathways have not been fully evaluated.[225] This also applies to the relative role of somatic versus autonomic afferent pathways (see above). Thus further data are needed on the role of pain stimuli versus other neural stimuli, and the role of afferent neural blockade versus blockade of efferent pathways to various organs. It is hoped that such data will clarify the reported discrepancies in the efficacy of neural blockade in altering the stress response to surgery and also point toward better techniques to obtain a more sufficient blockade of nociceptive stimuli and the stress response.

TABLE 5-6. INFLUENCE OF NEURAL BLOCKADE WITH LOCAL ANESTHETICS ON THE ENDOCRINE-METABOLIC RESPONSE TO MAJOR ABDOMINAL SURGERY

Author (Reference)	Technique of Regional Anesthesia	Extent of Sensory Blockade	Duration of Blockade or Study (h)	Surgical Procedure	Modification of Endocrine-Metabolic Response	
Bromage *et al.*[29] (1971)	Continuous epidural (intermittent inj.) lidocaine 2% or bupivacaine 0.5% with epinephrine	C6-L2/T4-L2	24	Thoracic/abdominal	B-glucose P-cortisol	↓ ↘
Menzies *et al.*[141] (1979)	Continuous epidural (intermittent inj.) plain bupivacaine 0.5%	T4-T12	48	Cholecystectomy	P-glucose P-cortisol P-aldosterone P-renin	→ ↘ ↘ ↕
Gelman *et al.*[73] (1980)	Continuous epidural (intermittent inj.) plain bupivacaine 0.5%	?	48-72	Gastric bypass	O_2 uptake	↓
Cochrane *et al.*[38] (1981)	Continuous epidural (intermittent inj.) plain bupivacaine 0.5%	T4-T12	48	Cholecystectomy	P-arginine vasopressin P-osmolality U-volume	→ → →
Kossman *et al.*[121] (1982)	Continuous epidural (infusion) plain bupivacaine 0.5%	T4-L1	72	Aorto-bifemoral bypass	P-glucose P-cortisol P-glucagon P-insulin	↘ → → →
Seeling *et al.*[187] (1982)	Continuous epidural (infusion) plain bupivacaine 0.5%; initially 0.2% during infusion	T4-L1	72	Abdominal/thoracic; aorto-bifemoral bypass colonic/rectal op.	B-glucose Glucose tolerance P-glycerol and FFA N-balance, U-creatinine and 3-m-histidine	↘ → → →
Traynor *et al.*[200] (1982)	Epidural (single dose) + vagal block (hiatus) plain bupivacaine 0.5%	T4-?	1	Cholecystectomy	P-glucose P-cortisol P-lactate P-FFA P-insulin	↓ → → → ↓
Tsuji and Shirasaka[202] (1982)	Continuous epidural (infusion) plain bupivacaine 0.5%	T3-4-L1-2	48	Gastrectomy	U-epinephrine U-norepinephrine	↘ ↓
Asoh *et al.*[8] (1983)	Continuous epidural (infusion) plain bupivacaine 0.5%	T3-4-L1-2	48	Gastrectomy	B-glucose B-lactate B-FFA P-insulin	↓ → ↘ ↘
Tsuji *et al.*[203] (1983a)	Continuous epidural (infusion) plain bupivacaine 0.5% ± vagal block (hiatus) or vagotomy	T3-4-L1-2	48	Gastrectomy	P-cortisol P-cortisol; addition of vagal block had no influence	↘ →
Tsuji *et al.*[204] (1983b)	Continuous (intermittent inj.) plain bupivacaine 0.5% + splanchnic blockade (single inj.) epidural morphine 4 mg/8 h	T3-4-L1-2	72	Gastrectomy	B-glucose P-cortisol P-FFA	↓ ↓ ↓

Bormann *et al.*[19] (1983)	Continuous epidural (intermittent inj.) plain bupivacaine 0.5%	?	?	Abdominal/thoracic	P-ADH	↓
Rutberg *et al.*[180] (1984)	Continuous epidural (intermittent inj.) plain bupivacaine 0.5% intraop.; 0.25–0.375% postop.	T4–L3	24	Cholecystectomy	P-cortisol P-epinephrine P-norepinephrine	↘ ↓ ↓
Delalande *et al.*[54] (1984)	Continuous epidural plain bupivacaine 0.5% + etidocaine 1% intraop.; bupivacaine 0.5% 12.5–25 mg/h postop.	T4–?	24	Abdominal	P-cortisol P-glucose P-prolactin Nitrogen balance	→ → → ↘
Hennek and Sydow[88] (1984)	Continuous epidural plain bupivacaine 0.5% intraop.; bupivacaine 0.25% 5–6 ml/h postop.	T2–T12 (intraop.) T4–T8 (postop.)	48–72	Thoracic	B-glucose P-cortisol	→ →
Seeling *et al.*[189] (1984)	Continuous epidural plain bupivacaine 0.5% intraop.; bupivacaine 0.125% 0.25–0.3 ml/kg/h postop.	T3-4–T11-12 (intraop.) ? (postop.)	96	Cholecystectomy	P-glucose P-cortisol P-ACTH P-T_3, T_4 +T_3	↓ ↘ → →
Tønnesen *et al.*[206] (1984)	Epidural (intraop.) plain bupivacaine 0.5%	T4–S5	Intraop.	Vagotomy	P-norepinephrine P-epinephrine P-cortisol P-prolactin	↓ ↘ → →
Hjortsø *et al.*[90] (1985)	Continuous epidural (intermittent inj.) etidocaine 1.5% intraop.; plain bupivacaine 0.5% postop. plus epidural morphine 4 mg/12 h.	T4–S5	72	Major gastrointestinal surgery	U-cortisol U-epinephrine U-norepinephrine, nitrogen balance	→ → ↘ →
Håkanson *et al.*[101] (1985)	Continuous epidural (intermittent inj.) plain bupivacaine 0.5% intraop.; 0.25–0.375% postop.	T4–L3	24	Cholecystectomy	B-glucose P-FFA B-glycerol B-lactate B-3-BOH O_2 uptake	↓ ↓ ↘ ↘ ↘ →
Rutberg *et al.*[181] (1985)	Continuous epidural (intermittent inj.) plain bupivacaine 0.5% intraop.; 0.25–0.375% postop.	T4–L3	24	Cholecystectomy	S-T_4, F-T_4 S-T_3, F-T_3 S-rT_3, TSH S-prealbumin S-TBG	→ → → → →

↓ = Pronounced reduction of response; ↘ = slight reduction of response; → = no influence of response; ↑ = amplification of response; P = plasma; B = blood; S = serum; U = urine.

ROLE OF PAIN STIMULI VERSUS OTHER NEURAL STIMULI

Although pain *per se* will elicit an endocrine metabolic response,[112] the inhibitory effect of neural blockade on the endocrine metabolic response to surgery is mediated not only through alleviation of pain. Thus a definite adrenocortical response to hysterectomy was observed in patients receiving epidural analgesia with sufficient pain alleviation.[41,63,129] Further, postoperative analgesia by epidural administration of a combination of local anesthetics and morphine[90] or morphine only did not result in a pronounced inhibition of the stress response to various procedures (see below).

AFFERENT VERSUS EFFERENT NEURAL BLOCKADE

The neural release mechanisms of the endocrine and metabolic responses to surgery may involve both afferent and efferent pathways but differ among the individual endocrine glands. Thus only afferent pathways are involved in the release of the pituitary hormone responses, whereas release of adrenocortical responses is more complex. The cortisol response is triggered by a dual mechanism involving an efferent neural limb to the pituitary and the humoral efferent limb to the adrenal cortex by ACTH. The aldosterone response may be mediated partly by the ACTH response, but afferent and efferent neural pathways are also involved in releasing the renin and angiotensin response. The epinephrine response is mediated by afferent neural pathways combined with efferent sympathetic pathways to the adrenal medulla. Further, afferent/efferent neural reflexes may directly affect various organs (*e.g.*, liver, kidney) independent of endocrine changes.[123,150]

The literature is conflicting with regard to the influence of neural blockade on the cortisol response to surgery, probably because of an insufficient afferent block in most studies (see Tables 5-2 and 5-6). Thus systematic studies on the influence of the extent of sensory analgesia on the cortisol response to lower abdominal surgery have shown that an extensive blockade from T4 to S5 must be achieved to prevent the cortisol response (Fig. 5-14).[63] These findings have been confirmed in other studies during hysterectomy under spinal anesthesia, where plasma cortisol did not increase intraoperatively in patients in whom analgesia did not regress below T4, whereas a progressive increase was observed with waning analgesia (Fig. 5-15).[152]

Afferent sensory blockade to T8 has no effect on the cortisol response to hysterectomy,[30,63] indicating that efferent pathways to the adrenal glands (T11–L1) are unimportant in this context. Also, a neural blockade from T3 to L1 has no influence on ACTH-stimulated cortisol secretion.[188]

The role of sympathetic and parasympathetic stimulation in initiating the endocrine metabolic responses has been discussed above, and it appears that sympathetic blockade may be more effective than parasympathetic blockade in reducing the response. The relative efficacy of somatosensory blockade versus sympathetic blockade has not been definitely assessed because no information is available on the influence of intercostal blockade on the stress response. Studies on coeliac plexus block suggest that a pure sympathetic block has only a minor modulating effect on the surgical stress response,[33,219] whereas a combination of sympathetic and somatic neural blockade by coeliac plexus and epidural blockade was most effective.[204]

In contrast to the changes in adrenocortical function, the adrenal medullary and hyperglycemic responses to surgery apparently are released through both afferent and efferent neural pathways, and these responses generally are more easily inhibited. Thus several studies have shown that a neural blockade, including efferent pathways to the adrenal glands (T11–L1), leads to an inhibition of the hyperglycemic response to lower abdominal surgery[30,63] and upper abdominal procedures[29,101,189,200] despite an unmodulated cortisol response. An additional factor to reduce the hyperglycemic response may be concomitant blockade of efferent sympathetic pathways to the liver.[102,123]

SPINAL ANALGESIA VERSUS EPIDURAL ANALGESIA

No systematic studies have been performed comparing endocrine metabolic responses to similar surgical procedures performed during either spinal (intrathecal) or epidural analgesia, except during hysterectomy, where no additional metabolic effect could be obtained by the more efficient blockade of efferent pathways with motor blockade during spinal analgesia.[63,152] Unfortunately, similar studies from upper abdominal procedures are not available.

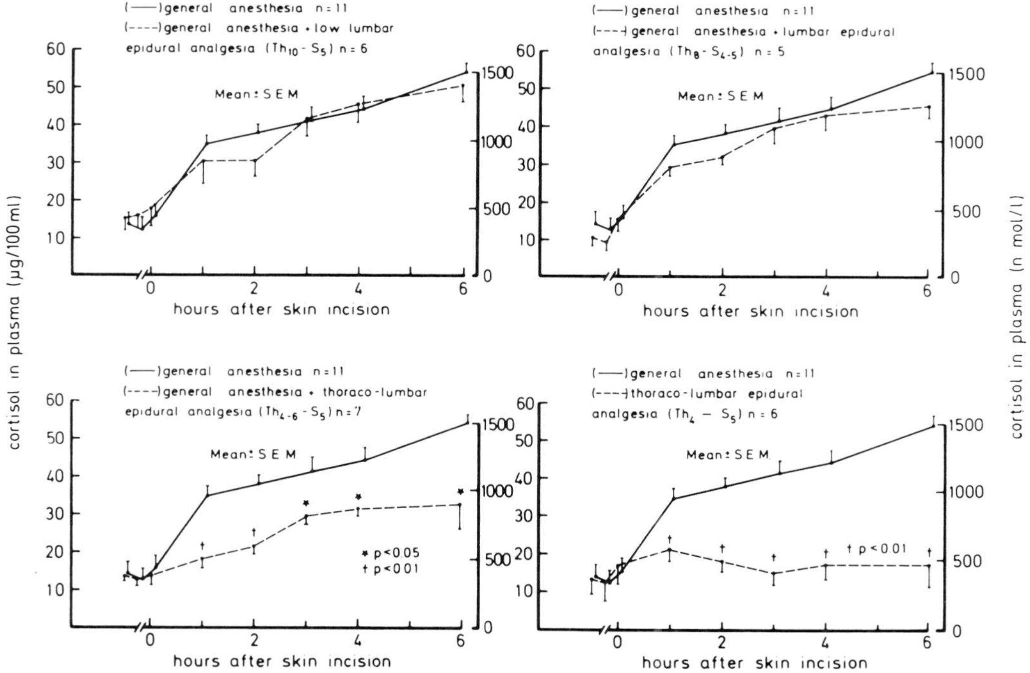

FIG. 5-14. Influence of varying sensory levels of analgesia during epidural analgesia with 0.5% plain bupivacaine in patients undergoing abdominal hysterectomies. Control patients received general anesthesia with halothane or enflurane. The results show that analgesia extending to T_{10} or T_8 has no effect on the plasma cortisol response to surgery despite postoperative pain relief. Further extension of levels of analgesia leads to a reduction in plasma cortisol during and after surgery, and when the fourth thoracic segment is included the response is blocked. Similar results were found in changes in plasma glucose. (Reproduced with permission from Engquist, A., Brandt, M.R., Fernandes, A., Kehlet, H.: The blocking effect of epidural analgesia on the adrenocortical and hyperglycemic response to surgery. Acta Anesthesiol. Scand., *21*:330, 1977.)

INFLUENCE OF DURATION OF NEURAL BLOCKADE

A single dose neural blockade by spinal analgesia[152,184] or epidural analgesia[74] has only a short-lasting (2–5 hours) inhibitory effect on the stress response (Fig. 5-16). There is a lack of data on the effect of an intermediate blockade (6–12 hours) on later postoperative responses, but in studies with maintenance of epidural analgesia for 24 hours a prolonged effect could be demonstrated as a reduction of nitrogen loss during the following 4 postoperative days[27] and a reduction in plasma creatinine phosphokinase in the later postoperative period.[173] Further data are needed before any conclusion can be given on the optimal duration of the neural block to inhibit the stress response.

DIFFERENTIAL MODIFYING EFFECT OF LOCAL ANESTHETICS

An increasing number of studies have demonstrated that the different local anesthetics may preferentially block some fibers compared to others (see Chaps. 2 and 4), but no data have shown whether any single agent or a mixture of local anesthetics provides a more complete block, and thereby a more pronounced reduction of the stress response.

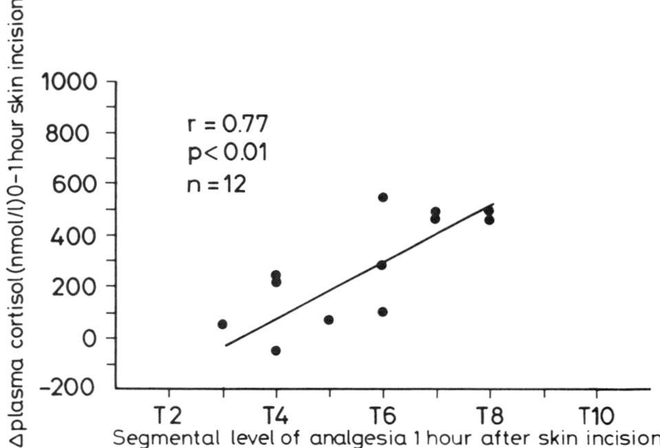

FIG. 5-15. Comparison between changes in analgesic level and plasma cortisol 1 hour after skin incision in patients undergoing abdominal hysterectomies under spinal anesthesia with 0.5% hyperbaric tetracaine or neuroleptanesthesia. Preoperative sensory level of analgesia to pinprick extended to at least T_4. The results show unchanged plasma cortisol levels with maintenance of analgesic level at T_4, while regression of analgesia leads to a progressive increase in plasma cortisol, in accordance, with systematic studies on the influence of sensory levels of analgesia during epidural analgesia on the adrenocortical and hyperglycemic response to hysterectomy (see Figure. 5-12). (Reproduced with permission from Møller, I.W., Hjortsø, E., Krantz, T., *et al.:* The modifying effect of spinal anesthesia in intra- and postoperative adrenocortical and hyperglycemic response to surgery. Acta Anesthesiol. Scand., *28:*266, 84.)

INFLUENCE OF POST-TRAUMATIC NEURAL BLOCKADE

In contrast to the vast amount of data on the influence of neural blockade in abating endocrine and metabolic changes to a subsequent surgical trauma, there is a paucity of data on the influence of post-traumatic application of neural blockade. Initiation of epidural analgesia half an hour after skin incision during abdominal hysterectomy prevented further amplification of the stress response to surgery as measured by changes in plasma cortisol and glucose, but preoperative levels in these stress parameters were not attained (Fig. 5-17).[151] The influence of neural blockade on the stress response to accidental trauma and burn injury has not been clarified. Spinal anesthesia had no influence on the increased energy consumption in one burn patient.[221]

MODULATING EFFECT OF COMBINED NEURAL BLOCKADE AND GENERAL ANESTHESIA

Although neural blockade alone was used in most of the above mentioned studies, the concomitant administration of general anesthesia has no additional inhibitory or stimulatory effects on endocrine metabolic function. Thus a pronounced inhibition of both cortisol and hyperglycemic response to hip replace-

FIG. 5-16. Comparison between the hyperglycemic response to abdominal hysterectomy in patients operated on under neuroleptanesthesia or spinal anesthesia with 0.5% hyperbaric tetracaine. Sensory level of analgesia extended to at least T_4 before skin incision. The results show a transient inhibition of the glucose response to surgery by spinal anesthesia, but parallel to regression of analgesia plasma glucose increased and attained levels as in the general anesthesia group 4 to 6 hours after skin incision. (Reproduced with permission from Møller, I.W., Hjortsø, E., Krantz T., *et al.:* The modifying effect of spinal anesthesia on intra- and postoperative adrenocortical and hyperglycemic response to surgery. Acta Anesthesiol. Scand., *28:*266, 1984.)

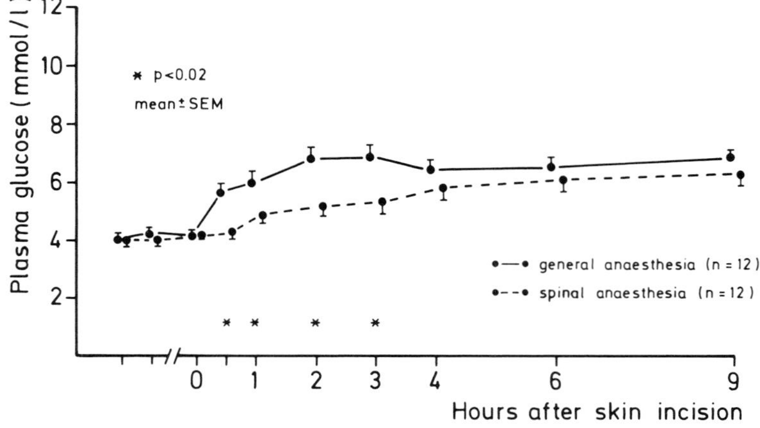

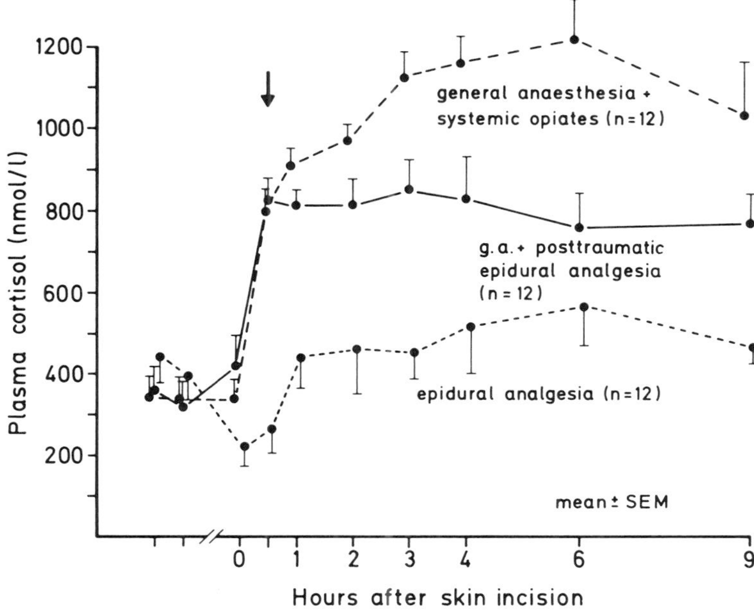

FIG. 5-17. Comparison of plasma cortisol response to abdominal hysterectomy in patients receiving general anesthesia (halothane) and systemic opiates for postoperative pain relief, and in patients receiving continuous epidural analgesia (T_4 to S_5) with intermittent injections of 0.5% plain bupivacaine. The third group was anesthetized with halothane but had an epidural catheter inserted before surgery; 30 minutes after skin incision an identical dose of bupivacaine (35 ml) was administered (indicated by ↓) as in the epidural group. The results show that epidural analgesia inhibits the plasma cortisol response to surgery. If administered postinjury, epidural analgesia prevented further amplification of the cortisol response, but levels did not attain preoperative levels within the 9-hour study period. Similar results were obtained by plasma glucose measurements. (Reproduced with permission from Møller, I.W., Rem, J., Brandt, M.R., and Kehlet, H.: Effect of posttraumatic epidural analgesia on the cortisol and hyperglycemic response to surgery. Acta Anesthesiol. Scand., *26*:56, 1982.)

ment was observed in patients receiving epidural analgesia alone or combined epidural analgesia and general anesthesia (Fig. 5-18).[177] Similarly, the intraoperative impairment in monocyte and lymphocyte function observed during general anesthesia was avoided by operating on patients both during epidural analgesia and combined epidural analgesia and general anesthesia.[95,97]

INFLUENCE OF EPIDURAL OR INTRATHECAL OPIATES ON THE STRESS RESPONSE

It is well documented that epidural or intrathecal opiate administration provides excellent postoperative pain relief. The modifying effect of this analgesic regimen on the stress response is less pronounced, however, compared to local anesthetics despite similar analgesia with the two techniques. Thus epidural morphine administration had no influence on the intraoperative response in cortisol and glucose[36] and either a slight or no effect on postoperative responses in cortisol, glucose, and fluid and electrolyte balance following hysterectomy.[36,48,106] Similarly, epidural morphine administration 4 mg twice daily for 3 days after various major abdominal procedures did not reduce urinary excretion of cortisol, catecholamines, or nitrogen to any major extent, despite superior pain relief compared to intermittent systemic morphine administration.[90] In a comprehensive comparison of the effect of epidural morphine versus bupivacaine and intermittent systemic morphine on the endocrine and metabolic changes following cholecystectomy,

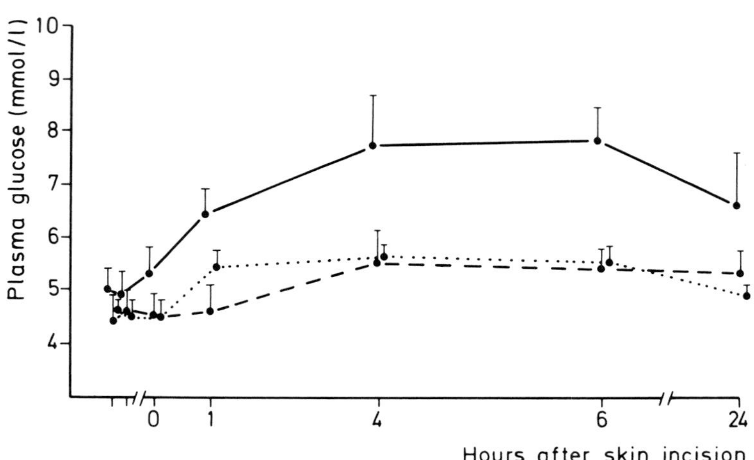

FIG. 5-18. Comparison of changes in plasma glucose in patients undergoing hip replacement who received general anesthesia (enflurane) (*unbroken line*, n = 10), general anesthesia plus epidural analgesia (T_8) with intermittent injections of 0.5% plain bupivacaine for 24 hours (*broken line*, n = 10), or epidural analgesia alone (*dotted line*, N = 10) (all values mean ± SEM). The results show that usual hyperglycemic response to hip replacement is abolished by neural blockade with epidural analgesia. This reduction of the hyperglycemic response (and adrenocortical, results not shown) is independent of concomitant administration of general anesthesia. (Reproduced with permission from Riis, J., Lomholt, B., Haxholdt, O., *et al.*: Immediate and long term mental recovery from general vs epidural anesthesia in elderly patients. Acta Anaesthesiol. Scand., *27*:44, 1983.)

epidural morphine was less effective in reducing the stress response compared to bupivacaine despite a similar degree of pain relief (Fig. 5-19).[101,180]

The influence of epidural opiates on plasma ADH response to surgery is debatable because fentanyl apparently reduced postoperative ADH concentrations,[19,20] while another study suggested that morphine increased ADH secretion.[120] In the latter study, however, patient groups were not comparable with regard to duration of surgery.[120]

Intrathecal diamorphine 0.5 mg/10 kg reduced the plasma cortisol but not the glucose response to colonic surgery.[34] The effect, however, was observed in the later postoperative period, and the mechanism may be a direct hypothalamic influence caused by rostrad spread of diamorphine within the cerebrospinal fluid, and not caused by a selective nociceptive blockade at the spinal level. Addition of 2.5 mg morphine to a single dose intrathecal cinchocaine led to a more pronounced inhibition of plasma cortisol following hip replacement than did cinchocaine alone.[149]

At present, no conclusion can be made as to a possible differential effect of the different opiates in reducing the stress response following epidural/intrathecal administration (see also Chap. 28).

INFLUENCE OF NEURAL BLOCKADE ON PERIOPERATIVE MORBIDITY

Despite an improved understanding of the physiologic changes resulting from anesthesia and surgery, major operative procedures may still be beset with morbidity such as myocardial infarction, pulmonary complications, thromboembolic complications, mental disturbances, and prolonged convalescence with fatigue and inability to work. It has been hypothesized that the occurrence of such complications may not necessarily be related to imperfections in surgical technique but rather to increased demands caused by the endocrine metabolic response to surgical trauma.[111] Neural blockade, which reduces the surgical stress response (see above), may therefore be expected to mitigate some aspects of perioperative morbidity. The following sections review information available from controlled studies on the effect of neural blockade on various parameters of perioperative morbidity.

NEURAL BLOCKADE WITH LOCAL ANESTHETICS

Mortality is a well-defined end-point parameter of postoperative morbidity, but the incidence of this complication is usually too low in modern anesthesia and surgery to allow any conclusion on the effect of a therapeutic regimen unless a very large number of patients are investigated. Accordingly, there is no conclusive evidence that neural blockade with local anesthetics reduces postoperative mortality following elective surgical procedures, either in single studies or after accumulation of all data.

An exception is the fair amount of data that has been collected from patients undergoing acute hip surgery for fracture (Table 5-7). In only two of the eight studies did early postoperative mortality appear

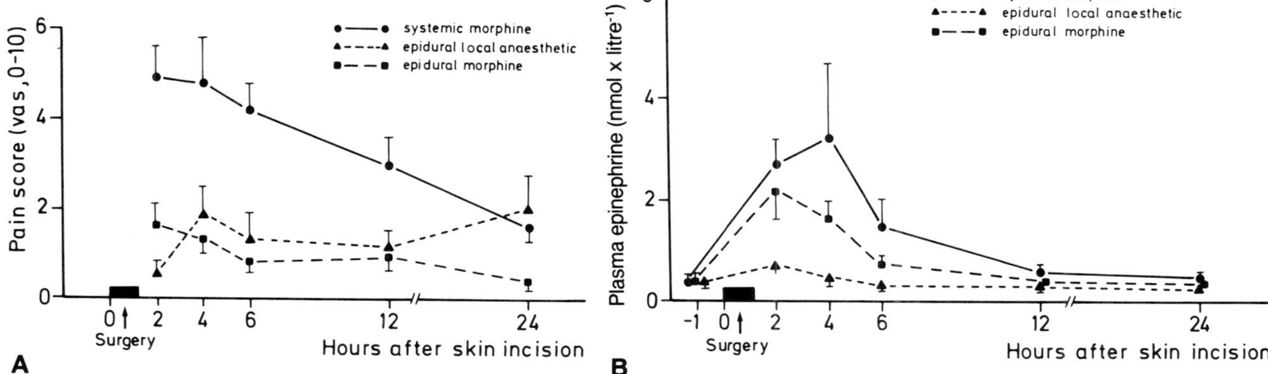

FIG. 5-19. Comparison of pain relief **(A)** and changes in plasma epinephrine **(B)** following cholecystectomy in patients receiving general anesthesia with nitrous oxide/oxygen, diazepam, and fentanyl and systemic opiates for postoperative pain relief (n = 8), general anesthesia plus epidural analgesia with 0.5% plain bupivacaine effective before surgery (T_4 to L_3) and continued with intermittent injections (0.25–0.375% bupivacaine for 24 hours) (n = 8), or general anesthesia plus epidural morphine 4 mg 1 hour before surgery and repeated every 10 hours (n = 8). The results show an improved postoperative pain relief by the two epidural regimens without differences between epidural local anesthetics and epidural morphine. Similar results were found in changes in plasma norepinephrine and in various metabolic responses.[101] Thus epidural analgesia with morphine is less efficient in reducing the surgical stress response than are epidural local anesthetics despite similar pain relief. (Reproduced with permission from Rutberg, H., Håkansson, E., Anderberg, B., *et al.*: Effects of the extradural administration of morphine, or bupivacaine, on the endocrine response to upper abdominal surgery. Br. J. Anaesth., 56:233, 1984.)

TABLE 5-7. INFLUENCE OF NEURAL BLOCKADE (SPINAL/EPIDURAL) ON MORTALITY AFTER ACUTE SURGERY FOR HIP FRACTURE (CONTROLLED STUDIES)

Authors (Reference)	Neural Blockade (n)	S/E	General Anesthesia (n)	Postoperative Observation (months)	p
Couderc *et al.*[44] (1977)	7/50	E	12/50	3	NS
McKenzie *et al.*[136] (1980)	5/49	S	8/51	1	NS
White *et al.*[216] (1980)	0/20	S	0/20	1	NS
Davis *et al.*[53] (1981)	3/64	S	9/68	1	NS
McLaren[138] (1982)	4/56	S	17/60	1	<0.05
Wickström *et al.*[218] (1982)	2/32	E	6/97	1	NS
McKenzie *et al.*[137] (1984)	3/73	S	12/75	½ (2)	<0.05
Valentin *et al.*[208] (1986)	17/281	S	24/297	1 (24)	NS
Total mortality	41/625 (6.6%)		88/718 (12.3%)		<0.002

S = spinal; E = epidural.

to be significantly reduced by neural blockade. In no study was mortality higher, however, than in the group receiving neural blockade. The data do not allow any conclusion as to whether epidural analgesia may be more effective in reducing mortality than is spinal anesthesia. The cumulated data show an almost 50% reduction in early mortality after acute surgery for hip fracture by neural blockade (6.6% versus 12.3%).

A reservation should be made, however, with regard to the final conclusion on the influence of neural blockade on mortality following surgery for hip fracture, because a follow-up in two studies[137,208] for 2 to 24 months postoperatively showed that the initial difference in mortality between neural blockade and general anesthesia disappeared (Fig. 5-20). The explanation of the identical survival rate during long-term postoperative follow-up,[137,208] despite an apparent initial reduction in mortality in patients operated on under neural blockade (Table 5-7), is not clear. Analysis of causes of death in the reported studies is not complete, but pulmonary complications (embolism, infections) counted for most fatalities. Retention of the early benefit of spinal/epidural block may depend on a vigorous program of activity after discharge home.

In summary, although the data are not conclusive, they strongly suggest that neural blockade reduces early postoperative mortality following acute hip surgery. Although further data are needed, long-term survival may be more dependent on factors other than choice of anesthesia.

Blood Loss. It is well documented that intraoperative blood loss is reduced by about 30% to 40% during elective hip replacement (Table 5-8). Accordingly, the need for blood transfusions was also reduced. The data are less consistent during acute surgery for hip fracture[44,53,137,208,216] probably because of the lower amount of blood loss during these procedures.

Neural blockade reduced blood loss by 37% ($p < 0.05$) during retropubic prostatectomy[84] and by 18% (insignificant) after transurethral prostatectomy.[135]

Results from differing abdominal procedures performed during thoracic or lumbar epidural analgesia could not demonstrate any significant reduction in intraoperative blood loss.[85,91,140,180,200,203] In one study spinal anesthesia reduced intraoperative blood loss by 45% ($p < 0.05$) during hysterectomy.[15] Spinal anesthesia also reduced blood loss by 51% ($p < 0.05$) during lower limb amputation.[131]

The mechanism of the apparent reduction in intraoperative bleeding during neural blockade in some operative procedures in debatable,[57] although hypotension usually has been quoted as the most important factor. Thus hypotensive anesthesia with halothane or nitroprusside also led to a similar reduction

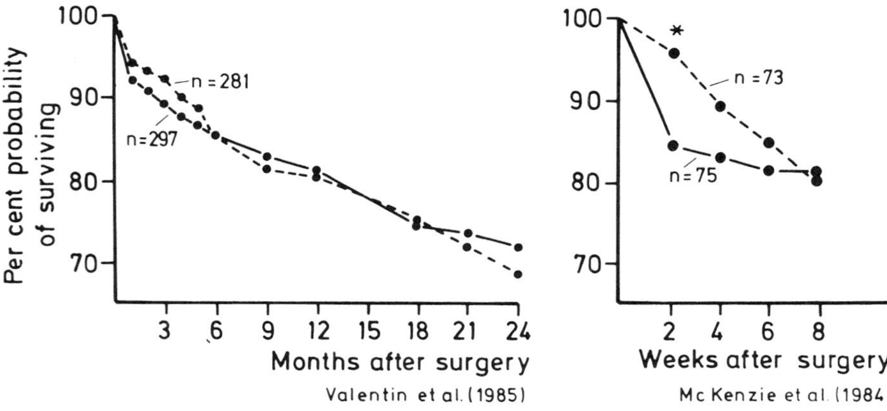

FIG. 5-20. Long-term survival in patients undergoing acute surgery for hip fracture who received spinal anesthesia or general anesthesia (controlled studies). Despite an initial reduction in early postoperative mortality (see also Table 5-7), no influence of spinal anesthesia was observed on long-term survival. (Reproduced with permission from Valentin, N., Lomholt, B., Jensen, J.S., *et al.*: Spinal or general anesthesia for surgery of the fractured hip? A prospective study of mortality in 578 patients. Br. J. Anaesth., *58*:284, 1986; and McKenzie, P.J., Wishart, H.Y., Smith, G.: Long term outcome after repair of fractured neck of femur. Comparison of subarachnoid and general anesthesia. Br. J. Anaesth., 56:581, 1984.)

TABLE 5-8. INFLUENCE OF NEURAL BLOCKADE (SPINAL/EPIDURAL) ON INTRAOPERATIVE BLOOD LOSS DURING HIP REPLACEMENT (CONTROLLED STUDIES)

Authors (Reference)	Neural Blockade/ General Anesthesia (n)	Reduction in Blood Loss (%)	p
Keith[114] (1977)	10/17	51	<0.01
Hole *et al.*[93] (1980)	29/31	20	NS
Modig *et al.*[145] (1981)	15/15	37	<0.001
Chin *et al.*[35] (1982)	21/21	39	<0.001
Hole *et al.*[94] (1982)	9/9	22	NS
Modig *et al.*[147] (1983)	30/30	28	<0.001
Mean		33%	

in intraoperative blood loss during hip replacement,[167,197] although others have failed to demonstrate a relation between arterial pressure and intraoperative blood loss.[57] Further, intraoperative blood loss during hip replacement under spinal anesthesia did not increase in patients receiving ephedrine to maintain systolic arterial pressure at or above 100 mm Hg.[198]

In summary, although the mechanism remains debatable, a fair amount of data suggests that intraoperative blood loss is reduced about 30% during operations in the lower part of the body, whereas no such advantage has been demonstrated during major (upper) abdominal procedures.

Thromboembolic Complications. The influence of neural blockade on postoperative thromboembolic complications has been investigated in seven controlled studies (Table 5-9). Thromboembolic complications in the lower extremities, verified by phlebography or ^{125}I-fibrinogen scan, were significantly reduced by about 50% in all three studies performed following hip surgery.[53,145,147] A pronounced reduction (77%) in thromboembolism was reported in patients undergoing retropubic prostatectomy under continuous epidural analgesia (24 hours).[84] In contrast, the three studies performed during abdominal surgery (Table 5-9) failed to show any influence of neural blockade on thromboembolism. In two of these studies, however, thoracic epidural analgesia was used, which may explain the lack of influence on thromboembolism (see below). In the third study[91] an extensive intraoperative neural blockade (T4–S5) was given but apparently without effect. This study, however, was noteworthy in that the control group received prophylactic thromboembolic treatment.[91]

The incidence of pulmonary embolism as assessed by perfusion lung scanning was reduced from 33% to 10% ($p < 0.05$) by continuous epidural analgesia (24 hours) after hip replacement.[147]

No information is available from controlled studies on the influence of neural blockade on graft patency rate in vascular procedures, but an advantageous effect might be expected owing to the demonstrated increase in graft blood flow.[45]

The relatively few studies on the influence of neural blockade on thromboembolic complications do not allow separation as to whether a single dose neural blockade is inferior to a continuous epidural analgesia technique. Addition of epinephrine to the local anesthetic solution during continuous epidural analgesia apparently does not prevent the reducing effect on thromboembolism.[147,148]

The eventual synergistic effect of neural blockade and low-dose heparin administration on postoperative thromboembolism has not been studied.

The mechanism of the observed reduction in thromboembolism by neural blockade is probably a modulation of several of the factors of the triad of Virchow (flow, vessel walls, coagulation/fibrinolysis). Thus a pronounced increase in blood flow to the lower extremities has been demonstrated after sympathetic blockade by neural blockade[45,144]; also, venous emptying rate and venous capacity were improved by continuous epidural analgesia.[144] Further, neural blockade may modify some of the postoperative changes in coagulation and fibrinolysis, although the data have not been ultimately conclusive (see Table 5-5). Finally, experimental and *in vitro* studies have suggested that local anesthetics *per se* may influence endothelial structure (see Fig. 5-11) and aspects of coagulation/fibrinolysis (see Table 5-5). A possible effect caused by a change in blood rheology cannot be excluded, but the pronounced

TABLE 5-9. INCIDENCE OF POSTOPERATIVE THROMBOEMBOLIC COMPLICATIONS (PHLEBOGRAPHY OR ^{125}I-FIBRINOGEN SCAN) IN PATIENTS OPERATED ON DURING NEURAL BLOCKADE (N) OR UNDER GENERAL ANESTHESIA (GA) (CONTROLLED STUDIES)

Surgery	Authors (Reference)	S/E	Prophylactic Antithrombotic Treatment in Control Group	Complications/ Number of Patients		Reduction of Complications in N-Group (%)	p
				N	GA		
Acute hip surgery	Davis *et al.*[53] (1981)	S	–	17/37	30/39	40%	<0.05
Elective hip replacement	Modig *et al.*[145] (1981)	E	–	3/15	11/15	73%	<0.05
Elective hip replacement	Modig *et al.*[147] (1983)	E	–	12/30	3/30	48%	<0.01
Prostatectomy	Hendolin *et al.*[84] (1981)	E	–	2/17	11/21	77%	<0.02
Cholecystectomy	Hendolin *et al.*[85] (1982)	E	–	4/56	5/40	46%	NS
Abdominal	Mellbring *et al.*[140] (1983)	E	–	8/21	9/24	0%	NS
Abdominal	Hjortsø *et al.*[91] (1985)	E	+	10/29	9/28	−6%	NS

S = spinal; E = epidural.

reduction in thromboembolism in the lower extremities and lungs was observed without any differences in hematocrit between patients receiving neural blockade or general anesthesia.[147]

Intravenous administration of lidocaine (2 mg/min) for 6 days after hip surgery has been reported to reduce thromboembolism,[40] whereas administration of an oral analogue of lidocaine (tocainide) did not reduce thromboembolism after hip replacement.[146]

Pulmonary Complications. It is well documented that neural blockade with local anesthetics may improve several parameters of pulmonary function postoperatively (see Chap. 26). Continuous postoperative epidural analgesia is apparently more effective than a single dose blockade.

In contrast to the plentiful data on the influence of neural blockade on postoperative pulmonary function, there is a paucity of data on the influence on postoperative pulmonary (infective) complications. Thus a significant reduction in pulmonary complications following a variety of elective surgical procedures could be demonstrated only in one[51a] of ten studies.[2,83,91,93,131,143,164,191,199] Accumulation of the data shows, however, that only 28 of 253 patients (11%) randomized to neural blockade developed pulmonary complications, in contrast to 57 of 283 patients (20%) randomized to general anesthesia ($p < 0.05$). This may suggest that neural blockade may reduce postoperative pulmonary infections, but obviously further data are needed in larger groups of patients and specific surgical procedures must be considered. It is also clear that the few data do not allow separation of a possible difference between the efficacy of a single dose block versus continuous epidural analgesia to reduce postoperative pulmonary complications (see also Chap. 26).

The use of a single dose infiltration anesthesia or intercostal block postoperatively reduced the incidence of postoperative atelectasis in two of three reported studies.[49,55,163]

In conclusion, the published data on postoperative pulmonary infective complications are insufficient to allow any conclusions as to whether neural blockade techniques may reduce this complication. This is unfortunate in view of the clinical importance and high incidence of postoperative pulmonary complications and the well-documented improvement in pulmonary function by neural blockade. Because the accumulated data suggest an advantageous effect, further data are urgently needed.

Cardiac Complications. The data on the influence of neural blockade on cardiovascular function in the perioperative period suggest that the normally increased demands are reduced (see Chap. 26), probably because of the concomitant inhibition of the catecholamine response to surgery. It might therefore be expected that neural blockade, and in particular continuous epidural analgesia, may favorably affect postoperative cardiac complications, and especially in high-risk patients. Unfortunately, the published studies do not allow any final conclusion on this important point.

Addition of thoracic epidural analgesia to general anesthesia reduced cardiovascular dysfunction as assessed by measurement of pulmonary arteriolar occlusion pressure, myocardial oxygen consumption, and ECG changes *intra*operatively (Fig. 5-21).[170] Although the patients were at high risk with a recent preoperative myocardial infarction, the postoperative mortality from reinfarction was only insignificantly reduced by epidural analgesia (epidural + general anesthesia, 1 of 23 patients; general anesthesia, 3 of 22 patients). It is not clear whether these results might have been improved if the epidural analgesia had been continued into the postoperative period.

Other studies, that included the postoperative period, could not demonstrate any advantageous effect of neural blockade either in the single studies or in the cumulated data that showed ECG abnormalities in 25 of 153 patients operated on under neural blockade and in 41 of 207 patients operated on under general anesthesia ($p < 0.5$).[44,83,135,199]

Cerebral Complications. Postoperative impairment of mental function is a well-recognized phenomenon, but the underlying mechanism leading to this complication is not completely understood.[142] The use of neural blockade might theoretically influence postoperative mental function by several mechanisms: [1] omission of general anesthetics may be advantageous because of their potential direct toxic effect on the cerebral cortex; and [2] neural blockade may lower metabolic demands concomitant to an inhibition of the endocrine metabolic response to surgery. Contrarily, the use of neural blockade may also adversely affect cerebral function, particularly in hypertensive patients with a blunted cerebrovascular autoregulation, although cerebral blood flow is not modified by a high spinal anesthesia in normotensive subjects.[118]

In one study,[93] a single dose epidural analgesia without concomitant administration of general anesthesia significantly reduced postoperative mental dysfunction as assessed by the patients' relatives or anesthesiologists. In a subsequent study, however, in elderly patients undergoing hip replacement and including patients operated on under general anesthesia alone, general anesthesia plus epidural analgesia (24 hours), and epidural analgesia alone (24 hours), no favorable effect of the two epidural regimens could be demonstrated despite an inhibition of the stress response.[177] Mental function was assessed by trained psychologists using elaborate psychological methods. It was concluded that the short-lasting (2 to 4 days) impairment of mental function is caused by factors other than general anesthetic agents and the endocrine metabolic response to surgery.[177] Similarly, no differences in postoperative mental function could be demonstrated in patients undergoing eye surgery under general anesthesia or topical regional

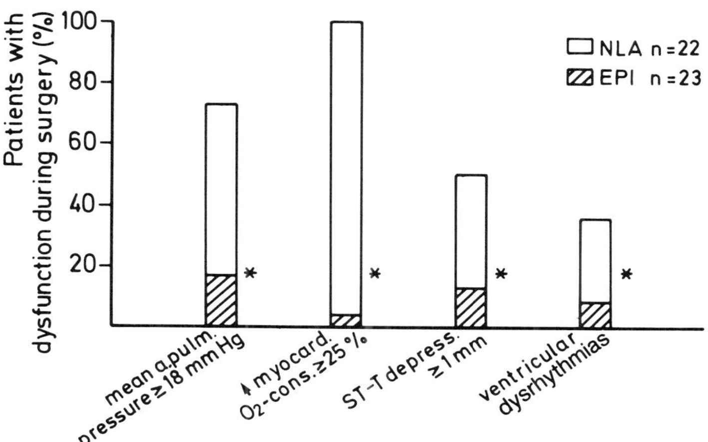

FIG. 5-21. Cardiac effects of thoracic epidural analgesia (0.5% plain bupivacaine) plus light balanced anesthesia or neuroleptanesthesia alone in patients undergoing major abdominal surgery. All patients had had a recent (less than 3 months) myocardial infarction. The results show a significant reduction in intraoperative hemodynamic, metabolic, and ECG changes in patients receiving epidural analgesia. Measurements were not performed in the postoperative period. Reinfarction rate was 1 of 23 in the epidural group and 5 of 22 in the neuroleptanesthesia group. (Modified from data by Reiz, S., Bålfors, E., Sørensen, M.B., *et al.*: Coronary hemodynamic effects of general anesthesia and surgery: Modification by epidural analgesia in patients with ischemic heart disease. Reg. Anaesth., 7:S8, 1982.)

anesthesia.[107] A mental status questionnaire performed 24 and 72 hours after lower limb amputation was not different between patients allocated to spinal anesthesia or to general anesthesia.[131]

In conclusion, the available data do not suggest that neural blockade may favorably affect postoperative mental function.

Gastrointestinal Function. Postoperative adynamic ileus is predominantly confined to the stomach and colon; the motility of the small intestine usually returns within a few hours postoperatively.[69] The mechanism leading to postoperative ileus has only partly been evaluated, but inhibitory neural reflexes mediated through the sympathetic nervous system play a major role.[69] Various measures to remove the sympathetic inhibition of the alimentary tract have had a variable success in relieving ileus both in experimental and clinical studies.[154]

Spinal analgesia and epidural analgesia have been reported to restore gastrointestinal motility in clinical studies,[1,65,132] but the design of these studies impedes final interpretation. Other studies, however, suggest that epidural analgesia may enhance postoperative gastric emptying rate assessed by paracetamol absorption.[156] The demonstration of an increased electrical activity of the stomach and intestines after cholecystectomy under epidural analgesia cannot be interpreted as a clinically advantageous effect of neural blockade on adynamic ileus. An intra-abdominal instillation of bupivacaine (2 mg/kg) significantly shortened transit time in the right part of the colon but did not affect total colonic transit or time for the first passage of flatus and feces postoperatively.[178] In contrast, continuous epidural analgesia for 3 days after left-sided colonic surgery led to a major reduction in total transit time of x-ray contrast from 150 hours in the control group to 35 hours in the epidural group ($p < 0.05$).[3]

Neural blockade has been reported to hasten postoperative oral intake after herniotomy[196] and lower limb amputation[131]; no data exist from abdominal procedures. The possible influence of neural blockade on the incidence of anastomotic breakdown in colonic surgery is unknown; however, three cases of very early, immediate postoperative presentation of a disruption of colonic anastomosis have been reported.[12,201] These reports hardly justify the recommendation that surgery on the colon should be considered to be a relative contraindication to epidural analgesia,[201] since it is highly unlikely that the resulting sympatheticolysis *per se* may precipitate the anastomic breakdown. Rather it may lead to an earlier presentation of a disruption already present and caused by failure of the surgical technique or other factors. Theoretically the increased tone of the bowel wall following neural blockade may impede the use of a stapling gun for colonic anastomosis, but no data are available to assess the magnitude of this problem.

In experimental studies spinal anesthesia led to a 44% decrease in colonic vascular resistance and a 22% increase in colonic blood flow.[4] This may be important for anastomotic healing but awaits documentation in clinical studies.

In summary, surgeons and anesthesiologists should be aware of the possible influence of anesthetic techniques on postoperative gastrointestinal function,[5] and further studies should be undertaken to evaluate the possible beneficial effect of neural blockade on postoperative gastrointestinal function.

Convalescence. Postoperative convalescence as assessed by ambulation has been reported to be shortened[158] or unchanged[49] by an intercostal block following renal surgery, and improved when hip surgery[164] and inguinal herniotomy[196] were performed under neural blockade. Similarly, postoperative hospital stay was shortened in all seven reported studies (Table 5-10) by an average of 1.3 days (16% of total postoperative hospital stay in the control groups). The reduction in hospital stay was only significant, however, in one study.[164] These studies (Table 5-10) represent a variety of surgical procedures, and different techniques of neural blockade were used. Cumulation of data as given in Table 5-10 therefore should not be considered as an indication of a shortened hospital stay following neural blockade but rather as a suggestion that this may be an important area for future research in selected groups of patients and operative procedures.

No data have been published on the influence of neural blockade on such variables as postoperative fatigue, muscle function, and return to work.

NEURAL BLOCKADE WITH EPIDURAL/INTRATHECAL OPIATES

The powerful, selective analgesia following epidural/intrathecal opiate administration is well established.[47] In addition to the advantages of this regimen in postoperative pain relief, a variety of both respiratory and nonrespiratory side-effects of epidural/intrathecal opiates have been described, including pruritus, nausea, vomiting, and urinary bladder dysfunction.[47] Besides the alleviation of postoperative

TABLE 5-10. DIFFERENCES IN POSTOPERATIVE HOSPITAL STAY BETWEEN PATIENTS OPERATED ON DURING NEURAL BLOCKADE (N) OR UNDER GENERAL ANESTHESIA (GA) (CONTROLLED STUDIES)

Surgery	Authors (Reference)	Technique of Neural Blockade	Hospital Stay (days) (N − GA)	p*
Combined hip + abdominal	Pflug *et al.*[164] (1974)	Cont. epi (72 h)	−3.0 (41%)	<0.05
Abdominal	Miller *et al.*[143] (1976)	Cont. epi (24 h)	−2.0 (18%)	NS
Abdominal	Patel *et al.*[163] (1983)	Single dose infiltration	−0.7 (11%)	NS
Prostatectomy	Hendolin[83] (1980)	Cont. epi (24 h)	−1.3 (12%)	NS
Prostatectomy	McGowan *et al.*[135] (1980)	Spinal	−1.4 (18%)	NS
Prostatectomy	Tolksdorf *et al.*[199] (1980)	Single dose spinal or epi	−0.5 (4%)	NS
Renal surgery	Crawford *et al.*[49] (1982)	Single dose intercostal block	−0.5 (6%)	NS
		Mean	−1.3 days (16% of hospital stay)	

Cont. = continuous; epi = epidural.
*Denotes level of significance.

pain, considerable uncertainty remains as to other advantageous effects of epidural/intrathecal opiates on postoperative morbidity parameters such as pulmonary, cardiac, or thromboembolic complications, postoperative recovery of gastrointestinal function, ambulation, and convalescence.

In the following sections the data from controlled studies on the influence of epidural/intrathecal opiate administration on postoperative morbidity will be discussed; the effects on pain *per se* and side-effects will be discussed in Chapter 28.

Mortality. Influence of pain relief by epidural/intrathecal opiate administration on postoperative *mortality* has not been assessed.

Pulmonary Complications. The effect of epidural/intrathecal opiates on postoperative *pulmonary complications* has not been completely evaluated. Several studies have reported an improvement in various parameters of postoperative pulmonary function (see Chap. 28). In one study postoperative pulmonary complications as assessed by x-ray changes 24 to 48 hours after abdominal surgery were significantly reduced from 67% to 21%, compared to complications in patients receiving i.m. morphine, but without differences between the number of pulmonary infections.[182] In a controlled study in 30 adipose patients undergoing gastroplasty, 6 of 15 patients receiving pain alleviation with i.m. morphine had pulmonary complications, versus 2 of 15 patients receiving epidural morphine ($p > 0.05$).[169] Finally, in a controlled study of 100 patients receiving either i.m. morphine or epidural local anesthetics during the initial 24 hours after surgery plus epidural morphine 4 mg every 12 hours during the first 3 postoperative days, the incidence of pulmonary infections was insignificantly reduced from 28% to 20% by the epidural analgesic regimen (Table 5-11).[91] Thus, in all reported studies on postoperative pulmonary complications, only an insignificant trend toward advantageous effect of epidural morphine administration could be demonstrated (see also Chap. 28).

Cardiac Complications. The effect of epidural/intrathecal opiate administration on postoperative *cardiac complications* is unknown but is not expected to be reduced to a major degree owing to the very minor effect of this regimen on endocrine metabolic responses to surgery (Tables 5-2 and 5-3). In the above-mentioned epidural analgesic regimen with combined local anesthetics and morphine epidurally for 3 days,[91] an insignificant reduction of cardiac dysrythmias from 10% to 4% was found compared with i.m. morphine (Table 5-11).

Blood Loss. No data have been published on *blood loss* in patients allocated to epidural/intrathecal opiates, but again blood loss should not be expected to be reduced because epidural opiate administration does not cause sympathetic depression and hypotension, which are considered to be mechanisms that diminish blood loss after epidural local anesthetics.

Thromboembolic Complications. Similar considerations are valid with regard to *thromboembolic complications,* since epidural/intrathecal opiates will not increase lower limb blood flow. Accordingly, no reduction in thromboembolism was observed in a limited number of adipose patients undergoing gastroplasty and allocated to either i.m. or epidural morphine for postoperative pain relief.[169] Similarly, 3 days of epidural morphine administration in addition to initial epidural local anesthetics in patients under-

TABLE 5-11. INFLUENCE OF EPIDURAL MORPHINE* (PLUS INITIAL, 24 H, POSTOPERATIVE EPIDURAL LOCAL ANESTHETICS) VERSUS PAIN RELIEF WITH SYSTEMIC MORPHINE† ON MORBIDITY AFTER ABDOMINAL SURGERY (CONTROLLED STUDY)[91]

Morbidity	General Anesthesia + Systemic Morphine (n = 50)	General Anesthesia + Epidural Analgesia (n = 44)	p	Risk of Type II Error (50% MIREDIF)
Mortality	3/50 (6%)	1/44 (2%)	>0.7	0.60
Pneumonia	14/50 (28%)	m 9/44 (20%)	>0.5	0.25
Dysrhythmia	5/50 (10%)	2/44 (5%)	>0.7	0.40
Venous thrombosis	9/28 (32%)	10/29 (34%)	>0.9	0.08
Wound complications	8/50 (14%)	5/44 (11%)	>0.9	0.30
Not recovered ≤ 10 days	12/38 (32%)	9/38 (24%)	>0.6	0.20
Blood transfusion	850 ± 15 ml	650 ± 15 ml	>0.3	
Flatus (mean ± SEM)	3.0 ± 0.2 days	3.1 ± 0.2 days	>0.7	
Feces (mean ± SEM)	4.4 ± 0.2 days	4.7 ± 0.2 days	>0.4	
Number of patients without complications	25/50 (50%)	22/44 (50%)	>0.8	0.01

*4 mg/12 h over 72 hours.
†4–8 mg/4–6 h.

going abdominal surgery did not reduce thromboembolic complications as verified by ^{125}I-fibrinogen scan and phlebography (Table 5-11).[91]

Cerebral Function. The effect of epidural/intrathecal opiates on postoperative *cerebral function* has been considered only in one study involving 20 patients allocated to i.m. morphine or epidural morphine for postoperative pain relief.[119] Postoperative sedation scores were significantly lower in the epidural morphine group.

Gastrointestinal Motility. Preliminary experimental studies have suggested that epidural fentanyl administration may inhibit the inhibitory gastrointestinal reflexes responsible for post-traumatic reduction of *gastrointestinal motility*[125]; however, in a study of 100 patients undergoing abdominal surgery and allocated to pain relief with i.m. morphine or epidural morphine 4 mg every 12 hours for 3 days plus epidural local anesthetics during the initial 24 hours, no effect was observed on the first appearance of flatus and bowel movement and intake of the first normal meal despite improved pain relief by the epidural regimen (Table 5-11).[91] In adipose patients undergoing gastroplasty, epidural morphine had a dual effect on gastrointestinal function, since the amount of gastric aspirate increased while the recovery period until first passage of flatus and feces was shortened.[159] The effect of epidural opiate administration on bile duct pressures is controversial.[186,209]

Immunofunction. An eventual modulation of postoperative *immunofunction* remains to be evaluated, but epidural morphine administration had no influence on postoperative depression of delayed hypersensitivity.[89]

Convalescence. As regards *convalescence* the few studies again do not allow any firm conclusion. The postoperative feeling of well-being was rated better after epidural morphine 0.1 mg/kg than after systemic morphine or epidural saline in patients undergoing orthopedic operations.[122] In 30 adipose patients undergoing gastroplasty, the 15 patients allocated to postoperative epidural morphine administration were ambulated earlier than those receiving i.m. morphine; in addition, their hospital stay was reduced from 9.0 to 7.1 days ($p < 0.05$).[169] In a study of 100 elderly patients undergoing major abdominal surgery and allocated to either systemic morphine or epidural analgesia with local anesthetics for 24 hours plus morphine epidurally 4 mg every 12 hours for 72 hours, no influence could be demonstrated on fatigue 10, 30, and 60 days postoperatively.[91] Further, no beneficial effects were found on postoperative weight loss, recovery of ambulation, and ability to take care of personal hygiene, and postoperative restoration of preoperative fitness score level was not accelerated by the epidural analgesic regimen (Table 5-11).[91]

Thus, despite the ample evidence that epidural/intrathecal opiate administration may provide sufficient postoperative pain relief after a variety of operative procedures, there is a disappointing paucity of information on other effects that might prove beneficial to postoperative recovery, and firm conclusions cannot be given at present. Obviously, more data are required, but it should be reiterated that pain relief by epidural/intrathecal opiate administration is not very effective in reducing the endocrine metabolic stress response to operative injury, and postoperative demands on various organs may therefore not be reduced by this regimen.

CONCLUSION

In summary, this review has revealed that neural blockade with local anesthetics may diminish a predominant part of the physiologic response to surgical procedures in the lower abdomen and to procedures on the lower extremities. The inhibitory effect is less pronounced during major (upper) abdominal and thoracic procedures probably because of insufficient afferent neural blockade by the current available techniques. To obtain a pronounced reduction of the surgical stress response, a continuous postoperative epidural technique should be used. Pain relief by epidural/intrathecal opiate administration is less efficient in reducing the stress response.

On the basis of controlled studies there is increased evidence that neural blockade may mitigate various aspects of postoperative morbidity. The evidence is only convincing, however, with regard to reduction in blood loss and thromboembolism, and then only in procedures such as hip replacement and prostatectomy. The data from other procedures similarly show an insignificant trend toward a reduction in most morbidity parameters in patients randomized to neural blockade. The studies on the effect of epidural/intrathecal opiate administration on postoperative morbidity do not allow any conclusion, but most probably an eventual effect is less consistent than following neural blockade with local anesthetic agents.

Future studies should focus on an evaluation of humoral mediators of the stress response and their release and inhibitory mechanisms; an evaluation of a more selective and sufficient nociceptive blockade (? combined epidural opiates and local anesthetics); and an evaluation of the optimal duration of nociceptive blockade in order to obtain a pronounced reduction of the surgical stress response. Studies should also focus on the effect of neural blockade on the stress response in traumatized patients.

Finally, controlled studies on clinical morbidity parameters should be performed when more efficient techniques have been evaluated to modulate the stress response. Such studies should focus on eventual differential effects of a single dose versus continuous neural blockade and on an identification of specific surgical procedures and patients who may or may not benefit from neural blockade.

REFERENCES

1. Acalovski, I., and Badea, G.: Efficiency of continued (intermittent) peridural anesthesia in the prevention of postoperative ileus. Rev. Chir., *27*:315, 1978.
2. Addison, N.V., Brear, F.A., Budd, K., and Whittaker, M.: Epidural analgesia following cholecystectomy. Br. J. Surg., *61*:860, 1974.
3. Ahn, H., Andåker, L., Bronge, A., Lindhagen, J., *et al.*: Effect of continuous epidural analgesia on gastrointestinal motility. Acta Anaesthesiol. Scand. (In Press).
4. Aitkenhead, A.R., Gilmour, D.G., Hothersull, A.P., and Ledingham, I.M.A.: Effects of subarachnoid nerve block and arterial P_{CO_2} on colon blood flow in the dog. Br. J. Anaesth., *52*:1071, 1980.
5. Aitkenhead, A.R.: Anaesthesia for bowel surgery. Ann. Chir. Gynaecol., *73*:177, 1984.
6. Altemeyer, K-H., Seeling, W., Breucking, E., Feist, H., *et al.*: Untersuchungen zur stressreaktion bei knieoperationen unter kontinuerlicher periduralanaesthesie im vergleich zur neuroleptanalgesie. Anaesthesist, *32*:219, 1983.
7. Annamunthodo, H., Keating, V.J., and Patrick, S.J.: Liver glycogen alterations in anaesthesia. Anaesthesia, *13*:429, 1958.
8. Asoh, T., Tsuji, H., Shirasaka, C., and Takeuchi, Y.: Effect of epidural analgesia on metabolic response to major upper abdominal surgery. Acta Anaesthesiol. Scand., *27*:233, 1983.
9. Bellmann, O., and Stoeckel, H.: The influence of anaesthesia on prolactin secretion in man. *In* Stoeckel, H., and Oyama, T. (eds.): Endocrinology in anaesthesia and surgery, p. 101. New York, Springer Verlag, 1980.
10. Bengtsson, M.: Changes in skin blood flow and temperature during spinal analgesia evaluated by laser Doppler flowmetry and infrared thermography. Acta Anaesthesiol. Scand., *28*:625, 1984.

10a. Bent, J.M., Paterson, J.L., Mashiter, K., and Hall, G.M.: Effects of high-dose fentanyl anaesthesia on the established metabolic and endocrine response to surgery. Anaesthesia, *39*:19, 1984.

11. Bessey, P.Q., Watters, J.M., Aoki, T.T., and Wilmore, D.W.: Combined hormonal infusion simulates the metabolic response to injury. Ann. Surg., *200*:264, 1984.

11a. Bevan, D.R.: Modification of the metabolic response to trauma under extradural analgesia. Anaesthesia, *26*:188, 1971.

12. Bigler, D., Hjortsø, N-C., and Kehlet, H.: A case of disruption of colonic anastomosis two hours postoperatively during continuous epidural analgesia. Anaesthesia, *40*:278, 1985.
13. Bigler, D., Hjortsø, N-C., and Kehlet, H.: Variation in spread of sensory and temperature analgesia during intermittent

postoperative epidural bupivacaine administration. Acta Anaesthesiol. Scand., *30*:289, 1986.

14. Bigler, D., Hjortsø, N-C., Edstrøm, H., Christensen, N.J., *et al.*: Comparative effects of intrathecal hyperbaric bupivacaine and tetracaine on sensory and cold analgesia, and cardiovascular and plasma catecholamine responses. Acta Anaesthesiol. Scand. (In Press).
15. Blunnie, W.P., McIlroy, P.D.A., Merrett, J.D., and Dundee, J.W.: Cardiovascular and biochemical evidence of stress during major surgery associated with different techniques of anaesthesia. Br. J. Anaesth., *55*:611, 1983.
16. Bonica, J.J.: Autonomic innervation of the viscera in relation to nerve block. Anesthesiology, *29*:793, 1968.
17. Bonnet, F., Harari, A., Thibonnier, M., and Viars, P.: Suppression of antidiuretic hormone hypersecretion during surgery by extradural anaesthesia. Br. J. Anaesth., *54*:29, 1982.
18. Borg, T., and Modig, J.: Potential anti-thrombotic effects of local anaesthetics due to their inhibition of platelet aggregation. Acta Anaesthesiol. Scand., *29*:739, 1985.
19. von Bormann, B., Weidler, B., Dennhardt, R., and Hempelmann, G.: Anaesthesieverfahren und postoperative ADH-secretion. Anaesthesist, *32*:177, 1983.
20. von Bormann, B., Weidler, B., Dennhardt, R., Sturm, G., *et al.*: Influence of fentanyl on stress-induced elevation of plasma vasopressin (ADH) after surgery. Anesth. Analg., *62*:727, 1983.
21. Boskovski, N.: The effects of epidural versus general anesthesia on perioperative water and electrolyte excretion. Reg. Anaesth., *9*:165, 1984.
22. Bovill, J.G., Sebel, P.S., and Stanley, T.H.: Opiod analgesics in anesthesia: with special reference to their use in cardiovascular anesthesia. Anesthesiology, *61*:731, 1984.
23. Brandt, M.R., Kehlet, H., Binder, C., Hagen, C., *et al.*: Effect of epidural analgesia on the glucoregulatory endocrine response to surgery. Clin. Endocrinol., *5*:107, 1976.
24. Brandt, M.R., Kehlet, H., Hansen, J.M., and Skovsted, L.: Serum triiodothyronine and surgery. Lancet, *1*:491, 1976.
25. Brandt, M.R., Kehlet, H., Skovsted, L., and Hansen, J.M.: Rapid decrease in plasma triiodothyronine during surgery and epidural analgesia independent of afferent neurogenic stimuli and of cortisol. Lancet, *2*:1333, 1976.
26. Brandt, M.R., Kehlet, H., Faber, O., and Binder, C.: C-peptide and insulin during blockade of the hyperglycemic response to surgery by epidural analgesia. Clin. Endocrinol., *6*:167, 1977.
27. Brandt, M.R., Fernandes, A., Mordhorst, R., and Kehlet, H.: Epidural analgesia improves postoperative nitrogen balance. Br. Med. J., *1*:1106, 1978.
28. Brandt, M.R., Ølgaard, K., and Kehlet, H.: Epidural analgesia inhibits the renin and aldosterone response to surgery. Acta Anaesthesiol. Scand., *23*:267, 1979.
29. Bromage, P.R., Shibata, H.R., and Willoughby, H.W.: Influence of prolonged epidural blockade on blood sugar and cortisol responses to operations upon the upper part of the abdomen and the thorax. Surg. Gynecol. Obstet., *132*:1051, 1971.
30. Buckley, F.P., Kehlet, H., Brown, N.S., and Scott, D.B.: Postoperative glucose tolerance during epidural analgesia. Br. J. Anaesth., *54*:325, 1982.
31. Cannon, W.B.: The Wisdom of the Body. New York, Norton, 1939.
32. Carli, F., Clark, M.M., and Woollen, J.W.: Investigation of the relationship between heat loss and nitrogen excretion in elderly patients undergoing major abdominal surgery under general anaesthetic. Br. J. Anaesth., *54*:1023, 1982.
33. Chari, P., Katariya, R.N., Dash, R.J., and Phanindranath, T.S.N.: Effect of coeliac plexus block on plasma cortisol in major abdominal surgery. Indian J. Surg., *42*:384, 1980.
34. Child, C.S., and Kaufman, L.: Effect of intrathecal diamorphine on the adrenocortical, hyperglycemic and cardiovascular responses to major colonic surgery. Br. J. Anaesth., *57*:389, 1985.
35. Chin, S.P., Abou-Madi, M.N., Eurin, B., Witvoët, J., *et al.*: Blood loss in total hip replacement: Extradural v. phenoperidine analgesia. Br. J. Anaesth., *54*:491, 1982.
36. Christensen, P., Brandt, M.R., Rem, J., and Kehlet, H.: Influence of extradural morphine on the adrenocortical and hyperglycaemic response to surgery. Br. J. Anaesth., *54*:24, 1982.
37. Christensen, T., Waaben, J., Lindeburg, T., Vesterberg, K., *et al.*: Effect of epidural analgesia on plasma and muscle amino acid pattern after surgery. Acta Chir. Scand., *152*:407, 1986.
38. Cochrane, J.P.S., Forsling, M.L., Menzies Gow, N., and Le Quesne, L.P.: Arginine vasopressin release following surgical operations. Br. J. Surg., *68*:209, 1981.
39. Colman, R.W.: Surface-mediated defense reactions. The plasma contact activation system. J. Clin. Invest., *73*:1249, 1984.
40. Cooke, E.D., Bowcock, S.A., Lloyd, M.J., and Pilcher, M.F.: Intravenous lignocaine in prevention of deep venous thrombosis after elective hip surgery. Lancet, *2*:797, 1977.
41. Cooper, G.M., Holdcroft, A., Hall, G.M., and Alaghband–Zadeh, J.: Epidural analgesia and the metabolic response to surgery. Can. Anaesth. Soc. J., *26*:381, 1979.
42. Cort, J.H.: Relief of post-traumatic anuria. Am. J. Physiol., *164*:686, 1951.
43. Cosgrove, D.O., and Jenkins, J.S.: The effect of epidural anaesthesia on the pituitary-adrenal response to surgery. Clin. Sci. Mol. Med., *46*:403, 1974.
44. Couderc, E., Mauge, F., Duwaldstein, P., and Desmonts, J-M.: Résultats comparatifs de l'anesthésia générale et péridurale chez le grand viellard dans la chirurgie de la hanche. Anesth. Anal. Réan., *34*:987, 1977.
45. Cousins, M.J., and Wright, C.J.: Graft, muscle and skin bloodflow after epidural block in vascular surgical procedures. Surg. Gynecol. Obstet., *133*:59, 1971.
46. Cousins, M.J., and Mazze, R.I.: Anaesthesia, surgery and renal function. Anaesth. Intensive Care, *1*:355, 1973.
47. Cousins, M.J., and Mather, L.E.: Intrathecal and epidural administration of opiods. Anesthesiology, *61*:276, 1984.
48. Cowen, M.J., Bullingham, R.E.S., Paterson, G.M.C., McQuay, H.J., *et al.*: A controlled comparison of the effects of extradural diamorphine and bupivacaine on plasma glu-

cose and plasma cortisol in postoperative patients. Anesth. Analg., *61*:15, 1982.
49. Crawford, E.D., and Skinner, D.G.: Intercostal nerve block with thoracoabdominal and flank incision. Urology, *14*:25, 1982.
50. Crile, G.W.: Phylogenetic association in relation to certain medical problems. Boston Med. Surg. J., *163*:893, 1910.
51. Cullen, B.F., and von Belle, G.: Lymphocyte transformation and changes in leukocyte count: Effects of anesthesia and operation. Anesthesiology, *43*:563, 1975.
51a. Cuschieri, R.J., Morran, C.G., Howie, J.C., and McArdle, C.S.: Postoperative pain and pulmonary complications: Comparison of three analgesic regimens. Br. J. Surg., *72*:495, 1985.
52. Cuthbertson, D.P.: The metabolic response to injury and its nutritional implications: Retrospect and prospect. J. Par. Ent. Nutr., *3*:108, 1979.
53. Davis, F.M., and Laurenson, V.G.: Spinal anaesthesia or general anaesthesia for emergency hip surgery in elderly patients. Anaesth. Intens. Care, *9*:352, 1981.
54. Delalande, J.P., Le Page, J.L., Perramant, M., Lozach, P., *et al.*: Influence of epidural analgesia on protein sparing in major visceral surgery. Ann. Fr. Anesth. Réanim., *3*:16, 1984.
55. Delilkan, A.E., Lee, C.K., Yong, N.K., Ong, S.C., *et al.*: Postoperative local analgesia for thoracotomy with direct bupivacaine intercostal blocks. Anesthesia, *28*:561, 1973.
56. Dinarello, C.A.: Interleukin-1. Rev. Infect. Dis., *6*:51, 1984.
57. Donald, J.R.: Induced hypotension and blood loss during surgery. J. R. Soc. Med., *75*:149, 1982.
58. Dworkin, L.D., Ischikawa, I., and Brenner, D.M.: Hormonal modulation of glomerular function. Am. J. Physiol., *244*:F95, 1983.
59. Ecoffey, C., Edouard, A., Pruszczynski, W., Taly, E., *et al.*: Effects of epidural anesthesia on catecholamines, renin activity and vasopressin changes induced by tilt in elderly men. Anesthesiology, *62*:294, 1985.
60. Edwards, A.E., Gemmel, L.W., Mankin, P.P., Smith, C.J., *et al.*: The effects of three differing anaesthetics on the immune response. Anaesthesia, *39*:1071, 1984.
61. Elfstrom, J.: Drug pharmacokinetics in the postoperative period. Clin. Pharmacokin., *4*:16, 1979.
62. Engquist, A., Askgaard, B., and Funding, J.: Impairment of blood fibrinolytic activity during major surgical stress under combined extradural blockade and general anaesthesia. Br. J. Anaesth., *48*:903, 1976.
63. Engquist, A., Brandt, M.R., Fernandes, A., and Kehlet, H.: The blocking effect of epidural analgesia on the adrenocortical and hyperglycemic response to surgery. Acta Anaesthesiol. Scand., *21*:330, 1977.
64. Engquist, A., Fog-Møller, F., Christiansen, C., Thode, J., *et al.*: Influence of epidural analgesia on the catecholamine and cyclic AMP responses to surgery. Acta Anaesthesiol. Scand., *24*:17, 1980.
65. Fasano, M., Waldvogel, H.H., and Muller, C.A.: Prophylaxie de l'ileus paralytique apres chirurgie du çolon par blocage sympatique peridural continu. Helv. Chir. Acta, *46*:245, 1979.
66. Finley, J.H., Cork, R.C., Hameroff, S.R., and Scherer, K.: Comparison of plasma beta-endorphine levels during spinal versus general anesthesia. Anesthesiology, *57*:A191, 1982.
67. Fournell, A., Wilhelmy, B., Falke, K., Sandmann, W., *et al.*: Kontinuerlische Messung der Sauerstofaufnahme bei postoperativer Periduralanalgesie. *In* Wüst, H.J., and Zindler, M. (eds.): Neue Aspekte in der Regionalanaesthesie 1. p. 54. Berlin, Springer Verlag, 1980.
68. Fragen, R.J., Shanks, C.A., Molteni, A., and Avram, M.J.: Effects of etomidate on hormonal responses to surgical stress. Anesthesiology, *61*:652, 1984.
69. Furness, J.B., Costa, M.: Adynamic ileus, its pathogenesis and treatment. Med. Biol., *52*:82, 1974.
70. Gelfand, R.A., DeFronzo, R.A., and Gusberg, R.: Metabolic alterations associated with major injury or infection. In: Kleinberger, G., and Deutsch, E. (eds.): New Aspects of Clinical Nutrition. p. 211. Basel, Karger, 1983.
71. Gelfand, R.A., Matthews, D.E., Bier, D.M., Sherwin, R.S.: Role of counterregulatory hormones in the catabolic response to stress. J. Clin. Invest., *74*:2238, 1984.
72. Gelman, S., Feigenberg, Z., Dintzman, M., and Levy, E.: Electroenterography after cholecystectomy — The role of high epidural analgesia. Arch. Surg., *112*:580, 1977.
73. Gelman, S., Laws, H.L., Potzick, J., Strong, S., *et al.*: Thoracic epidural vs. balanced anesthesia in morbid obesity: An intraoperative and postoperative hemodynamic study. Anesth. Analg., *59*:902, 1980.
74. Gordon, N.H., Scott, D.B., and Percy Robb, I.W.: Modification of plasma corticosteroid concentrations during and after surgery by epidural blockade. Br. Med. J., *1*:581, 1973.
75. Güllner, H-G.: Regulation of sodium and water excretion by catecholamines. Life Sci., *32*:921, 1983.
76. Hack, G., Marx, M., Witassek, F., and Vetter, H.: Zum Einfluss von Periduralanästhesie und Operation auf das Renin-Angiotensin-Aldosteron-System. *In* Wüst, H.J., and Zindler, M. (eds.): Neue Aspekte in der Regional-anaesthesie. 1st ed., p. 119. Berlin, Springer Verlag, 1980.
77. Hagen, C., Brandt, M.R., and Kehlet, H.: Prolactin, LH, FSH, GH and cortisol response to surgery and the effect of epidural analgesia. Acta Endocrinol., *94*:151, 1980.
78. Hallberg, D., and Orö, L.: Free fatty acids of plasma during spinal anaesthesia in man. Acta Med. Scand., *178*:281, 1965.
79. Halter, J.B., and Pflug, A.E.: Relationship of impaired insulin secretion during surgical stress to anesthesia and catecholamine release. J. Clin. Endocrinol., *51*:1093, 1980.
80. Halter, J.B., and Pflug, A.E.: Effects of anesthesia and surgical stress on insulin secretion in man. Metabolism, *29*:1124, 1980.
81. Halter, J.B., and Pflug, A.E.: Effect of sympathetic blockade by spinal anesthesia on pancreatic islet function in man. Am. J. Physiol., *239*:E151, 1980.
82. Hasselstrøm, L., Mogensen, T., Kehlet, H., and Christensen, N.J.: Effect of intravenous bupivacaine on cardiovascular function and plasma catecholamines in humans. Anesth. Analg., *63*:1053, 1984.
83. Hendolin, H.: The influence of continuous epidural analgesia and general anaesthesia on the peri- and postoperative

course of patients subjected to retropubic prostatectomy. Thesis. University of Kuopio, Finland, 1980.

84. Hendolin, H., Mattila, M.A.K., and Poikolainen, E.: The effect of lumbar epidural analgesia on the development of deep vein thrombosis of the legs after open prostatectomy. Acta Chir. Scand., *147*:425, 1981.

85. Hendolin, H., Tuppurainen, T., and Lahtinen, J.: Thoracic epidural analgesia and deep vein thrombosis in cholecystectomized patients. Acta Chir. Scand., *148*:405, 1982.

86. Hendolin, H., and Länsimies, E.: Skin and central temperatures during continuous epidural analgesia and general anaesthesia in patients subjected to prostatectomy. Ann. Clin. Res., *14*:181, 1982.

87. Hendolin, H., and Penttila, I.M.: Liver enzymes after retropubic prostatectomy in patients receiving continuous lumbar epidural analgesia or general anaesthesia. Ann. Clin. Res., *14*:1, 1982.

88. Hennek, K., and Sydow, F-W.: Die thorakale periduralanaesthesie zur intra- und postoperativen analgesie bei lungenresektionen. Reg. Anaesth. *7*:115, 1984.

89. Hjortsø, N.C., Andersen, T., Frøsig, F., Neumann, P., *et al.*: Failure of epidural analgesia to modify postoperative depression of delayed hypersensitivity. Acta Anaesthesiol. Scand., *28*:128, 1984.

90. Hjortsø, N.C., Christensen, N.J., Andersen, T., and Kehlet, H.: Effects of the extradural administration of local anaesthetic agents and morphine on the urinary excretion of cortisol, catecholamines and nitrogen following abdominal surgery. Br. J. Anaesth., *57*:400, 1985.

91. Hjortsø, N.C., Andersen, T., Frøsig, F., Lindhard, A., *et al.*: Influence of epidural analgesia with local anaesthetics and morphine on morbidity after abdominal surgery. Acta Anaesthesiol. Scand., *29*:790, 1985.

92. Holdcroft, A., Hall, G.M., and Cooper, G.M.: Redistribution of body heat during anaesthesia. Anaesthesia, *34*:758, 1979.

93. Hole, A., Terjesen, T., and Breivik, H.: Epidural versus general anaesthesia for total hip arthroplasty in elderly patients. Acta Anaesthesiol. Scand., *24*:279, 1980.

94. Hole, A., Unsgaard, G., and Breivik, H.: Monocyte functions are depressed during and after surgery under general anaesthesia but not under epidural anaesthesia. Acta Anaesthesiol. Scand., *26*:301, 1982.

95. Hole, A., and Unsgaard, G.: The effect of epidural and general anaesthesia on lymphocyte functions during and after major orthopaedic surgery. Acta Anaesthesiol. Scand., *27*:135, 1983.

96. Hole, A.: Depression of monocytes and lymphocytes by stress-related humural factors and anaesthetic-related drugs. Acta Anaesthesiol. Scand., *28*:280, 1984.

97. Hole, A.: Per- and postoperative monocyte and lymphocyte functions: Effects of combined epidural and general anaesthesia. Acta Anaesthesiol. Scand., *28*:367, 1984.

98. Hole, A., and Bakke, O.: T-lymphocytes and the subpopulations of T-helper and T-suppressor cells measured by monoclonal antibodies (T_{11}, T_4 and T_8) in relation to surgery under epidural and general anaesthesia. Acta Anaesthesiol. Scand., *28*:296, 1984.

99. Houghton, A., Hickey, J.B., Ross, S.A., and Dupre, J.: Glucose tolerance during anaesthesia and surgery. Comparison of general and extradural anaesthesia. Br. J. Anaesth., *50*:495, 1978.

100. Hume, D.M., and Egdahl, R.H.: The importance of the brain in the endocrine response to injury. Ann. Surg., *150*:697, 1959.

100a. Håkansson, E., Rutberg, H., Jorfeldt, L., and Wiklund, L.: Endocrine and metabolic responses after standardized moderate surgical trauma: Influence of age and sex. Clin. Physiol., *4*:461, 1984.

101. Håkansson, E., Rutberg, H., Jorfeldt, L., and Mårtensson, J.: Effects of extradural administration of morphine or bupivacaine on the metabolic response to upper abdominal surgery. Br. J. Anaesth., *57*:394, 1985.

102. Järhult, J., Falck, B., Ingemansson, S., and Nobin, A.: The functional importance of sympathetic nerves to the liver and endocrine pancreas. Ann. Surg., *189*:96, 1979.

103. Jenkins, J., Fox, J., and Sharwood-Smith, G.: Changes in body heat during transvesical prostatectomy. Anaesthesia, *38*:748, 1983.

104. Jensen, B.H., Berthelsen, P., and Bröchner-Mortensen, J.: Glomerular filtration rate during halothane anaesthesia and epidural analgesia in combination with halothane anaesthesia. Acta Anaesthesiol. Scand., *21*:395, 1977.

105. Jensen, C.H., Berthelsen, P., Kühl, C., and Kehlet, H.: Effect of epidural analgesia on glucose tolerance during surgery. Acta Anaesthesiol. Scand., *24*:472, 1980.

106. Jørgensen, B.C., Andersen, H.B., Engquist, A.: Influence of epidural morphine on postoperative pain, endocrine-metabolic, and renal responses to surgery: A controlled study. Acta Anaesthesiol. Scand., *26*:63, 1982.

107. Karhunen, U., and Jönn, G.: A comparison of memory function following local and general anaesthesia for extraction of senile cataract. Acta Anaesthesiol. Scand., *26*:291, 1982.

108. Kehlet, H., Brandt, M.R., Prange Hansen, A., and Alberti, K.G.M.M.: Effect of epidural analgesia on metabolic profiles during and after surgery. Br. J. Surg., *66*:543, 1979.

109. Kehlet, H.: The modifying effect of general and regional anesthesia on the endocrine-metabolic response to surgery. Reg. Anaesth., *7*:S38, 1982.

110. Kehlet, H., Wandall, J., and Hjortsø, N.C.: Influence of anesthesia and surgery on immunocompetence. Reg. Anaesth., *7*:S68, 1982.

111. Kehlet, H.: The stress response to anaesthesia and surgery: Release mechanisms and modifying factors. Clin. Anaesth., 2:315, 1984.

112. Kehlet, H.: Pain relief and modification of the stress response. *In* Cousins, M.J., and Phillips, G.D. (eds.): Acute Pain Management. Clin. Crit. Care Med., London, Churchill Livingstone 1986.

113. Kehlet, H., and Schulze, S.: Modification of the general response to injury—Pharmacological and clinical aspects. *In* Little, R.A., and Frayn, K.N. (eds.): The Scientific Basis of Care of the Critically Ill. Manchester, Manchester University Press, 1986.

114. Keith, I.: Anaesthesia and blood loss in total hip replacement. Anaesthesia, *32*:444, 1977.

115. Kent, J.R., and Geist, S.: Lymphocyte transformation during operations with spinal anesthesia. Anesthesiology, *42*:505, 1975.

116. Kinney, J.M., and Felig, P.: The metabolic response to injury and infection. *In* DeGrott, L.J., Cahill, G.F., and Odell, W.D. (eds.): Endocrinology. New York, Grune & Stratton, 1979.

117. Kinney, J.M., and Elwyn, D.H.: Protein metabolism and injury. Annu. Rev. Nutr., *3*:433, 1983.

117a. Kirkeby, O.J., and Risöe, C.: Influence of neural pathways on the pyrexial response to surgical trauma. Acta Chir. Scand., *151*:7, 1985.

118. Kleinerman, J., Sancetta, S.M., and Hackel, D.B.: Effects of high spinal anesthesia on cerebral circulation and metabolism in man. J. Clin. Invest., *37*:285, 1958.

119. Klinck, J.R., and Lindop, M.J.: Epidural morphine in the elderly. A controlled trial after upper abdominal surgery. Anaesthesia, *37*:907, 1982.

120. Korinck, A.M., Languille, M., Bonnet, F., Thibonnier, M., *et al.*: Effect of postoperative extradural morphine on ADH secretion. Br. J. Anaesth., *57*:407, 1985.

121. Kossman, B., Völk, E., and Spilker, E.D.: Influence of thoracic epidural analgesia on glucose, cortisol, insulin, and glucagon responses to surgery. Reg. Anaesth., *7*:107, 1982.

122. Lanz, E., Theiss, D., Riess, W., and Sommer, U.: Epidural morphine for postoperative analgesia: A double-blind study. Anaesth. Analg., *61*:236, 1982.

123. Lautt, W.W.: Afferent and efferent neural roles in liver function. Prog. Neurobiol., *21*:323, 1983.

124. Lewis, R.A., and Arturson, G.: How are prostaglandins and leukotrienes involved in immunological alterations? J. Trauma, *24*:S125, 1984.

125. Lisander, B., Stenqvist, O.: Extradural fentanyl and postoperative ileus in cats. Br. J. Anaesth., *53*:1237, 1981.

126. Little, R.A., and Frayn, K.N.: The Scientific Basis of the Care of the Critically Ill. Manchester, Manchester University Press, 1986.

127. Loft, S., Boel, J., Kyst, A., Rasmussen, B., *et al.*: Increased hepatic microsomal enzyme activity after surgery under halothane or spinal anesthesia. Anesthesiology, *62*:11, 1985.

128. Longnecker, D.E.: Stress free: To be or not to be? Anesthesiology, *51*:643, 1984.

129. Lush, D., Thorpe, J.N., Ricardson, D.J., and Bowen, D.J.: The effect of epidural analgesia on the adrenocortical response to surgery. Br. J. Anaesth., *44*:1169, 1972.

130. Löfström, J.B., Malmquist, L-Å., and Bengtsson, M.: Can the "sympathogalvanic reflex" (skin conductance response) be used to evaluate the height of the sympathetic block in spinal analgesia? Acta Anaesthesiol. Scand., *28*:578, 1984.

130a. MacGregor, R.R., Thorner, R.E., and Wright, D.M.: Lidocaine inhibits granulocyte adherence and prevents granulocyte delivery to inflammatory sites. Blood, *56*:203, 1980.

131. Mann, R.A.M., and Bisset, W.I.K.: Anaesthesia for lower limb amputation. Anaesthesia, *38*:1185, 1983.

132. Markowitz, J., and Campbell, W.R.: The relief of experimental ileus by spinal anesthesia. Am. J. Physiol., *81*:101, 1927.

133. Mather, L.E., Runciman, W.B., and Ilsley, A.H.: Anesthesia-induced changes in regional blood flow. Reg. Anaesth., *7*:S24, 1982.

134. McConn, R. (ed.): The Role of Chemical Mediators in the Pathophysiology of Acute Illness and Injury. New York, Raven Press, 1982.

135. McGowan, S.W., and Smith, G.F.N.: Anaesthesia for transurethral prostatectomy. Anaesthesia, *35*:847, 1980.

136. McKenzie, P.J., Wishart, H.Y., Dewar, K.M.S., Gray, J., *et al.*: Comparison of the effects of spinal anesthesia and general anaesthesia on postoperative oxygenation and perioperative mortality. Br. J. Anaesth., *52*:49, 1980.

137. McKenzie, P.J., Wishart, H.Y., and Smith, G.: Long-term outcome after repair of fractured neck of femur. Br. J. Anaesth., *56*:581, 1984.

138. McLaren, A.D.: Mortality studies. A review. Reg. Anaesth., *7*:S172, 1982.

139. Mehta, P., Theriot, E., Mehrotra, D., Patel, K., *et al.*: Shivering following epidural anesthesia in obstetrics. Reg. Anaesth., *9*:83, 1984.

140. Mellbring, G., Dahlgren, S., Reiz, S., and Sunnegårdh, O.: Thromboembolic complications after major abdominal surgery: Effect of thoracic epidural analgesia. Acta Chir. Scand., *149*:263, 1983.

141. Menzies Gow, N., and Cochrane, J.P.S.: The effect of epidural analgesia on postoperative sodium balance. Br. J. Surg., *66*:864, 1979.

142. Millar, H.R.: Psychiatric morbidity in elderly surgical patients. Br. J. Psychiatry, *138*:17, 1981.

143. Miller, L., Gertel, M., Fox, G.S., and MacLean, L.D.: Comparison of effect of narcotic and epidural analgesia on postoperative respiratory function. Am. J. Surg., *131*:291, 1976.

144. Modig, J., Malmberg, P., and Karlström, G.: Effect of epidural versus general anaesthesia on calf blood flow. Acta Anaesthesiol. Scand., *24*:305, 1980.

145. Modig, J., Hjelmstedt, Å., Sahlstedt, B., and Maripuu, E.: Comparative influences of epidural and general anaesthesia on deep venous thrombosis and pulmonary embolism after total hip replacement. Acta Chir. Scand., *147*:125, 1981.

146. Modig, J., Borg, T., Karlström, G., Sahlstedt, B., *et al.*: Effects of tocainide, an oral analogue of lidocaine, on thromboembolism after total hip replacement. Ups. J. Med. Sci., *86*:269, 1981.

147. Modig, J., Borg, T., Karlström, G., Maripuu, E., *et al.*: Thromboembolism after total hip replacement: Role of epidural and general anesthesia. Anesth. Analg., *62*:174, 1983.

148. Modig, J., Borg, T., Bagge, L., and Saldeen, T.: Role of extradural and of general anaesthesia in fibrinolysis and coagulation after total hip replacement. Br. J. Anaesth., *55*:625, 1983.

149. Moore, R.A., Paterson, G.M.C., Bullingham, R.E.S., Allen, M.C., *et al.*: Controlled comparison of intrathecal cinchocaine with intrathecal cinchocaine and morphine. Br. J. Anaesth., *56*:837, 1984.

150. Moss, N.G.: Renal function of renal afferent and efferent nerve activity. Am. J. Physiol., *243*:F425, 1982.

151. Møller, I.W., Rem, J., Brandt, M.R., and Kehlet, H.: Effect of posttraumatic epidural analgesia on the cortisol and hyper-

glycaemic response to surgery. Acta Anaesthesiol. Scand., *26*:56, 1982.

152. Møller, I.W., Hjortsø, E., Krantz, T., Wandall, E., *et al.*: The modifying effect of spinal anaesthesia on intra- and postoperative adrenocortical and hyperglycemic response to surgery. Acta Anaesthesiol. Scand., *28*:266, 1984.

153. Møller, I.W., Krantz, T., Wandall, E., and Kehlet, H.: Effect of alfentanil anaesthesia on the adrenocortical and hyperglycemic response to surgery. Br. J. Anaesth., *57*:591, 1985.

154. Neely, J., and Catchpole, B.: Ileus: The restoration of alimentary-tract motility by pharmacological means. Br. J. Surg., *58*:21, 1971.

155. Newsome, H.H., and Rose, J.C.: The response of human adrenocorticotrophic hormone and growth hormone to surgical stress. J. Clin. Endocrinol. Metab., *33*:481, 1971.

156. Nimmo, W.S., Littlewood, D.G., Scott, D.B., and Prescott, L.F.: Gastric emptying following hysterectomy with extradural analgesia. Br. J. Anaesth., *50*:559, 1978.

157. Nistrup Madsen, S., Brandt, M.R., Engquist, A., Badawi, I., *et al.*: Inhibition of plasma cyclic AMP, glucose and cortisol response to surgery by epidural analgesia. Br. J. Surg., *64*:669, 1977.

158. Noller, D.W., Gillenwater, J.Y., Howards, S.S., and Vaughan, E.D.: Intercostal nerve block with flank incision. J. Urol., *117*:759, 1977.

159. Oikkonen, M., Rosemberg, P.H., and Nwuvonen, P.J.: Hepatic metabolic ability during anaesthesia. Anaesthesia, *39*:660, 1984.

160. O'Shaughnessey, L., and Slome, D.: Etiology of traumatic shock. Br. J. Surg., *22*:589, 1934.

161. Oyama, T.: Influence of anaesthesia on the endocrine system. *In* Stoeckel, H., and Oyama, T. (eds.): Endocrinology in Anaesthesia and Surgery. p. 39. Heidelberg, Springer Verlag, 1980.

162. Oyama, T., and Matsuki, A.: Plasma cortisol level during epidural anaesthesia and surgery in man. Anaesthesist, *20*:140, 1971.

163. Patel, J.M., Lanzafame, R.J., Williams, J.S., Mullen, B.V., *et al.*: The effect of incisional infiltration of bupivacaine hydrochloride upon pulmonary functions, atelectasis and narcotic need following elective cholecystectomy. Surg. Gynecol. Obstet., *157*:338, 1983.

164. Pflug, A.E., Murphy, T.M., Butler, S.H., and Tucker, G.T.: The effects of postoperative peridural analgesia on pulmonary therapy and pulmonary complications. Anesthesiology, *41*:8, 1974.

165. Pflug, A.E., and Halter, J.B.: Effect of spinal anesthesia on adrenergic tone and the neuroendocrine response to surgical stress in humans. Anesthesiology, *55*:120, 1981.

166. Punnonen, R., and Viinamäki, O.: Vasopressin release following operation upon the vagina performed under general anesthesia or epidural analgesis. Surg. Gynecol. Obstet., *156*:781, 1983.

167. Qvist, T.F., Skovsted, P., and Bredgaard Sørensen, M.: Moderate hypotensive anaesthesia for reduction of blood loss during total hip replacement. Acta Anaesthesiol. Scand., *26*:351, 1982.

168. Ramus, G.V., Cesano, L., and Barbalonga, A.: Different concentrations of local anaesthetics have different modes of action on human lymphocytes. Agents Actions, *13*:333, 1983.

169. Rawal, N., Sjöstrand, U., Christoffersson, E., Dahlström, B., *et al.*: Comparison of intramuscular and epidural morphine for postoperative analgesia in the grossly obese. Anaesth. Analg., *63*:583, 1984.

170. Reiz, S., Bålfors, E., Bredgaard Sørensen, M., Häggmark, S., *et al.*: Coronary hemodynamic effects of general anesthesia and surgery. Reg. Anaesth., *7*:S8, 1982.

171. Rem, J., Kehlet, H., and Brandt, M.R.: Prevention of postoperative lymphopenia and granulocytosis by epidural analgesia. Lancet, *1*:283, 1980.

172. Rem, J., Saxtrup Nielsen, O., Brandt, M.R., and Kehlet, H.: Release mechanisms of postoperative changes in various acute phase proteins and immunoglobulins. Acta Chir. Scand. [Suppl.], *502*:51, 1980.

173. Rem, J., Møller, I.W., Brandt, M.R., and Kehlet, H.: Influence of epidural analgesia on postoperative changes in various serum enzyme patterns and serum bilirubin. Acta Anaesthesiol. Scand., *25*:142, 1981.

174. Rem, J., Feddersen, C., Brandt, M.R., and Kehlet, H.: Postoperative changes in coagulation and fibrinolysis independent of neurogenic stimuli and adrenal hormones. Br. J. Surg., *68*:229, 1981.

175. Renck, H.: The elderly patient after anaesthesia and surgery. Acta Anaesthesiol. Scand., *34*:44, 1969.

176. Richard, L.C., Büller, H.R., Bovill, J., and Ten Cate, J.W.: Influence of anaesthesia on coagulation and fibrinolytic proteins. Br. J. Anaesth., *55*:869, 1983.

177. Riis, J., Lomholt, B., Haxholdt, O., Kehlet, H., *et al.*: Immediate and long-term mental recovery from general versus epidural anesthesia in elderly patients. Acta Anaesthesiol. Scand., *27*:44, 1983.

178. Rimbäck, G., Cassuto, J., Faxén, A., Högström, S., *et al.*: The effect of intra-abdominal bupivacaine instillation on postoperative colonic motility. Gut, *27*:170, 1986.

179. Roizen, M.F., Horrigan, R.W., and Frazer, B.M.: Anesthetic doses blocking adrenergic (stress) and cardiovascular responses to incision—MAC BAR. Anesthesiology, *54*:390, 1981.

180. Rutberg, H., Håkansson, E., Anderberg, B., Jorfeldt, L., *et al.*: Effects of extradural morphine and local anaesthetics on the endocrine response to upper abdominal surgery. Br. J. Anaesth., *56*:233, 1984.

181. Rutberg, H., Anderberg, B., Håkansson, E., Jorfeldt, L., *et al.*: Influence of extradural blockade on serum thyroid hormone concentrations. Acta Chir. Scand., *151*:97, 1985.

182. Rybro, L., Schurizek, B.A., Petersen, T.K., and Wernberg, M.: Postoperative analgesia and lung function: A comparison of intramuscular with epidural morphine. Acta Anaesthesiol. Scand., *26*:514, 1982.

183. Ryhänen, P.: Effects of anesthesia and operative surgery on the immune response of patients of different ages. Thesis. University of Oulu, Finland, 1977.

184. Sandberg, A.A., Eik-Nes, K., Samuels, L.T., and Tyler, F.H.:

The effects of surgery on the blood levels and metabolism of 17-hydroxycorticosteroids in man. J. Clin. Invest., *33*:1507, 1954.

185. Saugbjerg, P., Asoh, T., Lund, C., Petrea, I., *et al.*: Effects of epidural analgesia on scalp recorded somatosensory evoked potentials to posterior tibial nerve stimulation. Acta Anaesthesiol. Scand., *30*:400, 1986.

186. Scheinin, B., Rosenberg, P.H.: Effect of prophylactic epidural morphine or bupivacaine on postoperative pain after upper abdominal surgery. Acta Anaesthesiol. Scand., *26*:474, 1982.

187. Seeling, W., Altemeyer, K-H., Berg, S., Feist, H., *et al.*: Die kontinuierliche thorakale periduralanaesthesie zur intra- und postoperativer analgesie. Anaesthesist, *31*:439, 1982.

188. Seeling, W., and Fehm, H.L.: Eine thorakale PDA mit 0.75%-igen bupivacain hat keinem einfluss auf die ACTH-stimulierte cortisolsekretion. Reg. Anaesth., *7*:11, 1984.

189. Seeling, W., Altemeyer, K-H., Butters, M., Fehm, H.L., *et al.*: Glukose, ACTH, kortisol, T_4, T_3 und rT_3 in plasma nach cholecystektomie. Reg. Anaesth., *7*:1, 1984.

190. Simpson, P.J., Radford, S.G., Forster, S.J., Cooper, G.M., *et al.*: The fibrinolytic effects of anaesthesia. Anaesthesia, *37*:3, 1982.

191. Spence, A.A., and Smith, G.: Postoperative analgesia and lung function: A comparison of morphine with extradural block. Br. J. Anaesth., *43*:144, 1971.

192. Stanley, T.H., Hill, G.E., and Hill, H.R.: The influence of spinal and epidural anesthesia on neutrophil chemotaxis in man. Anesthesiol. Analg., *57*:567, 1978.

193. Stefansson, T., Wickström, I., and Haljamäe, H.: Effects of neuroleptic and epidural analgesia on cardiovascular function and tissue metabolism in the geriatric patient. Acta Anaesthesiol. Scand., *26*:386, 1982.

194. Stewart, G.J.: Antithrombotic activity of local anesthetics in several canine models. Reg. Anaesth., *7*:S89, 1982.

195. Takagi, S., Kitagawa, S., Oshimi, K., Takaku, F., *et al.*: Effect of local anaesthetics on human natural killer cell activity. Clin. Exp. Immunol., *53*:477, 1983.

196. Teasdale, C., McCrum, A., Williams, N.B., and Horton, R.E.: A randomized controlled trial to compare local with general anaesthesia for short-stay inguinal hernia repair. Ann. R. Coll. Surg. Engl., *64*:238, 1982.

197. Thompson, G.E., Miller, R.D., Stevens, W.C., and Murray, W.R.: Hypotensive anesthesia for total hip arthroplasty: A study of blood loss and organ function (brain, heart, liver, and kidney). Anesthesiology, *48*:91, 1978.

198. Thorburn, J.: Subarachnoid blockade and total hip replacement; effect of epinephrine on intraoperative blood loss. Br. J. Anaesth., *57*:290, 1985.

199. Tolksdorf, W., Raiss, G., Striebel, J-P., and Lutz, H.: Intra- und postoperative Kardiopulmonale Komplikationen bei transurethralen Prostataresektionen in Intubationsnarkose und rückenmarksnaher leitungsanästhesie. *In* Wüst, H.J., and Zindler, M. (eds.): Neue Aspekte in der Regional-Anästhesie I. p. 146. Berlin, Springer Verlag, 1980.

200. Traynor, C., Paterson, J.L., Ward, I.D., and Hall, G.M.: Effects of extradural analgesia and vagal blockade on the metabolic and endocrine response to upper abdominal surgery. Br. J. Anaesth., *54*:319, 1982.

201. Treissmann, D.A.: Disruption of colonic anastomosis associated with epidural anesthesia. Reg. Anaesth., *5*:22, 1980.

202. Tsuji, H., and Shirasaka, C.: Inhibition of adrenergic response to upper abdominal surgery with prolonged epidural blockade. Japan. J. Surg., *12*:343, 1982.

203. Tsuji, H., Asoh, T., Takeuchi, Y., and Shirasaka, C.: Attenuation of adrenocortical response to upper abdominal surgery with epidural blockade. Br. J. Surg., *70*:122, 1983a.

204. Tsuji, H., Shirasaka, C., Asoh, T., and Takeuchi, Y.: Influences of splanchnic nerve blockade on endocrine-metabolic responses to upper abdominal surgery. Br. J. Surg., *70*:437, 1983b.

205. Tyler, E., Caldwell, C., and Ghia, J.N.: Transcutaneous electrical nerve stimulation: An alternative approach to the management of postoperative pain. Anesth. Analg., *61*:449, 1982.

206. Tönnesen, E., Hüttel, M.S., Christensen, N.J., and Schmitz, O.: Natural killer cell activity in patients undergoing upper abdominal surgery: Relationship to the endocrine stress response. Acta Anaesthesiol. Scand., *28*:654, 1984.

207. Ukai, M., Moran, W.H., and Zimmermann, B.: The role of visceral afferent pathways on vasopressin secretion and urinary excretory patterns during surgical stress. Ann. Surg., *168*:16, 1968.

208. Valentin, N., Lomholt, B., Jensen, J.S., Hejgaard, N., *et al.*: Spinal or general anaesthesia for surgery of the fractured hip? Br. J. Anaesth., *58*:284, 1986.

209. Vatashsky, E., Beilin, B., and Aronson, H.B.: Common bile duct pressure in dogs after opiate injections—Epidural versus intravenous route. Can. Anaesth. Soc. J., *31*:650, 1984.

210. Vaugham, M.S., Vaugham, R.W., and Cork, R.C.: Postoperative hypothermia in adults: Relationship of age, anesthesia and shivering to rewarming. Anesth. Analg., *60*:746, 1981.

211. Verhoef, J., and Sharmu, S.D.: Inhibition of human natural killer activity by lysosomotropic agents. J. Immunol., *131*:125, 1983.

212. Wagenknecht, L.V., Zamora, M., and Madsen, P.O.: Continuous recording of renal clearance by external monitoring during epidural anesthesia. Invest. Urol., *8*:540, 1971.

213. Wagner, R.L., and White, P.F.: Etomidate inhibits adrenocortical function in surgical patients. Anesthesiology, *61*:647, 1984.

214. Webb, P.J., James, F.M., and Wheeler, A.S.: Shivering during epidural analgesia in women during labour. Anesthesiology, *55*:706, 1981.

215. Whelan, P., and Morris, P.J.: Immunological responsiveness after transurethral resection of the prostate: General versus spinal anaesthetic. Clin. Exp. Immunol., *48*:611, 1982.

216. White, I.W.C., and Chapell, W.A.: Anaesthesia for surgical correction of fractured femoral neck. A comparison of three techniques. Anaesthesia, *35*:1107, 1980.

217. White, I.W.C., Gelb, A.W., Wexler, H.R., Stiller, C.R., *et al.*: The effects of intravenous anaesthetic agents on human neutrophil chemiluminiscence. Can. Anaesth. Soc. J., *30*:506, 1983.

218. Wickström, I., Holmberg, I., and Stefansson, T.: Survival of female geriatric patients after hip fracture surgery. A comparison of 5 anesthetic methods. Acta Anaesthesiol. Scand., *26*:607, 1982.

219. Wiklund, L.: Splanchnic oxygen uptake in relation to systemic oxygen uptake during postoperative splanchnic blockade and postoperative fentanyl analgesia. Acta Anaesthesiol. Scand., *19*:29, 1975.

220. Wiklund, L., and Jorfeldt, L.: Splanchnic turn-over of some energy metabolites and acid-base balance during intravenous infusion of lidocaine, bupivacaine, or etidocaine. Acta Anaesthesiol. Scand., *25*:200, 1981.

221. Wilmore, D.W.: Hormonal responses and their effect on metabolism. Surg. Clin. North Amer., *56*:999, 1976.

222. Wilmore, D.W., Long, J.M., Mason, A.D., and Pruitt, B.A.: Stress in surgical patients as a neurophysiologic reflex response. Surg. Gynecol. Obstet., *142*:257, 1976.

223. Wilmore, D.W.: Alterations in protein, carbohydrate and fat metabolism in injured and septic patients. J. Am. Coll. Nutr., *2*:3, 1983.

224. Wüst, H.J., Fiedler, H-W., Trobisch, H., and Richter, O.: Fibrinolyse—Und komplementsystem—profile während aortofemoraler bypassimplantation. Anaesthesist, *31*:564, 1982.

225. Yaksh, T.L., and Hammond, D.L.: Peripheral and central substrates involved in the rostrad transmission of nociceptive information. Pain, *13*:1, 1982.

part two
TECHNIQUES OF NEURAL BLOCKADE

6 PATIENT MANAGEMENT FOR NEURAL BLOCKADE: SELECTION, MANAGEMENT, PREMEDICATION, AND SUPPLEMENTATION

PHILLIP O. BRIDENBAUGH

Without regard to which nerve block technique might be considered or with which local anesthetic agent, the principles of general anesthesia are just as essential for a successful outcome of a neural blockade anesthetic. This includes the essential ingredients of a well-trained anesthetist working in a well-equipped anesthetizing location. There are additional requirements, however, for the successful practice of the subspecialty area of neural blockade. The anesthetist must be skilled, not just in the technical aspects of "how" to accomplish a selected technique, but also in its indications, contraindications, and proper intraoperative management. Initially, and hopefully during one's early training in anesthesia, these skills are taught and closely supervised by an expert in the subspecialty. From this beginning, the anesthetist who has a sincere interest in neural blockade and who is convinced of its efficacy will continue to use and polish these skills until they become an essential part of his anesthetic armamentarium. A thorough knowledge of the pertinent anatomy obtained from textbooks and atlases should be reinforced through visualization in both cadavers and surgical specimens. In addition, one should be familiar with the physiology and pharmacology of the local anesthetic agents themselves, as well as the physiologic effects and complications that accompany the various regional anesthetic techniques. One can therefore anticipate any changes in the patient's status and not only determine the suitability of a given technique for a specific patient undergoing a specific operation, but also be prepared to institute therapy if and when those changes occur.

Finally, this thorough knowledge of the requirements for successful neural blockade also requires that the anesthetist undertake his activities in a suitable anesthetizing location equipped not only with a block tray but also with other anesthetic and resuscitation drugs and equipment. Under all but the most unusual circumstances, an assistant to the anesthetist is essential for optimal patient care, and this applies as equally to regional anesthesia as it does to general anesthesia.

PREANESTHETIC MANAGEMENT

Most anesthetic selections begin with the notification of the anesthetist, usually through the operative schedule, to provide the anesthetic for a named patient scheduled to undergo a specific surgical procedure. That time is the first opportunity to determine, principally on the basis of the surgical procedure, whether certain regional anesthetic techniques can be used. Knowledge of the surgeon's abilities and personality will also, likely, play a role in that determination. With that degree of forethought, one is then in a better position to conduct the preanesthetic review of the patient's chart and to visit the patient.

PATIENT SELECTION

The most important, if not the final, determinant in the selection of a regional anesthetic technique is the suitability of that technique to the patient. Unless careful consideration is given to this aspect of the anesthetic management, all else will likely fail. Patient selection must give consideration to anatomy, pathophysiology, and psychological state.

Because nearly all regional anesthetic techniques are based on the identification and utilization of anatomic landmarks, it is essential that the patient be able to display those landmarks. Examples of anatomic impediments to the conduct of a successful block include morbid obesity, severe arthritis, and other limitations to accurate patient positioning to perform the block.

Pathophysiologic considerations may be either local or systemic. Local conditions such as infection, dermatitis, trauma, burns, or dressings could all preclude the opportunity to do a block. More subtle, and often more important, are the systemic problems of the patient. Clearly a severely hypovolemic patient should not be considered for a technique that involves major sympathetic neural blockade unless appropriate prophylaxis is accomplished beforehand. Patients with neurologic disease, coagulopathies, or severe cardiovascular disease all need to have careful laboratory documentation of their pathology. It may turn out that one type of block technique would be contraindicated whereas another might be perfectly acceptable. Coincident with this evaluation of patient physical status as it affects the selection of anesthesia techniques is the drug therapy the patient is receiving. Of special concern for centrally acting blocks (spinal, epidural, and celiac plexus) are the vasoactive drug such as antihypertensives, alpha-blocking agents, and beta-blocking agents. These drugs in combination with a major sympathetic nerve block can precipitate major management problems for the anesthetist.

Finally, the mental attitude or psychologic makeup of the patient will play a major role in determining the advisability of selecting a regional anesthetic technique. This is highly specific to the type of surgical and anesthetic technique being considered.

The patient who would accept a single venipuncture for a 45-minute Bier block might be hysterical at the thought of a spinal anesthetic for amputation of the leg. Equally as difficult to manage as the excitable patient is the disoriented patient. Mental disorientation, whether senile, pathologic, or pharmacologic, may not prevent the accomplishment of a successful nerve block but will likely commit the anesthetist to unconscious levels of sedation during the conduct of the operation. Clearly, nerve blocks that require patient cooperation with positioning or identification of paresthesias are difficult to accomplish in psychologically disturbed patients. Parenthetically, it may be noted that somnolent or comatose patients are ideal candidates for nerve block techniques that can be accomplished with a peripheral nerve stimulator, making patient participation unnecessary.

In addition to the aforementioned considerations that aid in selecting suitable patients for regional anesthetic techniques, the anesthetist must undertake the other aspects of the preanesthetic visit. This includes the history and chart review to determine whether the patient has major systemic disease, current medications, past operations and anesthetics, allergies, dental status, and family history of anesthetic problems. Further, all laboratory studies essential for the conduct of a general anesthetic must be accomplished before anesthesia. For purposes of the preanesthetic visit and evaluation, all patients must first be candidates for a general anesthetic before they are considered candidates for a regional block technique. It is a rare regional anesthetic that can be guaranteed as 100% satisfactory at zero percent risk of needing to medicate, anesthetize, or resuscitate the patient.

PATIENT INTERVIEW

Once the anesthetist has satisfied himself that the patient is a candidate for a regional anesthetic technique, he must so inform the patient. A general, but useful, definition of informed consent is the obligation to explain to the patient [1] the risks and benefits of your selected anesthetic as opposed to [2] the risks and benefits of an alternate technique. Clearly, the anesthetist must first be convinced in his own mind that regional anesthesia is the preferred technique before he can convince his patient.

A significant number of patients refuse a regional anesthetic because they "don't want to be awake during the operation." It is essential, therefore, that the anesthetist describe in chronological detail the fact that the patient will receive a "sleeping pill" the evening before surgery, a sedative an hour before surgery, and additional intravenous medications as needed and desired by the patient during both the induction of the anesthetic and the conduct of the operation. It is equally important that a detailed description of the performance of the block be given to the patient, including initiation of the intravenous line, position during the block, and any cooperative role required of him in identifying paresthesias or vascular reactions. As long as the patient knows what to expect and has the anesthetist's assurance that incremental sedation will be administered as required for patient comfort, most patients will consent to a regional anesthetic. Informing the patient about the rationale for neural blockade will further motivate patients toward acceptance. It is worth mentioning that neural blockade will greatly reduce the amount of anesthetic and muscle relaxant drugs required; that it may avoid endotracheal intubation; and that it will allow a painless transition during the recovery period and a more rapid return of normal mental function. In hip and prostatic surgery, blood loss may be greatly reduced and transfusion therefore avoided. Evidence now indicates that risk of venous thrombosis is less and the "stress response" of the body is reduced, so that there is less interference with important body functions. The amount of information given will vary for each patient; however, such discussion invariably increases the confidence of the patient and may influence his response postoperatively. Data in the psychology literature indicate that patients benefit considerably from good preparation for procedures[35] (see Chap. 25).

All that remains, then, is for the anesthetist to write that he has discussed the use of a selected regional anesthetic and that the patient understands what is to be done and agrees with the anesthetist's selection.

PREMEDICATION OF PATIENTS FOR NEURAL BLOCKADE TECHNIQUES

Just as the principles applied to selection of a regional anesthetic technique are primarily those used for general anesthetic, so too are the basic tenets in writing the preanesthetic orders. All patients who will receive anesthesia, without regard to choice of technique, should have nothing by mouth (NPO) from the evening before surgery or for a minimum of 6 hours, if possible. Similarly, most patients will appreciate receipt of a mild sleeping medication even if they do not use such in their daily lives. As long as the selected drug is not of inordinately long duration or given inordinately close to the conduct of anesthesia, there is nothing unique to regional anesthesia that makes the choice of a specific drug important. There are, however, opinions and controversies about the choice of the other drugs commonly used in premedicating patients for regional anesthesia and surgery.

ANTICHOLINERGICS

Most practitioners of regional anesthesia have now abandoned the routine use of anticholinergics unless they plan to supplement their blocks to levels of unconsciousness. Those abandoning the preoperative use of these drugs have considered primarily their antisialogogue effect; however, these drugs may be used in combination with other drugs to produce sedation and amnesia, to reduce reflex bradycardia, and to reduce gastric hydrogen ion secretion. Earlier practitioners of anesthesia frequently preferred scopolamine to atropine for its perceived amnesic effects. Frumin and colleagues, however, compared scopolamine alone in a dose of 0.4 mg with diazepam added in doses of 5 mg, 7.5 mg, and 10 mg.[14] Whereas patients had nearly total recall on three different tests with the scopolamine alone, they demonstrated maximum amnesia (67%) with the addition of 7.5 mg of diazepam. The 10 mg dose was no better than the 7.5 mg dose.

The remaining major indication for the anticholinergics was to provide a measure of vagal blockade deemed especially important if one planned a major sympathetic block such as high spinal, epidural, or a celiac plexus block. Current practice is to give incremental doses of atropine or glycopyrolate intravenously if and as needed to counteract reflex bradycardia. In general, patient discomfort in the form of an extremely dry mouth has convinced most practitioners of regional anesthesia to use intravenous vagolytics or antisialogogues if and when they are indicated.

NARCOTIC ANALGESICS

Inclusion of analgesic doses of a narcotic into the premedication of patients who will be undergoing a regional anesthetic should be given strong consideration. Whereas the patient who will receive routine general anesthesia may suffer no greater pain than the insertion of a single infusion needle before going to sleep, the patient who will receive regional anesthesia must receive several needle punctures and change positions on occasion. Further, the neural blockade renders only portions of the patient's anatomy analgesic. A narcotic premedicant will also provide analgesia for the nonblocked areas of the patient's body. Two major determinants for the inclusion of a narcotic include the type of nerve block and the mental attitude of the patient. Nerve blocks that require no paresthesias or multiple punctures may not require a narcotic. Conversely, the paravertebral blocks (intercostal, lumbar sympathetics or paramedian spinal and epidural) pass through significant areas of soft tissue and can be quite painful to the unmedicated patient. Similarly, the more apprehensive or excitable the patient, the greater is the need for higher doses of premedicant drugs. Although narcotics may do less to sedate or tranquilize a patient than those specific drugs, they still constitute an important part of the premedication.

Excitable or apprehensive patients heavily medicated with only nonanalgesic sedatives or tranquilizers tend to be drowsy or relaxed if not stimulated but will often over-react or react inappropriately and in an uncooperative way during administration of the nerve block.

As always, the selection of a specific narcotic in the appropriate premedicant dose must be individualized to the patient and to the procedure selected by the anesthesiologist. Some recent changes in our practices, however, should be noted. Contrary to times past, it is currently accepted that *oral* premedications may be given without increased risk and to the comfort of the patient over the earlier intramuscular route.[16] Kay and colleagues[18] conducted a double-blind study of the effect of oral controlled-release morphine, 30 mg, on preoperative anxiety, anesthetic requirements, and postoperative pain in patients undergoing cholecystectomy. Although the patients who received morphine were more sedated than the placebo group, there was no significant difference in the anxiety scores of the two groups. During anesthesia, there were also no significant differences between the groups, although the morphine patients required less anesthetic supplement and appeared to recover more slowly than did the placebo group.

Another advance in our practice is the availability of a variety of new premedicant drugs, which in the narcotic category include fentanyl and alfentanyl. These two drugs and a number of others still being studied represent a search for potent, short-acting analgesics. As premedicants, they have less to offer than their longer-acting predecessors. As will be noted in subsequent discussions of intraoperative supplementation of regional anesthesia, however, they play a major role, particularly for outpatient surgery.

SEDATIVES AND HYPNOTICS

Earlier practitioners of regional anesthesia combined short-acting barbiturates with narcotics as their premedicant of choice. Although the phenothiazine derivatives enjoyed some popularity, their effects on the circulation were such as to contraindicate their use in a number of situations in which either hypovolemia or high sympathetic blockade, or both, existed. Just as new narcotics have found their place in regional anesthesia, so have the newer sedatives and hypnotics, primarily butyrophenone or benzodiazepine derivatives. After some initial popularity as a premedicant, Innovar, the 50 : 1 mixture of droperidol and fentanyl, has gradually been replaced with longer-acting narcotics and a shorter-acting sedative, usually a benzodiazepine.

The perceived advantage of the butyrophenones is in their ability to produce a state of mental calm and indifference with little hypnotic effect. It was soon discovered, however, that larger doses, especially without analgesic or sedative drugs already present, could produce hallucinations, restlessness, and even extrapyramidal dyskinesias.[44] There has been a recent return of the use of droperidol in lower doses (2.5 – 5 mg) as a premedicant to exploit its antiemetic effects. Mortensen, using 2.5 mg or 5 mg doses of droperidol intravenously in a study of 300 women, showed a significant reduction from 34.4% (in controls) to 10.3% after droperidol in the frequency of nausea and vomiting postoperatively during the first 24 hours. Further, there was no difference between the 2.5 mg dose and the 5 mg dose.[31]

As is well known, however, no single factor is responsible for, nor any single drug capable of, preventing nausea or vomiting in the operative period. Palazzo and Strunin, in their review of anesthesia and emesis, noted that children and women were more susceptible to nausea and vomiting in the perioperative period.[34] It behooves the anesthetist to be aware of the many factors predisposing to these problems and to alter premedication accordingly.

Perhaps the most popular premedicant for patients undergoing neural blockade is diazepam, not only because of its potent amnesic properties but also because of its alleged anticonvulsant properties. deJong[6] first reported on the superiority of diazepam over barbiturates in preventing seizures from local anesthesia overdose in animals (see Chap. 2). As a result of those animal studies, diazepam has enjoyed widespread use in the prevention and treatment of toxic seizures with local anesthetic agents. A serious criticism needs to be given, however, against the use of diazepam as a prophylactic to allow use of greater than the recommended doses of local anesthetic agents. Many factors contribute to a given patient's toxic threshold to local anesthetics. It is important, therefore, that the selected dose of a local anesthetic be at or below that recommended. Giving a larger premedicant dose of diazepam will not guarantee against a seizure in the face of a local anesthetic overdose.

For those patients in whom amnesia is the desired effect, other benzodiazepines besides diazepam may be considered (*e.g.*, lorazepam, midazolam, flunitrazepam). Since the introduction of the benzodiazepines into clinical practice, there has been a constant search for a potent, short-acting amnesic. Diazepam has been the "standard" against which all of the other benzodiazepines have been compared. In early studies,[24] lorazepam in doses of 2 mg, 3 mg, and 4 mg as oral premedication for surgery and regional anesthesia was shown to produce a higher incidence of anterograde amnesia than diazepam. Both drugs provided adequate sedation without side-effects, but lorazepam did provide a higher incidence and degree of drowsiness. Because of its slow onset of effect, others have advocated using lorazepam for both nighttime sedation and premedication before surgery. Studd and Eltringham[43] compared lorazepam, 2.5 mg, with diazepam, 10 mg, in 50 healthy patients who would undergo surgery and found the quality of sleep the night before surgery superior in the lorazepam group. The frequency of effective preoperative sedation was similar in both groups. Although the incidence of amnesia for visual stimuli after lorazepam was higher than that after diazepam, there was no difference in the recall of auditory and painful stimuli. The overall incidence of side-effects was similar for each drug, although excessive salivation, as noted by other authors,[7] was more frequent after lorazepam but not statistically significant. Although there was no significant difference between the two with regard to time to awaken from anesthesia, the long duration of action of lorazepam and high blood levels even 24 hours after administration raise questions about its suitability as a drug for outpatients.[8] McKay and Dundee[28] not only focused on the amnesic properties of three different benzodiazepines (diazepam, flunitrazepam, lorazepam) in different doses, but also compared routes of administration. Although most clinicians have learned that these drugs are not only less effective but also painful when administered intramuscularly, they are less aware of the differences in onset and effectiveness of these drugs when given orally and intravenously. These investigators showed that all three drugs, when given orally in doses normally used for premedication, produced dose-related anterograde amnesia. This paralleled closely, both in extent and duration, their sedative action. No detectable amnesia was found, however, with minimal tranquilizing doses of diazepam (5 mg) or lorazepam (1 mg). Also in this study, *retrograde* amnesia was a sporadic occurrence that was neither drug- nor dose-related.

Finally, of importance in using these drugs as premedicants is the observation (Fig. 6-1) that the amnesic effects of diazepam intravenously are maximal in 2 to 3 minutes and nearly gone before the effects of the oral dose become apparent (20 minutes), with the latter having a peak effect at 60 minutes. This supports our common practice of administering oral diazepam as a premedicant not more than 60 minutes before inducing regional anesthesia, with subsequent intravenous doses during operation.

If the regional technique being planned does not require a significant degree of patient awareness or cooperation, then the benzodiazepine–narcotic combination is highly recommended. A random study of 120 surgical patients in four groups of 2 mg and 5 mg of lorazepam alone or in combination with 5 mg of morphine showed that the addition of morphine to lorazepam significantly improved sedation and relief of anxiety. Lack of recall was enhanced by increasing the dose of lorazepam from 2 mg to 4 mg. The only significant side-effect was restlessness, which occurred in 15% of patients receiving 4 mg of lorazepam alone and in 3% of patients receiving 2 mg of lorazepam alone.[23]

Pain on injection and venous thrombosis are un-

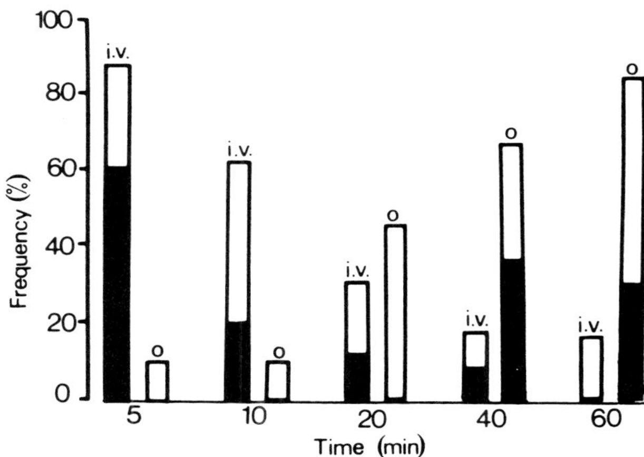

FIG. 6-1. Percentage frequency of complete *(solid)* and partial *(clear)* failure of recognition at the times shown following the i.v. and oral (*o*) administration of diazepam 10 mg. (McKay, A.C., Dundee, J.W.: Effect of oral benzodiazepines on memory. Br. J. Anaesth., *52:*1254, 1980.)

wanted side-effects of diazepam attributed to its poor water solubility and need for organic solvents. Recently midazolam, a water-soluble benzodiazepine with actions similar to those of diazepam, has been introduced. Early studies in surgical patients showed that it was about twice as potent (dose for weight) as diazepam and had neither pain on injection nor venous sequelae. Maximum amnesia after 5 mg doses intravenously occurred between 2 and 5 minutes after injection and had mainly subsided in 20 to 30 minutes (Fig. 6-2).[10]

Two generalizations regarding the premedication of patients for neural blockade should be stated: [1] Larger doses of sedatives and narcotics may be given to healthy and emotionally distraught patients, especially those scheduled for stimulating nerve blocks that do not require patient response to paresthesias or cooperation with changes in position; and [2] light doses or even no premedication should be given to the very elderly or poor-risk patient. Small increments of intravenous drug under the watchful eye of the anesthetist just before the block may be just as effective and far safer. This is also the recommended practice for outpatients receiving regional block procedures.

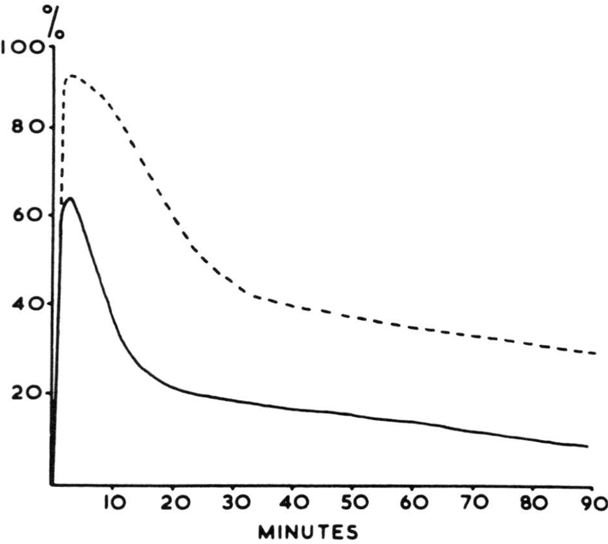

FIG. 6-2. Incidence of complete amnesia (—) and partial amnesia (- - -) following midazolam 6 mg i.v. (Dundee, J.W., Samuel, I.O., Toner, W., Howard, P.J.: Midazolam: A water-soluble benzodiazepine. Anaesthesia, *35*:460, 1980.)

MANAGEMENT OF THE PATIENT RECEIVING NEURAL BLOCKADE

One of the cardinal principles for the safe and efficient practice of anesthesia is a well-equipped anesthetizing location. Anesthetists accustomed to working in operating rooms are familiar with the insecurity and inadequacy of administering anesthesia in other areas of the hospital not routinely used or designed as anesthetizing locations, for example, radiology departments and dental clinics. It is equally important, therefore, that the anesthetist performing neural blockade have access to a suitable location—operating room or induction area of sufficient size to provide proper lighting, space, and equipment for administering his anesthetic. Induction areas are preferable to operating rooms in that they allow performance of regional anesthesia in a quieter (and frequently less expensive) environment and often can be accomplished while a preceding operative procedure is being completed or the operating room is being prepared for the forthcoming procedure.

Before discussing the special equipment and supplies required for neural blockade, it should be emphasized that all induction or anesthetizing areas must have as a minimum the basic resuscitation equipment required for airway management and intravenous therapy, and the monitors and equipment needed to complete cardiopulmonary resuscitation (see Chap. 4, Tables 4-9 and 4-10). Every practitioner of neural blockade, even those using infiltration or minor nerve blocks as part of office procedures, should have this basic equipment immediately available (Fig. 6-3). There are still too many anecdotes or case reports of serious complications as a result of inadequate treatment to recommend otherwise.

EQUIPMENT SPECIFIC TO NEURAL BLOCKADE

There are, naturally, extremes of anesthesia practice from the solo office practice to a large anesthesia teaching department. The necessary equipment will vary accordingly. Nonetheless, suggestions regarding basic equipment may be useful to most and can be modified to individual needs and desires.

Block Trays

Basically, two types of neural blockade techniques are performed by anesthetists: [1] central, that is, spi-

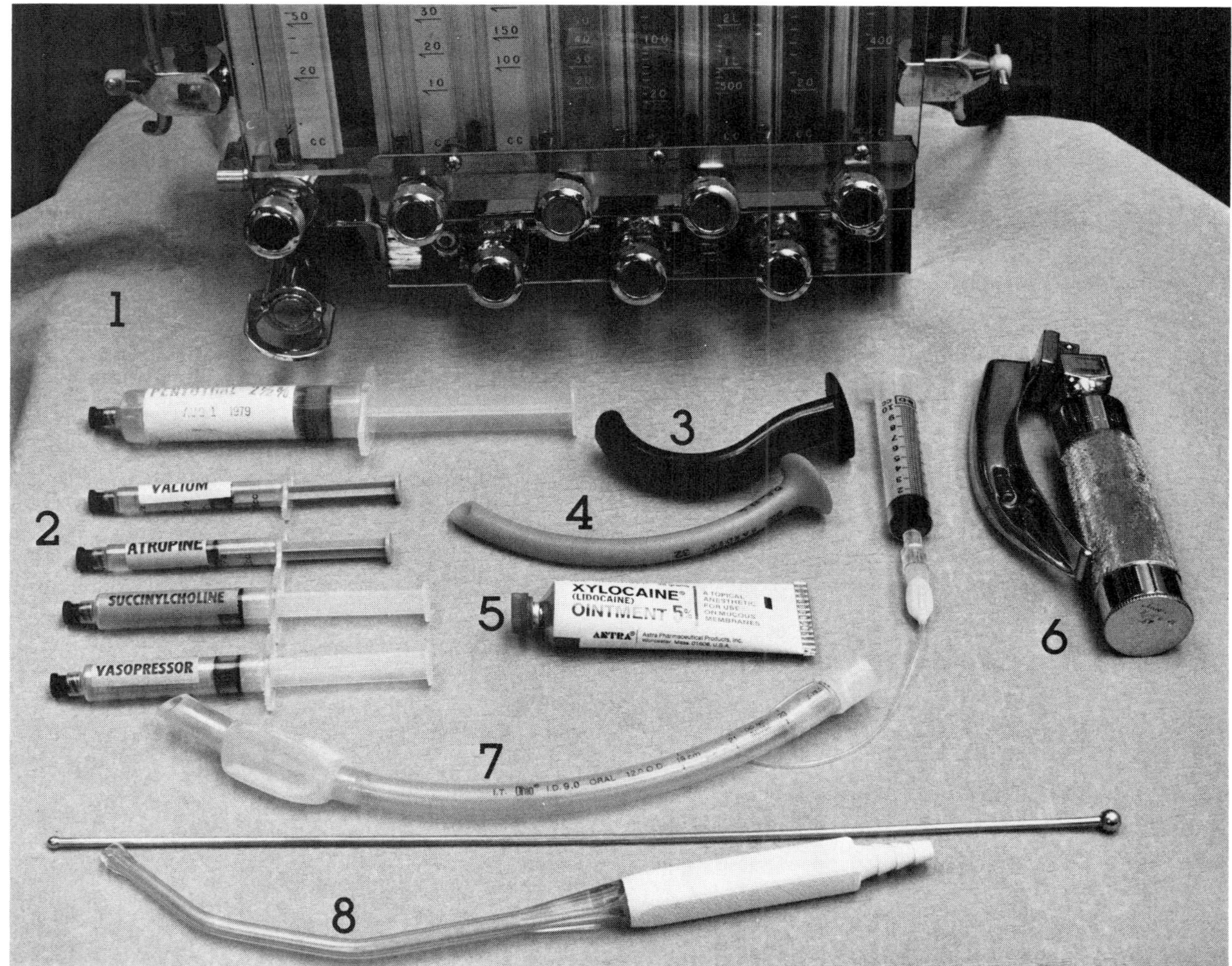

FIG. 6-3. Equipment for resuscitation and treatment of adverse reactions. (*1*) Anesthesia machine as source of oxygen and ventilation; (*2*) labeled syringes containing succinylcholine, atropine, vasopressor (ephedrine, 5 mg/ml), diazepam, and thiopental; (*3*) oropharyngeal airway; (*4*) nasopharyngeal airway; (*5*) topical anesthetic; (*6*) laryngoscope and blade; (*7*) endotracheal tube with stylet and cuff syringe; (*8*) Yankauer suction.

nal, epidural, and caudal, and [2] peripheral nerve blocks. Because the equipment required for epidural and spinal is sufficiently different, most departments will have separate trays for these two procedures (caudal usually being included in the epidural tray). The specific requirements of syringes, needles, and ancillary equipment will be discussed in the following chapters that describe each technique.

Apart from the specific needles and syringes, some basic components should be a part of all block trays, including [1] a liquid impermeable tray into which all components may be put for sterilization and storage; [2] a cup, sponges, and sponge forceps for receipt and application of the skin preparation solution (usually an iodine derivative such as povodone); [3] several additional sponges for wiping skin surfaces during the block; [4] several small towels for draping the area to be blocked; [5] frequently a medicine cup for containing the local anesthetic solution; and [6] a sterility indicator (Fig. 6-4).

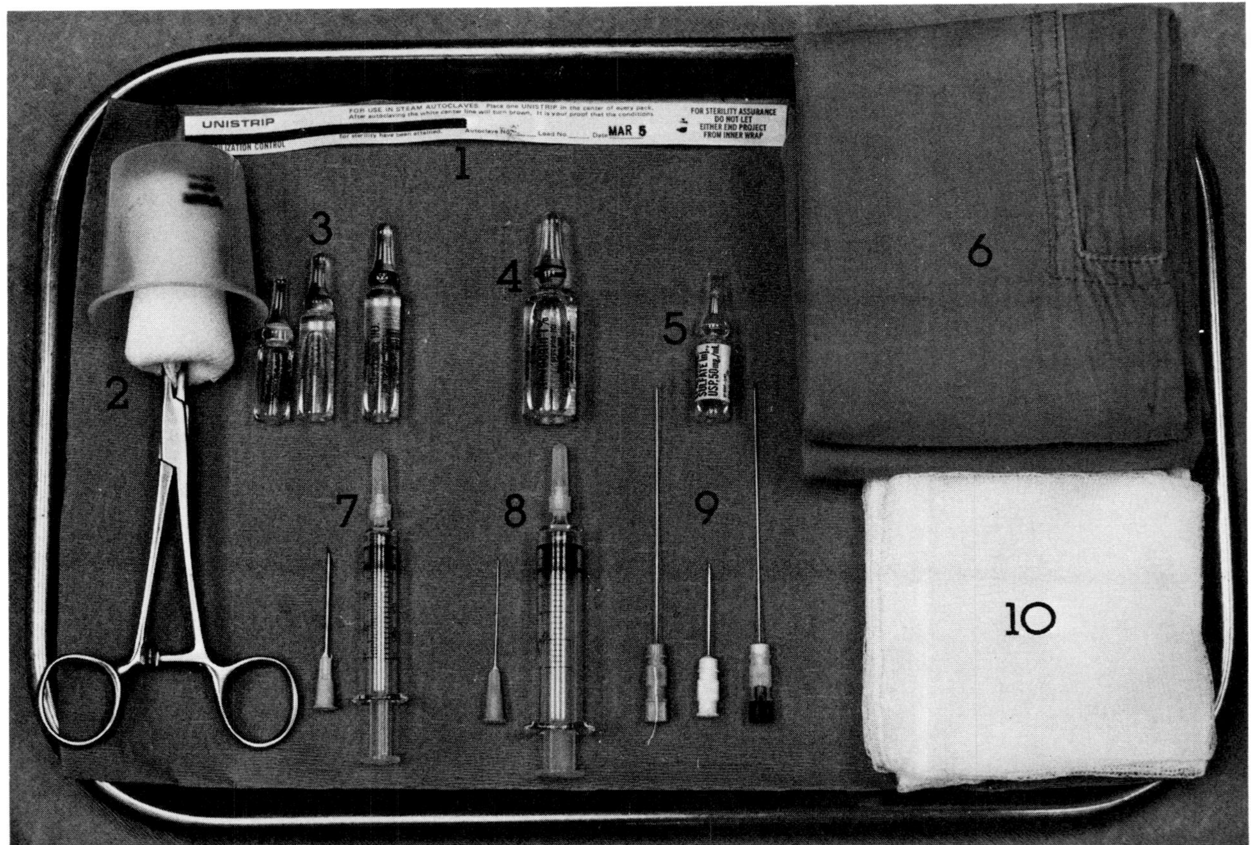

FIG. 6-4. Spinal tray, department-prepared with disposable components. (*1*) Sterility indicator; (*2*) Preparation sponge and forceps for antiseptic solution (iodine tincture, 1%, or povidone-iodine); (*3*) drugs for spinal anesthesia; (*4*) local anesthetic solution for infiltration; (*5*) vasopressor; (*6*) fenestrated drape; (*7*) mixing needle and disposable syringe for spinal anesthesia drugs; (*8*) disposable syringe and 25-gauge needle for local infiltration; (*9*) disposable needles for spinal anesthesia—22-gauge and 25-guage with 20-guage introducer: (*10*) sponges.

For the past two decades, there has been a gradual replacement, in many centers, of internally prepared block trays with disposable, commercially produced trays. The determination of which one to use is very subjective and relates to cost, convenience, reliability, and even locale. In an early comparison of hospital trays with disposable trays, no difference was found, either in quality of anesthesia or in frequency of complications. A summary of other consumers of disposable trays reported no neurologic complications for the use of 242,018 disposable spinal trays containing no drugs.[3] Since that early study, millions of commercially prepared disposable trays for all types of neural blockade techniques have been used without apparent problems. Just as with hospital trays, they do have a finite shelf life, albeit considerably longer, and should be checked periodically to be certain that they are not outdated. The use of outdated trays may not only increase the risk of possible contamination, but also increase the possibility that any drugs within the disposable tray will have exceeded their time for maximum efficacy. In summary, the strongest argument for the use of commercially prepared disposable trays is for the anesthesia department in which the volume of certain block techniques does not support the high cost of labor, stainless steel needles and trays, glass syringes, and so forth required for hospital prepared trays. What the disposable tray lacks in quality of equipment it provides in sterility, reliability, efficiency, and availability of equipment for a variety of neural blockade techniques to practitioners who do not have the time or the personnel to gather pieces of equipment on each occasion they want to perform a regional block technique. Some departments gather all the required neural blockade equipment on a purpose designed cart (Fig. 6-5).

Special Equipment

To improve the success rate of neural blockade or to make it possible in very difficult cases and extreme circumstances, special devices, needles, and pieces of equipment have been advocated or introduced. Most illustrative of this would be the various needles and modifications on the technique of epidural anesthesia, all aimed at making identification of the ligamen-

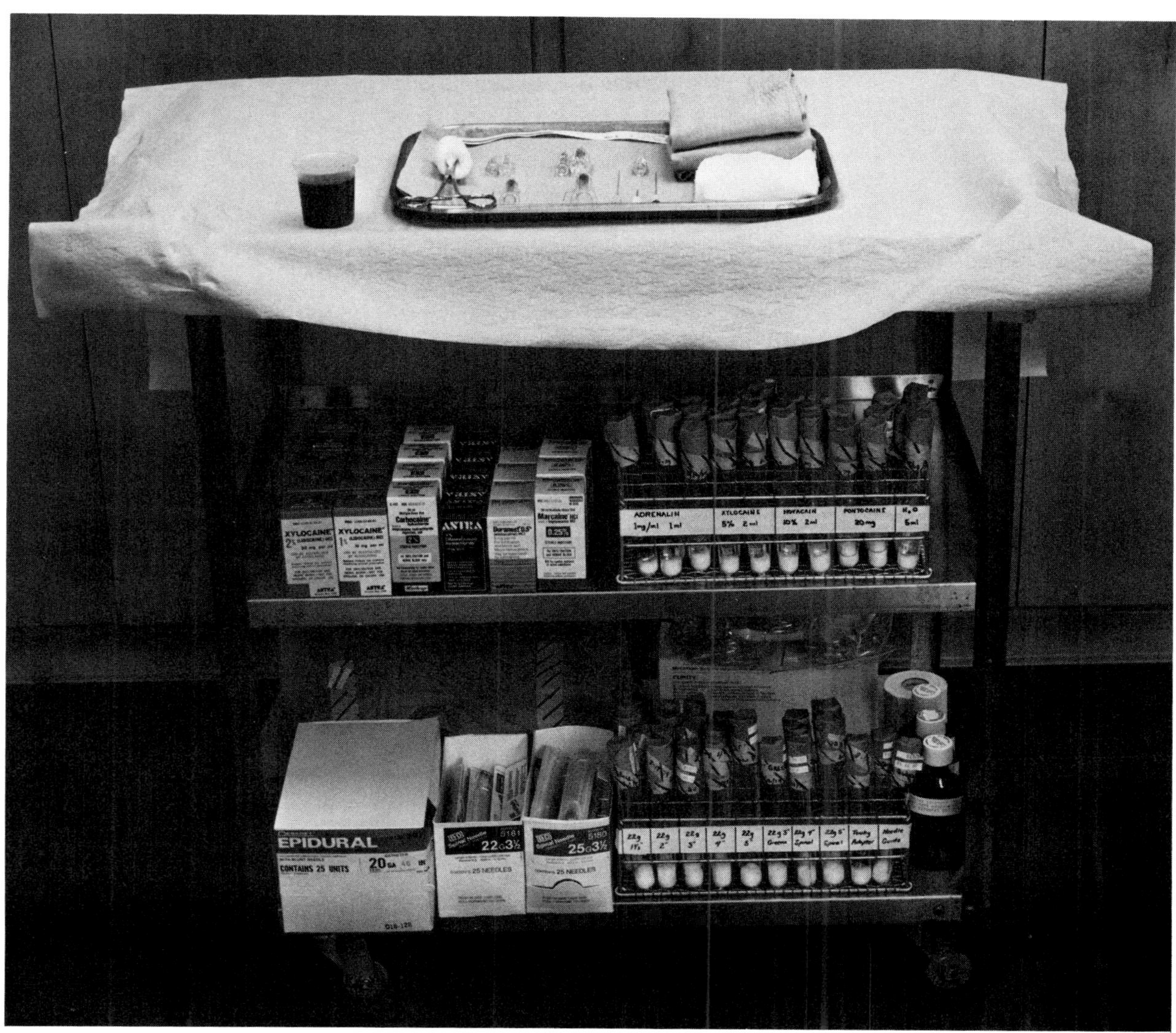

FIG. 6-5. Mobile regional anesthesia cart. Top shelf, work surface for block tray. Middle shelf, assortment of local anesthetic solutions for spinal, epidural, and caudal anesthesia and peripheral nerve blocks. Bottom shelf, disposable and reusable needles for spinal, epidural, and caudal anesthesia and peripheral nerve blocks, epidural catheters, block trays, tape, preparation solution, and nasal oxygen cannulae.

tum flavum or epidural space more certain (see Chap. 7). Many practitioners have advocated radiologic verification of needle placement as the surest way to succeed. Although this is probably true and has much to recommend it for very difficult blocks or those for the placement of neurolytic solutions, it is too expensive and time consuming to become a viable tool for the daily practice of neural blockade.

Peripheral Nerve Stimulators

The use of the peripheral nerve stimulator to locate nerves with motor fiber components has become increasingly popular. Although the original description of this technique has been ascribed to Von Perthes, it received little recognition until after the equipment for peripheral nerve stimulation became available to evaluate neuromuscular blockade. Although several early reports on the efficacy of such equipment appeared, they all recommended the use of sheathed needles. Montgomery and co-workers[29] acknowledged these contributions but reported that standard, unsheathed steel needles (as normally used for neural blockade) could also be used with the nerve stimulator. They showed that the current density was greatest at the tip of the needle (Fig. 6-6), although they did obtain tissue and nerve stimulation from the side of the needle as well. This made available to most clinicians a new technique of neural blockade without the need for unusual special equipment. Many refinements of this technique have been made over the past 15 to 20 years. More sophisticated nerve stimulators and specially prepared shielded needles are now readily available through various commercial outlets (see "Needles and Drugs" section in this chapter).

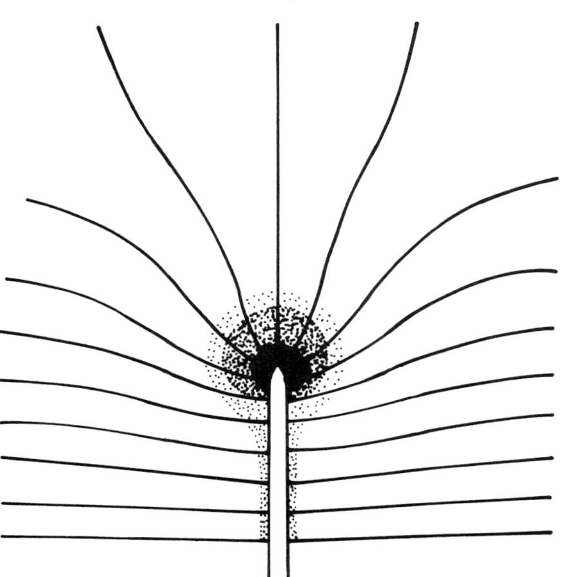

FIG. 6-6. Isocurrent lines from an unshielded needle. Stippling represents current density. (Montgomery, S.J. Raj, P.P., Nettles, D., Jenkins, M.T.: The use of the nerve stimulator with standard unsheathed needles in nerve blockade. Anesth. Analg. (Cleve), *52*:828, 1973.)

Although most of the peripheral nerve stimulators used to measure neuromuscular blockade will work, certain characteristics make some more suitable than others. Raj[37] evaluated five commercially available models and noted that the following characteristics are essential in such equipment: [1] voltage range from 1 to 10 V; [2] ampere range from 0.1 mA to 1.0 mA; and [3] one or two "H" toggle switches. The instruments should be pocket sized, easily stabilized on the table or intravenous pole, battery operated, and preferably able to be sterilized. The features and principles of use of a nerve stimulator are shown in Figure 6-7.

Ford and colleagues[12] compared the sheathed and unsheathed needles in a cat model to determine relative proximity of the needle tip to the nerve as measured by both muscle twitch and compound action potential of the nerve. Whereas stimulating current to the insulated needle was always least when the tip was closest to the nerve, the uninsulated needles displayed the least stimulating current when the tip of the needle was beyond the nerve by as much as 0.8 cm. Injecting saline, a recommended technique, did not assist in improving the placement of the needle. Ford and co-workers concluded that insulated needles are more precise in locating the peripheral nerve than are the standard uninsulated needles routinely used for neural blockade. In a further study, they ascertained the electrical characteristics of peripheral nerve stimulators that contributed to localization of a peripheral nerve.[13] The following characteristics were found to be important:

1. A *linear output,* that is, a plot of percent output versus percentage of meter scale, gives a straight line passing through zero and with 100% of the meter scale corresponding to 100% output.
2. *High and low output ranges.* Allows use of high output, if needed, when the needle is distant from the nerve; however, a good range of control in the low output range is essential when the needle tip is close to the nerve. Some stimulators developed for

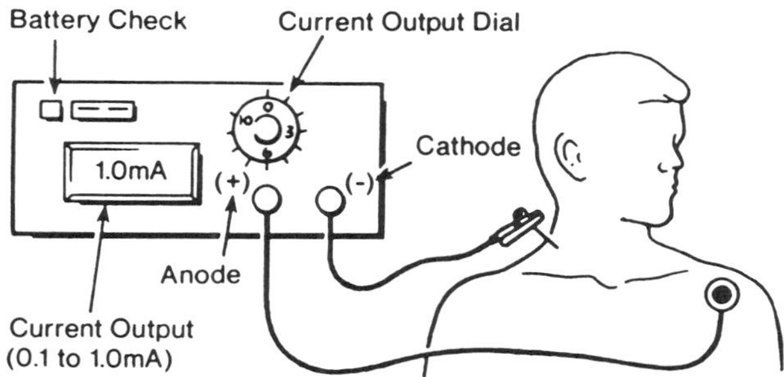

FIG. 6-7. Key features and illustration of use of nerve stimulator.

neuromuscular monitoring do not have the required control in the low output range, and thus are not suitable for location of peripheral nerves.

3. *Clearly marked polarity, extending to the ends of the connecting cords.* The stimulating needle must be attached to the cathode (−) and the surface of the patient to the anode (+). If the polarity is reversed, four times as much current is required to produce a muscle twitch as a result of nerve stimulation compared to when the polarity is correct. *Note:* On some stimulators, it is difficult to determine which is the cathode (−); indeed, on some, the anode (+) is marked red, whereas on others the cathode (−) is red.
4. *Constant current output,* that is, current output should remain the same regardless of different resistances applied to the output. In comparison, a constant voltage output instrument will decrease current output as resistance increases.
5. A *short stimulation pulse.* The shorter the pulse, the greater is the ratio of the current required to stimulate the nerve when the needle is 1 cm away compared to when the needle is on the nerve. For example, for a pulse width of 40 μsec, this ratio is 11, whereas for 1000 μsec it is only 5.
6. *Design features:* a) a large, easily turned current output dial; b) a *digital* current output meter; and c) a battery check.

Techniques for Use of a Nerve Stimulator

1. The anode (+) is connected by means of an alligator clamp to an electrode on the skin well clear of the block site.
2. The needle may be sheathed or unsheathed (but preferably sheathed). It is attached to an extension tubing and syringe of local anesthetic. It is then inserted in the usual manner, using the usual landmarks. As the needle approaches the depth at which the nerve is expected to be located, the stimulator is turned on to the low range at about the fourth mark on the scale. Local muscle contraction in the area of needle insertion should be minimal at this low range and should be ignored.
3. The area to be blocked is observed for muscle contraction, for example, muscles of the hand in a brachial plexus block. With a sheathed needle, muscle contractions will increase as the needle approaches the nerve and then decrease as the needle passes the nerve. If possible, the current should be turned to the minimum value and a point found at which maximum muscle movement still occurs; this indicates the needle tip is on the nerve. With unsheathed needles, it may be necessary to withdraw the needle to the point at which maximum stimulation still occurs, since marked muscle contraction sometimes occurs when the needle tip is past the nerve (see above).
4. One milliliter to 2 ml of local anesthetic is injected, which should immediately reduce or abolish muscle contraction. If it does not, the needle should be withdrawn slightly and the process repeated. A further test is to increase the output of the stimulator after the test dose. It should still be possible to produce some muscle movement at the higher output.
5. The full dose of local anesthetic is injected. *Note:* Paresthesiae are sometimes produced but are not specifically sought. Indeed, this is one of the values of the use of a stimulator because muscle movement can accurately guide the anesthetist while allowing the patient to be sedated and unaware of the block procedure.

Needles and Drugs

As might be expected, the major variation in what otherwise might be an "all purpose" block tray is the numbers and kinds of syringes, needles, and drugs that are included. Other than the personal preferences for glass versus plastic or three ringed versus plain syringes, there is little to choose among syringes.

Interest in size of needles has focused primarily on their role in inducing postlumbar puncture headache. Commensurate with the ability to aspirate blood as an indication of possible intravascular injection, the practice should be to use the smallest needle possible. Because most practitioners must do multiple needle insertions to accomplish a successful block, all patients deserve skin and subcutaneous infiltration with a 27-gauge or smaller needle. Moore[30] has always advocated the use of a needle with a security bead at its proximal shaft to preclude loss of broken needles. Today's technology and extensive use of disposable equipment make that practice unnecessary and expensive. The role of the needle, its size, and angle of bevel (*i.e.*, sharp point) in producing nerve injury have recently been studied by Selander and colleagues.[41] In a study of 433 patients comparing the "paresthesia" approach against the "transarterial" approach to the brachial plexus in the axilla, they reported a 2.8% incidence of neurologic symptoms after paresthesias and only 0.8% in the transarterial group (Table 6-1). To separate drug effects from needle trauma, they also compared, in isolated rat sciatic nerve, the neural damage resulting from a sharp, 14° needle bevel and a blunt, 45° needle bevel.[40] They found that the 45° needle produced significantly less damage than did the sharper needle (Table 6-2). Additional caution needs to be exercised on the use of the long bevel disposable needle. The metal with which these needles are made is relatively soft. After such a needle point strikes a bony surface (rib or spine) on one or more occasions, it develops a hook or barb at its tip (Fig. 6-8). This barb can cause significant damage as it passes through nerves, vessels, and tissue and should be discarded. Frequent wiping of the tip of the needle across sterile cotton or gauze will allow early recognition of this needle deformity.

Drugs are frequently added to the commercially prepared disposable trays that have been presterilized, usually with ethylene oxide. Bridenbaugh[2] demonstrated many years ago that it was not only safe but beneficial to autoclave the drugs to be used in neural blockade. This is usually done by adding the drugs to the hospital prepared trays so that all are sterilized together; however, ampules and vials of drugs may also be wrapped or packaged in test tubes and autoclaved to be added to the opened sterile tray at the time of use, much the same as extra needles and syringes are added. This not only ensures sterile drug within the container, but also allows the anesthetist freedom to handle the sterile outer container without benefit of an assistant. All local anesthetic drugs used for neural blockade may be safely steam autoclaved. Dextrose-containing solutions will often acquire a brownish discoloration if autoclaved more than once; if such occurs, they should be discarded.

In an effort to determine the safety of subjecting these drugs to gas autoclaving with ethylene oxide, Abrams[32] studied both ampules and vials of local anesthetic agents, some of which had intentionally been "pre-cracked." There was no evidence of ethylene oxide metabolites, ethylene glycol, in any of the intact ampules. Some of the vials (rubber stoppers) and precracked ampules had detectable ethylene glycol. In a separate animal study of the neurologic effect of ethylene glycol, Abrams found no effect in

TABLE 6-1. NUMBER OF PATIENTS WITH SYMPTOMS OF POSTANESTHETIC NERVE LESION

	Patients	Patients with Nerve Lesion	%
Paresthesia group	290	8	2.8
Artery group	243	2	0.8
Total	533	10	1.9

(Selander, D., Edshage, S., Wolff, T.: Paresthesiae or no paresthesiae? Acta Anesthesiol. Scand., *23*:29, 1979.)

TABLE 6-2. FASCICULAR INJURY AFTER INTRANEURAL INJECTIONS WITH NERVE *IN SITU*

	Long Bevel		Short Bevel	
n	15	15	15	15
Fascicular injury	9	5	0	3

(Selander, D., Dhuner, K.-G., Lundborg, G.: Peripheral nerve injury due to injection needles used for regional anesthesia. Acta Anesthesiol. Scand., *21*:186, 1977.)

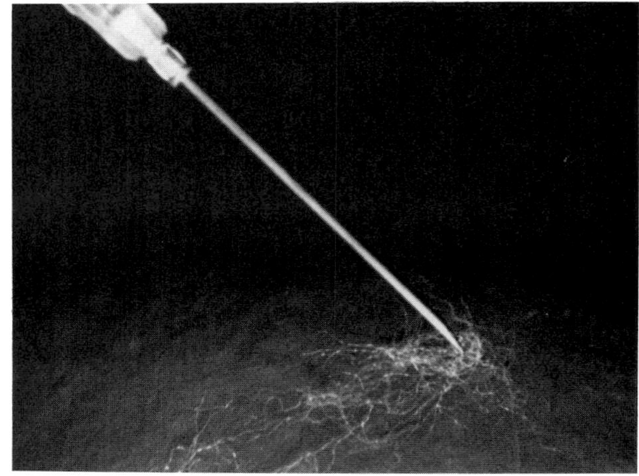

FIG. 6-8. Needle with barb or "fish hook."

doses severalfold greater. His conclusion was that it was safe to sterilize local anesthetic agents with ethylene oxide, especially those in snap-top ampules. It is important, however, that 24 to 72 hours be allowed for the exclusion of ethylene oxide if it is used to sterilize the entire block tray. Without regard to how hospital prepared trays are sterilized, there should be indicator tape or tags to ensure the anesthetist that his equipment has, in fact, been sterilized.

PERFORMANCE OF NEURAL BLOCKADE

Ideally, appropriately selected and premedicated patients will arrive at a well-equipped anesthetizing area, for example, induction room, for performance of the selected regional block technique. Hyperbaric or hypobaric spinals should be performed on a surface that can be put in Trendelenburg or reverse Trendelenburg positions, preferably the operating table. Other neural block procedures not affected by the patient's position can usually be done with the patient on a stretcher or bed, as long as it would allow appropriate resuscitation efforts should they be necessary.

Before starting to induce regional anesthesia, the anesthetist should check the patient's record to determine if and when the patient received the prescribed premedication and if it has — or has had time to have — the desired effect. Only then should the judgment be made for additional sedative or analgesic supplementation during the block itself.

The use of supplemental parenteral agents during the administration of regional anesthesia is actually a continuation of the philosophy of the preanesthetic indication previously discussed. The goal of the anesthetist is to provide the patient with a pleasant anesthetic experience throughout the entire operative period. The amount of additional supplementation required depends not only on the effect of the premedication but also on the degree of painful stimulation of the selected block technique. Most patients require little additional supplementation for the simple, single injection blocks such as spinal, epidural, and axillary block. In fact, patients often are more easily positioned and responsive to paresthesias if they are not heavily medicated. Conversely, deep paravertebral or multiple intercostal nerve blocks are quite stimulating and will likely require additional parenteral sedation. Nervous or hypersensitive patients will also benefit from such supplementation.

The selection of drugs for supplementing the administration of regional anesthesia is as individual as the choice of premedication. The common goal, however, is to either retain the patient's consciousness (albeit depressed) or have it restored very soon after the block has been completed. Excessive sedation incurs risks of respiratory obstruction or circulatory collapse and will also mask the early onset of complications of the block, such as high spinal or epidural or intravascular injection. Excessive doses of some of the psychotropic or dissociative drugs may also render a previously cooperative patient excitable or unmanageable. It should be apparent, therefore, that the ultra-short-acting intravenous drugs given in small doses or by slow continuous infusion will allow titration of the drug to the desired level of sedation and still ensure a rapid recovery at the conclusion of the block.

Both thiopentone and methohexital are satisfactory for this use. At any time supplemental intravenous agents are being used, it is doubly important that the anesthetist have an assistant to monitor the patient and ensure proper positioning. Small doses of benzodiazepines alone or in combination with ultrashort-acting narcotics such as fentanyl or alfentanyl are also effective. A marked advantage of the short-acting narcotics is not only their analgesic properties, but also their rapid reversibility should excess drug be given.

Fentanyl and diazepam are both clearance-limited drugs with respect to their long half-lives; for fentanyl, this is determined by liver blood flow but varies from 2 to 7 hours; for diazepam, it is determined by hepatic microsomal activity (capacity limited) and is much longer (24–48 hours). However, offset of sedation after small doses intravenously depends on redistribution and thus may be quite rapid (Fig. 6-9). Thus brief analgesia and sedation may be obtained by a combination of, for example, diazepam, 2 to 5 mg, and fentanyl, 25 to 50 micrograms i.v. The newer opioid alfentanil may be particularly suitable because of its smaller volume of distribution compared to other opioids.[25]

INTRAOPERATIVE SUPPLEMENTATION AND MANAGEMENT OF THE PATIENT WITH A NEURAL BLOCKADE

The most important and probably the most challenging aspect of the successful practice of regional anesthesia is the intraoperative management of the patient who has received a nerve block of some kind. Most patients refuse or are dissatisfied with regional

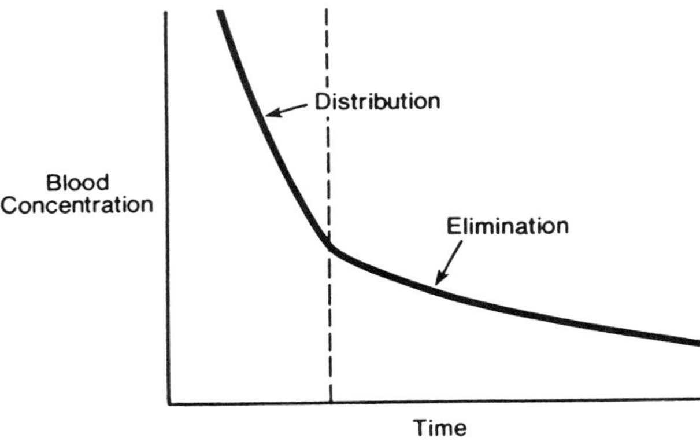

FIG. 6-9. Distribution and elimination phases of drugs given intravenously. Single doses of drugs such as diazepam and fentanyl have a short duration of action because blood concentration falls rapidly owing to distribution of the drug. Larger doses or prolonged administration produces a longer duration of effect because decline in blood concentration relies more on the much slower elimination phase.

anesthesia because they do not want to be "wide awake during surgery." This all too common approach to the management of patients with nerve blocks harkens back to the earliest days of surgery when there were no, or too few, anesthetists. Surgeons performed all of the nerve blocks and then left their patients wide awake (and unmonitored) while they proceeded with the operation. It is not surprising, then, that early anesthetists administered general anesthesia to those patients for procedures not amenable to surgical nerve blocks. It has taken decades for surgeons and anesthetists alike to accept the fact that it is not a sign of failure if a patient who has had a nerve block, which would provide 100% of the surgical anesthetic requirements, receives enough supplemental sedation to sleep lightly or rest quietly during the operative period.

Labat, a surgeon and the "father of regional anesthesia," in his early writings acknowledges the occasional importance of supplementation of regional anesthesia. Usually overlooked and even more important are his comments relating to excessive noise in the operating room, unnecessary conversation that might be misinterpreted by the patient, and avoidance of the surgeon asking the patient if he feels this or that stimulus.[22] Many patients would be content with little or no sedation if the environment during the operation were quiet and nonthreatening.

At present, more anesthetists and surgeons alike accept the philosophy that every patient deserves the same quality of anesthesia care (amnesia, analgesia, and so forth) without regard to which drugs are used and how, when, or where they are administered. It seems no more rational to say that a patient will have "a nerve block and nothing else" than it would be to say that a patient will have "only pentothal and nothing else." If one adopts this philosophy of patient-oriented total anesthesia care, then the intraoperative administration of supplemental drugs, in addition to the previously administered local anesthetic drugs, may be structured around a few basic principles unique to the use of neural blockade. Generally speaking, this involves consideration of the needs of not only the patient, but also the surgeon and anesthetist.

PATIENT CONSIDERATIONS

Often the compelling indication for a regional block technique rather than general anesthesia is the patient who should not be rendered unconscious because of a full stomach, difficult airway, or poor physical status, all features that impose serious risks to general anesthesia. Clearly, these patients should be awake or only very lightly sedated for apprehension. Specific techniques will be discussed subsequently, but this is a situation in which "vocal anesthesia" (friendly conversation) or music can be very helpful. The other extreme is the younger or extremely anxious patient who does need to be asleep before surgery can proceed peacefully. It is clear, therefore, that supplementation must be tailored from "none" to "a lot" depending on patient circumstances alone. It is a rare patient, however, who is healthy and undergoing elective surgery who must be denied *any* kind of supplemental sedation just as a matter of principle. Our armamentarium of drugs and techniques no longer makes this objection valid.

SURGICAL CONSIDERATIONS

Frequently the determinant of supplemental drugs and techniques is the location or anticipated duration of the surgical procedure, or both. In general, the closer the surgical procedure is to the head and neck, the more complex is the anesthetic management. Patients tend to be more apprehensive about operations in this area. The proximity of darkening and smothering drapes, retractors, and surgical manipulation around the eyes and airways may further enhance their apprehension and feelings of claustrophobia.

All of this mitigates for heavy sedation. Similarly, the anesthetist as protector of the airway has often been dislocated to a more distant site and his anxiety also increases. Certainly, he should not invoke sedation to the point of unconsciousness without first securing the airway.

Concurrent with these considerations is the duration of such procedures — or any other, for that matter. A brief or moderate length procedure can be carried out under supplemental sedation. Conversely, if the procedure exceeds 1 hour or more, all of the "nonblocked" areas of the patient's body can become progressively more uncomfortable. The rapidity with which this occurs is contingent upon the previously discussed premedication and supplemental drug given preoperatively, which have now begun to wear off. Anesthetists who work with otolaryngologists, ophthalmologists, and plastic surgeons in the infamous "local with standby" category appreciate all of the aforementioned pitfalls. For these reasons, many prefer to produce good topical anesthesia of the airway and supplement their blocks, or those of the surgeon, with light endotracheal general anesthesia, for example, nitrous oxide and oxygen.

ANESTHETIC CONSIDERATIONS

Finally, at least three features of regional anesthesia are, in and of themselves, indications for supplementation. First is the knowledge of the neural elements involved in the surgical procedure and the regional block that has been performed, that is, will the block provide anesthesia for all of the surgical stimulus? For example, the use of an intercostal nerve block is extremely beneficial as the anesthetic for a feeding gastrostomy. One must appreciate, however, that it provides only sensory and motor blockade of the abdominal wall. When the surgeon enters the abdomen, visceral pain will be noted by the patient and a modest amount of analgesia and sedation will be required for that portion of the operation. Second is the possibility that the neural elements one intended to block completely and for the full duration of the procedure are incompletely blocked, which could result from poor technique, improper selection of drug, volume, or concentration, or surgical intervention beyond the area of the block. Clearly, sedation or supplementation in the amount and duration to cover the inadequacy of the block will be required.

It is totally inappropriate, and unnecessary, to have a 90% successful regional anesthetic converted to a 100% general anesthetic because the patient responded in some fashion at some time during the procedure. One should supplement only to the degree necessary to obtain the maximum benefit from the neural blockade administered.

One final feature often overlooked by anesthesiologists was previously alluded to — that of total patient comfort. One may provide a perfectly anesthetized arm or leg with a good extremity block only to have the patient become progressively uncomfortable with immobility and aching joints on hard operating tables. A ready solution to this problem in healthy patients receiving spinal or epidural anesthesia is to anticipate patient discomfort and produce a higher level of blockade. For example, T11 spinal anesthesia would be sufficient for lower extremity surgery; however, if no significant adverse effects would ensue, then a T6 level would provide patient comfort up to the shoulders without additional analgesics. All too many "perfect blocks" have been abandoned because of poor management of the patient's other needs.

DRUGS AND TECHNIQUES

Selection of specific agents or techniques for intraoperative supplementation includes the entire gamut of anesthesia practice. Obviously, for a variety of surgical, anesthetic, and patient factors, every regional anesthetic could potentially become a full-fledged general anesthetic at a moment's notice, and the anesthetic preparations should have been made accordingly. Not withstanding that possibility, it might be appropriate to discuss methods of supplementation in ascending fashion, that is, from the least to the most, because in practice that is the progression that should occur if one is to enjoy maximum benefit from the regional anesthetic technique performed.

Nonpharmacologic Techniques

A surprising number of patients will actually request a nerve block because they are afraid of "going to sleep." Others are ambivalent but make no demands. Often, for these people, a thorough explanation of the anesthetic and surgical happenings is all they require. Patients should, however, be relatively unaware of the actual events of the operation. Scott[39] describes a method of mental distraction that he combines with low doses of intravenous diazepam. Techniques for distraction vary, but all are designed to prevent anticipation of pain and perception by the patient. Office practitioners who do procedures under local anesthesia become adept at these techniques of "vocal anesthesia." Clearly, the success of these techniques considerably depends on the cooperation of the surgeon and the operating room staff.

Intravenous Techniques

The report by Gjessing and Tomlin[15] provides evidence of the benefit of both a premedicant and an intravenous sedation. Forty of their study group of 229 patients received no premedication before outpatient surgery under regional anesthesia. The patients were then divided into a placebo group and a diazepam group. Of the unmedicated patients who received a placebo injection immediately after the block, 50% needed additional sedation within the first 15 minutes of the procedure. By contrast, of the unmedicated patients who received diazepam intravenously, only 1 of 13 needed additional sedative (Table 6-3). Of the premedicated patients who received a placebo, 36% required additional sedation, whereas if they received diazepam, the presence of premedication made little difference in the requirement for sedation but did deepen the level of sedation (Table 6-4). It may be concluded that while the use of intravenous diazepam reduces the need for premedication, the premedication does assist in producing an improved level of sedation.

Although diazepam has been used alone, it is more often combined with narcotics, pentazocine, or even ketamine, among others. The main advantage of diazepam in the doses used to supplement regional anesthesia include a relative absence of cardiovascular and respiratory effects, adequate sedation, and, most importantly, anticonvulsant properties. Its anterograde amnesic effect is of particular benefit in obtunding recall for the operative period; however, retrograde amnesia has never been proved conclusively. After intravenous doses of 0.24 mg/kg, peak amnesic action occurred in 10 minutes and declined over the ensuing 30 to 40 minutes.[4] Despite the amnesia, there was evidence of only slight reduction in the level of consciousness and also evidence of normal complex processing within 20 minutes of the injection. The major disadvantages of diazepam that have emerged with its extensive use include pain on injection and a venous thrombophlebitis rate as high as 40%, depending on the size of the vein and the speed of injection. Also, there is a large biological variation in patient response. Pharmacokinetic studies have corroborated the clinical observations of long-lasting residual effects of diazepam. The terminal half-life of diazepam may extend from 30 to 50 hours. Also, active metabolites are formed; these too may contribute to prolonged recovery, especially in the elderly.[19] For these reasons, the use of larger doses of diazepam as a supplement for outpatients should be avoided. Kortilla and colleagues[21] reported impairment of driving skills up to 10 hours after doses of 0.3 and 0.45 mg/kg of diazepam. The same effect was observed when diazepam was given in conjunction with narcotics.

Other benzodiazepines have followed diazepam,

TABLE 6-3. DISTRIBUTION OF NUMBERS OF PATIENTS REQUIRING ADDITIONAL SEDATION

	Diazepam	Placebo	
Unpremedicated			
Additional sedation	1	13	p = 0.0125
No additional sedation	14	12	
Premedicated			
Additional sedation	13	30	p = 2.005
No additional sedation	83	63	

(Gjessing, J., Tomlin, P.J.: Intravenous sedation and regional analgesia. Anaesthesia, *32*:66, 1984.)

TABLE 6-4. VALUE OF PREMEDICATION

	Reduced Need for Additional Sedation	
	Additional Sedation	No Additional Sedation
Diazepam group		
Unpremedicated	1	14
Premedicated	13	83
Total	14	97
p = 0.35 not significant		
Placebo group		
Unpremedicated	13	12
Premedicated	30	63
Total	43	75
p = 0.025 very significant		
	Deepened Level of Sedation (time only 15 minutes)	
	Unpremedicated	**Premedicated**
Diazepam group		
Asleep	1	41
Drowsy	6	17
Relaxed	7	18
Total	14	76
p = 0.005 very significant		

(Gjessing, J., Tomlin, P.J.: Intravenous sedation and regional analgesia. Anaesthesia, *32*:66, 1984.)

each in an effort to be less irritating to the veins, to provide better amnesia, and with a shorter biological half-life. Clinical trials with these drugs have usually included their similar efficacy in supplementing regional anesthesia. A newer benzodiazepine of benefit is the water-soluble derivative midazolam, which is shorter-acting than diazepam. McClure and coworkers compared midazolam and diazepam in emulsion as intravenous sedatives for spinal anesthesia.[27] Mean doses of midazolam, 12 mg, and diazepam, 27 mg, were needed to produce adequate sedation for periods of about 1 hour. Neither drug caused loss of airway or significant cardiorespiratory changes. The frequency of drowsiness following surgery was greater after sedation with diazepam, but objective testing of recovery showed no significant difference between the two drugs. The frequency of amnesia was greater after midazolam. No patient in either group had clinically significant venous sequelae. Dundee studied times of recovery and plasma levels in volunteers[9] and found that, in the doses he used, midazolam was a much shorter-acting drug than diazepam and there was no evidence of enterohepatic recirculation or tendency for subjects to fall asleep again. Individual variation to dose was the same as with diazepam. It appears from his work that midazolam is about twice as potent as diazepam and with similar amnesic properties.

Another benzodiazepine, lorazepam, was offered as a better amnesic than diazepam. After intravenous administration of lorazepam, a slower onset but longer amnesia has been reported, persisting up to 6 hours. There is a latent period of about 15 to 30 minutes after a dose of 2 to 4 mg before the beginning of the antirecall effect. Meperidine, but not morphine, has been shown to increase this effect. Both lorazepam and flunitrazepam have a significantly reduced venous irritation as compared to diazepam. The pharmacokinetic parameters of the more common benzodiazepines are listed in Table 6-5.[17]

Use of low-dose narcotics alone to supplement regional anesthesia is of limited value. Although their use will address the additional analgesic needs of the patient, most narcotics have little effect on the control of amnesia and wakefulness. Mather,[26] in a study of plasma concentrations after intramuscular injection of meperidine, 100 mg, reported subjective effects, including dryness of the mouth, drowsiness but not tranquility, visual disturbances, and loss of concentration and ability to keep track of time. This last feature could be a real asset in a supplemental agent because some volunteers believed only 10 minutes had passed when, in fact, 45 to 60 minutes had elapsed. The addition of an analgesic to benzodiazepine sedation has been shown to reduce the requirements of the latter. Corall and associates[5] showed that patients receiving 30 mg of pentazocine at the start of the operation needed about 25% less diazepam than did those receiving a placebo solution. Currently, the practice has shifted to the use of the shorter-acting narcotic analgesics, such as fentanyl and alfentanil. Fentanyl, a potent cogener of meperidine, has a very short redistribution half-life of about 15 minutes, with greater than 98% of the injected drug cleared from plasma in 60 minutes. It is usually given in 50 μg increments every 5 to 10 minutes until desired analgesia has been obtained. Additional doses may be given every 30 to 60 minutes as needed. The administration of fentanyl, even in doses as low as 1.3 μg/kg, results in respiratory depression comparable to 0.12 mg/kg of morphine and may remain below 80% of normal for 4 hours.[36] The hepatic metabolism and elimination half-life of fentanyl are delayed as long as 220 minutes. The anesthetist needs to be prepared for prolonged sleepiness or even delayed respiratory depression, especially for outpatient sur-

TABLE 6-5. PHARMACOKINETIC PARAMETERS OF DIAZEPAM, LORAZEPAM, MIDAZOLAM, AND FLUNITRAZEPAM

	$t_{1/2\alpha}$ (min)	V_1 (liters/kg)	$t_{1/2\beta}$ (h)	Vd_β (liters/kg)	Cl (ml/min)
Diazepam	9–130	0.31–0.41	31.3–46.6	0.9–1.2	26–35
Lorazepam	3–10	0.30–0.72	14.3–14.6	1.14–1.30	1.05–1.10 (ml/min/kg)
Midazolam	3–38	0.17–0.44	2.1–2.4	0.8–1.14	202–324
Flunitrazepam	15 ± 8	0.61 ± 0.36	25 ± 11	3.6 ± 1.3	94 ± 37

$t_{1/2\alpha}$ = half-life of distribution; V_1 = volume of the central compartment; $t_{1/2\beta}$ = elimination half-life; Vd_β = apparent volume of distribution; Cl = total plasma clearance.

(Kanto, J., Klotz, U.: Intravenous benzodiazepines as anaesthetic agents. Acta Anesthesiol. Scand., *26*:555, 1982.)

gery. This property of fentanyl has led to a greater trial of alfentanil as a supplement for short outpatient procedures. The pharmacokinetics of alfentanil include a rapid redistribution half-life of 11.6 minutes and an elimination half-life of 94 minutes. Alfentanil is said to be one fourth as potent as fentanyl and with a duration one third as long.[36]

Some reports have suggested that the use of a continuous infusion of narcotic supplements will provide equivalent analgesia with lower total doses of drug and fewer unwanted side-effects of prolonged somnolence or respiratory depression.[45] These studies, however, were done in conjunction with general anesthesia or have been used during the postoperative period. The difficulty with the use of continuous infusions during surgery with regional anesthesia is the relatively rapid nature in the degree and frequency of noxious stimuli. If surgical patients need additional sedation or analgesia, the response time of a change in infusion rate is inadequate, and one usually reverts to bolus injections. These, in addition to the calculated infusion dose, could conceivably result in greater doses and side-effects rather than fewer, as published.[45]

Ketamine, because it also possesses analgesic properties, would seem, in low doses, to be an attractive alternative to the combinations previously noted. Austin,[1] in unpremedicated patients, started with diazepam, 2.5 mg, followed by ketamine, 20 mg, into the infusion line. Supplemental doses of ketamine, 10 mg, or diazepam, 2.5 mg, were given as the need for analgesia or sedation was judged by the anesthetist. Mean age of the patient group was 84 years. No serious sequelae were noted. Titration of ketamine infusion to the desired effect should be equally effective.

Althesin, when it became familiar to practitioners, was also advocated for supplementation of regional anesthesia. Park and Wilson,[33] believing the short duration of action, noncumulation, and ease of hypnotic control of althesin, made it more suitable as a supplement for regional anesthesia than its predecessors methohexitone, propanidid, and chlormethiazole. Their conclusions of the above advantages were confirmed in the study, but they did notice transient depression of breathing and, in extreme cases, apnea if the infusion was given rapidly.

Seow and colleagues[42] compared bolus injections of diazepam with chloromethiazole infusion for sedation of patients with epidural blockade. A satisfactory state of sedation and amnesia was achieved rapidly with both agents in which patients lapsed into a sleeplike state when left undisturbed, yet spontaneously opened their eyes to make comments and cooperate with verbal commands. Both agents provided very good anterograde amnesia, without any retrograde amnesia. There was considerable postoperative somnolence, with a high incidence of relapse into amnesia and sedated states. When the total volume of chlormethiazole infused was less than 300 mg, however, a distinct advantage of a very abrupt and lucid recovery was apparent.

Inhalation Techniques

There are three major reasons for combining inhalation techniques with a regional anesthetic technique. First, there are procedures about the airway or in the upper abdomen that require endotracheal tube protection of the airway against obstruction or aspiration. Although patients in critical care areas tolerate endotracheal tubes with mild intravenous sedation, most surgical patients need to be anesthetized if the tube is to be tolerated. Second, procedures of very long duration can be done under regional anesthesia; however, the cumulative doses of the parenteral sedatives and narcotics can become very high over several hours of administration, leading to a prolonged postoperative recovery time. In these circumstances, basal sedation has been established with sedatives, and narcotics, and mask inhalation, or nasally insufflated agents (*e.g.*, N_2O) may be given for the duration of the procedure. Third, there is always the possibility that the regional block technique and the aforementioned intravenous techniques have not succeeded in meeting the needs of the patient or the surgeon. At that point, it is essential to proceed to an inhalation anesthetic technique to supply the missing elements of a successful anesthetic. Scott,[38] a strong advocate of general anesthesia supplement for extradural blockade during surgery, prefers the inhalation techniques as providing a more predictable effect and a more rapid recovery postoperatively than many of the intravenous drugs. His preference is pentothal induction followed by $N_2O:O_2$ or light halothane by mask with spontaneous ventilation.

For situations in which inhalation anesthesia is *not* required for airway management but rather as a form of sedation, nitrous oxide in low concentrations (25%–50%) may be used. Edmunds and Rosen[11] referred to this as "inhalation sedation" and reported on 394 patients who received 1005 outpatient dental treatments with the usual local anesthetic techniques plus a fixed concentration of 25% nitrous oxide administered by means of nasal mask. Ninety-nine percent of their patients were treated successfully without loss of consciousness. The change in anxiety level on subsequent treatments declined from the initial 86% who were "very anxious" to less than 10% on the fourth visit (Fig. 6-10). Kortilla and co-workers[20] studied the time-course of the effects of 30% nitrous oxide on selected cognitive and psychomotor tasks, clearly, a function of importance if used for outpatient anesthesia. They concluded that "the distinct impairment in hand–eye coordination 12 minutes after cessation of the (45-minute test period) administration of 30% nitrous oxide suggests that even in healthy young subjects, total recovery after its inhalation is *not* instantaneous and that outpatients need supervision for at least 20 to 30 minutes after administration. In a continued experiment, the trial was repeated to test for tolerance to nitrous oxide; none was noted. This evidence would seem to substantiate that, in select cases, nitrous oxide recovery is more rapid than prolonged administration of intravenous drugs.

SUMMARY

Two basic principles can be derived from the preceding material. First, the practice of neural blockade is merely a different or additional technique in the total armamentarium of the anesthetist. Just as he must be intellectually, psychologically, and technically prepared to do inhalation or intravenous anesthesia techniques, so must he be prepared to do regional anesthesia techniques. Similarly, because the successful outcome of those practices requires provision of adequate space, equipment, and assistance, so does the successful outcome of regional anesthesia have those requirements. Finally, just as he would not select either a single intravenous or inhalation agent for his sole management of the patient or else call it a failure, so should he not feel that if regional anesthesia cannot be used to the exclusion of all other anesthetic techniques and agents he has failed. To exploit to the maximum each alone or in combination is the ultimate in the consultant practice of anesthesia.

Second, it follows then that the use of regional anesthesia techniques is only a part of the total anesthetic care of the patient. The anesthetist must deal with the *whole* patient from the preanesthetic visit through the postanesthetic visits. The goal of correct premedication and supplementation of regional anesthesia is to maximize the benefits of what was, presumably, the appropriately selected and well-administered regional anesthetic technique. Empiric or premature oversupplementation will likely discourage many anesthetists from doing regional anesthesia because "they take too long to do and I put them all to sleep anyway." Conversely, refusing to supplement when and to the degree necessary will incur only the ill will of the patient and surgeon. The appropriate use of premedication and supplementation is the real key to an ever-increasing acceptance of the practice of regional anesthesia.

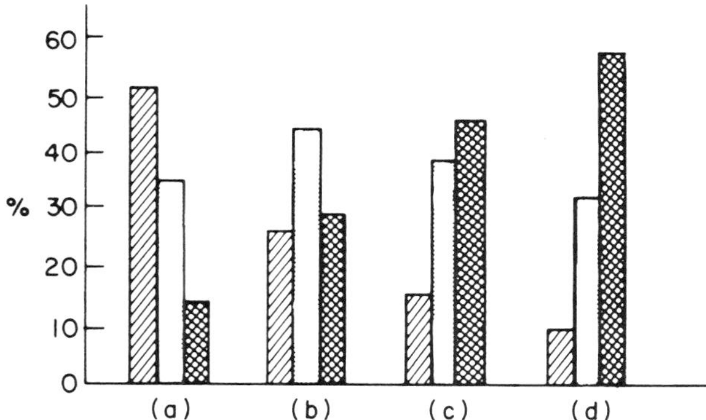

FIG. 6-10. Change in anxiety level as course of treatment proceeds, excluding patients who attended only once. ▨, extremely anxious; □, very anxious; ▩, slightly or not anxious. (*a*) First visit, n = 197; (*b*) second visit, n = 197; (*c*) third visit, n = 135; (*d*) fourth visit, n = 97. (Edmunds, D.H., Rosen, M.: Inhalation sedation with 25% nitrous oxide. Anaesthesia, *39*:140, 1984.)

REFERENCES

1. Austin, T.R.: Low dose ketamine and diazepam during spinal analgesia. Anaesthesia, *35*:391, 1980.
2. Bridenbaugh, L.D., and Moore, D.C.: Does repeated heat sterilization of local anesthetic drugs affect potency? Anesthesiology, *25*:372, 1964.
3. Bridenbaugh, L.D., Moore, D.C., and DeVries, J.C.: Sterile disposable spinal anesthesia trays: Fact or fancy? Anesth. Analg., *46*:191, 1967.
4. Clarke, P.R.F., Eccersley, R.S., Frisby, J.P., and Thornton, J.A.: The amnesic effect of diazepam. Br. J. Anaesth., *42*:690, 1970.
5. Corall, I.M., Strunin, L., Ward, M.E., Mason, S.A., *et al.*: Sedation for outpatient conservative dentistry. Anaesthesia, *34*:855, 1979.
6. deJong, R.H., and Heavner, J.E.: Diazepam prevents local anesthetic seizures. Anesthesiology, *34*:523, 1971.
7. Dodson, M.E., and Eastley, R.J.: Comparative study of two long-acting tranquilizers for oral premedication. Br. J. Anaesth., *50*:1059, 1978.

8. Dundee, J.W., Lilburn, J.K., Toner, W., Howard, P.J.: Plasma lorazepam levels. A study following single dose administration of 2 and 4 mg by different routes. Anaesthesia, *33*:15, 1978.
9. Dundee, J.W., Samuel, I.O., Turner, W., Howard, P.J.: Midazolam: A water soluble benzodiazepine. Anaesthesia, *33*:454, 1980.
10. Dundee, J.W., and Wilson, D.B.: Amnesic action of midazolam. Anaesthesia, *35*:459, 1980.
11. Edmunds, D.H., and Rosen, M.: Inhalation sedation with 25% nitrous oxide. Anaesthesia, *39*:138, 1984.
12. Ford, D.J., Pither, C., and Raj, P.P.: Comparison of insulated and uninsulated needles for locating peripheral nerves with a peripheral nerve stimulator. Anesth. Analg., *63*:925, 1984.
13. Ford, D.J., Pither, C.E., Raj, P.P.: Electrical characteristics of peripheral nerve stimulators: Implications for nerve localization. Reg. Anaesth., *9*:73, 1984.
14. Frumin, M.J., Herekar, V.R., Jarvik, M.E.: Amnesic actions of diazepam and scopolamine in man. Anesthesiology, *45*:406, 1976.
15. Gjessing, J., Tomlin, P.J.: Intravenous sedation and regional analgesia. Anaesthesia, *32*:63, 1977.
16. Hjortso, E., Mondorf, T.: Does oral premedication increase the risk of gastric aspiration? Acta Anaesthesiol. Scand., *26*:505, 1982.
17. Kanto, J., Klotz, U.: Intravenous benzodiazepines as anaesthetic agents: Pharmacokinetics and clinical consequences. Acta Anaesthesiol. Scand., *26*:554, 1982.
18. Kay, B., Healey, T.E.J.: Premedication by controlled release morphine. Anaesthesia, *39*:587, 1984.
19. Klotz, U., Avant, G.R., Hoyumpa, A., Schenker, S., Wilkinson, G.R.: The effects of age and liver disease on the disposition and elimination of diazepam in man. J. Clin. Invest., *55*:347, 1975.
20. Kortilla, K., Ghoneim, M.M., Jacobs, L., Mewaldt, S.P., Petersen, R.C.: Time course of mental and psychomotor effects of thirty percent nitrous oxide during inhalation and recovery. Anesthesiology, *54*:220, 1981.
21. Kortilla, K., Linnoula, M.: Recovery and skills related to driving after intravenous sedations: Dose-response relationship with diazepam. Br. J. Anaesth., *47*:457, 1975.
22. Labat, G.: Regional anesthesia. *In* Adriani J. (ed).: Regional Anaesthesia, ed. 3, p. 9. Philadelphia, W.B. Saunders Co., 1967.
23. L'Armand, J., Vredevoe, L.A., Conner, J.T., Herr, G.P., *et al.*: Lorazepam and morphine for IV surgical premedication. Br. J. Anaesth., *52*:1259, 1980.
24. Magbagbeola, J.A.O.: A comparison of lorazepam and diazepam as oral premedicants for surgery under regional anesthesia. Br. J. Anaesth., *46*:449, 1974.
25. Mather, L.E.: Clinical pharmacokinetics of fentanyl and its newer derivatives. Clin. Pharmacokinet., *8*:422, 1983.
26. Mather, L.E., Lindop, M.J., Tucker, G.T., Pflug, A.E.: Pethidine revisited: Plasma concentrations and effects after intramuscular injection. Br. J. Anaesth., *47*:1269, 1975.
27. McClure, J.A., Brown, P.T., Wildsmith, J.A.W.: Comparison of the IV administration of midazolam and diazepam as sedation during spinal anaesthesia. Br. J. Anaesth., *55*:1089, 1983.
28. McKay, A.C., Dundee, J.W.: Effect of oral benzodiazepines on memory. Br. J. Anaesth., *52*:1247, 1980.
29. Montgomery, S.J., Raj, P.P., Nettles, D., Jenkins, M.: The use of the nerve stimulator with standard unsheathed needles in nerve blockade. Anesth. Analg., *52*:827, 1973.
30. Moore, D.C.: Regional Block. Springfield, Illinois, Charles C. Thomas Publishers, 1965.
31. Mortensen, P.T.: Droperidol: Postoperative anti-emetic effect when given intravenously to gynaecological patients. Acta Anaesthesiol. Scand., *26*:48, 1982.
32. Noram, S.E., Ho, K., Doumas, B.T.: Ethylene oxide sterilization of local anesthetics: A potential hazard? Reg. Anaesth., *4*:2, 1979.
33. Park, G.R., Wilson, J.: Althesin infusion and regional blockade anaesthesia for major gynaecological surgery. Br. J. Anaesth., *50*:1219, 1978.
34. Palazzo, M.G.A., Strunin, L.: Anaesthesia and emesis: I. Etiology. Can. Anaesth. Soc. J., *31*:178, 1984.
35. Peck, C.: Pain management in critical care. *In* Cousins, M.J., Phillips, G.D. (eds.): Clinics in Critical Care Medicine. p. 251. W.B. Saunders, Philadelphia, 1985.
36. Philip, B.K.: Supplemental medication for ambulatory procedures under regional anesthesia. Anesth. Analg., *64*:1117, 1985.
37. Raj, P.P., Rosenblatt, R., Montgomery, S.J.: Use of the nerve stimulator for peripheral blocks. Reg. Anaesth., *5*:14, 1980.
38. Scott, D.B.: Management of extradural block during surgery. Br. J. Anaesth., *47*:271, 1975.
39. Scott, D.L.: Sedation for local analgesia. Anaesthesia, *30*:471, 1975.
40. Selander, D., Dhuner, K.G., Lundborg, G.: Peripheral nerve injury due to injection needles used for regional anesthesia. Acta Anaesthesiol. Scand., *21*:182, 1977.
41. Selander, D., Edshage, S., Wolff, T.: Paresthesiae or no paresthesiae? Acta. Anaesthesiol. Scand., *23*:27, 1979.
42. Seow, L.T., Mather, L.E., Cousins, M.J.: A comparison of the efficacy of chlormethiazole and diazepam as intravenous sedatives for supplementation of epidural anesthesia. Br. J. Anaesth., *57*:747, 1985.
43. Studd, C., Eltringham, R.J.: Lorazepam as night sedation and premedication: A comparison with diazepam. Anaesthesia, *35*:60, 1980.
44. Vickers, M.D., Wood-Smith, F.G., Stewart, H.C.: Central nervous system depressants. *In* Drugs in Anaesthetic Practice, 5th ed., p. 66. London, Butterworth & Co., 1978.
45. White, P.F.: Use of continuous infusion versus intermittent bolus administration of fentanyl or ketamine during outpatient anesthesia. Anesthesiology, *59*:294, 1983.

section A
CENTRAL NEURAL BLOCKADE

7 SPINAL (SUBARACHNOID) NEURAL BLOCKADE

PHILLIP O. BRIDENBAUGH
NICHOLAS M. GREENE

Spinal anesthesia consists of the temporary interruption of nerve transmission within the subarachnoid space produced by injection of a local anesthetic solution into cerebrospinal fluid. Used widely, safely, and successfully for almost 90 years, spinal anesthesia has many potential advantages over general anesthesia, especially for operations involving the lower abdomen, the perineum, and the lower extremities.

In this chapter we review the techniques of spinal anesthesia and its advantages and disadvantages based on anatomic, pharmacologic, and physiologic principles. Spinal anesthesia for diagnostic and therapeutic purposes, including differential spinal anesthesia, is discussed in Chapter 27. Intrathecal injection of opioids is discussed in Chapter 28.

Many terms have been used to describe the injection of local anesthetics into the subarachnoid space, including *spinal anesthesia, spinal* or *subarachnoid analgesia, spinal* or *subarachnoid block,* and *subarachnoid anesthesia. Subarachnoid* is semantically correct: The injection is made into the subarachnoid space, and that is where the neural response occurs. *Subarachnoid* is certainly clear and unambiguous to physicians. *Subarachnoid* is not equally clear to any but the patient with the most sophisticated knowledge of anatomy. In communicating with patients, *subarachnoid* is best avoided if truly informed consent is to be obtained for the type of anesthesia to be used. The term *block,* as in *spinal* or *subarachnoid block,* is incorrect. To neurologists, neurosurgeons, and other nonanesthesiologic physicians, *spinal block* means obstruction to the flow of CSF within the spinal subarachnoid space. *Analgesia* is also not entirely correct. Injection of local anesthetics (not local "analgesics") into CSF produces anesthesia, not analgesia in the operative field. All sensation is lost, not just the ability to feel pain. It is suggested that *spinal anesthesia,* the term used in this chapter, is preferable. It is accurate. It is unambiguous.

HISTORY

The history of anesthesia is not the story of random events. It was logical, almost predictable in fact, that anesthesia would be first introduced about 1846 and that, when introduced, the first anesthetic would be an inhalation agent of rather simple chemical structure.[43] It was equally logical, almost inevitable, that the next type of anesthesia to be introduced would be local, not intravenous, anesthesia. But other things had to take place before local anesthesia could be introduced. The needle and syringe had to be invented. The industrial evolution had to develop to the point where needles and syringes could be mass produced with accuracy great enough to assure a perfect match between barrels and plungers of the syringes. Above all, the germ theory of disease had to be introduced, and, after that, the ability to avoid infection by asepsis had to be proved. Invasive anesthetic techniques using needles were impossible until the fear of creating infection was resolved.

The prerequisites necessary for the introduction of local anesthesia were all realized by the 1880s, and in 1884 Koller reported that the topical application of cocaine to the eye produced anesthesia of the cornea and conjunctiva.[55] Again, there is a sense of inevitability about what Koller did, not only in its timing but also in the fact that cocaine was the first local anesthetic. The first local anesthetic almost had to be a naturally occurring compound. Industrial chemistry had not advanced in the 1880s to the point where compounds as chemically complex as local anesthetics could be synthesized. Also, doctors of the time had to know about and be acquainted with the first local anesthetic in the same way they had to be already familiar with the first inhalation anesthetic, ether.[43] Cocaine, identified in 1855 and isolated in 1860, was a naturally occurring alkaloid that, by the 1880s, had been purified and medically used for nonanesthetic purposes.

Within months of publication of Koller's paper, cocaine was being injected to produce regional anesthesia, not just topical anesthesia. In the same year, 1885, Halsted used cocaine to block the brachial plexus, and Corning, a neurologist in New York, injected cocaine intervertebrally in dogs and in patients.[23] As a neurologist, Corning's objective was to relieve chronic pain in his patients, not to produce operative anesthesia. Indeed, whether his injections were made into the subarachnoid or the epidural space is not clear. Corning thus cannot be considered as the one who introduced operative spinal anesthesia. In fact, spinal anesthesia could not become an acceptable means for use of cocaine until a safe, predictable means for performing lumbar punctures was described. Quincke did this in 1891, but even so it was not until 1899 that August Bier used Quincke's technique to inject cocaine in order to produce operative anesthesia in six patients, the first real spinal anesthesia.[9] Bier's report of his success with spinal anesthesia was rapidly seized upon by others. In the same year Matas in New Orleans and Tuffier in France also reported on the use of cocaine spinal anesthesia,[66,94] as did Tait and Cagliesi in San Francisco in 1900.[91] In 1901, there were no less than 27 papers published on cocaine spinal anesthesia.[5] In 1902, Morton, in New York,[73] reported a series of cocaine spinal anesthetics for operations on all portions of the body, including the head and neck.

The first phase in the history of spinal anesthesia, from 1899 to 1905, was characterized by the use of only cocaine for spinal anesthesia. The popularity of cocaine spinal anesthesia in the year following 1899 was, however, limited principally to a relatively few enthusiasts who, despite their almost evangelical fervor, were unsuccessful in convincing others of the advantages of their new-found technique. They were unable to do so mainly because of the high frequency of conspicuous central nervous system side-effects, including tremors, hyperreflexia, severe headaches, and muscle spasms and pains. By the turn of the century, however, the German chemical and pharmaceutical industry had advanced to the point where new and totally synthetic drugs were being developed. Among these was procaine, first synthesized by Einhorn in 1904. In 1905, Heinrich Braun, a German surgeon, reported the use of procaine for operative spinal anesthesia.[11] With the introduction of procaine, spinal anesthesia entered a new phase, an era of development, refinement, and widespread popularity. Procaine for spinal anesthesia initiated this new era because it was the first neurologically safe local anesthetic. Within an astonishingly brief time, spinal anesthesia became widely used, even though still not universally accepted as a safe, convenient, and effective anesthetic technique. It was, in the eyes of many, vastly superior to general anesthesia with ether or chloroform. It was also simpler than other more complex types of regional anesthesia. Equally important, thanks to the remarkably astute observations of clinicians like Babcock, Koster, Labat, and Pitkin,[4,56,59,80] came understanding of the causes of hypotension during spinal anesthesia and how to manage it. So, too, came refinements in the techniques of spinal anesthesia, including means for controlling levels of anesthesia by making procaine solutions hyperbaric by adding glucose, first reported by Barker in 1907,[6] or hypobaric, initially by adding alcohol. The popularity of spinal anesthesia was further advanced by the synthesis of tetracaine in 1931 and its introduction into clinical practice by Sise in 1935, as well as by the synthesis of dibucaine and its introduction into clinical practice by Jones in 1930.[50,88] These new local anesthetics provided longer duration of spinal anesthesia than did procaine. Duration of spinal anesthesia was further extended by the use of continuous spinal anesthesia by Lemmon in 1940 and Tuohy in 1945.[60,95] In 1945, Prickett and associates published their report on the neurologic safety of intrathecal epinephrine to prolong the duration of spinal anesthesia,[82] a practice introduced as early as 1903 by Braun[10] but never widely accepted because of the fear of neurologic complications.

By the mid-1940s spinal anesthesia had reached a peak of its popularity, a popularity soon followed by almost equally widespread avoidance and neglect.

The era of neglect of spinal anesthesia was brought about by a combination of circumstances, including the fear of neurologic complications, a fear based on widely publicized legal decisions, especially in the United Kingdom, and scientifically unsound but widely publicized articles on extraordinarily high incidences of neurologic sequelae. The demise of spinal anesthesia was further contributed to by the introduction and popularization of intravenous anesthetics, neuromuscular relaxants, and, somewhat later, modern halogenated inhalation anesthetics. The pharmacologic explosion in anesthesia between 1945 and 1965 made spinal anesthesia appear unnecessarily demanding, inconvenient, and tedious, as well as, at least medicolegally unsafe. To all of this was added the introduction of ever increasingly radical operations, the magnitude and duration of which were incompatible with spinal anesthesia.

Around 1965, spinal anesthesia began a recovery that has persisted and even accelerated over the last 20 years. One factor in this renaissance was the epidemiologically impeccable studies of Dripps and Vandam demonstrating that, when properly performed, spinal anesthesia is neurologically safe.[31] Another factor was the introduction of new amide-type local anesthetics. Finally, there was gradual acceptance of the fact that general anesthesia, too, has risks and hazards, a concept contributed to by the halothane hepatitis controversy of the 1960s and 1970s.

ANATOMY

Intimate knowledge of the anatomy of the vertebral column and its contents is the keystone to successful, safe spinal anesthesia, not only in terms of the performance of lumbar puncture but also in terms of the spread of local anesthetics in CSF and the level of anesthesia achieved.

VERTEBRAL COLUMN

The vertebral column, comprising 33 vertebrae (7 cervical, 12 thoracic, 5 lumbar, 5 fused sacral, and 4 coccygeal), has four curves (Fig. 7-1). The cervical and lumbar curves are convex anteriorly, whereas the thoracic and sacral curves are convex posteriorly. The curves of the vertebral column have a significant influence on the spread of local anesthetics in the subarachnoid space. In the supine position, the high points of the cervical and lumbar curves are at C5 and L5; the low points of the thoracic and sacral curves are at T5 and S2, respectively. The vertebral column is bound together by several ligaments, which give it stability and elasticity (Fig. 7-2).

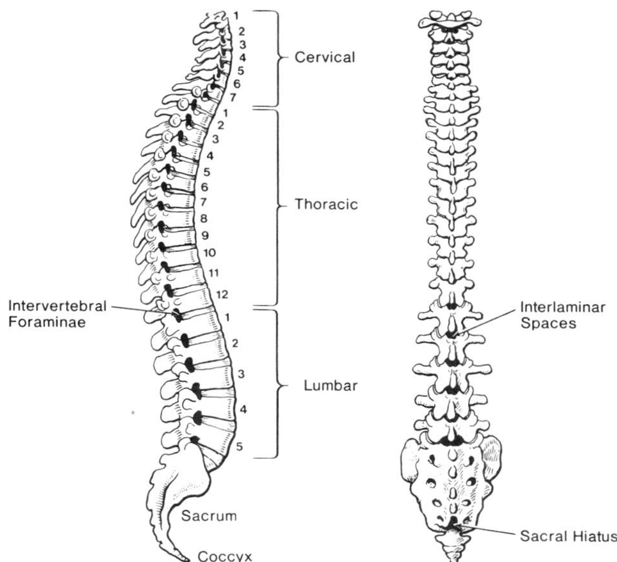

FIG. 7-1. Vertebral column, lateral *(left)* and posterior *(right)* views, illustrating curvatures and interlaminar spaces.

Supraspinous ligament is a strong fibrous cord that connects the apices of the spinous processes from the sacrum to C7, where it is continued upward to the external occipital protuberance as the ligamentum nuchae. It is thickest and broadest in the lumbar region and varies with patient age, sex, and body build.

Interspinous ligament is a thin, membranous ligament that connects the spinous processes, blending anteriorly with the ligamentum flavum and posteriorly with the supraspinous ligaments. Like the supraspinous ligaments, the interspinous ligaments are broadest and thickest in the lumbar region.

Ligamentum flavum, or the "yellow ligament," comprises yellow elastic fibers and connects adjacent laminae that run from the caudal edge of the vertebra above to the cephalad edge of the lamina below. Laterally, this ligament begins at the roots of the articular processes and extends posteriorly and medially to the point where the laminae join to form the spinous process. Here, the two components of the ligaments are united, thus covering the interlaminar space.

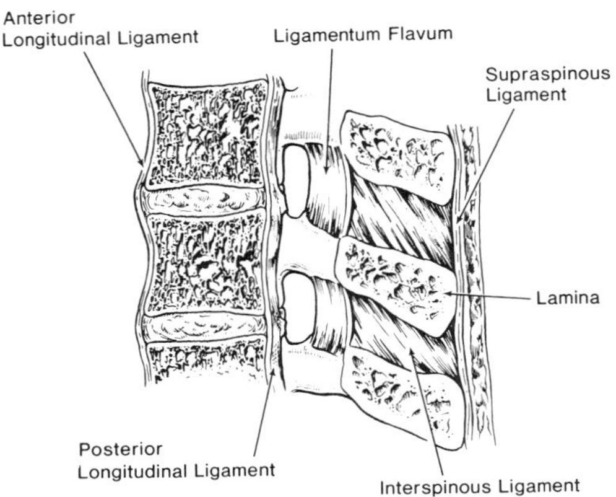

FIG. 7-2. Sagittal section of vertebral column, showing ligaments.

Longitudinal Ligaments. The anterior and posterior longitudinal ligaments bind the vertebral bodies together.

Epidural space surrounds the spinal meninges and extends from the foramen magnum, where the dura is fused to the base of the skull, to the sarcral hiatus, which is covered by the sacrococcygeal ligament (see Chap. 8). It is bounded anteriorly by the posterior longitudinal ligament, laterally by the pedicles and the intervertebral foramina, and posteriorly by the ligamentum flavum and the anterior surface of the lamina. The anterior epidural space is very narrow because of the proximity of the dura and the anterior surface of the vertebral canal. The epidural space is widest posteriorly and varies with the vertebral level, ranging from 1 to 1.5 mm at C5 to 2.5 to 3 mm at T6 to its widest point 5 to 6 mm at the level of L2. In addition to nerve roots that traverse the epidural space, the contents of the epidural space are fat, areolar tissue, lymphatics, arteries, and the extensive internal vertebral venous plexus of Batson.[7]

Spinal Meninges. The spinal cord is protected by both the bony vertebral column and three connective tissue coverings, the meninges (Fig. 7-3).

Dura mater, the outermost membrane, is a tough, fibroelastic tube the fibers of which run longitudinally. Although continuous, it can be described in two parts: the *cranial* and the *spinal.* The cranial dura consists of an outer layer (endosteal) that lines the skull, and an inner layer (meningeal), that invests the brain and folds inward to form the falx cerebri. The two layers are closely united except where they enclose the great venous sinuses that drain the blood from the brain (Fig. 7-4).

At the spinal level, the outer (endosteal) layer continues down the vertebral canal as periosteal lining. The inner (meningeal) layer continues caudad as the spinal dura, or *theca.* Superiorly, it is firmly attached to the circumference of the foramen magnum of the occipital bone. Inferiorly, or caudally, the dural sac ends at the lower border of S2, where it is pierced by the filum terminale. The filum terminale is the terminal thread of the pia mater, which extends from the tip of the spinal cord to blend with the periosteum on the back of the coccyx. The filum terminale anchors the cord and spinal dura, the latter being further steadied in the lower end of the vertebral column by a few fibrous strips from the posterior longitudinal ligament. The spinal dura also provides a thin cover for the spinal nerve roots, becoming progressively thinner near the intervertebral foramina, where it continues as epineural and perineural connective tissue of the peripheral nerves (Fig. 7-5).

Arachnoid mater is the middle of the three coverings of the brain and spinal cord. It is a delicate nonvascular membrane closely attached to the dura, and, with it, ends at the lower border of S2. There is a capillary interval or potential cavity between the dura and arachnoid mater called the subdural space: It contains a minute quantity of serous fluid that moistens the smooth surfaces of the opposed membranes. It does not communicate directly with the subarachnoid space but extends laterally over the nerve roots and ganglia. The subdural space is wider in the cervical region and more accessible than elsewhere in the spinal column. It is also wider laterally adjacent to the nerve roots, which can be shown after injection of radioactive dye (Fig. 7-6). In this situation, the injected solution curves downward between the arachnoid and dura to lymph spaces within root ganglia.[69] Analgesic solutions introduced into this space are said to ascend, but only very slowly in the cranial cavity with which this space communicates.

Although most subdural injections of local anesthetics are unintentional, Mehta[68] describes the technique for intentional entry into the space with x-ray control. He notes that if the needle enters the subarachnoid space with flow of CSF, one withdraws the needle until the flow stops, and at this point the bevel of the needle will likely rest in the subdural space. This could also allow CSF to flow into the subdural

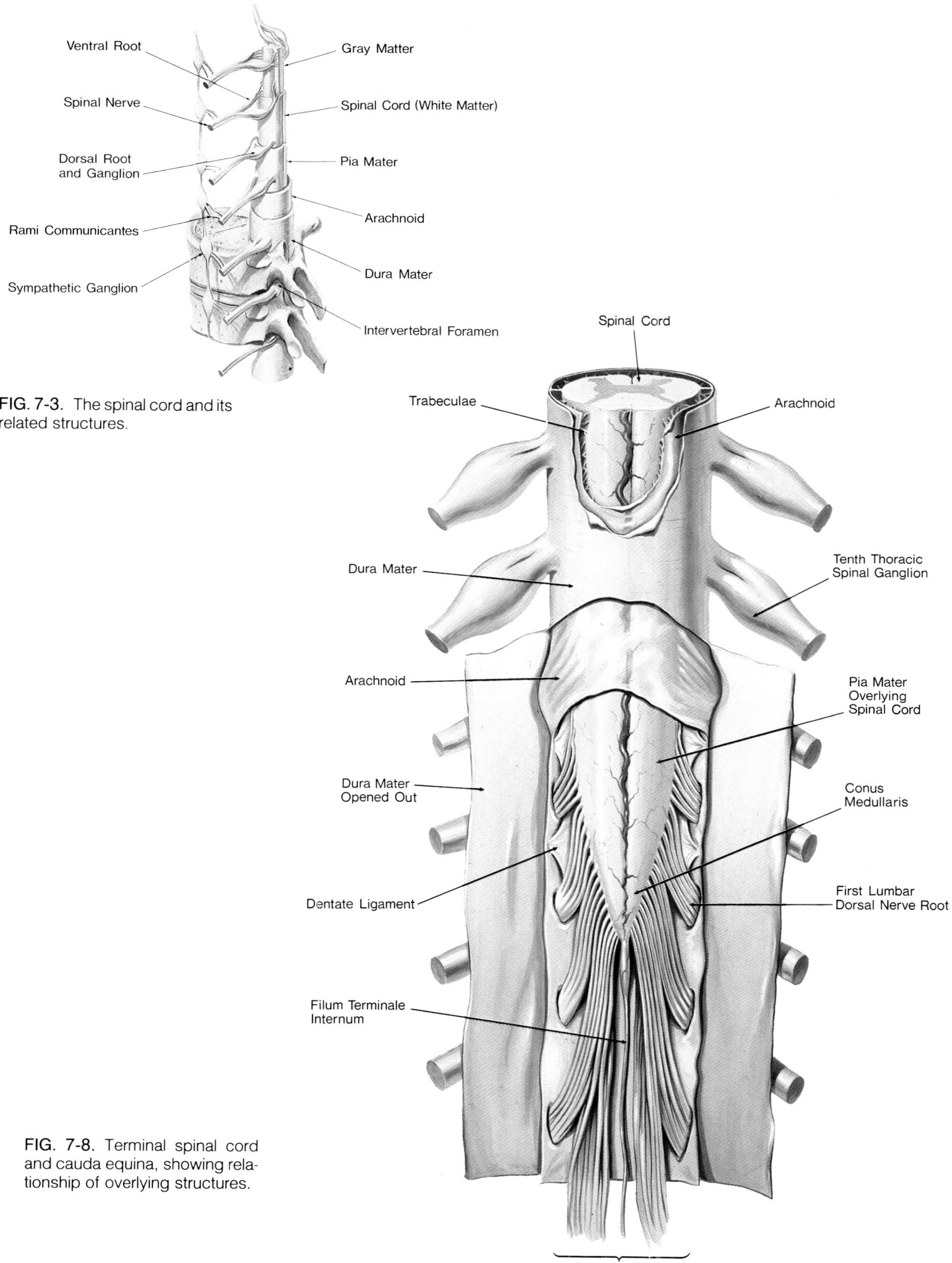

FIG. 7-3. The spinal cord and its related structures.

FIG. 7-8. Terminal spinal cord and cauda equina, showing relationship of overlying structures.

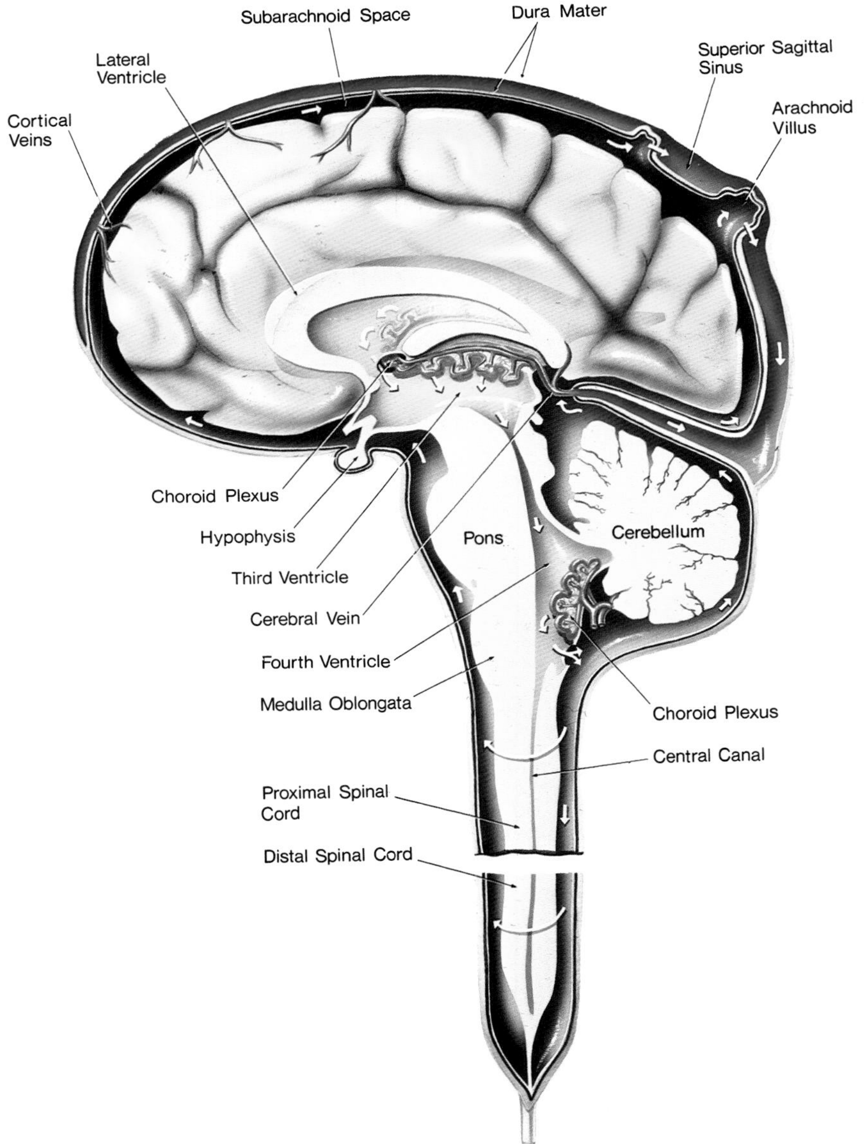

FIG. 7-9. Production, circulation, and resorption of cerebrospinal fluid.

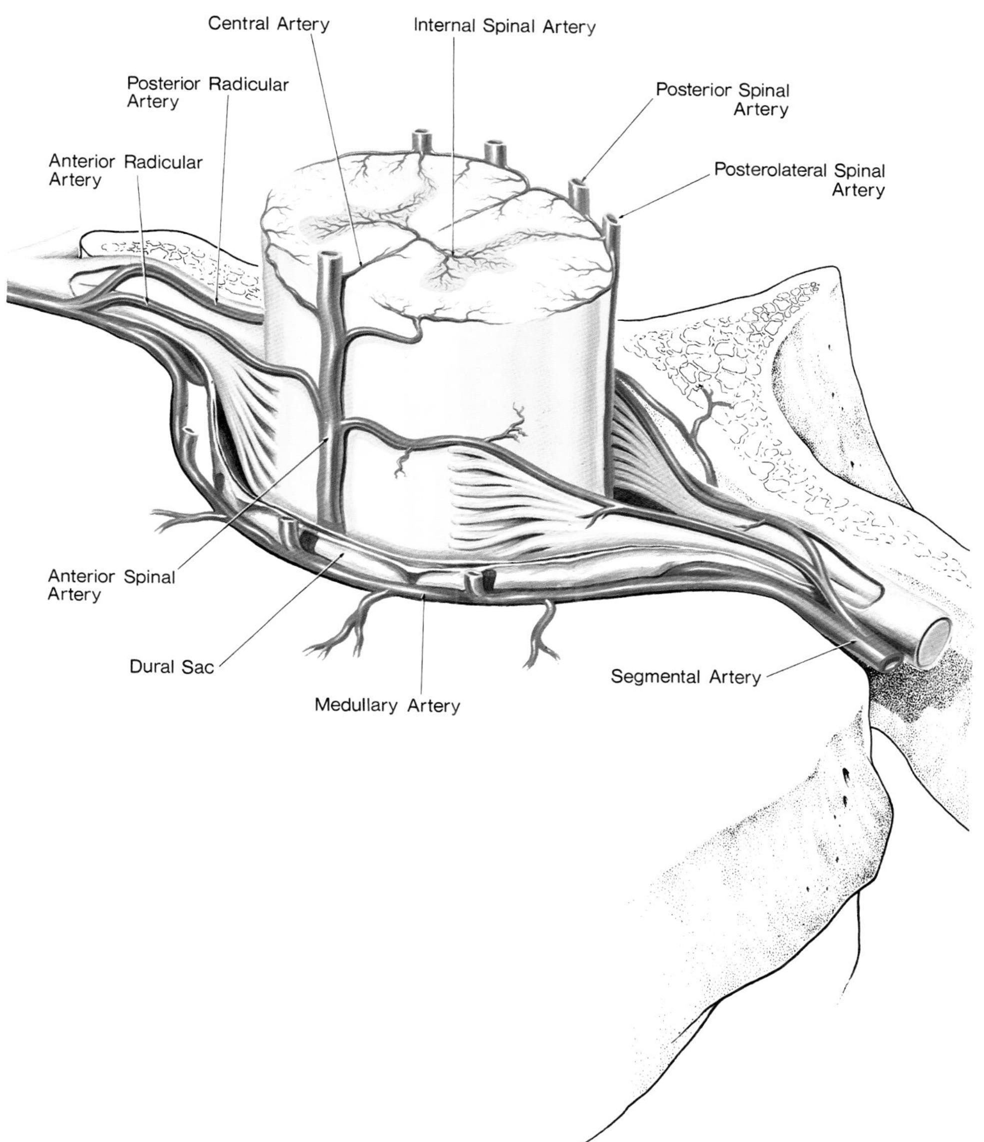

FIG. 7-10. Arterial supply of the spinal cord.

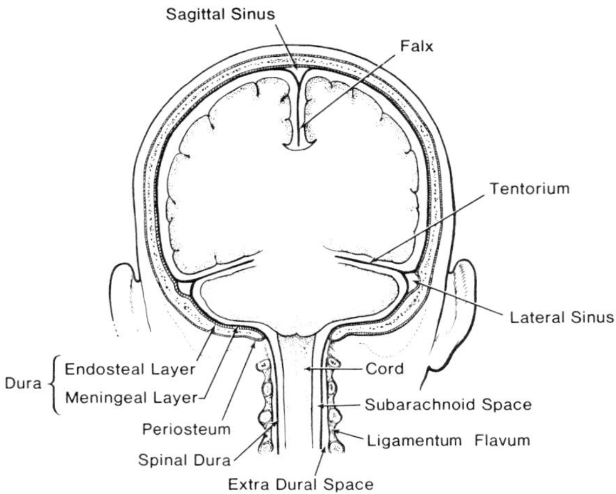

FIG. 7-4. Meningeal coverings of brain and proximal cord.

space. The subdural space has long been recognized by radiologists during the performance of a myelogram. If dye leaks through the needle puncture into the subdural space, it obscures the radiologic field for weeks, which may account for a few, but clearly not all, of the failed spinals despite aspiration of "some" spinal fluid. The case reports of subdural injection indicate unilateral or inordinately high levels of anesthesia, but usually after volumes of local anesthetic intended for epidural anesthesia.[65,78] This occasional phenomenon explains why the term "subdural block" is incorrect when referring to spinal anesthesia and explains the rare case of spinal subdural hematoma.

Pia mater is a delicate, highly vascular membrane closely investing the spinal cord and brain. It clings to the surface of both throughout their entire course. The space between the arachnoid and the pia is thus called the *subarachnoid space.* A large number of cobweblike trabeculae run between these two membranes, and, of course, the space contains the spinal nerves and the CSF as well. The many blood vessels that supply the spinal cord are also found in this space. Lateral projections of the pia, the denticulate ligaments, are attached to the dura and aid in supporting the spinal cord (Fig. 7-7).

Spinal cord, continuous above with the medulla oblongata, begins at the level of the foramen magnum and ends below as the conus medullaris. At birth, the cord ends at the level of L3 but rises to end in adult life at the lower border of L1 (Fig. 7-8).

Spinal Nerves. There are 31 pairs of symmetrically arranged spinal nerves, which are attached to the spinal cord by two roots. Both the anterior and posterior roots arise from the cord as several filaments, or rootlets. The lumbar and sacral nerve roots extending beyond the termination of the spinal cord at the lower border of L1 form the cauda equina. The greater surface area of nerves in the cauda equina as they traverse the subarachnoid space from their point of origin in the cord to their point of exit through the dura, together with the fact that they are covered by only a thin layer of pia, means that lumbar and sacral nerve roots are especially sensitive to the effects of local anesthetics in the CSF by which they are bathed.

Subarachnoid space, bounded internally by the pia and externally by the arachnoid, is filled with cerebrospinal fluid and contains numerous arachnoid trabeculae, which form a delicate, spongelike mass. This space has three divisions: cranial (surrounding the brain), spinal (surrounding the spinal cord), and root (surrounding the dorsal and ventral spinal nerve roots). All of these components are in "free communication" with each other. Again, as the dorsal and ventral nerve roots leave the spinal cord, they are covered only by pia and bathed in CSF (see Fig. 7-3). As these spinal nerve roots pass beyond the spinal dura and traverse the epidural space, they carry with them all three meningeal layers and have distinct epidural, subdural, subarachnoid, and subpial spaces. As indicated above, as the dura extends further out toward the intervertebral foramen, it becomes much thinner. The subarachnoid space extends separately along both the dorsal and ventral

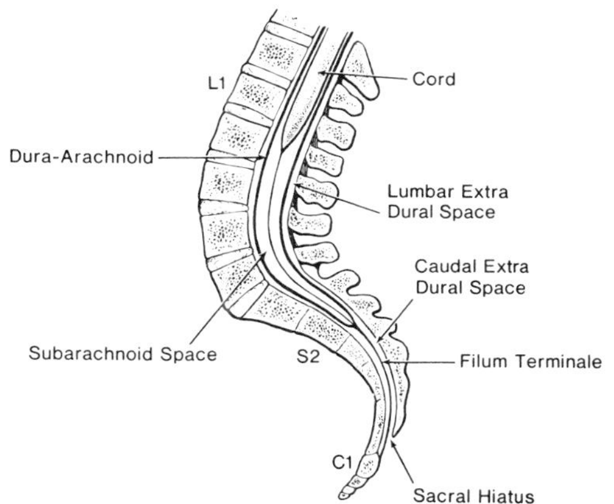

FIG. 7-5. Lumbosacral portion of vertebral column, showing terminal spinal cord and its coverings.

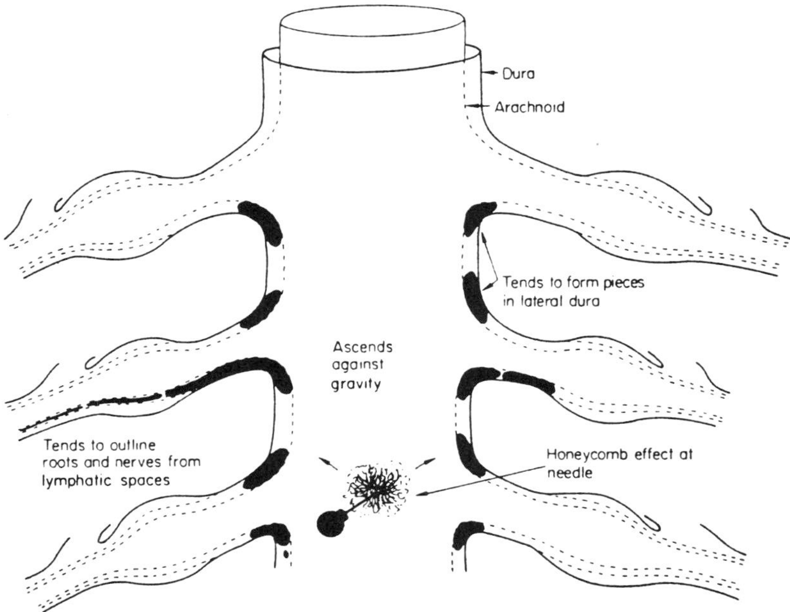

FIG. 7-6. Diagrammatic representation of the spread of radiopaque contrast medium injected into the cervical subdural space. The initial honeycomb effect at the injection site is replaced by the collection on either side of small pools or pieces in the lateral dura owing to outward spread of the solution. (Mehta, M., and Maher, R.: Injection into the extra-arachnoid subdural space. Anaesthesia, *32*:761, 1977.)

roots to the level of the dorsal root ganglion where the arachnoid and the pia continue as the perineural epithelium of the peripheral nerve. The spinal nerve root arachnoid contains proliferations of arachnoid cells, or villi, which have been identified in humans and other animals, along with dorsal and ventral roots.[86] These proliferations are of many shapes and sizes and may protrude into adjacent subdural spaces (see Chap. 8).

Cerebrospinal fluid is an ultrafiltrate of the blood plasma with which it is in hydrostatic and osmotic equilibrium. It is a clear, colorless fluid found in the spinal and cranial subarachnoid spaces and in the ventricles of the brain. At 37°C, the specific gravity ranges from 1.003 to 1.009, with a mean of 1.006. The total volume of CSF in the average adult ranges from 120 to 150 ml, of which 25 to 35 ml is in the spinal subarachnoid space. The majority of the spinal subarachnoid volume lies distal to the cord in the area of the cauda equina. In the horizontal position, the pressure of CSF ranges from 60 to 80 mm H_2O.

Acid–Base. In normal subjects, the *p*H of CSF is slightly lower than that of the arterial blood (7.32).

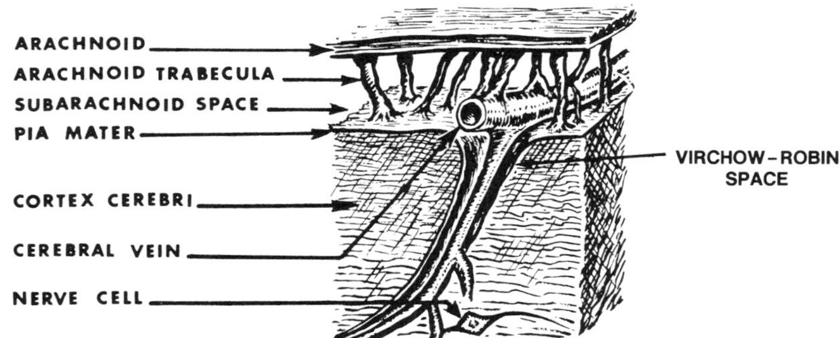

FIG. 7-7. Diagram of subarachnoid space showing blood vessels and arachnoid trabecula. (Redrawn after Strong, O.S., and Elwyn, A.: Human Neuroanatomy. Baltimore, Williams & Wilkins, 1959.)

The P_{CO_2} is higher (48 mm Hg) and the bicarbonate level about the same in both fluids (23 mEq/liter). Cisternal and lumbar CSF samples obtained at the same time in steady-state have very similar *p*H, P_{CO_2} and bicarbonate levels; however, during rapidly changing conditions, as in respiratory alkalosis or acidosis, the lumbar CSF is slow to respond, whereas cisternal values reflect changes in systemic acid–base parameters.[36]

Electrolytes. The concentrations of electrolytes in CSF are similar to, but vary from, those in serum. The sodium ion is the major cation present in plasma and CSF. Whereas the normal concentration range in both fluids is similar, varying between 133 and 145 mEq/liter, the absolute concentration is slightly greater in plasma. The CSF calcium levels vary between 2 and 3 mEq/liter and the total serum levels between 4 and 5 mEq/liter. Not only is CSF calcium not affected by diseases of the nervous system, but also it is even maintained postmortem. Thus there seems little basis for measuring CSF calcium in clinical practice. Similar stability occurs with CSF phosphorus (largely phosphate). The normal CSF level is about 60% of the serum level (1.6 mg/dl compared with 4.0 mg/dl). There has been more interest in the magnesium levels in CSF because magnesium is the sole cation in which the concentration in CSF is substantially greater (30%) than that in serum. The CSF level lies between 2.0 and 2.5 mEq/liter and the serum level between 1.5 and 2.0 mEq/liter.

Interest in the CSF chloride results from its role as the major anion of CSF and the fact that its concentration exceeds the plasma level. CSF chloride level is normally 15 to 20 mEq/liter higher than the serum level. It is slightly reduced in the presence of a very elevated CSF protein level and otherwise follows serum level, but absolute changes are less than those in serum. There seems to be no indication for measurement of CSF chloride in clinical practice.[36]

Proteins. In normal children and adults, there is a concentration gradient of protein from a low level in the ventricles (6–15 mg/dl) to an intermediate level in the cisterna magna (15–25 mg/dl) to the highest level in the lumbar sac (20–50 mg/dl). This gradient is best explained by the relatively increased permeability of the blood–CSF barrier to proteins in the spinal subarachnoid space. Normal values reported for the lumbar CSF total protein have varied. Normal patients and volunteers have mean values ranging from 23 to 28 mg/dl. Since the reported upper and lower limits vary from 9 to 58 mg/dl, it is essential that clinicians know the range of normal values for the laboratory doing the test.

Cerebrospinal fluid is formed by either secretion or ultrafiltration from the choroid arterial plexuses of the lateral, third, and fourth ventricles. The choroid plexus comprises invaginations of capillaries from the subarachnoid space (Fig. 7-9). These capillaries are supported in a flimsy connective tissue framework of pia mater, which, in turn, is in intimate contact with the ependyma, a single-layered epithelium lining the ventricle. It is presumed that these ependymal cells are primarily responsible for the secretion of CSF. Although it is possible, experimentally, to induce both increased and decreased rates of CSF formation, there is a great tendency for it to be maintained at a constant rate.[37] Cardiac glycosides in usual clinical doses probably have no measurable effect, whereas systemic administration to animals of acetazolamide, a carbonic anhydrase inhibitor, reduces the rate of CSF formation by as much as 50%. Furosemide, in large doses, may reduce the rate of CSF formation, whereas steroids have an inconsistent effect. Drugs such as norepinephrine, insulin, chlorothiazide, neostigmine, and phenytoin, among several others less used have no or an insignificant effect on CSF formation. Studies of the effect of hydrostatic pressure showed that CSF formation declines as intraventricular pressure increases to a sufficient degree and duration. CSF formation is reduced when serum osmolality increases, and increases when serum is made hypotonic. The relationship is approximately linear, with a 1% change in serum osmolality causing a 6.7% change in CSF formation. During equilibrium, the rate of absorption of CSF equals its rate of formation. These rates are about 0.35 ml/minute or 500 ml/day.

Composition of Cerebrospinal Fluid

Specific gravity, 1.006 (1.003–1.009)
Volume, 120–150 ml (25–35 ml spinal space)
CSF pressure (lumbar), 60–80 mm H_2O
*p*H, 7.32 (7.27–7.37)
P_{CO_2}, 48 mm/Hg
HCO_3^-, 23 mEq/liter
Sodium, 133–145 mEq/liter
Calcium, 2–3 mEq/liter
Phosphorus, 1.6 mg/dl
Magnesium, 2.0–2.5 mEq/liter
Chloride, 15–20 mEq/liter
Proteins (lumbar), 23–38 mg/dl

Spinal Arteries. The spinal cord receives its blood supply from arteries of the brain above, and from spinal branches of the subclavian, aorta, and iliac arteries below. These last-mentioned spinal arteries enter the intervertebral foramina, cross the epidural space, and enter the subarachnoid space in the region of the dural cuff of the spinal nerve roots to gain access to the spinal cord (Fig. 7-10). Although the major purpose of these branches is to serve as blood supply to the spinal nerve roots, only a few feed into the anterior spinal artery. It has been shown, however, that these "nonfeeder" arteries do actually penetrate into the spinal cord and contribute to the segmental nature of the blood supply to the cord.[24]

The paired posterior arteries arise from the posterior inferior cerebellar arteries and descend medially to the posterior nerve roots, sending penetrating vessels to the posterior white columns and the remainder of the posterior gray column. These arteries are fed by 25 to 40 radicular arteries.

The anterior spinal artery is a single, midline artery formed between the pyramids of the medulla oblongata by the union of a branch from the terminal part of each vertebral artery. It descends in front of the anterior longitudinal sulcus of the spinal cord and the corresponding vein to the filum terminale. It gives off numerous circumferential vessels that supply the periphery of the cord and send some 200 branches into the sulcus toward the center of the cord while also sending radiating twigs into the anterior and lateral gray and white columns and into the anterior part of the posterior gray column. As previously noted, these three longitudinal vessels (two posterior and a single anterior arteries) are "fed" by only a few of the spinal branches of the vertebral, deep cervical, ascending cervical, posterior intercostal, lumbar, and lateral sacral arteries. Only about 6 or 7 of these arteries make a significant contribution to the anterior artery, and a similar number make a contribution to the posterior arteries, but not at the same level. These feeders are broken into series of short lengths freely anastomosing posterior to anterior across the midline, providing adequate cord blood flow over three large and relatively discreet segments of spinal cord (Fig. 7-11). The largest of the feeder arteries is the radicularis magna (artery of Adamkiewicz), which supplies the anterior spinal artery in the area of the lumbar enlargement of the cord. It enters by way of a single intervertebral foramen (78% of the time on the left) between the T8 and L3 foramina. Damage to this artery by needle trauma or other means could result in ischemia in the lumbar area of the cord. This is possible because there is poor vertical anastomosis between cervical, thoracic, and lumbar segments of the anterior spinal artery. Anterior spinal artery ischemia results in a predominantly motor lesion, since the anterior two thirds of the spinal cord, including the anterior horn cells, is supplied almost exclusively by the anterior spinal artery. In a small percentage of cases (15%), the artery of Adamkiewicz takes off high (T5), and the usually slender contribution of iliac tributaries to the conus medullaris and lumbar cord enlarges; under these circumstances, iliac tributaries may feed the anterior spinal artery by means of vessels passing through low lumbar intervertebral foramina. Ligation of these iliac tributaries during pelvic surgery or trauma during epidural anesthesia may result in a lesion in the region of the conus medullaris. In the midthoracic region, relatively small feeder arteries reach the anterior spinal artery by way of intervertebral foramina between T4 and T9. In the cervical and upper thoracic regions, the anterior spinal artery begins with a contribution descending from both vertebral arteries and then receives feeder branches, through intervertebral foramina, from the subclavian artery to help maintain anterior spinal artery blood flow in the upper thoracic region, although this is reduced near T4. The T4 region appears to be the most tenuously supplied, since blood flow from the midthoracic region becomes sluggish near T4.

PHARMACOLOGY

The versatility of spinal anesthesia is afforded by a wide range of local anesthetics and additives that allow control over the level, the time of onset, and the duration of spinal anesthesia. A brief discussion of some of the more common local anesthetics used for spinal anesthesia (see Chap. 4) is followed by consideration of factors governing the distribution of local anesthetic solutions in CSF (*i.e.*, the level of anesthesia), the uptake of local anesthetics by neural elements within the subarachnoid space (*i.e.*, the types of nerves blocked), and the elimination of local anesthetics from the subarachnoid space (*i.e.*, duration of action).

DRUGS

Procaine produces spinal anesthesia with an onset of effect in about 3 to 5 minutes and a duration of 50 to 60 minutes. In the United States, procaine for spinal anesthesia is marketed in 2-ml ampules of 10% aqueous solution. The 10% solution, when diluted with an equal volume of CSF, produces a 5% solution of procaine that weighs about the same as CSF and,

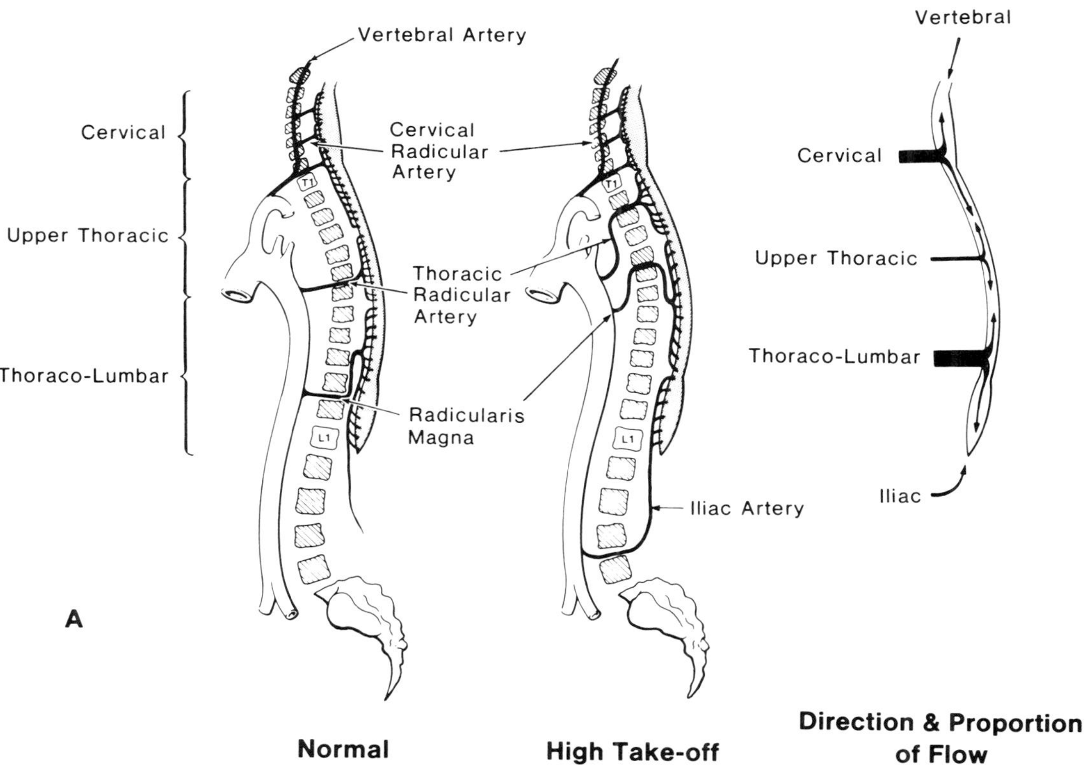

FIG. 7-11. **A.** Blood supply of spinal cord, vertical distribution; functional concept. *In "normal" situations,* note the following; relatively discrete vertical areas with little anastomosis; direction of flow dependent on relationship of area to major "feeder" artery; proportion of flow greatest from radicularis magna 'feeder' artery (artery of Adamkiewicz) to thoracolumbar region. *In abnormal situations* (*e.g.,* "high takeoff"), note the following: The iliac artery branch may supply the lower thoracolumbar region of cord entering by way of the intervertebral foramen in the vicinity of L4–5. **B.** Blood supply of spinal cord; anatomic description. This highlights recent demonstration of "segmental" anatomic distribution of spinal arteries; however, note that although all spinal arteries reach the spinal cord, many are extremely small and offer only a minimal contribution to nutritive blood flow. (Modified from data of Crock, H.V., and Yoshizawa, H.: The blood supply of the vertebral column and spinal cord in man. New York, Springer-Verlag, 1977.)

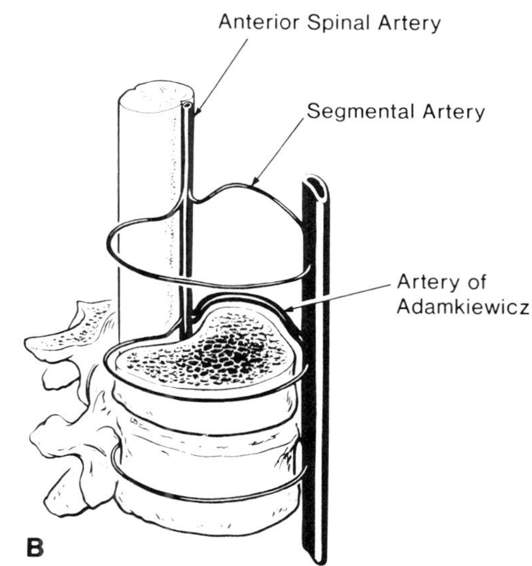

when mixed with an equal volume of 10% glucose, produces a 5% solution of procaine that is heavier than CSF. Aqueous solutions of 2.5% procaine, lighter than CSF, are used principally for differential or diagnostic rather than operative spinal anesthesia. Procaine should not be injected in concentrations exceeding 5%. The suggested dosage ranges from 50 to 100 mg for perineal and lower extremity surgery to 150 to 200 mg for upper abdominal surgery (Table 7-1).

Lidocaine also provides onset of anesthesia in 3 to 5 minutes and lasts slightly longer than procaine, 60 to 90 minutes. Lidocaine is almost universally used in spinal anesthesia as a commercial solution of 5% lidocaine in 7.5% glucose. It is also packaged in the United States as a 2-ml ampule of 1.5% concentration in 7.5% glucose for spinal anesthesia in obstetrics. Usual doses range from 25 to 50 mg for perineal surgery and saddle block anesthesia to 75 to 100 mg for upper abdominal surgery (Table 7-1).

Tetracaine (amethocaine) provides anesthesia with time to onset of 3 to 6 minutes but with a considerably longer duration of action (210–240 minutes) than procaine or lidocaine.[84] Tetracaine is marketed both in ampules that contain 20 mg of crystals and in ampules that contain 2 ml of a 1% aqueous solution of tetracaine. Solutions of 1% tetracaine diluted to 0.1% to 0.33% by the addition of distilled water are lighter than CSF. The 1% solution, when mixed with equal volumes of 10% glucose (0.5% tetracaine in 5% glucose), is widely used as a spinal anesthetic solution that is heavier than CSF. The suggested dosages for tetracaine spinal anesthesia range from 5 mg for perineal and lower extremity surgery to 15 mg for upper abdominal surgery (Table 7-1).

Bupivacaine produces onset of anesthesia in 5 to 8 minutes. Anesthesia lasts about as long as that produced by tetracaine.[57] At this writing, bupivacaine for spinal anesthesia is commercially available in the United States in a 2-ml ampule containing 0.75% bupivacaine in 8.5% glucose. In Australia and most European countries, the 0.5% concentrations, plain or with glucose, have been used for spinal anesthesia. The plain solutions of bupivacaine are very slightly lighter than CSF but can be treated as isobaric solutions. Recommended dosages of bupivacaine for spinal anesthesia range from 8 to 10 mg for perineal and lower extremity surgery and from 15 to 20 mg for upper abdominal surgery (Table 7-1).

Dibucaine (cinchocaine), like tetracaine, produces onset of anesthesia in about 3 to 6 minutes. Anesthesia lasts 210 to 240 minutes. A clinical double-blind study of glucose containing solutions of 0.25% dibucaine and 0.5% tetracaine demonstrated little difference in onset, spread, and duration of sensory analgesia. Tetracaine produced more profound motor blockade.[84]

Vasoconstrictors

Vasoconstrictors have been used for more than 75 years to prolong the duration of spinal anesthesia. Initially, there was concern that vasoconstrictors might produce ischemia of the spinal cord sufficient to cause postoperative neurologic complications. This fear has been proved to be groundless. Although none of several carefully controlled clinical studies[31,63,82] of spinal anesthesia with and without vasoconstrictors have shown that vasoconstrictors are associated with neurologic complications, there are conflicting animal data on the effect of vasoconstrictors on spinal cord blood flow. Studies using unmedicated dogs showed a dose-response reduction in spinal cord blood flow with the subarachnoid administration of phenylephrine.[30] Conversely, measure-

TABLE 7-1. DRUGS FOR SPINAL ANESTHESIA

Drug and Concentration	Dose (mg) To L4	To T10	To T4	Duration (min) Plain	With 0.2 mg Epinephrine
Procaine (5%)	50–75	100–150	150–200	40–55	60–75
Lidocaine (5%)	25–50	50–75	75–100	60–70	60–70
Tetracaine (0.5%)	4–6	6–10	12–16	60–90	120–180
Bupivacaine (0.75%)	4–8	8–12	14–20	90–110	90–110
Dibucaine (0.5%)	4–6	6–8	10–15	150–180	180–240

Bupivacaine 0.5% is available as an isobaric solution that is ideal for surgery below the level of T10, such as hip surgery. Motor block with solution is profound and long lasting in the legs. Doses are 10 to 15 mg for the L4 level and 15 to 20 mg for the T10 level. A heavy solution of bupivacaine 0.5% is also available and is suitable for abdominal surgery. Doses and effects are similar to those with the bupivacaine 0.75% solution.

ment of spinal cord blood flow in anesthetized cats after subarachnoid injection of lidocaine, mepivacaine, and tetracaine, with and without epinephrine, showed no changes.[81]

Epinephrine and phenylephrine are the vasoconstrictors most widely used to prolong the duration of spinal anesthesia. Dosages of epinephrine vary from 0.2 to 0.5 mg (0.2–0.5 ml of 1 : 1000 epinephrine). Dosages of phenylephrine range from 0.5 to 5 mg (0.05–0.5 ml of a 1% solution). Despite the wide range of doses, there is no discernible relationship in published reports between dose of vasoconstrictor and the extent to which duration of anesthesia is prolonged. When, for example, the dose of epinephrine is kept constant at 0.2 mg, the duration of hyperbaric tetracaine spinal anesthesia has been variously reported as being increased by 12%,[34] by 25%,[71] and by 53%.[77] Further, although 0.5 mg of epinephrine has been reported to increase the duration of tetracaine spinal anesthesia by only 27%,[34], 0.2 mg has been found to prolong tetracaine spinal anesthesia by 25%[71] to 53%.[77]

Failure to establish a clear relation between dose of epinephrine added and the magnitude of prolongation of spinal anesthesia can be ascribed to two factors: failure to control other determinants of duration of spinal anesthesia, including age of the patient, the amount of local anesthetic injected, and the area over which the anesthetic is distributed within the subarachnoid space (*i.e.*, level of anesthesia)[45]; and failure of past reports to use a clear, consistent, and logical definition of the duration of anesthesia.

Rigidly controlled double-blind clinical studies have recently evaluated the extent to which epinephrine and phenylephrine prolong spinal anesthesia while keeping constant the age of patients studied, the dose of local anesthetic used, and the level of anesthesia. Duration of anesthesia was defined as the time required for the maximum level of sensory anesthesia to decrease by a certain number of spinal segments. These clinical studies, subsequently confirmed by pharmacokinetic studies (see Elimination below), indicate that the effect of epinephrine or phenylephrine on duration of spinal anesthesia depends on the local anesthetic used. The addition of epinephrine or phenylephrine to lidocaine or bupivacaine, for example, produces no *clinically meaningful* prolongation of spinal anesthesia as determined by two-segment regression.[19,20,90] If, on the other hand, one compares duration of anesthesia at the lumbar with that at the sacral segment, as would be clinically relevant for perineal and lower extremity surgery, one sees longer anesthesia time with the epinephrine-containing solutions. As previously mentioned, it is important to note the measured end point when making judgments about the role of vasoconstrictors in prolonging clinical anesthesia. The time required for four-segment regression of lidocaine spinal anesthesia averaged 109 minutes without epinephrine and 100 minutes with 0.3 mg of epinephrine.[19] On the other hand, in equally well-controlled studies of tetracaine spinal anesthesia, both epinephrine and phenylephrine produced prolongation of duration of spinal anesthesia that was both clinically and statistically significant.[2,16,22] The time to regression of the sensory level to L1 following 12 mg of hyperbaric tetracaine, for example, averaged 171 minutes without epinephrine, 383 minutes with 0.3 mg of epinephrine, and 357 minutes with 1.0 mg of phenylephrine.[22] Epinephrine and phenylephrine prolong the duration of tetracaine spinal anesthesia and do so equally well when equipotent doses are used. Indeed, one of these studies was so rigidly controlled that a dose-response effect of epinephrine could be seen: The time to regression to L1 when 0.2 mg of epinephrine was added (272 minutes) was significantly less than when 0.3 mg was used (383 minutes).[22] There was, however, no significant difference between the time to regression to L1 when 1.0 mg of phenylephrine was used (357 minutes) and when 2.0 mg of phenylephrine was added (324 minutes).

Why vasoconstrictors prolong tetracaine differently from lidocaine spinal anesthesia remains unclear. A possible reason why the upper levels of regression (two-segment regression) are unaffected by vasoconstrictors may be the failure of the epinephrine to diffuse cephalad in CSF in sufficient concentrations to affect a clinical response, whereas at lower levels it may exert a clinically significant influence.

DISTRIBUTION

Distribution of local anesthetic solutions within the subarachnoid space determines the extent of the neural blockade produced by spinal anesthesia.

At one extreme, the distribution of a local anesthetic solution injected at the L3–L4 interspace may be limited to sacral roots only. At the other extreme, the local anesthetic solution may spread to produce blockade of sacral, lumbar, thoracic, and even cervical roots, even though injected at the same L3–L4 interspace. In either case, the local anesthetic injected at L3–L4 is not homogeneously distributed in CSF. Instead, the concentration of local anesthetic in CSF decreases as a function, not of distance from the site of injection, but of distance from the epicenter at which the concentration of local anesthetic is greatest. A spinal anesthetic solution injected at the L3 – L4 interspace may have an epicenter of greatest concentration in the sacral area, at the site of injection, or in the high thoracic area depending on where the solution has spread and been distributed after injection. Determinants of where the epicenter of concentration lies are discussed later, but the existence of a decrease in concentration of anesthetic in CSF on either side of the point of maximum concentration means that uptake of local anesthetic by neural elements within the subarachnoid space, a function of concentration of anesthetic in CSF, varies at different levels of the cord. The result is the existence of clinically important zones of differential block, as discussed in the following section on uptake.

At least 23 factors have been invoked as being involved in determining where and how far local anesthetic solutions spread in CSF (Table 7-2). Not all, however, are of demonstrable clinical importance. When all other factors that affect distribution are kept constant, factors that have no demonstrable significant effects on distribution include patient weight; composition of CSF; CSF circulation; concentration of local anesthetic in the solution injected; diffusion of local anesthetics in CSF independent of the effects of baricity; addition of vasoconstrictors to the local anesthetic solution; and circulation of CSF.[46]

TABLE 7-2. FACTORS CLAIMED TO INFLUENCE DISTRIBUTION OF LOCAL ANESTHETIC SOLUTIONS IN CEREBROSPINAL FLUID*

Patient characteristics
Age
Height
Weight
Gender
Intra-abdominal pressure
Anatomic configuration of spinal column
Position
Site of injection
Direction of needle bevel
Force of injection
Diffusion
Characteristics of spinal fluid
Characteristics of anesthetic solution
Density
Specific gravity
Baricity
Hypobaric solutions
Isobaric solutions
Hyperbaric solutions
Amount of anesthetic
Concentration of anesthetic
Volume injected
Vasoconstrictors

*Hypothetical or demonstrable.
(Reproduced with permission from Greene, N.M.: Anesth. Analg., *64*:715, 1985.)

The direction in which the bevel of the needle is facing during injection also plays no role in determining where the anesthetic solution goes. Nor, clinical impression to the contrary, does turbulence within CSF during injection affect distribution, except locally at the site of injection. That turbulence has no significant effect on distribution is shown by the fact that, under controlled conditions, differing the rate of injection of a spinal anesthetic solution through needles of the same size has no effect on the level of anesthesia achieved.[67,75] Not even deliberate production of considerable turbulence at the site of injection by barbotage affects distribution.[61,76] Finally, sudden increases in CSF pressure produced by coughing or straining fail to affect spread of local anesthetic solutions in CSF.[32]

Eleven of the 23 factors in Table 7-2 do, nevertheless, influence how far and in what direction a spinal anesthetic solution spreads during and after injection into CSF.[46] One of these — age — is only of minor importance. The level of anesthesia is, when everything else is kept constant, slightly but discernibly greater in older patients than in younger ones. The site of injection, especially if at a level other than the L3 – L4 interspace, is a more important determinant of spread. So, too, is anatomic configuration of the spinal column, particularly when pronounced, as in kyphosis. The height of a patient also affects spread: The taller that a patient is, the fewer the number of spinal segments blocked when a given amount of local anesthetic is injected at L3 – L4. The direction of the needle during injection also plays a role. If the long axis of the needle is pointing in a cephalad direction, the distribution will be more cephalad than if the long axis of the needle is at right angles to the spinal column or facing in a caudad direction during injection. So, too, the volume of CSF significantly affects distribution. Increased intra-abdominal pressure, as in term pregnancy or in patients with ascites or large intra-abdominal tumors, may often be associated with the development of collateral venous channels that pass through the lumbar epidural space because of obstruction of blood flow through the inferior vena cava. If chronic, epidural venous engorgement causes the dura to impinge upon the subarachnoid space with a consequent reduction in volume of CSF in the lumbar subarachnoid space. The decrease in lumbar CSF volume explains why otherwise normal doses of spinal anesthetics produce unexpectedly high levels of anesthesia in term parturients.

The most important factors in determining the spread of spinal anesthetic solutions and the factors most susceptible to manipulation in order to achieve predictable levels of spinal anesthesia are the weight of the anesthetic solution injected in relation to the weight of CSF, the dosage and volume of anesthetic solution injected, and the position of the patient during and immediately after injection.

The weights of spinal anesthetic solutions are expressed in terms of density. Density is the weight in grams of 1 ml of a liquid. The specific gravity of a solution is a ratio: the density of the solution divided by that of water. The baricity of a spinal anesthetic solution is also a ratio: the density of the anesthetic solution divided by that of CSF. Because density is inversely related to temperature, when it is involved in the calculation of specific gravity or baricity, it must be measured at the same temperature, preferably 37°C, if data are to be clinically meaningful. Baricity is the most useful index of determining how spinal anesthetic solutions distribute themselves when added to CSF. Being the ratio between density of the anesthetic solution and density of CSF, baricity is a more direct and simpler index than are calculations based on specific gravities that depend upon the ratio between two ratios, each of which has water as a common denominator. If the baricity of a solution is 1.0, it is by definition isobaric; if greater than 1.0 it is hyperbaric; if less than 1.0 it is hypobaric. The density of normal CSF varies, however, by 0.0003 (two standard deviations) above and below the mean value of 1.0003. For spinal anesthetic solutions to be predictably hypobaric or hyperbaric in all patients requires, therefore, that their baricities be, respectively, less than 0.9990 and greater than 1.0010. Representative densities, specific gravities, and baricities of solutions of importance are given in Table 7-3.

Hypobaric Solutions. Tetracaine and dibucaine are the local anesthetics most frequently used for hypobaric spinal anesthesia. Solutions of 0.1% to 0.33% tetracaine in water are reliably hypobaric in all patients (Table 7-3). Because of the high anesthetic potency and lipid solubility of tetracaine, even solutions of 0.1% to 0.33% in water provide good sensory anesthesia and motor relaxation for up to 2 hours. Such solutions are readily prepared by diluting commercially available 1% tetracaine for spinal anesthesia with sterile distilled water without preservatives or other additives. The commercially available 0.066% solution of dibucaine in 0.5% saline is equally satisfactory. Hypobaric solutions of bupivacaine with baricities substantially less than 0.9990 would also be expected to be equally effective but have not been studied extensively to date. Hypobaric solutions of procaine, lidocaine, and other local anesthetics with relatively low anesthetic potencies are generally unsuitable for operative hypobaric spinal anesthesia. When diluted in distilled water sufficiently to produce hypobaric solutions, they approach the minimum effective concentrations. When further diluted by CSF after intrathecal injection, their concentrations decrease to the point that muscle relaxation is usually incomplete and sensory anesthesia becomes too brief for most procedures.

TABLE 7-3. PHYSICAL CHARACTERISTICS* OF SPINAL ANESTHETIC SOLUTIONS AT 37°C

	Density	Specific Gravity	Baricity
Water	0.9934	1.0000	0.9931
CSF	1.0003	1.0069	1.0000
Tetracaine			
0.33% in water	0.9980	1.0046	0.9977
1.0% in water	1.0003	1.0007	1.0000
0.5% in 50% CSF	0.9998	1.0064	0.9995
0.5% in half normal saline	1.0000	1.0066	0.9997
0.5% in 5% dextrose	1.0136	1.0203	1.0133
Dibucaine			
0.066% in 0.5% saline	0.9970	1.0036	0.9976
Bupivacaine			
0.5% in water	0.9993	1.0059	0.9990
0.5% in 8% dextrose	1.0210	1.0278	1.0207
Procaine			
2.5% in water	0.9983	1.0052	0.9983
Lidocaine			
2% in water	1.0003	1.0066	1.0003
5% in 7.5% dextrose	1.0265	1.0333	1.0265

*Mean values.
(Reproduced with permission from Greene, N.M.: Anesth. Analg., *64*:715, 1985.)

The position of the patient during and for the first few minutes after intrathecal injection of hypobaric solutions determines spread in CSF. If the patient is in the head-up position during and after injection, the anesthetic ascends in a cephalad direction; if in the head-down position, the anesthetic solution spreads caudad. Hypobaric solutions are particularly useful for perineal and rectal operations performed in the prone, jack-knife position. In such cases, anesthesia is induced in the same position as that required for surgery, thus avoiding the need to change the position of the patient after induction of anesthesia. Hypobaric solutions are also useful for low unilateral anesthesia, especially operations on a lower extremity. Hypobaric solutions are not recommended for intra-abdominal procedures. The head-up position required to achieve high enough levels of anesthesia may be dangerous in the presence of extensive sympathetic denervation. Arterial hypotension may be severe in hypovolemic patients.

Isobaric Solutions. Isobaric solutions of tetracaine are readily prepared by mixing equal volumes of the commercial 1% tetracaine solution and either CSF or half normal saline (Table 7.3). The 1% tetracaine solution is itself isobaric but is too concentrated to allow wide enough distribution in CSF to produce levels of anesthesia sufficient for most procedures. Bupivacaine 0.5% in water is slightly hypobaric (Table 7-3), but so slightly that it has been widely and successfully used as an isobaric solution. The slight hypobaricity of 0.5% aqueous solutions of bupivacaine is demonstrated by the fact that lumbar injection of 0.5% bupivacaine in patients in the seated position and who remain seated for the next 2.5 minutes results in sensory levels of anesthesia about one to two segments higher than levels produced in patients in whom the same amount of the same solution is injected in the lateral horizontal position with the patients then being immediately placed in the supine horizontal position.[18,51,96] Isobaric solutions of lidocaine or procaine (Table 7-3) are easily prepared but are of limited value in operative spinal anesthesia for the same reasons as those mentioned previously for hypobaric solutions.

A major clinical advantage of isobaric spinal anesthetics is that position of the patient during and after injection has no effect on distribution of the anesthetic and thus no effect on the levels of anesthesia. Injection can be made with the patient in any position, and the patient can then be placed in the operative position without affecting the level of anesthesia. Isobaric spinals are particularly useful when levels of anesthesia to T10 or below are required. Isobaric solutions, to produce midthoracic or high thoracic levels of anesthesia, will require larger doses and volumes and are used less frequently.

Hyperbaric Solutions. The easiest, safest, and most widely used way to render spinal anesthetic solutions hyperbaric is by adding glucose. Commercially marketed hyperbaric solutions of bupivacaine and lidocaine contain 5% to 8% glucose. Commercial solutions of 1% tetracaine are usually made hyperbaric by mixing with equal volumes of 10% glucose to produce a 5% glucose solution to be injected intrathecally. Five percent to 8% glucose solutions have densities far in excess of those required to render them hyperbaric (Table 7-3). Once enough glucose has been added to increase the baricity of the solution above 1.0010, the concentration of glucose has no effect on distribution.[3,18,25]

Distribution of hyperbaric solutions is governed by position of the patient during injection and for the next 20 to 30 minutes. After that, distribution should no longer be significantly affected by position; however, sensory level should be monitored an additional 10 to 20 minutes, since occasional higher levels have been reported. The seated position during and after injection restricts distribution to lower lumbar and sacral roots. The head-down position results in thoracic levels of anesthesia, depending on the degree and duration of head-down position (see Techniques).

Concentration and the *amount* (dose) of local anesthetic injected, together with *volume* of injectate, have all been said to affect distribution. Separation of the individual effects on distribution of each of these three variables is difficult because changing one of the three affects either or both of the other two variables. This problem has, however, been resolved in a double-blind study by Shesky and colleagues, in which age, height, position, and other factors that affect distribution[87] were controlled. The 72 patients given glucose-free bupivacaine in this study were divided into six groups of 12 patients each with concentrations (5) of bupivacaine volumes (ml) injected, and amounts (mg) of bupivacaine injected being systematically altered as shown in Table 7-4. Levels of anesthesia were significantly higher (T2–T4) in patients given 15 or 20 mg of bupivacaine (groups II, III, V, and VI) than they were in patients given 10 mg (T5–T8; groups I and IV). Further, levels of anesthesia were similar in patients given the same amount of bupivacaine (groups I and IV) even though the con-

TABLE 7-4. CONCENTRATION AND DOSE OF GLUCOSE-FREE BUPIVACAINE AND VOLUME OF SOLUTION USED IN THE SIX GROUPS OF 12 PATIENTS EACH STUDIED BY SHESKY AND CO-WORKERS[87]

Group	Concentration (%)	Volume (ml)	Dose (mg)
I	0.5	2.0	10
II	0.5	3.0	15
III	0.5	4.0	20
IV	0.75	1.3	10
V	0.75	2.0	15
VI	0.75	2.7	20

centration of bupivacaine and the volume injected differed. Also, patients given the same volume of anesthetic solution (2 ml) had levels of anesthesia significantly higher when 0.75% bupivacaine was injected (group V) than when 0.5% was used (group I). The authors concluded that "total dosage of bupivacaine is more important than volume or concentration of anesthetic solution" in determining spread of local anesthetic solution in CSF. These results with slightly hypobaric solutions of bupivacaine may not be directly applicable to solutions that are more clearly hypobaric, more definitely isobaric, or strongly hyperbaric. These data demonstrate, nevertheless, that dosage significantly affects distribution independently of concurrent changes in baricity and volume. There is no evidence that concentration of the injectate *per se* has any influence on clinical spinal anesthesia. Once the selected dose of local anesthetic is injected into the CSF, it takes on a new concentration dependent upon the other factors of drug distribution within the CSF. The concentration of the drug in the injecting syringe has no relevance to any of these other factors. The adjective "more" in the conclusion that dosage is more important than volume is most appropriate. It does not preclude the possibility that volume is also a determinant of distribution, although probably of secondary importance compared to dosage.

UPTAKE

Uptake of local anesthetics into neuronal tissues within the subarachnoid space during spinal anesthesia depends on four factors: concentration of local anesthetic in CSF; surface area of nerve tissue exposed to CSF; lipid content of nerve tissue; and blood flow to nerve tissue.

Uptake of local anesthetics is greatest where the concentration of local anesthetic in CSF is greatest. Since concentration of local anesthetic in CSF decreases as a function of distance above and below the site of highest concentration, so too does uptake by neuronal tissue.

The surface area of nerve roots and their uptake of local anesthetics in CSF is considerable as they cross the subarachnoid space from the cord to their points of exit through the dura.[21] The spinal cord also takes up local anesthetics involving two processes: One is diffusion of local anesthetic along a concentration gradient from CSF through the pia mater directly into the cord. This is a slow process affecting only the most superficial portions of the cord; the other process involves extensions of the subarachnoid space, known as the spaces of Virchow–Robin, that accompany blood vessels penetrating the spinal cord from the pia mater. Through the spaces of Virchow–Robin, local anesthetics in CSF have access to deeper structures in the cord (Fig. 7-7). If accessibility were the only factor governing tissue levels of local anesthetics, concentrations in the spinal cord might be expected to be lower than those present in nerve roots traversing the subarachnoid space. This is not the case; concentrations of local anesthetics are greater in the spinal cord than in nerve roots[21] because of the role played by lipid content in determining uptake of local anesthetics.

Since local anesthetics are more soluble in lipids than in water, heavily myelinated tissues within the subarachnoid space, which have high lipid contents, would be expected to have high concentrations of local anesthetics. This is borne out by the observations of Cohen,[21] who found not only higher concentrations of local anesthetics in tracts within the spinal cord than in nerve roots, but also a correlation between concentrations of local anesthetics in spinal cord tracts and the degree of myelination of fibers within spinal cord tracts.

Tissue blood flow governs tissue concentrations of local anesthetics within subarachnoid nerve tissues because blood flow determines the rate at which local anesthetics are removed from tissue. Highly perfused areas of the cord may thus not always have high concentrations of local anesthetics even though they may contain more lipid and more spaces of Virchow–Robin, and thus greater accessibility to CSF than more poorly perfused areas.[45]

During spinal anesthesia, local anesthetics are found both in nerve roots and within the substance of the spinal cord.[21] The major cause of loss of sensation and muscle relaxation during spinal anesthesia is, however, the presence of local anesthetics in spinal nerve roots and in dorsal root ganglia, not within the spinal cord. The concentration of local anesthetics in nerve roots is, as mentioned above, a function of distance from the site of highest concentration of local anesthetic in CSF. This, combined with the fact that different types of nerve fibers differ in their sensitivities to the blocking effects of local anesthetics, gives rise to zones of differential blockade of great clinical and physiologic importance. These zones of differential blockade are most apparent and most readily measured above, that is, cephalad to, the site of highest concentration of local anesthetic in CSF. During hyperbaric tetracaine spinal anesthesia, for example, the concentration of tetracaine in CSF decreases in cephalad direction until it becomes so low that it is sufficient to block only those nerve fibers in the subarachnoid space that are most sensitive to local anesthetics. These are the preganglionic sympathetic nerves. Traditionally, there has been thought to be a zone of differential sympathetic denervation during anesthesia that averages two spinal segments above the level of sensory blockade.[42] This implies that with sensory analgesia above T4, all or nearly all of the sympathetic chain *should be* blocked; however, results of work done by Bengtsson and colleagues[8] showed that the extent and the intensity of sympathetic block during spinal analgesia were far less than the extent and intensity of sensory analgesia. In addition, the duration of sympathetic blockade was far shorter than either sensory or motor blockade. Their conclusion was that preganglionic sympathetic beta fibers or sympathetic spinal cord pathways, or both, seem to be *more* difficult to block than A fibers during spinal anesthesia.[8,62] Somatic sensory afferent fibers are more sensitive to local anesthetics than are somatic motor fibers. Therefore, a zone of differential motor blockade averaging two spinal segments below the level of sensory analgesia also exists.[38,97] In addition, there are zones of differential sensory blockade because different types of sensory afferent fibers have different sensitivities to local anesthetics. Thus, during hyperbaric tetracaine spinal, the level of analgesia (inability to appreciate pinprick) lies an average of two spinal segments higher than the level of anesthesia (inability to appreciate touch).[99]

The functional significance of the presence of local anesthetics within the spinal cord during spinal anesthesia remains unproven. The result is certainly not chemical transection of the cord. Some neural elements within the cord fail to absorb appreciable amounts of local anesthetics. The concentrations of local anesthetics in neural elements that do absorb local anesthetics vary widely.[21] That the spinal cord is itself relatively unaffected during spinal anesthesia is indicated, nevertheless, by the fact that it is possible, and indeed frequent, that segmental spinal anesthesia occurs, intentionally or not. In the presence of profound blockade of midthoracic sensory and motor fibers, it is also often possible to detect in lumbar and sacral areas normal or nearly normal motor function, as well as transmission of pain sensation in lumbar and sacral areas.

The uptake of local anesthetics by neuronal tissues and blood vessels within the subarachnoid space results in a decrease in concentration of local anesthetic in CSF. Figure 7-12 shows the decrease in CSF concentration of four solutions of lidocaine as a function of time after injection. The lowest concentration 5 minutes after injection occurred with an isobaric hypo-osmotic solution. After 10 minutes, however, disappearance curves of lidocaine from CSF became parallel for all solutions for the next 50 minutes and were not significantly different.[27] The initial sharp falloff in concentration is a result of two simultaneously operative processes: distribution of lidocaine in CSF away from the site of injection, and uptake of lidocaine from CSF into subarachnoid tissues. The initial sharp falloff is followed by a more gradual decrease in CSF concentration. This represents not only continued tissue uptake, but also elimination of procaine from the subarachnoid space. The result of distribution of lidocaine, uptake into subarachnoid tissue, and elimination from the subarachnoid space is that the concentration of lidocaine and glucose in CSF decreases to the point where the remaining solution, previously hyperbaric, approaches isobaricity. When this point is reached (about 30–35 minutes with lidocaine), changes in position of patients given hyperbaric spinal anesthetic solutions no longer influence distribution of the anesthetic solution in CSF. The level of anesthesia becomes "fixed." The position of the patient can be changed without changing the level of anesthesia[27] (see previous section on Hyperbaric Solutions).

ELIMINATION

The rate at which local anesthetics are removed or eliminated from the subarachnoid space determines the duration of spinal anesthesia. Elimination does not involve metabolism of local anesthetics within the subarachnoid space. Elimination is entirely by vascular absorption and is reflected by systemic blood levels of intrathecally injected local anesthetics.[15,26,27,28,39,83]

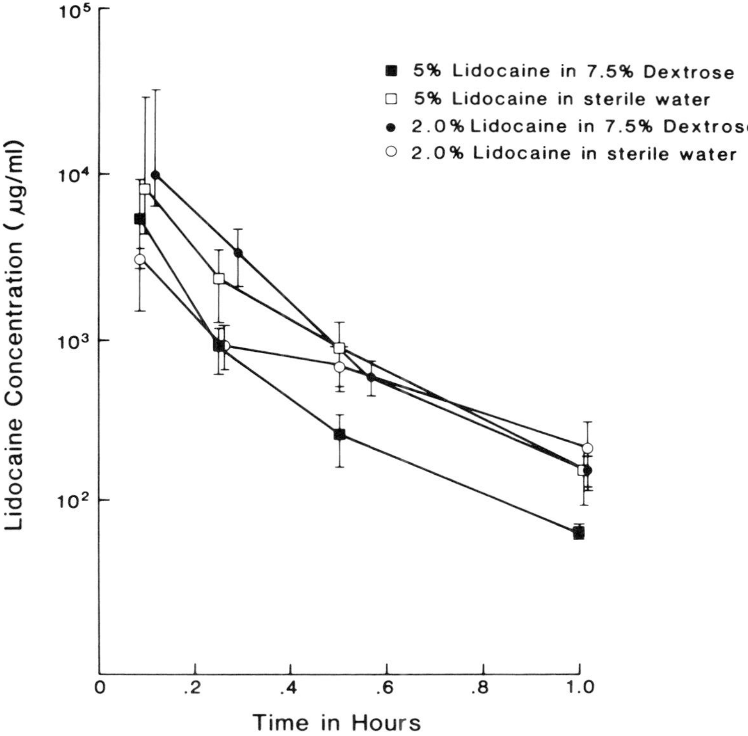

FIG. 7-12. Cerebrospinal fluid lidocaine concentrations as a function of time after injection of lidocaine solutions of different osmolalities and baricities. Data are presented as mean ± SD for the four animals in the Latin square study. (Denson, D.D., Bridenbaugh, P.O., Turner, P.A., *et al.:* Neural blockade and pharmacokinetics following subarachnoid lidocaine in the rhesus monkey: II. Effects of baricity, osmolality and volume. Anesth. Analg., *62*:1000, 1983.)

Elimination by vascular absorption occurs in two areas: the epidural space and the subarachnoid space. Just as local anesthetics pass through the dura into CSF after injection into the epidural space, so, too, do local anesthetics in CSF cross the dura as they move down the concentration gradient between CSF and the epidural space.[45] Movement of drugs across the dura is related to neither lipid solubility nor degree of ionization (and thus not to pKa).[72] Once in the epidural space, local anesthetics originally injected into CSF are again susceptible to vascular absorption. The blood supply in the epidural space is, in terms of ml blood flow $\cdot g^{-1} \cdot min^{-1}$, greater than in the subarachnoid space. Vascular absorption of local anesthetics from the epidural space, therefore, represents as important a route of elimination of local anesthetics from CSF as does vascular reabsorption from the subarachnoid space. Vascular absorption within the subarachnoid space is accomplished principally by vessels in the pia mater on the surface of the cord and by vessels within the cord. Because vascular perfusion of the cord varies in different areas, the rate of elimination, and thus the concentration of local anesthetics in the cord, also varies from one area to another.

The rate at which a given dose of local anesthetic is eliminated from the subarachnoid space in part depends on the vascular absorptive surface area to which that dose is exposed. For example, spinal anesthesia with 10 mg of tetracaine to a level of T12 lasts longer than with a sensory level of T3. It lasts longer because the absorptive surface to which the 10 mg of tetracaine is exposed is greater with T3 than with T12 levels. Differences in rate of vascular absorption as a function of differences in absorptive surface have yet to be pharmacokinetically proved. Burin and colleagues, however, made the interesting observation that times to peak plasma levels of bupivacaine are significantly shorter with 15 mg of hyperbaric bupivacaine than with 15 mg of isobaric bupivacaine, even though peak levels show no significant difference.[15] By contrast, primate studies of lidocaine spinal solutions of varying baricity show significantly faster rates of absorption of lidocaine in sterile water than do the corresponding dextrose solutions, suggesting that rate of absorption from CSF increases with decreasing baricity. There were no differences in height of block or time to two-segment regression among the test solutions.[27]

Lipid solubility would also be expected to determine the rate of elimination of intrathecal local anesthetics. Lipid solubility of local anesthetics is directly related to their duration of action. The more tightly a local anesthetic is bound to lipids, the less susceptible it is to vascular absorption, and the less susceptible it is to removal from its site of action. The rate of vascular absorption, and therefore plasma levels of long-acting, highly lipid-soluble local anesthetics, should be expected to differ from plasma levels of less lipid-soluble, shorter-acting local anesthetics injected intrathecally. This has not, however, been quantitated. Indeed, Burm and co-workers found that times to peak plasma levels of intrathecal hyperbaric lidocaine and bupivacaine were similar[15] despite the greater lipid solubility of bupivacaine.

Decreases in spinal cord blood flow would also be expected to decrease the rate of vascular absorption of intrathecal local anesthetics and thus prolong the duration of spinal anesthesia. This has been proposed as an explanation for the greater duration of spinal anesthesia in older patients, an explanation that has not, however, been quantitated by measurements of peak plasma levels of local anesthetics and times to peak plasma levels as a function of age.

Prolongation of spinal anesthesia by the addition of vasoconstrictors such as epinephrine and phenylephrine has also been ascribed to decreased rates of elimination of intrathecal local anesthetic as a consequence of intrathecal vasoconstriction. However, Kozody and colleagues found that neither 0.2 mg of epinephrine nor 5 mg of phenylephrine decreased spinal blood flow in dogs.[58] Pharmacokinetically more meaningful are data on plasma levels of lidocaine following the intrathecal injection of lidocaine with or without added epinephrine or phenylephrine in experimental animals.[26-28,83] In all of these studies, times to peak levels and peak levels of plasma lidocaine were similar with or without epinephrine or phenylephrine added to the injectate. The disparity between the lack of effect of vasoconstrictors on peak plasma levels of local anesthetics injected into CSF and conflicting reports on their clinical effects needs further study. It appears that local anesthetics placed into CSF are simultaneously and quickly being deposited into neural and vascular tissue. The rate and amount absorbed into the vascular bed is apparently unaffected by vasoconstrictors. There still remains, however, significant amounts of local anesthetic bound to neural tissue in equilibrium with CSF and which must be eliminated therefrom by continued vascular absorption. Here, apparently, factors such as total dose of drug, baricity, vasoconstrictors, cord blood flow, and lipid solubility may play a role in the intensity and duration of neural blockade.

PHYSIOLOGIC RESPONSES

The injection of local anesthetic solutions into the subarachnoid space produces important and often widespread physiologic responses. Understanding the etiology and significance of these physiologic effects is the key to the safe management of patients during spinal anesthesia and to understanding the indications and contraindications of spinal anesthesia.

CARDIOVASCULAR

The most important physiologic responses to spinal anesthesia involve the cardiovascular system.[44] They are mediated by the combined effects of autonomic denervation and, with higher levels of neural blockade, the added effects of vagal nerve intervention. The cardiovascular effects of spinal anesthesia are not due to the presence of local anesthetics in ventricular CSF adequate to produce direct depression of medullary vasomotor centers. Even the concentration of local anesthetics in cisternal CSF during cervical levels of anesthesia is below the concentration required to produce effects on medullary vasomotor centers when applied directly to the brain stem.[44] Similarly, plasma levels of local anesthetics during spinal anesthesia are below those required to produce direct effects on the myocardium or on peripheral vascular smooth muscles. Because of the primacy of sympathetic denervation in the genesis of cardiovascular changes during spinal anesthesia, the effect of spinal anesthesia on the sympathetic nervous system warrants discussion before consideration of the cardiovascular responses themselves.

Sympathetic Denervation. Because the level of sympathetic denervation determines the magnitude of cardiovascular responses to spinal anesthesia, it might be anticipated that the higher the level of neural blockade, the greater would be the change in cardiocirculatory parameters. The relationship is neither predictable nor precise. In the presence of partial sympathetic blockade, a reflex increase in sympathetic activity occurs in sympathetically intact areas. The result is vasoconstriction that tends to compensate for the peripheral vasodilation taking place in the sympathetically denervated areas. This can be seen in the changes in arterial pulse wave contours and in cutaneous blood flow in the upper extremities in the presence of low or midthoracic sensory levels of spinal anesthesia.[12] Of even greater importance is the fact that the most cephalad preganglionic sympathetic fibers come off the spinal cord at the level of T1. Existence of a zone of differential sympathetic denervation may mean that the level of sympathetic denervation is even higher than the level of sensory anesthesia. Since sympathetic denervation is complete at the T1 level, cardiovascular changes are no greater with midcervical sensory levels of anesthesia than they are with T1 levels. Finally, as will be seen below, with proper intraoperative management, vascular hypotension may be modest or even absent in the presence of total sympathetic denervation. The correlation of levels of anesthesia and changes in blood pressure is weak indeed.

Arterial Circulation. Sympathetic denervation produces arterial and, physiologically more important, arteriolar vasodilation. Vasodilation is, however, not maximal. Vascular smooth muscle on the arterial side of the circulation retains a significant degree of autonomous tone following acute, pharmacologically induced, sympathetic denervation. As a result, total peripheral vascular resistance (TPVR) decreases only modestly, about 15% to 18% in normal subjects even in the presence of total sympathetic denervation, providing that cardiac output, the other determinant of blood pressure, is kept normal.[44] Because TPVR decreases only 15% to 18%, mean arterial pressure decreases only 15% to 18% in the presence of a normal cardiac output.

Venous Circulation. Veins and venules, with only few smooth muscles in their walls, retain no significant residual tone following acute pharmacologic denervation. They can, therefore, vasodilate maximally. Whether they do so or not is determined by intraluminal hydrostatic pressure. Intraluminal hydrostatic pressure on the venous side of the circulation depends on gravity. If denervated veins lie below the level of the right atrium, gravity causes peripheral pooling of blood in these capacitance vessels. If the denervated veins lie above the level of the right atrium, gravity causes the blood to flow back to the heart. Preload, that is, venous return to the heart, therefore depends on position of the patient during spinal anesthesia, especially during high spinal anesthesia.

Cardiac Output. Preload determines cardiac output. During levels of spinal anesthesia high enough to produce total sympathetic denervation, cardiac output remains unchanged in normovolemic subjects as long as they are positioned with the legs elevated above the level of the heart. The head-up (legs down) position, on the other hand, leads to severe decreases in venous return to the heart, and thus to severe decreases in cardiac output.

Heart Rate. Heart rate characteristically decreases during spinal anesthesia in the absence of autonomically active drugs and medications. The bradycardia is due in part to blockade of preganglionic cardiac accelerator fibers arising from T1–T4 during high (*i.e.*, T3–T4) levels of anesthesia.[98] The bradycardia is also, however, mediated by significant decreases in right atrial pressure and pressure in the great veins as they enter the right atrium. This can be seen during fixed levels of high spinal anesthesia. Placing the patient in the modest head-down position (or legs elevated) increases venous return, which in turn increases right atrial pressure and thus heart rate at a time when blockade of cardiac accelerator fibers remains constant. The slight head-up position, on the other hand, further decreases venous return, right atrial pressure, and heart rate. The inverse relation between right atrial pressure and heart rate during high spinal anesthesia is mediated not only by the now generally discredited Bainbridge reflex but rather by intrinsic chronotropic stretch receptors located in the right atrium and adjacent great veins (see Chap. 8).

Hypotension. The preceding indicates that slight decreases in arterial pressure in the range of 15% or so during high spinal anesthesia in normovolemic patients can be ascribed to decreases in afterload, that is, decreases in TPVR. Severe hypotension, however, can be due only to decreases in cardiac output secondary to decreases in preload associated with peripheral pooling of blood in vasodilated capacitance vessels or to hypovolemia, or both.

The indications for treatment of arterial hypotension during spinal anesthesia and the methods to be used are best considered in light of what arterial hypotension caused by sympathetic denervation means in terms of oxygenation of the myocardium and the central nervous system (the organs most susceptible to diminution in oxygenation). The following discussion applies only to hypotension during spinal anesthesia in normovolemic subjects. Hypovolemic subjects are highly susceptible to the hypotensive effects of spinal anesthesia because, in the presence of hypovolemia, maintenance of cardiovascular function depends on compensatory reflex increases in sympathetic activity. Elimination of these compensatory reflexes by sympathetic denervation during spinal anesthesia can result in such catastrophic hypotension owing to decreases in TPVR and venous return to the heart that spinal anesthesia is contraindicated in the presence of hypovolemia, as is shown in the case of epidural block in Fig. 7-13.

Myocardial Oxygenation. A major determinant of coronary blood flow and, thus myocardial oxygen supply, is the perfusing pressure across the coronary vasculature. A decrease in mean arterial pressure during spinal anesthesia is therefore associated with a decrease in coronary flow. In normal subjects, Hackel and colleagues found that as mean arterial pressure decreased from 119.5 mm Hg before to 67.20 mm Hg during spinal anesthesia, coronary flow decreased from 153.2 ml to 73.6 ml • 100 g^{-1} • min^{-1}. The 48% decrease in myocardial oxygen supply was, however, associated with a parallel 53% decrease in myocardial oxygen requirements; myocardial oxygen consumption averaged 16.1 ml • 100 g^{-1} • min^{-1} before and 7.5 ml • 100 g^{-1} • min^{-1} during spinal anesthesia.[48] Similar data have also been reported in experimental animals.[33,89] Myocardial oxygen demands decrease during hypotension associated with spinal anesthesia for three reasons: First, afterload decreases. The resistance against which the left ventricle ejects blood during systole is diminished, and therefore left ventricular work decreases; second, preload decreases. As venous return and cardiac output decrease, so, too, does the work load of both ventricles because the amount of blood to be ejected per unit of time is lessened; and third, heart rate decreases. Ventricular work load is diminished as the frequency of contraction diminishes. Recognition of the fact that myocardial work and oxygen requirements diminish to essentially the same extent as does myocardial oxygen supply during moderate levels of arterial hypotension in normal subjects has altered past concepts of when and how hypotension should be treated during spinal anesthesia (see below).

Cerebral Blood Flow. Cerebrovascular autoregulatory mechanisms maintain cerebral blood flow in humans at constant levels even in the presence of wide fluctuations in mean arterial pressure. Not until mean arterial pressure decreases below about 55 mm Hg does cerebral blood flow become pressure dependent. Cerebrovascular autoregulation is independent of the sympathetic nervous system.

Cerebral blood flow remains unaffected, therefore, in normal persons even when mean arterial pressure decreases from control levels of 93 mm Hg to levels of 63 mm Hg during spinal anesthesia because cerebrovascular resistance decreases from 2.1 to 1.5 units.[54] Cerebrovascular autoregulatory mechanisms are, however, blunted in patients with essential hypertension. A decrease in mean arterial pressure in hypertensive subjects from 158 mm Hg before to 79 mm Hg during spinal anesthesia, a 50% decrease in pressure, is associated with a 17% decrease in cerebral flow, from 47 ml • 100 g^{-1} • min^{-1} to 38 ml • 100 g^{-1} • min^{-1}.[53,54] The levels of blood pressure during spinal anesthesia that require initiation of corrective measures are accordingly higher in hypertensive than in normotensive patients, both in absolute terms and in terms of percent decrease in pressure from preanesthetic control levels. In neither normotensive nor in hypertensive patients need arterial pressure be maintained exactly at preoperative control levels during spinal anesthesia in order to assure maintenance of adequate cerebral perfusion.

Regional Blood Flow. In addition to the effects of spinal anesthesia on cardiac and cerebral blood flow, it is of interest to know whether blood flow to other organs, such as kidney and liver, is affected and whether the changes are of a clinical magnitude. In awake, unrestrained sheep, the effects of five drugs with flow-limited characteristics on regional blood flow and organ oxygen tensions was compared with spinal anesthesia. Under spinal anesthesia, except for a 10% decrease in hepatic blood flow, there were no significant changes in any hemodynamic variable or in any of the arterial or venous oxygen tensions. The intravenous infusion of adequate volumes of saline at the time of the spinal blockade probably contributed to maintaining the normal variables (Fig. 7-14).[85]

Under general anesthesia (1.5 end tidal halothane), cardiac output and hepatic blood flow were decreased to 70% and renal blood flow to 50% of control values. Heart rate was unchanged and mean arterial pressure decreased by an average of 10%. Hepatic and renal oxygen tensions decreased significantly. If these findings are confirmed in humans, it would suggest that well-controlled spinal anesthesia may have much to commend it over general anesthesia with halothane, especially in patients with hepatic or renal disease (Fig. 7-14 *A, B*).[85]

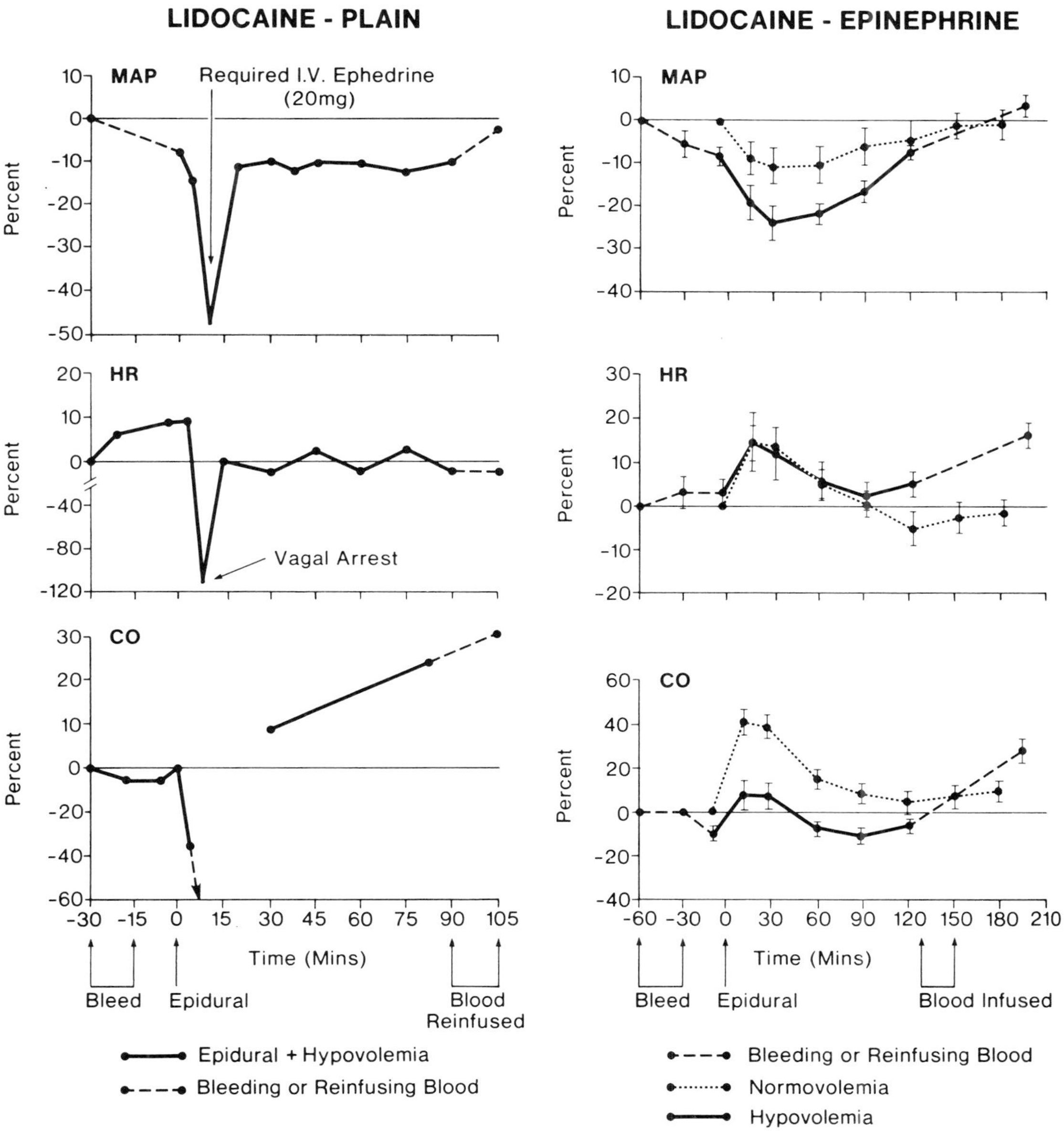

FIG. 7-13. Cardiovascular effects of epidural block, effect of hypovolemia in conscious volunteers; epidural block to T5 with plain and epinephrine-containing solutions. The mean percent changes are shown for each variable. Lidocaine-epinephrine *(right)*. The cardiovascular changes after lidocaine-epinephrine in the presence of normovolemia are compared with hypovolemia (− 13%). During normovolemia, note the marked increase in heart rate and cardiac output, lasting about 60 minutes. During hypovolemia, mean arterial pressure is significantly lower (− 23%), but cardiac output remains close to control levels as a result of an elevated heart rate. Lidocaine plain *(left)*. A representation of a typical response is shown. Severe bradycardia is associated with extreme hypotension, and in two subjects, vagal arrest occurred that required rapid resuscitation with ephedrine and oxygen. In only one subject was hypotension associated with increased heart rate, and this prevented the extreme hypotension seen in the other five subjects. (Modified from data of Bonica, J.J., Berges, P.U., and Morikawa, K.: Circulatory effects of epidural block: I. Effects of levels of analgesia and dose of lidocaine. Anesthesiology, *33*:1619, 1970; Bonica, J.J., Akamatsu, T.J., Berges, P.U., Morikawa, K., et al.: Circulatory effects of epidural block: II. Effects of epinephrine. Anesthesiology, *34*:514, 1971; and Bonica, J.J., et al.: Anesthesiology, *36*:219, 1972)

Management of Hypotension. Oxygenation of the two most critical organs, the brain and the myocardium, is now recognized as being maintained in normal subjects in the presence of moderate levels of hypotension during spinal anesthesia. It is thus no longer considered necessary or desirable to maintain blood pressure at "normal" levels during spinal anesthesia. There comes a point, nevertheless, at which hypotension becomes so great that decreases in cerebrovascular resistance and decreases in myocardial oxygen requirements are no longer able to compensate for decreases in cerebral and coronary artery perfusing pressures. Exactly what this critical pressure is has not been defined. Pragmatically, however, decreases in systolic blood pressure to levels 33% below resting control levels (preferably as measured before the patient gets out of bed in the morning) need not be treated during spinal anesthesia in normal asymptomatic patients. Although also not quantitated, equal levels of hypotension may be tolerated in patients with coronary arterial disease based on similar decreases in arterial blood pressure being deliberately induced in coronary care units by use of nitroprusside or nitroglycerin as a means of favorably affecting the ratio between myocardial oxygen supply and demand even in patients with demonstrable myocardial ischemia. Physiologic responses to nitroprusside or nitroglycerin are quite similar to those associated with spinal anesthesia. Pragmatically, it would appear prudent to initiate corrective measures in patients with essential hypertension when systolic blood pressure decreases more than 25% below resting control levels. Clearly, appropriate monitors to detect significant changes as well as enhanced F_{IO_2} *are to be recommended.*

Vasopressors are no longer routinely relied on in the management of hypotension during spinal anesthesia. Alpha-adrenoceptor agonists such as methoxamine and phenylephrine may so increase afterload that increases in left ventricular oxygen demand owing to the increased work load may exceed the increase in myocardial oxygen supply brought about by the increase in coronary perfusing pressure. Also, of course, the cause of hypotension great enough to require treatment during spinal anesthesia is not a decrease in TPVR, which alpha-adrenoceptor ago-

A

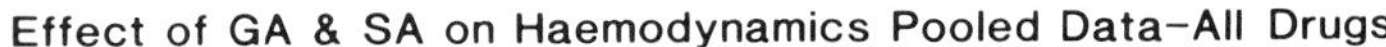

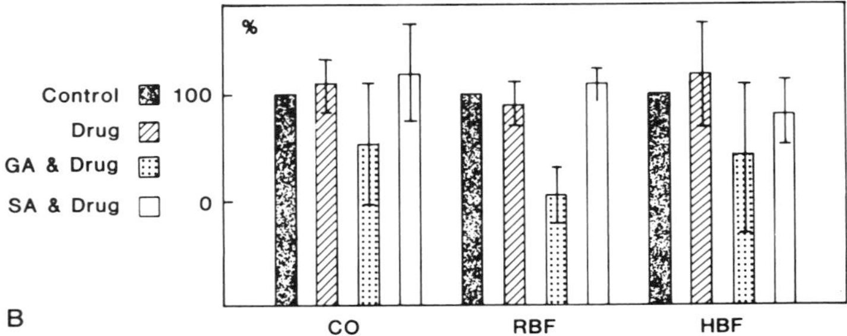

B

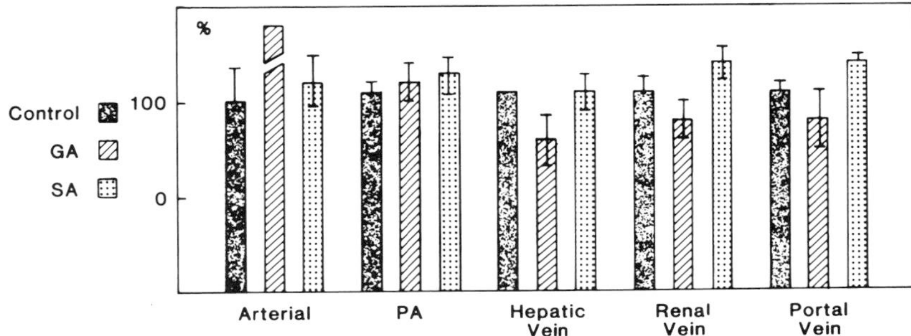

FIG. 7-14. Summary of blood flow **(A)** and oxygen tension data **(B)**. The mean value of each variable during control-drug, general anesthesia, or subarachnoid anesthesia studies has been expressed as a percentage of the mean value of the corresponding variable during the control preinfusion period on the same day. The mean and SD of these percentages for all five drugs studied are shown. Drug = control-drug study; GA & Drug = general anesthesia study; SA & Drug = subarachnoid anesthesia study; CO = cardiac output; RBF = renal blood flow; HBF = hepatic blood flow; PA = pulmonary artery. (Modified from Runciman, W.B., Mather, L.E., Ilsley, A.H., Carapetis, R.J., *et al.:* A sheep preparation for studying interactions between blood flow and drug disposition: III. Effects of general and spinal anaesthesia on regional blood flow and oxygen tensions. Br. J. Anaesth., *56:*1251, 1984.)

nists would correct, but rather decreases in preload and cardiac output, neither of which is favorably affected by alpha-adrenoceptor agonists. Proportionately greater increases in myocardial oxygen requirements than in myocardial oxygen supply may also result when positive chronotropic drugs, including atropine, are used to elevate blood pressure by increasing heart rate and thus cardiac output. Positive inotropic agents that increase cardiac output by increasing myocardial contractility may not be effective either. Myocardial contractility is not impaired by spinal anesthesia. Increasing ventricular contractility when end diastolic filling volumes are decreased because of decreased preload may be misguided. The ideal vasopressor for treatment of hypotension during spinal anesthesia would be one that acts selectively to produce venoconstriction without affecting afterload, heart rate, or myocardial contractility. Such an ideal vasopressor would selectively remedy the cause of severe hypotension during spinal anesthesia, decreased preload. Such an ideal vasopressor is, however, not available. The best means for treating hypotension during spinal anesthesia is thus physiologic, not pharmacologic. In instances in which physiologic measures (see below) need to be supplemented by vasopressors, the most useful are ephedrine and mephentermine. Both have at least some venoconstrictive effects without major undesirable effects on the ratio between myocardial oxygen supply and demand.

Physiologic treatment of hypotension during spinal anesthesia consists of restoration of preload by increasing venous return to the heart and thus restoring cardiac output. This is most simply and most effectively done by providing the patient with an internal autotransfusion: merely placing the patient in the slight head-down or legs up position. By doing so, cardiac output improves, and, in normovolemic patients, blood pressure returns to near normal levels. The remaining minor decrease in blood pressure represents the decrease in afterload secondary to arterial and arteriolar vasodilatation. The head-down position need not and should not exceed about 20°. Extreme Trendelenburg position may be counterproductive by increasing internal jugular venous pressure to such an extent that effective cerebral perfusion pressure and cerebral blood flow are diminished. Use of the head-down position to maintain blood pressure or to correct hypotension during hyperbaric spinal anesthesia may result in unnecessarily high levels of anesthesia if used before the level of anesthesia becomes fixed. This can be avoided by elevating the lower body above the level of the heart at the same time the upper thorax and cervical area are elevated at about the T4 level by placing a pillow or other support under the patient's shoulders. This arrests the rising spinal at the T4 level at the same time that venous return is being maximized. This technique also reduces the chance of producing significant respiratory depression.

Another means for restoration of venous return, preload, and cardiac output during spinal anesthesia consists of the rapid intravenous infusion of large volumes (1.5 – 2.0 liters) of electrolyte solutions such as lactated Ringer's. Restoration of blood pressure alone, however, is not the sole objective in treating hypotension during spinal anesthesia. The objective is restoration of tissue oxygenation, especially myocardial oxygenation. Vasoconstrictors restore blood pressure, too, as discussed above, but their adverse effects on the balance between myocardial oxygen supply and demand are so well recognized that they are today infrequently relied upon. Unquantitated by appropriately controlled physiologic studies of myocardial oxygen supply and demand are the effects of increasing preload by infusion of large volumes of crystalloid solutions in normovolemic subjects that develop hypotension during spinal anesthesia. Such data are desirable to prove whether such a practice is in fact associated with increases in coronary flow and decreased viscosity sufficient to offset the decrease in oxygen-carrying capacity of coronary blood secondary to the hemodilution associated with this form of treatment. Measurement of coronary flow alone is not sufficient. Measurement of coronary oxygen supply, including oxygen content of coronary arterial blood, is also required. Measurement of myocardial oxygen requirements is also necessary, since the increases in preload and cardiac output caused by infusion of large volumes of electrolyte solutions increase ventricular work. Is the increase in myocardial oxygen demand actually accompanied by a parallel increase in myocardial oxygen supply when large volumes of electrolyte solutions are used for maintenance of arterial pressure in patients during spinal anesthesia? Also to be quantitated is the effect of increases in left ventricular end diastolic filling pressure on subendocardial oxygenation that occurs when preload is increased in this way, especially since left ventricular is increased at the same time that there is hemodilution of coronary arterial blood. Such objective, quantitative data are needed to confirm the theoretical advantages of management of arterial pressure in normovolemic subjects by use of large volumes of electrolyte solutions. Already quantitated is one undesirable side-effect of treatment of hypotension during spinal anesthesia by infusion of large volumes of crystalloids in normovolemic subjects, namely, the increased frequency of urinary retention requiring catheterization in the immediate postoperative period owing to the diuresis that results from this form of therapy. Given the high incidence of lower urinary tract infections in hospitalized patients after bladder catheterizations, this is a complication that also deserves consideration. Another consideration in the use of this therapy in the elderly patient is the risk of inducing cardiac failure or pulmonary edema, or both. Careful monitoring of patients needs to be done in conjunction with fluid therapy.

VENTILATORY

Arterial blood gas tensions are unaffected during high spinal anesthesia in patients spontaneously breathing room air.[44] Resting tidal volume, maximum inspiratory volume, and negative intrapleural pressure during maximal inhalation are similarly unaffected.[34,38] They remain unaltered despite the intercostal paralysis associated with high thoracic sensory levels of spinal anesthesia because diaphragmatic activity is unimpaired. Maximum breathing capacity and maximum expiratory volumes are, on the other hand, significantly diminished during high thoracic levels of anesthesia, as are maximum intrapleural pressures during forced exhalation, including coughing. Pulmonary mechanics during exhalation are impaired because the muscles involved in forced exhalation, especially the anterior abdominal muscles, are denervated by high thoracic levels of spinal anesthesia. The effects of high spinal anesthesia on forced exhalation are of clinical importance in patients with tracheal or bronchial secretions in whom the ability to maintain clear airways depends on their ability to cough.

The phrenic nerves are unaffected by even midcervical levels of sensory anesthesia because the level of motor blockade is usually below the level of sensory anesthesia, as discussed previously. Respiratory arrest owing to phrenic paralysis secondary to excessively high or "total spinal" is relatively rare. Nor is respiratory arrest caused by the presence of local anesthetics in ventricular CSF in concentrations adequate to produce direct depression of medullary respiratory neurons. Even the concentration of local anesthetic in cisternal CSF during high spinal anesthesia, greater than that in ventricular CSF, is below the threshold concentration of local anesthetic required to produce depression of central respiratory neurons when applied directly to the medulla. The most likely cause of transient respiratory arrest during high spinal anesthesia is ischemia of medullary respiratory neurons secondary to decreases in blood pressure and cardiac output severe enough to impair cerebral blood flow. Medullary ischemia as the cause of apnea during high spinal anesthesia is evidenced by the fact that respiratory arrest rarely occurs in the absence of hypotension severe enough to be associated with impending loss of consciousness. Further, restoration of blood pressure and cardiac output in cases of respiratory arrest during spinal anesthesia is, if done promptly, associated with immediate return of spontaneous respirations. This would not happen if the respiratory arrest were caused by pharmacologic block of the phrenic nerves or central respiratory neurons.

The character of spontaneous respirations serves as a valuable indication of the adequacy of medullary blood flow during high spinal anesthesia. It is therefore advisable to let patients breathe spontaneously during high spinal anesthesia rather than to control ventilation. Elimination of the negative intrapleural pressure of spontaneous inhalation by positive pressure ventilation not only removes a valuable indication of the adequacy of cerebral blood flow, but also may further decrease venous return, cardiac output, and arterial blood pressure.

The frequency and the type of postoperative respiratory complications have been reported to be similar after spinal anesthesia, local infiltration anesthesia, and general anesthesia in normal patients, as well as in patients with preexisting respiratory disease, provided that all other factors involved in determining the incidence of postoperative respiratory complications are kept constant.[44] These other factors include the site and type of operation, age, sex, obesity, smoking history, and frequency with which narcotics are administered for relief of postoperative pain. In studies of spinal anesthesia, no special advantage has been reported in the respiratory cripple. There may be an advantage, however, in using saddle block or low spinal anesthesia for perineal, urologic, and other surgery in order to avoid general anesthesia and possible artificial ventilation in patients on the brink of respiratory failure, with severe bronchospasm, excessive amounts of sputum, or a very difficult airway. Data are lacking to document these theoretical advantages.

HEPATIC

Hepatic blood flow decreases during spinal anesthesia to the extent that arterial blood pressure decreases.[52,64,74] The decrease in hepatic blood flow is associated with an increase in the difference between systemic arterial and hepatic venous oxygen content. This reflects an increase in hepatic oxygen extraction, not hepatic hypoxia. The frequency and the magnitude of postoperative hepatic dysfunction are the same following spinal anesthesia in normal patients, as well as in patients with preexisting hepatic disease, as they are when similar operations are performed under general anesthesia. This is true not only when blood pressure is maintained at normal levels during spinal anesthesia but also when severe hypotension is intentionally produced, as with hypotensive spinal anesthesia.[47] Spinal anesthesia has not been proved to represent either an advantage or a disadvantage in patients with preexisting liver disease. Further data are needed. Spinal anesthesia, when possible, could avoid hepatotoxicity caused by halogenated anesthetics if susceptible patients were able to be identified preoperatively. Recent data from a sheep model with chronic vascular catheters indicate that spinal anesthesia to T4 is associated with minimal changes in hepatic blood flow, oxygenation, and drug metabolism. In contrast, general anesthesia with halothane resulted in reduced hepatic blood flow, decreased hepatic vein oxygen content, and decreased intrinsic clearance of drugs metabolized by the liver.[84]

RENAL

Renal blood flow, much like cerebral blood flow, is maintained by autoregulatory mechanisms through a wide range of changes in arterial perfusing pressure. In the absence of vasoconstriction, renal blood flow does not decrease until mean arterial pressure decreases below about 50 mm Hg. In the absence of severe hypotension, renal blood flow, and therefore urinary output, thus remain unaffected during spinal anesthesia. When spinal anesthesia is associated with mean arterial pressures below about 50 mm Hg, transient decreases in renal blood flow and urinary output occur. Even during severe, prolonged periods of hypotension, blood flow remains adequate to provide oxygenation of renal tissues so that renal function returns to normal as the blood pressure returns to normal in the postoperative period.[47]

ENDOCRINE AND METABOLIC

Spinal anesthesia blocks hormonal and metabolic responses to nociceptive stimuli arising from the operative site to a degree not observed with general anesthesia.[44] The effect is only transient, however. Soon after the spinal anesthesia wears off, metabolic and hormonal responses in patients having had spinal anesthesia for their operation become indistinguishable from those having had general anesthesia for the same operation. The value of temporary inhibition of these responses on ultimate outcome remains to be defined (see also Chap. 5).

GASTROINTESTINAL

Preganglionic fibers from T5 to L1 are inhibitory to the gut. The small intestine therefore contracts during midthoracic levels of spinal anesthesia owing to the relatively unopposed activity of the vagus nerve. Sphincters are relaxed, and peristalsis is normally active. The combination of a contracted gut and complete relaxation of the abdominal muscles provides exceptionally fine operating conditions for intra-abdominal procedures.

OBSTETRIC

The physiology of spinal anesthesia on mother, fetus, and neonate are discussed in Chapter 18.

TECHNIQUE

EQUIPMENT

The preference of the anesthesiologist can dictate whether disposable, commercially prepared, or reusable department-prepared spinal anesthesia trays are used. Reusable department-prepared trays must be meticulously prepared by conscientious, well-trained personnel, with care being taken to prevent chemical and bacterial contamination. Because the manufacturers of disposable trays have been able to duplicate almost completely the traditional reusable tray for spinal anesthesia, it appears that disposable spinal trays will eventually replace the traditional reusable tray (see Chap. 6).

Needles for Spinal Anesthesia. A needle with a close-fitting, removable stylet is essential. This will prevent coring of the skin and the rare, though possible, occurrence of epidermoid spinal cord tumors from the introduction of pieces of epidermis into the subarachnoid space. Over the years, a large number of spinal needles of various diameters with numerous types of points have been developed. In general, in order to keep the incidence of postpuncture headache to a minimum, needles either of small bore or with a rounded, noncutting bevel (Greene or Whitacre) should be used.

A description of a few of the more popular spinal needles follows (Fig. 7-15). The Quincke–Babcock spinal needle, the so-called standard spinal needle, has a sharp point with a medium-length cutting bevel. The Pitkin spinal needle has a sharp point but short bevel with cutting edges and a rounded heel. Despite Pitkin's original claims, the incidence of postpuncture headache with this needle is relatively high. The Greene spinal needle has a rounded point and a rounded noncutting bevel of medium length.

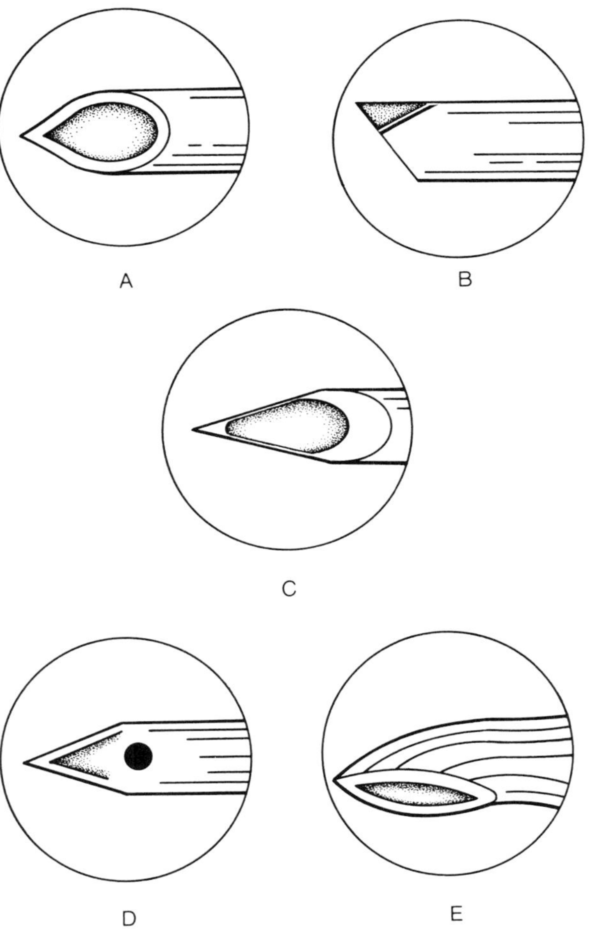

FIG. 7-15. Spinal needles. **A.** Quincke–Babcock. **B.** Pitkin. **C.** Greene. **D.** Whitacre. **E.** Tuohy.

The Whitacre spinal needle, or the pencil-point needle, has a completely rounded, noncutting bevel with a solid tip, the opening of the needle being on the side, 2 mm proximal to the tip of the needle.[35] The Huber point needle has a curved tip for introducing catheters into the subarachnoid space. For the inexperienced, the use of either a 22-gauge Greene needle or a 22-gauge Whitacre needle is recommended because the characteristic "feel" of the various structures can more readily be learned than with smaller-bore spinal needles, while simultaneously keeping the incidence of postpuncture headache low (2–7%).

Several combination, or double-needle, sets are available. One such set is composed of the standard 5 cm, 21-gauge Quincke–Babcock spinal needle with a stylet and a 9 cm, 26-gauge Quincke–Babcock needle with a close-fitting stylet. The 21-gauge introducer is inserted into either the ligamentum flavum or the epidural space, and puncture of the dura arachnoid is made with the fine 26-gauge needle.

Regardless of the size of the needle used, care must be taken so that the dural fibers that run longitudinally are separated rather than transected. With that in mind, the opening bevel is always on the side of the notch on the hub of the needle; the notch is then arranged so that the needle bevel is parallel to the longitudinal dural fibers.

Introducers. Various introducers have been developed both to facilitate the introduction of small-bore spinal needles, which are not easily directed, and to prevent contact of the spinal needle with the skin, hence reducing the incidence of coring and the introduction of pieces of epidermis or bacteria into the subarachnoid space. As an alternative, a disposable 18-gauge needle may be used. The use of an introducer is particularly helpful with 25-gauge or 26-gauge needles (Fig. 7-16).

POSITION OF THE PATIENT

Inasmuch as all conduction anesthetics may potentially become general anesthetics, the preparation for spinal anesthesia should be the same as that for general anesthesia. This includes a functional intravenous line, blood pressure monitor,and appropriate equipment for airway management. As in the management of any technique, the spinal anesthesia should be administered to a cooperative patient who is lying on a table that can be tipped upward or downward. The primary advantage of spinal over

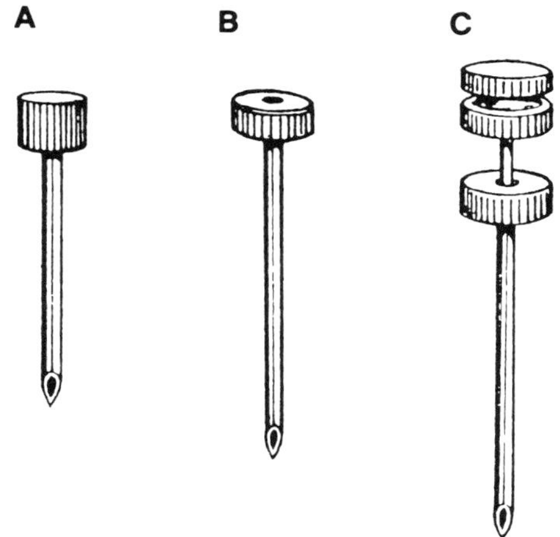

FIG. 7-16. Spinal needle guides and introducers. **A.** Pitkin guide. **B.** Sise introducer for 20-gauge or smaller spinal needles. **C.** Lundy modification of Sise with locking stylet. (Lung, P.C.: Principles and Practice of Spinal Anesthesia. Springfield, Ill., Charles C Thomas, 1971.)

epidural anesthesia is the ability to control the spread of the anesthetic by manipulation of the specific gravity of the solution and the position of the patient. Except when using isobaric solutions, failure to use a movable table will lead to a higher incidence of both unsatisfactory anesthetics and complications. Similarly, the anesthesiologist must be able to assess the spread if it is to be controlled. The spread in overly sedated or anesthetized patients is virtually impossible to assess, and, again, this will lead to a greater degree of failure or complications.

Lateral decubitus position is undoubtedly the most popular position for the performance of spinal anesthesia because of the comparative comfort it affords the patient (Fig. 7-17). The patient should be placed on the very edge of the table closest to the anesthesiologist. The vertebral column is then flexed to widen the interlaminal spaces, which is accomplished by drawing the knees up to the chest and putting the chin down on the chest, the head supported by a pillow. (Care must be taken that the vertebral column remains parallel with the edge of the table and the iliac crest and shoulders perpendicular to the table.) An assistant must stand in front of the patient to help the patient maintain the correct position. If the anesthesiologist is right-handed, the left lateral decubitus position should be used with the spinal anesthesia tray to the right of the anesthesiologist. If the patient is to be positioned prone or supine at the conclusion of administering the spinal anesthetic, the location of the operative site is irrelevant. If, on the other hand, unilateral or hypobaric techniques are being used, then position of the operative site appropriate to the relative baricity of solution is essential.

Sitting position is used less frequently than lateral decubitus, with the exceptions of low spinal anesthesia in obstetrics, certain gynecologic and urologic procedures, and certain hypobaric (and hyperbaric) techniques. The sitting position also facilitates lumbar puncture in obese patients. (Fig. 7-18). Precautions must be taken against hypotension when patients who have received moderate to heavy premedication or are prone to fainting are in the sitting position. As in the lateral decubitus position, the patient sits on the table as close to the anesthesiolo-

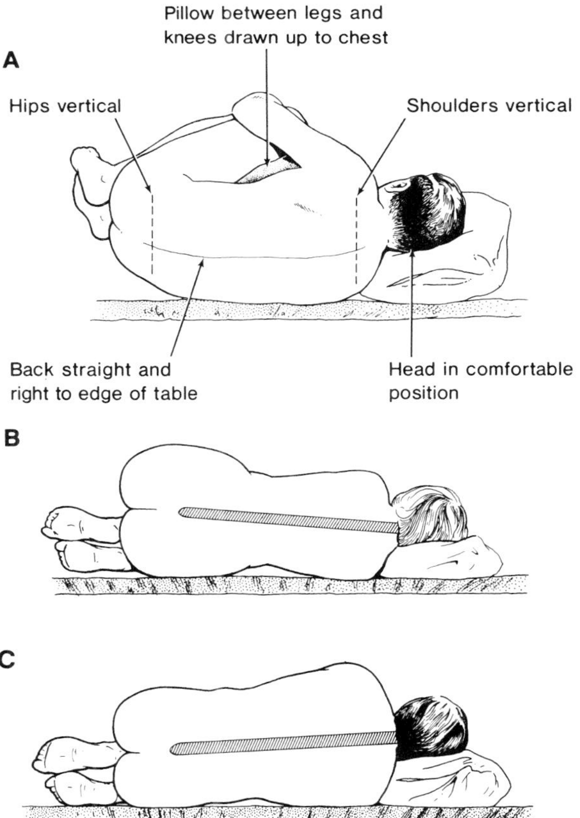

FIG. 7-17. Lateral decubitous position for spinal anesthesia. Note skeletal differences of female **(B)** and male **(C)** on level of subarachnoid space.

gist as possible, the feet supported by a stool. The patient's neck and back are flexed again to provide maximum opening of the interlaminal spaces. An assistant must stand in front of the patient at all times both to support and to maintain the correct position of the patient.

Prone position is used primarily for the hypobaric technique for procedures on rectum, sacrum, and lower vertebral column. Preferably, the patient is placed on his abdomen on the operating table to avoid repositioning after induction of spinal anesthesia. The technique is most easily accomplished if the lumbar curve is extended by flexion of the table or by placing a pillow under the patient's abdomen. The spinal fluid pressure is low in this position, and therefore aspiration may be necessary to obtain a free flow of spinal fluid. Flow of spinal fluid may be facilitated by elevating the head of the table. If this is to be done and the technique is hypobaric, it is critical that the table be repositioned before injection of the anesthetic so that the highest portion of the vertebral column is at the desired level of anesthesia.

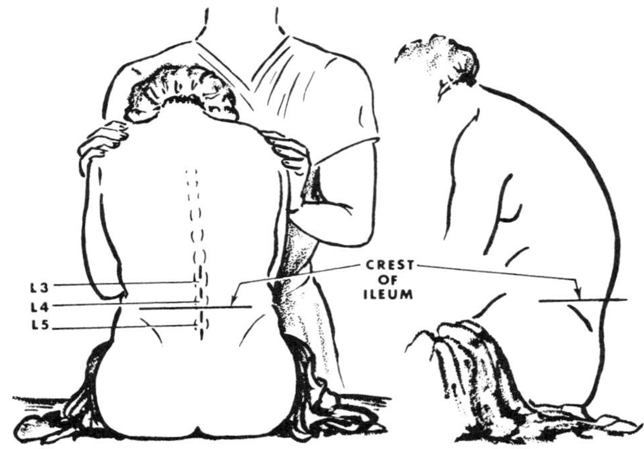

FIG. 7-18. Sitting position correctly demonstrated for spinal anesthesia. (Lund, P.C.: Principles and Practice of Spinal Anesthesia. Springfield, Ill., Charles C Thomas, 1971.)

PREPARATION

Before the induction of any major anesthetic technique, fundamental preparations must be accomplished. With rare exception, all patients who undergo a spinal anesthetic technique should initially have an intravenous cannula in place. Blood pressure and heart rate must be measured before anesthesia. The patient is then placed in the appropriate position and the puncture area (usually lumbar) exposed (see Chap. 6).

Preparation of Equipment and Puncture Site. A previously prepared tray (hospital or commercial) should then be opened, and its sterility noted by checking the sterilization indicator. All subsequent activity should be performed using careful septic technique. The patient's back is then widely prepared with an antiseptic solution and sterile drapes applied. After discarding the preparation solution, one should prepare the anesthetic drugs, being careful at all times to ensure no contamination of drugs or equipment with the preparation solution.

A line between the upper border of the iliac crest passes through either the spinous process of L4 or the interspace between L4 and L5. The anesthesiologist should be positioned with the tray on the right (if right-handed) and the patient as nearly at eye level as possible. One may sit or stand as desired. Before any injection, the spinal needle should be inspected to make certain the stylet fits properly and that there are no barbs or foreign material on the tip of the needle. Care is taken not to handle the plunger of the syringe, which contains the spinal anesthetic solution, or to touch the shaft of the spinal needle, which will subsequently be introduced into the subarachnoid space.

Depending on the interspace and approach selected, an intracutaneous skin wheal is made at the puncture site with a 25- to 27-gauge, 1-cm needle attached to a 2- to 5-ml syringe. One milliliter to 2 ml of 1% lidocaine is the usual dosage and drug for skin wheals. After this, subcutaneous infiltration of additional local anesthetic may be accomplished with a 2- to 3-cm, 22-gauge needle. The patient is then ready for the spinal needle to be introduced.

TECHNIQUE OF LUMBAR PUNCTURE

Midline. Traditionally, midline with the patient lateral is the most popular approach (Fig. 7-19). If an introducer is being used, it is inserted through the skin wheal firmly into the interspinous ligament. Then the spinal needle is held like a dart (*i.e.*, the hub is held between the thumb and index finger with the third finger along the proximal part of the shaft of the needle). If no introducer is used, the skin and soft tissues are fixed against the bony landmark by the second and third fingers of the left hand, which straddle the interspace.

The spinal needle is inserted through the same hole in the skin that was used to perform the intracutaneous wheal and subcutaneous infiltration. The bevel of the spinal needle should be directed laterally (notch facing upward), so that the dural fibers that run longitudinally are spread rather than transected. After traversing the skin and subcutaneous tissues, the needle is advanced in a slightly cephalad direction (100° – 105° on the cephalad side) with the long axis of the vertebral column, care again being taken to stay absolutely in the midline. (Even in the lumbar area where the spinous processes of the lumbar vertebrae are relatively straight, the interlaminal space is slightly cephalad to the interspinous space.) There is a characteristic change in resistance as the needle traverses the ligamentum flavum and the dura arachnoid, which becomes quite recognizable as experience is gained with this technique. The stylet is removed and CSF allowed to appear at the hub of the needle. If proper flow of spinal fluid does not occur, the needle is rotated in 90° increments until good flow is achieved. Occasionally, with patients in the prone position or if a small-bore spinal needle is being used, free flow of CSF will not be apparent. Gentle aspiration with a small, sterile syringe may then be used to obtain fluid.

With the hub of the spinal needle held firmly between the thumb and index finger of the left hand — the back of the left hand against the patient's back to prevent either withdrawal or advance of the spinal needle — the syringe containing the local anesthetic solution is firmly attached to the needle. Aspiration of spinal fluid is then performed, and if there is free flow the local anesthetic solution is injected. Before removing the spinal needle, one again performs aspiration and reinjection of a small amount of fluid to reconfirm that the tip of the needle is still in the subarachnoid space. The patient is then placed in the desired position; cardiovascular and respiratory functions are monitored frequently; and the analgesic level to pinprick or temperature level with alcohol is checked at 5-minute intervals until the desired level is achieved. The patient should be repositioned as necessary, according to the baricity of the injected solution to achieve this desired level; however, this must be accomplished within the "fixing time" of about 20 to 30 minutes for the local anesthetic.

Paramedian (Lateral) Approach. Many variations of the paramedian (lateral) approach avoid traversing

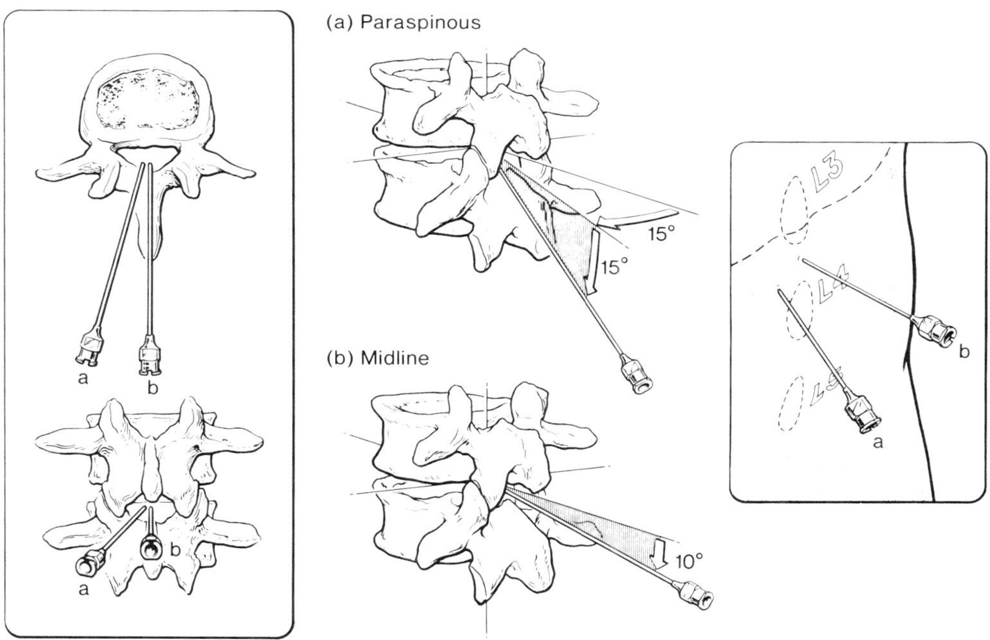

FIG. 7-19. Two common techniques of lumbar puncture for spinal anesthesia. **(a)** Paraspinous, paramedian, or lateral approach. **(b)** Midline.

the sometimes narrowed or calcified interspinous space. This approach is especially useful when degenerative changes are encountered in the interspinous structures (*e.g.*, in elderly patients) and when ideal positioning of the patient cannot be achieved, owing to pain (*e.g.*, fractures, and dislocations involving the hips and lower extremities).

The patient is placed in the flexed lateral decubitus position and a skin wheal raised 1.5 cm lateral to the midline directly opposite the cephalad tip of the spinous process below the selected interspace. The direction of the spinal needle is at an angle of about 15° to 20° with the midline and slightly cephalad, 100° to 105° on the cephalad side. As with the midline approach, there is a characteristic "feel" encountered as the needle passes through the ligamentum flavum and dura arachnoid. At this point, the advance is stopped and the stylet withdrawn to allow spinal fluid to appear in the hub of the needle. If periosteum rather than the subarachnoid space is encountered, the needle should be redirected slightly cephalad, thus walked off the laminae into the interspace. Anesthesiologists should remember that the interlaminal space is created by the failure of the laminae to unite in the midline. If the needle is walked off the laminae, it must enter the interlaminal space and go into the subarachnoid space. Once the tip of the needle lies within the subarachnoid space, the remainder of the technique for administering spinal anesthesia is identical to that described previously for the midline approach.

The Taylor approach is a special paramedian approach to enter the L5 interspace (the largest interlaminal space). It was originally described for urologic procedures but was subsequently used for other operations in the pelvis and perineum.[93] The patient is placed in the flexed lateral decubitus position and a 12-cm spinal needle inserted through a skin wheal made 1 cm medial and 1 cm caudad to the lowest part of the posterior–superior iliac spine. The needle is directed medially and cephalad at an angle of 55° into the subarachnoid space. Again, if periosteum is encountered, the needle is withdrawn and redirected slightly cephalad or walked into the correct location. Once the needle has been placed in the subarachnoid space, the remaining steps are identical to those described for the midline approach (Fig. 7-20).

The continuous catheter approach is a standard midline approach but with Tuohy-tip needle that will allow passage of a plastic catheter through its lumen. The bevel of the needle is most advantageously directed cephalad during the advancement of the needle through the interspinous ligament. The tip acts like a ski directing the needle between the spines along their natural slant, whereas if it were turned longitudinally the tendency would be to direct the needle laterally out of the interspinous ligament. Once the needle is on, or just through, the ligamentum flavum, the bevel is rotated 90° to be parallel to the dural fibers before entry into the subarachnoid space. Once free flow of CSF is observed, the needle should be advanced another 1 to 2 mm to ensure that the entire tip of the needle is within the subarachnoid space; otherwise, the catheter will impinge on the dura as it emerges from the tip of the needle. The threading and fixation of the catheter are identical to the technique used for epidural anesthesia (see Chap. 8). Because stimulation of the nerve roots by the catheter tip is painful and the catheter could conceivably enter a subarachnoid vessel, it is preferable to thread it only 2 to 4 cm beyond the tip of the needle. Once free flow of CSF through the catheter has been demonstrated, local anesthetic may be injected. The use of a Millipore filter at the injection end of the catheter is recommended for all doses not administered at the time of insertion of the catheter.

There is obviously no advantage to adding epinephrine to agents being injected through the cath-

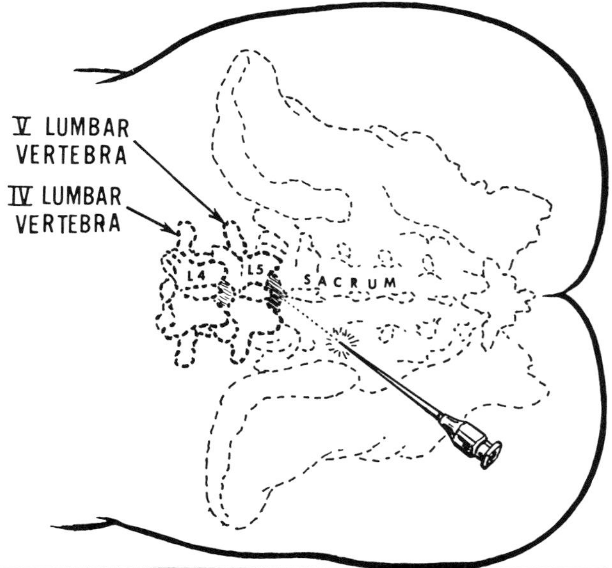

FIG. 7-20. Taylor approach to spinal anesthesia. (Lund, P.C.: Principles and Practice of Spinal Anesthesia. Sprinfield, Ill., Charles C Thomas, 1971.)

eter because the duration is limitless anyway. Subsequent doses through the catheter may be reduced by 30% to 50% from the original dose.

INTRAOPERATIVE AND POSTOPERATIVE MANAGEMENT

The first 5 to 10 minutes after administration of the spinal anesthetic are the most critical in adjusting the level of anesthesia when hyperbaric or hypobaric solutions are used. Levels of spinal anesthesia required for common surgical procedures are shown in Table 7-5. The first 10 to 20 minutes are also the most critical in assessing the cardiovascular responses to spinal anesthesia. Frequent measurements of blood pressure and heart rate will allow early recognition of any degree of hypotension. Indications and methods for treatment of hypotension have been previously described in this chapter (see Hypotension).

After surgical anesthesia levels and cardiovascular stability have been achieved, the anesthesiologist may evaluate whether supplemental drugs should be administered to make the patient comfortable. Sedation may be achieved with repeated small doses of an intravenous hypnotic. Pentobarbital or secobarbital have been used for many years, with considerable success. An initial dose of 50 mg/70 kg will produce a quietly sleeping but rousable patient without respiratory or cardiovascular depression, a state that can be maintained with subsequent injections of 25 mg doses every 45 to 60 minutes as required. Diazepam, 2.5 to 5 mg, produces much the same effect, but with repeat doses its duration of action is substantially longer. Geriatric patients especially often remain somnolent for many hours postoperatively when small doses are used. Midazolam may have a shorter duration of effect (see Chap. 6). If pain is severe because the level of spinal anesthesia is inadequate, light general anesthesia should be induced rather than relying upon large doses of opioids. Opioids during spinal anesthesia are best reserved for management of discomfort or slight pain from the operative site and for discomfort that occurs in the unanesthetized upper part of the body when patients lie immobile on the operating table for long periods. The low doses of opioids required for this type of analgesia will have minimal depressant effects on respiration. The amount of opioids given to produce satisfactory intraoperative analgesia during spinal anesthesia can be greatly decreased by administration of 50% nitrous oxide in oxygen by mask or by insufflation through a nasopharyngeal catheter (see Chap. 6).

TABLE 7-5. LEVEL OF SPINAL ANESTHESIA REQUIRED FOR COMMON SURGICAL PROCEDURES

Level	Surgical Procedure
T4-5 (nipple)	Upper abdominal surgery
T6-8 (xiphoid)	Intestinal surgery (including appendectomy),* gynecologic pelvic surgery, and ureter and renal pelvic surgery
T10 (umbilicus)	Transurethral resection, obstetric vaginal delivery, and hip surgery
L1 (inguinal ligament)	Transurethral resection, if no bladder distension; thigh surgery; lower limb amputations, and so forth
L2-3 (knee and below)	Foot surgery
S2-5 (perineal)	Perineal surgery, hemorrhoidectomy, anal dilation, and so forth

*Blockade to T10 is not adequate for appendectomy because of splanchnic supply to peritoneum (T6-L1).

Supplemental oxygen by mask or by nasopharyngeal insufflation is usually not necessary in normal patients with low levels of spinal anesthesia. Supplemental oxygen is, however, often used in patients with high thoracic levels. It is also often used if the patient's respirations are depressed by hypnotics, tranquilizers, or opioids. The anesthesiologist should bear in mind, however, that supplemental oxygen given to a hypoventilating patient may improve arterial oxygenation but it will not relieve the accompanying increase in arterial carbon dioxide tension, and may even aggravate it.

The anesthesiologist's role postoperatively can be divided into two periods. The first is actually a continued monitoring of the anesthetized patient in the recovery unit until complete cessation of the spinal anesthesia has occurred. Concerns during this period start with the careful movement and transport of the patient from the operating room to the unit. It is not uncommon for such activities to precipitate some degree of hypotension owing to redistribution of blood volume with movement; thus careful monitoring of the blood pressure is essential. If the patient does not have an indwelling urinary catheter, then recovery room personnel should be alert for a distended bladder. The voiding mechanism is mediated through sacral autonomic fibers, which are the last to regain function after spinal anesthesia. Even after patients are able to move their extremities and respond to sensory stimuli, they may have some residual autonomic blockade, and thus may not only be unable to void but may also become hypotensive in the sitting or standing position. Postspinal headache is related neither in severity nor in incidence to the patient's position while spinal anesthesia is wearing off and during the immediate postoperative period. Patients are kept flat in bed after spinal anesthesia only if necessary to avoid hypotension, not postoperative headaches.

The second phase of the postoperative period is the postanesthetic period. The role of the anesthesiologist becomes surveillance with special attention to the possible development of postanesthetic complications, which are discussed below. Equally as important as the detection of bona fide complications is good rapport with the patient, which will permit the explanation of postsurgical aches and pains and the appropriate dismissal of them when clearly not caused by spinal anesthesia.

INDICATIONS

Indications for spinal anesthesia are much the same as they are for any type of regional anesthesia. These include, for example, the presence of a full stomach. Vomiting and aspiration can occur during regional anesthesia, especially in overly sedated patients, but the likelihood of this happening is less with regional anesthesia. Anatomic distortions of the upper airway that might make maintenance of a clear airway difficult under general anesthesia also indicate use of regional anesthesia. Certain types of operations are also relative, although not usually absolute indications for regional anesthesia. Regional anesthesia is particularly indicated in operations such as rectal procedures. The area in which anesthesia and muscle relaxation are required is so circumscribed in rectal operations that the physiologic trespass associated with a small, discrete area of regional anesthesia is substantially less than that associated with general anesthesia. Operations such as transurethral resection of the prostate are also often relative indications for major regional (*i.e.*, epidural or spinal) anesthesia; not only is the physiologic trespass in geriatric patients having this procedure under regional anesthesia less than that associated with general anesthesia, but complications associated with this operation, including perforation of the bladder and hypervolemia with congestive heart failure secondary to vascular absorption of irrigating fluid, can be more rapidly recognized during regional anesthesia than during general anesthesia. As a general principle, however, the greater the extent of anesthesia required, the fewer are the indications for regional anesthesia. Certainly, cholecystectomies and gastrectomies can be, and in past years have been, successfully performed under spinal anesthesia. Upper abdominal operations require, however, T4 levels of sensory anesthesia. The physiologic trespass associated with such high levels of anesthesia is greater than that associated with use of modern general anesthetic techniques. Major regional anesthesia by itself is infrequently strongly indicated for operations above the level of the umbilicus. It may, however, be valuable as part of a "balanced" technique.

Indications for major regional anesthesia are especially frequent in obstetrics. The role of regional anesthesia in obstetrics is fully discussed in Chapter 18, but some of the advantages, and thus indications, for major regional anesthesia deserve emphasis. They include resolution of the problem associated with the fact that the mother almost invariably has a full stomach. Spinal anesthesia is also free of significant blood concentrations of drugs that can cross the placenta and affect the fetus. Early bonding between mother and neonate is not impaired by regional anesthesia. Finally, when properly managed, sensory anesthesia without major somatic motor paralysis can be provided during both labor and delivery. The mother is still able to participate in helping delivery, especially by bearing-down.

The relative merits of spinal and epidural anesthesia as forms of major regional anesthesia are considered later. The advantages of spinal anesthesia over major nerve blocks are most evident in operations involving the lower extremities. Either spinal anesthesia or nerve blocks can be used for operations below the knee. Spinal anesthesia has, however, the advantage of being simpler, more rapidly induced and, especially in untrained hands, more predictable for such procedures. For operations involving the knee and upper leg, these advantages become even more evident. The number and the complexity of nerve blocks needed for operations on the knees, the thigh, and the hip are so great that spinal anesthesia is usually the preferred technique.

CONTRAINDICATIONS

Contraindications to spinal anesthesia can be either usual or relative. *Usual contraindications* include the following:

1. Infections at the site of injection.
2. Dermatologic conditions (*e.g.*, psoriasis) that preclude aseptic preparation of the skin at the site of injection.

3. Septicemia or bacteremia.
4. Shock or severe hypovolemia.
5. Preexisting disease involving the spinal cord. This contraindication is based on the untested and untestable hypothesis that abnormal nervous tissue is more susceptible to the neurotoxicity of local anesthetics than is normal nervous tissue. Although there are no objective data to support this hypothesis, common sense and medicolegal considerations make it prudent to avoid spinal anesthesia in patients with progressive disease involving the cord lest the progression be blamed on the spinal anesthetic. Traumatic paraplegia and carcinoma of the prostate with metastases to lumbar vertebrae are, however, not necessarily absolute contraindications to spinal anesthesia when neurologic status is stable.
6. Increased intracranial pressure is a contraindication because of the risk of herniation of the medullary vasomotor and respiratory centers. Intracranial diseases without increased intracranial pressure, for example, cerebral arteriosclerosis, are, on the other hand, often indications for spinal anesthesia.
7. Gross abnormality of blood clotting mechanisms (see also minor abnormalities of blood clotting mechanisms under relative contraindications).
8. Patient refusal or patients who are psychologically or psychiatrically unsuited.
9. Lack of skill in, and experience with, spinal anesthesia. Spinal anesthesia is not for the unsupervised novice, nor is it for the anesthesiologist who, although skilled in general anesthesia, gives spinal anesthesia only rarely.
10. For the operating surgeon who cannot predictably complete the proposed operation in the time provided by spinal anesthesia or the surgeon who is unaccustomed to operating (especially intra-abdominally) under regional anesthesia.
11. Uncertainty about the extent or duration of the proposed operation, for example, "Exploratory laparotomy? Whipple."

Relative contraindications to spinal anesthesia include the following:

1. Major surgical procedures above the umbilicus, using spinal anesthesia as the sole technique.
2. Deformities of the spinal column, including severe arthritis, severe kyphoscoliosis, and fusion of lumbar vertebrae at several levels.
3. Chronic severe headache or backache.
4. Blood in the CSF that fails to clear after 5 to 10 ml of CSF have been aspirated.
5. Inability to achieve a spinal tap after three attempts; after unsuccessful attempts one should either abandon spinal anesthesia or obtain the help of a more experienced anesthesiologist.
6. Failure to obtain free flow of CSF through the lumbar puncture needle in all four quadrants during rotation of the needle; getting satisfactory spinal anesthesia in this situation is not impossible, but the chances of doing so are significantly diminished.
7. Minor abnormalities of blood clotting, including "mini" doses of heparin administered up to the time of surgery.

Cardiac disease, whether myocardial, valvular, or ischemic, is best considered a major contraindication to spinal anesthesia if sensory levels to T6 or above are required. On the other hand, spinal anesthesia is often indicated in patients with even severe cardiac disease if only perineal levels of anesthesia are required.

COMPLICATIONS

Intra-operative complications during spinal anesthesia involving respiration and the cardiovascular system was previously discussed in this chapter and also in Chapter 22. Another complication is complete failure of anesthesia to develop despite apparently correct injection of the local anesthetic solution into CSF. This is probably most frequently due to movement of the needle during injection but may occasionally be a result of subdural instead of subarachnoid injection, as discussed earlier in this chapter. Although often attributed to injection of pharmacologically inert local anesthetic solutions (*i.e.,* the failure is blamed on the drug manufacturer), this is rarely the case. If the anesthesiologist routinely retains a portion of the uninjected local anesthetic and performs a bioassay of its anesthetic potency by placing a drop or two of the solution on the tongue or by making an intracutaneous wheal with it, only rarely, if ever, will the commercially supplied preparation be found to be devoid of local anesthetic activity when apparent injection of local anesthetic solution into CSF has produced no anesthesia.

Backache is a frequent postoperative complaint after spinal anesthesia. Lund, in reviewing the literature, found an incidence of backache varying from 2% to

25%.[63] Although it is remotely possible that needle puncture of an invertebral disk might result in postanesthetic backache, the more likely and understandable cause is the flattening of the normal lordotic lumbar curve secondary to relaxation of the muscles and ligaments of the back. This, presumably, results in stretching of joint capsules, ligaments, and muscles beyond their normal "self-protective" range and results in pain. To this extent, it seems just as likely that a patient who receives paralyzing doses of muscle relaxants would suffer the same problem and that the lithotomy position might even exaggerate the condition. A study by Brown and Elman found the incidence of postoperative backache to be similar following general and spinal anesthesia.[13] A more recent clinical report recorded the incidence of transient (14%) and prolonged (3%) backache in 2046 patients receiving either epidural or spinal lumbar spine puncture in the usual way. They claimed that paraspinous infiltration of local anesthetic agent at the puncture site blocked the recurrent spinal nerves innervating the interspinous ligaments and muscles. In the succeeding 322 patients, the incidence of backache was reduced to 5.6% and to 0 for prolonged backache.[79]

Headache. The next most common complication of spinal anesthesia postoperatively is headache. This is more appropriately called postdural-puncture headache rather than spinal headache.

The incidence of postdural-puncture headaches over the years has varied from 0.2% to 24%.[40,41,49,92] They are more frequent in women and in younger patients. The highest incidence is in obstetric patients. Also, the larger the size of the needle, the more frequent and severer are the postdural-puncture headaches. Although headaches after spinal anesthesia can be a postspinal-anesthetic problem, diagnostic lumbar punctures and myelography are associated with an even higher incidence of headaches. Further, postoperative headaches occur after general anesthesia. Not all headaches after spinal anesthesia are due to the dural puncture. It is important, therefore, to be conversant with the diagnostic features that are unique to this complication.

Clinical Features. Although a history of dural puncture is helpful, the clinical features of postdural-puncture headache are still diagnostic. First, the onset of headache occurs a minimum of several hours after the puncture but usually in the first or second day postpuncture. A recent controlled study showed that bed rest did not prevent — merely postponed — the onset of headache.[17] The headache has been described[14] as invariably bifrontal and occipital, frequently involving the neck and upper shoulders. Severity varies from mild to incapacitating and may be aggravated, especially by the upright position and also by coughing and straining. The headache subsides dramatically to completely when the patient is lying down. Associated symptoms are related to the severity of the headache and may include nausea and loss of appetite, photophobia, changes in hearing acuity and tinnitus, and depression. Patients whose headache persists for any period of time feel miserable, tearful, bedridden, and dependent. In more severe cases, diplopia and cranial nerve palsies have been attributed to traction on those cranial nerves (Fig. 7-21).

Once the diagnosis of postdural-puncture headache has been established, prompt treatment is essential. Until the past few years, treatment was conservative and serially progressive to the point that therapeutic efficacy could not be separated from the self-limiting nature of the process itself. The earliest measure was prophylactic in the form of enforced flat bed rest for 24 to 48 hours. This, of course, became therapeutic once the headache had occurred. Symptomatic treatment with analgesics or sedatives is just that, and probably has no beneficial effect in reversing the process. The most popular current concept of the pathophysiology is loss of CSF through the puncture site with resultant intracranial tension on meningeal vessels and nerves. Therapeutic modalities have, therefore, been directed at restoring the pressure relationships in the peridural and subarachnoid spaces. This has included such measures as the following: abdominal binders to force more venous blood through epidural plexus, injection of saline in large volumes into the epidural space, overhydration of the patient — orally or intravenously — to stimulate production of CSF, and antidiuresis. In practical terms, many mild headaches may be resolved with forced fluid intake of 3 liters/day or more, plus the use of a tight abdominal binder when the patient is sitting or standing.

In 1970, DiGiovanni reported on 50 patients who received epidural injections of autologous blood as treatment for postlumbar-puncture headache.[29] Subsequently, and despite fears of infection and neurologic sequelae, the procedure has become an important therapy, employed progressively earlier. Abouleish summarized 524 cases reported by 11 centers.[1] He also reported a prospective study of an additional 118 patients. The technique of autologous blood patch is simply the insertion of a needle in the

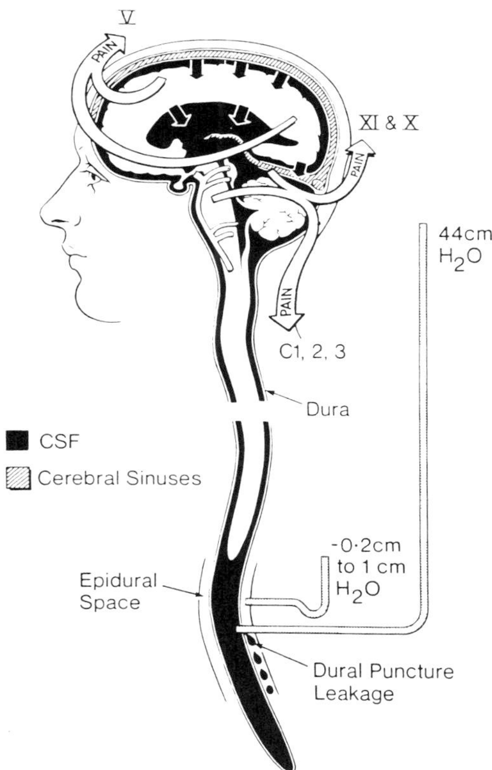

FIG. 7-21. Pathophysiology of dural puncture headache. Barometric figures are those to be expected in the subarachnoid and epidural spaces in the upright position at the site of lumbar puncture. The pressure differential favors CSF leakage. Note that CSF pressure is approximately atmospheric at the base of the brain. CSF leakage leads to descent of the brain in the upright position *(dark arrows)* on pain-sensitive intracranial vessels and the tentorium. Pain is referred *(open arrows)* above the tentorium via the trigeminal nerve *(V)* to the frontal region, and below the tentorium via the glossopharyngeal and vagal nerves *(IX, X)* to the occiput and via the upper cervical nerves *(C1, 2, 3)* to the neck and shoulders. (Brownridge, P.: The management of headache following accidental dural puncture in obstetric patients. Anaesth. Intensive Care, *11*:9, 1983.)

epidural space by the usual methods, followed by the injection of 5 to 10 mg of blood drawn aseptically from the patient's own antecubital vein. If patients are at all volume depleted, it is desirable to simultaneously infuse 1000 ml of intravenous fluid. Subsequent to the injection, the patient remains supine for 30 to 60 minutes. The success rate after the first injection varies from 89% to 95%. The procedure may be repeated 24 hours later and will provide equivalent success. Reported complications are few and mild but include backache (35%), neckache (0.9%), and transient temperature elevation (5%) of 24 to 48 hours' duration. It appears, then, that this is a worthwhile procedure with known minor risk that should be considered if early conservative measures fail.

Neurologic Sequelae. The remaining complications of postspinal anesthesia fall into the category of neurologic sequelae (see Chap. 22). Although these are the most feared and most serious of all complications, they are extremely rare.[31,70] Lund tabulated the major series of spinal anesthesia reported between 1948 and 1958.[63] Of these 582,190 cases of spinal anesthesia, he stated that "no incidence of permanent motor paralysis [was] reported" (Table 7-5). Nonetheless, cases have been reported. It is obviously important to both patient and anesthetist alike that every postanesthetic complication be examined critically with reference to prevention of similar complications. This is especially important with neurologic sequelae after spinal anesthesia.

Nowhere in the foregoing have any of these neurologic complications been identified as being caused by spinal anesthesia. This is not to say that it is not possible, but rather that not all postspinal-anesthetic neurologic complications are directly related to the anesthetic; perhaps they are not even indirectly related to the anesthetic, and, even more perplexing, may never have a proven etiology. Much of the negative image of spinal anesthesia has been a result of "speculative etiology by association."

It is important to keep the perspective that determination of etiology should not be fault-motivated but rather therapy-oriented. To that end, the important first step in any neurologic complication is early detection, diagnosis, and treatment. The degree of irreversibility of many of these complications is time related. Since most anesthesiologists are not trained neurologists, an early neurologic consultation is mandatory.

Anatomically, injuries may be categorized as peripheral nerve, cauda equina, spinal cord, and intracranial. Peripheral nerves usually have multiple nerve root origins. A complication in a unilateral peripheral nerve distribution (*e.g.*, hypoesthesia or weakness) is more likely secondary to trauma to the nerve, secondary to positioning, or secondary to operative trauma than to spinal anesthesia. The precise location, by a neurologist, of the neural distribution of the lesion is essential in arriving at an appropriate differential diagnosis and treatment. In contrast, bilateral involvement, whether cauda equina or higher up the spinal cord, would be more indicative of a peridural or subarachnoid injury with totally different therapeutic and prognostic implications. Anesthesiologists and surgeons alike should realize that patients who have complications are not interested in fault if they are assured that everyone is working together for an early diagnosis and treatment (see also Chap. 8).

From the prophylactic viewpoint, strict attention must be paid to the cleansing of the patient, particularly the locally or systemically infected patient. Care should be exercised to eliminate introduction of detergents or chemicals into the subarachnoid space and extreme caution to ensure use of the correct drugs and vasopressors in the correct concentrations. Traumatic complications can usually be avoided by careful and cooperative positioning of the patient by the surgeon and the anesthesiologist with awareness of the vulnerability of peripheral nerves for the particular surgical procedure. Certainly, the anesthesiologist always endeavors to use an atraumatic spinal technique but should be sensitive to early abandonment rather than perseverance in extremely difficult cases.

COMPARISON OF SPINAL AND EPIDURAL

Although spinal and epidural anesthesia are major regional anesthetic techniques, there are significant differences between them. Efforts to compare the upper levels of sensory and sympathetic block after epidural have not been done as carefully with spinal (see Chap. 8 for factors influencing level and degree of sympathetic blockade with epidural)[8,62]; however, obstetric anesthetists have the distinct clinical impression that the speed of onset of sympathetic block and therefore the adverse cardiovascular side-effects occur more rapidly with spinal anesthesia. They use the slower onset of side-effects and their ability to respond in time as a reason for preferring epidural for cesarean section.

An offsetting disadvantage of epidural anesthesia is the requirement for larger volumes and doses of local anesthetic agents that result in pharmacologically active plasma concentrations of local anesthetics. Equivalent levels of sensory analgesia with spinal anesthesia are accompanied by plasma levels of local anesthetics too low to have direct systemic effects (see Chap. 4). By acting directly on the myocardium and on peripheral vascular smooth muscles, epidural local anesthetics, with their varying systemic effects, produce cardiovascular changes that are often additive to those produced by high sympathetic blockade.

An additional problem with epidural anesthesia is that many of the local anesthetics have contained additives such as methylparaben and bisulfite, which, when unintentionally placed into the subarachnoid space, have produced major complications (see Chaps. 4 and 22). These same drugs in low doses and without additives or low *p*H have been used safely for spinal anesthesia. The effect of higher plasma levels of local anesthetics during epidural anesthesia also becomes important when comparing epidural and spinal anesthesia for obstetrics because local anesthetics pass from the maternal to the fetal circulation (see Chap. 18).

One major advantage of epidural or spinal anesthesia is that continuous epidural catheter techniques can extend the duration of anesthesia beyond that usually possible with spinal anesthesia. This difference is especially useful when continuous epidural analgesia is used for control of pain during labor. This difference is also particularly appreciated by those who are hesitant to use either intrathecal vasoconstrictors with spinal anesthesia or continuous spinal catheter techniques.

Many anesthesiologists believe that more predictable levels of anesthesia can be achieved with single injection spinal than with single injection epidural anesthesia. This advantage of spinal over epidural is lost when continuous epidural catheter techniques are used that allow one to increase or decrease the levels of epidural anesthesia when short-acting local anesthetics are applied. The potential benefit of epidural over spinal insofar as avoidance of postdural-puncture headaches is not always fully realized under clinical conditions. Even in the hands of experts, dural punctures do occur during planned epidural anesthesia. Given the size of epidural needles, especially those used for insertion of catheters, when this happens the likelihood of a postdural-puncture headache may be considerable.

Anesthesiologists equally well trained in epidural and spinal anesthesia realize that both techniques have advantages and both have disadvantages. Neither should be used to the exclusion of the other. Both should be used and the choice based upon advantages for individual patients.

REFERENCES

1. Abouleish, E., Vega, S., Blendinger, I., and Tio, T.: Long term follow-up epidural blood patch. Anesth. Analg., *54*:459, 1975.
2. Armstrong, I.A., Littlewood, D.G., and Chambers, W.A.: Spinal anesthesia with tetracaine—the effect of added vasoconstrictors. Anesth. Analg., *62*:793, 1983.
3. Axelsson, K., and Widman, B.: Clinical significance of specific

gravity of spinal anaesthetic solutions: Two double-blind studies with hyperbaric 5% lidocaine. Acta Anaesthesiol. Scand., *23*:427, 1979.

4. Babcock, W.W.: Spinal anaesthesia: A clinical study of 658 administrations. NY Med. J., *98*:897, 1913.
5. See 27 references to cocaine spinal anesthesia in Bibliographia Medica II, Paris. p. 855, 1901.
6. Barker, A.E.: Clinical experiences with spinal analgesia in 100 cases. Br. Med. J., *1*:665, 1907.
7. Batson, O.V.: The function of the vertebral veins and their role in the spread of metastases. Ann. Surg., *112*:138, 1940.
8. Bengtsson, M., Löfström, J.B., and Malmquist, L.A.: Skin conductance responses during spinal analgesia. Acta Anesthesiol. Scand., *29*:67–71, 1985.
9. Bier, A.: Versuche über Kokainisierung des Rückenmarks. Dtsch. Z. Chir., *51*:361, 1899.
10. Braun, H.: Üeber den Einfluss der Vitalität der Gewebe auf die örtlichen und allgemeinen Gifturkungen localanästhesirender Mittel und über die Bedeutung des Adrenalins für die Localanästhesis. Arch. F. Klin. Chir., *19*:541, 1903.
11. Braun, H.: Über einige neue örtliche Anästhetica (Stovain, Alypine, Novokain). Dtsch. Med. Wochenschr. *31*:1667, 1905
12. Bridenbaugh, P.O., Moore, D.C., and Bridenbaugh, L.: Capillary pO_2 as a measure of sympathetic blockade. Anesth. Analg., *50*:26, 1971.
13. Brown, E.M., and Elman, D.S.: Postoperative backache. Anesth. Analg., *40*:683, 1961.
14. Brownridge, P.: Management of headache following dural puncture in obstetric patients. Anaesth. Intensive Care *11*:4, 1983.
15. Burm, A.G., van Kleef, J.W., Gladines, M.P., Spierdijk, J., *et al.*: Plasma concentrations of lidocaine and bupivacaine after subarachnoid administration. Anesthesiology, *59*:191, 1983.
16. Caldwell, C., Nielsen, C., Baltz, T., Taylor, P., *et al.*: Comparison of high dose epinephrine and phenylephrine in spinal anesthesia with tetracaine. Anesthesiology, *62*:804, 1985.
17. Carbaat, P.A.T., Van Crevel, H.: Lumbar puncture headache: Controlled study of the preventive effect of 24 hours bedrest. Lancet, *2*:1133, 1982.
18. Chambers, W.A., Edström, H.H., and Scott, D.B.: Effect of baricity on spinal anaesthesia with bupivacaine. Br. J. Anaesth., *53*:279, 1981.
19. Chambers, W.A., Littlewood, D.G., Logan, M.R., and Scott, D.B.: Effect of added epinephrine on spinal anesthesia with lidocaine. Anesth. Analg., *60*:417, 1981.
20. Chambers, W.A., Littlewood, D.G., and Scott, D.B.: Spinal anesthesia with bupivacaine: Effect of added vasoconstrictors. Anesth. Analg., *61*:49, 1982.
21. Cohen, E.N.: Distribution of local anesthetic agents in the neuraxis of the dog. Anesthesiology, *29*:1002, 1968.
22. Concepcion, M., Maddi, R., Francis, D., *et al.*: Vasoconstrictors in spinal anesthesia. A comparison of epinephrine and phenylephrine. Anesth. Analg., *63*:134, 1984.
23. Corning, J.L.: Spinal anesthesia and local medication of the cord. NY State J. Med., *42*:483, 1885.
24. Crock, H.V., and Yoshizawa, H.: The Blood Supply of the Vertebral Column and Spinal Cord in Man. New York, Springer-Verlag, 1979.
25. Cummings, G.C., Bamber, D.B., Edström, H.H., and Rubin, A.P.: Subarachnoid blockade with bupivacaine: A comparison with cinchocaine. Br. J. Anaesth., *56*:573, 1984.
26. Denson, D.D., Bridenbaugh, P.O, Turner, P.A., Phero, J.C., *et al.*: Neural blockade and pharmacokinetics following subarachnoid lidocaine in the Rhesus monkey. I. Effects of epinephrine. Anesth. Analg., *61*:746, 1982.
27. Denson, D.D., Bridenbaugh, P.O., Turner, P.A., and Phero, J.C.: Comparison of neural blockade and pharmacokinetics after subarachnoid lidocaine in the Rhesus monkey. II. Effects of volume, osmolality, and baricity. Anesth. Analg., *62*:995, 1983.
28. Denson, D.D., Turner, P.A., Bridenbaugh, P.O., and Thompson, G.A.: Pharmacokinetics and neural blockade after subarachnoid lidocaine in the Rhesus monkey. III. Effects of phenylephrine. Anesth. Analg., *63*:129, 1984.
29. DiGiovanni, A.J., Dunbar, B.S.: Epidural injections of autologous blood for postlumbar puncture headache. Anesth. Analg., *49*:268, 1970.
30. Dohi, S., Matsumiya, N., Takeshima, R., and Naito, H.: Effects of subarachnoid lidocaine and phenylephrine on spinal cord and cerebral blood flow in dogs. Anesthesiology, *61*:238, 1984.
31. Dripps, R.D., and Vandam, L.D.: Long term follow-up of patients who received 10,098 spinal anesthetics. I. Failure to discover major neurological sequelae. J.A.M.A., *156*:1486, 1954.
32. Dubelman, A.M., and Forbes, A.R.: Does cough increase the spread of subarachnoid anesthesia? Anesth. Analg., *58*:306, 1979.
33. Eckenhofff, J.E., Hafkenschiel, J.H., Foltz, E.L., and Driver, R.L.: Influence of hypotension on coronary blood flow, cardiac work, and cardiac efficiency. Am. J. Physiol., *152*:545, 1948.
34. Egbert, L.D., and Deas, T.C.: Effect of epinephrine on the duration of spinal anesthesia. Anesthesiology; *21*:345, 1960.
35. Etherington-Wilson, W.: Intrathecal nerve root block: Some contributions and a new technique. Proc. R. Soc. Med. (Anaesth.), *27*:323, 1937.
36. Fishman, R.A.: Cerebrospinal Fluid in Diseases of the Nervous System. pp. 168-252. Philadelphia, W.B. Saunders, 1980.
37. Fishman, R.A.: Cerebrospinal Fluid in Diseases of the Nervous System. pp. 15-62. Philadelphia, W.B. Saunders, 1980.
38. Freund, F.G., Bonica, J.J., Ward, R.J., Akamatsu, T.J., *et al.*: Ventilatory reserve and level of motor block during high spinal and epidural anesthesia. Anesthesiology, *28*:834, 1967.
39. Giasi, R.M., D'Agostino, E., Covino, B.G.: Absorption of lidocaine following subarachnoid and epidural administration. Anesth. Analg., *58*:360, 1979.
40. Greene, B.A.: A 26-gauge lumbar puncture needle: Its value in the prophylaxis of headache following spinal analgesia for vaginal delivery. Anesthesiology, *11*:464, 1950.
41. Greene, H.M.: A technique to reduce the incidence of headache following lumbar puncture in ambulatory patients with a plea for more frequent examination of cerebrospinal fluids. Northwest Med., *22*:240, 1923.
42. Greene, N.M.: The area of differential block during spinal anesthesia with hyperbaric tetracaine. Anesthesiology, *19*:45, 1958.
43. Greene, N.M.: A consideration of factors involved in the discovery of anesthesia and their effect on subsequent development of anesthesia. Anesthesiology, *35*:515, 1971.

44. Greene, N.M.: Physiology of Spinal Anesthesia. ed. 3. Baltimore, Williams & Wilkins, 1981.
45. Greene, N.M.: Uptake and elimination of local anesthetics during spinal anesthesia. Anesth. Analg., *62*:1013, 1983.
46. Greene, N.M.: Distribution of local anesthetic solutions within the subarachnoid space. Anesth. Analg., *64*:715, 1985.
47. Greene, N.M., Bunker, J.P., Kerr, W.S., von Felsinger, J.M., *et al.*: Hypotensive spinal anesthesia: Respiratory, metabolic, hepatic, renal and cerebral effects. Ann. Surg., *140*:641, 1954.
48. Hackel, D.B., Sancetta, S.M., and Kleinerman, J.: Effect of hypotension due to spinal anesthesia on coronary blood flow and myocardial metabolism in man. Circulation, *13*:92, 1956.
49. Hart, J.R., and Whitacre, J.J.: Pencil-point needle in prevention of postspinal headache. J.A.M.A., *147*:657, 1951.
50. Jones, W.H.: Spinal analgesia: A new method and a new drug. Br. J. Anaesth., *7*:99, 1930.
51. Kalso, E., Tuominen, M., Rosenberg, P.H.: Effect of posture and some CSF characteristics on spinal anaesthesia with isobaric 0.5% bupivacaine. Br. J. Anaesth., *54*:1179, 1982.
52. Kennedy, W.F. Jr., Everett, G.B., Cobb, L.A., and Allen, G.D.: Simultaneous systemic and hepatic hemodynamic measurements during high spinal anesthesia in normal man. Anesth. Analg., *49*:1016, 1970.
53. Kety, S.S., King, B.D., Horvath, S.M., Jeffers, W.A., *et al.*: The effects of acute reduction in blood pressure by means of differential spinal sympathetic block on the cerebral circulation of hypertensive patients. J. Clin. Invest., *29*:40, 1950.
54. Kleinerman, J., Sancetta, S.M., and Hackel, D.B.: Effects of high spinal anesthesia on cerebral circulation and metabolism in man. J. Clin. Invest., *37*:285, 1958.
55. Koller, C.: Über Verwendung des Kokains zur Anästhesierung am Auge. Wien. Med. Wochenschr., *43*:46, 1884.
56. Koster, H.: Spinal analgesia with special reference to its use in surgery of the head, neck and thorax. Am. J. Surg., *5*:554, 1928.
57. Koster, H., Shapiro, A., and Leikensohn, A.: Spinal anesthesia: Procaine concentration changes at site of injection in subarachnoid anesthesia. Am. J. Surg., *33*:245, 1936.
58. Kozody, R., Palahniuk, R.J., Wade, J.G., and Cumming, M.O.: The effect of subarachnoid epinephrine and phenylephrine on spinal cord blood flow. Can. Anaesth. Soc. J., *31*:503, 1984.
59. Labat, G.: Regional Anesthesia: Its Technique and Clinical Application. Philadelphia, W.B. Saunders, 1922.
60. Lemmon, W.T.: A method of continuous spinal anaesthesia. Ann. Surg., *111*:140, 1940.
61. Levin, E., Muravchick, S., and Gold, M.I.: Isobaric tetracaine spinal anesthesia and the lithotomy position. Anesth. Analg., *60*:810, 1981.
62. Lofstrom, J.B., Malmquist, L.A., and Bengtsson, M.: Can the "sympatho-galvanic reflex" be used to evaluate sympathetic block in spinal analgesia? Acta Anaesthesiol. Scand., *28*:578, 1984.
63. Lund, P.C.: Principles and Practice of Spinal Anesthesia. Springfield, IL, Charles C. Thomas, 1971.
64. Lynn, R.B., Sancetta, S.M., Simeone, F.A., and Scott, R.W.: Observations on the circulation during high spinal anesthesia. Surgery, *32*:195, 1952.
65. Manchanda, V.N., Murad, S.H.N., Shilyansky, G., and Mehringer, M.: Unusual clinical course of accidental subdural local anesthetic injection. Anesth. Analg., *62*:1124, 1983.
66. Matas, R.: Report of successful spinal anesthesia. Medical News. J.A.M.A., *33*:1659, 1899.
67. McClure, J.H., Brown, D.T., Wildsmith, J.A.W.: Effect of injected volume and speed of injection on the spread of spinal anaesthesia with isobaric amethocaine. Br. J. Anaesth., *54*:917, 1982.
68. Mehta, M., and Maher, R.: Injection into the extra-arachnoid subdural space. Anaesthesia, *32*:760, 1977.
69. Møller, I.W., Fernandes, A., and Edstrom, H.H.: Subarachnoid anaesthesia with 0.5% bupivacaine: Effects of density. Br. J. Anaesth., *56*:1191, 1984.
70. Moore, D.C.: Complications of Regional Anesthesia. Springfield, IL, Charles C. Thomas, 1955.
71. Moore, D.C.: Spinal anesthesia: Bupivacaine compared with tetracaine. Anesth. Analg., *59*:743, 1980.
72. Moore, R.A., Bullingham, R.E.S., McQuay, H.J., Hand, C.W., *et al.*: Dural permeability to narcotics: In vitro determination and application to extradural administration. Br. J. Anaesth., *54*:1117, 1982.
73. Morton, A.W.: The subarachnoid injection of cocaine for operations on the upper part of the body. J.A.M.A., *39*:1162, 1902.
74. Mueller, R.P., Lynn, R.B., and Sancetta, S.M.: Studies of hemodynamic changes in humans following induction of low and high spinal anesthesia. II. The changes in splanchnic blood flow, oxygen extraction and consumption and splanchnic vascular resistance in humans not undergoing surgery. Circulation, *6*:894, 1952.
75. Neigh, J.L., Kane, P.B., and Smith, T.C.: Effects of speed and direction of injection on the level and duration of spinal anesthesia. Anesth. Analg., *49*:912, 1970.
76. Nightingale, P.J.: Barbotage and spinal anaesthesia. Anaesthesia, *38*:7, 1983.
77. Park, W.Y., Balingot, P.E., and McNamara, T.E.: Effects of patient age, *p*H of cerebrospinal fluid and vasopressor on onset and duration of spinal anesthesia. Anesth. Analg., *54*:455, 1975.
78. Pearson, A.: A rare complication of extradural analgesia. Anaesthesia, *39*:460, 1984.
79. Peng, A.T.C., Behar, S., and Blancato, L.S.: Reduction of postlumbar puncture backache by the use of field block anesthesia prior to lumbar puncture. Anesthesiology, *63*:227, 1985.
80. Pitkin, G.P.: Controllable spinal anesthesia. Am. J. Surg., *5*:537, 1928.
81. Porter, S.S., Albin, M.S., Watson, W.A., and Bugengin, L.: Spinal cord and cerebral blood flow responses to subarachnoid injection of local anesthesia with and without epinephrine. Acta Anaesth. Scand., *29*:330, 1985.
82. Prickett, M.D., Gross, E.G., and Cullen, S.C.: Spinal anesthesia with solutions of procaine and epinephrine: Preliminary report of 108 cases. Anesthesiology, *6*:469, 1945.
83. Ravindran, R.S., Viegas, O.J., Pantazis, K.L., and Baldwin, S.J.: Serum lidocaine levels following spinal anesthesia with lidocaine and epinephrine in dogs. Reg. Anaesth *8*:6, 1983.
84. Rocco, A.G., Frances, D., Wark, J.A., Conception, M.A., *et al.*: A clinical double blind study of dibucaine and tetracaine in spinal anesthesia. Anesth. Analg., *61*:133, 1982.

85. Runciman, W.B., Mather, L.E., Ilsley, A.H., *et al.*: A sheep preparation for studying interactions between blood flow and drug disposition. III: Effect of general and spinal anesthesia on regional blood flow. Br. J. Anaesth., *56*:1267, 1984.
86. Shantha, T.R., Evans, J.A.: The relationship of epidural anesthesia to neural membranes and arachnoid villi. Anesthesiology, *37*:543, 1972.
87. Shesky, M.C., Rocco, A.G., Bizzarri-Schmidt, M., Francis, D.M., *et al.*: A dose-response study of bupivacaine for spinal anesthesia. Anesth. Analg., *62*:931, 1983.
88. Sise, L.F.: Pontocaine-glucose solution for spinal anesthesia. Surg. Clin. North Am., *124*:1501, 1935.
89. Sivarajan, M., Amory, D.W., Lindbloom, L.E., and Schwettman, R.S.: Systemic and regional blood-flow changes during spinal anesthesia in the Rhesus monkey. Anesthesiology, *43*:78, 1975.
90. Spivey, D.L.: Epinephrine does not prolong lidocaine spinal anesthesia in term parturients. Anesth. Analg., *64*:468, 1985.
91. Tait, D., Caglieri, G.: Experimental and clinical notes on the subarachnoid space. Trans. Med. Soc. Calif., *30*:266, 1900.
92. Tarrow, A.B.: Solution to spinal headaches. Int. Anesthesiol. Clin., *1*:877, 1963.
93. Taylor, J.A.: Lumbosacral subarachnoid tap. J. Urol., *43*:561, 1940.
94. Tuffier, *et al.*: Analgesie chirurgicale per l'injection sous-arachnoidienne lombarie de cocaine. C.R. Soc. Bull. (Paris), *51*:882, 1899.
95. Tuohy, E.B.: Continuous spinal anesthesia: Its usefulness and technic involved. Anesthesiology, *5*:142, 1944.
96. Tuominen, M., Kalso, E., and Rosenberg, P.H.: The effects of posture in the spread of spinal anaesthesia with isobaric 0.75% or 0.5% bupivacaine. Br. J. Anaesth., *54*:313, 1982.
97. Walts, L.F., Koepke, T., and Margules, R.: Determination of sensory and motor levels after spinal anesthesia with tetracaine. Anesthesiology, *25*:634, 1964.
98. Ward, R.J., Bonica, J.J., Freud, F.G., and Akamatsu, T.: Epidural and subarachnoid anesthesia: Cardiovascular and respiratory effects. J.A.M.A., *191*:275, 1965.
99. Wildsmith, J.A.W., McClure, J.H., Brown, D.T., and Scott, D.B.: Effects of posture on the spread of isobaric and hyperbaric amethocaine. Br. J. Anaesth., *53*:273, 1981.

8 EPIDURAL NEURAL BLOCKADE

MICHAEL J. COUSINS
PHILIP R. BROMAGE

Although techniques of epidural anesthesia do not offer the economy of drug dosage or degrees of blockade of spinal anesthesia, they are currently more versatile and better studied. No other neural blockade techniques are used as extensively in each of the fields of surgical anesthesia, obstetric anesthesia, and diagnosis and management of acute and chronic pain. Epidural blockade is also unique because of special features of the anatomic site of injection and the resultant diverse sites of action of the local anesthetic solution (see below).

The most practical and widely used continuous method of neural blockade is spinal epidural blockade; pharmacokinetic data have helped to increase the efficacy and safety of epidural infusion techniques (see Chap. 26). Continuous caudal blockade has useful but limited applications, and continuous spinal anesthesia is now seldom used. As indicated in Chapters 24 and 28, new developments in the understanding of pain conduction have extended the use of continuous epidural blockade to the administration of drugs that selectively block pain conduction, while leaving sensation, motor power, and sympathetic function essentially unchanged. The safety and the reliability of spinal epidural catheter techniques, with the addition of bacterial filters, have permitted relief of acute pain (see Chaps. 18 and 26) and chronic pain (see Chaps. 27 and 28) for many days, often with patients remaining ambulatory. This has heralded an even more vigorous and fruitful era of investigation and clinical application of epidural blockade than did the unprecedented development of the past 20 years.

HISTORY AND RECENT DEVELOPMENT

The study of epidural blockade sustained interest in neural blockade techniques in the 1940s and 1950s, when they seemed doomed to obscurity, and it played an important part in a recent resurgence of interest. By a coincidence, the introduction of curare in 1946 and its meteoric rise of popularity in the 1950s occurred at a similar time to the rise in popularity of obstetric caudal analgesia.[117,259] For many years, however, caudal rather than lumbar epidural blockade was the preferred method of obstetric and postoperative pain relief.[201,259] The adaptation of Tuohy's subarachnoid needle[497] for use with epidural blockade in 1949[155] and the use of continuous catheter techniques, both caudal[260] and lumbar epidural,[116] played a major part in enabling improvements to be made in epidural neural blockade with respect to its efficacy, safety, and duration of action for surgical analgesia, postoperative pain management, and obstetric pain relief. Although lumbar epidural anesthesia, by continuous catheter techniques, was first used extensively in surgical operations and for postoperative pain,[116] it was the obstetric application of this technique that most sustained its use in the 1950s. A gradual recognition of the greater anatomic difficulty of caudal block in adults,[90,493] the higher dose required, and the "nonselective" nature of this block in obstetric applications[67] increased the popularity of lumbar epidural block over caudal block. In the early 1950s, the availability of a new drug, lidocaine,[328] with rapid onset and superior neural penetration, greatly increased enthusiasm for use of epidural block. More important, detailed studies of the spread of analgesia and site of action of epidural blockade supported and rationalized the use of the technique.[69,70,76] During the 1960s, epidural blockade became the most widely used technique of neural blockade for pain relief in obstetrics in Canada,[67] in the United States,[253] and in other countries, such as Australia[399] and New Zealand[278]; it was used in Britain initially in surgery and postoperative pain relief by Dawkins.[162,163]

By the early 1970s, there was an increased understanding of the advantages of segmental blockade, with minimal local anesthetic dosage, and thus reduced toxicity. Controlled clinical studies had clearly demonstrated the long duration of action of the new drug bupivacaine, originally introduced in the early 1960s (see Chap. 4). This now made prolonged segmental blockade a practical reality. Previous attempts to provide long-duration epidural analgesia with lidocaine alone often led to tachyphylaxis and sometimes caused toxicity (see below). The addition of small doses of long-acting agents such as tetracaine to solutions of lidocaine was said to be successful in some institutions,[363] but tetracaine is not available throughout the world. Prolonged pain relief with bupivacaine by continuous catheter epidural blockade became very attractive when it was demonstrated that excellent analgesia after surgery, or in obstetrics, could be obtained with minimal motor blockade.[74,175] Detailed pharmacokinetic studies of local anesthetic drugs administered by infusion and by single or repeated epidural injection,[496] and comparative studies of toxic blood concentrations of local anesthetics in humans,[48,445] permitted meaningful estimations of toxicity ratios for the various local anesthetics in the clinical application of epidural blockade (see also Chaps. 3, 4, and 26).[496] Concurrently, detailed studies of the cardiorespiratory effects of epidural blockade[37,38–40,515,516] provided important information to increase the safety of the technique by careful attention to level of blockade, maintenance of blood volume, and other factors. New knowledge of the cardiac effect of local anesthetics has helped prevent and treat such effects, if they occur (see Fig. 8-4).

APPLIED ANATOMY OF EPIDURAL BLOCKADE

The reader should review the description of the anatomy of bony spine, ligaments, meninges, cerebrospinal fluid (CSF), and spinal arteries in Chapter 7, since this is directly applicable to epidural blockade.

The epidural space is not as voluminous as the subarachnoid space. Nevertheless, it extends from the base of the skull to the sacrococcygeal membrane and has complicated direct communications with the paravertebral space and indirect communications with the CSF. It also leads directly to the vascular system by way of its large epidural veins, which have no valves and connect with the basivertebral venous plexus, intracranial veins, and the azygos vein (see Fig. 28-15); this is a potential direct route to the brain and heart for drugs, air, or other material inadvertently injected into an epidural vein. Within the cranium, there is no epidural space, as the meningeal dura and endosteal dura are closely adherent, except where they separate to form the venous sinuses. At the foramen magnum, these two layers separate: the former becomes the spinal dura, and the latter becomes the periosteum of the spinal canal (Figs. 8-1, 8-2, 8-3). Thus, although local anesthetics cannot enter between the endosteal and meningeal layer of the cerebral dura, they can diffuse across the spinal dura at the base of the brain into the CSF and, thence, to the brain (Fig. 8-3). Between the spinal dura and the spinal periosteum lies the epidural space. The ligamentum flavum completes the posterior wall in direct continuity with the periosteum of the spinal canal (Fig. 8-1). Because the spinal canal is approximately triangular in cross section and the articular processes indent the triangle (Fig. 8-4), the epidural space narrows posterolaterally and then widens again laterally toward the intervertebral foramina (Fig. 8-5). Thus, the safest point of entry into the epidural space is in the midline.

Resin injection studies in cadavers have confirmed that the epidural space is predominantly located in dorsomedial and dorsolateral regions of the spinal canal. Thin ventral spread occurred in 40% of cases.[251] The narrowness of the ventral epidural space was confirmed in other studies using injection of iodized oil and examination by x-ray.[416a]

The *shape* of the dorsal epidural space was studied with computed tomography of T8–12 in patients. This revealed a sawtooth shape, with the dorsal epidural space narrowest near the rostral lamina (1.3–1.6 mm) and widest near the caudad lamina (6.9–9.1 mm) of each interspace[416a] (see Fig. 8-9). This is in keeping with the attachment of ligamentum flavum to the *anterior* surface of the rostral lamina and the *posterior* surface of the caudad lamina. It emphasizes the desirability of not entering the epidural space close to the rostral lamina. Further information about the anatomy of the epidural space is likely to be provided by studies with nuclear magnetic resonance

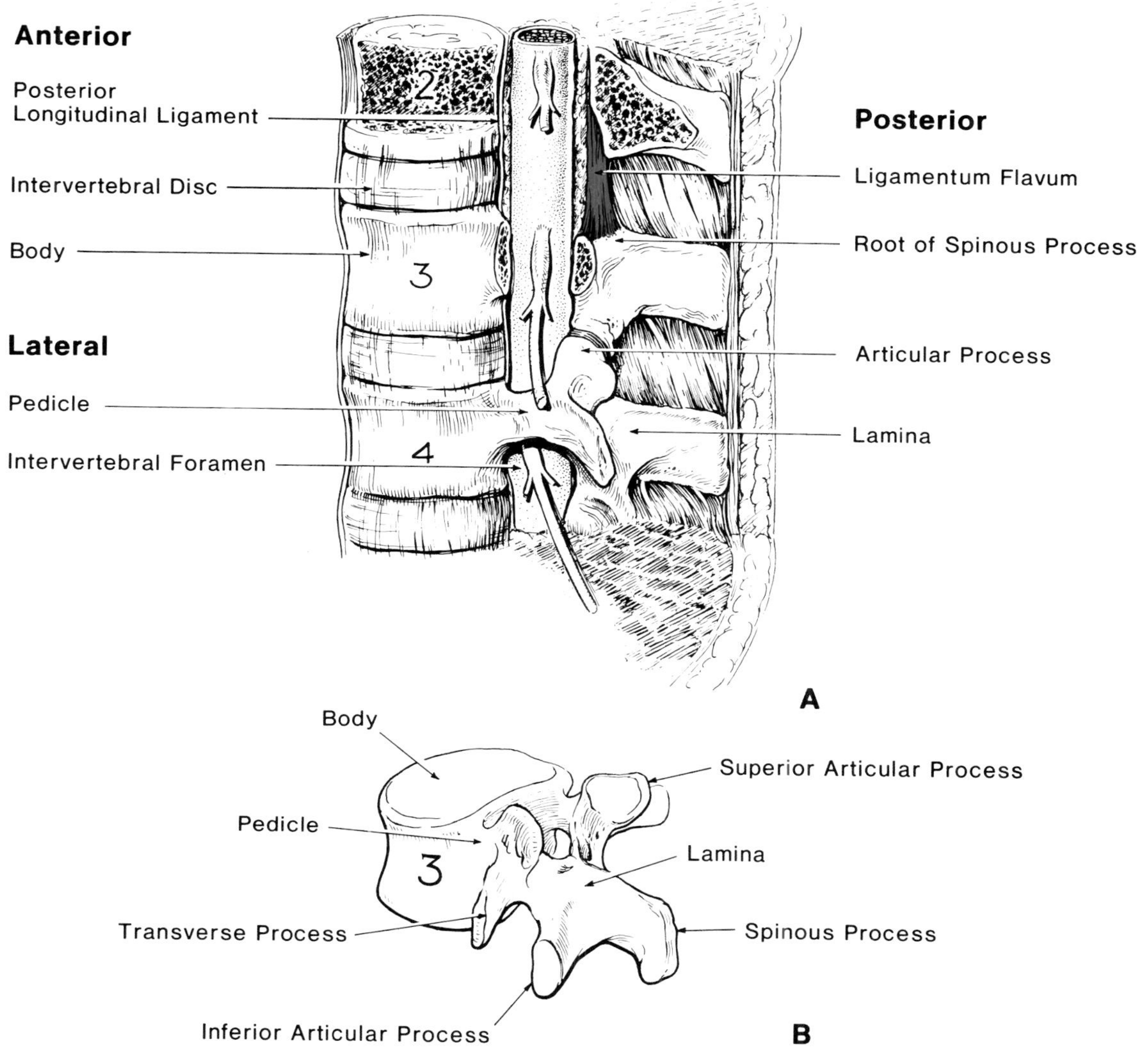

FIG. 8-1. **A.** Boundaries of the epidural space. Note the superior portion of ligamentum flavum, hidden from posterior view because of attachment to the anterior aspect of the lamina, and the inferior attachment of the ligamentum flavum to the posterior aspect of the lamina (see also Fig. 8-9). **B.** Lumbar vertebra. (Macintosh, R.R.: Lumbar Puncture and Spinal Analgesia. Edinburgh, E. & S. Livingstone, 1957.)

equipment and with fine fiber-optic scopes that can be threaded through a 16-gauge epidural needle.[32a] (see below).

Surface Anatomy

The key anatomy for safe placement of a needle in the epidural space is summarized in Tables 8-1 to 8-3 on pages 260 and 261. However, before considering deep structures, the anesthesiologist should be certain of the level and direction of insertion of the needle; thus, surface anatomy is important. Because the easiest and safest point of entry into the epidural space is in the midlumbar region, a reliable surface marking for this level is important: The line drawn between the highest point of the two iliac crests usually passes through the spinous process of the fourth lumbar vertebra (Fig. 8-7A). The interspinous

(*Text continues on p. 258*)

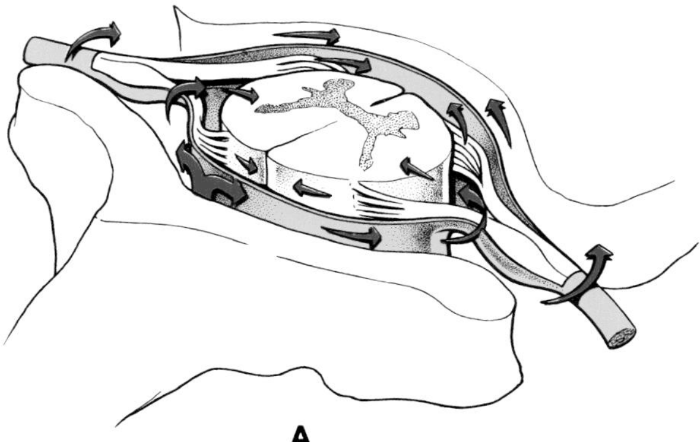

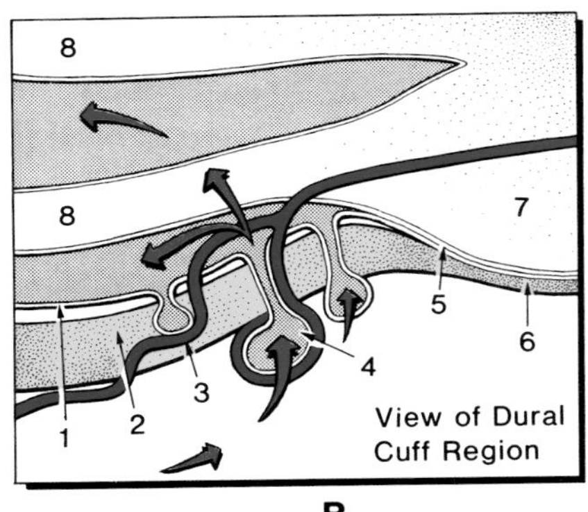

FIG. 8-2. **A.** Horizontal spread of local anesthetic in epidural space. Major spread posteriorly to the region of "dural cuff" (root sleeve) region is shown, with subsequent entry to cerebrospinal fluid (CSF) and spinal cord. Minor spread into anterior epidural space is also shown. **B.** Enlarged view of dural cuff region shows rapid entry of local anesthetic into CSF by way of arachnoid granulations: *1,* arachnoid membrane; *2,* dura; *3,* epidural vein; *4,* arachnoid "granulation" protruding through dura and contacting epidural vein; *5,* perineural epithelium of spinal nerve in continuity with arachnoid; *6,* epineurium of spinal nerve in continuity with dura; *7,* dorsal root ganglion; *8,* intradural spinal nerve roots.

Summary of Boundaries of the Epidural Space

Superior
- The foramen magnum where the periosteum of the spinal canal and the spinal dura fuse together to form the endosteal and meningeal layer of the cerebral dura (Fig. 8-3)

Inferior
- The sacral hiatus and sacrococcygeal membrane (Fig. 8-3)

Lateral
- The periosteum of the pedicles of the vertebrae and the intervertebral foramina (Fig. 8-1)

Anterior
- The posterior longitudinal ligament covering the vertebral bodies, and intervertebral disks (Fig. 8-1)

Posterior
- The periosteum of the anterior surfaces of the laminae, the articular processes, and their connecting ligaments, the roots of the vertebral spines, and the interlaminar spaces filled by the ligamenta flava (Figs. 8-1, 8-6).

Summary of Spread of Injected Solutions in Epidural Space

Contrast medium, local anesthetic, or other agent injected into the spinal (or caudal) epidural space may potentially spread as follows:
- Superior and inferior spread is mainly in posterior portion of epidural space between dura and ligamentum flavum (Fig. 8-3).
- Superiorly to foramen magnum. Note the possibility of diffusion of drugs of low molecular weight across dura at base of brain to cerebral CSF, with possibility of access to cranial nerves, vasomotor and respiratory centers, and other vital centers.
- Inferiorly to sacral hiatus, caudal canal, and through anterior sacral foramina (Fig. 8-3).
- Laterally through intervertebral foramina to paravertebral space, to produce paravertebral neural blockade. Note rapid access to CSF at "dural cuff" region (Figs. 8-1, 8-2) to produce spinal nerve root blockade, and subsequent access to spinal cord (see below).
- Anteriorly in thin epidural space between dura and anterior longitudinal ligament (Fig. 8-2).

Note also:

Access to CSF by slow diffusion across spinal dura, subdural space, and subarachnoid membrane into subarachnoid space

Vascular absorption by way of epidural veins may convey drug to heart and brain (see below).

Profuse epidural fat may take up drug (see below).

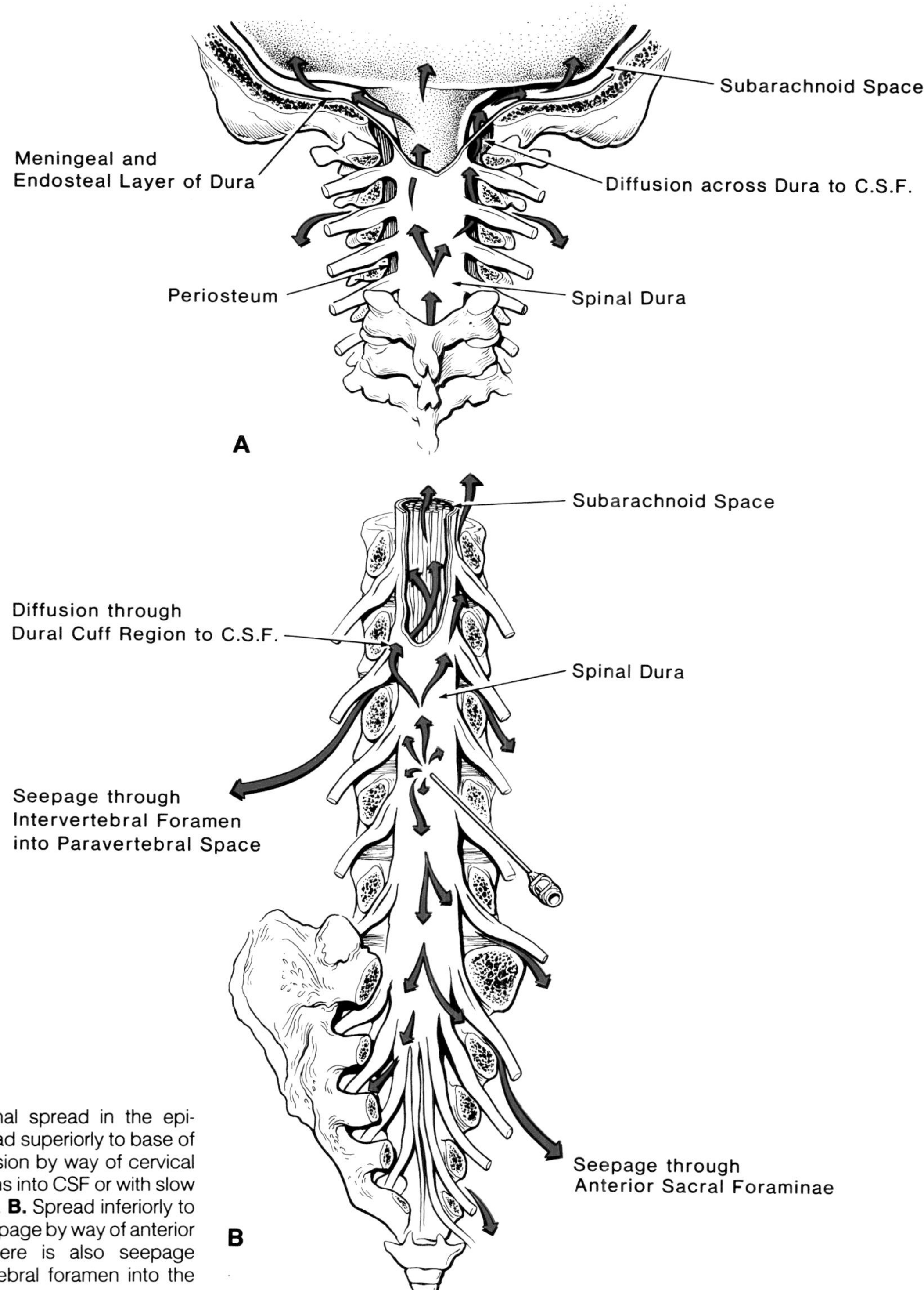

FIG. 8-3. Longitudinal spread in the epidural space. **A.** Spread superiorly to base of skull, with rapid diffusion by way of cervical arachnoid granulations into CSF or with slow diffusion across dura. **B.** Spread inferiorly to caudal canal with seepage by way of anterior sacral foramina. There is also seepage through the intervertebral foramen into the paravertebral space.

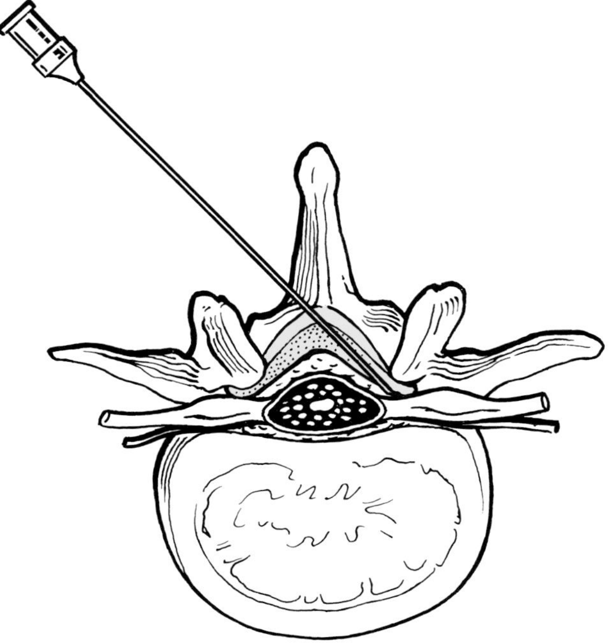

FIG. 8-4. Ligamentum flavum, cross-sectional view. The triangular shape of each half of the ligament is apparent. They narrow toward the articular processes, as does the underlying epidural space. Also, incorrect extreme lateral angulation of a needle is shown. Oblique penetration of the ligamentum flavum results, with continued resistance for several millimeters and eventual loss of resistance in the dural cuff region, where there are two main hazards: The epidural space is very narrow and the dura is thin (see also Fig. 8-2); the needle is close to spinal nerve and vessels. (Macintosh, R.R.: Lumbar Puncture and Spinal Analgesia. Edinburgh, E. & S. Livingstone, 1957.)

space above this spinous process (L3–4) or one higher (L2–3) is the standard site of needle insertion for epidural block in adults, since the spinal cord usually ends at the lower border of vertebra L1. As noted in Chapter 21, this is not the case in children and is one reason why the caudal route of entry is preferred to the lumbar route in young children. Also, the dural sac terminates at the level of S2 in adults (S3 in small children): A line through the posterior superior iliac spines crosses this level. As noted in Table 8-1, puncture below L4 increases the difficulty of "midline" epidural block because of the ill-defined interspinous ligament; also, puncture above L2 increases the risk of damage to the conus medullaris, so that the interspaces of L2–3 and L3–4 are both the safest and the easiest; identification of L4 reassures that an easy entry may be achieved. Identification of L1 acts as a double check and confirms that the point of entry is safely below the conus medullaris. There is no difference in the potential danger of damaging the cord if one chooses the T12–L1 interspace or the C7–T1 interspace, both of which can often be technically easy; however, the spinal cord lies directly beneath the epidural space in both instances. Thus, only anesthesiologists experienced with epidural techniques require the anatomic landmarks above L1: the inferior angle of scapula (T7), the root of the spine of the scapula (T3), and the vertebra prominens (C7).

Because of the extreme angulation of the spinous processes in the midthoracic region, midline puncture is difficult, and the paraspinous (paramedian) approach is preferable. In contrast, there is excellent access to the interlaminar space in the midline at C7–T1 and T1–2; the same applies in the low thoracic region. However, it should be noted that anatomic differences, such as a narrower epidural space (Tables 8-2, 8-3), require greater technical skill at these levels and a technique somewhat different from that usually used for lumbar epidural block.

In the lumbar region, correct needle insertion takes full advantage of the fact that it is both easier and safer to insert the needle at the L2–3 or L3–4 interspace, with the needle entering the epidural space in the midline. The latter does not necessarily imply that the needle must start in the midline, although in most cases that is an easy approach. As shown in Figures 8-1 and 8-12B, the inferior aspects of the spinous processes, in the midlumbar region, lie opposite the line across the widest lateral extent of the interlaminar space. Thus, needle insertion should be close to the superior spinous process, since the upper border of the inferior spine lies over the lamina of its underlying vertebral body. A needle inserted with due regard to this requires very slight upward angulation to give an unobstructed approach to the interlaminar space (see Fig. 8-30). A surface anatomic aid that is often neglected involves checking that the needle is inserted in the center of a line running through the middle of the superior and inferior aspects of the spinous processes: that is, in the center of the supraspinous ligament. This is best achieved by grasping the spinous processes adjacent to the site of puncture between thumb and forefinger, while needle is inserted through skin and subcutaneous tissue into the supraspinous ligament (Fig. 8-7B). If this is done, the needle should sit firmly in the supraspinous ligament without angulation to one side. Obese subjects may require additional maneuvers (see section on technique).

Segmental Levels

In assessing the level of epidural blockade, it is important for the anesthesiologist to have a method of using simple surface landmarks to indicate level of dermatomal blockade and, thus, segmental spinal nerve (and sympathetic blockade). Table 8-4 lists the key levels (see Fig. 8-35).

There is no point in testing for blockade of T1 – 2 by testing above the nipple line, since this area has double innervation from T1 – 2 and C3 – 4, so that normal sensation remains even when T1 – T2 are blocked. Thus, residual activity in the important cardiac sympathetics T1 and T2 is checked by testing skin sensation on the inside of the arm above the elbow (T2) and below the elbow (T1). Residual motor activity in T1

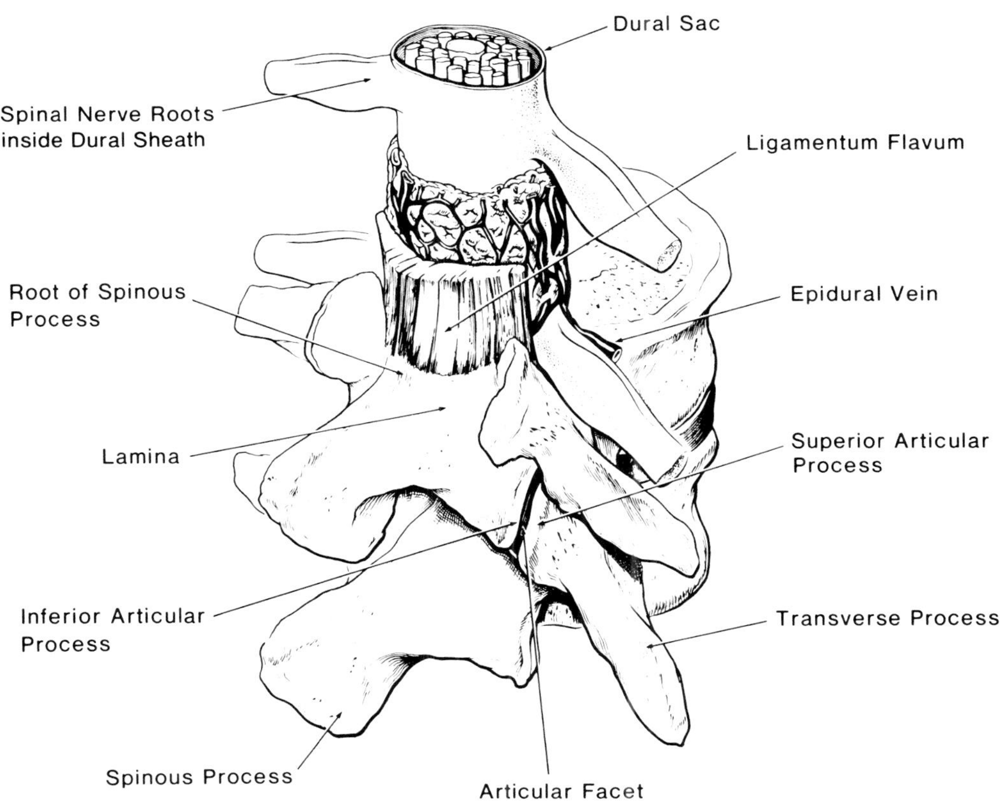

FIG. 8-5. Epidural space, relationships from the posterior view. Note the increased prevalence of epidural veins lateral to the midline; narrowing of the ligamentum flavum and epidural space laterally; slight downward slope of spinous processes; proximity of articular facets at lateral aspect of lamina (see also Fig. 8-12*B*). (Macintosh, R.R.: Lumbar Puncture and Spinal Analgesia. Edinburgh, E. & S. Livingstone, 1957.)

TABLE 8-1. KEY ANATOMIC FEATURES FOR ADMINISTRATION OF LUMBAR EPIDURAL ANESTHESIA

Spine and Ligaments

Spinous process
- Widest in midlumbar region
- Only slight downward angulation (see Fig. 8-1)
- Inferior border opposite widest point of interlaminar space (see Fig. 8-12B)
- Superior border over upward-sloping lamina (see Fig. 8-12B)
- Narrower superiorly. Needle inserted beside spinous process guided into midline by lateral aspect of spinous process (see Fig. 8-30A)

Interspinous ligament
- Well defined above L4. Below L4 narrower and loose—may offer less resistance

Lamina
- Posterior surface slopes down and back
- Needle may strike lamina superficially at inferior aspect of slope or deep at superior aspect of slope (see Fig. 8-5)

Interlaminar space
- Increased by flexing lumbar spine
- Larger "target" area in midline and in midlumbar region
- Smaller target laterally (see Fig. 8-12B)

Articular facets
- Needle directed past lateral aspect of interlaminar space may impinge on articular facets, causing severe radiating pain and muscle spasm (see Fig. 8-12B)

Ligamentum flavum
- Thickest in midlumbar region in midline (see Fig. 8-8)
- Attached to anteroinferior aspects of lamina above and posterosuperior aspects of lamina below; thus, needle entering at inferior aspect may be held up by lamina (see Fig. 8-9).

Relationships of Epidural Space

Epidural space
- Widest in midlumbar region in midline (5–6 mm), narrower next to articular processes where ligamentum flavum and dura almost touch (see Fig. 8-4)
- Widens laterally where spinal nerve surrounded by dural cuff (see Fig. 8-2A)
- Communicates with paravertebral space by way of intervertebral foramen (see Fig. 8-1); therefore, epidural catheter may stimulate spinal nerve—unisegmental paresthesia.

Spinal nerve
- Needle inserted past depth of lamina with lateral angulation on *same* side may penetrate past spinous process to spinal nerve (Fig. 8-5).
- Needle angled across midline to *opposite* side may run in substance of ligamentum flavum laterally to reach spinal nerve and/or dural cuff (see Fig. 8-4).

Arterial supply of spinal cord (see Figs. 7-10 and 7-11)
- Only one anterior spinal artery
- In thoracolumbar region fed mainly by "Radicularis Magna," which usually enters by way of an intervertebral foramen on left side at T11–12 (may be at other interspaces T8–L3).
- Supply to anterior thoracolumbar cord is discontinuous with higher levels.
- Sharp demarcation between anterior and posterior spinal artery territory

Epidural veins
- Prominent in lateral portion of epidural space (see Fig. 8-5)
- Drain to azygos vein and connect to pelvic veins, providing an alternative route from pelvis to right heart. Therefore, they become distended when inferior vena cava is obstructed (see Fig. 8-13).
- Also connect to cerebral venous sinuses by way of basivertebral veins (see Fig. 28-15).

can also be checked by testing the ability of the patient to hold a sheet of paper between the outstretched fingers (interossei C8, T1). In a lightly anesthetized patient, spinal reflexes may be useful for testing level of blockade: epigastric (T7–8); abdominal (T9, T12), cremasteric (L1, L2), plantar (S1, S2), knee-jerk (L2–4), ankle-jerk (S1, S2).

Structures Encountered During Midline Insertion of Epidural Needle

If *correct* use of surface anatomy described above is observed and prior skin puncture is made with a larger needle (introducer), an epidural needle should encounter no resistance in the skin and subcutaneous

TABLE 8-2. KEY ANATOMIC FEATURES FOR ADMINISTRATION OF MIDTHORACIC EPIDURAL ANESTHESIA

Spinous process
- Extreme downward slope, inferior border opposite midpoint of *lamina* below.
- Small posterior surface, processes close together and difficult to identify
- Therefore, the paraspinous (paramedian) technique is easier (see Fig. 8-30B)

Interspinous ligament
- Difficult to identify because spinous processes close to one another.

Lamina
- Broader than lumbar laminae, but shorter in vertical dimension
- Large area available for location of depth of ligamentum flavum with less fear of accidental puncture of dura

Ligamentum flavum
- Thick but less so than midlumbar

Epidural space
- In midline 3–5 mm, narrow laterally

TABLE 8-3. KEY ANATOMIC FEATURES FOR ADMINISTRATION OF CERVICOTHORACIC EPIDURAL ANESTHESIA

Spinous process
- At C7 (vertebra prominens) and T1, direction is almost horizontal
- Inferior border C7 opposite widest point of C7–T1 interlaminar space

Lamina
- Shaped like narrow rectangle

Interlaminar space
- Accessible with midline puncture if neck flexed

Ligamentum flavum
- Thinner than at any other level

Epidural space
- Width at first thoracic interspace is 3 to 4 mm (note width at C3–6 is 2 mm)
- Increased width if neck flexed
- Usually marked negative pressure (increased if sitting)

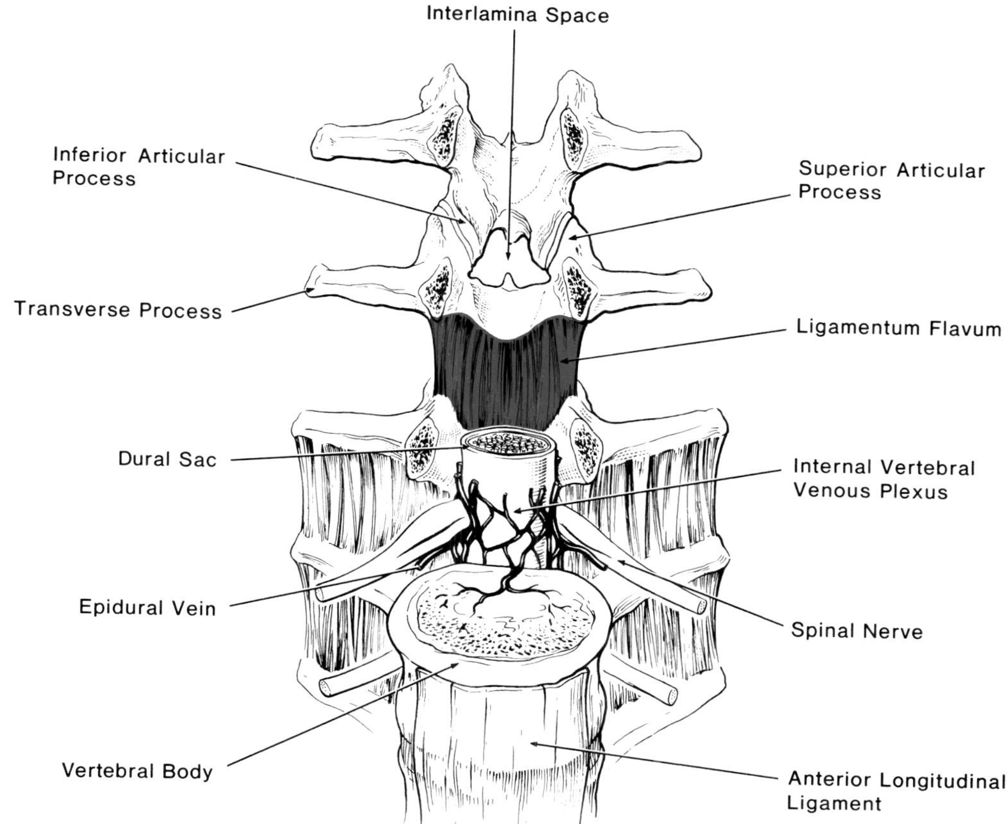

FIG. 8-6. Epidural space, relationships from anterior view. Note "interlaminar space" at one level and covered by ligamentum flavum at the level below. Epidural veins are in continuity with veins draining vertebral body ("internal vertebral venous plexus"). (Macintosh, R.R.: Lumbar Puncture and Spinal Analgesia. Edinburgh, E. & S. Livingstone, 1957.)

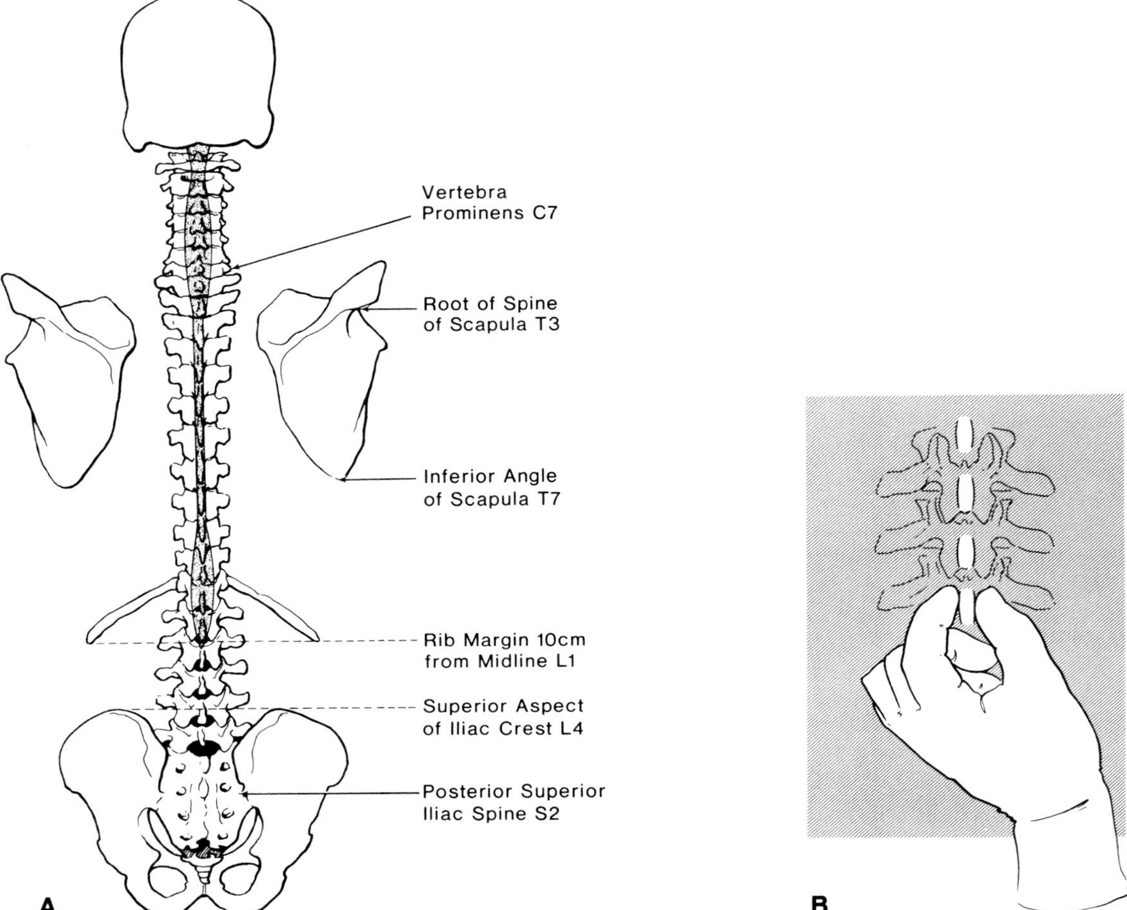

FIG. 8-7. **A.** Surface anatomy and landmarks for epidural blockade. The spinous process (vertebra prominens) at C7 is the most prominent spinous process when the neck is flexed. The spinous process at T3 lies opposite the root of the spine of the scapula (arm by side). The spinous process at T7 lies opposite the inferior angle of the scapula (arm by side). For puncture between C7 and T1 there is direct access to the interlaminal space, but there are other hazards (see text). Puncture below T3 and above T7 is difficult because of angled spinous processes. Puncture below T7 becomes progressively similar to L2–3. Other hazards are the same as those for high puncture (see text). The spinous process at L1 (lower border) is noted by a line meeting the costal margin 10 cm from the midline. The spinous process at L4 *(center)* lies at the top of the iliac crests. S2 is noted by the posterior superior iliac spines. Puncture is *safest* and *easiest* in the lumbar region. L2–3 and L3–4 are the preferred levels. **B.** Method of checking midline. Labat's method of checking center of spinous processes uses the thumb and forefinger to grasp the spinous processes above and below the site of the needle puncture.

tissue, but should then penetrate the tough supraspinous ligament (Fig. 8-8), which will support it at right angles to the skin in all directions; the *interspinous* ligament then offers continued resistance to advancing the needle; an increase in resistance to advancement of the needle signals that the needle tip has entered the thick, elastic ligamentum flavum; after only a few millimeters of advancement, a sudden loss of all resistance occurs as the needle tip enters the epidural space.

TABLE 8-4. KEY LEVELS OF DERMATOMAL BLOCKADE

Cutaneous Landmark	Segmental Level	Significance
Little finger	C8	All cardioaccelerator fibers (T1-T4) blocked
Inner aspect of arm and forearm	T1 and T2	Some degree of cardio-accelerator blockade
Apex of axilla	T3	Easily remembered landmark
Nipple line (midway sternal notch and xiphisternum)	T4-5	Possibility of cardioaccelerator blockade
Tip of xiphoid	T7	Splanchnics (T5-L1) may become blocked
Umbilicus	T10	Sympathetic blockade limited to lower limbs
Inguinal ligament	T12	
Outer side of foot	S1	No lumbar sympathetic blockade Most difficult nerve root to block

The distance of the epidural space from the skin varies widely. It is most commonly 4 cm (50%) and is 4 to 6 cm in 80% of the population according to detailed records of 3200 cases.[244] In obese patients, however, this distance may be greater than 8 cm but is less than 3 cm in thin patients.

Incorrect procedure (Tables 8-5, 8-6) or sometimes inadvertent aberrant needle placement owing to anatomic difficulties may result in quite a different sequence of events than that described earlier and contact with different anatomic structures. Failure to clearly define the midline results in needle entry beside the supraspinous ligament. If the anesthesiologist persists with this unsatisfactory start, it is likely that the needle will next enter the interspinous ligament obliquely, resulting in only a transient resistance, followed by loss of resistance; or, it may miss the ligament completely, resulting immediately in a feeling of no resistance, in the paravertebral muscles. Both of these situations may be interpreted as rapid entry into the epidural space. However, injection of local anesthetic is followed by marked "drip back," and subsequent attempts to thread an epidural catheter will be met with considerable resistance. If the needle is inserted too close to the spinous process (or during any attempt at midline puncture in the midthoracic region), it is not uncommon for the needle to contact the spinous process. Perhaps the most common obstruction to the needle is the lamina of the vertebral body. Because the posterior surface of the lamina slopes gently down and back from its anterior end to its posterior end (see Fig. 8-5), an epidural needle inserted too far laterally may encounter lamina either at a superficial depth or deeper, close to its junction with the ligamentum flavum (Fig. 8-9). Even more extreme lateral insertion or lateral angulation of the needle may result in the needle point contacting the superior or inferior articular processes or the joint space (Fig. 8-12B), where their articular facets meet. The latter can be particularly painful, since the articular facets have a rich nerve supply, and needle trauma may result in sudden severe localized pain on one side of the back with accompanying paravertebral muscle spasm on that side. This pain is not dissimilar to that caused by direct contact with a nerve root: "radicular pain." Both may result in pain that radiates into the leg. Radicular pain is usually more discreet with only one area involved (*e.g.*, the inside of the knee for L3 or inside of the leg for L4). Facet pain may radiate but is somewhat more diffuse.

The ligamentum flavum should be entered in the center of the interlaminar gap, regardless of where the needle enters the skin (midline or paraspinous). Even with midline puncture, failure to control the

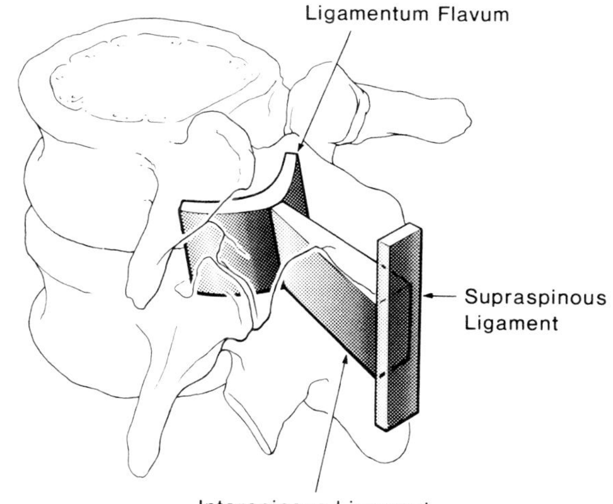

FIG. 8-8. Ligaments encountered during a midline puncture.

TABLE 8-5. STRUCTURES ENCOUNTERED DURING EPIDURAL BLOCK

Structure	Comment
With Correct Procedure (Midline Technique)	
Skin	Prior puncture with 19-gauge needle should ensure no "drag" on epidural needle
Supraspinous ligament	Needle sits *firmly* in midline
Interspinous ligament	Clear-cut resistance to syringe plunger (above L4) ? Poorly defined resistance (below L4, or sometimes at other levels, ? choose another interspace)
Ligamentum flavum	Increase in resistance to syringe plunger, with marked "elastic" quality Increased resistance to advancing needle
Epidural space	*Controlled* and well-defined loss of resistance No resistance to injected solution No, or minimal, "drip back" of injected solution Catheter passes easily
Incorrect Procedure or Unintentional Misplacement of Needle	
Skin	Lack of prior puncture causes marked "drag" on epidural needle
Supraspinous ligament	Entered to one side, causes needle to angle laterally Missed completely, causes needle to flop to one side and appear to have no support
Interspinous ligament	Entered obliquely, results in transient resistance, then loss of resistance, which is interpreted as entrance to epidural space; however, there is marked run back of injected solution, and catheter will not thread Missed completely, results in low resistance—needle in paravertebral muscles
Spinous process	Very superficial contact: interspace not marked ?; spine flexed? (see Fig. 8-12B) Deep contact: needle angled much too acutely?
Lamina	Posterior end of slope: superficial obstruction to needle advancement Anterior end of slope: deep obstruction (see Fig. 8-9)
Articular processes	Sudden pain in back Muscle spasm on one side of back
Ligamentum flavum (LF)	
LF pierced midline but with poor control of entry	Needle "overshoots" through epidural space and punctures dura (see Table 8-6)
LF pierced to side of midline where dura close and veins prominent	Dural puncture ± CSF flow; or cannulation of epidural vein, +/− bleeding
Failure to identify LF with subsequent entry into subdural space	No CSF aspirated Some resistance to injected solution and "drip back," which is local anesthetic Catheter passes with difficulty Small dose of local anesthetic results in widespread block with bizarre distribution
Needle enters lateral aspect from opposite side and continues within ligament to region of spinal nerve (see Fig. 8-4)	Continued "elastic resistance" for several millimeters and then sudden unisegmental paresthesia May be followed by CSF flow if dural cuff entered
Epidural space	
Entry uncontrolled, needle against dura, no solution injected to expand epidural space	Catheter threads with difficulty or sudden loss of resistance—CSF in catheter
Entry to side of midline into epidural vein or CSF	Blood or CSF via needle or bleeding as catheter threaded—clot in catheter unless flushed with saline
Entry at extreme inferior aspect of ligamentum flavum at attachment to lamina of lower vertebra	Loss of resistance to syringe plunger but needle progress halted by upper edge of lamina and catheter will not thread
Entry at extreme superior aspect with only tip of needle piercing ligament	Loss of resistance to syringe plunger but some resistance to injected solution and catheter will not thread Further progress of needle easy
Entry at lateral aspect	Catheter may impinge on spinal nerve

penetration of the ligament results in a second loss of resistance, signaling dural puncture. Entry at the lateral aspect of the interlaminar gap may also result in dural puncture, since the epidural space is narrow at this point (Fig. 8-4); there is also an increased risk of puncturing an epidural vein with return of blood from the epidural needle.

The epidural space should permit easy injection of solution and easy threading of an epidural catheter, if it is entered in the midline in a controlled manner. Uncontrolled entry or failure to fix the needle securely during subsequent injections or catheter insertions may result in pushing the needle tip forward until it touches the dura. This results in some resistance to injected local anesthetic and may cause the epidural catheter to puncture the dura if undue force is used when catheter insertion becomes difficult. Many textbooks fail to explain why catheter insertion is impossible, and why further progress of the needle is obstructed immediately after an otherwise impeccably correct loss of resistance through the ligamentum flavum. The explanation lies in the anatomy of the lamina and ligamentum flavum; the latter attaches to the anteroinferior aspects of the lamina below (Figs. 8-1, 8-6). Thus, a needle piercing the ligamentum flavum at its extreme inferior aspect may be held up by the upper edge of the sloping lamina (see also Fig. 8-9). Usually reinsertion of the needle, more to the center of the interlaminar space, is then necessary. Less commonly, a needle angled sharply upward may undergo a clear-cut loss of resistance as its tip penetrates the ligamentum flavum, but attempts to pass a catheter meet with bony resistance. In this case, the recurved tip of an epidural needle still lies partially in the ligamentum flavum immediately adjacent to its attachment to the lamina above. If the epidural needle can be advanced without further resistance, and the catheter then threads easily without aspiration of CSF, this confirms a high entry through the interlaminar gap. More rarely, but of great importance, a needle angled acutely laterally may penetrate the ligamentum flavum close to a spinal nerve. Subsequent attempts to pass a catheter may lead to resistance and the immediate report of a unisegmental paresthesia. This calls for repositioning of the needle, since persistence may lead to spinal nerve trauma.

It is unusual not to obtain a jet of CSF back through an 18-gauge (or larger) needle if it enters the subarachnoid space. Thus, the syringe should always be disconnected as soon as the loss of resistance through the ligamentum flavum is obtained, or if a subsequent second loss of resistance is noted. The width of the posterior epidural space, beneath the ligamentum flavum, varies considerably, depending on the level of the bony spine at which it is approached and the horizontal point of needle entry (see Tables 8-1, 8-2, 8-3); it is widest in the midline in the midlumbar region (5–6 mm) but narrows next to the articular processes (see Fig. 8-4). In the midthoracic region, it is

TABLE 8-6. SUSPECTED DURAL PUNCTURE

Sign	Cause	Management
Second loss of resistance and fluid flows from needle	Dural puncture	Convert to spinal anesthetic or move to higher interspace for epidural
Second loss of resistance after identifying ligamentum flavum and no fluid flows from needle, but injected solution → some "drip back"	? Entry into subdural space ? Dural puncture	Test "drip back" on arm: Cold = LA; warm = CSF Drip into container with etidocaine in it: CSF → precipitate† With glucose test tape: CSF → color change If drip back only LA, withdraw needle and reidentify epidural space If drip back = CSF ± LA, move to a rostrad* interspace or convert to spinal anesthetic
One loss of resistance only; however, "drip back" at: A shallow level	Interspinous ligament pierced and needle in paravertebral muscle	Reinsert needle in midline
A deeper level	Low compliance of epidural fat	Test as above, if drip back only LA: Attempt to pass catheter → easy passage
	Needle only partially through ligamentum flavum	Attempt to pass catheter → does not pass: Superiorly needle can be advanced and then catheter threaded Inferiorly needle will not advance
	Needle in CSF	Test for CSF, if positive move to rostrad interspace or convert to spinal

LA = Local anesthetic CSF = Cerebrospinal fluid.
*Do not attempt to withdraw needle into *epidural* space at the same level, as this may result in subdural cannulation.[483]
†Anaesthetist, *29*:570, 1980.

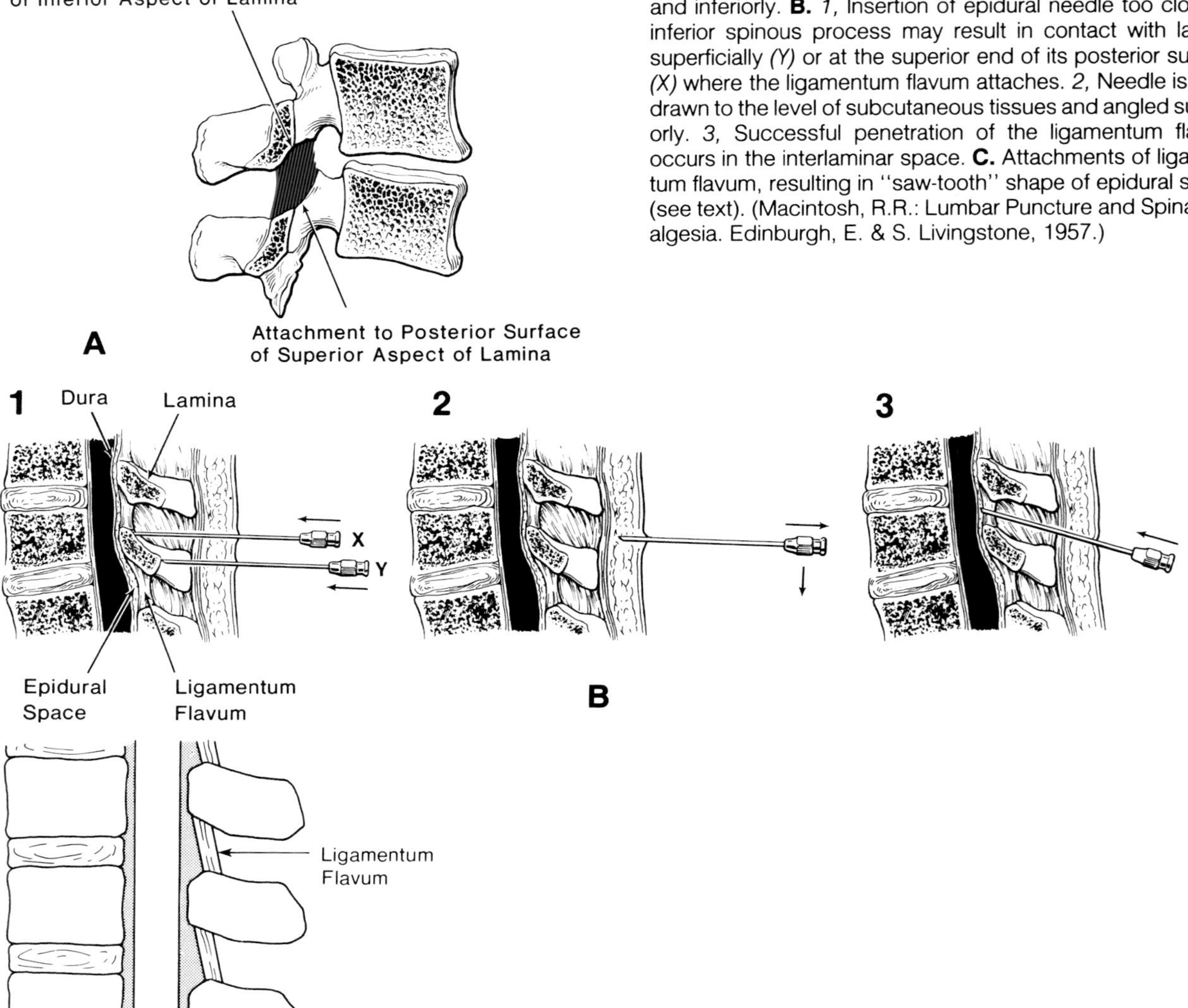

FIG. 8-9. **A.** Attachment of ligamentum flavum, superiorly and inferiorly. **B.** *1*, Insertion of epidural needle too close to inferior spinous process may result in contact with lamina superficially *(Y)* or at the superior end of its posterior surface *(X)* where the ligamentum flavum attaches. *2*, Needle is withdrawn to the level of subcutaneous tissues and angled superiorly. *3*, Successful penetration of the ligamentum flavum occurs in the interlaminar space. **C.** Attachments of ligamentum flavum, resulting in "saw-tooth" shape of epidural space (see text). (Macintosh, R.R.: Lumbar Puncture and Spinal Analgesia. Edinburgh, E. & S. Livingstone, 1957.)

3 to 5 mm in the midline and very narrow laterally. In the lower cervical region, the distance between ligamentum flavum and dura is only 1.5 to 2 mm in the midline; however, this increases below C7 to 3 to 4 mm, particularly if the neck is flexed.

The epidural veins are most prominent along the lateral walls of the spinal canal in the lateral portion of the epidural space.

The spinal arteries reach the spinal cord by way of the intervertebral foraminae and enter the epidural space to reach spinal nerve roots in the region of the dural cuffs (see Figs. 8-2, 8-4). It is thus possible to cause spinal cord ischemia if a spinal artery is traumatized by a needle inserted toward a spinal nerve root. The spinal cord territory supplied by the anterior spinal artery is most vulnerable, since there is only one anterior artery (Fig. 8-10) and since the major feeder to this artery usually enters unilaterally (on the left in 75%) by way of a single intervertebral foramen, between T5 and L3 (see Fig. 7-11). This further supports the practice of ensuring that the needle enters the epidural space in the midline and suggests that the L3–4 interspace is the best choice for beginners.

Aspects of Individual Anatomic Structures with Relevance to Epidural Block

The description given of applied anatomy of epidural puncture highlights relevant aspects of the anatomy of the bony spine, ligaments, meninges, spinal nerves, and blood vessels. Anesthesiologists are strongly advised to study the detailed anatomy of the individual lumbar vertebrae, as well as the articulated skeleton, with the aid of an atlas of anatomy.

Only by direct handling of the bony spine and its articulations will the reader fully appreciate the important relationships discussed (see Tables 8-1, 8-2, 8-3).

The vertebrae and vertebral column hold the key to both spinal subarachnoid and epidural blockade (see Figs. 8-1, 8-11, 8-12, and 8-30). These are also discussed in Chapter 7. However, the following are of particular importance to epidural blockade. The spinous processes are widest in the midlumbar region and have only slight angulation, making insertion of the 16- to 18-gauge Tuohy needle into the center of the supraspinous ligament relatively easy compared with elsewhere in the spine. The inferior border of the spinous process lies over the widest part of the interlaminar space (Fig. 8-12). The process becomes somewhat narrower superiorly, so that a needle can be guided by the lateral aspect of the spinous process to enter the midpoint of the ligamentum flavum. In the midthoracic region, the spinous processes are much narrower, closer together, and angulated sharply downward, thus obscuring the interlaminar space (see Fig. 7-1). The inferior border of spinous processes in this region lies opposite the lamina of the vertebral body below. Insertion of an epidural needle may necessitate a paraspinous (paramedian) approach. If the needle is inserted beside the lower border of the spinous process and angled upward at 130 degrees, the lateral aspect of the process can once again be used to guide the needle inward 15 degrees toward the center of the ligamentum flavum (see Fig. 8-30). In the cervical region, the spinous processes widen and become bifid with a wide supraspinous ligament. They are almost horizontal in the lower cervical region and permit easy access to the interlaminar space (see Fig. 8-11).

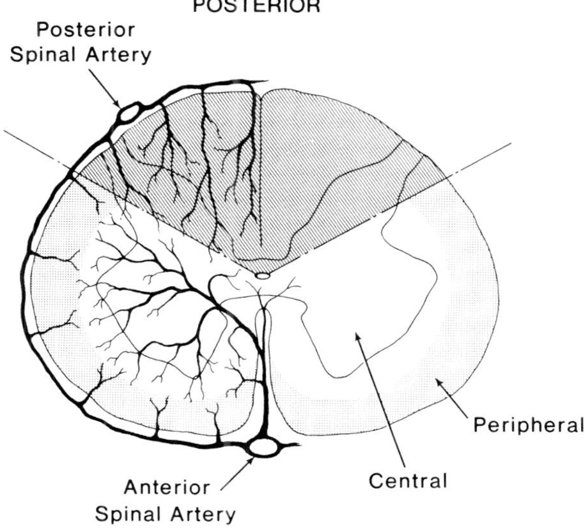

FIG. 8-10. Blood supply of spinal cord, horizontal distribution. The "central" area, supplied only by anterior spinal artery, is predominantly a motor area (see text).

The supraspinous ligament runs vertically between the apices of the spinous processes of lumbar and thoracic vertebrae and continues above as ligamentum nuchae. It varies in width directly with the width of the spinous process; in the lumbar region, it may be as much as 1 cm wide (see Fig. 8-8). In persons who engage in heavy physical activity and in laborers and the aged, the ligament may become ossified, making midline puncture impossible.

The interspinous ligament runs obliquely between the spinous processes and is continuous anteriorly with the ligamentum flavum and posteriorly with the supraspinous ligament. As indicated in Tables 8-1, 8-2, and 8-3, its thickness is greatest above L4 in the lumbar region. Although it is a thin ligament, its fibers are attached along the entire superior and inferior surfaces of the spinous processes; thus, in the lumbar region, the ligament is rectangular and provides an identifiable resistance to injected air or solution (see Fig. 8-8).

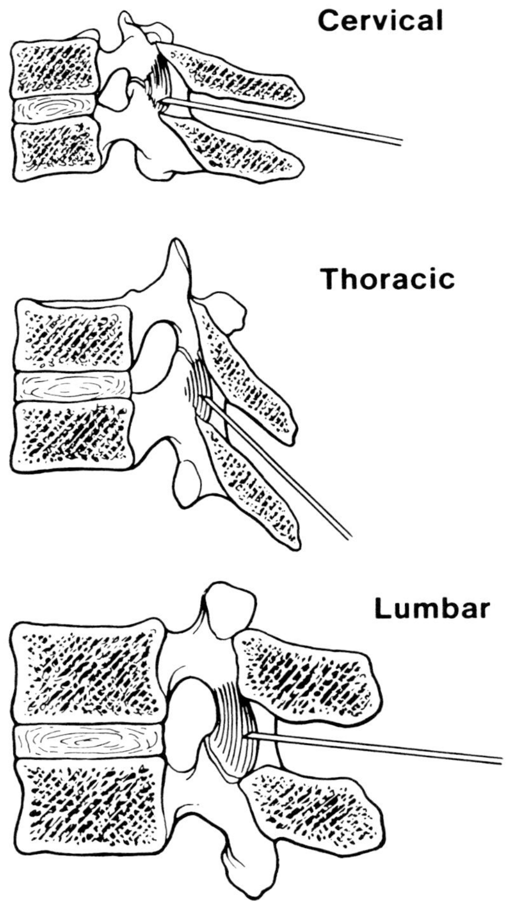

FIG. 8-11. Ligamentum flavum in lumbar, thoracic, and cervical regions.

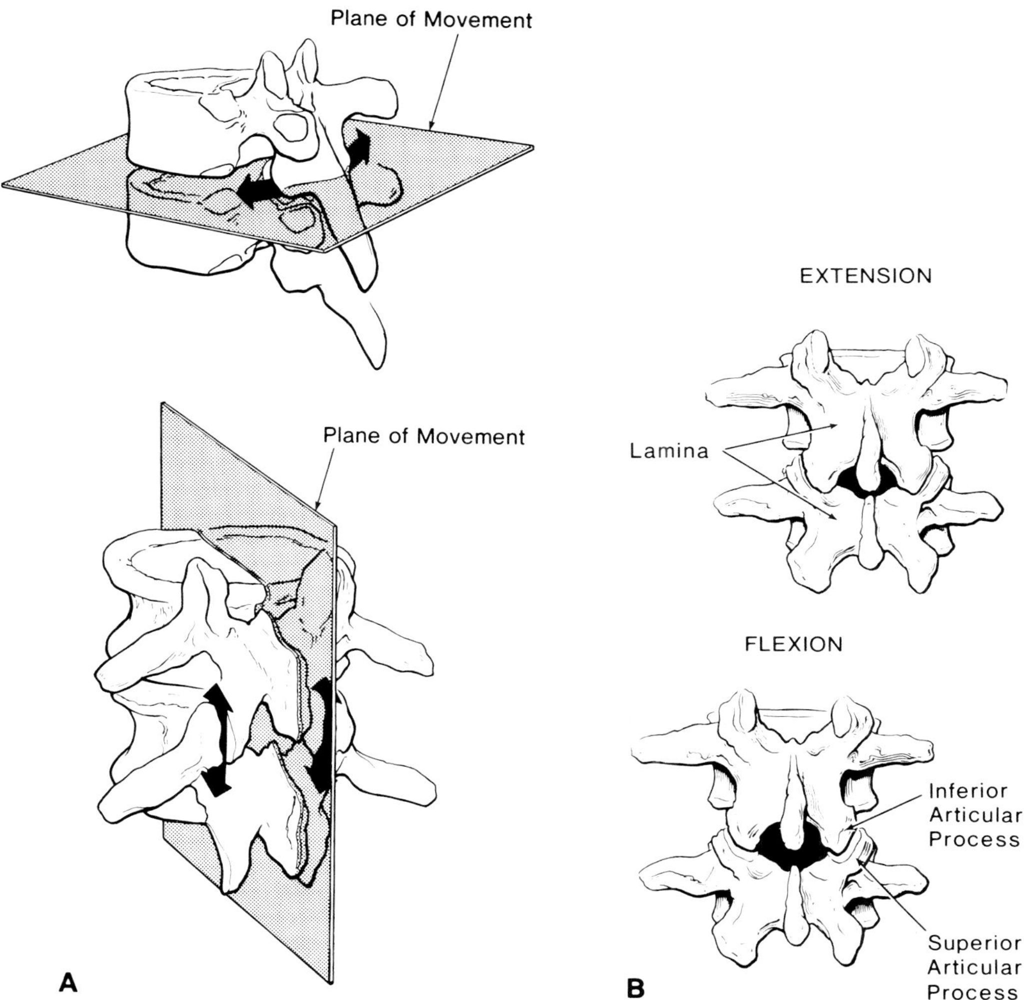

FIG. 8-12. **A.** Articular facets, plane of rotation. In the thoracic region, the plane through the facets is a horizontal circle, so that lateral rotation can occur. In the lumbar region, the plane through the facets is a vertical circle, so that lateral rotation cannot occur and the only possible movement is flexion and extension. (Arrows indicate direction of movement.) **B.** Interlaminar space, lumbar region, in extension and flexion. In extension, the boundaries are roots of spinous processes and laminae. With flexion, articular processes form the lateral boundary, and articular facets are exposed at the lateral extremity of the interlaminar space. (Part B modified from Macintosh, R.R.: Lumbar Puncture and Spinal Analgesia. Edinburgh, E. & S. Livingstone, 1957.)

The laminae and articular processes form the boundaries of the interlaminar foramen. In the lumbar region, the foramen is triangular when the lumbar spine is extended, with the base being formed by the upper borders of the laminae of the lower vertebra and the sides, by the medial aspects of the inferior articular processes of the vertebra above. However, if the lumbar spine is flexed, the inferior articular processes glide upward by means of the synovial joints between facets of articular processes, thus enlarging the interlaminar foramen to a diamond shape (Fig. 8-12B); borders of the superior articular process of the vertebra below now form the lower part of the lateral boundaries of the foramen. It is worth noting that, in the lumbar region, the facets of the articular processes articulate at right angles to a circle with its center in the middle of the vertebral body, so that rotation cannot take place; by contrast, in the thoracic region, the facets articulate in the same plane as such a circle, so that rotation of one vertebra on another readily occurs.[336] This further indicates the potential increased difficulty of puncture in the thoracic compared with the lumbar region (Fig. 8-12A).

The lamina itself slopes down and back on its posterior surface, so that it may be contacted by a needle either superficially or deep (see Figs. 8-5, 8-9B). As indicated above, the lamina forms only the wide base of the interlaminar space. The remaining boundaries are formed laterally and superiorly by the articular processes (see Fig. 8-6).

The ligamentum flavum is composed almost entirely of elastic fibers and is aptly named, since it is indeed yellow. Because of its tough elasticity and its thickness of several millimeters in the lumbar region, the ligament imparts a characteristic "springy" resistance, particularly to a large-bore needle with an upturned end (Tuohy needle). The ligament runs from the anterior and inferior aspects of the lamina above to the posterior and superior aspects of the lamina below. Laterally, the ligament narrows as it blends with the capsule of the joint between the articular processes (see Figs. 8-4, 8-5, 8-6). Because developmentally two laminae fuse at each level to form the root of the spinous process, two ligamenta flava meet in the median plane and here become continuous with the deep fibers of the interspinous ligament (see Fig. 8-8). Thus, an epidural needle advancing in the midline encounters continuing resistance that increases immediately as the needle passes into the ligamentum flavum. There is evidence from cadaver dissections that the ligamentum flavum may retain a midline cleft or sulcus in a high percentage of cases.[223] This raises the interesting possibility that the loss of resistance felt before entering the epidural space in the midline may be deep fibers of the interspinous ligament. This may provide support for the paramedian approach, since the depth of lamina can be positively identified and the resistance of the ligamentum flavum may be more reliably located by this approach. However, in life it is likely that the elastic ligamenta flava come tightly together in the midline in cases when the two "halves" remain potentially separated.

The pedicles that join the laminae to the vertebral bodies complete the bony spinal canal that protects the dural sac. Each pedicle is notched, so that pedicles of adjacent vertebral bodies form the intervertebral foramen. The inferior pedicle of each foramen is notched more deeply. The intervertebral foramina are completed posteriorly by the capsule surrounding the articular processes of adjoining vertebrae and anteriorly by an intervertebral disk and the lower part of the body above it (see Fig. 8-1). Because the epidural space is continuous with the paravertebral space, it is possible to produce an epidural block by injection close to an intervertebral foramen (see Chap. 10), or to penetrate the dura at the dural cuff region if a needle is inserted into an intervertebral foramen. The degree of patency of intervertebral foramina is thought to influence the spread of local anesthetics and contrast media injected into the epidural space[458]; it has been shown that extensive "leakage" of local anesthetic occurs through intervertebral foramina.[203,337,465] There are a total of 58 foramina, so the potential for "leakage" is considerable. However, the density of areolar tissue around the foramina varies considerably, and with advancing age it forms a recognizable "operculum" that effectively blocks off foramina.[203] This appears to play a part in the declining dose requirements with advancing age,[73,458] although a declining neural population may also contribute.[128] Similar mechanisms probably result in reduction in dose requirements in atherosclerosis.[70]

The contents of the epidural space are also discussed in Chapter 7. However, several aspects deserve further comment with relation to epidural block.

The epidural fat is semifluid lobulated areolar tissue that extends throughout the spinal and caudal epidural space. It is most abundant posteriorly, diminishes adjacent to the articular processes, and then increases laterally around the spinal nerve roots, where it is continuous with the fat surrounding the spinal nerves in the intervertebral foramina and thence with the fat in the paravertebral space. Anteriorly, it is sparse, and thus the dura may lie close to the posterior longitudinal ligament. Overall, the amount of fat in the epidural space tends to vary in direct relation to that present elsewhere in the body, so that obese patients may have epidural spaces that are occupied by generous amounts of fat. Mostly, the epidural fat lies free in the epidural space except near the nerve roots, where connective tissue tends to tether the fat in the intervertebral foramina. The epidural fat is surprisingly vascular, with small capillaries that form a rich network in its substance.[410,490] The fat itself has a great affinity for drugs with high-lipid solubility, such as bupivacaine and etidocaine, which may remain in epidural fat for long periods (see Chap. 3); uptake of local anesthetic into epidural fat competes with vascular and neural uptake. The compliance of the epidural fat varies considerably between persons and with increasing age.[507,508] In children and young adults, it offers little resistance to injection, but in some adults, a low compliance may result in considerable "drip back" of injected local anesthetic. A fiberoptic endoscopy study of 48 cadavers reported a dorsomedian connective tissue band, of varying thickness, in every case.[32a]

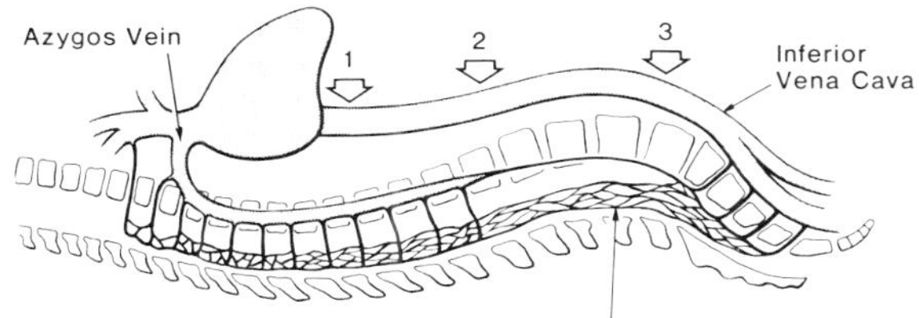

FIG. 8-13. Epidural veins (vertebral venous plexus) and their connections with inferior vena cava (IVC) and azygos vein. Epidural veins are protected from compression by the vertebral canal; thus, obstruction to IVC results in rerouting of venous return by way of epidural veins, and thence to the azygos vein above the level of obstruction. Some common sites of IVC obstruction are shown: *(1)* below the liver (*e.g.*, severe ascites); *(2)* thoracolumbar junction (*e.g.*, abdominal pressure) in prone position; *(3)* pelvic brim (*e.g.*, pregnancy). (Modified from Bromage, P.R.: Epidural Analgesia. Philadelphia, W.B. Saunders, 1978.)

Epidural Veins. The large valveless epidural veins are part of the internal vertebral venous plexus,[17,18] which drains the neural tissue of spinal cord, the CSF, and the bony spinal canal. The major portion of this plexus lies in the anterolateral part of the epidural space,[44] out of reach of a correctly placed epidural needle (see Figs. 8-5, 8-6). The plexus has rich segmental connections at all levels within intervertebral foramina and epidural space, and within the body of the vertebrae (the basivertebral veins). Superiorly, the plexus communicates with the occipital, sigmoid, and basilar venous sinuses within the cranium. Inferiorly, anastomoses by way of the sacral venous plexus link the vertebral plexus to uterine and iliac veins. By way of the intervertebral foramina at each level, the vertebral plexus communicates with thoracic and abdominal veins,[533] so that pressure changes in these cavities are transmitted to the epidural veins but not to the supporting bony elements of the neural arch and the vertebral bodies. Thus, marked increases in intra-abdominal pressure may compress the inferior vena cava while distending the epidural veins and increasing flow up the vertebrobasilar plexus. This increased flow is accommodated mostly by means of the azygos vein, which ascends in the right chest over the root of the right lung into the superior vena cava (Fig. 8-13). However, it is also possible for a small dose of local anesthetic injected rapidly into an epidural vein to be channeled directly up the basivertebral system to a cerebral venous sinus; this is most likely to occur in a pregnant woman in the supine position when the inferior vena cava is obstructed, and intrathoracic pressure rises during active bearing down, so that the azygos flow is temporarily increased. Clearly, local anesthetic should not be injected into the epidural space under such conditions. More likely, distention of epidural veins, owing to direct inferior vena caval obstruction (*e.g.*, by the uterus) or owing to increased thoracicoabdominal pressure, will also diminish the effective volume of the epidural space, with the result that injected local anesthetics spread more widely up and down the epidural space. In addition, the potential absorptive area of venules and capillaries is increased, with increased drug reaching the heart by way of the azygos vein. The impressive size of the epidural veins on the lateral wall of the spinal canal (see Figs. 8-5, 8-6) can be confirmed by epidural phlebography during a Valsalva maneuver.[221,437] Three important aspects of safety emerge:

The epidural needle should pierce the ligamentum flavum in the midline to avoid the large laterally placed epidural veins.

Insertion of epidural needles or catheters or injection of local anesthetic should be avoided during episodes of marked increase in size of epidural veins, such as that which occurs with increased thoracicoabdominal pressure during straining.

The presence of vena caval obstruction calls for a reduction in dose, a decreased rate of injection, and increased care in aspirating for blood (see below) before epidural injection.

An intriguing feature of the epidural veins is of importance in draining CSF and in the transfer of local anesthetic to the CSF. In the region of the dural cuffs, bulbs of arachnoid mater protrude through the dura into the epidural space, where they often invaginate the walls of epidural veins that drain the spinal cord and nerve root area.[458,524] Although the primary function of these arachnoid granulations is to drain CSF[161] and remove debris from the CSF into the vascular system,[274] they also provide a favorable site for transfer of local anesthetic into the spinal fluid (see Fig. 8-2).

Spinal Arteries. The spinal cord receives its blood supply from arteries on the surface of the brain above or from arteries that enter the intervertebral foramina and then gain access to the spinal cord by way of the spinal nerve roots (see Figs. 7-10 and 7-11).

It is of significance to epidural block that the spinal branches of the subclavian, aortic, and iliac arteries cross the epidural space and enter the subarachnoid space in the region of the dural cuffs (see Fig. 8-2). The anterior spinal artery territory supplying the anterior horn or motor area of the spinal cord is most vulnerable[226] (see Fig. 8-10). Details of spinal arterial supply are given in Figure 7-11 and described in Chapter 7, pages 219–220.

Epidural Lymphatics. The dural cuff region is supplied with a rich lymphatic network that rapidly conveys debris from arachnoid villi out through intervertebral foramina to reach lymph channels in front of the vertebral bodies.[56,532] It is reassuring that foreign material can be carried away rapidly by an efficient system that runs in a direction away from spinal fluid and the spinal cord.

Dural sac, containing dura, arachnoid, spinal fluid, pia, spinal nerves, and spinal cord, is, strictly speaking, contained within the annular epidural space. A detailed description of the meninges and CSF is given in Chapter 7. For the purposes of this chapter, it is important to examine some aspects of the anatomy of the dura, arachnoid, and spinal nerves in the region adjacent to the intervertebral foramina, the so-called dural cuff region.

The dura can be considered as a protective tube that is pierced by and gives a short "cuff" to each pair of spinal nerves; at this point, the dura becomes markedly thinner and is closely adherent to the dorsal surfaces of the dorsal root ganglia as far as the point where anterior and posterior roots fuse to form the spinal nerve. Within these dural cuffs, there is a small blind pocket of CSF, which is separated from the epidural space only by the greatly thinned dura (see Fig. 8-2). Here, the dura is pierced by veins, arteries, and lymphatics, running to and from the underlying subarachnoid space. Also, the arachnoid membrane pushes small "granulations"[458] through the dura; these may either indent epidural veins or come into contact with epidural lymphatics, to facilitate drainage of CSF and elimination of foreign material.[56,532] This region also provides a ready route for passage of local anesthetics into the spinal fluid. Although the dura and arachnoid are usually in close apposition, they are easily separated, and it is possible to inadvertently insert an epidural catheter into the subdural space[45,483] (see Fig. 7-6).

Arachnoid Membrane. It is now known that the arachnoid membrane is metabolically active[513] and is capable of forming giant vacuoles, which may temporarily communicate with the subdural space or, in the dural cuff region, directly with the epidural space. This probably provides a system for rapid drainage of CSF and clearance of debris from the CSF.[491,492]

Spinal Nerves. Some advances in neuroanatomy have helped to explain the segmental onset of epidural blockade. Studies of the size of dorsal roots indicate a considerable variation in size, with large roots at C8 and S1 and a "valley" between these two peak sizes in the thoracic region.[217,280] Studies of the number of myelinated and nonmyelinated fibers in ventral roots also reveal a peak at S1 and in the lower cervical region at C5–8.[118] This is in keeping with the relative resistance of the lower cervical region and S1 to neural blockade. Anatomic studies suggested that the pia of the spinal cord and spinal nerve roots is continuous with the perineurium of the spinal nerves. Because the epineurium of spinal nerves is continuous with the dura, this raises the possibility of continuity between the subarachnoid space and a subepineurial space.[459] This would explain reports of transverse myelitis after injection of neurolytic agents directly beneath spinal nerve epineurium.[364] All that is required for rapid spread of injected solution from spinal nerve to CSF is accurate needle placement beneath the spinal nerve epineurium (see Fig. 8-2).

Spinal Cord. It is known that local anesthetics, injected into the epidural space, can subsequently be detected in spinal nerve roots and the peripheral areas of the spinal cord[82] in concentrations sufficient to block nerve conduction.[209] The peripheral part of the spinal cord in the dorsolateral funiculus contains descending excitatory sympathetic fibers, the descending pyramidal tracts, and medullary reticulospinal fibers. The pyramidal tract synapses in Rexed's laminae IV, V, and VI, which are involved in the modulation of sensory input (see Chap. 24). It has been hypothesized that local anesthetics with a high propensity to penetrate the spinal cord may produce a rapid and long-lasting sympathetic blockade, followed closely by motor blockade owing to the superficial placement of the appropriate tracts. At the same time, the modulating influences on lamina V and VI may be blocked, with a resultant expansion of segmental receptive fields[517] and a relative "antianalgesic" state.[511] This anatomic basis may emerge as an explanation for the "sensory motor dissociation" exhibited by drugs such as bupivacaine and etidocaine (see below). Currently no data support differential penetration of the spinal cord for the various local anesthetics (see also Chap. 3). Recent support for rapid transport of drugs from epidural space to spinal fluid and spinal cord as provided by studies of epidural narcotics (see Chap. 28).[142]

Epidural Pressures

In the **lumbar region,** the major cause of generation of a negative pressure lies in "coning" of the dura by the advancing needle point. Since Janzen's original observation of negative pressure in the lumbar epidural space, a number of studies have substantially agreed with his conclusions regarding the etiology of this negative pressure.[42,62,89,180,255,507,508]

The negative pressure increases as the needle advances across the epidural space toward the dura.

Blunt needles with side openings produce the greatest negative pressure: they produce a good "coning" effect on the dura without puncturing it and transmit the negative pressure well because of their side opening.

Slow introduction of the needle produces the greatest negative pressure. Even if the needle is halted and the pressure equalized, further advances of the needle will continue to produce a negative pressure until the dura is eventually punctured.

Greater negative pressure can be obtained if the dura is not distended (*e.g.,* by gravity in the sitting position or by high abdominal or thoracic pressure).

Eaton[180] provided key data when he showed that tenting the dura with a blunt stylet in the interspace above an epidural needle caused negative pressures of up to -14 cm H_2O, which were recorded by means of the epidural needle. The pressure could be returned to zero by withdrawing the stylet from the dura, and then the same level of negative pressure could be obtained by advancing the stylet again. Despite the convincing nature of these data, Bryce-Smith[89] was able to record an increase in negative pressure in the epidural space during deep inspiration with no associated change in CSF pressure. In all four patients studied, the epidural pressure was zero at rest and varied from -2 to -8 cm H_2O with deep inspiration. It is noted that the contribution of negativity from deep inspiration was small compared with the potential effect of tenting the dura. Of further interest, it was shown that coughing caused a small positive swing in epidural pressure. Thus, although under resting conditions any negativity in the lumbar epidural space is produced by tenting of the dura, it appears that large changes of intrathoracic pressure are transmitted to the lumbar epidural space. Care was taken in the studies of Bryce-Smith[89] and in many hundreds of measurements by Usubiaga and colleagues,[507,508] to ensure that pressure was measured as soon as the needle entered the epidural space. These results then should apply to a carefully performed epidural block, in which the needle is immediately halted when it enters the epidural space. Bromage[47] measured pressure immediately on entering the lumbar epidural space with the patient sitting and during expiration. His results agreed with those of Usubiaga.[507,508] There was still a recordable negative pressure in 10 of 16 cases, pointing to a tenting effect on the dura in 60% of cases, even with careful entry into the epidural space. Our view is that the absence of initial negative pressure in Bryce-Smith's studies, and in at least 12% of Usubiaga's patients in the lying position, means that negative pressure is an unreliable sign of *initial entry* into the lumbar epidural space. Further advancement of the needle in the epidural space may be able to demonstrate negativity where it is initially absent, as reported in the studies of Janzen[283] and Eaton.[180] This appears to conflict with the optimal clinical technique of halting the epidural needle as soon as it enters the epidural space. Techniques of lumbar epidural puncture that are based on "loss of resistance" tests through ligamentum flavum with air-filled or fluid-filled syringes offer a more reliable means of achieving this optimal technique in the lumbar area (see below). If the anesthesiologist finds it easier to use the two-handed grip in the "hanging-drop" negative pressure test, then it is important to ensure that pressure in the lumbar epidural space is as low as possible by arranging for the patient to be in the lateral position, with a slight head-down tilt, to lower intra-abdominal pressure as the diaphragm moves upward.[42]

In the **thoracic region** the major determinant of negative pressure is the transmission of negative respiratory pressures from the thorax by way of the paravertebral space and intervertebral foramina to the epidural space. The direct communication between adjacent and contralateral paravertebral spaces by way of the epidural space was strikingly demonstrated by injecting dye from one paravertebral space and showing its distribution by way of the epidural space to other paravertebral spaces on the same and opposite sides.[337] Because the mean intrapleural pressure is -7 cm H_2O (-5 to -10 cm H_2O), it is not surprising that Usubiaga and others found thoracic epidural pressures of -1 to -9 cm H_2O at the point of needle entry into the epidural space.[507,508] In contrast to the lumbar region, they found negative pressure in the thoracic epidural space in 100% of patients, regardless of whether the patients were sitting or lying; there was a slight increase in negative pressure on moving from a lying to a sitting position. The same results were obtained in the cervical region, except that a larger increase in negative pressure was obtained in the sitting position. Because the needle is inserted obliquely in the midthoracic region, it is less likely that the dura will be tented, and negative pressure effects are predominantly caused by transmitted intrathoracic negative pressure. The reliability of a negative pressure sign in the thoracic region implies that the "hanging-drop" test is appropriate for cervicothoracic punctures in cases in which a true negative intrapleural pressure can be assured.[77] The narrowness of the epidural space in this region and the excellent control afforded by the two-handed grip of the winged "hanging-drop" needle give strong support to this recommendation (however, see also pp. 324–325).

If one routinely uses a *negative pressure test* for epidural puncture, it is important to be aware of factors that result in marked changes in epidural pressure.

In severe lung diseases such as emphysema, epidural negative pressure may be abolished, particularly if the patient is lying down.[206,403]

Any factor that increases abdominal pressure and/or occlusion of the inferior vena cava may distend the epidural veins (see earlier) and increase pressure in the lumbar epidural space. This results in only slight changes in the thoracic epidural space, particularly if the patient is sitting.[507]

During labor, baseline lumbar epidural pressures are higher in women in the supine position compared with those in the lateral position. As labor progresses, baseline pressures increase to as high as $+10$ cm H_2O at full dilatation.[216] Also, there are peaks of epidural pressure during each uterine contraction, with increases of 8 to 15 cm H_2O.[67]

Coughing or a Valsalva maneuver increases both intrathoracic and intra-abdominal pressure, so that pressure in thoracic and lumbar epidural space increases,[507,508] resulting in high positive pressures being recorded throughout the epidural space.

Changes in pressure in the epidural space also have implications for the ease of injection into the epidural space and the spread of local anesthetic solutions. Studies by Usubiaga[507,508] have helped to explain why successful entry into the epidural space is sometimes followed by "drip back" when local anesthetic is subsequently injected; classic pressure-volume compliance studies showed that compliance decreased with increasing age and that residual pressure after injection of 10 ml of solution at a standard rate had a positive correlation with age. Thus, some patients with a low compliance in the epidural space will be unable to accommodate a large volume of solution if it is injected rapidly; "drip back" will be less common in young patients and if injection is made slowly because, although there was a transient increase in epidural pressure in young patients, Usubiaga found that pressure was essentially back to baseline in 30 seconds.

As expected from the data, Usubiaga found that spread of analgesia was positively correlated with residual epidural pressure and, in turn, with age. These studies tend to support radiologic studies, in which "peridurograms" with water-soluble contrast media showed a reduced longitudinal spread of injected solutions in young patients purportedly because of widely patent intervertebral foramina.[78,458,466] In contrast, in old patients with relatively obstructed foramina, longitudinal spread was increased. More recent radiologic studies have shown minimal leakage of contrast media through intervertebral foraminae in young patients. Thus, soft tissue (fat) in the epidural space seems most important in the spread of epidural solutions.

PHYSIOLOGIC EFFECTS OF EPIDURAL BLOCKADE

With currently available local anesthetic agents, spinal epidural neural blockade implies sympathetic blockade accompanied by somatic blockade, which may involve sensory and motor blockade alone or in combination. Although it is possible to avoid blockade of "peripheral" lumbar sympathetic fibers if only sacral segments are blocked by a caudal approach to the epidural space, spinal epidural blockade almost invariably results in some degree of sympathetic blockade (Fig. 8-14A). Some of the most important (but not all) of the physiologic effects of epidural blockade can be discussed in relation to either sympa-

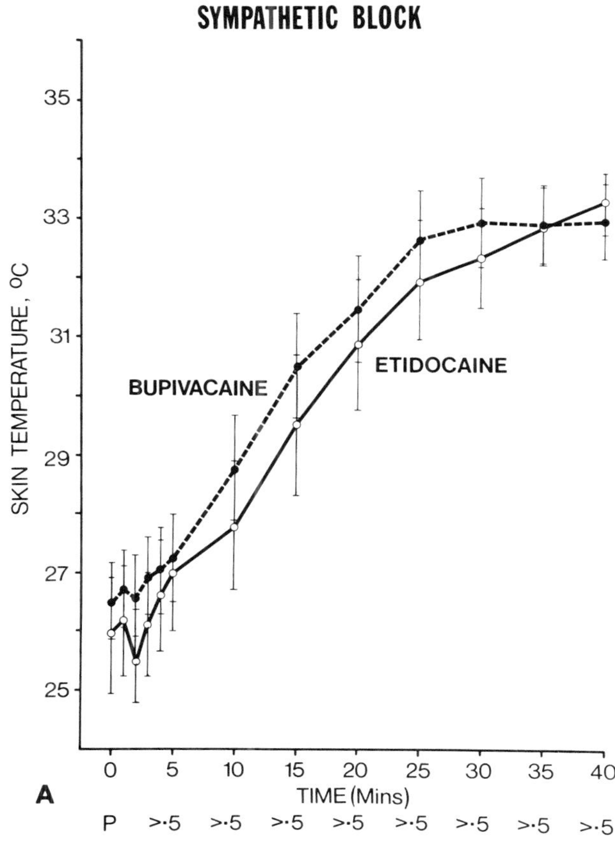

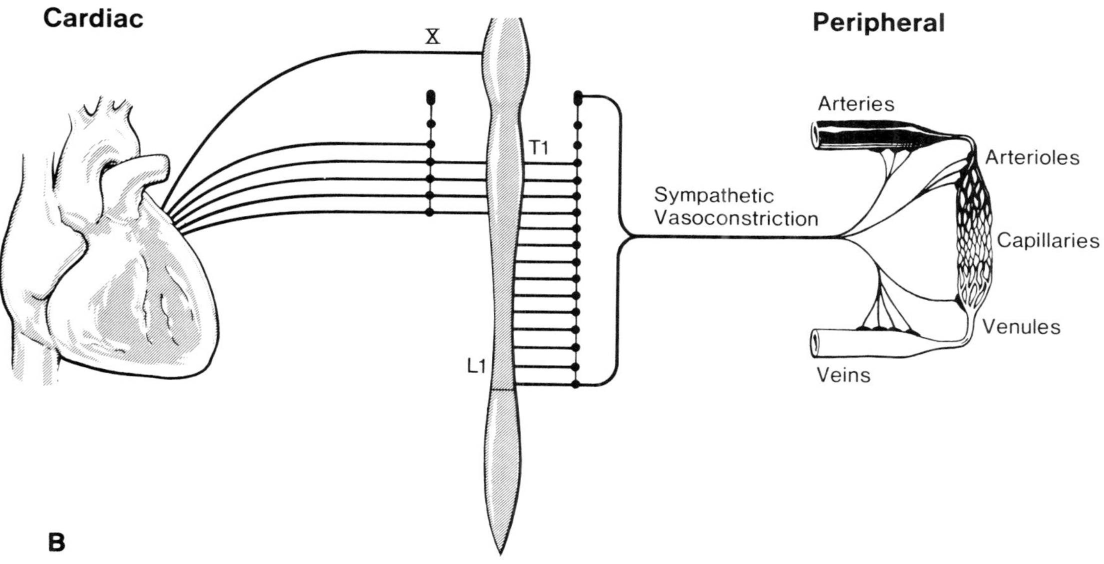

FIG. 8-14. **A.** Sympathetic blockade. Onset profile of "peripheral" sympathetic blockade is indicated by skin temperature measurements in the lower limbs. **B.** Sympathetic blockade: "central" (cardiac) and "peripheral" components. These consist of T1–4 cardiac sympathetic fibers and T1–L2 "peripheral" sympathetic fibers. Note important innervation of veins and venules. Vagal cardiac fibers are also shown. (Part A from Cousins, M.J., *et al.*: Anaesth. Intens. Care, *21*:108, 1978.)

thetic blockade only of vasoconstrictor fibers (below T4) and/or of cardiac sympathetic fibers (T1–4; Fig. 8-14B). Many clinicians prefer to have a wide margin of safety if they are intent on avoiding major sympathetic blockade. Thus, they aim to restrict the level of analgesia to T10. Studies discussed in Chapter 13, however, indicate that the level of sympathetic block with epidural anesthesia may be lower than the level of sensory block and more incomplete in terms of the quality of block.[22] This concept of sympathetic blockade is still a practical approach in considering the physiologic effects of epidural blockade because inguinal, perineal, urological, and lower limb surgical procedures can be carried out with blockade to T10 or lower, which at most will produce only a "peripheral" sympathetic blockade. However, lower abdominal surgery (such as appendectomy, gynecologic surgery, and cesarean section) necessitates blockade to T4. Thus, the most frequent use of epidural block will be to either T4 or T10 level. Occasionally, a T1 level is needed for chest injury or thoracotomy. We will consider the cardiovascular effects of epidural block with respect to the degree of sympathetic block (and its effects) with sensory blockade to T1, T4, or T10.

Subtler and somewhat more indirect is the reduced input to the central nervous system (CNS), which accompanies various levels of sensory blockade. This "deafferentation" has long been thought capable of exerting a "protective" effect that reduces the efferent neurohumoral response to surgical stimulation or trauma. Objective data have now become available to support this hypothesis (see Chap. 5).

Finally, it is important to remember that extensive epidural blockade often requires large doses of local anesthetic (with or without epinephrine). Large doses themselves may cause physiologic changes as a result of the direct pharmacologic effects of circulating blood concentrations. These are an inevitable outcome of vascular absorption from the epidural space. Because of the unique epidural venous system (see earlier), direct intravascular injection may result in the rapid attainment of high concentrations of local anesthetic in the brain and/or heart with the potential for convulsions and/or sudden depression of cardiac output (see Chaps. 2–4). Also, important changes in vagal tone accompany sympathetic block (see Fig. 8-21). The various mechanisms for physiologic effects of epidural block are summarized in Table 8-7.

TABLE 8-7. MECHANISMS FOR PHYSIOLOGIC EFFECTS OF EPIDURAL ANALGESIA

By Way of Vascular Absorption of Local Anesthetic (LA) or Epinephrine (EPI)	By Way of Direct Neural Blocking Effects or Indirect Results of Blockade
Receptor	Spinal nerves (roots and trunks) by axonal blockade
β-stimulation by EPI	*Sympathetic*
α-stimulation by EPI	Efferent blockade
or phenylephrine	Peripheral (T1–L2) vasoconstrictor
Smooth muscle	"Adrenal" (T6–L1)
Blood vessels, LA or EPI	"Central" (T1–4) cardiac sympathetic
Heart, LA or EPI	*Sensory*
Other organs, LA or EPI	Afferent blockade
Cardiac muscle	Reduced peripheral sensation
By LA or EPI	Blockade of visceral pain fibers
Neural tissue	Reduced efferent neurohumoral response to surgical or other
CNS, by LA	stimulus within the blocked area
Conducting system of	*Motor*
heart, by LA	Efferent blockade
Miscellaneous	Varying degrees of motor paralysis
Neuromuscular	Reflex muscle relaxation without paralysis (Deafferentation)
junction by LA	Spinal cord
	Axons
	Superficial, sensory tracts blocked (*e.g.*, bupivacaine, lidocaine, and etidocaine)
	Deep motor paths blocked (*e.g.*, etidocaine)
	Dorsal horn modulation of pain transmission (? axons, ?cells)
	Possibility of "antianalgesic" effect owing to block of inhibitory paths
	Cell Bodies: "selective" blockade, by opioids (see Chap. 28)
	Secondary changes in parasympathetic activity
	Sympathetic block to T5 + ↓ venous return may → ↑↑ vagus
	Sympathetic block to T1 → unopposed vagus (see Fig. 8-21)

CARDIOVASCULAR EFFECTS OF EPIDURAL BLOCKADE

In order to understand the cardiovascular effects of epidural blockade, a sound knowledge of the autonomic control of circulation is required (see Chap. 13).[323,347] Although it has been claimed that epidural block results in a lesser degree of sympathetic block and much greater cardiovascular stability than subarachnoid block,[162,172] there are no controlled data to support this. In general, cardiovascular depression may occur with both epidural and subarachnoid blockade (Fig. 8-15) and is at least partly related to the level of sympathetic blockade (see Figs. 8-14, 8-16; see also Chap. 7).[38,40,302,303] While the potential for cardiovascular changes owing to sympathetic block is present for epidural and subarachnoid blockade,* vascular absorption of local anesthetic and vasoconstrictor may result in significant hemodynamic changes after epidural but not after subarachnoid blockade; the reason for this lies predominantly in the much larger doses of drugs used in epidural blockade and in the proximity of the large epidural veins, which, owing to their anatomy, have considerable potential for rapid transport of drug to heart (Table 8-8) and CNS. The more gradual onset of sympathetic blockade after epidural analgesia (Fig. 8-14A) compared with subarachnoid block may provide a mechanism for initial responses that are less severe for epidural block.[463] When used for epidural block, lidocaine, chlorprocaine, and etidocaine have a rapid onset of sympathetic block (especially etidocaine). This is even more evident if epinephrine-containing solutions are used. In comparison, onset of sympathetic block is slower with bupivacaine and there is a lesser tendency for rapid development of hypotension; indeed, sympathetic block may take 25 to 30 minutes to develop and even then may be only a "partial" block (see Chap. 13). Animal studies have shown that autoregulation at the level of the precapillary sphincters develops within 30 minutes of complete ablation of neural activity.[233]

Although controlled studies are not available, experience with large series of thoracic epidural blocks administered in intensive care units by continuous catheter techniques further supports the allowance of adequate time for autoregulation. A common management protocol for "topping up" thoracic epidural blockade for chest trauma involves keeping the patient supine during and for 20 to 30 minutes after "top-up." Using this procedure, serious hypotension is uncommon, whereas topping up in the semirecumbent position or allowing inadequate time in the supine position after blockade may result in large reductions in blood pressure (see Chap. 26).

*Level of sympathetic block is the same as (or lower than) sensory with epidural blockade. In comparison, sympathetic block is two to three segments higher than sensory level with subarachnoid block.

Blockade Below T4

Epidural blockade that is restricted to the level of the low thoracic and lumbar region (T5 – L4) results in a "peripheral" sympathetic blockade with vascular dilatation in the pelvis and lower limbs; if all splanchnic fibers are blocked (T6 – L1), then pooling of blood in the gut and abdominal viscera also may occur. This "peripheral" blockade has been demonstrated by measurements of large increases in lower limb blood flow owing to arteriolar vasodilation[38,145,470] and "pooling" of blood in the venous capacitance vessels.[463] Because the latter contain 80% of blood volume, venodilatation has a potential for dramatic changes in venous return, reduction in right atrial pressure, and reduced cardiac output. The decrease in venous return has been shown to result in increased cardiac vagal tone. This explains why heart rate remains unchanged or decreased despite hypotension and activation of cardiac sympathetic accelerator fibers.[15] In healthy unmedicated subjects, there is a potential for at least an eightfold increase in skin blood flow in the lower limbs[351] and the possibility of pooling up to 1 L of blood in the venous capacitance vessels. The magnitude of this change can be appreciated by observing the increase of great toe skin temperature of more than 8°C that often accompanies onset of lumbar epidural sympathetic blockade (see Fig. 8-14A). A precise quantitative measurement of increased venous capacitance requires venous occlusion plethysmography of the calf.

Distribution of blood to the splanchnic area was studied by Arndt and co-workers in healthy young volunteers after injection of 20 ml of plain 2% lidocaine in the lumbar region.[11] Sympathetic block was not assessed independently; however, it is unlikely that it spread much higher than the lower thoracic segments[22] (see Chap. 13). In all eight subjects except two, splanchnic blood volume decreased as assessed by distribution of radioactively labeled red cells. Radioactivity also decreased in thorax and upper limbs, indicating compensatory vasoconstriction.[11] It is possible that the two subjects with increased splanchnic region blood volume did achieve blockade of the T6 – L1 splanchnic sympathetic fibers.

Compensatory Mechanisms. *Peripheral Sympathetic Activity.* Even without intravenous "rehydra-

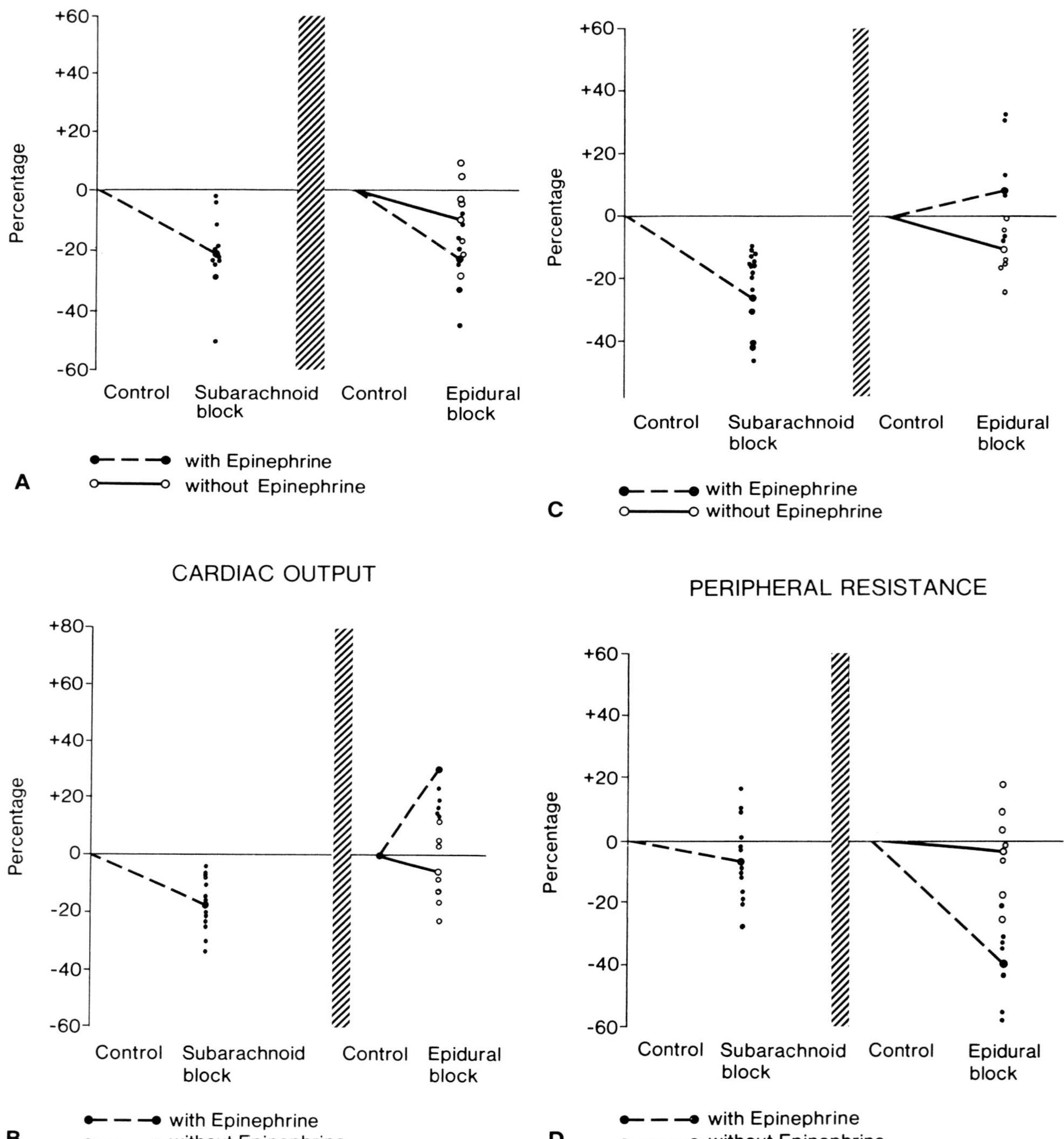

FIG. 8-15. Cardiovascular effects of epidural block to T5 level, with and without epinephrine. **A.** Mean arterial pressure. **B.** Cardiac output. **C.** Stroke volume. **D.** Peripheral resistance. Percentage changes for each variable are shown after epidural block, with a comparison given for a similar level of subarachnoid block. (Ward, R.J., *et al.:* Epidural and subarachnoid anesthesia. Cardiovascular and respiratory effects. J.A.M.A., *25*:275, 1965. Copyright © 1965, American Medical Association.)

TABLE 8-8. CARDIOVASCULAR EFFECTS OF EPIDURAL BLOCKADE

Mechanism	Effect
Neural Effects	
"Peripheral" sympathetic block (T10–L2)	
Blockade of vasoconstrictor fibers to lower limbs	Arteriolar dilatation. Increased venous capacitance and pooling of blood in lower limbs → decreased venous return → ↓ CO
Reflex increase in vasoconstrictor fiber activity in upper limbs via baroreceptors	Increased vasomotor tone in upper limbs → ↑ venous return → ↑ CO
Reflex increase in cardioaccelerator nerve activity	↑ HR ↑ CO
Reduced right atrial pressure, due to ↓ venous return*	? ↓ HR (Note ↓↓ RA pressure → ↓↓ HR*; see Fig. 8-21)
Adrenal medullary sympathetic block (T6–L1)	
(Blockade of splanchnic nerves)	
Vasoconstrictor fibers to abdominal viscera	Pooling of blood in gut → decreased venous return
Adrenal medullary catecholamine secretion	Decreased levels of circulating catecholamines → ↓ HR ↓ CO
"Central" sympathetic block (T1–4)	
Blockade of	
Cardiac sympathetic outflow from vasomotor center	↓ HR ↓ CO
Cardiac sympathetic reflexes at segmental level	
Vasoconstrictor fibers to head, neck, and arms	Vasodilatation in upper limbs. Blockade of compensatory lower limb vasoconstriction if T5–L1 is also blocked
Vagal predominance	"Inappropriate bradycardia"; "sudden bradycardia"; vagal arrest (see Fig. 8-21 and Table 8-11)
Effects of Drug Absorption	
Absorbed local anesthetic	Usually no measurable effects on HR, CO, MAP, or TPR even in patients with vascular disease
Moderate blood levels	
Antiarrhythmic	Lidocaine may → ↑ CO, which is balanced ↓ TPR, so that MAP is unchanged
Maintenance of normal CO	
Minimal reduction in vascular tone	
High blood levels *(toxic)*	↓ CO ↓ HR
Decreased contractility	↓ MAP
If convulsions occur hypoxia results in further reduction in CO	
Cardiac conducting tissue,? unidirectional blockade	Bupivacaine (very high levels) may → VT, VF, and cardiac arrest
Vascular dilatation	↓ TPR
Absorbed epinephrine	↑ CO ↑ HR ↓ TPR
β-stimulation	MAP may be unchanged or slightly reduced Antagonism of reflex vasoconstriction above level of blockade because of β-effects on muscle vasculature (→ ↓ TPR)

CO = Cardiac output, HR = heart rate, MAP = mean arterial pressure, TPR = total peripheral resistance, VT = ventricular tachycardia, VF = ventricular fibrillation.

*Decreased venous return was associated with increased vagal activity in one study. This may offset any increases in sympathetic activity.[15]

tion," healthy subjects in the supine position compensate for a decrease in mean arterial pressure with a reflex increase in efferent sympathetic vasoconstriction above the level of the block. Thus, blood flow and venous capacitance are reduced in the head, neck, and upper limbs.[38,463,470] This increased efferent sympathetic activity is mediated predominantly (by means of the baroreceptors) by those sympathetic vasoconstrictor nerves (T1–5) that remain unblocked and by circulating catechloamines released from the adrenal medulla owing to increased activity in any unblocked fibers in the splanchnic nerves (T6–L1). Although blood vessels in some viscera, such as the kidney, appear to be more responsive to direct neural stimuli,[2] in other vascular beds both neural and hormonal influences have major effects, although at different levels of the vasculature. Major arterioles respond mostly to neural stimuli, while small arterioles and venules near the capillary bed respond predominantly to circulating catecholamines. Thus, while any splanchnic fibers remain unblocked, there is a potential for vasoconstrictor activity below (as well as above) the level of blockade, by release of catecholamines from the adrenal medulla. Finally, the ability of precapillary sphincters to achieve autoregulation within a short time of cessation of neural activity[233] provides a further mechanism for regaining vascular tone and minimizing vascular pooling below the level of blockade.

Increased activity in cardiac sympathetic fibers (T1–4) may result in increased cardiac contractility and increased heart rate; similar effects are produced by increased levels of circulating catecholamines. Evidence that the latter are important in maintaining homeostasis in some clinical situations is provided by the surprisingly small changes in heart rate and cardiac output (−16%) with blockade of C5–T4, but with splanchnic fibers to the adrenal medulla (T6–L1) intact (Fig. 8-16).[391] Although quite large compensatory cardiac effects may be observed in unmedicated volunteers (*e.g.*, a 20% increase in heart rate and cardiac output[38]), these changes are not seen in premedicated patients (Table 8-9).[225] In premedicated patients, despite decreased peripheral resistance, an unchanged heart rate, and cardiac output, mean arterial pressure was reduced by only 10%, since changes in total vascular resistances were held to only a 25% reduction by increased sympathetic activity in unblocked areas (see Fig. 8-20).

The studies by Germann and colleagues[225] and Sjögren and Wright[470] report changes that are close to those that the anesthesiologist may anticipate in clinical practice, although patients in the latter study were not rehydrated. The practice of preblock "rehydration" with intravenous balanced salt solution is capable of maintaining mean arterial blood pressure close to preblock levels in healthy patients, including parturients, provided the level of blockade is below T4 and inferior vena caval obstruction is avoided.[38,530]

Is there any reason to believe that blockade to T10 is any safer than extending up to T5? Data available from studies in healthy volunteers[38] and healthy patients[225,470] indicate that, even with block to T5, changes are minimal, provided bradycardia is avoided. There are, however, several inescapable differences if blockade is extended right up to T5: [1] A larger number of vasoconstrictor fibers are blocked; [2] the level of blockade is close to the cardiac sympathetics, so that any "overshoot" with initial or "top up" doses will produce changes similar to those shown for blockade to T1 in Figure 8-16; and [3] the splanchnic nerves T6–L1 may be blocked—thus varying degrees of blockade of visceral pain are provided, but also blockade of adrenal medullary activity and splanchnic vasoconstrictor fibers may be produced.

The combination of [1] and [3] may become important if a patient's state of hydration has been wrongly assessed, if blood volume is reduced,[39] owing to occult blood loss or disease states, or if compensatory mechanisms are for any other reason impaired. It is to be expected that the cardiovascular effects of other sedative and narcotic drugs will be additive. Such effects are mild if anesthesia is light and patients are healthy (see Fig. 8-20); however, the additional cardiovascular depression can be clearly documented even in healthy patients[225,482] and may be much greater in ill patients (Table 8-9). It seems wise, then, to be most cautious about the level of blockade and the dose of sedative/narcotic in patients with any compromise of compensatory mechanisms.

Although the benefits of retaining activity in vasoconstrictor fibers are fairly clear, what evidence is there that splanchnic neural activity may produce significant cardiovascular effects? The potential for circulating catecholamines to provide cardiovascular activity and overshoot hypertension is seen most dramatically in patients with pheochromocytoma (see Fig. 8-33). Although in routine surgery there is recent support for the modification of the stress response in suitable patients,[86] the removal of this emergency response in a patient whose compensatory mechanisms are impaired may be undesirable. Direct stimulation of the splanchnic nerve in cats results in a 20-fold increase in catecholamine secretion,[109] and in humans, catecholamine secretion is thought to increase by at least this amount during emergency situations.[112] Thus, although volunteers and healthy patients appear to be able to maintain cardiovascular stability after blockade to T5, which is similar to that seen with more limited blockade to T10, it should not be assumed that this can be extrapolated to patients with varying degrees of pathology.

The role of the splanchnic blood vessels in hypotension after epidural blockade has not been clearly defined. It is well known that blockade of the celiac plexus may produce marked pooling of blood in the splanchnic region, which receives 25% of cardiac output ("splanchnicectomy faint"), although this pooling is no greater than in the limbs; the potential for hypotension owing to both these mechanisms is markedly accentuated in patients with hypovolemia.

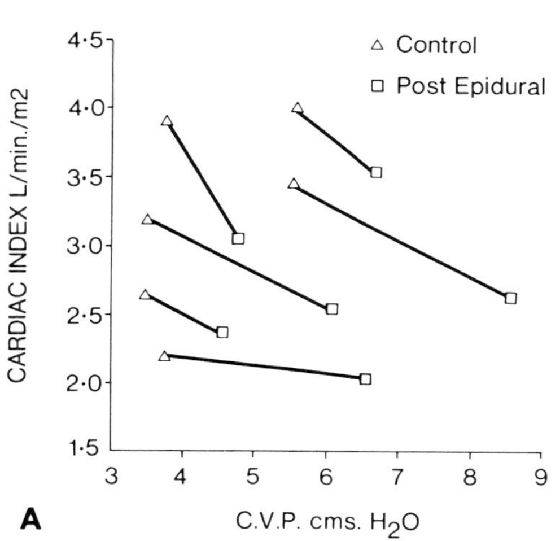

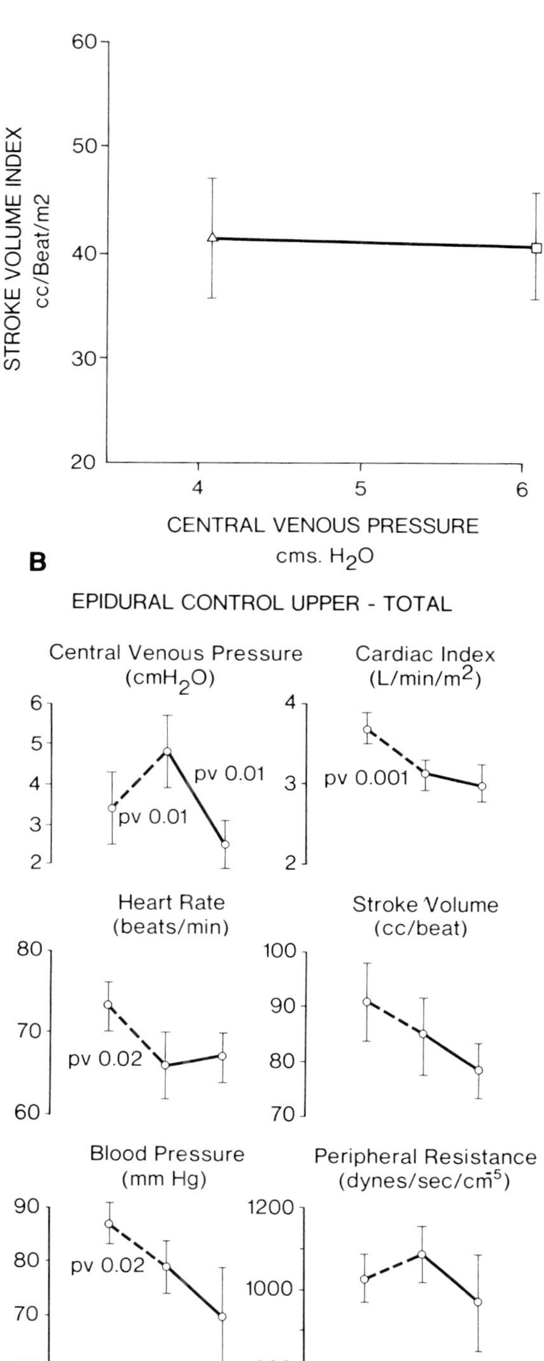

FIG. 8-16. Cardiovascular effects of epidural block. **A, B.** Blockade of T1–4 alone compared with control measurements (control). **C.** Blockade of T1–4 alone (upper) is compared with total blockade of T1–S5 (total) and control measurements (control). *Note:* Block of T1–4 alone results in reductions in blood pressure, heart rate, and cardiac index, accompanied by a rise in central venous pressure. Extension of block to T1–S5 results in a further fall in CVP and cardiac index. (Parts A and B from Otton, P.E., and Wilson, E.J.: The cardiocirculatory effects of upper thoracic epidural analgesia. Can. Anaesth. Soc. J., *13*:541, 1966; Part C from McLean, A.P.H., Mulligan, G.W., Otton, P., and MacLean, L.D.: Hemodynamic alterations associated with epidural anesthesia. Surgery, *62*:79, 1967.)

TABLE 8–9. CARDIOVASCULAR EFFECTS OF EPIDURAL BLOCKADE BY LEVEL OF BLOCKADE WITH PLAIN SOLUTIONS

		Change from Control Value (%)										
Extent of Block	Dose of Local Anesthetic	Venous Capacitance	Cardiac Output	HR	MAP	SV	CVP	TPR	dp/dt	Arm Flow	Leg Flow	Reference
	Lower abdominal block											
T10–S5	20–25 ml 1.5% lidocaine				−6*							167
T10–S5	10 ml 2% lidocaine		0	+5	0	0	0	0	−25	+300	+300	38
	Upper abdominal block											
T4/5–S5	20–25 ml 1.5% lidocaine				−21*							167
T4/7–S5	30 ml 1.5% lidocaine	+20	0	0	−16	0		0		0	+64	463
T5–S5	25–40 ml 2% lidocaine		−5	+7	−9		−10	−3				520
T3–S5	20–35 ml 2% lidocaine⁺		+21	+22	+5	+1	+13	−17	+23	−51	+287	38
T4–L4	15 ml 2% lidocaine		+7	+3	−1	+6	+6	−13		−35	+510	470
T7–S5	15–20 ml 1.5% lidocaine		0	0	−20	0		−24				225
	High thoracic block											
C5–T4	6–8 ml 1% mepivacaine		−17	−17	−8	0	+45	+8				391
C8–S5	30–40 ml 2% lidocaine⁺		+2	+6	−17	−3	+26	−21	−12	+91	+177	38
C5–S5	24–32 ml 1% mepivacaine		−19	−8	−20	−13	−27	−6				338
T2–12	8 ml 2% lidocaine		−1	−7	−12	+10	−3	−3		+47	+21	470
T3–	20–25 ml 1.5% lidocaine				−23*							167

*Systolic pressure
⁺Incremental doses

In a study of blood volume distribution after epidural block, two subjects with increases in splanchnic blood volume had substantial decreases in thoracic blood volume and arterial blood pressure. In one subject this was accompanied by a low heart rate and incipient faint reaction.[11] This is in keeping with the evidence of increased vagal tone in response to reduced venous return (see earlier).[15]

Blockade Above T4 (High Thoracic Block)

"Total Sympathetic Blockade" (T1 - L4). It has been thought that control of cardiac rate (chronotropy) and force of contraction (inotropy) resided in the vasomotor center and was mediated by means of the cardiovascular sympathetic fibers (T1 – 4). Although this is substantially true, it now appears that changes of cardiovascular sympathetic activity of approximately 20%[342] can be accomplished at a spinal cord level by reflex activity in the upper four or five thoracic segments, without vasomotor center control[26,127,473]; this can still be overridden by changes in parasympathetic activity.[323] Thus, epidural blockade of T1 – 5 segments has the following effects on cardiac sympathetic activity: blockade of segmental cardiac reflexes in segments T1 – 4; blockade of outflow from vasomotor center to cardiac sympathetic fibers (T1 – 4); vasoconstrictor nerve blockade in head, neck, and upper limbs.

If, as is often the case, blockade extends from T1 to L4, the following effects will be added to the above: splanchnic nerve blockade (T6 – L1) with resultant blockade of adrenal medullary secretion of catecholamines and blockade of splanchnic vasoconstrictor fibers; blockade of vasoconstrictor fibers in the lower part of the body, most important the capacitance vessels of the lower limbs (see Table 8-8).

The magnitude of cardiovascular changes has been documented in unmedicated volunteers[37,38] and in unmedicated patients[459,470] (Fig. 8-16). In general, the mean arterial blood pressure was reduced approximately 20%, with a similar reduction in total peripheral resistance. Although Bonica and colleagues found that cardiac output was increased slightly or unchanged, McLean and colleagues found a 15% to 20% reduction.[338] Bonica and colleagues found that central venous pressure was markedly raised (26%).[37,38] Because only the studies of McLean and Bonica achieved blockade above T1, their results are more indicative of the effects of complete cardiac sympathetic block. Most surprising was the minimal change in heart rate observed despite blockade of C5 – S5, that is, complete blockade of cardioaccelerator fibers and adrenal medullary catecholamine secretion. Because changes in cardiac rate are known to be controlled chiefly by the balance of sympathetic and parasympathetic tone at any moment, it must be assumed that parasympathetic tone was reduced to almost the same degree as sympathetic tone to maintain heart rate at a normal or near normal level (see Table 8-11). This small change in heart rate gives a deceptive picture of cardiac sympathetic activity, since Otton and Wilson have shown that blockade of T1 – 4 alone produced an increase in central venous pressure (CVP) without an increase in stroke volume output of the heart (Fig. 8-16).[391] That is, the heart did not empty as well as before blockade — a reduced response of the Frank – Starling mechanism. Because the other major determinant of stroke volume is catecholamine stimulation determining the level of Frank – Starling response, the patient with blockade extending from T1 to L2 potentially has both mechanisms obtunded. Thus, one may view the rise in CVP in Bonica's study[38] as a warning sign that the myocardium has exhausted its compensatory mechanisms. Although the associated changes in mean arterial pressure and cardiac output were surprisingly small in the studies of T1 blockade (see Table 8-9), the cardiovascular system has essentially no further mechanisms to respond if called on to do so. In this situation, the anesthesiologist has "assumed control of the circulation" and must be prepared to make rapid adjustments in body position, blood volume, vascular tone, cardiac rate, and cardiac contractile state; this may require administration of various combinations of crystalloids, colloids, atropine, ephedrine, catecholamines. Although such control can (see Table 8-21) and has been accomplished, it is by no means easy to mimic the subtle interbalance achieved by the vasomotor center.

Absorbed Local Anesthetics

Plain Solutions. Pharmacokinetic studies (see Chap. 3) have provided a precise picture of the blood concentration profile resulting from absorption of local anesthetics from the epidural space.[496] This formed the basis for determining systemic effects after intravenous infusion of local anesthetics to achieve blood concentrations similar to those occurring with epidural block. Early observations came from intravenous use of lidocaine in the treatment of cardiac arrhythmias.[250] At blood concentrations of lidocaine similar to those resulting from epidural blockade (3–5 μg/ml), Harrison reported excellent cardiovascular stability, even in patients with severe myocardial disease. Subsequent studies in healthy patients reported minimal changes in cardiovascular function with blood concentrations of lidocaine of 4 to 8 μg/ml.[288] Indeed, there was even some evidence of cardiovascular stimulation. The latter was postulated as the cause of surprising increases in cardiac output, cardiac rate, and mean arterial pressure associated with thoracic epidural block accomplished with large incremental doses of lidocaine (1500 mg). Because these changes were not reported by other studies of thoracic blockade, Bonica and colleagues postulated that the high blood concentrations of lidocaine (4–7 μg/ml) resulted in stimulatory effects on the circulation.[38] Such stimulation was thought to be caused by a central effect of lidocaine enhancing sympathetic activity by means of remaining cardiac sympathetic fibers. An alternative peripheral mechanism would have to invoke potentiation of peripheral sympathetic activity. Although local anesthetics can exert a biphasic effect on vascular smooth muscle (see Chap. 3), it seems unlikely that a peripheral mechanism is responsible for the changes observed by Bonica and colleagues.[38]

Studies of bupivacaine and etidocaine administered intravenously to volunteers failed to show significant cardiovascular changes when blood concentration profiles were carefully matched to those expected for epidural block.[350] However, rapid intravascular injection of lidocaine and bupivacaine may result in brief reductions in cardiac contractility (see Fig. 4-12A). Rapid intravascular injection of larger doses of bupivacaine may be followed by profound and long-lasting depression of myocardial contractility and depression of the cardiac conducting system, leading to cardiac arrest ("cardiac toxicity"; see Fig. 4-12C). Severe and persistent bradycardia may precede ventricular arrhythmias and then ventricular fibrillation. Attempts at resuscitation may result in a poor response of the myocardium to ionotropes and a slow cardiac rate. Vigorous resuscitation, including large doses of epinephrine, may be required[416] (see Chap. 4). In some cases, transvenous cardiac pacing may be necessary. The initial bradycardia may sometimes raise a problem in differentiating "cardiac toxicity" from high epidural block with vagal dominance.

Epinephrine-Containing Solutions. The preceding discussion has focused on studies using plain solutions of local anesthetic. Vascular absorption of added epinephrine does result in systemic actions on β-adrenergic receptors. It is now well established that the cardiovascular effects of low-dose epinephrine are quite different from its traditional picture of tachycardia, hypertension, and peripheral ischemia. Systemic effects of doses of epinephrine in the range of 80 to 130 μg, as used in epidural block, are a moderate increase in heart rate, increased cardiac output, decreased peripheral resistance, and decreased mean arterial pressure. Bonica and colleagues[37] attribute these effects solely to β-adrenergic stimulation. In order to investigate this hypothesis, they administered epinephrine epidurally without local anesthetic in doses similar to those usually incorporated in local anesthetic solutions (80–130 μg). The epinephrine *per se* produced changes similar to those seen with epinephrine-containing local anesthetics, except that the changes were of lesser magnitude and shorter lived. Also Bromage[77] has postulated that the epinephrine-containing solutions result in more profound sympathetic neural blockade, in a manner similar to the increase in intensity of motor blockade that results from epinephrine-containing solutions.[80] There is direct evidence that epidural and subarachnoid local anesthetic blockade may produce a variable degree of sympathetic blockade. Using the skin conductance response and laser Doppler flowmetry, sympathetic blockade was much lower in segmental level, and of briefer duration, than sensory block[22] (see Chap. 13). Indirect support is provided by Bonica's observation that two out of ten of his subjects failed to develop evidence of sympathetic blockade despite sensory analgesia to T1.[38] Also Cousins and Wright[145] observed that, in patients with postoperative pain, abolition of vasoconstrictor responses sometimes did not occur with 1% plain lidocaine but appeared more satisfactory with 2% plain lidocaine. They attributed this effect to more profound sensory blockade with better "deafferentation" of the operative site and prevention of adrenal medullary release of catecholamines; level of blockade was only from T7 to T10 in these studies (*i.e.*, incomplete denervation of adrenal medulla). However, it is entirely possible that the stronger solution produced more effective sympathetic nerve penetration over the same number of segments or over a more extensive area. The latter may be important, since there is ample evidence of large individual variations in extent of sympathetic innervation of upper and lower limbs.[202]

The most likely explanations for the more pronounced cardiovascular effects of epinephrine-containing local anesthetic solutions appear to be as follows:

1. Systemic absorption of epinephrine: β-adrenergic effects on the heart, resulting in increased heart rate and cardiac output; peripheral vascular β-adrenergic effects, resulting in further vasodilatation within the area of sympathetic block and antagonism of compensatory vasoconstrictor responses outside the area of blockade. Thus, total peripheral resistance falls and mean arterial blood pressure is reduced to a comparable degree to that seen with equivalent levels of subarachnoid blockade (Fig. 8-15).
2. More intense neural penetration or more extensive spread of neural blockade, resulting in more reliable sympathetic block.

Hypovolemia and Epidural Block

It has long been said that subarachnoid or epidural neural blockade may result in dangerously accentuated cardiovascular depression in the presence of uncorrected hypovolemia. However, this was largely anecdotal until the studies of Bonica and colleagues: Healthy volunteers received epidural block to T5 with and without epinephrine. Subjects were normovolemic or had undergone withdrawal of 13% of blood volume.[37-39] In comparison to the mild cardiovascular changes at normovolemia, major reductions in heart rate, cardiac output, and mean arterial pressure occurred in the presence of hypovolemia; in five out of seven patients who had received plain solutions of lidocaine, vigorous resuscitation, including ephedrine administration, was required. Cardiovascular homeostasis was better maintained with epinephrine-lidocaine blockade. However, marked reductions in mean arterial blood pressure still occurred (Fig. 8-17). Because cardiac sympathetic fibers were thought not to be blocked in these patients, an explanation was sought for the large reductions in heart rate and cardiac output. Morikawa and colleagues repeated the same studies of plain lidocaine in anesthetized dogs.[366] Although they recorded large reductions in mean arterial pressure and cardiac output, heart rate was not reduced and cardiovascular collapse did not occur in the presence of withdrawal of 13% of blood volume. It thus seemed likely that the sudden bradycardia resulting in cardiovascular collapse in human subjects may have been due to parasympathetic activity similar to that seen in the "faint" response to decreased venous return.[57] This sudden increase in parasympathetic activity is a vagal response to marked reductions in venous return[15] (Tables 8-10, 8-11; see Fig. 8-21). Usually this response occurs only in conscious humans (and in no other species) and is abolished by general anesthesia.[460] It is worth emphasizing that severe reductions in venous return, such as those observed in Bonica's study,[39] result in a sudden large increase in vagal activity[238,384-387] (see Fig. 8-21). Thus, a patient's condition may suddenly deteriorate to the point of loss of consciousness and perhaps asystole. This situation may be confused with "cardiac toxicity" if bupivacaine is the local anesthetic used. However, "cardiac toxicity" usually occurs soon after injection of the local anesthetic, whereas there is a time lag for the response described above.

What factors were responsible for the somewhat less pronounced cardiovascular depression in hypovolemic subjects receiving epidural block with lidocaine-epinephrine? It has already been noted that absorbed lidocaine-epinephrine results in increased heart rate and cardiac output, but a lower mean arterial pressure, owing to decreased peripheral resistance, compared with plain lidocaine; however, the higher cardiac rate may protect the heart from increases in vagal activity, although it has been noted that a high level of sympathetic activity may accentuate cholinergic effects in patients with poor venous return.[387] It is also possible that peak arterial blood concentrations of lidocaine were higher after plain lidocaine in patients with hypovolemia, owing to decreased cardiac output and, thus, a smaller volume of distribution (see Table 3-16). In this situation, the myocardium receives a larger percentage of cardiac output and, thus, is potentially exposed to higher concentrations of local anesthetics (see Fig. 4-19). Any coexistent hypercapnia or acidosis would tend to accentuate the depressant effects of local anesthetic on the myocardium (see Chap. 3). The moral of Bonica's study is clear[39]: Epidural block should be avoided or used with great care in patients with uncorrected hypovolemia or in any other patient in whom venous return is markedly impaired (*e.g.*, patients with large intra-abdominal masses in whom the pressure of the mass on the vena cava cannot be relieved before blockade; see Fig. 8-13).

Epidural Block in Patients with Pain

Cardiovascular effects of epidural block in such patients are not necessarily the same as in healthy volunteers or in patients before surgery.[43] Also, critical care units and "high dependency" units often use continuous infusion techniques—either *high concen-*

(*Text continues on p. 289*)

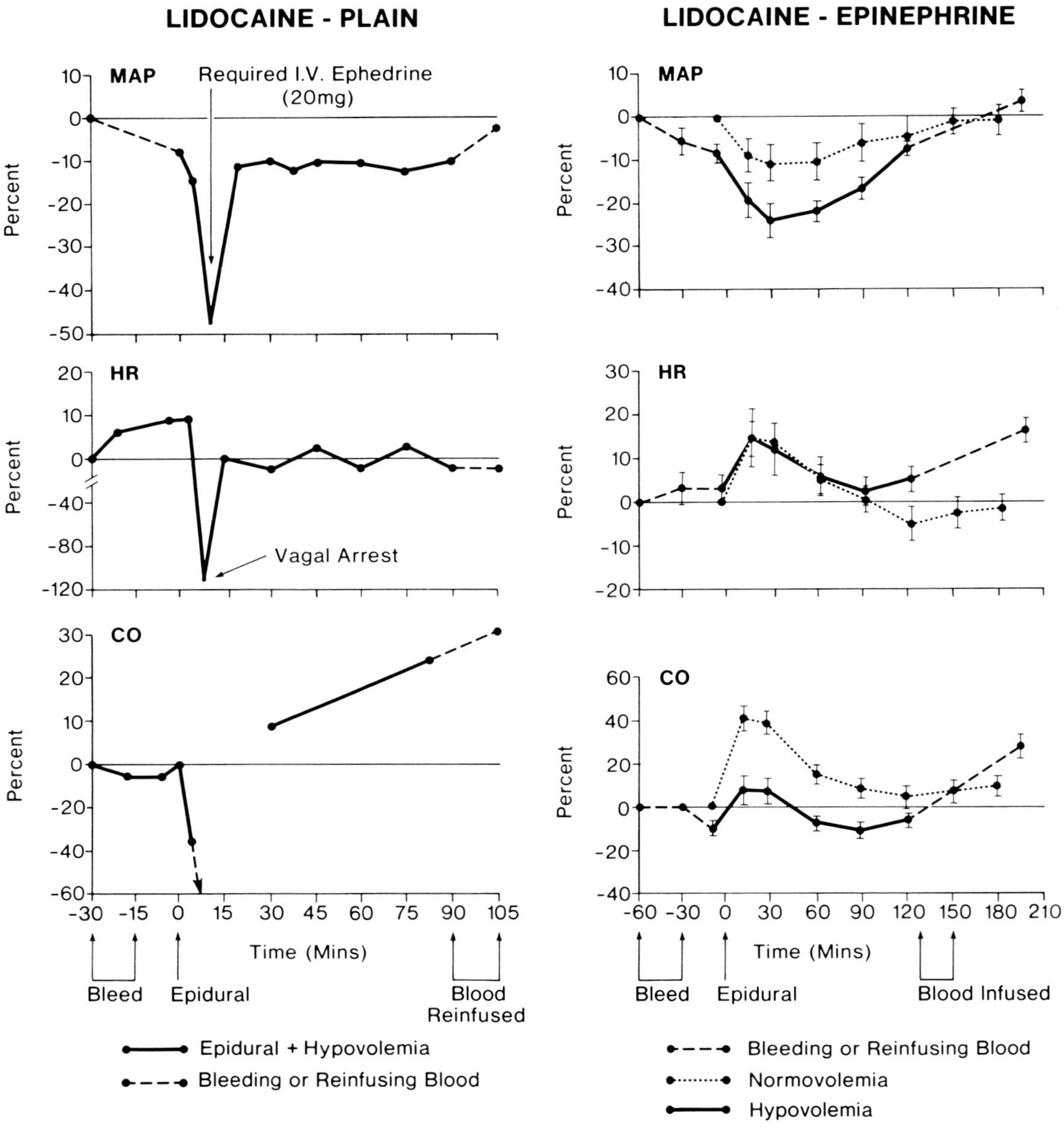

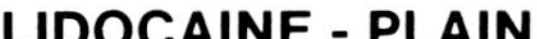

FIG. 8-17. Cardiovascular effects of epidural block, effect of hypovolemia in conscious volunteers; epidural block to T5 with plain and epinephrine-containing solutions. The mean percentage of change is shown for each variable. **Right.** Lidocaine–epinephrine. The cardiovascular changes after lidocaine–epinephrine in the presence of normovolemia are compared with hypovolemia (−13%). During normovolemia, note the marked increase in heart rate and cardiac output, lasting about 60 minutes. During hypovolemia, mean arterial pressure is significantly lower (−23%), but cardiac output remains close to control levels as a result of an elevated heart rate. **Left.** Lidocaine plain. A representation of a typical response is shown. Severe bradycardia is associated with extreme hypotension, and, in two subjects, vagal arrest occurred that required rapid resuscitation with ephedrine and oxygen. In only one subject was hypotension associated with increased heart rate, and this prevented the extreme hypotension seen in the other five subjects. (Modified from data of Bonica, J.J., Berges, P.U., and Morikawa, K.: Circulatory effects of epidural block: I. Effects of levels of analgesia and dose of lidocaine. Anesthesiology, *33*:1619, 1970; Bonica, J.J., Akamatsu, T.J., Berges, P.U., Morikawa, K., *et al.:* Circulatory effects of epidural block: II. Effects of epinephrine. Anesthesiology, *34*:514, 1971 and Bonica, J.J., et al.: Anesthesiology, *36*:219, 1972.)

TABLE 8-10. DANGER SIGNALS: CARDIOVASCULAR EFFECTS OF EPIDURAL BLOCK

Signal	Mechanisms and Potential Sequelae	Treatment
↑ HR ↓ BP in supine parturient with sensory level T11–L4 or ↓ HR ↓ BP—a more dangerous sign	Inferior vena caval occlusion + venodilatation in lower limbs → ↓ Venous return, ↓ CO, ↓ organ perfusion (incl. fetus) → Epidural vein engorgement → ↓ spinal cord perfusion → "spinal stroke" → ↑ Sympathetic → ↑ HR (baroreceptors) + vasoconstriction activity (above level of block) in upper limbs → ↓ RA pressure → ↓ HR (↑ vagal tone) (Note ↓↓ RV pressure may → ↓↓ HR; see Table 8-11 and Fig. 8-21)	Lateral position i.v. fluids, oxygen until MAP normal May require atropine and/or ephedrine if above measures fail
Gradual ↓ HR ↓ BP with level above T4	Venodilatation (as above) + ↓ cardiac sympathetic activity → ↓ CO ↓ HR ↓ MAP → ↓ Cardiac sympathetic activity initially accompanied by ↓ parasympathetic (see also Fig. 8-21). → However, ↓↓ venous return → ↑ vagal activity. Therefore, ↓↓ HR may occur before blockade of all T1–4	i.v. fluids. Elevate legs. Atropine. Oxygen until MAP normal. Vasopressor (ephedrine) if required.
"Sudden bradycardia" in either condition above	↓↓ Venous return may result in sudden ↑ parasympathetic tone ("faint response"); see Table 8-11; Fig. 8-21) ↓↓ HR → cardiac arrest	As above, but emphasis on sequence: elevate legs, oxygen, i.v. atropine, i.v. fluids–ephedrine rapidly if no response to above. May need epinephrine*
"Inappropriate" bradycardia (*i.e.*, "normal" HR in face of ↓ MAP with sensory level T3–4)	Peripheral vasodilatation should evoke an ↑ HR. But ↓ venous return → ↑ vagal tone, so HR remains at preblock rate but is "inappropriately" slow	i.v. atropine if MAP does not respond to fluids and elevation of legs, and relief of venous obstruction
Reduced blood volume or known obstruction of inferior vena cava	Hemorrhage Increased intra-abdominal pressure (see Fig. 8-13)	Restore blood volume; Relieve vena caval obstruction } Before epidural block
↓ HR with visceral traction in presence of blockade to T1	Total sympathetic block Unopposed vagus Changes in vagal tone → profound changes in HR; may → transient asystole (see Table 8-11 and Fig. 8-21)	i.v. atropine(?) Local infiltration to block vagal stimulus Ensure venous return adequate + arterial PO_2 adequate since ↑ HR (atropine) → ↑ myocardial oxygen demand

*Sudden bradycardia and hypotension may also result from **cardiac toxicity** of local anesthetics (see p. 284). This may require rapid resuscitative measures, including large doses of epinephrine.

TABLE 8-11. VAGAL AND SYMPATHETIC ACTIVITY: EFFECTS ON HEART RATE

	Venous Return "Sensors" in Great Veins, Atria, Ventricles	Arterial Pressure "Sensors" in Carotid Sinus and Aortic Arch
Afferent path	Vagus	Vagus, glossopharyngeal
Efferent path	Vagus	Sympathetic
Effect of increased venous return + ↑ BP	↑ Venous return ↘ ↓ Vagal activity → ↑ HR	↑ BP ↘ ↓ sympathetic activity → ↓ HR
Effect of decreased venous return + ↓ BP		
Mild ↓: (? ↓ atrial *volume*)	↑ Vagal activity → ↓ HR ↓ HR (vagus) balanced by ↑ HR (sympathetic).: HR unchanged	↑ sympathetic activity → ↑ HR
Severe ↓↓: (? ↓ ventricular *pressure*)	↑↑ Vagal activity → ↓↓ HR If cardiac sympathetics blocked, vagus is unopposed, and with sensitized vagal receptors (serum catecholamines) → ↓↓ HR and possible cardiac arrest	↑↑ Sympathetic activity ? Accentuates activation of vagal receptors in ventricle†

†↓↓ BP also → ↓ carotid body oxygen supply. This initiates a "hypoxic" reponse and further increases vagal efferent activity.

tration of local anesthetic/low hourly volume or *low concentration/high hourly volume.* Once these infusions are established, cardiovascular effects usually become stable and appear to be less for a given level of block than for a "bolus" injection technique[43] (see Chap. 26).

Epidural Block and General Anesthesia

It has been a standard practice in many institutions to use a combination of light general anesthesia and epidural block for lower abdominal and pelvic surgery.[444] Despite anecdotes suggesting that the combination has dangerous hemodynamic consequences, there are few objective data available. Stephen and colleagues studied the combination of epidural block administered approximately 20 minutes after the induction of light general anesthesia consisting of thiopentone-nitrous oxide-oxygen.[482] In 6 of the 11 patients studied, there were no significant hemodynamic changes resulting from the epidural injection of 30 ml of 2% plain lidocaine at the L3 interspace. The remaining five patients had significant reductions of mean arterial blood pressure (−30%). However, only one of these five also had a reduced cardiac output (−40%) that was associated with bradycardia (−25%). Unfortunately, level of blockade could not be recorded in this study, although it was likely to be in the region of T5, considering the dose of local anesthetic used (Fig. 8-18). Interesting additional observations were made by Stephen and colleagues in patients given epidural block and general anesthesia[482]: Elevation of the legs resulted in increased mean arterial pressure, central venous pressure, and peripheral resistance, but no change in cardiac output; intravenous ephedrine (10 mg) was more effective in producing the same changes and increased cardiac output (Fig. 8-19). Scott's group extended the study to epidural block with lidocaine and epinephrine (1 : 200,000).[450] Although hemodynamic changes were quite variable, their findings were similar to those of Bonica and colleagues in conscious subjects.[37] In particular, total peripheral resistance was much lower than when plain solutions were used. Germann and colleagues addressed themselves to important gaps in knowledge of the cardiovascular effects of epidural block combined with general anesthesia (thiopentone-nitrous oxide-oxygen-succinylcholine)[225]: precise documentation of level of epidural block and hemodynamic effects of superimposed general anesthesia; the effect of order of performance of epidural block either before or after general anesthesia; the comparative effects of 10-degree, head-down tilt and intravenous atropine during established epidural block and general anesthesia.

Epidural block was carried out in healthy patients by using an indwelling epidural catheter (L3–4), with a dose of 15 to 20 ml of 1.5% plain lidocaine. Level of analgesia extended to T6 (± two segments) in patients who received epidural block before general anesthesia, and it was assumed that similar levels were achieved in those who had general anesthesia induced first. Because the protocol for this study was complicated, a summary of the sequence of events is given in Table 8-12. In patients receiving general anesthesia first (group A), epidural block resulted in reductions of mean arterial pressure (−22%), which were the only significant changes (Fig. 8-20; Table 8-13). In those receiving epidural block first (group B), mean arterial pressure was reduced by 20% from awake control values after epidural block, and there was a further reduction to 35% below control values when general anesthesia was induced (Table 8-13). Heart rate and cardiac output were not significantly changed. However, it seems reasonable to postulate that a heart rate of approximately 60 beats per minute is *inappropriately slow* in the face of reduced mean arterial pressure and reduced peripheral vascular resistance. (Other studies showed that decreased venous return with this level of epidural block results in increased vagal activity.[15]) Subsequent administration of 0.6 mg intravenous atropine returned mean arterial blood pressure to control values in both groups and was associated with a heart rate of approximately 110 beats per minute. Head-down tilt (10°) resulted in a small increase in stroke volume but no other significant hemodynamic changes in either group. Right atrial pressure was not significantly altered at any stage of the studies. Blood gases were not significantly altered, except that Pa_{O_2} was reduced when epidural block was added to established general anesthesia; however, there was no change in oxygen consumption (Table 8-13). When the sequence of performance of epidural block and general anesthesia was examined, no significant differences in hemodynamics or blood gases were found; these findings indicated that order of performance of epidural block did not affect hemodynamic variables. However, technical and anatomic considerations also influence the decision, since the awake patient can signal contact of needle with nerve root, facet, and other important structures (see Table 8-20). Also, the ability to determine level of blockade before induction of anesthesia permits more informed decisions

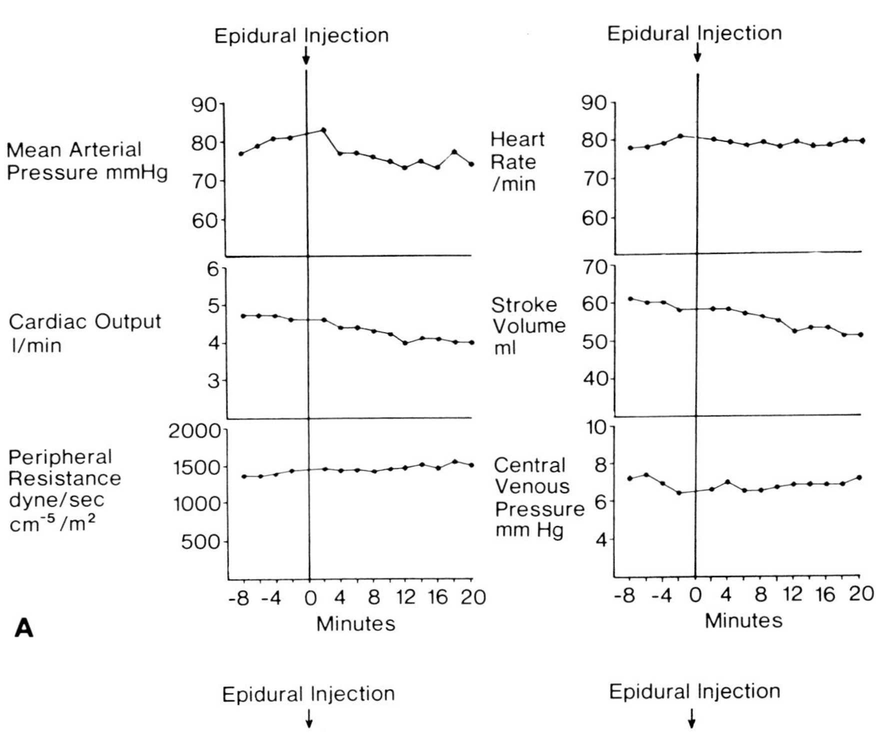

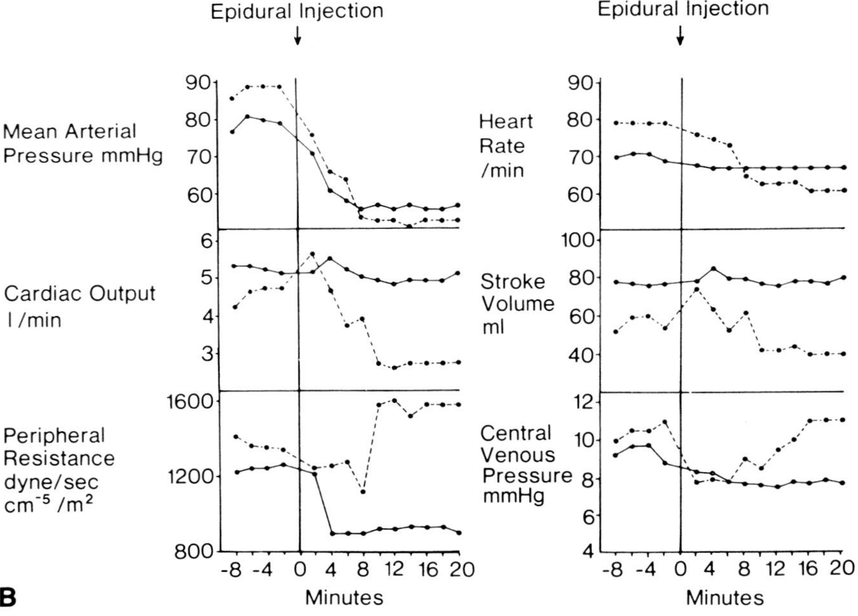

FIG. 8-18. Cardiovascular effects of epidural block and general anesthesia. **A.** Patients (n = 6) who did not become markedly hypotensive maintained normal heart rate and cardiac output. **B.** Patients (n = 5) who developed marked hypotension. Four of the patients *(continuous line)* had cardiac output and heart rate that were essentially unchanged so that hypotension was due to the marked reduction in peripheral resistance. In one patient *(dotted line)* cardiac output fell coincident with reduced heart rate. (Stephen, G.W., Lees, M.M., and Scott, D.B.: Cardiovascular effects of epidural block combined with general anaesthesia. Br. J. Anaesth., *41*:933, 1969.)

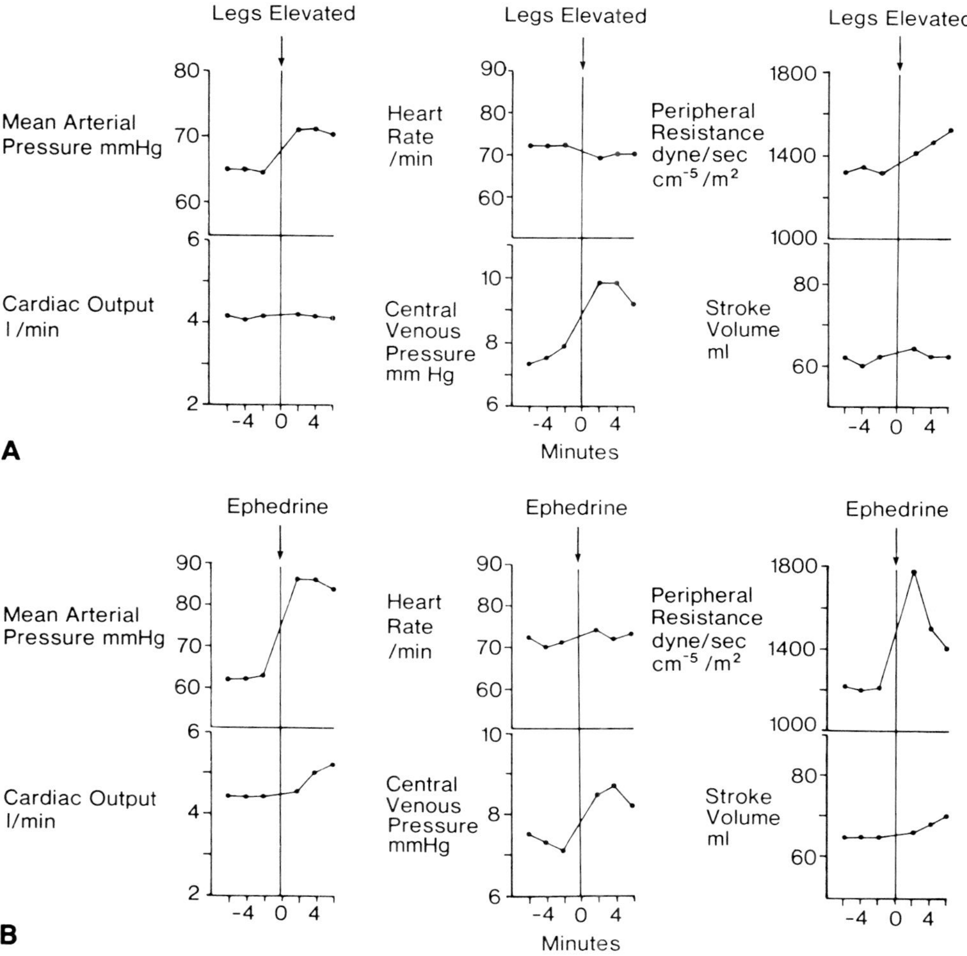

FIG. 8-19. CVS changes with epidural block and general anesthesia; effect of ephedrine and leg elevation. **A.** Leg elevation results in increased mean arterial blood pressure and central venous pressure but no change in cardiac output. **B.** Ephedrine (10 mg i.v.) results in increased mean arterial blood pressure initially due to increased peripheral resistance and subsequently due to increased cardiac output. (Stephen, G.W., Lees, M.M., and Scott, D.B.: Cardiovascular effects of epidural block combined with general anaesthesia. Br. J. Anaesth., *41*:933, 1969.)

about cardiovascular support and confirms adequacy of blockade of operative field. Nancarrow and associates[374] compared the cardiovascular effects of epidural block to T5 level, given before nitrous oxide-halothane (0.35% end-tidal) general anesthesia, with the same general anesthesia minus epidural block. Decreases in mean arterial pressure were significantly greater in the epidural group; however, decreases in liver blood flow and reductive metabolism of halothane were similar in both groups.

In summary it appears that light general anesthesia can be safely combined with epidural block to the level of T5 in healthy patients. The studies of Stephen and colleagues,[482] Germann and colleagues,[225] and Baron and colleagues[15] recommend the use of small incremental doses of atropine in this situation to maintain heart rates of approximately 90 beats per minute. If additional cardiovascular support is required, elevation of the legs, increased intravenous fluid administration, or ephedrine should be used

TABLE 8-12. SUMMARY OF PROTOCOL FOR STUDY OF EPIDURAL BLOCK AND GENERAL ANESTHESIA

Stage	Time (min)	Procedure
	0	Insertion of epidural and vascular catheters
		20-minute rest period
1	20	Hemodynamic and blood gas measurements
	30	Group A receives general anesthesia
		Group B receives epidural block
		20-minute stabilization
2	60	Hemodynamic and blood gas measurements
	65	10° head-down tilt
3	70	Hemodynamic and blood gas measurements (patient returned to horizontal position)
	75	Group A epidural block
		Group B general anesthesia
		20-minute stabilization
4	100	Hemodynamic and blood gas measurements
	105	10° head-down tilt
5	110	Hemodynamic and blood gas measurements
		Groups A and B
	115	Return to horizontal position
	125	Atropine (0.6 mg i.v.)
6	130	Hemodynamic and blood gas measurements

(Germann, P.A.S., Roberts, J.G., and Prys-Roberts, C.: The combination of general anesthesia and epidural block. I: The effects of sequence of induction on haemodynamic variables and blood gas measurements in healthy patients. Anaes. Intens. Care, 7:229, 1979)

depending on each patient's cardiovascular status and likely response to such maneuvers. Although significant changes in Pa_{O_2} were only observed by Germann and colleagues with the sequence of general anesthesia followed by epidural block, it seems wise to administer at least 30% inspired oxygen whenever epidural block is combined with general anesthesia or with intravenous sedation.

IMPORTANT ASPECTS OF VENOUS RETURN AND EPIDURAL BLOCKADE

As indicated in Tables 8-10, 8-11, and Figure 8-21, reduced venous return may play a dominant role in initiating sudden reductions in cardiac rate, which should be viewed as a danger signal that venous return is markedly reduced and oxygenation of the myocardium is at risk. There is no doubt that obstruction to venous return, by whatever means, must be avoided in patients being given epidural block. If postural changes are added to obstruction in the presence of the increased venous capacitance of epidural block, then serious impairment of venous return will follow. In addition, pressure in epidural veins will rise owing to channeling of blood from the pelvis by way of the alternative route of the vertebral venous plexus and azygos vein to the right atrium; this has important consequences for increased spread of segmental analgesia and may impair arterial blood flow to the spinal cord.[468] Partial occlusion of the inferior vena cava in dogs has been reported to markedly decrease cardiac output and increase the resuscitation time for cardiac toxicity resulting from intravascular injection of bupivacaine. Also, much larger doses of epinephrine and bicarbonate were required for resuscitation.[297] Although not measured, presumably peak arterial concentrations of bupivacaine were much higher in animals with inferior vena caval occlusion.

Situations in which venous return may be compromised may be summarized (see Fig. 8-13):

Supine hypotensive syndrome in pregnancy resulting from uterine compression of the vena cava is accentuated by increased venous capacitance owing to sympathetic block of epidural analgesia and postural changes favoring pooling of blood in the lower limbs.[270,442,443,448]

Uterine contraction during labor in supine position. Mean brachial arterial pressure may be maintained at deceptively normal levels because of simultaneous compression of vena cava and aorta (Poseiro effect). However, mean femoral arterial pressure drops precipitously, as does uterine blood flow.[31] These effects are accentuated by epidural block if the patient is allowed to remain supine.

Intestinal obstruction, ascites, and large intra-abdominal tumors may compress the vena cava at three main sites: *below the liver,* owing to abdominal distention, by intestinal obstruction,[21] or by ascites[412] (this site is also commonly occluded by overenthusiastic retraction or by abdominal packs during upper abdominal surgery); *in the upper lumbar region,* by large intra-abdominal tumors (including the uterus); *at the pelvic brim,* by stretching of the iliac vessels owing to extreme backward tilting of the pelvis. This is sometimes an accompaniment of later pregnancy and may also result from extreme lordotic posturing on the operating table. The "extended lordotic posture" may occlude the vena cava below the liver as well—with potential for venous congestion in the kidney and resultant proteinuria.[94]

The most common causes of vena caval obstruction in surgical applications of epidural block are poor posturing, heavy-handed retraction, and incorrect use of abdominal packs. Extreme postures, such as the jackknife prone, lateral "kidney," and hyperflexed lithotomy, should be avoided in association with any anesthetic and with epidural block in particular.[340,442] Whenever possible, caval obstruction should be relieved before epidural block or carefully avoided after epidural block. If it occurs and cannot be corrected for a period of time, then venous return may be assisted by restoring venous capacitance to normal levels by using carefully titrated doses of ephedrine (5–10 mg), intravenously. In some patients with large abdominal tumors, the aorta and vena cava may both be partially obstructed, but with maintenance of sufficient venous return to keep mean arterial pressure normal, with a partly occluded aorta. Sudden relief of the aortic obstruction as the tumor is removed may cause a precipitous fall in blood pressure owing to the reactive hyperemia below the level of obstruction. This situation may be avoided by ensuring adequate hydration and perhaps by using appropriate amounts of colloid before tumor removal. Also, one should be prepared to use small doses of ephedrine until reactive hyperemia subsides.

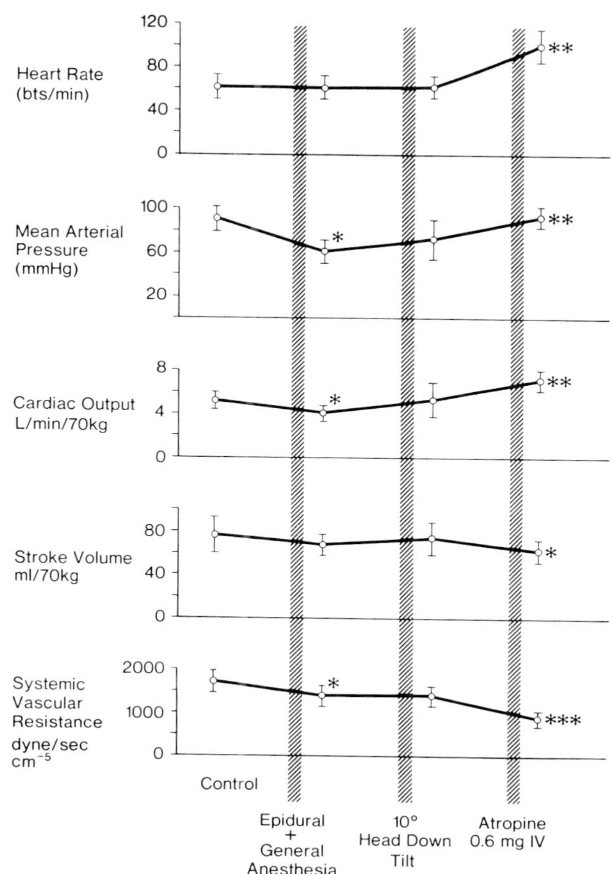

FIG. 8-20. CVS effects of epidural block and general anesthesia; effect of sequence of block, atropine, and 10° head-down tilt. Epidural block (to T6) plus general anesthesia results in a similar degree of reduction in mean arterial blood pressure (MAP) whether epidural block is induced before or after general anesthesia. Administration of atropine (0.6 mg i.v.) returned MAP to control values in both groups. Head-down tilt (10°) was not effective in reversing hemodynamic changes. (Germann, P.A.S., Roberts, J.G., and Prys-Roberts, C.: The combination of general anaesthesia and epidural block: I. The effects of sequence of induction on haemodynamic variables and blood gas measurements in healthy patients. Anaesth. Intens. Care, 7:229, 1979.)

Epidural Blockade and Reduction of Blood Loss

Although initial emphasis on methods to reduce operative blood loss focused on reduction of arterial blood pressure,[185,237] it was also well known that posture played an important part.[185]

TABLE 8-13. EPIDURAL BLOCK AND GENERAL ANESTHESIA, HEMODYNAMICS

		Stage 1 (Control)	Stage 2 (GA or Epidural)	Stage 4 (GA + Epidural)
Heart rate (beats/min)	A (GA 1st)	67 ± 18	63 ± 11	63 ± 8
	B (epidural 1st)	60 ± 4	64 ± 8	57 ± 13
Mean arterial pressure	A	82 ± 10	75 ± 6	*64 ± 5
	B	89 ± 10	*71 ± 18	*58 ± 16
Cardiac output (liters/min/70 kg)	A	4.95 ± 0.70	4.35 ± 0.90	4.25 ± 0.75
	B	4.35 ± 0.90	4.50 ± 1.00	3.60 ± 1.00
Stroke volume (ml)	A	79 ± 19	70 ± 10	68 ± 11
	B	73 ± 14	70 ± 9	64 ± 11
Systemic vascular resistance	A	1487 ± 277	1528 ± 305	1344 ± 206
(dyn • sec • cm − 5)	B	1889 ± 239	*1428 ± 177	*1447 ± 233

*Significant change ($p < 0.05$) versus control.
There were no significant differences when stage 4 was compared with stage 2.
(Germann, P.A.S., Roberts, J.G., and Prys-Roberts, C.: The combination of general anaesthesia and epidural block. I: The effects of sequence of induction on haemodynamic variables and blood gas measurements in healthy patients. Anaesth. Intensive Care, 7:229, 1979)

There has been a gradual recognition of the importance of avoidance of venous obstruction and the use of posture in combination with sympathetic blockade to aid venous pooling away from the operative site. Thus, although epidural blockade has been used to produce hypotension and, in turn, control operative blood loss,[502,503] others have found that blood loss can be reduced *without* the levels of hypotension commonly required if general anesthesia and ganglion blockade are used.[198,300,330,358,489,539] Keith deliberately avoided arterial hypotension in a randomized prospective study of blood loss using epidural or general anesthesia for surgery for total hip replacement.[300] Blood loss intraoperatively was determined by a colorimetric technique and postoperatively, by closed suction drains. Patients receiving epidural block had operative blood losses that were half those associated with general anesthesia. In contrast, there was no difference in postoperative blood losses between the two groups. Other studies reported a reduction in blood loss by 30% to 40% if epidural block is used for hip surgery.[356,478] Thus, it appears that epidural block may reduce operative blood loss by factors other than a mild reduction in arterial blood pressure, increased venous capacitance,[463] and the use of appropriate posture. Additional factors may include the prevention of high venous pressure in response to sympathetic activity resulting from pain,[77] avoidance of "reactive arterial hypertension,"[262] and avoidance of increased airway pressure with resultant effects on venous pressure[357] (see also Chap. 5 and Table 5-8).

FUNCTION OF HOLLOW VISCERA AFTER EPIDURAL BLOCKADE

The Bladder

One of the most commonly observed sequels of lumbar epidural block is temporary atonia of the bladder owing to blockade of sacral segments S2–4. This is similar to lower motor neuron lesions in which bladder sensation is lost. Fortunately, this type of effect after epidural blockade is usually short-lived and causes no or minimal increases in post-block bladder dysfunction.[149,359]

When continuous epidural techniques are used, however, catheterization of the bladder may be necessary.[269] On the other hand, segmental thoracic epidural block (*e.g.*, T5–L1) may spare the sacral segments, and thus leave bladder sensation intact. In addition, relief of severe abdominal pain by epidural block from T5 to L1 may prevent reflex sympathetic activity (via T12–L1 spinal segments), which increases bladder sphincter tone and may predispose to acute retention.

The Gut

Epidural block extending from T6 to L1 effectively denervates the splanchnic sympathetic supply to the abdominal viscera (see Figs. 13-1, 13-2). The sympathetic blockade results in a small contracted gut owing to parasympathetic dominance. This may greatly enhance access during surgery. However, the question has been raised whether this predisposes to postoperative ileus. In 1977 electroenterographic studies were carried out in patients after cholecystectomy under general anesthesia, with or without thoracic epidural blockade.[224] The electrical activity of the stomach and intestine decreased after surgery in all patients and did not return to normal until the third or fourth postoperative day. However, a marked increase in amplitude and frequency of electrical oscillations was recorded in 80% of patients, who received epidural block. Also, eating resulted in markedly increased electrical activity in patients whose postoperative pain was treated by epidural block, whereas eating in association with systemic nicomorphine injection resulted in no change in electrical activity. These interesting results suggest that intraoperative and postoperative epidural block may be useful in preventing and treating postoperative adynamic ileus. However, a note of caution is necessary: The use of epidural block should not distract attention from the treatment of important causes of ileus, such as obstruction and peritonitis. Further work to elucidate the effects of epidural block on gut motility is warranted.

Gastric emptying, as assessed by paracetamol absorption, was much closer to normal after epidural block compared with the use of systemic morphine for postoperative pain.[380]

The integrity of gut anastomotic suture lines has been questioned in patients receiving epidural block. Some surgeons have been concerned that the small contracted bowel may make the surgery more difficult and may later compromise the suture line. There is no evidence for either of these fears. To the contrary, *increased* sympathetic activity may contribute to bowel distention, endangering anastomoses. Patients anesthetized with general anesthesia, including opioids, are likely to have uncoordinated peristalsis and "segmentation" that results in high intraluminal pressure.[6] This may be accentuated if neostigmine is given in large doses to antagonize neuromuscular blocking drugs. Thus, epidural block poses a *lesser* potential for anastomotic breakdown than does general anesthesia.[6]

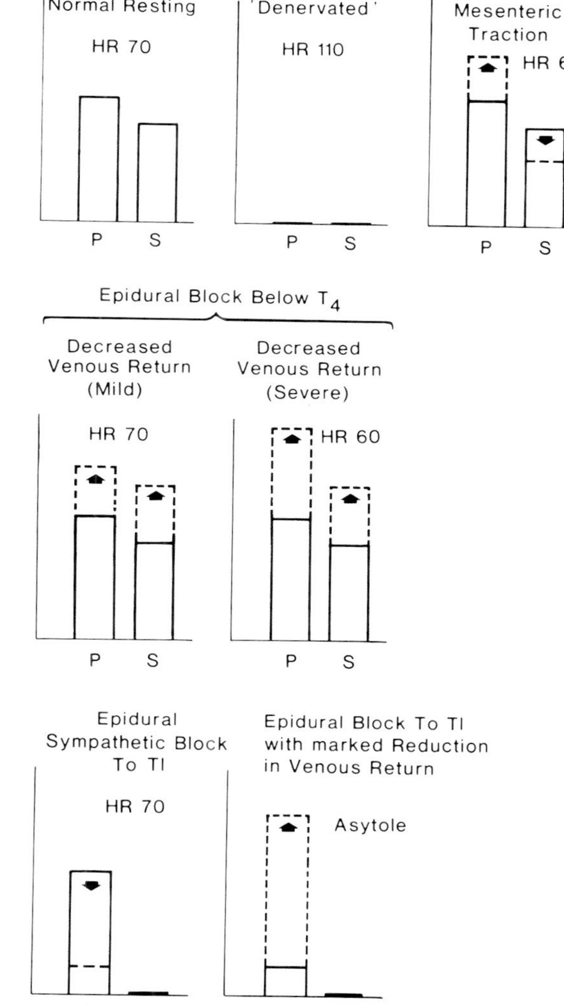

FIG. 8-21. Vagal effects of epidural block. **Top, left.** The balance of cardiac parasympathetic *(P)* activity and sympathetic *(S)* activity is shown with a normal resting heart rate of 70. **Top, middle.** The presence of a heart rate of 110 following complete "denervation" of the heart emphasizes the dominant action of the vagus. **Top, right.** Autonomic reflexes such as mesenteric traction usually result in bradycardia by an opposite change in P and S. **Center.** Epidural block to T4. **Center, left.** A mild reduction in venous return results in increased vagal tone,[15] which may offset the increase in sympathetic tone (arterial baroreceptors) so that heart rate is unchanged or slightly decreased. **Center, right.** Marked reduction in venous return stimulates a marked increase in P, and S increases in an attempt to minimize the bradycardia. **Bottom.** Epidural block to T1. **Bottom, left.** Usual situation, in which P has diminished to compensate for a blocked S. A heart rate of 70 is the result of the same dominance of P over S that exists at rest; however, P is now completely unopposed. **Bottom, right.** Marked reduction in venous return (or other stimulus to P) results in unopposed increase in P, which may lead to asystole. Such responses are much more likely in the conscious patient.

THERMOREGULATION, SHIVERING, AND MALIGNANT HYPERPYREXIA

The vasodilatation of extensive epidural block may predispose to hypothermia if vasodilated areas of the patient are left exposed in a cold environment. However, this reduction in body temperature occurs slowly and does not explain the rapid onset of shivering that sometimes immediately follows the injection of local anesthetic solutions into the epidural space.[175]

Various causes of shivering in association with epidural blockade have been proposed:

a. a decrease in *core temperature* owing to peripheral vasodilatation caused by sympathetic blockade;
b. an effect of the local anesthetic absorbed into the circulation on temperature *regulatory centers;*
c. a differential inhibition of *spinal cord* afferent *thermoreceptor fibers* (loss of warm sensation before cold sensation), causing an erroneous indication of a fall in peripheral temperature[211,375];
d. a direct effect of cold local anesthetic solutions on thermosensitive structures within the spinal cord. Such structures have been demonstrated in animals,[308] but not in humans.

The strongest evidence supports *d*: Injecting boluses of cold local anesthetic solutions was associated with marked reductions (below 20°C) in epidural temperature at the site of injection, which remained low for more than 10 minutes. Shivering occurred within a few minutes of injection in a high percentage of patients and in 50% of those was reduced or stopped by injection of local anesthetic warmed to 41°C. These results support the hypothesis that early shivering after epidural injection is due to stimulation of cold-sensitive structures in the spinal canal by cold local anesthetic solutions.[519] Injection of epidural meperidine (50 mg) has been reported to abolish shivering in a high percentage of patients during epidural local analgesia in labor.[88a] It appears that shivering is more common after bupivacaine, and the slow onset of blockade would certainly permit a longer period of differential loss of warm sensation with associated shivering. A controlled study comparing incidence of shivering with saline, lidocaine, and bupivacaine, all at a similar temperature, is not available.

Malignant Hyperthermia

Malignant hyperthermia (MH) is a pharmacogenetic disorder of skeletal muscle.[368] Inheritance is autosomal dominant with variable penetrance.[184] Abnormalities in calcium flux appear to be important.[184] A primary or secondary role for changes in sympathetic activity has not been determined.[239] However, Kerr and colleagues reported that porcine MH could be prevented by epidural block: Surprisingly, if epidural block involved only the hind limbs, these remained flaccid while the rest of the body became rigid and the temperature rise was prevented.[304]

In contrast, spinal cord transection in the cervical region delayed the rise in temperature but did not prevent it. Thus, it appears that maintenance of some spinal cord activity is necessary, but modification of sensory, sympathetic, and perhaps efferent motor activity is somehow involved in preventing the explosive temperature rise of malignant hyperpyrexia. Further investigations are required to determine the implications of these observations for human malignant hyperpyrexia.

The use of amide local anesthetics in MH-susceptible patients has now been shown to be safe.[24] For example, femoral nerve block with mepivacaine has been repeatedly and safely used for muscle biopsy in patients susceptible to MH.[24] Supplementation of local anesthesia should avoid volatile anesthetics, nitrous oxide, and ketamine. Other triggering agents should also be avoided, including calcium, potassium, and calcium channel blockers. It may be wise to avoid epinephrine-containing local anesthetic solutions, since epinephrine may alter calcium flux and there is still a question about the role of catecholamines in MH.[239] Although local anesthetics do not trigger MH, there is no guarantee that the use of a neural blockade technique will *prevent* the development of an episode of MH during surgery. Thus, the use of dantrolene before and/or during surgery must be considered and the drug must be readily available.[184]

NEUROENDOCRINE EFFECTS OF EPIDURAL BLOCKADE

Does "deafferentation" of the surgical field by epidural block favorably modify the "stress" response to surgery[106]? The difficulty in answering this question has been twofold: methodological problems in measuring neuroendocrine responses and uncertainty about the clinical significance of changes that have been observed. In interpreting the results of such studies, it should be remembered that epidural block to T5 level may abolish efferent splanchnic outflow to the adrenal medulla as well as noxious afferent somatic and visceral impulses, provided blockade extends outside the upper and lower limits of the operative field. A sensory level of T5 may not be associated with complete sympathetic block to T5 level,[22] and thus visceral afferents and efferents to the adrenal medulla may not be blocked. Also, epidural block does not block vagal afferent fibers from the upper abdominal viscera, and this may be responsible for afferent stimulation of release from the hypothalamus of hormones (*e.g.*, ADH) or of humoral "trophic" hormones (*e.g.*, ACTH), which in turn may result in humoral release from target organs (*e.g.*, cortisol from adrenal cortex). The relative importance of the various components of the neurohumoral "stress" response in the surgical patient has not been elucidated, so that it is not possible to say if the failure of epidural block to obtund vagal afferents negates its favorable effect on adrenal medullary function[84,144] and hepatic release of blood glucose.[86] However, a gross indication that the net effect may be favorable is a markedly diminished hospital stay of patients who received continuous epidural block for perioperative management of upper abdominal surgery compared with those who received general anesthesia and narcotic medication.[401] Further evidence is provided by a favorable influence of epidural block on incidence of deep vein thrombosis after hip replacement[356] and prostatectomy[256] (see Chap. 5). However, a controlled study in upper abdominal surgical patients reported no difference between epidural and general anesthesia, except for superior pain control with postoperative epidural block.[261]

Adrenal Medulla

Although it is known that surgery and pain increase sympathetic activity with resultant rises in circulating catecholamine levels,[379] precise quantitation has had to await the development of assay techniques capable of measuring basal levels of catecholamines in humans.[101] These techniques are currently being applied to investigate the perioperative changes in catecholamine output associated with general and/or regional anesthesia.

Early animal studies indicate that during surgery, general anesthesia alone may be sufficient to dampen catecholamine release.[176,423] Some studies in humans report that insignificant changes in serum catecholamine levels occur during surgery under general anesthesia.[97] However, studies with sensitive assays indicate that high doses of volatile anesthetics or opioids are necessary to suppress the surgically induced increases in plasma catecholamines.[422] Indirect evidence, from measurement of cardiovascular variables,[262,470] indicates that catecholamine levels are high in the postoperative period if opioids are used for analgesia. Epidural block modifies the pentazocine-stimulated increase in catecholamines.[487] Because epidural block prevents catecholamine release owing to surgical stimulus in patients with pheochromocytoma,[84,144] it is likely that it is capable of preventing intraoperative catechol release in normal patients. Studies of the antihypertensive effects of epidural block after cardiac surgery[262] indicate that postoperative catecholamine release and associated reduction in myocardial oxygen delivery may also be prevented by the "deafferentation" of epidural block. In patients with ischemic heart disease undergoing major upper abdominal surgery, the addition of epidural block to general anesthesia decreased the incidence of ST–T segment depression and cardiac arrhythmias and prevented increases in myocardial oxygen consumption.[415] Obstetric studies indicate that epidural block prevents increased catecholamine secretion[464] and resultant reductions in uterine blood flow that are associated with severe pain[534] (see Chap. 18). Further circumstantial evidence of reduced catecholamine secretion by epidural block is the maintenance of normal blood sugar response and glucose tolerance during surgery under epidural block[86,272] (see Figs. 5-8, 5-16).

Adrenal Cortex

It is well known that adrenal cortical output of cortisol may be increased up to ten times by surgical trauma[276] to result in fivefold rises in plasma cortisol levels.[86] Epidural or subarachnoid blockade may delay the normal increase in cortisol secretion[246,510]; however, even in lower abdominal surgery, epidural block provides only a temporary effect, and cortisol levels may eventually reach the same concentration as with general anesthesia, even if postoperative analgesia is managed with epidural block.[52,134,188,231,334] Gordon and colleagues interpreted their results,[231] in gynecological surgery, as an indication that cortisol response could be prevented if complete deafferentation of the lower abdomen was obtained and continued into the postoperative period. They reported that patients with satisfactory "continuous" blockade did not manifest an increase in plasma cortisol in the perioperative period. Only patients with unsatisfactory or discontinuous block developed a delayed increase in plasma cortisol. Studies by Kehlet and

Brandt's group and others have confirmed these results[299] (see Fig. 5-7 and Chap. 5).

Upper abdominal and thoracic surgery show a more consistent picture. There is little difference in plasma cortisol levels between general anesthesia alone and/or epidural block.[51,86] In the study by Bromage and colleagues, epidural block was maintained above T4 during and for 19 hours after abdominal surgery and above T1 in association with thoracic surgery.[86] Despite meticulous attention to adequate blockade, plasma cortisol levels increased as much as with general anesthesia, presumably because vagal afferents were unblocked (Fig. 8-22). It was suggested that vagal impulses to the hypothalamus initiated ACTH release, which then produced a humoral release of cortisol from the adrenal cortex. Studies of the effect on cortisol secretion of celiac plexus or splanchnic nerve blockade combined with epidural block[495] are discussed in Chapter 5.

Blood Sugar Level

In animals epidural block, which abolishes reflex efferent stimuli to the adrenal medulla and liver, usually prevents increased blood glucose during surgical stress under general anesthesia, provided the entire splanchnic outflow is blocked.[286] Bromage and colleagues[86] and Brandt and colleagues[51] were able to show complete abolition of blood glucose response if effective blockade was maintained during and after upper abdominal and thoracic surgery (Fig. 8-22).

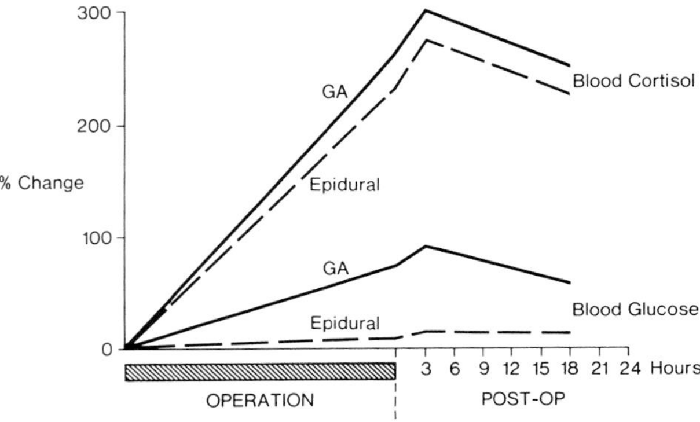

FIG. 8-22. Upper abdominal surgery: neuroendocrine effects of epidural block. The blood sugar response to surgery is completely abolished by epidural block, which "deafferents" the operative site. The increase in plasma cortisol is little affected by epidural block in upper abdominal and thoracic surgery, presumably because afferent vagal impulses to the hypothalamus release cortisol by means of blood-borne ACTH.

Houghton and colleagues[272] reported that epidural block maintained normal glucose tolerance and insulin release during surgery, whereas general anesthesia resulted in decreased insulin release and glucose tolerance. Because sympathetic stimulation may occur under general anesthesia, the finding of decreased insulin release by Houghton and colleagues[272] is supportive of animal studies, in which sympathetic stimulation reduced insulin secretion[405] and resulted in increased glucagon secretion. However, other studies in humans have failed to measure a decrease in insulin secretion during surgery under general anesthesia.[49,51] On the contrary, Brandt and colleagues reported that insulin secretion remained low and unchanged during both general and epidural anesthesia.[49] Thus, the "inappropriately" low insulin secretion in the face of hyperglycemia during general anesthesia and surgery indicates that the secretion of insulin in response to hyperglycemia is blocked during general anesthesia. The abolition of the hyperglycemic response by epidural analgesia is not caused by an increased insulin secretion. It is still possible that glucagon secretion is increased by general anesthesia, thus raising blood sugar, and that this increase is prevented by epidural block. It is more likely, however, that abolition of reflex sympathetic activity during surgery by epidural block prevents sympathetic neural and humoral effects on the liver, which would otherwise result in glycogenolysis and increased blood glucose (see Chap. 5).

Important clinical implications of the effect of epidural block on blood sugar are as follows:

Diabetic patients may be managed satisfactorily by this method, provided that insulin is not given to such patients unless added glucose is administered intravenously; otherwise, blood sugar levels may become dangerously low. Unintentional hypotension caused by epidural block with reduced oxygen delivery to the brain and the added insult of hypoglycemia may have disastrous effects on cerebral function.

If insulin is administered on the basis of a high blood glucose measurement, it should be remembered that the subsequent reduction in blood glucose may be much greater than that without epidural block, since additional factors, such as increased catecholamine levels, that usually elevate blood glucose are probably not present.

Other Hormonal Effects

Some hormonal effects of epidural block are as follows:

Reduced epinephrine and cyclic AMP[339] response to surgery (see Chap. 5).
Cyclic AMP rises after epidural block during the first stage of labor, possibly because of decreased uterine contraction.[289]
Reduced intraoperative and postoperative changes in plasma aldosterone and renin, in patients subjected to hysterectomy and hip surgery.[53]
Reduced concentrations of renin and angiotensin II during labor in patients with epidural block compared with controls.[332]
Suppression of increases in prolactin during surgery.[50]
Inhibition of growth hormone and ACTH responses to surgery.[50]
Suppression of the increase in plasma cortisol response during late stages of labor.[92]
Thyroid hormone concentration in plasma is not influenced by epidural block (see Chap. 5).
Inhibition of intraoperative lipolysis (see Chap. 5).
Reduction of normal perioperative increase in blood lactate and 3-hydroxy butyrate (see Chap. 5).
Improved amino acid and nitrogen balance (see Chap. 5).

The clinical implications of these observations are not clear. However, they may be evidence of a favorable modification of the "stress" response to surgery and may influence recovery from surgery (see Chap. 5). For example, urinary nitrogen losses from catabolic breakdown of proteins are significantly reduced by prolonged epidural block after lower abdominal surgery[299] (see Fig. 5-9).

EFFECTS OF EPIDURAL BLOCKADE ON RESPIRATION

Two important questions concerning respiration and epidural blockade require an answer: Does epidural block interfere with respiration? Is the ability to cough impaired?

The following aspects of epidural blockade may influence respiration:

Aspects of Epidural Blockade That May Influence Respiration

Sensory ("afferent") neural blockade reduces nociceptive afferent drive to respiratory center
Motor ("efferent") neural blockade of intercostal muscles, abdominal muscles, and diaphragm (rarely)
Sympathetic neural blockade with resultant changes in cardiac output and pulmonary blood flow
Vagal dominance in the presence of complete sympathetic blockade
Effects of systemically absorbed epinephrine and local anesthetic on:
- Respiratory control center in midbrain and on chemoreceptors in medulla and carotid bodies
- Myoneural junction
- Metabolism of succinylcholine in serum

The potential for phrenic (C3–5) palsy is extremely low with epidural block, since even blockade to T1 produces motor blockade to only the T4–5 level. The only exception may be intentional epidural block at the cervical level or inadvertent epidural block during interscalene brachial plexus block (see Chap. 10).

Respiratory arrest during high epidural blockade is not usually the result of the effects of sensory or motor blockade, nor is it due to depressant effects of local anesthetic in the CSF; the concentrations attained in the brain by means of this route are insufficient to depress neuronal activity unless gross overdosage is administered.[82] The most common causes of the rare instances of respiratory arrest associated with epidural block are extensive sympathetic blockade, reduced cardiac output, and reduced oxygen delivery to the CNS. It cannot be overemphasized that meticulous attention to maintenance of organ perfusion, by means of the clinical measures described earlier, should ensure that respiratory arrest in association with epidural block occurs extremely seldom and that such an occurrence should be rapidly reversible, with proper management.

It has been claimed that extensive sensory blockade may result in loss of consciousness owing to lack of input to the reticular activating system. However, epidural block to T1 does not cause loss of consciousness.[144] This requires complete afferent blockade, including blockade of cervical nerve roots and the cranial nerves.[77] Although it is likely that such loss of consciousness would interfere with respiratory drive, cardiovascular depression associated with this level of blockade poses an even greater potential for respiratory depression unless appropriate supportive measures are applied; this classically occurs in patients with hypovolemia and with attempts to limit the spread of analgesia by use of the "head-up" position. However, even patients with sensory loss extending to the level of the chin may have normal respiration and may be fully conscious, provided that cardiovascular homeostasis is maintained.[144]

Many factors may contribute to the respiratory effects of epidural block. At present, our knowledge in this area is meager. However, the documented changes produced by epidural block *per se* appear to be mild. For example, a sensory level of T3, associated with a motor level of T8, may be expected to result in essentially no change in vital capacity (VC) and functional residual capacity (FRC) in normal patients, so that respiration and the ability to cough are not impaired.[208,335,515] In patients with severe pain, epidural block probably improves VC and FRC as well as Pa_{O_2}, at least in the early postoperative period (see also Chap. 26); this may result in improved respiratory exchange and more effective coughing (Fig. 8-23).[64,77,269,354,469,470,475,516]

EPIDURAL BLOCK AND MOTOR FUNCTION

Clinical Applications of Deliberate Preservation of Motor Function

With respect to respiratory function, it is clear from the previous section that the aim is to use the appropriate drug and regimen to preserve motor function, and thus to permit deep breathing and coughing. In postoperative patients, continuous infusion of bupivacaine has proved to be an attractive method of achieving this goal. This method is described in detail

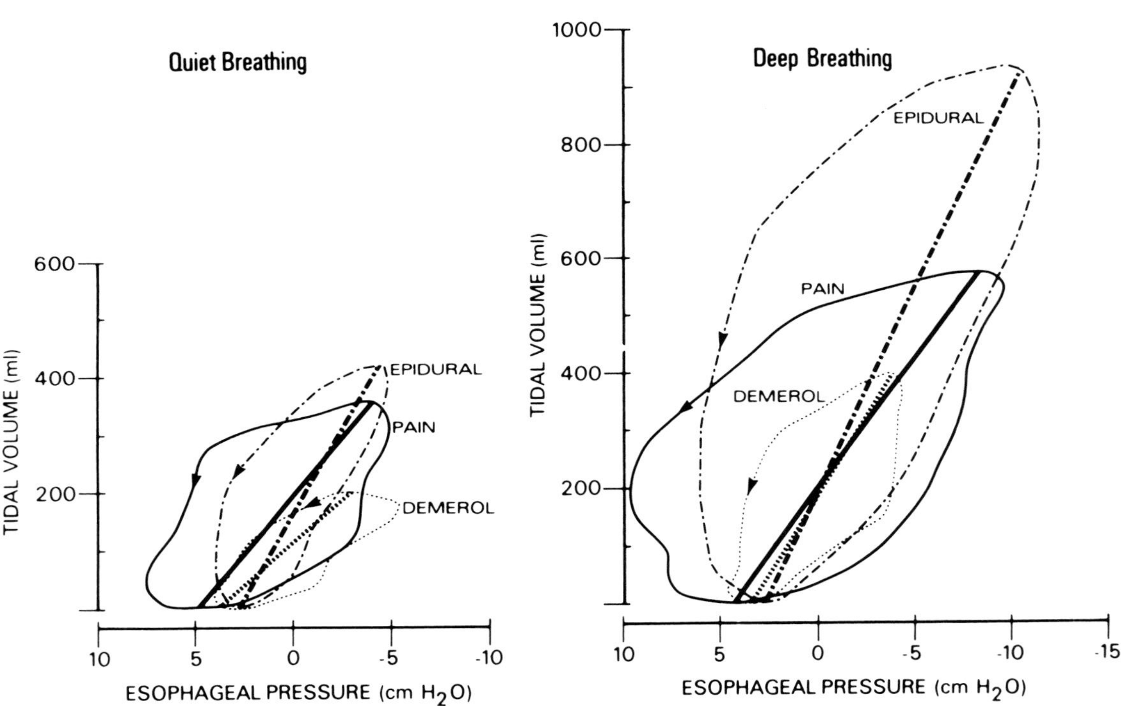

FIG. 8-23. **Effect of pain and analgesia on thoracic pressure volume relationships.** Pressure volume loops are shown 2 to 6 hours after cholecystectomy during quiet breathing **(left)** and deep breathing **(right)**. Pain is associated with decreased tidal volume, which is marked when deep breathing is attempted. During expiration there is high positive pressure, particularly during deep breathing. Such high pressure would be associated with glottic closure, abdominal splinting, and grunting type of respiration. Demerol decreases tidal volume but decreases the high pressure during expiration; thus grunting diminishes, an apparent and deceptive improvement. Epidural blockade increases tidal volume, particularly during deep breathing. This is achieved with much lower positive pressure during expiration and would be accompanied by elimination of grunting and abdominal splinting. A tidal volume of nearly 1000 ml would be associated with effective coughing. (Reproduced with permission from Bromage, P.R.: Epidural Analgesia. Philadelphia, W.B. Saunders, 1978.)

in Chapter 26. Preservation of motor function also permits ultra-early ambulation, since patients who are pain-free are able to ambulate soon after surgery.[77] It may be necessary to use vasopressors if epidural block is continued with only local anesthetic. Alternatives are to use dilute bupivacaine plus opioid (some risk of hypotension) or opioid alone (no risk of hypotension) as described in Chapter 28. Ultra-early ambulation probably decreases the risk of venous thrombosis and may decrease the hospitalization time.[77,401] More controlled data are required (see also Chap. 5).

In normal labor, preservation of motor function is highly desirable. Although this is possible with infusions of weak concentrations of bupivacaine (*e.g.*, 0.125%),[324] these do not always give acceptable analgesia. A combination of weak bupivacaine plus low-dose opioid infusion appears to offer good analgesia with good preservation of motor function (*e.g.*, 0.125% bupivacaine and 0.25% meperidine). Such a mixture may provide good analgesia, high acceptance by patients, and a forceps rate that is lower than with local anesthetic alone (Brownridge, P.: Personal communication; see also Chap. 18).

Clinical Applications of Motor Function Depression

In abdominal and hip surgery, depression of motor function is necessary *during* surgery. In this situation, the powerful motor blockade of etidocaine or lidocaine may be used (see pharmacology section and Fig. 8-25). Some of the motor effects are obtained by "deafferentation," preventing reflex muscle contraction by blocking nociception before it reaches the spinal cord (see Fig. 8-23).

Factors determining motor effects of epidural block are as follows (see pharmacology section):

1. *The local anesthetic drug:* Bupivacaine has the least motor effects; etidocaine has the most potent effects.
2. *Dose of drug:* Degree of motor blockade is increased as dose of drug increases.
3. *Repeated doses of drug:* With "top-up" techniques, both motor and sensory blockade tend to become more intense with repeated doses; however, if dilute solutions of bupivacaine are used by controlled continuous infusion, motor blockade can be kept to a minimum.
4. *Epinephrine as an adjuvant,* increases the degree of motor blockade (see pharmacology section).

NEURAL EFFECTS OF EPIDURAL BLOCKADE

The differential neural effects of epidural block on motor, sensory, and sympathetic function are discussed in the context of the pharmacology of the local anesthetics used for epidural block. Although epidural blockade aims to produce a reversible blockade of axonal activity, it has sometimes been questioned whether more permanent interference with the integrity of the nervous system may result. Depressed rapid axonal transport[194,196] does result from high concentrations of local anesthetics. This indicates reduced oxidative metabolism in the axoplasm of nerves. However, this is a reversible process, and the margin of safety appears to be large for local anesthetics compared with drugs producing an irreversible block (*e.g.*, batrachotoxin). (See also Chap. 29.1 for a discussion of circumstances that may lead to neurotoxic effects of local anesthetics.) It is not known whether some people have genetic abnormalities in neural structure that make them more susceptible to irreversible blockade or whether regenerating neurons are at greater risk. There is some evidence that the developing nervous system may be quite susceptible to some local anesthetics, since neurobehavioral changes in the newborn have been observed after obstetrical epidural block with mepivacaine in relatively high dosage.[436] However, such changes are not seen with bupivacaine[129] or chloroprocaine[263] (see Chap. 18).

Spinal cord effects of epidural blockade have been proposed by Bromage[75] after his observations of changes in lower limb reflexes in association with thoracic epidural blockade. This is supported by autoradiographic studies: Quite high concentrations of radioactively labeled local anesthetic were found in or close to the peripheral areas of the spinal cord.[82] Thus, it appears likely that epidural block results in blockade of long tracts in the spinal cord and possibly in cell bodies. Further evidence for blockade of cell bodies is given in Chapter 27.1.

The brain is not immune from local anesthetic penetration, since local anesthetics reach the CSF by way of dural cuffs and are then conveyed to the brain (see Figs. 8-2, 8-3).[76] High-dosage epidural block thus exposes the brain to local anesthetic in significant amounts by means of vascular absorption and by diffusion up the CSF. Although concentrations in the brain are usually below C_m*, it is possible for neural

*C_m, minimum concentration resulting in blockade (see Chap. 2).

blocking concentrations to be reached if large doses are used epidurally or accidentally injected into the subarachnoid space.

Another neural effect of epidural analgesia relates to the deprivation of afferent input that results. Bromage and Melzack reported that patients often experienced "phantom" limb phenomena during epidural blockade, presumably owing to the loss of normal afferent input from body surface, joints, and other structures.[83]

Electromyographic (EMG) recording in animals after application of high concentrations of local anesthetic to the muscle's nerve supply shows temporary abolition of EMG activity. However, ischemic and toxic effects on nerves may result in permanent or semipermanent abolition of normal EMG activity. Denervation results in the development of a low-voltage "fibrillation" pattern in the muscle(s) supplied by the damaged nerve. Recording from appropriate muscle groups can be helpful in determining whether only a single spinal nerve is involved distal to the intervertebral foramen. In such a situation, it is unlikely that epidural injection of local anesthetic results in nerve damage.[343,344] At the present time, there is no evidence that permanent changes in EMG occur after the use of appropriate clinical concentrations of local anesthetics for epidural blockade. A more detailed examination of the potential for complications in association with epidural blockade reveals, however, that other factors, such as direct trauma by the needle, may result in neural damage.

Studies in humans, using intra-arterial injection of lidocaine, indicate a significant reduction in response as assessed by evoked EMG.[486] The pattern of response indicated that the results may be attributable to an effect of lidocaine on the motor nerve terminal. Thus, high blood concentrations of lidocaine might be expected to produce additive effects with both depolarizing and nondepolarizing muscle relaxants.

Analgesic effects of epidurally administered local anesthetics may also be produced by drug absorbed into the circulation. Systemic administration of local anesthetics has been reported to cause a selective depression of C-afferent fiber evoked activity in the spinal cord.[531]

EPIDURAL BLOCKADE AND PREGNANCY

The known and potential physiologic effects of epidural block on mother, placenta, and fetus must be viewed in the light of contemporary knowledge of the physiology and pathophysiology of pregnancy,[34] fetal physiology,[197] and pharmacology.[355,409,435] The detailed implications for regional anesthesia are discussed further in Chapter 18 (see Figs. 18-3 through 18-7 and 18-12).

There are important changes in respiration[29] with implications for the fetus[409] and for the management of epidural block and use of supplemental agents.[394] Maternal cardiovascular changes are also critical in the safe management of epidural block[150,267] (see Figs. 18-3 through 18-7 and 18-12). Of crucial importance is the avoidance of the supine position throughout labor (by use of the lateral position) and at vaginal delivery and cesarean section, where the lateral tilt of the table or use of a wedge is mandatory (see Chap. 18). Uteroplacental circulation and fetal oxygen delivery may be influenced by the management of epidural block[16,99-100,235,290,305,346,409,518,522,534] (see Figs. 18-4 through 18-7 and 18-12). Management of the patient with preeclampsia requires special knowledge of the complex pathophysiology of the condition, to safely manage epidural block (see Fig. 18-12). Gastrointestinal changes and other factors contribute to the statistic that acid aspiration syndrome is still the most common cause of maternal death related to anesthesia (see Chap. 18).

Major physiologic changes secondary to pain in labor can be partially or often completely reversed by epidural block (see Fig. 18-5). Some of the sequelae of unrelieved pain produce adverse changes in fetal physiology, and drugs used to produce and supplement epidural block may affect the fetus.[3,30,267,355,409,435] Thus, fetal monitoring is as important as monitoring of the mother during epidural block.

Perinatal pharmacology is also pertinent to epidural block management.[3,30,267,355,409,435] The controversy surrounding local anesthetics and neurobehavioral effects on the fetus has been resolved.[3] It is clear that mepivacaine is not suitable for obstetrics, but lidocaine, bupivacaine, and chloroprocaine are satisfactory options for appropriate situations (see Chap. 18). Avoidance of maternal hypotension is more important than the effects of local anesthetics.[267]

Large doses of salicylates may depress platelet function (but not the platelet count) and predispose to increased bleeding. It is prudent in such cases to obtain a coagulation screen and do a simple Lee–White bleeding time at the bedside, before epidural block.

If magnesium is used in large doses to treat preeclampsia, it should be noted that it may cause maternal hypotonia and respiratory depression, and cardiovascular depression in the newborn. These effects may be additive with those of local anesthetics, which have crossed the placenta.

Safe management of epidural block in parturients

requires that the anesthesiologist be part of the obstetric team and be fully informed of the preexisting physiologic status of mother and fetus. He should fully understand the significance of changes in maternal and fetal physiology. With careful attention to such considerations, epidural block with lidocaine, bupivacaine, and/or chloroprocaine has minimal effects on the fetus. In some patients it may *improve* oxygen delivery to the fetus, reduce maternal cardiac work, and permit an otherwise distressed mother to remember her delivery as a satisfying and fulfilling experience. This may enable her to look forward to a further delivery with confidence rather than with dread (see Chap. 18).

PHARMACOLOGY OF EPIDURAL BLOCKADE

The essence of the clinical pharmacology of epidural block is the provision of safe and effective neural blockade. To safely institute an epidural block, a knowledge of the physiology of epidural block is necessary, as well as a revision of the pharmacokinetics of local anesthetics as related to their administration by means of the epidural route. The efficacy of epidural block depends on this and on the clinical effects of the local anesthetics used.

Factors in "Safety" of Epidural Blockade. The majority of studies of absorption and disposition of local anesthetics have been carried out in patients receiving epidural blockade. Thus, this aspect of the pharmacology of epidural analgesia is discussed in detail in Chapter 3. Also, much of the work on local anesthetic toxicity has been obtained with reference to the epidural route of administration of local anesthetics; this is presented in Chapter 4. It is worth emphasizing that epidural blockade often entails the use of maximum clinical doses of local anesthetic, with resultant blood levels that are nearly toxic.[496] Thus, a thorough knowledge of the pharmacokinetics and toxicity of local anesthetics is a prerequisite to the safe use of epidural analgesia.

The discussion below summarizes some important aspects that are covered in detail in Chapters 2, 3, and 4.

ABSORPTION

Epidural injection deposits local anesthetic some distance from the neural target, so that diffusion across tissue barriers is of great importance. Thus, local anesthetics with excellent qualities of penetration of lipid are desirable for rapid and effective epidural analgesia. Because a major site of action is within the dural sac, water solubility is of equal importance (see Tables 3-1, 3-2, 3-11). Thus, agents with a *p*Ka close to physiologic *p*H (*e.g.*, lidocaine, *p* Ka = 7.87) are most effective, in that they are able to readily exhibit both lipid and water solubility. Procaine and tetracaine, with a high *p*Ka (9.05 and 8.46), suffer in this respect and perform poorly in epidural blockade.

Epidural fat provides a potential "reservoir" for deposition of fat-soluble local anesthetics. Thus, accumulation of long-acting fat-soluble agents, such as bupivacaine, occurs in epidural fat. This is not so for less fat-soluble agents, such as lidocaine (see Table 3-11). Thus, with repeated injections of bupivacaine, epidural fat concentrations rise but blood concentrations tend to remain the same, provided that dosage is appropriate. Repeated injections of lidocaine result in little accumulation in epidural fat, but progressive accumulation in the blood, with a potential for gradually increasing blood concentration (see Figs. 3-12, 3-14, 3-15).

The epidural venous system provides a rich network for rapid absorption of local anesthetic (see Fig. 8-13). Rapid injection into an epidural vein may dispatch local anesthetic directly to the brain by way of the basivertebral venous system. Another risk of rapid intravascular injection is high peak concentrations of local anesthetic in the myocardium. With bupivacaine this may lead to serious and prolonged "cardiac toxicity" and possibly ventricular fibrillation and/or cardiac arrest (see Chap. 4, Figs. 4-12, 4-13, and Tables 4-4, 4-5).

The inclusion of epinephrine in local anesthetic solutions may greatly reduce vascular absorption (see Tables 3-7 to 3-10 and Figs. 3-13, 3-17), and thus enhance neural blocking properties and reduce the likelihood of systemic toxicity after epidural injection.[349]

The time profile of local anesthetic absorption indicates a peak blood level at 10 to 20 minutes after injection, so that surveillance is necessary for at least 30 minutes after injection (see Fig. 3-13).

Acidic solutions, containing antioxidants to stabilize epinephrine, may release local anesthetic base with difficulty, and thus spread poorly across lipid barriers. Carbonated solutions release base readily and have superior penetrating ability.[107]

Plasma protein binding may influence the amount of free local anesthetic available for placental transfer or for action on the CNS after systemic absorption from the epidural space (see Table 3-1 and Figs. 3-21, 3-22, and 3-32).

Hyaluronidase does not improve onset time of epidural block and reduces efficacy of motor and sensory block.[79]

Potassium additives to local anesthetics reduce sensory onset time but are not clinically acceptable for epidural block because of depolarizing phenomena that may cause distressing muscle spasms.[79]

DISPOSITION

Disposition is influenced by distribution, metabolism, and renal excretion.

Distribution

Distribution of local anesthetics after epidural injection depends initially on the "initial dilution volume" (V), which reflects dilution of the dose in blood, and the "buffering" action of uptake of local anesthetic by the lung and transit time through the lung. Bupivacaine and etidocaine have higher values for V than do mepivacaine and lidocaine.[496] Subsequent distribution of "unbound" drug is by the "volume of distribution" at steady-state (V_{SS}), which reflects total distribution through the body tissues. This provides an approximate indication of tissue affinities, including epidural fat, plasma protein binding, and red cell uptake. Etidocaine has a large V_{SS} (1478 liters), followed by bupivacaine (1028 liters), mepivacaine (382 liters), and lidocaine (253 liters). Surprisingly, a value is not yet available for prilocaine (see Table 3-13 and Figs. 3-10, 3-11, 3-18, 3-19, 3-20, 3-21, 3-22, 3-24).

Metabolism and Excretion

Metabolism of ester agents procaine and chloroprocaine takes place at rapid rates in the serum. Chloroprocaine is effective in producing satisfactory epidural block, while procaine is not. Thus, the rapid plasma clearance of chloroprocaine combines with its efficacy to give it a high therapeutic index.

Metabolism of the amide agents in the liver is much slower. Hepatic extraction ratios are as follows: etidocaine, 0.74; bupivacaine, 0.39; mepivacaine, 0.52; and lidocaine, 0.63. Decreased hepatic blood flow in association with epidural block may reduce the clearance of amide agents[406,488]; the greatest effect is on slowly cleared agents, such as bupivacaine. Enhanced liver blood flow, after ephedrine administration, increases hepatic clearance (see Chap. 3, Table 3-13 and Figs. 3-25 through 3-31, 3-33).

Clearance is determined by the sum of values for distribution, metabolism, and renal excretion. Thus, total clearance values are highest for etidocaine (1.11 liters/min), followed by lidocaine (0.95 liters/min), mepivacaine (0.78 liters/min), and bupivacaine (0.58 liters/min). However, since V values are similar for all four drugs, initial half-lives are quite similar (etidocaine = 2 min, bupivacaine = 3 min, mepivacaine = 1 min, lidocaine = 1 min). Maximum arterial concentrations following equipotent doses are summarized in Tables 3-6 through 3-12. The larger V_{SS} and higher clearance of etidocaine contribute to a shorter intermediate half-life compared with bupivacaine (etidocaine = 18 min, bupivacaine = 29 min), so that duration of a toxic reaction should be shorter for etidocaine compared with bupivacaine after slow absorption from the epidural space (however, see also Chap. 4). It would be expected that duration of toxicity for mepivacaine and lidocaine will be similar and much shorter than for the long-acting amides because of shorter intermediate half-lives (lidocaine = 7 min, mepivacaine = 10 min). Because etidocaine must be used in twice the dose of bupivacaine for effective epidural block, direct injection of etidocaine intravascularly is more likely to produce toxicity; under these circumstances, the rapid clearance and large V_{SS} of etidocaine are insufficient to compensate for the twofold increase in blood concentration compared with bupivacaine. Etidocaine also poses a risk of cardiac toxicity (see Chap. 4).

Clearance of mepivacaine in neonates appears to be halved, and there is a prolonged half-life compared with adults, whereas lidocaine clearance is the same as in adults (see Fig. 3-33). Thus, mepivacaine appears less attractive for obstetric patients. In aged patients, the volume of distribution of lidocaine is reduced and half-life is increased,[376] so that epidural dosage should be reduced if toxicity is to be avoided.

Biotransformation of lidocaine results in at least one active metabolite: monoethylglycylxylidide (MEGX). The half-life of MEGX may be greater than lidocaine, and its CNS toxicity is additive to that of lidocaine. Thus, prolonged administration of lidocaine into the epidural space may result in accumulation of MEGX, particularly in patients with cardiac disease, where clearance of MEGX may be reduced.[406] MEGX is broken down to glycylxylidide (GX), which has a much longer half-life than lidocaine. Thus, GX has a high potential for accumulation and is capable of CNS toxicity after prolonged administration of lidocaine. These two compounds may be responsible for a delayed onset of convulsions during the course of continuous epidural block with lidocaine (see Fig. 3-27).

Prilocaine biotransformation results in formation of *o*-toluidine and subsequent formation of an *N*-hydroxy metabolite (Fig. 3-28). The latter causes methemoglobinemia if the dose of prilocaine exceeds 600 mg. Single-dose epidural block can almost always be accomplished with a dose of prilocaine of less than 400 mg. Because blood concentrations of prilocaine after equipotent doses are 50% of those of lidocaine (see Fig. 3-16), prilocaine is an attractive alternative for single-shot epidural blockade, except in obstetric patients. The drug is not suitable for continuous epidural block.

Clearance data from local anesthetics give important insights into the safety of various dose regimens (see below).[168,169]

ALTERATIONS IN ABSORPTION AND DISPOSITION

Age and Weight of Patient

As discussed in Chapter 3, plasma concentrations of local anesthetic after epidural block do not correlate well with age or weight. However, because dose requirements for epidural block diminish at the extremes of age, it is necessary to reduce dosage for this reason and because clearance of local aesthetics may be reduced in very young (see also Chap. 21) or in aged people.

Pathophysiologic Changes

Acidosis, Hypoxia, and Hypercarbia. Tissue (metabolic) acidosis would be expected to result in increased uptake of local anesthetic into that tissue (*e.g.*, brain), as shown in Figure 3-24. However, the converse is true in general systemic acidosis (see Fig. 3-20). This complex situation is discussed in Chapter 3. However, by whatever mechanism, there is no doubt that local anesthetic toxicity is enhanced in the presence of acidosis as well as hypoxia[432] and hypercarbia (see Chap. 4 and Table 4-3).

Hypothermia may result in tissue acidosis, as well as reduced hepatic biotransformation of local anesthetics, so that amide-type local anesthetics may be more toxic in patients with hypothermia. The vasodilatation accompanying epidural block may predispose to hypothermia in surgical or obstetric patients; with regard to the latter, neonates are also susceptible to hypothermia unless they are rapidly dried and warmed.

Heart Disease. Clearance of amide agents may be greatly reduced owing to low hepatic blood flow. In addition, reduced cardiac output may result in higher peak arterial blood concentrations of local anesthetic (Fig. 4-19). This is particularly important when using amide local anesthetics, such as lidocaine, for continuous epidural block, when the cumulative dosage may be large (see also Tables 3-16 and 3-18).

Liver Disease. Reduced hepatic clearance of the amide agents suggests that long-acting amide agents should be used for continuous epidural block, so that cumulation of blood concentration does not occur; the large V_{SS} of etidocaine and bupivacaine may act as a buffer if hepatic metabolism is reduced, provided that injection is not made directly intravascularly (see Tables 3-16 and 3-18).

Kidney Disease. Likelihood of local anesthetic toxicity is increased because of several contributing factors, such as acidosis and reduced plasma protein binding. Also, duration of action of local anesthetics is reduced probably because of increases in cardiac output and tissue perfusion associated with incipient renal failure. Thus, there is an increased risk of cumulative toxicity during continuous epidural block with short-acting agents, such as lidocaine. Long-acting agents, such as bupivacaine, may be a better choice in these patients if continuous epidural block is used (see also Tables 3-15, 3-16, and 3-18).

Lung Disease. Despite the frequent use of epidural block in patients with pulmonary disease, little is known about potential changes in drug kinetics and toxicity. Because the lung acts as an important "buffer" during absorption of local anesthetics, it is possible that pulmonary disease may increase the risk of acute toxicity (see Chap. 3, p. 92).

FACTORS ASSOCIATED WITH ADMINISTRATION OF EPIDURAL BLOCKADE

Dosage

If dosage is kept constant, blood concentrations of local anesthetic are similar within the range of concentrations used for epidural block (*e.g.*, 40 ml of 1% lidocaine compared with 20 ml of 2% lidocaine) (see Tables 3-6 through 3-12). However, at high concentrations, the same dose (*e.g.*, 10 ml of 4% lidocaine) results in disproportionately higher blood concentrations.[47,48]

Thus, the use of high concentrations of local anesthetic for epidural block should be avoided; previously, viscous "plombes" of concentrated agent were used in the mistaken belief that they would increase effectiveness of block without increasing toxicity (see also Chap. 29.1).

Epinephrine

In general, epinephrine lowers peak plasma concentrations after epidural block. However, the effect is most pronounced with lidocaine. For other drugs, rather complex effects are produced by the local anesthetic concentration and the agent used (see Tables 3-6 through 3-12). No benefit results from use of epinephrine concentrations in excess of 1 : 200,000.

Speed of Injection

Braid and Scott showed that peak venous plasma concentration of lidocaine was slightly higher after epidural injection over 15 seconds compared with 60 seconds. If injection is made directly into a blood vessel, peak arterial blood concentrations are much higher if injection is rapid (see Figs. 4-10, 4-19). The other advantage of a slow injection is the detection of impending toxicity, before all of the dose has been injected. Furthermore, rapid injection may be painful for the patient and cause serious increases in CSF pressure.

Tachyphylaxis

Increasing dose requirements for maintenance of the same segmental spread of blockade (see Fig. 8-29) may result in a high potential for cumulative toxicity. This is most likely to occur with short-acting agents; they are more likely to be associated with tachyphylaxis and accumulation in epidural fat is minimal, thus drug cumulates in the blood (see Figs. 3-14, 3-15).

"EFFICACY" OF EPIDURAL BLOCK

Site of Action

Before discussing factors that influence the clinical efficacy of epidural blockade, it is helpful to summarize current data concerning the site(s) at which local anesthetics act after their injection into the epidural space. The anatomic spread of local anesthetic is summarized in Figures 8-2 and 8-3. It can be seen that local anesthetic comes into contact with the following structures, which are potential candidates for a site of action.

Spinal Nerves in Paravertebral Spaces. Local anesthetic readily seeps out through the intervertebral foramina (see Fig. 8-3).[190,336]

Dorsal Root Ganglia Immediately Adjacent to the "Dural Cuff" Region. The dura is thin in this region (see Fig. 8-2B).

Individual Anterior and Posterior Spinal Nerve Roots Within Their Dural Root "Sleeves" or "Cuffs." Local anesthetic diffuses rapidly into adjacent CSF in this region by way of "arachnoid granulations" (see Fig. 8-2A,B).

Spinal nerve "rootlets" are fine nerve filaments and have a large surface area, exposed to local anesthetic reaching the CSF by way of the adjacent dural cuff region (see Fig. 8-2A).

Peripheral regions of the spinal cord are bathed by CSF, with local anesthetic crossing from nearby dural cuffs (see Fig. 8-2A).

The Brain. By way of spread of local anesthetic upward in the CSF or, indirectly, up the epidural space and then across dural cuffs in the upper cervical region (see Fig. 8-3), the brain is exposed to local anesthetic.

Studies to Determine Sites of Action

The key data were provided by injecting [^{14}C]-labeled lidocaine into the epidural space of dogs and then carrying out autoradiography and tissue assays.[82] These data suggested that rapid diffusion of local anesthetic into the CSF at the dural cuff region is the most important determinant of onset of epidural block: Peak local anesthetic concentrations in the CSF are reached within 10 to 20 minutes of epidural injection, and concentrations are high enough to produce blockade in the spinal nerve roots and "rootlets."[82,214] This coincides with clinical onset of epidural block. The same study also showed that by 30 minutes after injection, the C_m for lidocaine (0.28 μg/mg) had been exceeded in the peripheral spinal cord (1.38 μg/mg) as well as in spinal nerves in the paravertebral space (1 μg/mg). Data from other studies in which local anesthetic was injected directly into the CSF indicate that C_m is not exceeded in the dorsal root ganglion or in the more central parts of the spinal cord.[120,273]

These studies also demonstrated local anesthetic in the brain but in insufficient concentrations to produce neural blockade. However, it seems likely that large overdoses of local anesthetic may be capable of achieving C_m in brain tissue.[82]

It is most likely that diffusion into intradural spinal nerve roots (see Fig. 8-2) plays a major role during the early stages of epidural block. This is in keeping with the rapid *onset* of a segmental pattern of blockade. Subsequently, local anesthetic seepage through intervertebral foramina may contribute by producing "multiple paravertebral block" (see Fig. 8-3). After lumbar epidural block, diffusion through the CSF to the spinal cord (see Fig. 8-2) is probably a secondary phenomenon, although it may occur more rapidly when local anesthetic is injected closer to the spinal cord in thoracic blockade. Urban has reported that *regression* of analgesia after epidural block follows a circumferential pattern in the sagittal plane, rather than the classic segmental pattern seen during onset of epidural block.[499] This is consistent with a persisting action of local anesthetic on the peripheral spinal cord after the initial effects on spinal nerve roots have abated. Also, Bromage has shown reflex changes in lower limbs during thoracic epidural blockade that spares the lumbar segments.[75] Changes typical of an upper motor neuron (long tract) lesion were seen: increased deep tendon reflexes and an upgoing toe on Babinski's reflex.

Differences in vascularity of dorsal and ventral nerve roots have been found not to be a significant factor in uptake of local anesthetic,[193] and thus do not offer an explanation for the "differential" block of weak solutions of local anesthetics, especially bupivacaine, on sensory and sympathetic, rather than motor, fibers. However, Fink reported that the lengths of human dural root sleeves (approximately 5 mm) were less than three times the length of a large (motor) fiber internode. This is less than the minimum length of fiber necessary for local anesthetic blockade. Because internodal distance is directly proportional to fiber size, a larger number of internodes from sensory fibers would be exposed to local anesthetic in the dural sleeve region.[193] This tends to support an action of local anesthetics on intradural spinal nerve roots, since "differential" block with weak local anesthetic solutions can be persistent. However, local anesthetic diffuses rapidly into the CSF,[82] and thus could reach motor fibers in ventral roots by an alternative route (see Fig. 8-2).

Penetration of spinal cord depends on the local anesthetic used and its concentration. This has been confirmed by electrophysiologic studies in monkeys[156,157] (see Chap. 3). Thus, important effects of local anesthetics on the spinal cord may follow initial actions on dorsal roots and explain differences in sensory and motor blockade. Bromage's data[82] indicate that all local anesthetics reach the spinal cord in significant "blocking" concentrations. Penetration to different structures in the cord then depends on physicochemical and perhaps other properties. Thus, drugs with low lipid solubility, such as lidocaine, penetrate predominantly to superficial areas of the spinal cord, such as spinothalamic tracts and sympathetic excitatory tracts.[77] Highly lipid-soluble etidocaine could penetrate to deeply placed long motor tracts (upper motor neuron type of block).[77] If etidocaine reached the dorsal motor horn in high concentrations, it could abolish descending modulation of pain—thus producing an antianalgesic effect (see Fig. 24-3).

Evidence from pharmacokinetic and analgesic efficacy studies of epidural opioids give further insights, since molecular weights and physicochemical properties of opioids have similarities to local anesthetics (see Table 28-3). Epidural opioids have their predominant site of action in the superficial layer of dorsal horn (substantia gelatinosa). Lipid-soluble drugs, such as sufentanil, have an almost immediate onset of action in animal studies[141] and an onset time of 5 to 15 minutes in humans.[305a] This implies that the drug reaches the lamina II region of the dorsal horn almost instantaneously. Diffusion across the dural cuff into the CSF and then the spinal cord may be rapid for a highly lipid-soluble drug of opioid or local anesthetic class. However, another possibility is that fine posterior radicular arteries convey drug by way of branches that penetrate directly into the dorsal horn (see Fig. 28-12). Future developments may permit design of local anesthetic drugs with physicochemical properties that permit them to selectively reach the dorsal horn in high concentrations[140] and block axonal conduction of nociceptive impulses either before reaching the "transmission (T) cell" or in the axons of the T cell (see Chap. 24.2). Other drugs may be designed to combine block of nociception and motor power. These developments will depend on precise pharmacokinetic and drug effect data and on modern methods of molecular engineering. Collaboration between anesthesiologists and basic scientists with highly developed skills in structural design could yield exciting new methods of "selective" blockade of axons. Such methods are likely to be more potent for surgical and postoperative pain than spinal opioids and other drugs that act by way of inhibitory systems (see Chaps. 24.2 and 28). Also, "selective axonal blockade" would avoid the respiratory depressant effects of spinal opioids.[140]

The most likely mechanisms for rapid appearance of local anesthetic in the CSF relates to the unique anatomy of the dural cuff region. This is extensively reviewed by Shantha and Evans,[458] who point out that arachnoid proliferations and villi are plentiful along both dorsal and ventral roots. Although these "granulations" are frequently found in quadrupeds, their importance in humans is not certain. They are most plentiful in the region of the dural root sleeves ("cuffs"), immediately proximal to the dorsal root ganglion, where the dura becomes thin and is continuous with the epineurium of spinal nerves (see Fig. 8-2B). Shantha and Evans described at least five types of villi; three are shown in Figure 8-2B. They provide a mechanism by which arachnoid protrudes either partially or completely through the dura into adjacent subdural and epidural spaces. This implies that local anesthetics may only have to diffuse across a layer of arachnoid epithelial cells to reach CSF.

Even if the granulations are sparse in humans, the dura is thin in the root sleeve area and it is clear from local anesthetic[82] and opioid[141,142] studies that these drugs rapidly gain access to CSF (see also Chap. 28). These anatomic and pharmacological data provide strong evidence that the major sites of action of local anesthetics after epidural block are the spinal nerve roots and spinal cord. It seems likely that future research in the epidural administration of drugs will indeed support the results of Corning's original experiment of 1885 (see Chap. 1).[131] He inadvertently injected anesthetic into the epidural space and claimed that he had produced "spinal anesthesia and local medication of the cord" (see also Chap. 32).

Longitudinal Spread of Solutions in the Epidural Space

Studies using radiological contrast media and radioactively labeled solutions have mostly shown that these solutions tend to spread more in a cranial than a caudal direction.[96,111,213,381,466,508] However, radiological contrast media cannot be expected to accurately reflect the spread of a local anesthetic drug; mixtures of local anesthetics and radioactive substances, such as ^{131}I, may result in different rates of diffusion of the local anesthetic and the radioactive substance. Because access to the CSF is important in determining clinical effects of local anesthetics, studies that determine only longitudinal spread in the epidural space may have limited value. More useful would be studies with labeled local anesthetics in which autoradiographs were taken at different levels to determine concentrations in epidural space, CSF, spinal roots, spinal cord, and so forth.

CLINICAL CONSIDERATIONS FOR THE EFFICACY OF EPIDURAL BLOCKADE

There is no question now that epidural block can be effective in nearly all cases if attention is paid to the anatomy, physiology, and pharmacology of the technique. Yet there are still many major medical centers throughout the world that hold the belief that epidural blockade has a high failure rate compared with subarachnoid blockade. This merely serves to underline the relatively recent acquisition of relevant data on which to base the effective use of epidural block.

Assessment of Epidural Blockade

In defining important factors in effective epidural block, the development of standardized methods of assessment of epidural block has been essential:

Sensory block is graphed by testing for loss and return of pinprick sensation *(partial sensory block)* in each dermatome on both sides of the body (Fig. 8-24). An alternative method of testing initial onset is to use an alcohol swab to assess loss of temperature sensation, which is the most sensitive indicator of initial onset of sensory block (see Table 2-1). *Complete* loss of touch sensation may also be charted.[138,454]

From a "time-segment" graph, the following can be obtained: time to initial onset and complete spread of analgesia; time to regression of two segments and complete regression of analgesia (Fig. 8-24); total number of segments blocked on both sides of the body; milliliters of local anesthetic per mean segmental spread (total segments R + L divided by two); and area of the segment-time diagram (segment minutes), which can be related to the dose of local anesthetic, in segment minutes per dose. The latter expression is used to assess the development of tachyphylaxis (see below).

Sympathetic block is assessed by measuring skin temperature with a telethermometer (see Fig. 8-14), thermography, or temperature-sensitive papers. Al-

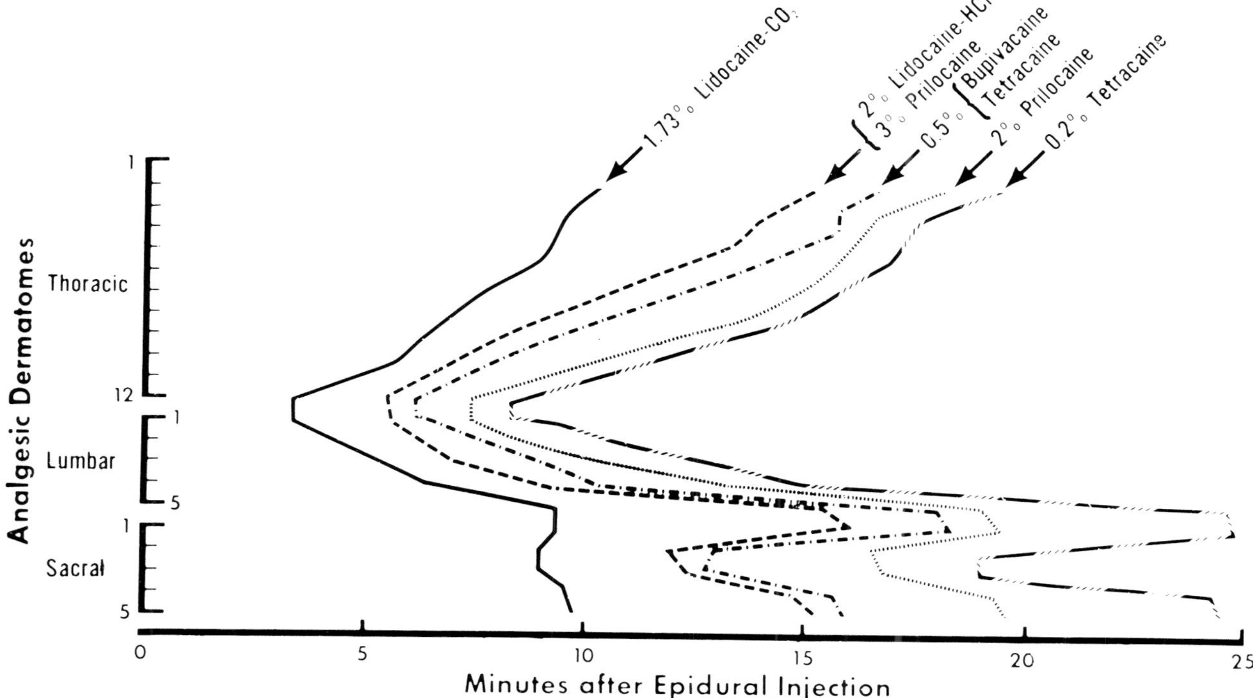

FIG. 8-24. *Sensory blockade.* Mean latency profile of 1.73% carbonated lidocaine contrasted with 2% lidocaine HCl, 2 and 3% prilocaine, 0.5% bupivacaine, and 0.2% tetracaine. All solutions contained 1:200,000 epinephrine. Injection was given at the second lumbar interspace. (Reproduced with permission from Bromage, P.R.: Epidural Analgesia. Philadelphia, W.B. Saunders, 1978.)

ternatively, a digital plethysmogram may be used (see Fig. 13-6). Skin conductance can be measured in the clinical setting by use of the psychogalvanic response; reliable measurements are much more difficult than usually acknowledged. More precise, but of research application only, are the use of various sweat tests, such as cobalt blue and starch iodine, or the response of skin plethysmography to ice during venous occlusion plethysmography (see Figs. 13-6, 13-14). A full discussion of the clinical and laboratory tests of sympathetic block is given in Chapter 13.

Motor block is usually assessed by use of the Bromage scale for motor blockade in the lower limbs.[72]

Bromage Scale

No block (0%)	Full flexion of knees and feet possible
Partial (33%)	Just able to flex knees, still full flexion of feet possible
Almost complete (66%)	Unable to flex knees. Still flexion of feet
Complete (100%)	Unable to move legs or feet

Motor blockade in the lower limbs can be assessed with reference to specific myotomes (*e.g.*, L2 hip flexion).[454] A score of 0 is assigned for no block, and 1 for complete block (no movement) at each joint, on each side. Thus maximal motor block is present bilaterally with a score of 10:

	Right	Left	
Hip flexion (L2)	1	1	
Knee extension (L3)	1	1	
Ankle dorsiflexion (L4)	1	1	
Great toe dorsiflexion (L5)	1	1	
Ankle plantar flexion (S1)	1	1	
	5 +	5 = 10	(complete motor block)

This test removes some observer error because only a "move" (0) or "no move" (1) decision needs to be made at each joint.

An onset profile for motor blockade can be presented as a "myotome score/time" diagram.

For research purposes, Axelsson reported an apparatus that measures maximal isometric strength by a force transducer, at ankle, knee, and hip. This provides objective, reproducible measurements of muscle power.[12]

Abdominal muscle power may be assessed by the rectus abdominus muscle (RAM) test.[509] This is useful in abdominal surgery when abdominal muscle blockade is required rather than lower limb muscle blockade. On the other hand, the Bromage scale is useful for lower limb surgery. Both scales may be used when a comprehensive picture is required: RAM-test (T5–T12) and Bromage scale (L1–S2).

"RAM" Test of Abdominal Muscles

100%	Able to rise from supine to sitting position with hands behind head
80% power	Can sit only with arms extended
60% power	Can lift only head and scapulae off bed
40% power	Can lift only shoulders off bed
20%	An increase in abdominal muscle tension can be felt during effort. No other response.

Testing of 100% and 80% power has limitations in patients with vasodilation; blood pressure and pulse rate must be carefully monitored if these tests are to be used.

A broad comparison of agents used for epidural block can be compiled based on their "success rate" in producing motor and sensory block. Because different methods of testing have been used in many studies, the comparisons are only qualitative (Fig. 8-25).

EMG. Few studies have used the more quantitative method of electromyography (EMG), although this would provide more sensitive assessment.

Reflex Response. Under general anesthesia without muscle relaxation, sensation can still be crudely assessed by use of reflex response to pinch by a forceps at appropriate segmental levels. Alternatively, the tendon reflexes in the lower limbs give a gross index of both motor and sensory block, while reflexes such as those of the cremaster, anal, and abdominal may also be useful as a gross guide to adequacy of blockade.

FACTORS AFFECTING EPIDURAL BLOCKADE

Many factors may affect the efficacy, spread of blockade, fiber types blocked, and other aspects of epidural blockade. These are summarized in Table 8-14 and are discussed below.

Site of Injection and Nerve Root Size

It can readily be seen from the time-segment diagram in Figure 8-24 that blockade tends to be most intense and has the most rapid onset close to the site of injection. The subsequent spread of analgesia depends to some extent on whether the injection is made in thoracic or lumbar regions.

After *lumbar epidural* injection, analgesia spreads in the manner shown in Figure 8-24. There is a somewhat greater cranial than caudal spread and there may be a delay in the L5 and S1 segments. The delay in onset at these segments appears to be due to the large size of these nerve roots.[217]

After *midthoracic epidural* injection, analgesia spreads quite evenly from the site of injection. However, the upper thoracic and lower cervical segments are resistant to blockade because of the large size of the nerve roots and the large number of nerve fibers within them. Repeated doses by the midthoracic route eventually may cause analgesia to spread into lumbar and sacral segments, with the expected lag in onset at L5–S1. Careful control of dose in the thoracic region permits sparing of the lumbar segments and, thus, avoidance of sympathetic block in the lower limbs and maintenance of normal bladder function—that is, a true segmental block. Similarly, a small dose injected at L2–3 for labor pain may block only T11 and L3–4 segments, while it spares the sacral segments.

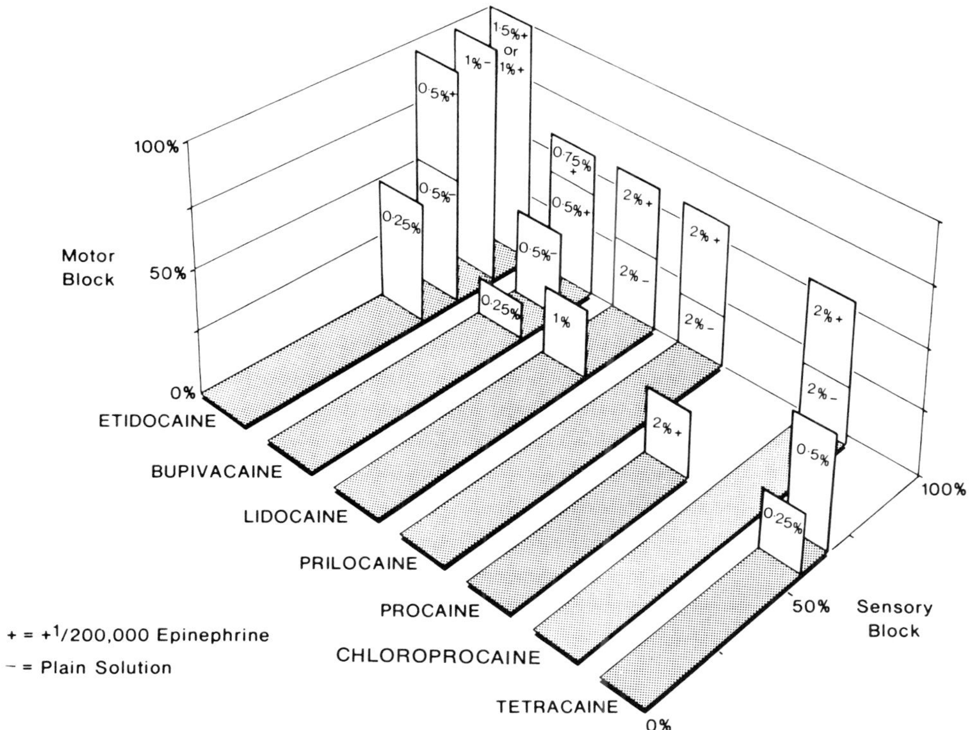

FIG. 8-25. Motor and sensory block percentage success rate. Comparison of agents, concentrations, and addition of epinephrine are based on subjective data, so that only approximate comparisons can be made.

The profile of onset of *caudal* epidural block spreads upward from S5, and the S1 segment is the last to be blocked, as expected (see Fig. 9-9).

Weight, Age, and Height

There appears to be no correlation between spread of analgesia and weight in adults. However, Bromage found a correlation between age and dose requirements when more than 2000 patients between ages 4 and 102 years were assessed by a standard technique[69,76]: An increase in dose requirements was found from ages 4 to 18, and a gradual decrease in dose requirements from ages 19 to 104. The increasing dose requirements from childhood to adulthood has been confirmed by Schulte-Steinberg and Rahlfs.[439,440] However, if one examines the data for dose requirements between ages 20 and 40, there is a variation of 1 to 1.6 ml of 2% lidocaine per segment. This variation shows little difference in this age-group. At the extremes of age, it does seem necessary to reduce dosage. However, this is more predictable in children (see Chap. 21) on the basis of age; in adults, other factors, such as the presence of pregnancy[67,81,242] and arteriosclerosis,[70,240] also require consideration. Interestingly, a recent study showed high levels of blockade in patients 60 to 80 years of age regardless of dose.[461]

TABLE 8-14. FACTORS AFFECTING EPIDURAL BLOCKADE

Site of injection and nerve root size
Weight (? no), age, height
Posture — sitting (? minimal)
— lateral (? yes)
Local anesthetic agent
Dose (? volume/concentration)
Addition of epinephrine
Carbon dioxide solutions
Number and frequency of injections
? Injection by needle compared with catheter

Increases in longitudinal spread (and duration) of analgesia, with increasing age, have been attributed to reduced lateral leakage of solution, owing to progressive sclerotic closure of intervertebral foramina[76] (see Fig. 8-3). This is supported by measurements of epidural pressure that were found to be higher after epidural injection in old patients; by evidence from epidurograms showing more extensive spread in the elderly; by external counting of a mixture of lidocaine and ^{131}I solution injected epidurally.[76,77,381] However, Burn and co-workers[96] did not find a consistent correlation between reduced lateral spread of solution and greater longitudinal flow. Other studies have, in general, supported the relationship of declining dose requirements with increasing age. However, it has been shown that the relationship is more complex than originally proposed.[240,241,397,398,461]

In practical terms, a range of 1 to 1.6 ml of 2% lidocaine per segment can be used in adults between ages 20 and 40 years, and further adjustments are then made on the basis of height, site of injection (Table 8-15), and pathophysiologic state.

Bromage reported a trend to increasing dose requirements with increased height, although the correlation is weak when injections are made in the lumbar region.[69] A dose of 1 ml per segment is adequate for most patients 5 feet tall (150 cm), whereas a dose of 1.6 ml per segment is sufficient for most patients 6 feet tall (180 cm; Table 8-15). A simple rule of thumb is to use 1 ml per segment for 5 feet of height, and then to add 0.1 ml per segment for each 2 inches (each 5 cm) over 5 feet.

It is wise to check that the dosage to be delivered is safe (see Table 4-1), and one should reduce dosage to about 50% for aged patients. Thus, 500 mg plain lidocaine or 600 mg with epinephrine is acceptable in a healthy adult, while 200 to 250 mg of plain lidocaine is a reasonable dose in an 80-year-old. As noted below, 30% reductions are recommended for pregnancy, and 50% reductions for severe arteriosclerosis.

TABLE 8-15. DOSE CALCULATION FOR EPIDURAL BLOCK WITH 2% LIDOCAINE IN NORMAL ADULTS

Site of Injection	Height	Volume	Maximum Dose*
Lumbar region	5 feet (150 cm)	1 ml/segment	(Lidocaine) or equipotent dose of other agent
	+2 inches (5 cm)	Add 0.1 ml/segment for each 2 inches (5 cm) above 5 feet	500 mg at 20 yr 200 mg at 80 yr
Midthoracic region		70% of above	

*Caution should be taken with dosage in obstetrics. A 30% reduction may be required.[67,81] In patients with arteriosclerosis, a 50% reduction may be needed.[70] In both of these situations, *incremental* doses are advised. A further "rule of thumb" for 2% lidocaine solution (+ epi) or eqivalent: 20–40 years: 1 to 1.5 ml/segment, adjusted for height; 40–60 years: 0.5 to 1 ml/segment, adjusted for height; 60–80 years: 0.3 to 0.6 ml/segment, adjusted for height.

Posture

Comparison of *sitting and lateral positions* for epidural block reveals no significant differences in cephalad spread.[353,396] An exception is the obese patient, who achieves a lower level of block when seated.[264] Caudad spread of block in seated patients was reported to be marginally less in one study;[353] another reported that caudad spread of analgesia was slightly favored by the sitting position.[69] From these studies it seems that the differences between sitting and lateral position are small. The *lateral position* favors spread of analgesia to the dependent side in both pregnant and nonpregnant patients,[10,160,241,277,353,454] but the differences are small. In surgical patients, however, Seow and associates found that onset of sensory and motor block was significantly more rapid on the dependent side and had a longer duration (Fig. 8-26A). In addition to being more rapid in onset, motor blockade was greater on the dependent side at all time intervals tested out to 40 minutes after injection (Fig. 8-26B). Onset time for sympathetic block was not faster on the dependent side, but duration of maximum elevation of skin temperature was greater on the dependent side.[454] The differences in sensory and motor block are great enough to indicate an advantage in lying patients on the operative side during epidural block before lower limb surgery.[454]

Speed of Injection

Increasing the speed of injection has no effect on bulk flow of solutions in the epidural space.[96,381] Also, spread of analgesia is only minimally influenced. However, rapid injection of large volumes of solution may increase CSF pressure,[230] decrease spinal cord blood flow, increase intracranial pressure, and pose a risk of spinal or cerebral complications. In susceptible patients sudden increases in CSF pressure may compromise spinal cord blood flow (see Chap. 29.1), and this may increase susceptibility to neurotoxicity[230] or, in atherosclerotics, may possibly cause "spinal stroke." There is evidence that nutritive vessels crossing the perineurium of nerves are subject to a pathologic "valve" mechanism initiated by perineur-

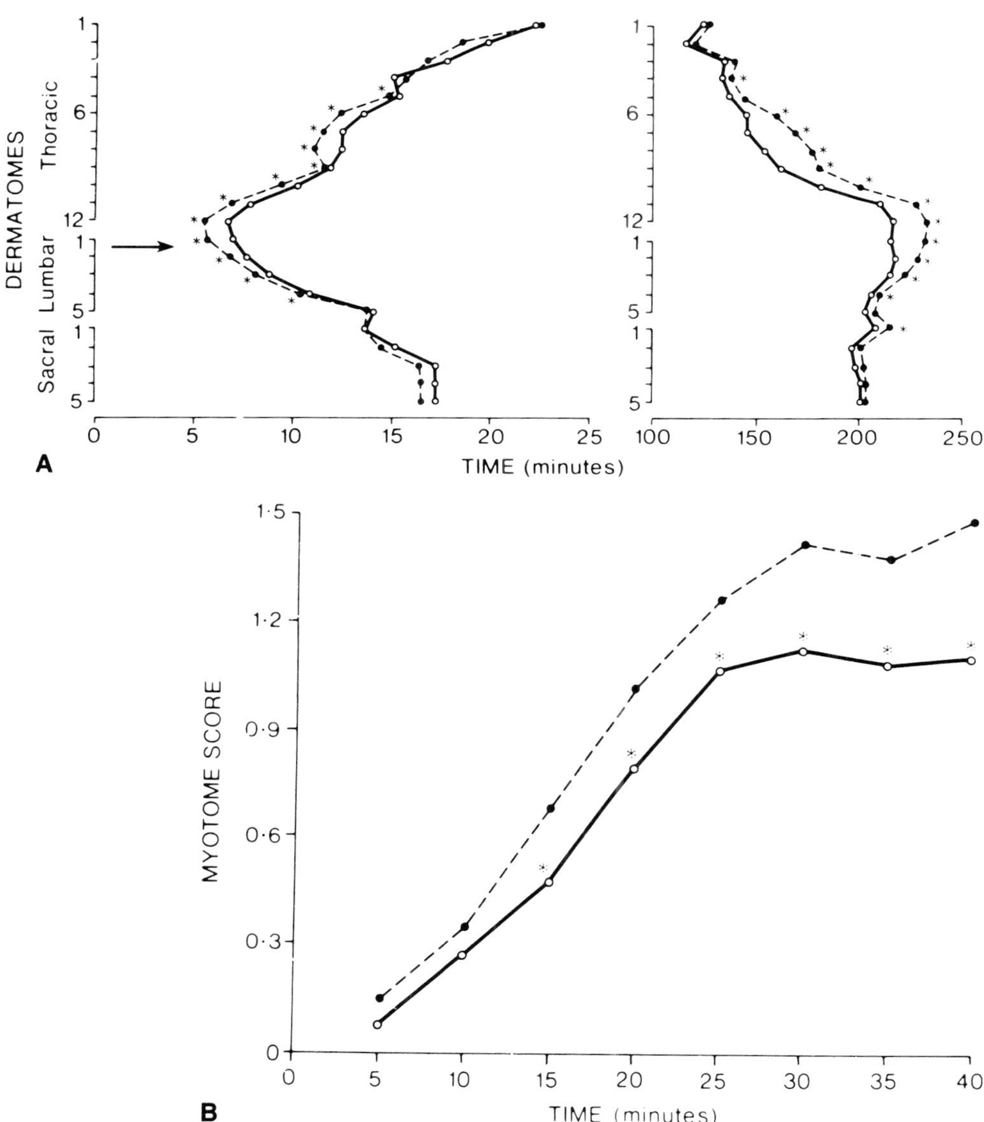

FIG. 8-26. **A.** Mean time-segment diagram for partial sensory blockade at each dermatome level. Data points plotted are mean values. → Site of injection of local anesthetic; *Denotes significant difference between the (● - - ●) dependent and (O—O) nondependent sides ($p < 0.05$). A similar time-segment diagram for complete sensory blockade was obtained, with significant difference between the two sides for dermatomes T8–L4 inclusive for onset profile and T8–L3 inclusive for sensory regression profile. **B.** Mean myotome score for total number of myotomes with complete motor blockade at each time interval after administration of epidural blockade (maximum possible number = 10 myotomes, that is, five for each right and left side). *Denotes significant difference between (● - - ●) dependent and nondependent (O—O) sides ($p < 0.05$). (Reproduced with permission from Seow, L.T., Lips, F.J., and Cousins, M.J.: Effect of lateral posture on epidural blockade for surgery. Anaesth. Intensive Care, *11*:97, 1983.)

ial edema.[331] This edema could be initiated by sudden increases in CSF pressure. Subsequent hypotension owing to sympathetic block may decrease spinal cord flow if CSF pressure and perineurial pressure remain high. A combination of these effects could result in neural damage (see also Chap. 29.1).

Sudden increases in intracerebral pressure may cause headache, cerebral hemorrhage, or isolated hemorrhage in a small vessel, such as a retinal vessel. Headache is commonly reported if epidural solutions are injected rapidly. Intraocular hemorrhage has been described after rapid epidural injection of 30 ml of solution of local anesthetic.[114] Thus, rapid injection is not only ineffective in "forcing solution up the epidural space," but also potentially dangerous. Local anesthetics should be injected into the epidural space slowly and preferably in incremental doses.

Volume, Concentration, and Dose of Local Anesthetic

Early concepts of epidural block as a "multiple paravertebral block" led to a firmly held view that the local anesthetic solution had to diffuse widely up and down the epidural space if extensive blockade was required. Thus, the early proponents of high epidural block used large volumes (60 – 100 ml) of dilute local anesthetic (1.0% – 1.5% procaine).[172,244]

Extensive studies by Bromage indicated that the dose of drug (concentration × volume) determined the spread of analgesia,[76] at least between the concentrations of 2% and 5% lidocaine and 0.2% and 0.5% tetracaine. However, data were not obtained to compare 0.5% lidocaine with a range of 1% to 2%, which is a typical clinical range of concentrations. It did appear from Bromage's data that dose requirements diminished from about 30 mg per segment to 20 mg per segment when concentration was reduced from 2% to 1% lidocaine. Erdmeir and colleagues have shown that 30 ml of 1% lidocaine produced a higher sensory level than 10 ml of a 3% solution.[189] Burn and colleagues showed that large volumes of contrast media (40 ml) were more likely to spread into cervical regions compared with higher concentrations and smaller volumes (20 ml).[96]

With regard to motor blockade, dosage becomes less important when dilute solutions are used. Below concentrations of 1% lidocaine, motor block is minimal regardless of dose, unless injections are repeated at intervals. Then intensity of sensory and motor block increases with each successive injection. Dr. Robert Hingson used the analogy of "repainting the fence" to describe the gradual ripening and deepening of blockade with successive epidural doses. This mechanism is important in obstetric analgesia when using dilute solutions of 0.125% or 0.065% bupivacaine.

Increasing dosage results in a linear increase in degree of *sensory block* and duration of epidural block, while increasing concentration results in a reduction in onset time and intensity of motor blockade (see also Fig. 8-25). A general summary of the effects of local anesthetic dose and added epinephrine is given in Table 4-2. However, it should be recognized that choice of drug influences these effects.

Choice of Local Anesthetic

The concept of a "spectrum" of local anesthetics depicted in Figure 4-8 relates significantly to epidural block. The great flexibility of sensory and motor block that can be obtained by careful choice of drug is seen in Figure 8-25. For example, 0.25% bupivacaine may provide satisfactory analgesia for acute pain with close to zero motor block, while 0.25% etidocaine results in close to 50% motor block, but variable analgesia.

If more potent analgesia with minimal motor block is required, then 0.5% bupivacaine or 2% plain lidocaine may be chosen, although the former is the best choice for continuous techniques. The requirements of profound sensory block and excellent muscle relaxation (*e.g.*, for surgery or operative obstetrics) are best met by 2% lidocaine with epinephrine or 1.5% etidocaine (if long duration is required).[329]

Procaine, dibucaine, and tetracaine are not usually chosen for epidural block because of their rather inferior sensory and motor blocking properties. An exception may be the use of tetracaine if chloroprocaine is unavailable and amides are thought to be contraindicated.

Chloroprocaine has become an attractive alternative for short procedures and for obstetric analgesia; it is a safe drug because of its high rate of metabolism (however, see Table 4-7 and Chap. 4).

Use of prilocaine for epidural block is worthy of consideration. It is still the safest amide agent when used in a dose of less than 600 mg and should be considered for single-shot epidural block, except in obstetrics. Of practical use, the 2% plain solution provides intense sensory block and minimal motor block which is associated with plasma levels similar to the 2% epinephrine-containing solution, provided dose is below 400 mg. This solution has appeal for outpatient caudal blocks or for single-shot epidural block for brief procedures. Alternatively, the 3% solution may be used if rapid onset is required, although a 20-ml dose produces some degree of motor block even with the plain solution (Table 8-16).

Differential Block. The differential capabilities of local anesthetics to block sensory and motor fibers has been referred to as "sensory-motor dissociation" (see Fig. 8-25). The basis for this phenomenon is unknown: Different *rates* of development of sensory and motor block for different local anesthetics seems to be important, as discussed below. Differential penetration of spinal cord also seems likely to play a part[75] (see "Site of Action" above). This could be in keeping with observations of sensory-motor dissociation in peripheral nerve block where access to motor fibers may also play a part. Wildsmith and others[528] reported that, as lipid solubility increased within a series of amino-ester local anesthetics, the *rate* of development of A (motor) fiber blockade increased. At equipotent concentrations of the various drugs, A (motor) fibers were *more sensitive* than C (pain) fibers.[528] These results agree with those of Gissen and

TABLE 8-16. CHOICE OF AGENT FOR EPIDURAL BLOCK

Application and Requirements	Agent(s)	Comment
Surgical analgesia (medium to long duration) Sensory +++ Motor +++	2% Lidocaine (HCl or CO_2) +	Rapid onset, excellent analgesia and motor block, medium duration
	3% Chloroprocaine	For brief procedures only. Rapid onset.
	1.5%–1% Etidocaine ±	Rapid onset, profound analgesia and motor block, long duration
	0.5%–0.75% Bupivacaine	Slow onset, good analgesia, moderate motor block, long duration
	2% Mepivacaine	Similar to lidocaine. Can be used for medium duration if epinephrine is undesirable.
	3% Prilocaine –	Single-shot techniques. Dose of <600 mg, low toxicity
Postoperative or post-trauma pain (long duration) Sensory +++ Motor O	0.25%–0.5% Bupivacaine –	Slow onset, long duration of sensory analgesia with little motor blockade (0.25%)
Obstetric analgesia (long duration) Sensory ++ Motor O	0.125%–0.5% Bupivacaine –	0.125%–0.25% may be brief duration
	1% Lidocaine-CO_2 +	Useful for resistant "missed segments" Rapid onset, medium duration
Obstetric surgery or instrumental delivery (medium to long duration) Sensory +++ Motor ++	3% Chloroprocaine + 2% Lidocaine +	Considerations similar to surgical analgesia (Note: 0.25% bupivacaine is not potent enough and 0.5% bupivacaine provides inadequate analgesia in 5%–10% of patients. Bupivacaine 0.75% not recommended for obstetrics.
Diagnostic and therapeutic neural blockade Range of blockade from sympathetic to motor	0.5%–2% Lidocaine	0.5%– sympathetic, 1%– sensory, 2%+ motor blockade, for diagnostic blockade
	0.25% Bupivacaine	May be useful for diagnostic blockade requiring long-duration sensory block with no motor block, also used for "therapeutic block" (see Chap. 27)

+ = with epinephrine; – = without epinephrine.
Note: This table does not (and cannot) cover all the shades of difference between agents. See also Tables 3-1 and 4-1 and Chapter 4.

associates[229] and Fink[193,195] for amino-amide local anesthetics as far as *sensitivity* is concerned. However, Wildsmith and co-workers[528] stressed that *rate of onset* of motor block varied greatly, so that drugs of relatively low lipid solubility (*e.g.*, procaine) had a slow *onset* of motor blockade compared with sensory blockade. In contrast, highly lipid-soluble amethocaine blocked A fibers more rapidly than it blocked C fibers. This explains the confusion aroused by these new studies (differences in onset of sensory and motor block *for different agents*) and old studies using only procaine (sensory fibers always blocked before motor fibers). This is discussed in an excellent review by Wildsmith.[527]

The phenomenon of "frequency dependent conduction block" (see Fig. 2-8) is discussed in Chapter 2.

Exciting new possibilities for providing selective blockade of pain conduction[142] while sensory, motor, and sympathetic function remain intact are presented in Chapter 28.

Local Anesthetic Mixtures. Amide–amide and amide–ester mixtures enjoyed a period of popularity because of perceived improvement in rapidity of onset combined with increased duration of analgesia. However, there are no well-documented advantages in the use of such mixtures for epidural blockade. Thus, there is no rationale for use of mixtures, particularly when an epidural catheter is used and a rapid-acting agent can be used initially followed by a long-acting agent if desired.

A time-honored mixture of an ester and an amide has been 0.2% tetracaine and 1.5% lidocaine; it is claimed to have rapid onset and long duration,[363] but objective data are lacking. In the obstetric setting, Cohen and Thurlow found that the solution of a mixture of chloroprocaine–bupivacaine had a duration of analgesia that was *shorter* than that of a solution of bupivacaine alone.[124] This reduced duration has been attributed in part to a decrease in *p*H of approximately 3.0[219] (see also Chap. 4 and Table 4-7). Decreased *p*H would decrease the amount of bupivacaine available in the uncharged base form, thus decreasing the concentration gradient from outside to inside neurons and decreasing number of molecules penetrating into the neuron. If *p*H is corrected, duration of block with chloroprocaine–bupivacaine increases.[219] Also, data from isolated nerve studies suggest that a metabolite of chloroprocaine may inhibit the binding of bupivacaine to membrane receptor sites.[130] Mixtures of amides also offer little advantage in epidural block. In a randomized prospective double-blind study of mixtures of various concentrations of lidocaine and bupivacaine, no significant differences in onset of blockade were observed among the solutions tested (see Fig. 8-24).[454] Time to regression of blockade was positively correlated with increasing dosage of bupivacaine in the solutions. However, duration of regression of two segments of sensory blockade with a 50% mixture of lidocaine–bupivacaine (89 minutes) was only marginally greater than for lidocaine alone (76 minutes). Onset of complete motor blockade was fastest and the degree of motor blockade most profound with the mixture containing equal proportions of lidocaine and bupivacaine (see Fig. 8-27). Pharmacokinetics of individual drugs were unaltered in any of the mixtures (see Fig. 8-27). The authors concluded that there seemed to be little advantage of any of these mixtures if a catheter technique were to be used. Only when a single-dose (through the needle) technique is used does the 1 : 1 mixture of lidocaine–bupivacaine have some merit in achieving rapid onset of profound motor blockade, followed by some increases in duration of analgesia compared with lidocaine alone; however, the gains are small.[454]

The potential for amide agents to produce CNS toxicity and cardiovascular depression is generally similar for equipotent doses. Because pharmacokinetics are not altered in amide mixtures toxic potential would seem to be additive, as indicated in animal studies[369] (see Chap. 4). However, large doses of bupivacaine given rapidly intravascularly pose a greater risk of "cardiac toxicity" than do large doses of lidocaine (see Fig. 4-12 and Table 4-5). In theory, reducing the dose of bupivacaine by "making up" the total dose with lidocaine may reduce the risk of cardiac toxicity; however, there are no data to support this approach. More important is use of the appropriate single agent and dose and *slow, incremental* injection.

Epinephrine

There is general agreement that addition of epinephrine reduces vascular absorption to a variable extent (Tables 3-6 through 3-12 and Figs. 3-16, 3-18) and enhances the efficacy of epidural blockade. However, with respect to efficacy, the following distinctions must be drawn: Enhancement of blockade is much less marked with the longer-acting agents bupivacaine and etidocaine; addition of fresh epinephrine in a concentration of 1 : 200,000 may enhance the intensity of motor block, quality of sensory blockade, and duration of blockade at least for lidocaine and prilocaine.[72,80]

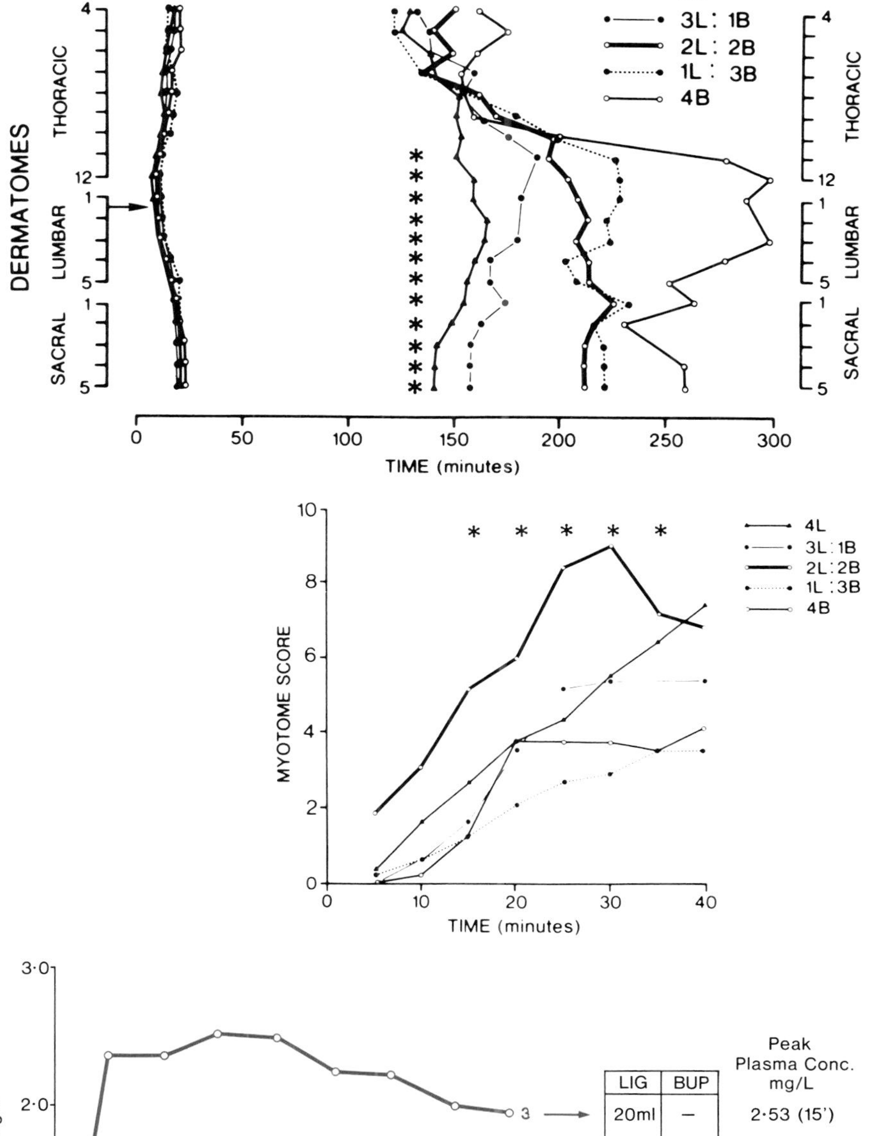

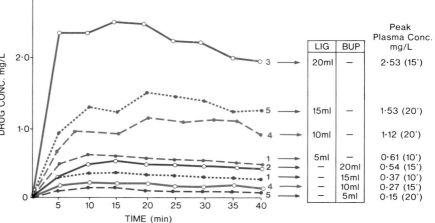

FIG. 8-27. Epidural block and local anesthetic mixtures. **Upper Panel.** Mean time-segment diagram for partial sensory blockade at each dermatome level. Data points plotted are mean values. (→) = site of injection of local anesthetics; *denotes significant difference among groups ($p < .05$). A similar time-segment diagram for complete sensory blockade was obtained. **Middle Panel.** Mean myotome score at each time-interval after epidural injection. **Bottom Panel.** Epidural block and local anesthetic mixtures: pharmacokinetics. The solutions are the same as in the upper panel. Peak blood concentrations from components of mixtures are almost identical to those anticipated from injection of the same dose of the component by itself. However, the time to achievement of peak blood concentration is altered by mixtures of short- and long-acting agents. (Reproduced with permission from Seow, L.T., Lips, F.J., Mather, L.E., and Cousins, M.J: Lidocaine and bupivacaine mixtures for epidural blockade. Anesthesiology, *56*:177, 1982.)

As indicated in Table 3-3, the combination of local vasoconstriction owing to epinephrine and acidity owing to antioxidants in premixed epinephrine-containing solutions may lower tissue *p*H below 7 for more than 90 minutes. This theoretically would result in reduced release of local anesthetic base and reduced penetration of neural tissue. It has been proposed that this may be responsible for increased latency to onset of sensory blockade.[80]

Despite these considerations, addition of fresh epinephrine to local anesthetic, *at the time of injection,* does not prolong the onset of clinical epidural or subarachnoid neural blockade with lidocaine or buipvacaine. In fact, with lidocaine of etidocaine the opposite has been reported[55,370] (Fig. 8-28). A controlled study comparing commercially prepared epinephrine-containing solutions with solutions containing freshly added epinephrine is not available. However, reduced tissue *p*H results from epinephrine-containing solutions regardless of whether the solution has a *p*H of 3.5 or 6.5, so that adding epinephrine freshly may not have a great advantage. Another effect of epidurally administered epinephrine has become apparent: inhibitory receptors in the dorsal horn of the spinal cord are responsive to epidural or subarachnoid administration of α-agonists.[414] In one study in dogs, clonidine was as effective as epinephrine in prolonging duration of sensory blockade of subarachnoid tetracaine. Interestingly, clonidine was more effective in prolonging motor blockade.[19] Because clonidine does not produce vasoconstriction, it seems that at least part of the enhancement of analgesia seen with epinephrine is due to activation of dorsal horn inhibitory systems (see Chap. 28).

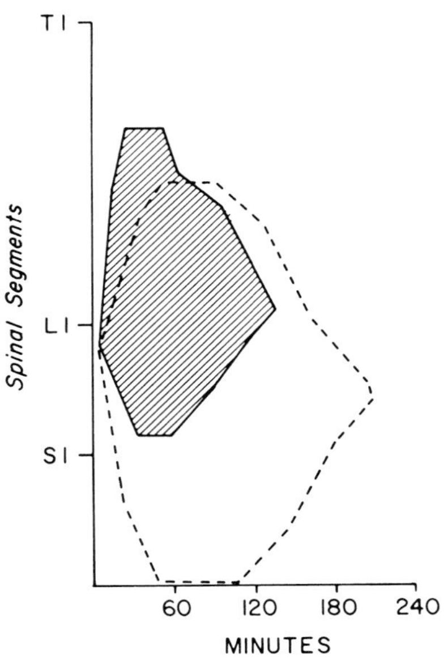

FIG. 8-28. Effect of epinephrine; segmental spread and duration of sensory blockade for lidocaine. Segmental spread and duration of analgesia are enhanced by addition of epinephrine. Caudad spread of analgesia is also markedly improved with epinephrine-containing solutions. *Broken line*, + epinephrine (5 μg/ml); *solid line*, plain solution. (Murphy, T.M., Mather, L.E., Stanton-Hicks, M.D.A., Bonica, J.J., *et al.*: Effects of adding adrenaline to etidocaine and Lignocaine in extradural anaesthesia: I. Block characteristics and cardiovascular effects. Br. J. Anaesth., *48*:893, 1976.)

Carbon Dioxide Salts

In vitro data indicate a tenfold increase in uptake of lidocaine base into neural tissue when the same dose of lidocaine–carbon dioxide base is compared with lidocaine–hydrochloric acid base.[107] Open clinical comparisons using lumbar epidural block and caudal block show a shortened latency to onset and a more extensive spread of analgesia when lidocaine–carbon dioxide is compared with lidocaine–hydrochloric acid.[72,139] Double-blind investigations reported that carbonation improved the quality of epidural analgesia but did not affect onset of action of lidocaine or bupivacaine.[345,367] However, these studies are in contrast to double-blind studies of brachial plexus block (see Chap. 3, p. 58) and epidural block[377a] in which carbonation does enhance the onset of action. Peak blood lidocaine concentrations are slightly higher when lidocaine–carbon dioxide is used for epidural block.[345] The cost of manufacturing carbon dioxide salts of local anesthetics has so far precluded their release except in Canada.

Number and Frequency of Local Anesthetic Injections

Whether augmentation or diminution of neural blockade occurs after repeated epidural injection of local anesthetics depends on the local anesthetic agent, the number of injections, and the timing between injections (Fig. 8-29).

A single "repeat" dose (20% of total dose) given approximately 20 minutes after the main dose of local anesthetic has been said to consolidate blockade, within the level of blockade already established.

Thus, "missed segments" may be "filled in," but the level of blockade may not be extended.[63]

A second dose of approximately 50% of initial dosage will maintain the initial segmental level of analgesia if given when the upper level of segmental analgesia has receded one to two dermatomes. On the other hand, administration of the same dose as given for induction of block will result in augmentation of level of blockade at this time. Clinical practice relies on either mean duration times (Table 8-17) or careful monitoring for signs of regression of blockade, to determine the need for a second or refill dose.

A "refill" dose given more than 10 minutes outside regression of analgesia (the "interanalgesic interval") may result in tachyphylaxis. That is, an *increase* in dosage is required to maintain a constant level of blockade. Tachyphylaxis increases with the length of interanalgesic interval up to 60 minutes, but then it remains constant; at 60 minutes there is a 30% to 40% decrease in effect of a repeated dose (see Fig. 8-29).[85]

Tachyphylaxis has been most clearly demonstrated in association with "continuous" epidural block in patients in whom repeated injections of the short-acting amides, lidocaine, prilocaine, or mepivacaine, are used. Because the interanalgesic interval seems so important, it is not surprising that tachyphylaxis has been much less of a problem with the longer-acting agents, such as bupivacaine (see Fig. 8-29).

Bromage found that tachyphylaxis increased with the number of injections administered. This again indicates the desirability of using long-acting agents. Finally, it should be recalled that bupivacaine and etidocaine have a lesser tendency to accumulate in the blood, whereas the short-acting agents are associated with gradually increasing blood concentrations with increased risks of toxicity (see Figs. 3-14, 3-15).

The mechanism of tachyphylaxis is not known. It may be partly explained by *p*H changes[105] in spinal fluid with repeated injections; however, this is not an adequate explanation on its own (see Chap. 3, p. 58).

Injection by Needle or Catheter

Is there any difference in the spread of analgesia when injection is made with an epidural needle or catheter? Before answering this question, it should be noted that there is undoubtedly an increased incidence of outright failure with epidural catheter techniques and a higher incidence of complications. For example, Cousins and Mazze found a failure rate of 10%,* using catheters without stylets in 80 patients. This compares with a rate of failure of 1.2% in 84 cases when injection was made by needle. The major causes of "catheter failures" were complete inability to thread the catheter (5%); inability to clear the catheter of blood (2.5%); and threading the catheter through an intervertebral foramen (1.3%; see Table 8-18). The use of stylets to introduce catheters may reduce the incidence of failure to thread the catheter but may increase vascular cannulation. Other studies report a similar failure rate for the use of a catheter.[54,254,434,457,505]

In individual cases, failure to thread a catheter can usually be overcome (see Table 8-6 and Figs. 8-1 through 8-9), thus 5% of such "failures" should be retrievable. Even if a catheter does not completely clear of blood, a small test dose of epinephrine-containing solution can be injected to test whether the catheter is placed inside a vessel or outside a vessel that has been traumatized. Threading through a foramen can be minimized by only inserting a minimal amount of catheter. Overall the irretrievable failure

*Unpublished data.

TABLE 8-17. CLINICAL EFFECTS OF LOCAL ANESTHETIC SOLUTIONS COMMONLY USED FOR EPIDURAL BLOCKADE

Drug	Time Spread to ± Four Segments ± 1 SD (min)	Approximate Time to Two-Segment Regression ± 2 SD* (min)	Recommended "Top-Up" Time from Initial Dose* (min)
Lidocaine, 2%	15 ± 5	100 ± 40	60
Prilocaine, 2% -3%	15 ± 4	100 ± 40	60
Chloroprocaine, 2%-3%	12 ± 5	60 ± 15	45
Mepivacaine, 2%	15 ± 5	120 ± 150	60
Bupivacaine, 0.5%-0.75%	18 ± 10	200 ± 80	120
Etidocaine, 1%-1.5%	10 ± 5	200 ± 80	120

*Note top-up time is based on duration −2 SD, which encompasses the likely duration in 95% of the population. In a conscious, cooperative patient, an alternative is to use frequent checks of segmental level to indicate need to "top up." All solutions contain 1 : 200,000 epinephrine. (Data from studies of Allen, P. R., and Johnson, R. W.[7]; Cohen, S. E., and Thurlow, A.;[1,24] Bromage, P. R.;[77] Cousins, M. J., et al.[142]; Murphy, T. M., et al.[370]; and Seow, L. T., et al.[454]

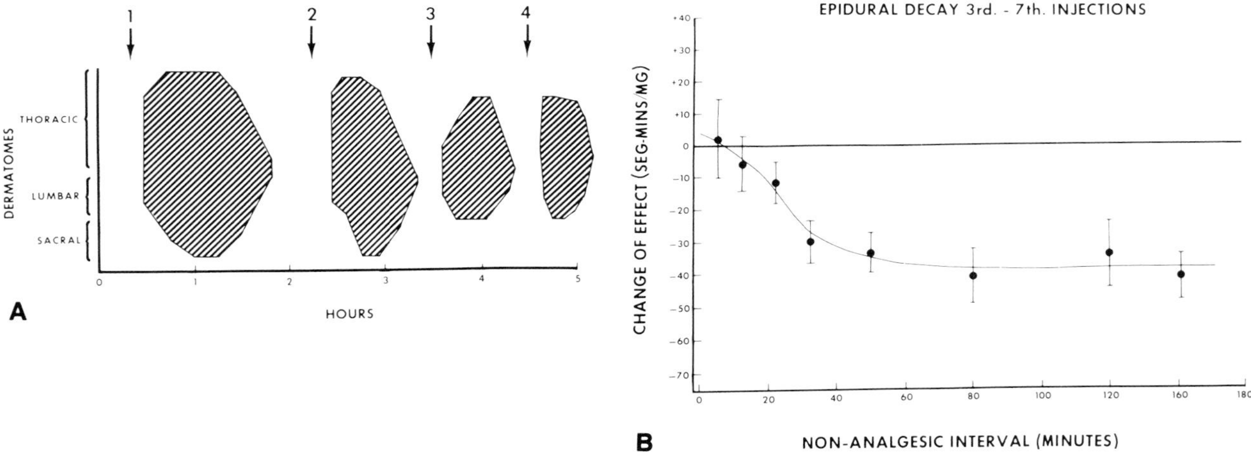

FIG. 8-29. Tachyphylaxis. **A.** Diminished segmental spread and duration of action of repeated epidural injections of the same dose of local anesthetic, injected at each arrow. Note reinjection has been made at least 30 minutes after analgesia has regressed two segments. **B.** "Nonanalgesic interval." As the time lag from loss of analgesia to reinjection exceeds 10 to 15 minutes, there is a progressive reduction in analgesic effect that reaches a maximum reduction of about 35% to 40% at 60 minutes. (Bromage, P.R., Pettigrew, R.T., and Crowell, D.E.: Tachyphylaxis in epidural analgesia: I. Augmentation and decay of local anesthesia. J. Clin. Pharmacol., 9:30, 1969.)

rate owing to catheters should be close to 1 in 100. Catheters inserted via upward slanted needles in the thoracic region tend to travel straight up the epidural space without deviating through an intervertebral foramen. Thus no catheter failures were encountered in a series of 160 blocks performed between T8 and L1 (Bromage, P.R.: Unpublished data).

TECHNIQUE OF EPIDURAL BLOCKADE

Epidural Trays

There are now a large number of commercially prepared disposable epidural trays that contain a variable number of the ideal components for epidural blockade. Individual preference plays a considerable part in choice of a tray. However, there are several desirable features:

Separation of a preparation section from the equipment section of the tray is desirable.

Glass syringes for testing loss of resistance should be of highest quality, with freely moving, snug-fitting plungers.

Disposable epidural needles should not have the "chisel" tip of the original Tuohy needle, since this increases the risk of dural puncture. Some disposable epidural needles are dangerously sharp (Fig. 8-30A).

Epidural needle stylets should fit the needle precisely, particularly at the needle tip.

Epidural catheters should be of clear material so that aspirated blood can be clearly seen in the catheter. Also, catheters should be strong and flexible, should be inert, and should not have sharp tips capable of tearing blood vessels or puncturing dura. They should also be marked for roentgenographic detection.

Local anesthetics to be used in disposable trays should be packed in sterile protective covering on the tray or in individual sterile containers. Single-use vials are available with a "top hat"-shaped cap that can easily be grasped and pulled off without contaminating the solution with particles of glass or rubber as may occur with ampuls and some types of vials.

Mixing cups should be free of any particulate matter.

Unfortunately, many disposable trays fall short of these ideals. However, sterility is guaranteed by the manufacturer, and needles and syringes should be free of imperfections.

Many anesthesiologists still prefer department-prepared trays, which contain all items decided on by that particular group. This works well in a practice in which all can agree on a "standard" tray and a dedicated and skilled staff prepare the trays to ensure sterility and exclusion of chemical materials that may

TABLE 8-18. EPIDURAL FAILURES: LUMBAR INJECTION BY NEEDLE COMPARED WITH CATHETER

	Injection by Needle	Injection by Catheter	
Number	84	80	
Total failures	2 (2.4%)*	12 (15%)*	
Cause of failure	Inadequate dose, 1	Catheter unable to thread	4†
	Incorrect needle placement, 1	Catheter threaded, but no analgesia	3
		Patchy block	1
		Blood in catheter, unable to clear	2
		Unisegmental block	1
		Dural tap in effort to pass catheter	1
Irretrievable failure	1 (1.2%)	8 (10%)†	

*$p < 0.001$: Mann-Whitney U test for nonparametric data (Cousins, M. J., and Mazze, R. I.: Unpublished data).

†A catheter stylet may improve the success rate for threading catheters but may also increase other complications, such as vascular cannulation. The group of catheter threading failures were potentially retrievable by injecting the whole dose by way of the needle or by moving to another interspace, thus necessitating a further needle insertion with its potential complications.

be neurolytic. In smaller hospitals that use epidural trays infrequently, commercial trays may be a valuable insurance against chemical and bacterial contamination. Larger units may prefer to design their own trays and use carefully maintained, reusable, high-quality needles and syringes. The following "traps" should be avoided.

Syringe barrels and plungers should be kept together, since "odds" may not fit with the precision required for loss of resistance testing. Powder or other material on syringe plungers may result in sticking, which can be dangerous if entry into the epidural space is missed, particularly above the level of L1.

Epidural needles should be skillfully machined and maintained, so that rough and sharp edges are avoided. Stylets must fit perfectly to avoid tissue damage or plunges in the end of the needle.

Epidural local anesthetics must be carefully sterilized, using a technique approved by a trained pharmacist, so that sterility, potency, and freedom from chemical contamination are ensured.

Hospital prepared anesthetic trays should have the date of sterilization marked on the outside of the pack and a sterilization indicator included inside the pack.

Epidural Needles

As for spinal analgesia, a close-fitting removable stylet is essential for epidural anesthesia, to prevent plugging of the needle tip with skin and failure to recognize loss of resistance. The possibility of a large epidermal plug being carried into the epidural or subarachnoid space must also be avoided. The epidural space can also be identified by compression of a 10- to 20-ml air-filled syringe attached to a 22-gauge Greene or Whitacre spinal needle; this is a useful teaching aid while performing lumbar puncture and may also be an alternative technique for single-shot epidural block. The "standard" Tuohy needle has a gentle curve of the "Huber" tip but with a rather sharp point at the end and this is favored by some experienced epiduralists. For the novice, a rounded blunt needle end of the Huber tip is less likely to puncture the dura[497] (Fig. 30A). This type of needle end also permits easier identification of the ligamentum flavum, sometimes requiring considerable force to penetrate the ligament. Some authorities like to teach with a 16-gauge needle and then let the novice "graduate" to an 18-gauge needle.

A useful refinement is the Scott needle, which has the shaft protruding from the hub.[141] This permits easier threading and advancement of epidural catheters, particularly with 18-gauge catheters, which sometimes kink and curl within the standard hub. Calibrated needles with centimeter markings also are available.[174,319]

The 18-gauge Crawford, thin-walled needle is often used for the paramedian, "paraspinous" (lateral) approach, since a catheter threads directly up the epidural space if the needle is angled at 45° to 60° upward. With a Tuohy needle, the catheter is sometimes difficult to thread with this approach, since the recurved needle tip is angled back against the ligamentum flavum or lamina. However, the Crawford needle with its "front end" orifice is more likely to penetrate the tissues, like an "apple corer," and to become plugged with tissue fragments than is the

Tuohy needle with its recured orifice. Other needles, such as the large Cheng[110] and Crawley needles[131] and the fine 22-gauge Wagner needle,[437] are less commonly used, since they have little advantage over standard needles.

"Winged needles" are ideal for "hanging-drop" techniques, since the grip on the needle should be well away from the fluid drop on the hub of the needle. Many variants of the original Labat winged needle are available, and detachable wings made of plastic have also been designed[529] for use with standard Tuohy needles. Some anesthesiologists prefer more versatile and more solid "spool"-type needles with a Barker style of hub, (*e.g.*, the Bromage needle).[68]

Epidural Catheters

Plastic epidural catheters have replaced those made of other materials. There are various plastic materials and no systematic study has been made of the requirements for epidural catheters and the features of different plastic materials. Sporadic information only is available. For example, some Teflon catheters were found to kink and this led to breakages in the wall. Bromage has summarized ideal characteristics: biochemical inertness, low coefficient of friction, high tensile strength, maneuverable rigidity, kink resistance, atraumatic tip, depth indicators, radiopacity. A stylet is not recommended, since it increases the risk of trauma to blood vessels, nerve roots, and so on. One catheter (the Racz catheter) has a stainless steel coil at the tip that makes the tip flexible. This is reported to decrease the chance of penetrating an epidural vein (see Chap. 29.2).

Epidural Cannulas

In an attempt to overcome the risk of pulling a catheter back through a Tuohy needle and shearing it off, epidural "cannula-over-needle" equipment was developed—analogous to intravascular equipment. This includes the Winnie–Jelco cannula, the Henkin–Bard cannula, and others (see Ref. 77). They all suffer from the need to connect the cannula to a catheter after it is advanced over the straight epidural needle. In our view this equipment is not an advantage over standard equipment.

Epidural equipment should be simple. A steady pair of hands with a highly trained feel for loss of resistance, a freely running glass syringe, and a high-quality epidural needle are far superior to the multitude of mechanical devices offered as aids to identify the epidural space.[164]

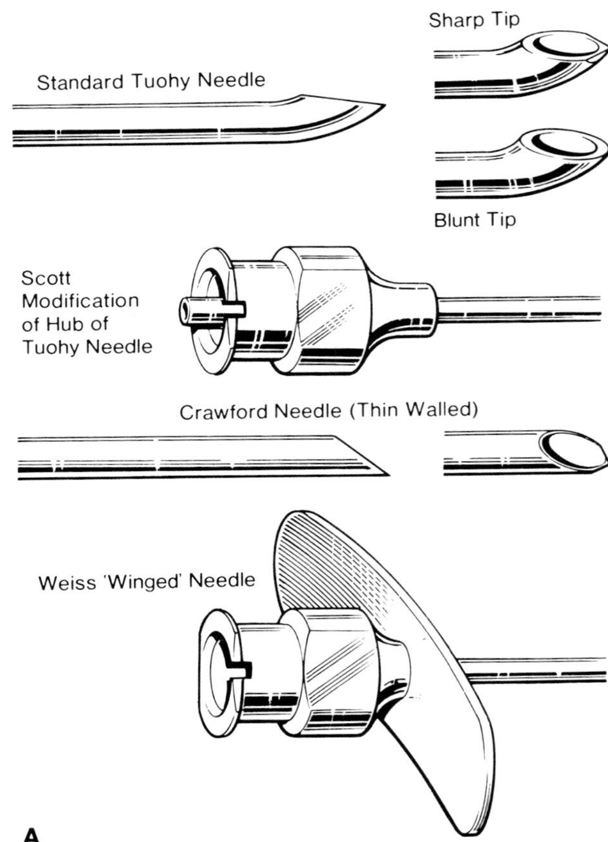

FIG. 8-30. **A.** Epidural needles.

Required Equipment for Epidural Blockade

A satisfactory preparation section of tray (sterilizing fluid cup, swabs, swab holder, sterile towels)
1 × 2.5-cm, 25-gauge needle for skin analgesia
1 × 4-cm, 22-gauge needle for deep infiltration
1 × 18-gauge needle for drawing up epidural solutions and then piercing skin* before inserting the epidural needle.
Epidural needle (Tuohy, Crawford)
Epidural catheter
1 × 2-ml, glass syringe for infiltration, syringe mount
2 × 10-ml, all-glass syringes for loss of resistance tests and drawing up local anesthetic
Local anesthetic mixing cup
Normal saline
Local anesthetics
Filters and caps for epidural catheter
Sterility indicator

*Alternatively a small scalpel blade is used.

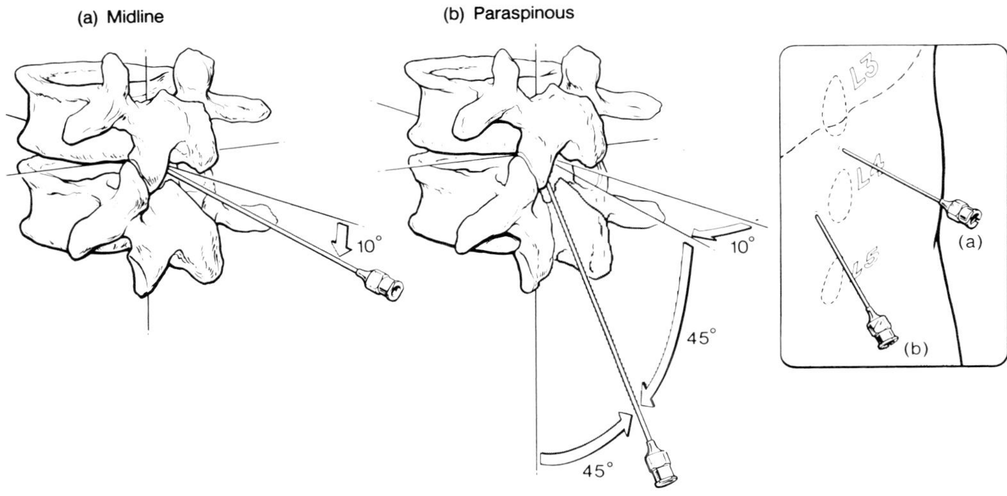

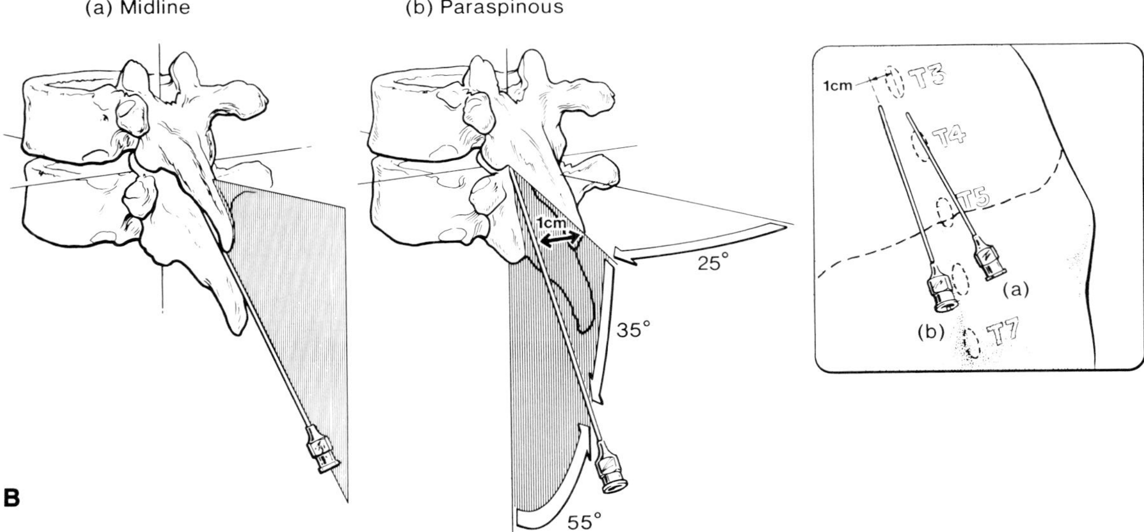

B

FIG. 8-30. *(Continued).* **B. Lumbar epidural. Sites of needle insertion.** *Upper panel,* Lumbar epidural. *(a)* Midline. Note insertion closer to the superior spinous process and with a slight upward angulation; *(b)* paraspinous (paramedian). Note insertion beside caudad edge of "inferior" spinous process, with 45° angulation to long axis of spine below. *Lower panel.* Thoracic epidural. *(a)* Midline. Note extreme upward angulation required in midthoracic region. Therefore, a paraspinous approach may be easier: *(b)* paraspinous. Note needle insertion next to caudad tip of the spinous process above interspace of intended level of entry through ligamentum flavum. Upward angulation is 55° to long axis of spine below and inward angulation is 10° to 15°.

Some practitioners prefer to have sterilized vials of local anesthetic on the tray and to draw them up into 10-ml glass syringes, rather than using a "mixing" container and exposing the solution to possible contamination. Although Millipore filters have not been conclusively shown to reduce the incidence of epidural infection, they may have other advantages. Particulate matter has been reported from mixing containers and "snap-neck" glass ampuls.[298] The Millipore filter offers some protection against this material reaching the epidural space. (Chap. 6 should be consulted for general information regarding equipment for neural blockade and preparation of the patient.)

Patient Evaluation and Preparation

As in any preanesthetic evaluation, certain essential information should be obtained. Its implications must be considered before selecting epidural blockade as part of the anesthetic regimen. If epidural block seems appropriate, then the necessary preoperative steps should be taken: The minimum entails adequate psychological preparation, adequate baseline data (*e.g.*, blood sugar levels in a diabetic), and correction of reversible abnormalities, such as dehydration (Table 8-19). Informed consent is obtained.

Preoperative Discussion with Medical Staff

A discussion with the medical staff should not be omitted because the choice of anesthesia is considered the province of the anesthesiologist. Consultation with the surgeon is necessary to help determine the precise nature of operative approach and, therefore, the level of blockade required, the need for supplementation, and the necessity for intubation if exploration will markedly impinge on upper abdominal areas. Preoperative communication with nursing staff can be accomplished by a telephone call, to inform them beforehand of requirements for special equipment, timing of transportation of the patient to the operating room, and the need for assistance during positioning of the patient for a block (Table 8-19).

Planning for Technique of Block and Drug Dose

Choice of patient posture for puncture follows the same principles outlined in Figures 7-17 and 7-18. Although the effect of gravity may be debatable, reliability of blockade of S1 is probably increased in the sitting position. Also, it is easier to enter the epidural space in obese patients if the sitting position is used.On the other hand, patients who have a history of fainting or who are heavily premedicated should have their block induced in the lateral position. Site of puncture is usually at L2–3 or L3–4 (see Fig. 8-7A), unless the anesthesiologist is an experienced epiduralist; puncture at L5–S1 aids in ensuring blockade of the resistant S1 segment for ankle or knee surgery. At higher levels, experienced epiduralists may choose an interspace close to the center of the dermatomal segments required.[269] However, the degree of difficulty of needle insertion should also be considered. Thus, one may choose T9–10 for a thoracic operation, even though the more difficult T5–6 level may be closer to the center of the required dermatomes. Similarly, C7–T1 level may be chosen for an upper thoracic procedure rather than the more difficult T3–4 level. We believe that the midline approach should be learned thoroughly before using the paraspinous (lateral) approach, since the chance of needle entry into the lateral aspects of the ligamentum flavum (see Fig. 8-4) may be greater if inexperienced attempts are made to "angle" the needle toward the midline. However, careful use of the spinous process to guide the needle for a paraspinous approach to a midline entry through the ligamentum flavum can be extremely reliable and easy in the hands of an experienced epiduralist (see Table 8-1), and this feature is helpful in the midthoracic region (see Table 8-2). In the cervical region, midline puncture becomes more reliable again, and it is best to choose the C7–T1 level, since the epidural space is wider than at higher cervical levels, and access between the spinous processes is easy if the neck is flexed (see Table 8-3).

The technique chosen for identification of epidural space depends largely on personal preference and familiarity with technique.[238,362] We prefer the technique of loss of resistance, using an air-filled syringe at all levels, provided that the firm "Bromage" grip is used.[77] Certainly, the two-handed grip of the "hanging-drop" technique ensures excellent control; however, the slight risk that there may be a plug in the needle tip and the occurrence of low or no negative pressure tends to outweigh the benefits of the "hanging-drop," or "Gutierriez," technique. We prefer to use the midline approach (Fig. 8-30), with an air-filled syringe (Figs. 8-31, 8-32) at lumbar, low-thoracic, and C7–T1 levels, unless midline entry

TABLE 8-19. CHECKLIST: A SAFETY PROCEDURE BEFORE SPINAL EPIDURAL BLOCKADE

Patient Evaluation

Psychological suitability
Physical suitability with emphasis on the following:
  Obesity and/or bony spine abnormalities
  Preexisting neurologic disease
  Cardiorespiratory function (*e.g.*, ability to withstand sympathetic blockade)
  Blood volume
  Drug factors:
    Anticoagulants, aspirin and other anti-platelet drugs, sensitivity to local anesthetics, antihypertensive agents, monoamine oxidase inhibitors (and other drugs interferring with sympathetic function)
  History of previous anesthetic and other drug administration
  Family history of adverse drug effects

Patient Preparation

Explanation of blockade procedure and its benefits (intraoperative and postoperative)
Inquiry as to patient's desire for sedation or full unconsciousness
Baseline information
  Spine radiograph for undefined pathology, blood sugar level for diabetics
  Correction of reversible abnormalities (*e.g.*, dehydration)
  Informed consent is obtained.
  Record history and management plan in notes
Order
  Changes (if any) in current medication
  Premedication

Preoperative Discussion

Operative details with surgeon to determine the following:
  Level of blockade required
  Appropriate supplementation
  Necessity for intubation
Management plan with surgical staff: equipment and drug requirements
  Timing for patient transport to operating room
  Assistance from nursing staff

proves difficult; then a paraspinous approach is used. In the midthoracic region, the paramedian, paraspinous (lateral) approach (see Fig. 8-30) is routinely used with an air-filled syringe.

A special plea for avoiding air-filled syringes may be made in patients presenting for ablation of renal stones by extracorporeal shock wave lithotripsy.[1] The focused shock waves set up turbulence and tissue damage at air–water or air–tissue interfaces, and so epidural or paravertebral bubbles of air might conceivably predispose to local neural damage if traversed by the shock beam. Thus, there are theoretical grounds for using saline-filled syringes for loss of resistance in such cases.[1] The chances of problems arising from epidural bubbles would seem to be extremely remote if puncture is made in the thoracic region and above the path of the shock beam.*

It is desirable when puncture is made above the L2 level to routinely infiltrate down beside the spinous process and check the depth of the lamina as a guide to the depth of the interlaminar space. This avoids the danger of continuing to advance a needle with a plug in the end. Experience with the use of the Bromage grip develops a keen sense of resistance in the hand advancing the needle and the hand compressing the syringe plunger. Unfortunately, the "hanging-drop" is not under the anesthesiologist's control; it may impart a visual sign only on entry into the epidural space without premonitory sign of increased plunger resistance, which becomes highly developed during routine use of lumbar epidural block. Nevertheless, many anesthesiologists find that the two-handed grip of the "hanging-drop" technique gives them greater control. If this technique is used, the stylet must not be withdrawn until the needle is close to the ligamentum flavum. It should be reinserted if the needle contacts periosteum and requires repositioning. Also, it is preferable to advance the needle only during inspiration so that negative pressure in the epidural space is maximal.[77]

*Air-filled syringes have been used for placement of thoracic epidural needles in 300 cases of lithotripsy, without ill effects. However, care was taken to limit the volume of injected air to minimal amounts. (Bromage, P.R.: Unpublished observations.)

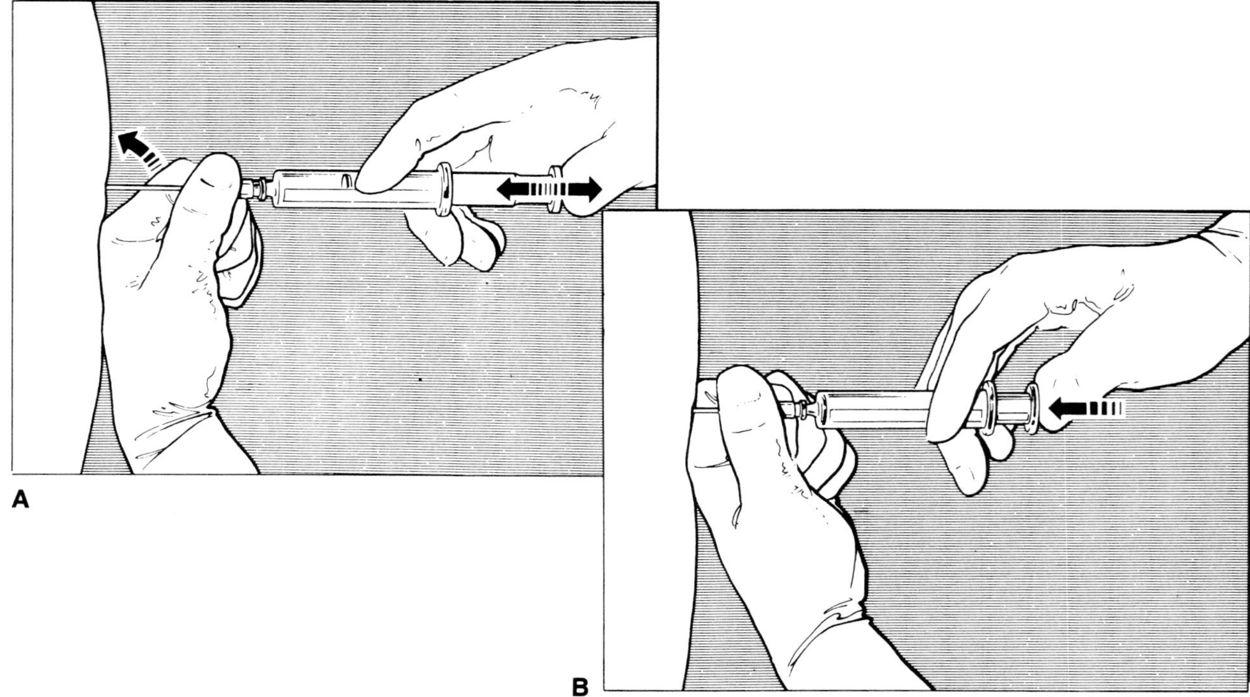

FIG. 8-31. "Bromage" grip for loss of resistance technique. **A.** Note the vicelike grip of needle between thumb and *entire fist*. Metacarpal heads are braced against the back. The needle is advanced by rotation of the entire hand around the metacarpal heads; only a small, highly controlled movement is possible without repositioning the hand on the needle. There is continual compression of syringe plunger, with a "bouncing" movement. **B.** As soon as the ligamentum flavum is pierced, resistance to syringe plunger is lost, and the needle is immediately halted. (This sequence is seen from above.)

The choice of single-shot or catheter technique depends on the patient and the type of operation. Catheter techniques are useful in debilitated and aged patients, since level of blockade can be gradually extended to the required level; this is also a wise approach in operative obstetrics. Prolonged surgery requires catheter techniques. Healthy patients undergoing brief procedures can be adequately managed with a single shot by the needle; even if it is planned to thread a catheter for "insurance." In this situation we prefer to inject the dose by way of the needle, since catheters may malfunction owing to transforaminal escape or superficial placement,[54,254] "curling up,"[434] or, sometimes, passage into the anterior epidural space.[505] Threading catheters only 3 to 4 cm into the epidural space reduces, but does not eliminate, malfunction.[457]

Dosage calculation and choice of agent depend on factors discussed on page 314. Single-shot techniques depend on a generous calculation of dose requirements (see Table 8-15), so that catheter techniques are preferable if it is essential to restrict dose and level of blockade. Considerations of the most appropriate drug and concentration, and addition of epinephrine are also discussed on pages 314 and are outlined in Table 8-16.

Needle insertion under general anesthesia is certainly more comfortable for the patient. However, comfort is bought at the price of safety, since valuable signs of contact with neural tissue and of intravascular, or subarachnoid injection may be lost, so that considerable experience or supervision by an experienced epiduralist is required.

CONDUCT OF EPIDURAL BLOCKADE

Epidural neural blockade should be viewed as part of a complete anesthetic procedure (Table 8-20), which includes preparative steps, continuous surveillance, and appropriate responses (*e.g.*, supplementation if indicated). It should be stressed that technical expertise in inserting an epidural needle is insufficient, by itself, to safely manage epidural block. Reports of anesthetic mortality committees[474] have drawn attention to

1. deficiencies in knowledge of physiology and pharmacology of epidural blockade and treatment of altered physiology and of pharmacologic side-effects;
2. inadequate preparation (*e.g.*, lack of restoration of blood volume);
3. inadequate monitoring before, during, and after surgery;
4. inadequate supplementation and general management (*e.g.*, artificial ventilation in situations where it is required);
5. slowness and inappropriate responses to sudden changes in physiology;
6. lack of appropriate resuscitative skills.

All of the above have parallels in the safe administration of *general* anesthesia. Somehow some individuals attempting to use epidural block have failed to realize that the same level of knowledge, surveillance, and technical skill is required for epidural block and its management.

Initial steps in the operating room must always include preparation of drugs and equipment for life support, the means of supplementation, and provision of a contingency plan for general anesthesia, to provide complete coverage for the operative procedure if the epidural block is inadequate. There should be no delay in deciding whether epidural block can

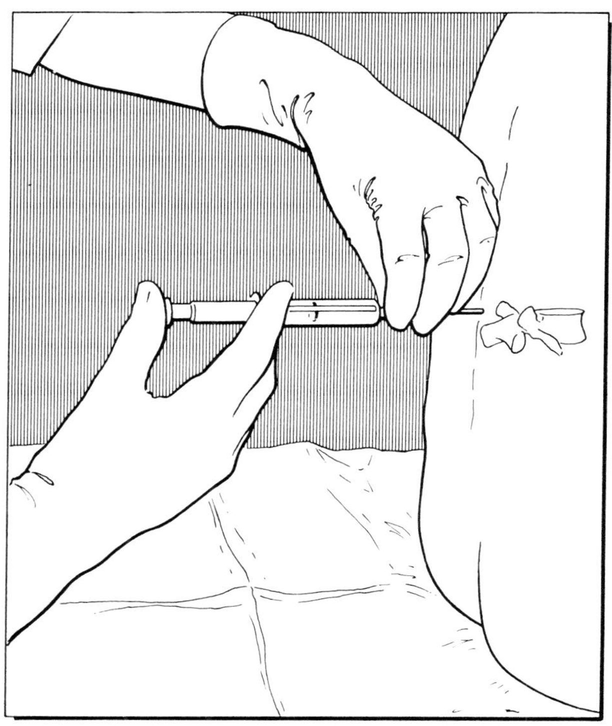

A

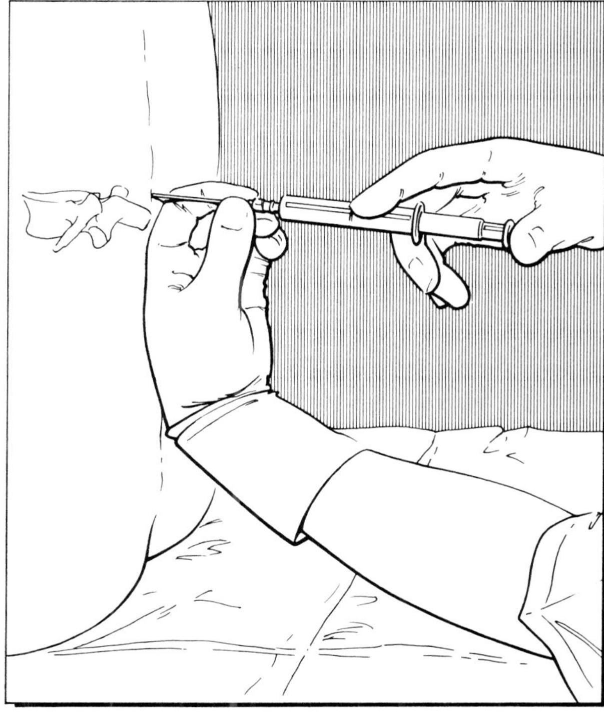

B

FIG. 8-32. Alternative, less-controlled grips. **A.** Hand gripping needle from above. **B.** Hand gripping needle from below. Note that in both **A** and **B** the hand holding the needle is braced against the patient's back at all times, and the needle is advanced by forward movement of the forefinger and thumb.

TABLE 8-20. THERAPEUTIC PROCEDURES* FOR EPIDURAL BLOCK

Initial Steps in the Operating Room

Preparation
Resuscitative drugs and equipment (see Table 4-9). Monitoring equipment.
Plastic oxygen mask and appropriate connection to anesthetic machine
Supplementation: drugs and equipment
  Opioid, sedative requests from drug "safe"
  Stereo headphones
  Screen (to be erected *as soon as* patient is in operating room)
  Contingency plan for general anesthesia if needed, equipment and drugs prepared
The patient
  Inquire about adequacy of sedation and other problems
  Insert i.v. line and rehydrate
  Position correctly but *comfortably*
  Reiterate step of procedure
  Mark landmarks with skin marker or other means
  Check blood pressure, heart rate. Attach ECG electrodes. Monitor ECG continuously.

Skin Preparation and Preparation of Neural Block Tray

Equipment physically separated from all other drugs
  Sterile tray
  Sterile wrapped drugs
Check sterility control indicator
Skin preparation
  Keep equipment and drugs covered and separated from cleansing solutions during skin preparation
  Discard cleansing solution and equipment before uncovering block equipment
  Discard entire block tray if cleansing solution splashed onto drugs/needles
  Allow at least 3 minutes for solution to act (draw up drugs during this time)
Preparation of drugs and equipment
  Discard drug solutions that are cloudy or have crystals
  Double check identity of drugs
  Check dose of local anesthetic (and vasoconstrictor)
  Draw up solution for epidural block in 10-ml syringes (to facilitate aspiration)
  Draw up infiltration solution
  Check fit of stylet, tip of epidural needle, fit of catheter through needle, patency of catheter
  Check that "loss of resistance" syringe operates without sticking

Insertion of Needle (Midline Technique)

Infiltrate skin and interspinous region (then recheck epidural equipment)
Puncture skin with 18-gauge needle or scalpel blade
Check that epidural needle insertion is midline by "Labat" palpation of spinous process
Maintain constant pressure on "testing" syringe
Control needle advancement in vicelike grip with hand braced against patient at all times (see Fig. 8-31)
Halt needle immediately if resistance is lost or if there is any doubt about position (see Table 8-5)
Aspirate gently and then immediately inject "test dose," 4 ml of prepared solution, again with hand holding needle braced against back
Disconnect syringe and check temperature of any backflow solution on arm (? cold = LA; ? warm = CSF)
Question patient about warmth or numbness in lower limbs
Maintain constant verbal contact; check heart rate, blood pressure, ECG
Single shot
  Inject (<0.3 ml/sec) one-half the full dose, aspirate; then disconnect syringe, check as above, and inject remainder of dose if no adverse sequelae
Catheter technique
Insert catheter and inject 4-ml dose through catheter; wait 5 minutes; check level, blood pressure, heart rate, aspirate; then inject remainder of dose (use Millipore filters)
Caution: Reposition needle/catheter if the following occur:
  Paresthesia during insertion in a conscious patient
  Muscle twitching in segmental nerve distribution
  Excessive force appears necessary
  CSF or blood are aspirated
  Onset of analgesia appears excessively prolonged

(continued)

TABLE 8-20. THERAPEUTIC PROCEDURES* FOR EPIDURAL BLOCKADE (Continued)

Insertion of Needle (Midline Technique)

No resistance is felt in interspinous ligament (? below L4) Choose another interspace or use paraspinous approach to check depth of lamina and ligamentum flavum

Insertion of Needle (Paraspinous)

Infiltrate skin, 0.5–1 cm lateral to caudad edge of spinous process
Using 22-gauge "spinal needle," infiltrate at 90° to skin down to lamina; note depth
Insert epidural needle *beside* spinous process (see Fig. 8-30) and angle toward midline 10–15°

Lumbar epidural

Epidural needle angled at 45° to long axis of spine, caudad to point of insertion
Needle beside spinous process, caudad to intended level of entry

Thoracic epidural

Epidural needle angled at 55° to long axis of spine, caudad to point of insertion
Needle beside spinous process *above* intended level of entry

Further steps in techniques are same as those for midline, except that little resistance is encountered until ligamentum flavum is engaged
Epidural needle should enter epidural space in midline

Continuing Management

Monitor

By constant verbal contact (if patient conscious). Continuous ECG, end-tidal CO_2, and pulse oximetry are desirable additions.
Cardiorespiratory systems for "danger signals" (see Table 8-10)
Level of blockade

Respond to altered physiology

(See Tables 8-7 through 8-11 and Figs. 8-14 through 8-21)

Diagnose and treat local anesthetic "reactions"

(See Tables 4-8 and 4-10)

Supplement as needed

With additional opioid or sedative agents
By superimposed general anesthesia if operative or patient requirements warrant it

Maintain adequate epidural block

Check for "missed" segments
Top up at mean duration minus 2 SD (see Table 8-17) or when measured segmental level regresses two segments, or use continuous infusion (see Chap. 26)
Diagnose and treat problems such as tachyphylaxis, vascular cannulation, delayed dural puncture

Follow-up

Early
- Arrange continuing postoperative epidural analgesia if needed
- Prevent infection

Late
- Check for any sequelae and, if present, participate in diagnosis and management

*The term "therapeutic procedure" is used to include the planning and preparation, the technical procedure, monitoring, and prompt responses to adverse effects.

be counted on to provide analgesia and muscle relaxation (if required). Inadequate or patchy blockade should be swiftly covered by appropriate supplementation, and this should be done in a manner that is not discernible to the patient or the surgeon. This is extremely important in maintaining acceptability of the technique to patient, surgeon, and other medical staff. Also, emphasis is placed on erecting a screen as soon as the patient is placed on the operating table.

Supplementation agents are discussed in Chapter 6. Some practitioners have a preference for supplementation with low-dose opioid infusion (*e.g.*, pethidine[479]) or with low-dose infusion of rapidly cleared drugs, such as methohexitone, hexobarbital, midazolam, low-dose ketamine, etomidate, propofol, or chlormethiazole (hemineurin).[348,441,455] The aim of "low-dose" sedative infusion is to produce "natural" sleep with maintenance of an unobstructed airway, even in the prone position. This technique permits patients to tolerate uncomfortable positions without the long-standing problems associated with induction of general anesthesia and an obstructed airway. Because such drugs are rapidly cleared from the body, cessation of infusion may result in a rapid recovery from sedation within a few minutes.[348]

Once the patient arrives in the operating room, all of the above should be ready, and activity should then concentrate on aspects relating directly to the patient (Table 8-20). For example, adequacy of sedation before needle insertion should be assessed. Any recent untoward events, such as severe angina during the night, should be elicited. The medical record should be checked. In particular, drug therapy should be scrutinized to determine whether prescribed drugs (*e.g.*, insulin) have been given and undesired drugs (*e.g.*, heparin) have been discontinued. The steps of the procedure should be reassuringly outlined for the patient, and any changes in patient requirements determined (*e.g.*, a desire to be completely asleep rather than lightly sedated).

Although there are many approaches to *locating the desired interspace,* we prefer to make an indentation with the thumbnail in the chosen interspace, to leave a mark at the level of the anterior superior iliac crest with the skin preparation solution, and then finally to palpate the rib margin as a guide to location of L1 (see Fig. 8-7A). With this approach, the landmarks can be identified immediately before needle insertion. In contrast, marking with a skin "pen" is carried out before skin preparation, and the patient may move in the interim. Baseline blood pressure and heart rate should always be recorded on the anesthetic record before blockade.

Skin preparation and preparation of the neural block tray should require two separate steps. Also, it should be stressed that the neural block tray must be kept separate from all other drugs, since human error may result in injection of inappropriate agents into the epidural space with potentially disastrous sequelae.[504] It is preferable to complete the skin preparation before uncovering the epidural needles and drugs. In any event, splashing of preparatory solutions on neural block equipment must be avoided (Table 8-20).

Except for skin infiltration, complete preparation of neural block equipment should take place before commencing the block. The remaining steps are completed while skin analgesia ensues. It should be noted that the local anesthetic to be used for epidural block is drawn up, ready to inject, and the catheter (if used) has been checked and is ready to thread. Care should be taken that glove powder or other material does not soil the barrel of the "loss of resistance" syringe, since this may result in dangerous sticking of the barrel.

Midline Technique

The essential anatomy of needle insertion in the midline is described in detail in the text accompanying Tables 8-1, 8-2, 8-3, 8-5, 8-6, and 8-7 (see also Figs. 8-30, 8-31). The anesthesiologist should constantly think of the structures the needle encounters. The practical steps are outlined in Table 8-20, and the following aspects should be emphasized: Needle insertion should be in the center of the interspace; deep infiltration with a 22-gauge needle is important to "explore" the anatomy and to make subsequent insertion of the epidural needle comfortable; the skin should be punctured with a large-bore (18- or 19-gauge) needle or scalpel blade to avoid "drag" on the epidural needle or carriage of an epidermal "plug" into the epidural space; if the midline approach is used, the spinous processes should be gripped as shown in Figure 8-7B, to assist in identification of the midline; constant pressure on the testing syringe should be maintained (Fig. 8-31A), and the epidural needle should be held in a vicelike grip that permits only a small forward movement at a time; the hand holding the needle must be braced firmly against the patient at all times; even in the lumbar region, a slight upward angulation is required to reach the interlaminar space (see Figs. 8-8, 8-9). If the "Bromage" grip shown in Figure 8-31 is used, it is possible to readily identify changes in resistance, transmitted by the hand holding the needle and the syringe plunger, as the needle enters supraspinous, interspinous, and ligamentum flavum (see Fig. 8-8). Constant pressure on the syringe plunger permits immediate recognition of loss of resistance as the needle tip enters the epidural space, and the vicelike grip on the needle permits immediate halting of needle progress (Table 8-20). Gentle aspiration or, preferably, mere disconnection of the syringe is carried out to check for flow of CSF or blood. If neither is present, 4 ml of solution is immediately injected to push the dura away from the needle tip. Two points require emphasis: The injected solution should meet no resistance and the hand holding the needle must remain braced against the patient's back; otherwise, the needle may be advanced as the solution is injected. The syringe is disconnected again and any drip back is tested as in Table 8-6 while the patient is questioned about warmth and numbness in lower limbs; a subarachnoid injection results in almost immediate onset of blockade of β-fibers (Table 2-1, Chap. 2). If no evidence of onset of a subarachnoid block is present, one may proceed to inject the calculated epidural dose as follows:

Single-Shot Techniques. After gentle aspiration, a *test dose* of 5 ml (preferably epinephrine-containing) local anesthetic solution is injected at 10 ml min^{-1}. The syringe is disconnected and any drip back is tested (see Table 8-6). The patient is observed for increased heart rate owing to intravascular injection of epinephrine and is questioned about sudden onset of warmth or numbness in the legs. If the response to these is negative, further 5-ml increments are injected until the full dose has been given. It should be noted that a "negative" response to a test dose does not provide absolute proof of correct placement.

Catheter Techniques. The catheter is inserted 3 to 4 cm while the hand holding the needle is braced against the patient's back to ensure that the needle does not move. After removal of the needle and careful aspiration, a 5-ml test dose (see above) is then injected through the catheter. After 5 to 10 minutes, the level of blockade, heart rate, and blood pressure are checked; if satisfactory, a careful aspiration test is carried out, and then the remainder of the dose is injected. Alternatively, the remainder of the dose can be injected slowly in 5-ml increments. As noted in Table 8-20, needle or catheter insertion should be halted if undue force is required or if paresthesias or muscle twitches are elicited. If blood flows freely from an epidural needle, it may be necessary to move to an adjacent interspace and ensure that the subsequent entry through the ligamentum flavum is in the midline (see Figs. 8-5, 8-6). If clear solution drips back or is aspirated from needle or catheter, then the steps outlined in Table 8-6 must be taken to determine whether the fluid is local anesthetic or CSF.[108,222] Aspiration of blood from the epidural catheter may be overcome by withdrawing the catheter *(provided that the catheter is not still in the epidural needle)* or by injecting some saline. The catheter must not be left with blood in it, since it may rapidly become occluded. If blood aspiration does not cease, then the catheter should be reinserted at another level. Two further signs to reposition needles or catheters are important: If resistance is poorly defined at any level, then it is often helpful to either try another interspace or to choose the paraspinous (lateral) approach, which permits checking of the depth of the lamina by an exploring needle; if onset of analgesia is excessively prolonged, it is likely that injection has not been made into the epidural space.

Paraspinous Techniques ("Paramedian")

Paraspinous, paramedian (lateral) insertion is a useful alternative technique. The term *paraspinous* is favored for the following reasons:

The needle should be inserted close to the spinous process because in both lumbar and thoracic regions, the spinous process narrows superiorly and thus guides the needle to a midline entry through the ligamentum flavum.

Extreme lateral angulation of the needle should be avoided, since it may result in oblique penetration of the ligamentum flavum (see Fig. 8-4) and vascular or neural damage. In most instances, the needle need not be angulated and merely follows the spinous process; thus, "paraspinous" describes the essence of the technique.

Techniques with extreme angulation of the needle should be disgarded in favor of the safer paraspinous approach (see Fig. 8-30).

In the lumbar region infiltration is made 1 to 1.5 cm lateral to the caudad tip of the inferior spinous process of the chosen interspace.[33] A 9- to 10-cm, 22-gauge spinal needle is then used to infiltrate perpendicular to the skin beside the spinous process; this enables the depth of the lamina to be determined before inserting the epidural needle. It is worth noting that the epidural space can be identified, for single-shot techniques, if an air-filled syringe is attached to the 22-gauge needle and constant pressure is applied to the plunger. However, in most patients an 18-gauge epidural needle is next inserted beside the spinous process and angled upward at 45° to the skin (Fig. 8-30B); often the spinous process carries the needle slightly inward 10° to 15° to the sagittal plane. This may not always be so, and the needle may pass directly to the ligamentum flavum without any necessity for inward angulation. With this technique, resistance to the advancing needle and syringe plunger is encountered only when the needle tip enters the ligamentum flavum. Thus, careful location of the depth of ligamentum flavum is essential; from this point the technique is identical to that at the midline.

In the thoracic region skin infiltration is made 1 to 1.5 cm lateral to the caudad tip of the spinous process, *cephalad to* the intended level of needle insertion (see Fig. 8-30B). Infiltration down to the level of the lamina is carried out as described above. The epidural needle is inserted beside the spinous process and 55° to 60° to the skin (sagittal plane); that is, a *steep* angle is required to reach ligamentum flavum *caudad to* the chosen spinous process (Fig. 8-30B). For both thoracic and lumbar paraspinous approaches, the Crawford 18-gauge thin-wall needle is an option for single-shot and catheter techniques. The angulation of the needle may permit easier threading of a catheter if a straight-tip Crawford needle is used rather than the Huber tip of the Tuohy needle (but see p. 321).

Technique for Obese Subjects and Those with Impalpable Spinous Processes

If preoperative evaluation determines that the patient is obese, of a very "squat" stature, or bony landmarks are impalpable for other reasons, additional maneuvers may be required. In this situation it may be helpful to plan to carry out the epidural block with the patient in the sitting position, since landmarks may be more readily palpable and epidural puncture is often easier than in the lateral position.

At the time of epidural block, absence of bony landmarks need not cause dismay, since they can be identified during gentle infiltration with local anesthetic. A 5-cm, 22-guage needle is used to infiltrate the deeper tissues in the region where the spinous processes are judged to lie. The needle is used to probe gently for the underlying spine.[77] Each time the needle touches bone, the depth is noted and the needle is systematically redirected medially or laterally until bone is located at the most superficial depth (i.e., the spinous process).* At this stage it may be necessary to infiltrate a new "track" directly toward the spinous process. The epidural needle is then inserted as for the "midline technique" above. Alternatively the lamina may also be located and the "paramedian" approach used as above.

Continuing Management

As indicated in Table 8-20, monitoring and response to altered physiology are important aspects of the conduct of epidural block. The management of sudden reactions to injection of local anesthetic requires a sound knowledge of the differential diagnosis of local anesthetic reactions[445] (Table 4-8) and their treatment, as well as detailed knowledge of the cardiovascular effects of epidural block (Tables 8-7 through 8-13). Only with constant monitoring can the appropriate responses to physiologic changes be made (Table 8-21). Atropine is often used for situations of vagal dominance (see Table 8-10). Ephedrine is useful for cardiovascular support if it is desired to use bolus injections of a medium-durataion drug. Ephedrine is not useful in patients with depleted norepinephrine in sympathetic nerve endings, such as some elderly and debilitated patients and those under treatment with drugs that chronically deplete norepinephrine stores. In this situation, direct-acting drugs, such as epinephrine and norepinephrine, are required. Both of these drugs have a brief duration of action, and thus it is more rational to use them by intravenous infusion, with careful titration against response. Surveillance also permits appropriate supplementation with sedative-opioid or anesthetic agents and also appropriately timed "top-up" doses for the epidural block.

Maintenance of effective epidural block may entail overcoming common deficiencies in blockade and problems in the management of epidural catheters.

*It may be helpful to leave the infiltration needle *in situ* and to use this as a guide to the location of the spinous process, when the epidural needle is inserted by means of a separate "track."

TABLE 8-21. CARDIOVASCULAR SUPPORT—EPIDURAL BLOCK: CARDIOACTIVE DRUGS (70-KG ADULT)

Drugs of Choice	
Atropine	0.3 mg i.v. increments[225]
Ephedrine	5–10 mg i.v. increments[39,61,186,187,482,521]
Epinephrine	1 mg in 500 ml solution (2 μg/ml) Infuse at rate 2–4 μg/min* Titrate against heart rate, mean arterial blood pressure, improved tissue perfusion At low rates of infusion mainly β-effects at higher rates, increasing α-effects
Norepinephrine	1 mg in 500 ml solution (2 μg/ml) Infuse at rate 2–4 μg/min Titrate as above At <6 μg/min β- as well as α-effects, and thus perfusion (*e.g.*, urine flow) not reduced 2–4 μg/min usually sufficient to maintain blood pressure in presence of total sympathetic block
Metaraminol	100 mg in 500 ml solution (0.5 μg/ml) Infuse at rate 30–60 μg/min Titrate as above Both α- and β-effects May be given as a bolus of 5–10 mg if a long-acting agent (1–2 h) of indirect activity is needed
Other Drugs	
Dopamine and *dobutamine*[9] are alternatives to epinephrine; however, dopaminergic receptors are blocked by butyrophenones and phenothiazines. *Isuprel* (β) is usually inadequate alone, since both α- and β-effects are needed.[351] *Methoxamine* produces mainly α-effects with reflex slowing of the heart and decreased cardiac output.[326]	

*Resting catechol output of 70-kg man is 3–4 μg/min.[122] This can be replaced exogenously by 3–10 μg/min epinephrine.[480] Note, however, that these requirements need verification by modern catecholamine assay techniques.[101]

Problems in Epidural Blockade

Blockade Too Low at Upper Level or Inadequate Blockade at Lower Level. Approximately one-half the initial dose is administered 30 minutes after the first dose. However, if the initial dose was small (*e.g.*, 4–8 ml), it may be necessary to repeat the initial dose. This is particularly so in the region of L5–S1, which is difficult to block.

"Missed Segments." Manage missed segments as above, depending on the size of initial dose and size of nerve root of "missed segment(s)." If a segment is missed on one side, it is worthwhile turning the patient on to that side before injection.[453] Epinephrine-containing solutions are the most effective, particularly 2% lidocaine with 1:200,000 epinephrine, in dealing with missed segments or inadequate block. This is a useful practice even if another agent has been used for the initial injection. If available, 2% lidocaine–carbon dioxide is the best choice for such problems.

Inadequate motor block within the segmental area blocked requires further injection, 30 minutes after the initial dose, of approximately half this dose, preferably as 2% lidocaine with epinephrine.

Level Too High but Inadequate Sacral Analgesia. Careful monitoring of the physiologic effects of the high block and appropriate treatment are essential. Approximately 30 to 60 minutes after the initial dose, a small dose of 8 to 10 ml may be injected by a separate single-shot caudal needle. Such a dose will reliably block sacral segments without extending the upper level of lumbar epidural block. If access to the sacral hiatus is impossible, then it is preferable to wait as long as possible (approximately 60 minutes) and inject a small increment (*e.g.*, 5–8 ml by the epidural catheter), since blockade tends to spread progressively into the sacral segments with each repeat injection. Careful monitoring is required for signs of total epidural block.

"Visceral" Pain During Lower Abdominal Surgery. It is not commonly recognized that peritoneal stimulation during appendectomy and sometimes during a difficult herniorrhaphy may require blockade to the level of T5–6. Thus, adequate provision should be made to block to this level or, alternatively, to "top-up" to this level if required. If there is a delay in onset of T5 block, then intravenous or epidural opioid or light general anesthesia may be required.

Inability to Thread Epidural Catheter. This is often a confirmatory sign that a false loss of resistance has been encountered in a tissue space dorsal to the ligamentum flavum and that the needle has been halted superficial to the ligamentum flavum. Clearly injection of local anesthetic at this point will be ineffectual. The most prudent course is to withdraw the needle and catheter together, after noting the depth of the needle. The needle is then redirected in the midline and maintained in resistant ligamentous tissues until a convincing loss of resistance is achieved.

On the other hand if the anesthetist is firmly convinced, by all the evidence available, that the needle is properly sited and if the planned operative procedure is likely to be accomplished within the duration of a long-acting local anesthetic, then it may be reasonable to proceed with a "single shot" injection through the needle, using bupivacaine or etidocaine. However, the latter course of action involves two assumptions: that the needle is properly sited and that the operation will not extend longer than expected. One or both of these assumptions may be wrong; thus the unpredictability of this course is not recommended.

Dural Puncture. Often it is feasible to convert to a subarachnoid block merely by maintaining the needle in position and injecting the appropriate intrathecal dose of tetracaine, dibucaine, or bupivacaine. If the anesthesiologist wants to persevere with epidural block, then another interspace should be chosen (preferably above) and a catheter should be threaded upward. Injection should be made entirely by the catheter and should be slow. A test dose is essential (see above).

Subarachnoid cannulation may occur at the time of initial insertion of needle or epidural catheter.[245,294,360] It has an incidence of 0.2% to 0.7%.[294,360] Failure to recognize malplacement of needle or catheter and injection of the usual epidural dose would result in a total spinal anesthesia (see Table 4-8). Epidural catheters have also been found to penetrate the dura at the time of a "top-up" dose, having initially functioned as if normally placed in the epidural space.[402] Thus, a small test dose administered by an epidural catheter is always advisable.

Subdural cannulation results from perforation of the dura without penetration of the underlying arachnoid membrane. This is a rare result of intended epidural cannulation.[45,483] It occurs quite frequently during myelography[119] and in spinal anesthesia, with an incidence of up to 1 in 100. Spread of analgesia is patchy, markedly asymmetrical, and sometimes quite extensive.[45,483] Replacement of the epidural catheter at a more rostrad interspace level is required.

Cannulation of an epidural vein is a greater hazard, especially in pregnant women because of epidural venous distention during labor, particularly if the needle or catheter enters the epidural space other than in the midline (see Fig.8-5). Usually the risk of epidural venous cannulation is small.[177,279,537] The best treatment is *prevention,* which depends on gentle insertion of catheters that do not have sharp ends, and avoidance of use of stylets; insertion of only 3 to 4 cm of the catheter length; aspiration before injection by way of an epidural catheter; use of a test dose, preferably with epinephrine (injected into an epidural vein results in a rapid increase in heart rate and blood pressure) (see also Table 8-18).

Injection of a small amount of saline and withdrawal of the catheter by 1 to 2 cm usually permits retrieval of the catheter from the vein; if not, then the catheter should be reinserted at another level. Delayed entry of a catheter into a vein may occur at the time of a "top-up" dose, with resulting CNS toxicity.[431] Once again, the catheter must be withdrawn, or if it is inaccessible, then epidural block must be discontinued.

Venous cannulation is less likely to occur if the catheter is inserted into a "wet" epidural space, expanded by prior injection of local anesthetic, rather than into a dry one.[509a] The practice of injecting a "priming" dose of local anesthetic through the needle is therefore a logical precaution against venous cannulation. Expansion of the epidural space can be accomplished by using a test dose of 4 ml via the needle, before inserting the catheter.

Epidural Hematoma. Needle or catheter trauma to epidural veins may result in bleeding, but this is usually minimal and stops rapidly; it is rare for an epidural hematoma and neurologic symptoms to arise if coagulation is normal. Only one case is currently recorded.[321] However, patients on anticoagulant therapy may develop large epidural hematomas and, possibly, paraplegia if either an epidural needle or catheter is inserted.[166,212,228]

It should be remembered that more than 100 cases of spontaneous epidural hematoma have occurred in patients on anticoagulant therapy unassociated with epidural block.[248,476] Thus, spontaneous epidural hematoma may sometimes be erroneously attributed to epidural block. It is not known whether the tendency toward epidural hematoma in patients on anticoagulants is accentuated by the use of epidural block. Because there is still doubt, it is best to carefully weigh the benefits of epidural block against the risks of epidural hematoma.[137] In the majority of cases, alternative means of providing most of the beneficial effects of epidural block are now available if anticoagulation is felt to be essential. For example, epidural block increases graft blood flow in association with vascular procedures on the lower limb.[145] However, limb blood flow may also be increased by prior sympathetic blockade using long-acting local anesthetics or intravascular reserpine injected into the affected limb, or even surgical sympathectomy (see Chap. 13). It is also important to note that surgical procedures involving the abdominal aorta may cause paraplegia. This may be the result of prolonged clamping of the aorta[135] or sectioning of nutrient arteries to nerve plexuses and the spinal cord.[506] Thus, while in lower limb vascular surgery, anticoagulation or epidural block, or both, may lead to epidural hematoma and paraplegia; in aortic surgery, direct cord ischemia must be added to the differential diagnosis of postoperative paraplegia.

Despite the theoretical risks, epidural block has been used extensively for lower extremity vascular surgery, with controlled heparin therapy during and after surgery. In two series with a combined total of 4164 patients, none developed an epidural hematoma.[387,413] A protocol was used that involved insertion of the epidural catheter the night before surgery. If any bleeding resulted from epidural needle insertion, the epidural and surgery were aborted for 24 hours.[387,413]

The risk-benefit ratio of epidural block in these categories of patients need to be better defined. In the meantime, the indication for epidural block in each patient should be carefully assessed. If epidural block is used, postoperative neurologic deficits should be viewed in the light of the differential diagnosis discussed above, and when it is necessary, surgical intervention should be early.

In particular, it is important to allow a continuous epidural block to wear off for long enough to assess as soon as possible after the surgery. Failure to recover function fully and, in some cases, severe lumbar pain indicate the possibility of epidural hematoma. Anticoagulants should then be stopped and myelography and/or CT scan carried out immediately because most patients who have recovered from epidural hematoma have been decompressed within 12 hours of the onset of symptoms.[32] The variability in individual response to "low-dose" heparin therapy means that some patients may still develop epidural hematomas, and this risk will not be obviated until rapid methods are available to measure plasma levels of heparin and to assess the effect of heparin therapy on coagulation[536] (see below). Patients with potential interference with normal hemostatic mechanisms include those with disease (*e.g.,* severe preeclampsia, intrauterine death) or medication (*e.g.,* heparinization or oral warfarin, aspirin and other nonsteroidal anti-inflammatory drugs). Epidural puncture should be avoided if the platelet count falls below 100,000/mm^3. However, aspirin-like drugs do not change platelet *count;* they alter platelet *function*. A bedside template bleeding time (*e.g.*, Lee–White) should be performed if there is any concern about platelet function (bleeding time should be less than 8 minutes). In patients with preeclampsia and other conditions likely to alter the coagulation cascade, a full range of clotting studies should be performed in consultation with a hematologist.

Tachyphylaxis. Tachyphylaxis is discussed above (see Fig. 8-29) and in Chapter 3. The most important methods of avoiding the problem are as follows: use of long-acting local anesthetic for continuous catheter techniques; "topping-up" before analgesia wears off — usually at a time for mean duration — "2 SD" for the agent used or at the first sign of two-segment regression (see Table 8-17); use of continuous infusion; sometimes changing to an alternative agent is said to help.

MANAGEMENT OF EPIDURAL CATHETERS

Accurate placement of a minimal length of catheter is described in the foregoing discussion as an essential aid to successful "continuous" catheter epidural blockade. The problems of patchy blockade, missed segments, intravascular cannulation, and subarachnoid and subdural cannulation can usually be effectively managed if the "correct procedure" is carefully followed and close monitoring is carried out (see Table 8-20). The long-term complications of catheter placement, owing to damage to neural tissue, should be avoidable if catheters are withdrawn at the first sign of pain or paraesthesias on insertion or on reinjection. The complications of epidural hematoma are mostly (but not always) avoidable.

Prevention of Infection

Perhaps the most important aspect of management of epidural catheters is the avoidance of infections:

A strict antiseptic routine should always be carried out during catheter insertion. Adequate time should be allowed for the skin preparation to exert its antibacterial effect, and great care should be taken not to contaminate the epidural catheter before insertion.

Multidose local anesthetic vials should not be used: Preservative-free, single-use local anesthetic solutions should be used, and any residuum should be discarded after injection.

Local anesthetics should not be aspirated through "rubber bungs" in tops of local anesthetic vials; the top should be removed and the vial discarded after single use.

Glass syringes should be used only once and then resterilized, since the outside of the plunger may be contaminated during use. Many hospitals now use plastic single-use syringes.

During "top-up," the syringe nozzle and epidural catheter connection must not be contaminated, and if they are touched directly, then the appropriate components should be changed. Wiping with alcohol swabs is not advised, since it is possible that neurolytic alcohol solution may then be carried into the epidural space.

The use of micropore (Millipore) filters has been shown in one study to reduce catheter contamination.[282] Although other studies have not substantiated this finding,[4] it seems reasonable to recommend the use of such filters. They provide at least some protection against infection and reduce the chance of contamination with particulate matter.[298]

If reasonable precautions are taken, the risk of infection from contamination of epidural catheters or local anesthetic solution should be small (*e.g.*, 30,000 epidurals without a single infection[77]). However, endogenous infection owing to bloodborne spread from a preexisting focus on infection may be a hazard.[14] Also, patients with septicemia clearly pose a considerable risk of metastatic epidural infection, and insertion of an epidural catheter is best avoided in such patients. Infection in the pelvic region could possibly spread to the epidural space by way of the venous connections to epidural veins (see Fig. 8-13); thus, the use of epidural catheters should be avoided unless the pelvic infection has been treated adequately with antibiotics. The risk of metastatic infection is even further increased in diabetics and in patients with suppressed immune responses.[438] The diabetic patient has proven to be a problem with long-term epidural catheters in treatment of cancer pain. However, immunosuppressed patients with cancer have been safely managed with long-term totally implanted epidural systems (see Chap. 28).

More complex measures to combat contamination at reinjection include the enclosure of large-volume syringes in sterile bag.[77] and the use of continuous drips and syringe pumps.[95,450]

PROCEDURE FOR "TOP-UP" AND CATHETER REMOVAL

In conscious and cooperative patients, careful monitoring for signs of segmental regression will indicate the need for "top-up." In other situations, it is most convenient to top-up at the approximate time of regression of analgesia (minus 2 SD) as determined in clinical studies (see Table 8-17), provided that this timing coincides with safe blood concentrations of local anesthetic (see Fig. 3-14). The mean −2 SD predicts the duration in 95% of patients. In practice, injection of one-half the initial dose of lidocaine approximately every hour results in maintenance of blockade associated with a small but significant gradual increase in blood lidocaine concentration (see Fig. 3-14). This is usually not of importance during surgery, when one to two top-ups are often sufficient. In contrast, with the long-acting agents bupivacaine and etidocaine, topping up with half the initial dose every 2 hours maintains level of blockade without appreciable increase in blood concentration over many successive top-ups. Thus, for long-term catheter techniques, bupivacaine is preferable with respect to toxicity and because the generous margin between top-up and two-segment regression lessens the chance that tachyphylaxis may occur. It should be clearly understood that we are interested in duration of blockade from time of complete spread to regression of two segments, provided an appropriate level of blockade is achieved with the initial dose; duration to two-segment regression is considerably shorter than complete duration. If initial level of blockade is much too high, then initial top-up should be appropriately delayed, and size of top-up dose should be reduced in proportion to the level of "overshoot." A routine for topping-up is important.

Topping-Up Routine

Check level if possible: pinprick or ice in conscious patients, reflexes, and presence or absence of bradycardia (? level above T2) in anesthetized patients. Do not top-up if a high level is suspected.

Aspirate for CSF or blood.

Inject a small test dose (3–4 ml) of epinephrine-containing solution and check heart rate and blood pressure: Intravascular injection results in rapid increase in heart rate and blood pressure; subarachnoid injection results in extensive blockade with hypotension and sometimes bradycardia.

Inject remainder of top-up dose *slowly* with frequent aspiration, only if no complications ensue after the step above.

Monitor closely for one-half hour after top-up. If the patient is conscious and mobile, he should lie flat during top-up and for one-half hour afterward. In any patient, be prepared to increase rate of intravenous infusion or to manage local anesthetic reactions or extensive sympathetic blockade (see Table 4-8).

Durations of maintenance of epidural catheters for more than 2 weeks have been reported. Bromage advocates replacement of catheters at a different site every 72 hours,[77] and this is supported on the grounds that epidural catheters become walled off by fibrous tissue reaction after about 72 hours.[178] However, if a catheter is functioning satisfactorily with no sequela, it is reasonable for it to remain *in situ* for approximately 1 week (see also Chap. 28). Catheters should be removed gently, and the end of the catheter should be carefully checked for completeness. If difficulty is experienced in withdrawing the catheter, the spine should be flexed and gentle continuous traction exerted. There is a remote possibility that a knot may form in the catheter if excessively long lengths have been inserted; this is impossible if only 3 to 4 cm of catheter is inserted into the epidural space. There is an even remoter possibility that a catheter may loop around a spinal nerve if excess lengths are inserted; pain on removal of catheter should alert the anesthesiologist to this possibility. If subsequent radiographs, after injection of 0.3 ml of contrast media into the catheter, show that it is located in the region of a spinal nerve, removal by laminectomy may have to be considered. Sequestration of a small amount of catheter in the epidural space should be noted, and the patient must be carefully assessed over the ensuing weeks. However, it is usually not necessary to remove this foreign body, nor is it technically easy to locate it at laminectomy. Thus, in general, laminectomy is reserved for situations associated with symptoms or signs.

LOW-DOSE HEPARIN THERAPY AND IMPLICATIONS FOR EPIDURAL BLOCKADE

A major international multicenter study of low-dose heparin prophylaxis for postoperative deep venous thrombosis (DVT) reported the following impressive results: Only two patients receiving heparin (n = 2045) developed fatal pulmonary embolus (0.09% of all patients), and there was a 7.7% incidence of DVT detected by ^{125}I fibrinogen scanning; 16 control patients (n = 2076) developed fatal pulmonary embolus (0.7% of all patients), and there was a 24.0% incidence of DVT.[292] The incidence of deaths from hemorrhage was the same in both groups, but a breakdown of morbidity owing to hematoma formation was not given. Despite these impressive results, too little attention was paid to the variability in plasma heparin concentration, with the risk of either ineffective prophylaxis or overdose with hematoma formation; also there was insufficient emphasis on the increased risks of heparin therapy in some surgical procedures, such as prostatectomy, hip surgery, and thoracotomy.

Nevertheless, an initial wave of enthusiasm for low-dose heparin therapy led to its almost routine use in some hospitals. Their aim was to lower a rather alarming rise in postoperative pulmonary embolism.[265,418] More objective assessment of benefits and risks of this treatment for surgical patients has gradually confirmed an approach directed at at-risk groups,[293] in which the heparin treatment *per se* does not result in significant problems.[378] For example, the risk of hematoma and hemarthrosis in major orthopedic surgery far outweighs the benefits of low-dose heparin. Risks of excessive bleeding in pulmonary and prostatic surgery have resulted in a similar reluctance to use heparin. On the other hand, patients with cancer requiring major surgery are at considerable risk of postoperative thrombosis.[420] This risk has to be carefully weighed against potential problems of heparin therapy for the proposed surgery. Unfortunately, even the responses to the low-dose regimen proposed by Kakkar and colleagues[292] vary considerably and unpredictably; this indicates the possibility of hematoma formation in susceptible patients. This may occur in major joints, behind the peritoneum, and in other concealed sites, causing occult blood loss and acting as a site for infection. They may also result in neurologic deficits (*e.g.*, from an epidural hematoma).

In consultation with a hematologist experienced in heparin prophylaxis,[220] we have developed the following approach to the conflict of interest of use of epidural block and heparin prophylaxis: The risks and benefits of epidural block are compared with low-dose heparin for the patient under consideration and the proposed operation; if the benefits of heparin are minimal and epidural block is the anesthetic technique of choice, then heparin therapy is omitted; on the other hand, if heparin prophylaxis is strongly indicated and is practicable for the proposed surgery, then a single-shot epidural technique with long-acting local anesthetic may be used before starting heparin — in this situation, epidural catheters are not used, since there is a small chance that they may cause subsequent trauma or dislodge a previously formed clot on an epidural vein with resultant fresh bleeding. In some patients, heparin therapy should be started before the patient is brought to the operating room. In such a patient, epidural block is not used in any form. Another approach has been used in vascular surgery whereby an epidural catheter is inserted the night before surgery and low-dose heparin is used during and after surgery[388,413] (see above).

If the patient is at a high risk for venous thrombosis, but heparin therapy is incompatible with the proposed surgery (*e.g.*, total hip replacement, prostatic surgery), then epidural block may be chosen in an attempt to modify the stress response and reduce coagulation changes. Also, the analgesia and freedom from sedation associated with epidural block are used to facilitate early and vigorous postoperative mobilization.

APPLICATIONS OF EPIDURAL BLOCKADE

A discussion of the "indications" and "contraindications" of epidural block is not the scope of this section. The preceding material in this chapter has provided a broad anatomic, technical, pharmacologic, and physiologic basis on which to answer two important questions: Does epidural blockade offer significant benefits to the *individual* patient under consideration for the proposed operative or other application? Do the benefits outweigh the risks owing to factors peculiar to the patient and/or procedure?

When viewed in this context, lists of "indications" and "contraindications" can be misleading and dangerous, since they cannot take into consideration factors that vary in individual patients. The only absolute *contraindications* to epidural blockade are patient refusal, major coagulation defects, uncorrected hypovolemia, infection in the area of proposed needle insertion, or severe systemic infection. As with spinal anesthesia, the benefits of epidural blockade in patients with neurologic disease should be carefully weighed; it appears wise, although there is no clear evidence, to avoid blockade in patients with unstable neurologic disease, particularly if the spinal cord is involved. However, if epidural block offers significant benefits in patients with stable "peripheral" neurologic disease, such as diabetic neuropathy, then its use may be considered in light of individual patients and procedures. The use of epidural block in many thousands of patients with back pain and neurologic deficit after back surgery (see Chap. 27) attests to its safety in carefully selected patients with stable neurologic signs. Abnormalities of the bony spine may increase the difficulty of epidural block, although by no means do they make it impossible; this difficulty must be weighed against the skill of the anesthesiologist and the risk-benefit ratio for the patient and procedure; both anteroposterior and lateral radiographs of the lumbar spine should be available to assist in making such a decision.

Other anatomic, pharmacologic, and physiologic factors in individual patients may lead to a decision not to use epidural block. However, they cannot be merely "listed" here, since the balance of risk to benefit must be decided for each patient. For example, a patient with a low fixed cardiac output owing to constrictive pericarditis may be better managed during a perineal procedure by a saddle-block spinal anesthetic rather than an epidural anesthetic. A patient with severe congestive cardiac failure may be safely managed by epidural block for lower abdominal surgery, provided that incremental doses are used by a catheter and the "internal phlebotomy" owing to sympathetic block has a slow onset. In addition, the vasodilation must be carefully balanced by titrating a slow vasopressor infusion, as shown in Table 8-21, to prevent the blood pressure from falling more than 30% below the preblock mean. The vasopressor must be given with great caution, since hypertension is more harmful than a little hypotension in congestive cardiac failure. Indeed, mild hypotension may be beneficial.

The considerations above enable the anesthesiologists to determine which benefits epidural blockade offers to each patient in each clinical setting. The potential applications may include operative surgery; postoperative pain management; posttrauma pain management (see also Chap. 26); obstetric analgesia and operative obstetrics (see also Chap. 18); chronic pain diagnosis and management (see also Chaps. 24–29); and special applications in the management of particular medical and surgical conditions (*e.g.*, Fig. 8-33) (see Table 8-22).

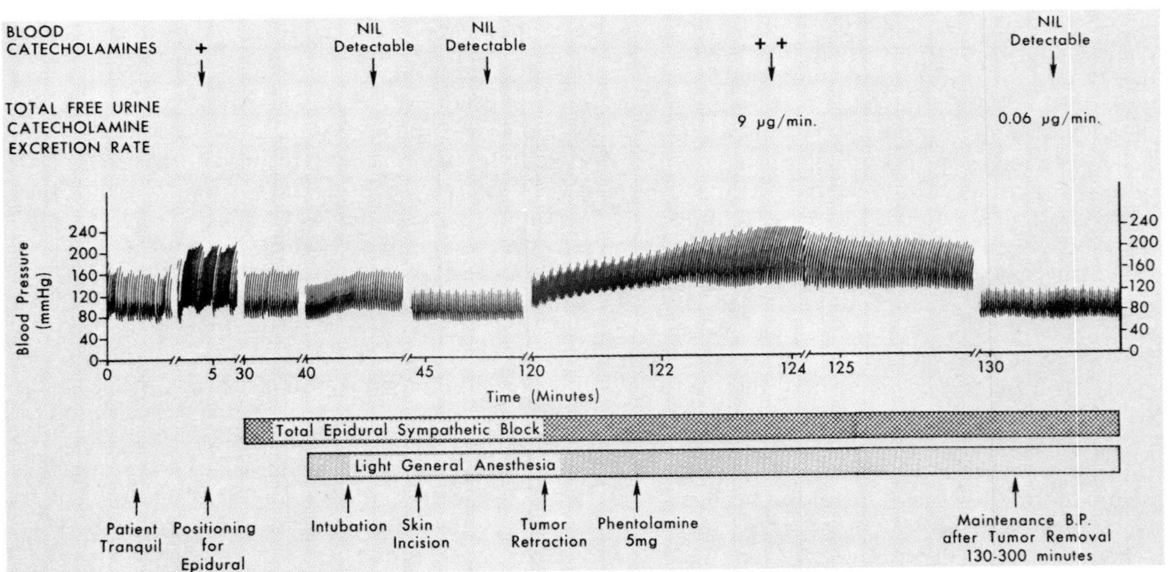

FIG. 8-33. Pheochromocytoma and total epidural blockade. Radial artery blood pressure and urine and serum catecholamine levels were determined during surgery. Total epidural blockade was gradually accomplished by incremental doses of 1.5% mepivacaine administered by an epidural catheter, with essentially no change in blood pressure. Only a small change in blood pressure resulted from intubation, and there was no response to skin incision. Direct manipulation of the tumor required phentolamine to control the blood pressure rise. (Cousins, M.J., and Rubin, R.B.: The intraoperative management of phaeochromocytoma with total epidural sympathetic blockade. Br. J. Anaesth., *46*:78, 1974.)

COMPLICATIONS OF EPIDURAL BLOCKADE

The problems discussed on pages 332–333 may be considered minor complications. Any complication should be viewed in the light of a sound knowledge of the anatomy, pharmacology, and physiology of epidural block.

Complications Relating to Anatomic or Technical Problems

Several problems were discussed elsewhere: inadvertent dural puncture and total spinal blockade; massive subdural spread; total epidural blockade; epidural venous injection; epidural hematoma; epidural abscess; anterior spinal artery syndrome; ligation of spinal cord blood supply during major vascular surgery; injection of local anesthetics contaminated with neurolytic agents; injection of the "wrong drug" (*e.g.*, thiopentone); broken epidural catheters; and local anesthetic toxicity.

Rigid adherence to a "therapeutic procedure," as outlined in Table 8-20, greatly reduces the risks of major complications.

The occurrence and management of postdural puncture headache are discussed in Chapter 7. Unfortunately, the incidence of headache is high (70%–80%) if the dura is punctured with a 16- to 18-gauge epidural needle.[147,148] Thus, routine prophylaxis is advisable if the dura is punctured with an epidural needle; this includes use of the supine posture, increased oral and intravenous fluid intake, the use of abdominal binders, and systemic analgesics. If an epidural catheter has been inserted at another level, it should be left *in situ* and 1500 ml of saline should be infused over 24 hours.[147,148] The use of epidural blood patch is discussed in Chapter 7 (see also Fig. 7-21).

Backache is supposed to be severer when large epidural needles (compared with spinal needles) are used. However, there are no data to support this. In obstetrics, the incidence of backache appears to be the same after delivery with or without epidural block.[149,232,291,359]

Bladder dysfunction is a distinct possibility if blockade of the sacral segments continues into the postoperative period. As discussed in more detail in Chapter 26, it is important to attempt to restrict epidural block to the required segments, which often do not include S2–5. Also, it is vital to ensure that the bladder does not become overdistended if epidural block extends into the sacral segments during surgery; this is particularly important in aged men with incipient prostatic obstruction. Careful management of level of blockade in obstetric patients results in a similar incidence of catheterization, whether or not epidural block is used.[148,359]

TABLE 8-22. SOME APPLICATIONS OF EPIDURAL BLOCKADE

1. Surgery
   - Upper and lower abdominal surgery,[77,275,444] urologic surgery,[191,539] pelvic surgery,[358] hip surgery,[300,357,478] vascular surgery,[145] surgery in the obese patient,[205] thoracic surgery,[151,215] surgery of the neck and upper limb, radical mastectomy[486a]
   - Surgery in patients with medical conditions (see Chap. 7), *e.g.*, buccal pemphigus,[285] malignant hyperthermia[303]
   - Specialized surgical procedures
     - Pheochromocytoma[77,84,144]
     - Surgery of spine[451]
     - Bladder distention for bladder cancer
     - Extracorporeal shock wave lithotripsy[179]
2. Postoperative and post-trauma pain relief
   - See Chapter 26.
3. Obstetrics (see also Chap. 18)
   - *e.g.*, for patient comfort, to avoid incoordinate uterine action,[360] to minimize fetal acidosis,[382,425] to reduce use of "urgent" instrumental delivery or "painful delivery" needing general anesthesia,[35,170,327] to relieve pain during labor for *medical*[181] indications, preeclampsia,[360] for cesarean section.[88,149,150]
4. Diagnosis and management of chronic pain
   - "Differential" epidural block (see Chap.27)
   - "Diagnostic epidural opioid blockade" (see Chap. 28)
   - Epidurography with metrizamide[78,452]
   - Neurolytic epidural block[77] (see Chap. 29)
   - **Pain due to** vasospasm due to ergot poisoning,[8,452] cold injuries of extremities,[44,312] Raynaud's disease or phenomenon and other vasospastic problems,[320] phantom limb pain and causalgia,[352] postherpetic neuralgia,[125,400] pancreatitis,[389] renal colic,[326,424] acute priapism.[307]
5. New epidural techniques
   - Epidural electrical stimulation[462,500] (see Chap. 30)
   - Epidural narcotics[142] (see Chap. 28)

Major neurologic sequelae of epidural block are potentially the same as for spinal anesthesia (see Chap. 7). It was initially thought that these sequelae followed spinal anesthesia and not epidural block, but this has been disproved. In a major world review of the use of epidural blockade, Usubiaga uncovered a number of cases of neurologic sequelae that were purportedly caused by epidural block.[504] However, the retrospective nature of the documentation in many of these cases often make it impossible to determine the relative contribution of preexisting medical factors, the surgical procedure itself, and the epidural block. As with spinal anesthesia, several large epidural case series report no neurologic sequelae in major hospitals where a standard procedure is followed: Bromage reports more than 40,000 epidural blocks without major neurologic sequelae.[77] The majority of cases of serious neurologic sequelae occur in small hospitals or occur after epidural block by an inexperienced operator who violates some aspect of a reasonable therapeutic regimen. Even so, there is a *potential* for neurologic sequelae resulting from anatomic, technical, physiologic, and pharmacologic factors associated with epidural block (see Fig. 8-34) and the surgery, obstetric delivery, or other procedure for which the epidural block is used (see also Chap. 22). A survey of the literature revealed only a small number of cases of neurologic deficit in association with epidural block.[295] Some of these have subsequently been shown to be due to inadvertent subarachnoid injection of large volumes of a preparation of chloroprocaine that had a low *p*H and contained bisulfite in a concentration now recognized as being higher than desirable (see Chap. 4 and Tables 4-6, 4-7). Many anesthesiologists were not aware of the precise composition of this preparation of the drug, and indeed it has been changed over the years as the manufacture of the drug changed hands. There is an important lesson in this story: Subtle changes in the formulation of local anesthetic solutions may have vital importance, *particularly* for spinal anesthesia and epidural anesthesia (see also Chap. 29.1). Unfortunately, history tends to repeat itself. In the 1930s, solutions of procaine were prepared with 15% ethanol and glycerine; cauda equina syndromes resulted and it was concluded that procaine was the causative factor, the other ingredients apparently being regarded as harmless (see Ref. 295). The same situation arose with the use of amylocaine) (Stovaine) and piperocaine solutions containing neurolytic components.[295] Local anesthetic solutions for epidural block should, as far as possible, contain only local anesthetic with *p*H adjusted as close as possible to normal *p*H. The precise solution to be used clinically should be tested under the most extreme conditions that could be experienced clinically (see also Chap. 29.1). Changes in formulation should not occur without repeating this testing, approval by drug regulatory bodies, and full information of the medical community.

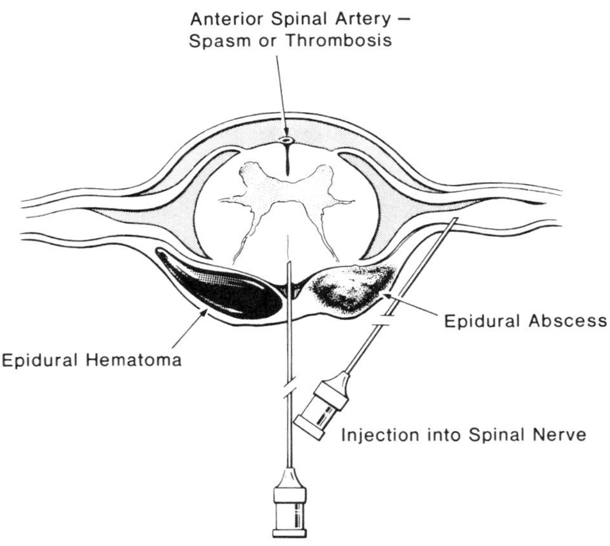

FIG. 8-34. Complications of epidural block (see text).

Possible causes of neurologic sequelae are summarized in Tables 8-23, 8-24, in Figure 8-34.

Direct trauma to the spinal cord can be eliminated if puncture is below L2. In all reported cases in which the patient was conscious, insertion of needle or catheter was followed by *severe lancinating pain* in dermatomes adjacent to or below the site of puncture.[77,271]

Epidural hematoma is discussed on page 334.[137,212,228] This complication can be prevented if the combination of coagulation defects or complete heparinization and epidural block is avoided. It is remotely possible for epidural hematoma to occur in patients without coagulation defects. Constant surveillance and early investigation are most important. In all reported cases, there is a rapid onset of signs of neurologic deficit or severe back pain, or both. These signs should always be rapidly investigated by myelography and/or CT scan, and if necessary, laminectomy should be performed within a maximum of 12 hours, since recovery is unlikely if decompression is delayed beyond this time.[32] Note that uncommon arteriovenous abnormalities of the spinal cord may pose a risk of excessive bleeding into epidural or subarachnoid space either because of or associated with epidural block (see Table 8-24).

Epidural Abscess

In a series of 39 cases of epidural abscess, Baker and colleagues found that 38 cases were associated with endogenous infection.[14] In this series, an epidural abscess occurred in association with epidural block in only one case. Important diagnostic features present in all cases were severe back pain, local back tenderness, fever, leukocytosis, and abnormal myelogram with obstruction to flow of contrast medium. As for epidural hematoma, rapid investigation and laminectomy are essential for complete recovery. Because *Staphylococcus aureus* is the most common infecting organism,[247] antibiotic administration should include treatment for a staphylococcus infection if positive cultures are not available. The majority of reported cases of epidural abscess have followed continuous caudal blockade before the emphasis on sterile technique.[87,182,467] However, a disturbing case of extensive epidural empyema has been reported after midthoracic epidural blockade.[192] It should be noted that epidural abscess may occur in association with general systemic infection,[341] which reinforces the view that epidural block should be avoided in this situation. Epidural corticosteroid administration may result in immune suppression. For example, epidural methylprednisolone 80 mg results in significant suppression of adrenal function for about 3 weeks.[281] Theoretically, this could pose a risk of epidural infection. To date, epidural abscess has not been reported in association with epidural steroids; however, meticulous care with sterility should be observed when epidural steroids are injected.

Subarachnoid infection has also been reported after epidural block, and contamination of equipment or drugs appears to be responsible.[46,284]

Trauma to Spinal Nerves or Blood Vessels in Dural Cuff Region

Oblique lateral entry into the ligamentum flavum may direct the needle into the dural cuff region (Fig. 8-34). This may result in direct trauma to a nerve root, with resultant unisegmental paresthesia; such a sign should warn the anesthesiologist not to persist with needle insertion in this position and not to attempt to thread a catheter. It is also possible that a major "feeder" artery to the anterior spinal artery may be damaged as it enters by way of an intervertebral foramen (see Fig. 7-11), resulting in the so-called anterior spinal artery syndrome, or possibly in a large epidural hematoma (even in a patient with normal coagulation).

TABLE 8-23. POSSIBLE FACTORS IN NEUROLOGIC SEQUELAE IN PATIENTS RECEIVING EPIDURAL BLOCK

1. Direct trauma to spinal nerve roots, spinal cord
2. Compression of spinal cord or nerve roots
   - Epidural hematoma
   - Epidural abscess
   - Postpartum paresis owing to cephalopelvic disproportion (may also compress spinal cord "feeder" vessels)
3. Neurotoxicity
   - Low *p*H, high concentration of antioxidants (*e.g.*, bisulfite) (see Chap. 4 and Chap. 29.1)
   - Neurotoxic additives (*e.g.*, ethanol, benzyl alcohol, chlorocresol, methylparaben)*
   - Injection of "wrong drug" (*i.e.*, *not* a local anesthetic)
4. Ischemia
5. Anterior spinal artery spasm or thrombosis
   - Trauma by needle
   - Spasm ? by epinephrine or other factors
   - Thrombosis owing to very low blood pressure (*e.g.*, only in those with vascular disease)
   - ? Combination of hypotension and injection of large volume of local anesthetic raising CSF pressure (see Chap. 29.1).
6. Ischemia *within* spinal cord
   - ? "Neurotoxic" effects by way of reduced perineurial blood flow —Only with neurotoxic additives and inappropriate use of local anesthetics (see Chap. 29.1).
7. Factors unrelated to epidural may frequently be found to be the causative factors *e.g.*, preexisting disease (see Table 8-24), surgical factors

*Such additives should never be used in epidural solutions (they have been in some multiple-use solutions in the past).

TABLE 8-24. ASSOCIATED BUT UNRELATED NEUROLOGIC SEQUELAE IN PATIENTS RECEIVING EPIDURAL BLOCK*

Anatomic abnormalities
- "High take off" of artery radicularis magna and supply of lumbosacral area of cord by sacral branches of internal iliac artery (15% of population). Ligation or compression of this artery at surgery (? incidence 1 : 20,000).

Undiagnosed neurologic disease
- A-V abnormalities of spinal cord—1 : 15,000
- Vertebral angioma—1 : 4–6,000
- Atherosclerotic "spinal stroke"—1 : 20,000
- Unrecognized prolapsed intervertebral disk— ? 1 : 6000
- Unrecognized spinal metastases (=5% of all cancer cases)
- Unrecognized primary spinal cord tumor— ? undiagnosed incidence

Damage to neuraxis during surgery
- Compression of pelvic nerves (lumbosacral trunk) ? incidence 1 : 4000 (in labor related to duration and difficulty of labor)
- Ligation or compression of spinal arteries during aortic surgery— ? incidence
- Compression of peripheral nerves by retraction, pressure on operating table
- Stretching of peripheral nerves by extreme postures

*Incidence of condition is given where known (see also Chap. 22).

Unexplained Causes of Anterior Spinal Artery Syndrome

The most likely explanations for unexplained cases of anterior spinal artery syndrome are direct trauma and reduced perfusion pressure and/or venous congestion. The contribution of the small doses of epinephrine (1 : 200,000) in modern epidural local anesthetic solutions is doubtful, except perhaps in patients with severe arteriosclerosis if epidural block has been used in association with hypotension (see also Chap. 7). Studies of spinal cord blood flow, with concentrations of epinephrine in local anesthetic solutions, have not shown deleterious reductions in blood flow[309] (see also Chap. 7). Spinal cord ischemia and anterior spinal artery syndrome may result from low spinal cord perfusion unassociated with epidural block.[204] It is not known whether epidural block increases the risk of low spinal cord perfusion. However, it is certain that the same precautions should be taken, whether or not epidural block is used.

It should be noted that angiomas of vertebrae or the spinal cord are relatively common and may compress the spinal cord, particularly if intraspinal pressure is increased (*e.g.*, during labor).[377] Once again, investigation by myelography and CT scan, and rapid exploration, if indicated, must be carried out if permanent sequelae are to be avoided.

Unexplained Arachnoiditis and Transverse Myelitis

Arachnoiditis and transverse myelitis are discussed in Chapter 7. Meticulous precautions must be taken to ensure that chemical agents capable of causing these lesions[306] are excluded from epidural block equipment and drugs (see Table 8-20). Only preservative-free local anesthetics from sterile single-use containers should be used for epidural block. The lack of neurotoxicity of any agent should be established before it is injected epidurally. Previous tragedies have occurred with the neurolytic carriers present in the so-called long-acting local anesthetic "efocaine."[115] As is the case with paraplegia after spinal anesthesia, it seems likely that reported cases of adhesive arachnoiditis after epidural blockade are due to chemical contamination.[77] However, the features of adhesive arachnoiditis may be produced by infection, trauma, and hemorrhage in the region of the arachnoid. Perhaps the best example of the latter is adhesive arachnoiditis after laminectomy or spinal fusion for "back pain." We have seen a number of these patients, who were neurologically normal before laminectomy, apart from symptoms of back pain; they developed classic signs of adhesive arachnoiditis after operation. Subsequent reexploration revealed no infective process, but signs of extensive tissue trauma and classic features of adhesive arachnoiditis were present.

Partial or complete lesions of the cauda equina resulting in loss of bladder function, incontinence of feces, and sacral analgesia are sometimes attributed to epidural block. Although these lesions are possible, owing to abscess, hematoma, or chemical contamination, a more widespread neurologic deficit would be expected, considering the usual level of needle insertion. More likely causes are ligation of nutrient iliac vessels supplying the distal spinal cord in some patients or, alternatively, compression of sacral nerve roots or the pudendal nerve during pelvic surgery.

Complications Relating to Altered Physiology

The potential for complications owing to alteration in oxygen delivery to vital organs is outlined in detail in Tables 8-10 and 8-11. Thus, like general anesthesia, it is possible for epidural block to result in compromise of oxygen delivery to heart, brain, liver, or kidney, with sequelae that depend on the degree and duration of compromise. Full knowledge of preexisting physical status and careful monitoring throughout the use of epidural block are essential to avoid such complications.

Complications of epidural block are given further consideration in Chapters 22 and 23.

DIFFERENTIAL DIAGNOSIS OF POSTOPERATIVE NEUROLOGIC SEQUELAE

It is all too easy to attribute a serious neurologic deficit after anesthesia and surgery to epidural block if the latter has been used as part of the anesthetic regimen. This is comforting for the surgical team, but it has no greater validity than does labeling all cases of postoperative jaundice as "halothane hepatitis." Factual evidence that links epidural blockade with neurologic sequelae is scarce: Local anesthetics in clinical concentrations do not cause neural damage or meningeal irritation; a properly placed epidural needle or catheter with no evidence of contact with nerve root during insertion does not damage spinal nerves or spinal cord, unless gross infection or epidural hematoma results, usually from associated medical or surgical problems; epinephrine used in a concentration of 1 : 200,000 almost certainly does not result in anterior spinal artery spasm.[309]

There are a large number of common causes of neurologic deficit after anesthesia and surgery, just as there are common causes of postoperative jaundice. The medical team must consider a differential diagnosis with these common causes at the top of the list and must ensure that a readily treatable condition is not overlooked.

"Associated but unrelated" cases of spastic paraplegia may occur after childbirth in patients who received epidural block. This is strongly supported by the report of five cases of spastic paraplegia in parturients who did *not* have epidural block.[13] All were associated with spontaneous vertex deliveries, two of which had a forceps delivery. All five had features in keeping with anterior spinal artery ischemia, with sparing of the posterior columns (Bademosi, O.: Personal communication) (see Table 8-24).

The effective management of postoperative neurologic sequelae requires the collaboration of the anesthesiologist, the surgeon, and a neurologist. The assistance of a radiologist and neurosurgeon may well also be required. A frank discussion aimed at defining etiology rather than fault should take place after each physician has had an opportunity to examine the patient and history. The investigative steps are as listed in Table 8-25.

Anesthesiologists should have a thorough knowledge of the causes of postoperative **neurologic sequelae that have been reported in patients who did not receive epidural block (see Table 8-24):** [1] *Spinal cord lesions* resulting from ligation of nutrient spinal cord vessels during abdominal surgery[506] or during pelvic surgery (iliac vessels, see anatomy section and Fig. 7-11); prolonged clamping of the aorta[135]; extreme posture and severe retraction causing epidural venous congestion, combined with low cardiac output and leading to "spinal stroke"; [2] *lesions of the cauda equina or spinal nerve roots:* "Adhesive arachnoiditis" has been found at reexploration after major back surgery, and damage to spinal nerve roots has also resulted from surgery in the paravertebral region. Epidural hematoma associated with coagulation defects and systemic heparinization are discussed on page 334. Bladder dysfunction or complete loss of bladder and bowel control is a difficult diagnostic problem. Careful neurologic examination, including cystometry, EMG, and, sometimes,myelography, is required to determine etiology. Ligation of

TABLE 8-25. INVESTIGATIVE STEPS IN THE MANAGEMENT OF POSTOPERATIVE NEUROLOGIC SEQUELAE

1. Thorough review of preexisting medical problems and drug therapy (preexisting signs and symptoms of a spinal cord tumor may be elicited or a family history of neurologic problems, or drug therapy capable of causing neurologic side-effects)
2. Review of anesthetic management and surgical procedure (*e.g.*, evidence of poor spinal cord perfusion; see physiology section): dangerous posturing during surgery? surgical section of nutrient vessels to spinal cord? surgical section or retraction of spinal nerves or peripheral nerves?
3. An attempt to anatomically localize the lesion (see Fig. 8-35)
4. Consideration of most likely causes of a lesion located at such a level
5. Appropriate further investigations, such as blood culture, coagulation studies, myelography, CT scan, NMR scan, EMG
6. Careful surveillance for signs of progression of the lesion or associated medical problems
7. Rapid response to significant abnormalities (*e.g.*, progressive neurologic deficit, back pain, pyrexia, and leukocytosis require myelogram to identify possible epidural abscess, and urgent laminectomy)
8. Follow-up documentation of outcome with appropriate investigation of progress of lesion (*e.g.*, repeated EMG, serial cystometric measurements to document return or otherwise of bladder function)
9. Careful postmortem examination of nervous system by a skilled neuropathologist, if possible in conjunction with the anesthesiologist and surgeon involved. The pertinence of the pathologist's examination is greatly enhanced by firsthand information, and the education of medical staff is best served by direct participation in examining the morbid anatomy of such major complications
10. Precise reporting in the medical literature, avoiding misleading titles. For example, an excellent report by Usubiaga[506] provided clear evidence that paraplegia after vascular surgery under epidural block was due to ligation of nutrient vessels to the spinal cord during the surgery; unfortunately, the title of this article was "Neurological Complications of Prevertebral Surgery Under Regional Anesthesia." This implies that the regional anesthesia was to blame.

nutrient "iliac" supply to sacral segments of spinal cord may result in a clinical picture that mimics a cauda equina lesion. Severe retraction of sacral nerve roots during pelvic surgery may also result in such a lesion; [3] *peripheral nerve lesions* are the most common neurologic sequelae[58] and should be carefully distinguished from more "central" causes on the basis of distribution of sensory, motor, and autonomic deficit and EMG to determine pattern of "muscle denervation" (if present) and timing of onset of denervation. This assists in determining whether spinal root(s) or peripheral nerves are involved and whether the lesion predates or postdates the operation or is consistent with an intraoperative episode.[343] However, such data alone are not definitive and provide only a guide.[77] Knowledge of potential sites of

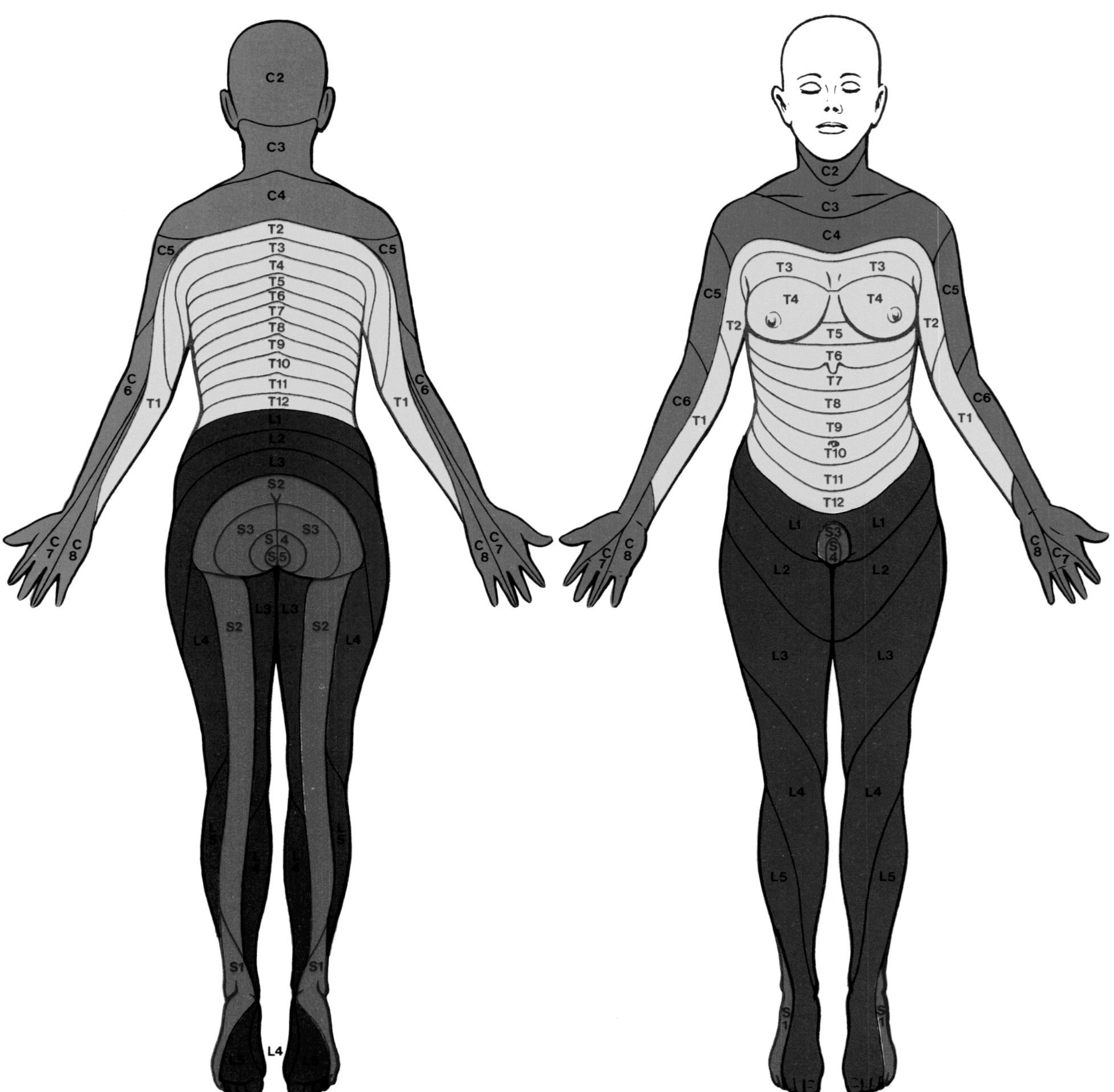

FIG. 8-35. Dermatomal chart. The segmental areas are illustrated to emphasize the most reliable cutaneous area to test for blockade of individual spinal cord segments.

peripheral nerve injury during surgery and a tendency for such lesions to be unilateral also serve as a basis for differentiation.

Examples of sites of peripheral lesions are *lumbosacral trunk* (L4–5): compression on the ala of the sacrum during pregnancy, with resultant footdrop and weakness or analgesia[371] at L4–5; *sacral nerves:* during delivery or pelvic surgery; *femoral nerve* (L2–4): during pelvic surgery; *lateral femoral cutaneous nerve* (L2–3): commonly damaged in the lithotomy position or because of direct pressure or retraction close to the inguinal ligament; *lateral popliteal nerve* (L4–S2): pressure over the head of the fibula. It should be noted that patients with preexisting neurologic disease, such as diabetic neuropathy, are at greater risk.[103]

CONCLUSION

Epidural neural blockade is capable of great diversity in terms of its range of neural blocking effects and the clinical applications of these effects. It is undoubtedly a most complex technique in terms of its anatomy, site of action, physiology, and pharmacology. Because of this, it is a technique for the specialist—the anesthesiologist. However, if used with due attention to the data presented in this chapter, it can be done with a high degree of safety and efficacy.

APPENDIX

EPIDURAL BLOCK—FUTURE DEVELOPMENTS

Review of the physiology of epidural block points to a number of areas in which basic information or further development of current data is indicated. A brief summary with some appropriate references is given in this appendix. References refer to studies of epidural block and relevant source information where no studies of epidural block have yet been reported. It is encouraging to note that many of the questions raised in this section of the first edition have been addressed and a number have been successfully answered.

CARDIOVASCULAR PHYSIOLOGY

Myocardium??Cardiac effects of absorbed local anesthetics enhanced in the presence of general anesthesia, hypovolemia, acidosis, hyperkalemia.[39,416,432,446,481]

??Most effective resuscitation regimen for bupivacaine cardiotoxicity.[297,416]

??Precise mechanism of bupivacaine cardiotoxicity and relative toxicity of other long-acting agents, such as etidocaine and other newly developed drugs[416] (see Chaps. 2, 4).

??Most useful indices of myocardial oxygenation in patients with ischemic heart disease or hypertension receiving epidural block.[267,415,429]

??Does thoracic epidural block improve myocardial oxygenation[93,160a,262,417] and morbidity/mortality in patients with ischemic heart disease undergoing surgery.[415]

??Effects of α-stimulation during epidural block on coronary vascular resistance[429] and coronary blood flow.[428]

??Usefulness of ECG monitoring for myocardial ischemia during epidural block.[296,310,408]

??Effects of epidural block on myocardial irritability.[39,218,446,481]

Venous Return Decreased venous return (VR) increases vagal tone during epidural block[15]: ?Mild reductions in VR, owing to receptors in great veins. ?Severe reductions in VR, owing to ventricular receptors, potentiated by norepinephrine.[238,384–387]

??What role does reduced oxygen delivery to carotid bodies play in states of low VR.[158,159,314,526]

EFFICACY OF EPIDURAL SYMPATHETIC BLOCK

?? Level of sympathetic block lower than sensory level and patchy in distribution.[22]

DISTRIBUTION OF BLOOD VOLUME

??Splanchnic vasoconstriction compensates for lower limb vasodilatation in blocks below T5 level?[11]

??Loss of splanchnic vasoconstrictor tone with *complete* sympathetic block of T5–L2 outflow results in marked increases in splanchnic blood volume and large reductions in VR?

LIVER BLOOD FLOW (LBF) AND LIVER FUNCTION

??LBF reduced by epidural block only if perfusion pressure reduced[302,303,430] or increased catecholamine secretion.[315]

??Is sympathetic block by epidural techniques capable of protecting the liver from toxic injury[59,374] or shock.[395]

RENAL BLOOD FLOW (RBF) AND RENAL FUNCTION

??RBF reduced by epidural block only if perfusion pressure reduced or catecholamine secretion increased.[26,142a,315,374,494]

??Sympathetic denervation by epidural block prevents renal changes associated with anesthesia.[26,512]

??When total RBF maintained under normotensive epidural block,[301] is the "key" inner cortical area normally perfused.[41,404]

??Epidural block prevents renal failure after trauma[132] or medical conditions such as pancreatitis.[525]

CENTRAL NERVOUS SYSTEM

BRAIN

??Safe reductions in cerebral blood flow in normal patients and those with diseased vessels.[484]

??Do rapid reductions in cerebral perfusion pressure with epidural block initiate neurogenic cerebral vasoconstriction that initially overcomes local vasodilatory mechanisms?[249]

??Usefulness of supplementation with moderate doses of thiopentone to reduce cerebral metabolic rate of oxygen consumption.[472]

??Analgesic effects of absorbed local anesthetic at level of brain and spinal cord.[297]

SPINAL CORD

??Is autoregulation present in humans to maintain normal flow when epidural block reduces perfusion pressure?[307,309,471]

??Are clinical doses of epinephrine in local anesthetics responsible for spinal cord ischemia?[309,501]

THERMOREGULATION

??Shivering prevented by warmed local anesthetic solutions[519] and/or epidural opioid.[88a]

??Malignant hyperthermia response in humans modified by prior epidural block.[239,304]

"STRESS RESPONSE"

??Modification of neurohumoral response associated with reduced morbidity and mortality[261,299,313,401]

GUT

??Epidural block is not associated with delayed gastric emptying in patients with acute pain.[380]

??Epidural block does not increase risk of rupture of bowel anastomoses.[6]

HEMATOLOGIC EFFECTS

??Is reduced platelet aggregation[373] clinically significant after epidural block?

??Is increased lower limb blood flow after epidural block a significant factor in reducing venous thrombosis?[143,313,372,463]

??In major surgery of long duration is adjunctive epidural block useful in preventing the initiation of venous thrombosis?[200,257,356,477]

??In reducing venous thrombosis as judged by ^{125}I fibrinogen scanning,[419] which treatment(s) are most effective or in combination: ?epidural block,[313,478] ?electrical calf stimulation,[426] ?calf compression with a pump,[102,257,421] ?dextran, ?heparin.[27,287]

RESPIRATORY EFFECTS

??Changes in central and peripheral control of respiration after epidural block.[64a,65,66,383,433,456]

??Compliance changes.[64a,65,66,151,215]

??Precise pathways of afferents for noxious stimuli.[151,215,311]

??Changes in functional residual capacity and airway closure.[20,173,210,483a]

??Reduced ability to cough owing to motor block.[183,207,208]

??Blood gas changes and oxygen flux with epidural and general anesthesia.[77,275,365]

?Respiratory effects of relief of severe pain such as acute pancreatitis.[252]

??Does epidural block relieve asthma[23,25,77,104,113,199,322,538] or does it cause exacerbation?

REFERENCES

1. Abbott, M.A., Samuel, J.R., and Webb, D.R.: Anaesthesia for extracorporeal shock wave lithotripsy. Anaesthesia, *40*:1065, 1985.
2. Abboud, F.M.: Control of the various components of the peripheral vasculature. Fed. Proc., *31*:1226, 1972.
3. Abboud, T.K., David, S., Nagappala, S., *et al.*: Maternal, fetal and neonatal effects of lidocaine with and without epinephrine for epidural anesthesia in obstetrics. Anesth. Analg., *63*:973, 1984.
4. Abouleish, E., Amortegui, A.J., and Taylor, F.H.: Are bacterial filters needed in continuous epidural analgesia for obstetrics? Anesthesiology, *46*:351, 1977.
5. Adamkiewicz, A.: Die blutgefasse des menschlichen ruckenmarkes. II. Die gefasse der ruckenmarksoberflache. S.B. Heidelberg Akad. Wiss., *85*:101, 1882.
6. Aitkenhead, A.R.: Anaesthesia and bowel surgery. Br. J. Anaesth., *56*:95, 1984.
7. Allen, P.R., and Johnson, R.W.: Extradural analgesia in labor. A comparison of 2-chloroprocaine hydrochloride and bupivacaine hydrochloride. Anaesthesia, *34*:839, 1979.
8. Andersen, P.K., *et al.*: Sodium nitroprusside and epidural blockade in the treatment of ergotism. N. Engl. J. Med., *296*:1271, 1977.
9. Andy, J.J., *et al.*: Cardiovascular effects of dobutamine in severe congestive heart failure. Am. Heart J., *94*:175, 1977.
10. Apostolou, G.A., Zarmakoupis, P.K., and Mastrokostopoulos, G.T.: Spread of epidural anesthesia and the lateral position. Anesth. Analg. (Cleve.), *60*:584, 1981.
11. Arndt, J., Hock, A., Stanton-Hicks, M., and Stuhmeier, K.D.: Peridural anesthesia and the distribution of blood in supine humans. Anesthesiology, *63*:616, 1985.
12. Axelsson, K.H.: A double-blind study of motor blockade in the lower limbs. Studies during spinal anaesthesia with hyperbaric and glucose-free 0.5% bupivacaine. Br. J. Anaesth., *57*:960, 1985.
13. Bademosi, O.: Obstetric neuropraxia in the Nigerian African. Int. J. Gynaecol. Obstet., *17*:611, 1980.
14. Baker, A.S., Ojemann, R.G., Swartz, M.N., and Richardson, E.P.: Spinal epidural abscess. N. Engl. J. Med., *293*:463, 1975.
15. Baron, J.F., Decaux-Jacolot, A., Edouard, A., Berdeaux, A., *et al.*: Influence of venous return on baroreflex control of heart rate during lumbar epidural anesthesia in humans. Anesthesiology, *64*:188, 1986.
16. Barton, M.D., Killam, A.P., and Meschia, G.: Response of ovine uterine blood flow to epinephrine and norepinephrine. Proc. Soc. Exp. Biol. Med., *145*:996, 1974.
17. Batson, O.V.: The function of the vertebral veins and their role in the spread of metastases. Ann. Surg., *112*:138, 1940.
18. ———: The vertebral vein system, A. J. R., *128*:195, 1957.
19. Bedder, M.D., Kozody, R., Palahniuk, R.J., *et al.*: Clonidine prolongs tetracaine spinal anesthesia in dogs. Anesth. Analg., *65*:S14, 1986.
20. Beecher, H.K.: The measured effect of laparotomy on the respiration. J. Clin. Invest., *12*:639, 1933.
21. Bellis, C.J., and Wangensteen, O.H.: Venous circulatory change in the abdomen and lower extremities attending intestinal distention. Proc. Soc. Exp. Biol. Med., *41*:490, 1939.
22. Bengtsson, M.: Changes in skin blood flow and temperature during spinal analgesia evaluated by laser Doppler flowmetry and infra-red thermography. Acta. Anaesthesiol. Scand., *28*:625, 1984.
23. Benumof, J.L., and Wahrenbrock, E.A.: Blunted hypoxic pulmonary vasoconstriction by increased lung vascular pressures. J. Appl. Physiol., *38*:846, 1975.
24. Berkowitz, A., and Rosenberg, H.: Femoral block with mepivacaine for muscle biopsy in malignant hyperthermia patients. Anesthesiology, *62*:651, 1985.
25. Bergren, D.R., and Beckman, D.L.: Pulmonary surface tension and head injury. J. Trauma., *15*:336, 1975.
26. Berne, R.M.: Haemodynamics and sodium excretion of denervated kidney in anaesthetized and unanaesthetized dog. Am. J. Physiol., *171*:148, 1952.
27. Berquist, E., Berquist, D., Bronge, A., Dahlgreen, S., and Lindquist, B.: An evaluation of early thrombosis prophylaxis following fracture of the femoral neck. Acta Chir. Scand., *138*:689, 1972.
28. Bevan, D.R.: The sodium story: Effects of anaesthesia and surgery on intrarenal mechanisms concerned with sodium homeostasis. Proc. R. Soc. Med., *66*:1215, 1973.
29. Bevan, D.R., *et al.*: Closing volume and pregnancy. Br. Med. J., *1*:13, 1974.
30. Biehl, D.B., Shnider, S.M., Levinson, G., and Callender, K.: Placental transfer of lidocaine: Effects of fetal acidosis. Anesthesiology, *48*:409, 1978.
31. Bieniarz, J., *et al.*: Aortocaval compression by the uterus in late human pregnancy. II: An arteriographic study. Am. J. Obstet. Gynecol., *100*:203, 1968.
32. Binnert, D., Thierry, A., Michiels, R., Soichot, P., and Perrin, M.: Presentation d'un nouveau cas d'hematome extradural rachidien spontane observe au cours d'un accouchement. J. Med. Lyon, *52*:1307, 1971.

32a. Blomberg, R.: The dorsomedian connective tissue band in the lumbar epidural space of humans. Anesth. Analg., *65*:747, 1986.

33. Bonica, J.J.: Continuous epidural block. Anesthesiology, *17*:626, 1956.
34. ———: Maternal physiologic changes during pregnancy and anesthesia. In Shnider, S.M., and Moya, F. (eds.): The Anesthesiologist, Mother and Newborn. pp. 3–19. Baltimore, Williams & Wilkins, 1974.
35. ———: Principles and Practice of Obstetric Analgesia and Anesthesia. pp. 725, 745. Philadelphia, F.A. Davis, 1967.
36. Bonica, J.J., *et al.*: Peridural block: Analysis of 3637 cases and a review. Anesthesiology, *18*:723, 1957.
37. Bonica, J.J., Akamatsu, T.J., Berges, P.U., Morikawa, K., and Kennedy, W.F.: Circulatory effects of peridural block. II. Effects of epinephrine. Anesthesiology, *34*:514, 1971.
38. Bonica, J.J., Berges, P.U., and Morikawa, K.: Circulatory effects of peridural block. I. Effects of levels of analgesia and dose of lidocaine. Anesthesiology, *33*:619, 1970.
39. Bonica, J.J., Kennedy, W.F., Akamatsu, T.J., and Gerbershagen, H.U.: Circulatory effects of peridural block. III. Effects of acute blood loss. Anesthesiology, *36*:219, 1972.

40. Bonica, J.J., Kennedy, W.F., Ward, R.J., and Tolas, A.G.: A comparison of the effects of high subarachnoid and epidural anesthesia. Acta Anaesthesiol. Scand., *23*[*Suppl.*]:429, 1966.
41. Bonjour, J.P., Churchill, P.C., and Malvin, R.L.: Change of tubular reabsorption of sodium and water after renal denervation in the dog. J. Physiol. (Lond.), *204*:571, 1969.
42. Bonniot, A.: Note sur la pression epidurale negative. Bull. Soc. Nat. Chir., *60*:124, 1934.
43. Bowler, G.M., Wildsmith, J.A., and Scott, D.B.: Epidural administration of local anesthetics. *In* Acute Pain Management. pp 187–235. Cousins, M.J., and Phillips, G.D. (eds). New York, Churchill Livingstone, 1986.
44. Bowsher, D.: A comparative study of the azygos venous system in man, monkey, dog cat, rat and rabbit. J. Anat., *88*:400, 1954.
45. Boys, J.E., and Norman, P.F.: Accidental subdural analgesia. Br. J. Anaesth., *47*:1111, 1975.
46. Braham, J., and Saia, A.: Neurological complications of epidural anaesthesia. Br. Med., J., *2*:657, 1958.
47. Braid, D.P., and Scott, D.B.: The systemic absorption of local analgesic drugs. Br. J. Anaesth., *37*:394, 1965.
48. ———: Dosage of lignocaine in epidural block in relation to toxicity. Br. J. Anaesth., *38*:596, 1966.
49. Brandt, M.R., *et al.*: C-Peptide and insulin during blockade of the hyperglycaemic response to surgery by epidural analgesia. Clin. Endocrinol. (Oxf)., *6*:167, 1977.
50. Brandt, M.R., Kehlet, H., Binder, C., *et al.*: Effect of epidural analgesia on the glucoregulatory endocrine response to surgery. Clin. Endocrinol., *5*:107,1976.
51. Brandt, M.R., Kehlet, H., Binder, C., Hagen, C., and McNeilly, A.S.: Effect of epidural analgesia on the glycoregulatory endocrine response to surgery. Clin. Endocrinol. (Oxf.), *5*:107, 1976.
52. Brandt, M.R., Kehlet, H., Skovsted, L., and Hansen, J.M.: Rapid decrease in plasma-triiodothyronine during surgery and epidural analgesia independent of afferent neurogenic stimuli and of cortisol. Lancet, *2*:1333, 1976.
53. Brandt, M.R., Olgaard, K., and Kehlet, H.: Epidural analgesia inhibits the renin and aldosterone response to surgery. Acta Anaesthesiol. Scand., *23*:267, 1979.
54. Bridenbaugh, L.D., Moore, D.C., Bagdi, P., and Bridenbaugh, P.O.: The position of plastic tubing in continuous-block techniques: An X-ray study of 552 patients. Anesthesiology, *29*:1047, 1968.
55. Bridenbaugh, P.O., *et al.*: Role of epinephrine in regional block anesthesia with etidocaine: A double-blind study. Anesth. Analg. (Cleve.), *53*:430, 1974.
56. Brierley, J.B., and Field, E.J.: The connexions of the spinal sub-arachnoid space with the lymphatic system. J. Anat., *82*:153, 1948.
57. Brigden, W., Howarth, S., and Sharpey-Schafer, E.P.: Postural changes in the peripheral blood-flow of normal subjects with observations on vasovagal fainting reactions as a result of tilting, the lordotic posture, pregnancy and spinal anaesthesia. Clin. Sci. Mol. Med., *9*:79, 1950.
58. Britt, B.A., and Gordon, R.A.: Peripheral nerve injuries associated with anaesthesia. Can. Anaesth. Soc. J., *11*:514, 1964.
59. Brody, T.M., Calvert, D.N., and Schneider, A.F.: Alteration of carbon tetrachloride induced pathologic changes in the rat by spinal transection, adrenalectomy and adrenergic blocking agents. J. Pharmacol. Exp. Ther., *131*:341, 1961.
60. Bromage, P.R.: Vascular hypotension in 150 cases of epidural analgesia. Anaesthesia, *6*:26, 1951.
61. ———: Comparison of vasoactive drugs in man, Br. Med. J., *2*:72, 1952.
62. ———: The "hanging-drop" sign. Anaesthesia, *8*:237, 1953.
63. ———: Spinal epidural analgesia. Edinburgh, E. & S. Livingstone, 1954.
64. ———: Spirometry in assessment of analgesia after abdominal surgery. A method of comparing analgesic drugs. Br. Med. J., *2*:589, 1955.
64a. ———: Hypotension and vital capacity. Anaesthesia, *11*:139, 1956.
65. ———: The phrenic reflex in epidural analgesia. Can. Anaesth. Soc. J., *5*:29, 1958.
66. ———: Total respiratory compliance in anaesthetized subjects and modifications produced by noxious stimuli. Clin. Sci., *17*:217, 1958.
67. ———: Continuous lumbar epidural analgesia for obstetrics. Can. Med. Assoc. J., *85*:1136, 1961.
68. ———: Epidural needle. Anesthesiology, *22*:1018, 1961.
69. ———: Spread of analgesic solutions in the epidural space and their site of action: A statistical study. Br. J. Anaesth., *34*:161, 1962.
70. ———: Exaggerated spread of epidural analgesia in arteriosclerotic patients. Dosage in relation to biological and chronological ageing. Br. Med. J., *2*:1634, 1962.
71. ———: A comparison of the hydrochloride salts of lignocaine and prilocaine for epidural analgesia. Br. J. Anaesth., *37*:753, 1965.
72. ———: A comparison of the hydrochloride and carbon dioxide salts of lidocaine and prilocaine in epidural analgesia. Acta Anaesthesiol. Scand., *16*[*Suppl.*]:55, 1965.
73. ———: Ageing and epidural dose requirements. Segmental spread and predictability of epidural analgesia in youth and extreme age. Br. J. Anaesth., *41*:1016, 1969.
74. ———: An evaluation of bupivacaine in epidural analgesia for obstetrics. Can. Anaesth. Soc., J., *16*:46, 1969.
75. ———: Lower limb reflex changes in segmental epidural analgesia. Br. J. Anaesth., *46*:504, 1974.
76. ———: Mechanism of action of extradural analgesia. Br. J. Anaesth., *47*:199, 1975.
77. ———: Epidural Analgesia. Philadelphia, W.B. Saunders, 1978.
78. Bromage, P.R., Bramwell, R.S.B., Catchlove, R.F.H., Belanger, G., and Pearce, C.G.A.: Peridurography with metrizamide: Animal and human studies. Radiology, *128*:123, 1978.
79. Bromage, P.R., and Burfoot, M.F.: Quality of epidural blockade. II. Influence of physico-chemical factors: Hyaluronidase and potassium. Br. J. Anaesth., *38*:857, 1966.
80. Bromage, P.R., Burfoot, M.F., Crowell, D.F., and Pettigrew, R.T.: Quality of epidural blockade. I. Influence of physical factors. Br. J. Anaesth., *36*:342, 1964.

81. Bromage, P.R., Datta, S., and Dunford, L.A.: Etidocaine: An evaluation in epidural analgesia for obstetrics. Can. Anaesth. Soc. J., *21*:535, 1974.
82. Bromage, P.R., Joyal, A.C., and Binney, J.C.: Local anesthetic drugs: Penetration from the spinal extradural space into the neuraxis. Science, *140*:392, 1963.
83. Bromage, P.R., and Melzack, R.: Phantom limbs and the body schema. Can. Anaesth. Soc. J., *21*:267, 1974.
84. Bromage, P.R., and Millar, R.A.: Epidural blockade and circulating catecholamine levels in a child with phaeochromocytoma. Can. Anaesth. Soc. J., *5*:282, 1958.
85. Bromage, P.R., Pettigrew, R.T., and Crowell, D.E.: Tachyphylaxis in epidural analgesia. I. Augmentation and decay of local anesthesia. J. Clin. Pharmacol., *9*:30, 1969.
86. Bromage, P.R., Shibata, H.R., and Willoughby, H.W.: Influence of prolonged epidural blockade of blood sugar and cortisol responses to operations upon the upper part of abdomen and the thorax. Surg. Gynecol. Obstet., *132*:1051, 1971.
87. Brown, W.W.: Meningitis following continuous caudal anesthesia. Am. J. Obstet. Gynecol., *53*:682, 1947.
88. Brownridge, P.: Central neural blockade and caesarian section. I. Review and case series. Anaesth. Intens. Care, *7*:33, 1979.
88a. Brownridge, P.: Shivering related to epidural blockade in labor, and the influence of epidural pethidine. Anesth. Intens. Care, *14*:412, 1986.
89. Bryce-Smith, R.: Pressures in the extradural space. Anaesthesia, *5*:213, 1950.
90. ———: The spread of solutions in the extradural space. Anaesthesia, *9*:201, 1954.
91. Bryce-Smith, R., and Williams, E.O.: The treatment of eclampsia (imminent or actual) by continuous conduction analgesia. Lancet, *1*:1241, 1955.
92. Buchan, P.C., Milne, M.K., and Browning, M.C.K.: The effect of continuous epidural blockade of plasma 11-hydroxycorticosteroid concentrations in labour. Br. J. Obstet. Gynaecol., *80*:974, 1973.
93. Buckberg, G.D., Fixler, D.E., Archie, J.P., and Hoffman, J.I.E.: Experimental subendocardial ischemia in dogs with normal coronary arteries. Circ. Res., *30*:67, 1972.
94. Bull, G.M.: Postural proteinuria. Clin. Sci. Mol. Med., *7*:77, 1948.
95. Burn, J.M.B.: A method of continuous epidural analgesia. Anaesthesia, *18*:78, 1963.
96. Burn, J.M., Guyer, P.B., and Langdon, L.: The spread of solutions injected into the epidural space: A study using epidurograms in patients with the lumbosciatic syndrome. Br. J. Anaesth., *45*:338, 1973.
97. Butler, M.J., *et al.*: Plasma catecholamine concentrations during operation. Br. J. Surg., *64*:786, 1977.
98. Calder, A.A., Moar, V.A., Qunsted, M.K., and Turnbull, A.C.: Increased bilirubin levels in neonates after induction of labour by intravenous prostaglandin E_2 or Oxytocin. Lancet, *2*:1339, 1974.
99. Caldeyro-Barcia, R., *et al.*: Effects of position changes on the intensity and frequency of uterine contractions during labor. Am. J. Obstet. Gynecol., *80*:284, 1960.
100. Caldeyro-Barcia, R., and Poseiro, J.J.: Physiology of the uterine contraction. Clin. Obstet. Gynecol., *3*:386, 1960.
101. Callingham, B.A., and Barrand, M.A.: Catecholamines in blood. J. Pharm. Phrmacol., *28*:356, 1976.
102. Calnan, J.S., and Allenby, F.: The prevention of deep vein thrombosis after surgery. Br. J. Anaesth., *47*:151, 1975.
103. Calverley, J.R., and Mulder, D.W.: Femoral neuropathy. Neurology, *10*:963, 1960.
104. Campbell, E.J.M.: The relationship of the sensation of breathlessness to the act of breathing. *In* Howell, J.B.L., and Campbell, E.J.M.: Breathlessness. pp. 55-64. Oxford, Blackwell Scientific Publications, 1966.
105. Campbell, H.H., and Walker, F.G.: Continuous epidural analgesia in the treatment of frostbite. A report of three cases. Can. Med. Assoc. J., *84*:87, 1961.
106. Carrom, H., and Covino, B.G.: Symposium: Influence of anaesthetic procedures on surgical sequelae. Reg. Anesth. *7*[*Suppl.*]:S1-S193, 1982.
107. Catchlove, R.F.H.: The influence of CO_2 and *p*H on local anesthetic action. J. Pharmacol. Exp. Ther., *181*:298, 1972.
108. Catterberg, J.: Local anesthetic vs. spinal fluid. Anesthesiology, *46*:309, 1977.
109. Celander, O.: The range of control exercised by the sympathico-adrenal system. A quantitative study on blood vessels and other smooth muscle effectors in the cat. Acta Physiol. Scand., *32*[*Suppl. 116*]:1, 1954.
110. Cheng, P.A.: Blunt-tip needle for epidural anesthesia. Anesthesiology, *19*:556, 1958.
111. ———: The anataomical and clinical aspects of epidural anesthesia. Anesth. Analg. (Cleve.), *42*:398, 1963.
112. Christensen, N.J., and Brandsborg, O.: The relationship between plasma catecholamine concentration and pulse rate during exercise and standing. Eur. J. Clin. Invest., *3*:299, 1973.
113. Christensen, V., Ladengaard-Pedersen, H.J., and Skovsted, P.: Intravenous lidocaine as a suppressant of persistent cough caused by bronchoscopy. Acta Anaesthesiol. Scand., *67*[*Suppl.*]:84, 1978.
114. Clarke, C.J., and Whitewell, J.: Intradural haemorrhage after epidural injection. Br. Med. J., *2*:1612, 1961.
115. Clarke, E., Morrison, R., and Roberts, H.: Spinal cord damage by Efocaine. Lancet, *1*:896, 1955.
116. Cleland, J.G.P.: Continuous peridural and caudal analgesia in surgery and early ambulation. Northwest. Med. J., *48*:26, 1949.
117. ———: Continuous peridural and caudal analgesia in obstetrics. Anesth. Analg. (Cleve.), *28*:61, 1949.
118. Coggeshall, R.E., Coulter, J.D., and Willis, W.D.: Unmyelinated axons in the ventral roots of the cat lumbosacral enlargement. J. Comp. Neurol., *153*:39, 1974.
119. Cohen, C.A., and Kallos, T.: Failure of spinal anesthesia due to subdural catheter placement. Anesthesiology, *37*:352, 1972.
120. Cohen, E.N.: Distribution of local anesthetic agents in the neuraxis of the dog. Anesthesiology, *29*:1002, 1968.
121. Cohen, E.N., Levine, D.A., Colliss, J.E., and Gunther, R.E.: The role of pH in the development of tachyphylaxis to local anesthetic agents. Anesthesiology, *29*:994, 1968.

122. Cohen, G., Holland, B., Sha, J., and Goldenberg, M.: Plasma concentrations of epinephrine and norepinephrine during intravenous infusions in man. J. Clin. Invest., *38*:1935, 1959.
123. Cohen, S., Luykx, W.M., and Marx, G.F.: High versus low flow rates during lumbar epidural block. Reg. Anaesth., *9*:8, 1984.
124. Cohen, S.E., and Thurlow, A.: Comparison of a chloroprocaine–bupivacaine mixture with chloroprocaine and bupivacaine used individually for obstetric epidural analgesia. Anesthesiology, *51*:288, 1979.
125. Colding, A.: The effect of regional sympathetic blocks in the treatment of herpes zoster. A survey of 300 cases. Acta Anaesthiol. Scand., *13*:133, 1969.
126. Corbett, J.L., Frankel, H.L., and Harris, P.J.: Cardiovascular reflex responses to cutaneous and visceral stimuli in spinal man. J. Physiol. (Lond.), *215*:395, 1971.
127. ———: Cardiovascular responses to tilting in tetraplegic man. J. Physiol. (Lond.), *215*:411, 1971.
128. Corbin, K.B., and Gardner, E.D.: Decrease in number of myelinated fibers in human spinal roots with age. Anat. Rec., *68*:63, 1937.
129. Corke, B.C.: Neurobehavioral responses of the newborn. The effect of different anaesthesia. Anaesthesia, *32*:539, 1977.
130. Corke, B.G., Carlson, C.G., and Dettbarn, W.D.: The influence of 2-chloroprocaine on the subsequent analgesic potency of bupivacaine. Anesthesiology, *60*:25, 1984.
131. Corning, J.L.: Spinal anaesthesia and local medication of the cord. N.Y. Med. J., *42*:483, 1885.
132. Cort, J.H.: Relief of post-traumatic anuria. Am. J. Physiol., *164*:686, 1951.
133. ———: Effect of nervous stimulation on the arterio-venous oxygen and carbon dioxide differences across the kidney. Nature, *171*:784, 1953.
134. Cosgrove, D.O., and Jenkins, J.S.: The effects of epidural anaesthesia on the pituitary-adrenal response to surgery. Clin. Sci. Mol. Med., *46*:403, 1974.
135. Coupland, G.A.E., and Reeve, T.S.: Paraplegia: A complication of excision of abdominal aortic aneurysm. Surgery, *64*:878, 1968.
136. Cousins, M.J.: Vascular responses in arteriosclerotic patients. Anesthesiology, *35*:99, 1971.
137. ———: Hematoma following epidural block. Anesthesiology, *37*:263, 1972.
138. Cousins, M.J., *et al.*: Epidural block for abdominal surgery: Aspects of clinical pharmacology of etidocaine. Anaesth. Intens. Care, *6*:105, 1978.
139. Cousins, M.J., and Bromage, P.R.: A comparison of the hydrochloride and carbonated salts of lignocaine for caudal analgesia in out-patients. Br. J. Anaesth., *43*:1149, 1971.
140. Cousins, M.J., Gourlay, G.K., and Mather, L.E.: Axon, spinal cord, brain: Targets for acute pain control. *In* Scott, D.B., McClure, J., Wildsmith, J.A. (eds.): Regional Anaesthesia 1884–1984. Denmark, J.H. Schultz, 1984.
141. Cousins, M.J., and Mather, L.E.: Intrathecal and epidural administration of opioids. Anesthesiology, *61*:276, 1984.
142. Cousins, M.J., Mather, L.E., Glynn, C.J., Wilson, P.R., and Graham, J.R.: Selective spinal analgesia. Lancet, *1*:1141, 1979.
142a. Cousins, M.J., Skowronski, G., and Plummer, J.L.: Anaesthesia and the kidney. Immediate and delayed effects. Anaesth. Intens. Care, *11*:292, 1983.
143. Cousins, M.J., and Phillips, G.D. (eds): Acute pain management. *In* Clinics in Critical Care Medicine. Edinburgh, Churchill Livingstone, 1986.
144. Cousins, M.J., and Rubin, R.B.: The intraoperative management of phaeochromocytoma with total epidural sympathetic blockade. Br. J. Anaesth., *46*:78, 1974.
145. Cousins, M.J., and Wright, C.J.: Graft, muscle, skin blood flow after epidural block in vascular surgical procedures. Surg. Gynecol. Obstet., *133*:59, 1971.
146. Covino, B.G., and Scott, D.B.: Handbook of Epidural Anaesthesia and Analgesia. Orlando, Grune & Stratton, 1985.
147. Craft, J.B., Epstein, B.S., and Coakley, C.S.: Prophylaxis of dural-puncture headache with epidural saline. Anesth. Analg. (Cleve.), *52*:228, 1973.
148. Crawford, J.S.: The prevention of headache consequent upon dural puncture. Br. J. Anaesth., *44*:598, 1972.
149. ———: Principles and Practice of Obstetric Anaesthesia. ed. 4. Oxford, Blackwell Scientific Publications, 1978.
150. Crawford, J.S., Burton, M., and Davies, P.: Time and lateral tilt at caesaren section. Br. J. Anaesth., *44*:477, 1972.
151. Crawford, O.B.: The technic of continuous peridural anesthesia for thoracic surgery. Anesthesiology, *14*:316, 1953.
152. Crawley, B.E.: Catheter sequestration. A complication of epidural analgesia. Anaesthesia, *23*:270, 1968.
153. Crock, H.V., and and Yoshizawa, H.: The blood supply of the Vertebral Column and Spinal Cord in Man. New York, Springer-Verlag, 1977.
154. Cullen, M.L., Staren, E.D., El-Ganzouri, A., *et al.*: Continuous epidural infusion for analgesia after major abdominal operations: A randomized, prospective, double-blind study. Surgery, *98*:718, 1985.
155. Curbelo, M.M.: Continuous peridural segmental anesthesia by means of a ureteral catheter. Anesth. Analg. (Cleve.), *28*:13, 1949.
156. Cusick, J.F., Myklebust, J.B., and Abram, S.E.: Differential neural effects of epidural anesthetics. Anesthesiology, *53*:299, 1980.
157. Cusick, J.F., and Davidson, A.: Altered neural conduction with epidural bupivacaine. Anesthesiology, *57*:31, 1982.
158. Daly, M. de B., *et al.*: Cardiovascular-respiratory reflex interactions between carotid bodies and upper-airways receptors in the monkey. Am. J. Physiol., *234*:H293, 1978.
159. Daly, M. de B., and Scott, M.J.: An analysis of the primary cardiovascular reflex effects of stimulation of carotid body chemoreceptors in the dog. J. Physiol. (Lond.), *162*:555, 1962.
160. Datta, S., Alper, M.H., Ostheimer, G.W., *et al.*: Effects of maternal position on epidural anesthesia for cesarean section, acid base status, and bupivacaine concentrations at delivery. Anesthesiology, *50*:205, 1979.
160a. Davis, R.F., DeBoer, W.V., and Maroko, P.R.: Thoracic epidural anesthesia reduces myocardial infarct size after coronary artery occlusion in dogs. Anesth. Analg., *65*:711, 1986.
161. Davson, H., Demer, F.R., and Hollingsworth, J.R.: The mechanism of drainage of the cerebrospinal fluid. Brain, *96*:329,1973.

162. Dawkins, C.J.M.: Discussion on extradural spinal block. Proc. R. Soc. Med., *38*:299, 1945.
163. ———: Discussion of anaesthesia for caesarean section. Proc. R. Soc. Med., *40*:564, 1947.
164. ———: The identification of the epidural space. A critical analysis of the various methods employed. Anaesthesia, *18*:66, 1963.
165. ———: The relief of pain in labour by mean of continuous-drip epidural block. Acta Anaesthesiol. Scand., *37*[*Suppl.*]:248, 1970.
166. de Angelis, J.: Hazards of subdural and epidural anesthesia during anticoagulant therapy: A case report and review. Anesth. Analg. (Cleve.), *51*:676, 1972.
167. Defalque, R.J.: Compared effects of spinal and extradural anesthesia upon the blood pressure. Anesthesiology, *23*:627, 1962.
168. Denson, D.D., Raj, P.P., Saldahna, F., Finnsson, R.A., Ritschel, W.A., *et al.*: Continuous perineural infusion of bupivacaine for prolonged analgesia: Pharmacokinetic considerations. Int. J. Clin. Pharmacol., *21*:591, 1983.
169. Denson, D., Thompson, G., Raj, P., Finnsson, R.A., *et al.*: Continuous perineural infusions of bupivacaine for prolonged analgesia — a rapid two-point method for estimating individual pharmacokinetic parameters. Int. J. Clin. Pharmacol., *22*:552, 1984.
170. Dinnick, O.P.: Discussion on general anaesthesia for obstetrics: An evaluation of general and regional methods. Some aspects of general anaesthesia. Proc. R. Soc. Med., *50*:547, 1957.
171. Dogliotti, A.M.: Segmental peridural anaesthesia. Am. J. Surg., *20*:107, 1933.
172. ———: Anesthesia. p. 537. Chicago, S.B. Debour, 1939.
173. Don, H.F., Wahba, M., Caudrado, L., and Kelkar, K.: The effects of anesthesia and 100 per cent oxygen on the functional residual capacity of the lungs. Anesthesiology, *32*:521, 1970.
174. Doughty, A.: A precise method of cannulating the lumbar epidural space. Anaesthesia, *29*:63, 1974.
175. Downing, J.W.: Bupivacaine: A clinical assessment in lumbar extradural block. Br. J. Anaesth., *41*:427, 1969.
176. Dreyer, C., Bischoff, D., and Gothert, M.: Effects of methoxyflurane anesthesia on adrenal medullary catecholamine secretion: Inhibition of spontaneous secretion and secretion evoked by splanchnic-nerve stimulation. Anesthesiology, *41*:18, 1974.
177. Duncalf, D., and Foldes, F.F.: The use of radioiodinated serum albumin to confirm accidental intravascular insertion of epidural catheters. Anesthesiology, *25*:564, 1964.
178. Durant, P.A., Yaksh, T.L.: Epidural injections of bupivacaine, morphine, fentanyl, lofentanil, and DADL in chronically implanted rats: a pharmacologic and pathologic study. Anesthesiology, *64*:43–53, 1986.
179. Duval, J.O., and Griffith, D.P.: Epidural anesthesia for extracorporeal shock wave lithotripsy. Anesth. Analg., *64*:544–546, 1985.
180. Eaton, L.M.: Observations on the negative pressure in the epidural space. Mayo Clin. Proc., *14*:566, 1939.
181. Editorial: A time to be born. Lancet, *2*:1183, 1974.
182. Edwards, W.B., and Hingson, R.A.: The present status of continuous caudal analgesia in obstetrics. Bull. N.Y. Acad. Med., *19*:507, 1943.
183. Egbert, L.D., Tamersoy, K., and Deas, T.C.: Pulmonary function during spinal anesthesia: The mechanism of cough depression. Anesthesiology, *22*:882, 1961.
184. Ellis, F.R., Heffron, J.J.: Clinical and biochemical aspects of malignant hyperthermia. In: Recent Advances in Anesthesia and Analgesia, Ed. by R.S. Atkinson and A.P. Adams. Churchill Livingstone, New York, 1985 pp 173–207.
185. Enderby, G.E.H.: Controlled circulation with hypotensive drugs and posture to reduce bleeding in surgery. Preliminary results with pentamethonium iodide. Lancet, *1*:1145, 1950.
186. Engberg, G., and Wiklund, L.: The use of ephedrine for prevention of arterial hypotension during epidural blockade. A study of the central circulation after subcutaneous premedication. Acta Anaesthesiol. Scand., *66*[*Suppl.*]:1, 1978.
187. ———: The circulatory effects of intravenously administered ephedrine during epidural blockade. Acta Anaesthesiol. Scand., *66*[*Suppl.*]:27, 1978.
188. Engquist, A., Askgaard, B., and Funding, J.: Impairment of blood fibrinolytic activity during major surgical stress under combined extradural blockade and general anaesthesia. Br. J. Anaesth., *48*:903, 1976.
189. Erdemir, H.A., Soper, L.E., and Sweet, R.B.: Studies of factors affecting peridural anesthesia. Anesth. Analg. (Cleve.), *44*:400, 1965.
190. Evans, J.A., Dobben, G.D., and Gay, G.R.: Peridural effusion of drugs following sympathetic blockade. J.A.M.A., *200*:573, 1967.
191. Evans, T.I.: Regional anaesthesia for trans-urethral resection of the prostate — which method and which segments. Anaesth. Intens. Care, *2*:240, 1974.
192. Ferguson, J.F., and Kirsch, W.M.: Epidural empyema following thoracic extradural block. J. Neurosurg., *41*:762, 1974.
193. Fink, B.R. Mechanism of differential epidural block. Anesth. Analg. (Cleve.), *65*:325, 1986.
194. Fink, B.R., Aasheim, G., Kish, S.J., and Croley, T.S.: Neurokinetics of lidocaine in the infraorbital nerve of the rat in vivo: Relation to sensory block. Anesthesiology, *42*:731, 1975.
195. Fink, B.R., and Cairns, A.M.: Differential peripheral axon block with lidocaine: Unit studies in the cervical vagus nerve. Anesthesiology, *59*:182, 1983.
196. Fink, B.R., and Kish, S.J.: Reversible inhibition of rapid axonal transport in vivo by lidocaine hydrochloride. Anesthesiology, *44*:139, 1976.
197. Finster, M., and Petrie, R.H.: Monitoring of the fetus. Anesthesiology, *45*:198, 1976.
198. Fisher, A., and James, M.L.: Blood loss during major vaginal surgery. Br. J. Anaesth., *40*:710, 1968.
199. Fishman, A.P.: Pulmonary edema: The water-exchanging function of the lung. Circulation, *46*:390, 1972.
200. Flanc, C., Kakkar, V.V., and Clarke, M.B.: The detection of venous thrombosis of the legs using 125 I-labelled fibrinogen. Br. J. Surg., *55*:742, 1968.

201. Flowers, C.F.: Continuous peridural analgesia in obstetrics. Anaesthesia, *9*:146, 1954.
202. Folkow, B.: Nervous control of blood vessels. Physiol. Rev., *35*:629, 1955.
203. Forestier, J.: Le trou de conjugaison vertebral et l'espace epidural. p. 105. Paris, Jouve et Cie, 1922.
204. Forrester, A.C.: Mishaps in anaesthesia. Anaesthesia, *14*:388, 1959.
205. Fox, G.S.: Anaesthesia for intestinal short circuiting in the morbidly obese with reference to the pathophysiology of gross obesity. Can. Anaesth. Soc. J., *22*:307, 1975.
206. Frank, N.R., Mead, J., and Ferris, B.G.: The mechanical behaviour of the lungs in healthy elderly persons. J. Clin. Invest., *36*:1680, 1957.
207. Freund, F., Roos, A., and Dodd, R.B.: Expiratory activity of the abdominal muscles in man during general anesthesia. J. Appl. Physiol., *19*:693, 1964.
208. Freund, F.G., *et al.*: Ventilatory reserve and level of motor block during high spinal and epidural anesthesia. Anesthesiology, *28*:834, 1967.
209. Frey, H.H., and Soehring, K.: Untersuchungen uber die Durchlassigkeit der Dura Mater des Hundes fur Procain. Arch. Exp. Veterinaermed., *8*:804, 1954.
210. Froese, A.B., and Bryan, A.C.: Effects of anesthesia and paralysis on diaphragmatic mechanics in man. Anesthesiology, *41*:242, 1974.
211. Fruhstorfer, H., Zenz, M., Nolte, H., and Hensel, H.: Dissociated loss of cold and warm sensibility during regional anaesthesia. Pflugers Arch., *349*:73, 1974
212. Frumin, M.J., and Schwartz, H.: Continuous segmental peridural anesthesia. Anesthesiology, *13*:488, 1952.
213. Frumin, M.J., Schwartz, H., Burns, J.J., Brodie, B.B., and Papper, E.M.: Sites of sensory blockade during segmental spinal and segmental peridural anesthesia in man. Anesthesiology, *14*:576, 1953.
214. ———: The appearance of procaine in the spinal fluid during peridural block in man. J. Pharmacol. Exp. Ther., *109*:102, 1953.
215. Fujikawa, Y.F., Neves, A., Brasher, C.A., and Buckingham, W.W.: Epidural anesthesia in thoracic surgery: A preliminary report. J. Thorac. Surg., *17*:12W, 1948.
216. Galbert, M.W., and Marx, G.F.: Extradural pressures in the parturient patient. Anesthesiology, *40*:499, 1974.
217. Galindo, A., Hernandez, J., Benavides, O., Ortegon de Munoz, S., and Bonica, J.J.: Quality of spinal extradural anaesthesia: The influence of spinal nerve root diameter. Br. J. Anaesth., *47*:41, 1975.
218. Galindo, A., and Sprouse, J.H.: The influence of epidural anaesthesia on cardiac excitability in profound hypothermia. Can. Anaesth. Soc. J., *11*:614, 1964.
219. Galindo, A., and Witcher, T.: Mixtures of local anesthetics: bupivacaine-chloroprocaine. Anesth. Analg., *56*:683, 1980.
220. Gallus, A.S., *et al.*: Small subcutaneous doses of heparin in prevention of venous thrombosis. N. Engl. J. Med., *288*:545, 1973.
221. Gargano, F.P., Meyer, J.D., Sheldon, J.J.: Transfemoral ascending lumbar catheterization of the epidural veins in lumbar disk disease. Radiology, *111*:329, 1974.
222. Gavin, R.: Continuous epidural analgesia, an unusual case of dural perforation during catheterisation of the epidural space. N.Z. Med. J., *64*:280, 1965.
223. Gaynor, P.A.: The anatomy of the ligamentum flavum and its clinical applications. Br. J. Anaesth. (In Press)
224. Gelman, S., Feigenberg, Z., Dintzman, M., and Levy, E.: Electroenterography after cholecystectomy. The role of high epidural analgesia. Arch. Surg., *112*:580, 1977.
225. Germann, P.A.S., Roberts, J.G., and Prys-Roberts, C.: The combination of general anaesthesia and epidural block. I. The effects of sequence of induction on haemodynamic variables and blood gas measurements in healthy patients. Anaesth. Intens. Care, *7*:229, 1979.
226. Gilles, F.H., and Nag, D.: Vulnerability of human spinal cord in transient cardiac arrest. Neurology, *21*:833, 1971.
227. Gillies, I.D.S., and Morgan, M.: Accidental total spinal analgesia with bupivacaine. Anaesthesia, *28*:441, 1973.
228. Gingrich, T.F.: Spinal epidural hematoma following continuous epidural anesthesia. Anesthesiology, *29*:162, 1968.
229. Gissen, A.J., Covino, B.G., and Gregus, J.: Differential sensitivity of mammalian nerves to local anesthetic drugs. Anesthesiology, *53*:467, 1980.
230. Gissen, A.J., Datta, S., and Lambert, D.: The chloroprocaine controversy. Reg. Anesth., *9*:124, 1984.
231. Gordon, N.H., Scott, D.B., and Robb, I.W.P.: Modification of plasma corticosteroid concentrations during and after surgery by epidural blockade. Br. Med. J., *1*:581, 1973.
232. Gove, L.H.: Backache, headache and bladder dysfunction after delivery. Br. J. Anaesth., *45*:1147, 1973.
233. Granger, H.J., and Guyton, A.C.: Autoregulation of the total systemic circulation following destruction of the central nervous system in the dog. Circ. Res., *25*:379, 1969.
234. Greene, N.M.: Area of differential block in spinal anesthesia with hyperbaric tetracaine. Anesthesiology, *19*:45, 1958.
235. Greiss, F.C., and Gobble, F.L.: Effect of sympathetic nerve stimulation on the uterine vascular bed. Am. J. Obstet. Gynecol., *97*:962, 1967.
236. Griffiths, D.P.G., Diamond, A.W., and Cameron, J.D.: Postoperative extradural analgesia following thoracic surgery: A feasibility study. Br. J. Anaesth., *47*:48, 1975.
237. Griffiths, H.W.C., and Gillies, J.: Thoraco-lumbar splanchnicectomy and sympathectomy: Anaesthetic procedure. Anaesthesia, *3*:134, 1948.
238. Grodner, A.S., *et al.*: Neurotransmitter control of sinoatrial pacemaker frequency in isolated rat atria and in intact rabbits. Circ. Res., *27*:867, 1970.
239. Gronert, G.A., Theye, R.A., Milde, J.H., *et al.*: Role of sympathetic activity in porcine malignant hyperthermia. Anesthesiology, *47*:411, 1977.
240. Grundy, E.M., *et al.*: Extradural analgesia revisited. A statistical study. Br. J. Anaesth., *50*:805, 1978.
241. Grundy, E.M., Rao., L.N., and Winnie, A.P.: Epidural anesthesia and the lateral position. Anesth. Analg. (Cleve.), *57*:95, 1978.
242. Grundy, E.M., Zamora, A.M., and Winnie, A.P.: Comparison of spread of epidural anesthesia in pregnant and nonpregnant women. Anesth. Analg. (Cleve.), *57*:544, 1978.
243. Gutierrez, A.: Valor de la aspiracion liquida en el espacio

peridural en la anestesia peridural. Review Circulation Buenos Aires, *12*:225, 1933.
244. ———: Anestesia Extradural. Review Cirugie Buenos Aires, p. 34, 1939.
245. Hamelberg, W., Siddall, J., and Claassen, L.: Perforation of dura by a plastic catheter during continuous caudal anesthesia. Arch. Surg., *78*:357, 1959.
246. Hammond, W.G., *et al.*: Studies in surgical endocrinology. IV. Anesthetic agents as stimuli to change in corticosteroids and metabolism. Ann. Surg., *148*:199, 1958.
247. Hancock, D.O.: A study of 49 patients with acute spinal extradural abscess. Paraplegia, *10*:285, 1973.
248. Harik, S.I., Raichle, M.E., and Reis, D.J.: Spontaneously remitting spinal epidural hematoma in a patient on anticoagulants. N. Engl. J. Med., *284*:1355, 1971.
249. Harper, A.M., Deshmukh, D., Rowan, J.O., and Jennett, W.B.: The influence of sympathetic nervous activity on cerebral blood flow. Arch. Neurol., *27*:1, 1972.
250. Harrison, D.C., Sprouse, J.H., and Morrow, A.G.: The antiarrhythmic properties of lidocaine and procaine amide. Clinical and physiologic studies of their cardiovascular effects in man. Circulation, *28*:486, 1963
251. Harrison, G.R., Parkin, I.G., and Shah, J.L.: Resin injection studies of the lumbar extradural space. Br. J. Anaesth., *57*:333, 1985.
252. Hayes, M.F., Rosenbaum, R.W., Zibelman, M., and Matsumoto, T.: Adult respiratory distress syndrome in association with acute pancreatitis. Evaluation of positive end expiratory pressure ventilation and pharmacologic doses of steroids. Am. J. Surg., *127*:314, 1974.
253. Hehre, F.W., and Sayig, J.M.: Continuous lumbar peridural anesthesia in obstetrics. Am. J. Obstet. Gynecol., *80*:1173, 1960.
254. Hehre, F.W., Sayig, J.M., and Lowman, R.M.: Etiologic aspects of failure of continuous lumbar peridural anesthesia. Anesth. Analg. (Cleve.), *39*:511, 1960.
255. Heldt, J.H., and Moloney, J.C.: Negative pressure in the epidural space. Am. J. Med. Sci., *175*:371, 1928.
256. Hendolin, H., Mattila, M.A., and Poikolainen, E.: The effect of lumbar epidural analgesia on the development of deep venous thrombosis of the legs after prostatectomy. Acta Chir. Surg., *147*:425, 1981.
257. Hills, N.H., Pflug, J.J., Jeyasingh, K., Boardman, L., and Calnan, J.S.: Prevention of deep vein thrombosis by intermittent pneumatic compression of calf. Br. Med. J., *1*:131, 1972.
258. Hindmarsh, T.: Methiodal sodium and metrizamide in lumbar myelography. Acta Radiol. (Stockh.), *355*[*Suppl.*]:359, 1973.
259. Hingson, R.A., and Edwards, W.B.: An analysis of the first ten thousand confinements managed with continuous caudal analgesia with a report of the authors' first one thousand cases. J.A.M.A., *123*:538, 1943.
260. Hingson, R.A., and Southworth, J.L.: Continuous caudal anesthesia. Am. J. Surg., *58*:93, 1942.
261. Hjorts, N.C., Neumann, P., Frsig, F., *et al.*: A controlled study on the effect of epidural analgesia with local anesthetics and morphine on morbidity after abdominal surgery. Acta Anaesthesiol. Scand., *29*:790, 1985.
262. Hoar, P.F., Hickey, R.F., and Ullyot, D.J.: Systemic hypertension following myocardial revascularization. A method of treatment using epidural anesthesia. J. Thorac. Cardiovasc. Surg., *71*:859, 1976.
263. Hodgkinson, R., *et al.*: Neonatal neurobehavioural tests following vaginal delivery under ketamine thiopental and extradural anesthesia. Anesth. Analg. (Cleve.), *56*:548, 1977.
264. Hodgkinson, R., and Husain, F.J.: Obesity gravity and spread of epidural anesthesia. Anesth. Analg. (Cleve.), *60*:421, 1981.
265. Hodgson, D.C.: Venous stasis during surgery. Anaesthesia, *19*:96, 1964.
266. Hoffman, J.I.E., and Buckberg, G.D.: Transmural variations in myocardial perfusion. *In* Yu, P., and Goodwin, J. (eds.): Progress in Cardiology. Vol. V. pp. 37–89, Philadelphia, Lea & Febiger, 1976.
267. Hollmen, A.I., *et al.*: Neurologic activity of infants following anesthesia for cesarean section. Anesthesiology, *48*:350, 1978.
268. Hollmen, A., and Saukkonen, J.: The effects of postoperative epidural analgesia versus centrally acting opiate on physiological shunt after upper abdominal operation. Acta Anaesthesiol. Scand., *16*:147, 1972.
269. Holmdahl, M.H., Sjorgren, S., Strom, G., and Wright, B.: Clinical aspects of continuous epidural blockade for postoperative pain relief. Ups. J. Med. Sci., *77*:47, 1972.
270. Holmes, F.: Spinal analgesia and caesarean section. Maternal mortality. Br. J. Obstet. Gynaecol., *64*:229, 1957.
271. Honkomp, J.: Zur Begutachtung Bleibender Neurologischer Schaden nach Periduralanaesthesie. Der Anaesthesist, *15*:246, 1966.
272. Houghton, A., Hickey, J.B., Ross, S.A., and Dupre, J.: Glucose tolerance during anaesthesia and surgery. Comparison of general and extradural anaesthesia. Br. J. Anaesth., *50*:495,1 978.
273. Howarth, F.: Studies with a radioactive spinal anaesthetic. Br. J. Pharmacol., *4*:333, 1949.
274. ———: Observations on the passage of a colloid from cerebrospinal fluid to blood and tissues. Br. J. Pharmacol., *7*:573, 1952.
275. Howat, D.D.C.: President's address. Anaesthesia for biliary and pancreatic surgery. Proc. R. Soc. Med., *70*:152, 1977.
276. Hume, D.M., Bell, C.C., and Bartter, F.M.: Direct measurement of adrenal secretion during operative trauma and convalescence. Surgery, *52*:174, 1962.
277. Husemeyer, R.P., and White, D.C.: Lumbar extradural injection pressures in pregnant women. An investigation of relationships between rate of injection, injection pressures and extent of analgesia. Br. J. Anaesth., *52*:55, 1980.
278. Hutchinson, B.R.: Caudal analgesia in obstetrics. N.Z. Med. J., *65*:224, 1966.
279. Hylton, R.R., Eger, E.I., and Rovno, S.H.: Intravascular placement of epidural catheters. Anesth. Analg. (Cleve.), *43*:379, 1964.
280. Ingbert, C.: An enumeration of the medullated nerve fibers in the dorsal roots of the spinal nerves of man. J. Comp. Neurol., *13*:53, 1903.
281. Jacobs, S., Pullan, P.T., Potter, J.M., and Shenfield, G.M.:

Adrenal suppression following extradural steroids. Anaesthesia, *38*:953, 1983.

282. James, F.M., George, R.H., Haiem, H., and White, G.J.: Bacteriologic aspects of epidural analgesia. Anesth. Analg. (Cleve.), *55*:187, 1976.

283. Janzen, E.: Der Negative Vorschlag bei Lumbalpunktion. Dtsch. Z. Nervenheilk., *94*:280, 1926.

284. Jenicek, J.A.: Aseptic meningitis following lumbar epidural block: Case report. Anesthesiology, *16*:464, 1955.

285. Jeyaram, C., and Torda, T.A.: Anesthetic management of cholecystectomy in a patient with buccal pemphigus. Anesthesiology, *40*:600, 1974.

286. Johnson, S.R.: The mechanism of hyperglycemia during anesthesia: An experimental study. Anesthesiology, *10*:379, 1949.

287. Johnsson, S.R., Bygdeman, S., and Eliasson, R.: Effect of dextran on postoperative thrombosis. Acta Chir. Scand., *387*[*Suppl.*]:80, 1968.

288. Jorfeldt, L., *et al.*: The effect of local anaesthetics on the central circulation and respiration in man and dog. Acta Anaesthesiol. Scand., *12*:153, 1968.

289. Jouppila, R., *et al.*: Cyclic amp and segmental epidural analgesia during labour. Acta Anaesthesiol. Scand., *21*:95, 1977.

290. Jouppila, R., *et al.*: Effect of segmental extradural analgesia on placental blood flow during normal labour. Br. J. Anaesth., *50*:563, 1978.

291. Jouppila, R., *et al.*: Segmental epidural analgesia and postpartum sequelae. Ann. Chir. Gynaeacol., *67*:85, 1978.

292. Kakkar, V.V., *et al.*: Prevention of fatal postoperative pulmonary embolism by low doses of heparin. An international multicentre trial. Lancet, *2*:45, 1975.

293. Kakkar, V.V., Howe, C.T., Nicolaides, A.N., Renney, J.T.G., and Clarke, M.B.: Deep vein thrombosis of the leg. Is there a "high risk" group? Am J Surg., *120*:527, 1970.

294. Kalas, D.B., and Hehre, E.W.: Continuous lumbar peridural anesthesia in obstetrics. VIII. Further observations on inadvertent lumbar puncture. Anesth. Analg. (Cleve.), *51*:192, 1972.

295. Kane, R.F.: Neurologic deficits following epidural or spinal anesthesia. Anesth. Analg., *60*:150, 1981.

296. Kaplan, J.A., and King, S.B.: The precordial electrocardiographic lead (V5) in patients who have coronary-artery disease. Anesthesiology, *45*:570, 1976.

297. Kasten, G.W., and Martin, S.T.: Resuscitation from bupivacaine-induced cardiovascular toxicity during partial inferior vena cava occlusion. Anesth. Analg., *65*:341, 1986.

298. Katz, H., Borden, H., and Hirscher, D.: Glass-particle contamination of color-break ampules. Anesthesiology, *39*:354, 1973.

299. Kehlet, H.: The stress response to anaesthesia and surgery: Release mechanisms and modifying factors. Clin. Anaesth., *2*:215, 1984.

300. Keith, I.: Anaesthesia and blood loss in total hip replacement. Anaesthesia, *32*:444, 1977.

301. Kennedy, W.F., Jr.: Effects of spinal and peridural blocks on renal and hepatic functions. *In* Clinical Anesthesia Series. pp. 110–121. F.A. Davis, Philadelphia, 1969.

302. Kennedy, W.F., Everett, G.B., Cobb, L.A., and Allen, G.D.: Simultaneous systemic and hepatic hemodynamic measurements during high spinal anesthesia in normal man. Anesth. Analg. (Cleve.), *49*:1016, 1970.

303. ———: Simultaneous systemic and hepatic hemodynamic measurements during high peridural anesthesia in normal man. Anesth. Analg. (Cleve.), *50*:1069, 1971.

304. Kerr, D.D., Wingard, D.W., and Gatz, E.E.: Prevention of porcine malignant hyperthermia by epidural block. Anesthesiology, *42*:307, 1975.

305. Khazin, A.F., Hon, E.H., and Hehre, F.W.: Effects of maternal hyperoxia on the fetus. I. Oxygen tension. Am. J. Obstet. Gynecol., *109*:628, 1971.

305a. Klepper, I.D., Sherril, D.L., Boetger, C.L., and Bromage, P.R.: The analgesic and respiratory effects of epidural sufentanil in volunteers and the influence of adrenaline as an adjunct. Br. J. Anaesth. (In Press).

306. Kliemann, F.A.D.: Paraplegia and intercranial hypertension following epidural anesthesia. Report of four cases. Arq. Neuropsiquiatr., *33*:217, 1975.

307. Kobrine, A.I., Doyle, T.F., and Rizzoli, H.V.: Spinal cord blood flow as affected by changes in systemic arterial blood pressure. J. Neurosurg., *44*:12, 1976.

308. Kosaka, M., Simon, E., and Thauer, R.: Shivering in intact and spinal rabbits during spinal cord cooling. Experientia, *23*:385, 1966.

309. Kosody, R., Palahniuk, R.J., Wade, J.G., and Cumming, M.O.: The effect of subarachnoid epinephrine and phenylephrine on spinal cord blood flow. Can. Anaesth. Soc. J., *31*:503, 1984.

310. Kossman, C.E., *et al.*: Recommendations for standardisation of leads and of specifications for instruments in electrocardiography and vectorcardiography. Circulation, *35*:583, 1967.

311. Kostreva, D.R., Zuperku, E.J., Hess, G.L., Coon, R.L., and Kampine, J.P.: Pulmonary afferent activity recorded from sympathetic nerves. J. Appl. Physiol., *39*:37, 1975.

312. Kyosola, K.: Clinical experiences in the management of cold injuries: A study of 110 cases. J. Trauma, *14*:32, 1974.

313. Lahnborg, G., and Bergstrom, K.: Clinical and haemostatic parameters related to thromboembolism and low-dose heparin prophylaxis in major surgery. Acta Chir. Scand., *141*:590, 1975.

314. Landgren, S., and Neil, E.: The contribution of carotid chemoceptor mechanisms to the rise of blood pressure caused by carotid occlusion. Acta Physiol. Scand., *23*:152, 1951.

315. Larson, C.P., Mazze, R.I., Cooperman, L.H., and Wollman, H.: Effects of anesthetics on cerebral, renal and splanchnic circulations. Anesthesiology, *41*:169, 1974.

316. Lassen, N.A.: Control of cerebral circulation in health and disease. Circ. Res., *34*:749, 1974.

317. Lazorthes, G., *et al.*: La vascularisation arterielle du renflement lombaire. Etude des variations et des suppleances. Rev. Neurol. (Paris), *114*:109, 1966.

318. Lazorthes, G., Poulhes, J., Bastide, G., Chancolle, A.R., and Zadeh, O.: Le vascularisation de la moelle epiniere (etude anatomique et physiologique). Rev. Neurol. (Paris), *106*:535, 1962.

319. Lee, J.A.: Specially marked needle to facilitate extradural block. Anaesthesia, *15*:186, 1960.

320. Leriche, R.: Resultat eloigne de la ganglionectomie lombaire dans les troubles trophiques et vasomoteurs de la poliomyelite infantile. Lyon Chir., *44*:399, 1949.
321. Lerner, S.M., Gutterman, P., and Jenkins, F.: Epidural hematoma and paraplegia after numerous lumbar punctures. Anesthesiology, *39*:550, 1973.
322. Levin, G.L.L.: Treatment of bronchial asthma by dorsal perisympathetic injection of absolute alcohol. Lancet, *2*:249, 1934.
323. Levy, N.M.: Sympathetic-parasympathetic interactions in the heart. Circ. Res., *29*:437, 1971.
324. Li, D.F., Rees, G.A.D., and Rosen, M.: Continuous extradural infusion of 0.0625% or 0.125% bupivacaine for pain relief in primigravid labour. Br. J. Anaesth., *57*:264, 1985.
325. Li, T.-H., Shimosato, S., and Etsten, B.E.: Methoxamine and cardiac output in nonanesthetised man and during spinal anesthesia. Anesthesiology, *26*:21, 1965.
326. Lloyd, J.W., and Carrie, L.E.S.: A method of treating renal colic. Proc. R. Soc. Med., *58*:634, 1965.
327. Lock, R.F., Greiss, F.C., and Winston-Salem, N.C.: The anesthetic hazards in obstetrics. Am. J. Obstet. Gynecol., *70*:861, 1955.
328. Löfgren, N.: Studies on Local Anaesthetics. Xylocaine. A New Synthetic Drug. Stockholm, Haegggstroms, 1948.
329. Löfström, B.: Blocking characteristics of etidocaine (Duranest). Acta Anaesthesiol. Scand., *60*[*Suppl.*]:21, 1975.
330. Loudon, J.D.O., and Scott, D.B.: Blood loss in gynaecological operations. Br. J. Obstet. Gynaecol., *67*:561,1 960.
331. Low, P.A.: Endoneural fluid pressure and microenvironment of nerve. p 599. *In* Peripheral Neuropathy. Dyck, P.J., Thomas, P.K., Lambert, E.H., and Bunge, R. (eds), Philadelphia, W.B. Saunders, 1984.
332. Lumbers, E.R., and Reid, G.C.: Effects of vaginal delivery and caesarian section on plasma renin activity and angiotensin II levels in human umbilical cord blood. Biol. Neonate, *31*:127, 1977.
333. Lund, P.C.: Peridural Analgesia and Anesthesia. pp. 71, 93. Springfield, Charles C Thomas, 1966.
334. Lush, D., Thorpe, J.N., Richardson, D.J., and Bowen, D.J.: The effect of epidural analgesia on the adrenocortical response to surgery. Br. J. Anaesth., *44*:1169, 1972.
335. McCarthy, G.S.: The effect of thoracic extradural analgesia on pulmonary gas distribution. Functional residual capacity and airway closure. Br. J. Anaesth., *48*:243, 1976.
336. Macintosh, R.R.: Lumbar Puncture and Spinal Analgesia. Edinburgh, E. & S. Livingstone, 1957.
337. Macintosh, R.R., and Mushin, W.W.: Observations on the epidural space. Anaesthesia, *2*:100, 1947.
338. McLean, A.P.H., Mulligan, G.W., Otton, P., and MacLean, L.D.: Hemodynamic alterations associated with epidural anesthesia. Surgery, *62*:79, 1967.
339. Madsen, S.N., Brandt, M.R., Endquist, A., Badawi, I., and Kehlet, H.: Inhibition of plasma cyclic AMP, glucose and cortisol response to surgery by epidural analgesia. Br. J. Surg., *64*:669, 1977.
340. Malatinsky, J., and Kadlic, T.: Inferior vena caval occlusion in the left lateral position. Br. J. Anaesth., *46*:165, 1974.
341. Male, C.G., and Martin, R.: Puerperal spinal epidural abscess. Lancet, *1*:608, 1973.
342. Malliani, A., Peterson, D.F., Bishop, V.S., and Brown, A.M.: Spinal sympathetic cardiocardiac reflexes. Circ. Res., *30*:158, 1972.
343. Marinacci, A.A.: Applied electromyography. pp. 163–180. Philadelphia, Lea & Febiger, 1968.
344. Marinacci, A.A., and Courville, C.B.: Electromyogram in evaluation of neurological complications of spinal anesthesia. J.A.M.A., *168*:1337, 1958.
345. Martin, R., Lamarche, Y., and Tetreault, L.: Comparison of the clinical effectiveness of lidocaine hydrocarbonate and lidocaine hydrochloride with and without epinephrine in epidural anaesthesia. Can. Anaesth. Soc. J., *28*:217, 1981.
346. Marx, G.F., and Greene, N.M.: Lactate-pyruvate ratio of umbilical vein blood. Am. J. Obstet. Gynecol., *92*:548, 1965.
347. Mason, D.T.: The autonomic nervous system and regulation of cardiovascular performance. Anesthesiology, *29*:670, 1968.
348. Mather, L.E., and Cousins, M.J.: Low-dose chlormethiazole infusion as a supplement to epidural blockade: Blood concentrations and clinical effects. Anaesth. Intens. Care, *8*:421, 1980.
349. Mather, L.E., Tucker, G.T., Murphy, T.M., Stanton–Hicks, M.D'A., and Bonica, J.J.: The effects of adding adrenaline to etidocaine and lignocaine in extradural anaesthesia. II. Pharmacokinetics. Br. J. Anaesth., *48*:989, 1976.
350. Mather, L.E., *et al.*: Cardiovascular and subjective central nervous system effects of long-acting local anaesthetics in man. Anaesth. Intens. Care, *7*:215, 1979.
351. Mellander, S., and Johansson, B.: Control of resistance, exchange and capacitance functions in the peripheral circulation. Pharmacol., Rev., *20*:117, 1968.
352. Melzack, R.: Phantom limb pain: Implications for treatment of pathologic pain. Anesthesiology, *35*:409, 1971.
353. Merry, A.F., Cross, J.A., Mayaded, S.V., and Wild, C.J.: Posture and spread of extradural analgesia in labour. Br. J. Anaesth., *53*:303, 1983.
354. Miller, L., Gertel, M., Fox, G.S., and MacLean, L.D.: Comparison of effect of narcotic and epidural analgesia on postoperative respiratory function. Am. J. Surg., *131*:291, 1976.
355. Mirkin, B.L.: Perinatal Pharmacology and Therapeutics. New York, Academic Press, 1976.
356. Modig, J., Borg, T., Karlstrom, G., Maripuu, E., and Sahltedt, B.: Thromboembolism after total hip replacement: Role of epidural and general anesthesia. Anesth. Analg., *62*:174, 1983.
357. Modig, J., and Malmberg, P.: Pulmonary and circulatory reactions during total hip replacement surgery. Acta Anaesthesiol. Scand., *19*:219, 1975.
358. Moir, D.D.: Blood loss during major vaginal surgery. A statistical study of the influence of general anaesthesia and epidural analgesia. Br. J. Anaesth., *40*:233, 1968.
359. Moir, D.D., and Davidson, S.: Postpartum complications of forceps delivery performed under epidural and pudendal nerve block. Br. J. Anaesth., *44*:1197, 1972.
360. Moir, D.D., and Willocks, J.: Epidural analgesia in British obstetrics. Br. J. Anaesth., *40*:129, 1968.

361. Moloney, P.J., Elliott, G.B., and Johnson, H.W.: Experience with priapism. J. Urol., *114*:72, 1975.
362. Moore, D.C.: Regional Block. ed. 4. Springfield, Charles C Thomas, 1976.
363. Moore, D.C., Bridenbaugh, L.D., Bridenbaugh, P.O., Thompson, G.E., and Tucker, G.T.: Does compounding of local anesthetic agents increase their toxicity in humans? Anesth. Analg. (Cleve.), *51*:579, 1972.
364. Moore, D.C., Hain, R.F., Ward, A., and Bridenbaugh, L.D.: Importance of the perineural spaces in nerve blocking. J.A.M.A., *156*:1050, 1954.
365. Morgan, M., and Norman, J.: The effect of extradural analgesia combined with light general anaesthesia and spontaneous ventilation on arterial blood-gases and physiological deadspace. Br. J. Anaesth., *47*:955, 1975.
366. Morikawa, K.-I., Bonica, J.J., Tucker, G.T., and Murphy, T.M.: Effect of acute hypovolaemia on lignocaine absorption and cardiovascular response following epidural block in dogs. Br. J. Anaesth., *46*:631, 1974.
367. Morison, D.H.: A double blind comparison of carbonated lidocaine and lidocaine hydrochloride in epidural anaesthesia. Can. Anaesth. Soc. J., *28*:387, 1981.
368. Moulds, R.F.W., and Denborough, M.A.: Biochemical basis of malignant hyperpyrexia. Br. Med. J., *2*:241, 1974.
369. Munson, E.S., Paul, W.L., and Embro, W.J.: Central-nervous-system toxicity of local anesthetic mixtures in monkeys. Anesthesiology, *46*:179, 1977.
370. Murphy, T.M., Mather, L.E., Stanton-Hicks, M.D'A., Bonica, J.J., and Tucker, G.T.: Effects of adding adrenaline to etidocaine and lignocaine in extradural anaesthesia. I. Block characteristics and cardiovascular effects. Br. J. Anaesth., *48*:893, 1976.
371. Murray, R.R.: Maternal obstetrical paralysis. Am. J. Obstet. Gynecol., *88*:399, 1964.
372. Mustard, J.F., and Murphy, E.A., Rowsell, H.C., and Downie, H.G.: Factors influencing thrombus formation in vivo. Am. J. Med., *33*:621, 1962.
373. Nachmias, V.T., Sullender, J.S., and Fallon, J.R.: Effects of local anesthetics and human platelets. Filopodial suppression and endogenous proteolysis. Blood, *53*:63, 1979.
374. Nancarrow, C., Plummer, J.L., Ilsley, A.H., McLean, C.F., and Cousins, M.J.: Effects of combined extradural blockade and general anaesthesia on indocyanine green clearance and halothane metabolism. Br. J. Anaesth., *58*:29, 1986.
375. Nathan, P.W.: Observations on sensory and sympathetic function during intrathecal analgesia. J. Neurol. Neurosurg. Psychiatry, *39*:114, 1976.
376. Nation, R.L., Triggs, E.J., and Selig, M.: Lignocaine kinetics in cardiac patients and aged subjects. Br. J. Clin. Pharmacol., *4*:439, 1977.
377. Nelson, D.A.: Spinal cord compression due to vertebral angiomas during pregnancy. Arch. Surg., *11*:408, 1964.
377a. Nickel, P.M., Bromage, P.R., Sherrill, D.L.: Comparison of hydrochloride and carbonated salts of lidocaine for epidural analgesia. Reg. Anaesth., *11*:62, 1986.
378. Nicolaides, A.N., *et al.*: Small doses of subcutaneous sodium heparin in the prevention of deep vein thrombosis after elective hip operations. Br. J. Surg., *62*:348, 1975.
379. Nikki, P., Takki, S., Tammisto, T., and Jaattela, A.: Effect of operative stress on plasma catecholamine levels. Ann. Clin. Res., *4*:146, 1972.
380. Nimmo, W.S., *et al.*: Gastric emptying following hysterectomy with extradural analgesia. Br. J. Anaesth., *50*:559, 1978.
381. Nishimura, N., Kitahara, T., and Kusakabe, T.: The spread of lidocaine and 1-131 solution in the epidural space. Anesthesiology, *20*:785, 1959,
382. Noble, A.D., *et al.*: Continuous lumbar epidural analgesia using bupivacaine: A study of the fetus and newborn child. Br. J. Obstet. Gynaecol., *78*:559, 1971.
383. Nunn, J.F.: Applied respiratory physiology with special reference to anesthesia. *In* Control of Breathing. London, Butterworth, 1969.
384. Oberg, B., and Thoren, P.: Studies on left ventricular receptors signalling in non-medullated vagal afferents. Acta Physiol. Scand., *85*:145, 1972.
385. ———: Increased activity in left ventricular receptors during hemorrhage or occlusion of caval veins in the cat. A possible cause of vaso-vagal reaction. Acta Physiol. Scand., *85*:164, 1972.
386. Oberg, B., and White, S.: Circulatory effects of interruption and stimulation of cardiac vagal afferents. Acta Physiol. Scand., *80*:383, 1970.
387. ———: The role of vagal cardiac nerves and arterial baroreceptors in the circulatory adjustments to hemorrhage in the cat. Acta Physiol. Scand., *80*:395, 1970.
388. Odoom, J.A., Sih, I.L.: Epidural analgesia and anticoagulant therapy. Experience with 1,000 cases of continuous epidurals. Anaesthesia *38*:254, 1983.
389. Orr, R.B., and Warren, K.W.: Continuous epidural analgesia in acute pancreatitis. Lahey Clin. Bull., *6*:204, 1950.
390. Ottesen, S., Renck, H., and Jynge, P.: Cardiovascular effects of epidural analgesia. An experimental study in sheep of the effects on central circulation, regional perfusion and myocardial performance during normoxia, hypoxia and isoproterenol administration. Nunt. Radiol., *69*:2, 1978.
391. Otton, P.E., and Wilson, E.J.: The cardiocirculatory effects of upper thoracic epidural analgesia. Can. Anaesth. Soc. J., *13*:541, 1966.
392. Oyama, T., and Matsuki, A.: Serum levels of thyroxine in man during epidural anesthesia and surgery. Der Anaesthetist, *19*:298, 1970.
393. Pages, F.: Anestesia metamerica. Rev. Sanid. Mil. (Madr.), *11*:351, 1921.
394. Palahniuk, R.J., Shnider, S.M., and Eger, E.I. II: Pregnancy decreases the requirement for inhaled anesthetic agents. Anesthesiology, *41*:82, 1974.
395. Palmeiro, C., *et al.*: Denervation of the abdominal viscera for the treatment of shock. N. Engl. J. Med., *269*:709, 1963
396. Park, W.Y., Hagins, F.M., Massengale, M.D., and MacNamara, Y.: The sitting positions and anesthetic spread in the epidural space. Anesth. Analg (Cleve.), *63*:863, 1984.
397. Park, W.Y., Hagins, F.M., Rivat, E.L. and MacNamara, T.E.: Age and epidural dose response in adult men. Anesthesiology, *56*:318, 1982.
398. Park, W.Y., Massengale, M., Kin, S.I., *et al.*: Age and the spread of local anesthetic solutions in the epidural space. Anesth. Analg (Cleve.), *59*:768, 1980.

399. Paton, A.S.: Lumbar epidural analgesia in obstetrics. Med. J. Aust., *2*:449, 1966.
400. Perkins, H.M., and Hanlon, P.R.: Epidural injection of local anesthetic and steroids for relief of pain secondary to herpes zoster. Arch. Surg., *113*:253, 1978.
401. Pflug, A.E., Murphy, T.M., Butler, S.H., and Tucker, G.T.: The effects of postoperative peridural analgesia on pulmonary therapy and pulmonary complications. Anesthesiology, *41*:8, 1974.
402. Philip, J.H., and Brown, W.U.: Total spinal anesthesia late in the course of obstetric bupivacaine epidural block. Anesthesiology, *44*: 340, 1976.
403. Pierce, J.A., and Ebert, R.V.: The elastic properties of the lungs of the aged. J. Lab. Clin. Med., *51*:63, 1958.
404. Pomeranz, B.H., Birtch, A.G., and Barger, A.C.: Neural control of intrarenal blood flow. Am. J. Physiol., *215*:1067, 1968.
405. Porte, D., Girardier, L., Seydoux, J., Kanazawa, Y., and Posternak, J.: Neural regulation of insulin secretion in the dog. J. Clin. Invest., *52*:210, 1973.
406. Prescott, L.F., Adjepon-Yamoah, K.K., and Talbot, R.G.: Impaired lignocaine metabolism in patients with myocardial infarction and cardiac failure. Br. Med. J., *1*:939, 1976.
407. Price, H.L., *et al.*: Can general anesthetics produce splanchnic visceral hypoxia by reducing regional blood flow? Anesthesiology, *27*:24, 1966.
408. Prys-Roberts, C.: Monitoring of the cardiovascular system. *In* Saidman, L.J., and Smith, N.T. (eds.): Monitoring in Anesthesia. pp. 53-83. New York, John Wiley and Sons, 1978.
409. Ralston, D.H., and Shnider, S.M.: The fetal and neonatal effects of regional anesthesia in obstetrics. Anesthesiology, *48*:34, 1978.
410. Ramsey, H.J.: Fat in the epidural space of young and adult cats. Am. J. Anat., *104*:345, 1959.
411. Ramsey, R., and Doppman, J.L.: The effects of epidural masses on spinal cord blood flow. An experimental study in monkeys. Radiology, *107*:99, 1973.
412. Rannigner, K., and Switz, D.M.: Local obstruction of the inferior vena cava by massive ascites. A. J. R., *93*:935, 1965.
413. Rao, T.L.K., and El-Etr, A.A.: Anticoagulation following placement of epidural and subarachnoid catheters: An evaluation of neurologic sequelae. Anesthesiology, *55*:618, 1981.
414. Reddy, S.V.R., and Yaksh, T.L.: Spinal noradrenergic terminal system mediates antinociception. Brain Res., *189*:391, 1980.
415. Reiz, S., Balfors, E., Sorensen, M.B., *et al.*: Coronary hemodynamic effects of general anesthesia and surgery: Modification by epidural analgesia in patients with ischemic heart disease. Reg. Anaesth. 7[*Suppl.*]:S8, 1982.
416. Reiz, S., and Nath, S.: Cardiotoxicity of local anesthetic agents. Br. J. Anaesth., *58*:736, 1986.
416a. Reynolds, A.F., Roberts, P.A., Pollay, M., and Stratemeier, P.H.: Quantitative anatomy of the thoracolumbar epidural space. Neurosurgery, *17*:905, 1985.
417. Risk, C., Rudo, N., and Falltrick, R.: Comparison of right atrial and pulmonary capillary wedge pressures. Crit. Care Med., *6*:172, 1978.
418. Roberts, V.C.: Thrombosis and how to prevent it. New Scientist and Science Journal, September 16, p. 620, 1971.
419. ———: Fibrinogen uptake scanning for diagnosis of deep vein thrombosis: A plea for standardization. Br. Med. J., *3*:455, 1975.
420. Roberts, V.C., and Cotton, L.T.: Prevention of postoperative deep vein thrombosis in patients with malignant disease. Br. Med. J., *1*:358, 1974.
421. ———: Failure of low-dose heparin to improve efficacy of preoperative intermittent calf compression in preventing postoperative deep vein thrombosis. Br. Med. J., *3*:458, 1975.
422. Roizen, M.F., Horrigan, R.W., and Frazer, B.M.: Anaesthetic doses blocking adrenergic (stress) responses to incision—MacBar. Anesthesiology, *54*:390, 198.
423. Roizen, M.F., Moss, J., Henry, D.P., and Kopin, I.J.: Effects of halothane on plasma catecholamines. Anesthesiology, *41*:432, 1974.
424. Romagnoli, A., and Batra, M.S.: Continuous epidural block in the treatment of impacted ureteric stones. Can. Med. Assoc., J., *109*:968, 1973.
425. Rooth, G., McBride, R., and Ivy, B.J.: Fetal and maternal *p*H measurements—a basis for common normal values. Acta Obstet. Gynecol. Scand., *52*:47, 1973.
426. Rosenberg, I.L., Evans, M., and Pollock, A.V.: Prophylaxis of postoperative leg vein thrombosis by low dose subcutaneous heparin or preoperative calf muscle stimulation: A controlled clinical trial. Br. Med. J., *1*:649, 1975.
427. Rosenberg, P.H., Saramies, L., and Alila, A.: Lumbar epidural anaesthetic with bupivacaine in old patients: Effect of speed and direction of injection. Acta Anaesth. Scand., *25*:270, 1981.
428. Ross, G.: Adrenergic responses of coronary vessels. Circ. Res., *39*:461, 1976.
429. Rowe, G.G.: Responses of the coronary circulation to physiologic changes and pharmacologic agents. Anesthesiology, *41*:182, 1974
430. Runciman, W.B., Mather, L.E., Ilsley, A.H., *et al.*: A sheep preparation for studying interactions between blood flow and drug disposition. III. Effects of general and spinal anaesthesia on regional blood flows and oxygen tensions. Br. J. Anaesth., *56*:1247, 1984.
431. Ryan, D.W.: Accidental intravenous injection of bupivacaine: A complication of obstetrical epidural anaesthesia. Br. J. Anaesth., *45*:907, 1973.
432. Sage, D.J., Feldman, H.S., Arthur, G.R., *et al.*: Influence of lidocaine and bupivacaine on isolated guinea pig atria in the presence of acidosis and hypoxia. Anesth. Analg. (Cleve.), *63*:1, 1983.
433. Salmoiraghi, G.C.: Functional organization of brain stem respiratory neurones. Ann. N.Y. Acad. Sci., *109*:5771, 1963.
434. Sanchez, R., Acuna, L., and Rocha, F.: An analysis of the radiological visualization of the catheters placed in the epidural space. Br. J. Anaesth., *39*:485, 1967.
435. Scanlon, J.W.: Effects of local anesthetics administered to parturient women on the neurobehavioural and behavioural performance of newborn children. Bull. N.Y. Acad. Med., *52*:231, 1976.

436. Scanlon, J.W., Brown, W.U., Weiss, J.B., and Alper, M.H.: Neurobehavioral responses of newborn infants after maternal epidural anesthesia. Anesthesiology, *40*:121, 1974.
437. Schobinger, R.A., Krueger, E.G., and Sobel, G.L.: Comparison of intraosseous vertebral venography and pantopaque myelography in the diagnosis of surgical conditions of the lumbar spine and nerve roots. Radiology, *77*:376, 1961.
438. Schreiner, E.J., Lipson, S.F., Bromage, P.R., and Camporesi, E.M.: Neurological complications following general anaesthesia. Anaesthesia, *38*:226, 1983.
439. Schulte-Steinberg, O., and Rahlfs, V.W.: Caudal anaesthesia in children and spread of 1 per cent lignocaine. A statistical study. Br. J. Anaesth., *42*:1093, 1970.
440. ———: Spread of extradural analgesia following caudal injection in children. A statistical study. Br. J. Anaesth., *49*:1027, 1977.
441. Schweitzer, S.A.: Chloremethiazole (Hemineurin) infusion as supplemental sedation during epidural block. Anaesth. Intens. Care, *6*:248, 1978.
442. Scott, D.B.: Inferior vena caval pressure. Changes occurring during anaesthesia. Anaesthesia, *18*:135, 1963.
443. ———: Inferior vena caval occlusion in late pregnancy. Clinical Anesthesia. Philadelphia, F.A. Davis, *10*:37, 1973.
444. ———: Management of extradural block during surgery. Br. J. Anaesth., *47*:271, 1975.
445. ———: Evaluation of the toxicity of local anesthetic agents in man. Br. J. Anaesth., *47*:56, 1975.
446. Scott, D.B., Davie, I.T., and Stephen, G.W.: Cardiovascular effects of intravenous lignocaine during nitrous oxide/halothane anaesthesia. Br. J. Anaesth., *43*:595, 1971.
447. Scott, D.B., Jebson, P.J.R., and Boyes, R.N.: Pharmacokinetic study of the local anaesthetics bupivacaine (Marcaine) and etidocaine (Duranest) in man. Br. J. Anaesth., *45*:1010, 1973.
448. Scott, D.B., and Kerr, M.G.: Inferior vena caval pressure in late pregnancy. Br. J. Obstset. Gynaecol., *70*:1044, 1963.
449. Scott, D.B., Littlewood, D.G., Drummond, G.B., Buckley, P.F., and Covino, B.G.: Modification of the circulatory effects of extradural block combined with general anaesthesia by the addition of adrenaline to lignocaine solutions. Br. J. Anaesth., *49*:917, 1977.
450. Scott, D.B., and Walker, L.R.: Administration of continuous epidural analgesia. Anaesthesia, *18*:82, 1963.
451. Scoville, W.B.: Epidural anesthesia and lateral position for lumbar disc operations. Surg. Neurol., *7*:163, 1977.
452. Semb, B.K., *et al.*: Ergot-induced vasospasm of the lower extremities treated with epidural anaesthesia. Scand. J. Thorac. Cardiovasc. Surg., *9*:254, 1975.
453. Seow, L.T., Lips, F.J., and Cousins, M.J.: Effect of lateral posture on epidural blockade for surgery. Anaesth. Intens. Care, *11*:97, 1983.
454. Seow, L.T., Lips, F.J., Cousins, M.J., and Mather, L.E.: Lidocaine and bupivacaine mixtures for epidural blockade. Anesthesiology, *56*:177, 1982.
455. Seow, L.T., Mather, L.E., and Cousins, M.J.: Comparison of the efficacy of chlormethiazole and diazepam as I.V. sedatives for supplementation of extradural anaesthesia. Br. J. Anaesth., *57*:747, 1985.
456. Severinghaus, J.W., *et al.*: Respiratory control at high altitude suggesting active transport regulation of CSF *p*H. J. Appl. Physiol., *18*:1155, 1963.
457. Shanks, C.A.: Four cases of unilateral analgesia. Br. J. Anaesth., *40*:999, 1968.
458. Shantha, T.R., and Evans, J.A.: The relationship of epidural anesthesia to neural membranes and arachnoid villi. Anesthesiology, *37*:543, 1972.
459. Shanthaveerappa, T.R.., and Bourne, G.H.: Perineural epithelium: A new concept of its role in the integrity of the peripheral nervous system. Science, *154*:1464, 1966.
460. Sharpey-Schafer, E.P.: Syncope. Br. Med. J., *1*:506, 1956.
461. Sharrock, N.E.: Epidural anesthetic dose responses in patients 20 to 80 years old. Anesthesiology, *49*:425, 1978.
462. Shimoji, K., *et al.*: Spinal hypalgesia and analgesia by low-frequency electric stimulation in the epidural space. Anesthesiology, *41*:91, 1974.
463. Shimosato, S., and Etsten, B.E.: The role of the venous system in cardiocirculatory dynamics during spinal and epidural anesthesia in man. Anesthesiology, *30*:619, 1969.
464. Shnider, S.M., Abboud, T.K., Artal, R., Henrikson, E.H., Stefani, S.J., and Levinson, G.: Maternal catecholamines decrease during labor after lumbar epidural anesthesia. Am. J. Obstet. Gynecol., *147*:13, 1983.
465. Sicard, J.A., and Forestier, J.: Radiographic method for exploration of the extradural space using lipiodol. Rev. Neurol. (Paris), *28*:1264, 1921.
466. ———: The Use of Lipiodol in Diagnosis and Treatment. p. 178. London, Oxford University Press, 1932.
467. Siever, J.M., and Mousel, L.H.: Continuous caudal anesthesia in three hundred unselected obstetric cases. J.A.M.A., *122*:424, 1943.
468. Silver, J.R., and Buxton, P.H.: Spinal stroke. Brain, *97*:539, 1974.
469. Simpson, B.R., Parkhouse, J., Marshall, R., and Lambrechts, W.: Extradural analgesia and the prevention of postoperative respiratory complications. Br. J. Anaesth., *33*:628, 1961.
470. Sjögren, S., and Wright, B.: Circulation, respiration and lidocaine concentration during continuous epidural blockade. Acta Anaesthesiol. Scand., *16*[*Suppl.*]:5, 1972.
471. Smith, A.L., Pender, J.W., and Alexander, S.C.: Effects of PCO_2 on spinal cord blood flow. Am. J. Physiol., *216*:1158, 1969.
472. Smith, A.L., and Wollman, H.: Cerebral blood flow and metabolism: Effects of anesthetic drugs and techniques. Anesthesiology, *36*:378, 1972.
473. Smith, O.A.: Reflex and central mechanisms involved in the control of the heart and circulation. Annu. Rev. Physiol., *36*:93, 1974.
474. South Australian Health Commission, 1985. Report of the Anaesthetics Mortality Committee. Anaesthetic Deaths in South Australia, 1974-1983.
475. Spence, A.A., and Smith, G.: Postoperative analgesia and lung function: A comparison of morphine with extradural block. Br. J. Anaesth., *43*:144, 1971.
476. Sreerama, V., Ivan, L.P., Dennery, J.M., and Richard, M.T.: Neurosurgical complications of anticoagulant therapy. Can. Med. Assoc. J., *108*:305, 1973.
477. Sripad, S., Antcliff, A.C., and Martin, P.: Deep-vein throm-

bosis in two district hospitals in Essex. Br. J. Surg., *58*:563, 1971.

478. Stanton–Hicks, M.D'A.: A study using bupivacaine for continuous peridural analgesia in patients undergoing surgery of the hip. Acta Anaesthesiol. Scand., *15*:97, 1971.

479. Stapleton, J.V., Austin, K.L., and Mather, L.E.: A pharmacokinetic approach to postopertive pain: Continuous infusion of pethidine. Anaesth. Intens. Care, *7*:25, 1979.

480. Steen, P.A., *et al.*: Efficacy of dopamine, dobutamine and epinephrine during emergence from cardiopulmonary bypass in man. Circulation, *57*:378, 1978.

481. Steinhaus, J.E., and Howland, D.E.: Intravenously administered lidocaine as a supplement to nitrous oxide-thiobarbiturate anesthesia. Anesth. Analg. (Cleve.), *37*:40, 1958.

482. Stephen, G.W., Lees, M.M., and Scott, D.B.: Cardiovascullar effects of epidural block combined with general anaesthesia. Br. J. Anaesth., *41*:933, 1969.

483. Stevens, R.A., and Stanton–Hicks, M.D.'A.: Subdural injection of local anesthetic: A complication of epidural anesthesia. Anesthesiology, *63*:323, 1985.

483a. Sundberg, A., Wattwil, M., and Arvill, A.: Respiratory effects of high thoracic epidural anaesthesia. Acta Anaesthesiol. Scand., *30*:215, 1986.

484. Sundt, T.M., *et al.*: Cerebral blood flow measurements and electroencephalograms during carotid endarterectomy. J. Neurosurg., *41*:310, 1974.

485. Sutton, J.R., Cole, A., Gunning, J., Hickie, J.B., and Seldon, W.A.: Control of heart-rate in healthy young men. Lancet, *2*:1398, 1967.

486. Suzuki, H., *et al.*: Neuromuscular effects of i.a. infusion of lignocaine in man. Br. J. Anaesth., *49*:1117, 1977.

486a. Takeshima, R., and Dohl, S.: Cervical epidural anesthesia and surgical blood loss in radical mastectomy. Reg. Anaesth., *11*:171, 1986.

487. Takki, S., Nikki, P., Tammisto, T., and Jaattela, A.: Effect of epidural blockade on the pentazocine-induced increase in plasma catecholamines and blood pressure. Br. J. Anaesth., *45*:376, 1973.

488. Thomson, P.D., *et al.*: Lidocaine pharmacokinetics in advanced heart failure, liver disease, and renal failure in humans. Ann. Intern. Med., *78*:499, 1973.

489. Thorud, T., Lund, I., and Holme, I.: The effect of anesthesia on intraoperative and postoperative bleeding during abdominal prostatectomies: A comparison of neurolept anesthesia, halothane anesthesia and epidural anesthesia. Acta Anaesthesiol. Scand., *57*[*Suppl.*]:83, 1975.

490. Tretjakoff, D.: Das Epidurale Fettgewebe. Z. Anat., *79*:100, 1926.

491. Tripathi, R.C.: Ultrastructure of the arachnoid mater in relation to outflow of cerebrospinal fluid. Lancet, *2*:8, 1973.

492. Tripathi, B.J., and Tripathi, R.C.: Vacuolar transcellular channels as a drainage pathway for cerebrospinal fluid. J. Physiol., *239*:195, 1974.

493. Trotter, M.: Variations of the sacral canal: Their significance in the administration of caudal analgesia. Anesth. Analg. (Cleve.), *26*:192, 1947.

494. Trueta, J., Barclay, A.E., Daniel, P.M., Franklin, K.J., and Prichard, M.M.L.: Studies of the Renal Circulation. Oxford, Blackwell Scientific Publications, 1948.

495. Tsuji, H., Shirasaka, C., Asoh, T., and Takeuchi, Y.: Influences of splanchnic nerve blockade on endocrine metabolic responses to upper abdominal surgery. Br. J. Surg., *70*:437, 1983.

496. Tucker, G.T., and Mather, L.E.: Pharmacokinetics of local anaesthetic agents. Br. J. Anaesth., *47*:213, 1975.

497. Tuohy, E.B.: Continuous spinal anesthesia: A new method of utilising a ureteral catheter. Surg. Clin. North. Am., *25*:834, 1945.

498. Turnbull, I.M.: Blood supply of the spinal cord: Normal and pathological considerations. Clin. Neurosurg., *20*:56, 1973.

499. Urban, B.J.: Clinical observations suggesting a changing site of action during induction and recession of spinal and epidural anesthesia. Anesthesiology, *39*:496, 1973.

500. Urban, B.J., and Nashold, B.S.: Percutaneous epidural stimulation of the spinal cord for relief of pain: Long term results. J. Neurosurg., *48*:323, 1978.

501. Urquhart–Hay, D.: Paraplegia following epidural analgesia. Anaesthesia, *24*:461, 1969.

502. Urquhat–Hay, D., Marshall, N.G., and Marsland, J.M.: Comparison of epidural and hypotensive anaesthesia in open prostatectomy. Series 1. N.Z. Med. J., *69*:280, 1969.

503. ———: Comparison of epidural and hypotensive anaesthesia in open prostatectomy. Series 2. N.Z. Med. J., *70*:223, 1969.

504. Usubiaga, J.E.: Neurological complications following epidural anesthesia. Int. Anaesthesiol. Clin., *13*:2, 1975.

505. Usubiaga, J.E., Dos Reis, A., and Usubiaga, L.E.: Epidural misplacement of catheters and mechanisms of unilateral blockade. Anesthesiology, *32*:158, 1970.

506. Usubiaga, J.E., Kolodny, J., and Usubiaga, L.E.: Neurological complications of prevertebral surgery under regional anesthesia. Surgery, *68*:304, 1970.

507. Usubiaga, J.E., Moya, F., and Usubiaga, L.E.: Effect of thoracic and abdominal pressure changes on the epidural space pressure. Br. J. Anaesth., *39*:612, 1967.

508. Usubiaga, J.E., Wikinski, J.A., and Usubiaga, L.E.: Epidural pressure and its relation to spread of anesthetic solutions in epidural space. Anesth. Analg. (Cleve.), *46*:440, 1967.

509. Van Zundert, A., Vaes, L., Van Der Aa, P., *et al.*: Motor blockade during epidural anesthesia. Anesth. Analg., (Cleve.), *65*:333, 1986.

509a. Verniquet, A.J.W.: Vessel puncture with epidural catheters. Experience in obstetric patients. Anaesthesia, *35*:660, 1980.

510. Virtue, R.W., Helmreich, M.L., and Gainza, E.: The adrenal cortical response to surgery. I. The effect of anesthesia on plasma 17-hydroxycorticosteroid levels. Surgery, *41*:549, 1975.

511. Vogt, M.: The effect of lowering the 5-hydroxytryptamine content of the rat spinal cord on analgesia produced by morphine. J. Physiol., *236*:483, 1974.

512. Wagenknecht, L.V., Zamora, M., and Madsen, P.O.: Continuous recording of renal clearance by external monitoring during epidural anesthesia. Invest. Urol., *8*:540, 1971.

513. Waggener, J.D., and Beggs, J.: The membranous coverings of

neural tissues: An electron microscopy study. J. Neuropathol. Exp. Neurol., *26*:412, 1967.
514. Wagner, R.S.: A needle for single-dose peridural anesthesia. Anesth. Analg. (Cleve.), *36*:31, 1957.
515. Wahba, W.M., Craig, D.B., Don, H.F., and Becklake, M.R.: The cardio-respiratory effects of thoracic epidural anaesthesia. Can. Anaesth. Soc. J., *19*:8, 1972.
516. Wahba, W.M., Don, H.F., and Craig, D.B.: Post-operative epidural analgesia: Effects on lung volumes. Can. Anaesth. Soc. J., *22*:519,1975.
517. Wall, P.D.: The laminar organization of the dorsal horn and effects of descending impulses. J. Physiol., *188*:403, 1967.
518. Wallis, K.L., Shnider, S.M., Hicks, J.S., and Spivey, H.T.: Epidural anesthesia in the normotensive pregnant ewe: Effects on uterine blood flow and fetal acid-base status. Anesthesiology, *44*:481, 1976.
519. Walmsley, A.J., Giesecke, A.H., and Lipton, J.M.: Epidural temperature: A cause of shivering during epidural anesthesia. Anesth. Analg. (Cleve.), *65*:S1, 1986.
520. Ward, R.J., *et al.*: Epidural and subarachnoid anesthesia. Cardiovascular and respiratory effects. J.A.M.A., *191*:275, 1965.
521. Ward, R.J., *et al.*: Experimental evaluation of atropine and vasopressors for the treatment of hypotension of high subarachnoid anesthesia. Anesth. Analg. (Cleve.), *45*:621, 1966.
522. Weaver, J.B., Pearson, J.F., and Turnbull, A.C.: The effect upon the fetus of an oxytocin infusion in the absence of uterine hypertonus. Br. J. Obstet. Gynaecol., *81*:297, 1974.
523. Weil, J.V., McCullough, R.E., Kline, J.S., and Sodal, I.E.: Diminished ventilatory response to hypoxia and hypercapnia after morphine in normal man. N. Engl. J. Med., *292*:1103, 1975.
524. Welch, K., and Pollay, M.: The spinal arachnoid villi of the monkeys *Cercopitheus aethiops sabaeus* and *Macaca irus.* Anat. Rec., *145*:43, 1963.
525. Werner, M.H., Hayes, D.F., Lucas, C.E., and Rosenberg, I.K.: Renal vasoconstriction in association with acute pancreatitis. Am. J. Surg., *127*:185, 1974.
526. White, S.W., Traugott, F.M., and Quail, A.W.: Arterial chemoreflex in unanesthetized man, monkey and rabbit: Circulatory-respiratory interactions during severe arterial hypoxia. Proc. Aust. Phys. Pharmacol. Soc., *10*:1979.
527. Wildsmith, J.A.W.: Peripheral nerve and local anaesthetic drugs. Br. J. Anaesth., *58*:692, 1986.
528. Wildsmith, J.A.W., Gissen, A.J., Gregus, J., and Covino, B.G.: Differential nerve blocking activity of amino-ester local anesthetics. Br. J. Anaesth., *57*:612, 1985.
529. Winnie, A.P.: A grip to facilitate the insertion of epidural needles. Anesth. Analg. (Cleve.), *50*:23, 1971.
530. Wollman, S.B., and Marx, G.F.: Acute hydration for prevention of hypotension of spinal anesthesia in parturients. Anesthesiology, *29*:374, 1968.
531. Woolf, C.J., and Wiesenfeld–Hallin, Z.: The systemic administration of local anesthetics produces a selective depression of c-afferent fiber evoked activity in the spinal cord. Pain, *23*:361, 1985.
532. Woollam, D.H.M., and Millen, J.W.: An anatomical approach to poliomyelitis. Lancet, *1*:364, 1953.
533. ———: The anatomical background to vascular disease of the spinal cord. Proc. R. Soc. Med., *51:540, 1958.*
534. Wright, R.G., *et al.*: The effect of maternal stress on plasma catecholamines and uterine blood flow in the pregnant ewe. Abstracts of Scientific Papers. p. 17. Memphis. Society of Obstetric Anesthesia and Perinatology. 1978.
535. Wugmeister, M., and Hehre, F.W.: The absence of differential blockade in peridural anaesthesia. Br. J. Anaesth., *39*:953, 1967.
536. Yin, E.I., Wessler, S., and Butler, J.V.: Plasma heparin: A unique, practical, submicrogramsensitive assay. J. Lab. Clin. Med., *81*:298, 1973.
537. Youngman, H.R.: Toxic reactions in epidural anesthesia. Anesthesiology, *17*:632, 1956.
538. Zapol, W.M., and Snider, M.T.: Pulmonary hypertension in severe acute respiratory failure. N. Engl. J. Med., *296*:476, 1977.
539. Zorgniotti, A.W., Narins, D.J., and Dell'Aria, S.L.: Anesthesia, hemorrhage and prostatectomy. J. Urol., *103*:774, 1970.

9 CAUDAL EPIDURAL BLOCKADE

RICHARD J. WILLIS

Local anesthetic injection into the sacral canal by way of the sacral hiatus, or caudal anesthesia as it is now known, was first introduced in 1901[15] and was used as the only available form of epidural anesthesia until the lumbar approach was described by Pagés in Spain in 1921. Since that time, caudal epidural blockade has consistently suffered from comparison with central neural blockade induced at a higher level by both lumbar epidural and subarachnoid spinal techniques.

The reasons for these unfavorable comparisons are clear. First, there is considerable variation in the anatomy of the tissues near the sacral hiatus, in particular, the bony sacrum. Frequently, the bony landmarks are to a greater or lesser extent obscured both by asymmetric bony overgrowth and by the overlying fibrous or fatty soft tissues. Attempts have been made to assess the incidence of sacral bony features that would make caudal blockade "impossible." One old study quoted an incidence of 7.7% of "absent hiatus."[7] This pessimistic figure takes no account of differences with advancing age, it being well accepted that distorted anatomy is less common in younger patients and quite rare in children. It is difficult to correlate this figure with some modern success rates of 94% and greater.[19,49] Whether this represents a difference in the age distribution of the population studied or whether a modern study of bony abnormalities would reveal a lesser incidence of "impossible" anatomy remains conjectural. There is certainly no doubt that the failure rate with caudal blockade decreases markedly with greater experience. Another reason for the unfavorable comparison of caudal with lumbar block is also anatomic, relating to the dermatomal distribution of the nerve roots, the site of the entry hiatus at the exit of the most terminal roots, and the frequency of minor bony obstructions in the sacral canal. In the lumbar region, spread of anesthetic solution can occur both cephalad and caudad, giving rise to a wide dermatomal distribution of anesthesia. Clearly, with caudal entry to the epidural space, spread can only be cephalad and may be limited by minor bony obstructions such that the total number of segments blocked is bound to be less. To predictably achieve a wide distribution of anesthesia with marked cephalad spread of solution, a large dose of local anesthetic drug must be used with its inherent risk of drug toxicity and occasional excessive spread. Although single-dose caudal anesthesia has been and still is used to block thoracic segments, it seems to be an inappropriate use of the technique and partly to blame for the block's poor reputation. When an indwelling catheter is inserted via the sacral hiatus and freely introduced in the line of the canal such that the tip of the catheter lies closer to the lumbosacral junction, there is a greater likelihood of cephalad spread with a moderate dose. This is a worthwhile technique as long as the primary requirement for anesthesia is still in the lumbosacral distribution.

If one viewed the caudal approach merely as the lowest of segmental approaches to the epidural space and restricted the block to the dermatomes supplied by lumbosacral roots, the technique would achieve much greater popularity and a much lower failure rate.

ANATOMY

The key to success in any regional anesthetic technique is a clear understanding of the normal anatomy of the region and an appreciation of variations of normality that may be encountered. This is possibly more relevant to the success of caudal blockade than of most other techniques. Wide variations of normality in the region can readily lead the unwary into needle misplacement which, at best, results in failed block and at worst may contribute to undesirable complications.

THE SACRUM

The sacrum is a triangular bone, dorsally convex, that consists of the fused five sacral vertebrae and that articulates cephalad with the fifth lumbar vertebra and caudad with the coccyx. Detailed descriptions of the bone can be found in standard textbooks of anatomy and should be studied by all trainees unfamiliar with the technique. Only those features of the bone relevant to caudal blockade will be discussed in this chapter.

The concave anterior surface features four pairs of large anterior sacral foramina that provide passage from the midline sacral canal for the anterior rami of the upper four sacral nerves. In contrast with their posterior counterparts, the anterior foramina are unsealed and provide a ready passage for escape of local anesthetic solution injected into the sacral canal (Figs. 9-1, 9-2).

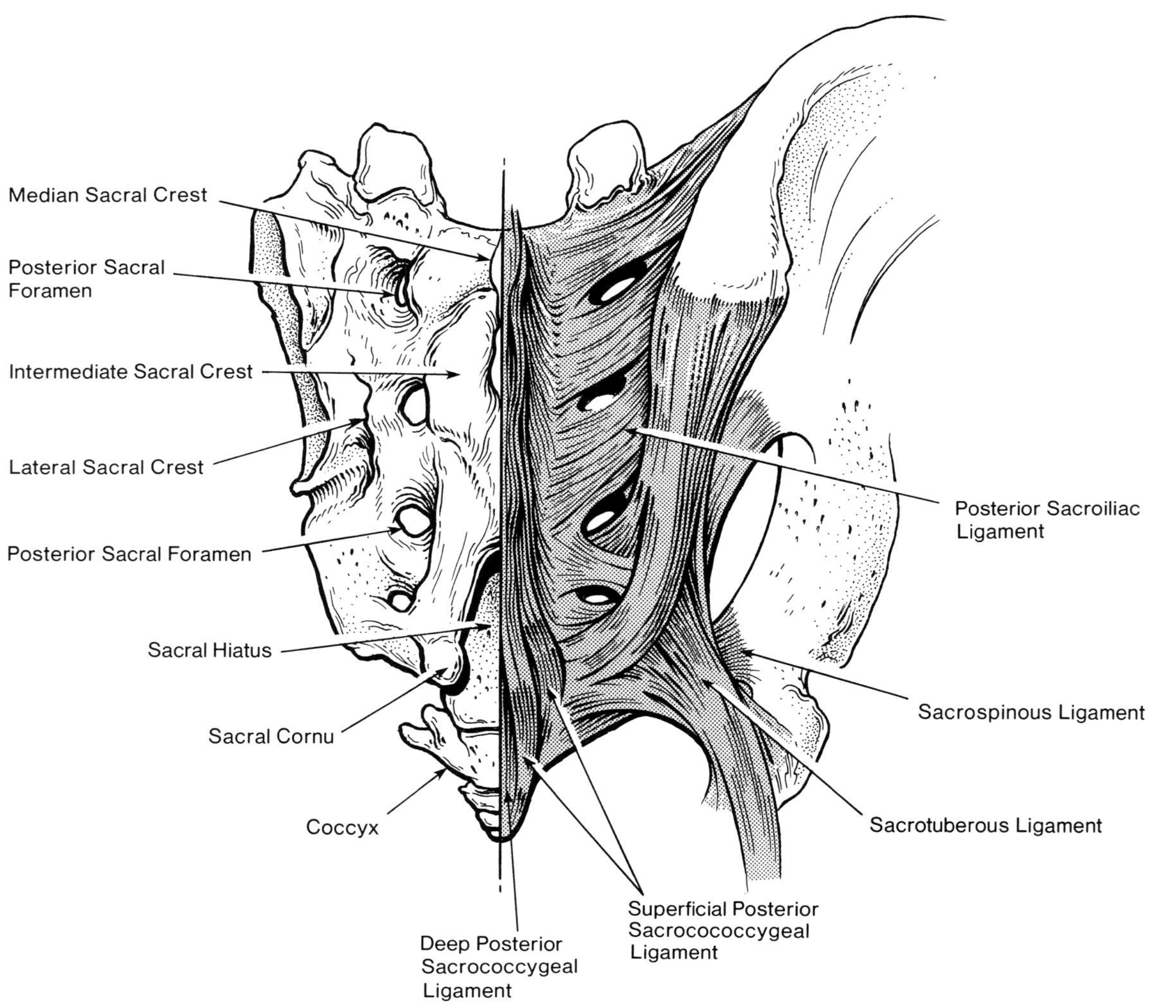

FIG. 9-1. The sacrum, dorsal aspect. Anatomy of bone structures and ligaments shown.

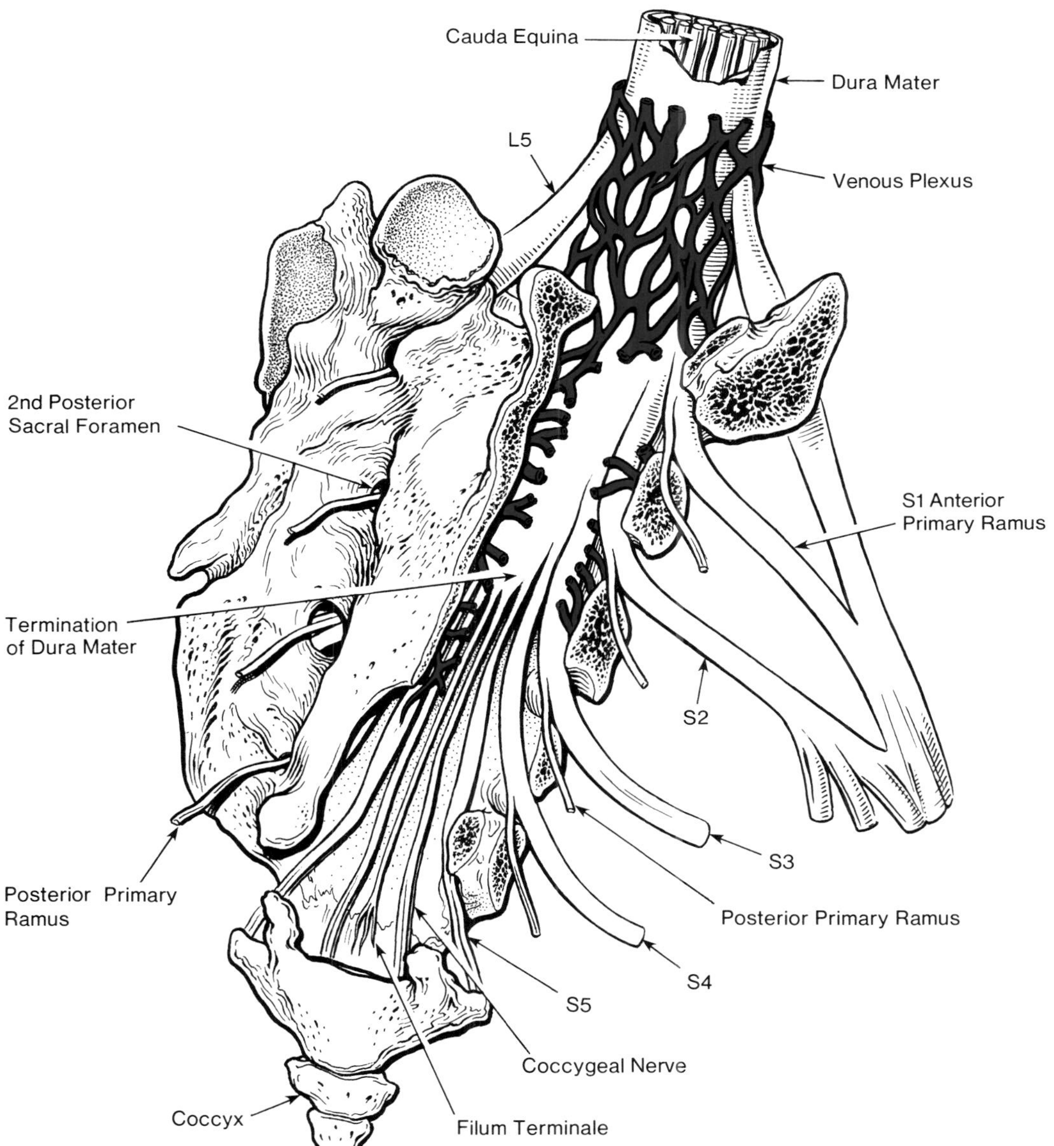

FIG. 9-2. Sacral canal, sacral nerves, and sacral venous plexus. The posterior wall of the sacral canal has been removed on the right side. *Note:* Posterior sacral foramina and small posterior primary rami; large anterior sacral foramina through which pass relatively large anterior primary rami; extensive venous plexus; termination of dural sac near S2 posterior sacral foramen; continuity of sacral epidural space with lumbar epidural space.

The anesthetically important dorsal surface of the sacrum is variably convex and irregular with important prominences representing the fused elements of the sacral vertebrae. In the midline there is a median crest with three, or more commonly four, variably prominent tubercles representing the sacral spinous processes. Lateral to this crest and medial to the four posterior sacral foramina is the intermediate sacral crest with a row of four tubercles representing the upper four sacral articular processes. The posterior sacral foramina are smaller than their anterior counterparts and are effectively sealed by multifidus and sacrospinal muscles. The remnants of the S5 inferior articular processes are free, prominent, and flank the sacral hiatus. They constitute the sacral cornua and, together with the adjacent coccygeal cornua to which they abut, are key landmarks for identification of the sacral hiatus and successful caudal blockade. The fused sacral transverse processes give rise to a variably raised lateral sacral crest with transverse tubercles, the most caudad of which occurs where the lateral border of the sacrum deviates more medially at the inferior lateral sacral angle. This is clinically important because it may be confused with one of the cornua (Figs. 9-1, 9-2).

The shape of the sacrum varies somewhat between sexes and different races. In the female, the bone is shorter and wider, with the curvature being less in the upper part and more acute in the lower part. The anterior concave surface faces more downward than in the male. The angle of the sacral canal varies between the white and black populations of North America, giving rise to a steeper angle of needle insertion and a slightly easier procedure in black patients.[56]

COCCYX

The coccyx is a small triangular bone consisting of three to five fused rudimentary vertebrae; it attaches by means of its upper articular surface to the lower articular surface of the sacrum. It has two prominent coccygeal cornua that abut their sacral counterparts. The bone tends to be angulated forward from the sacrococcygeal junction with its pelvic surface facing anteriorly and upward. This angulation can be quite marked, making palpation difficult, but the bone should be sought because its tip is a useful confirmatory landmark for the midline of the sacrum (Figs. 9-1, 9-2, and 9-6).

SACRAL HIATUS

The sacral hiatus is a defect in the lower part of the posterior wall of the sacrum, formed by the failure of the laminae of S5 and usually part of S4 to meet and fuse in the median plane. This leaves a space of variable dimension, often described as being like an inverted U or V, which is covered by the thick fibrous posterior sacrococcygeal ligament, part of a network of fibrous ligaments covering the sacroiliac and sacrococcygeal areas (see Fig. 9-1). Penetration of this ligament by a needle yields direct access to the caudal limit of the epidural space in the sacral canal. It is in this area that there is considerable variation in "normal" anatomy.[73] Anatomic studies of sacra of mixed sex and race[7,44,76] have confirmed this variability (Fig. 9-3). Relevant findings are as follows.

1. The hiatus varies widely in size and shape from the "normal" inverted U (Fig. 9-3*a*) to longitudinal (*e.g.*, Figs. 9-3*b* and *g*) or horizontal slits (*e.g.*, Figure 9-3*d*).
2. The apex of the hiatus lies higher than the lower one third of S4 in about 50% of specimens. (*e.g.*, Figs. 9-3*g,h,i*).
3. The distance between the tip of the dural sac and the apex of the hiatus, obviously important in order to avoid dural puncture, is variable but almost always exceeds 20 mm and is usually closer to 45 mm.
4. In about 1% of specimens, however, there is total sacral spina bifida (Fig. 9-3*i*), and there is at least one recorded case of the dura directly underlying the hiatus at a distal level.
5. The hiatus is absent in up to 7.7% of specimens.
6. The anteroposterior diameter of the canal at the apex of the hiatus is less than 2 mm in 5% of specimens.

Some of these features of variable anatomy will make the procedure easier rather than more difficult. It is really only item 5 that makes the block impossible, and reasons have already been given as to why the quoted incidence of 7.7% may be excessive.

SACRAL CANAL AND ITS CONTENTS

The sacral canal is the continuation of the lumbar spinal canal. It communicates laterally with the anterior and posterior sacral foramina. Inferiorly it terminates at the sacral hiatus. The volume of the sacral

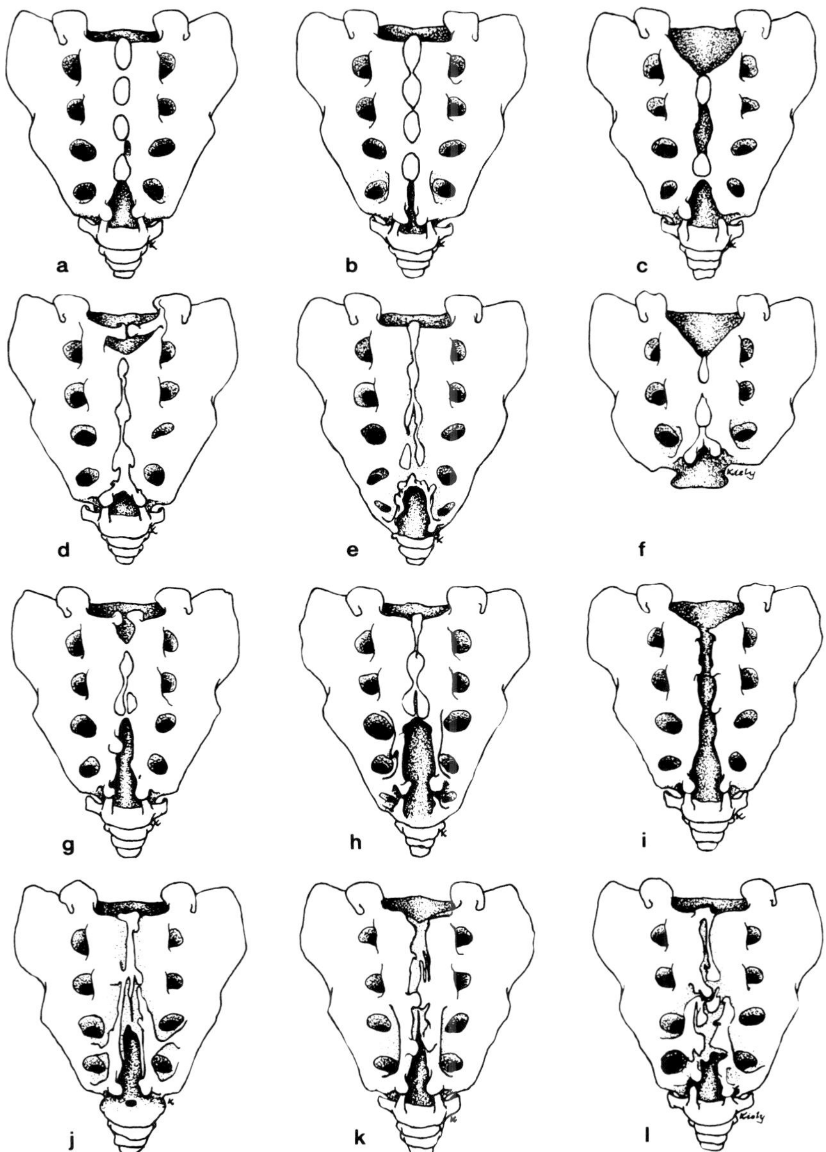

FIG. 9-3. Anatomic variants of dorsal wall of sacrum and sacral hiatus. **Dorsal Wall:** Despite its many structural variations, the sacral canal is open at the lower half of S5 and the hiatus is invariably in line with the median sacral crest (where present and palpable). **Sacral Hiatus: (a)** normal; **(b)** longitudinal slit-like hiatus; **(c)** second midline hiatus; **(d)** transverse hiatus; **(e)** large hiatus with absent cornua; **(f)** transverse hiatus with absent coccyx and two prominent cornua, with two proximal "decoy" hiatuses lateral to the cornua; **(g,h,i)** large midline defects in posterior sacral wall continuous with sacral hiatus; **(j,k,l)** enlarged longitudinal hiatuses, each with an overlying "decoy hiatus." In **(l)** the "decoy hiatus" is large and is surrounded by "cornua-like" structures, which could lead to needle insertion through posterior sacral ligaments but not into sacral canal. Also in **(l)** the sacral cornu is absent on the left side; this could lead to identification of the right S4 posterior sacral foramen as the sacral hiatus.

canal, including the sacral foraminal extensions, has been measured to vary between 12 and 65 ml, with a mean of about 30 to 34 ml.[75] These volumes were measured in dried specimen bones; they therefore are of little use in estimating *in vivo* dose requirement and serve only to underline its great variability.

The canal contains the terminal part of the dural sac, ending between S1 and S3, generally at S2 on a line joining the posterior superior iliac spines. The five sacral nerve roots and the coccygeal nerve, constituting the cauda equina, all transit the canal. The sacral epidural venous plexus, a part of the valveless internal vertebral venous plexus, generally ends at S4 but may extend throughout the canal. It tends to lie against the anterior wall of the canal, but this is an inconstant feature. It is very much at risk from needle or catheter puncture. Also found in the canal is the filum terminale, the non-nervous terminal filament of the spinal cord, which exits through the sacral hiatus to attach to the back of the coccyx (see Fig. 9-2). The remainder of the canal is filled with epidural fat, the character of which changes from a loose texture in children to a more fibrous close-meshed texture in adults. It has been suggested that it is this difference that gives rise to the predictability of caudal local anesthetic spread in children and its unpredictability in adults.[62]

SACRAL AND COCCYGEAL NERVES

The anterior and posterior primary rami of S1–S4 exit from the sacral canal by way of the anterior and posterior foramina, respectively. S5 and the minute coccygeal nerve exit laterally through the sacral hiatus and wind laterally around the sacrum and coccyx, respectively (see Fig. 9-2).

These roots give rise to the following nerves: posterior cutaneous nerve of the thigh (subdividing into gluteal, perineal, and terminal branches to the back of the thigh and leg), perforating cutaneous nerve (inconstant), pudendal nerve (subdividing into inferior rectal nerve, perineal nerve, scrotal or labial branches, nerve to urethral bulb, and dorsal nerve of penis or clitoris), anococcygeal nerves, pelvic splanchnic nerves, and various muscular branches. These nerves relay total sensory input from the vagina, anorectal region, floor of the perineum, anal and bladder sphincters, urethra, and scrotal skin. The vulva is sacrally innervated except for its most anterior margin (see Fig. 18-2). Likewise with the penis, only the base is not sacrally innervated. Sacral nerves also innervate a narrow band of skin extending from the posterior aspect of the gluteal region to the plantar and lateral surface of the foot.

In addition to these areas that have exclusive sacral innervation, several organs on the pelvic floor and perineum have multiple innervation through preaortic and sacrococcygeal nerve groups (see Fig. 18-1), including the uterus, uterine tubes, bladder, and possibly prostate. Although unsupplemented caudal blockade may not provide full pain control for operations on these structures, it can provide a major component of a combined anesthetic sequence (see also Chap. 18, Part 2).

PHARMACOLOGY

Various studies have attested to the safety of caudal anesthesia in terms of the local anesthetic blood levels attained. As would be expected, there is such wide variation between the doses, concentrations, and drugs used in the different studies that comparisons are difficult to make.

In addition, some of these studies have measured the time of onset of the block and the duration. This information has been tabulated in Tables 9-1–9-3. The following generalizations can be made from this information.

1. Plasma levels for all local anesthetic drugs tend to be low after caudal administration.[24,29,52] Even very large doses in children have given plasma levels well below the accepted adult toxic levels.[72]
2. Onset time or latent interval seems to be longer with caudal than with lumbar epidural anesthetic.[30] Etidocaine and carbonated lidocaine have the shortest time of onset.[19,30,67]
3. The time to attainment of maximum spread is variable and takes longer than for lumbar epidural block, on occasions taking up to 40 minutes.[19]
4. Block of the large diameter S1 root is less predictable than it is after lumbar epidural block when moderate doses are used.[30]
5. Concentrations of solution that are adequate to block sensory fibers are bupivacaine 0.25%, etidocaine 1%, mepivacaine 1%, lidocaine 1%, prilocaine 1%, and chloroprocaine 2%. Increased concentration will increase the degree of motor block and possibly improve speed of onset. The addition of epinephrine will increase the degree of motor block, decrease plasma levels, and increase the duration of the shorter acting drugs (see Chap. 3).

TABLE 9-1. PHARMACOKINETICS AND CAUDAL BLOCK

Study	Drug	Dose	Mean Peak Blood Concentration and Range	Mean Time to Peak Blood Concentration	Comments
Mazze, et al., 1966[52] Young adults	1.5% lidocaine with epinephrine 1:200,000	5.8–7.5 mg/kg mean 428 mg = 28.5 ml	1.4 μg/ml (0.5–2.9)	30 min	Lower blood levels with caudal than with lumbar epidural or i.v. regional
Cousins and Bromage, 1971[19] Adults	Lidocaine HCl and CO_2 lidocaine 1.75% base	About 17 ml	CO_2 lidocaine 3.1 μg/ml (2.6–3.8), lidocaine HCl 2.7 μg/ml (1.5–4.2)	CO_2 lidocaine 7 min, lidocaine HCl 12 min	
Moore, et al., 1968[54] Obstetric patients with caudal catheter	1.5% mepivacaine	300–450 mg = 20–30 ml	About 3.0 μg/ml	Not stated; 40 min for one patient	Blood levels rose after equivalent top-up doses to reach 7–9 μg/ml in four of five patients at delivery
Freund, et al., 1984[29] Young males < 40 years compared with older males > 55 years; caudal catheters inserted to 10 cm	2% lidocaine or 0.75% bupivacaine, both with epinephrine 1:200,000	Lidocaine 6 mg/kg, bupivacaine 2.2 mg/kg	Lidocaine <40 2.47 μg/ml ±0.23 lidocaine >55 2.61 μg/ml ±1.45 bupivacaine <40 0.86 μg/ml ±0.22 bupivacaine >50 0.69 μg/ml ±0.25	Lidocaine <40 45 min, lidocaine >55 25 min, bupivacaine <40 30 min, bupivacaine >55, 20 min	No significant difference between peak plasma lidocaine or bupivacaine levels with age; no significant difference in dermatomal levels for the four groups
Eyres, et al., 1978[25] Children	1% lidocaine, 0.5% bupivacaine	Lidocaine 4 mg/kg, bupivacaine 2 mg/kg	Lidocaine 2 μg/ml, bupivacaine ?0.7 μg/ml	Lidocaine 10–20 min, bupivacaine ?about 15 min	
Ecoffey, et al., 1984[24] Children	1% lidocaine	5 mg/kg	2.05 ± 0.08 μg/ml	28.2 ± 2.9 min	Long terminal half-life in children attributed to larger volume of distribution
Takasaki, 1984[71] Children	1.5% lidocaine, 1.5% mepivacaine, 0.5% bupivacaine, all with epinephrine	Lidocaine 11 mg/kg, mepivacaine 11 mg/kg, bupivacaine 3.7 mg/kg	Lidocaine 2.2 μg/ml, mepivacaine 2.53 μg/ml, bupivacaine 0.67 μg/ml	45 min 45 min 45 min	Low blood concentrations with slow decrease in concentrations

TABLE 9-2. DOSE REGIMENS FOR CAUDAL BLOCK

Study	Formula	Indication	Comments
Schulte-Steinberg and Rahlfs, 1977[64]	0.1 ml/segment/year + 0.1 ml/segment	Adapt to number of segments required	Gives rise to low doses
Armitage, 1979[5]	0.5 ml/kg 0.25% bupivacaine 1 ml/kg 1.25 ml/kg	For circumcision For inguinal herniotomy For umbilical herniorraphy or orchidopexy	
Kay, 1974[43]	0.5 ml 0.5% bupivacaine with epinephrine per year of age	Circumcision	Similar to Schulte-Steinberg and Rahlfs
Takasaki, et al., 1977[72]	ml/segment = 0.056 × weight (kg)	Adapt to number of segments required	Very slow speed of injection 0.15 ml/sec
Yeoman, et al., 1983[83]	1 ml 0.5% bupivacaine/year + 2 ml (max 20 ml)	Circumcision	
Lourey and McDonald, 1973[45]	3-4 mg 1% lidocaine/kg, 1.0 mg 0.5% bupivacaine/kg	Lower abdominal and urogenital operations	
McGown, 1982[49]	To S3: 0.55 ml/kg 1-2% lid. + epinephrine; to L2: 1.1 ml/kg 1-2% lid. + epinephrine; to T11: 1.7 ml/kg 1-2% lid. + epinephrine	Areas innervated by these nerve roots	Dose of 1.7 ml/kg is unacceptable even with 1% lidocaine with epinephrine
Spiegel, 1962[70]	$\text{Volume (ml)} = 4 + \frac{D - 15}{2}$ D = distance between C7 and sacral hiatus in cm	? upper abdominal surgery	
Satoyoshi and Kamiyama, 1984[61]	Volume (ml) = D − 13 (ml) D = distance between C7 and sacral hiatus in cm	Upper abdominal surgery, T4-T5	Excessive dose
Hassan, 1977[35]	7 mg/kg 1.5% lidocaine or mepivacaine	"Routine surgical procedures"	
Touloukian, et al., 1971[74]	2.7-7.6 mg/kg of 0.5-1% lidocaine	Neonatal surgery no higher than inguinal herniotomy	Seems satisfactory
Fortuna, 1967[28]	To T 12: 10 mg/kg 0.5-2% lidocaine; to T 10: 12.5 mg/kg 0.5-2% lidocaine; to T 6: 15 mg/kg 0.5-2% lidocaine	Areas innervated by these nerve roots	High to excessive dose

DOSE AND SPREAD

Many factors have, over the years, been implicated in influencing the spread of a standard dose of local anesthetic solution injected into the caudal canal. Such factors as age, weight, height, dose (both volume and mass of drug), and speed of injection will be known or controllable. Their influences have been studied by a number of investigators. There are, however, a number of other factors, the influences of which will remain both unknown and uncontrollable, and which must inevitably give rise to the significant unpredictability of all epidural spread, but particularly that in the sacral canal. Such factors follow.[58]

1. The size of the caudal epidural space.
2. The size and patency of the sacral canal and the anterior sacral foramina.
3. The amount of bony distortion of the sacral canal.
4. The presence of septa in the epidural space.
5. The amount and nature of the soft tissues in the epidural space, especially fatty tissues.
6. The permeability of the neural tissue and dural cuffs to the drug.

Adults

The only two factors that have been shown to affect caudal spread in adults are dose and speed of injection.[58]

In a study comparing the maximum spread of either lidocaine 2% with epinephrine 1:200,000 or bupivacaine 0.5% with epinephrine 1:200,000 in volumes of 20 ml, 10 ml, or 5 ml, there was a highly significant difference between the spread achieved with the three different volumes.[82] There was no dif-

TABLE 9-3. ONSET AND DURATION OF CAUDAL BLOCK

Study	Drug	Onset (min)	Spread (segments)	Two-Segment Regression (min)	Total Regression (min)	Comments
Cousins and Bromage, 1971[19] Adult outpatients	2% lidocaine HCl, 17 ml	14.4 (3-32)	6.8 in 24.8 ± 6.4 min	At 67	At 87	Very rapid onset confirmed for carbonated lidocaine
	CO_2 lidocaine 1.75% base, 17 ml	3.2 (1-8)	9.6 in 12.8 ± 5.8 min	At 66	At 94	
Seow, et al., 1976[67] Adults	1% etidocaine with epinephrine 1:200,000, 25 ml	7.06 SD = 4.54	11.7 SD = 3.9	Not measured	Not measured	Rapid onset but persisting motor block noted with etidocaine
	1.5% lidocaine with epinephrine 1:200,000, 25 ml	12.44 SD = 6.14	12.7 SD = 5.8	Not measured	Not measured	
Park, et al., 1979[58]	30 ml 1.5% lidocaine with 1:200,000 epinephrine					Several instances of acute hypertension >200/100 in 1 min injection group
	Injection over 1 min	3.9 (2-15)	17 (8-22)		203 ± 5.3	
	Injection over 2 min	3.6 (2-12)	12 (3-21)	Not measured	192 ± 11	
Willis and Macintyre, 1986[82] Young female adults	2% lidocaine with 1:200,000 epinephrine					
	20 ml		9.5 (range 6.5-13)			
	10 ml		7 (4-13)			
	5 ml		4 (3-5)			
	0.5% bupivacaine with 1:200,000 epinephrine					
	20 ml		9 (4-12.5)			
	10 ml		6.5 (3-10)			
	5 ml		4 (3-5)			
			Block of S1 Root			
			Delay (min)	Failure (%)		
Galindo, et al., 1978[30]	1.5% chloroprocaine	4.8 SD = 1.5	20 (8.6)	20	All onset times are similar and very low. The delay in the block of the large S1 root is very variable. Because individual doses range from 10-20 ml, it is difficult to assess the significance of this.	
	3% chloroprocaine	5.5 (0.7)	24.3 (6.7)	25		
	2% mepivacaine	5.9 (2.6)	27 (8.4)	23		
	0.75% bupivacaine	4.9 (2.0)	17.9 (5.6)	13		
	1% etidocaine	4.9 (1.4)	17.8 (3.5)	0		
	1.5% etidocaine	4.2 (2.5)	15 (3.8)	0		
	All with epinephrine 1:200,000—dose range, 10-20 ml					

ference in spread between the two different drugs when the same volume was used.

The mean spread measured in dermatomes and the range are shown below.

	20 ml	10 ml	5 ml
Lidocaine 2% with epinephrine	9.5 (6.5–13)	7 (4–13)	4 (3–5)
Bupivacaine 0.5% with epinephrine	9 (4–12.5)	6.5 (3–10)	4 (3–5)

When dermatomal levels were different on each side, the mean was recorded.

In another study, 30 ml of 1.5% lidocaine with epinephrine 1 : 200,000 injected over 1 minute gave a mean upper level of T6–T7 (L3–T1), whereas a similar volume injected over 2 minutes gave a mean upper level of T11 (S2–T2).[58] There was, incidentally, an 8% incidence of transient acute hypertension and tachycardia in the more rapid injection group. The lack of influence of age in adults is well shown in a study in which the dose of anesthetic per spinal segment is plotted against age for both lidocaine HCl and carbonated lidocaine[19] (Fig. 9-4). In the same study there was also no correlation with height or weight. In another study comparing spread with both lidocaine and bupivacaine in a group of older and a group of younger adult males, there was no significant difference between any of the four groups.[29]

Children

In children, the situation is different: Schulte-Steinberg and Rahlfs in 1970 established that there was a high correlation between dose and age.[63] There were lesser degrees of correlation between dose and weight and dose and height in children. In 1977, the same authors produced a single regression line for three drugs (1% lidocaine, 1% mepivacaine, and 0.25% bupivacaine, all with epinephrine) showing in children the linear relation between age and spread (measured in ml/spinal segment).[64] Reference to this study shows that an adequate dosing schedule would be

$$0.1 \text{ ml/segment/yr} + 0.1 \text{ ml/segment}$$

(see Chap. 21).

There is strong agreement between this work and that done by Bromage with lumbar epidural anesthesia.[14]

Despite the academic appeal of the above dosing schedule, it has been challenged by a number of authors. This has given rise to a bewildering collection of formulae, some for specific purposes, and some for

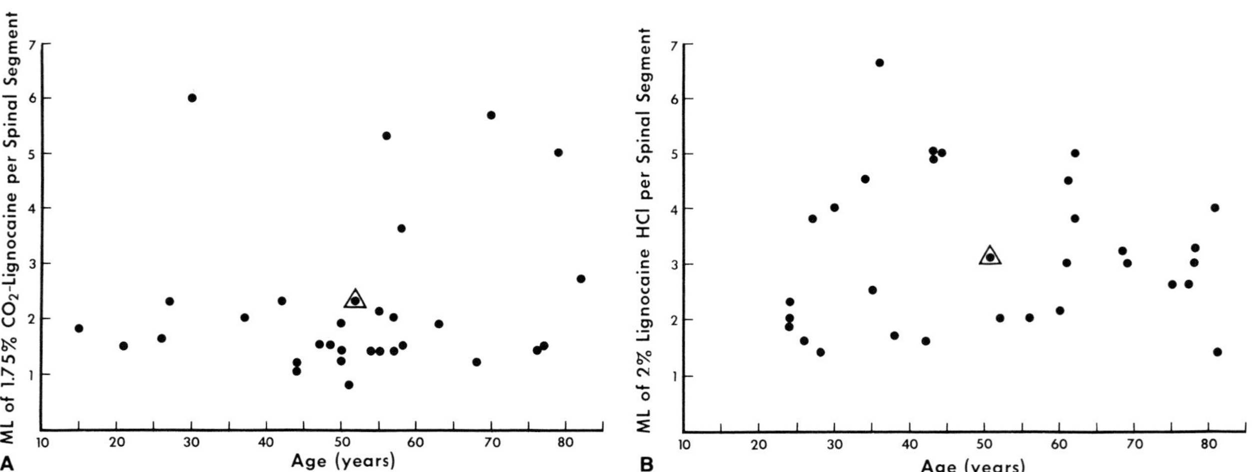

FIG. 9-4. Caudal blockade in adults: segmental spread analgesia with advancing age. **A.** 1.75% lidocaine carbonate. **B.** 2% lidocaine hydrochloride. Dose requirements in milliliter per spinal segment are plotted against age, with the mean dose indicated by a dot in a triangle. There is no consistency in spread of analgesia at any age or any correlation between age and segmental spread. (Cousins, M.J., and Bromage, P.R.: Br. J. Anaesth., *43:*1149, 1971.)

such vague indications as "routine surgical procedures." These are summarized in Table 9-2.

Two dosing schedules are worthy of further mention. The Armitage formula of 0.5 ml of 0.25% bupivacaine/kg for circumcision and anal surgery (low sacral) is easy to use, reliable, and safe but gives rise to much larger doses of drug.[5] The same author recommends 1 ml/kg of 0.25% bupivacaine to block the lower thoracic nerves and 1.25 ml/kg to block the midthoracic nerves (*e.g.*, for orchidectomy or umbilical herniorrhaphy). This latter dose is high but seems to have been proved to be safe in children.

The second study[49] is notable in the extent of the detail presented. It states that with at least 97% confidence, 0.55 ml of 1% to 2% lidocaine/kg will produce a block to S3 or higher, 1.1 ml/kg will produce a block to L2 or higher, and 1.7 ml/kg will produce a block to T11 or higher. These doses gave rise to some excessively high blocks, and there was an alarmingly high incidence of respiratory or cardiac arrest (2.8%), or both, which one must deduce was at least contributed to by the very high doses of drug given. Such large doses should not be given.

Dose by Means of Caudal Catheter

As previously stated, the tip of a caudal catheter may be as high as the L5–S1 level. The block then tends to behave more like a lumbar epidural. Estimation of dose can be done using the criteria that one uses for this latter block. "Top-up" doses should be scaled down, as with lumbar epidural "top-ups." Accumulation of mepivacaine during labor with steadily rising blood levels and toxicity has occurred where caudal top-up doses have been the same as the initial dose.[54]

ONSET AND DURATION

To understand and rationally use any regional anesthetic technique, it is important to know the following time-intervals: the time to achieve maximum spread of block and the duration (usually measured for a central block as the time from onset to regression of two spinal segments). It is useful also to know the onset interval (latency) and the time to total regression of the block. Only a limited amount of data are available on this subject, and its most notable feature is its great variability, particularly with regard to onset interval (see Table 9-3). This would seem to result from different methods used as criteria for "onset." In most studies time of onset is the period from injection until the patient first notices loss of sensation to pinprick or other stimulus.

Probably the most useful clinical information comes from the study by Cousins and Bromage[19] in which 1.75% carbonated lidocaine was compared with 2% lidocaine HCl. Although this study confirmed the usefulness of carbonated lidocaine, a drug not generally available, it also showed that the time to attain total sacral anesthesia with 2% lidocaine HCl was 21 minutes (mean), with some taking more than 30 minutes (Fig. 9-5). Two-segment regression took 67 minutes (mean), and total duration was 87 minutes (mean).

PHYSIOLOGIC EFFECTS

The physiologic changes associated with epidural anesthesia are well documented in Chapter 8. A limited sacral block from a caudal epidural would be expected to cause minimal physiologic trespass.

As well as the sensory and motor block of the sacral roots, one could expect a degree of autonomic block. The sacral component of the parasympathetic craniosacral outflow (the pelvic splanchnic nerves) will be blocked, causing loss of visceromotor function in the bladder and bowel distally from the splenic flexure of the colon. There should, in theory also be an increase in anal and bladder sphincter tone, but this is seldom seen in practice because of a coexistent sympathetic

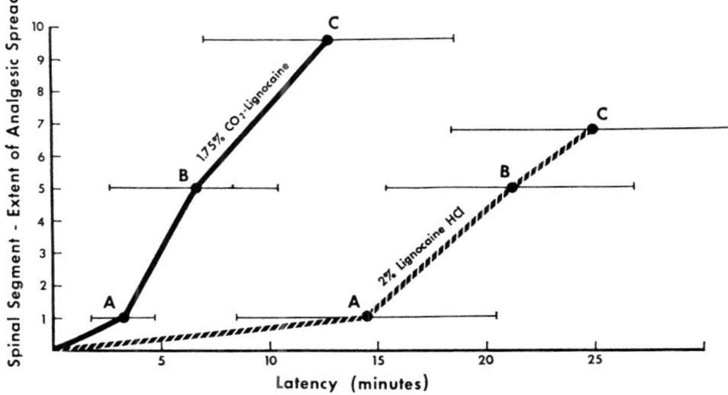

FIG. 9-5. Caudal blockade: latency of onset and spread of complete blockade (*i.e.*, "surgical" analgesia). Two percent lidocaine hydrochloride is compared to 1.75% lidocaine carbonate. Onset of blockade and complete loss of sensation are much more rapid with lidocaine carbonate. Even with the lidocaine carbonate solution, blockade of five segments may require nearly 10 minutes, whereas with the lidocaine hydrochloride solution it may require in excess of 20 minutes. (Cousins, M.J., and Bromage, P.R.: Br. J. Anaesth., *43:*1149, 1971.)

block as outlined below. Since the sympathetic outflow from the spinal cord ends at L1 level, a limited caudal block should theoretically avoid any sympathetic block. It would seem in practice, however, that this is not necessarily so. Vascular dilatation in the lower limb is often seen with a low level of caudal block. There seems no doubt that the level of sympathetic block is higher than that of sensory block, although there is very little "hard" evidence in the literature to confirm this (see Chap. 7). An oft-quoted study[53] has shown evidence of sympathetic block of the eye in 17 of 20 consecutive obstetric patients having caudal analgesia. Although the dose of drug and supine positioning of the patient have been rightly criticized in this study, nevertheless the upper level of sensory block was dramatically lower than T1 in all patients. It would seem, therefore, that at least the potential exists for a degree of unwanted sympathetic block. Of course, if an extensive sensory block occurs (intentional or otherwise), a similarly extensive sympathetic block will inevitably occur, with all the consequences outlined in Chapter 8. Likewise, similar respiratory and neuroendocrine effects of high epidural anesthesia would be expected with an extensive caudal block.

The effects of caudal analgesia on respiratory parameters were measured in children undergoing lower abdominal and genital procedures with halothane general anesthesia and spontaneous ventilation. Those children receiving caudals had significantly lower minute ventilations and respiratory rates than those having only general anesthesia. End tidal CO_2 concentration was the same in both groups, indicating improved efficiency of ventilation in the caudal group.[36] The ventilatory responses to hypospadias surgery in children under light halothane or enflurane anesthesia have been compared. With coexistent caudal anesthesia, no changes were measured between the two general anaesthetic groups.[16]

Changes in ACTH, immunoreactive beta-endorphin, ADH, and cortisol levels were measured in children undergoing minor surgery with either halothane anesthesia or caudal anesthesia. There was a rapid and major increase in hormone levels with general but not with caudal anesthesia.[31]

TECHNIQUE OF CAUDAL BLOCK

As in the preparation for any major regional anesthetic technique, all equipment must be assembled and checked, including block tray, resuscitation equipment, and suction. Secure intravenous access must be obtained (see Chap. 6).

The needles used for this procedure will depend to some extent on the clinical circumstances. For single-injection caudal block in a child, a 2- to 3-cm disposable 23- to 25-gauge needle should be used. In an adult, the slightly greater rigidity of a 22-gauge needle may make the procedure easier. The needles should all be short-beveled if these are available because they give a better feel when different tissues are penetrated, they have less tendency to form barbs if bone is struck, the bevel is more likely to fully enter the canal if it is very shallow, and they cause less trauma to nerves.[66] If a catheter is to be inserted, a short 5- to 7-cm 18T-gauge Crawford-tip needle and a standard epidural catheter are recommended. Some operators prefer to use a Teflon intravenous needle of small caliber.[57] Although this has some advantages, it has a tendency to kink and seems to be less reliable. A large-gauge i.v. needle can be used to insert a standard epidural catheter. The use of a Tuohy needle to insert a catheter is not recommended. The needle will lie in the long axis of the canal, and the Tuohy tip will therefore direct the catheter toward the wall rather than in the axis of the canal, as with a Crawford or an i.v. needle.

Positioning of the patient can be in one of three ways: The preferred position is the lateral Sim's position (left side down for a right-handed operator) with the lower leg only slightly flexed at the hip and the upper leg more flexed such that it lies over and above the lower leg and also in contact with the bed. This maneuver tends to separate the buttocks. In contrast to lumbar epidural block, excess hip flexion is unnecessary and may on occasion stretch the skin to such an extent that palpation of the landmarks may become more difficult. This position has the advantages of comfort for the patient, a familiar working position for the anesthesiologist, and easy access to the airway if the patient is sedated or in the event of an adverse reaction. Sagging of the gluteal cleft occasionally may cause some confusion in confirming landmarks in inexperienced hands but can be readily corrected by an assistant holding the upper buttock to reposition the gluteal cleft in the median plane of the sacrum. This is in accordance with the general principle that skin creases are poor landmarks for regional anesthesia (see Fig. 9-6*A*).

The prone position with a pillow under the pelvis is still popular with some anesthetists. Both legs are rotated so that the toes of both feet are facing medially. This again separates the buttocks. In this position there is no distortion from movement of the gluteal cleft, but difficulty can be experienced if urgent access to the mouth and airway is required.

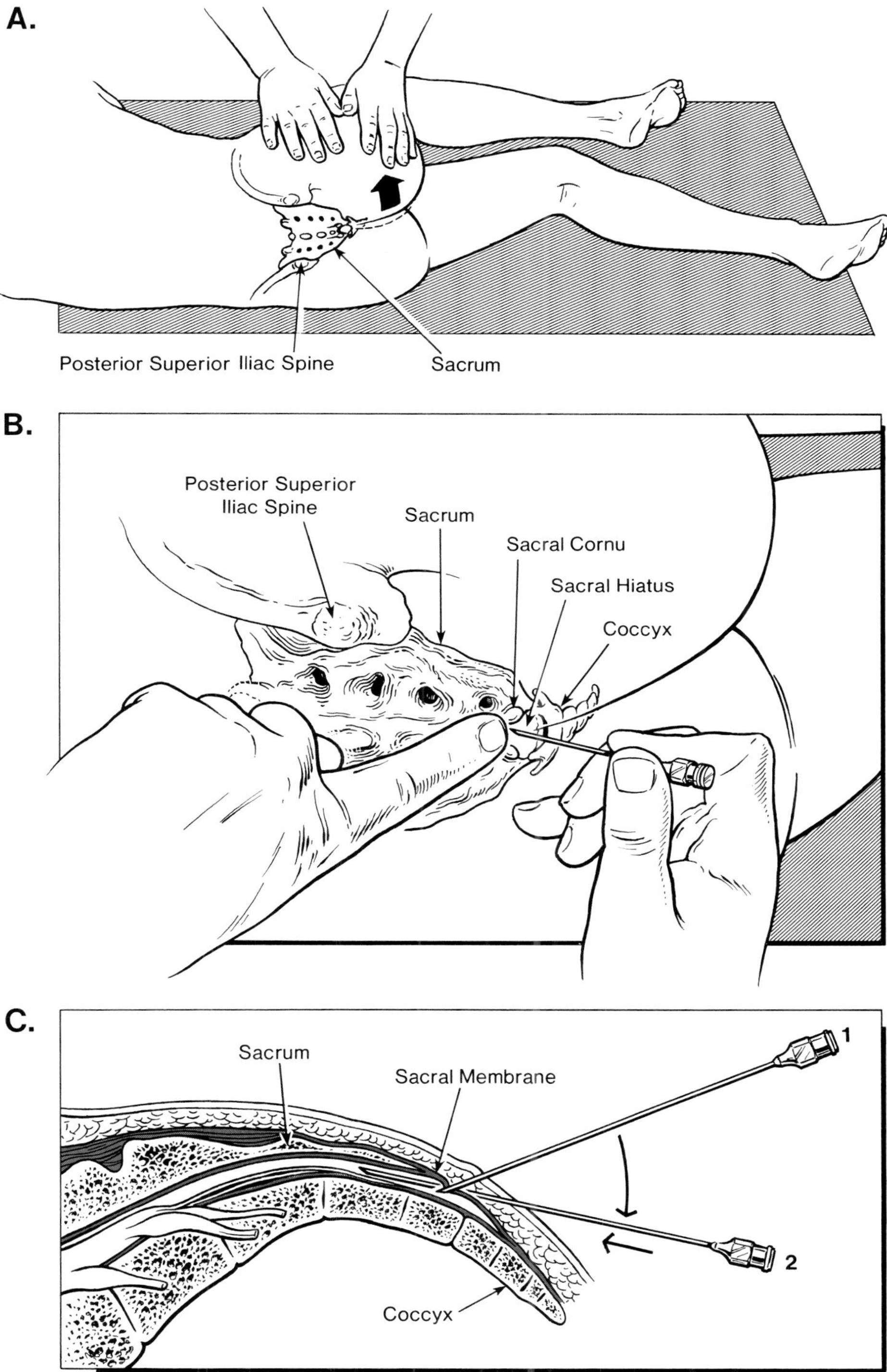

FIG. 9-6. Technique of caudal block (see text). **A.** Positioning for caudal block. **B.** Palpation of landmarks and needle insertion. **C.** Needle insertion through sacrococcygeal (sacral) membrane.

The less popular knee–chest position still may be useful, particularly for the pregnant patient.

Skin preparation should be over a large area such that all the landmarks can be palpated aseptically. If alcoholic solutions are used, a swab should be placed deep in the gluteal cleft to prevent pain in the exposed sensitive perineal area.

Confirmation of bony landmarks is the key to success. In the thin young patient, the protrusions of the sacral cornua can be seen without palpation, and the shallow depression over the sacral hiatus can be seen between them. Successful needle placement in these circumstances is exceedingly easy; however, the vast majority of patients have less obvious surface anatomy and require very careful palpation of all the bony landmarks. Needle penetration of a posterior sacral foramen may mimic the feel of entering the sacral hiatus. Often closed bony depressions covered by fibrous ligament can also mimic the sacral hiatus, although injection is impossible (see Fig. 9-7*B*). Only the most meticulous attention to the landmarks can prevent needle entry into these "decoy hiatuses."

It is important, initially, to identify the midline positively. This can be achieved by palpating the tip of the coccyx with the finger and moving cephalad about 4 to 5 cm in an adult until the fingertip lies over the sacral hiatus with the prominent sacral cornua palpable on each side by moving the fingertip from side to side (Fig. 9-6*B*). The use of excessive pressure while moving the finger in this latter manner can be painful. Considerable variability occurs in the prominence of the cornua, causing problems for the unwary. If one cornu is much less obvious than the other, there may be a tendency to palpate further laterally until a prominent tubercle of the lateral sacral crest at the inferior lateral sacral angle is felt. The importance of establishing the midline of the sacrum cannot be overemphasized. Palpation of the median sacral crest in a caudad direction can also lead to the sacral hiatus but is a less reliable method. The posterior superior iliac spines form an equilateral triangle with the sacral hiatus. This should be used as a confirmatory landmark for correct needle placement. Unfortunately these spines are not always readily palpable. It is useful to remember that the line joining these spines is an approximate indication of the level of termination of the dural sac (S2 level). In patients in whom landmark palpation is difficult, digital examination with one finger inserted per rectum may be performed to help select a point of needle entry. A useful alternative method of palpating the cornua and hiatus using the thumb of each hand has been described.[47]

Having found the area of the suspected hiatus, it is well to keep the palpating hand in position until after the needle insertion because the landmarks can be quickly obscured, especially in the obese patient. Because the canal has a tendency to become deeper as one progresses cephalad, canal entry is facilitated if a point of needle entry is chosen toward the upper end of the hiatus. The initial angle of needle insertion should be about 120° to the back (Fig. 9-6C). Penetration of the sacrococcygeal ligament has a characteristic feel to it. This "pop" can be learned only by practice. There is a feeling of emptiness after penetration of the ligament in most patients until the anterior wall is contacted. This contact should not be sought. The needle, both hub and shank, should then be depressed toward the skin to align the needle approximately in the long axis of the canal. It may then be inserted a further centimeter (Fig. 9-6C). On occasion, further needle insertion is not possible because of the size of the canal. This should be accepted and, after aspiration, a test dose of the local anesthetic drug injected at this point.

SIGNS OF CORRECT NEEDLE PLACEMENT

The following are the objective and subjective signs of accurate needle positioning, and those that appear appropriate should be elicited before completion of injection; the first four should be regarded as essential (modified from McCaul, 1980[47]).

1. Presence of sacral bone on each side of, in front of, and behind the needle at its point of insertion does not exclude the possibility of entry into a decoy hiatus but does protect against injection lateral to the sacral or coccygeal margins or into the presacral tissues or rectum.
2. The lack of CSF, air, or blood on aspiration is important. Light blood staining is not uncommon and indicates that entry into the sacral canal has been achieved and that repeat aspiration should be attempted during the injection of solution.
3. There should be no subcutaneous bulge or superficial crepitus after injection of 2 or 3 ml of anesthetic solution or air.
4. There should be no tissue resistance to injection; the force required to inject should not exceed that necessary to overcome syringe and needle resistances and should be constant throughout. Injection should feel like any other injection into the epidural space.
5. When correctly positioned, the needle should be

able to move in the canal, pivoting at the point of penetration of the sacrococcygeal ligament. Eliciting this sign may, however, cause trauma to the tissues in the canal, particularly blood vessels, and is usually not necessary.

6. There should be no local pain during injection of solution; pain indicates misplacement of the needle, and injection should stop.
7. Paresthesia or a feeling of fullness that extends from the sacrum to the soles of the feet is common during injection but ceases on completion and portends successful blockade.
8. The feeling of grating as the needle moves along the anterior wall of the sacral canal indicates accurate positioning but should not be purposefully elicited lest the sacral venous plexus be damaged.
9. A useful test when substantial doubts about needle position cannot be resolved is to inject 2 to 4 ml of air while listening with ear or stethoscope over the lumbar vertebrae for transmitted sound.
10. There should be ease of threading a short Teflon cannula over an intravenous needle, if such a needle is used for caudal blockade.
11. If an epidural catheter is inserted, it should enter the canal freely with the same or greater ease than in the lumbar epidural space.

It is recommended that one use a test dose before the full dose. Because of the proximity of needle and catheter to venous plexuses, there is a risk of a local anesthetic toxic reaction.

CATHETER TECHNIQUES

The epidural catheter should enter the canal without difficulty. Because of the angle of insertion, it will probably progress cephalad more predictably[8,84] than in the lumbar region. Fixation of the epidural catheter to prevent soiling is important. One secure method is to spray the area lightly with an adhesive such as tincture of benzoin compound and apply a sterile adhesive plastic dressing initially into the previously separated gluteal cleft and then directly over the site of insertion of the catheter. Because many of these patients will have surgery in the lithotomy position, the aim is to have a very adherent dressing in the gluteal cleft that will *not* form a pocket to collect fluids from the operative site, which may run down directly over the anus.

MONITORING

Despite the limited extent of block anticipated with caudal anesthesia, it is still mandatory to monitor the patient. Intravenous or intraosseous misplacement of the needle or excessive spread of block may give rise to unwanted effects. Maintaining verbal communication with the patient is the simplest, and in some ways the most reliable, method; however, blood pressure and pulse should be measured frequently and the progress of the block plotted.

INDICATIONS

OBSTETRIC ANESTHESIA AND ANALGESIA

The widespread and safe use of epidural analgesia to control the pain of labor has been a major factor in increasing the popularity of regional anesthesia for elective and emergency surgery. Although the lumbar approach is now used as the technique of choice in most obstetric units, it should be remembered that it was the report in 1943 by Hingson and Edwards entitled "Continuous Caudal Analgesia — An Analysis of the First 10,000 Confinements Thus Managed with the Report of the Authors' First 1,000 Cases"[39] that first popularized the method. The advantages were immediately obvious: high-quality analgesia with a low incidence of complications and a low failure rate for that time of only 7%.

In later years, clinical studies confirmed some of the advantages.[26,38] Most, but not all,[4] studies showed that caudal analgesia had essentially no effect on uterine activity during labor. Local anesthetic blood levels did not correlate with any measured changes in uterine activity.[77] Cardiac output increases during labor were decreased, and the tachycardia of the second stage and the early postpartum period was prevented by caudal analgesia.[34,78] One study demonstrated the prolongation of analgesia achieved by adding epinephrine to the caudal local anesthetic.[33] It also reported that epinephrine, 25 ml of 1 : 200,000 dilution, significantly prolonged labor; however, "top-up" doses of 15 to 20 ml were given in this study and patients were supine; thus the epinephrine dose was large, and some supine hypotension may have occurred.

As regional anesthetic techniques became more refined, it became apparent that there were significant objections to the use of the caudal route for routine analgesia in labor. The pathways for the pain of first stage labor are by way of T10–L1 (see Chap. 18). Thus a technique that initially and predominantly blocked sacral roots was less effective for early labor. Large doses of local anesthetic drug needed to be given. Admittedly the caudal approach offered superb management of the sacrally mediated pain of second stage, but it did so for what could be a lengthy period of first stage when it was not required. What was previously a tolerable failure rate of 7% became no longer acceptable. An unfortunate objection was the report of four cases in which local anesthetic drugs were injected into the fetus during attempted caudal injection.[27,69] For these reasons, continuous caudal analgesia in labor has fallen into disuse in most obstetric units to an extent that facility in performing the technique has now been largely lost. There is still a place for continuous caudal analgesia in labor in those cases in which lumbar epidural analgesia is contraindicated because of anatomic abnormalities or localized infection. On rare occasions, sacral analgesia is either required early in labor or cannot be obtained from a lumbar catheter.

A two-catheter technique, one lumbar and one caudal, has been used in an effort to lower the total dose of local anesthetic drug.[1,18] This would seem to compound the likelihood of complications without a sufficiently significant positive advantage. The technique of using a lumbar catheter for first-stage analgesia supplemented late in labor by single-injection caudal block is popular in some centers.[47] Single-injection caudal is useful as an alternative to saddle-block spinal anesthesia for forceps delivery. In these circumstances the proximity of the needle to the presenting part of the fetus must be remembered. The procedure is safe if bone of the sacrum and coccyx is palpable on all sides of the needle. Rectal examination is advised when there is any doubt. It has been stated that caudal block should not be performed if the presenting part is at the perineum.[47]

PEDIATRIC ANESTHESIA

Caudal block has been used successfully for anesthesia in children since about 1960,[70] with many studies attesting to its success. In children, the sacral hiatus is usually very easy to palpate, thus making the procedure very simple, quick, and reliable.[49] Because of the ease of its performance in children, the block has been recommended for a wide variety of surgical procedures, both as the sole anesthetic and in combination with light general anesthesia (see Chap. 21). In summary, the surgical indications for the block divide into three groups: sacral block (*e.g.*, circumcision, anal surgery), lower thoracic block (*e.g.*, inguinal herniotomy), and upper thoracic block.

The significance of these three groups relates to the doses of local anesthetic drug required to consistently achieve the desired spread. This subject has been discussed at length in a previous section, but it should be reemphasized here that there is no justification for the use of doses of lidocaine in excess of 10 to 12 mg/kg, despite the allegations of safety by some authors. Midabdominal or upper abdominal surgery is *not* an indication for caudal block.

For surgery in the groin, lower limbs, and perineum, caudal anesthesia is excellent. Young children do not, however, tolerate well the frightening environment of the operating room, let alone a caudal needle. Although many techniques have been used to enable the procedure to occur under calm conditions, light general anesthesia seems to be the preferred technique for both insertion of the block and the duration of surgery; however, awake caudal anesthesia has been used for surgery on restrained neonates[74] and on other children of various ages.[28,35,49]

A specific indication for caudal anesthesia in children is surgery in patients with congenital dystrophia myotonica. Regional anesthesia enables the anesthesiologist to avoid the respiratory depression associated with general anesthetic agents.[3,11]

Relief of pain in the early postoperative period is probably the major advantage of caudal anesthesia in children. Several studies have confirmed the benefit of caudal anesthesia for the control of postoperative pain following circumcision.[43,46,50,51,83] It would seem to be better than i.m. morphine,[46] i.m. buprenorphine,[51] and i.m. dihydrocodeine[10] and at least equivalent to penile block.[83] The coexistent motor block has, however, been considered a disadvantage by some authors,[81,83] and a significantly higher incidence of vomiting was reported in one study.[79]

ADULT ANESTHESIA

Caudal blockade can be used whenever the area of surgery is primarily innervated by the sacral and lumbar nerve roots. When the area is innervated from a higher level, lumbar epidural blockade and spinal subarachnoid block are preferable procedures. The following procedures are appropriate indications: anal surgery, especially hemorrhoidectomy and anal dilatation, surgery on the vulva and vagina, surgery on the scrotal skin and penis, and surgery of the lower limb. If a caudal catheter is used with its tip positioned near the lumbosacral junction, a higher level of anesthesia can be assured and more extensive surgery accommodated. Such procedures could include vaginal hysterectomy and inguinal herniorrhaphy. The use of caudal blockade for relief of postoperative pain following hemorrhoidectomy is well documented.[6]

CHRONIC PAIN MANAGEMENT

The caudal approach to the epidural space has been used for many years by pain-control physicians to both diagnose and treat a variety of largely unspecified low back pain syndromes. In the main, the therapeutic techniques have involved injecting large volumes (up to 64 ml) of diluted procaine, lidocaine, or bupivacaine with or without steroid at a fairly rapid rate.[20,32,55,68] Cure or improvement rates of more than 50% have been claimed[32,37] (see Chap. 27.2 for further information). Rapid injection of large volumes of any solution into the epidural space is *not* recommended. Such practice can result in large increases in spinal CSF pressure, with a risk of cerebral hemorrhage, visual disturbances, headache, or compromised spinal cord blood flow (spinal stroke). Central nervous system vascular catastrophies are particularly a hazard in patients with atherosclerosis.

CAUDAL OPIOIDS

The caudal epidural route has been used for the administration of opioids with varying claims of success.[9,41,42,50,60] Although there is some current doubt about the limitation of action of epidural opioids to a local segmental area, most caudal studies have been restricted to perineal surgery.

When caudal morphine is compared with caudal bupivacaine, a similar duration of action is claimed by some authors,[50,60] whereas in one study, morphine analgesia clearly outlasted bupivacaine analgesia.[41] Caudal morphine was better than i.m. morphine for the first 12 postoperative hours for subumbilical surgery,[42] whereas caudal bupivacaine with or without morphine was no better than systemic diamorphine for postcircumcision pain in children.[50]

On balance, it would seem that the addition of morphine (4 mg in an adult) to the caudal bupivacaine solution may prolong analgesia following perineal surgery to a significant degree in some patients. From the limited amount of information available, it would appear to be more effective in children.

One would expect that the side-effects of caudal epidural opioids would be similar to those of the more common lumbar epidural route. Certainly itching has been reported and claimed in a single report to be dose related.[40]

COMPLICATIONS

The range of complications seen with caudal anesthesia is predictable and, in common with most other regional anesthetic procedures, decreases markedly with experience and with meticulous attention to technique (see Chap. 22).[22]

IMPROPER NEEDLE PLACEMENT

It is not unexpected that in this region of renowned variability of anatomy, malpositioning of the caudal needle, particularly by novices, is not uncommon. There is no substitute for practical experience coupled with a sound knowledge of the possible anatomic variants. The possible consequences of improper needle placement follow.

Absent or Patchy Block

Particularly in an obese patient, the needle may come to lie in the soft tissues superficial to the sacrum. The experienced hand can often detect the absence of firm fixation of the needle that is present when the needle has correctly penetrated the sacrococcygeal ligament. Palpation over the needle tip during injection of air or fluid will detect the appearance of a subcutaneous lump (Fig. 9-7*B*). With malplacement of the needle under periosteum either outside the canal or inside the canal anteriorly or posteriorly, the needle will be "fixed," but there will be considerable resistance to injection (Fig. 9-7*C*).

If the needle is malplaced laterally, it may penetrate a posterior sacral foramen, or it may miss any hiatus and lie in the presacral soft tissues (Figs. 9-7*E*, 9-7*F*). In either case, injection may be easy, but absent or patchy block will result. Penetration of a ligament-covered sealed depression (decoy hiatus) may sometimes give the "correct feel," but injection will be impossible (see Figs. 9-3*I* and 9-7D). With any malplacement where periosteum is needled or

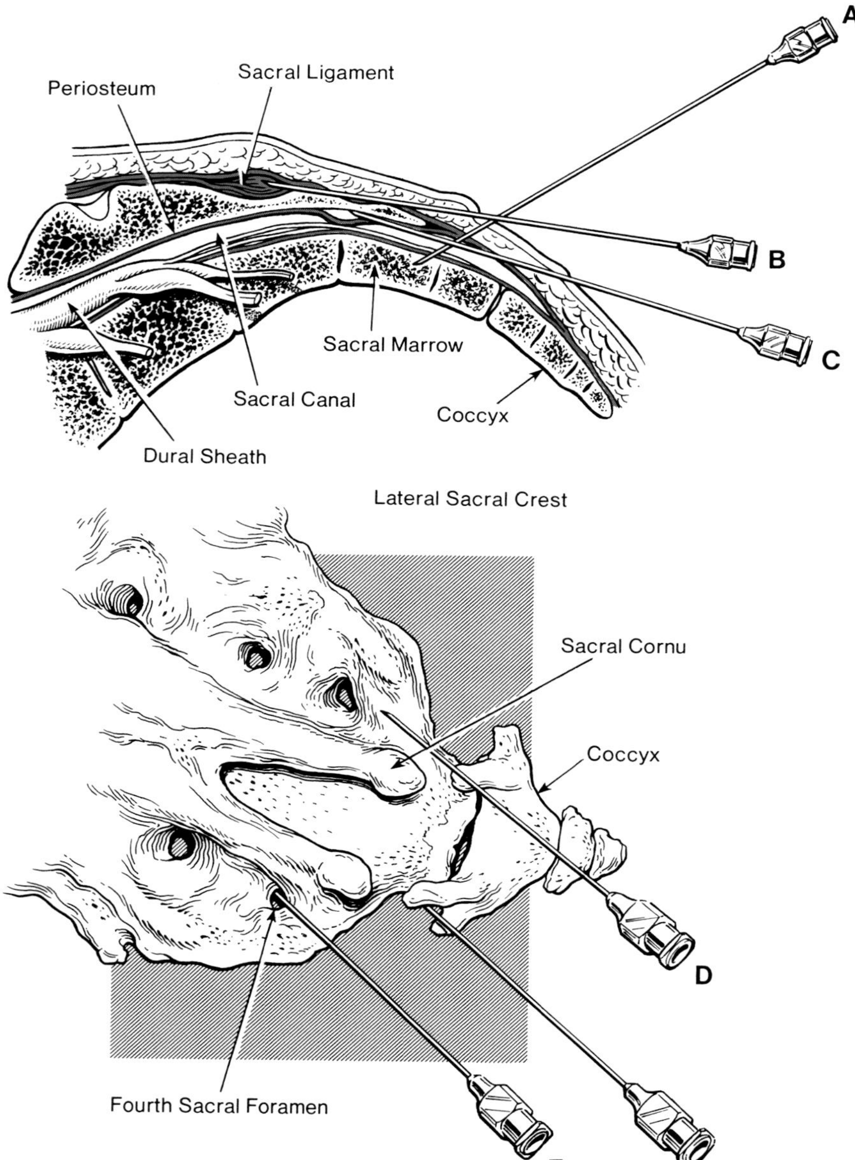

FIG. 9-7. Misplacement of needle during attempted caudal block. *Note:* injection into posterior sacral ligaments *(B)*; subperiosteal injection *(C);* and injection into marrow *(A);* lateral injection into a "decoy hiatus" *(D)* (see also Fig. 9-3); injection lateral to coccyx and toward anterior sacral wall *(E)*, with a risk of damaging intrapelvic structures (including a fetus); injection into 4th sacral foramen *(F)*, perhaps one of the most common causes of a unilateral limited block.

stretched, the awake patient will feel pain that can be severe. This pain may continue into the postoperative period and give rise to patient complaints. There is no place for persistent clumsy attempts to locate the correct hiatus.

Intravenous or Intraosseous Placement

Claims for a high incidence of local anesthetic toxic reactions during caudal anesthesia are not substantiated by studies.[21] Nevertheless, the potential exists for producing early onset high blood levels by either intravenous or intraosseous injection.[59] The venous plexus of the caudal canal has already been described (see Fig. 9-2). When a fine needle is used, free aspiration of blood on entering an epidural vein may not be obvious, suggesting the desirability of using a test dose.

Of at least equal importance in toxicity potential is the possibility of intraosseous injection, produced by penetrating the thin layer of cortical bone of the anterior wall of the sacral canal in those circumstances in which the ligament penetration has not been felt (Fig. 9-7*A*). The feeling of bone penetration may be confused with that of ligament penetration, and injection of local anesthetic drug into the marrow is possible. The result is similar to an intravenous injection with the rapid attainment of a high blood level and again supports the need for use of a test dose. This was reported following the aspiration of marrow cells during clinical caudal anesthesia[23,48] and reproduced in animal studies.[23] A further recent case has been reported.[80] Any suggestion of "granularity" during needle insertion or during attempted aspiration should alert one to the possibility of this hazard; however, the test dose provides the only practical protection against this complication.

Dural Puncture

With the dural sac ending at S2 level or approximately on a line joining the posterior–superior iliac spines, dural puncture should be exceedingly rare. An incidence of more than 1% has, however, been quoted,[21] although the rate of consequent accidental spinal block was much lower at 0.1%. A knowledge of the variable distance from the tip of the sac to the apex of the sacral hiatus should warn one of the possibility of dural puncture. Advancement of the needle more than 1 to 2 cm in the sacral canal should be avoided.

Injection into Fetus

Four cases of fetal intoxication by local anesthetic drug injected into the fetal scalp during attempted caudal injection have been reported.[27,69] Two babies died. Unfortunately, these isolated reports have done much to discourage the use of caudal anesthesia during labor despite the fact that the risk only exists when the presenting part has descended to the perineum and questionable techniques are used.

EXCESSIVE SPREAD

Unpredictability of spread of the local anesthetic solution, especially in adults,[19] has already been mentioned. Although *limited* cephalad spread is a more common problem with caudal, on rare occasion *excessive* spread may occur to a high thoracic level, even in the absence of a subarachnoid injection.[21] This extensive region of blockade is of itself no particular problem. After all, such levels are deliberately sought with lumbar epidural anesthesia for a variety of surgical procedures, and the physiologic changes that result are well controlled by simple standard measures. There is, however, a difference in the degree of expectation of these changes occurring, often resulting in a lesser degree of vigilance by the anesthesiologist. One must not forget that the potential exists for a caudal to give rise to a somatic and sympathetic block at least as extensive as a lumbar epidural block, albeit less commonly. Secure intravenous access, adequate monitoring, and normal resuscitation equipment must be assured (see Chap. 8 for details of management of extensive epidural or total spinal block).

CATHETER PROBLEMS

Problems from caudal epidural catheters are no different from those that occur with lumbar insertion. Catheter insertion when the needle is correctly placed is generally very easy, occurring more readily than with lumbar insertion. Early resistance to insertion is usually an indication that the needle is incorrectly placed. The catheter should never be withdrawn through the needle because of the risk of shearing it off. Shearing has also been reported when a properly placed needle was being withdrawn over the catheter in the accepted fashion.[17] This was caused by a barb directed toward the lumen, which had developed during a difficult insertion. Dural puncture by the catheter is possible, particularly with older, more rigid catheters with sharper tips. There has also been a case report of a catheter knotting in the caudal canal, requiring neurosurgical exploration for its removal.[17]

POSTOPERATIVE PROBLEMS

Pain

Pain at the injection site is the most common postoperative complaint. Ligament penetration without periosteal trauma will give rise to only minimal pain both during insertion and postoperatively. On the other hand, a periosteal hematoma may cause pain that lasts several weeks. There is no substitute for careful technique, using the information from all landmarks before needle insertion. It is worth remembering that coccygodynia resulting from the stress of childbirth may be erroneously blamed on the caudal block.

Urinary Retention

There seems little doubt that some increased risk of urinary retention occurs after epidural block of the sacral segments, especially when a long-acting local anesthetic drug is used.[12] The likelihood of retention may be greater in those patients who would normally be considered "at risk," that is, elderly men, puerperal women, and after perineal surgery. These groups, of course, make up the bulk of the indications for caudal blockade. A single bladder catheterization should not cause significantly increased morbidity if proper technique is followed.[12]

Infection

Intuitively, one would think that the infection rate would be significantly higher with caudal block than with lumbar epidural block. In a bacteriologic comparison between simultaneous caudal and lumbar epidural catheters (two-catheter technique) during childbirth, cultures were taken from skin at the puncture site, catheter tip, catheter fluid, and catheter subcutaneously.[2] Specimens from the skin surface in the caudal area produced a significantly larger number of positive cultures than did those from the epidural area. This result was repeated when a more extensive skin preparation, including povidone–iodine ointment, was used in the caudal area; however, there were no clinical infections, and in fact all cultures in both areas taken from sites deep to the skin were negative. The study indicates that the risk of infection, although remote, does exist. Compromises in sterile technique have no place in regional anesthesia.

Neurological Complications

In common with lumbar epidural and subarachnoid anesthesia, caudal epidural anesthesia is inevitably associated with some slight risk of neurologic damage. In his analysis of complications, Dawkins mentions one permanent lesion in nearly 23,000 cases, but the details are not specified.[21] Whatever the true incidence it must be very small. Of greater significance is the likelihood that a coexistent neurologic lesion will be blamed on the block. Neurologic sequelae of traumatic vaginal delivery notoriously fall into this group. As anesthesiologists, we need to ensure that our medical colleagues maintain a balanced view of regional anesthetic techniques and that any neurologic lesions be thoroughly examined and investigated. In almost all cases, such investigations will reveal the coincident nature of the lesion (see Chap. 22).

CONCLUSION

Objective data obtained from randomized prospective controlled studies are still needed for many aspects of caudal blockade. Such data as are available indicate that caudal block can provide safe, effective analgesia of lumbosacral spinal segments.

The caudal route to the epidural space is particularly attractive in children (see Chap. 21) and in adults in whom mainly sacral block is required. In children, the technique is reliable and easy to perform and has a consistent dose/spinal segment response relationship. In adults, there is an inevitable failure rate that is higher than that for lumbar epidural block, but with a knowledge of pertinent anatomy and with practical experience it can be reduced to an acceptable level.

REFERENCES

1. Abouleish, E.: Pain Control in Obstetrics, p. 285. Philadelphia, J.B. Lippincott, 1977.
2. Abouleish, E., Orig, T., and Amortegui, A.J.: Bacteriologic

comparison between epidural and caudal techniques. Anesthesiology, *53*:511, 1980.

3. Alexander, C., Wolf, S., and Ghia, J.N.: Caudal anesthesia for early onset myotonic dystrophy. Anesthesiology, *55*:597, 1981.
4. Alexander, J.A., and Franklin, R.R.: Effects of caudal anesthesia on uterine activity. Obstet. Gynecol., *27*:436, 1966.
5. Armitage, E.N.: Caudal block in children. Anaesthesia, *34*:396, 1979.
6. Berstock, D.A.: Haemorrhoidectomy without tears. Ann. R. Coll. Surg. Engl., *61*:51, 1979.
7. Black, M.G.: Anatomic reasons for caudal anesthesia failure. Anesth. Analg (Cleve.), *28*:33, 1949.
8. Bonica, J.J.: Principles and Practice of Obstetric Analgesia and Anesthesia. Philadelphia, F.A. Davis, 1967.
9. Boskovski, N., Lewinski, A., Xuereb, J., and Mercieca, V.: Caudal epidural morphine for postoperative pain relief. Anesthesia, *36*:67, 1981.
10. Bramwell, R.G., Bullen, C., and Radford, P.: Caudal block for postoperative analgesia in children. Anaesthesia, *37*:1024, 1982.
11. Bray, R.J., and Inkster, J.S.: Anaesthesia in babies with congenital dystrophia myotonica. Anaesthesia, *39*:1007, 1984.
12. Bridenbaugh, L.D.: Catheterization after long- and short-acting local anesthetics for continuous caudal block for vaginal delivery. Anesthesiology, *46*:357, 1977.
13. Bromage, P.R.: Ageing and epidural dose requirements: Segmental spread and predictability of epidural analgesia in youth and extreme age. Br. J. Anaesth., *41*:1016, 1969.
14. Bromage, P.R.: Epidural Analgesia. Philadelphia, W.B. Saunders, 1978.
15. Cathelin, M.F.: Une nouvelle voie d'injection rachidienne. Methode des injections epidurales pas le procede du canal sacre. C.R. Soc. Biol. Paris, *53*:452, 1901.
16. Charlton, A.J., and Lindahl, S.G.E.: Ventilatory response during halothane and enflurane anaesthesia. Anaesthesia, *40*:18, 1985.
17. Chun, L., and Karp, M.: Unusual complications from placement of catheters in caudal canal in obstetrical anesthesia. Anesthesiology, *27*:96, 1966.
18. Cleland, J.G.P.: Continuous peridural and caudal analgesia in obstetrics. Anesth. Analg., *28*:61, 1949.
19. Cousins, M.J., and Bromage, P.R.: A comparison of the hydrochloride and carbonated salts of lignocaine for caudal analgesia in outpatients. Br. J. Anaesth., *43*:1149, 1971.
20. Cyriax, J.H.: Textbook of orthopaedic medicine. Vol 1. Diagnosis of soft tissue lesions. Ch. 19. London, Bailliere Tindall, 1978.
21. Dawkins, C.J.M.: An analysis of the complications of extradural and caudal block. Anaesthesia, *24*:554, 1969.
22. DeJong, R.H.: Anesthetic complications during continuous caudal analgesia for obstetrics: Analysis of 826 cases. Anesth. Analg. (Cleve), *40*:384, 1961.
23. DiGiovanni, A.J.: Inadvertent intraosseous injection — A hazard of caudal anesthesia. Anesthesiology, *34*:92, 1971.
24. Ecoffey, C., Desparmet, J., Berdeaux, A., and Maury, M., *et al.*: Pharmacokinetics of lignocaine in children following caudal anaesthesia. Br. J. Anaesth., *56*:1399, 1984.
25. Eyres, R.L., Kidd, J., Oppenheim, R., and Brown, T.C.K.: Local anaesthetic plasma levels in children. Anaesth. Intensive Care, *6*:243, 1978.
26. Fernandez-Sepulveda, R., and Gomez-Rogers, C.: Single dose caudal anesthesia. Its effect on uterine contractility. Am. J. Obstet. Gynecol., *98*:847, 1967.
27. Finster, M., Poppers, P.J., Sinclair, J.C., Morishima, H.O., *et al.*: Accidental intoxication of the fetus with local anesthetic drug during caudal anesthesia. Am. J. Obstet. Gynecol., *92*:922, 1965.
28. Fortuna, A.: Caudal analgesia: A simple and safe technique in paediatric surgery. Br. J. Anaesth., *39*:165, 1967.
29. Freund, P.R., Bowdle, T.A., Slattery, J.T., and Bell, L.E.: Caudal anesthesia with lidocaine or bupivacaine: Plasma local anesthetic concentration and extent of sensory spread in old and young patients. Anesth., Analg., *63*:1017, 1984.
30. Galindo, A., Benavides, O., Ortega De Munos, S., Bonilla, O., *et al.*: Comparison of anesthetic solutions used in lumbar and caudal peridural anesthesia. Anesth. Analg., *57*:175, 1978.
31. Giaufre, E., Conte-Devolx, B., Morisson-Lacombe, G., Boudouresque, F., *et al.*: Caudal epidural anesthesia in children. Study of endocrine changes. Presse Med., *14*:201, 1985.
32. Gordon, J.: Caudal extradural injection for the treatment of low back pain. Anaesthesia, *35*:515, 1980.
33. Gunther, R.E., and Bellville, J.W.: Obstetrical caudal anesthesia: II. A randomized study comparing 1 per cent mepivacaine with 1 per cent mepivacaine plus epinephrine. Anesthesiology, *37*:288, 1972.
34. Hansen, J.M., and Ueland, K.: The influence of caudal analgesia on cardiovascular dynamics during normal labour and delivery. Acta Anaesthesiol. Scand., *23*[*Suppl.*]:449, 1966.
35. Hassan, S.Z.: Caudal anesthesia in infants. Anesth. Analg., *56*:686, 1977.
36. Hatch, D.J., Hulse, M.G., and Lindahl, S.G.: Caudal analgesia in children. Influence on ventilatory efficiency during halothane anaesthesia. Anaesthesia *39*:873, 1984.
37. Hauswirth, R., and Michot, F.: Sacral epidural anesthesia in the treatment of lumbosacral backache. Schweiz Med. Wochenschr., *112*:222, 1982.
38. Hingson, R.A., Cull, W.A., and Benzinger, M.: Continuous caudal analgesia in obstetrics: combined experience of a quarter of a century in clinics in New York, Philadelphia, Memphis, Baltimore and Cleveland. Anesth. Analg. (Cleve.), *40*:119, 1961.
39. Hingson, R.A., and Edwards, W.B.: Continuous caudal analgesia. An analysis of the first ten thousand confinements thus managed with the report of the authors' first thousand cases. J.A.M.A., *123*:538, 1943.
40. Hirlekar, G.: Is itching after caudal epidural morphine dose related? Anaesthesia, *36*:68, 1981.
41. Jensen, B.H.: Caudal block for post operative pain relief in children after genital operations. A comparison between bupivacaine and morphine. Acta Anaesthesiol. Scand., *25*:373, 1981.
42. Jensen, P.J., Siem-Jorgensen, P., Nielsen, T.B., Wichmand-Nielsen, H.: Epidural morphine by the caudal route for post operative pain relief. Acta Anaesthesiol. Scand., *26*:511, 1982.

43. Kay, B.: Caudal block for postoperative pain relief in children. Anaesthesia, *29*:610, 1974.
44. Letterman, G.S., and Trotter, M.: Variations of the male sacrum. Their significance in caudal analgesia. Surg. Gynecol. Obstet., *78*:551, 1944.
45. Loury, C.J., and McDonald, I.H.: Caudal anaesthesia in infants and children. Anaesth. Intens. Care, *1*:547, 1973.
46. Lunn, J.N.: Post operative analgesia after circumcision. A randomized comparison between caudal analgesia and intramuscular morphine in boys. Anaesthesia, *34*:552, 1979.
47. McCaul, K.: Caudal blockade. In Cousins M.J., and Bridenbaugh, P.O. (eds.): Neural Blockade in Clinical Anesthesia and Management of Pain. 1st ed. pp. 275–293. Philadelphia, J.B. Lippincott, 1980.
48. McGown, R.G.: Accidental marrow sampling during caudal anaesthesia. Br. J. Anaesth, *44*:613, 1972.
49. McGown, R.G.: Caudal analgesia in children. Anaesthesia, *37*:806, 1982.
50. Martin, L.V.: Post-operative analgesia after circumcision in children. Br. J. Anaesth., *54*:1263, 1982.
51. May, A.E., Wandless, J., and James, R.H.: Analgesia for circumcision in children. A comparison of caudal bupivacaine and intramuscular buprenorphine. Acta Anaesthesiol. Scand., *26*:331, 1982.
52. Mazze, R.I., and Dunbar, R.W.: Plasma lidocaine concentrations after caudal, lumbar epidural, axillary block, and intravenous regional anesthesia. Anesthesiology, *27*:574, 1966.
53. Mohan, J., and Potter, J.M.: Pupillary constriction and ptosis following caudal epidural analgesia. Anaesthesia, *30*:769, 1975.
54. Moore, D.C., Bridenbaugh, L.D., Bagdi, P.A., and Bridenbaugh, P.O.: Accumulation of mepivacaine hydrochloride during caudal block. Anesthesiology, *29*:585, 1968.
55. Natelson, S.E., Gibson, C.E., and Gillespie, R.A.: Caudal block: Cost effective primary treatment for back pain. South Med. J., *73*:286, 1980.
56. Norenberg, A., Johanson, D.C., and Gravenstein, J.S.: Racial differences in sacral structure important in caudal anesthesia. Anesthesiology, *50*:549, 1979.
57. Owens, W.D., Slater, E.M., and Battit, G.E.: A new technique of caudal anesthesia. Anesthesiology, *39*:451, 1973.
58. Park, W.Y., Massengale, M., and MacNamara, T.E.: Age, height and speed of injection as factors determining caudal anesthetic level, and occurrence of severe hypertension. Anesthesiology, *51*:81, 1979.
59. Prentiss, J.E.: Cardiac arrest following caudal anesthesia. Anesthesiology, *50*:51, 1979.
60. Pybus, D.A., Dubras, B.E., Goulding, G., Liberman, H., *et al.*: Post-operative analgesia for haemorrhoid surgery. Anaesth. Intensive Care, *11*:27, 1983.
61. Satoyoshi, M., and Kamiyama, K.: Caudal anaesthesia for upper abdominal surgery in infants and children: A simple calculation of the volume of local anaesthetic. Acta Anaesthesiol. Scand. *28*:57, 1984.
62. Schulte-Steinberg, O.: Spread of extradural analgesia following caudal injection in children. Br. J. Anaesth., *50*:973, 1978.
63. Schulte-Steinberg, O., and Rahlfs, V.W.: Caudal anaesthesia in children and spread of 1 per cent lignocaine. A statistical study. Br. J. Anaesth., *42*:1093, 1970.
64. Schulte-Steinberg, O., and Rahlfs, V.W.: Spread of extradural analgesia following caudal injection in children: A statistical study. Br. J. Anaesth., *49*:1027, 1977.
65. Schulte-Steinberg, O., and Rahlfs, V.W.: Caudal anaesthesia in children. Anesthesiology, *49*:372, 1978.
66. Selander, D., Dhuner, K.G., and Lundborg, G.: Peripheral nerve injury due to injection needles used for regional anaesthesia. Acta Anaesth. Scand., *21*:182, 1977.
67. Seow, L.T., Chiu, H.H., and Tye, C.Y.: Clinical evaluation of etidocaine in continuous caudal analgesia for pelvic floor repair and post operative pain relief. Anaesth. Intensive Care, *4*:239, 1976.
68. Sharma, P.K.: Indications, technique and results of caudal epidural injection for lumbar disc retropulsion. Postgrad. Med. J., *53*:1, 1977.
69. Sinclair, J.C., Fox, H.A., Lentz, J.F., Fuld, G.L., *et al.*: Intoxication of the fetus by a local anesthetic. A newly recognized complication of maternal caudal anesthesia. N. Engl. J. Med., *273*:1173, 1965.
70. Spiegel, P.: Caudal anesthesia in pediatric surgery: A preliminary report. Anesth. Analg., *41*:218, 1962.
71. Takasaki, M.: Blood concentrations of lidocaine, mepivacaine and bupivacaine during caudal analgesia in children. Acta Anaesthesiol. Scand., *28*:211, 1984.
72. Takasaki, M., Dohi, S., Kawabata, Y., and Takahashi, T.: Dosage of lidocaine for caudal anesthesia in infants and children. Anesthesiology, *47*:527, 1977.
73. Thompson, J.E.: An anatomical and experimental study of sacral anaesthesia. Ann. Surg., *66*:718, 1917.
74. Touloukian, R.J., Wugmeister, M., Pickett, L.K., and Hehre, F.W.: Caudal anesthesia for neonatal anoperineal and rectal operations. Anesth. Analg. (Cleve.), *50*:565, 1971.
75. Trotter, M.: Variations of the sacral canal: Their significance in the administration of caudal analgesia. Anesth. Analg., *26*:192, 1947.
76. Trotter, M., and Letterman, G.S.: Variations of the female sacrum. Their significance in continuous caudal anaesthesia. Surg. Gynecol. Obstet., *78*:419, 1944.
77. Tyack, A.G., Parsons, R.J., Millar, D.R., and Nicholas, A.D.G.: Uterine activity and plasma bupivacaine levels after caudal epidural analgesia. J. Obstet. and Gynaecol. Br. Comm., *80*:896, 1973.
78. Ueland, K., and Hansen, J.M.: Maternal cardiovascular dynamics III. Labour and delivery under local and caudal analgesia. Am. J. Obstet. Gynecol., *103*:8, 1969.
79. Vater, M., and Wandless, J.: Caudal or dorsal nerve block? A comparison of two local anaesthetic techniques for postoperative analgesia following day case circumcision. Acta Anaesthesiol. Scand., *29*:175, 1985.
80. Weber, S.: Caudal anesthesia complicated by intraosseous injection in a patient with ankylosing spondylitis. Anesthesiology, *63*:716, 1985.
81. White, J., Harrison, B., Richmond, P., Proctor, A., *et al.*: Postoperative analgesia for circumcision. Br. Med. J., *286*:1934, 1983.

82. Willis, R.J., and Macintyre, P.E.: The effect of dose and drug on the spread of caudal anaesthesia. (in preparation).
83. Yeoman, P.M., Cooke, R., and Hain, W.R.: Penile block for circumcision. A comparison with caudal blockade. Anaesthesia, *38*:862, 1983.
84. Zaaijman, J. DuT., and Slabber, C.F.: The position of epidural catheters in obstetric regional anaesthesia. S. Afr. Med. J., *55*:915, 1979.

section B
EXTREMITIES

10 THE UPPER EXTREMITY: SOMATIC BLOCKADE

L. DONALD BRIDENBAUGH

All of the deep structures of the upper extremity and the skin distal to the middle of the upper arm are rendered insensitive by blocking the nerves making up the brachial plexus. The nerves of the plexus may be blocked anywhere along their course: from their emergence from intervertebral foramina and entrance into the sheath between the anterior and middle scaleni muscles until they terminate in the specific nerves in the hand. Techniques for blocking of the plexus involve infiltration at one of five anatomic areas — that is, paravertebral, supraclavicular, infraclavicular, in the axilla, and by blocking the specific terminal nerves. Thus, any surgical procedure on the arm — for example, reduction of fractures or dislocations, suturing of tendons, or repair of lacerations — is an indication for the use of this kind of anesthesia. However, frequently the primary indication for the choice of brachial plexus nerve block versus general anesthesia is the wish of the patient, the surgeon, or the skill of the anesthesiologist.

History

Brachial plexus nerve block was reportedly first accomplished by Halsted in 1884 when he "freed the cords and nerves of the brachial plexus — after blocking the roots in the neck with cocaine solution." In 1887 Crile disarticulated the shoulder joint after rendering the arm insensitive by blocking the "brachial plexus by direct intraneural injection of each nerve trunk with 0.5 percent cocaine under direct vision."[13] In 1911 Hirschel and Kulenkampff, working independently, were the first to inject the brachial plexus blindly through the skin without exposure of the nerves.[23,28] Subsequently, there have been many advocated modifications of these original techniques. These modifications vary mostly according to site and include the following: infraclavicular, supraclavicular, axillary, and perivascular infiltration and the sheath technique.[8,14,17,20,23,25,27,28,30,31,34,38,39,45,47,56,59-61] With the advent of barbiturates and cyclopropane, the enthusiasm for block anesthesia waned in the early 1940s. It has, in current years, however, enjoyed somewhat of a rejuvenation.

Each of the modifications previously noted has specific advantages and disadvantages. These will be discussed individually along with the techniques for performing each of the blocks.

Advantages

Brachial plexus block, like all other regional anesthetic procedures, offers certain advantages to the patient, surgeon, and anesthesiologist that may not be associated with general anesthesia. These include the following:

1. *The anesthesia is limited to the restricted portion of the body on which it is proposed to operate,* leaving the other vital centers intact. The physiology of the patient is taxed less than with general anesthesia because metabolism of the rest of the body is undisturbed. This consideration is important in

the poor-risk patient who cannot tolerate the stress imposed by general anesthesia. Patients who present complicating conditions such as heart, renal, and pulmonary disease; chest injuries; diabetes; and so forth are able to withstand surgery performed with brachial block anesthesia without aggravation of the disease. This does not imply that the technique should be reserved only for poor-risk patients. On the contrary, nearly all patients who present themselves for surgery of the upper extremity could be afforded the benefits of this form of regional anesthesia.

2. *It is possible and desirable for the patient to remain ambulatory.* Outpatients may be sent home after procedures such as closed reduction of fractures or repair of lacerations. Brachial plexus block is also of great benefit in aged patients in whom early ambulation is necessary to prevent complications.
3. *Whenever fluoroscopy is a necessary adjunct to the surgical procedure, brachial plexus block eliminates the potential general anesthesia dangers of explosions, respiratory depression, or obstruction in a darkened room* in which the patient cannot readily be observed. It also permits the patient to cooperate with the surgeon or the radiologist.
4. *Postanesthetic nausea, vomiting, and other complications of general anesthesia, such as atelectasis, hypotension, ileus, and dehydration, are reduced.* This allows the patient to maintain a regular diet and, thus, to benefit from oral feeding earlier in the postoperative period.
5. *Prolonged operations on the upper extremity, if they are performed with general anesthesia, are sometimes followed by postoperative depression* because of the comparatively large doses of drugs required. Operations such as tendon repairs and plastic procedures can, therefore, have complications out of proportion to the surgical procedure.
6. *Brachial block anesthesia allows patients who dread losing consciousness to be awake.* If it is properly performed, brachial plexus block provides a minimum degree of discomfort to the patient.
7. *Patients who arrive at surgery in genuine or impending shock may improve as soon as the pain has been relieved by the block.* The improved circulation resulting from the sympathetic blockade may be a positive factor in the prognosis of the traumatized upper extremity, which has areas of severely compromised circulation and questionable tissue viability.
8. *Any patient who arrives at surgery with a full stomach presents less danger of aspiration if he vomits.*
9. *Ideal operating conditions can be obtained to meet surgical requirements.* Complete motor relaxation can be accomplished. If it is desirable to have the patient move and cooperate — such as for surgical repair of tendons — this can also be accomplished by using a weaker concentration of the local anesthetic drug.
10. *If an anesthesiologist is not present, such as in rural regions or during wartime, brachial block anesthesia permits the maximum utilization of available personnel.* The surgeon can perform the block and then perform the operation, or one anesthesiologist can furnish anesthesia for more than one patient.
11. *Ward nurses particularly appreciate the use of regional anesthesia.* Patients who return to the wards awake, without nausea and vomiting, and are able to help themselves immediately, enable the nursing staff to care for many more patients at one time.

Anatomy

The brachial plexus supplies all of the motor and almost all of the sensory function of the upper extremity. The remaining area — the skin over the shoulder — is supplied by the descending branches of the cervical plexus, and the posterior medial aspect of the arm extending nearly to the elbow is supplied by the intercostobrachial branch of the second intercostal nerve. The plexus is formed from the anterior primary rami of the fifth, sixth, seventh, and eighth cervical and the first thoracic nerves and frequently receives small contributing branches from the fourth cervical and second thoracic nerve (Fig. 10-1).

After these nerves leave their respective intervertebral foramina, they proceed anterolaterally and inferiorly to occupy the interval between the anterior and middle scalene muscles, where they unite to form three trunks, thus initiating the formation of the plexus proper. These trunks emerge from the interscalene space at the lower border of these muscles and continue anterolaterally and inferiorly to converge toward the upper surface of the first rib, where they are closely grouped. (It is to be noted that, as the newly formed trunks approach the first rib, they are arranged according to their designation "superior," "middle," and "inferior" — *i.e.*, one above the other vertically, not next to the others horizontally as is depicted in so many texts.) At the lateral edge of the rib, each trunk divides into an anterior and posterior division, which pass inferior to the midportion of the clavicle to enter the axilla through its apex. These divisions, by which fibers of the trunk reassemble to gain the ventral and dorsal aspect of the limb, reunite within the axilla to form three cords—the lateral, medial, and posterior—named because of their relationship with the second part of the axillary artery.

At the lateral border of the pectoralis minor, the three cords break up to give rise to the peripheral nerves of the upper extremity. The lateral cord gives off the lateral head of the median nerve and the musculocutaneous nerve; the medial cord gives off the medial head of the median nerve, the ulnar, the medial antebrachial, and the medial brachial cutaneous nerves; and the posterior cord terminates as the axillary and radial nerves (Fig. 10-2).

In its course, the brachial plexus is in close relationship to certain structures, some of which serve as important landmarks during the injection of the anesthetic. In its position between the anterior and middle scalene muscles, the plexus lies superior and posterior to the second and third parts of the subclavian artery, which is also located between the two muscles. Anteromedial to the lower trunk and posteromedial to the artery lies the dome of the pleura.

Livingston and Werthein originally pointed out, and Winnie has refocused our attention on, the fascial barriers that surround these structures.[31,56,61] The prevertebral fascia divides to invest the anterior and middle scalene muscles and then fuses at the lateral margins to form an enclosed interscalene space. Therefore, as the nerve roots leave the transverse processes, they emerge between the two walls of fascia that cover the anterior and middle scalene muscles, and, in their descent toward the first rib to form the trunks of the plexus, the roots may be considered to be "sandwiched" between the anterior and middle scalene muscles, the fascia of which serves as a "sheath" of the plexus (Fig. 10-3). As the roots pass down through this space, they converge to form the trunks of the brachial plexus and, together with the subclavian artery, invaginate the scalene fascia, which forms a subclavian perivascular sheath, which, in turn, becomes the axillary sheath as it passes under the clavicle (Fig. 10-4). It is important for the anesthesiologist to recognize a continuous fascia-enclosed space extending from the cervical transverse process to several centimeters beyond the axilla and enclosing the entire brachial plexus from the cervical roots to the great nerves of the upper arm. All the techniques for blocking the brachial plexus involve the location of the nerves and injection of the local anesthetic within the fascial sheath.

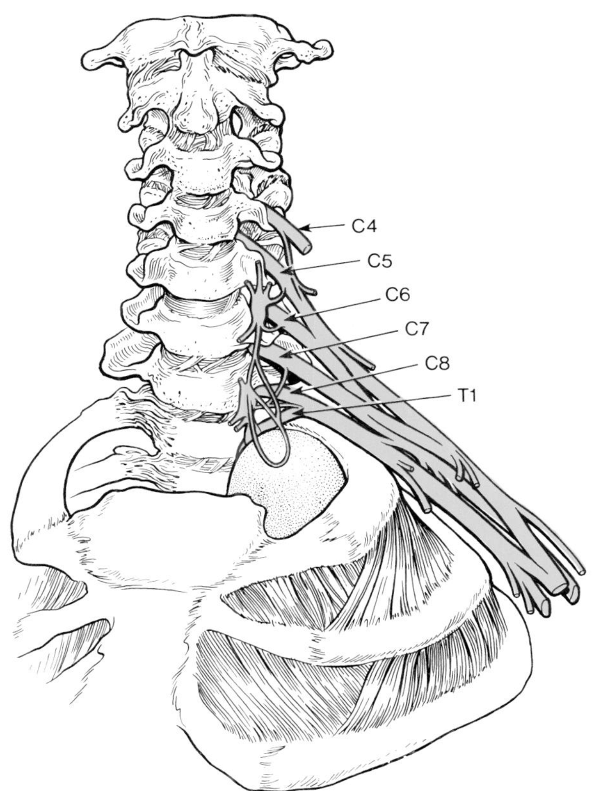

FIG. 10-1. Brachial plexus. Note the components of the plexus and relationship to intervertebral foramina and "gutters" of transverse processes.

PATIENT CARE, DRUGS, AND EQUIPMENT

Premedication

A high proportion of patients presenting for upper extremity block may be accident cases in whom opportunities for formal preparation and premedication may not be possible. Accordingly, the following points should be noted. First, the best way to achieve adequate pain relief is to insert a block as quickly as possible. Second, people who have suffered from injuries to their hands are especially anxious about the outcome. Third, fractures are most common in children and the elderly. Fourth, many patients can be treated as outpatients, and last, because paresthesias are sought to facilitate many upper limb blocks, cooperation of the patient is required.

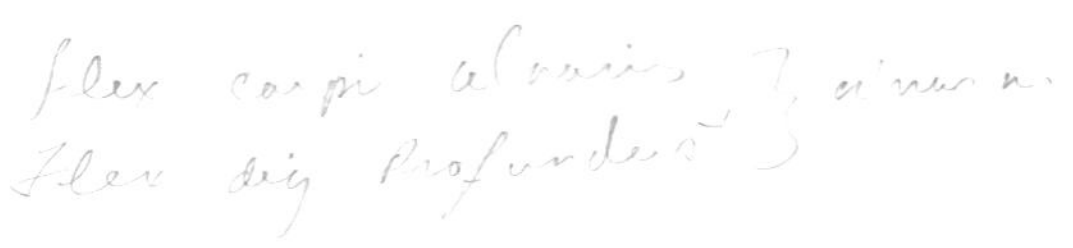

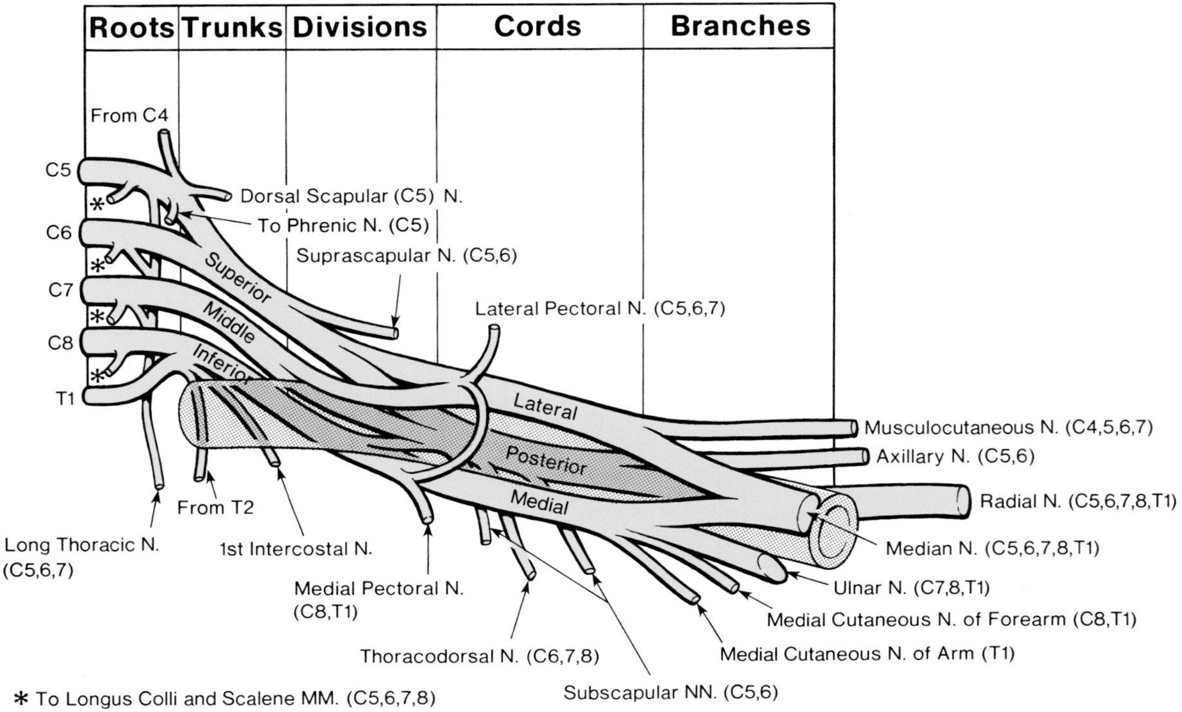

FIG. 10-2. Roots, trunks, divisions, cords, and branches of brachial plexus. Note also relationship to subclavian artery. Note that the intercostobrachial nerve is not shown in this diagram.

For both elective surgery and, where practicable, with emergencies, premedication is strongly recommended, preferably a narcotic combined with a small dose (0.2 – 0.3 mg) of hyoscine or another mild sedative. It is important that the patient be alert and cooperative enough for the block procedure but not distressed by it (see Chap. 6).

Intraoperative Analgesia and Sedation

Requirements for intraoperative analgesia and sedation depend on the patient's preference, the effects of premedication, the duration of the surgical procedure, additional stimuli such as a tourniquet, and the possibility of need for active tendon movement during stages of the operation. Even though complete analgesia is provided by nerve block, a narcotic and tranquilizer combination, such as fentanyl and diazepam, is recommended (see Chap. 6).

Postoperative Analgesia

Pain is not prominent after surgery on the upper limb. It is usually relieved by simple oral analgesics and the release of compression dressings if this is appropriate.

Except in a few cases of extensive surgery or trauma, when stronger analgesics may be required for a short time, severe pain should be regarded as a sign of possible surgical complication. Because of this, the use of bupivacaine for nerve blocks may not be appropriate. However, many surgeons consider that after hand surgery, the prolonged period of immobility, together with functional sympathectomy and good pain relief from a long-acting block, outweighs the potential disadvantage of removing pain that might have indicated complications.

Posture of the Blocked Arm

Special care must be taken with the anesthetized limb. The arm must not be allowed to fall onto the face; this may occur when the patient attempts to move his half-paralyzed limb. Second, it is important that the arm should not be put into a position that would stretch the brachial plexus (*i.e.*, extended further than 90° or displaced posteriorly).[27] Third, the ulnar nerve at the elbow should be properly padded,

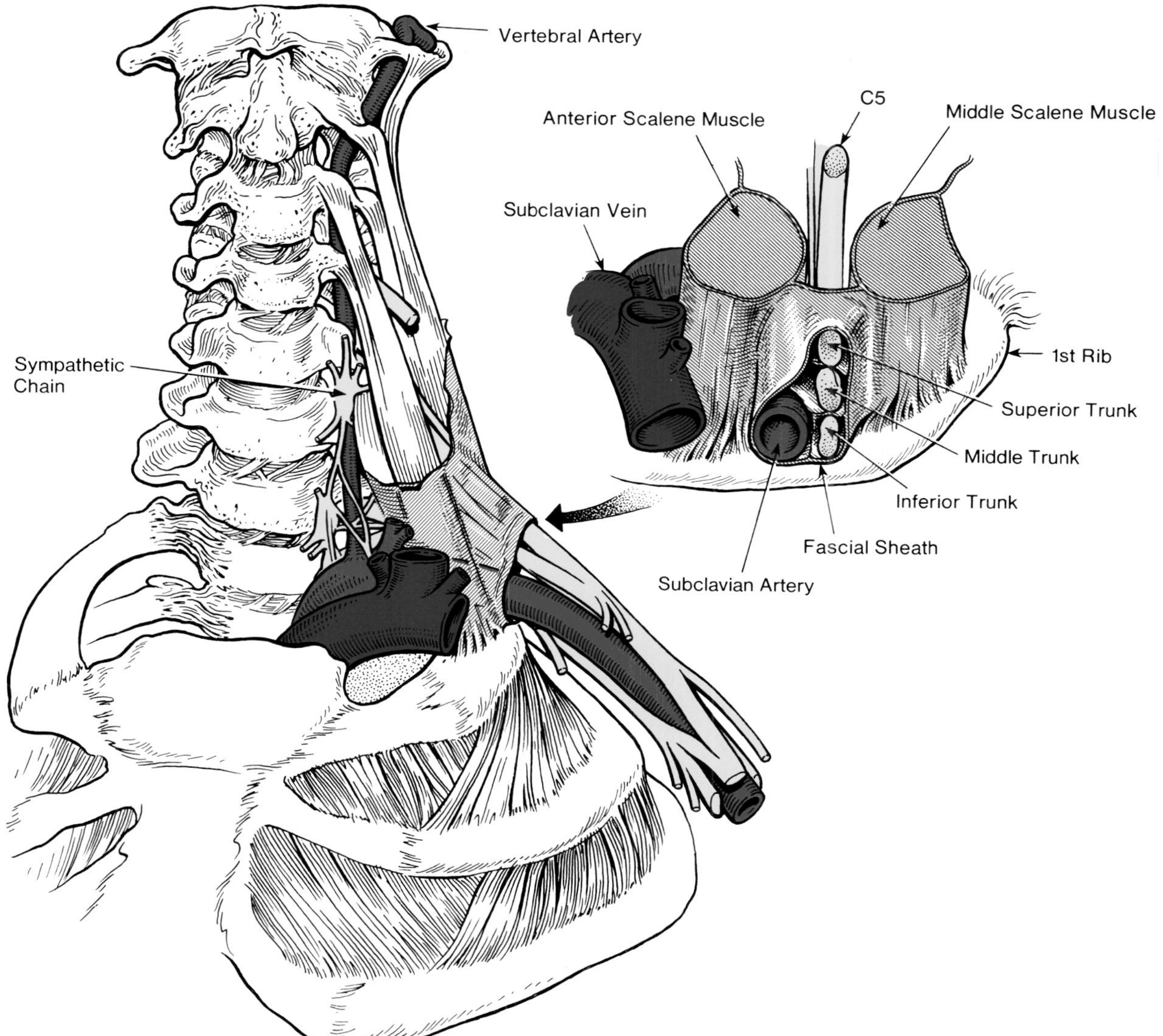

FIG. 10-3. Brachial plexus sheath and scalene muscles. Note brachial plexus "sandwiched" between anterior and middle scalene muscles, prevertebral fascia splitting to enclose scalenes and then forming a fascial sheath around the brachial plexus. Note also relationships to vertebral artery, subclavian artery, and sympathetic chain.

particularly if the forearm is pronated. Last, the arm should be properly supported during movement of the patient, transit from the operating table, and at all other times, until power and sensation return.

Local Anesthetic Drugs

At present, all upper extremity block techniques may be adequately performed with any of the local anesthetic drugs approved for peripheral nerve block (see Chap. 4). For emergency room use, practitioners may desire a short-acting drug with rapid onset, such as 2-chloroprocaine or lidocaine. As has been previously noted, a long-acting drug like bupivacaine or etidocaine will not only provide anesthesia for long operative procedures, but will also ensure a prolonged period of postoperative analgesia and sympathetic blockade. In general, a short-acting drug, a

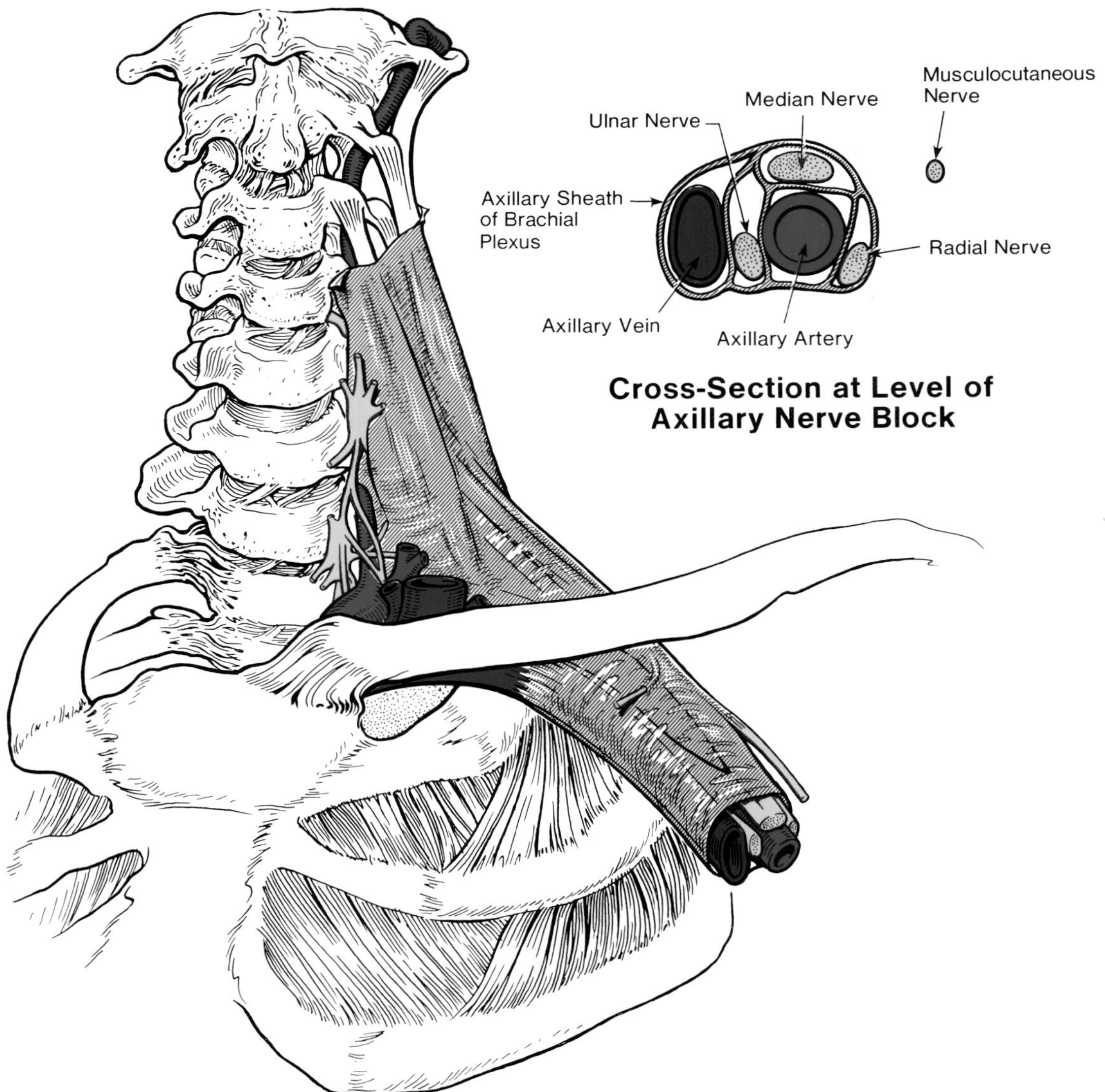

FIG. 10-4. Brachial plexus sheath extending from interscalene to subclavian and axillary regions. Note the brachial plexus enclosed in a vertical tube (the interscalene fascia or sheath), which is invaginated to form a horizontal tube (the subclavian and axillary sheath). A cross-section at the level of an axillary nerve block shows the relationships of major nerves to the axillary artery and axillary vein. Small fascial septa may subdivide the main sheath to enclose each of these structures. The role of these septa as diffusion barriers to local anesthetics is controversial.

drug of intermediate action, and a long-acting drug will suffice to meet the needs of most practitioners.

As in other peripheral nerve blocks, the use of epinephrine-containing solutions depends generally on the agent to be used, the total dose of drug being contemplated, and the duration of the block desired. Epinephrine-containing solutions should not be used on the digital nerves of the hands.

Concentration of the drug required depends primarily on the size of the nerve trunk, the modalities required to be blocked (*i.e.,* fiber size), and the disposition of these fibers within the nerve trunk (see Chap. 2).

Muscle relaxation is important for shoulder surgery, particularly the reduction of dislocations. Although the brachial plexus trunks are quite large, the actual nerve fibers that supply the shoulder are thought to be distributed in their periphery as "mantle fibers," so that they are quickly and relatively easily blocked. In contrast, hand surgery requires little muscle relaxation but a profound degree of sensory anesthesia. The nerves to the hand at the brachial plexus level are centrally situated within the nerve trunks, thus they are more difficult to block and may require a stronger concentration of local anesthetic despite relatively small fiber size.

Equipment

In institutions where many regional blocks are performed and in which adequate preparation and sterilization can be assured, packs of appropriate syringes, needles, and other equipment can be assembled for various kinds of blocks. Finger control Luer-Lok glass syringes and stainless steel needles of appropriate length, bore, and bevel can be provided.

In other situations it may be better to rely on disposable syringes and needles, which are quite satisfactory for upper extremity blocks. However, there is not the same variety of needles available, and their long bevels may "spur" if contact with bony surfaces occurs.

For the nerve blocks described in this chapter, either 23-gauge, 32-mm or 25-gauge, 16-mm needles are suitable. Some anesthesiologists prefer stouter needles in order to be more certain of eliciting paresthesias and aspirating blood if the needle is within a vessel; others favor fine needles in the hope that they will do less damage.

SUPRACLAVICULAR BLOCK

Advantages

There are several advantages to the use of the supraclavicular block. The brachial plexus is blocked where it is most compactly arranged—at the level of the three trunks. A low volume of solution is required and quick onset is achieved. Also, the technique can be performed with the arm in virtually any position, and all of the brachial plexus is reliably blocked. There is no danger of missing peripheral or proximal nerve branches because of failure of local anesthetic spread.

Limitations and Problems

Supraclavicular block has certain drawbacks. A reliable quick-onset block is achieved only if paresthesias are elicited. Furthermore, the technique is rather difficult to describe and teach. (What is anterior, posterior, backward, above, below, the length not breadth of the rib, and so forth?) Therefore, considerable experience is required to master it and this is best accomplished by personal observation of an experienced anesthesiologist or by time spent in the postmortem room. In addition, there is the risk of pneumothorax.

Contraindications

This approach to the brachial plexus is best avoided in the following patients: those who are uncooperative; those of difficult stature in which bony and muscular landmarks are not clear; the respiratory cripples in whom pneumothorax or even phrenic block would result in significant dyspnea. Patients who require bilateral block should not have both performed by this technique to avoid the risk of bilateral phrenic nerve paralysis, pneumothoraces, or a combination of the two. In addition, supraclavicular block should not be performed by a person who is unfamiliar with the technique or has not performed the block under the supervision of an experienced colleague.

Anatomy

The following are important points in the descriptive and topographic anatomy (Fig. 10-5*A*,*B*). First, the component parts of the plexus unite in a bundle that lies inferior to the clavicle at about its midpoint, on the posterior and lateral aspect and superior to the subclavian artery. Second, the artery can often be palpated as a valuable landmark. Third, the first rib is an important landmark to prevent the needle from passing medially and entering the pleural dome. The rib is short, broad, and flat. It slopes downward as it passes forward. Although it is deeply curved, that small portion in relation to the subclavian artery and the brachial plexus is primarily anteroposterior in the body plane.

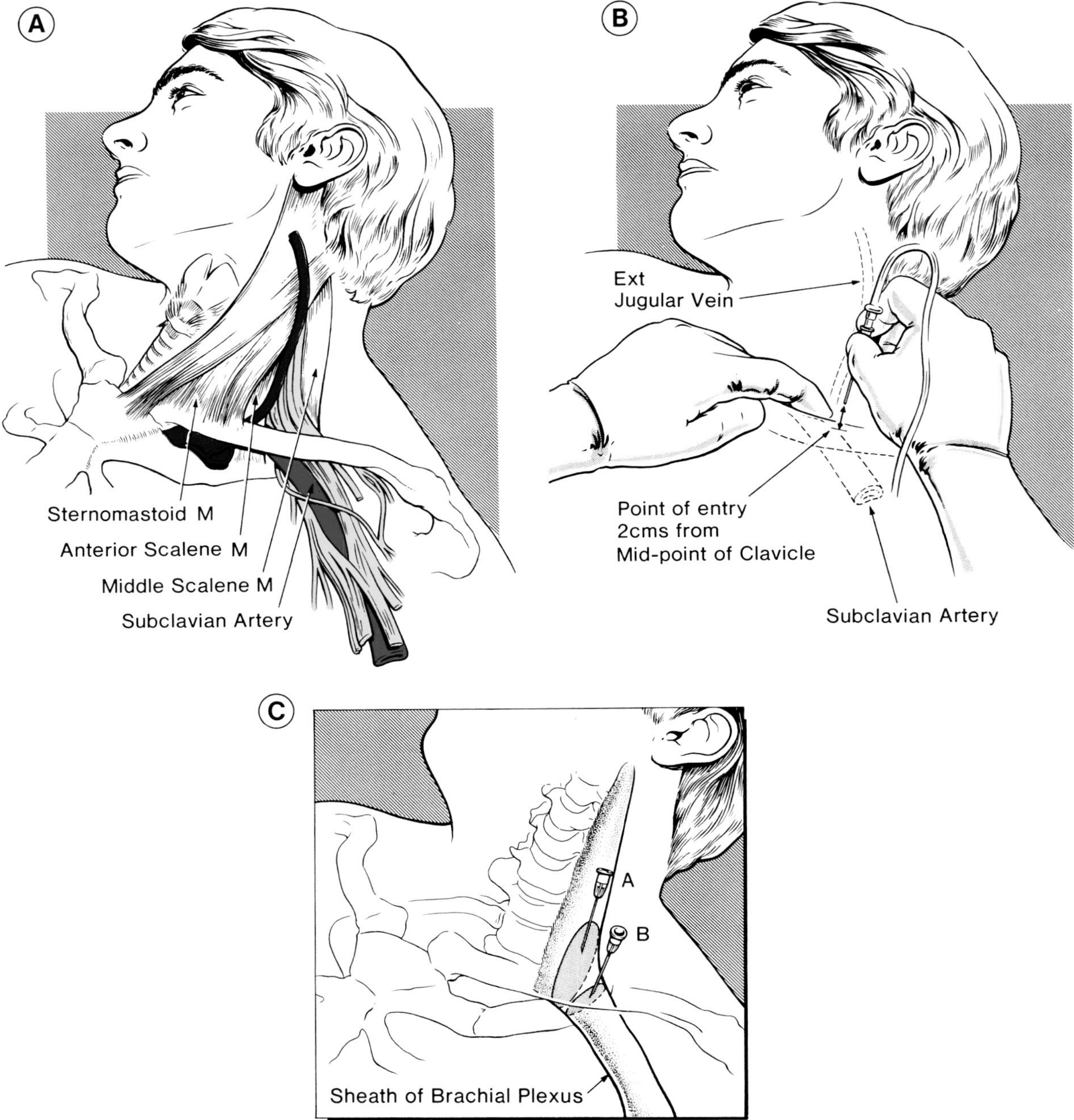

FIG. 10-5. **A.** Supraclavicular block. Anatomic landmarks. **B.** Supraclavicular block. Technique of needle insertion. **C.** Supraclavicular block. Note that the brachial plexus sheath becomes deeper as one moves medially and further back from the clavicle *(position A)* than it is at the lateral margin of the first rib immediately behind the clavicle *(position B).*

Technique

The classic approach for supraclavicular block of the brachial plexus should be regarded as a combination of the early published techniques. It calls for a downward, backward, and inward direction for insertion of the needle from a point just (or 1 cm) behind the midpoint of the clavicle (Fig. 10-5*C*). This is generally satisfactory; however, strict interpretation may not always be appropriate.

In some patients, beginning at a point just behind the clavicle results in a backward (posterior) direction of the needle. A starting point 2 to 3 cm behind the clavicle may make it easier to locate the interscalene groove and the nerve trunks above the first rib.

If a point is taken directly behind the clavicle, it will almost certainly lie outside the lateral margin of the rib. Inward (medial) inclination of the needle can easily penetrate the pleura. The more lateral the starting point, and the *more medial the inclination,* the more likely this is to occur.

"Rib walking" to achieve paresthesias, if they are not more simply obtained, is important for a satisfactory block. However, rib seeking or further "rib walking" after eliciting paresthesias would seem unnecessary and only increase the risk of pneumothorax.

The pulsation of the subclavian artery against the palpating finger or needle is the surest guide to the brachial plexus. It may not be felt if the clavicle is raised, if the platysma muscle is tense, or if the patient is obese.

An additional guide to locating the midpoint of the clavicle is finding the point where the straight portion of the external jugular vein, if continued, would cross the clavicle. Asking the patient to "blow out his cheeks" will frequently make the external jugular vein prominent.

Positions and Landmarks. The patient should lie supine without a pillow, arms at the side, and head turned slightly to the opposite side. The shoulder should be depressed downward (caudad) and posterior by gentle pressure on the relaxed shoulder and by asking the patient to touch his knee. This posterior displacement of the shoulder can be exaggerated by molding the shoulders over a roll placed between the scapulae. The patient is then instructed to raise his head approximately 20° from the table, putting strain on the neck muscles. This permits the clavicular head of the sternocleidomastoid muscle to be palpated and marked. The interscalene groove is palpated by rolling the finger back from the posterior border of the lower end of the identified sternocleidomastoid muscle and over the belly of the anterior scalene muscle. Because the brachial plexus makes its exit at the lateral border of the anterior scalene muscle, the skin is marked at this point immediately above the clavicle. Usually this point lies approximately at the middle of the clavicle, 1.5 to 2 cm from the lateral border of the clavicular head of the sternocleidomastoid muscle. The subclavian artery can often be clearly palpated in the supraclavicular fossa because it also emerges from the lower end of the interscalene groove. This serves as a check on the other landmarks.

Despite the multiple landmarks, this block is one of the simplest to perform if the subclavian artery can be palpated easily because the needle is inserted directly down from the tip of the palpating finger. If neither the artery nor the interscalene groove can be clearly felt, a point is taken approximately 2 cm along a line marked behind the midpoint of and perpendicular to the clavicle (Fig. 10-5*B*). In a patient with a protuberant clavicle or in whom it is difficult to achieve adequate posterior displacement of the shoulder, this point should be taken nearer to 3 cm behind the clavicle.

Procedure. The area should be aseptically prepared and draped. The anesthesiologist stands at the side of the patient to be blocked, facing the head of the table, since this position allows better control of the needle. An intradermal wheal is raised at the previously determined point. If the anesthesiologist is right-handed, a filled 10-ml syringe with a 23-gauge, 32-mm needle attached is held in the right hand and the patient is instructed to say "now" and not move as soon as he feels a "tingle" or "electriclike shock" going down his arm. This initial technique varies slightly, depending on whether or not the subclavian artery is palpable. If the artery is palpable, the tip of the index finger is rested in the supraclavicular fossa directly over the arterial pulsation. The needle is inserted through the skin wheal and advanced slowly downward (caudad), rolled slightly inward (medially) and slightly backward (posteriorly) so that the shaft of the needle and syringe are almost parallel to the patient's head (Fig. 10-5*B,C*). The index finger and thumb of the left hand firmly hold the hub of the needle and control the movement of the needle at all times.

Paresthesias will usually be immediately elicited. If so, the needle is fixed in position, and 15 to 25 ml of the local anesthetic drug is injected. If paresthesias are not immediately elicited, then one should proceed onto the rib and either deposit all the solution on or slightly superficial to the rib, in this position just behind the artery, or make further attempts to seek paresthesias by gentle reinsertions posteriorly for an estimated 2 cm along the length (not breadth) of the rib. After the rib is encountered, the anesthesiologist, by gently tapping it with the point of the needle, "walks" the needle forward (anteriorly) along the rib for approximately 1.5 cm, maintaining the initial plane of direction of the needle and seeking paresthesias. With each insertion of the needle, aspiration tests should be undertaken to see that the needle point is not in the subclavian artery. If it is, the anesthesiologist should not become alarmed; he has found a valuable landmark. By withdrawing the needle and reinserting it posterolaterally to the subclavian artery, paresthesias will usually be elicited as the needle is slowly advanced. If no paresthesias are elicited, but the rib is contacted, a barrage of solution between the skin and the rib behind the artery can be used. This is the principle of the Patrick technique.

If the artery is not palpable and has not been located, the previously located point 2 cm behind the midpoint of the clavicle can be used and will more certainly be placed over the rib. The needle is inserted directly downward (caudad) until paresthesias are elicited or the rib is contacted, and again, if necessary, the needle should be "walked" anteroposteriorly along the rib to seek the plexus. In a robust patient, occasionally the rib cannot be contacted at the full depth of this needle. Under these circumstances, the anesthesiologist should make a sweep with gentle reinsertions posteriorly as before, each time to the depth of the needle, in an attempt to elicit paresthesias superficial to the rib. If no paresthesias or rib are encountered at full depth of the needle, it may be advisable to choose another method. If the patient is properly positioned and all of the available landmarks are used and checked against one another, the need to change techniques will be rare.

Complications

Pneumothorax. Serious complications seldom ensue. The most specific complications of the supraclavicular approach for blocking the brachial plexus is pneumothorax. The frequency of occurrence is between 0.5% and 6.0% and decreases as the anesthesiologist becomes more skilled. Tall, thin patients, who characteristically have a high apical pleura, usually account for the greater number of these complications. Some authorities believe that the pneumothorax results from the piercing of the pleura, with air entering through the open needle. This is unlikely, since many of the pneumothoraces seen after this block have not occurred for some hours after the procedure, and a syringe is kept on the end of the needle at all times. Most likely the pneumothoraces are caused by the needle piercing the lung as exhalation occurs and the lung surface is torn by the needle point. The pneumothorax that results is then caused by air escaping from the lung. The risk of pneumothorax can be minimized by careful attention to detail, taking time, and being gentle; by the avoidance of multiple indiscriminate probings; and by the use of short and relatively fine needles. Fine needles limit the ability to elicit paresthesias and detect intravascular injections, but they are less damaging to the lung.

A pneumothorax must be suspected when there is dyspnea, cough, or pleuritic chest pain, but the diagnosis can be confirmed only by chest x-ray. It is important to realize in assessing the size of a pneumothorax that there is apparent exaggeration on a film taken in full expiration.

A minority of the pneumothoraces become obvious within a few hours. These are usually extensive and accompanied by symptoms. The majority of pneumothoraces take up to 24 hours to develop, are usually small to moderate, and may or may not cause symptoms, so there is little point in routine x-rays in the hours immediately after the block. It is also encouraging to note that it is most unusual for a "brachial block" pneumothorax to get any larger after 24 hours.

The treatment of pneumothorax depends on the extent and symptoms. In the early, more extensive pneumothorax (*i.e.*, greater than 50%), the patient should be admitted to the hospital and the air removed. Under these circumstances a continuous drainage system for 24 to 48 hours is preferable to simple aspiration.

With lesser degrees of pneumothorax, usually diagnosed the next day, the air should be removed only if it is causing symptoms. In this case, aspiration with a small catheter, syringe, and three-way stopcock is all that is required, provided proper surgical sterility is observed.

Pneumothoraces that are asymptomatic and not extensive can usually be followed on an outpatient basis with suitable advice and warnings. Analgesics, such as codeine and aspirin, may be prescribed for pain and discomfort if indicated. Serial films of the chest should be taken to assure that expansion of the lung is proceeding. However, there is no point in daily films when it may take weeks for the air to absorb completely.

Other complications seen with the supraclavicular brachial plexus block include the following.

Block of the phrenic nerve occurs in 40% to 60% of cases and usually causes no symptoms. However, if a bilateral phrenic block occurs in a patient with underlying chest disease, signs of hypoxia may result. Ordinarily, no treatment is necessary for the unilateral phrenic nerve block. Symptoms, if present, clear as the block dissipates. If signs of hypoxia occur, oxygen should be given by bag and mask or by other forms of oxygen therapy.

Horner's syndrome (stellate ganglion block) occurs in approximately 70% to 90% of the brachial plexus blocks when large volumes of solution (50 ml or more) of the local anesthetic drug are injected. The symptoms clear as the block is dissipated, and no treatment is necessary. These signs and symptoms should be explained to the patient, with assurance that they will disappear as the local anesthetic wears off.

Nerve damage or neuritis is an uncommon but possible complication of all peripheral blocks, including the supraclavicular technique for blocking the brachial plexus. When it occurs, the most frequent reason is faulty positioning of the anesthetized arm during surgery or in the immediate postoperative period rather than the block technique itself. Occasional trauma by the needle, prolonged ischemia of the nerve owing to vasoconstrictor drugs, or too concentrated an anesthetic solution may also be potential offenders. Treatment usually consists of "tincture of time." These injuries may last for days or even months. Physiotherapy by trained technicians and exercise at home are invaluable to prevent muscle atrophy. A neurologic consultation should be obtained to establish the level, extent, and treatment of the lesion as well as to avoid and protect against medicolegal action.

Toxic Reactions Owing to High Blood Level of the Local Anesthetic Drug. The cause and treatment of toxic reactions to the local anesthetic drugs are discussed in detail in Chapter 4. The most common reason for its occurrence in supraclavicular brachial plexus block is an unintentional intravascular injection of the local anesthetic drug or use of an excessive amount of solution. Properly treated, it should not be a serious complication.

Comments

It is strongly advised that paresthesias be obtained, since they denote contact with the plexus, assuring a successful block with quicker onset. Signs of injury after these blocks that could be attributed to paresthesias have not been observed. On the other hand, promiscuous probing should be avoided. If, after five or six careful insertions, a paresthesia is not obtained, one of the other techniques should be used.

One of the most certain causes of presumed failure of the block is to commence the operation before the anesthesia has had time to become complete. This interval may be as brief as 5 minutes or as long as 30 minutes. The custom of promiscuously sticking needles throughout the limb immediately after the injection for the purpose of testing the degree of anesthesia cannot be condemned too strongly. The patient's confidence is, too often, utterly destroyed by this method. An excellent rule is to keep the patient quiet for 15 minutes and make the first tests for anesthesia no sooner than at the termination of this period.

Because the trunks of the brachial plexus are so compact at the point of crossing the first rib, 15 to 25 ml of solution is usually sufficient to produce a total brachial plexus block even in the robust patient. If no paresthesias are obtained, larger volumes are often required and even then a delay in onset and possibly patchy anesthesia is likely.

A common error in locating the midpoint of the clavicle is to assume that the tip of the acromion is the lateral end. The "midpoint" will then be too far lateral. The accurately selected medial starting point and direct insertion toward the flat surface of the rib are important factors in avoiding missing the rib on either its *inner or outer* borders.

INTERSCALENE BLOCK

The interscalene block was developed and later described as an alternative to the supraclavicular approach to the brachial sheath.[30,31,56]

Advantages

Interscalene block is suitable when a proximal block is required, such as for shoulder surgery when it is often necessary to block the cervical plexus. In addition, it can be performed with the arm in virtually any position, and the pneumothorax risk is reduced. Finally, the landmarks are usually clear even in patients of stout build.

Limitations and Problems

It is essential to elicit paresthesias. Also, unless large volumes are used, lower trunk anesthesia may be missed; supplementary ulnar block may then be required. Uncommon but potentially serious complications can occur.

Anatomy

The cervical nerves of the brachial plexus, after leaving their respective intervertebral foramen, pass laterally in a deep groove or "gutter" in the superior surface of the transverse process of the cervical vertebrae. This groove separates the transverse process into anterior and posterior tubercles, which give origin to the scalenus anterior and scalenus medius muscles, respectively (see Fig. 10-4). After leaving the transverse processes, the nerve roots of the brachial plexus pass immediately into a plane between the two scalene muscles — the paravertebral or interscalene space (see Fig. 10-3). The direction of the "gutters" in the lower cervical vertebrae is primarily lateral but also slightly forward and almost 45 degrees downward, as if they were drawn down by the scalene muscles.

Although transverse processes in this region tend to overlap, it must be remembered that they are quite short and offer little protection to the intervertebral foramina from a horizontally directed needle.

Before attempting this block, the anesthesiologist should closely examine the skeleton of the cervical vertebral column with particular regard to the intervertebral foramina and the shape and direction of the transverse processes.

Technique

Position and Landmarks. The patient lies supine with the neck straight but the head turned slightly to the side opposite to the side to be treated. The arm is placed by the side with the shoulder depressed as for supraclavicular block. The right-handed operator stands at the head of the table for a right arm block and by the patient's shoulder for a left arm block.

The head is temporarily lifted in order to palpate the posterior border of the sternomastoid muscle. The interscalene groove is palpated by rolling the fingers back from the border of the sternomastoid over the belly of the scalenus anterior to the groove, which is then marked. A line is extended directly laterally from the cricoid cartilage to intersect the interscalene groove. The point of entry is at this intersection, which should be directly opposite the transverse process of C6. The external jugular vein may overlie this point (Fig. 10-6*A*,*B*).

Needle Insertion and Injection. After suitable preparation and the insertion of a skin wheal, with the index and middle fingers of the left hand still palpating the groove, a 23-gauge, 32-mm needle is inserted in a direction almost perpendicular to the floor of the "gutter" on the superior aspect of the transverse process (Fig. 10-6*B*,*C*). The anesthesiologist should visualize the transverse process as being directed primarily laterally but also downward and slightly forward. The direction of the needle, therefore, is mainly inward but also 45° caudad and slightly backward.

The needle is advanced until paresthesias are elicited. Injection is then made of the full volume of solution. To avoid the problem of needle displacement, it should be held firmly by the hub during the period of injection. The transverse process is surprisingly superficial in the normal patient, no more than 1.5 to 2 cm. If bone is encountered at this depth but no paresthesias, one should "walk" the needle across the transverse process, and thus across the path of the nerve.

If bony contact is made only on deep insertion, it is likely that the transverse process has been missed and what has been reached is the vertebral body. If no bony contact is made near full depth of the needle, the vertebral column has been missed, probably anteriorly, and a more posterior direction should be undertaken.[51]

In the vast majority of cases, paresthesias are easily obtained superficially. If a blunt bevel needle is used, the anesthesiologist may also feel the penetration of the fascia.

Ten milliliters to 40 ml of solution is injected, depending on the extent of the block required as well as the condition and stature of the patient. Volume to anesthesia relationships have been studied with radiopaque contrast, and these suggest that 20 ml of solution will anesthetize the lower cervical nerves and most of the brachial plexus; however, with this volume the lower trunk is often spared.[56] Forty milliliters of solution blocks all of the cervical and the

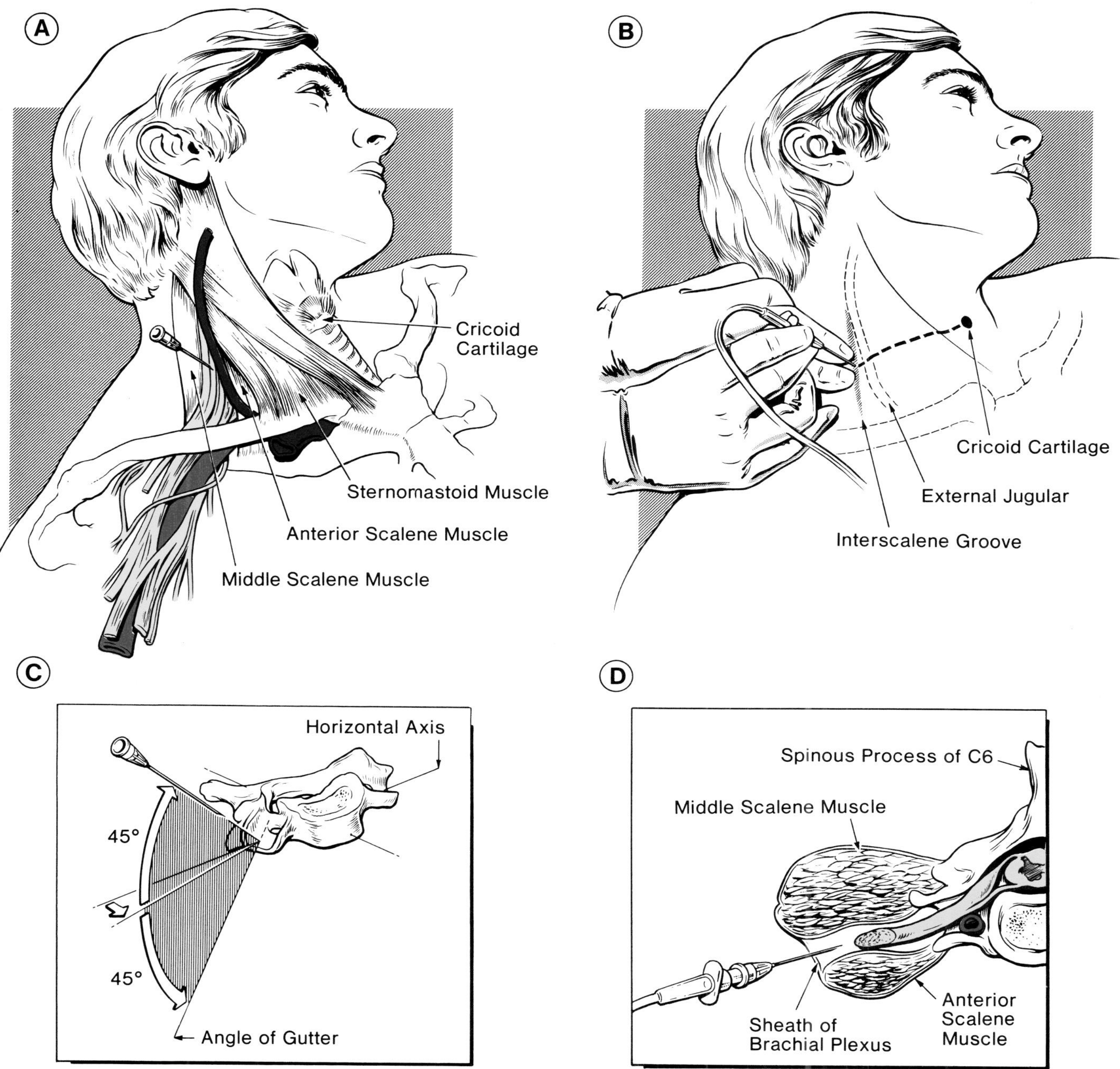

FIG. 10-6. **A.** Interscalene block. Anatomic landmarks. **B.** Interscalene block. Method of palpating interscalene groove and inserting needle. Note hand holding needle braced against clavicle. **C, D.** Interscalene block. Needle direction in relation to spine from anterolateral view *(C),* from above *(D).*

brachial plexuses. Digital pressure during injection and massage after helps downward spread.

Comments

Anesthesia of the cervical plexus can also be readily obtained by this single injection into the interscalene groove.[60] The C4 level can be identified by extending a line laterally from the upper border of the thyroid cartilage. Injection of 10 to 15 ml is made in identical fashion to that for interscalene brachial plexus block.

Complications

As with any paravertebral technique, inadvertent epidural or spinal anesthesia is always possible and has been reported with this block.[29,42] Also, the vertebral artery is close to the point of even a correctly placed needle.

The phrenic nerve must frequently be blocked because of either C4 root involvement or anterior spread under the prevertebral fascia in front of the scalenus anterior muscle, but this is seldom significant, at least in unilateral blocks. Vagus, recurrent laryngeal, and cervical sympathetic nerves are sometimes involved, but these are of no significance except that it may be important to reassure the patient.

AXILLARY BLOCK

The perivascular axillary infiltration has become one of the most popular techniques for blocking the nerves of the arm.

Advantages

Axillary block provides excellent operating conditions for surgery of the forearm and hand with less risk of major complications than is associated with alternative supraclavicular methods. This makes it suitable for emergency department and outpatient use. It is an easy technique to master and probably the safest and most reliable for the patient of stout build. It is not imperative to seek paresthesias, and fine needles are quite satisfactory. The block is, therefore, particularly useful in children (*e.g.*, for the reduction of fractures[11,22]).

Limitations and Problems

The axillary approach does have certain limitations, the first of which is that the arm must be abducted in order to perform the block. The extent of anesthesia also is insufficient for shoulder or upper arm surgery without using large volumes of solution. The circumflex and musculocutaneous nerves are sometimes missed because they have left the sheath proximal to the point of injection. The musculocutaneous nerve is most important because of its extensive area of innervation on the radial side of the forearm extending onto the thenar eminence.

Anatomy

A cross section of the arm at the level of the anterior axillary fold demonstrates several anatomic points, including the compact, axillary neurovascular bundle (Fig. 10-7*B*). On its medial (superficial) aspect, the axillary sheath is covered only by connective tissue, being behind the biceps/coracobrachialis and in front of the triceps muscles. On its lateral or deep aspect, the sheath lies close to the neck of the humerus. In the sheath, the median nerve tends to lie anterior to the axillary artery (as did the musculocutaneous nerve higher up the sheath), the ulnar nerve, posterior, and the radial nerve, posterior and somewhat lateral. The medial antebrachial cutaneous nerve and the medial brachial cutaneous nerves are medial to the artery. The axillary vein overlies the artery on its medial aspect. The musculocutaneous nerve has already left the sheath and is now in the substance of the coracobrachialis muscle.

Technique

Position and Landmarks. The patient is placed in a supine position, with the head turned away from the side to be blocked. The arm is abducted to approximately 90° and the forearm flexed to 90° and externally rotated, so the dorsum of the hand lies on the table and the forearm parallel to the long axis of the patient's body. Although it is tempting to have the patient's hand under the head, it should not be done because frequently the hyperabduction obliterates the brachial artery pulse.

The brachial artery is identified and the pulse followed as far proximally as possible, ideally to the pectoralis major muscle.

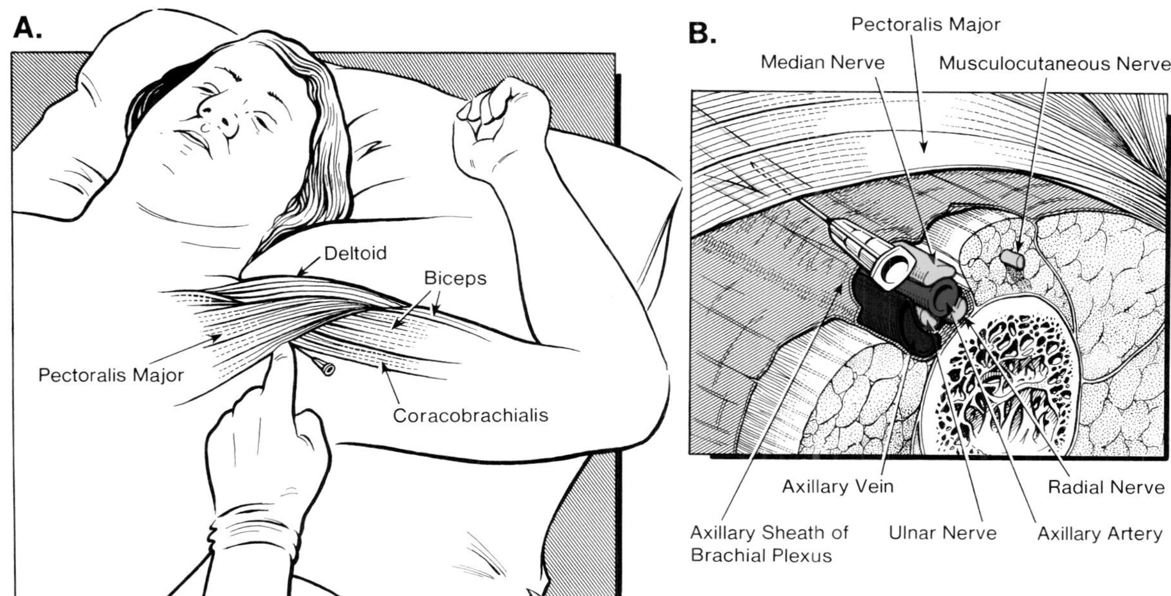

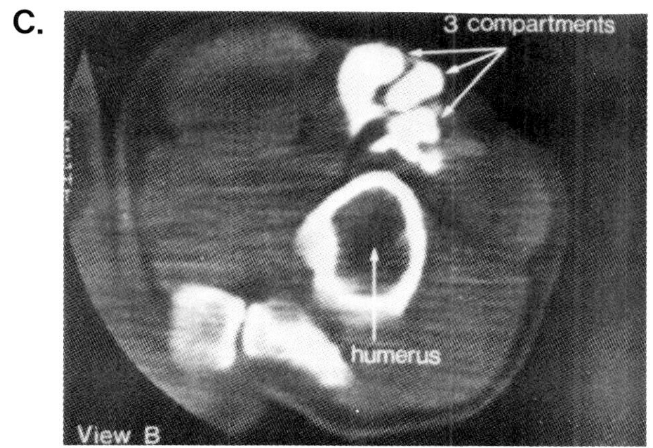

FIG. 10-7. Axillary block. **A, B.** Technique of needle insertion. *(A)* Note forefinger palpating axillary artery. Hand holding needle (not shown) should be braced against arm. Needle insertion is adjacent to coracobrachialis and pectoralis major muscles, immediately superior to tip of forefinger (see text). *(B)* Note direction of needle toward apex of axilla, in same direction as neurovascular bundle. Needle enters neurovascular sheath and may run inside sheath to a higher level. The medial head of triceps, lying between the neurovascular sheath and the humerus, has been compressed by the palpating finger and is not shown in this cross-section. **C.** Computer tomogram, after axillary block with bupivacaine 0.5% and iodothalamate. Separate injections of 10-ml solution were made after obtaining paresthesias in median and radial nerves and also on passing a needle through the axillary artery. Contrast medium apparently remained in three discrete compartments; it is not certain whether these relate to major branches of brachial plexus. Also local anesthetic may diffuse in a different manner to contrast medium. (Part *C* reproduced with permission from Thompson, G.E., and Rorie, D.H.: Functional anatomy of brachial plexus sheaths. Anesthesiology, *59*:117–122, 1983.)

Point of Entry. The artery is fixed against the humerus by the index and middle fingers of the left hand, and a skin wheal is raised directly over the arterial pulse (Fig. 10-7).

Needle Insertion and Injection. With the index finger still on the pulse of the axillary artery, a skin wheal is raised directly over the pulse (Fig. 10-7). A 25 mm or 32 mm, 22-gauge short-bevel needle is inserted just superior to the fingertip, directing the needle toward the apex of the axilla in almost the same direction as the neurovascular bundle. The needle may be either bare or attached to an anesthetic-filled extension tubing or syringe. As the needle is advanced, evidence of entering the sheath is sought by the feel of the "fascia click" as the needle penetrates the fascia; paresthesias, blood flow back, or oscillation of a free needle.

The feeling of penetrating the sheath is facilitated by the use of a short-bevel needle and the elimination of skin drag. The simple expedient of first puncturing the skin with a larger needle helps, but it can be further reduced by a needle-through-needle hole technique.[53]

The eliciting of paresthesias is encouraging and reliable evidence of correct position but is not essential for a satisfactory block, and it may be distressing. Recent studies by Selander and associates[44] indicate that this practice may carry an increased incidence of postanesthetic neuropathy; and, if so, the production of paresthesias should be avoided. The use of the nerve stimulator as described in Chapter 6 may obviate the need for paresthesias.

The flow or aspiration of blood, particularly arterial blood, strongly suggests that the needle tip is within the sheath. The needle can then be either just withdrawn from the vessel or pushed on through to the other side before injection. Although it cannot be recommended, it is the practice of some anesthesiologists to set out deliberately to puncture the artery as their means of identifying the sheath.

Oscillation of the needle produced by arterial pulsation indicates that the needle is at least near the artery, and thus probably within the sheath.

Single-Injection Technique. After aspiration, which is particularly important in this site, the entire volume of local anesthetic may be injected. On the basis of sheath volume and assuming equal up and down spread, de Jong calculated that 42 ml of solution was necessary to fill the adult sheath sufficient to reach the coracoid process, which is the approximate level at which the musculocutaneous nerve leaves the sheath.[14] This kind of volume to anesthesia relationship has been confirmed with radiopaque contrast studies.[61] Recent studies by Vester-Andersen and others,[50] however, showed that increasing the volume of the injected local anesthetic drug above 40 ml did not improve spread to the musculocutaneous or radial nerve area.

Although the solution tends to spread up rather than down the sheath, and measures can be taken to increase this rostral spread, 40 ml of solution is required to block, consistently, all of the brachial plexus. This is scaled downward in children and when other circumstances call for a reduction in dose.

Prevention of needle movement during injection may be a little awkward in the axilla but is absolutely essential with this technique. It can be aided by fixing the needle hub with the thumb and index finger of the left hand, if using direct syringe attachment, or the right hand, if using a needle attached to extension tubing. This "immobile needle" helps to prevent movement during syringe removal and reattachment.[55]

A few milliliters of solution are deposited in the subcutaneous tissue on withdrawal, to block the intercostobrachial nerve and its communications with the medial cutaneous nerve of the arm (Fig. 10-7*B*).

Double-Injection Technique. Nearly all earlier descriptions of axillary block have used the technique of injection on both sides of the artery.[8,14,20,35,52] Most believed that if the first insertion is correct and the needle is not moved, the second injection should not be necessary, provided sufficient volume is used. Thompson and Rorie,[48] however, have demonstrated that the sheath may be divided into a fascial compartment created for each nerve, which functionally limited the circumferential spread of injected solutions of local anesthetic (Fig. 10-7*C*). They recommend a double- or triple-injection technique.

There are some advantages of a double-injection technique. If the anesthesiologist is prepared to disregard the musculocutaneous nerve or routinely block it separately, the volume of solution can be significantly reduced—10 to 15 ml with each injection is quite sufficient to block the other nerves within the sheath. Also, there are two chances to enter the sheath. On some occasions the areolar septa within the sheath may act as a barrier to the spread of a single injection.[14]

The double-injection technique can be performed with one or two needles. With a single needle, half the total volume of local anesthetic solution is injected anterior to (above) the artery; the needle is then withdrawn from the fascia and redirected posterior to (below) the artery, and the remainder of the solution is injected. When two needles are used, they are inserted through the same skin wheal, but one is directed anterior and the other posterior to the artery, before injecting through each needle.[25] Again, subcutaneous injection on withdrawal may be indicated.

Promotion of Central Flow Within the Sheath. With the single-injection, high-volume technique, measures should be taken to promote proximal flow within the sheath. Digital pressure should be applied immediately distal to the needle with the index and middle fingers, both during and immediately after injection. If these fingers are required for fixation of the needle hub, pressure on the distal sheath can be applied with the ulnar side of the hand. The application of the distal tourniquet frees the left hand but is of doubtful effectiveness and causes some discomfort.[21] Directing the needle toward the apex of the axilla has also been used in an effort to gain more proximal spread and higher block. Winnie has suggested the use of a 37-mm needle directed centrally at approximately 20° to the artery.[57] Hopcroft uses a 21-gauge, 50-mm needle directed centrally along the axis of the artery.[24] These techniques no doubt achieve the desired goal, but at some point the pneumothorax problem must again arise. As soon as the injection is completed and while still applying some form of distal pressure, the arm should be adducted. This removes the effect of pressure of the humeral head, which may be a factor in limiting proximal spread.[58]

Comments

Axillary block is probably the most widely used technique for brachial plexus block today. More modifications, technical variations, and "tricks of the trade" are associated with this technique than with any other. Some actually decrease the effectiveness of the block.

In children particularly, a standard 23- or 25-gauge scalp vein set can be useful. Paresthesias can be an essential part of this method, particularly in a large arm with vague arterial pulsation or when there is difficulty in identifying the sheath. A nerve stimulator may be essential in such circumstances or when patients are unresponsive or uncooperative. Another method is to infiltrate local anesthetic from skin to humerus on either side of the axillary artery.

Continuous Axillary Block. Continuous axillary block has been advocated as the anesthesia of choice for prolonged surgical procedures, such as reimplantations.[43] Toxic reactions to the local anesthetic drugs used in this manner have not been seen.[49] Pharmacokinetic data indicate that a continuous infusion of 0.25% bupivacaine at a rate of 20 to 30 mg/h (*e.g.*, 10 ml) is effective and does not result in cumulative increases in blood concentration[15a] (see Chap. 3). In practice a standard bolus dose is given to establish the block (see above), and about 1 hour later the infusion is started.[15a]

Complications and Contraindications

There are no complications or contraindications specific to this block; however, the risk of intravascular injection, particularly into the overlying vein, must always be kept in mind, and the patient with a bleeding diathesis is probably at an increased risk of incurring a hematoma with this approach.

INFRACLAVICULAR BRACHIAL PLEXUS BLOCK

Several recent modifications of the original infraclavicular approach to the brachial plexus (Raj and others,[40] Sims,[46] Whiffler[54]) suggest that the perivascular sheath may be injected in this area as an alternative to other more popular approaches.

Advantages

While maintaining the advantage of the interscalene or axillary sheath blocks, injection of the local anesthetic drug in the sheath above the level of the formation of the musculocutaneous and axillary nerves would block these nerves frequently missed on an axillary approach. Blocking lower than the first rib would eliminate the potential for pneumothorax or missing the ulnar segment of the medial cord, sometimes missed on a supraclavicular technique, as well as block the intercostobrachial nerve, which is not blocked on any of the other approaches. Also, it does not require positioning of the arm, as does the axillary block.

Limitations and Problems

The infraclavicular approach is limited in that to be effective, it requires a nerve stimulator to locate the plexus. Because the palpating finger cannot identify the arterial pulse in that area, the needle must be advanced blindly, increasing the likelihood of vascular puncture or more pain to the patient. If the needle point should rest distal to the coracoid process, most of the solution will move distally and the musculocutaneous and axillary nerves will be missed, as on the axillary approach.

Anatomy

Because this is essentially a sheath block of the plexus in the upper axilla from an infraclavicular approach, the axillary landmarks are [a] the outer border of the first four ribs, [b] the posterior surface of the clavicle, [c] the pectoralis major and minor anteriorly, and [d] the subscapularis, teres major, and latissimus dorsi muscles posteriorly (Fig. 10-8). The contents of the axilla are the axillary vessels, the brachial plexus with its branches, some branches of the intercostal nerves, lymph glands and fat, and loose areolar tissue.

Technique

Position and Landmarks. The patient lies supine with his head turned away from the arm to be blocked. If possible, the arm is abducted to 90° and allowed to rest comfortably. The physician stands on the opposite side from the arm to be blocked.

The whole length of the clavicle is marked after palpation. The subclavian artery is palpated where it dips under the clavicle and marked; it is usually at the midpoint of the clavicle. If the subclavian artery is not palpable, the midpoint of the clavicle is marked. The brachial artery is palpated in the arm and marked, and the C6 tubercle on the same side is palpated and marked. A line is drawn from the C6 mark to the brachial artery in the arm. This line should go through the midpoint of the clavicle and is the surface marking of the brachial plexus (Fig. 10-8).

Needle Insertion and Injection. The ground electrode of a peripheral nerve stimulator is attached to the opposite shoulder (see Fig. 6-7). A skin wheal is

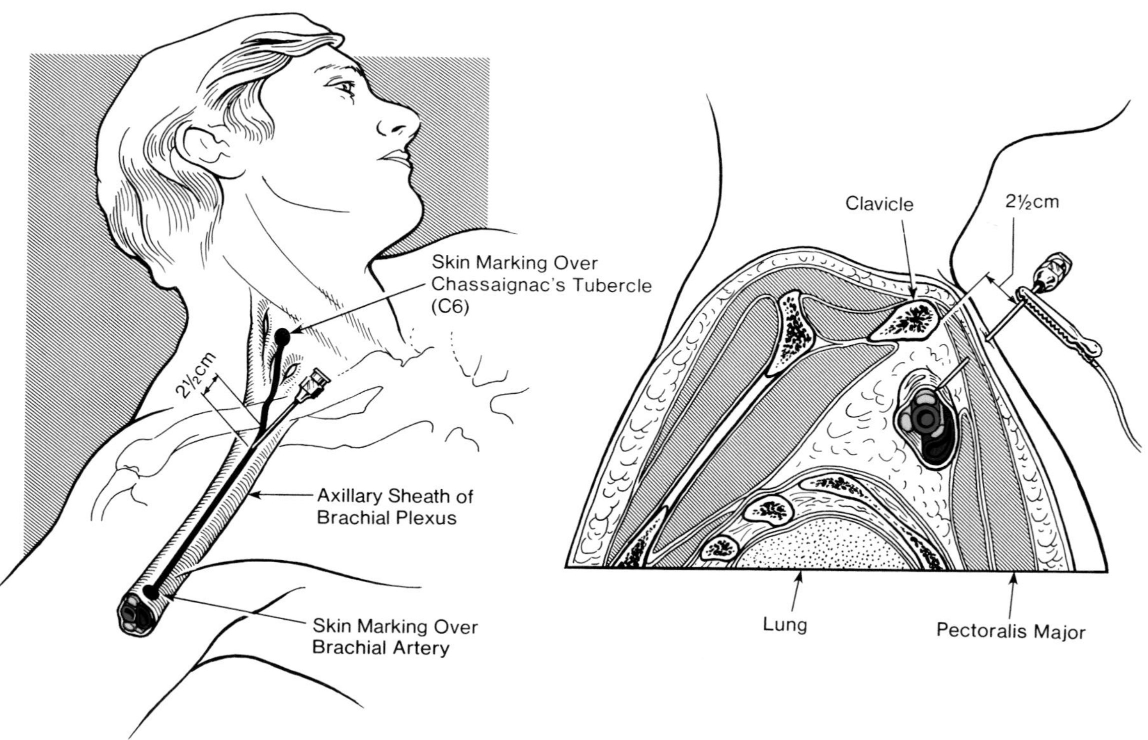

FIG. 10-8. Infraclavicular brachial plexus block (see text). Note position of arm abducted to 90° and supinated. Point of insertion is 2.5 cm below clavicle, along a line from C6 tubercle across clavicle to brachial artery. Note direction of needle laterally, inferiorly, and posteriorly toward brachial artery.

raised 1 inch below the inferior border of the clavicle at its marked midpoint or where the subclavian artery dips under the clavicle. A 22-gauge unsheathed standard 80-mm spinal needle is introduced through the skin wheal. The needle point is directed laterally toward the brachial artery (Fig. 10-8). The exploring electrode is then attached to either the stem or the hub of the needle with a sterile alligator clip. The voltage control of the peripheral nerve stimulator is set to deliver 6 to 8 volts, and the needle is advanced at an angle of 45 degrees to the skin. As the needle approaches the fibers of the brachial plexus, movements of the muscles supplied by those fibers will confirm that the needle point is in proximity to the nerve fibers of the brachial plexus. The voltage is decreased to 2 to 4 volts. The needle is then advanced. The muscle movements previously seen increase as the needle tip moves closer to the brachial plexus, so the needle is advanced until the muscle movements start to decrease. Withdraw the needle slowly until the maximum muscle movements are again observed. Hold the needle in that position as 2 ml of 2% lidocaine is injected through the needle with the one-impulse-per-second button on the nerve stimulator turned on. If the needle is located correctly, within 30 seconds there is loss of the previously seen muscle movements. If the needle is not located correctly, it may have been pushed through the nerve. It should then be withdrawn and the process repeated. When the needle tip is properly located, 20 to 30 ml of local anesthetic drug is then injected at that site. (The use of sheathed needles and other modifications on the use of the nerve stimulator are described in Chapter 6.) As with the axillary block, digital pressure in the axilla distal to the injection site can increase the central flow of the local anesthetic drug.

Comments

The success of neural blockade of the arm by injection of the local anesthetic drug into the perivascular spaces in the axilla or interscalene area and the confirming of continuity of the perivascular sheath suggests a logical compromise or alternative to the two techniques that might preserve the advantages and overcome the disadvantages. This approach to the plexus is at a higher level than that of the axillary approach, to assure blockade of all the nerves derived from the plexus, but at a lower level than that of the supraclavicular approach, to minimize the risk of pleural injury. Although such an *infraclavicular* approach was originally suggested by Bazy and coworkers[4] in 1917, it did not gain much popularity because the available equipment and technology did not give anesthesia comparable to the classic Kulenkampff technique and still resulted in pleural trauma. In 1977 Raj and associates[40] modified the infraclavicular technique by a lateral direction of the needle, thus avoiding the potential pneumothorax and using the nerve stimulator to make the technique of locating the plexus more acceptable to the patients. It is still not widely used because it does require the use of a nerve stimulator and a long needle that penetrates both the pectoralis major and minor muscles, causing significantly greater patient discomfort than other perivascular techniques that block the plexus at points where it is superficial. It has recently gained favor in patients in whom a continuous block technique is desired. Experience with catheters for hyperalimentation has conclusively demonstrated that maintaining a catheter in position is most readily done if it is inserted infraclavicularly. This is also true of catheters for perivascular infiltration for continuous neural blockade of the arm.

USE OF A NERVE STIMULATOR FOR ARM BLOCKS

The availability of high-quality insulated needles and stimulators designed for peripheral nerves now provides a practical adjunct to plexus and peripheral nerve blocks in the arm and elsewhere in the body. It is important that the characteristics of the stimulator are suitable and that it is applied correctly as described in Chapter 6 and Figure 6-7. Use of a nerve stimulator is no substitute for anatomic knowledge and the use of appropriate landmarks as described in the foregoing sections. The stimulator should not be turned on until the needle is approaching the "target," having first used standard technique. It is vital that a motor response be obtained at only minimal current output; otherwise, the tip of the needle may be still some distance from the nerve. Although uninsulated needles can at times be successfully used, it is now clear that accuracy increases with coated needles (see Chap. 6). It is important to be sure that the *cathode* (−) of the stimulator is attached to the needle; otherwise, four times as much current is needed to stimulate the nerve (see Fig. 6-7). Because current output is what stimulates the nerve, this is what the operator wants to be displayed (from 0.1 to 1.0 mA) on the stimulator. With precise needle placement, a motor response should be obtained with close to 0.1

mA of current output. With a sheathed needle, muscle contraction will increase as the needle nears the nerve and then decrease as the needle moves past the nerve. The use of anatomic landmarks to position the needle close to the "target" nerve or plexus obviates the need to turn on the stimulator with a superficially placed needle and high current output. Such a practice is to be condemned, since it produces confusing and painful local muscle contractions.

The major muscle responses obtained for a needle located close to radial, ulnar, median, and musculocutaneous nerves are shown in Figure 10-9.

PERIPHERAL BLOCKS

With safe and reliable brachial plexus anesthesia, and particularly with the more widespread use of axillary block, the need for distal nerve blocks has diminished; however, at times these can be of considerable value. Peripheral block can be useful when circumstances such as infection, difficult anatomy, bilateral surgery, or an anesthesiologist's inexperience may preclude the use of plexus blocks. Also, it can be used for surgery on the hand that is of limited extent and duration, when it is on a part supplied by individual nerves, or as an alternative to digital, particularly multiple digital, blocks.

With nerve block at the wrist, long flexor motor power is retained and this is of considerable value in certain kinds of hand procedures, such as tenolysis.[12,26] Peripheral block is always available to supplement patchy brachial plexus anesthesia, and furthermore, the ulnar nerve is the most reliable model for testing local anesthetic drugs.[32]

GENERAL CONSIDERATIONS

Tourniquet

An upper arm tourniquet is usually applied before surgery on the limb, and this has often been said to contraindicate peripheral blocks as the method of anesthesia. Up to 30 minutes of tourniquet time is well tolerated by most patients even when they are unpremedicated, and this can easily be extended to an hour with suitable analgesic sedation.[18] A sterile Esmarch bandage should be available for the surgeon to apply *after* skin preparation and marking. The method of application of the tourniquet may also be a factor in patient tolerance.[19] The use of circumferential subcutaneous infiltration, although it is extensively used, would appear to be unnecessary and of doubtful value.[35]

Elbow or Wrist?

There is little to be gained by blocking the nerves at the elbow as opposed to the wrist. Only hand anesthesia results from blocking the three major nerve trunks at the elbow because the forearm cutaneous nerves arise in the upper arm and are quite separate at this level. The wrist block is usually simpler to per-

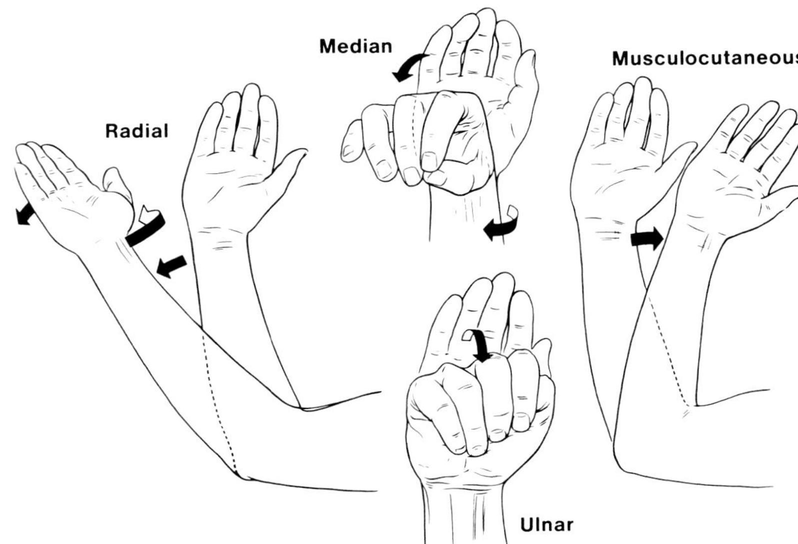

FIG. 10-9. Some characteristic movements of fingers, wrist, and elbow in response to nerve stimulation. *Radial:* Note extension at elbow, supination of arm, and extension at wrist and of fingers. *Median:* Note pronation of arm, flexion of wrist, opposition of middle, forefinger, and thumb, and flexion of lateral three fingers. *Ulnar:* Note flexion of wrist, adduction of all fingers (clenched together), and flexion and opposition of lateral two fingers toward thumb. *Musculocutaneous:* Note flexion at elbow. In general, it is not always possible to obtain stimulation of each major nerve or all components of that nerve. Thus motor responses vary considerably.

form, but it is sometimes preferable to use a combination of the two levels (see Fig. 10-16 for areas of sensory supply of individual nerves of arm).

Paresthesias

As a general rule, anesthesia is quicker in onset and more reliable if paresthesias are sought when blocking the median and ulnar nerves at either elbow or wrist. Care should be taken, however, to avoid injecting the solution intraneurally. Intense paresthesias on injection of a small volume would tend to suggest intraneural placement, and the needle should be either advanced or withdrawn slightly (or both) as the injection is made.

Another method of avoiding intraneural injection is to keep moving the needle in and out while injecting; this will deposit solution superficial and deep to the nerve but has the potential disadvantage of greater needle trauma.[36]

Paresthesias, if they are not elicited on initial insertion, are sought by gentle fanwise insertions across the path of the nerve. If no paresthesias are found, the anesthesiologist should retrace the fan and inject as the needle is moved gently in and out, the aim being to lay down a wall of solution over an area of approximately 2 cm^2 across the path of the nerve.

MEDIAN NERVE BLOCK

Median nerve block is applicable for surgery on the radial side of the palm and three and one-half digits and for reduction of fractures, particularly the first metacarpal. It is usually combined with either ulnar or radial nerve blocks, depending on whether surgery extends to the ulnar side or to the back of the hand. There is also occasional variation in innervation, which may necessitate multiple blocks.

Technique for Blocks at Elbow

The arm is abducted on a board with the elbow extended and the forearm supinated. One should stand beside the radial side of the forearm. The intercondylar line between medial and lateral epicondyles of the humerus is drawn across the cubital fossa and the brachial artery is palpated and marked at this level (Fig. 10-10). A 23-gauge, 32-mm needle is inserted at

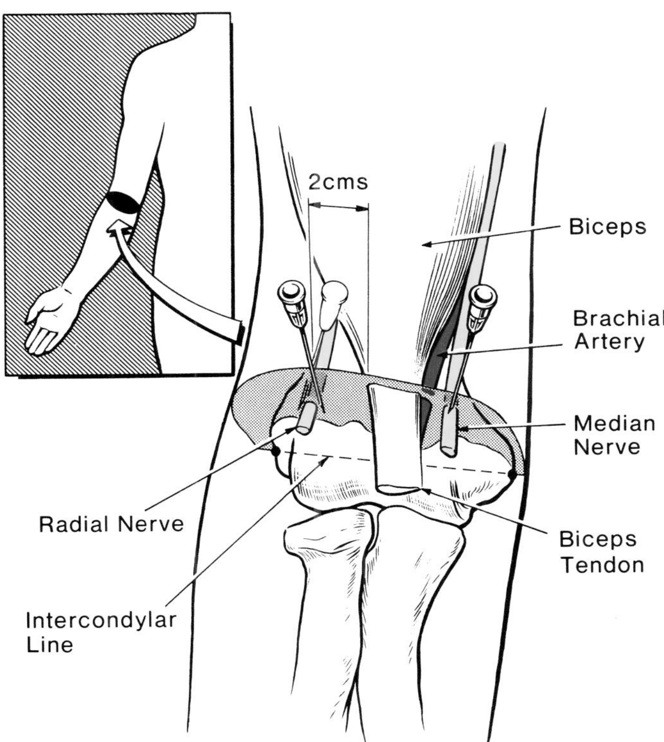

FIG. 10-10. Anatomic landmarks for median and radial nerve block at elbow.

a point just medial to the artery and directed perpendicular to the skin (Fig. 10-11). Three milliliters to 5 ml should be injected after eliciting paresthesias. If no paresthesias are obtained on initial insertion, the needle should be moved fanwise medially from the artery across the path of the nerve.

Technique for Block at Wrist

The arm is abducted on a board with the elbow extended and the forearm supinated. One should sit beside the ulnar side of the hand for right arm block and the radial side for left arm block.

The palmaris tendon should be made prominent by flexing the wrist against resistance with the fingers extended. The radial border of the tendon should be marked at a point approximately 2 cm proximal to the most distal wrist crease. If the tendon is absent, the point will be approximately 1 cm medial to the ulnar edge of the flexor carpi radialis tendon (Fig. 10-12).

With the wrist slightly extended, a 25-gauge, 16-mm needle is inserted perpendicular to the skin. The nerve is contacted on penetration of the deep fascia, usually at a depth of less than 1 cm (Fig. 10-13).

Three milliliters to 5 ml should be injected after eliciting paresthesias. If paresthesias are not obtained on initial insertion, they should be sought in a more ulnar direction under cover of the palmaris tendon. One milliliter of solution is deposited in the subcutaneous tissue on withdrawal to block the palmar cutaneous branch.

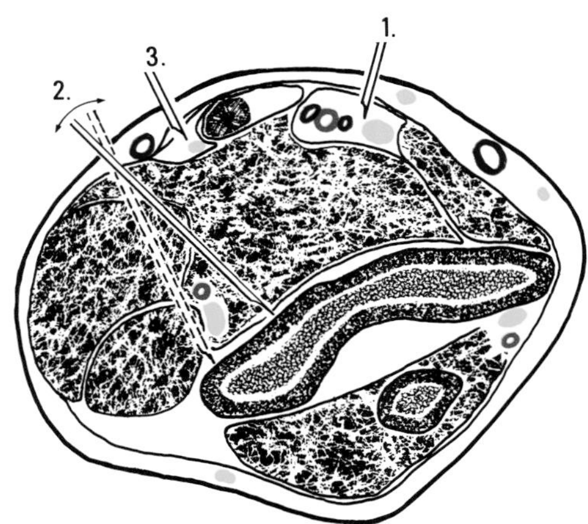

FIG. 10-11. Cross-section of arm at elbow. *(1)* Median nerve block. *(2)* Radial nerve block. *(3)* Lateral cutaneous nerve block. (Note nerve under deep fascia and close to biceps tendon.)

ULNAR NERVE BLOCK

This anesthetic technique is applicable for surgery of the ulnar side of the hand and one and one-half (usually) digits and for reduction of fractures of the fifth digit, commonly the neck of the metacarpal. It is often used on its own but may be combined with median and radial nerve blocks. Block of the ulnar nerve at the elbow is often said to lead to residual neuritis. This is probably because where the nerve is palpable, it is well protected by fibrous tissue, and a total intraneural injection is required for success. This approach is quite satisfactory, provided it is performed with a fine needle and only a small volume, such as 1 ml, is injected.[32] However, it may be preferable to block the nerve 2 to 3 cm proximal to the medial epicondyle with 5 to 8 ml of solution.

Technique for Block at Elbow

With the patient lying supine, the elbow is flexed, with the forearm across the chest. One should stand beside the patient on the side of the arm to be blocked. The medial epicondyle and ulnar groove are palpated and a point taken 2 to 3 cm proximal and along the line of the nerve. A 23-gauge, 32-mm needle is introduced perpendicular to the skin and advanced gently until a paresthesia is obtained or periosteum encountered (Fig. 10-14). Five milliliters to 8 ml should be injected after paresthesias. If no paresthesias are obtained on initial insertion, the needle should be moved fanwise across the path of the nerve until they are elicited. No paresthesias will probably result in a long delay or inadequate anesthesia.

Technique for Block at Wrist

Ulnar block at the wrist is more reliable and carries less risk of complications than block of the ulnar nerve at the elbow. The arm is abducted on a board with the elbow extended and the forearm supinated. One should sit beside the ulnar side of the hand.

At the wrist, the ulnar nerve is blocked where it lies under cover of the flexor carpi ulnaris tendon just proximal to the pisiform bone before the nerve bifurcates into its terminal deep (motor) and the superficial (sensory) branches. At this point, the nerve lies on

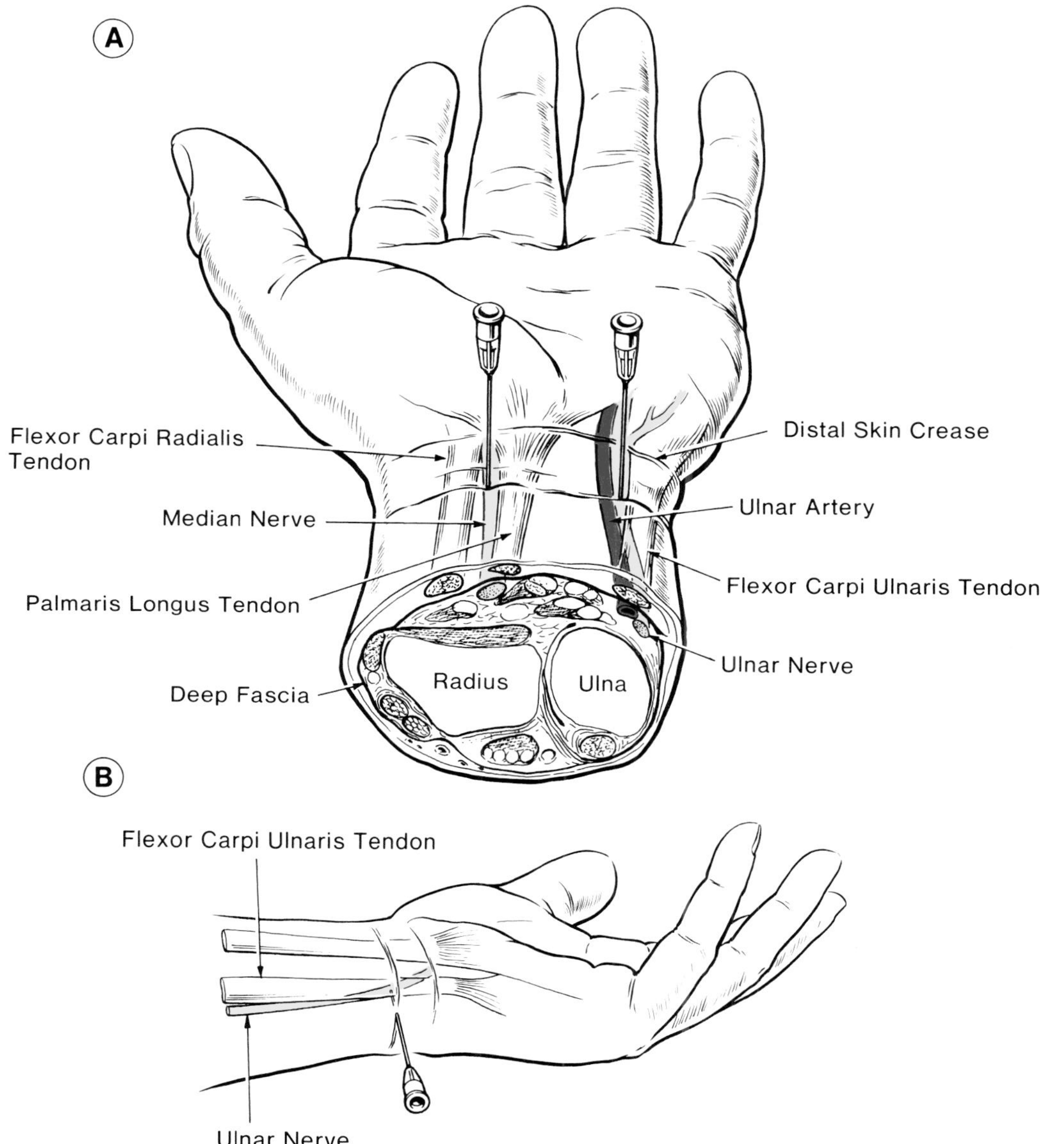

FIG. 10-12. **A.** Landmarks and technique of needle insertion for median and ulnar nerve block at wrist. **B.** Alternative method of ulnar nerve block, from ulnar side of wrist.

the ulnar side of, but deep to, the ulnar artery, and it has already given off its palmar cutaneous and dorsal branches (see Fig. 10-13).

The nerve may be approached either from the volar aspect of the wrist, with the needle directed dorsally from the radial side of the flexor carpi ulnaris tendon, or preferably from the ulnar side of the tendon with the needle directed radially for a distance of approximately 1.5 cm (see Fig. 10-12). A 25-gauge, 16-mm needle is again most suitable, and 3 to 5 ml is injected after eliciting of paresthesias. It is important to seek paresthesias with this second approach in case the needle comes into a plane anterior to the neurovascular bundle, and thus anterior to a thick

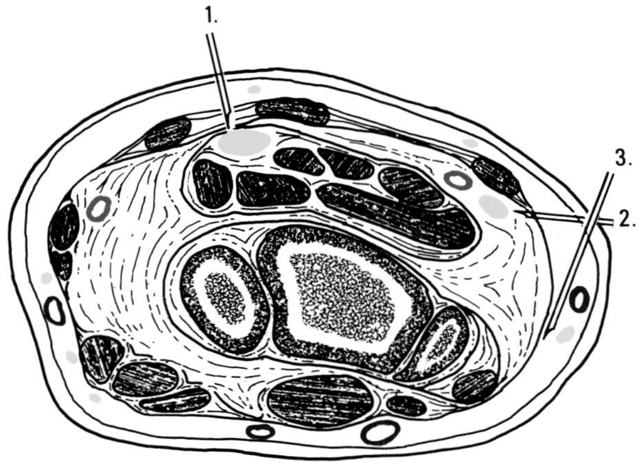

FIG. 10-13. Cross-section of forearm at wrist showing alternative method of ulnar nerve block *(2)* from ulnar side of flexor carpi ulnaris tendon. The dorsal cutaneous branch of the ulnar nerve can also be blocked by redirecting the needle superficially in a dorsal direction *(3)*. Median nerve block *(1)* is also shown. Note necessity to pierce the deep fascia; however, median nerve lies less than 1 cm below the skin.

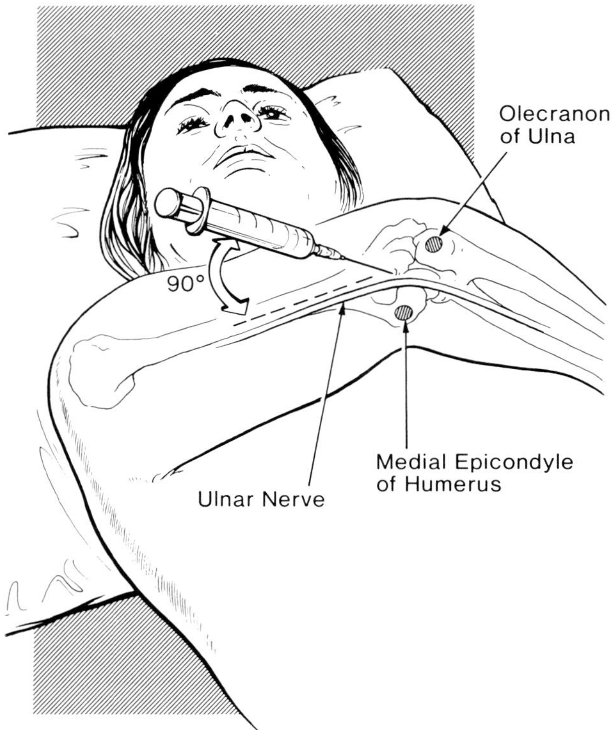

FIG. 10-14. Anatomic landmarks for ulnar nerve block at elbow. Note direction of needle at 90° to humerus.

fascial layer. The approach from the side of the wrist is preferred because it is possible to block the cutaneous branches from the same site of entry. Also, there is probably less chance of damaging the ulnar artery.

If necessary, the two cutaneous branches may be blocked before completely removing the needle: the dorsal branch by subcutaneous infiltration of 2 to 3 ml back along the ulnar border of the carpus and the palmar branch by directing the needle onto the volar aspect of the wrist as far as the radial side of the flexor carpi ulnaris tendon and injecting 1 to 2 ml (see Fig. 10-13).

RADIAL NERVE BLOCK

This is an easy and useful block at the wrist to interrupt the terminal cutaneous branches that supply the radial side of the dorsum of the hand and proximal parts of the radial three and one-half (usually) digits. It is often combined with a median nerve block.

Block at the elbow is more difficult and uncertain and has limited application. It may be combined with block of the lateral cutaneous nerve of the forearm for arteriovenous fistula surgery at the wrist, and it may be needed to supplement inadequate plexus block, particularly when fractures of the radius are involved.

Technique for Block at Elbow

The radial nerve is blocked as it passes over the anterior aspect of the lateral epicondyle, close to the bone (see Fig. 10-10). The arm is abducted on a board with the elbow extended and the forearm supinated. One should stand beside the ulnar side of the arm for left arm block and the radial side for right arm block.

The intercondylar line is marked and the biceps tendon palpated at this level. From a point along the intercondylar line 2 cm lateral to the biceps tendon, a longer (4 – 5 cm) 23-gauge needle is inserted directly backward onto the bone of the lateral epicondyle toward its lateral margin (see Figs. 10-10, 10-11). The palpating index finger of the left hand on the posterior aspect of the epicondyle is used as a guide to direction. Two milliliters to 4 ml is injected as the needle is withdrawn 0.5 to 1 cm. The needle is withdrawn almost to the skin and redirected twice, slightly more medially each time but again onto bone, and further injections are made in the same fashion.

Technique for Block at Wrist

Radial nerve block at the wrist is a field block of the superficial terminal branches as they pass in a variable manner over the radial side of the carpus.

The anatomic "snuffbox" is made prominent by extension of the thumb. The extensor pollicis longus and brevis tendons are both marked. A point is taken over the extensor longus tendon opposite the base of the first metacarpal. A 23-gauge, 32-mm needle is directed proximally along the tendon as far as the dorsal radial tubercle as 2 ml is injected subcutaneously. The needle is withdrawn almost to the skin and redirected at a right angle across the snuffbox to a point just past the brevis tendon as a further 1 ml is injected (Fig. 10-15).

MUSCULOCUTANEOUS NERVE BLOCK

Block of the musculocutaneous nerve is usually performed as a supplement to axillary plexus block, but it may be indicated as an independent procedure or in combination with block of the radial nerve.

First, it may be blocked as the main nerve trunk in the substance of the coracobrachialis muscle from the same point of entry as in the axillary block procedure.[15] Second, it may be blocked 5 cm proximal to the elbow crease, where the terminal sensory lateral cutaneous nerve of the forearm is said to emerge from between the brachialis and biceps muscles.[15] Third, a more recent technique has been described in which the block is performed just lateral to the tendon of the biceps muscle at the level of the intercondylar line. Olson has shown in 64 cadaver dissections that the nerve, rather than emerging from the brachialis biceps groove and running down over the cubital fossa superficially and somewhat lateral to the biceps tendon, stays deep to the fascia and close in under cover of the lateral side of the tendon before it becomes superficial at a variable distance distal to the elbow crease.[37] Last, the musculocutaneous nerve may be blocked as a subcutaneous field block.

Technique for Blocking Lateral to the Tendon of the Biceps Muscle

The arm is abducted on a board with the elbow extended and the forearm supinated; the intercondylar line and biceps tendon are marked. A 25-gauge, 16-mm needle is inserted at the point at which the intercondylar line crosses the lateral border of the biceps tendon, and 2 ml of anesthetic is injected deep to the fascia, just lateral to the tendon. Failures of block result from too deep an insertion (see Fig. 10-11).

This method is more definitive than block in the biceps brachialis groove, much less solution is required, and it can be performed in a few seconds.

FIELD BLOCK OF THE CUTANEOUS NERVES OF THE FOREARM

The *lateral cutaneous nerve* often does not pierce the deep fascia until it is distal to the elbow crease (see

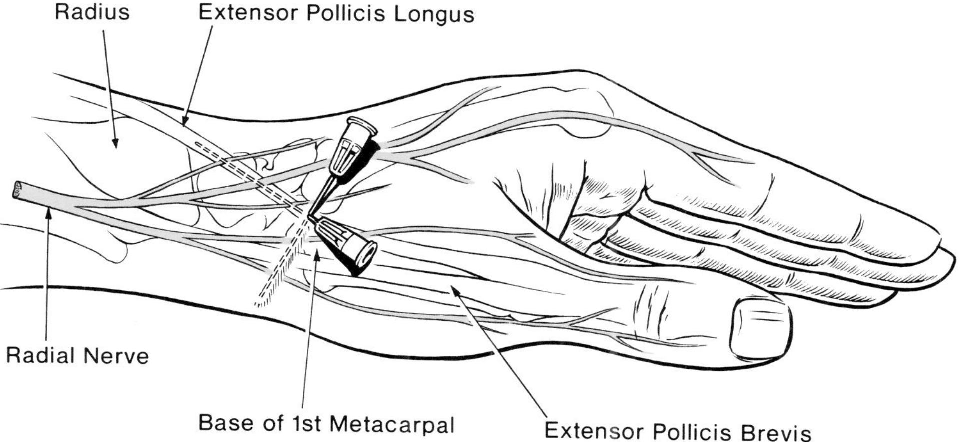

FIG. 10-15. Landmarks and method of needle insertion for radial nerve block at the wrist.

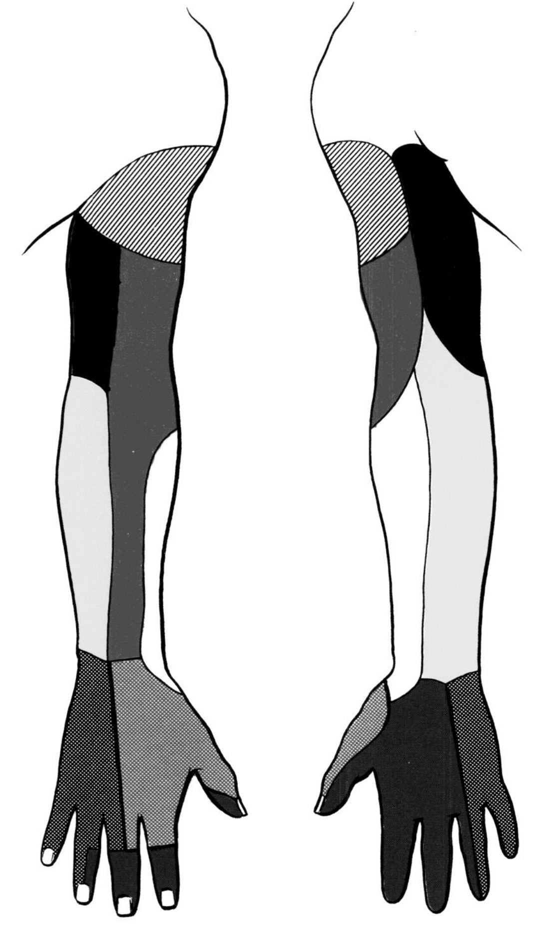

FIG. 10-16. Cutaneous nerve supply of upper limb.

- Upper Lateral Cutaneous Nerve of Arm
- Medial Cutaneous Nerve of Arm and Intercosto-Brachial
- Cutaneous Branches of Radial Nerve (lower lateral cutaneous nerve of forearm & posterior cutaneous nerves of arm and forearm)
- Superficial Radial Nerve
- Lateral Cutaneous Nerve of Forearm
- Medial Cutaneous Nerve of Forearm
- Median Nerve
- Ulnar Nerve

above). Subcutaneous infiltration should begin from a point 5 cm distal to the crease and in line with the biceps tendon and then directed laterally for a distance of 3 to 4 cm.

The *medial cutaneous nerve of the forearm* arises from the medial cord of the brachial plexus in the axilla. It pierces the deep fascia in company with the basilic vein in the midarm and then bifurcates. Its anterior, or volar, branch passes down over the front of the cubital fossa medial to the biceps tendon to supply the anteromedial aspect of the forearm. The smaller posterior, or ulnar, branch passes downward farther back just in front of the medial epicondyle to supply the posteromedial aspect (Fig. 10-16). Subcutaneous infiltration should extend from the biceps tendon to the medial epicondyle (see Fig. 10-11).

The *posterior cutaneous nerve of the forearm* arises from the radial nerve and pierces the deep fascia above the elbow. It descends along the lateral side of the arm and then along the back of the forearm to the wrist. From a point directly over the lateral epicondyle of the humerus with the elbow slightly flexed, subcutaneous infiltration should extend for 3 to 4 cm toward the olecranon.

LOCAL ANESTHETIC BLOCK OF THE DIGITAL NERVES

Digital nerve block is a commonly used and effective method of anesthesia for a wide variety of minor outpatient surgical procedures on the digits. However, because of the uncommon but serious complications of ischemia and necrosis, it should not be undertaken lightly; alternatives such as nerve block at the wrist should be considered, particularly when more than one digit is involved. When digital nerve block is used, certain aspects of technique must be strictly followed.

Anatomy

The common digital nerves are derived from the median and ulnar nerves and divide in the distal palm into the volar digital nerves to supply adjacent sides of the fingers, palmar aspect, tip and nail bed area. These main digital nerves are accompanied by digital vessels and run on the ventrolateral aspect of the finger beside the flexor tendon sheath. Small dorsal digital nerves derived from the radial and ulnar nerves supply the back of the fingers as far as the proximal joint. These run on the dorsolateral aspect of the finger.

Techniques

Block of Both Volar and Dorsal Digital Nerves at Each Side of the Base of the Finger. A 25-gauge, 16-mm needle is inserted at a point on the dorsolateral aspect of the base of the finger and directed anteriorly to slide past the base of the phalanx (Fig. 10-17*A*). The needle is advanced until the anesthesiologist feels the resistance of the palmar dermis or the pressure on a "protective" finger placed under the patient's finger and directly opposite the needle path. One milliliter of solution is injected as the needle is withdrawn 2 to 3 mm to block the volar nerve, and 0.5 ml is injected just under the point of entry to block the dorsal nerve. The volar digital nerves can also be approached from the side of the finger.

Block of the Common Volar Digital Nerves near Their Bifurcation Between the Metacarpal Heads. With the fingers widely extended, a 25-gauge, 16-mm needle is inserted into the web 2 to 3 mm dorsal to the junction of the web and palmar skin. It is directed straight back toward the hand in line with the extended fingers, and 2 ml of solution is injected when the needle almost reaches the hub (Fig. 10-17*B*).

Redirection from the same point of entry to the region of the dorsal nerves on each side can easily be performed, if necessary.

A metacarpal approach may also be performed either from the dorsal aspect and inserting the needles between the bones almost as far as the palmar skin or from the palmar aspect at the level of the distal crease and inserting a short fine needle just through the palmar aponeurosis[9,10,41] (Fig. 10-17*B*). This second approach would seem to be unnecessarily painful. For these digital blocks, lower concentrations of local anesthetics are satisfactory and *must be used without vasoconstrictors.*

THUMB BLOCK

The thumb is supplied by superficial branches of the radial nerve (see Fig. 10-15) and by digital branches of the median nerve (see Fig. 10-16). Thus, complete sensory block of the thumb is produced by median nerve block at the wrist (see Fig. 10-12A) and radial nerve block at the wrist (see Fig. 10-15). The thumb can also be blocked by circumferential infiltration at the base of the thumb ("ring block"), using a non-epinephrine-containing solution.

INFILTRATION OF FRACTURE SITES

The principle of this technique is to render insensitive the periosteum in the region of the bony fracture. It has most commonly been applied in the treatment of Colles' fractures. The results under expert, careful, and patient hands would appear to be satisfactory.[16]

Technique. Under very strict aseptic conditions 10 to 15 ml (in the case of Colles) of 1% lidocaine or prilocaine without adrenaline are injected into the periosteum at and around the fracture site from the dorsal aspect. At least 10 minutes must then elapse before the fracture is gently manipulated.

This technique is not recommended for routine use, not only because of the risk of infection and the possibility of rapid uptake of the local anesthetic, but also because it often does not produce the satisfactory analgesia or muscle relaxation.

COMPLICATIONS AND CONTRAINDICATIONS

The only complication specific to these peripheral blocks, apart from those already mentioned, is vascular insufficiency and gangrene after digital nerve block. This catastrophe is a result of digital artery occlusion together with failure of adequate collateral circulation and a number of causative factors may be involved.

Epinephrine-containing Solutions. Although not the only cause of gangrene, vasoconstrictor solutions in this region have undoubtedly been responsible for many cases in the past and should never be used.

Volume of Solution. The mechanical pressure effects of injecting solution in a relatively confined space should always be borne in mind, particularly in blocks at the base of the digit. Maximum volumes of 2 ml on each side should not be exceeded.

Tourniquets are commonly applied to produce a bloodless field (and perhaps in the hope that it would both hasten and prolong anesthesia). Bradfield, in a report on 44 cases of gangrene, could not exonerate the tourniquet but recommended that an upper limit of 15 minutes' duration could be set and that it never be used in patients with Raynaud's phenomena.[7] Bunnell has condemned the use of rubber band-type tourniquets at the base of the digit and has stated that

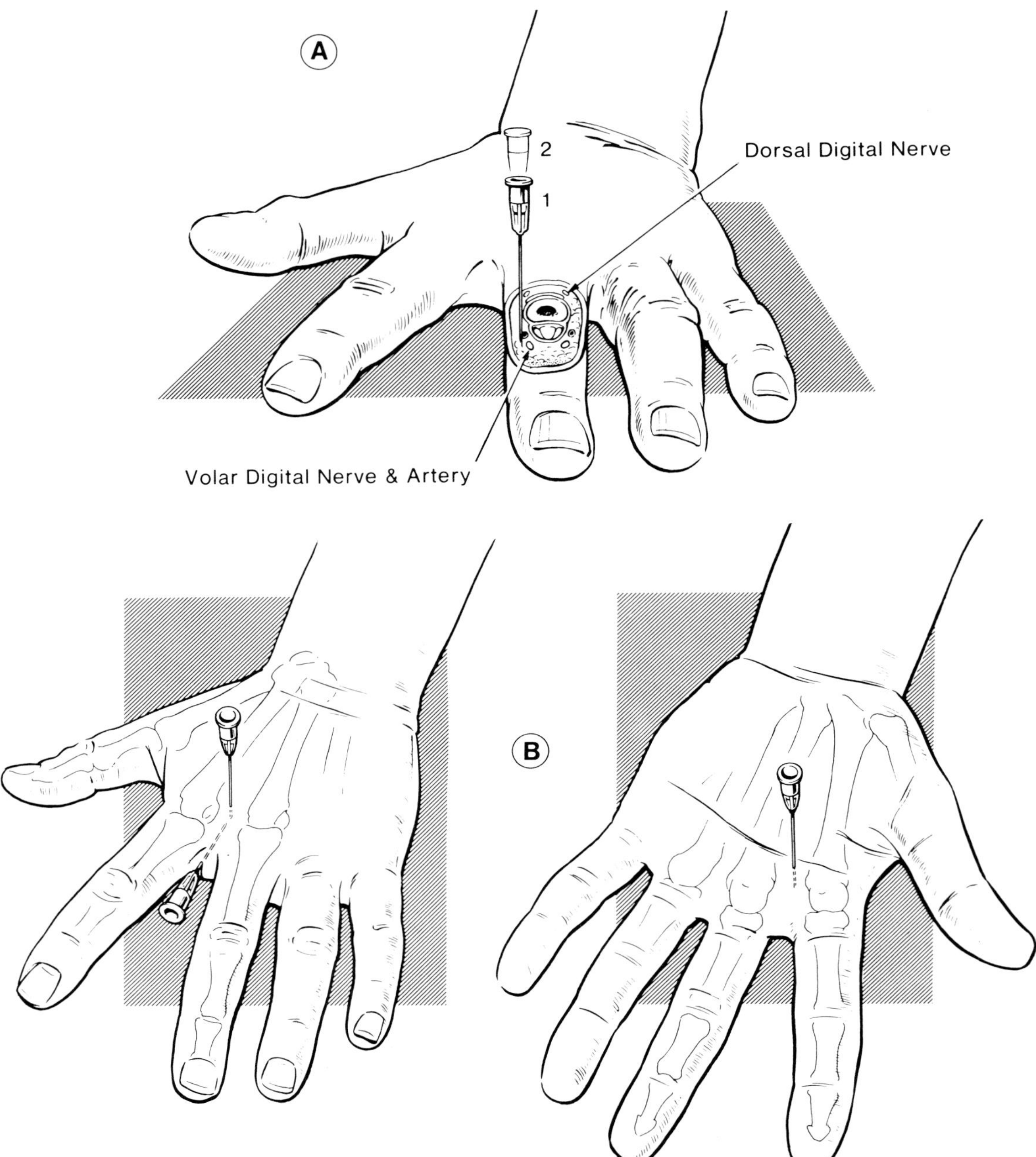

FIG. 10-17. **A.** Technique of digital nerve block at base of finger. **B.** Techniques of block of common volar digital nerves between metacarpal heads.

whenever a tourniquet is needed, a proper upper arm tourniquet should be applied.[6]

Peripheral Vascular Disease. In patients with small vessel disease, perhaps an alternative method should be sought in addition to avoidance of digital tourniquet.

Direct vascular damage by the needle may contribute to the complication.

The incidence of digital gangrene is unknown. Even in reported cases, the duration of the tourniquet and other important facts are often not recorded. With the current level of knowledge, it would seem wise to avoid vasoconstrictors; avoid a digital tourniquet, or certainly limit its duration to 15 minutes; use small volumes of solution; avoid digital blocks in patients whose vessels may be suspect; and, as with all nerve blocks, be gentle and patient.

A source of infection proximate to the proposed site of injection is probably the main contraindication to nerve blocks on the upper limb.

The excellent contribution of Dr. Fred Berry to material in this chapter derived from the first edition is gratefully acknowledged.

REFERENCES

1. Accardo, N.J., and Adriani, J.A.: Brachial plexus block—a simplified technique using the axillary route. South. Med. J., *42*:920, 1949.
2. Babitski, P.: A new method of anesthetizing the brachial plexus. Zentralbl. Chir., *45*:215, 1918.
3. Bazy, L., and Blondin, S.: L'anesthesie du plexus brachial. Anesth. Analg. (Paris), *1*:190, 1935.
4. Bazy, L., Pouchet, V., Sourdat, P., and Laboure, J.: Anesthesie Regionale. pp 222–225. Philadelphia, W.B. Saunders, 1917.
5. Bonica, J.J., Moore, D.C., and Orlov, M.: Brachial plexus block anesthesia. Am. J. Surg., 65, 1949.
6. Boyes, J.H.: Bunnell's Surgery of the Hand, 5th ed. Philadelphia, J.B. Lippincott, 1970.
7. Bradfield, W.J.D.: Digital block anesthesia and its complications. Br. J. Surg., *50*:495, 1962.
8. Burnham, P.J.: Simple regional nerve block for surgery of the hand and forearm. J.A.M.A., *169*:109, 1959.
9. ———: Regional block anaesthesia for surgery of the fingers and thumb. Industrial Med. Surg., *27*:67, 1958.
10. Chase, R.A.: Atlas of Hand Surgery. Philadelphia, W.B. Saunders, 1973.
11. Clayton, M.L., and Turner, D.A.: Upper arm block anesthesia in children with fractures. J.A.M.A., *169*:99, 1959.
12. Conolly, W.B., and Berry, F.R.: Selective peripheral nerve blocks for reconstructive hand surgery. Med. J. Aust., 2:94, 1974.
13. Crile, G.W.: Anesthesia of nerve roots with cocaine. Cleve. Med. J., 2:355, 1897.
14. de Jong, R.H.: Axillary block of the brachial plexus. Anesthesiology, *22*:215, 1961.
15. ———: Modified axillary block. Anesthesiology, *26*:615, 1965.

15a. Denson, D.D., Raj, P.P., Saldahna, F., *et al.*: Continuous perineural infusion of bupivacaine for prolonged analgesia: Pharmacokinetic considerations. Int. J. Clin. Pharmacol. Ther. Toxicol., *21*:591, 1983.

16. Dinley, R.J., and Michelinakis, E.: Local anaesthesia in the reduction of Colles' fracture. Injury, *4*:345, 1972–1973.
17. Dogliotti, A.M.: Anesthesia: Narcosis, Local, Regional, and Spinal. (Authorized English translation by Scuderi, C.S.) Chicago, S.B. Debour, 1939.
18. Dupont, C., *et al.*: Hand surgery under wrist block and local infiltration anesthesia using an upper arm tourniquet. Plast. Reconstr. Surg., *50*:532, 1972.
19. Dushoff, I.M.: Letters to the editor. Plast. Reconstr. Surg., *51*:685, 1973.
20. Eather, K.F.: Axillary brachial plexus block. Anesthesiology, *19*:683, 1958.
21. Erikkson, E.: A simplified method of axillary block. Nord. Med., *68*:1325, 1962.
22. ———: Axillary brachial plexus anaesthesia in children with Citanest. Acta Anaesth. Scand., *16*[*Suppl.*]:291, 1965.
23. Hirschel, G.: Die Anasthesierung des Plexus Brachialis fur die Operataionen an der oberen Extremitat. Munchen. Med. Wochenschr., *58*:1555, 1911.
24. Hopcroft, S.C.: The axillary approach to brachial plexus anaesthesia. Anaesth. Intensive Care, *1*:232, 1973.
25. Hudon, F., and Jacques, A.: Block of the brachial plexus by the axillary route. Can. Anaesth. Soc. J., *6*:400, 1959.
26. Hunter, J.M., *et al.*: A dynamic approach to problems of hand function. Clin. Orthop., *104*:112, 1974.
27. Jackson, L., and Keats, A.S.: Mechanism of brachial plexus palsy following anesthesia. Anesthesiology, *26*:190, 1965.
28. Kulenkampff, D.: Die anasthesierung des Plexus Brachialis. Zentralbl. Chir., *38*:1337, 1911.
29. Kumar, A., *et al.*: Bilateral cervical and thoracic epidural blockade complicating interscalene brachial plexus block. Anesthesiology, *35*:650, 1971.
30. Labat, G.: Brachial plexus block: Details of technique with lantern slides. Br. J. Anaesth., *4*:174, 1926–1927.
31. Livingston, E.M., and Werthein, H.: Brachial plexus block: Its clinical application. J.A.M.A., *88*:1464, 1927.
32. Lofstrom, J.B.: Ulnar nerve blockade for the evaluation of local anaesthetic agents. Br. J. Anaesth., *47*:297, 1975.
33. Lofstrom, J.B., *et al.*: Late disturbance in nerve function after block with local anaesthetic agents. Acta Anaesth. Scand., *10*:111, 1966.
34. Macintosh, R.R.: and Mushin, W.W.: Local Anesthesia: Brachial Plexus. Oxford, Blackwell Scientific Publishers, 1944.
35. Moir, D.D.: Axillary block to the brachial plexus. Anaesthesia, *17*:274, 1962.
36. Neuhof, H.: Supraclavicular anesthetization of the brachial plexus. J.A.M.A., *62*:1629, 1914.

37. Olson, I.A.: The origin of the lateral cutaneous nerve of the forearm and its anesthesia for modified brachial plexus block. J. Anat., *105*:381, 1969.
38. Patrick, J.: The technique of brachial plexus block anesthesia. Br. J. Surg., *27*:734, 1939–1940.
39. Pitkin, W.M., Southworth, J.L., and Hingson, R.A.: Conduction Anesthesia. Philadelphia, J.B. Lippincott, 1953.
40. Raj, P.P., Montgomery, S.J., Nettles, D., and Jenkins, M.T.: Infraclavicular brachial plexus block—a new approach. Anesth. Analg., *52*:897, 1973.
41. Rank, B.K., Wakefield, A.R., and Hueston, J.T.: Surgery of Repair as Applied to Hand Injuries, 4th ed., p. 88. Edinburgh, E. & S. Livingstone, 1973.
42. Ross, S., and Scarborough, C.D.: Total spinal anesthesia following brachial plexus block. Anesthesiology, *39*:458, 1973.
43. Selander, D.: Catheter technique in axillary plexus block. Acta Anaesth. Scand., *21*:324, 1977.
44. Selander, D., Edshage, S., and Wolff, T.: Paresthesiae or no paresthesiae? Nerve lesions after axillary block. Acta Anaesth. Scand., *23*:27, 1979.
45. Sherwood-Dunn, B.: Regional Anesthesia. p. 242. Philadelphia, F.A. Davis, 1920.
46. Sims, J.K.: A modification of landmarks for infraclavicular approach to brachial plexus block. Anesth. Analg., *56*:554, 1977.
47. Strachauer, A.C.: Brachial plexus anesthesia: A complete local anesthesia of upper extremities permitting all major surgical procedures. Lancet, *34*:301, 1914.
48. Thompson, G.E., and Rorie, D.H.: Functional anatomy of the brachial plexus sheaths. Anesthesiology, *59*:117, 1983.
49. Tuominen, M., Rosenberg, P., and Kalso, E.: Blood levels of bupivacaine after single dose, supplementary dose, and continuous infusion in axillary plexus block. Acta Anaesth. Scand., *27*:303, 1983.
50. Vester-Andersen, T., *et al.*: Perivascular axillary block: II. Influence of injected volume of local anaesthetic on neural blockade. Acta Anaesth. Scand., *27*:95, 1983.
51. Ward, M.E.: The interscalene approach to the brachial plexus. Anaesthesia, *29*:147, 1974.
52. Webling, D.D.: Anaesthesia of the upper limb for casualty procedures. Med. J. Aust., *2*:496, 1960.
53. Wen-Hsien, W.U.: Brachial plexus block. J.A.M.A., *215*:1953, 1971.
54. Whiffler, K.: Coracoid block—a safe and easy technique. Br. J. Anaesth., *53*:845, 1981.
55. Winnie, A.P.: An "immobile" needle for nerve blocks. Anesthesiology, *31*:577, 1969.
56. ———: Interscalene brachial plexus block. Anesth. Analg. (Cleve.), *49*:455, 1970.
57. ———: The perivascular techniques of brachial plexus anaesthesia. ASA Refresher Courses in Anesthesiology, *2*:151, 1974.
58. ———: Recent developments in anesthesia. Surg. Clin. North Am., *55*:878, 1975.
59. ———: Plexus anesthesia: I. Perivascular Techniques of Brachial Plexus Block. Philadelphia, W.B. Saunders, 1983.
60. Winnie, A.P., *et al.*: Interscalene cervical plexus block. Anesth. Analg. (Cleve.), *54*:370, 1975.
61. Winnie, A.P., and Collins, V.J.: The subclavian perivascular technique to brachial plexus anaesthesia. Anesthesiology, *25*:353, 1964.

11 THE LOWER EXTREMITY: SOMATIC BLOCKADE

PHILLIP O. BRIDENBAUGH

Although there are many anatomic similarities between the innervation and bony landmarks of the upper and lower extremities, there are fewer techniques for peripheral neural blockade of the lower extremity than for the upper extremity, and the enthusiasm for performing them is not as great. It is very probable that peridural or subarachnoid anesthesia, which provides rapid, complete, safe anesthesia of the lower extremities, is more easily accomplished by anesthesiologists than is lower extremity peripheral neural blockade. Further, although it is possible to accomplish complete anesthesia of the upper extremity with a single injection, that is still not the case with the lower extremity. Nonetheless, peripheral neural blockade of the lower extremity is easily accomplished with a minimum of side-effects and should have a place in the armamentarium of the anesthesiologist who uses regional anesthesia as part of his overall practice.

Like other forms of neural blockade, lower extremity techniques are not new. Braun mentions that blockade of the lateral cutaneous femoral nerve was described by Nystrom in 1909.[3] Laewen expanded on this by describing the additional blockade of the anterior crural nerve, and Keppler improved both techniques by advocating the elicitation of paresthesias. Earlier than all of this—around 1887—Crile performed amputations by exposing the sciatic nerve in the gluteal fold and the femoral nerve in the inguinal fold and injecting cocaine intraneurally. Subsequently, no fewer than six others advocated percutaneous approaches to the sciatic nerve alone. Some of these same authors wrote about blockade of other nerves of the leg as well (see Chap 1).

Not only is this old concept still valid today, but also many of the techniques are nearly identical to the original descriptions. This emphasizes remarks made by Labat that "Anatomy is the foundation upon which the entire concept of regional anesthesia is built"; that "Landmarks are anatomic guideposts of the body which are used to locate the nerves"; that "Superficial landmarks are distinguishing features of the surface of the body which can be easily recognized and identified by sight or palpation. Bones and their prominences, blood vessels and tendons serve as deep landmarks. Deep landmarks can be defined only by the point of the needle. They are the only reliable guide for advancing the needle in attempting to reach the vicinity of the nerve"; and that "The anesthetist should attempt to visualize the anatomic structures traversed by the needle and utilize the tactile senses to determine the impulses transmitted by the point of the needle as it approaches a deep landmark (*e.g.*, bone)."[17]

Illustrative of the importance of bony landmarks are the many approaches proposed for blockade of the sciatic nerve. The course of the nerve through the pelvis and medial to the femoral head provides a plethora of bony landmarks, all at some time in the past 100 years having been advocated by someone in his favorite technique.

NERVE SUPPLY

The nerve supply to the lower extremity is composed of the lumbar and sacral plexuses. The lumbar plexus is formed in the psoas muscle by the anterior rami of the first four lumbar nerves, including, frequently, a branch from the 12th thoracic nerve and occasionally one from the 5th lumbar nerve. The sacral plexus is derived from the anterior rami of the 4th and 5th lumbar and the first two or three sacral nerves.

While the lumbosacral plexus as a whole contributes to the nerve supply of the lower extremities, the upper part of the lumbar division supplies the iliohypogastric and ilioinguinal nerves, which are in series with the thoracic nerves and innervate the trunk above the level of the extremity (see Chap. 14). Specifically, the iliohypogastric nerve provides cutaneous innervation to the skin of the buttock and the muscles of the abdominal wall. The ilioinguinal nerve supplies the skin of the perineum and adjoining portion of the inner thigh. A third nerve, the genitofemoral, arises from the first and second lumbar nerves. It supplies filaments to the genital area and adjacent parts of the thigh. It also gives off a lumboinguinal branch, which supplies the skin over the area of the femoral artery and femoral triangle (see Fig. 14-9).

Caudad to these nerves are the major nerves that supply all of the lower extremity. Details of their course and distribution will be covered individually.

In brief, there are five major nerves to the lower extremity. The *lateral femoral cutaneous nerve,* the *femoral nerve* (sometimes called the *anterior crural nerve*), and the *obturator nerve* are derived from the lumbar plexus, along with minor contributions from the iliohypogastric, ilioinguinal, and genitofemoral nerves. The two remaining nerves are the *posterior cutaneous nerve of the thigh* and the *sciatic nerve* (see Fig. 11-5). The posterior cutaneous nerve has sometimes been referred to as the "small sciatic" nerve. It derives from the first, second, and third sacral nerves, as does the larger sciatic nerve, which also receives branches of the anterior rami of the fourth and fifth lumbar nerves. Inasmuch as the two nerves course through the pelvis together and out through the greater sciatic foramen, they are considered together when techniques for blocking the sciatic nerve are discussed.

The sciatic nerve is really an association of two major nerve trunks. The first is the tibial, derived from the ventral branches of the anterior rami of the fourth and fifth lumbar and first, second, and third sacral nerves. The second is the common peroneal, derived from the dorsal branches of the anterior rami of the same five nerves. These two major nerve trunks pass as the sciatic to the proximal angle of the popliteal fossa, where they separate with the tibial portion passing medially and the common peroneal (lateral popliteal) laterally.

The smaller branches of these nerves, which provide distal innervation of the lower extremity, are discussed in detail in conjunction with techniques for nerve block at the knee and ankle.

LUMBAR SOMATIC NERVE BLOCK

ANATOMY

In considering neural blockade of the lower extremity at the lumbar level, the bony, muscular, and fascial relationships to the emerging nerves must be recalled. The spinal nerve that comes off the spinal cord at each level is formed by the union of a ventral motor root with a dorsal sensory root. This mixed spinal nerve gives off a dorsal ramus, a ventral ramus, and a ramus communicans, the latter which contributes to the formation of the sympathetic ganglion and trunk. The lumbar plexus, as previously noted, is formed by the anterior (ventral) divisions of the 1st, 2nd, 3rd, and 4th lumbar nerves with about 50% inclusion of a branch from the 12th thoracic nerve and occasionally from the 5th lumbar. The lumbar plexus is formed in front of the transverse processes of the lumbar vertebrae into a series of oblique loops that lie deep in the substance of the psoas major muscle and at the medial border of the quadratus lumborum muscle. From here, the individual nerves form and course in the direction of their terminal innervation.

The relation of the lumbar somatic plexus to the sympathetic chain should be remembered, since each may be blocked separately but with a similar approach. The first and second lumbar spinal nerves, frequently the third, and sometimes the fourth send communicating rami to form the lumbar portion of the sympathetic trunk. The sympathetic trunk lies on the ventrolateral surface of the lumbar and sacral bodies medial to the anterior foramina. It is apparent, therefore, that although these two nerve systems are separated by distance, muscle, and tissue planes, they have considerable intercommunication (Fig. 11-1).

TECHNIQUE

The standard approach to blockade of the lumbar somatic nerves is paravertebral (see also Chap. 14). The original writings of Labat and Pitkin advocate

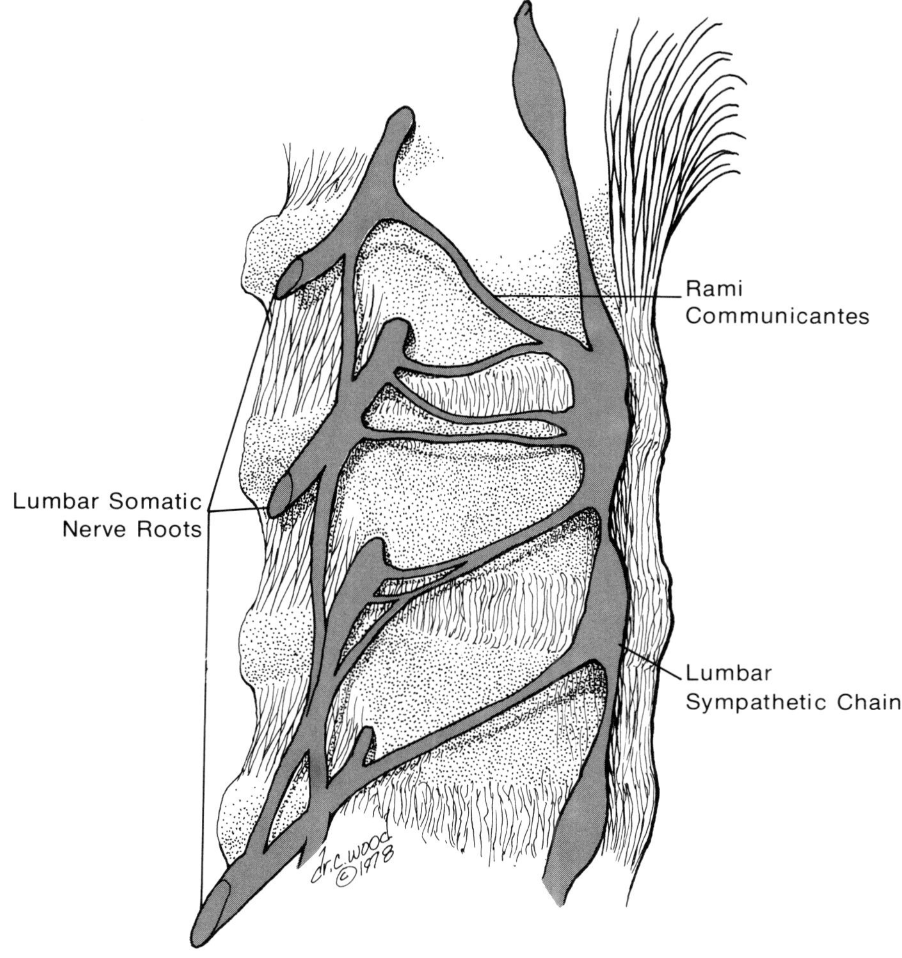

FIG. 11-1. Relationship of lumbar sympathetic chain to the somatic nerve roots. (Drawn by Dr. Charles D. Wood)

having the patient lie on the side opposite the one to be blocked. Additionally, a soft roll placed between the iliac crest and the costal margin will minimize the lateral spinal curvature. A preferred position, in the healthy patient, is that of having the patient lie prone over a soft pillow, which will flatten (or elevate) the lumbar curve. Regardless of position, the landmarks used are the spinous processes of the lumbar vertebrae. Skin wheals are raised opposite the cephalad aspect of the spinous processes, on a line 3 to 4 cm laterally from and parallel to the midline of the back (Fig. 11-2). Depending on the size of the patient, an 8- or 10-cm needle is inserted through each of the skin wheals and advanced perpendicular to the surface of the skin until its tip comes in contact with the transverse process of the vertebral body, usually at a depth of 4 to 5 cm. The needle is then partially withdrawn and reintroduced slightly more cephalad and medially, making an angle of about 25° with the sagittal plane of the body. This should allow the needle to pass just tangential to the superior aspect of the transverse process and to be advanced an additional 2 to 3 cm. Paresthesias may frequently be elicited. If so, 8 to 10 ml of the selected local anesthetic solution should be injected. If no paresthesias are elicited, the solution is distributed in front of the transverse process.

It should be remembered that the spinous processes of the lumbar vertebrae do not slope downward as do the thoracic spines, their upper and lower borders being more nearly horizontal. Their average

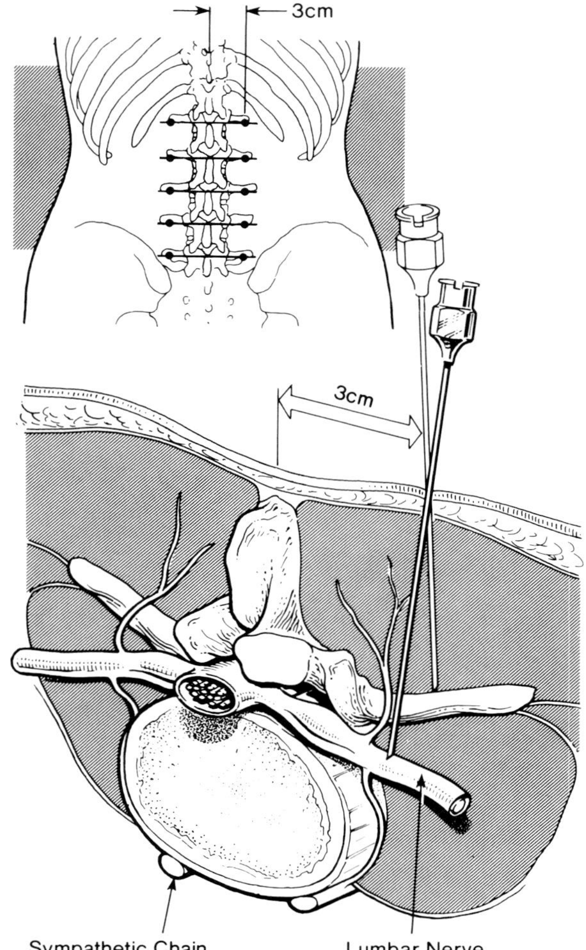

FIG. 11-2. Paravertebral lumbar somatic nerve block. **Upper Panel.** Skin markings are made by drawing lines across the cephalad aspect of spinous processes and then drawing vertical lines 3 cm from the midline. **Lower Panel.** A needle inserted perpendicular to the skin will contact the cephalad edge of a spinous process. Angulation of the needle in a cephalad direction to slide superior to the transverse process will reach the spinal nerve 2 to 3 cm deeper than the transverse process.

thickness is from 0.5 to 1 cm. The distance between the tip of the spine and its attachment to the vertebral lamina is approximately 3 to 4 cm. A horizontal line drawn tangential to the superior aspect of the spine will overlie the transverse process of that vertebrae. The transverse processes of the lumbar vertebrae are short, accounting for the paravertebral skin wheal being only 2 to 3 cm from the midline. The average depth of the transverse process to the skin is 5 cm, which varies with the size of the patient and the paraspinous musculature. The transverse processes of L4 and L5 are more deeply situated than are those of the vertebrae above. When the needle passes superior to the transverse process, it is in proximity to the somatic nerve of the preceding segment (*e.g.*, the needle passing over the transverse process of L1 injects the T12 nerve root). The L5 root is blocked through the same skin wheal as L4, by redirecting the needle in a caudad direction until it passes from the lower border of the L4 transverse process and by injecting the nerve root in a manner similar to the technique used in other roots (Fig. 11-2).

A more peripheral approach to the major branches of the lumbar plexus that supply the leg has been described by Winnie.[38] His *inguinal paravascular* technique of lumbar plexus block utilizes the fascial envelope around the femoral nerve as a conduit, which carries injected anesthetic superiorly to the level where the lumbar plexus forms (Fig. 11-3).

As previously noted, the lumbar plexus lies between the quadratus lumborum muscle posteriorly and the psoas major muscle anteriorly, being invested, therefore, by the fasciae of those two muscles. Although the other nerves to the leg take divergent courses through the pelvis, the femoral nerve descends from under the psoas muscle and remains in the groove between the psoas and iliacus muscle. Superior to the inguinal ligament, the femoral nerve is then in a fascial sheath, with the anterior covering being provided by the transversalis fascia.

INGUINAL PARAVASCULAR BLOCK

The technique for inguinal paravascular block is very similar to that for femoral nerve block. The patient lies supine with the anesthesiologist standing next to the side that is to be blocked. After careful palpation, a skin wheal is raised just lateral to the femoral artery, where it emerges distal to the inguinal ligament. A short-bevel 22-gauge needle connected to a syringe filled with anesthetic is inserted just over the tip of the palpating finger in a cephalad direction. A paresthesia of the femoral nerve must be produced as an indication that the tip of the needle is within the fascial sheath. The needle is then fixed and the desired volume of local anesthetic injected while firm digital pressure is applied just distal to the needle in an attempt to force the flow of local anesthetic proximally into the area of the lumbar plexus. A volume of 25 to 30 ml of local anesthetic should be injected.

INDICATION

The lumbar plexus and its somatic nerves supply the cutaneous nerves not only to the upper thigh but also to the lower abdominal area. (Analgesia for the abdomen is covered more completely in Chapter 14.) Lumbar somatic block is indicated in patients who for some reason cannot be given a spinal or epidural anesthetic for operations of the hip, thigh, or upper leg.

Branches of the first three lumbar nerves provide cutaneous distribution to the inner and outer aspects of the thigh and the anterior gluteal region along with adjacent perineal and suprapubic areas. With lumbar plexus block, it is possible to block these fibers. If the five major peripheral nerve blocks are performed, however, and procedures proximal to the midthigh are anticipated, then paravertebral blockade of the appropriate nerves is indicated. In contrast, lumbar somatic blockade alone will not be sufficient for complete anesthesia of the lower extremity because it cannot achieve blockade of the sacral roots that supply the sciatic nerve.

SIDE-EFFECTS AND COMPLICATIONS

For purposes of clarification, *side-effects,* as the word is used here, are physiologic occurrences that result from a particular technique or local anesthetic agent, which may not be desirable in a particular patient. The classic example is sympathetic nerve blockade. In theory, a carefully performed paravertebral lumbar somatic nerve block should not give rise to blockade of the lumbar sympathetic fibers. Nonetheless, in clinical practice, local anesthetic may reach the sympathetic chain, and the anesthesiologist should watch for such side-effects, especially in the hypovolemic patient in whom the magnitude of response (usually hypotension) may be exaggerated.

A rare complication of the paravertebral approach to neural blockade is that of epidural or subarachnoid injection. In a large patient with considerable soft tissue overlying the paraspinous area, a needle introduced at a slight medial angle can pass quite easily through the interspace and accomplish what is referred to in anesthesia terms as a *paramedian approach* to the epidural or subarachnoid space (see Chap. 7).

Finally, anterior to the vertebral column are major blood vessels. If caution is not observed in recalling or marking the depth of the transverse process when the anesthesiologist is advancing the needle to the level of the lumbar plexus, the needle may be inserted too

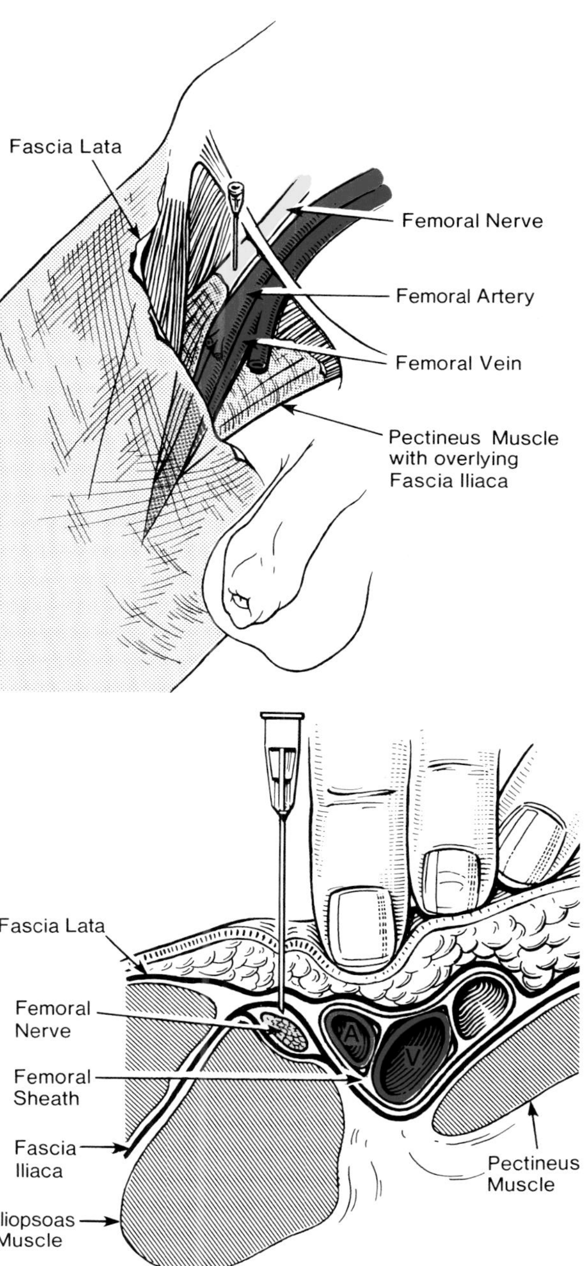

FIG. 11-3. Inguinal structures showing fascial envelope around femoral nerve and relationships for inguinal paravascular femoral nerve block techniques.

deeply and these vessels entered. Careful aspiration before injection of local anesthetic solutions should prevent the serious complication of direct intravascular injection, with a likely systemic toxic reaction. Mere needle entry into a normal blood vessel without injection of drug is usually of no consequence. The most frequently encountered vessel with the right paravertebral approach is the inferior vena cava—and on the left, of course, is the aorta.

SACRAL PLEXUS NERVE BLOCK

Since the derivation of the sciatic nerve comes in part from spinal roots S1–S3, it is apparent that blockade of these roots must be combined with the aforementioned lumbar somatic block if complete anesthesia of the lower extremity is to be obtained by paravertebral blockade.

ANATOMY

The sacral plexus is formed by the union of the first three sacral nerves and the fourth and fifth lumbar nerves. It also connects with the ascending division of the fourth sacral nerve. The sacral plexus is located on the anterior surface of the sacrum and is separated from the sacrum by the piriformis muscle. It is covered by the parietal portion of the pelvic fascia. In front of it lie the ureter, the pelvic colon, part of the rectum, and the iliac artery and vein. The plexus gives off two sets of branches: the collateral and the terminal. The collateral branches (anterior and posterior) supply the pudendal plexus, the hip joint, the gluteal structures, and the adductor and hamstring muscles. More pertinent to this discussion, the terminal branches supply the greater and lesser sciatic nerves.

The sacrum is the wedge-shaped, fused lower five sacral vertebrae attached by joints and ligaments to the iliac bones. On its posterior surface are two rows of openings—the posterior sacral foramina, present on each side of the fused spinous processes (see Fig. 9-1). The posterior divisions of the sacral nerves pass through these foramina to the soft tissues of the sacral region at the back. Although these rows of foramina are not exactly parallel, angling toward the midline, they are not as steeply angulated as the edges of the sacrum. This is an important point to remember when surface landmarks are plotted (Fig. 11-4).

Another important anatomic relationship is that of the anterior sacral foramina to the homologous posterior foramina, thereby constituting the transacral

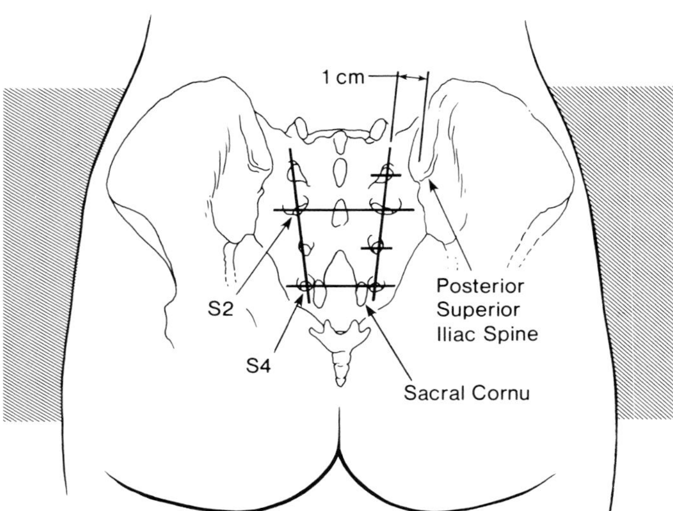

FIG. 11-4. Landmarks for sacral plexus nerve block.

canal. The depth of the canal varies from 2.5 cm at the level of S1 to 0.5 cm at S4 (see Fig. 9-7). It is important to have these figures in mind when blocking the sacral nerves by the transsacral method; otherwise, the needle may be introduced into the pelvis.

TECHNIQUE

For transsacral block, the patient is prone over a pillow placed under the hips. The posterior superior iliac spine and the sacral cornu are both palpated and marked. A skin wheal is raised immediately lateral to and above the sacral cornu, and another placed 1 cm medial to and below the posterior superior iliac spine of the side to be blocked. The distance between the wheals is bisected, and an additional wheal is raised at this site. Those three wheals thus identify the second, third, and fourth sacral foramina. The first sacral foramen is found by placing a wheal 1 to 2 cm above the second and on the same line as the others. There is no fifth sacral foramen. The fifth sacral nerves lie 1 to 2 cm caudad to the fourth foramen on the lines marked. The thickness of the soft tissues overlying the sacrum is greater superiorly—and, therefore, requires longer needles—than the lower segments. An 8- to 10-cm, 22-gauge needle is satisfactory for S1 and S2 and a 5-cm needle for the lower segments. The second foramen is often easiest to locate and thus usually attempted first. This helps in locating the others. The needle is inserted toward the posterior aspect of the sacrum, inclined slightly medially until striking bone. The needle is then withdrawn and reintroduced until it enters the respective transsacral canal. The needle is advanced approximately 2 to 2.5 cm into the first sacral canal and in 0.5-cm decrements for each succeeding canal. Similarly, 5 to 7 ml of solution should be injected into the first sacral foramen, the volume being reduced by 1 to 1.5 ml for each subsequent injection. The precision of this block is aided by use of a peripheral nerve stimulator.

SIDE-EFFECTS AND COMPLICATIONS

Since the sacral nerves represent the parasympathetic portion of the autonomic nervous system, sympathetic blockade and its potential for hypotension are not seen with transsacral block unless excessive volumes of solution spread proximally to the lumbar sympathetic fibers. Loss of parasympathetic function to bowel, bladder, and sphincters may, however, occur. Injection of local anesthetic through misdirected needles into the subarachnoid or vascular compartments is a remote risk. Classically, the dural sac is said to terminate at the lower border of S2; however, there are enough clinical reports of subarachnoid puncture with a 6- to 7-cm caudal needle to suggest individual variations below this "classic" location. Finally, an appreciation of the pelvic contents, especially colon, rectum, and bladder, is important; should a deeply inserted needle enter the colon or rectum and not be noticed, it could result in seeding fecal material into the sacral canals.

INDICATIONS

The combined lumbosacral paravertebral approach to neural blockade of the lower extremity conserves neither the number of needle insertions nor the total volume of solution used, compared to the more traditional "four-nerve block" approach to be described. It does offer the benefit of anesthesia over the upper thigh, hip, and perineum, which the peripheral nerve blocks do not. It may thus be used for high amputations and for the relief of sciatic pain. It is also useful when immediate access to the individual nerves is not possible; for example, owing to trauma or infection.

SCIATIC NERVE BLOCK

ANATOMY

The largest of the four major nerves supplying the leg is the sciatic nerve (L4–L5, S1–S3). The sciatic nerve, as previously noted, arises from the sacral plexus where it is nearly 2 cm in width as it leaves the pelvis in company with the posterior cutaneous nerve of the thigh. It passes from the pelvis through the sacrosciatic foramen beneath the lower margin of the piriformis muscle, and between the tuberosity of the ischium and the greater trochanter of the femur. The nerve becomes superficial at the lower border of the gluteus maximus muscle. From there, it courses down the posterior aspect of the thigh to the popliteal fossa, where it divides into the tibial and common peroneal nerves. Branches supplying the posterior thigh are given off during the descent of the nerve to the popliteal space. The sciatic nerve supplies sensory innervation to the posterior thigh and entire leg and foot from just below the knee.

TECHNIQUE

Several approaches to blockade of the sciatic nerve have been proposed, primarily to avoid positioning problems that are difficult for trauma patients and the elderly.

Classic Approach of Labat. The classic approach to the sciatic nerve block is with the patient lying on the side opposite the one to be blocked, rolled forward onto the flexed knee with the heel in opposition to the knee of the outstretched dependent leg (Fig. 11-5).

After careful palpation, a line is drawn between points made over the upper aspect of the greater trochanter of the femur and the posterior superior iliac spine. This line should coincide with the upper border of the piriformis muscle and also the upper border of the sacrosciatic foramen (sciatic notch). A line perpendicular and bisecting this is then drawn downward 3 cm and represents the point for injection. A second verification of this point may be made by projecting a line from the greater trochanter to a point 1 to 2 cm below the sacral cornua. This line crosses the perpendicular at about 3 cm and also rep-

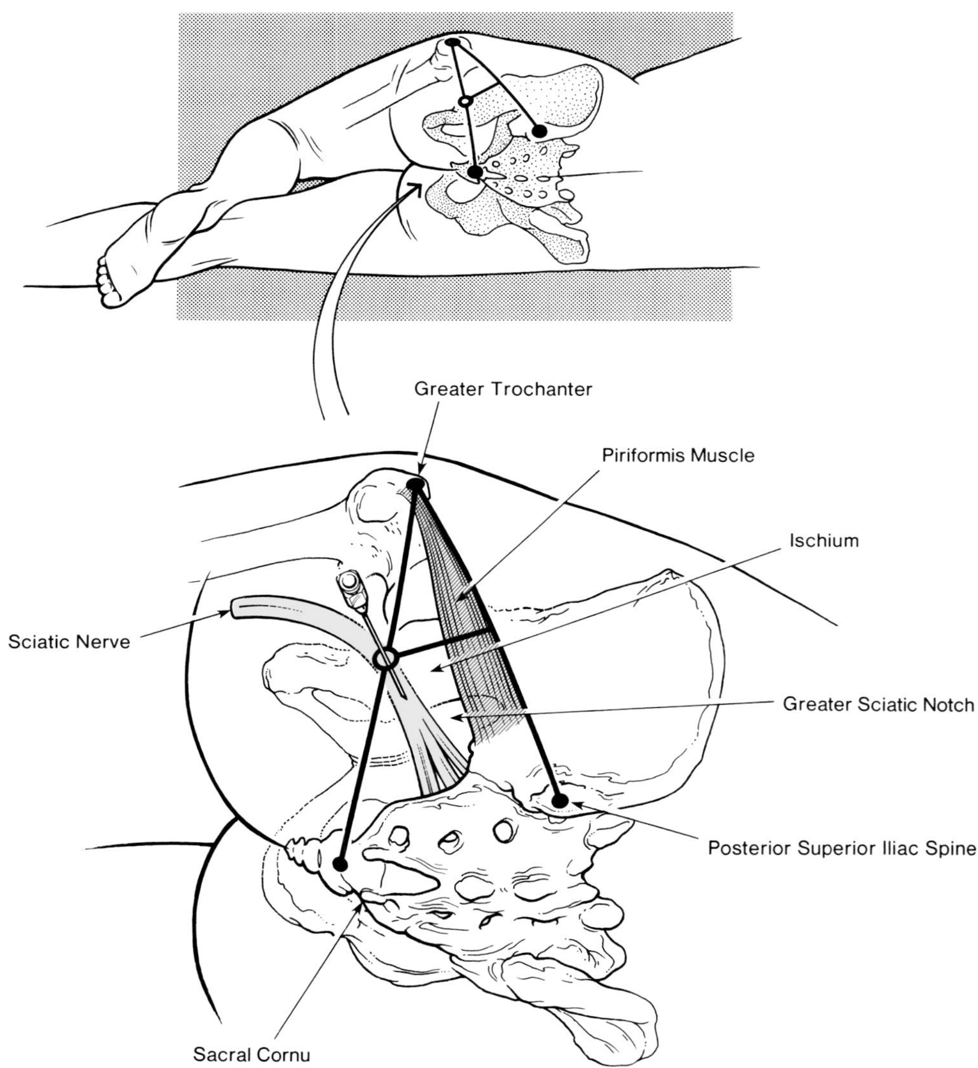

FIG. 11-5. **A.** Landmark anatomy of sciatic nerve components.

resents a point overlying the sciatic nerve where it exits from the pelvis.

A 10- to 12-cm needle is inserted through a wheal made at this point in a direction perpendicular to the skin until it strikes bone. Usually this will occur at 6 to 8 cm in a patient of average stature. Occasionally, the needle will pass into the sciatic notch when it is first introduced. If this occurs, it should be withdrawn nearly to the skin and the tip redirected more cephalad along the perpendicular line until bone is contacted. Determination of the depth of the bony pelvis assists in the correct evaluation of paresthesias, which must be elicited in the leg below the level of the thigh. A geometric-grid approach in searching the notch for sciatic paresthesias will also ensure greater success, compared to random thrusts up and down through the notch. Some also advocate the use of a nerve stimulator (see Chap. 6). Although successful blockade may be accomplished by injecting 10 ml of local anesthetic solution after one paresthesia, the sciatic is a large nerve, and it is often helpful to seek additional paresthesias and inject a total volume of

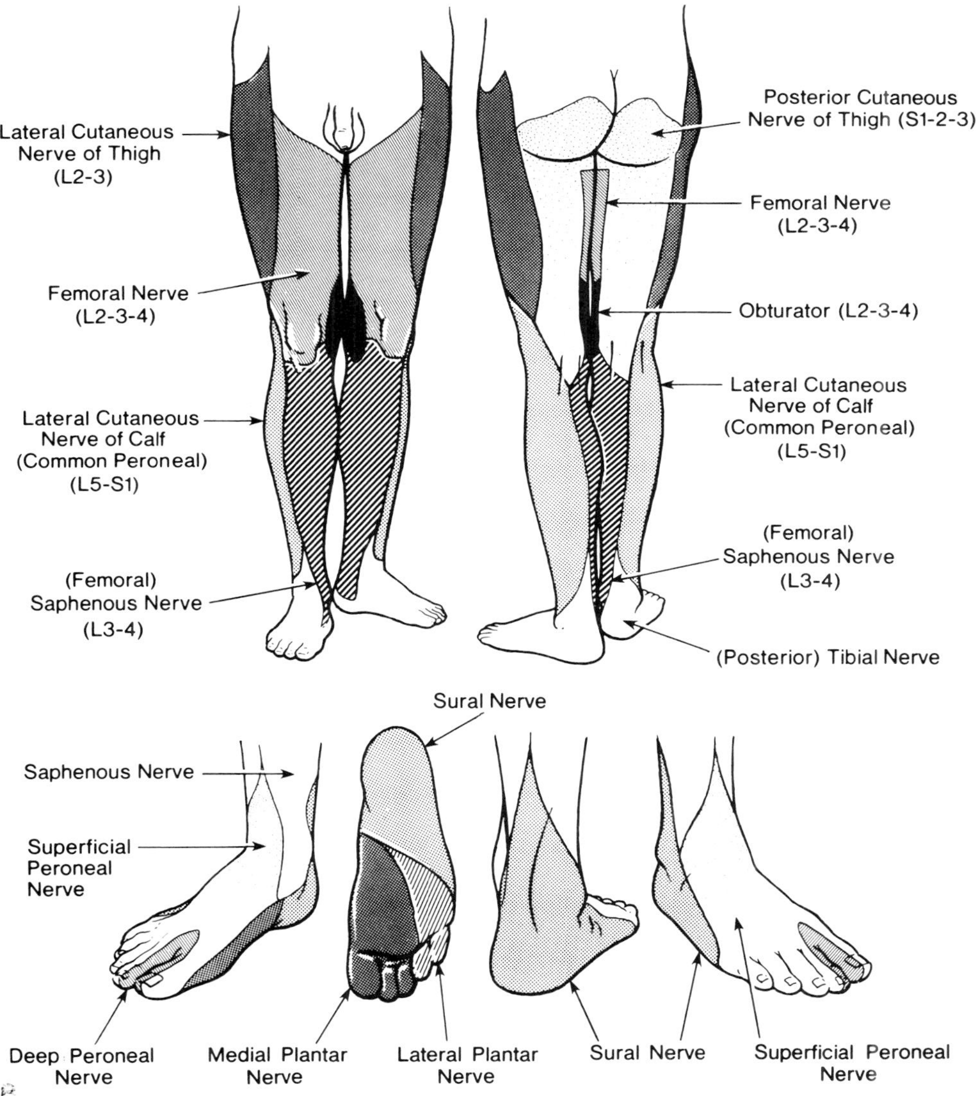

FIG. 11-5. **B.** Cutaneous nerve distribution of the lower limb.

20 to 30 ml of solution. Conceivably, a single paresthesia at the edge of the nerve and injection there would not provide complete anesthesia over the entire nerve.

Recently a technique of continuous sciatic nerve block was described to relieve pain from ischemic gangrene of the foot. This was subsequently combined with a continuous inguinal paravascular block (described later in this chapter) to provide regional anesthesia for the operative procedure and for postoperative pain relief for the first few postoperative days.[36]

The standard posterior approach was used except that the sciatic nerve was identified with a nerve stimulator attached to a standard 16-gauge intravenous infusion cannula. An epidural type catheter was passed through the cannula and advanced about 6 cm into the neurovascular space. Correct catheter placement was verified with radiologic contrast medium. Continuous infusion of a local anesthetic agent with the use of a continuous infusion device connected to the well-anchored catheter should then provide continuous analgesia.

Other Approaches. Labat also describes an *anterior approach* to the sciatic nerve. The nerve passes from the lower border of the gluteus maximus where it is bounded medially by the hamstring muscles. It runs down the thigh, lying on the medial surface of the femur. The posterior femoral cutaneous nerve sometimes branches away from the greater sciatic nerve above the level of blockade and may be missed with this approach.

The patient is placed supine with the lower extremity in a neutral position. A line that represents the inguinal ligament is trisected, and a perpendicular line from the junction of the middle and medial thirds of this line is extended downward and laterally on the anterior aspect of the thigh. The greater trochanter is located by palpation and a line extended from its tuberosity medially across the anterior surface of the thigh parallel to the inguinal ligament. The point of intersection of this line and the perpendicular line from the inguinal ligament represents the point of injection (Fig. 11-6). A 10- to 12.5-cm needle is inserted through a wheal at this point and directed slightly laterally from a plane perpendicular to the skin. The needle is advanced until bone is contacted, then withdrawn and redirected medially and more perpendicular to pass 5 cm beyond the femur, where it should be resting slightly posterior and medial to the femur within the neurovascular compartment (containing the sciatic nerve). After aspiration,

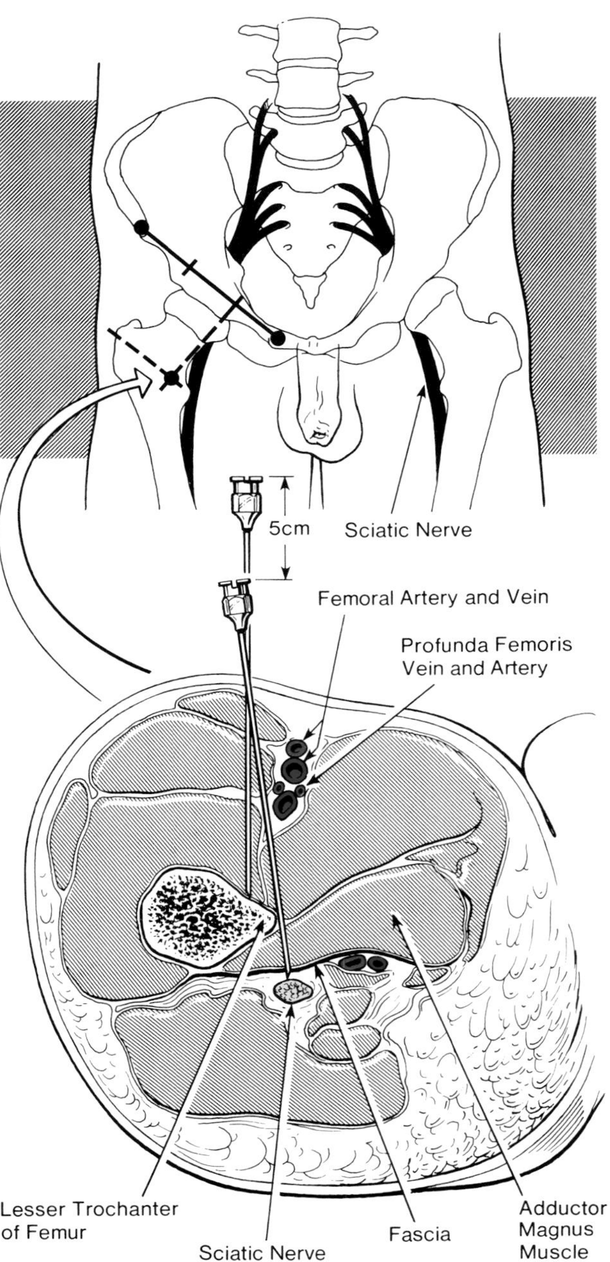

FIG. 11-6. Anterior approach to sciatic nerve block (see text). Cross-section of the leg at the level of the lesser trochanter to show the relationship between the sciatic nerve and the femur, and the fascia separating it from adductor magnus.

a small test dose should be injected to determine ease of injection — whether the needle lies in a muscle bundle or fascial space. The former offers firm resistance to injection, and the needle should be advanced until minimal resistance to injection indicates correct placement. Paresthesias, although not sought, would prove to be helpful. The use of a nerve stimulator would also assist in locating the nerve in this approach. A modification of the anterior approach has been described to aid in locating the neurovascular compartment in children.[23] In adults, the average distance from the femoral surface to the sciatic neurovascular compartment varies little from 4.5 to 6 cm. In pediatric practice, the depth varies with the age and size of the child. It proved helpful to use a "loss of resistance" technique similar to that used for identifying the epidural space. The needle chosen was one removed from a standard 16-gauge intravenous catheter. It was always attached to a 10-ml syringe without regard to the volume of solution intended for injection. The needle with syringe attached was inserted through the skin wheal in the traditional manner until it struck the surface of the femur. It was then "walked off" the medial edge of the femur until it entered the thigh muscles. Continuous pressure was applied to the plunger of the syringe and the needle advanced through the muscle mass. At the point where the needle entered the neurovascular compartment, a sudden loss of resistance occurred similar to that encountered when performing an epidural block. Following aspiration to exclude an intravascular injection, the predetermined amount of solution to be given was injected and the needle removed. It should be noted that smaller bore needles may have too much internal resistance to clearly reflect loss of resistance upon entry into the neurovascular compartment. Once mastered, the success rate with this technique is said to be 95.2%.[23] Fifteen milliliters to 30 ml of local anesthetic solution should then be injected.

The *lithotomy position* has also been advocated to facilitate approaching the sciatic nerve.[29] The anatomy is nearly identical to that in the aforementioned anterior approach. After the sciatic nerve passes between the ischial tuberosity and the greater trochanter, it lies just anterior to the gluteus maximus muscle. The nerve is accompanied at this point by the sciatic artery and the inferior gluteal veins, but they are relatively small vessels and add little risk to the procedure.

The patient is placed supine, and the extremity to be blocked is flexed at the hip as far as possible (90–120°). The extremity may be supported by stirrups, mechanical devices, or an assistant. In this position, the gluteus maximus muscle is flattened and the sciatic nerve relatively more superficial. A line is drawn between the ischial tuberosity and the greater trochanter and a wheal raised at its midpoint. A 12- to 15-cm needle is inserted perpendicular to the skin and advanced until paresthesias are elicited. (A peripheral nerve stimulator has been advocated but is seldom necessary unless the patient is unable to respond to paresthesias.) Twenty milliliters to 25 ml of a local anesthetic solution is then injected.

A lateral approach to the sciatic nerve has also been described.[10] The sciatic nerve is approached from the lateral thigh with the patient lying supine. The earliest report of a lateral approach was by Ichiyanaghi in 1959 but was thought by many to be "extremely difficult."[13] The quadratus femoris is the lowermost of the short rotators of the hip crossed by the sciatic nerve on its way to the posterior compartment of the thigh. The subgluteal space, wherein lies the sciatic nerve as it crosses this muscle, can be identified in relation to the femur and the ischial tuberosity.

The block is performed with a 15-cm needle and uses the nerve stimulator (see Chap. 6). The patient lies supine with the whole limb exposed and with the hip held in the natural position. After appropriate skin preparation and drape, the needle is inserted through a skin wheal made 3 cm distal to the point of maximum lateral prominence of the trochanter, along the posterior profile of the femur (Fig. 11-7). Upon striking the bone of the femoral shaft, the needle is redirected to slide under the femur and is advanced to a total depth of 8 to 12 cm to reach the sciatic nerve. The nerve stimulator may elicit response from any of the three motor components of the sciatic. After correct identification of the nerve, a minimum of 20 ml of local anesthetic is injected.

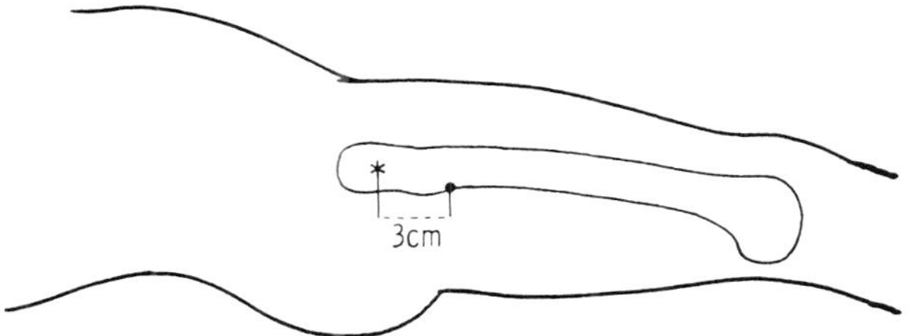

FIG. 11-7. Landmarks for insertion of the needle for lateral approach to sciatic nerve. (Guardini, R.: Acta Scand, *29*:516, 1985.)

SIDE-EFFECTS AND COMPLICATIONS

Sciatic nerve block is primarily a somatic nerve block. It does carry some sympathetic fibers to the extremity, however, and may therefore allow pooling of small quantities of blood—usually insufficient to cause significant hypotension. On some occasions, this sympathetic block may be therapeutically exploited. The effect of compensatory vasoconstriction on the opposite extremity should, however, be considered. There is some evidence that tissue oxygenation may be further reduced during this period of compensation, although it is unlikely that this is of clinical significance.[4]

No significant complications secondary to this block have been documented. Residual dysesthesias for periods of 1 to 3 days are reported by some patients but are usually self-remitting.[34] It is reported that these minor problems may result from the use of long-bevel needles, producing damage to nerve fascicles.

INDICATIONS

As one considers the sensory and cutaneous distribution of the sciatic nerve, it is not surprising that few surgical procedures could be accomplished using sciatic nerve block as the sole anesthetic (perhaps operations on the sole of the foot and the digits). More frequently, however, it is combined with one or more of the nerve blocks yet to be described to provide a significantly larger field of surgical anesthesia.

In recent times with increasing emphasis on pain relief, sciatic nerve block has been advocated for children for postoperative pain relief.[23] Although blocks were done before surgery but after induction of anesthesia, general anesthesia was maintained during surgery and the effectiveness of the block evaluated in providing postoperative pain relief. In a series of 82 patients, the analgesic success rate was 95.2%. The use of sciatic block, either single injection or with the continuous infusion technique, for treatment of long-term pain, acute or chronic, secondary to ischemia or causalgia has also been reported.[10,36] Certainly when there are contraindications to epidural or lumbar paravertebral blocks in the treatment of these pain syndromes, one should consider the use of sciatic nerve blocks.

A few surgical procedures may be accomplished under sciatic nerve block alone. The block is, however, usually combined with femoral, obturator, or lateral femoral cutaneous nerve block to provide complete anesthesia of the lower extremity.

FEMORAL NERVE BLOCK

The femoral nerve (L2–L4) proceeds from the lumbar plexus in the groove between the psoas major and iliac muscles, where it enters the thigh by passing deep to the inguinal ligament. At the level of the inguinal ligament, the femoral nerve lies anterior to the iliopsoas muscle and slightly lateral to the femoral artery (see Fig. 11-3). It is important to remember that at or even above the level of the inguinal ligament, the femoral nerve divides into an anterior and posterior bundle. The anterior branches innervate the skin that covers the anterior surface of the thigh along with the sartorius muscle; the posterior branches innervate the quadriceps muscles, the knee joint, and its medial ligament and give rise to the saphenous nerve, which descends over the medial side of the calf to supply the skin down to the medial malleolus. Another classification of the divided femoral nerve is into superficial and deep, which correspond to the aforementioned anterior and posterior. It may be helpful to recall that, in general, the deep branches are chiefly motor in function with articular branches to the hip and knee joints. The superficial branches are chiefly sensory and cutaneous in their distribution. They supply the anterior, anteromedial, and medial aspects of the thigh, the knee, and the upper portion of the leg.

TECHNIQUE

Classic Approach of Labat. The patient lies supine and may be sedated, since paresthesias are helpful but not essential to this particular method. The femoral artery is palpated immediately below the inguinal ligament, and a wheal raised immediately lateral to the artery. A line drawn from the anterior superior iliac spine to the symphysis pubis will approximate the inguinal ligament, with the wheal adjacent to the femoral artery being approximately 1 to 2 cm below this line (see Fig. 11-3). A 3- to 4-cm needle, without syringe, is advanced perpendicular to the skin until a paresthesia is elicited or the needle undergoes maximum lateral pulsation from its position adjacent to and slightly deep to the artery. It should be repositioned until one of these two indicators has been achieved. If paresthesias occur, 10 to 20 ml of local anesthetic solution should be injected, after careful aspiration, to ensure against intravascular injection. If no paresthesias occur, then 7 to 10 ml of local anesthetic is deposited fanwise lateral to the artery. The needle should then be carefully repositioned adjacent to the artery and the injection repeated.

An alternate technique uses a single needle placement similar to the paravascular inguinal technique previously described.[15] This technique is based on the fact that two fascial layers can be identified by the use of a short beveled needle. Recall that the femoral triangle is covered by the fascia lata; however, in contrast to the femoral vessels that are in a plane between the fascia lata and the underlying fascia iliaca, the femoral nerve lies deep to both.

The fundamental technique is the same as the others previously described; however, the advancing needle is felt to "pop" through the two layers of fascia, that is, a sudden loss of resistance upon passing through each fascial layer. Paresthesias need not be elicited. The needle is aspirated and 20 to 30 ml of local anesthetic solution is injected.

Paravascular Approach. An alternate technique for femoral nerve block has been noted in conjunction with blockade of the lumbar plexus (see Fig. 11-3).[38] This paravascular technique requires elicitation of paresthesias and a cooperative patient or, failing that, a nerve stimulator.

COMPLICATIONS AND SIDE-EFFECTS

As with the sciatic nerve block, some of the sympathetic fibers to the lower extremity are blocked with the femoral procedure; however, with femoral block this is more likely to be advantageous to blood flow without being of a magnitude likely to produce systemic hypotension. Inasmuch as the site of blockade is adjacent to a major artery and vein, hematoma at the site is a possibility. Although this probably occurs, it is seldom if ever a complication of clinical significance. With the advent of vascular surgery,the anesthesiologist should be alert to the presence of vascular grafts of the femoral artery, which would be a relative contraindication for elective femoral nerve block.

Residual nerve involvement—dysesthesias or paresis—is remotely possible, but trauma to the nerve from these techniques is minimal, and such complication therefore highly unlikely.

INDICATIONS

Surgical use of femoral nerve block includes operations of the anterior portion of the thigh, both superficial and deep. As with sciatic nerve block, the femoral nerve block is usually part of the combined block approach, incorporating not only sciatic but also lateral femoral cutaneous and obturator nerves.

Recently, additional uses for femoral nerve block have been recommended. Despite earlier concerns regarding the use of local anesthetic agents in patients suspected of malignant hyperthermia, femoral nerve block combined with lateral femoral cutaneous nerve block was used successfully in 103 patients, ranging in age from 4 to 76 years, undergoing muscle biopsy as the diagnostic test for the suspected disease.[1]

The analgesic role of femoral nerve block was noted to be effective in patients with a fractured shaft of the femur[2] and has now been expanded to the total perioperative period. Orthopedic surgeons evaluating acute knee injuries in outpatients used a combination of sciatic and femoral nerve blocks to examine patients in whom clinical examination under local infiltration was considered totally unreliable secondary to severe pain. They achieved a 96% successful examination rate and suggested its potential for outpatient arthroscopy.[31] Not surprising, then, that there has appeared a report comparing the paravascular inguinal technique alone and in combination with the lateral femoral cutaneous nerve block with traditional general anesthesia for outpatient knee arthroscopy.[27] Both regional techniques were deemed better than general anesthesia, but inclusion of the lateral femoral cutaneous nerve block improved analgesia on the lateral side of the knee. Recovery time for general anesthesia was significantly longer than with either regional technique.

Femoral nerve blocks alone have also been shown to be an effective adjunct to general anesthesia for knee joint surgery.[30] It was also noted that blocks performed before surgery were more effective than those done after surgery. Postoperative opiate administration was reduced by 80% in the recovery room and by 40% in the first 24 hours postoperatively in patients receiving nerve blocks. Although this study was done in adults, similar work has been performed in a group of 50 children undergoing procedures on the lower limbs who would require postoperative narcotic analgesia.[24] After induction of general anesthesia, a combination of femoral and lateral femoral cutaneous nerve block was performed. There was a 96% success rate with a significant reduction in postoperative narcotic analgesia.

LATERAL FEMORAL CUTANEOUS NERVE BLOCK

The lateral femoral cutaneous nerve (L2–L3) emerges at the lateral border of the psoas muscle at a level lower than the ilioinguinal nerve. It passes obliquely under the iliac fascia and across the iliac muscle to enter the thigh deep to the inguinal ligament at a point approximately 1 to 2 cm medial to the anterior superior iliac spine. It then crosses or passes through the tendonous origin of the sartorius muscle and courses downward beneath the fascia lata. It emerges from the fascia lata at a point 7 to 10 cm below the anterior superior iliac spine where it branches into anterior and posterior branches. The anterior branch supplies the skin over the anterolateral aspect of the thigh as low as the knee. The posterior branch pierces the fascia lata and passes backward to supply the skin on the lateral side of the thigh from just below the greater trochanter to about the middle of the thigh (Fig. 11-8).

TECHNIQUE

The patient is placed in the supine position. After palpation of the anterior superior iliac spine, a skin wheal is placed 2 to 3 cm inferior and 2 to 3 cm medial to it. A 3- to 4-cm needle with syringe attached is then inserted through the wheal and perpendicular to the skin surface. Soon after passing through the skin, the firm fascia lata is felt and then a sudden release as the needle passes through. Ten milliliters of a local anesthetic solution should be deposited fanwise as the needle is moved upward and downward, depositing solution both above and below the fascia, most of it below (Fig. 11-8).

An alternate technique is to direct the needle through the skin wheal in a slightly lateral and cephalad direction to strike the iliac bone just medial and below the anterior superior iliac spine. Since the nerve emerges here, the deposition of 10 ml of local anesthetic solution in a medial fanwise fashion will also accomplish satisfactory blockade of the nerve. If the volume of the solution is of no concern to the total dose of drug administered, then the nerve could be blocked in both places on the same patient to doubly ensure success.

Another modification of this technique attempts to locate the fascial canal in which the nerve lies as it passes under the inguinal canal. Reportedly this allows a single injection of a lesser volume of local anesthetic, an important consideration in nerve blocks for children.[7] A short beveled needle is inserted just medial to the anterior superior iliac spine and advanced until the loss of resistance ("pop") is felt as the needle passes through the external oblique aponeurosis. With syringe attached, the needle is advanced through the second loss of resistance of the

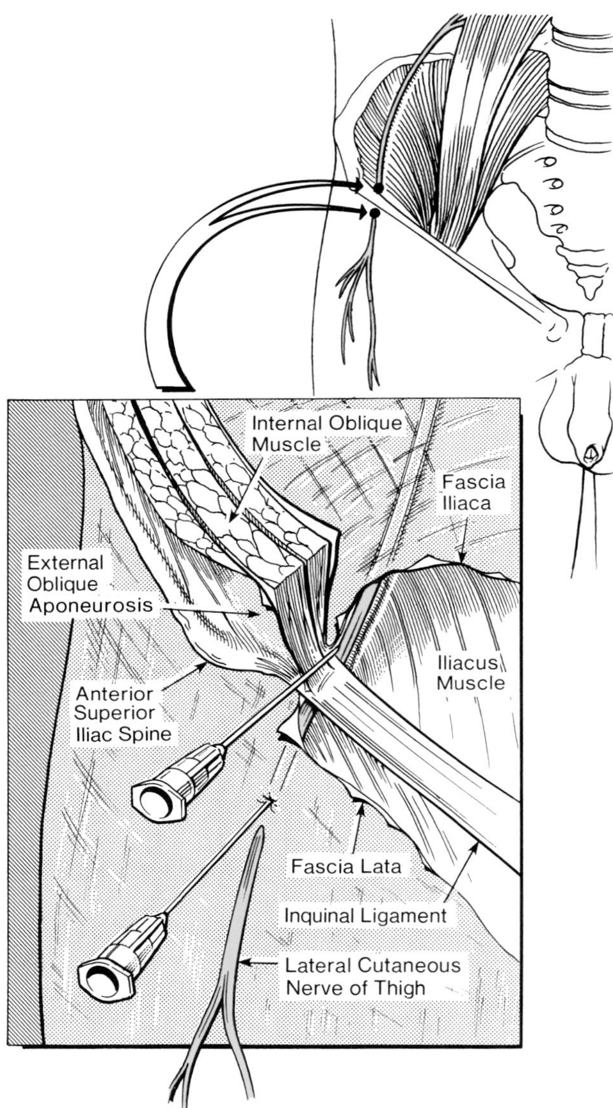

FIG. 11-8. Lateral cutaneous nerve block (see text). The lateral cutaneous nerve of the thigh passes inferiorly on iliacus muscle covered by iliacus fascia. Just medial to the anterior superior iliac spine it turns anteriorly to pass just below the inguinal ligament and runs deep to the fascia lata until it emerges subcutaneously. The lateral cutaneous nerve can be blocked just medially to the anterior superior iliac spine or 1 to 2 cm below it.

internal oblique muscle and the underlying fascia iliacus. At this point, the 5- to 10-ml volume of local anesthetic should be injected easily (Fig. 11-8).

COMPLICATIONS AND SIDE-EFFECTS

With the exception of a remotely possible dysesthesia or hypoesthesia, there are no known risks to this nerve block technique.

INDICATIONS

Lateral femoral cutaneous nerve block by itself is extremely suitable for anesthetizing the donor site before the removal of small skin grafts. Its primary indication as a supplement to the femoral and sciatic nerve blocks for operating on the lower extremity is the provision of analgesia for tourniquet pain. Since one of the terminal anterior branches forms part of the patellar plexus, it must be included with the other nerve blocks for operations on the knee, with or without tourniquet.

OBTURATOR NERVE BLOCK

The obturator nerve (L2–L4) derives its major source from L3–L4—the portion coming from L2 is very small and sometimes even lacking. The nerve appears at the medial border of the psoas muscle, covered anteriorly by the external iliac vessels, and passes downward in the pelvis. It continues with the obturator vessels along the obturator groove and passes through the obturator foramen into the thigh. As the nerve passes through the obturator canal, it divides into posterior and anterior branches. The anterior branch supplies an articular branch to the hip joint, the anterior adductor muscles and cutaneous branches, to the lower inner thigh. The size or existence of this cutaneous innervation is small and variable depending on which anatomic reference material is quoted. The posterior branch innervates the deep adductor muscles and frequently sends an articular branch to the knee joint, which may be important in providing analgesia for knee surgery.

Some anatomy books describe an accessory obturator nerve that leaves the medial border of the psoas muscle in company with the obturator nerve. It has been said to be incorrectly named, having much more in common with the femoral nerve.[18] Like the femoral nerve, it passes over, not under, the pubic ramus where it supplies the pectineus muscle. It is present in about one third of individuals.

TECHNIQUE

The patient is placed supine with the leg to be blocked in slight abduction. Caution should be taken to protect the skin of the genitalia from irritating antiseptic solutions used in preparing the area. It should not be necessary to shave the pubic area to be blocked.

The pubic tubercle is palpated and a skin wheal raised 1 to 2 cm below and 1 to 2 cm lateral to it. A 7- to 8-cm needle, without syringe attached, is introduced through the wheal in a slight medial direction to strike the horizontal ramus of the pubis. It is then withdrawn and redirected approximately 45° in a cephalad direction to identify the superior bony portion of the obturator canal. The depth at which the needle strikes bone in each direction should be noted. The needle is again withdrawn and the point redirected slightly laterally and inferiorly and passes into the obturator canal. It should be advanced 2 to 3 cm beyond the previously noted depth of bone where, after careful aspiration to ensure the obturator vessels have not been entered, 10 to 15 ml of local anesthetic is injected. Only by identifying the bony wall of the canal can the anesthesiologist be certain that the needle has passed into the canal rather than into the soft tissues (*e.g.*, bladder or vagina) medially or superiorly (Fig. 11-9). The presence of successful obturator nerve block is determined by demonstrating paresis of the adductor muscles, since the cutaneous distribution is small and inconstant.

A modification of this technique advocates searching for paresthesias to the area of the inner thigh.[26] If paresthesias are not elicited, then it is suggested that a fan-like wall of anesthesia be deposited. The major difference in the two techniques lies in a greater attempt to palpate the tendon of the adductor longus muscle, which constitutes the upper medial aspect of the obturator foramen. With gentle deep palpation, one may be able to palpate the entire foramen and, placing the skin wheal inferior to the midpoint of the superior pubic ramus, gain a more precise location of the obturator nerve.

COMPLICATIONS AND SIDE-EFFECTS

Obturator nerve block has vascular and neural complications and side-effects nearly identical to those of the femoral nerve. Similarly, these represent remote

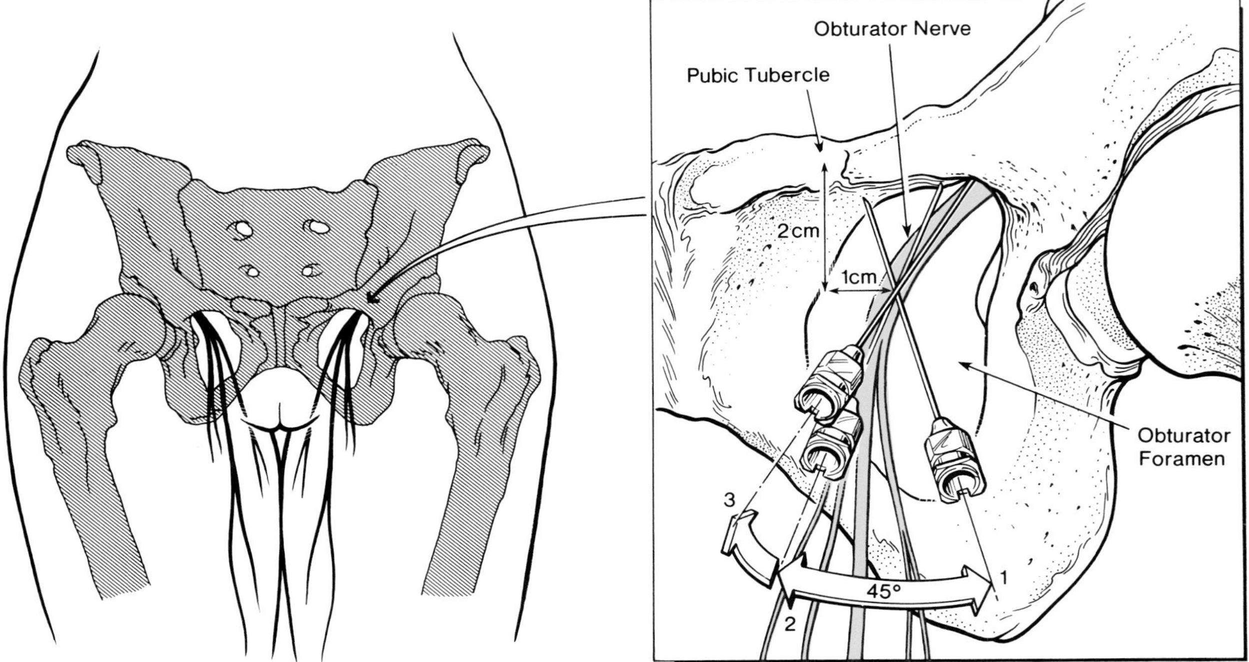

FIG. 11-9. Anatomy of obturator nerve, showing bony landmarks used in nerve block technique (see text).

possibilities rather than clinically important considerations.

INDICATIONS

Obturator nerve block is a valuable technique in diagnosing painful conditions of the hip and in the relief of adductor spasm of the hip. It is also necessary as a supplement to sciatic, femoral, and lateral femoral cutaneous nerve blocks for surgery on or above the knee.

NERVE BLOCKS AROUND THE KNEE

Three major nerve trunks can be blocked at the level of the knee: the saphenous, the common peroneal, and the tibial.

ANATOMY

The *saphenous nerve* is the cutaneous and terminal extension of the femoral nerve. It supplies the skin over the medial, anteromedial, and posteromedial aspects of the leg, extending from above the knee as far distal as the ball of the great toe.

The common peroneal and tibial nerves are extensions from the sciatic nerve. The *tibial nerve* arises at the upper end of the popliteal fossa and is the larger of the two terminal branches of the sciatic nerve. It has both a muscular branch to the back of the leg and cutaneous branches in the popliteal fossa and down the back of the leg to the ankle. The *common peroneal nerve* is about one half the size of the tibial nerve, being the other portion of the sciatic nerve when it bifurcates at the upper end of the popliteal space. It contains articular branches to the knee joint and cutaneous nerves to the lateral side of the leg, heel, and ankle (see Figs. 11-5B and 11-10).

TECHNIQUES

One of the unexplained phenomena of regional blockade is the uniform lack of enthusiasm for, and even less advocacy of, blockade of individual nerves

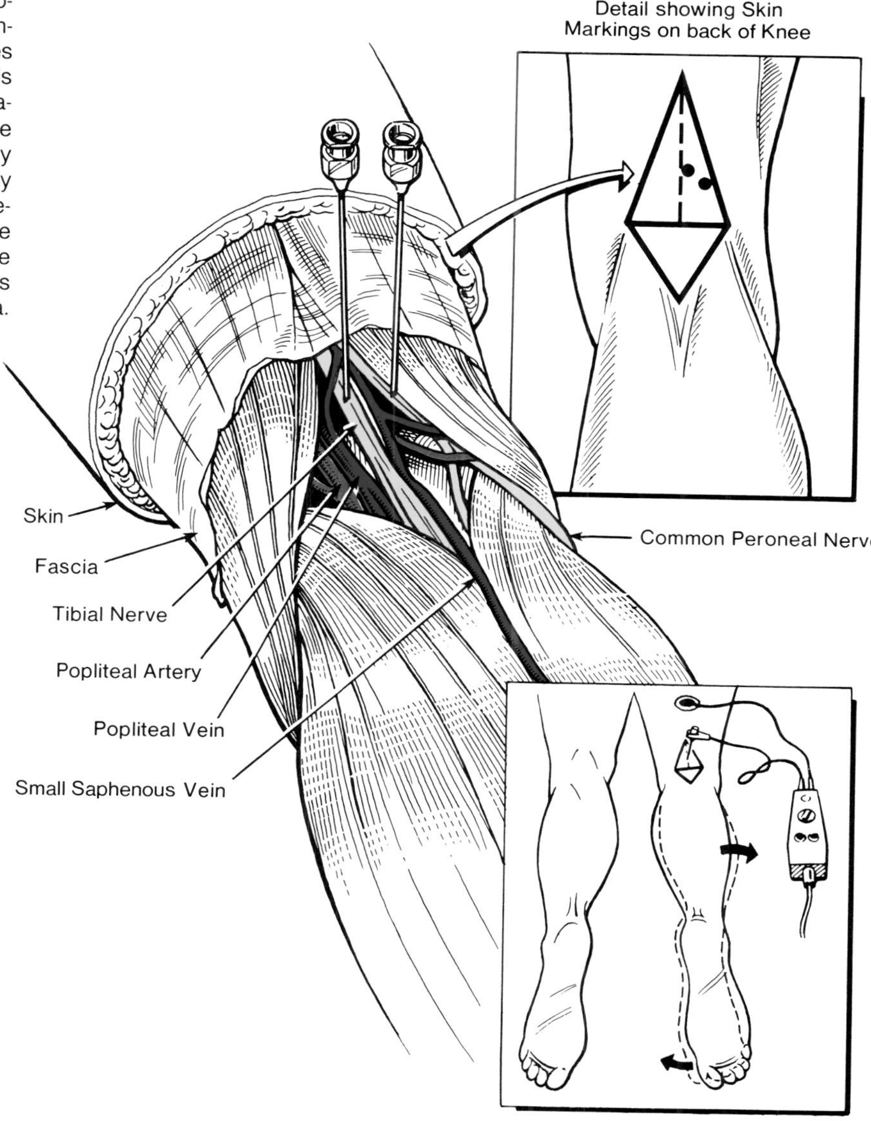

FIG. 11-10. Tibial and common peroneal nerve block. The tibial and common peroneal (lateral popliteal) nerves diverge in the popliteal fossa, which is bounded by biceps femoris muscle laterally and semimembranosus muscle medially. They can be blocked as they pass through the triangle formed by these muscles and a line drawn between the femoral condyles. As the needle is inserted, a loss of resistance should be felt as the needle penetrates the fascia overlying the popliteal fossa.

at the level of the knee by any of the authors of studies on regional anesthesia (Braun, Labat, Pitkin, Sherwood–Dunn, Eriksson, and Moore). Some have reluctantly recommended circular infiltration at the thigh, and Löfström advocates only a block of the saphenous nerve, stating that ". . . tibial nerve block is difficult to perform and peroneal nerve block, though simple to carry out where the nerve winds round the head of the fibula, may carry a considerable risk of postanesthetic neuritis."[20] Documentation of these criticisms, however, seems lacking in the literature. It is important, therefore that the anesthesiologist wishing to pursue nerve blocks of the knee undertake a careful review of the associated anatomy. More recently, there have been reports in the literature advocating nerve blocks in this area with documentation of both efficacy and safety.[14,16,32]

The popliteal fossa is a diamond-shaped area bounded inferiorly by the medial and lateral heads of the gastrocnemius muscles and superiorly by the long head of the biceps femoris laterally and the superimposed tendons of the semitendinosus and semimembranosus medially. As the sciatic nerve bifurcates, the larger tibial nerve goes medially and the common peroneal nerve laterally. Because the popliteal fossa is filled with fat, diffusion of injected local anesthetics may be impaired and requires that the needle tip be as close as possible to the nerve before injection. This is usually achieved by the use of paresthesias or the nerve stimulator. It is particularly important to know that the nerves are superficial to the popliteal vessels and are located about midway between the skin and the posterior surface of the femur. The distance from skin to nerve in the average adult is 1.5 to 2.0 cm.[32]

The patient, in the prone position, is asked to lift (flex) the leg, which allows the upper borders of the popliteal fossa to become more palpable. Once outlined, the popliteal fossa is divided into equal medial and lateral triangles, with the base of the two triangles being the skin crease behind the knee joint (Fig. 11-10). A skin wheal 5 cm superior to the skin crease and 1 cm lateral to the midline of the triangles should lie over the tibial and common peroneal nerves. Insert a 6- to 7.5-cm, 22-gauge needle at an angle of 45° to 60° to the skin with the tip in an anterior and superior direction. The needle is advanced until a paresthesia is obtained and 35 to 40 ml of local anesthetic solution is injected. The saphenous nerve block is performed by injecting 5 to 10 ml of local anesthetic solution deeply subcutaneously in a 5-cm area just below the medial surface of the tibial condyle.[32]

INDICATIONS

The paucity of reports on nerve blocks at the knee may be due to the relative narrow area of analgesia provided when compared to the more proximal nerve blocks previously described or to blockade of nerves at the ankles. Even so, lack of access to these nerves proximally and reduced dose of local anesthetic drugs in blocks at the knee justify familiarity with these techniques. Kofoed[16] reported 284 outpatients receiving peripheral nerve blocks at the knee and ankle for a variety of operations such as hallux valgus, suture of ligaments and tendons, removal of soft tissue and bony tumors, synovectomy of metatarsal joints, and toe amputations. Kempthorne and Brown[14] noted the benefit of these blocks in children as an adjunct to surgical anesthesia as well as for postoperative analgesia. Block of the tibial nerve has also been used as a diagnostic block in a child with myotonia and as an adjunct to physiotherapy for treatment of severe equinus deformity in children.

COMPLICATIONS AND EFFICACY

The satisfactory response to these blocks is similar to other peripheral nerve blocks and likely reflects appropriate management of the patient and satisfactory performance of the block (see Chap. 6). Rorie and associates reported 82% success in 130 patients, with 6.2% requiring general anesthesia. Four patients reported postoperative symptoms similar to dysesthesias, all spontaneously remitting in less than 1 month.[32] Kofoed[16] reported a 95% success rate without any complications, whereas Kempthorne[14] did not quote a success rate but noted no complications after 50 nerve blocks at the knee.

NERVE BLOCKS AT THE ANKLE

Five branches of the principal nerve trunks supply the ankle and foot: posterior tibial, sural, superficial peroneal (musculocutaneous), saphenous, and deep peroneal (anterior tibial).[22] These nerves are relatively easy to block at the ankle (Fig. 11-11).

TIBIAL NERVE BLOCK

The tibial nerve (L4–L5, S1–S3), the larger of the two branches of the sciatic nerve, reaches the distal part of the leg from the medial side of the Achilles tendon, where it lies behind the posterior tibial artery. The nerve then gives off the medial calcaneal branch to the inside of the heel, after which it divides at the back of the medial malleolus into the medial and lateral plantar nerves, both under the abductor hallucis running to the sole of the foot. The medial branch supplies the medial two thirds of the sole and plantar portion of the medial three and one-half toes up to the nail. The lateral branch supplies the lateral one third of the sole and plantar portion of the lateral one and one-half toes.

The patient lies prone with the ankle supported by a pillow. A skin wheal is raised lateral to the posterior tibial artery, if the artery is palpable. If the artery is not palpable, then the wheal is placed to the medial side of the Achilles tendon, level with the upper border of the medial malleolus. A 1- to 3-cm needle is advanced through the wheal at a right angle to the posterior aspect of the tibia, lateral to the artery. Shifting the needle in a mediolateral position may elicit a paresthesia, and then 3 to 5 ml of local anesthetic solution should be injected. If paresthesias are not obtained, 5 to 7 ml of local anesthetic solution is

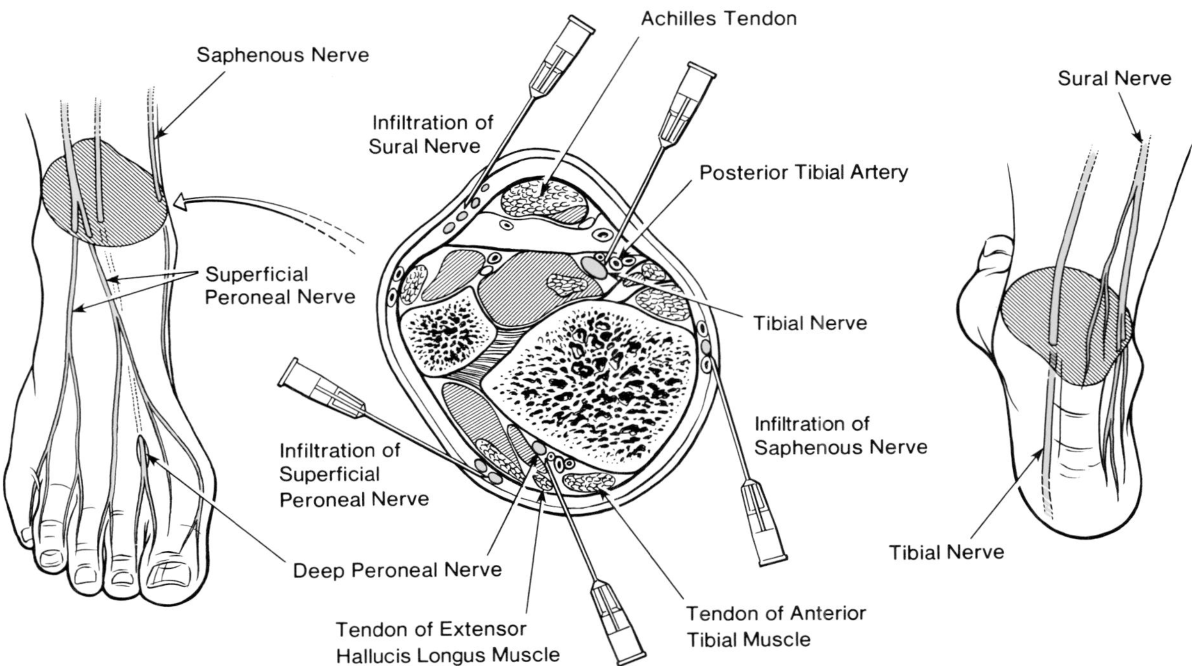

FIG. 11-11. Anatomy and technique of neural blockade for nerves at the ankle.

injected against the posterior aspect of the tibia while the needle is withdrawn 1 cm.

SURAL NERVE BLOCK

The sural nerve is a cutaneous nerve that arises through the union of a branch from the tibial nerve and one from the common peroneal nerve. It becomes subcutaneous somewhat distal to the middle of the leg and proceeds along with the short saphenous vein behind and below the lateral malleolus to supply the lower posterolateral surface of the leg, the lateral side of the foot, and the lateral part of the fifth toe (Fig. 11-11).

With the patient in the same position as for tibial nerve block, a skin wheal is raised lateral to the Achilles tendon at the level of the lateral malleolus. A 1- to 3-cm needle in inserted through the wheal approximately 1 cm and angled toward the fibula, where paresthesias may be sought. If no paresthesias occur, infiltration is accomplished from the Achilles tendon to the outer border of the lateral malleolus. Three milliliters to 5 ml of local anesthetic solution injected fanwise is usually sufficient to produce analgesia. Often the tibial and sural nerves are blocked at the same time with the same needles and equipment.

SUPERFICIAL PERONEAL NERVE BLOCK

The superficial peroneal nerve (L4–L5, S1–S2) perforates the deep fascia on the anterior aspect of the distal two thirds of the leg and runs subcutaneously to supply the dorsum of the foot and toes, except for the contiguous surfaces of the great and second toes.

The superficial peroneal nerve is blocked immediately above and medial to the lateral malleolus. A subcutaneous infiltration of 5 to 10 ml of local anesthetic solution is spread from the anterior border of the tibia to the superior aspect of the lateral malleolus (Fig. 11-11).

DEEP PERONEAL NERVE BLOCK

The deep peroneal nerve (L4–L5, S1–S2) courses down the anterior aspect of the interosseus membrane of the leg and continues midway between the malleoli onto the dorsum of the foot. Here, it innervates the short extensors of the toes as well as the skin on the adjacent areas of the first and second toes. At the level of the foot, the anterior tibial artery lies medial to the nerve, as does the tendon of extensor hallucis longus muscle.

The deep peroneal nerve is blocked in the lower portion of the leg by placing a wheal between the tendons of the anterior tibial and extensor hallucis longus muscles at a level just superior to the malleoli. Often the anterior tibial artery may be palpated. If this is possible, the skin wheal and nerve should be just lateral to the artery. The needle is advanced toward the tibia, and 3 to 5 ml of local anesthetic solution is injected (Fig. 11-11).

SAPHENOUS NERVE BLOCK

The saphenous nerve, which is the sensory terminal branch of the femoral nerve, becomes subcutaneous at the lateral side of the knee joint. It then follows the great saphenous vein to the medial malleolus and supplies the cutaneous area over the medial side of the lower leg anterior to the medial malleolus and the medial part of the foot as far forward as the midportion. Occasionally, its innervation extends to the metatarsophalangeal joint.

To block the saphenous nerve, a skin wheal is raised immediately above and anterior to the medial malleolus, and 3 to 5 ml of local anesthetic solution is infiltrated subcutaneously around the great saphenous vein (Fig. 11-11).

It is apparent that all five nerve blocks at the ankle, undertaken simultaneously, would produce a ring of infiltration around the ankle at the level of the malleoli. Such an approach has, in fact, been advocated by more than one textbook of regional anesthesia; it is possible and usually successful at the distal extremes of all extremities and digits. Nonetheless, with circular infiltration there is the hazard of vascular occlusion if large volumes of anesthetic solutions are injected, especially if they contain epinephrine. In general, block to a specific nerve, such as one of those just described, with smaller quantities of non-epinephrine-containing solutions of local anesthetic agents has a higher success rate with less risk.

Recently a technique has been reported for a "midtarsal" approach to nerve block of the forefoot.[35] Injections are made immediately distal to the ankle joint where the nerves are accessible without having to reposition the patient.

Posterior Tibial Nerve. With the patient in the supine position, the leg is rotated externally. The posterior tibial artery is palpated where it passes behind the medial malleolus. Three milliliters to 5 ml of local anesthesia is injected on either side of the artery. If no pulse is palpable, local anesthesia is still injected at this point and deep to the fascia (Fig. 11-11).

Deep Peroneal Nerve. The patient lying supine is asked to extend the great toe to facilitate palpation of the extensor hallucis longus tendon. The dorsalis pedus artery is usually palpable several millimeters lateral to the tendon. Two milliliters or 3 ml of local anesthesia is injected deep to the fascia and on either side of the artery and distal to the extensor retinaculum (Fig. 11-11).

Saphenous, Superficial Peroneal, and Sural Nerves. The technique for these nerves is the same as previously described. A total of 15 ml of local anesthetic per foot is acceptable; however, this can be reduced to 10 ml for bilateral foot procedures once the necessary skills are obtained.

Still another modification of nerve block at the ankle has been proposed while leaving the patient in the supine position.[33] The foot is extended to 90° relative to the leg and propped up on sheets or some other lift for easier access. Flexing and supporting the knee also improve access to the posterior tibial nerve. This nerve can also be blocked at a more proximal site—two fingerbreaths proximal to the medial malleolus with the needle inserted tangential to the medial border of the Achilles tendon and perpendicular to the tibia. The remainder of the nerves are approached as previously noted.

INDICATIONS AND COMPLICATIONS

Ankle block is indicated on nearly all surgical procedures of the foot. In the two series previously noted, these included such procedures as Morton's neuroma, operations on the great toe, including bunionectomy and amputation, amputation of midfoot and toes for peripheral vascular disease, metatarsal osteotomy, incision, drainage, and debridement procedures.

No major complications have been reported. Patients did not even complain significantly of tourniquet pain in one series.[35] One patient complained of dysesthesia for 3 to 4 weeks.

METATARSAL AND DIGITAL NERVE BLOCK

The relationship of the terminal nerves to the metatarsal bones and the toes is very similar to that of the structures of the hand, with the nerve fibers passing through the intermetatarsal space and alongside each toe, where they become the digital nerves.

Nerve block in the intermetatarsal space is very similar to the metacarpal block. Skin wheals are raised on the dorsum of the foot over the proximal aspect of each metatarsal space that bounds the toes to be blocked. Local anesthetic solutions are then infiltrated in a fanwise direction between the two wheals, taking care not to pierce the sole of the foot. Solution should be injected carefully around the plantar surface of the metatarsal bone as well. Digital block alone can be accomplished by injecting through the wheals at the webs of the toes, depositing 2 to 3 ml of local anesthetic solution along either side of the toes to be blocked. Use of epinephrine in the anesthetic solutions and excessive volumes should be avoided in these blocks (Fig. 11-12).

INTRAVENOUS REGIONAL AND INTRA-ARTICULAR BLOCKS

Although intravenous regional anesthesia in the upper extremity is a widely used technique, it has not been reported extensively for use in the lower limbs (see Chap. 12). When a tourniquet is applied to the thigh, a large dose of local anesthetic agent is required, with resultant failures and occasional reports of toxicity. The tourniquet may be placed either proximally on the thigh or at the ankle.

One prospective study of 58 consecutive unselected patients requiring anesthesia of the lower extremity employed placement of the tourniquet at the thigh.[19] The technique is fundamentally the same as that for intravenous regional anesthesia of the arm. A 7-cm pneumatic tourniquet should be used for adults with an occlusion pressure of 300 mm Hg. Use of the smaller 5-cm tourniquet may fail to provide complete arterial occlusion with pressures in excess of 450 mm Hg.[11] The greater saphenous vein just anterior to the medial malleolus can usually be cannulated with a 20- to 22-gauge needle and secured for vascular access of the local anesthetic agent.

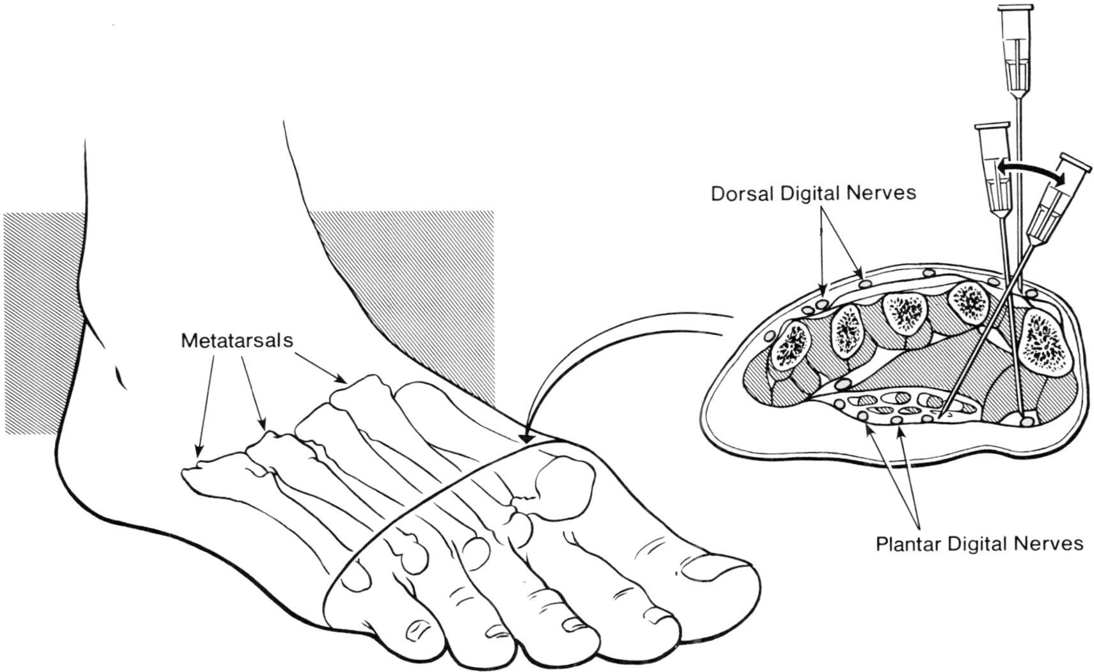

FIG. 11-12. Anatomic relationships and needle placement for metatarsal nerve block.

With the tourniquet placed at the thigh, larger volumes of more dilute solutions are advocated. Lidocaine 0.25% to a total dose of 3.3 mg/kg is recommended.[19] This will provide the 75 to 100 ml of solution desired.

Use of the lower limb tourniquet just above the ankle has also been reported.[8] A double-cuff tourniquet was used and arterial occlusion pressures measured before the start of anesthesia. Cuffs were then inflated 100 mm Hg above occlusion pressure. A maximum volume of 40 to 50 ml of a dilute solution of local anesthetic agent was used (0.25–0.5% lidocaine or mepivacaine). No major complications were noted,[8,11,19] but occasional cases of tinnitus or signs of transient vascular absorption were noted.

Because intravenous regional anesthesia is effective only during the period of tourniquet inflation, it, like general anesthesia, provides no postoperative analgesia. Recently there have been conflicting reports regarding postoperative pain relief achieved by the intra-articular injections of local anesthetic agents. In a comparison of femoral nerve block, intra-articular injection, or nothing, there was no difference in pain relief between intra-articular bupivacaine and the control, whereas only one of ten patients receiving a femoral nerve block had pain.[12] In a prospective study of patients undergoing bilateral Keller's arthroplasty, however, the foot into which bupivacaine was placed into the pseudoarthrosis was significantly more pain-free than was the placebo side.[28] Clearly, additional studies with other procedures and techniques will need to be undertaken before the efficacy of this analgesic technique can be appreciated.

LOCAL ANESTHETIC AGENTS

Although patient selection and regional block equipment have been discussed in Chapter 6, there are some considerations of local anesthetic agents that apply specifically to regional blockade of peripheral nerves. The extremes of the volume–concentration relationships that provide satisfactory anesthesia depend on the knowledge and technical expertise of the anesthesiologist.

Certain properties of the available local anesthetic agents must be exploited if the use of regional block of the lower extremity is to be maximally effective. Some of the more important of these properties are duration, concentration, toxicity, metabolism, and additives, such as epinephrine, carbon dioxide, and hyaluronidase (see Chap. 4).

Consideration of the appropriate agent, concentration, and perhaps an additive should allow the anesthesiologist to provide an optimal nerve block of the lower extremity. In general, because many of the surgical procedures on the lower extremity require little or no muscle relaxation, weaker concentrations of solutions may be used to reduce total dose while providing sufficient volume. For example, with the combined four-nerve block of the leg, it would be possible to use stronger concentrations on the sciatic and femoral blocks and dilute to a weaker solution for primary sensory blockade of the lateral femoral cutaneous and obturator nerves.

It is equally important that the duration of analgesia be selected according to need. For example, a short surgical outpatient procedure may well be performed with 2-chloroprocaine, which would restore the patient to early ambulation, whereas bupivacaine or etidocaine might well be used for a patient who would benefit from prolonged analgesia and the sympathetic block of a sciatic nerve block. Residual neurologic involvement (hypoesthesia and dysesthesia) is not uncommon after nerve block with the very long-acting agents. This should be kept in mind in certain orthopedic procedures, especially those with plaster casts in which postsurgical neural involvement must be recognized.

DURATION

The currently available local anesthetic agents may be separated into three general—albeit overlapping—categories: short-acting, intermediate-acting, and long-acting. The short-acting agents include procaine; 2-chloroprocaine, with or without epinephrine; lidocaine, without epinephrine; and prilocaine, without epinephrine. The intermediate group includes epinephrine-containing solutions of lidocaine and prilocaine; mepivacaine, with or without epinephrine; and perhaps tetracaine without epinephrine. The long-acting agents are effective over a longer period. They include dibucaine and tetracaine, with epinephrine, having a relatively long duration and bupivacaine and etidocaine, a very long duration. It should be recalled that very weak concentrations of a local anesthetic agent have a much shorter duration and that the very concentrated solutions have the longest duration of action.[9]

Perhaps the most complete data on peripheral nerve block, compiled by a single investigator, can be found in the work of Löfström, who used ulnar nerve blockade to evaluate the duration of local anesthetic agents.[21] In clinical studies from other investigators, there were longer durations of cutaneous hypoesthesia to pinprick or pinch with both bupivacaine and etidocaine. Wencker and colleagues report analgesia of 770 minutes with bupivacaine and 764 minutes with etidocaine for axillary nerve block.[37] This study also showed that motor anesthesia exceeded analgesia with both agents. It must be noted that duration of surgical anesthesia — or postsurgical pain relief, for that matter — will be considerably shorter than the analgesia to pinprick quoted in most studies. In general, 45 to 90 minutes of surgical anesthesia can be achieved with the short-acting agents, 90 to 120 minutes with the intermediate agents, and 120 to 748 minutes with the long-acting group — although, of course, individual patient variables contribute to this parameter in many situations.

CONCENTRATION

Traditionally, it was thought that the very weak concentrations would block only the smallest nonmyelinated fibers and provide mostly sympathetic nerve blockade or partial sensory analgesia and that the strongest concentrations provided blockade of major motor fibers, with excessive concentrations producing neuritis or other nerve toxicity. It is now appreciated, primarily through recent controlled studies with the newest long-acting agents, that this traditional concept of concentration effect is invalid. Despite the difficulties inherent in arriving at clinically equipotent doses of local anesthetic agents, the work of Wencker, which noted differences in the motor blocking properties of bupivacaine and etidocaine, has been confirmed by others.[37] Another observation by these investigators was that the sympathetic blockade by these agents varied, not only from agent to agent but also in degree of sensory and motor blockade — the sympathetic block with etidocaine apparently being of shorter duration than either its motor or its sensory blockade.

TOXICITY

In practice, the maximum recommended dose of most local anesthetic agents has been the dose that was, presumably, safe to administer to a patient without fear of central nervous system (CNS) toxicity (*i.e.*, seizures). This recommendation was based on animal studies. Although there is variability in the blood concentration at which seizures will occur, it is known that the site of administration does affect blood levels and therefore the hazard of toxicity (see Chaps. 3 and 4). Many investigators have shown that levels are highest after intercostal nerve block, that levels after epidural block are 40% to 50% lower, and that extremity blocks (arm and leg) produce intermediate levels. The risk of toxicity is especially increased after the combined nerve block of the lower extremity, chiefly through the relatively larger volumes of local anesthetic required to accomplish the block. That is why it is extremely important that the anesthesiologist initially determine the total volume required for the block, in conjunction with the maximum total dose recommended for the agent, and then dilute the concentration to comply with these requirements.

METABOLISM

The metabolism of local anesthetic drugs has little specific application to nerve block of the lower extremity other than the fact that certain conditions, such as hypercapnia and acidosis, have been shown to increase the likelihood of CNS toxicity for a particular dose of local anesthetic. Therefore, when maximum volume and total dose are determined, the systemic health of the patient should be noted carefully and dosage reduced accordingly. A more detailed discussion of toxicity and metabolism may be found in Chapters 3 and 4.

ADDITIVES

Epinephrine has been used with local anesthetic agents since the early 1900s because it was assumed that duration of action would be extended and the blood concentration of the local anesthetic would be reduced, owing to delayed absorption. Recent work indicates that the beneficial effects of epinephrine for both duration and blood concentration depend on which local anesthetic is being used. Certainly, epinephrine is not necessary to extend the duration of etidocaine and bupivacaine. On the other hand, etidocaine and bupivacaine are used in high total doses for leg blocks, and, if epinephrine reduces blood levels at all, that is probably sufficient justification for its use.[5]

Hyaluronidase has been advocated to prevent large hematomas at the site of injection in arm and leg blocks.[25] Although no apparent problems have been reported from this use, there are also no reports of significant hematoma formation so that its benefit, if any, is difficult to evaluate. Also undocumented is the effect that this additive may have on blood levels of the administered local anesthetic agents. Since its action is to allow diffusion of blood (or drugs) through tissue planes, it is conceivable that this might increase vascular absorption of drug and further increase marginally safe blood levels of local anesthetics.

Bromage has been especially enthusiastic about the addition of carbon dioxide to solutions of local anesthetic in order to hasten their clinical effectiveness.[6] Although carbon dioxide has been advocated primarily in epidural anesthesia, it is also effective for peripheral nerve block. Clinically, the speed of onset of nearly all of the local anesthetic agents, with the possible exception of 0.25% bupivacaine, is sufficiently rapid to provide surgical analgesia within the usual surgical preparation time—10 to 15 minutes.

REFERENCES

1. Berkowitz, A., and Rosenberg, H.: Femoral block with mepivacaine for muscle biopsy in malignant hyperthermia patients. Anesthesiology, *62*:651–652, 1985.
2. Berry, F.R.: Analgesia in patients with fractured shaft of femur. Anaesthesia, *32*:576, 1977.
3. Braun, H.: Anesthesia—Its Scientific Basis and Practical Use, 2nd ed., p. 380. Philadelphia, Lea & Febiger, 1924.
4. Bridenbaugh, P.O., Moore, D.C., and Bridenbaugh, L.D.: Capillary P_{O_2} as a measure of sympathetic blockade. Anesth. Analg., *50*:26, 1971.
5. Bridenbaugh, P.O., et al.: Role of epinephrine in regional block anesthesia with etidocaine: A double-blind study. Anesth. Analg., *53*:430, 1974.
6. Bromage, P.R.: A comparison of the hydrochloride and carbon dioxide salts in lidocaine and prilocaine in epidural analgesia. Acta Anaesthesiol. Scand., *9*:55, 1965.
7. Brown, T.C.K., and Dickens, D.R.V.: A new approach to lateral cutaneous nerve of thigh block. Anaesth. Intensive Care, *14*:126–127, 1986.
8. Davies, J.A.H., and Walford, A.J.: Intravenous regional anaesthesia for foot surgery. Acta Anaesth. Scand., *30*:145–147, 1986.
9. De Jong, R.H.: Physiology and Pharmacology of Local Anesthesia. pp. 132–136. Springfield, Ill., Charles C Thomas, 1970.
10. Guardini, R., and Waldrom, B.A., and Wallace, W.A.: Sciatic nerve block: A new lateral approach. Acta Anaesthesiol. Scand., *29*:515–519, 1985.
11. Hagenouw, R.P.M., Bridenbaugh, P.O., van Egmond, J., and Stuebing, R.: Tourniquet pain: A volunteer study. Anesth. Analg., *65*:1175–1180, 1986.
12. Hughes, D.G.: Intra-articular bupivacaine for pain relief in arthroscopic surgery. Anaesthesia, *40*:84, 1985.
13. Ichiyanaghi, K.: Sciatic nerve block: Lateral approach with patient supine. Anesthesiology, *20*:601–604, 1959.
14. Kempthorne, P.M., and Brown, T.C.K.: Nerve blocks around the knee in children. Anaesth. Intensive Care, *12*:14–17, 1984.
15. Khoo, S.T., and Brown, T.C.K.: Femoral nerve block: The anatomical basis for a single injection technique. Anaesth. Intensive Care, *11*:40–42, 1983.
16. Kofoed, H.: Peripheral nerve blocks at the knee and ankle in operations for common foot disorders. Clin. Orthop., *168*:97–101, 1982.
17. Labat, G.: Regional Anesthesia: Its Technic and Clinical Application. p. 45. Philadelphia, W.B. Saunders, 1924.
18. Last, R.J.: Anatomy: Regional and Applied, Section 5, p. 342. New York, Churchill Livingstone, 1978.
19. Lehman, W.L., and Jones, W.W.: Intravenous lidocaine for anesthesia in the lower extremity. J Bone Joint Surg. [Am.], *66*:1056–1060, 1984.
20. Löfström, B.: Nerve Block at the Knee-Joint. Illustrated Handbook in Local Anaesthesia. Chicago, Year Book Medical Publishers, 1969.
21. Löfström, B.: Ulnar nerve blockade for the evaluation of local anaesthetic agents. Br. J. Anaesth., *47*:297, 1975.
22. McCutcheon, R.: Regional anesthesia for the foot. Can. Anaesth. Soc. J., *12*:465, 1965.
23. McNicol, L.R.: Sciatic nerve block for children. Anaesthesia, *40*:410–414, 1985.
24. McNicol, L.R.: Lower limb blocks for children. Anaesthesia, *41*:27–31, 1986.
25. Moore, D.C.: Regional Block, 4th ed. Springfield, Ill., Charles C Thomas, 1975.
26. Parks, C.R., and Kennedy, W.F.: Obturator nerve block: A simplified approach. Anesthesiology, *28*:775–778, 1967.
27. Patel, N.J., Flashburg, M.H., Paskin, S., and Grossman, R.: A regional anesthetic technique compared to general anesthesia for outpatient knee arthroscopy. Anesth. Analg., *65*:185–187, 1986.
28. Porter, K.M., and Davies, J.: The control of pain after Keller's procedure—A controlled double blind prospective trial with local anesthetic and placebo. Ann. R. Coll. Surg., *67*:243–294, 1985.
29. Raj, P.P., Parks, R.I., Watson, T.D., and Jenkins, M.T.: New single position supine approach to sciatic–femoral nerve block. Anesth. Analg., *54*:489, 1975.
30. Ringrase, N.H., and Cross, M.J.: Femoral nerve block in knee joint surgery. Am. J. Sports Med., *12*:398–402, 1984.
31. Rooks, M., and Fleming, L.L.: Evaluation of acute knee injuries with sciatic/femoral nerve blocks. Clin. Orthop., *179*:185–188, 1983.
32. Rorie, D.K., Byer, D.E., Nelson, D.O., Sittipong, R., et al.: Assessment of block of the sciatic nerve in the popliteal fossa. Anesth. Analg., *59*:371–376, 1980.
33. Sarrafian, S.K., Ibrahim, I.N., and Breihan, J.H.: Ankle-foot peripheral nerve block for mid- and forefoot surgery. Foot Ankle, *4*:86–90, 1983.
34. Selander, D., Dhuner, K.E., and Lundberg, E.: Peripheral

nerve injury due to injection needles used for regional anesthesia. Acta Anaesthesiol. Scand., *21*:182, 1977.

35. Sharrock, N.E., Waller, J.F., and Fiero, L.E.: Midtarsal block for surgery of the forefeet. Br. J. Anaesth., *58*:37–40, 1986.
36. Smith, B.E., Fischer, A.B.J., and Scott, P.U.: Continuous sciatic nerve block. Anaesthesia, *39*:155–157, 1984.
37. Wencker, K.H., Nolte, H., and Fruhstorfer, H.: Brachial plexus blockade for evaluation of local anaesthetic agents. Br. J. Anaesth., *47*:301, 1975.
38. Winnie, A.P., Ramamurthy, S., and Durrani, Z.: The inguinal paravascular technic of lumbar plexus anesthesia. "The 3-in-1 block." Anesth. Analg., *52*:989, 1973.

12 INTRAVENOUS REGIONAL NEURAL BLOCKADE

C. McK. HOLMES

Intravenous regional anesthesia is a method of producing analgesia of part of a limb with an intravenous injection of a local anesthetic while the circulation to the limb is occluded.

HISTORY

The history of anesthesia of the arm has been reviewed in published reports.[42,43] Although both Halsted and Crile had blocked the brachial plexus by local infiltration under direct vision, intravenous regional anesthesia was the first method whereby anesthesia of the arm could be easily achieved. This method was discovered by August Bier in 1908.[5] Bier was Professor of Surgery in Berlin, and he is best remembered as the first to make regular use of spinal anesthesia. His method of intravenous analgesia consisted of occluding the circulation in a segment of the arm with two tourniquets and then injecting a solution of 0.5% procaine into a vein in the isolated segment. Many of the details mentioned by Bier in his paper are still relevant and are worth noting:

> It is important to empty the blood from the region to be anesthetised. This is done by winding an Esmarch bandage proximally up the arm. The circulation is then occluded above the level of the operation by many turns of a soft rubber bandage. A similar bandage is applied below the site of the operation. A cannula is inserted in a suitable vein between the two tourniquets [Fig. 12-1]. A 0.25% or 0.5% procaine solution in physiologic saline is used. Using the 0.5% strength, direct anesthesia (*i.e.*, between the two bandages) comes on very rapidly. In the distal part of the limb, below the distal bandage, one gradually obtains conduction (indirect) anesthesia. After removal of the bandages, motor and sensory paralyses disappear within a few minutes. The onset of anesthesia in the deeper tissues is as rapid as in the skin, or sometimes more so. The procaine in physiologic saline passes rapidly through the vein walls and is absorbed (into the tissues); after reestablishment of the circulation it only slowly enters the general circulation. Only once was a slight reaction to procaine observed on removing the bandages. To minimize the risk of reactions one may loosen the proximal bandage to permit arterial inflow and thereby flush the procaine out by way of the wound. [See also Chap. 1.]

This method enjoyed wide popularity for a time, and somewhat similar intra-arterial and even intraosseous methods were also described. However, it was not long before simple and reliable techniques for brachial plexus block were developed, and the intravenous method declined in popularity. It was revived in 1963 by Holmes,[41] who used lidocaine, which appeared to give more reliable anesthesia than procaine. Currently, Bier block is regarded as one of the several alternative techniques for arm anesthesia.

ADVANTAGES AND DISADVANTAGES

ADVANTAGES

Reliability. Correctly performed, the method is reliable and its success rate is high. Thorn-Alquist[72] has reported unsatisfactory analgesia in only 1% of 967 patients; Dunbar and Mazze[18] had a 96% success rate in 779 patients; and smaller series have reported 100% success rates (*e.g.*, Tryba *et al.*[75] in 60 cases). In

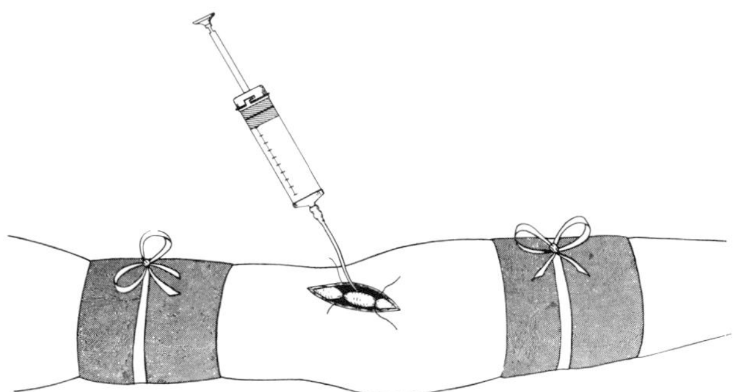

FIG. 12-1. Diagram of Bier's original method.

contrast, other methods of obtaining arm analgesia do not have such high success rates. In a retrospective study of 368 patients,[22] the success rates of four other methods were as shown in Table 12-1.

Ease of Performance. In contrast to the various techniques of brachial plexus block, for which specific skills and anatomical understanding are required, the intravenous regional technique requires only that the anesthesiologist be able to insert a needle or cannula into a suitable vein. However, as with any other method involving the use of local anesthesia, the anesthesiologist carrying out the intravenous regional technique must be thoroughly familiar with its potential risks and complications and must know how to manage them. He must also be skilled in the techniques of resuscitation and have all the necessary equipment readily available. It goes without saying that the person performing the anesthetic block should devote his full attention to the patient and should not himself perform the surgery.

Safety. The reported incidence of adverse side-effects is low, and there is certainly no risk of such complications as total spinal anesthesia, phrenic nerve block (see Table 12-1); or pneumothorax. However, there is a risk of systemic toxicity, but this is no greater than with other arm block techniques, provided that correct procedures are followed.

Onset of analgesia is rapid, so that surgery or manipulation may begin within 5 to 10 minutes.

Muscular relaxation is good, so that reduction of a fracture or dislocation is facilitated.

Controllable Duration of Action. The duration of action of the block is governed not by the duration of action of the local anesthetic agent being used, but rather by the time for which the tourniquet is kept inflated. Operations as long as 6 hours have been described,[46] and it would seem that there is no diminution of the block until the tourniquet is released.

Controllable Extent of Analgesia. The extent of the analgesia is limited proximally by the position of the tourniquet. The closer the tourniquet is to the periphery, the smaller the quantity of local anesthetic solution required. Thus, in order to produce analgesia of only the hand or the foot, the tourniquet can be placed on the forearm or lower calf, respectively, and less solution used.

Rapidity of Recovery. Normal sensation and motor power return rapidly after cuff release, even if the cuff is released well before the expiration of the agent's usual duration of nerve-blocking action. This rapid return to normal function is important because it facilitates reevaluation of neurologic signs after fracture reduction. Also, the patient who has had outpatient surgery will not be leaving the hospital with an anesthetized limb and thus will not be faced with the hazards of accidental injury, burns, and the like.

TABLE 12-1. SUCCESS RATES OF FOUR METHODS OF OBTAINING ARM ANALGESIA IN 368 PATIENTS (%)

Method	Perfect Result	Fair Result	Failure	Complication	Phrenic Nerve Block
Axillary	76	19	5	9	–
Kulenkampff (supra-clavicular)	73	19	8	10	38
Perivascular (subclavian)	76	23	1	8	36
Interscalene	74	15	11	–	35

DISADVANTAGES

A tourniquet must be used. As a result, the method cannot produce analgesia of the entire limb but only of that portion of the limb that is below the tourniquet. The tourniquet must be kept inflated continuously; it is not possible to release it to enable bleeding vessels to be identified unless more local anesthetic is injected after the tourniquet is reinflated.[8] The tourniquet may cause pain. The duration of surgery is limited by the time for which an arterial tourniquet is safe.

Exsanguination. It is generally considered desirable to exsanguinate the limb as completely as possible. This cannot always be done with an Esmarch bandage, for example, when there is a fracture or laceration of the limb. In such cases, however, elevation of the limb for 2 to 3 minutes or use of an air-inflated splint will usually be satisfactory.[83]

Toxic Reactions. There is the possibility of a systemic reaction to the local anesthetic agent when it is released into the general circulation, and in some cases, there may be a risk even *before* the tourniquet is released. The risk tends to be greater when larger quantities of local anesthetic agent are used, which, in turn, depends on the size of the limb and the position of the tourniquet. For this reason, analgesia of the whole leg with the use of a thigh tourniquet is not recommended because the quantity of anesthetic solution required would be in excess of acceptable maximum doses. An exception to this would be an amputation, in which case only a small amount of the anesthetic remains to reenter the circulation.

Inability to Provide a Bloodless Field. When analgesia of the hand is produced with a tourniquet on the forearm, there is likely to be a gradual vascular engorgement of the hand, owing to intraosseous blood flow. If necessary, this may be controlled by a second tourniquet on the upper arm.

Rapidity of recovery with loss of analgesia may be considered a disadvantage in major surgical cases, and parenteral narcotic analgesics may be required early in the postoperative period.

SELECTION OF CASES

Intravenous regional analgesia is most suited for surgery of the forearm and hand, including the manipulation of forearm fractures. It may be used for supracondylar fractures of the humerus but may sometimes be unsatisfactory because of the presence of the inflated cuff close to the fracture site. Similarly, other lesions above the elbow are usually better managed with some type of brachial plexus block. The intravenous regional method is also often unsatisfactory for anesthetizing the knee and calf region of the leg because of the large quantity of solution required; however, the foot may safely be anesthetized.

Tourniquet pain is seldom a problem in short procedures but may become a problem if the operation is prolonged. Methods of alleviating this discomfort, as will be discussed later in this chapter, are not without some disadvantages. It is this author's opinion that intravenous regional analgesia is therefore best suited for operations of relatively short duration.

CONTRAINDICATIONS

Disease processes in which prolonged tourniquet times are contraindicated (*e.g.*, sickle cell disease or trait, cellulitis, and so forth) would also be contraindications to the use of the intravenous regional technique. In addition, patients with a known hypersensitivity to a local anesthetic agent or with a history of certain cardiac diseases may be considered unsuitable candidates for intravenous regional anesthesia. In particular, untreated heart block is a relative contraindication, since sudden release of local anesthetic into the circulation may convert a partial heart block to a complete one or may precipitate asystole. Bradycardia has been recorded following cuff release when lidocaine was used for intravenous regional block, even in normal patients.[18,49]

TECHNIQUE

In this section, brief details of technique as preferred by the author will be set out. Many of the points advocated will be examined in detail later in this chapter.

STANDARD METHOD FOR THE ARM

Premedication. In emergency or outpatient cases, premedication may be omitted, particularly if the proposed operation is likely to be of short duration. However, some form of sedation is desirable for longer operations. Just prior to the performance of the block, an appropriate dose of a sedative, such as diazepam,[16] or a neuroleptanalgesic may be given intravenously. This will help to reduce the patient's awareness of the operation and the inflated cuff and may raise the threshold for toxic effects.[16] Additional small intravenous increments of narcotics and sedatives may be given during long operations (see Chap. 6).

Preparation of the Patient. The patient should be fasted as for general anesthesia, since vomiting could represent a hazard in the event of any complications such as convulsions. Having ascertained that the patient accepts this form of analgesia and has no history of allergic reactions to local anesthetic drugs or other contraindications, the anesthesiologist should explain the technique and should check the blood pressure on the side of the operative site to demonstrate the sensation of the cuff to the patient. This also enables the cuff to be inflated to the correct pressure later, after exsanguination. The pneumatic tourniquet should be an orthopaedic type, rather than a conventional sphygmomanometer (*i.e.,* a secure method of fastening the tourniquet is needed rather than relying on a Velcro-type adhesive material, which may slip). The pressure gauge should be reliable: it is recommended that all such gauges be checked regularly against a mercury manometer. It is the author's preference not to use an automatic gas-powered tourniquet, nor to use one of the double-cuff tourniquets originally designed for use with this method. Great care should be taken to ensure that the cuff is applied smoothly and snugly around the arm. A further safeguard is to wrap a bandage around the tourniquet to reduce the risk of it becoming loose or slipping. After the blood pressure has been checked, the cuff may be left temporarily inflated above the diastolic pressure in order to distend the veins for insertion of the needle. As with any anesthetic administration, it should be routine to secure a route for intravenous fluids and supplemental drugs, usually in the other arm, and also to place a blood pressure cuff on that arm so that the blood pressure can be monitored during the procedure.

Choice of Vein. Usually a vein on the dorsum of the hand is selected. However, if no veins are visible in this region, a vein on the forearm or even at the antecubital fossa may be chosen. There is, however, some evidence that failure to obtain analgesia, or "patchy" analgesia, is more likely to occur when proximal veins are used.[70] A "butterfly" needle with a short extension tube or a plastic cannula is used for the venipuncture. A long intravenous catheter should not be used, however, because there is at least one recorded case in which the end of such a catheter was actually above the inflated cuff, resulting in an injection directly into the general circulation.[2] The needle or cannula is placed in the vein, flushed with saline and/or heparin saline, and taped securely. Care must be taken not to dislodge it during the exsanguination or subsequent injection. As with any venipuncture, there should be careful palpation for superficial arteries to avoid intra-arterial injection.

Exsanguination. It has frequently been stated that exsanguination of the limb assists in the production of complete analgesia. However, not all workers agree.[15,73] The usual method is to wrap an Esmarch bandage snugly up the arm, starting, where possible, just proximal to the needle in the hand (Fig. 12-2). If this method is undesirable because of a fracture or wound, elevation of the arm or use of an air-inflated splint is an acceptable alternative.

The tourniquet is inflated to a pressure above the patient's systolic value. Although high pressures might be assumed to confer greater safety from leakage past the cuff, the discomfort is also likely to be related to the pressure. Therefore, the exact amount by which the tourniquet pressure should exceed the systolic pressure cannot clearly be stated because the patient's blood pressure may rise during the injection or during the operation. Some authors[25,55] advise a tourniquet pressure of 200 to 250 mm Hg, although a pressure of 150 mm Hg above systolic has also been recommended.[23] However, in all cases the disappearance of the radial pulse should be checked. The practice of cross-clamping the tubing of the cuff after inflation is not recommended; should the cuff have a small leak, it might not be detected. It is better to

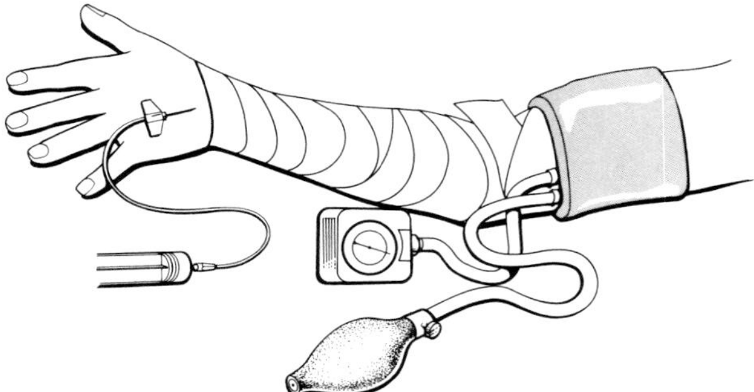

FIG. 12-2. Exsanguination with an Esmarch bandage before the injection.

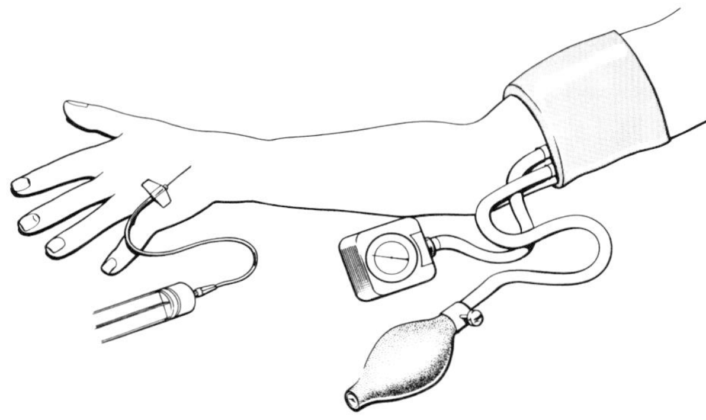

FIG. 12-3. The injection has been completed. The needle may be removed at this stage. Note the tourniquet tubing not clamped; the pressure is visible on the dial.

observe the cuff pressure at all times on the aneroid dial (Fig. 12-3).

Injection. Using a 50-ml disposable syringe, 40 ml of 0.5% prilocaine, without epinephrine or other vasoconstrictor, is injected *slowly.* The quantity may be varied according to the mass of tissue below the tourniquet even though the mass may not correlate well with the patient's overall weight. It may be necessary to use 50 ml for the muscular forearm of a slim patient, whereas the slim forearm of an obese patient may be satisfactorily anesthetized with a smaller amount. As the drug is injected, the skin usually becomes mottled, and analgesia develops rapidly. Muscular relaxation, usually quite profound, appears at the same time. If sufficient analgesia is not present 5 minutes after the injection of 40 ml, a further 10 ml should be given before removing the needle.

Tourniquet Discomfort. During the operation, the tourniquet must be kept inflated above the systolic value. After a time, particularly in the unsedated patient, discomfort may develop at the site of the tourniquet. This may respond to a small intravenous dose of diazepam or an analgesic drug. An alternative or additional maneuver is to place another cuff below the first and to inflate it over the analgesic part of the arm, after which the upper cuff is deflated. Although this method is facilitated if the double-compartment cuff[39,45] is used, for reasons that will be discussed later in this chapter, this device is not favored by the author. Another method that is said to relieve tourniquet discomfort is to apply a vibratory massager to the inflated cuff.[31]

Minimum tourniquet time is subject to some debate and will be discussed further. It is usually assumed that deflating the tourniquet soon after the injection would be equivalent to a rapid intravenous infusion of local anesthetic and could produce a toxic reaction. Without any direct evidence to the contrary, it is therefore recommended that the cuff remain inflated for a minimum of 15 minutes.

Tourniquet Release. The tourniquet is released at the end of the operation (and not before, since sensation returns rapidly). It has been suggested that the cuff be released and then reinflated immediately, to release a "test dose" of local anesthetic into the general circulation. However, pharmacokinetic data indicate that reinflation must occur within seconds of deflation to have an appreciable effect.[76] In any event, it is at the time of release that adverse reactions may occur, so the patient's pulse, blood pressure, and electrocardiogram (ECG) should be monitored closely during the first few minutes after tourniquet release (see Fig. 12-7). Appropriate resuscitation equipment should be available, and the patient should be warned to expect transient generalized paresthesia and, sometimes, tinnitus. There appears to be no risk of delayed after-effects.

MODIFIED METHOD FOR THE HAND

The cuff is placed on the forearm, taking care to keep it below the head of the radius (Fig. 12-4). About 10 ml of solution will usually provide complete analgesia. A difficulty sometimes encountered with this method is that blood flow through the radius and

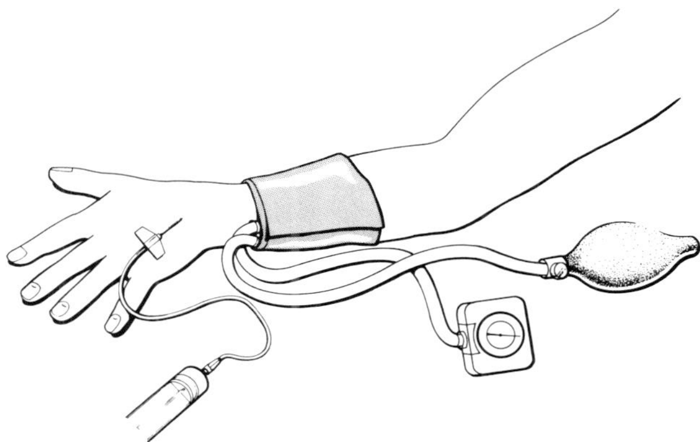

FIG. 12-4. The modified method for the hand. A second tourniquet might be placed on the upper arm, if necessary.

ulna causes gradual vascular congestion of the hand if the operation is other than quite short. Of course, since the quantity of solution is so small, the tourniquet could be released safely at any time, so a short procedure is quite feasible. For a longer operation, a second tourniquet on the upper arm may be needed to prevent this congestion. An interesting variation of this is the method of digital regional anesthesia described by Ryding.[67] He showed that if a vein on the dorsum of a finger can be cannulated with a fine needle, very good analgesia of the finger can be achieved with a small quantity of anesthetic, using a rubber tourniquet around the base of the finger. This method is quite appropriate for the treatment of conditions such as paronychia.

MODIFIED METHOD FOR THE FOOT

The same principles apply as for the hand (Fig. 12-5). The tourniquet should be well below the knee to avoid compressing the peroneal nerve on the neck of the fibula.

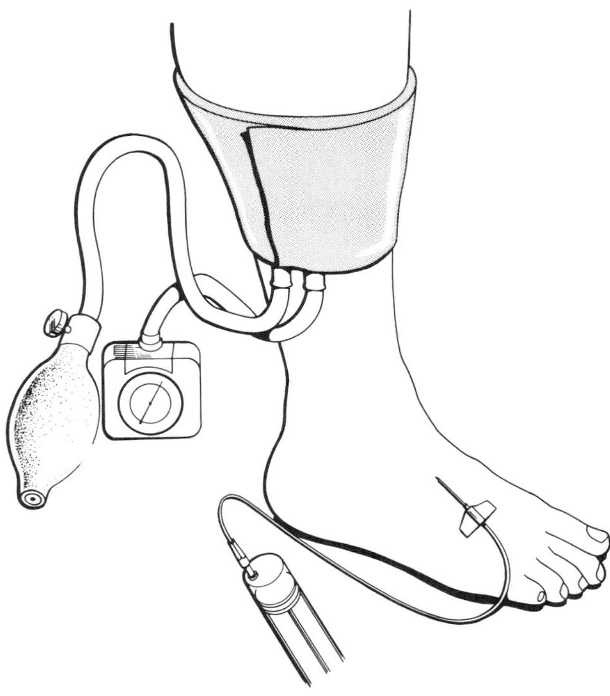

FIG. 12-5. The modified method for the foot.

PROLONGED INTRAVENOUS REGIONAL ANALGESIA

As mentioned above, intravenous regional anesthesia is better suited for short procedures. However, it is suitable for prolonged operations if the patient is well sedated. The technique described by Brown[8] consists of inserting an indwelling plastic catheter into a suitable vein away from the operation site and leaving it *in situ* during the operation. After about one hour, the tourniquet is deflated, and bleeding vessels may be secured during the short interval before sensation returns. The arm is then elevated, the tourniquet reinflated, and another dose of the local anesthetic injected. Brown found that to produce adequate analgesia, this dose may be only one-half the volume of the first. The procedure may be repeated if necessary. If this intermittent method is not used, the governing factor in long operations is the time for which it is considered safe to leave a tourniquet inflated.

PEDIATRIC USE

The method is readily applicable to children who are old enough to comprehend a simple explanation of the procedure.[9,24,28] It is a very valuable procedure for reduction of the common forearm fractures and similar lesions. The standard method is used, making sure the tourniquet is of an appropriate size for the circumference of the child's arm. Elevation is used for exsanguination, in preference to an Esmarch bandage, to avoid any discomfort. The dose of prilocaine may be calculated on the basis of 3 mg/kg.

CHOICE OF LOCAL ANESTHETIC AGENT

All the common local anesthetic agents have been used, including even cocaine. Procaine was, of course, the standard drug used by the early researchers, but it is undoubtedly less effective than the modern agents. Lidocaine was used first by Holmes,[41] and many large series in which this agent was used have since been reported. Equally satisfactory analgesia is likely obtainable with all current local anesthetic drugs. However, it should be noted that the duration of action does not depend on the drug but on the time for which the tourniquet is kept inflated. Patchy analgesia is sometimes seen for a varying time after tourniquet release; this analgesia has been shown to correlate with the known duration of action of the agent used.[21]

It is also of interest to note that quite satisfactory analgesia can be obtained with 2-chloroprocaine, even though this agent is normally hydrolyzed rapidly in the blood. This agent is, of course, the least toxic agent and would, in theory, be the ideal choice. Unfortunately, there is a higher incidence of thrombophlebitis with this agent and therefore it is not recommended.[34]

Prilocaine is the most rapidly metabolized of the amides, and given its efficacy by the intravenous route and the low incidence of thrombophlebitis associated with its use, it appears to have the most appeal of the drugs available (see Chap. 4). Prilocaine was first used by Hooper[44] in 64 cases and subsequently by many others. In a double-blind trial, Kerr[50] studied 22 patients who were given 0.5% prilocaine and 20 patients who were given 0.5% lidocaine. Nearly half the patients who received lidocaine had neurologic side-effects (dizziness, tinnitus, muscular twitching), whereas there was only one minor episode of dizziness among the patients who received prilocaine. Eriksson[20] demonstrated that the effects seen on the electroencephalograms (EEGs) of patients given 200 mg of lidocaine i.v. (40 ml of 0.5%), although smaller in magnitude, were similar to those seen after direct intravenous injection of the same solution over a period of 2.3 minutes. Subjective symptoms could be correlated with the EEG changes and occurred in all subjects. With a similar amount of prilocaine, the EEG changes were considerably reduced, and there were no subjective symptoms. This could be explained partly by the lower plasma levels that occur after the administration of prilocaine and partly by its lower inherent toxicity. Eriksson also showed that when intravenous regional analgesia was produced with a mixture of 0.25% lidocaine and 0.25% prilocaine, the maximum plasma concentration of the prilocaine was less than that of the lidocaine. This effect has also been demonstrated by Thorn-Alquist.[71]

Prilocaine must therefore be considered superior to lidocaine. However, most discussion now centers around the relative merits of prilocaine and bupivacaine, and here the question of superiority is not as clear-cut. Bupivacaine was first used in intravenous regional analgesia by Ware,[78,79] who recorded 14,000 cases without a single mishap.[81] Other authors have also used bupivacaine without problems.[29,48] A prospective double-blind trial[40] comparing prilocaine and bupivacaine showed no major side-effects in any of the 200 patients included in the study, but 20% of the patients in the bupivacaine group had minor side-effects compared with 12% in the prilocaine group. Another double-blind trial of these two drugs was carried out by McKeown, Meiklejohn, and Scott,[57] in which six volunteers underwent intravenous regional analgesia on four occasions each. Since bupivacaine has an *in vivo* potency four times that of prilocaine, 0.5% prilocaine was compared with 0.125% bupivacaine, and, since Ware recommends 0.2% bupivacaine, this was compared with 0.8% prilocaine. On each occasion, 40 ml of one of these solutions was injected, and the results were compared. The authors found that although the higher doses gave more rapid onset and more profound blocks, they were associated with more marked toxicity (though no serious side-effects were observed). These authors concluded that bupivacaine had no advantages and that there was little to be gained by using the higher concentrations of either drug. Bupivacaine is now no longer recommended for this technique in Britain or the United States.

Dose and Concentration. The dose of local anesthetic agent should be calculated according to the mass of tissue below the tourniquet. A 40-ml dose is appropriate for an average-size arm with the tourniquet above the elbow, but this quantity may be altered proportionately for larger or smaller arms. However, since the incidence of toxic reactions is related to the blood level of the agent and since this in turn depends on, among other factors, the dose given in proportion to the total body weight, maximum doses according to body weight have been recommended (lidocaine, 1.5–3 mg/kg; prilocaine, 3–4 mg/kg; bupivacaine, 0.75–1.5 mg/kg).[18,34,56,79]

Preinjection ischemia of 15 to 20 minutes' duration has been shown by Bell and co-workers[4] and Harris[34] to result in a significant reduction in the amount of solution required for satisfactory analgesia, but this modification does not appear to have achieved widespread popularity.

Varying concentrations from 0.15% up to 2% prilocaine have been used successfully. However, for a given total dose, a smaller volume would have to be used with the stronger solutions, which may result in rather patchy analgesia. However, few dose–response studies have been performed. In a prospective double-blind study of 60 patients, Tryba, Zenz, and Hausmann[75] compared 4 mg/kg of prilocaine in concentrations of 0.8%, 1.5%, and 2.0%. They found that after the administration of the higher concentrations, analgesia persisting after tourniquet release was greater, the blood level of the agent was lower, and no side-effects were observed. It should be noted that in this study the operations were around the wrist and that a tourniquet on the forearm was used in addition to the upper arm tourniquet. Hooper[44] recommended 20 ml of 1% prilocaine, but most workers have favored the 0.5% concentration.

Additives. It is important that all solutions of local anesthetic agents be free of additives or preservatives (single-dose ampules). Thrombophlebitis has occurred from use of preservative-containing solutions. A note of caution is important to those practitioners who provide their own dilute solutions of local anesthetics by adding normal saline to stronger concentrations of local anesthetic drugs. Many vials of normal saline contain preservatives or benzyl alcohol. Thus, it is just as important that diluents also be free of additives.

COMPLICATIONS

". . . The most important requirement for avoiding untoward sequelae with any regional block is not the technique or the drug used but by whom and in what circumstances they are used."*

In the first edition of this book, it was possible to write that "it is noteworthy that no fatalities have been reported with this technique." Sadly, this statement cannot be made in the current edition. There have been seven known fatalities (all with bupivacaine), and numerous other untoward reactions have been reported. Although these will be discussed further, it should be stressed at the outset that many of these adverse reports relate to failure to adhere to the correct technique or to apply the appropriate resuscitative measures, or to some other factors not directly attributable to the method itself. Also, these adverse reports must be set against the figure of "14,000 cases without mishap" mentioned by Ware,[81] and the "10,000 cases without fatality" quoted by Colbern.[10] The complications of intravenous regional anesthesia are caused entirely by the systemic toxicity of the agent used (see Chap. 4). Local anesthetics affect principally the central nervous system (CNS), where they may be either stimulant or depressant, and the cardiovascular system, where they are depressant (see Chaps. 2 and 4). A problem unique to prilocaine may be methemoglobinemia. A possible factor in some fatalities, and certainly documented in some cases of convulsions,[14,66] is leakage of the local anesthetic while the tourniquet is still apparently or actually inflated. Because of the adverse reactions that have been reported, two measures have been taken in Britain. First, the use of automatic gas-operated tourniquets has been advised against, and a "hazard notice"[17] has been issued. Second, it has been recommended that bupivacaine be no longer used.[11]

*Moore, D.C.: Correspondence. Anesthesiology, *61*:782, 1984.

Deaths. Seven deaths attributed to bupivacaine were reported in Britain over the period 1979 to 1983.[37] Not all are well documented, but some common facts are known for some of the cases:[36] the patients were healthy, automatic tourniquets were used, bupivacaine was the drug, and the attending physician was not an anesthesiologist. Moreover, after having performed the block, the physician went on to perform the surgery himself. The mode of death is not clearly known in these cases, but early cardiac depression was apparently a factor in some, raising the question of the relative cardiotoxicity of bupivacaine. This topic is discussed in Chapter 4.

Central nervous system symptoms and signs range from mild, transient giddiness, dizziness, or tinnitus to more serious phenomena such as muscular twitching, convulsions, and loss of consciousness. These latter signs are not common, however. In one series of 1400 patients,[77] only 8 patients had CNS stimulation sufficient to require the administration of a barbiturate and only three of these had frank convulsions. All these patients had received a dose of lidocaine in excess of 5 mg/kg. Fleming[25] records "5 or 6" convulsions in another large series, again with lidocaine. Convulsions have been reported in many instances in which bupivacaine has been used;[13,14,32,38,66] but no convulsions have been reported with prilocaine.[82]

The highest frequency of minor CNS toxicity has been recorded by Harris,[34] who reported an incidence of 67.3% with 5 mg/kg of prilocaine in a group of volunteers. A 50% incidence of CNS toxicity with lidocaine, 3 mg/kg, was recorded by Bell, Slater and Harris[4] in a small group of volunteers. Most other workers have reported a lower incidence of 10% or less. Dunbar and Mazze have recorded an incidence of 2.1% in 779 patients, with lidocaine or prilocaine.[18]

Cardiovascular system symptoms and signs are usually also mild and transient. In 779 patients, Dunbar and Mazze[18] found no arrhythmias and only a slight drop in blood pressure or a slight bradycardia on release of the tourniquet. This is in keeping with the observations of most other workers. By contrast, however, Kennedy, Duthie, Parbrook, and Carr,[49] who monitored the ECG in all their 77 patients, found a 15% incidence of ECG changes, mostly of a minor nature, but recorded one cardiac arrest (successfully treated) that was preceded by bradycardia. They did not feel justified in continuing to use the technique (with lidocaine).

Methemoglobinemia is known to occur after the administration of prilocaine and may cause cyanosis (see Chap. 4). A significant rise in serum methemoglobin levels is not usually seen below a total dose of 600 mg of prilocaine, which is above the dose required for intravenous regional analgesia.[53] Harris, Cole, Mital, and Laver[35] studied 58 volunteers given 5 mg/kg of prilocaine for intravenous regional analgesia and found a small rise in methemoglobin from 0.33 ± 0.11 g per 100 ml (control) to 1.02 ± 0.33 g per 100 ml after tourniquet release. No cyanosis was observed. McKeown and co-workers[56] report that they have "been using 0.5% prilocaine . . . in IVRA [intravenous regional analgesia] for 15 years and have never seen methaemoglobinaemia as a complication."

FACTORS THAT INFLUENCE THE INCIDENCE OF TOXIC REACTIONS

Leakage of Local Anesthetic Before Tourniquet Release. Many studies have now demonstrated that there may be leakage of anesthetic into the general circulation even in the presence of an apparently well-inflated tourniquet cuff. There may be several reasons for this:

1. Leakage through intraosseous veins
2. Leakage through ordinary veins
3. Malfunctioning tourniquet

Leakage Through Intraosseous Veins. This was postulated by Shamay and Robin[68] to explain leakage of ^{14}C-labeled lidocaine, and also by Hanton and Punchihewa[32] in a clinical case in which convulsions developed. However, no direct evidence has been produced.

Leakage Through Ordinary Veins. For this to occur in the presence of a correctly inflated cuff, the venous pressure caused by the cuff must presumably exceed the pressure in the tissues. This was first shown by Raj and associates[64] in a study with radiopaque solutions and has since been demonstrated by others.[66] Lawes and co-workers[51] measured pressures in a cephalic vein just below the cuff when injections were made in the dorsum of the hand. They found that rapid injection could often cause venous pressures exceeding cuff pressure. However, Finegan and Bukht,[23] although demonstrating pressures as high as 190 mm Hg in a similar experiment, found none higher than the cuff pressure when this was set at 150 mm Hg above systolic. Nevertheless, they felt it desirable to advise the use of wide cuffs that should fully encircle the arm (with a recommended width-to-length ratio of 1:3), that injections be made distally, that volumes of solution not exceed 60 ml, and that the injection be made slowly. Therefore, there is probably also an argument to avoid the saline "chasers" that some advocated in the past.[10] Additionally, Reynolds[65] recommends that exsanguination be as complete as possible. Finegan and Bukht point out that as veins are filled, their cross-sectional shape changes from oval to circular, at which point they become relatively indistensible and pressure rises rapidly. Therefore, the more completely veins are emptied before the injection commences, the more volume they can accommodate without pressure rise.

In contrast to these studies, however, Lillie and co-workers,[52] using 40 ml of technetium-labeled saline and a cuff pressure of 300 mm Hg, found no evidence of leakage in 5 volunteers. Injections were made at the antecubital fossa, but the injection speed and pressure were not stated.

Ogden[63] describes a case where, probably as a result of calcification of the vessels combined with the patient's obesity, the arm became congested despite a cuff pressure (double-cuff) of 320 mm Hg. The patient's blood pressure had been measured at 180/90 immediately beforehand using an ordinary cuff. This problem is also discussed in more detail by Jeyaseelam and co-workers.[47] Davies and associates[14] studied the relation between the "occlusion pressure" (*i.e.*, the cuff pressure at which the radial pulse disappears) and the systolic pressure. They found that in many cases the narrow-cuffed double tourniquets did not occlude the artery even at pressures 100 mm Hg greater than the systolic. Furthermore, "occlusion pressures" were usually different depending on whether the proximal or distal cuff was inflated. This difference was as great as 45 mm Hg. They therefore concluded that "occlusion pressure" should be measured with the same tourniquet and gauge that will be used for the procedure. A wide cuff is better than a double-cuff, but if the latter is used, "occlusion pressure" should be measured with both cuffs in turn, and the higher reading should be chosen as the reference point. The pressure then used to inflate the cuff for the procedure must exceed the "occlusion pressure" by a margin that allows for rises in blood pressure during surgery.

Malfunctioning Tourniquet. This has certainly been a problem with the automatic gas-operated tourniquets. Whether the problem has been mechanical or caused by operator error is not known in all cases, but, as mentioned earlier, these devices have been advised against by a "hazard notice" in Britain.[17] Heath[36] states that they "are expensive and have if anything increased the incidence of tourniquet failure. . . ." For this reason they cannot be recommended unconditionally but, if chosen, must be used with care and only after becoming fully conversant with the operating instructions.

Plasma levels of local anesthetic after tourniquet release have been studied by several authors. Using 0.5% lidocaine in a dose of 2.5 mg/kg and in most cases releasing the tourniquet after only 5 minutes, Hargrove, Hoyle, Parker, Beckett, and Boyes[33] found that maximum levels of anesthetic in venous blood from the other arm did not exceed 2 μg/ml. A similar figure of 1.5 ± 0.2 μg/ml was found by Mazze and Dunbar[54] following 3 mg/kg of 0.5% lidocaine. They found considerably higher levels after axillary block and after lumbar epidural block (Fig. 12-6; Table 12-2).

Tucker and Boas, who studied the plasma concentration of lidocaine in the contralateral artery, observed that the peak levels were 20% to 80% lower than those found after direct intravenous infusion of the same dose over 3 minutes.[76] They also found the levels were lower (by about 40%) when the same dose was used for intravenous regional anesthesia in a 0.5% solution rather than in a 1% solution. If a cuff time of 10 minutes is assumed, pharmacokinetic calculations from this data indicate that after cuff release the drug reaches the systemic circulation in the following biphasic manner: there is an initial fast release of 30% of the dose, which is so rapid that reinflation of the cuff would only retard systemic uptake if it were performed within 30 seconds of cuff release, and then there is a slower washout of the remainder of the dose, so that up to 30 minutes after cuff release half the dose would still be retained in the limb.

These findings are supported by recent clinical data that indicate sustained high local anesthetic concentrations in the venous drainage from the blocked arm.[21] Thus, it is possible to reestablish anesthesia for approximately 10 to 30 minutes after cuff release by injecting half the original dose after reinflation of the cuff.

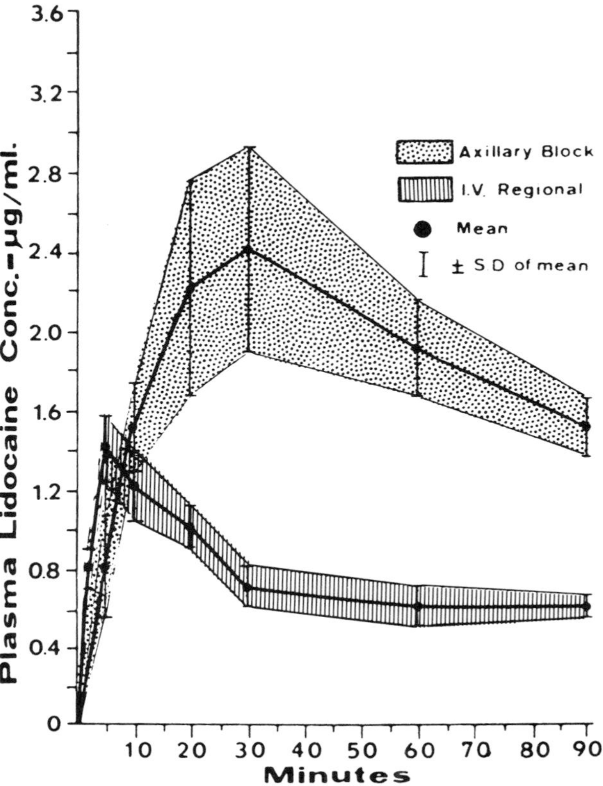

FIG. 12-6. A comparison of the blood levels of lidocaine after intravenous regional analgesia and axillary block. The horizontal axis refers to the time after tourniquet release for intravenous regional analgesia and time after injection of lidocaine for axillary block. (Mazze, R.I., and Dunbar, R.W.: Plasma lidocaine concentrations after caudal, lumbar epidural, axillary block and intravenous regional anesthesia. Anesthesiology, *27*:574, 1966)

TABLE 12-2. PLASMA LEVELS AFTER TOURNIQUET RELEASE

Block	Dose of Lidocaine (mg/kg)	Mean Peak Plasma Level (μg/ml)
Intravenous regional anesthesia	3, 0.5%	1.5 ± 0.2
Axillary block	6–6.8, 1.5%*	2.5 ± 0.5
Lumbar epidural block	4.7–6.5, 1.5%*	3.1 ± 0.7
Caudal epidural block	5.8–7.5, 1.5%*	1.4 ± 0.6

*With 1:200,000, epinephrine.
(Mazze, R. I., and Dunbar, R. W.: Plasma lidocaine concentrations after caudal, lumbar epidural, axillary block and intravenous regional anesthesia. Anesthesiology, *27*:574, 1966)

Eriksson[20] studied 5 volunteers who received intravenous regional anesthesia on two occasions, once with prilocaine and once with lidocaine (40 ml of 0.5% in each case). The tourniquet was left inflated for 30 minutes after all injections. Sampling was from the contralateral brachial artery. The results are shown in Figure 12-7, which demonstrates the consistently lower blood levels of prilocaine. These levels are lower than those usually considered toxic. Englesson, Eriksson, Wahlqvist, and Ortengren[19] found that symptoms were noted at a mean plasma level of 4.4 μg/ml in awake patients who received intravenous infusions of lidocaine, while Foldes, Molloy, McNall, and Koukal[27] found that toxic symptoms occurred at a plasma level of 5.3 μg/ml. In anesthetized patients, signs of toxicity were not seen below plasma levels of 10 μg/ml.[6]

Blood levels of bupivacaine were measured by Kalso and associates[48] following a mean dose of 1.8 mg/kg (range, 1.4–2.6/kg) of 0.25% bupivacaine. They found mean levels generally below 1.6 μg/ml (toxic level, 4–5 μg/ml[62]), but even in some individuals with higher levels (maximum, 2.72 μg/ml) there were no CNS side-effects. Ware and Caldwell,[80] in a study of 50 patients given 1.5 mg/kg of 0.2% bupivacaine, found that the highest mean venous level was 840 ± 164 ng/ml, well below toxic levels. They saw no side-effects other than transient drowsiness in one patient.

By contrast, however, Tryba and co-workers,[74] in a prospective randomized study comparing 1 mg/kg bupivacaine with 4 mg/kg prilocaine, found that the plasma levels of bupivacaine were 3 times higher than those of prilocaine when expressed as a percentage of the toxic level. In one case the bupivacaine level reached 85% of the toxic level. They suggest that their figures support their contention that bupivacaine not be used for intravenous regional analgesia.

The following factors may affect the peak blood level after tourniquet release: whether or not exsanguination is performed, time from injection to tourniquet release, mode of release of tourniquet, and arm movement after tourniquet release.

Exsanguination has been insufficiently studied. Adams, Dealy, and Kenmore[1] suggested that the more complete the exsanguination, the smaller would be the "reservoir" of lidocaine-containing blood to be flushed into the general circulation. Eriksson,[20] however, studied a few cases in which exsanguination had been performed with an Esmarch bandage, and he found no difference in plasma lidocaine level in these cases compared with those in which the arm had only been elevated.

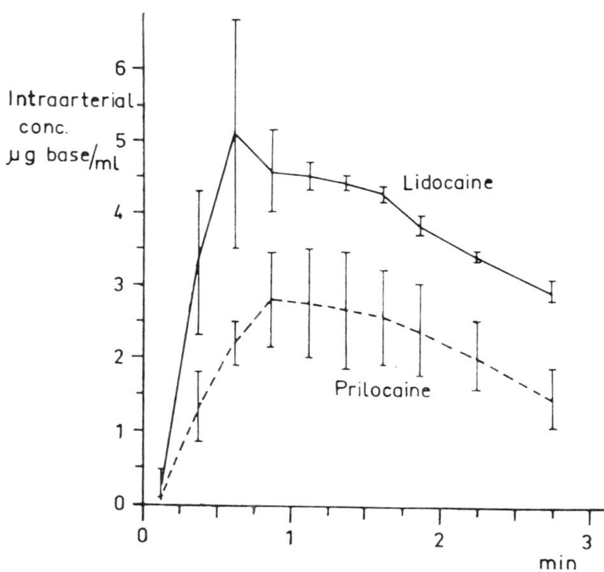

FIG. 12-7. The blood levels of lidocaine and prilocaine in the contralateral brachial artery after intravenous regional analgesia with a mixture of the two agents. (Eriksson, E.: The effects of intravenous local anesthetic agents on the central nervous system. Acta Anaesthesiol. Scand., *36[Suppl.]*:79, 1969.)

Time to tourniquet release has been studied by several workers, but their findings have been variable. Mazze and Dunbar[54] found no correlation between peak venous levels and tourniquet time; indeed, the patient who had the longest tourniquet time had the third highest plasma lidocaine concentration (Fig. 12-8). However, this may have been related to errors inherent in venous sampling. Comparing tourniquet times of 15 and 30 minutes, Thorn-Alquist[71] found no differences in peak levels when sampling from the contralateral artery. Both of these studies used rather insensitive colorimetric assays for lidocaine. By contrast, Tucker and Boas,[76] again using arterial sampling, did find an inverse relationship between tourniquet time and peak plasma level (Fig. 12-9). This study used a sensitive gas chromatography assay for lidocaine.

Mode of Release of Tourniquet. Holmes suggested that release and rapid reinflation of the tourniquet several times would lessen the incidence of symptoms.[41] This maneuver has also been recommended by other workers. Merrifield and Carter[58] found a mean peak

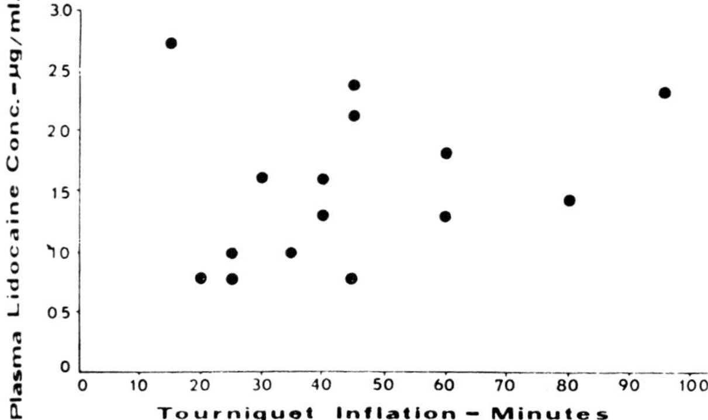

FIG. 12-8. Maximum plasma lidocaine concentration after tourniquet release, measured in venous blood, in relation to duration of tourniquet inflation. (Mazze, R.I., and Dunbar, R.W.: Plasma lidocaine concentrations after caudal, lumbar epidural, axillary block and intravenous regional anesthesia. Anesthesiology, *27*:574, 1966.)

venous lidocaine level of 5.9 ± 5.7 μg/ml when this procedure was performed, while with half the dose of lidocaine and without intermittent tourniquet release, the level was 4.7 ± 0.2 μg/ml, which indicates a definite protective effect. This method is perhaps less important if prilocaine is used; however, since it is simple to perform, it is wise to employ it as a safety measure.

Arm movement immediately after tourniquet release should be discouraged because it has been shown to result in increased plasma levels of the drug.[33]

Complications Related to the Use of a Tourniquet. When use of intravenous regional anesthesia is considered, the fact that a tourniquet must be used for the entire duration of the operation must be taken into account. There may be operations in which this is undesirable or even impossible, so that other methods of regional analgesia might be more appropriate. Also, there may be operations where the duration is considered too long for a tourniquet, although this is controversial because there does not appear to be any clear relationship between tourniquet time and complications.

Middleton and Varian[59] reviewed an estimated 630,000 tourniquet applications, and found an incidence of peripheral nerve damage of 1 : 8,000. The incidence was higher in procedures involving the upper limb (1 : 5,000) than in those involving the lower limb (1 : 13,000). In the upper limb, there were 27 patients with total palsy, 8 following the use of a pneumatic tourniquet and 19 following the use of an Esmarch bandage. All recovered. The tourniquet time varied from 20 minutes to 2½ hours. There were 19 patients with radial nerve palsy, in whom the tourniquet applications varied from 15 minutes to 1½ hours. All but one of these patients recovered. In the lower limb, there were 30 patients with palsy, all following the use of an Esmarch bandage. The tourniquet time varied from 30 minutes to 4½ hours, and all but one patient had an eventual full recovery. These authors studied the pressures that could be produced with an Esmarch bandage and found them variable and usually higher than supposed. How-

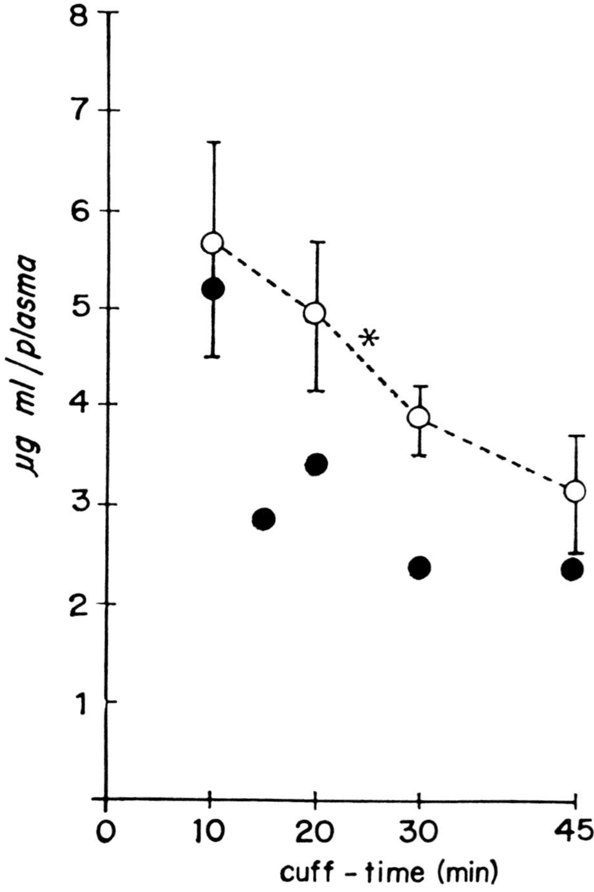

FIG. 12-9. Relation between cuff time and arterial plasma level of lidocaine, 1 minute after tourniquet release. Open circles represent mean data ± SD, solution; asterisk represents the difference significant at $p < 0.05$; closed circles indicate individual data with 0.5% solution. (Tucker, G.T., and Boas, R.A.: Pharmacokinetic aspects of intravenous regional anesthesia. Anesthesiology, *34*:538, 1971.)

ever, they were not able to draw definite conclusions about the etiology of tourniquet paralyses. There did not seem to be any common factor in any of their cases. Moldaver[61] believed that direct mechanical pressure was more likely to be a factor than ischemia, and he cautioned against using a tourniquet in any area where a nerve could be compressed against bony structures.

The following general recommendations can therefore be made:

A pneumatic tourniquet of a size appropriate to the arm circumference should be chosen.

The tourniquet should be applied where the nerves are best protected in the muscles.

Excessive tourniquet pressure should be avoided by measuring the "occlusion pressure" before the operation and by maintaining a tourniquet pressure of at least 50 mm Hg above the systolic.

The tubing should not be clamped between the cuff and the gauge because this would prevent a leaking cuff from being detected.

The duration of application of the tourniquet should be as short as possible.

MODE OF ACTION

The mode of action of the local anesthetic agents in intravenous regional analgesia has been the subject of much debate. There has been difficulty in separating the effects of the local anesthetic from those of ischemia alone. Direct pressure on nerves can cause anesthesia, and Miles, James, Clark, and Whitwam[60] and Shanks and McLeod[69] found quite marked effects from ischemia alone. In fact, Shanks and McLeod found that anesthesia, preceded by dysesthesia, usually developed in 5 to 30 minutes with ischemia alone, along with variable muscle weakness. However, all agree that the onset of anesthesia is much more rapid and complete when a local anesthetic is added.

Miles and colleagues[60] demonstrated that the latency of action potential in muscle was increased 55% by ischemia and 180% by ischemia plus lidocaine. They believed their results indicated that lidocaine acts on the peripheral part of the neuron. They showed that the muscle weakness was not reversible by neostigmine.

Shanks and McLeod,[69] however, using 1% lidocaine, concluded that the block was in the nerve trunks. They considered that the more pronounced effect of lidocaine on conduction in proximal segments of the nerve was the result of a greater concentration of the agent in the forearm, which would be in keeping with the radiographic studies of Fleming, Veiga-Pires, McCutcheon, and Emanuel[26] and Sorbie and Chacha,[70] who demonstrated that the local anesthetic proceeds rapidly in a proximal direction when it is injected in the dorsum of the hand.

Cotev and Robin,[12] in biopsy studies on dogs injected with ^{14}C-labeled lidocaine, showed a selective accumulation of the agent in nerves and relatively little accumulation in muscle. They noted a biphasic washout of the drug, which they attributed to reactive hyperemia. In an elegant series of experiments, Raj, Garcia, Burleson, and Jenkins[64] demonstrated, by means of a lidocaine–Renografin-60 mixture, that the contrast concentrated principally around the elbow. No contrast was seen distal to the proximal phalanges. Anesthesia developed from the fingertips upward, reaching the elbow last. Contrast material confined to the hand, injected by way of the radial artery, did not produce anesthesia. When the block was established between two tourniquets, as in the original Bier method, nerve conduction above the block (median nerve in the axilla to thenar muscles) was decreased, whereas nerve conduction below the block (ulnar nerve at the wrist to hypothenar muscles) was unaltered. Anesthesia tended to develop earlier in the anteromedial aspect of the forearm and later in the posterolateral aspect.

Raj and colleagues believe that these results show that the mode of action is on the larger nerve trunks. At the elbow, the median and ulnar nerves are fairly close together and surrounded by large venous channels. The radial nerve is posterolateral and has fewer large vessels near it. Histologically, the peripheral nerve shows a thick perineurium, but with many vascular channels in the core of the nerve in close proximity to the nerve fibrils. It would seem that these vascular channels carry the drug to the core of the nerve, from which it would diffuse toward the periphery. The greater number of venous channels close to the median and ulnar nerves, compared with the radial nerve, would explain the earlier onset of analgesia on the anteromedial aspect of the forearm (Fig. 12-10).

On the other hand, the speed of onset and, particularly, the rapidity of spread of analgesia are not like those seen with the block of a major nerve trunk.[7] Also, cases have been reported in which analgesia was complete everywhere except in a digit in which the local circulation was impaired; this does not support nerve trunk block.[3]

Furthermore, in a series of studies with techne-

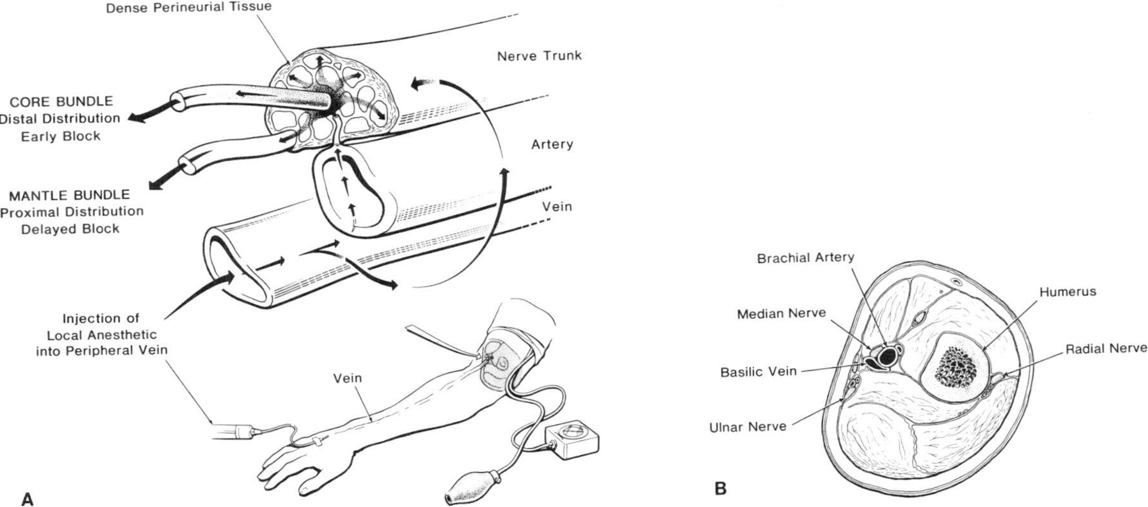

FIG. 12-10. Proposed mechanism of intravenous regional anesthesia. **A.** Local anesthetic injected into a dorsal hand vein travels to the large venous channels at the elbow. Here, it is transferred by arteries through the thick perineurium into the core of the major nerve trunks. From here, it diffuses outward so that the core bundles are blocked, initially resulting in "early distal block," and the mantle bundles (supplying proximal areas) are bocked last, resulting in "delayed proximal block." **B.** Note that, in a cross-section of the arm at the elbow, the median and ulnar nerves on the anteromedial aspect have rich vascular channels nearby. The radial nerve, on the posterolateral surface, has less vascularity in its vicinity. This may explain the later onset of analgesia in radial nerve distribution.

tium-labeled saline, Lillie and co-workers showed that when the injection was made at the antecubital fossa, all the arm veins apparently filled, but hand filling could be prevented with a forearm cuff. When prilocaine was injected, no analgesia of the hand was produced except in a small area corresponding to the distribution of the radial nerve. They argue that these results support the theory of block of small nerve endings, since no block of the major (median and ulnar) trunks was seen during the 20-minute duration of the study.

Perhaps Bier should have the last word: ". . . [this] new method uses the vascular bed to bring the anesthetic agent to the nerve endings as well as the nerve trunks."[5]

INTRAVENOUS REGIONAL SYMPATHETIC BLOCK

Intravenous regional sympathetic block is similar to the intravenous regional anesthesia technique. The method was devised by Hannington-Kiff,[30,31] whose papers should be consulted for further details.

Premedication is usually unnecessary, but all the usual precautions should be taken. The blood pressure should be monitored, an intravenous infusion should be running, and the patient should be on a table capable of being tilted. If there is marked sympathetic dystrophy, there is often severe pain on injection, so much so that general anesthesia is preferred on the first occasion. However, general anesthesia is not usually required on subsequent occasions, provided the block is repeated before its effect has fully worn off. Nor is general anesthesia commonly necessary in cases where the block is being performed for Raynaud's disease.

The agent usually used is guanethidine, which is strongly bound to sympathetic nerve endings. An alternative method, which reduces the pain of injection, is to mix the guanethidine with 0.5% prilocaine. The butterfly needle is placed in a hand vein, and the tourniquet is placed on the upper arm. Elevation is used for exsanguination, and the tourniquet is inflated to 50 to 100 mm Hg above the systolic pressure. The solution consists of 20 mg of guanethidine in 20 to 25 ml of physiologic saline. (For the leg, 40 mg of the drug is given in 40 ml of saline.) The tourniquet is kept inflated for 10 minutes and then released and reinflated several times while the blood pressure is monitored in the other arm. (A slight fall in blood pressure may occur.) Patients should be warned of the possibility of postural hypotension, which can occur for up to 48 hours postblock. When guanethidine is not available, reserpine has been used effectively.

The effectiveness of the sympathetic block may be checked with a temperature probe. The advantages of this method are that it may be used after "postsympathectomy escape," that it may be used in patients who are taking anticoagulants, and that the potential complications of stellate ganglion block are avoided. Also avoided are the adhesions that can result from lumbar sympathetic block with phenol, which may render subsequent surgery difficult. The duration of effect is often as long as 4 to 6 weeks, and the block can be repeated (see also Chap. 13).

REFERENCES

1. Adams, J.P., Dealy, E.J., and Kenmore, P.I.: Intravenous regional anesthesia in hand surgery. J. Bone Joint Surg., *46A*:811, 1964.
2. Anesthesia Conference (Clinical). N.Y. State J. Med., *66*:1344, 1966.
3. Atkinson, D.I.: The mode of action of intravenous regional anaesthetics. Acta Anaesthesiol. Scand., *36*[*Suppl.*]:131, 1969.
4. Bell, H.M., Slater, E.M., and Harris, W.H.: Regional anesthesia with intravenous lidocaine. J.A.M.A., *186*:544, 1963.
5. Bier, A.: Ueber einen neuen Weg Lokalanasthesie an den gliedmassen zu Erzeugen. Verh. dtsch. Ges. Chir., *37(2)*:204, 1908.
6. Bromage, P.R., and Robson, J.G.: Concentrations of lignocaine in the blood after intravenous, intramuscular, epidural and endotracheal administration. Anaesthesia, *16*:461, 1961.
7. Brown, B.R.: Discussion on: The site of action of intravenous regional anesthesia. Anesth. Analg. (Cleve.), *51*:776, 1972.
8. Brown, E.M., and Weissman, F.: A case report: Prolonged intravenous regional anesthesia. Anesth. Analg. (Cleve.), *45*:319, 1966.
9. Carrell, E.D., and Eyring, E.J.: Intravenous regional anesthesia for childhood fractures. J. Trauma, *11*:301, 1971.
10. Colbern, E.C.: The Bier block for intravenous regional anesthesia. Anesth. Analg. (Cleve.), *49*:935, 1970.
11. Committee on Safety of Medicines: Bupivacaine (Marcain Plain) in intravenous regional anaesthesia (Bier's Block). Current Problems, *12*, 1983.
12. Cotev, S., and Robin, G.C.: Experimental studies on intravenous regional analgesia using radioactive lidocaine. Acta Anaesthesiol. Scand., *36*[*Suppl.*]:127, 1969.
13. Davies, J.A.H., Gill, S.S., and Weber, J.C.P.: Intravenous regional analgesia using bupivacaine. Anaesthesia, *36*:331, 1981.
14. Davies, J.A.H., *et al.*: Intravenous regional analgesia. Anaesthesia, *39*:416, 1984.
15. Dawkins, O.S., *et al.*: Intravenous regional anaesthesia. Can. Anaesth. Soc. J., *11*:243, 1964.
16. De Jong, R.H., and Heavner, J.E.: Diazepam prevents local anesthetic seizures. Anesthesiology, *34*:523, 1971.
17. Department of Health and Social Security: Automatic Tourniquets 1982. HN(Hazard) (82)7.
18. Dunbar, R.W., and Mazze, R.I.: Intravenous regional anesthesia. Anesth. Analg. (Cleve.), *46*:806, 1967.
19. Englesson, S., Eriksson, E., Wahlqvist, S., and Ortengren, B.: Differences in tolerance to intravenous Xylocaine and Citanest (L67), a new local anaesthetic. A double-blind study in man. Proc. First Eur. Congr. Anaesth., *2*:206. 1, 1962.
20. Eriksson, E.: The effects of intravenous local anesthetic agents on the central nervous system. Acta Anaesthesiol. Scand., *36*[*Suppl.*]:79, 1969.
21. Evans, C.J., Dewar, J.A., Boyes, R.N., and Scott, D.B.: Residual nerve block following intravenous regional anaesthesia. Br. J. Anaesth., *46*:668, 1974.
22. Farrar, M.D., Scheybani, M., and Nolte, H.: Upper extremity block: Clinical effectiveness and complications. Anaesthesia, *37*:368, 1982.
23. Finegan, B.A., and Bukht, M.D.: Venous pressures in the isolated upper limb during saline injection. Can. Anaesth. Soc. J., *31*:364, 1984.
24. Fitzgerald, B.: Intravenous regional anaesthesia in children. Br. J. Anaesth., *48*:485, 1976.
25. Fleming, S.A.: Safety and usefulness of intravenous regional anaesthesia. Acta Anaesth. Scand., *36*[*Suppl.*]:21, 1969.
26. Fleming, S.A., Veiga-Pires, J.A., McCutcheon, R.M., and Emanuel, C.I.: A demonstration of the site of action of intravenous lignocaine. Can. Anaesth. Soc. J., *13*:21, 1966.
27. Foldes, F.F., Molloy, R., McNall, P.G., and Koukal, L.R.: Comparison of toxicity of intravenously given local anesthetic agents in man. J.A.M.A., *172*:1493, 1960.
28. Gingrich, T.F.: Intravenous regional anesthesia of the upper extremity in children. J.A.M.A., *200*:405, 1967.
29. Gooding, J.M., Tavakoli, M.M., Fitzpatrick, W.O., and Bagley, J.N.: Bupivacaine: Preferred agent for intravenous regional anesthesia. South. Med. J., *74*:1282, 1981.
30. Hannington-Kiff, J.G.: Intravenous regional sympathetic block with guanethidine. Lancet, *1*:1019, 1974.
31. Hannington-Kiff, J.G.: Pain Relief, p. 70. London, Heinemann Educational Books, 1974.
32. Hanton, R.J., and Punchihewa, V.G.: Intravenous regional analgesia using bupivacaine. Anaesthesia, *36*:350, 1981.
33. Hargrove, R.L., *et al.*: Blood lignocaine levels following intravenous regional analgesia. Anaesthesia, *21*:37, 1966.
34. Harris, W.H.: Choice of anesthetic agents for intravenous regional anesthesia. Acta Anaesthesiol. Scand., *36*[*Suppl.*]:47, 1969.
35. Harris, W.H., Cole, D.W., Mital, M., and Laver, M.B.: Methemoglobin formation and oxygen transport following intravenous regional anesthesia using prilocaine. Anesthesiology, *29*:65, 1968.
36. Heath, M.L.: Deaths after intravenous regional anaesthesia. Br. Med. J., *285*:913, 1982.

37. Heath, M.L.: Bupivicaine [sic] toxicity and Bier blocks. Anesthesiology, *59*:481, 1983.
38. Henderson, A.M.: Adverse reaction of bupivacaine: Complication of intravenous regional analgesia. Br. Med. J., *281*:1043, 1980.
39. Hoffman, S., Simon, B.E., and Hartley, J.: A new tourniquet for intravenous regional anesthesia. Plast. Reconstr. Surg., *40*:243, 1967.
40. Hollingworth, A., Wallace, W.A., and Dabir, R.: Comparison of bupivacaine and prilocaine used in Bier's Block: A double-blind trial. Injury, *13*:331, 1982.
41. Holmes, C. McK.: Intravenous regional analgesia. Lancet, *1*:245, 1963.
42. Holmes, C. McK.: Anaesthetising the arm. N.Z. Med. J., *63*:24, 1964.
43. Holmes, C. McK.: The history and development of intravenous regional anaesthesia. Acta Anaesthesiol. Scand., *36*[*Suppl.*]:11, 1969.
44. Hooper, R.L.: Intravenous regional anaesthesia: A report of a new local anaesthetic agent. Can. Anaesth. Soc. J., *11*:247, 1964.
45. Hoyle, J.R.: Tourniquet for intravenous regional analgesia. Anaesthesia, *19*:294, 1964.
46. Ishibashi, T., Onchi, Y., and Okuda, T.: New method of local anaesthesia for operations on the upper extremity [in Japanese]. Jpn. J. Anesthesiol., *15*:239, 1966.
47. Jeyaseelam, S., Stevenson, T.M., and Pfitzner, J.: Tourniquet failure and arterial calcification. Anaesthesia, *36*:48, 1981.
48. Kalso, E., Tuominen, M., Rosenberg, P.H., and Alila, A.: Bupivacaine blood levels after intravenous regional anesthesia of the arm. Reg. Anaesth., *5*:81, 1982.
49. Kennedy, B.R., Duthie, A.M., Parbrook, G.D., and Carr, T.L.: Intravenous regional analgesia: An appraisal. Br. Med. J., *1*:954, 1965.
50. Kerr, J.H.: Intravenous regional analgesia. Anaesthesia, *22*:562, 1967.
51. Lawes, E.G., Johnson, T., Pritchard, P., and Robbins, P.: Venous pressures during simulated Bier's block. Anaesthesia, *39*:147, 1984.
52. Lillie, P.E., Glynn, C.J., and Fenwick, D.G.: Site of action of intravenous regional anesthesia. Anesthesiology, *61*:507, 1984.
53. Lund, P.C., and Cwik, J.C.: Propitocaine (Citanest) and methemoglobinemia. Anesthesiology, *26*:569, 1965.
54. Mazze, R.L., and Dunbar, R.W.: Plasma lidocaine concentrations after caudal, lumbar epidural, axillary block and intravenous regional anesthesia. Anesthesiology, *27*:574, 1966.
55. Mazze, R.L., and Dunbar, R.W.: Intravenous regional anaesthesia: Report of 497 cases with a toxicity study. Acta Anaesthesiol. Scand., *36*[*Suppl.*]:27, 1969.
56. McKeown, D.W., *et al.*: Which agent for intravenous regional anesthesia? Lancet, 1503, 1983.
57. McKeown, D.W., Meiklejohn, B., and Scott, D.B.: Bupivacaine and prilocaine in intravenous regional anaesthesia. Anaesthesia, *39*:150, 1984.
58. Merrifield, A.J., and Carter, S.J.: Intravenous regional analgesia: Lignocaine blood levels. Anaesthesia, *20*:287, 1965.
59. Middleton, R.W.D., and Varian, J.P.: Tourniquet paralysis. Aust. N.Z. J. Surg., *44*:124, 1974.
60. Miles, D.W., James, J.L., Clark, D.E., and Whitwam, J.G.: Site of action of "intravenous regional anaesthesia." J. Neurol. Neurosurg. Psychiatry, *27*:574, 1964.
61. Moldaver, J.: Tourniquet paralysis syndrome. Arch. Surg., *68*:136, 1954.
62. Moore, D.C., Mather, L.E., and Bridenbaugh, L.D.: Bupivacaine (Marcaine): An evaluation of its tissue and systemic toxicity in humans. Acta Anaesthesiol. Scand., *21*:109, 1977.
63. Ogden, P.N.: Failure of intravenous regional analgesia using a double-cuff tourniquet. Anaesthesia, *39*:456, 1984.
64. Raj, P.P., Garcia, C.E., Burleson, J.W., and Jenkins, M.T.: The site of action of intravenous regional anesthesia. Anesth. Analg. (Cleve.), *51*:776, 1972.
65. Reynolds, F.: Editorial. Anaesthesia, *39*:105, 1984.
66. Rosenberg, P.H., Kalso, E.A., Tuominen, M.K., and Linden, H.B.: Acute bupivacaine toxicity as a result of venous leakage under the tourniquet cuff during a Bier block. Anesthesiology, *58*:95, 1983.
67. Ryding, F.N.: Digital regional analgesia. Anaesthesia, *36*:969, 1981.
68. Shamay, C., and Robin, G.C.: Experimental studies on intravenous regional anaesthesia using radioactive lignocaine. Br. J. Anaesth., *38*:936, 1966.
69. Shanks, C.A., and McLeod, J.G.: Nerve conduction studies in regional intravenous analgesia using 1% lignocaine. Br. J. Anaesth., *42*:1060, 1970.
70. Sorbie, C., and Chacha, P.: Regional anaesthesia by the intravenous route. Br. Med. J., *1*:957, 1965.
71. Thorn-Alquist, A-M.: Blood concentration of local anaesthetics after intravenous regional anaesthesia. Acta Anaesthesiol. Scand., *13*:229, 1969.
72. Thorn-Alquist, A-M.: Intravenous regional anaesthesia. Acta Anaesthesiol. Scand., *15*:23, 1971.
73. Trias, A.: The use of intravenous regional anaesthesia in orthopaedic surgery. Acta Anaesthesiol. Scand., *36*[*Suppl.*]:35, 1969.
74. Tryba, M., Hausmann, E., Zenz, M., and Wellhorner, H.H.: Toxizitat von Prilocain und Bupivacain in der intravenosen Regionalanasthesie. Anasth. Intensivther. Notfallmed., *17*:207, 1982.
75. Tryba, M., Zenz, M., and Hausmann, E.: Prolonged analgesia after cuff release following I.V. regional analgesia with prilocaine. Br. J. Anaesth., *55*:631, 1983.
76. Tucker, G.T., and Boas, R.A.: Pharmacokinetic aspects of intravenous regional anesthesia. Anesthesiology, *34*:538, 1971.
77. Van Niekerk, J.P., and Tonkin, P.A.: Intravenous regional analgesia. S. Afr. Med. J., *40*:165, 1966.
78. Ware, R.J.: Intravenous regional analgesia using bupivacaine. Anaesthesia, *30*:817, 1975.
79. Ware, R.J.: Intravenous regional analgesia using bupivacaine: A double-blind comparison with lignocaine. Anaesthesia, *34*:231, 1979.
80. Ware, R.J., and Caldwell, J.: Clinical and pharmacological studies of intravenous regional analgesia using bupivacaine. Br. J. Anaesth., *48*:1124, 1976.

81. Ware, R.J.: Intravenous regional analgesia: The debate continues. Anaesthesia, *37*:958, 1982.
82. Wildsmith, J.A.W.: Intravenous regional analgesia: Essential safeguards. Anaesthesia, *37*:959, 1982.
83. Winnie, A.P., and Ramamurthy, S.: Pneumatic exsanguination for intravenous regional anesthesia. Anesthesiology, *33*:664, 1970.

SUGGESTED READING

D'Amato, H., and Wiedling, S.: Intravenous regional anaesthesia: An international conference. Acta Anaesthesiol. Scand., *36*[*Suppl.*]:36, 1969.

Dundee, J.W., and Wyant, G.M.: Intravenous Anesthesia, Chap. 16, London, Churchill-Livingston, 1974.

Thorn-Alquist, A-M.: Intravenous regional anaesthesia. Acta Anaesthesiol. Scand., *40*[*Suppl.*]:40, 1971.

13 SYMPATHETIC NEURAL BLOCKADE OF UPPER AND LOWER EXTREMITY

J. BERTIL LÖFSTRÖM
MICHAEL J. COUSINS

HISTORY AND GENERAL CONSIDERATIONS

The effects of sympathetic nerves in maintaining normal constrictor tone in the blood vessels of the skin have been known since the classic work of Claude Bernard in 1852. The well-known observation of increased skin temperature of the foot after surgical lumbar sympathectomy was first made by Hunter and Royle (see Ref. 19). Surgical sympathectomy has been performed at some clinics, as reported by De Bakey in 1950, to promote healing of ischemic cutaneous ulcers and to relieve pain in the foot at rest (*rest pain*)[93]; however, at many vascular clinics today more emphasis is placed on vascular grafting procedures, and the refined surgical techniques undoubtedly have greatly improved the prognosis of the patient with occlusive vascular disease. Despite this movement away from sympathetic ablation, there is considerable potential benefit from sympathetic neural blockade as an adjunct to vascular surgery or as primary treatment for patients with rest pain who are not fit for, or not amenable to, vascular reconstruction. The large series of 1666 patients with neurolytic lumbar sympathetic blocks reported in 1970 by Reid and colleagues bears testimony to this, and it is surprising that many clinics have largely neglected this important option in the treatment of vascular disease.[75]

Mandl first described the technique of lumbar sympathetic neural blockade in 1926, and his technique was clearly very similar to that for celiac plexus blockade described by Kappis in 1919.[44,64] A similar neglect of celiac plexus block for upper abdominal cancer has been apparent (see Chap. 30). The classic "anterior" approach to stellate ganglion blockade was initiated by Leriche in 1934 and forms the basis of the technique described in this chapter; the use of this technique is still largely supported only by anecdotal information.

It is clear, then, that these techniques have all been available for well over 50 years. Surprisingly, precise documentation of their place in clinical medicine is only now becoming available, and much information remains to be obtained.

Sympathetic blockade is often produced as an accompaniment to motor and sensory blockade during regional block for operative surgery (*e.g.*, spinal and epidural anesthesia, brachial plexus block). It is maintained that "differential" sympathetic blockade without sensory and motor block can be produced with low concentrations of local anesthetic by means of epidural or spinal subarachnoid block (see below and Chap. 27). This has its most common use in the diagnosis of chronic pain, although we believe that selective sympathetic ganglion block provides more reliable information (see Chap. 27). In the management of acute pain, epidural block has been said to be capable of relieving labor pain and the pain of renal colic (see below and Chap. 8); however, the best application of sympathetic blockade appears to be in the use of selective blockade of the sympathetic ganglia (see below).

Because the sympathetic ganglia are, except in the thoracic region, relatively safely separated from somatic nerves, it is possible to achieve sympathetic blockade without loss of sensory or motor function. This offers the possibility of treating a variety of conditions in which reduced sympathetic activity might be beneficial. With careful technique, it is even possible to achieve permanent neurolytic blockade with essentially no loss of sensory and motor function. Thus, sympathetic blockade, at the three major levels indicated in Figure 13-2, is regarded as potentially one of the most rewarding series of techniques for diagnosis and management of acute and chronic pain syndromes and other conditions (see list on p. 473). Our clinical experience has been that, of all neural blockade techniques, lumbar sympathetic block for rest pain and celiac plexus block for upper abdominal cancer offer the most benefit at the lowest risk.

Celiac plexus blockade is described in Chapters 14 and 29, and lumbar sympathetic block and the remaining sympathetic ganglion blocks (stellate and thoracic) are described in this chapter, as is intravenous regional sympathetic block. At present, it is capable of a duration of only up to 2 weeks; however, often it is an attractive alternative to the higher-risk technique of thoracic sympathetic block or thoracic surgical sympathectomy. Advances in producing "immune" lesions in the sympathetic nervous system may eventually make it possible to perform a selective intravenous regional immunosympathectomy.

The contribution of lumbar sympathetic blockade to the management of pain in the pelvic region requires further investigation. As outlined below, initial information indicates that it may be possible to use either unilateral or bilateral lumbar sympathetic block for some kinds of pelvic pain (particularly urogenital). This, of course, poses a much lesser risk than the alternative of neurolytic subarachnoid block, with its possibility of loss of bladder function (see Chap. 30).

In order to take full advantage of sympathetic neural blockade, it is essential to bear in mind the general features of the anatomy and physiology of the peripheral sympathetic nervous system, as described in the next section, and the regional anatomy, as described with each of the techniques of sympathetic blockade. It is also important to use objective methods to evaluate the completeness of sympathetic blockade and its clinical effects, as shown on pages 474 and 475.

SYMPATHETIC NERVOUS SYSTEM

ANATOMY AND PHYSIOLOGY

The peripheral sympathetic nervous system begins as efferent preganglionic fibers in the intermediolateral column of the spinal cord, passing in the ventral roots from T1 to L2 (and perhaps some cervical roots) out of the spinal canal to run separately as white rami communicantes to the sympathetic chain, at the side of the vertebral bodies (Fig. 13-1). In the lower cervical region, the chain lies at the anterolateral aspect of the vertebral body and in the thorax is adjacent to the neck of the ribs, still relatively close to somatic roots (see Fig. 13-21). In the lumbar region, however, the chain angles forward to lie anterolateral to the body of the vertebra and is now separated from somatic roots by psoas muscle and psoas fascia (see Fig. 13-22). The preganglionic fibers pass a variable distance in the sympathetic chain to reach ganglia in the chain, or they may pass further to peripherally located ganglia (*i.e.*, in the gut; Fig. 13-1). The inconstant level of relay in the chain itself may be responsible for a number of disappointing results from an apparently technically successful block. Sympathetic ganglia are segmentally located in the chest (T1–11;T12). There are also three cervical ganglia, four to five lumbar ganglia, four sacral ganglia, and one coccygeal ganglion. The postganglionic fibers are widely distributed, partly to join peripheral nerves (the gray communicantes) and partly to join vessels in different organs. The sympathetic chain not only receives efferent preganglionic but also afferent visceral fibers, which conduct pain from head, neck, and upper extremity (cervicothoracic ganglia); abdominal viscera (see Chap. 14) (celiac plexus); and urogenital system and lower extremity (lumbar ganglia; Fig. 13-2).

Sympathetic Efferents to Blood Vessels

The great vessels (carotids, aorta, vena cava) receive direct postganglionic filaments from adjacent sympathetic ganglia (Fig. 13-3) and from plexuses (see Fig. 13-2). The main outflow of preganglionic fibers by means of the ventral roots may subsequently follow

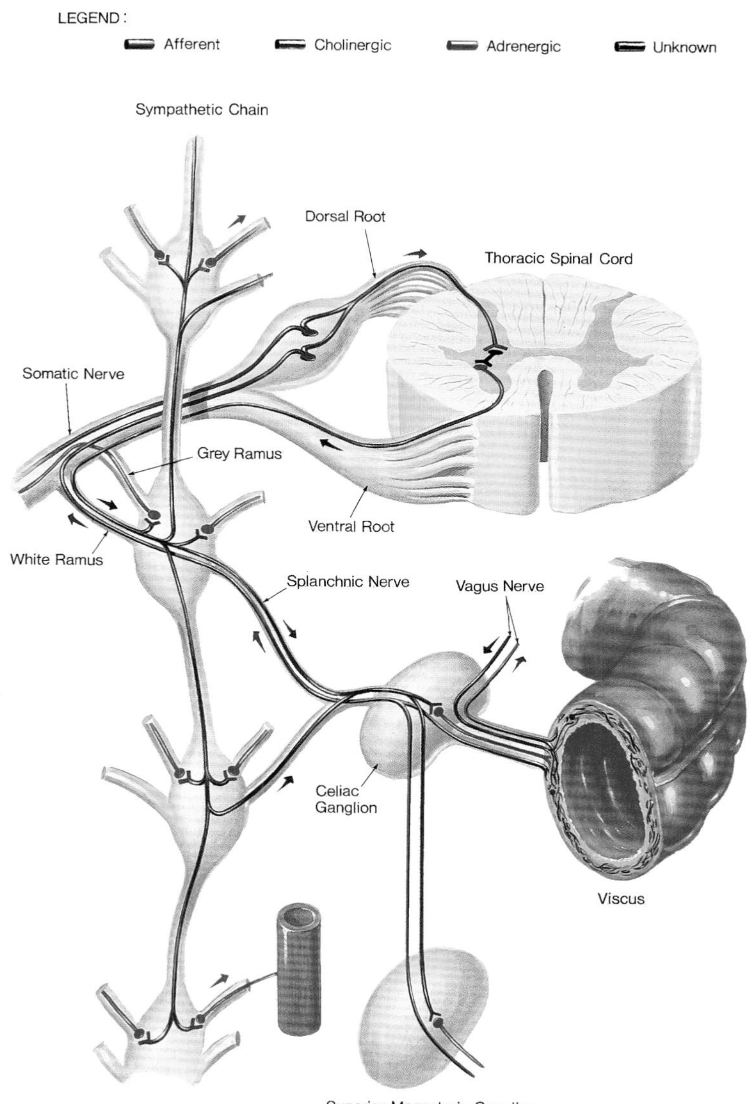

FIG. 13-1. Peripheral sympathetic nervous system. Cell bodies are located in the intermediolateral cell column of T1–L2 spinal segments. Efferent fibers (cholinergic) pass by way of the ventral root to a white ramus communicans and then to the paravertebral sympathetic ganglia or to more remotely located ganglia, such as the celiac ganglion. From each ganglion, they give rise to adrenergic fibers to supply viscera (celiac ganglion) or to join somatic nerves (from lumbar sympathetic ganglion) to supply efferent fibers to the limbs (sudomotor and vasomotor effects). In the case of lumbar sympathetic ganglia, the adrenergic fibers swing backward by a gray ramus communicans to join the somatic nerve. Afferent fibers travel by way of ganglia, such as celiac and lumbar sympathetic, without synapsing and reach somatic nerves and then their cell bodies in the dorsal root ganglia. They then pass to the dorsal root and synapse with interneurons in the intermediolateral area of the spinal cord. These afferent fibers convey pain impulses from the viscera and are similar to nociceptive afferents except that they pass without synapsing through sympathetic ganglia.

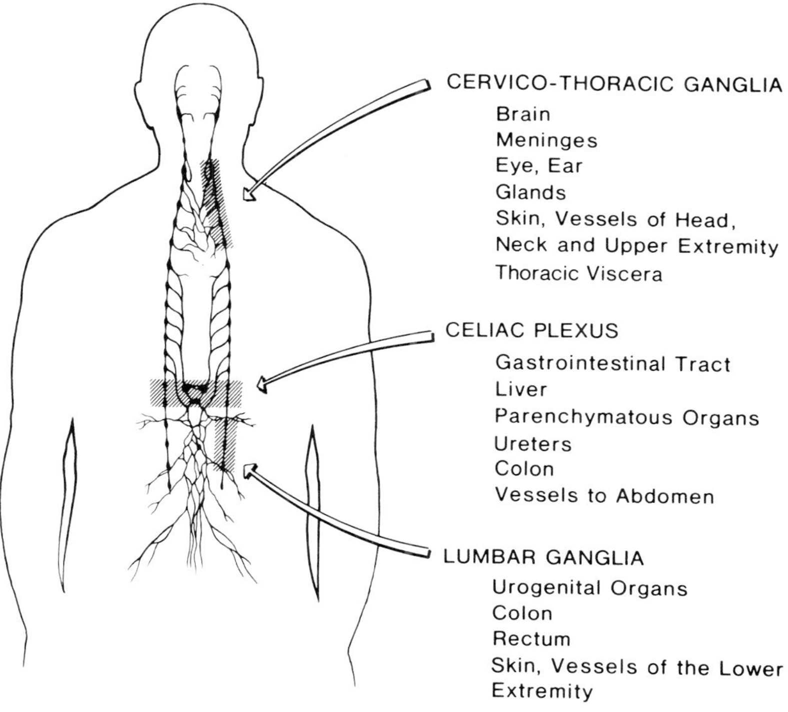

FIG. 13-2. An outline of the sympathetic nervous system. The three main levels of sympathetic blockade are shown along with major clinical uses. (Redrawn after Bonica, J.J.: The Management of Pain. Philadelphia, Lea & Febiger, 1953.)

alternative courses: [1] synapse in the same level or adjacent ganglia and pass in somatic nerves to vessels; [2] synapse in ganglia and pass directly to vessels via filaments; [3] pass directly through sympathetic ganglia and synapse in prevertebral plexuses and then pass to vessels (Fig. 13-3); or [4] pass through sympathetic ganglia and ascend or descend to synapse in ganglia above (*e.g.*, cervical) or below (*e.g.*, lower lumbar).

Vascular nerves and filaments from these diverse sources are united around individual vessels in extensive "perivascular adventitial plexuses," which in turn ramify into plexuses between adventitia and media and between media and intima. Plexuses are augmented by branches from nearby cranial or spinal nerves. Thus, there is great overlap from several spinal cord segments. Arteries and arterioles are more richly supplied than veins and venules. Although nerve fibers accompany venules, it is not known whether they serve a vasoconstrictor role.

Sympathetic fibers are generally found in a deep fascial plane and are less accessible than segmental nerves. Interruption of sympathetic nerve fibers by neural blockade can be achieved in the following ways: at the sympathetic chain by a sympathetic blockade, at peripheral nerves by a nerve block, or at a vessel by perivascular infiltration, or to some extent by intradural or extradural injection of local anesthetic (see below). Sympathetic activity can also be blocked pharmacologically by an alpha-receptor blocker (phentolamine, dibenzyline); by a "depleter" of norepinephrine activity in sympathetic nerve ending (guanethidine or reserpine); or by a beta-receptor blocker, propranolol (β_1- and β_2-) or practolol (mainly β_1-receptor). Sympathetic nerve endings have both presynaptic and postsynaptic receptors (Fig. 13-4). Until recently, available alpha-receptor blockers acted upon both presynaptic and postsynaptic receptors. Blockade of presynaptic receptors interrupted the negative feedback that modifies norepinephrine (NE) release. More selective postsynaptic blockers (*e.g.*, prazocin) are now available which have a much more sustained degree of alpha-blockade (Fig. 13-4).

FUNCTION

Vasoconstriction by Alpha Receptors. Arterioli (in the skin and in the splanchnic area), smaller arteries, and, in particular, peripheral veins are normally

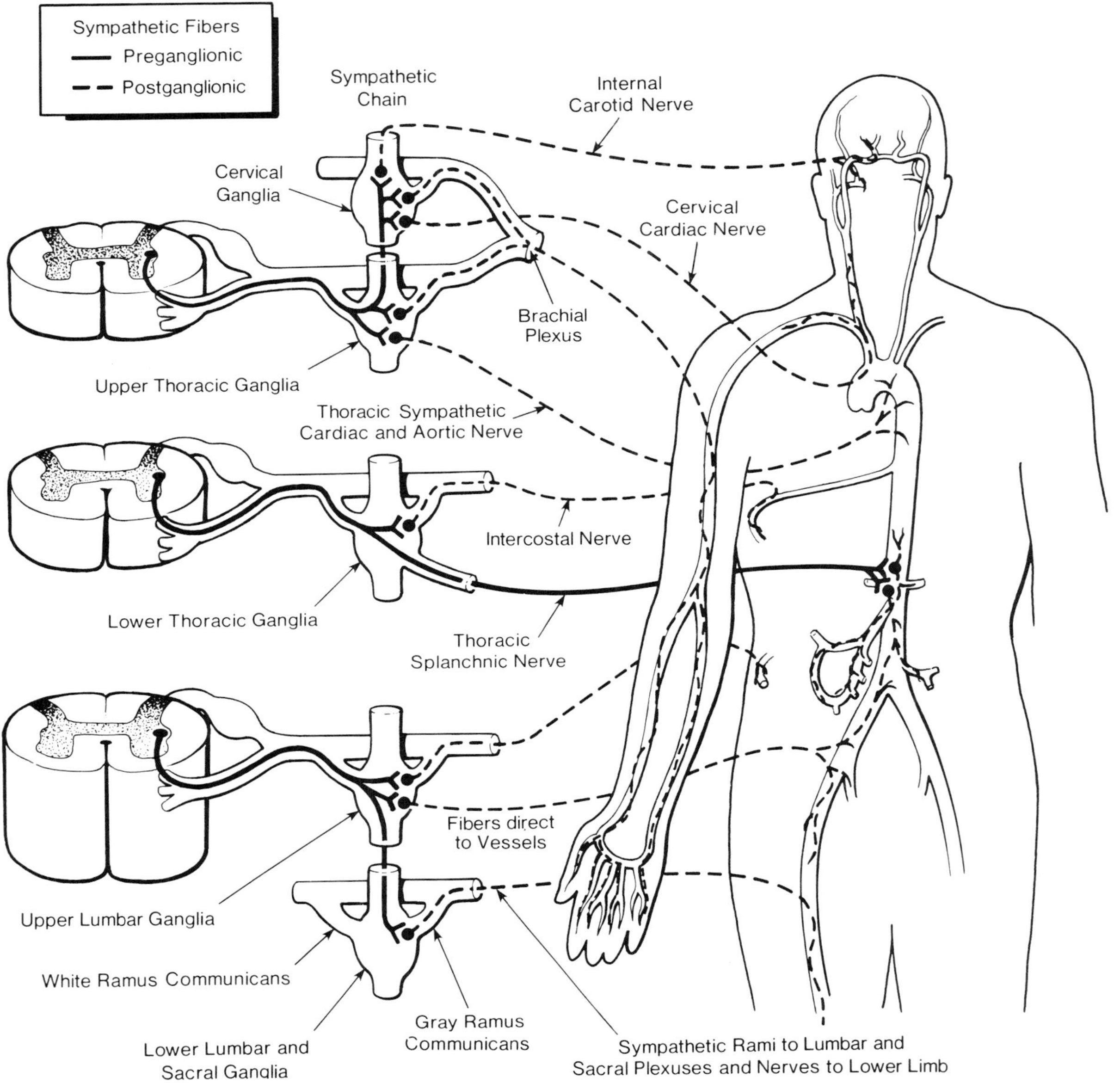

FIG. 13-3. Sympathetic nerve supply to blood vessels (see text).

under moderate vasoconstrictor influence. Pain, anxiety, and blood loss can provoke a very marked increase in arteriolar vasoconstrictor tone, mediated by the sympathetic nervous system; this change results in increased resistance, particularly in skin vessels, and thus influences the distribution of blood flow. In addition, there is an associated increase in venous tone, which decreases the compliance of the venous system, reducing its blood content and increasing the venous pressure.

Heart Muscle Activity (Chronotropic and Inotropic Effect). β_1-stimulation causes increased heart rate and increased cardiac contractility; thus high

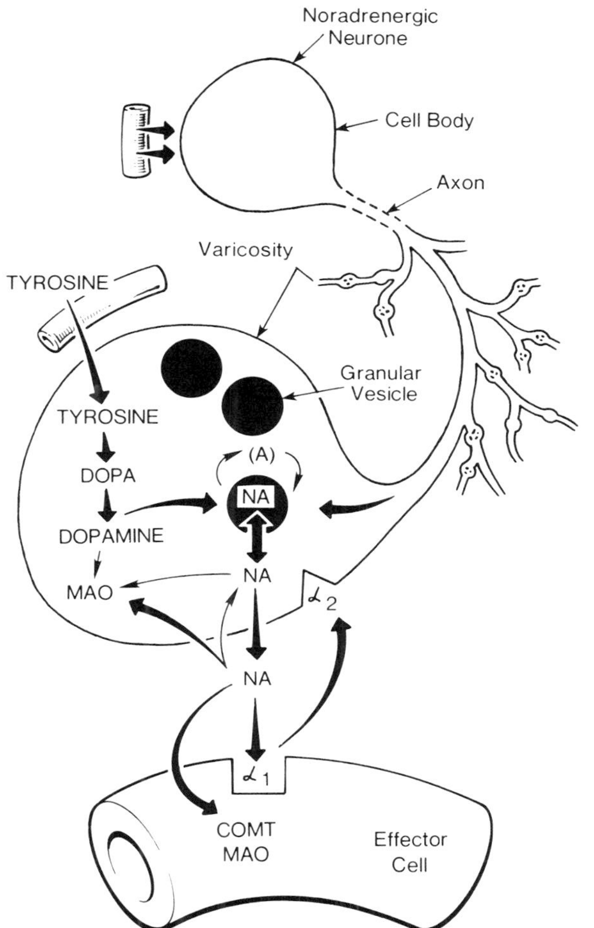

FIG. 13-4. Sympathetic nerve endings and receptors (see text). Diagram of synapse between a postganglionic sympathetic neuron and postsynaptic receptors on effector cells (*e.g.*, smooth muscle of vessel wall). Stimulation of presynaptic (α_2) receptors by previously released norepinephrine (noradrenaline, *NA*) results in inhibition of further release of N from the sympathetic neuron. Stimulation of α_1-receptors results in smooth muscle contraction. MAO, monoamine oxidase; COMT, catechol-o-methyl-transferase.

(T1–4) thoracic sympathetic blockade may cause a marked reduction in cardiac output.

Bronchial Tone. β_2-stimulation causes bronchodilation, so that it is theoretically possible for thoracic sympathetic blockade to cause bronchoconstriction, although this does not appear to be the case (see Chap. 8).

Vasodilatation. β_2-stimulation causes vasodilatation in some vascular beds (*e.g.*, muscle); however, this is a minor effect and is overridden by local metabolic effects (see below).

Smooth Muscle Tone (*e.g.*, in the Gut and in the Bladder). β_2-stimulation causes smooth muscle relaxation and sphincter contraction. Thus, sympathetic blockade results in smooth muscle contraction (a small contracted gut) and sphincter relaxation. These effects provide excellent surgical access during procedures such as abdominoperineal resection. **Sudomotor** (sweat glands) and **hair follicles** have the same postganglion efferents as blood vessels; however, the neurotransmitter in sweat glands is **acetylcholine**.

Metabolic. The sympathetic nervous system has a metabolic effect that is said to explain the relaxation of smooth muscle in vessels (β_2) and in the gut and its effect on the heart muscle. This metabolic effect is widespread and also affects carbohydrate and lipoid distribution and utilization.[25]

Pain may be mediated through the sympathetic nervous system. Labor pain is transmitted by *afferent fibers* that traverse the lower thoracic sympathetic ganglia, whereas pain from upper abdominal viscera and the gut as far as the descending colon can adequately be relieved by celiac ganglion block. Pain from some pelvic viscera may be transmitted by the lumbar sympathetic ganglia (see Fig. 13-2). Recent evidence suggests that sympathetic *efferents* may influence pain perception in the limbs. Release of neurotransmitters such as norepinephrine, and more likely dopamine, from sympathetic nerve endings increases the sensitivity of peripheral nociceptors. Also, microcirculatory changes caused by intense sympathetic activity may alter the biochemical environment and enhance nociceptor activity (Fig. 13-5). Sympathetic blockade may reverse such effects, provided it is done before abnormal nociceptive activity is initiated rostral to the spinal cord (see below).

PHYSIOLOGIC EFFECTS ON PERIPHERAL BLOOD FLOW

A regional sympathetic block has its primary and most obvious effect on vasomotor activity. In a normal subject, this leads to dilatation of veins, promoting an accumulation of blood in the veins, and dilatation of the arterial vessels, which leads to a fall in the peripheral resistance and thus, if the perfusion pres-

(Text continues on p. 468)

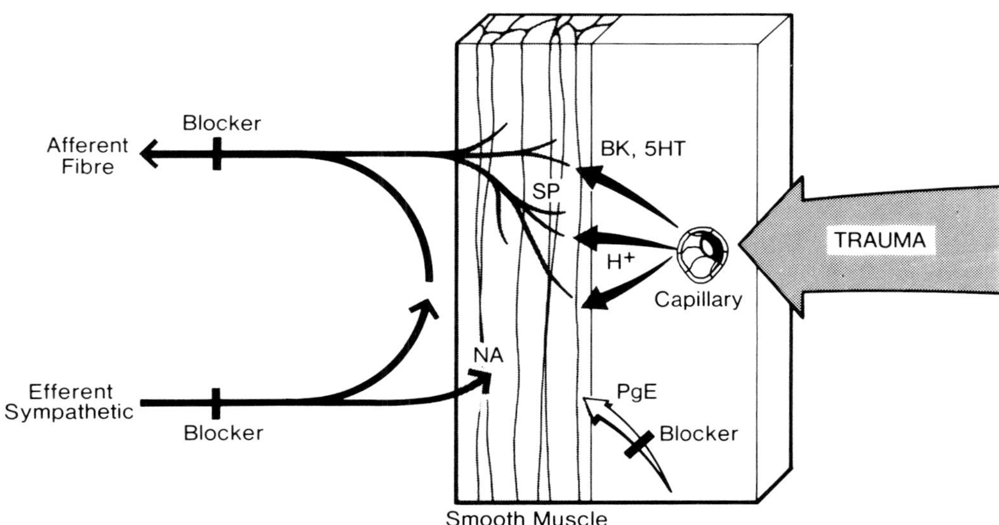

FIG. 13-5. Peripheral mechanisms of pain, sympathetic activity, and microcirculatory changes. Physical stimuli (*e.g.*, trauma), the chemical environment (*e.g.*, H^+ changes), algesic substance (*e.g.*, serotonin *[5HT]* and bradykinin *[BK]*), and microcirculatory changes (*e.g.*, edema) may all modify peripheral nociceptor sensitivity. Increased nociceptor activity increases afferent fiber activity, with resultant increases in efferent sympathetic vasoconstriction, and also norepinephrine (noradrenaline *[NA]*) release with further increases in nociceptor sensitivity. Thus a repetitive cycle is set up. Substance P *(SP)* is probably the peripheral pain transmitter. Prostaglandins *(PgE)* also increase nociceptor sensitivity. *Points of blockade of pain* (shaded and marked "blocker") are as follows: *1.* Afferent fibers (local anesthetics); *2.* efferent sympathetic fibers (local anesthetics); and *3.* prostaglandin synthesis (*e.g.*, nonsteroidal anti-inflammatory drugs given orally). All three may relieve pain and produce an associated improvement in microcirculation by breaking the repetitive cycle. *New approaches to pain* relief include substance P depletion (*e.g.*, by capsaicin). *Additional points of blockade to produce vasodilatation include* the following: *1.* Norepinephrine depletion at sympathetic nerve endings; *2.* norepinephrine receptor blockade (see Fig. 13-32); *3.* selective increase in levels of the prostaglandins PGE and PGE_1 (by intravascular infusion); and *4.* calcium channel blockade (see Fig. 13-32).

FIG. 13-6. Skin plethysmography and ice response: Effect of sympathetic block. **A.** Before sympathetic block. Skin blood flow is similar (2 ml/100 ml/min) in both limbs, and the response to ice *(arrow)* is a similar reduction in the height of the pulse wave in both limbs. **B.** After sympathetic block. The blocked limb *(right)* shows a marked increase in the slope of the upward deflection of the pulse wave and an increase in height of the pulse wave; this reflects a tenfold increase of skin blood flow to 22 ml/100 ml/min. There is no change in blood flow in response to ice. In contrast, the unblocked limb *(left)* shows the same shape and height of the pulse wave, and there is a similar marked reduction in blood flow (40% decrease) in response to ice. (Cousins, M.J., Reeve, T.S., Glynn, C.J., Walsh, J.A., *et al.*: Neurolytic lumbar sympathetic blockade: Duration of denervation and relief of rest pain. Anaesth. Intensive Care, 7:121, 1979). **C.** Apparatus for venous occlusion skin plethysmography *(VOP)*. The foot is enclosed in a constant temperature water bath, which surrounds a plethysmograph attached to a pressure transducer. A venous occlusion cuff is placed above the ankle. A typical trace is shown above. Application of ice to the side of the neck results in a marked increase in sympathetic tone, with a decrease both in the upslope and in the area under the curve. (Reproduced with permission from Walsh, J.A., Glynn, C.J., Cousins, M.J., and Basedow, R.W.: Blood flow, sympathetic activity and pain relief following lumbar sympathetic blockade or surgical sympathectomy. Anaesth. Intens. Care, *13:*18–24, 1984.)

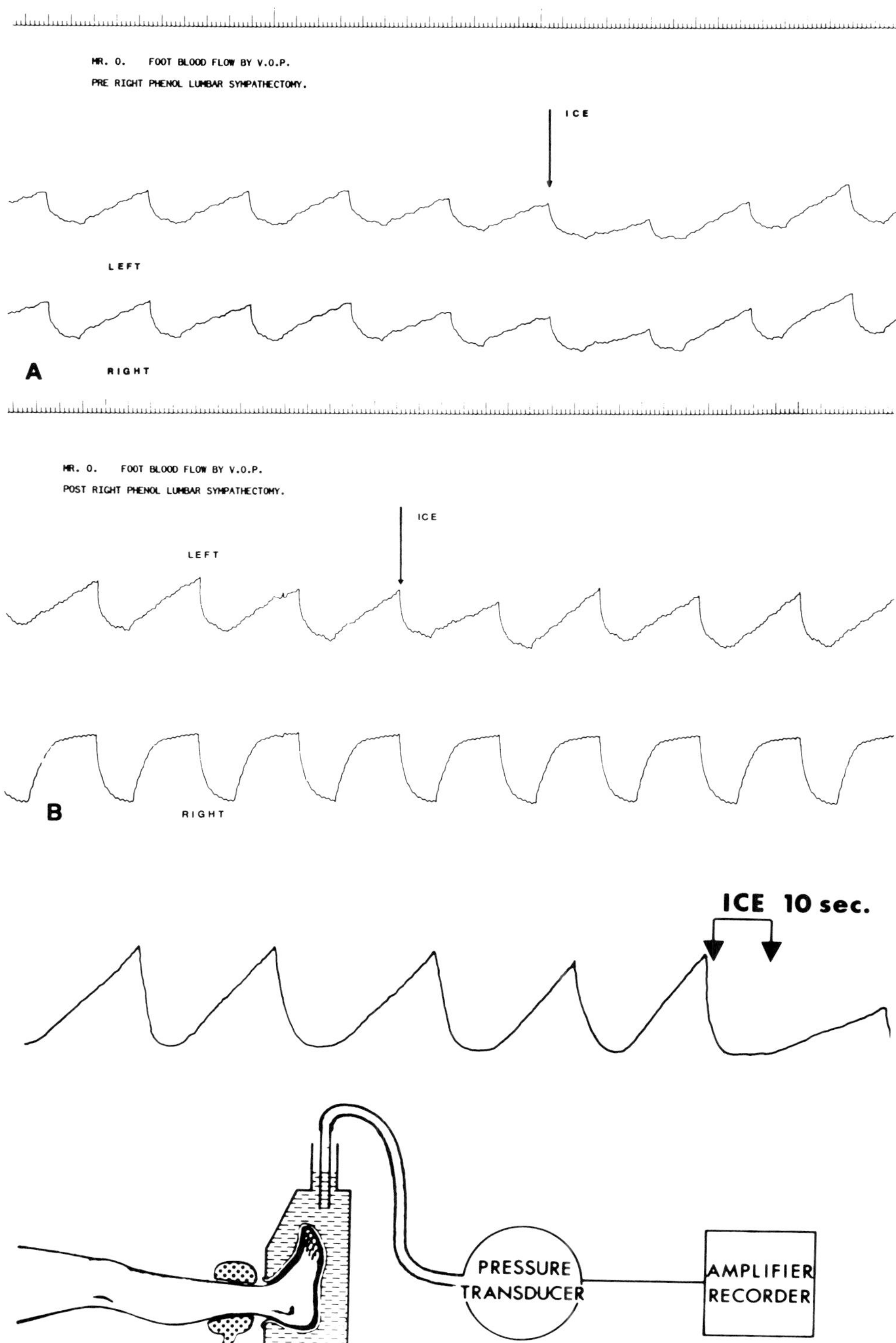
MR. O. FOOT BLOOD FLOW BY V.O.P.
PRE RIGHT PHENOL LUMBAR SYMPATHECTOMY.
ICE
LEFT
A
RIGHT
MR. O. FOOT BLOOD FLOW BY V.O.P.
POST RIGHT PHENOL LUMBAR SYMPATHECTOMY.
ICE
LEFT
B
RIGHT
ICE 10 sec.
PRESSURE
TRANSDUCER
AMPLIFIER
RECORDER
C

sure has not been altered, to an increased capillary blood flow.

In a normal subject, complete sympathetic block will be followed by visibly dilated veins or by increased blood flow, seen clinically in reduced capillary refill time or measured by plethysmography (Figs. 13-6 and 13-7), laser Doppler flowmetry,[3,4] or ^{133}Xe clearance, which measures capillary blood flow accurately (see below). Oscillometrically recorded, the peripheral pulse waves will be enlarged. Vasoconstrictor responses such as the "ice response" are abolished (Fig. 13-6). The blood flow increase will, to a large extent, be restricted to the skin, followed by an increase in skin temperature and a marked feeling of warmth in the extremity (Fig. 13-8).[93] Skin capillary oxygen tension and venous oxygen tension and saturation are also raised (see list on pp. 474–475). A widespread block will cause a peripheral pooling of blood, diminishing the venous return and producing a fall in cardiac output and blood pressure.

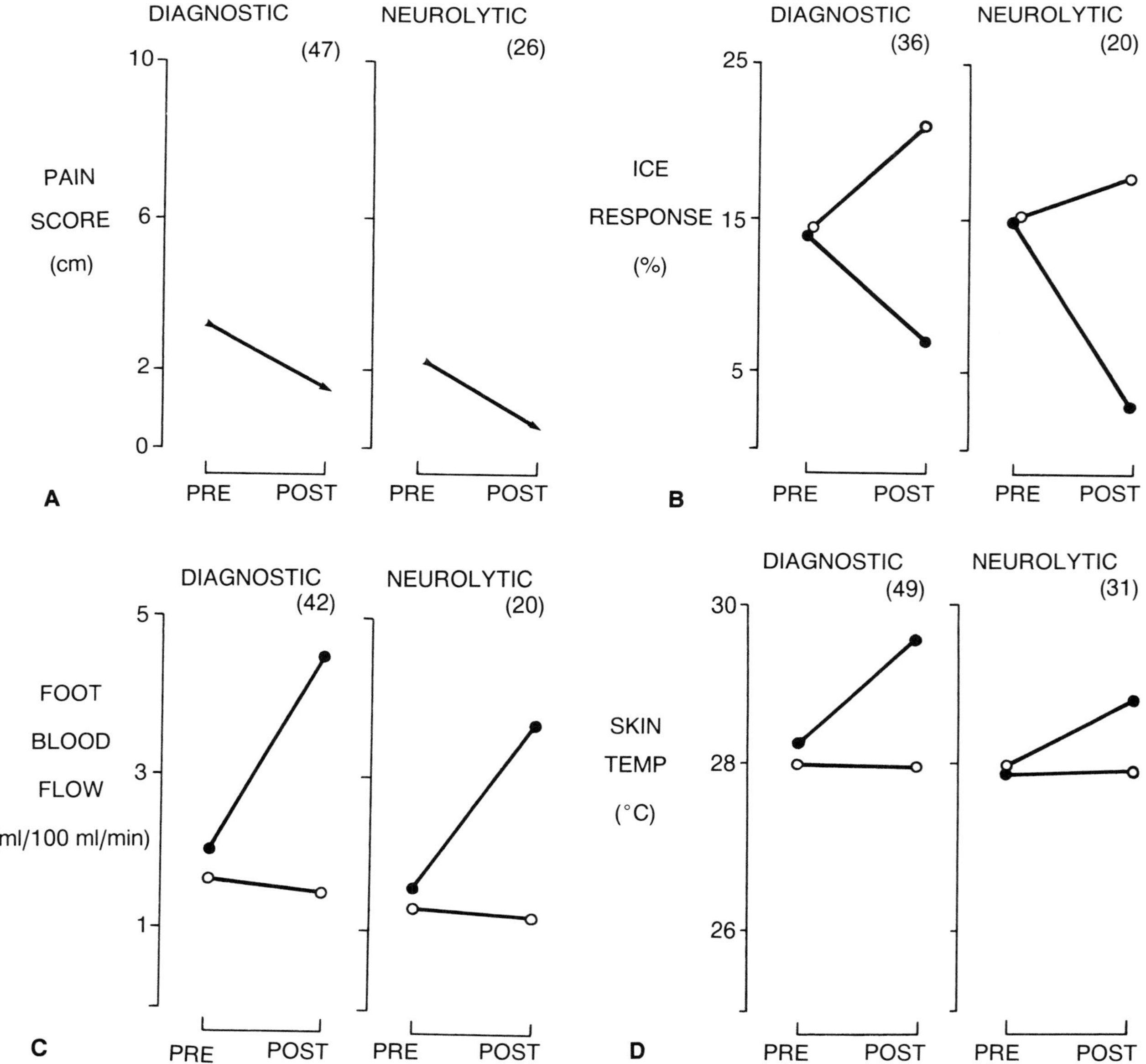

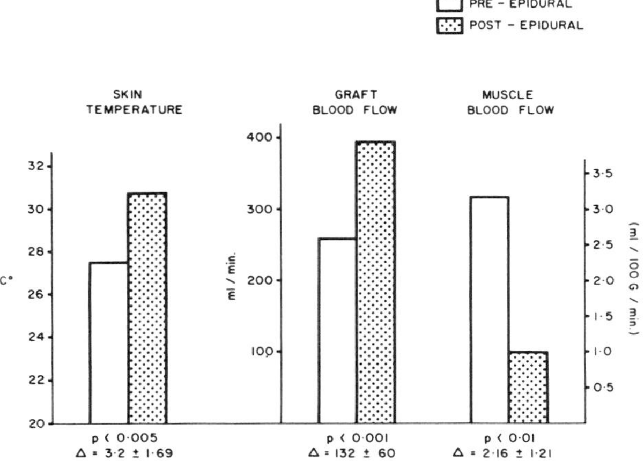

FIG. 13-8. Blood flow distribution after lumbar sympathetic blockade in arteriosclerotic patients at rest. Blood flow in the femoral artery (electromagnetic flow meter) is increased, as is skin blood flow (skin temperature); however, muscle blood flow (^{133}Xe clearance) is reduced. Note that this is a widespread sympathetic block (both lower limbs), which may sometimes even reduce the skin blood flow through diseased vessels (see Fig. 13-12). (Cousins, M.J., and Wright, C.J.: Graft muscle skin blood flow after epidural block in vascular surgical procedures. Surg. Gynecol. Obstet., *133*:59, 1971).

Muscle blood flow, being automatically regulated according to muscle metabolism, should not be affected by a sympathetic blockade at rest, at work, or after ischemia.[19] Thus reduced muscle flow (claudication) may not be helped by sympathetic block (Fig. 13-8). From what has been stated, it seems logical to use sympathetic blockade to improve the blood flow in a patient with insufficient peripheral skin blood flow because of vasospasm or arterial disease (*i.e.*, rest pain) (Fig. 13-8).[18,19] It is not possible, however, to predict the effect of a sympathetic blockade in a patient with a diseased vascular system, as can be explained with the aid of the following illustrations. In Figure 13-9, an artery divides into two smaller branches. The total flow (Q_A) in the artery is proportionate to the perfusion pressure (P) and inversely proportionate to the peripheral resistance (PR). In each branch (*B* and *C*) the flows (Q_B and Q_C) are affected by the perfusion pressures, almost the same as in the artery (*A*) and inversely related to the regional resistance (RR_B and RR_C) in each branch. A blockade of the sympathetic fibers to branch B alone will have very little effect on the perfusion pressure (Fig. 13-10). As the regional resistance decreases in branch B, the flow through this vessel will increase. A unilateral sympathetic blockade (in humans) is generally followed by a slight increase in vasomotor tone in the contralateral side, thus increasing the regional

FIG. 13-7. A. Pain score. Pain score (mean on 10-cm analogue scale) prediagnostic and postdiagnostic local anesthetic (bupivacaine) and neurolytic (phenol) sympathetic blockade in 47 and 26 patients, respectively. Significant decreases in pain score resulted from diagnostic ($p < 0.001$) and neurolytic ($p < 0.001$) block. **B.** Vasoconstrictor ice response. Effect of diagnostic local anesthetic (bupivacaine, 36 patients) and neurolytic (phenol, 20 patients) sympathetic blockade on vasoconstrictor ice response (%) on treated (●) and control (O) limb (mean values). Significant decreases in ice response resulted from diagnostic ($p < 0.04$) and neurolytic ($p < 0.01$) block. **C.** Blood flow. Effect of diagnostic local anesthetic (bupivacaine, 42 patients) and neurolytic (phenol, 20 patients) sympathetic blockade on foot blood flow (ml/ 100 ml/min) on treated (●) and control (O) limb (mean values). Significant increases in blood flow resulted from diagnostic ($p < 0.001$) and neurolytic ($p < 0.02$) block. **D.** Skin temperature. Effect of diagnostic local anesthetic (bupivacaine, 49 patients) and neurolytic block (phenol, 31 patients) on foot skin temperature (°C) on treated (●) and control (O) limbs (mean values). Significant increases in skin temperature resulted from diagnostic ($p < 0.001$) and neurolytic ($p < 0.01$) block. (Parts A–D are reproduced with permission from Walsh, J.A., Glynn, C.J., Cousins, M.J., and Basedow, R.W.: Blood flow, sympathetic activity and pain relief following lumbar sympathetic blockade or surgical sympathectomy. Anaesth. Intens. Care, *13:*18–24, 1984)

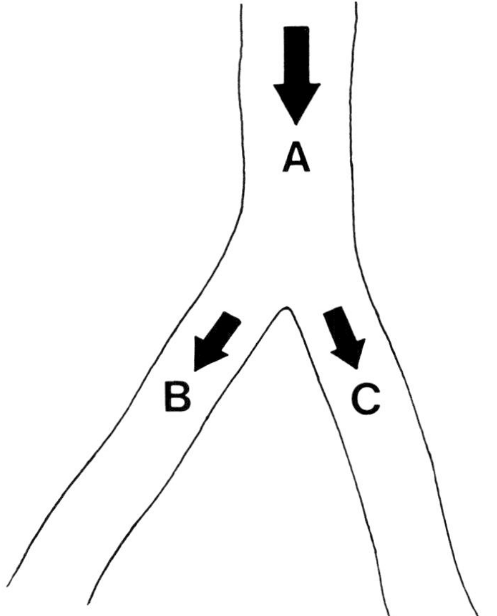

FIG. 13-9. The blood flows through an artery *(A)* or its branches *(B and C)* are proportionate to the perfusion pressures and inversely proportionate to total and regional resistances, respectively (see text).

resistance and reducing the blood flow through this part of the vascular system.

In Figure 13-11, an arterial obstruction in branch B is shown. Such an obstruction will in itself diminish the blood flow by mechanically increasing the regional resistance; however, this might at least be compensated by an increase in the collateral blood flow. A widespread sympathetic blockade, as illustrated in Figure 13-12, will diminish the regional resistance, mainly in branch C with its undamaged vessels. The blood flow will be diverted into this part of the vascular tree, and thus blood will be stolen from the diseased part (branch B). Such stealing of blood is known to occur in patients with advanced arterial disease. In theory, stealing can occur at three different levels: A generalized vasodilatation in the body will steal blood from, for instance, one extremity; increased blood flow around the hip and in the pelvis will diminish the blood flow to the peripheral part of the lower extremity; or increased skin blood flow might steal blood from the muscles (see Fig. 13-8).[19,22,95]

In contrast, a localized vasodilatation that affects the collaterals to branch B and vessels beyond the arterial obstruction should increase blood flow to this region (Fig. 13-13).

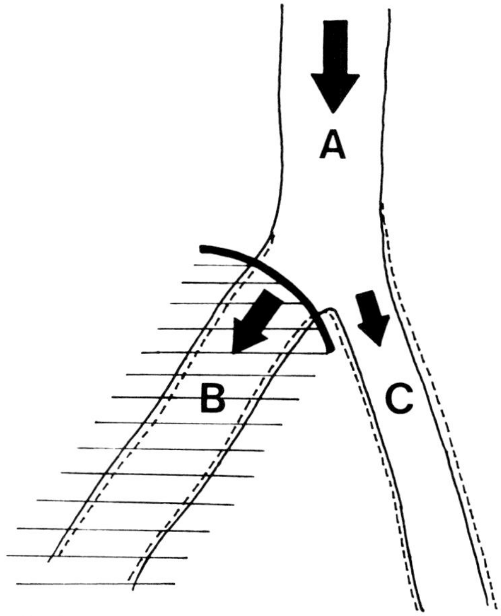

FIG. 13-10. A limited sympathetic blockade of fibers to branch B alone will little affect perfusion pressure. The flow in branch B will increase as the regional resistance is diminished. In branch C the flow will be slightly reduced as compensatory vasoconstriction occurs.

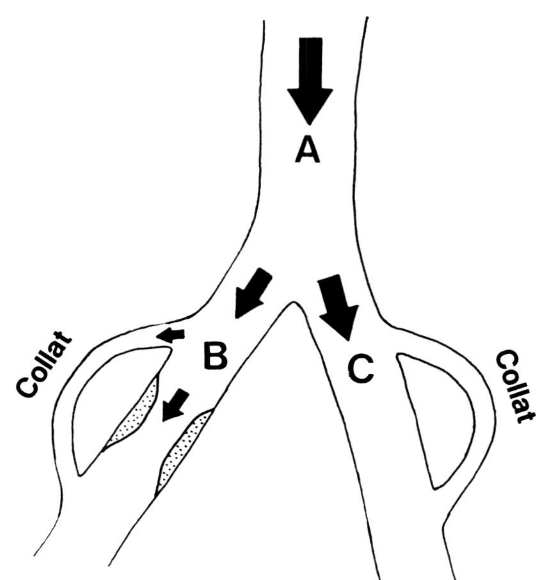

FIG. 13-11. An arterial obstruction in branch B will increase the resistance and thus hamper the blood flow. An increased flow through collaterals *(Collat)* may compensate for a fall in blood flow through the main channel (see text).

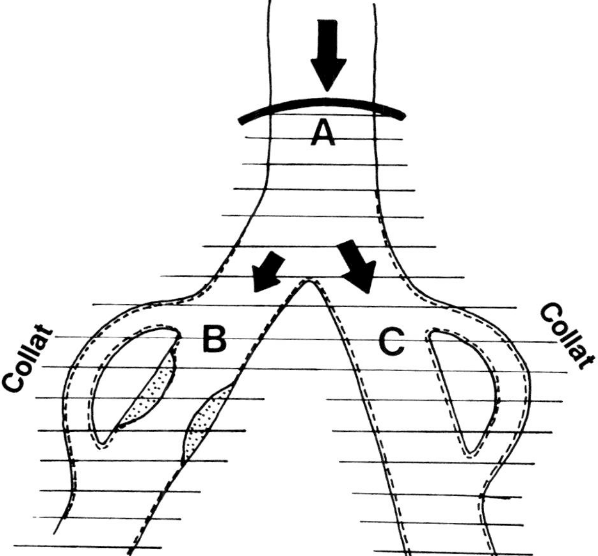

FIG. 13-12. A widespread sympathetic blockade of fibers to branches B and C will diminish resistance in undamaged vessels *(C)*, thereby potentially stealing blood from a diseased part *(B)* of the vascular tree.

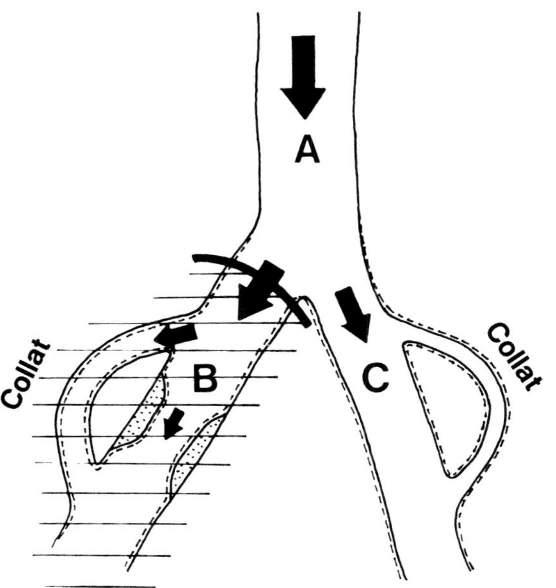

FIG. 13-13. A vasodilatation restricted to branch B and its collaterals *(Collat)* and vessels beyond the arterial obstruction should increase blood flow to this region.

If a decrease in vasomotor tone in the collaterals cannot be achieved, the maintenance of a good perfusion pressure is essential, as stressed by Lassen and Larson.[52,53]

From this discussion, it is obvious that the clinical effect of a sympathetic block cannot easily be predicted. Only physiologic studies in patients and clinical experience will identify when a sympathetic block is indicated.

In patients with occlusive vascular disease, the prime indication for surgical or chemical sympathectomy is "rest pain in a limb not amenable to direct arterial reconstruction."[94] Because of associated coronary artery disease, pulmonary disease, and other physical conditions, many of these patients are poor candidates for surgery and are thus better candidates for neurolytic sympathectomy.[18] However, the clinical results of both surgical and neurolytic sympathectomy, as reported in the literature, are contradictory. This might be explained by a poor selection of patients or by a lack of use of independent assessment of successful sympathetic ablation and its separate effects on blood flow and pain. This task may be simplified if one of the methods of evaluation in each category depicted in the list on pages 474–475 is used.

The detrimental effects of generalized vasodilatation in patients with arteriosclerotic vascular disease that causes rest pain or intermittent claudication have been well described and are generally accepted today.[95]

It has been suggested that an increased skin blood flow should always occur in the presence of regional vasodilatation. This has also been reported in patients with obliterative arterial disease.[50,67,86]

Although skin blood flow is markedly under the control of sympathetic activity, a decreased blood flow has been demonstrated in patients with severe arteriosclerosis and, in particular, in patients with lower limb vascular disease who have a low ankle blood pressure before lumbar sympathetic blockade (below 60/20 mm Hg).[49,70,71,86,88,89] In these patients, the vascular lesions in the periphery are so extreme that, hypothetically, a "proximal stealing" always occurs, and thus a fall in the perfusion pressure peripherally is followed by a vasodilatation in vessels located proximally. Although rare, there are reports of worsening of pain and gangrene.[31] Remarkably enough, an increase in skin temperature is not always related to an increase in blood flow through the skin and may merely reflect venous pooling and local inflammatory changes.[89] During spinal anesthesia, changes in skin temperature are not closely correlated to changes in skin blood flow, as evaluated by laser Doppler flowmetry.[4]

The blood flow through muscle is automatically regulated according to metabolic needs. Thus, in intermittent claudication, the muscle tissue hypoxia and accumulation of metabolites at exercise should be followed by maximal dilatation of the muscle blood vessels, and therefore a sympathetic blockade should be of no value or may even worsen the symptoms because of "stealing" blood flow to the skin.[19,32,90] However, this is not necessarily so. Pain is a primary factor in provoking increased sympathetic activity. Hypothetically, this could result in vasoconstriction in the collateral vessels that supply the affected muscle (see Fig. 13-4). Sympathetic blockade under these circumstances may improve blood flow to muscle and thus explain why a beneficial effect of sympathectomy is observed in some patients with intermittent claudication.[50,69,75] This assumption and the clinical experience of several investigators are supported by a metabolic study in which deep venous blood was drawn before and at the maximum of a one-leg bicycle ergometer test in patients with intermittent claudication.[62] In one group of patients with fairly high and segmentally located arterial lesions who received sympathetic block (Group I), the rise in femoral venoartrial lactate difference during exercise was not as marked as before their sympathetic block, indicating an improvement in nutrient blood flow. In contrast, in a group of patients with multiple vascular lesions (Group II), no improvement in nutrient blood flow was achieved by sympathetic blockade. In Group I, eight of ten also experienced less ischemic pain on exercise during the sympathetic blockade. No patients in Group II experienced such pain relief. The most important effect of sympathetic blockade in Group I seemed to be pain relief during exercise, at least partly because of an improved blood flow and also enhancement of the development of collateral vessels, which is known to occur over time, providing opportunities for revascularization (see Table 13-3). It should be acknowledged that, with respect to pain evaluation, a placebo effect may occur, which has been reported with lumbar sympathetic blockade.[33]

Lumbar sympathetic blockade in connection with vascular surgery improves the flow through reconstructed vessels and should be of value in the immediate postoperative period.[20,48,50,76,92] Although less selective, this effect can also be achieved with epidural sympathetic block; however, the ganglion blockade is preferable, as discussed on page 470.[19]

The blockade of beta-fibers (sympathetic preganglionic fiber) during spinal and epidural blockade has recently been questioned.[5,61] Thus efferent sympathetic change has been studied with the help of skin conductance response (SCR) in which different stimuli (*e.g.*, electrical stimulus, short deep breath, verbal stimulation) have been used. In spinal analgesia, the sympathetic blockade starts at a level much lower than that of analgesia in contrast to what has been stated previously in the literature.[37] Even at T1 blockade (which should have blocked all preganglionic fibers), an SCR response is often seen in the foot. This seems to indicate that the beta-fibers are not blocked as easily as previously thought. In most cases, when a T6 blockade has been achieved, a marked depression of the sympathetic responses is seen mainly in the foot (T12–L1). This partial sympathetic blockade, however, disappears much earlier than the analgesia, in most cases starting 20 to 40 minutes after the injection of the spinal anesthetic. Similar results have been seen when the skin blood flow has been studied with the help of laser Doppler flowmetry.[3,4] Also here, with a high blockade (T4–T6), an increased blood flow was seen only in the foot and in the thigh, at segment levels far below that of analgesia. A very high spinal analgesia is thus needed to make sure that marked depression of sympathetic activity in the lower extremity is produced. Changes in SCR response related to the height of an epidural blockade are very similar to those seen in spinal analgesia (Malmquist, L.A.: Personal communication).

The increase in limb blood flow resulting from epidural blocks has been clinically related to a lower incidence of postoperative thrombosis (see Chap. 8). This effect is most likely correlated with an increase in cardiac output, provoked by the local anesthetic itself (see Chap. 3, 4, and 8). The local anesthetics lidocaine and mepivacaine, when applied directly into the resistance vessels, produce a contraction, in contrast to what is seen during an i.v. infusion.[60]

The poor blocking of sympathetic fibers produced by an epidural blockade also explains the fact that a very high epidural blockade is required to ablate the stress responses during and after lower abdominal surgery. In upper abdominal surgery, epidural blockade is less effective in blocking the stress response. This can be markedly improved if a splanchnic blockade is added (see Chap. 5).

Thus there is a variable degree of sympathetic blockade achieved by an intradural or extradural injection of a local anesthetic. In contrast, in most instances, it is fairly easy to obtain a complete sympathetic blockade by an injection of the local anesthetic at sympathetic ganglia or postganglionic fibers.

From the discussion above, it is obvious that a proper selection of patients for sympathetic blockade is of great importance. Because the number of patients with vascular disease is very large, complicated and time-consuming physiologic studies are not always feasible. The use of continuous catheter sympathetic blockade that lasts for 5 days is one method of obtaining a clinical evaluation of the effect of the blockade, which should at least detect patients whose symptoms are exacerbated after blockade.[63] A selective alternative is intravenous regional sympathetic block, which can eliminate technical failure and is a useful preliminary test for whether surgical sympathectomy or permanent blockade by chemical sympathectomy will be successful.[39] The prolonged duration (1–3 weeks) of intravenous sympathetic block allows adequate time for clinical assessment. A third alternative is to perform diagnostic block with long-acting local anesthetic mixed with contrast medium and to check adequacy of coverage of sympathetic chain under image intensifier; however, this has proved the least reliable of the three.[18,91]

In a clinical series, Kövamees and Löfström found that the most beneficial effect of sympathetic blockade was relief of rest pain (19/23, or 83%) with a somewhat lesser effect of improved healing of ulcers (23/55, or 42%) see Table 13-2.[49] Increased walking tolerance (7/16, or 44%) was of significant benefit in a small group of patients with intermittent claudication. Sympathetic blockade was part of a general treatment program that included mobilization and wound treatment and sometimes infusion of low molecular weight dextran. It was not possible to attribute an improvement to the sympathetic blockade alone. In a recent study, however, Cousins and colleagues reported that duration of relief of rest pain was similar to duration of lumbar sympathetic blockade, strengthening the relation between pain relief and sympathetic denervation.[18] In one study, pain relief was accompanied by increased skin temperature and skin blood flow (venous occlusion plethysmography), whereas sweating and vasoconstrictor ice response were decreased (see Fig. 13-7).[91] Another study indicated that nutritive blood flow was not increased but pain was relieved in a high percentage of patients.[20b] Good results with relief of rest pain in the lower limbs have been reported by others.[8,20b,42,75] Very little data are available on upper limb vascular disease, although case reports indicate beneficial results with sympathetic block in vasospastic disorders such as those in the list on this page.

Thus it would appear that the primary benefits that result from sympathetic blockade are pain relief and improved healing of skin lesions; however, controlled studies of efficacy of sympathetic block are required to define better its role in the treatment of vascular disease of the lower and the upper limbs.

The pain-relieving effect of a sympathetic block in a patient with peripheral arterial disease is said to follow improved blood flow. Good pain relief often occurs, however, when no improvement in peripheral circulation can be noted;[20b] possible mechanisms are discussed below (see also Fig. 13-6).

Clinical Conditions That Sympathetic Blockade May Benefit

To produce pain relief
- Renal colic (lumbar sympathetic block)
- Obliterative arterial disease (lumbar sympathetic block)
- Acute pancreatitis and pancreatic cancer (celiac plexus block)
- Cancer pain from upper abdominal viscera (celiac plexus block)
- Cardiac pain (thoracic sympathetic or stellate ganglion block)
- Paget's disease of bone (stellate ganglion or lumbar sympathetic block)
- Reflex sympathetic dystrophy (stellate or lumbar sympathetic block)
  - Major causalgia, phantom limb, central pain
  - Minor post-traumatic syndrome, postfrostbite syndrome, shoulder/hand syndrome, Sudeck's atrophy

To improve blood flow in vasospastic disorders (stellate or lumbar sympathetic block)
- Raynaud's disease
- Accidental intra-arterial injections of thiopentone
- Early frostbite
- Obliterative arterial disease not suitable for vascular surgery
- Vascular surgery (to improve postoperative blood flow)

To improve drainage of local edema (stellate or lumbar sympathetic block)

INDICATIONS FOR SYMPATHETIC BLOCKADE

The precise mechanism whereby the sympathetic nervous system is involved in peripheral pain has not yet been fully elucidated (see above). It has been suggested that the cutaneous pain threshold, by means of a negative feedback loop, is influenced by sympathetic efferents (Fig. 13-5).[73] This may explain the often remarkable pain relief seen after sympathetic blocks in patients with threatening gangrene, despite a lack of improvement in skin blood flow. It is possible that increased efferent sympathetic activity increases activity in pain receptors by way of sympathetic fibers that are prevalent in proximity to sensory receptors. This provides an explanation of pain relief that may follow stellate ganglion block in patients with arteriopathy (*e.g.*, associated with scleroderma) in the upper limb despite the lack of change in blood flow.

There are also clinical observations that early herpes zoster pain and skin vesicles respond favorably to sympathetic blockade (see list on p. 480).[17,65] That they also respond well to a block of the appropriate somatic nerve is well established, and it is uncertain whether there is any specific sympathetic involvement in this condition. The results of sympathetic block in the treatment of postherpetic neuralgia are uniformly disappointing.

It is, of course, well established that the pain of uterine contraction and cervical dilatation can be abolished by sympathetic blockade of afferents* entering the spinal cord at T11–12. This is usually achieved by extradural sympathetic blockade (see Chap. 18). Also, in a small series of patients with renal colic treated with extradural sympathetic block at L1, 9 of 14 patients passed their stone in 10 days and all were pain-free from the start of treatment; this series has now been increased to 32, all of whom obtained complete pain relief.[58] This compares favorably with other methods, and it has been suggested that the relief of pain and the reduction of ureteral spasm are brought about by sympathetic blockade of the first lumbar segmental outflow. Chronic pain from the urogenital tract has, in a few cases, been eliminated with chemical lumbar sympathectomy.[43] Cervicothoracic sympathetic blockade is also of value in the treatment of patients with severe angina pectoris, provided that the block extends down to the level of T4. The hazards, however, may often outweigh the benefits.

In post-traumatic syndrome, a sympathetic blockade is often followed by relief of the burning pain in the injured extremity and a feeling of softening of the tissues, primarily around the joints.[6,23,78] The symptoms of post-traumatic syndrome might be caused by hyperactivity in the sympathetic nervous system, producing vasoconstriction, decrease in capillary surface area, redistribution of blood flow, fall in oxygen uptake (tissue hypoxia), increased vascular permeability, and lack of fluid mobilization.[56] A sympathetic blockade should then improve nutrient blood flow and decrease the accumulated fluid in the tissue, which explains the increased warmth and the rapid disappearance of tissue edema often seen during this form of treatment. Conclusive evidence, however, is lacking. Sympathetic block only produces significant residual clinical improvements if used early in this syndrome.

*These fibers are better classified as visceral nociceptive **afferents,** leaving sympathetic fibers only as **efferents.**

TESTING THE COMPLETENESS OF SYMPATHETIC BLOCKADE

In a patient with a healthy vascular system, a sympathetic blockade produces clear-cut subjective and objective effects on the peripheral circulation, as has been discussed in the previous section. In a patient with severe arterial disease, however, a complete sympathetic blockade can have been achieved with little or no demonstrable effect on the peripheral circulation.

The venous circulation is generally not involved in the disease process, and swelling of the veins can be a valuable indication of a successful block. Listed below are objective tests that can be used to provide an assessment of completeness of sympathetic block.

Independent Tests of Sympathetic Function, Blood Flow, and Pain

Method of Evaluation
- *Sympathetic function*
  - Skin conductance response (SCR)[5,16,30,55,61]
  - Sweat test
    - Ninhydrin[24]
    - Cobalt blue[18]
    - Starch iodine
  - Skin plethysmography and "ice response"[18]
- *Blood flow*[35]
  - Plethysmography (muscle and skin)[67,68]
  - Xenon-133 clearance (muscle and skin)[36,41,90]
  - Sodium-24 clearance (muscle and skin)[40]
  - Antipyrine clearance[95]
  - Doppler technique (whole limb)[84,85]
  - Electromagnetic flow meter (whole limb)[19,20,50,76,92]
  - Laser Doppler flowmetry[3,4]
  - Pulse wave (skin)[2,35]
  - Temperature (skin)[62,63,70,71,86,89]

Size of ulcer (skin)[18]
Distal perfusion pressure[49,70,71,86–88,89]
Capillary oxygen tension (muscle or skin)[12]
Venous oxygen tension, saturation (muscle)[62]
Metabolism (muscle)[62]

Pain
Pain score[18]
Analgesic requirements
Activity (*e.g.*, claudication distance)

SKIN CONDUCTANCE RESPONSE

Skin conductance response (SCR) was previously called the sympathogalvanic response (SGR). SCR tests not only efferent sympathetic activity but also afferent sensory activity and spinal and supraspinal interneurons. Increased sympathetic activity, which in many people can be evoked by a short deep breath or by pinching the skin, is followed by a change in skin conductance that can be recorded with a simple electrocardiograph. One ECG electrode is placed on the front and one on the back of the hand or foot (*i.e.*, where sweat glands are abundant). A third grounding electrode is placed anywhere on the body. It is important that before the electrodes are placed the skin is scrubbed free of epithelial cells. In most patients, there will be a slow change in the baseline, which will come to rest after a few minutes. A short deep breath or pinching will now, with a 1- to 2-second delay, be followed by a marked deflection that lasts for 4 to 5 seconds. This deflection does not occur if the sympathetic fibers of the extremity are blocked. A partial block of the response will be seen if the patient is atropinized (in clinically used doses). It is preferable to perform separate tests on two limbs simultaneously, thus making it possible to compare the blocked side with the unblocked side. This is essential if the SGR deflections are to be measured in the evaluation of indications for another sympathetic blockade (Fig. 13-14). It is well known that the baseline is far less stable and that the deflections much more marked in young patients than in elderly patients. In elderly patients, it is also more difficult to provoke a sympathetic response, particularly in depressed people and in people who are freezing. Also, the SCR undergoes marked habituation, that is, each stimulus has a tendency to be followed by a smaller and

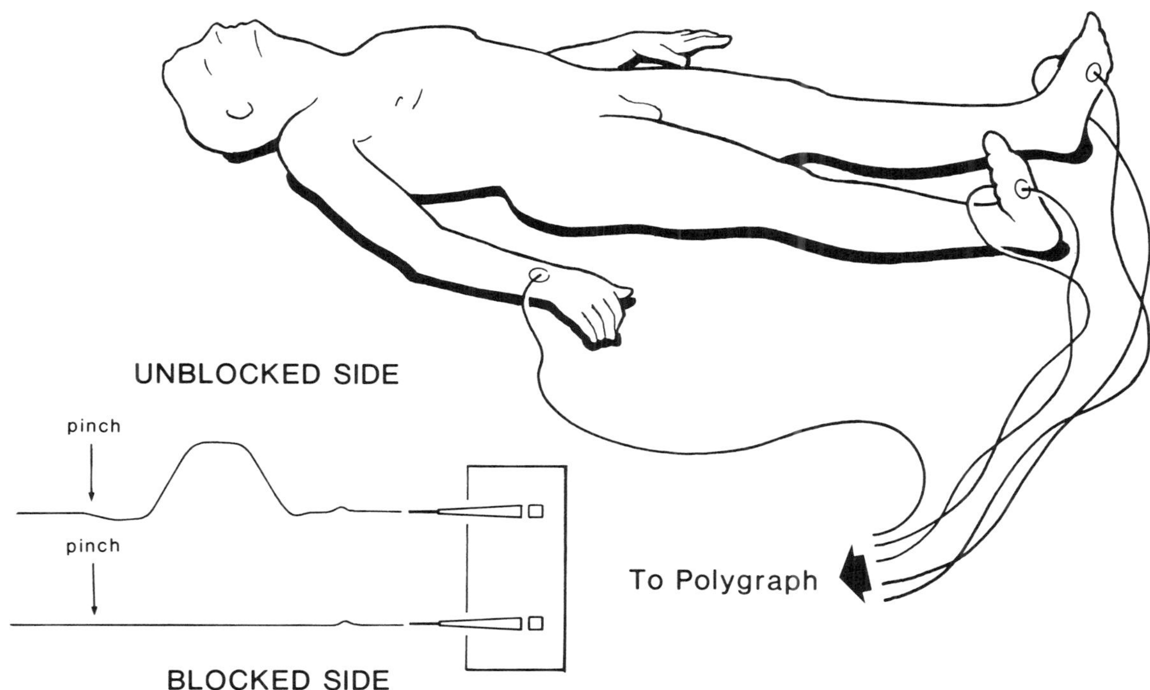

FIG. 13-14. Sympathogalvanic response. Electrodes are placed on the front and back of hands or feet, and a ground electrode is placed elsewhere on the body. Changes in baseline level on an ECG recorder indicate changes in sweat gland activity.

smaller deflection. Each stimulus should therefore be 2 to 3 minutes apart. When habituation occurs, waiting for a few minutes, putting a warm blanket over the patient, and changing the stimulus from a deep short breath to pinching or to verbal stimulation or, if available, to a more painful electrical stimulation usually brings back a good response.

Ample experience with SCR has made it clear that it is not always possible to obtain a complete abolition of the SCR with a sympathetic blockade, even though the vascular response seems to be maximal. It has been suggested that SCR can be used to predict the value of a sympathetic blockade in patients with arterial disease.[11] In this study, most patients with a good to moderate deflection on stimulation benefited from a sympathetic block. This was not seen in patients with little or no deflection. The SCR has also been used by us to check the completeness of sympathetic denervation following local anesthetic or chemical sympathectomy. When a permanent sympathetic blockade is under consideration and no or only weak skin resistance deflections are seen following SCR, a continuous sympathetic blockade is unlikely to be followed by any improvement in the peripheral circulation, although in some cases it may offer pain relief.

SKIN POTENTIAL RESPONSE

The skin potential response (SPR) is an alternative to the SCR.[20a] The SPR, like the SCR, has a rise time of 1 to 2 seconds and a fall time of 10 to 15 seconds. SPR has an amplitude of 5 mV. Like SCR, SPR is due to an increase in sympathetic activity and subsequent changes in sodium chloride flux in sweat gland ducts. The benefits claimed for SPR are that electrode size and placement are less critical than for SCR and no external signal source is required. However, a modified ECG recording equipment is needed because [1] most ECG machines have a frequency response of 0.1 to 100 Hz whereas SPR requires 0.03 to 2 Hz. Also, 50 Hz interference may occur; [2] SPR requires a wider range of input sensitivity than in standard ECG machines; [3] ECG recorder paper speed of 25 mm/sec is too fast for SPR; and [4] pre-gelled Ag-Agcl electrodes are required ("Red Dot"—3M). A positive electrode is placed over palm or sole and a negative electrode over back of hand or foot. An indifferent electrode is attached at the wrist or ankle. Spontaneous changes in sympathetic tone result in negative, then positive, swings on the SPR recording. As with SCR, several factors influence the response: [1] degree of arousal—CNS depression abolishes the response; [2] drugs that alter sympathetic activity, for example, opiates and tranquilizers; [3] anticholinergic drugs abolish the response since acetylcholine is the sudomotor transmitter; [4] steroids interfere with sodium flux in sweat glands; and [5] ouabain effects sodium pumping in sweat glands.

SWEAT TEST

The sweat test is perhaps the most practicable test of sympathetic activity.

Ninhydrin Method. Fingerprints are taken (at intervals) before and after blockade.[24] After suitable preparation, which includes heating, the fingerprints are developed, and each functioning sweat gland can be seen and counted. This test is very accurate and its results reproducible; however, it is time-consuming and does not provide the clinician with an answer at the bedside.

Cobalt Blue Filter Paper Test. Filter papers are soaked in cobalt blue and then dried in an oven, after which they are kept in a desiccator until needed. Two filter papers are removed from the desiccator with forceps and placed on a clean dry surface so that the patient can press both feet or hands onto the papers. Sweating is registered on the paper by a change in color from blue to pink. A limb with complete sympathetic block usually shows no color change (Fig. 13-15). Details for preparation of the filter papers are found in Appendix A of this chapter.

Starch-Iodine Test. The starch-iodine test works on a principle similar to that of the cobalt blue test. It has

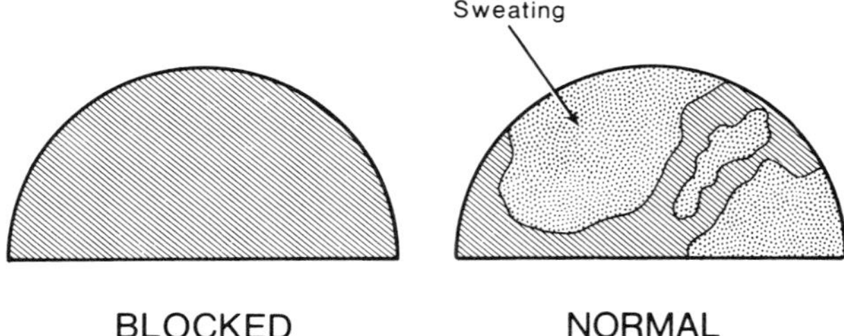

FIG. 13-15. Cobalt blue sweat test. The papers are blue *(shaded)* before the test. Sweating from the unblocked limb changes the color to pink *(stippled)*.

the advantage that the material can be spread over a complete limb. It is a messy technique, however, and not popular with patients.

Having ensured that sympathetic block is adequate, an independent assessment can then be made of the effect on blood flow. If this is combined with the ice test (see Fig. 13-6), a further evaluation of sympathetic function can be obtained and, if pain was present before blockade, pain relief can be independently assessed (see Fig. 13-7).

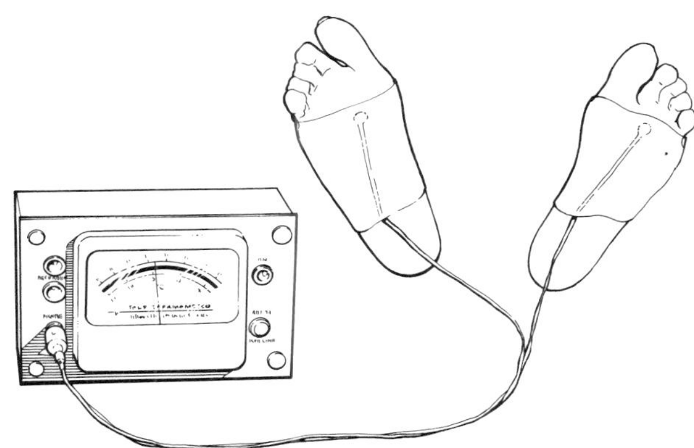

FIG. 13-17. Skin thermocouple probe and telethermometer. Simultaneous measurements are made on treated and untreated limb.

ASSESSMENT OF BLOOD FLOW CHANGES

Whole Limb Blood Flow

Indirect. *Doppler Ankle/Brachial Index.*[94] An ultrasound probe is used to facilitate blood pressure measurement with a standard cuff at brachial artery and also at the ankle. An ankle to brachial index is then calculated as follows:

$$\frac{\text{ankle}}{\text{brachial}} = \frac{80/50}{120/80} = 0.65$$

This reading is then repeated after sympathetic block.

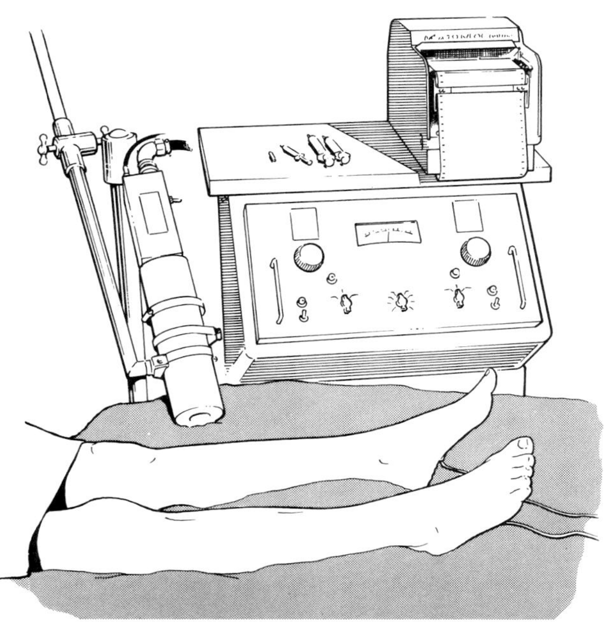

FIG. 13-16. Xenon-133 clearance technique for leg muscle blood flow. Xenon-133 is injected into the anterior tibial muscle and its clearance detected with a portable scintillation detector.

Impedance plethysmography is a new technique which attempts to correlate the changes in electrical impedance with blood flow. At this stage, it is not clear whether it provides an accurate estimate of limb blood flow under the whole range of clinical conditions.

Direct. *Electromagnetic flowmeter* can be applied either directly to the blood vessel during surgery or percutaneously using a "catheter tip" version.

Ultrasonic Flowmeter. Very small probes are now available that can be placed on the vessel wall at operation and left *in situ* postoperatively.

Muscle Blood Flow

Venous occlusion plethysmography has been used in the calf area under the assumption that the calf is mosty muscle with much less skin.

Clearance of radioactive substances after direct injection (*e.g.*, ^{133}Xe) provides one of the best measurements of nutritive blood flow (Fig. 13-16).[19]

Arterial oxygen concentration in blood from deep calf veins has also been used for an indirect estimate of oxygen delivery to calf muscle.[62] Recently, a *mass spectrometer probe* has been developed to measure muscle tissue P_{O_2} directly.

Skin Blood Flow

Clearance of radioactive substances injected directly into the skin has been used (*e.g.,* ^{133}Xe, ^{124}Na).

Laser Doppler flowmeters provide a noninvasive assessment of changes in skin blood flow.[3,4]

Mass spectrometer microprobes and skin "cups" are also being used in this situation to measure changes in skin Po_2 with different forms of treatment.

Occlusion skin plethysmography has also been used in the area of the foot, hand, and digits, as described above (see Fig. 13-6).[18]

Skin temperature measurements, using a telethermometer and thermistor or thermocouple skin probes, provide an indirect but easily obtained estimate of changes in skin blood flow (Fig. 13-17). Liquid thermal crystals and heat-sensitive papers are also available.

Optical Density Skin Plethysmography (or Pulse Monitor). Several quite sensitive finger "pulsemeters" are now available and use several different wavelengths of light directed into the skin capillary bed. Capillary blood flow results in a cyclical change in optical density, yielding a wave form similar to that shown in Figure 13-6, and its amplitude is proportional to sympathetic activity.

Measurement of Size of Skin Ulcers. Progressive documentation of change in ulcer size is a very simple, practical method of checking progress after sympathetic block in patients with ischemic skin lesions.

Transcutaneous oxygen electrodes and oximeters also provide an indirect assessment of skin blood flow by changes in oxygenation.

PAIN ASSESSMENT

As discussed in Chapters 24 and 25, there is still no objective method of pain assessment. Indirect methods such as the pain score (visual analogue scale), analgesic requirements, and improved level of activity are used; wherever possible these should be performed by an independent observer with a "double-blind" study design (see Chap. 25).

A baseline measurement/assessment before sympathetic block should be performed in each case for sympathetic activity, blood flow, and pain score by one of the methods described above. After sympathetic blockade, the completeness of sympathetic block, its effect on blood flow, and any effects on pain should be ascertained.

General Clinical Applications

The clinical situations in which sympathetic blockade may be considered are summarized in the list on page 473. The present lack of definitive data makes it highly desirable to carry out a diagnostic block before considering permanent blockade. In addition, any of the methods of independently assessing blockade, blood flow, and pain relief should be used.

General Contraindications

Patients on Heparin. Severe bleeding has been observed, particularly after lumbar sympathetic blockade in a heparinized patient. The bleeding occurs within the psoas fascia, producing minimal symptoms until frank shock occurs. Early symptoms are pain in the groin or pain when the leg is actively lifted and rotated outward. A hematoma may also pass through an intervertebral foramen into the spinal canal, after stellate or lumbar sympathetic block, causing pressure on nerves and vessels followed by neurologic symptoms (see also Chap. 8). Hematoma after stellate block has been reported to interfere with carotid blood flow (see Chaps. 22 and 23).

Bilateral injection during one treatment session should probably be avoided. Dosage tends to be high, and vascular responses may be a significant problem for this class of patient. Various side-effects may pose an increased hazard if both sides are blocked. For example, bilateral recurrent laryngeal block after stellate block may cause stridor (see Chap. 22).

Bilateral injection in the lumbar region for permanent blockade may cause loss of ejaculation and should be avoided in young persons; however, impotence does not occur, and the patient does not become sterile.

AGENTS FOR SYMPATHETIC BLOCKADE

For short-term block, any of the conventional local anesthetics can be used. Addition of epinephrine to the local anesthetic solution will, to some extent, prolong the duration of action; however, the use of epinephrine in patients with severe vascular disease or vasospasm is questionable. Mepivacaine and bupivacaine, without epinephrine, have durations of 1½ to 3 and 3 to 10 hours, respectively. These durations are influenced only marginally by the addition of epinephrine, and therefore plain solutions are the solutions of choice.[12,72] It is useful to add contrast medium (2 ml of Conray-420), as this allows confirmation of the adequacy of spread of solution (*e.g.*, over L2–4 ganglia; see Fig. 13-31).

The amount of local anesthetic agent needed in, for example, lumbar sympathetic blockade (1–5 ml, 0.5% mepivacaine or 0.25% bupivacaine at each level), even without epinephrine, poses a relatively small risk of a toxic reaction owing to local anesthetic absorption. There is, however, the ever-present risk of acute intravascular injection and the other adverse effects of local anesthetic injection (see Table 4-8).

For a permanent block (chemical sympathectomy), 6% to 7% phenol in water, 7% to 10% phenol in water-soluble (*e.g.*, Angiographin) contrast medium, or 50% to 100% alcohol may be used. The last yields the highest incidence of neuralgia, and most authorities now prefer 7% to 10% phenol in Angiographin because it poses minimal resistance to injection, and its spread can be viewed under radiographic control.[8,18,27,91]

TECHNIQUES

STELLATE GANGLION BLOCK (CERVICOTHORACIC SYMPATHETIC BLOCK)

Regional Anatomy

The cervical sympathetic chain lies in the fascial space, which is limited posteriorly by the fascia over the prevertebral muscles and anteriorly by the carotid sheath (Fig. 13-18).

Although the sympathetic preganglionic fibers for the head, neck, and upper limb leave the spinal cord from segments as widely separated as T1 to T6, pathways converge and pass anteriorly to the neck of the first rib. Here, the first thoracic and inferior cervical ganglion may be separated or fused to form the stellate ganglion. In the latter case, the ganglion lies over the neck of the first rib. The ganglion is covered anteriorly in its lower part by the dome of the pleura, and in its upper part by the vertebral artery. Block of the stellate ganglion alone may provide disappointing results despite the correct anatomic placement of solution. This may be explained by the diverse origin of the sympathetic fibers in the thoracic cord and also the fact that some thoracic preganglion fibers lie in other sympathetic ganglia and may bypass the stellate ganglion completely on their way into the head, neck, and upper extremity.[66] For best results, the local anesthetic solution has to fill the space in front of the prevertebral fascia down to at least T4. This can be achieved by an injection of 15 to 20 ml of weak local anesthetic solution in front of the transverse process of C6 (see Fig. 13-20). It is obvious that there is little advantage to be gained by needle placement at C7 and there is a greater risk of pneumothorax at this level. The term "cervicothoracic sympathetic block" thus seems more appropriate than "stellate ganglion block."

Procedure

A large number of techniques have been described. If the needle is aimed at C7 or the neck of the first rib, the risk of pneumothorax is considerable. On the other hand, the needle may be kept well above the pleura and reliance placed on the spread of a large volume of solution. This is the basis of the anterior approach first described by Leriche.[54]

"Paratracheal" (Anterior) Technique

The patient lies supine with the head slightly lifted forward on a thin pillow and tilted dorsally to stretch the esophagus away from the transverse processes on the left side. The mouth should be slightly opened to relax the neck muscles.

The trachea and the carotid pulse are gently palpated by inserting two fingers between the sternocleidomastoid muscle and the trachea to find the most prominent cervical transverse process, C6—the Chassaignac tubercle, which lies at the level of the cricoid cartilage (Fig. 13-18). A skin wheal is raised with a fine needle over this transverse process. Two fingers are now gently pressed down to the C6 tubercle, pushing away the carotid artery laterally and the trachea toward the midline with the fingers slightly separated so that the tubercle lies just in between them (Fig. 13-18).

A 22-gauge, short-bevel, 4- to 5-cm-long needle, with a 20-ml syringe attached, is advanced through the skin and underlying tissues until it hits bone, that is, rests on the junction of C6 body and transverse process. The palpating fingers maintain their position; the hand holding the needle is kept braced against the patient, and the needle is withdrawn about 2 mm and fixed (Fig. 13-18).

An aspiration test is performed before and after turning the needle 90°. If no blood enters the syringe, a test dose of 2 ml is injected. Injection of even this small dose directly into the vertebral artery can result in a convulsion (see Chap. 4). A high resistance to injection may indicate periosteal injection, and a significant but lesser resistance indicates that the needle is still in prevertebral muscle, while radiating pain means the needle is too deep, that is, has penetrated a nerve root. While the needle is *in situ*, it is important that the patient not talk. If aspiration tests are negative and no sequelae follow, the full dose, 15 to 20 ml of local anesthetic, is injected (Fig. 13-19). In most instances, the patient will feel a lump in the throat and may often be temporarily hoarse; he should be warned beforehand about these events. Because of these effects, patients are more comfortable sitting up. Fluids and food should be withheld while laryngeal reflexes are impaired.

Continuous Technique

A continuous technique has been described in which a thin radiopaque Teflon catheter is introduced under x-ray control with the paratracheal technique described above. The stylet is withdrawn and the catheter properly fixed.[57] It should be recognized, however, that movement of the catheter into proximity with vertebral artery, dural cuff, or other structures is possible.

Intravenous sympathetic block may be a more attractive technique when prolonged effect is required (see Chap. 12 and below).

Signs of a Successful Block

Horner's syndrome (Fig. 13-19) results if the cervical sympathetic fibers are successfully blocked: ptosis (drooping upper eyelid), myosis (small pupil), and enophthalmos (sinking of the eyeball). In addition, other features have been described, such as unilateral blockage of the nose (owing to engorgement of nasal mucosa), flushing of conjunctiva and skin, and anhydrosis (lack of sweating). The ptosis and conjunctival engorgement can be relieved by eyedrops of the alpha agonist Neosynephrine. It should be noted that these signs may be present without complete sympathetic denervation of the upper limb, which may receive sympathetic supply from as far down as T9. The cobalt blue sweat test or SCR is the most useful in this situation (see list on pp. 474–475) (see also Chap. 27).

Indications

The clinical indications for cervicothoracic sympathetic blocks are listed below.

Clinical Conditions That Cervicothoracic Sympathetic Blockade May Benefit

Circulatory insufficiency in the arm, due to
- Traumatic or embolic vascular occlusion or impaired circulation
- Postembolectomy vasospasm
- Raynaud's disease, scleroderma and other arteriopathies, frostbite*
- Occlusive vascular disease: "acute or chronic" episodes

Pain
- Post-traumatic syndrome (causalgia)
- Causalgia following abdominal injury[80]
- Herpes zoster
- Phantom limb
- Paget's disease
- Neoplasm
- Tropic changes in skin
- Pain due to lesions in the CNS[59]

Other
- Hyperhidrosis
- Shoulder/hand syndrome
- Miscellaneous conditions in head region: stroke, Meniere's disease, tinnitus
- Sudeck's atrophy[26]
- Amblyopia due to quinine poisoning[83] (also causes retinal artery spasm and thrombosis)

*All three of these conditions should be treated at an early stage, for "acute or chronic" episodes.

These indications are based largely on anecdotal case reports so that an initial diagnostic blockade should always be accompanied by a separate assessment, by one of the methods in the list on pages 474–475, for sympathetic ablation, blood flow, and pain.

The most controversial indications are stroke and other conditions in the cranial distribution of the sympathetic chain, such as Meniere's disease. At

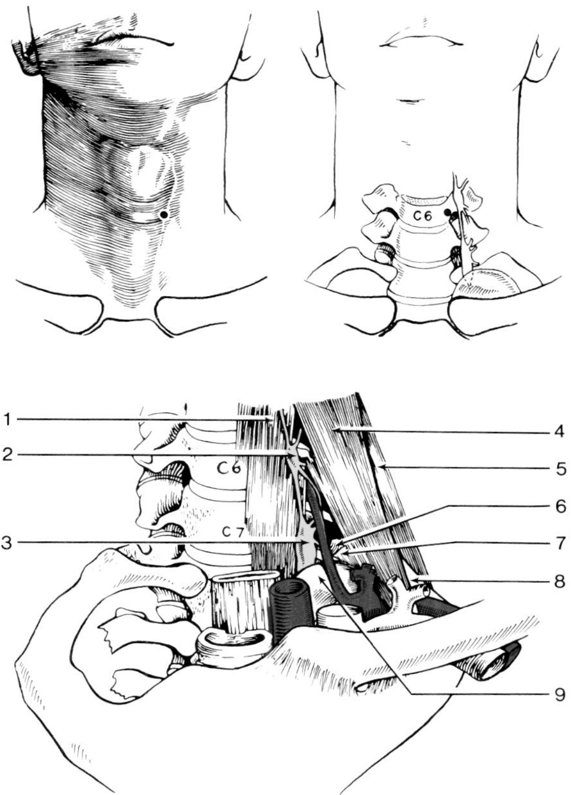

1. Longus Colli Muscle
2. Middle Cervical Ganglion
3. Stellate Ganglion
4. Scalenus Anterior Muscle
5. Scalenus Medius Muscle
6. Transverse Process of First Thoracic Vertebra
7. Tubercle of First Rib
8. Brachial Plexus
9. Dome of Pleura

FIG. 13-18. Cervicothoracic sympathetic chain: regional anatomy. **I.** Anterior view. Note stellate ganglion on neck of first rib and extending up to transverse process of C7. At this level, the cervicothoracic sympathetic chain has the vertebral artery on its anterolateral aspect with the pleura covering the lower third of the stellate ganglion. At the level of C6, the vertebral artery has dived posteriorly into the foramen intertransversarium and the pleura is well below. Note also that even at C6, a large volume of solution may diffuse posteriorly between the slips of origin of scalenus anterior to the roots of the brachial plexus. **II.** Cross-section. Note the importance of lateral retraction of the carotid and extension of the neck to draw the esophagus medial to the needle path on the left side. It is necessary to withdraw the needle 2 to 5 mm after contacting the transverse process in order to clear the anterior aspect of the longus colli muscle. Correct needle direction onto the transverse process is very important, as is the avoidance of force with the risk of penetration of prevertebral fascia and intertransverse ligaments leading to entry into vertebral artery or dural cuff. (Modified from Bryce-Smith et al.[14])

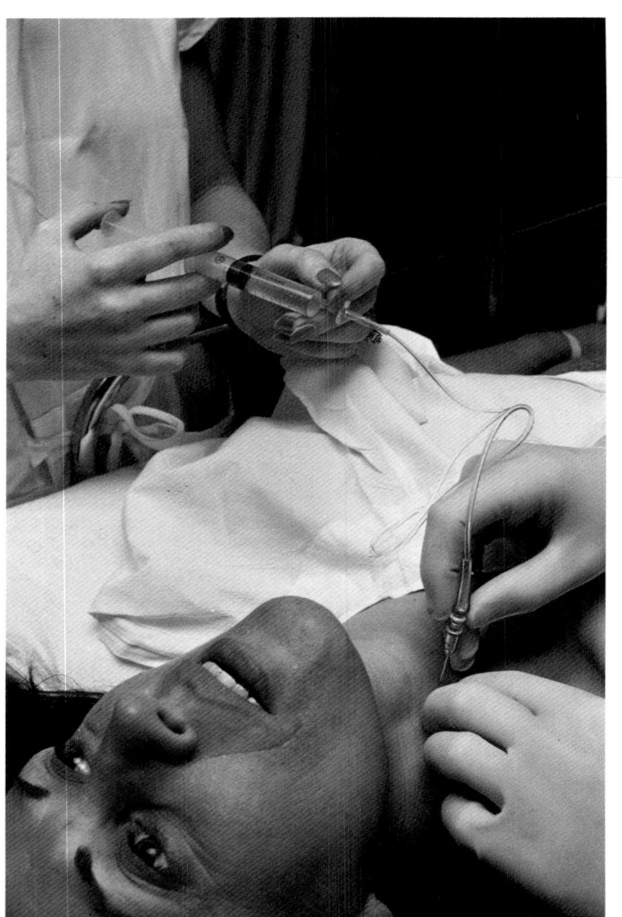

A

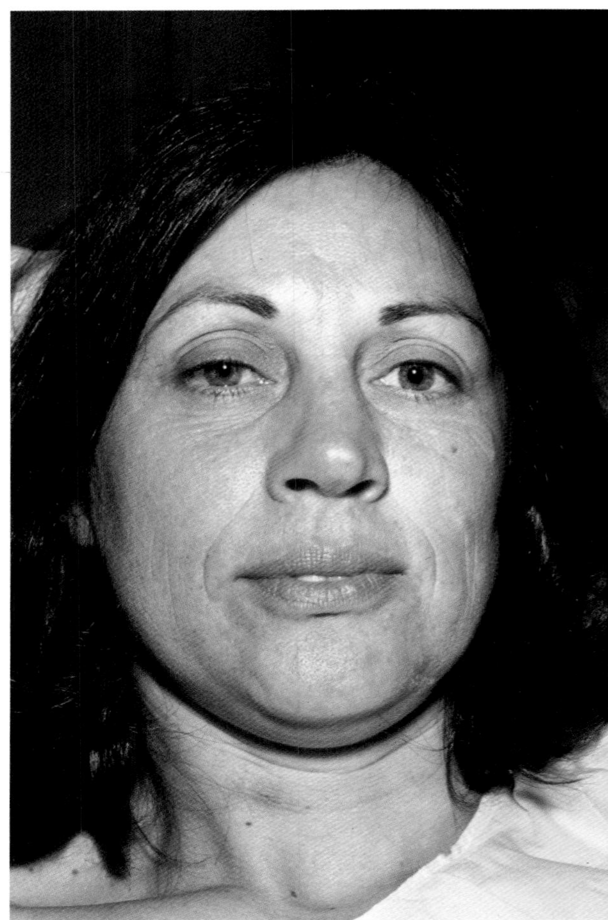

B

FIG. 13-19. **A.** Stellate ganglion block needle correctly placed. Note palpating hand *(left)* retracting carotid sheath laterally and hand holding needle *(right)* braced against clavicle. An extension tubing is used so that an assistant may aspirate and inject. **B.** Horner's syndrome *(right)*. Note ptosis, miois, anhydrosis, and unilteral conjunctival engorgement.

present, no definitive data are available to demonstrate any benefit from sympathetic blockade.

Complications

Intra-arterial and intradural injections are dangerous complications (see below). It should be firmly stated that the negative aspiration test, as described above, does not exclude an intra-arterial or an intradural injection. To prevent the occurrence of these complications, one must realize that the needle should not meet any resistance after it has passed through the skin until it rests on what is obviously bone. If the needle is pushed through the prevertebral fascia and the ligaments connecting the transverse processes (this fascia and the ligament can usually be felt), the tip of the needle might be in or close to the vertebral artery or the dural sheath enclosing the cervical nerve roots. Spinal analgesia follows dural sheath injection.

Complications of Cervicothoracic (Stellate Ganglion) Sympathetic Blockade

Common
- Temporary hoarseness and feeling of a lump in the throat (recurrent laryngeal nerve block)
- Unpleasant effects of Horner's syndrome
- Hematoma may occur
- Neuralgia along chest wall and inner aspect of upper arm

Uncommon
- Brachial plexus, rarely affected
- Phrenic nerve block
- Pneumothorax
- Osteitis — transverse process

Severe
- Injection into the vertebral artery — immediate CNS effects
- Intradural injection — slow onset of symptoms

An injection of local anesthetic solution into the paravertebral fascia may also spread along the fascial plane to involve the brachial plexus.[15] Bilateral injection is inadvisable since inadvertent bilateral recurrent laryngeal nerve block may result in airway problems (loss of laryngeal reflex). Also, loss of cardioaccelerator activity may result in bradycardias and hypotension.

If a hematoma occurs, it might be necessary to inject below C6. This can usually be accomplished because it is possible to feel the prevertebral fascia and the ligaments over C7, after which the needle should be withdrawn several millimeters and the block completed as described above; the risk of pneumothorax increases.

Osteitis of the transverse process has been described after a stellate ganglion block, possibly because the needle traversed the esophagus before it reached the transverse process.[66]

Chemical Stellate Ganglion Block

An injection of 1 to 2 ml of 6% aqueous phenol or 10% phenol in Conray dye (see below) at C6 will interrupt the cervical chain but not produce a complete cervicothoracic sympathetic blockade. The arm may partially escape, and in these cases an injection of the sympathetic chain at T2 and T3 can be used as a supplement; however, this technique is not commonly practiced because of the proximity of pleura and somatic nerves (see also Chap. 29.2). A dural sheath may be entered, and injected solutions may migrate by means of the CSF to the nearby medulla, with its important control centers.

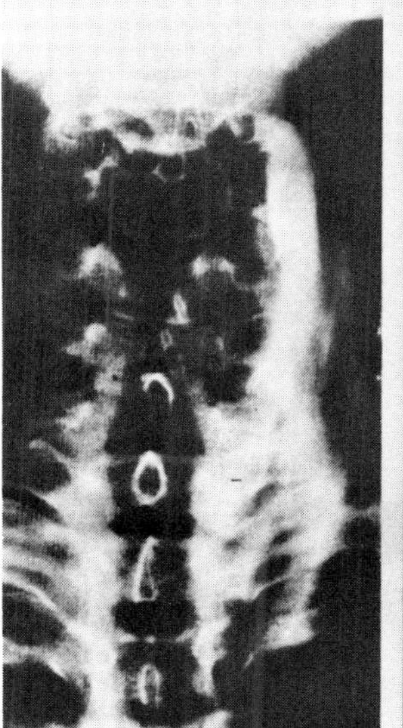
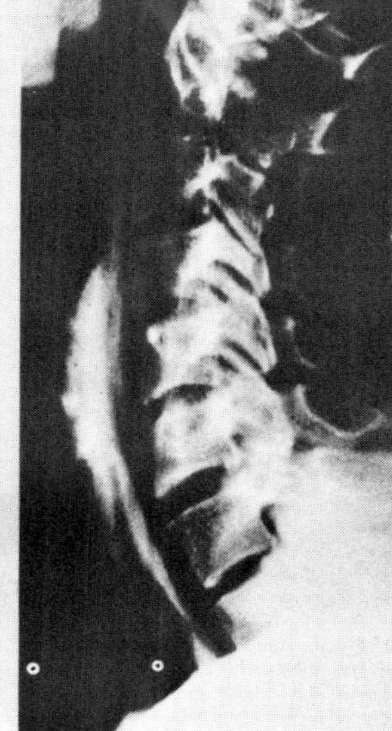

FIG. 13-20. The spread of 20 ml of local anesthetic solution injected in front of the prevertebral fascia at the 6th transverse process.

THORACIC SYMPATHETIC BLOCK

Regional Anatomy

As noted on page 462, the sympathetic chain in the thoracic region lies close to the neck of the ribs, and thus it is very close to the somatic roots (Fig. 13-21). In the cervical region, the sympathetic chain is separated from somatic roots by longus colli and anterior scalene muscles and, in the lumbar region, by psoas major. In contrast, no such muscle is present in the thoracic region, and the proximity of the pleura to the sympathetic chain adds a second hazard (Fig. 13-21).

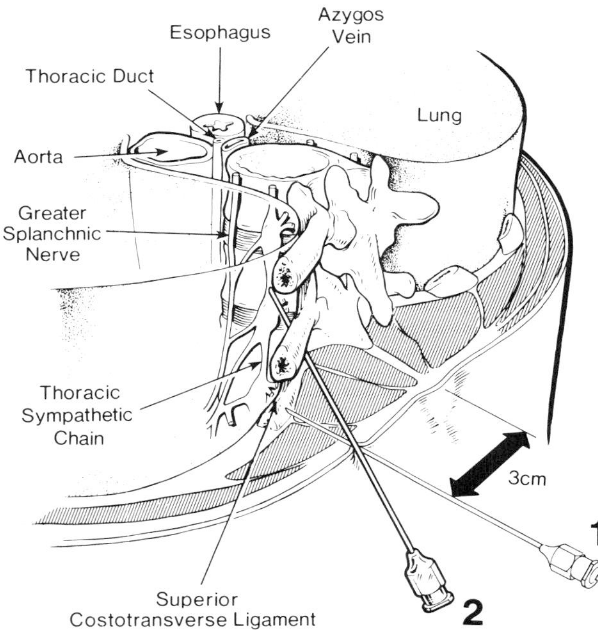

FIG. 13-21. Thoracic sympathetic (paravertebral) block. Needle insertion is 3 cm from the midline, opposite cephalad aspect of spinous process. Needle is initially inserted perpendicular to skin in all planes to reach rib or transverse process at a depth of about 2.5 to 3.5 cm. Sometimes needle may need to be angled slightly superiorly or inferiorly to locate rib or transverse process. Needle is then directed cephalad above the rib, and a loss of resistance may be detected, with an air-filled syringe, as the needle penetrates the costotransverse ligament. At this point the needle tip lies in the paravertebral space where both sympathetic and somatic thoracic nerves are located. Careful aspiration must be carried out for air (intrapleural), blood (intravascular), or CSF (intradural).

Technique

A 10-cm needle is introduced and angled toward the vertebral body three fingerbreadths (6 cm) from the midline opposite the T2 spinous process. As the needle is advanced, it either strikes rib or passes through the intercostal space and continues until it is held up by the body of the vertebra in the true para-vertebral space (Fig. 13-21). It is generally easy to decide whether the bone encountered is rib or vertebral body because the rib is more superficial and transmits through the needle a feeling of smoothness in contrast to the gritty roughness of the vertebral body; because of the anatomic problems outlined above, confirmation of position by image intensifier is highly desirable. When the needle reaches the vertebra, it is angled to pass less than 1 cm behind the crest of the vertebral body (Fig. 13-21). An injection of 2 ml of local anesthetic or, for permanent block, 6% phenol or alcohol is made at this point, and a successful result is indicated if the patient has a warm dry hand and no evidence of Horner's syndrome. The use of image intensifier and injection, under direct vision, of 10% phenol dissolved in Conray-420 (or Angiographin) greatly increases the safety of this technique.

Indications

Some possible indications for permanent neurolytic sympathectomy for the upper limb syndromes are given in the list on page 480. Many clinics still prefer surgical sympathectomy, although a transaxillary (thoracic) approach is necessary to obtain complete sympathetic denervation of the upper limb. The results and complications of the neurolytic technique with an image intensifier remain to be assessed. Intrathoracic pain, such as status anginosus, has been treated by sympathetic block (by either stellate or thoracic approach); however, the availability of beta-blockers has diminished the appeal of sympathetic block because the potential complications are very serious in a patient with severe myocardial disease.

Complications

The two principal complications of this technique are pneumothorax and intrathecal injection[77] by way of the intervertebral foramen. Because of these two complications, this technique was used only minimally, until recent application of image-intensifier techniques allowed direct viewing of needle placement and appropriate spread of solution.

LUMBAR SYMPATHETIC BLOCK

Regional Anatomy

The lumbar part of the sympathetic chain and its ganglia lies in the fascial plane close to the anterolateral side of the vertebral bodies, separated from somatic nerves by the psoas fascia and psoas muscle (Figs. 13-22 and 13-23). An injection of a large volume of fluid (*e.g.*, 25 ml) anywhere in this space will, in most instances, fill the whole space. Theoretically, one injection at L2 or L3 should be enough to achieve adequate longitudinal spread. This single injection technique is now used by a number of experienced specialists in pain clinics (see below). However, in other clinics, injections are performed at two different levels, particularly with a neurolytic agent such as phenol, to limit lateral spread at any one level, since this poses a risk of spread across psoas to the genitofemoral nerve, perhaps by a fibrous tunnel to a somatic nerve or, worse still, to a dural cuff region and thence to subarachnoid space (see Fig 13-24).[14] When continuous blockade with catheters is used, it is also preferable to have two catheters because there is a tendency for one of the catheters to slide dorsally out of position.

In an anatomic study, lumbar sympathetic blocks were performed "blind" in cadavers to investigate the frequency of puncture of a major organ.[16a] The technique of inserting the needles was based on that of Mandl (see below). With the cadaver in the lateral position, three 22-gauge, 15-cm needles were inserted about 10 cm (4 in) from the midline at the approximate levels of L1, L2, and L3. In thin cadavers, the distance of insertion of the needles from the midline was less, about 7.5 cm, whereas in obese subjects the distance was greater (up to 12.5 cm). Each needle was advanced onto the vertebral body, gradually positioned more anteriorly until it slipped beyond the anterolateral aspect of the vertebral body (see Fig. 13-22), and then advanced to the "hilt" to allow the cadaver to be positioned supine. The cadaver was then rolled over and the performance repeated on the other side.

Eighty needles were inserted in the direction of the lumbar sympathetic chain, and 95% passed either throughout the lumbar sympathetic chain or within 0.5 cm of it. In 90% of those occasions on which the chain was not traversed, the needles were lateral to the chain.

One needle passed through the hilum of the kid-

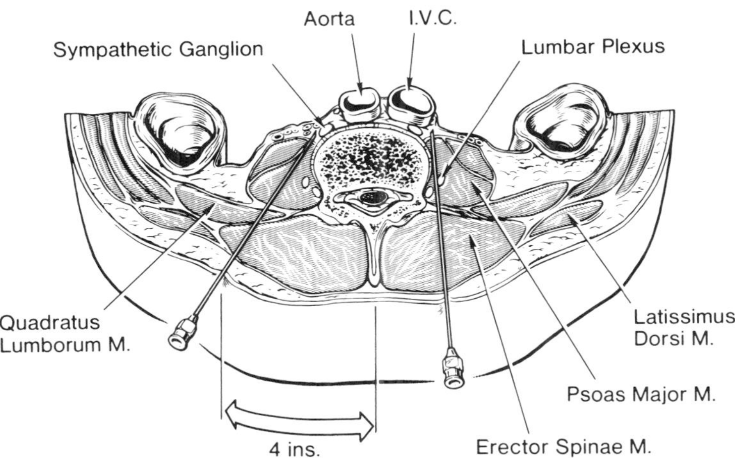

FIG. 13-22. Lumbar sympathetic block. Note that insertion of needle 10 cm from the midline enables the needle to reach the anterolateral angle of the vertebral body. Insertion of needle closer to the midline takes needle path close to somatic nerve roots and lateral to sympathetic chain. (Reproduced with permission from Cherry, D.A., Rao, D.M.: Lumbar sympathetic and coeliac plexus blocks—An anatomical study in cadavers. Br. J. Anaesth., *54*:1037, 1982.)

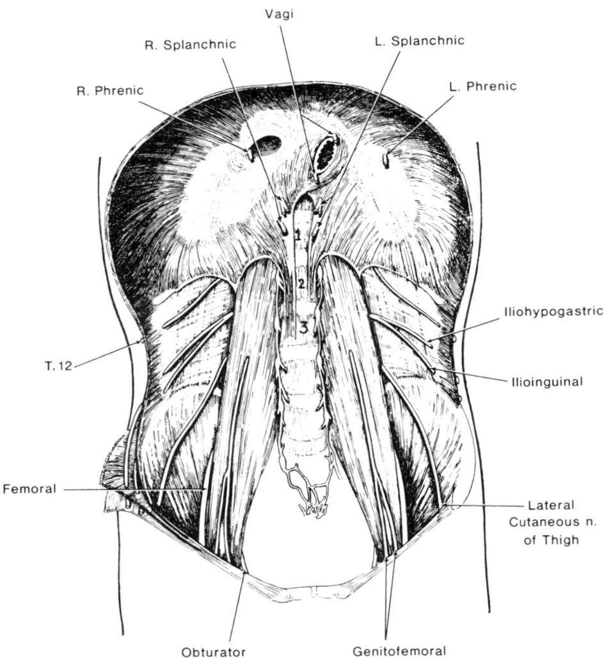

FIG. 13-23. Posterior abdominal wall, genitofemoral nerve. Note its course anterior to psoas major, thus being more vulnerable to neurolytic solution spreading laterally from the sympathetic chain. (Modified from Bryce-Smith et al.[14])

ney, although in that cadaver there was a large osteophyte over an intervertebral disk that displaced the needle laterally. Two needles were found embedded in grossly osteoporotic vertebral bodies. All three of these placements would doubtless have been prevented by using a *c*-arm *i*mage *i*ntensifier as is used routinely in clinical practice. The position of the lumbar sympathetic chain was found to be remarkably constant on the anterolateral aspect of the vertebral bodies.

Almost all of the needles passed either through the sympathetic chain or lateral to it. As Figure 13-22 shows, the more lateral the insertion of the needle, the closer the tip should be to the lumbar sympathetic chain. There is also a lesser risk of piercing roots of the lumbar plexus or of contracting the transverse process.

Technique (Mandl) with Two Needles

The method of blocking the lumbar sympathetic chain was first introduced by Mandl in 1926 and was similar to that used by Kappis for injecting the celiac plexus.[44,64]

The spinous processes of L1 and L4 are marked as reference points. L1 is level with the line between the two points where the lateral side of the erector spinae muscles meets the 12th ribs; a line joining the posterior superior iliac crests passes through the lower part of the spine at L4 (see Fig. 13-25).

A subcutaneous wheal is raised about 8 to 10 cm laterally to the middle of the spinous processes of L2 and L4. Local anesthetic solution is injected subcutaneously (and with an intramuscular needle, against the transverse process above or below the site of injection by directing the needle 45° cranially or caudally and in between the transverse processes, if these are to be contacted).

A 19- to 20-gauge needle of approximately 12 cm in length (or an 18-gauge needle for continuous blockade) with a rubber marker is introduced through the skin until the tip of the needle has reached a transverse process. The marker is pushed down to the skin and the needle withdrawn. The distance from the skin to the transverse process is, in the normal adult, roughly half the distance from the skin to the lateral side of the vertebral body (10 cm). This may be a shorter distance if the patient has thin back muscles, and longer if the muscles are thick. The marker on the needle is moved toward the hub of the needle so that the distance from the tip to the marker is roughly twice the first marked distance.

The needle is reintroduced and directed slightly medially to pass between the transverse processes. When bone is reached, the marker should be almost flush with the skin, the bevel of the needle being directed toward the lateral side of the vertebral body. A slight change in angle of the needle will allow the tip of the needle to slide off the vertebra and to reach the sympathetic chain on the ventrolateral aspect of the vertebral body (see Fig. 13-22).[29] Correct position can be verified by using a loss-of-resistance test with a syringe filled with air or saline. Penetration of the psoas fascia gives a resistance change not dissimilar to that of epidural block. Some specialists prefer to avoid the transverse process, so that the needle proceeds directly to the lateral aspect of the vertebral body (see below). A loss of resistance, at a shallower level, is often obtained between psoas and quadratus lumborum in the region of the transverse process (see Fig. 13-22). Placement of solution at this level would result in lumbar plexus block—highly undesirable if a neurolytic solution is used.

In clinical practice, the anesthesiologist often starts at L2 and, in a second step, introduces the needle at

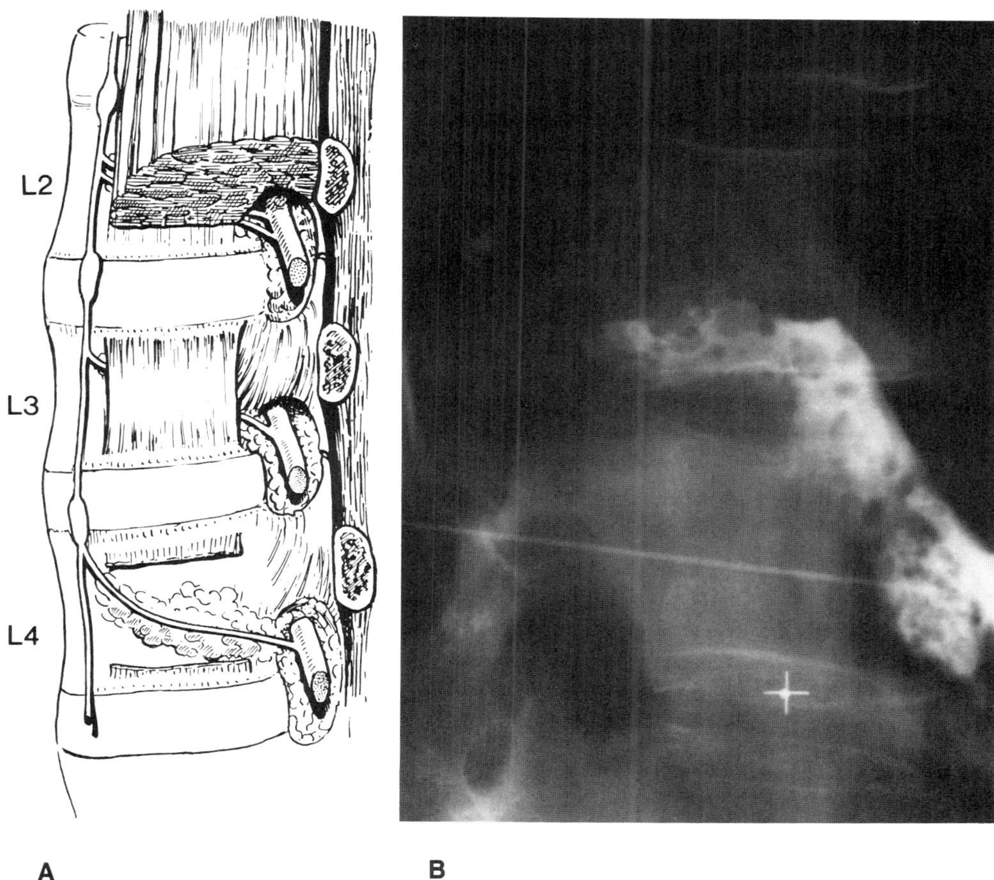

FIG. 13-24. **A.** Fibrous arch between paravertebral space and lumbar sympathetic chain. This pathway poses a potential for spread of neurolytic solution to somatic nerve roots, resulting in possible sensory loss or neuralgia. (Modified from Bryce-Smith et al.[14]) **B.** Contrast medium injected too close to side of vertebral body spreading via fibrous arch.

L4. When the needle is correctly placed at L2, the part of the needle outside the skin should be measured and the marker for L4 properly placed. In most patients, owing to the lumbar lordosis at L4, the distance from the skin to the vertebral body is usually a little greater than at L2. It is vitally important to aspirate to ensure that neither blood nor CSF is present and to check that there is no resistance to injection; resistance could be due to the needle being in the wall of the aorta or vena cava, an abdominal viscus, or an intervertebral disk. Once again, radiographic confirmation (local anesthetic mixed with contrast medium) and injection under direct vision increase safety.[8,18,27,91]

In the most simple cases (*e.g.*, renal colic), one injection of 20 to 30 ml, preferably of 0.25% bupivacaine with epinephrine, 1 : 200,000 (5×10^{-6} g/ml), at L2 will completely eradicate pain. In patients with obliterative arterial disease, a diagnostic block with 1 to 5 ml of local anesthetic mixed with contrast me-

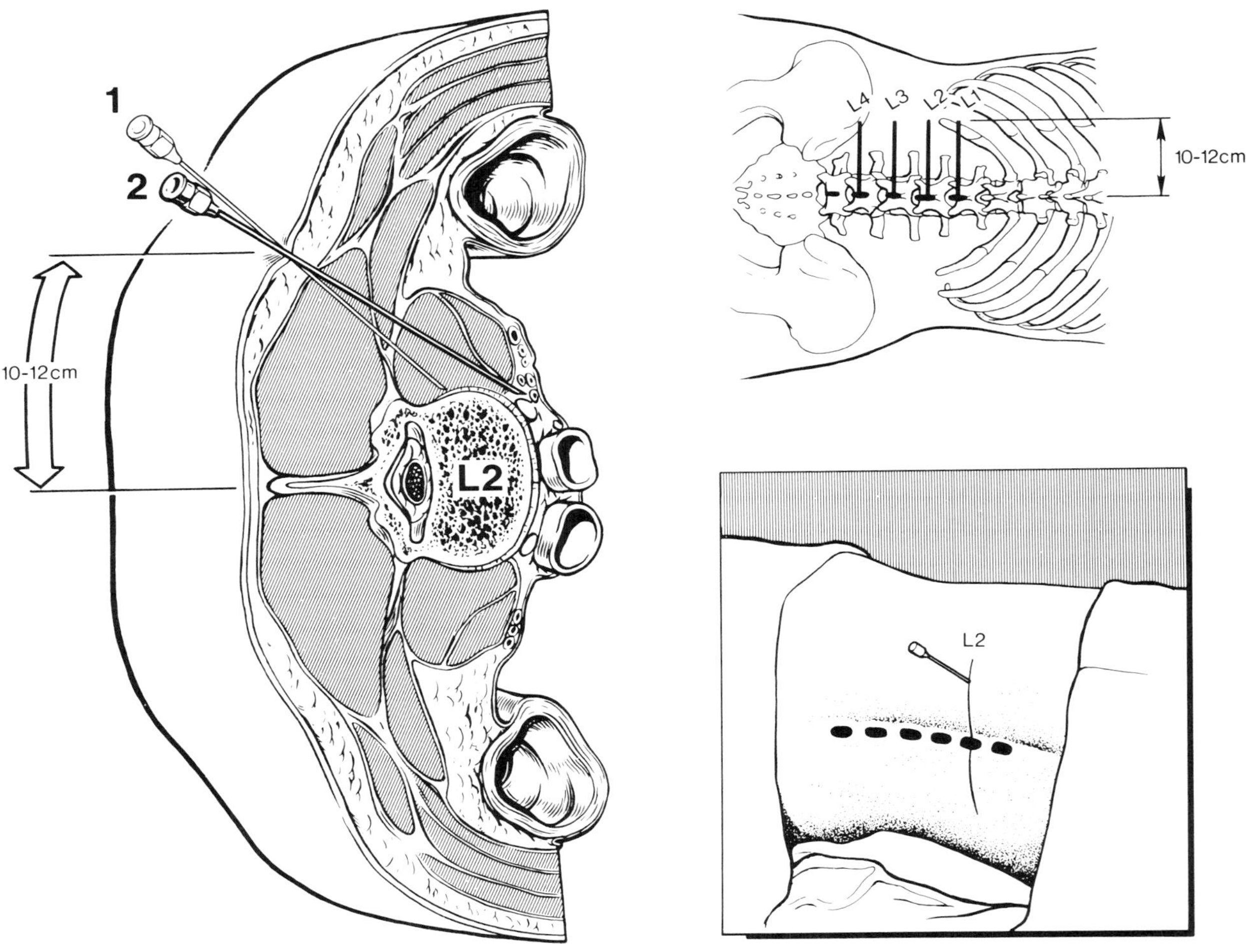

FIG. 13-25. Technique of lumbar sympathetic block. Note location of skin marks for L1 and L4 spinous processes, which then permit identification of L2 and L3. A line is drawn through the center of the spinous processes; this will lie below the transverse process of that vertebra. Needle insertion is at the lateral margin of the erector spinae muscle (approximately 10–12 cm from midline). If it is desired to check the depth of the transverse process, the needle must be angled cephalad. Otherwise the needle is inserted approximately 45° toward the vertebral body until this structure is located. Then the needle is angled more steeply until it slips just past the vertebral body and through the psoas fascia *(2)* (see text). A single needle can be used instead of two or three needles; however, an increased volume must be injected.

dium may be made at L2 and L4 under radiographic control. The continuous blockade technique is also very useful; needles are placed at L2 and L4, and, after the proper positioning of each needle, catheters are passed through the needles, which are then withdrawn over the catheters. The catheters are fixed along the erector spinae muscles. The cranial ends of the catheters, each with a needle and a Millipore filter, are placed in a sterile sponge in the supraclavicular fossa. The time-interval between injections may be increased to 6 hours if bupivacaine is used. The continuous blockade is maintained for 5 days, during which the clinical effects of the blockade should be evaluated. In the case of the single-shot diagnostic block, the volume of local anesthetic in contrast medium should be the same as that proposed for neurolytic block. Also, a method of assessment from each category on the list on page 474 should be used immediately after the block. Often, diagnostic blocks are repeated if there is any doubt about results.[10]

In most instances, the procedure is short (<30 min) and fairly free of pain. Heavy premedication or general anesthesia is not necessary. Now and then, however, a needle may pass close to a segmental nerve, provoking "lightening" pain. The needle should always be advanced slowly and redirected slightly if paresthesia should occur. The needle should not be directed too much toward the midline. We believe that it is better to be able to detect that the needle is close to a nerve in a lightly medicated patient than to accept the risk of laceration of the nerve with a fairly large needle. One case of severe segmental neuralgia, most likely the result of a nerve injury, supports this view.[18]

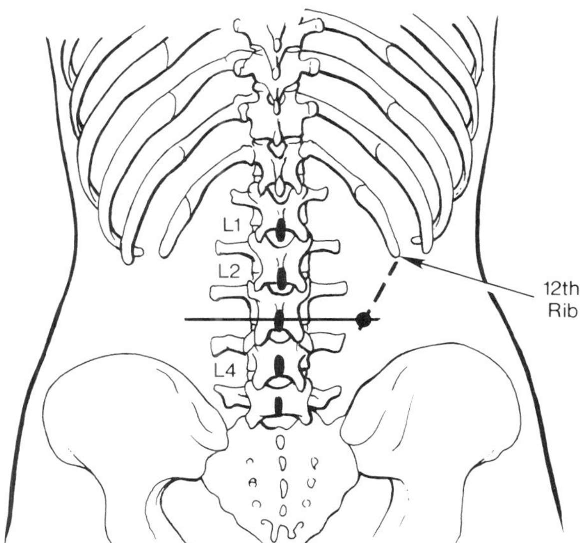

FIG. 13-26. Single needle technique of lumbar sympathetic block (see text). Note needle insertion 2 to 3 cm below and medial to the tip of the 12th rib. This should lie on a line through the center of L3 spinous process (see text). (Hatangdi, V.S., and Boas, R.V.: Lumbar sympathectomy: A single needle technique. Br. J. Anaesth., *57*:285, 1985.)

Single Injection Technique for Local Anesthetic or Neurolytic Block

Hatangdi and Boas describe the use of the tip of the 12th rib to act as a marker for needle insertion 2 to 3 cm below and medial to that point.[39a] This allows easy access to the L3 vertebral body, and then placement next to sympathetic chain is verified, as above. Sufficient solution is injected (mixed with contrast medium) to cover L2, L3, and L4 levels. An alternative is to use the 12th rib to intersect a line drawn through the middle of the L2 spinous process. Needle insertion at this point should be sufficiently lateral to obtain easy access to the L3 level. If desired, the transverse process can be avoided and the needle inserted directly onto the lateral aspect of the vertebral body. Sufficient solution is then injected to cover the sympathetic chain (Fig. 13-26).

Technique of Bryce-Smith

An alternative approach to **local anesthetic** lumbar sympathetic blockade has been described by Bryce-Smith (1951).[13]

Because of the anterolateral position of the ganglia in the lumbar region, the course of the rami communicantes is long and winds around the vertebral body in a fibrous tunnel. This arch forms one of the origins of the psoas muscle and provides indirect access to the lumbar sympathetic chain (Fig. 13-27).

A wheal is raised three fingerbreadths lateral to the tip of the spinous process of L3 and a 12-cm needle is introduced at 70° and advanced toward the body of the vertebra; when the point of the needle reaches the body of the vertebra, it lies within the fibrous tunnel (Fig. 13-27). Fifteen milliliters to 20 ml of solution are deposited here, and this tracks forward to reach the sympathetic chain. This approach should not be used when neurolytic solutions are employed because some of the fluid backtracks and causes a neuritis of the third lumbar nerve or enters a dural cuff and causes paraplegia.

Because this technique frequently leads to somatic block and does *not* provide a selective sympathetic block, it is also not indicated for diagnosis of pain syndromes.

LUMBAR SYMPATHECTOMY WITH NEUROLYTIC AGENT

Neurolytic lumbar sympathectomy should be used for the treatment of vascular disease in consultation with a vascular surgeon. It is clear that even a successful sympathetic block in a patient with rest pain may result sometimes in demarcation of a nonviable area, such as a distal phalanx of a toe. This will require

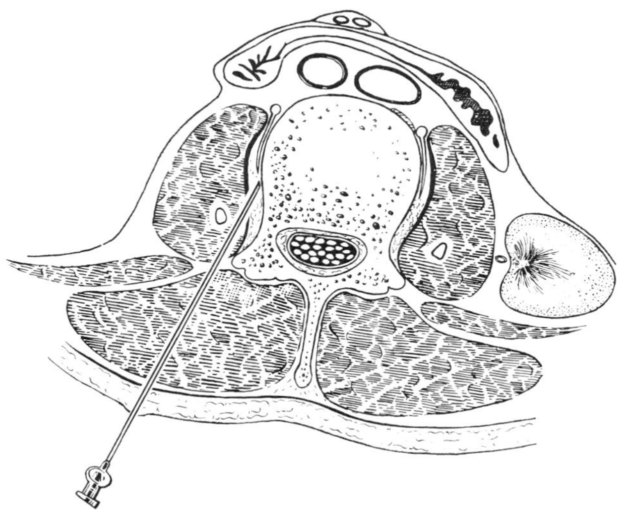

FIG. 13-27. Alternative technique for local anesthetic lumbar sympathetic block (see text). (Modified from Bryce-Smith et al.[14])

appropriate surgical treatment and should not be viewed as a disappointing side-effect of the block but as a necessary part of a rational treatment regimen.

The use of lumbar sympathetic block with proper collaboration offers the following very considerable advantages.

Symptoms can be ameliorated without risk of surgery and anesthesia in a group of patients with a high incidence of severe ischemic heart disease, pulmonary disease, and other problems of old age. In the series reported by Reid and colleagues there was a mortality of 1 : 1666 injections (less than 0.1%); this compares favorably with surgical sympathectomy, which has a mortality rate of at least 6% and as much as 20% in patients with severe vascular disease.[75] In a recent series of 386 blocks, there was only 1 death within 1 week of blockade, and this patient had severe ischemic heart disease with congestive cardiac failure prior to blockade.[18]

Outpatient Treatment. Treatment may be performed on an outpatient basis, and elderly patients (usually 60–80 years of age) can be released after a short stay. This allows for considerable economy in hospital-bed use; surgical sympathectomy often requires 6 to 10 days in the hospital when there are no complications.

Fewer Postoperative Thrombotic Phenomena. Such complications are reduced in the elderly because an operation and bed rest are avoided.

A large turnover of patients is possible (as many as eight to ten procedures in a single-day session).

If necessary, a bilateral procedure can be performed, with the second side blocked 1 week later, also on an outpatient basis.

Duration. Because the duration of sympathetic ablation is similar with surgical or neurolytic sympathectomy (mean, 6 months), the neurolytic technique offers an advantage. It can be repeated with very minimal morbidity. Nevertheless, the natural history of occlusive vascular disease is such that in one series only 5% required repeated blockade.[18]

Agents

Absolute alcohol has been used by several groups; however, it has a higher incidence of L1 neuralgia (see Chap. 29.2).[18] Seven percent phenol in water was used by Reid and colleagues in a very large series because of the low viscosity of the solution and ease of injection.[75] Seven percent to 10% phenol in Conray-420 dye or Angiographin has a similar low resistance to injection and the added advantage of being visible under image intensifier (see Fig. 13-29).[8,18,27,91] When the patient is placed on his side under a vertical radiographic beam, it is also of value to tilt him slightly ventrally and dorsally to check that the needle is fairly close to the vertebral column. One report advocates the semi-prone position with vertical x-ray screening to give a more precise view of needle position relative to vertebral body anterolateral aspect, with a single x-ray view.[47] If a biplanar image intensifier is available, then both lateral and anteroposterior views should be obtained (see Fig. 13-28). A convenient way to determine the spread is to dissolve phenol in an aqueous radiographic contrast medium (Conray-420 or Angiographin) and to inject it under direct radiographic control. This often allows confirmation of complete coverage of the lumbar sympathetic chain with as little as 3 to 4 ml of solution (see Fig. 13-31).

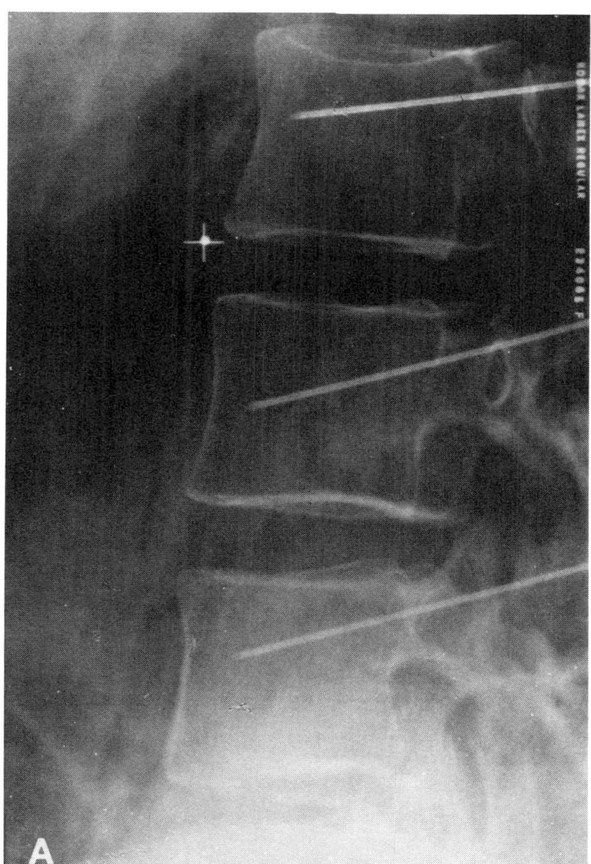

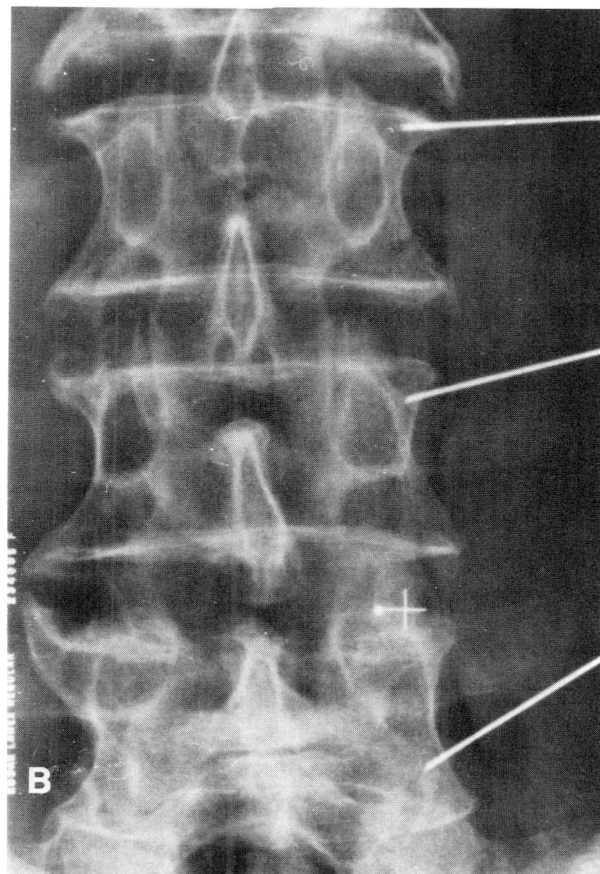

FIG. 13-28. **A.** X-ray: Needle placement, lateral view. **B.** X-ray: Needle placement, anteroposterior view.

Technique

The following modifications of local anesthetic blockade are advisable when neurolytic agents are used.

1. A radiopaque marker is placed on the skin,[39] and the level of needle insertion is checked under image intensifier. Needle position in the center of L2 and L4 vertebral bodies is checked with a lateral view (Fig. 13-28). Proximity of the needle to the disk space is avoided.
2. Needle position at the anterolateral angle of the L2 and L4 bodies is also checked in the lateral view (Fig. 13-28). Lack of movement of the needle during deep inspiration and expiration is checked carefully. With correct placement in psoas, needle tips should be immobile. Movement on respiration indicates placement lateral to psoas—possibly in the kidney.
3. An anteroposterior view is taken to check that each needle is close to the lateral aspects of the vertebral bodies (see Fig. 13-28).
4. Initially, 0.5 ml of contrast medium is injected and confirmation obtained that a sharp linear spread is occurring (Fig. 13-29). Resistance to injection and the appearance of a "blob" or fuzzy patch of contrast medium indicate injection into muscle or fascia, and injection is ceased (see Fig. 13-30).
5. As soon as linear spread is obtained, the injection

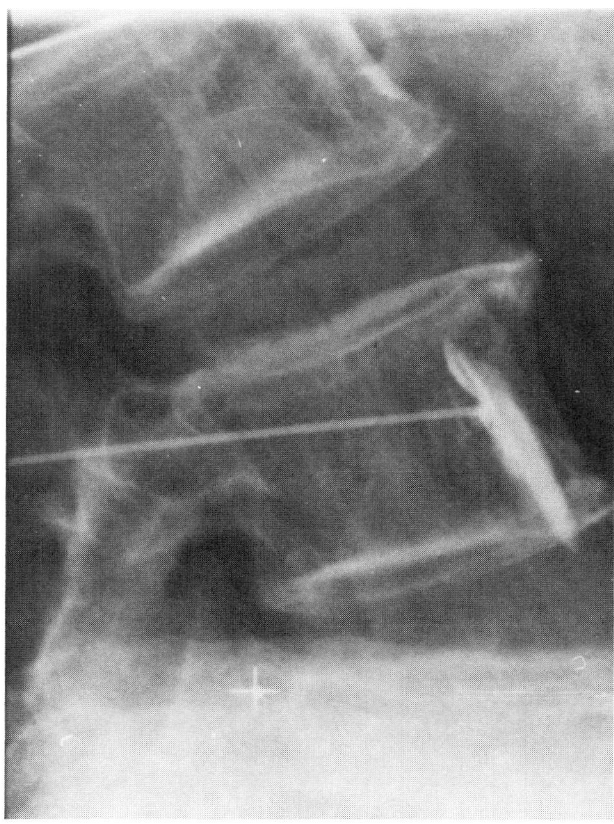

FIG. 13-29. Injection of 0.5 ml of contrast medium, showing correct linear spread along anterior aspect of psoas fascia.

is continued with neurolytic solution until each level has linear coverage. In most instances this requires no more than 2 ml and often as little as 1 ml of solution (see Fig.13-31).

6. At the completion of the injection, an anteroposterior view is taken to confirm the spread of solution along the line of the psoas muscle (see Fig. 13-31).
7. Finally, 0.5 ml of air is injected immediately before removing each needle to prevent the needle's depositing neurolytic solution on somatic nerve roots during removal.

Patients are kept on their sides for 5 minutes to prevent the solution from spreading laterally toward the genitofemoral nerve or posteriorly between the slips of origin of the psoas major and along the fibrous tunnel occupied by the rami communicantes, toward somatic nerve roots.[13,14] Patients are then turned supine but instructed not to raise their heads for 30 minutes. Observations of skin temperature, blood pressure, and pulse are continued.

Recovery Procedure

Observations are continued for 1 hour in a recovery room, and, if stable, patients are permitted to sit to 45° and begin oral intake again. Blood pressure is checked sitting and then standing, and, if unchanged, patients are allowed to ambulate and the intravenous line is removed. Most outpatients are then able to go home, accompanied by a friend or relative. Patients with highly unstable cardiovascular disease are maintained on an observation chart for at least 24 hours postblock.

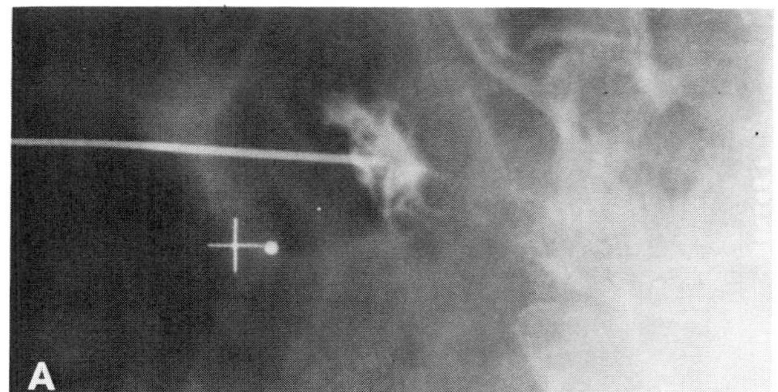

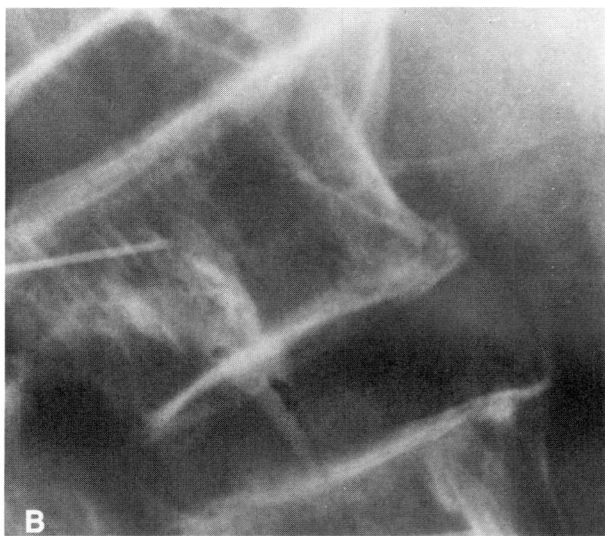

FIG. 13-30. **A.** X-ray showing injection of contrast medium into psoas major. **B.** X-ray showing injection too far posteriorly, probably into psoas sheath.

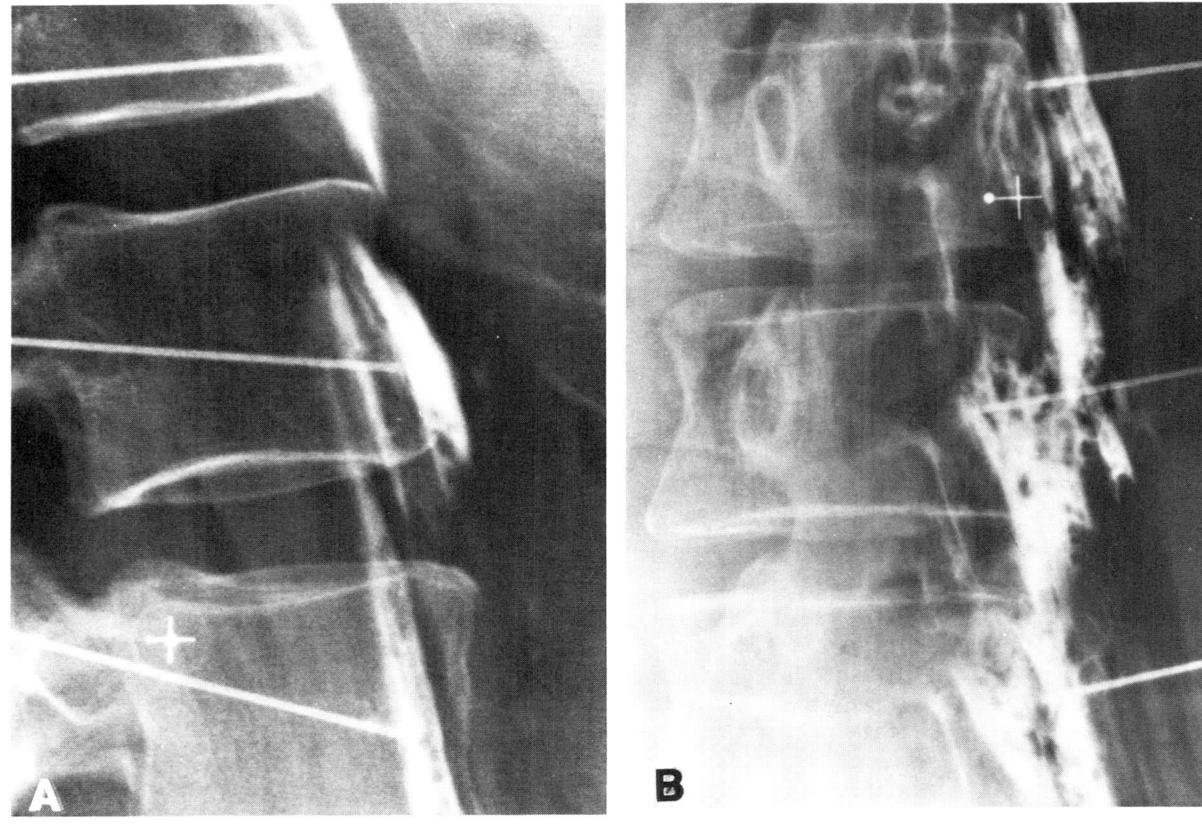

FIG. 13-31. **A.** Lateral view. Complete coverage of L2 and L4 vertebral body levels with injection of only 1 ml of 10% phenol on Conray 420 at each level. **B.** Anteroposterior view to show spread of solution following line of psoas muscle. Note limitation of lateral spread to reduce risk of genitofemoral nerve involvement.

Indications

The most common clinical indications for lumbar sympathetic blocks are listed as follows.

Clinical Conditions That Lumbar Sympathetic Blockade May Benefit

Circulatory insufficiency in the leg

- Arteriosclerotic disease, severe pain +++, gangrene ++; intermittent claudication* ++ in selected cases; diabetic gangrene +, Buerger's disease +
- After reconstructive vascular surgery
- Arterial embolus

Pain

- Renal colic
- Post-traumatic syndrome, causalgia†
- Herpes zoster
- Intractable urogenital pain in selected cases
- Sudeck's atrophy†
- Phantom limb†
- Amputation stump pain†
- Chill blains
- T8

General

- Hyperhidrosis — reduced sympathetic activity to reduce sweating
- White leg phlegmasia alba dolens‡

Trench foot‡
Erythromelalgia‡
Acrocyanosis‡

*Aortoiliac (small percentage responding) and femoropopliteal (higher percentage responding)
†See Chapter 27; only useful **early** in these conditions.
‡Miscellaneous conditions in which reduced sympathetic activity may help to correct an abnormality in nutritive blood flow or venous or lymphatic drainage.

Some clinics have stopped using diagnostic blocks for patients with atherosclerotic vascular disease and rest pain, skin ulcers, or gangrene. Their rationale is that the incidence of adverse effects is extremely low and many of these patients tolerate multiple procedures poorly. In a recent series with measurement of pain, blood flow, and sympathetic activity, the results of diagnostic and neurolytic sympathetic blocks were essentially the same in every patient studied (see Fig. 13–7).[91] In younger patients with less well-defined chronic pain syndromes, however, diagnostic blocks should be performed before neurolytic sympathetic block. As discussed in the section on physiologic effects of sympathectomy, the best rationale for the use of lumbar sympathectomy in arterial disease is to obtain improved skin blood flow; however, pain relief may occur even without improved blood flow (see p. 473). Tables 13-1 to 13-3 summarize available clinical data on the use of lumbar sympathectomy for pain and skin ulcers as well as other conditions in which its efficacy is more difficult to determine except by diagnostic block in each case.

TABLE 13–1. LUMBAR SYMPATHETIC BLOCK: EXAMPLES OF USES AND RESULTS IN THREE CLINICAL SERIES

Study*	Number of Cases
After vascular surgery (''continuous'' local anesthetic lumbar sympathetic block)	70
Arterial embolism—no surgery	13 (7 improved)
Cytostatic perfusion (melanoma)	4
Frostbite	2
	89
Obliterative arterial disease (local anesthetic block followed by chemical sympathectomy in 72 cases)	122 (see Table 13-2)
Diagnostic local anesthetic followed by neurolytic agent†	
Rest pain and ischemic ulcers	386 (80% relieved)
Gangrene of lower extremity (pain relief and speeding up demarcation)	50 (55% relieved)
Reflex sympathetic dysfunction	12 (50%) relieved—those treated early)
Claudication	12 (50% relieved; only those with response to local anesthetic block received neurolytic block)
Neurolytic agent over 10-year period‡	
Rest pain	194 (80% relieved)
Gangrene of lower extremity	40 (50% relieved)
Reflex sympathetic dysfunction (post-traumatic)	42 (45% relieved—those treated early)
Phantom limb	19 (60% relieved)

*Data from Löfström, B., and Zetterquist, S.: Lumbar sympathetic blocks in the treatment of patients with obliterative arterial disease of the lower limb. Int. Anesthesiol. Clin., 7:423, 1969.
†Data from Cousins, M.J., Reeve, T.S., Glynn, C.J., Walsh, J.A., *et al.*: Neurolytic lumbar sympathetic blockade: Duration of denervation and relief of rest pain. Anaesth. Intensive Care, 7(2):121–135, 1979.
‡Unpublished data from Lloyd, J.W., *et al.*

Complications

Complications of lumbar sympathetic blocks are extremely rare; however, a needle directed too far medially may pass into an intervertebral foramen, causing paraplegia. This may be recognized by the flow of CSF, but it is not always the case. Thus, confirmation of correct placement by radiography is highly desirable (see also Chap. 23).

Complications of Lumbar Sympathetic Blockade*

Puncture of major vessel or renal pelvis
Subarachnoid injection
Neuralgia—genitofemoral nerve (5–10% pain in the groin)
Somatic nerve, damage—neuralgia (1%)
Perforation of a disk
Stricture of the ureter after phenol or alcohol injection
Infection from catheter technique (extremely rare)
Ejaculatory failure (bilateral block in young males)
Chronic back pain

*Pain in the groin following injection is the most common untoward sequel. Subarachnoid tap is occasionally seen but easily recognized and should not constitute a hazard. The remaining complications are very rare, when image intensifier control is used.

After surgical and chemical sympathectomies, a pain or discomfort in the groin is often seen, hypothetically attributed to a genitofemoral nerve neuritis. The discomfort may last 2 to 5 weeks.[8,18,21,74] This is so-called L1 neuralgia and is characterized by hyperesthesia in L1 distribution and a burning pain. The patient often says that it is unbearable even to have

TABLE 13-2. RESULTS OF LUMBAR SYMPATHETIC BLOCKADE IN PATIENTS WITH OBLITERATIVE ARTERIAL DISEASE

Primary Symptoms	Number of Patients		Results of Initial Continuous Local Anesthetic and Neurolytic Block			
			Pain Relief 2+	1+	0	–
Gangrene arteriosclerotic	55	LA*	28		27	0
			∴ 28 phenol blocks			
			14	9	5	0
Diabetic	28	LA	14		14	
			∴ 14 phenol blocks			
			8	4	2	0
Severe rest pain	23	LA	19	4	0	0
			23			
			∴ 18 phenol blocks (5 resolved with LA)			
			18	0	0	0
Intermittent claudication	16	LA	7	6	2	1
			12			
			∴ 12 phenol blocks (1 resolved with LA)			
			7		9	

*LA = initial local anesthetic block. (Kövames, A., and Löfström, B.: Continuous lumbar sympathetic blocks in the treatment of patients with ischemic lower limbs. Tenth Congress of Int. Cardiovascular Soc., 1971)

clothes touch the thigh and may also describe the leg as "feeling as though it will explode." The condition responds well to transcutaneous electrical stimulation. The incidence is much higher with alcohol and appears to be least when the volume injected at any one level is the minimal amount necessary to achieve coverage of sympathetic ganglia, as checked by image-intensifier.[18]

TABLE 13-3. PERCENTAGE OF PATIENTS WITH OCCLUSIVE VASCULAR DISEASE WHO RESPONDED TO LUMBAR SYMPATHETIC BLOCK

Rest Pain (%)	Skin Lesions (%)	Claudication (%)	References
	55	13	34,35
	60	41	82
	64		7
57	45		46
71	55	20	38
62	100(5/5)		67
63–51	35		81
48 (some)	33		32
57	43		79
	6		31
49 (complete relief)	50	–	18
80 (complete or partial relief)		–	18
–	–	0	33
–	–	0	68

INTRAVENOUS REGIONAL SYMPATHETIC BLOCK

SITE OF ACTION AND EFFICACY

Intravenous regional sympathetic block is based on the "Bier block," a local anesthetic intravenous regional block described in Chapter 12. The sympathetic blocking drug guanethidine (Ismelin) has a high affinity for sympathetic nerve endings, where it displaces norepinephrine (NE) from presynaptic vesicles and prevents reuptake of NE. This causes a brief initial release of NE, followed by NE depletion (see Fig. 13-4), which results in long-lasting intravenous regional sympathetic blocks (IVRS) when the "Bier block" technique is used. Guanethidine has an advantage over reserpine, which has a similar action, except that reserpine crosses the blood–brain barrier and produces CNS effects whereas guanethidine does not. Controlled studies have now documented the efficacy of i.v. regional guanethidine in increasing blood flow[8a,36a,65a,89a] and skin temperature[8a,65a] while decreasing the vasoconstrictor ice response[36a] and reducing pain[8a,36a,65a] in vascular disease[36a] and reflex sympathetic dystrophies.[8a,25a,36a] Sweating is not reduced[36a,65a] because it is mediated by cholinergic postganglionic sympathetic fibers.

A controlled study in volunteers compared guanethidine and reserpine and found that only guanethidine significantly increased temperature after cold challenge and that this effect lasted 3 days.[65a]

Duration of effect and efficacy of guanethidine was compared with stellate ganglion block in a randomized trial in patients with reflex sympathetic dystrophies.[8a] In patients treated with stellate ganglion blocks, skin temperature and skin plethysmography measurements were significantly increased at 1 hour but not at later times. In patients treated with guanethidine, skin temperature was increased at 1 hour, 24 hours, and 48 hours postblock. Skin plethysmography measurements were significantly increased at 24 hours and remained so at 48 hours.[8a]

Stellate blocks every other day (up to total of eight blocks) produced similar clinical effects to i.v. guanethidine block every 4 days (up to total of four blocks) in terms of pain score and clinical signs, when assessed at 1 month and 3 month follow-up.[8a]

In a within-patient study of i.v. guanethidine blocks compared to placebo, skin temperature and hand blood flow were significantly increased at 1 hour postblock.[36a] At seven days postblock, hand blood flow, but not skin temperature, was increased. Vasoconstrictor response to ice was decreased at 1 hour and 7 days postblock.[36a]

Thus there is good evidence that an intravenous regional sympathetic block offers the following: [1] It is less "invasive" and uncomfortable for patients; [2] it results in significant modification of noradrenergic activity, that is, increased blood flow and decreased pain; and [3] effects are longer lasting than those of stellate blocks, 4 to 7 days compared with less than 1 day. However, cholinergic activity is *not* modified.

A further application of i.v. sympathetic block is in (upper) limb angiography, where the vasodilatation greatly facilitates delineation of the vasculature.[89a] It is also suggested as an aid to maintaining tissue perfusion in tissue grafting operations.[89a] In patients with severe vascular disease, in whom inflation of a tourniquet may be dangerous, guanethidine can be infused slowly into an artery by means of a narrow gauge needle, with effects similar to those of the i.v. technique.

CURRENT AND FUTURE OPTIONS

In some countries, for example, the United States, an i.v. preparation of guanethidine is no longer available* since the drug has ceased to be of value, by this route, for hypertension. Thus it is necessary to examine other potential candidates for use in this valuable technique. Figure 13-32 gives a summary of sympathetic nerve transmission at the adrenergic nerve terminal, sites of action of neurotransmitters, and other factors influencing smooth muscle cells of the vasculature.

*In the United States and some other countries, guanethidine is available for "investigational" use by the i.v. route.

Interference with NE Synthesis. Methyldopa (Aldomet) was previously thought to have a predominantly peripheral action leading to formation of a "false transmitter" α-methylnorepinephrine. It now seems, however, that this is metabolized to a powerful *agonist* methylepinephrine. Thus methyldopa is not an attractive choice for i.v. regional block.

Storage Vesicle Depletion and Block of NE Reuptake. Guanethidine and reserpine are the only drugs that have been evaluated and the only clinical options, where approved. Guanethidine and also bretylium block coupling of the action potential to NE release. Bretylium also blocks NE reuptake.

Reserpine is relatively ineffective and produces many side-effects. Bretylium does not appear to have been evaluated for IVRS. Many drugs prevent NE reuptake, but none have been used for IVRS (*e.g.*, tricyclic antidepressants, cocaine, bretylium).

Block of Presynaptic (α_2) and Postsynaptic (α_1) Receptors. Phentolamine (Regitine) has been given in a dose of 10 mg i.v. for IVRS (Cousins, M.J.: Unpublished data). Precise data on duration of effect are not available; however, a sympathetic block of at least 24 hours' duration can be obtained.

Block of Postsynaptic Receptors (α_1). Prazocin (Minipress) is a relatively pure α_1-blocker. It does not interfere with the negative feedback on NE release that is mediated by means of α_2-receptors. Thus there is no increase in NE release and no compensatory tachycardia seen with phentolamine. Duration of effect with IVRS is not known because an i.v. preparation has not been approved.

Other α_1-blockers are under development and include trimazosin and tarazosin. The latter may be of interest because of its reported long duration of effect. All of these drugs pose a potential for postural hypotension and water retention.

Block of NE Activity at Level of Vascular Smooth Muscle. This is a complex area, and precise sites of action are not delineated.

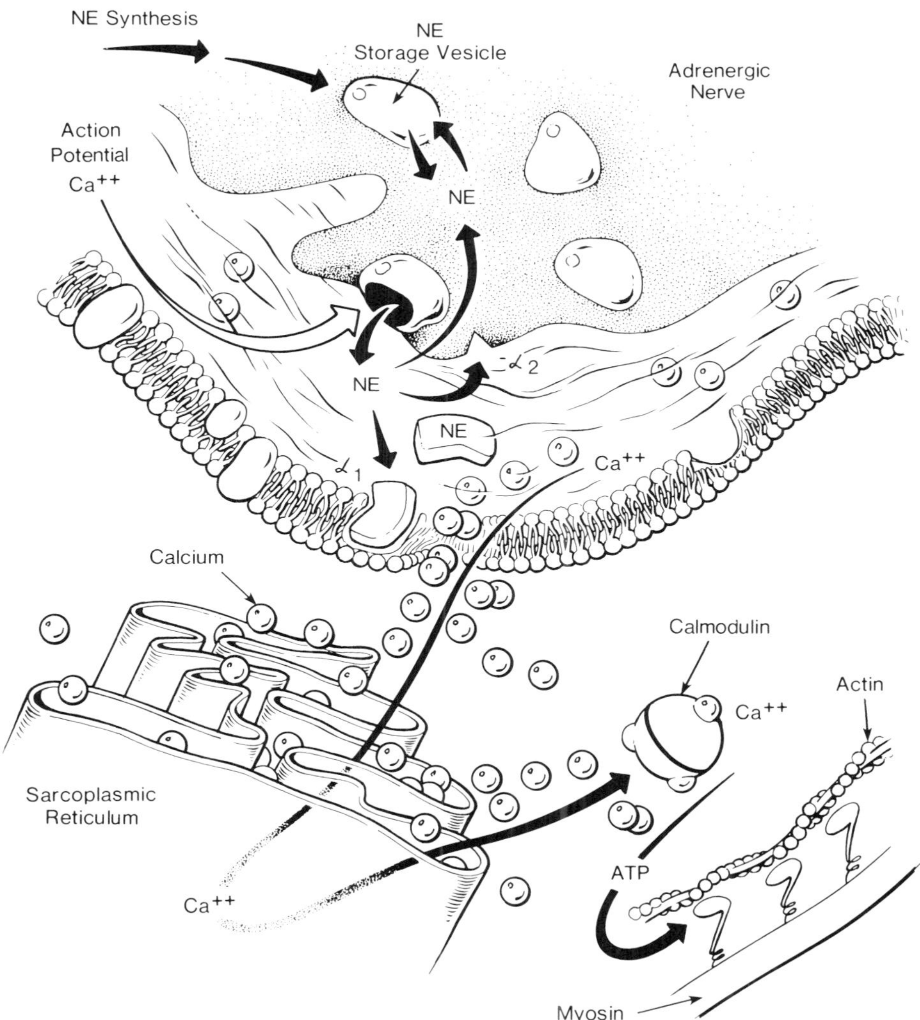

FIG. 13-32. Peripheral sympathetic neuroeffector synapse and potential sites of action of drugs for "intravenous regional sympathetic block" *(IVRS)*. A sympathetic nerve ending (adrenergic nerve terminal), synaptic cleft, cell membrane of smooth muscle of blood vessel wall, calcium channels, and contractile mechanism are shown. An action potential causes an influx of Ca^{++} into the nerve terminal, and the norepinephrine *(NE)* storage vesicle fuses with the plasma membrane to release NE. NE then activates α_1-excitatory receptors on smooth muscle (postsynaptic) and α_2-inhibitory receptors on plasma membrane (presynaptic). $Alpha_1$-receptor activation in the smooth muscle cell membrane results in an influx of Ca^{++}, which binds to calmodulin. This regulatory protein molecule then binds to myosin, causing phosphorylation (via ATP) and initiation of the actin–myosin contractile process. *Potential sites of action for IVRS* are as follows: *1. Norepinephrine synthesis:* No drugs currently available for IVRS; *2. blockade of NE release and reuptake:* Guanethidine and bretylium block NE reuptake (also block coupling of action potential to NE release), resulting in storage granule depletion. Reserpine also blocks NE reuptake. *Note:* Tricyclics and cocaine block NE reuptake at plasma membrane of sympathetic nerve ending—NOT useful for IVRS. Also, other drugs may inhibit NE release into synaptic cleft: prostaglandin (PGE_1) and adenosine triphosphate (ATP); *3. block of α_2- and α_1-receptors* (*e.g.,* phentolamine); *4. selective block of α_1 receptors.* Prazocin—not available yet as i.v. preparation. Trimazosin and tarazosin (long-acting) are under development; *5. effects on vascular smooth muscle* (*e.g.,* diazoxide and hydralazine ? action); *6. calcium channel blocking drugs;* verapamil, nifedipine, diltiazem.

Prostaglandins (e.g., *PGI_2*). In most vascular beds there is a balance between dilatation effects produced by molecules such as PGE_1 and PGI_2 and vasoconstriction effects produced by thromboxanes. PGI_2 is five times more potent than PGE_1 in producing vasodilatation in coronary, renal, mesenteric, and skeletal muscle beds. Effects on arterioles are much greater than on veins. It is possible that the vascular effects are produced by inhibition of NE release from sympathetic nerve endings. There may also be a direct effect on smooth muscle. Both PGI_2 and PGE_1 inhibit platelet aggregation. It should be noted that PGE_1 causes uterine contraction and is used to produce abortion. Both PGE_1 and PGI_2 have been used by IVRS in patients with severe peripheral vascular disease. Both were reported to give significant and long-lasting improvement in blood flow and tissue oxygenation.[72a,79a] No preparations of these drugs are currently available for IVRS.

Hydralazine (Apresoline) and Diazoxide (Hyperstat I.V.). These two drugs have a direct effect on vascular smooth muscle that is as yet poorly defined. Effects on arterioles are greater than on veins. Experimental work has shown a greater effect after intra-arterial than after intravenous infusion with respect to increased skin temperature and blood flow in limbs.

Neither drug has been evaluated by IVRS. Hydralazine can cause some serious side-effects with high-dose and long-term administration, for example, drug-induced lupus erythematosus, peripheral neuropathy, and pancytopenia. Both drugs produce a reflex increase in sympathetic activity as a result of hypotension. This has precipitated angina in susceptible patients.

Diazoxide is a relatively weak antagonist to NE and may have its action mediated by blocking calcium-dependent activation of action potentials in smooth muscle.

Calcium Entry ("Calcium Channel") Blocking Drugs. A very large number of drugs of this type are now available or under development. In general, they interfere with the flux of calcium ion through smooth muscle cellular membranes or with the uptake and release of calcium by intracellular membranes. Currently available drugs include verapamil, nifedipine, and diltiazem; however, many more drugs of very diverse structure are being investigated. Nifedipine appears to be more potent as a vasodilator than the other two but has potent effects on myocardial muscle. It remains to be ascertained whether any of these drugs will bind firmly enough to vascular smooth muscle with IVRS technique to produce long-lasting vasodilatation but with minimal cardiac effects. There are differences in site of action and physiochemical properties among these drugs that may influence their peripheral effects by IVRS technique. For example, nifedipine is a relatively pure slow channel (Ca^{++}) blocker acting at the "outer gate." Both verapamil and diltiazem appear to act on myosin kinase phosphorylation of myosin at the "inner gate." This prevents myosin-actin cross-bridging and thus prevents muscle contraction.

Diltiazem may stimulate Ca^{++} extrusion from the cell, thus lowering sarcoplasmic Ca^{++}. Because of its deeper site of action and dual action, diltiazem may be more effective for IVRS. However, none of these drugs is approved for IVRS. Because of the role of Ca^{++} in secretory physiology, endocrine side-effects may occur, in addition to cardiovascular side-effects resulting from relative overdose.

TECHNIQUE OF INTRAVENOUS REGIONAL SYMPATHETIC BLOCK (IVRS)

Guanethidine 10 to 20 mg is dissolved in 25 ml of normal saline, and 500 units of heparin is added. An i.v. cannula is placed in the nonaffected arm to be used in treatment of side-effects. A second cannula is placed in the affected arm. A double cuff, or appropriate equipment, is used to exsanguinate the arm (see Chap. 12). The guanethidine is injected slowly and the cuff kept inflated for 10 to 15 minutes. The cuff is then slowly deflated while monitoring the blood pressure. The patient remains supine until the blood pressure has been stabilized.

Some clinics dilute guanethidine in 20 ml of 0.5% prilocaine to make the injection more comfortable. An alternative technique is to infuse the guanethidine solution slowly into a peripheral artery over 10 to 15 minutes. The results are similar to IVRS, and the technique may be preferable if severe peripheral vascular disease is present.

APPENDIX A

COBALT BLUE SWEAT TEST

General Requirements*

Whatman no. 41 filter papers 5.5 cm (halved) × 100
Cobalt chloride crystals (500 g)
Silica-gel crystals
Thermometer (and antiseptic)
Distilled water
Dressing forceps
Oven and tray
Blankets
Infrared lamps × 2 (or heat cradle)

Filter paper preparation

Dissolve 10 g of cobalt chloride in 100 ml of distilled water
Dip and drain halved filter papers, using forceps
Place on tray in oven at approximately 150° for 20 minutes (avoid excessive drying)
Remove with forceps from oven when pink color changes to bright blue
Seal in airtight jar with silica-gel crystals

Procedure

Record patient's oral temperature
Apply lamp for 30 minutes to trunk and arms (take care not to burn patient or heat face excessively)
Using forceps, place filter paper on firm dry surface, and apply both palms or plantar surfaces of feet, ensuring application as airtight as possible
Rerecord oral temperature, aiming to increase it by 0.3°F
Cease heat application if the above is recorded or if frank sweating is present

*Available from any large chemical supplyhouse.

Comments. The procedure should be performed preblock and postblock because some patients have decreased sweating preblock (not including diabetic patients).

Ideally an area is also needed whereby the patient may bathe after treatment because a profuse sweating reaction is desired to ensure that adequate heating of the patient has been achieved before adequate denervation exists.

Response	*Filter Paper*
Normal response (profuse sweating)	Blue → pink
Slight reduction (moderate sweating)	Blue → mottled pink/blue small area
Moderate reduction (slight sweating)	Blue → mottled pink/blue large area
Complete reduction (no sweating)	Remains blue

APPENDIX B

Name of preparation
10% phenol in Conray-420 (or Angiographin)
Ingredients
100 g of phenol A.R. (crystals)
IL Conray-420 (or Angiographin)
Equipment
1-liter glass measuring cylinder with stopper
1-liter vacuum flask
Scintered glass filter
Tufryn 0.45 μm 7-mm (Gelmann HT-450) membrane filter mounted in a Millipore swinnex 47-mm holder
Sterile disposable 50-ml syringe
Connector tube (about 9 in) for outlet of filter
Identity number
All washed with pyrogen-free water for injections filtered through a 0.2 μm filter, then dried in hot air oven, with all exposed outlets covered with aluminum foil.
Method of manufacture
Weigh phenol into 1-liter measuring cylinder
Remove outer seals of Conray-420 bottles, leaving stoppers in place
Rinse exterior of these bottles with filtered water for injections
Place bottles in laminar flow cabinet after rinsing, and allow to dry in air stream
Remove stoppers with rinsed forceps
Pour Conray-420 into graduated cylinder containing phenol
Shake to dissolve phenol; make to volume and mix

Container/closure description
Container, 20-ml antibiotic vial
Stopper, red merco lacquered to suit
Crimp cap, gold aluminum long skirt to suit
Packing—equipment and method
Laminar flow cabinet
Filter through scintered glass into 1-liter vacuum flask
Pour into pyrex dish and load 50-ml syringe
Filter from syringe through 47-mm Tufryn filter with connector tube attached to outlet of filter holder and leading to vials
Pack 20-ml per vial; insert stoppers and seal
Example label
Injection solution: PHENOL 10% IN CONRAY 420 OR ANGIOGRAPHIN
20 ml. PROTECT FROM LIGHT

Prepared by Flinders Medical Centre Pharmacy, Bedford Park, South Australia, 5042, Australia

Batch:
Expiry: (6 months from manufacture)

REFERENCES

1. Baxter, A.D., and O'Kafo, B.A.: Ejaculatory failure after chemical sympathectomy. Anesth. Analg., *63*:770, 1984.
2. Beene, T.K., and Eggers, G.W.N., Jr.: Use of the pulse monitor for determining sympathetic block of the arm. Anesthesiology, *40*:412, 1974.
3. Bengtsson, M.: Changes in skin blood flow and temperature during spinal analgesia evaluated by laser Doppler flowmetry and infra-red thermography. Acta Anaesthesiol. Scand., *28*:625, 1984.
4. Bengtsson, M., Nilsson, G.E., and Lofstrom, J.B.: The effect of spinal analgesia on skin blood flow, evaluated by laser Doppler flowmetry. Acta Anaesthesiol. Scand., 17:206, 1983.
5. Bengtsson, M., Lofstrom, J.B., and Malmqvist, L.-A.: Skin conductance responses during spinal analgesia. Acta Anaesthesiol. Scand., *29*:67, 1985.
6. Bergan, J.J., and Conn, J., Jr.: Sympathectomy for pain relief. Med. Clin. North Am., *52*:147, 1968.
7. Blain, A., Zadeh, A.T., Teves, M.L., and Bing, R.J.: Lumbar sympathectomy for arteriosclerosis obliterans. Surgery, *53*:164, 1963.
8. Boas, R.A., Hatangdi, V.S., and Richards, E.G.: Lumbar sympathectomy—A percutaneous chemical technique. Advances in Pain Research and Therapy, *1*:685, 1976.

8a. Bonelli, S., Conoscente, F., Movilia, P.G., Restelli, L., *et al.*: Regional intravenous guanethidine vs. stellate ganglion block in reflex sympathetic dystrophies: A randomized trial. Pain, *16*:297, 1983.

9. Bonica, J.J.: The Management of Pain. Philadelphia, Lea & Febiger, 1953.
10. Bonica, J.J.: Clinical Application of Diagnostic and Therapeutic Nerve Blocks. Oxford, Blackwell Scientific Publications, 1958.
11. Boucher, J.R., Falardeau, M., Plante, R., Audet, J., *et al.*: Le reflexe sympatho-galvanique (RSG) et la sympathectomie. Can. Anaesth. Soc. J., *17*:504, 1970.
12. Bridenbaugh, P.O., Moore, D.C., and Bridenbaugh, L.D.: Capillary Po_2 as a measure of sympathetic blockade. Anesth. Analg. (Cleve.), *50*:26, 1971.
13. Bryce-Smith, R.: Injection of the lumbar sympathetic chain. Anaesthesia, *6*:150, 1951.
14. Bryce-Smith, R., and Macintosh, R.R.: Local Analgesia: Abdomen. Edinburgh, Livingstone Press, 1962.
15. Carron, H., and Litwiller, R.: Stellate ganglion block. Anesth. Analg. (Cleve.), *54*:567, 1975.
16. Christie, M.J.: Electrodermal activity in the 1980's: A review. J.R. Soc. Med. *74*:616, 1981.

16a. Cherry, D.A., and Rao, D.M.: Lumbar sympathetic and coeliac plexus blocks—An anatomical study in cadavers. Br. J. Anaesth. *54*:1037, 1982.

17. Colding, A.: Treatment of pain. Organization of a pain clinic: Treatment of acute herpes zoster. Proc. R. Soc. Med., *66*:541, 1973.
18. Cousins, M.J., Reeve, T.S., Glynn, C.J., Walsh, J.A., *et al.*: Neurolytic lumbar sympathetic blockade: Duration of denervation and relief of rest pain. Anaesth. Intensive Care, *7*(2):121, 1979.
19. Cousins, M.J., and Wright, C.J.: Graft muscle skin blood flow after epidural block in vascular surgical procedures. Surg. Gynecol. Obstet., *133*:59, 1971.
20. Cronestrand, R., Juhlin-Dannfeldt, A., and Wahren, J.: Simultaneous measurements of external iliac artery and vein blood flow after reconstructive vascular surgery: Evidence of increased collateral circulation during exercise. Scand. J. Clin. Lab. Invest., *31*[*Suppl. 128*]:167, 1973.

20a. Cronin, K.O., and Kirsner, R.L.: Assessment of sympathectomy—the skin potential response. Anaesth. Intens. Care, *7*:353, 1979.

20b. Cross, F.W., Cotton, L.T.: Chemical lumbar sympathectomy for ischemic rest pain. A randomized, prospective controlled clinical trial. Am. J. Surg., *150*:341, 1985.

21. Dam, W.H.: Therapeutic blockade. Acta Chir. Scand., *343*[*Suppl.*]:89, 1965.
22. DeBakey, M.E., Burch, G., Ray, T., and Ochsner, A.: The "borrowing-lending" hemodynamic phenomenon (hemometakinesia) and its therapeutic application in peripheral vascular disturbances. Ann. Surg., *126*:850, 1947.
23. Detakats, G.: Sympathetic reflex dystrophy. Med. Clin. North Am., *49*:117, 1965.
24. Dhuner, K.G., Edshage, S., and Wilhelm, A.: Ninhydrin test —objective method for testing local anaesthetic drugs. Acta Anaesthesiol. Scand., *4*:189, 1960.

25. Dollery, C.T., Paterson, J.W., and Conally, M.E.: Clinical pharmacology of beta-receptor-blocking drugs. Clin. Pharmacol. Ther., *10*:765, 1969.
25a. Driessen, J.J., Van Der Werken, C., Nicolai, J.P.A., and Crul, J.F.: Clinical effects of regional intravenous guanethidine (Ismelin) in reflex sympathetic dystrophy. Acta Anaesthesiol. Scand., *27*:505–509, 1983.
26. Dunningham, T.H.: The treatment of Sudeck's atrophy in the upper limb by sympathetic blockade. Injury, *12*:139, 1980.
27. Eaton, A.C., Wright, M., and Callum, K.G.: The use of the image intensifier in phenol lumbar sympathetic block. Radiography, *46*:298, 1980.
28. Eriksen, S.: Duration of sympathetic blockade. Stellate ganglion versus intravenous regional guanethidine block. Anaesthesia, *36*:768, 1981.
29. Eriksson, E.: Illustrated Handbook in Local Anaesthesia. Copenhagen, Munksgaard, 1969.
30. Fowles, D.C., Christie, M.J., and Edelberg, R., *et al.*: Publication recommendations for electrodermal measurements. Psychophysiology, *18*:232, 1981.
31. Froysaker, T.: Lumbar sympathectomy in impending gangrene and foot ulcer. Scand. J. Clin. Lab. Invest., *31*[*Suppl. 128*]:71, 1973.
32. Fulton, R.L., and Blakeley, W.R.: Lumbar sympathectomy: A procedure of questionable value in the treatment of arteriosclerosis obliterans of the legs. Am. J. Surg., *116*:735, 1968.
33. Fyfe, T., and Quin, R.O.: Phenol sympathectomy in the treatment of intermittent claudication: A controlled clinical trial. Br. J. Surg., *62*:68, 1975.
34. Gillespie, J.A.: Future place of lumbar sympathectomy in obliterative vascular disease of lower limbs. Br. Med. J., *2*:1640, 1960.
35. Gillespie, J.A.: Late effects of lumbar sympathectomy on blood flow in the foot in obliterative vascular disease. Lancet, *1*:891, 1960.
36. Gillespie, J.A.: An evaluation of vasodilator drugs in occlusive vascular disease by measurement. Angiology, *17*:280, 1966.
36a. Glynn, C.J., Basedow, R.W., and Walsh, J.A.: Pain relief following post-ganglionic sympathetic blockade with I.V. guanethidine. Br. J. Anaesth., *53*:1297, 1981.
37. Greene, N.M.: Preganglionic sympathetic blockade in man: A study of spinal anesthesia. Acta Anaesthesiol. Scand. *25*:463, 1981.
38. Haimovici, H., Steinman, C., and Karson, J.H.: Evaluation of lumbar sympathectomy in advanced occlusive arterial disease. Arch. Surg., *89*:1089, 1964.
39. Hannington-Kiff, J.G.: Pain Relief, p. 68. London, Heinemann Press, 1974.
39a. Hatangdi, V.S., and Boas, R.V.: Lumbar sympathectomy: A single needle technique. Br. J. Anaesth. *57*:285, 1985.
40. Herman, B.E., Dworecka, F., and Wisham, L.: Increase of dermal blood flow after sympathectomy as measured by radioactive sodium uptake. Vasc. Surg., *4*:161, 1970.
41. Hoffman, D.C., and Jepson, R.P.: Muscle blood flow and sympathectomy. Surg. Gynecol. Obstet., *127*:12, 1968.
42. Hughes-Davies, D.J., and Redman, L.R.: Chemical lumbar sympathectomy. Anaesthesia, *31*:1068, 1976.
43. Johansson, H.: Chemical sympathectomy with phenol for chronic prostatic pain. A case report. European Urology, *2*:98, 1976.
44. Kappis, M.: Sensibilitat und lokale Anasthesia im chirurginchen Gebiet der Bauchhohle mit besonderer Berucksichtigung der Splanchnicus-Anasthesie. Beitr. Z. Klin. Chir., *115*:161, 1919.
45. Kim, J.M., Arakawa, K., and von Linter, T.: Use of the pulse-wave monitor as a measurement of diagnostic sympathetic block and of surgical sympathectomy. Anesth. Analg. (Cleve.), *54*:289, 1975.
46. King, R.D., Kaiser, G.C., Lempke, R.E., and Shumacker, H.B.: Evaluation of lumbar sympathetic denervation. Arch. Surg., *88*:36, 1964.
47. Klopfer, G.T.: Neurolytic lumbar sympathetic blockade: A modified technique. Anaesth. Intens. Care *11*:43, 1983.
48. Kovamees, A.: Skin blood flow in obliterative arterial disease of the leg. Effect of vascular reconstruction examined with xenon and iodine antipyrine clearance and skin temperature measurements. Acta Chir. Scand. [*Suppl. 397*], 1968.
49. Kovamees, A., Lofstrom, B., McCarthy, G., and Aschberg, S.: Continuous lumbar sympathetic blocks in the treatment of patients with ischemic lower limbs. Tenth Congress of Int. Cardiovascular Soc., 1971.
50. Kovamees, A., Lofstrom, B., McCarthy, G., and Aschberg, S.: Continuous lumbar sympathetic blocks used to increase regional blood flow after peripheral vascular reconstruction. Eighteenth Congress Eur. Soc. Cardiovascular Surg., 1974.
51. Langer, J., and Matthes, H.: Blockaden mit Lokalanasthetika im Bereich der Sympathikuskette. Z. Prakt. Anaesth. Wiederbeleb., *8*:93, 1973.
52. Larsen, O.A., and Lassen, N.A.: Medical treatment of occlusive arterial disease of the legs. Walking exercise and medically induced hypertension. Angiologia, *6*:288, 1969.
53. Lassen, N.A., *et al.*: Conservative treatment of gangrene using mineralocorticoid-induced moderate hypertension. Lancet, *1*:606, 1968.
54. Leriche, R., and Fontain, R.: L'anesthesie isolee du ganglion etoile: Sa technique ses indications ses resultatas. Presse Medicale, *42*:849, 1934.
55. Lewis, L.W.: Evaluation of sympathetic activity following chemical or surgical sympathectomy. Anesth. Analg. (Cleve.), *34*:334, 1955.
56. Linde, B.: Studies on the vascular exchange function in canine subcutaneous adipose tissue with special reference to effects of sympathetic nerve stimulation. Acta Physiol. Scand., *433* [*Suppl.*] 1976.
57. Linson, M.A., Leffert, R., and Todd, D.P.: The treatment of upper extremity reflex sympathetic dystrophy with prolonged continuous stellate ganglion blockade. J. Hand Surg. *8*:153, 1983.
58. Lloyd, J.W., and Carrie, L.E.S.: A method for treating renal colic. Proc. R. Soc. Med., *58*:634, 1965.
59. Loh, L., Nathan, P.W., and Schott, G.D.: Pain due to lesions of central nervous system removed by sympathetic block. Br. Med. J., *282*:1026, 1981.
60. Lofstrom, J.B., Thorborg, P., and Lund, N.: Direct and indirect effect of some local anesthetics on muscle blood flow–tissue oxygen pressure. Reg. Anaesth., *10*:82, 1985.
61. Lofstrom, J.B., Malmqvist, L.-A., and Bengtsson, M.: Can the

"sympatho-galvanic reflex" (skin conductance response) be used to evaluate the extent of sympathetic block in spinal analgesia? Acta Anaesthesiol. Scand., *28*:578, 1984.

62. Lofstrom, B., and Zetterquist, S.: The effect of lumbar sympathetic block upon nutritive blood-flow capacity in intermittent claudication. A metabolic study. Acta Med. Scand., *182*:23, 1967.
63. Lofstrom, B., and Zetterquist, S.: Lumbar sympathetic blocks in the treatment of patients with obliterative arterial disease of the lower limb. Int. Anesthesiol. Clin., *7*:423, 1969.
64. Mandl, F.: Die Paravertebrale Injektion. Vienna, Springer-Verlag, 1926.
65. Masud, K.Z., and Forster, K.J.: Sympathetic block in herpes zoster. Am. Fam. Physician, *12*:142, 1975.
65a. McKain, C.W., Bruno, J.U., and Goldner, J.L.: The effects of intravenous regional guanethidine and reserpine. J. Bone Joint Surg., *6*:808, 1983.
66. Moore, D.C.: Stellate Ganglion Block. Springfield, Charles C Thomas, 1954.
67. Myers, K.A., and Irvine, W.T.: An objective study of lumbar sympathectomy: II. Skin ischaemia. Br. Med. J., *1*:943, 1966.
68. Myers, K.A., and Irvine, W.T.: An objective study of lumbar sympathectomy. I. Intermittent claudication. Br. Med. J., *1*:943 1966.
69. Nielsen, J.: Thrombangiitis obliterans (Buerger's disease). A study of the prognosis. Ugeskr. Laeger., *131*:1740, 1969.
70. Nielsen, P.E., Bell, G., Augustenborg, G., and Lassen, N.A.: Reduction in distal blood pressure by sympathetic nerve block in patients with occlusive arterial disease. Scand. J. Clin. Lab. Invest., *31[Suppl. 128]*:59, 1973.
71. Nielsen, P.E., Bell, G., Augustenborg, G., Paaske–Hansen, O., *et al.*: Reduction in distal blood pressure by sympathetic block in patients with occlusive arterial disease. Cardiovasc. Res., *7*:577, 1973.
72. Nolte, H., Ahnefeld, F.W., and Halmagyi, M.: Die lumbale Grenzstrangblockad zur Beurteilung der Wirkungsdauer von Lokalanaesthetika. Acta Anaesthesiol. Scand., 23[*Suppl.*]: 618, 1966.
72a. Olsson, A.G., and Carlsson, A.L.: Clinical, hemodynamic and metabolic effects of intra-arterial infusions of prostaglandin E_1 in patients with peripheral vascular disease. Adv. Prostaglandin Thromboxane Res., *1*:429, 1976.
73. Procacci, P., Francini, F., Zoppi, M., and Maresca, M.: Cutaneous pain threshold changes after sympathetic block in reflex dystrophies. Pain, *1*:167, 1975.
74. Raskin, N.H., Levinson, S.A., Hoffman, P.M., Pickett, J.B.E., III,, *et al.*: Postsympathectomy neuralgia amelioration with diphenylhydantoin and carbamazepine. Am. J. Surg., *128*:75, 1974.
75. Reid, W., Watt, J.K., and Gray, T.G.: Phenol injection of the sympathetic chain. Br. J. Surg., *57*:45, 1970.
76. Scheinin, T.M., and Inberg, M.V.: Intraoperative effects of sympathectomy on ipsi-and contralateral blood flow in lower limb arterial reconstruction. Ann. Clin. Res., *1*:280, 1969.
77. Selander, D., and Sjostrand, J.: Longitudinal spread of intraneurally injected local anesthetics. Acta Anaesth. Scand., *22*:622, 1978.
78. Sternschein, M.J., Myers, S.J., Frewin, D.B., and Downey, J.A.: Causalgia. Arch. Phys. Med. Rehabil., *56*:58, 1975.
79. Strand, L.: Lumbar sympathectomy in the treatment of peripheral obliterative disease. An analysis of 167 patients. Acta. Chir. Scand., *135*:597, 1969.
79a. Szczeklik, A., Nizankowski, R., Splawinski, J., *et al.*: Successful therapy of advanced arteriosclerosis obliterans with prostacyclin. Lancet, *1*:1111, 1979.
80. Szeinfeld, M., Saucedo, R., and Pallares, V.S.: Causalgia of vascular etiology following an abdominal injury. Anesthesiology, *57*:46, 1982.
81. Szilagyi, D.E., Smith, R.F., Scerpella, J.R., and Hoffman, K.: Lumbar sympathectomy. Current role in the treatment of arteriosclerotic occlusive disease. Arch. Surg., *95*:953, 1967.
82. Taylor, G.W., and Calo, A.R.: Atherosclerosis of arteries of lower limbs. Br. Med. J., *1*:507, 1962.
83. Thomas, D.: Forced acid diuresis and stellate ganglion block in the treatment of quinine poisoning. Anaesthesia *39*:257, 1984.
84. Thulesius, O.: Beurteilung des schwergrades arterieller Durchblutungsstorungen mit dem Doppler-Ultraschallgerat. Angiologie, 13. Bern, Hans Huber, 1971.
85. Thulesius, O., and Gjores, J.E.: Use of Doppler shift detection for determining peripheral arterial blood pressure. Angiology, *22*:594, 1971.
86. Thulesius, O., Gjores, J.E., and Mandaus, L.: Distal blood flow and blood pressure in vascular occlusion: Influence of sympathetic nerves on collateral blood flow. Scand. J. Clin. Lab. Invest., *31[Suppl. 128]*:53, 1973.
87. Tsuji, H., Shirasaka, C., Asoh, T., and Takeuchi, Y.: Influences of splanchnic nerve blockade on endocrine-metabolic responses to upper abdominal surgery. Br. J. Surg. *70*:437, 1983.
88. Uhrenholdt, A.: Relationship between distal blood flow and blood pressure after abolition of the sympathetic vasomotor tone. Scand. J. Clin. Lab. Invest., *31[Suppl. 128]*:63, 1973.
89. Uhrendholdt, A., Dam, W.H., Larsen, O.A., and Lassen, N.A.: Paradoxical effect on peripheral blood flow after sympathetic blockades in patients with gangrene due to arteriosclerosis obliterans. Vasc. Surg., *5*:154, 1971.
89a. Vaughan, R.S., Lawrie, B.W., and Sykes, P.J.: Use of intravenous regional sympathetic block in upper limb angiography. Annals of the Royal College of Surgeons of England, *67*:309, 1985.
90. Verstraete, M.: A critical appraisal of lumbar sympathectomy in the treatment of organic arteriopathy. Angiologia, *5*:333, 1968.
91. Walsh, J.A., Glynn, C.J., Cousins, M.D., and Basedow, R.W.: Blood flow, sympathetic activity and pain relief following lumbar sympathetic blockade or surgical sympathectomy. Anaesth. Intens. Care, *13*:18–24, 1984.
92. Weale, F.E.: The hemodynamic assessment of the arterial tree during reconstructive surgery. Ann. Surg., *169*:484, 1969.
93. Wright, C.J., and Cousins, M.J.: Blood flow distribution in the human leg following epidural sympathetic blockade. Arch. Surg., *105*:334, 1972.
94. Yao, J.S.T., and Bergan, J.J.: Predicting response to sympathetic ablation (quoted in editorial). Lancet, *1*:441, 1974.
95. Zetterquist, S.: Muscle and skin clearance of antipyrine from exercising ischemic legs before and after vasodilating trials. Acta Med. Scand., *183*:487, 1968.

section C
THORAX AND ABDOMEN

14 CELIAC PLEXUS, INTERCOSTAL, AND MINOR PERIPHERAL BLOCKADE

GALE E. THOMPSON
DANIEL C. MOORE

In 1953, Sir Robert Macintosh introduced his book *Local Analgesia: Abdominal Surgery* with the following paragraph: "A local analgesic can provide ideal operating conditions when used alone; a fortiori* it will afford ideal conditions if a general anesthetic is given at the same time. Local analgesia, alone or combined with light general anesthesia, is therefore theoretically justified in every abdominal operation."[21] Now, more than 4 decades later, it is even more credible that Sir Robert's admonitions should provoke the common practice of routine, daily use of the nerve blocks described in this chapter. In one form or another, they are indeed applicable to *every* abdominal surgical procedure.

There are several reasons for the tendency to pay lip service to regional anesthesia and then fail to use it. First, among many anesthesiologists, surgeons, and patients there is an element of bias and emotion that has some of its origin in fact but is perpetuated by fallacy. A single untoward event such as the famous Wooley and Roe cases in England (1948) casts a pall over the practice of regional anesthesia for many years. This same kind of emotional over-reaction to an untoward event has been played out in many countries in many slightly different ways. Ultimately it tends to lead to a halting, lame conceptual approach to regional anesthesia. Second, there are really very few training environments in which one can develop expertise in performing nerve blocks. Regional anesthesia is not just a medical curiosity, and it is not to be practiced only infrequently on the high-risk patient. To be performed well, it must be used routinely! Thus, each time a surgical anesthetic is being selected, the anesthesiologist should first consider what kind of regional anesthetic technique might be adaptable to the case. Training programs must accentuate this kind of thinking and practice. Finally, there is a tendency to evaluate the outcome of an anesthetic or surgical procedure in terms of survival. Survival is of basic importance, of course, but there are various routes to any goal and the choice or type of anesthetic may be equally important. The patient may remember very little of the surgical scenario and be aware only that the "operation was a success." New data from many sources are showing us, however, that regional anesthesia can provide a basic foundation resulting in a considerably less stressful operation.

In summary, certain basic precepts are essential to the successful use of the peripheral nerve blocks described herein. These are as follows:

- A personal conviction on the part of the anesthesiologist that regional anesthesia is indeed a safe, viable choice of anesthetic technique for any given surgical procedure.
- A thorough knowledge of anatomy.
- A thorough knowledge of the pharmacology of local anesthetic drugs.
- Adequate training in the use of regional anesthesia.

*"All the more said of a conclusion that follows with even greater logical necessity than another already accepted in the argument"—*Webster's New World Dictionary,* College Edition.

A philosophy of using supplemental drugs at appropriate times and in adequate amounts.
A perceptive awareness of the possible side-effects and complications of regional anesthesia. (*Note:* Side-effects are *not* complications.)
An enlightened patient who has been counseled on the benefits and nature of regional anesthesia. (*Note:* An enlightened surgeon is also desirable but not an absolute necessity. Confidence and competence in one's own role will stand on its own merit!)

RATIONALE

Three fundamental arguments might be used to support the routine use of regional anesthesia:

It is the ideal form of *balanced anesthesia.*
It provides the best means of protection from the stress of surgery.
It is the optimum method of providing pain relief in the postanesthetic period.

BALANCED ANESTHESIA

The term "balanced anesthesia" has many connotations. It commonly implies that several different drugs are used to achieve hypnosis, amnesia, analgesia, muscle relaxation, or other conditions that we recognize as separate components of the phenomenon of anesthesia. The general tendency today is to consider only inhaled or intravenous drugs when defining balanced anesthesia. The term was actually introduced by Lundy in 1926, and regional anesthesia played the key role in his description.[20] Elements of the concept were emphasized as early as 1915 by Crile.[8] It is therefore historically most reasonable to consider regional anesthesia as the foundational component of balanced anesthesia. For instance, peripheral nerve block of the abdomen and chest can be considered the primary ingredient of a total anesthetic regimen because it provides most of the analgesia and muscle relaxation objectives of the total anesthetic. The addition of appropriate and complementary doses of either inhaled or intravenous drugs will then be dictated by such additional factors as the nature and duration of the surgical procedure, the patient's safety and desires, and operating room environmental considerations, including noise, temperature, teaching, or other conversations.

Many anesthesiologists react negatively to the concept of combining regional nerve block with light general anesthesia. "Why give two anesthetics when one will do?" "You are doubling the risks of anesthesia!" "It takes too much time." "It's not worth it." These are frequently heard criticisms. Surprisingly, though, the same comments are not expressed about the potpourri of drugs used to accomplish general anesthesia. Often, these expressions merely reflect a lack of expertise or inclination to use regional anesthesia. In recent years there have been numerous reports and findings that help restore balance to this controversy. There has been an increasing focus, for instance, on the potential dangers of general anesthetic drugs. Ecologic hazards, renal and hepatic problems, induced enzyme changes, and the possibility of increased malignancies have been acknowledged.[39] Until the fabled "ideal" or complete anesthetic agent is found, a variety of drugs will continue to be used to produce anesthesia. In practical terms, the local anesthetic drugs still should play the primary role in providing truly balanced anesthesia.

PROTECTION FROM SURGICAL STRESS

Sir William Thompson once stated that a phenomenon that "cannot be quantitated, cannot be studied." Pain and stress are obvious examples of such phenomena. Surgical stress is not truly measurable, although we are slowly zeroing in on quantification of this elusive entity. Historically, George Crile's book *Anoci-association* contained many ideas about stress that were based on rudimentary knowledge. In simplified terms he proposed that the use of local anesthetic drugs prevented noxious stimuli from invading the central nervous system. This was thought to prevent surgical shock. In contrast, he believed that general anesthesia allowed such impulses to penetrate the CNS but obtunded the body's ability to respond. Intense central neuronal activity occurred, manifested by marked changes in vital signs and other stress indicators. Such changes were greatly modified or even lacking in patients administered regional anesthesia. As a result of this reduced stress, the patient appeared less fatigued and therefore better suited to deal with other postoperative stresses. Clinically, we continue to form impressions about the degree of physiologic insult to patients during surgery. Many appear "washed out" or "beaten down" by the experience. This, of course, may be due to several factors, including the primary disease process, the surgical technique, or the conduct of the anesthetic. Whatever the stimulus and the response, it is important to consider possible ways to reduce the insult. In one study, Katz reported that most anesthesiologists would favor regional anesthesia if surgery were to be performed on themselves.[17] It is likely that such opinions are shaped from clinical experiences that suggest that regional anesthesia is indeed the least stressful technique.

ANALGESIA IN THE POSTANESTHETIC RECOVERY PERIOD

It is just as important to achieve freedom from pain in the postoperative period as it is to control pain during surgery (see also Chap. 26). Anesthesiologists are increasingly concerned and involved in postoperative pain management despite their more classic role of relieving pain only during surgery. Patients have many fears about their surgical procedure, but they equally dread the thought of pain following surgery. They can be reassured to an amazing degree if the anesthesiologist offers them a basic regional anesthetic technique whereby they will be able to regain consciousness but remain relatively pain-free in the immediate postoperative period. Currently available local anesthetic drugs will give analgesia for only 8 to 12 hours. It is hoped that drugs will be developed with durations of action of 24 to 48 hours and with the characteristic of preferentially blocking only sensory nerves. Then the slight pain and time involved in performing one or two blocks in the postoperative period would be more than offset by the benefits and duration of pain relief. This approach would tend to avoid the problems of apnea, hypotension, immobility, tachyphylaxis, fear of subarachnoid injection, and urinary retention encountered with continuous catheter epidural injections of local anesthetics or narcotics. Even with currently available drugs, intercostal nerve blocks have been repeated as many as 14 times in the postoperative period.[3] Despite the discomforts of turning and the multiple needle-sticks involved in this procedure, patients consistently preferred repeated blocks rather than sedation with narcotics. There is no doubt that analgesia is more profound and pain therapy more specific with intercostal blocks than with narcotics. Pa_{O_2} values are slightly better in patients treated with repeated blocks, and the ability to cough and ambulate is especially impressive. The total hospital stay has been shortened in patients who received blocks as compared to those who were treated with narcotics for pain relief.

Other studies have examined the effects of intercostal blocks on lung volumes and gas flow rates following either abdominal or thoracic surgery. Unfortunately, it is often difficult to evaluate these studies and impossible to compare them because of differences in methodology. These differences include the site of incision, the number of nerves blocked, and the temporal relation of the blocks to the time of surgery. A few gross generalizations can, however, be made. Most authors have used peak expiratory flow as a measure of the maximal expiratory effort that can be generated by a patient. When compared with opioid analgesia, intercostal block results in higher peak expiratory flows.[32] This is true whether measured immediately after surgery or on the following day. In healthy volunteers, Jakobson found that bilateral intercostal nerve blocks with 0.25% bupivacaine or 0.5% etidocaine caused no change in the normal pattern of breathing.[16] There were minor changes in several of the lung capacities and flows. Vital capacity decreased by 7%, functional residual capacity decreased 8%, peak expiratory flow decreased 6%, and peak expiratory airway pressure decreased 7%. Interestingly, there was no difference in the effects of 0.25% bupivacaine and 0.5% etidocaine even though one might have expected a greater effect from etidocaine because of its more potent motor blocking effects. In general, intercostal nerve blocks are extremely effective in blocking motor function because of the small caliber of the nerves and because of the great length of the nerve in contact with the drug. When intercostal block does lead to respiratory failure, it is generally because pain relief from the block unmasks the ventilatory depression of previously administered narcotics.[7]

A fascinating new approach to postoperative pain control has been reported by Kvalheim and Reiestad.[19] They conceived the idea of injecting large doses of local anesthetic drug through an interpleural catheter. Much remains to be learned about this technique, but it would appear that multiple intercostal nerves are blocked by absorption of local anesthetic through the parietal pleura. Details of the technique include placement of an epidural-type catheter via a Touhy needle at the 8th intercostal space. Twenty milliliters to 30 ml of 0.5% bupivacaine is then injected by means of the catheter at intervals of 4 to 18 hours. Thus far, it has been used for surgical procedures such as cholecystectomy, nephrectomy, and thoracotomy, which require only unilateral incisions. The catheter may be left in place for several days as necessary for pain relief. Caution is warranted to avoid pneumothorax, but this potential problem is apparently rare.

PAIN PATHWAYS

Noxious stimuli from the thoracic and abdominal cavities are transmitted by nerve impulses carried along afferent fibers of the somatic, sympathetic, and parasympathetic divisions of the nervous system. The afferent somatic and sympathetic pain fibers converge on cells of secondary afferent neurons in the posterior horn of the spinal cord. After synapsing, they ascend in the spinothalamic tracts. Afferent vagal impulses from the abdominal viscera pass through the celiac plexus and by way of the vagus nerve to the medulla. Complete sensory anesthesia of thoracic and abdominal contents can be achieved only by blocking all afferent impulses from each of these three divisions of the nervous system. This is a formidable task to achieve with regional anesthesia alone. It is technically easier to block somatic nerve fibers, which are anatomically precise, as compared to autonomic pain fibers, which are diffuse, often ill-defined, and more difficult to isolate. Table 14-1 lists some of the anatomic sites at which peripheral nerve block might be attempted for deafferentation of the thorax and abdomen.

Pain from abdominal viscera can be perceived through sympathetic or parasympathetic fibers. Physiologists and anatomists have difficulty in precisely locating or describing such fibers, but the clinical response of many patients demonstrates their existence. For instance, patients may respond to surgical manipulation of abdominal viscera even though they have spinal anesthesia to upper thoracic levels. Similarly, female patients may respond to uterine manipulation while under an epidural anesthetic that is perfectly adequate for skin incision and abdominal wall relaxation. Vagal afferent nerves must convey many of these impulses to brain stem levels and thence to the cerebral cortex. Although pain defies description, there appear to be differences in pain perceived by the autonomic nervous system as compared to pain perceived by means of the somatic nervous system.[14] The following list provides a way to characterize these differences.

Differences in Pain Experienced by the Somatic and Autonomic Divisions of the Nervous System

Somatic

- Precisely localized
- Sharp and definite
- Hurts where the stimulus is
- Associated with external factors
- Represented at cortical levels
- Increases with increasing intensity of stimulus (*e.g.*, to cut or burn skin will produce pain)

Autonomic

- Poorly localized
- Vague—may be colicky, cramping, aching, squeezing, and so forth
- May be referred to another part of the body
- Associated with internal factors
- Primarily reflex or cord levels
- Intensity of stimulus important but quality of stimulus also important (*e.g.*, to cut or burn bowel will produce no pain, but distension of bowel will produce pain)

Regardless of the character of the pain that a patient perceives or what neural pathway is involved, the anesthesiologist must respond to a patient's surgical pain on a moment-to-moment basis. It is often difficult to identify precisely which nerve or nerves are transmitting noxious impulses to the patient's level of perception. Regional anesthetic techniques may leave certain pain pathways open, either by design or by default. Only by close observation and anticipation of difficulties can the basic regional an-

TABLE 14-1. ANATOMIC SITES AT WHICH PERIPHERAL NERVE BLOCK MAY BE PERFORMED TO PRODUCE SENSORY ANESTHESIA OF ABDOMEN AND THORAX

Component Portion of Nervous System	Specific Nerves	Possible Site of Block
Parasympathetic	Vagus	Neck, esophageal hiatus, celiac plexus
	S2,3,4	Pudendal, trans-sacral
Sympathetic	Thoracolumbar	Stellate ganglion
	Sympathetic chain	Paravertebral sympathetic chain, celiac plexus
Somatic	T1–12 intercostal	Posterior angle of rib
	Lumbar somatic	Paravertebral

esthetic be properly complemented with some form of supplementary drug.

There may be significant side-effects from blocking autonomic nerves.[5] When the balance between sympathetic and parasympathetic tone is upset, the ensuing functional changes in heart, lung, and gut may be quite disturbing. Therefore, bilateral vagus nerve block or major sympathetic nerve blocks are better avoided or at least undertaken with caution.[30] For abdominal surgery, intercostal nerve block may be combined with blockade of the visceral pain pathways at the level of the celiac plexus. Although celiac plexus blockade of sympathetic fibers may result in pooling of blood in the mesenteric vessels, it avoids interference with cardiac and pulmonary autonomic fibers.

PREMEDICATION AND SUPPLEMENTATION

The anesthesiologist who routinely advocates regional anesthesia will tend to use heavy premedication (see also Chap. 12). It is desirable to have a relaxed, analgesic, and amnesic patient during the performance of many nerve blocks. Likewise, most patients desire to sleep during the course of an operation. Sights, sounds, and conversations in the surgical suite that escape the attention of medical personnel may leave vivid impressions in the mind of a wide-eyed alert patient. There is also a need to create an operating room environment in which teaching and other professional conversation can take place without unduly alarming patients.

All peripheral nerve block procedures for thoracic and abdominal analgesia utilize bony or vascular anatomic landmarks, and hence require no patient participation for proper execution of the block. Likewise, performance of these blocks may elicit significant skin and periosteal stimulation that can be obtunded easily by light sleep or sedation. This is not to say that these nerve blocks cannot be performed without sedation! In fact, that may be mandatory when their purpose is diagnostic or when these blocks are performed on seriously ill surgical patients. For routine surgery, however, the nerve blocks described in this chapter are best performed on patients who will not be able to recall the event. Therefore, it is a challenge to achieve the proper degree of sedation for execution of the block while maintaining the patient in a stable and amnesic state.

For premedication, surgical patients may be given a combination of narcotic and anticholinergic drugs 1 hour before performance of the nerve block. In healthy patients below age 60, this might be 10 to 15 mg of morphine sulfate and 0.4 to 0.6 mg of scopolamine hydrobromide. Scopolamine is generally omitted in patients over 60 and the morphine dosage appropriately decreased. Atropine may be substituted for scopolamine in a patient of any age or added intravenously should vagal reflexes be evidenced during surgery. The state of calmly detached consciousness produced by scopolamine is an ideal complement to regional anesthesia. The occasional disturbing central side-effects of this drug can be readily controlled with physostigmine.

After the patient's arrival in the operating suite, an intravenous line should be established that supplies fluid and caloric requirements but, in addition, serves as a means of titrating supplementary sedative drugs. These may be indicated to accentuate premedication effects, to produce loss of awareness briefly during completion of the nerve block, or to produce sleep during the operation. Some drugs commonly used for these purposes are diazepam, fentanyl, ketamine, and the barbiturates. The clinical situation dictates which one or ones should be used, depending on the need for hypnosis, analgesia, tranquilization, or some combination of effects. A wide variety of other drugs may be used, but it is important to titrate them in small intravenous doses while observing closely for the desired action.

The drugs and techniques used, if one wishes to produce loss of consciousness during intercostal and celiac plexus nerve block, deserves special comment. Ideally, these blocks should be performed in an induction or other room that is separate from the noise and confusion of the operating room. It should be equipped with appropriate monitors and resuscitation materials. Upon completion of the nerve block, the patient will usually quickly regain awareness, which allows questioning and testing of the block while initiating additional monitoring procedures before the operation. A most satisfactory drug for patient sedation during this block is methohexitone. When it is prepared in 0.2% solution and administered intravenously, it affords a convenient means of titrating sedation to an appropriate level. The effects are rapidly reversible. It is helpful to have an assistant administer the drip and observe the patient's vital signs during performance of block. Ketamine, diazepam, althesin, and tentanyl have also been used for the same purpose.[37] Intravenous benzodiazepines may be doubly effective, first as sedative and amnesia-producing agents, and second as a potential prophylactic against toxic effects of the local anesthetics. Large dosages of local anesthetics are used for the blocks described in this chapter, and de Jong has shown that the threshold for toxic effects of local anesthetic drugs can be raised by pretreatment with diazepam. In cats pretreated with 0.25 mg/kg of intramuscular diazepam, the mean convulsant dose of intravenous lidocaine was raised from 8.4 mg/kg to 16.8 mg/kg.[10] In later work, he also demonstrated a protective effect of nitrous oxide on the lidocaine seizure threshold. Seventy percent nitrous oxide raised the threshold from 7.6 mg/kg to 11.4 mg/kg intravenous lidocaine.[11] Although these studies show that diazepam and nitrous oxide may protect from local anesthetic toxicity in animals, one should not be deceived or deluded into a careless disrespect for that potential problem. Early recognition is the key, and prompt use of resuscitation measures, especially oxygenation, must always remain the first priority.

Inhalation agents must be used intraoperatively to supplement most regional nerve blocks used for thoracic and intra-abdominal surgery. In the great majority of patients, a combination of nitrous oxide and oxygen will ensure toleration of the endotracheal tube, adequate ventilation, oxygenation, and loss of consciousness. The anesthesiologist should not be chagrined at having to administer low, supplementary concentrations of more potent inhalation agents or neuromuscular blocking drugs should it become necessary. This does not detract from the advantages to the patient of the nerve block because one still avoids the need for large doses of relaxants or high concentrations of the inhalation agents. Again, regional nerve block should be considered a component of balanced anesthesia with the required supplementation varying on a case-by-case basis. Music delivered by individual headphones is also an effective alternative to chemical or drug sedation in many patients.

LOCAL ANESTHETIC DRUGS

There are many ways to classify anesthetic drugs. They may be viewed, for instance, from a perspective of history, chemical structure, metabolism, dosage, or duration of action. The last is of utmost importance for the nerve blocks discussed in this chapter. Historically, the lack of effective long-acting local anesthetic drugs has been a major deterrent to the usefulness and application of many of the more important peripheral regional anesthetic techniques.[22] As stated earlier, among the pharmacologic achievements of the future one would hope for development of a local anesthetic agent with a predictable duration of action of 48 to 72 hours. There are problems in developing such drugs, chief among them being concerns about cardiac depression and neurotoxicity. Other features of the long-acting local anesthetic drugs are widespread variation in duration of block and the potential for tachyphylaxis.[9] Once such difficulties are overcome, however, anesthesia, which includes the postoperative as well as the intraoperative period, can be seriously considered.[26]

At present, there are short-acting (*e.g.*, procaine), intermediate-acting (*e.g.*, lidocaine), and long-acting (*e.g.*, bupivacaine) local anesthetic drugs. When ultra-long-acting drugs come into widespread use, the clinical role of the nerve blocks described herein will be greatly enhanced.

CHOICE AND DOSAGE OF DRUG

Before starting any regional anesthetic, the purpose or goal of the block must be determined by asking questions such as the following: "Do I want profound motor block, or is sensory anesthesia adequate?" "How many nerves are to be blocked?" "Is the patient going to be further anesthetized following the block, or will no supplementary drugs be given?" "Does the patient have major cardiovascular, respiratory, hepatic, or renal disease?" "What is the patient's size, body build, and age?" "Are there any special demands of this surgeon or of the surgical procedure?" Only when such questions have been answered can the anesthesiologist determine the proper volume, concentration, and dosage of local anesthetic drug.[25] For instance, in preparing a solution of local anesthetic for bilateral intercostal and celiac plexus nerve block, the following calculations are made:

Total volume of solution
Effective concentration of drug
Total (mg) dosage of drug
Volume of epinephrine to be added
Total dosage (μg) of epinephrine

There are safe or ideal limits for each of these factors. It is obvious that all are related. Volume multiplied by concentration determines total dose. Excesses of volume or concentration may possibly be tolerated by a particular patient, but toxic effects are more likely to occur. On the other hand, small volumes or low concentrations of drug will result in ineffective regional anesthesia. Any block might be inadequate in area,

TABLE 14-2. SOME POSSIBLE DRUG COMBINATIONS FOR PERIPHERAL NERVE BLOCKS OF ABDOMEN AND THORAX

Drug	Volume (ml)	Concentration (%)
Bupivacaine	60	0.5
Bupivacaine	60–100	0.25
Etidocaine	60–80	0.5
Tetracaine	60–100	0.15
Mepivacaine	60	1.0

inadequate in duration, or inadequate in extent of motor or sensory fiber blockade. The drug must be *tailored* to the block. This requires more than just a vague knowledge of local anesthetic drug dosages and effective concentrations.

The total volume of drug necessary for bilateral intercostal nerve block varies from 40 to 80 ml of solution. This allows for deposition of 3 to 5 ml of solution under each of the lower ribs. The effective concentration will primarily depend on the drug used and the desired degree of motor nerve blockade. Some commonly used combinations are provided in Table 14-2.[4,24]

For each local anesthetic there are approved recommendations for maximum total dose. These recommendations may vary from country to country or region to region according to the prevailing bias or custom. It is foolhardy to proceed to use any local anesthetic without an understanding of these limits. Many regional techniques (*e.g.*, subarachnoid block) involve drug dosages that do not even begin to approach the maximum recommended dose. To perform the nerve blocks considered in this chapter, however, the anesthesiologist will often need to approach the maximum recommended dose to achieve a successful block.

SYSTEMIC ABSORPTION

Blood levels of a local anesthetic are higher after intercostal nerve block than after any other of the commonly used regional anesthetic procedures. Tucker measured arterial plasma levels after epidural, caudal, intercostal, brachial plexus, and sciatic/femoral nerve block with a single injection of 500 mg of mepivacaine.[38] These blocks were performed with both 1% and 2% mepivacaine, with and without epinephrine. The highest plasma concentrations (5–10 μg/ml) were observed after intercostal nerve blocks without epinephrine. When a 1:200,000 concentration of epinephrine was added to the injected solution, plasma levels fell to the range of 2 to 5 μg/ml. These lower blood levels were similar to those found with all the other regional procedures he measured (see Chap. 3).

Systemic absorption of epinephrine may have a significant effect on both alpha- and beta-receptors and result in tachycardia, hypertension, and arrhythmias. Such changes are usually of little consequences in healthy patients if the total dose of epinephrine does not exceed 0.25 mg (Table 14-3). In patients with coronary artery disease and hypertension, the total dose should be limited to no more than 0.25 mg or avoided completely. On the other hand, it is arguable that epinephrine is an immediately available antidote to the cardiovascular depressant effects of local anesthetic drugs with which they are mixed.[28] Some authors include epinephrine in every nerve block for this reason. Likewise, one can use epinephrine as a probe or tracer drug to identify impending intravascular injections. This is perhaps most pertinent to epidural anesthesia, but the principle can be applied to any regional technique. Ideally, epinephrine should be added fresh to the local anesthetic solution just before the time of injection. This ensures optimum *p*H of the final solution. Commercial preparations of local anesthetics that already contain epinephrine are strongly acidic. This is attributable to the addition of sodium bisulfite as an antioxidant for the epinephrine in the local anesthetic solution. Acidity promotes the ionized form of local anesthetic drugs and inhibits passage of drug molecules into the nerve cell membrane where block occurs.

TECHNIQUES OF NERVE BLOCK

There are specific techniques of performing peripheral nerve blocks to produce anesthesia of the thorax and abdomen. Proper technique begins with a thor-

TABLE 14-3. FINAL CONCENTRATION OF EPINEPHRINE DERIVED FROM TOTAL DOSE AND THE VOLUME WITH WHICH IT IS MIXED

Epinephrine	Total Volume of Dilution	Final Concentration
0.1 mg in	20 ml =	1:200,000
0.2 mg in	40 ml =	1:200,000
0.25 mg in	50 ml =	1:200,000
0.25 mg in	60 ml =	1:240,000
0.25 mg in	70 ml =	1:280,000
0.25 mg in	80 ml =	1:320,000
0.25 mg in	90 ml =	1:360,000
0.25 mg in	100 ml =	1:400,000

ough knowledge of anatomic relationships. To this foundation is applied the technical expertise required to do the block. The need to tailor the choice of local anesthetic to the contemplated nerve block has previously been emphasized. In a similar manner, the anesthesiologist can choose various combinations of peripheral nerve blocks to tailor the anesthetic to the requirements of the surgical procedure. The most useful combination for upper abdominal surgery is that of intercostal nerve block and celiac plexus block. It is possible, however, to mix any of the following blocks in any manner suited to the anesthetic goal. The imaginative anesthesiologist will recognize many different situations in which one or more of these blocks might be of value.

INTERCOSTAL NERVE BLOCK

Anatomy

The intercostal nerves are the primary rami of T1 through T11. In the most accurate sense of the word, T12 is not an intercostal nerve because it does not run a course between two ribs; it might be more appropriately termed a thoracic or subcostal nerve.[12,13] Some of its fibers unite with other fibers from the first lumbar nerve and are terminally represented as the iliohypogastric and ilioinguinal nerves. Likewise many fibers from T1, at the opposite end of the thoracic group, unite with fibers from C8 to form the lowest trunk of the brachial plexus. These latter fibers leave the intercostal space by crossing the neck of the first rib, while a smaller bundle continues on a genuine intercostal course. The only other notable variation in intercostal nerves is the contribution of some fibers from T2 and T3 to the formation of the intercostobrachial nerve. Terminal distribution of this nerve is to the skin of the medial aspect of the upper arm.

A typical intercostal nerve has four significant branches (Fig. 14-1): The first branch is the gray rami communicans, which passes anteriorly to the sympathetic ganglion; the second branch arises as the posterior cutaneous branch. This nerve supplies skin and muscles in the paravertebral region; the third branch is the lateral cutaneous division, which arises just anterior to the midaxillary line. This branch is of most concern to the anesthesiologist because it sends subcutaneous fibers coursing both posteriorly and anteriorly to supply skin of much of the chest and abdominal wall; and the fourth and terminal branch of an intercostal nerve is the anterior cutaneous branch. In the upper five nerves, this branch terminates after penetrating the external intercostal and pectoralis major muscles to innervate the breast and front of the thorax. The lower six anterior cutaneous nerves terminate after piercing the sheath of the rectus abdominis muscle to which they supply motor branches. Some final branches continue anteriorly and become superficial near the linea alba to provide cutaneous innervation to the midline of the abdomen.

Medial to the posterior angles of the ribs, the intercostal nerves lie between the pleura and the internal intercostal fascia. This fascial layer is also known as the posterior intercostal membrane. In the paravertebral region, there is only fatty tissue between nerve and pleura. At the angle of the rib (6–8 cm from the spinous processes), the nerve comes to lie between the internal intercostal muscle and the intercostalis intimus muscle. At this point the costal groove is broadest and deepest. The nerve is accompanied by an intercostal vein and artery, which lie superior to the nerve in the inferior groove of each rib (Fig. 14-2). The location of these vessels explains the tendency to high blood levels of local anesthetic agents following intercostal block. The costal groove becomes a sharp inferior edge of the rib, about 5 to 8 cm anterior to the angle of the rib. At this point the intercostal groove ceases to exist, the lateral cutaneous branch is given off (see Fig. 14-1), and the intercostal nerve lies more inferiorly and moves toward the center of the intercostal space.

Technique

Intercostal nerve block may be performed at several possible sites along the course of the nerve. The most common site is in the region of the angle of the ribs just lateral to the sacrospinalis group of muscles. For technical ease of performance and for an optimal teaching or learning experience, the patient is best placed in a prone position, a position that facilitates performance of celiac plexus block, which is frequently combined with bilateral intercostal nerve block for abdominal surgery. The premedicated patient is turned to a prone position after establishment of an intravenous infusion. A pillow or roll of some kind is placed under the midabdomen to straighten the lumbar curve and to increase the intercostal spaces posteriorly.

The next step greatly facilitates nerve block and should be a routine part of nearly every regional anesthetic. This is the process of using skin markings to force a review of anatomic details and to define the site of needle insertion and direction for each block

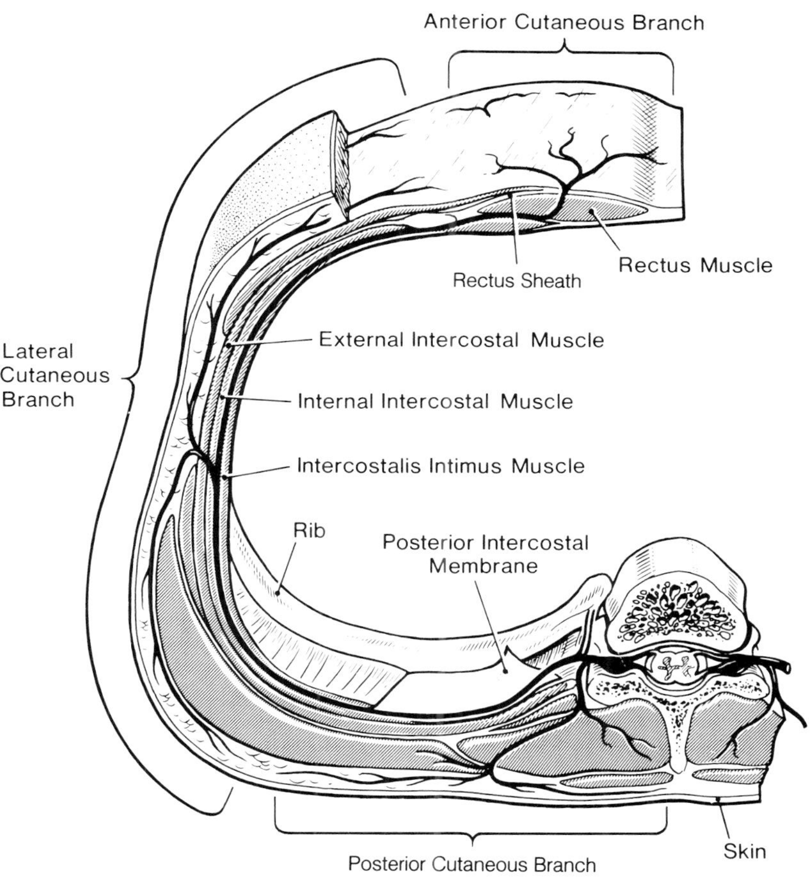

FIG. 14-1. An intercostal nerve and its branches. Approximate area of skin supplied by branches is also shown. There is evidence, however, that local anesthetic injected near the lateral cutaneous branch diffuses posteriorly to reach the posterior cutaneous branch (see also Fig. 14-4). Note also [a] the spinal nerves and dorsal root ganglia in the region of intervertebral foramen, with risk of perineurial spread into spinal fluid after intraneural injection in this region; [b] direct injection into an intervertebral foramen may reach spinal fluid by means of a dural cuff; [c] local anesthetic may gain access to epidural space by diffusing into an intervertebral foramen; and [d] close to the midline the intercostal nerve lies directly on the posterior intercostal membrane and pleura.

(Fig. 14-3). First, a vertical line should be drawn along the posterior vertebral spines. The next step is to palpate laterally to the edge of the sacrospinalis group of muscles where the ribs are most superficial. This distance is somewhat variable depending on body size, muscle mass, and physique but is usually 6 to 8 cm from the midline. Vertical lines are drawn somewhat parallel to the first line, but with a tendency to angle medially at the upper levels so as to avoid the scapulae. The caudal end of the line should cross near the end of the shortened 12th rib. Then, by successively palpating and marking the inferior edge of each rib along these two vertical lines, a diagram is completed (Fig. 14-3*A*). For abdominal surgery, six or seven ribs on each side are marked. For thoracic or other unilateral chest wall surgery, only the appropriate side and ribs are marked.

After positioning and marking of the patient, the local anesthetic solution is prepared. Epinephrine should be added to achieve a final concentration of 1:200,000 *or less* if the total dose of epinephrine required would exceed 0.25 mg (Table 14-3). The final solution is best prepared in a large mixing cup to afford ready access for refilling of the syringe during performance of the block.

Before starting the block, intravenous sedation should be given to allow for patient comfort. Barbiturates, benzodiazepines, ketamine, and short-acting narcotics are commonly used either alone or in combination. Obviously, attention must be given to airway maintenance and ventilatory adequacy in the prone patient. After an adequate level of sedation has been achieved, skin wheals are raised at each of the previously marked sites of injection. A disposable 30-gauge needle is ideal for raising these wheals. For maximal patient comfort, procaine or lidocaine might be chosen for the skin wheals because these drugs, injected subcutaneously, cause less pain than do the long-acting local anesthetics.

Finally, the intercostal nerve blocks are performed

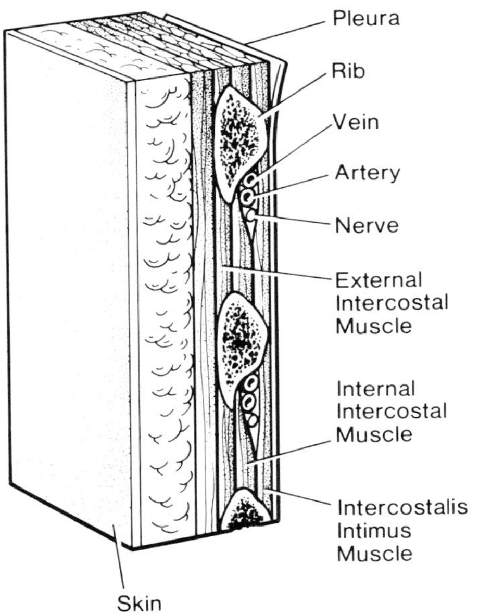

FIG. 14-2. Cross-section of rib and intercostal space. Section is shown in region of costal groove, which extends from near the head of the rib to 5 to 8 cm anterior to the angle of the rib. At the level of the angle of the rib, the intercostal nerve lies inferior to vein and artery in the intercostal groove.

successively at each of the skin wheal sites. To do this, a 3- to 4-cm, 22- or 23-gauge needle is attached to a full 10-ml Luer-Lok syringe. Reusable security bead needles offer some safety and hardness advantages. Disposable needles are of softer metal, and the tip may be bent with the repeated bony contact characteristic of this block, although they will more easily penetrate the thick skin of the back. A barbed needle will increase the risk of vascular or nerve damage.

In the following sequence, hand and finger position is of utmost importance (Fig. 14-3*B*–*E*). Beginning at the lowest rib, the index finger of the left hand is used to pull the skin at the lower edge of the rib up and over the rib. The needle is then introduced through the skin immediately off the tip of this retracting finger. While holding the syringe in the right hand, which rests on the patient's back, the anesthesiologist advances the needle to contact the rib. Should there be difficulty in contacting the rib with the needle, the palpating left index finger should be used to redefine its depth and position. Care should be taken not to allow the needle to penetrate beyond this palpated depth. The right hand maintains firm contact between needle and rib while the left hand is shifted to hold the needle's hub and shaft between thumb, index, and middle fingers. Of utmost importance is the firm placement of the left hand's hypothenar eminence against the patient's back. This allows total control of needle depth as the *left* hand "walks" the needle off the lower edge of the rib. At that point, it is advanced 2 to 5 mm and controlled by the left hand while the right hand merely squeezes to inject the solution. A very slight jiggling motion may decrease the risk of significant intravascular injection and help ensure proper spread of solution into the fascial plane containing the nerve. The above process is repeated for each of the nerves to be blocked. In certain patients with severe barrel chest deformity or neurasthenic habitus, the intercostal injection may best be done with an even shorter 23- or 25-gauge needle.

The success rate of intercostal nerve block should approach 100%. Failure is usually due to too superficial an injection of solution. Another common error is to rotate the long axis of the syringe as it is being walked off the rib (Fig. 14-4). A consequence of this is to inject solution superficially and inferiorly in the intercostal space where it will not bathe the nerve. When the technique described above is followed correctly, the firmly retracted skin over the rib will serve to ease the needle off the rib without need to resort to this rotary motion.

Intercostal nerve blocks can also be done at the midaxillary line while the patient is lying supine. This position is considerably more convenient in many situations. One concern with this approach is that the lateral cutaneous branch of the nerve could be missed by injected solution. Computed tomography studies show, however, that solutions spread readily along the subcostal groove for several centimeters and can come in contact with the origin or takeoff of this large branch (see Figs. 14-1 and 14-4).

Another variation is to consider intercostal nerve block by jet injection.[34] Seddon used such a technique but found that present jet guns deliver only 1 ml at a time. Using that volume of a 1.5% bupivacaine solution gave considerable postoperative analgesia. It is perhaps worthy of further study.

Surgical Applications

Relatively few surgical procedures can be performed under intercostal nerve block alone. It is possible to perform minor procedures on the chest or abdominal wall, but in general some degree of supplemental anesthesia must complement the block. For intra-ab-

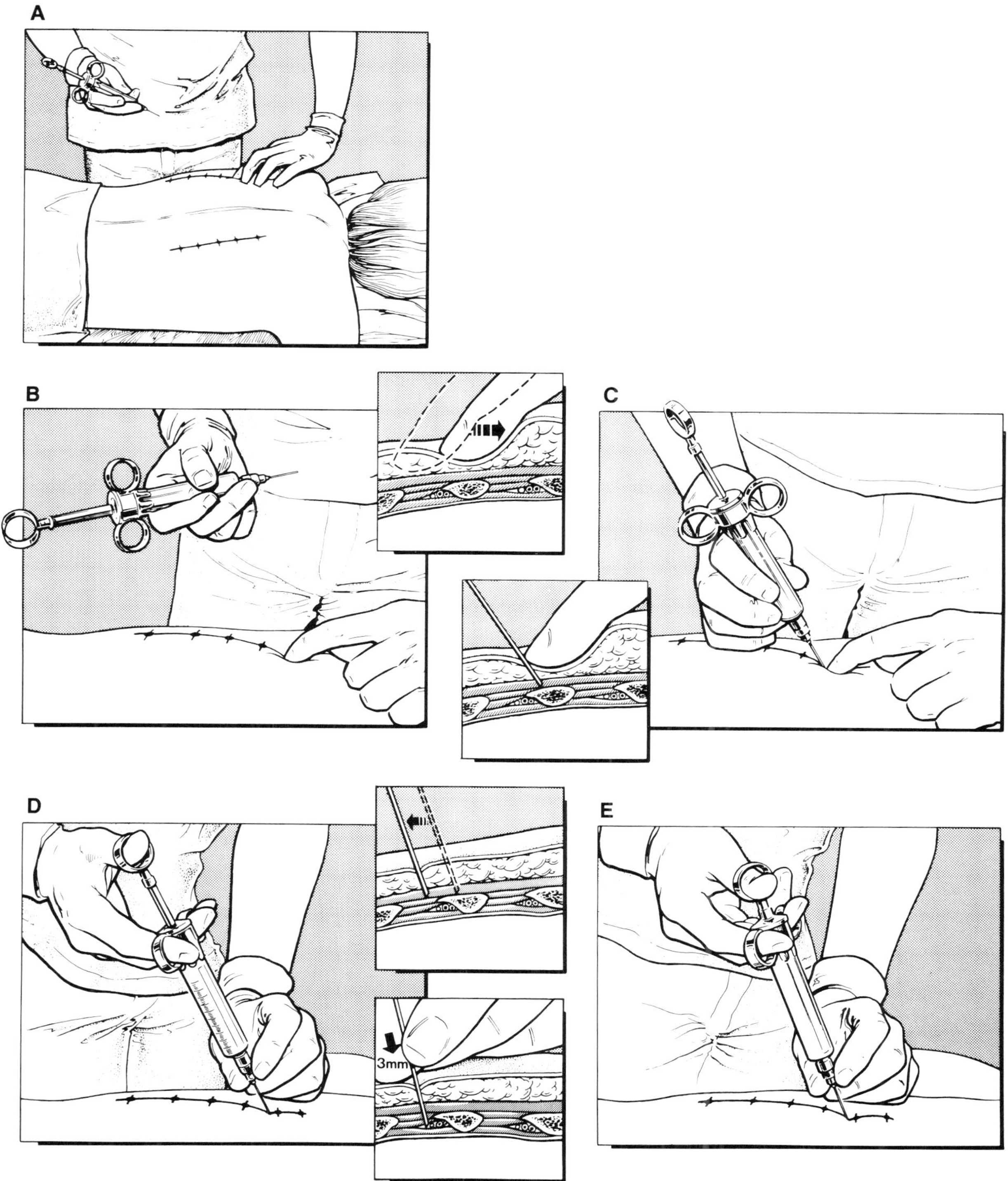

FIG. 14-3. Technique for intercostal block and corresponding deep anatomy (see text). **A.** Skin markings at lateral edge of sacrospinalis muscle (6–8 cm from midline). Note the medial curve of the line superiorly to avoid the scapulae. Ribs and interspaces are palpated. The lowest (most inferior) intercostal nerve is blocked first because the lower ribs are easy to palpate. (In **A–E** the diagrams show the second last intercostal nerves to be blocked in this patient.) **B.** Skin at lower edge of rib retracted superiorly onto rib. **C.** Needle inserted onto rib (see also inset). Note finger palpating rib still in place and hand holding syringe firmly braced against back. **D.** The position of the hands now change. Note *left* hand now rests against the back and holds the needle as it is walked off the inferior edge of the rib and advanced 3 mm. Right hand is free to aspirate and inject. **E.** Injection completed with left hand still firmly against patient's back and controlling the needle.

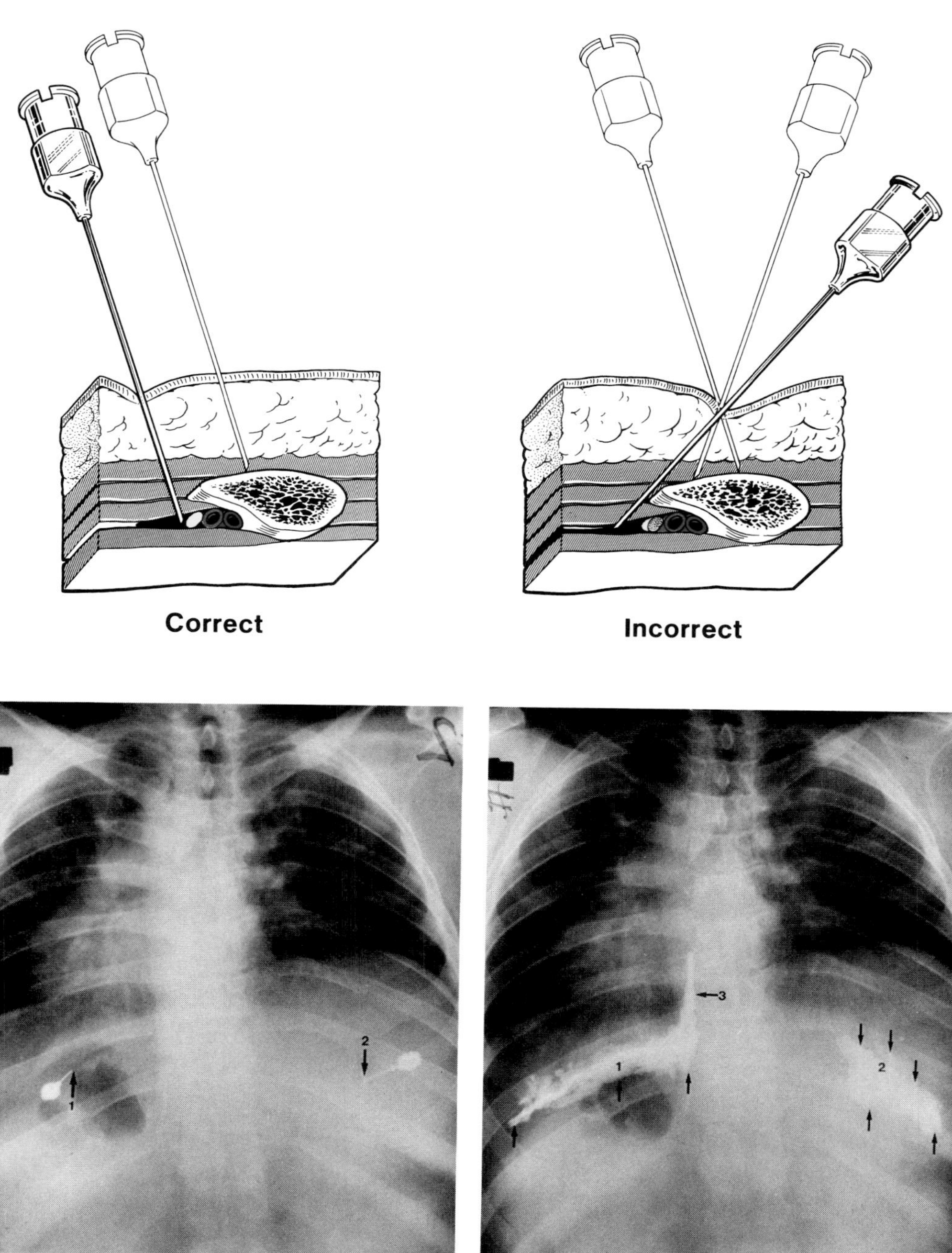

FIG. 14-4. **Upper Panel.** Comparison of correct *(left)* and incorrect *(right)* technique (see text). **Lower Panel.** *(Left)* X-ray showing correct needle insertion *(1)* compared to incorrect position *(2)*. *(Right)* X-ray showing injection of x-ray contrast medium. Injection from correctly placed needle results in spread along intercostal groove *(1)* and also into paravertebral space *(3)*. Injection from incorrectly placed needle results in a localized "blob" in intercostal muscles.[2] Arrows indicate extent of spread of solution.

dominal procedures, celiac plexus block may be added to provide visceral anesthesia. Intercostal block may also be combined with brachial plexus block for operations on the breast, upper extremities, and axilla. For intrathoracic procedures, stellate ganglion block may be a nice addition to obtund visceral pain from lung parenchyma. Pain from pelvic structures is not relieved by intercostal block, and operations in that region are better done with spinal, caudal, or lumbar epidural techniques.

Nonsurgical Applications

Intercostal nerve block is extremely effective in providing pain relief for fractured ribs. Pleuritic pain and pain from flail chest can also be relieved. Blockade of two or three nerves is a simple way to prepare for insertion of thoracostomy or feeding gastrostromy tubes. Herpes zoster pain may be relieved and even treated in this way. Intercostal nerve block can be helpful in the differential diagnosis of visceral versus abdominal wall pain. The most effective but least exploited use of this block is for postoperative control of pain (see Chap. 25).

Complications

The most feared complication of intercostal nerve block is pneumothorax. The actual incidence is extremely low, but many physicians avoid this block because of an imagined high frequency. Physicians in all stages of training performed more than 10,000 individual nerve blocks with a reported incidence of pneumothorax of only 0.073%.[23] An earlier study on silent pneumothorax done by obtaining routine postoperative chest films showed a 0.42% incidence. Further retrospective analysis forces one to conclude that the true risks and mechanisms of pneumothorax have been greatly exaggerated. For instance, Moore reported the unexpected finding of contrast material within the pleural cavity in a roentgenographic study of block technique.[27] Further evidence of parietal pleural penetration is noted in two papers on continuous intercostal nerve blockade.[1,29] The authors were surprised to find catheters within the pleural space in cadaver studies and in cardiac surgical patients. Surgeons observed the catheter tip from within after midline sternotomy. Nunn's observations of multiple dermatome block after a single injection might also be explained on this same basis.[31] Finally, there is the unorthodox and purposeful use of an interpleural catheter for postoperative pain control.[19] This internal pleural space approach to intercostal block forces us to re-evaluate our more traditional perspectives.

Treatment of pneumothorax by needle aspiration or merely by careful observation is usually all that is needed. Reabsorption of a small pneumothorax is also aided by administration of oxygen. Chest tube drainage should be performed only if there is failure to re-expand the lung with these preliminary maneuvers. Overzealous surgical treatment has often compounded an initial problem that might well have resolved with simple measures.

A second complication relates to the toxic effects of absorbed local anesthetic and epinephrine following intercostal block. As previously mentioned, blood levels of the anesthetic drug are higher after this block than after any other regional anesthetic procedure. Systemic toxic reactions rarely occur in patients having diagnostic or therapeutic blocks because smaller volumes of more dilute solution of drug are used. Greater amounts of more concentrated drug are injected to provide complete motor and sensory block in the surgical patient. These greater doses may result in delayed systemic toxicity, so that patients should be monitored closely for 15 to 20 minutes after completion of the block.

Any regional anesthetic procedure, and especially intercostal nerve block, can lead to complications if the anesthesiologist becomes so involved in the mechanics of administering the nerve block that he neglects total patient care. The beginning practitioner of regional anesthesia tends to become so engrossed in technique and methods that he fails to see the patient as more than a portion of anatomic detail through which a needle is being inserted. Vital signs may not be heeded! This is especially dangerous when depressant drugs have been administered before the block. Complications from inattentiveness are not those of the nerve block *per se,* although respiratory embarrassment or cardiovascular problems are often wrongly ascribed as toxic effects of the local anesthetic.[2] The American Society of Anesthesiologists motto, "Constant vigilance," is extremely appropriate for proper use of any nerve block.

CELIAC PLEXUS NERVE BLOCK

Of the many regional block techniques available to the anesthetist, blockade of the celiac plexus is potentially one of the more valuable and probably very underused. The reason for this lack of use is because it is exclusively an autonomic blockade and, in most surgical situations, must be combined with other somatic nerve blocks. Most anesthetists would prefer the "all-inclusive" spinal or epidural block. Most anesthetists view celiac plexus block as valuable only in large pain clinics. Fortunately, recent research work has focused on the role of autonomic blockade in mediating stress and endocrine response of surgery. This has rekindled interest in this block technique.

Anatomy

There seems to be significant confusion relating to the nomenclature of this portion of the autonomic nervous system. Different textbooks have used terms such as solar plexus, the abdominal brain (of Bichat), celiac ganglia, and splanchnic plexus to describe some or all of the same anatomy. As one wishes to evaluate the clinical and physiologic results of these nerve blocks, it is important to know whether the blocked structures are preganglionic or postganglionic and which target organs will be affected by the block.

The celiac plexus is the largest of the great plexuses of the sympathetic nervous system. The cardiac plexus innervates primarily thoracic structures, the celiac plexus innervates abdominal organs, and the hypogastric plexus supplies pelvic organs. All three contain visceral afferent and efferent fibers. In addition, they contain parasympathetic fibers that pass through these ganglia after originating in cranial or sacral areas of the nervous system. Although these latter fibers may be found in these plexuses, all are primarily sympathetic nervous system structures. They contain no somatic fibers but do innervate most of the abdominal viscera to include stomach, liver, biliary tract, pancreas, spleen, kidneys, adrenals, omentum, and small and large bowel. Although the terms plexus and ganglion are often used interchangeably, it is important to realize that plexus is a more inclusive term. A plexus is composed of a number of ganglion and nerve fibers that converge in a fairly well-defined anatomic location.

According to most standard anatomic textbooks, there are three splanchnic nerves—great, lesser, and least. The *great splanchnic nerve* arises from the roots of T5 or T6 to T9 or T10, running paravertebrally in the thorax through the crus of the diaphragm to enter the abdominal cavity, ending in the celiac (or semilunar) ganglion on that side. The *lesser splanchnic nerve* arises from T10 to T11 segments and passes lateral to, or with, the great nerve to the celiac ganglion. It sends postganglionic fibers to celiac and renal plexuses. The *least splanchnic nerve* arises from T11 and T12 segments and passes through the diaphragm to the celiac ganglion. It is worth remembering that all three splanchnic nerves are preganglionic, that the paired celiac (or semilunar) ganglia are where they synapse, and that the postganglionic fibers radiate from the ganglia to celiac, aortic, renal, and hypogastric plexuses, which in turn give off the sympathetic fibers to the abdominal viscera (Fig. 14-5).

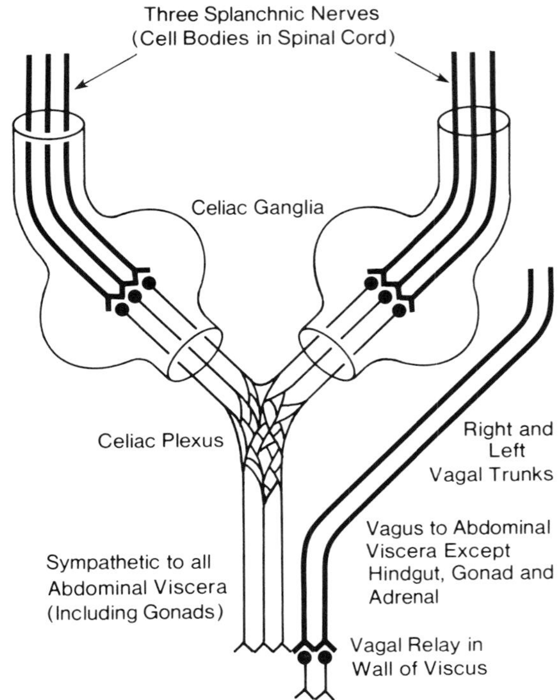

FIG. 14-5. Constituents of celiac plexus (see text). (Redrawn and reproduced with permission from Last, R.J.: Anatomy, Regional and Applied, 6th ed., p. 315. Edinburgh, Churchill Livingstone, 1978.)

Of more importance to performance of celiac plexus block is an understanding of the anatomy of the surrounding structures that will be subjected to the potential trauma of needles and drug. The celiac ganglia are situated in close relation to the first lumbar vertebrae. On the right side and anterior is the vena cava, and on the left, anteriorly, is the aorta. The kidneys are lateral on either side. The paired ganglia are close to the midline on each side between the adrenal glands and immediately above the pancreas. The postganglionic nerves are flat and rest against the crus of the diaphragm. They are partially covered by the vena cava on the right and pancreas on the left.

They become interconnected to form plexuses. The plexus anterior to the aorta, around the base of the celiac artery and superior mesenteric artery, is referred to as the solar (or celiac plexus). From it arise subplexuses such as gastric, hepatic, splanchnic, and renal.

In the past decade, some additional studies have further clarified the anatomy of this region. Ward and colleagues, in 1979, performed x-ray and careful autopsy examinations of 20 adult bodies.[40] The celiac ganglia were found to vary in number, size, and location. On either side, the number varied from one to five and size from 0.5 to 4.5 cm in diameter. Ganglia on the left were uniformly lower than on the right by an average of less than one vertebral level; the extreme was one and one-half vertebral levels. On both sides, the ganglia were 0.6 to 0.9 cm below the celiac artery. The most consistent relationship of the ganglia was to the anterior vertebral margin, most frequently less than 1.5 cm anterior to this margin.

In 1981, Moore and associates[27a] verified needle placement and spread of injected solution by conventional x-ray and by CT scan in 20 cancer patients. They noted that spread of the solution tended to be confined to the sides of the injection. They also noted that the anterior portion of the aortic plexus was 2 to 2.5 cm anterior to the anterior vertebral margin.

Technique

Celiac plexus nerve block is of special interest in that both bony and vascular landmarks can be used to good advantage in the performance of this block.[36] As with any nerve block, it is advisable to mark out a diagram on the skin that, projected mentally, can yield three-dimensional perspective for the ultimate placement of the needles. The easiest and most useful avenue of approach to the well-guarded celiac plexus is posterolateral. The patient is placed in a prone position with pillow under the abdomen, head turned flat to the table or cart, and arms dangling down at each side. The primary external topographic features are the 12th ribs and the inferior aspects of T12 and L1 spinous processes (Fig. 14-6). The figure formed by connecting the spine of T12 and L1 with points 7 to 8 cm lateral at the lower edges of the 12th ribs is that of a flattened isosceles triangle. The equal sides of this triangle serve as directional guides for the two needles. They are passed under the edge of each of the 12th ribs to approach the midline anterior to the body of L1. A 10- to 15-cm 20-gauge needle is used as dictated by either the frailty or obesity of the patient. Skin wheals are raised 7 to 8 cm from the midline at the inferior edge of the 12th rib. Infiltration with a small amount of local anesthetic solution can be carried deeper for 1 to 3 cm. The awake patient should be warned about brief twinges of pain, which result from the advancing needle coming in contact with periosteum or lumbar nerves.

At first insertion, the needle is tilted about 45° from the horizontal so that contact can be made with the lateral body of L1 at an average depth of 7 to 9 cm (Fig. 14-6). Bony contact at a more superficial level indicates that a vertebral transverse process has been encountered. This must be recognized for what it is, because an incorrect judgment might lead to a superficial injection of anesthetic solution just 2 to 3 cm deep to the transverse process. An ensuing epidural block or psoas muscle injection would result in a widespread somatic nerve paralysis. This point is of special importance when neurolytic solutions are to be used. The depth of L1 will depend on the patient's size and on the location on the vertebral body at which contact is made (*i.e.*, posterolateral or anterolateral). Once the vertebral body is identified at a usual depth of 8 to 10 cm, the needle is withdrawn to a subcutaneous level and its angle increased to allow the tip of the needle to pass 2 to 3 cm deeper than the previous point of bony contact. The needle's angle may have to be readjusted two or three times until it slides off the anterolateral side of the vertebral body. Determining the precise depth to which the needle should be advanced is of major importance. The simplest method is to advance the left-sided needle slowly until sensitive fingertips feel aortic pulsations transmitted up the shaft (Fig. 14-6). Once this aortic depth is discovered, the right-sided needle can be inserted and readily advanced to a similar depth. Problems caused by bleeding from penetration of either aorta or inferior vena cava are extremely rare.

Once the needles have been positioned in the periaortic region, other confirmatory tests of needle placement should be performed to rule out improper position of the needle tip. For instance, leakage of blood, urine, or cerebrospinal fluid (CSF) will usually be spontaneous. If not, aspiration should be performed in four quadrants. Should this prove negative, a 3-ml test dose of anesthetic solution is injected. This will provide additional confirmation of needle placement, since paralysis would rapidly follow unintended subarachnoid or epidural injection. The final confirmatory test depends on the "feel" that the anesthesiologist senses while injecting the final volume of anesthetic solution. In this regard, the difference between a 20- and a 22-gauge needle is very

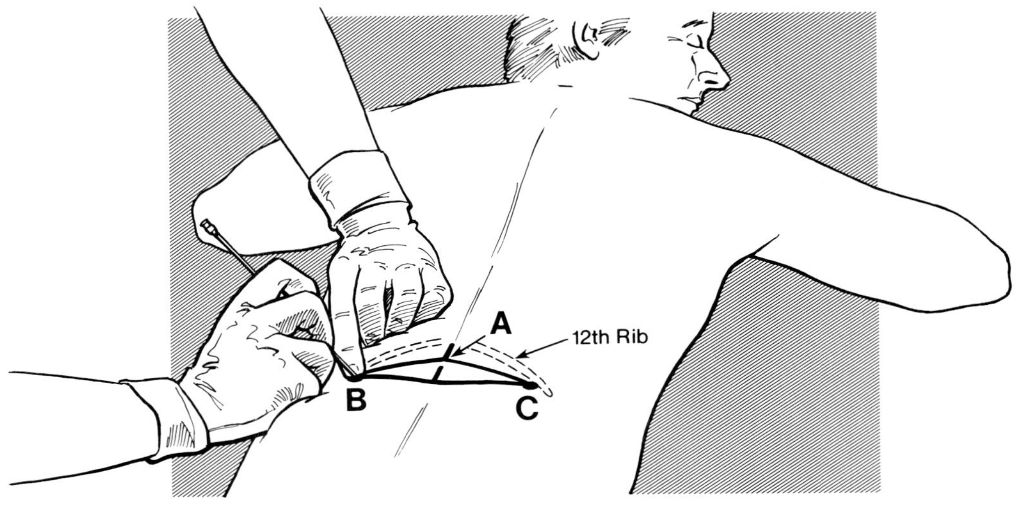

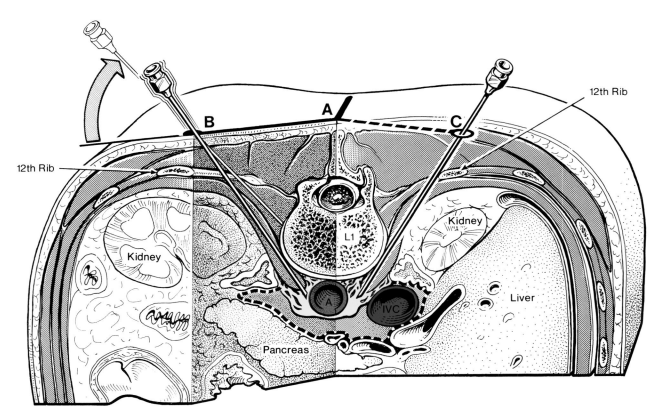

FIG. 14-6. Celiac plexus block. **Upper Panel.** Skin markings, position of patient, and initial insertion of needle. *Note:* Triangle formed by skin marks on lower border of 12th ribs (*B* and *C*) in line with inferior border of L1 spinous process and joined to inferior border of T12 *(A)*. **Lower Panel.** Needle insertion and deep anatomy (see text). Skin markings and triangle *(A, B, C)* are still shown. Needle initially is directed in the plane of the line BA or CA, and at 45° to the horizontal axis of the body, to contact the lateral aspect of the L1 vertebral body. It passes inferior to the 12th rib and medial to the kidney. The angle of insertion to the *horizontal* axis of the body is then increased until the needle slips past the lateral aspect of the vertebral body, still in the line BA or CA to reach the anterolateral aspect. On the left side the aortic pulsations will be detected at the needle hub before puncturing the artery. Spread of a test dose of contrast medium (in the approximate area indicated by the light blue color) is a valuable guide to correct needle placement prior to diagnostic or therapeutic celiac block.

pronounced. A 12-cm, 22-gauge needle requires such firm pressure during injection that it is difficult to appreciate whether resistance is due to the small-needle bore or whether the site of injection is subperiosteal or otherwise abnormal. On the other hand, injection of 20 to 25 ml of solution through a 20-gauge needle affords little resistance. This is to be expected if the injection is being properly performed in the loose retroperitoneal area where nerve fibers of the celiac plexus are located. Intraperitoneal injections could possibly occur, but this would require extremely lateral and deep placement of the needles.*

There have been reports of a number of other techniques for celiac plexus nerve block. Perhaps the most bold is the transaortic method of Ischia.[15] Using a combination of fluoroscopy and fingertip feel, the 20-gauge needle is advanced to penetrate the aorta and rest directly in the preaortic nerve network of the celiac plexus. Although this would seem to guarantee correct placement of local anesthetic or neurolytic solutions, these solutions would obviously be diluted by extravasated blood. Postblock CT scans showed no retroperitoneal hematoma in six patients. Long-term efficacy, side-effects, and complications have not, however, been thoroughly evaluated with this technique. Other authors have described variations of needle placement that emphasize the differences between transcrural celiac block and retrocrural splanchnic nerve block.[35] Anatomic variations make precise needle placement a difficult matter even though fluoroscopy, standard x-rays, or CT guidance may be used (Fig. 14-7).[6] It is possible that the block may actually occur at nerve, ganglion, or plexus sites with any of the described techniques, and the reported results are quite similar for any of these various combinations (see also Chap. 29.2).

*When neurolytic solutions are to be injected, the use of contrast media and an image intensifier is highly desirable (see also Chap. 29.2).

Surgical Applications

The combination of intercostal and celiac plexus nerve block is ideal for surgery of the upper abdomen. Usually these two blocks are supplemented

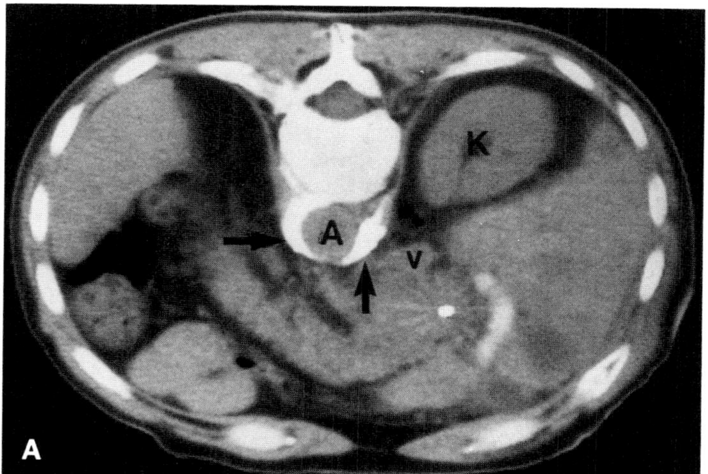

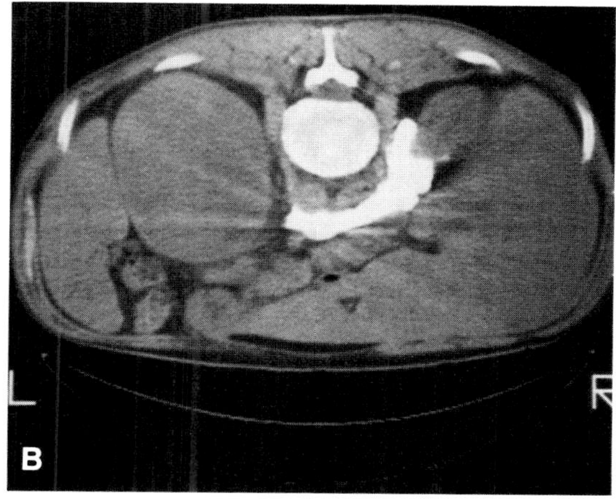

FIG. 14-7. Computed tomography scan of injection of contrast media during celiac plexus block. **A.** Needles have been inserted through the crus of the diaphragm (on right and left) and contrast medium injected. (In this case 25 ml of a solution of 50% alcohol containing iothalamate was injected through each needle.) Note contrast almost surrounding aorta in a similar distribution to that shown in Figure 14-6. A, aorta; V, vena cava; K, kidney; arrows, spread of contrast media. **B.** Patient with large metastasis in left adrenal gland, seen as large mass to the left of vertebral body. The kidney and liver are seen on the right. L, left; R, right. In this situation only one needle has been inserted through the crus of the diaphragm on the right side. Injection of 50 ml of the solution used in *A* results in an acceptable spread of solution. Insertion of a needle through the diaphragm on the left side would have a high chance of piercing the aorta. (Reproduced with permission from Moore, D.C.: Intercostal Nerve Block and Celiac Plexus Block for Pain Therapy. Advances in Pain Research and Therapy, Vol. 7. New York, Raven Press, 1984.)

with light general anesthesia, since celiac block does not provide total anesthesia of all upper abdominal visceral sensation or reflexes. One special advantage to the surgeon is the diminution in bowel diameter caused by block of sympathetic fibers and relative vagal overactivity with increased peristalsis and gut constriction.

As with spinal or epidural anesthesia, there is a tendency for the sympathetic block of celiac plexus anesthesia to produce a fall in blood pressure. This is neither as frequent nor as severe as the hypotension following high spinal anesthesia; however, hypotension can persist into the postoperative period if long-acting local anesthetics are used. This potential problem can be treated by using a shorter-acting local anesthetic for the celiac block than for the intercostal block, by adequate replacement of blood and fluid losses during surgery, or by small doses of vasopressors. In general, the supine patient will be asymptomatic and physiologically stable even at pressures as low as 70 mm Hg systolic.

Nonsurgical Application

Celiac plexus block can be used alone or in various combinations with intercostal nerve block to help in the differential diagnosis of visceral versus abdominal wall pain (see Chap. 27.1). The block can be of therapeutic value in acute pancreatitis by relieving spasm of ducts and sphincters in the pancreatic system.[18] When used in this regard, methylprednisolone may be mixed and injected along with the local anesthetic solution. Alcohol celiac plexus block is the most effective of all therapeutic endeavors commonly used in the treatment of pancreatic cancer pain.[36] In contrast, alcohol celiac block does not lead to good, prolonged pain relief in patients with chronic pancreatitis.

Complications

Possible complications of celiac plexus block include hypotension; subarachnoid, epidural, intraosseous, or intrapsoas injection; intravascular injection; retroperitoneal hematoma secondary to bleeding from aorta or vena cava; and puncture of viscera, abscess, or cysts. Other complications reported after neurolytic blocks include paralysis, lower extremity dysesthesias, and sexual dysfunction. In such cases, the solution had obviously spread to contaminate the lumbar plexus or central neuraxis. Another more remote possibility is the impairment of blood supply from hematoma or perivascular pressure of injected solution. Some drop in blood pressure will occur in 30% to 60% of patients, depending on blood volume and physical status. It is usually not abrupt in onset. Misplaced injections are best prevented by experience, drawing the proper skin markings, and having the patient fully prone for the injection. Although celiac block can be performed on patients who are in a lateral or semiprone position, these positions make it more difficult to ensure proper orientation to anatomic details. Initial aspiration and the use of a test dose of local anesthetic solution are other precautionary measures against the complications of misplaced injections.

SPLANCHNIC NERVE BLOCK

The anatomy of the splanchnic nerves is described above.

Technique

The splanchnic nerves can be blocked above the diaphragm, at the upper border of T12, with a technique similar to celiac plexus block.[2a] The needle is directed, however, to the anterolateral angle of the vertebral body of T12, to the same point on the vertebral body as in lumbar sympathetic block (see Chap. 13). This block is not recommended for surgical application. For diagnosis and treatment of chronic abdominal pain, it is possible to obtain pain relief with a much smaller volume of solution than is the case with celiac block. Needle insertion is carried out under image intensifier control (Fig. 14-8*A*). Then a small volume (1 ml) of contrast media (*e.g.*, angiographin) is injected to check that a linear spread is obtained, in anteroposterior and lateral views, along the anterolateral aspects of vertebral bodies immediately above the diaphragm (Fig. 14-8*B*). Then either local anesthetic or neurolytic solution may be injected for diagnostic or therapeutic block, respectively. The neurolytic solution of choice is phenol in contrast media (*e.g.*, 10% phenol in angiographin), which can be viewed directly as it spreads. Usually only 3 to 4 ml is required on each side.

Complications

Complications of this technique are similar to those of celiac block. Postural hypotension is less, however,

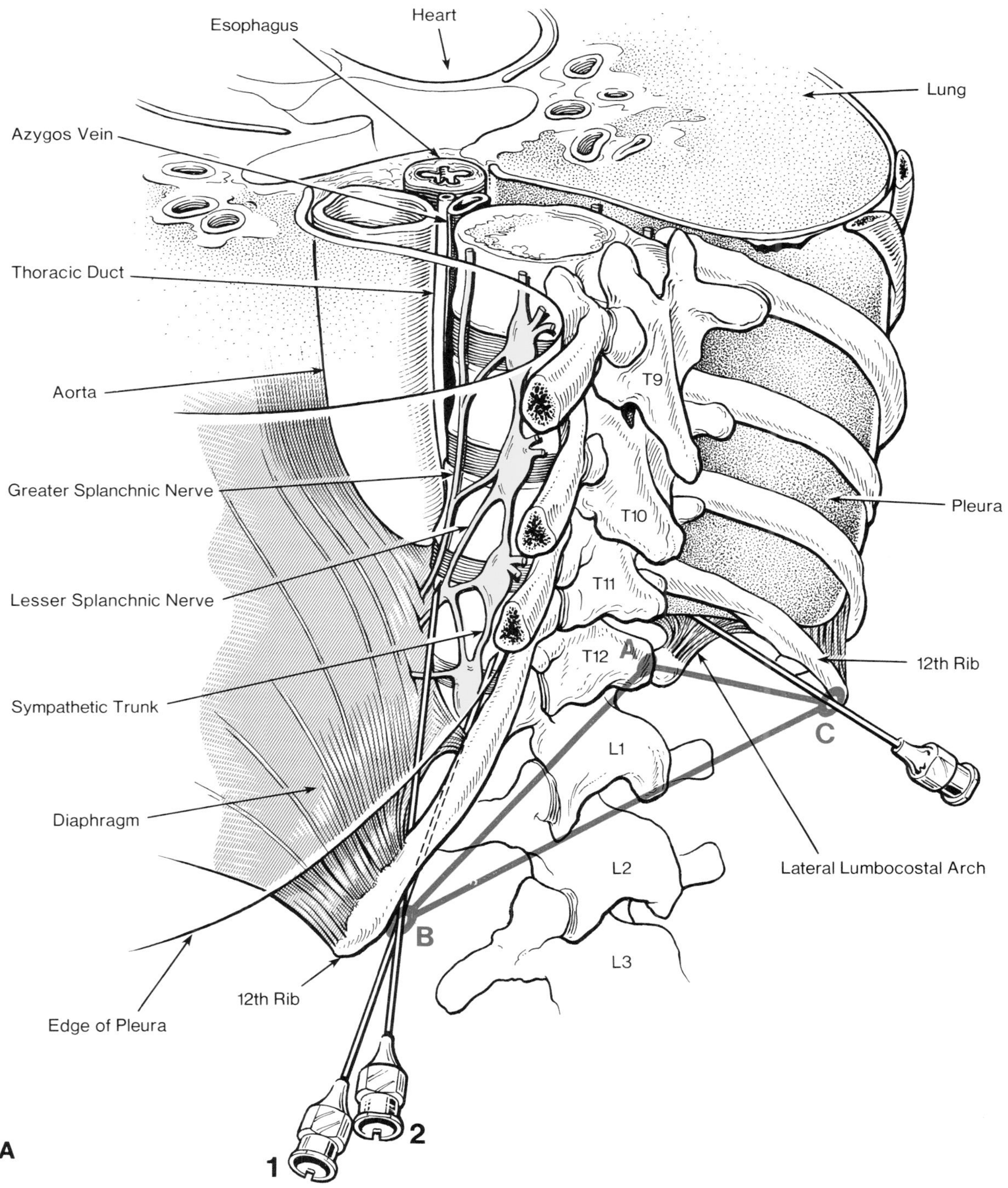

FIG. 14-8. **A.** Splanchnic nerve block, posterolateral view. Skin markings B and C are as in Figure 14-7. A is marked at the superior aspect of T12 spinous process. The technique of needle insertion is similar to that in Figure 14-7 but aimed along BA and CA to the superior aspect of T12. Note the proximity of pleura, and also the thoracic duct on left side. *(continued).*

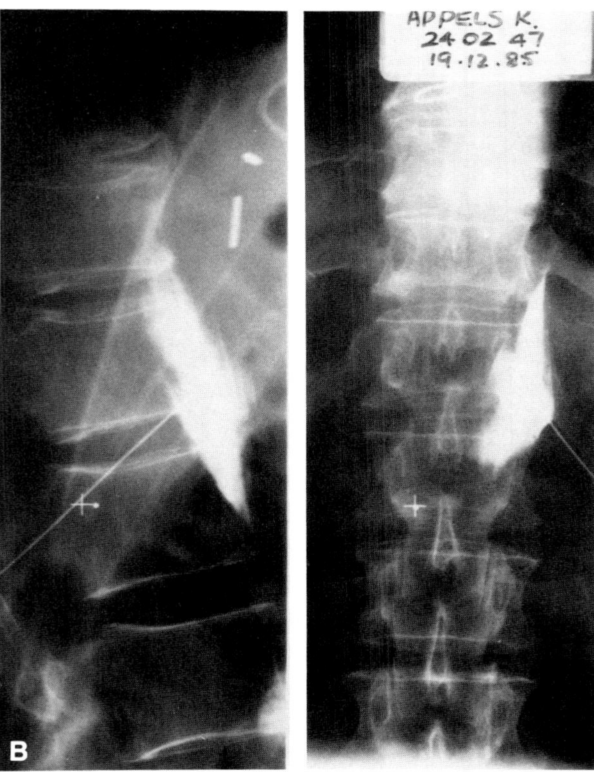

FIG. 14-8. *(Continued)* **B.** Splanchnic nerve block: x-ray of spread of contrast medium, lateral view *(left)* and anteroposterior view *(right)*. See text for details of block.

because lumbar sympathetic ganglia are not blocked. The risk of pneumothorax is considerable, and it is important to keep the needle as close as possible to the vertebral body. The thoracic duct may be damaged, leading to a chylothorax, or it may become obstructed, leading to lymphedema. Vascular puncture and hematoma formation may occur as in celiac block.

PARAVERTEBRAL LUMBAR SOMATIC NERVE BLOCK

Anatomy

When lumbar somatic nerve block is performed paravertebrally, it has many similarities to intercostal nerve block. Instead of using the ribs as bony landmarks, however, the primary bony guide becomes the transverse process of the lumbar vertebral body —a "rudimentary" rib. The lumbar nerves exit their respective intervertebral foramina just inferior to the caudad edge of each transverse process. These nerves divide immediately into anterior and posterior branches. The small posterior branches supply the skin of the lower back and the paravertebral muscles. Of primary interest, however, are the anterior branches of the first four lumbar nerves. These nerves, together with a small branch from the 12th thoracic nerve, form the lumbar plexus. This plexus is largely conceived within the substance of the psoas major muscle, and most of the peripheral branches exit laterally in a plane between the psoas and quadratus lumborum muscles.

The major branches of the lumbar plexus (*i.e.*, the iliohypogastric, ilioinguinal, and lateral femoral cutaneous nerves) continue laterally around the rim of the pelvis. Their terminal branches approach and pass near the anterior superior iliac spine. The femoral nerve passes almost directly caudad after emerging from the lateral edge of psoas major. The obturator nerve emerges from the medial edge of psoas major, descends under the common iliac vessels, and finally emerges from the pelvis through the obturator foramen. The ultimate cutaneous distribution of each of these nerves is quite variable in the groin and anterolateral leg. There is also considerable overlap of cutaneous branches of individual nerves. The primary peripheral branches of the lumbar plexus are listed in Table 14-4 and illustrated in Figure 14-9. It is apparent that paravertebral nerve block of L1–L4 will result in sensory and motor block of the groin and much of the leg. For intra-abdominal, pelvic, or groin operations, it is necessary to block only the upper two lumbar segments.

In general, the lumbar nerves tend to slope sharply caudad as they emerge from the intervertebral foraminae. In doing so, they tend to course anterior to the tips of the transverse processes of the next lower lumbar vertebral bodies. A needle placed at the inferior edge of a transverse process will be close to nerves from two lumbar segments: Medially, it will

TABLE 14-4. ORIGINS AND DISTRIBUTION OF THE LUMBAR PLEXUS

Peripheral Nerve	Root Segments
Iliohypogastric	T12, L1
Ilioinguinal	L1
Genitofemoral	L1, L2
Lateral femoral cutaneous	L2, L3
Femoral	L2, L3, L4
Obturator	L2, L3, L4

be close to the nerve exiting the vertebral foramen; laterally, it will be near the nerve from the next most cephalad vertebral level. Hence, local anesthetic solution injected at the proper depth inferior to one lumbar vertebral process can actually result in nerve block of two or more root segments.

Technique

The patient's prone position is unchanged from that described for intercostal and celiac plexus nerve block. The injection sites are marked while keeping in mind that "the cephalad edge of a lumbar posterior spinous process lies opposite the caudad edge of its homologous transverse process." The distance between any two lumbar transverse processes is about 2 cm. Visualizing and then locating the transverse process is fundamental to a successful block. After palpating and marking each of the lumbar vertebral spinous processes, the anesthesiologist draws horizontal lines at the cephalad edge of each one and projects them laterally. Two vertical lines should then be drawn parallel to, and 3 to 5 cm lateral from, the midline. The points of intersection of the vertical and horizontal lines mark the sites where skin wheals are raised (Fig. 14-10). In surgical patients, the block can be performed under the same sedation used for intercostal and celiac plexus block. An 8-cm, 22-gauge needle is inserted perpendicular to the skin until it contacts the transverse process at a depth of 3 to 5 cm. The needle should then be withdrawn to a subcuta-

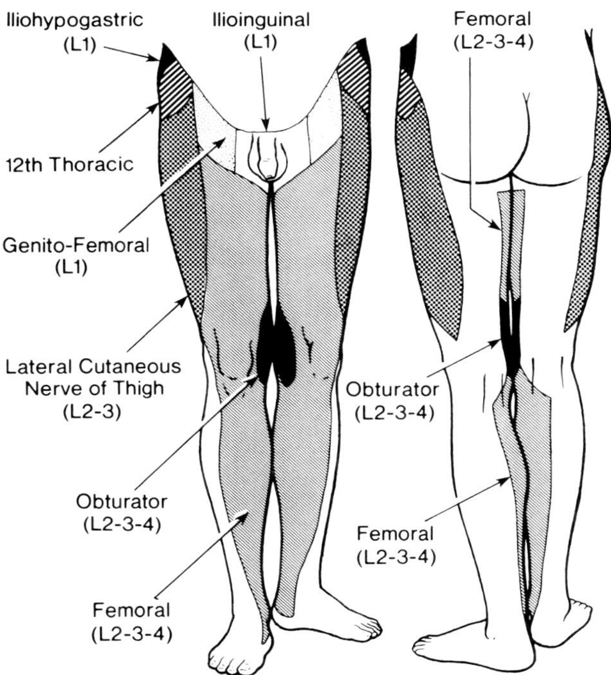

FIG. 14-9. Cutaneous branches of lumbar plexus and the areas of skin that they supply.

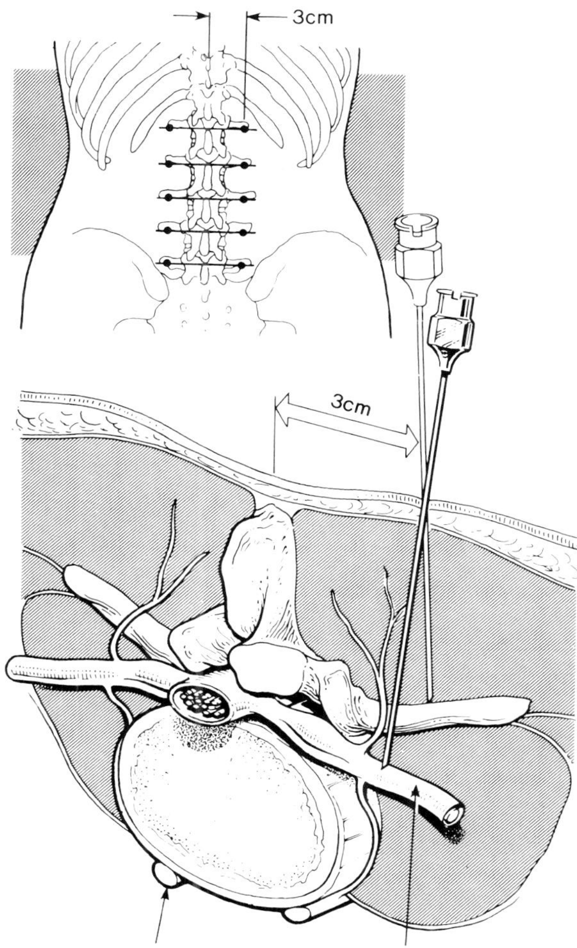

FIG. 14-10. Paravertebral lumbar somatic nerve block. **Upper Panel.** Skin markings are made by drawing lines across the cephalad aspect of spinous processes and then drawing vertical lines 3 cm from the midline. **Lower Panel.** A needle inserted perpendicular to the skin will contact the caudad edge of a spinous process. Angulation of the needle in a caudad direction to slide caudad to the transverse process will reach the spinal nerve 1 to 2 cm deeper than will the transverse process.

neous level and redirected to slide off the caudad edge of the transverse process. As the needle is advanced 1 to 2 cm beyond the point where it previously made contact with bone, 6 to 10 ml of local anesthetic solution is injected. This process is repeated at each of the lumbar levels at which anesthesia is desired. The useful concentrations of local anesthetic are the same as those used for intercostal block.

Surgical Application

Lumbar paravertebral nerve block can rarely be used as the sole anesthetic for surgery. It effectively complements intercostal and celiac plexus block for intra-abdominal and pelvic procedures. Groin operations such as herniorrhaphy can be performed with lumbar block, but supplementation with local infiltration or intravenous drugs is usually necessary.

Nonsurgical Application

When the block is used for diagnostic purposes, it is preferable to use only small volumes of local anesthetic solution so as to limit spread centrally or to adjacent lumbar nerves. Some physicians use fluoroscopy or a nerve stimulator to position the needle precisely and then inject only 0.5 to 1 ml of drug. This technique may be especially helpful in evaluating patients with back pain, in which the recurrent meningeal nerve may play a role. This branch is highly variable but tends to arise from the main nerve root just before separating into anterior and posterior parts. Another diagnostic use of paravertebral lumbar block is in evaluating groin or genital pain, such as the nerve entrapment syndromes that sometimes follow herniorrhaphy.

Complications

It is possible to inject into intravascular, epidural, or subarachnoid spaces during performance of this block. Should the needle be inserted too far medially, it could enter a vertebral foramen or penetrate a dural sleeve to produce spinal anesthesia. Likewise, there could be perineural spread of solution into the epidural space with a consequent variable degree of anesthesia over the lower extremities. Intravascular injection can be minimized by aspiration tests and by avoiding large volume injections. The lumbar sympathetic chain may be anesthetized either from local block of gray and white rami communicantes or by deeper penetration of local anesthetic drug down to the sympathetic chain itself. Intraperitoneal injection or puncture of retroperitoneal or intra-abdominal organs is possible, although only as a result of gross error.

MISCELLANEOUS NERVE BLOCKS OF THE ABDOMEN AND CHEST

The three nerve blocks previously described in this chapter are performed at anatomic sites near the central neuraxis. There are many more peripheral sites along these nerve pathways for nerve block, but all are merely variations. The more distal the site on a peripheral nerve, the greater is the chance for incomplete block, because of factors such as spatial distribution, overlap of nerve territories, and the difficulty of reaching each of the multiple branches of an arborizing nerve with injected local anesthetic solution. These factors can be partially overcome by using large volumes of solution, by using multiple injections, and by selecting local anesthetic agents with high penetrability; however, it is easier to hit the trunk of a tree than to touch each of its branches, and the previously described blocks are therefore more useful and predictable. A small amount of anesthetic injected at a primary nerve trunk will provide the best quality anesthesia. The following blocks are described primarily for the sake of completeness of information, historical perspective, and to improve appreciation of anatomic detail of nerve distribution.

RECTUS BLOCK

Anatomy

As the lower five intercostal nerves course anteriorly, they eventually surface and terminate after penetrating the rectus abdomonus muscle. These nerves enter the rectus sheath at the posterolateral border of the body of that muscle. The tendinous intersections of the rectus tend to create segmental distribution of individual intercostal nerves, but there is some overlap of adjacent fibers. Anteriorly, the rectus sheath is tough and fibrous from pubis to xiphoid. Posteriorly, it is strong and readily identifiable down to the level of the umbilicus, but then it fades into a thin sheath of transversalis fascia, which is closely adherent to peritoneum below the semicircular line of Douglas. The posterior rectus sheath above the umbilicus is quite substantial and can serve as a "backboard" for injecting local anesthetic solution. This solution will be confined by the tendinous intersections but within those limits will spread up and down to anesthetize the peripheral motor and sensory branches of the intercostal nerves.

Technique

The patient lies supine, and the anesthesiologist may stand at either side. Usually four to six sites are injected, depending on the location and size of surgical incision (Fig. 14-11). Skin wheals are raised at the middle of each segment of the rectus muscle body that can be palpated between tendinous intersections. A reusable or short bevel 5-cm, 22-gauge needle is passed through skin and subcutaneous tissue until it meets the firm resistance of the anterior rectus sheath. The block should be discontinued unless this sheath can be convincingly demonstrated by pushing on the needle. With controlled steady pressure, the needle is pushed to penetrate this sheath with a definite snap and then passed on through the softer belly of the muscle. As the needle approaches the posterior rectus sheath, a firm resistance will again become apparent. Using this posterior sheath as a backboard, 10 ml of local anesthetic solution is injected. The process is repeated at each injection site. Blocks above the umbilicus should be performed first and needle depth noted before attempting any additional blocks below the umbilicus.

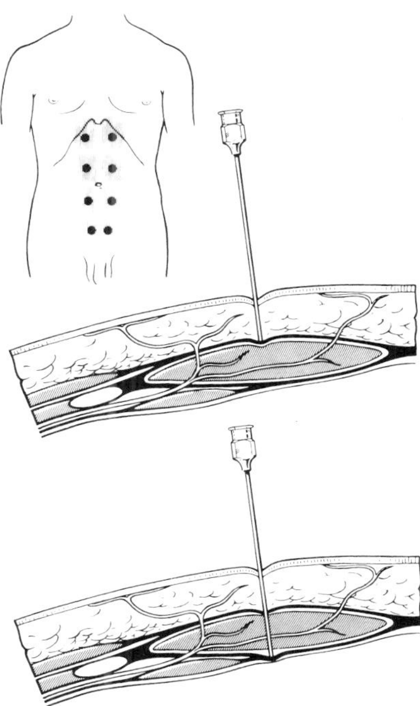

FIG. 14-11. Rectus block. **Upper.** Skin wheals are raised in the center of rectus segments. These are delineated by a vertical line through umbilicus and horizontal lines at umbilical level, and midway between umbilicus and xiphisternum, respectively. **Middle.** Short bevel needle contacts resistance of anterior rectus sheath. **Lower.** Needle penetrates rectus muscle and is halted by resistance of posterior rectus sheath. Note the latter structure is absent below the line midway between umbilicus and pubis. Thus these two rectus injections are made last.

Surgical Application

The block may be used for surgical pain from a midline incision. It requires supplementation if the abdominal cavity is to be explored.

Nonsurgical Application

Rectus block may be useful in diagnosing abdominal nerve entrapment syndromes or localized myofascial problems (see Chap. 26).

Complications

Near the xiphoid and pubis, it is difficult to identify the posterior rectus sheath. Attempting this block at these levels may result in penetration of peritoneum and underlying organs such as intensive, bladder, or uterus. In the patient with a distended abdomen, the thinly stretched rectus may prevent clear identification of anterior and posterior sheaths. A visible bulge in the abdominal wall upon injection indicates that the needle is too superficial, and a poor block will result. The block is difficult in the obese, cachectic, or elderly patient with poor abdominal muscle tone.

ILIAC CREST BLOCK

The peripheral extensions of the ilioinguinal, iliohypogastric, and 12th thoracic nerves follow a circular course that is somewhat determined by the bowl-like shape of the ilium. In sweeping around anteriorly, these branches pass near the anterior superior iliac spine — a prominent landmark even in the obese patient. At or near the level of the anterior superior iliac

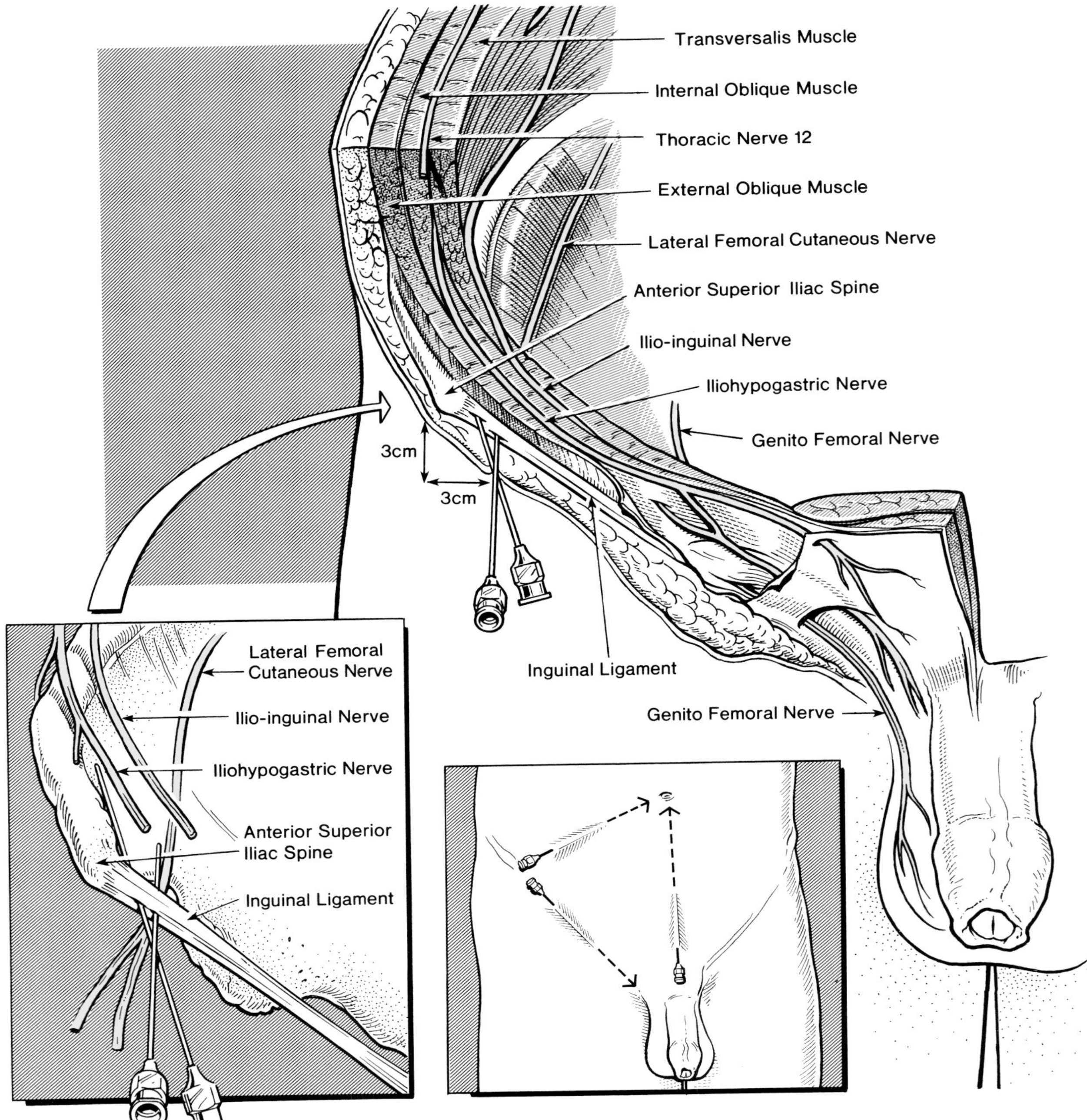

FIG. 14-12. Iliac crest block. **Upper Panel.** Note point of needle insertion 3 cm caudad to and 3 cm medial to anterior superior iliac spine (ASIS). Initial direction of needle is superolateral to reach the inner aspect of iliac bone. Then the needle is redirected approximately perpendicular to the long axis of the body (see also Fig. 14-13*A*). Note the locations of nerves in relation to muscles of the abdominal wall (see text). An alternative technique is to insert the needle 3 cm along a line from ASIS to umbilicus (see Fig. 21-17). **Lower Panel.** *(Left)* Bone and ligamentous landmarks in relation to nerves. *(Right)* Superficial infiltration for herniorrhaphy (see text).

spine, the 12th thoracic and iliohypogastric nerves lie between the internal and external oblique muscles. The ilioinguinal nerve lies between transversus abdominis and internal oblique muscles initially and then penetrates internal oblique a variable distance medial to the anterior superior iliac spine (Fig. 14-12). They continue anteromedially and become superficial as they terminate in branches to skin and muscles of the inguinal region. Using the anterior superior iliac spine as a primary point of orientation, the anesthesiologist can perform an infiltration block known as iliac crest block. Success depends on spreading a large volume of anesthetic solution between abdominal-wall muscle layers. The block is inadequate to provide total anesthesia for inguinal herniorraphy because structures that enter the inguinal canal through the internal inguinal ring will not be anesthetized. These can, however, be very adequately anesthetized by direct infiltration of the spermatic cord by the surgeon (see below).

Technique

The patient lies in the supine position. A point is marked on the skin roughly 3 cm medial and 3 cm inferior to the anterior superior iliac spine (Fig. 4-12). A skin wheal is raised and an 8-cm, 22-gauge needle inserted in a superolateral direction to contact the inner surface of the ilium (Fig. 14-12). Ten milliliters of local anesthetic solution is injected as the needle is slowly withdrawn. Then the needle should be reinserted at a somewhat steeper angle to ensure penetration of all three lateral abdominal muscles. The injection is again repeated as the needle is withdrawn. In the obese or heavily muscled patient, a third injection may be necessary at an even steeper angle. Subcutaneous infiltration superior to the skin wheal, from anterior superior iliac spine to umbilicus, will give a broader area of skin anesthesia as it catches some cutaneous branches of the last two or three intercostal nerves (Fig. 14-12). Infiltration is also extended along the line of the incision. Finally, midline infiltration, from umbilicus to pubis, may be used to block overlapping fibers from the opposite side (Fig. 14-12).

If herniorraphy is to be performed, a second skin wheal may be raised 2 to 3 cm above the midinguinal point. A 5-cm needle is inserted, perpendicular to the skin, to a depth of 3 to 5 cm. Ten milliliters to 15 ml of local anesthetic solution should be injected in fanwise fashion. This produces anesthesia of the genitofemoral nerve, sympathetic fibers, and peritoneal sac. However, there is a risk of hematoma owing to trauma to the femoral artery. Thus it is preferable for the surgeon to inject 2 to 3 ml of local anesthetic directly into the covering of the spermatic cord as soon as it is exposed.

Surgical Application

Iliac crest block is an excellent first maneuver for the surgeon or anesthesiologist who performs infiltration anesthesia for inguinal herniorrhaphy.[33] Although the two injection sites described above may be adequate for herniorrhaphy, additional direct local infiltration may be needed to have a completely pain-free operation. It is especially difficult to anesthetize all the structures in the internal ring or the pubic ramus with a percutaneous injection.

Nonsurgical Application

Iliac crest block may be useful in diagnosing nerve entrapment syndromes following herniorrhaphy.

Complications

Fairly large volumes of local anesthetic solutions can be injected with this block, and the anesthesiologist must use more dilute concentrations of drug as well as watching for signs and symptoms of systemic toxic reaction. It is possible to penetrate peritoneum, intestine, or blood vessels. Aspiration should be performed before each injection. The solution can spread to produce anesthesia of the lateral buttocks, thigh, and front of the leg in the distribution of the femoral nerve. This can interfere with ambulation and complicate an anticipated outpatient procedure.

CAVE OF RETZIUS BLOCK

Anatomy

The variable space located between urinary bladder and symphysis pubis is known as the cave of Retzius. This space contains a great venous plexus, as well as many terminating nerve fibers of the sacral plexus. An infiltration block of this area can be a useful adjunct to anesthesia for prostatectomy or bladder procedures. It will provide analgesia, decrease bleeding if vasoconstrictors are used, and facilitate the surgical dissection.

Technique

A skin wheal is raised 2.5 cm superior to the pubic symphysis. Subcutaneous infiltration can be performed laterally in the line of skin incision for retropubic prostatectomy. A 7- to 8-cm needle is then directed to the posterior aspect of the os pubis and anterior to the bladder. Ten milliliters of local anesthetic solution is injected as the needle reaches its maximum depth and is slowly withdrawn. This process is repeated with two lateral injections made through the same skin wheal (Fig. 14-13).

Surgical Application

The block may be combined with rectus block and infiltration of the incision in the poor-risk patient for prostatectomy.

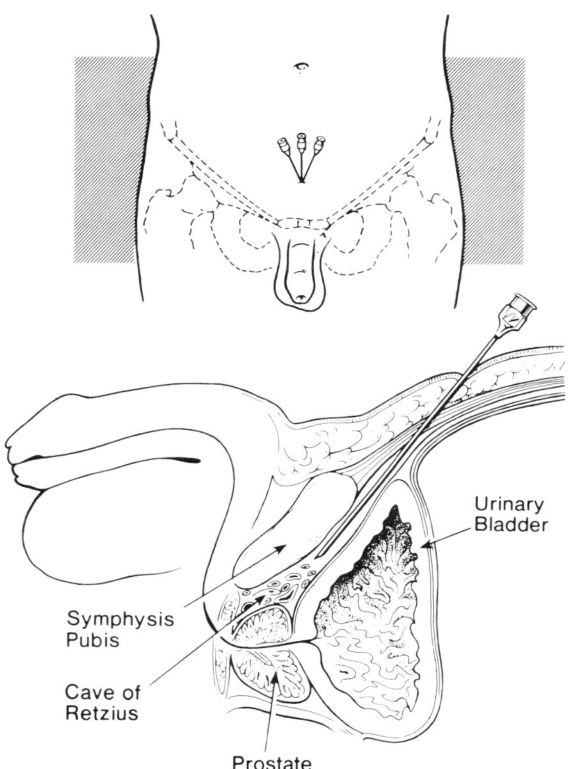

FIG. 14-13. Cave of Retzius' block. **Upper Panel.** Needle insertion immediately superior to pubis, in midline and then with angulation to each side. **Lower Panel.** Lateral view, with patient supine. Note cave to Retzius, containing sympathetic nerves and pampiniform plexus of veins, at posteroinferior aspect of pubis. Note also angulation of needle at approximately 45° to long axis of body.

Nonsurgical Application

There are few useful nonsurgical applications for cave of Retzius block.

Complications

The chief concern is for excessive intravascular injection. Bladder puncture may occur, but it is unlikely unless the block is performed in a patient with distended bladder.

INTRA-ABDOMINAL NERVE BLOCK

Many anesthesiologists become frustrated with regional anesthesia for intra-abdominal operations because the patient experiences pain from manipulation of viscera or from the surgeon's exploring hands. This can occur even if the patient has evidenced no response to skin incision or dissection through the anterior abdominal wall. Once the peritoneal cavity has been entered, there are additional pathways over which pain is transmitted. As previously discussed, these are the afferent pain fibers of the sympathetic and parasympathetic nervous systems. Light general anesthesia, heavy intravenous sedation, and rapid delicate surgical technique are measures calculated to offset the problem. In addition, the surgeon might conceivably be persuaded to inject additional local anesthetic solution to provide the necessary anesthesia. A major drawback to this is that the surgeon must inject and wait when he has an almost irresistible urge to proceed with the operation. Also, potentially toxic amounts of local anesthetic may be used and pain relief may still be incomplete. Despite these objections, the following three procedures might prove useful during the course of laparotomy.

Peritoneal Lavage

Local anesthetic solutions are readily absorbed from mucosal surfaces. Lavage of the peritoneal cavity with large volumes of local anesthetic solution will result in analgesia; however, it is difficult to lavage all peritoneal surfaces. One hundred milliliters to 300 ml of solution (*e.g.*, 0.15% lidocaine or 0.10% bupivacaine) are instilled into the peritoneal cavity. Slight jostling of the abdomen may aid distribution. The Trendelenburg position aids the flow of the solution over the celiac area and often improves analgesia.

Some authors have observed marked shrinking of the intestine after this maneuver. Use of a laparoscope also provides an additional port of entry for the lavage solution and might be a useful adjunct when laparoscopy is being performed.

Vagus Nerve Block

The familiar abbreviation LARP (left anterior, right posterior) indicates that the left vagus is anterior and the right vagus is posterior at the esophageal hiatus. It is possible for the surgeon to infiltrate these nerves directly from the inferior side of the diaphragm. They are deep within the abdomen, and access is not simple; however, infiltration of 10 to 20 ml of dilute anesthetic solution at or near the level of the hiatus will provide marked diminution of sensation from the abdominal cavity.

Celiac Plexus Block

Numerous reports and observations have been made of the celiac plexus reflex during laparotomy. Burstein has vividly described the clinical features of this reflex.[5] It is possible to infiltrate the celiac plexus directly with local anesthetic solution (20–40 ml). The surgeon may not always find this technically easy. Tumor masses, obesity, and the high posterior location of the celiac plexus in the abdomen make direct visualization a challenge. In this situation, however, infiltration of a large volume of solution near the plexus may result in an adequate nerve block. A variation is to wash 40 to 60 ml of anesthetic solution into the upper posterior abdominal cavity. Dilute concentrations of local anesthetic are quite adequate and should be used as previously described.

REFERENCES

1. Baxter, A.D., Flynn, J.F., and Jennings, F.O.: Continuous intercostal nerve blockade. Br. J. Anaesth., *56*:665, 1984.
2. Benumof, J.L., and Semenza, J.: Total spinal anesthesia following intrathoracic intercostal nerve blocks. Anesthesiology, *43*:124, 1975.
2a. Boas, R.A.: Sympathetic blocks in clinical practice. *In* Stanton-Hicks, M. d'A. (ed.): Regional Anesthesia: Advances and Selected Topics, Vol. 16, International Anesthesiology Clinics, pp. 149–182. Boston, Little, Brown, 1978.
3. Bridenbaugh, P.O., DuPen, S.L., Moore, D.C., Bridenbaugh, L.D., *et al.*: Postoperative intercostal nerve block analgesia versus narcotic analgesia. Anesth. Analg. (Cleve.), *52*:81, 1973.
4. Bridenbaugh, P.O., Tucker, G.T., Moore, D.C., Bridenbaugh, L.D., *et al.*: Etidocaine: Clinical evaluation for intercostal nerve block and lumbar epidural block. Anesth. Analg. (Cleve.), *52*:407, 1973.
5. Burstein, C.L.: Fundamental Considerations in Anesthesia, 2nd ed. New York, Macmillan, 1955.
6. Cherry, D.A., and Rao, D.M.: Lumbar sympathetic and coeliac plexus blocks: An anatomical study in cadavers. Br. J. Anaesth., *54*:1037, 1982.
7. Cory, P.C., and Mulroy, M.F.: Postoperative respiratory failure following intercostal block. Anesthesiology, *54*:418, 1981.
8. Crile, G.W., and Lower, W.E.: Anoci-Association. Philadelphia, W. B. Saunders, 1915.
9. deJong, R.H., and Cullen, S.C.: Buffer-demand and pH of local anesthetic solutions containing epinephrine. Anesthesiology, *24*:801, 1963.
10. deJong, R.H., and Heavner, J.E.: Diazepam prevents local anesthetic seizures. Anesthesiology, *34*:523, 1971.
11. deJong, R.H., Heavner, J.E., and deOliveira, L.F.: Effects of nitrous oxide on the lidocaine seizure threshold and diazepam protection. Anesthesiology, *37*:299, 1972.
12. Ellis, H., and McLarty, M.: Anatomy for Anesthetists. Philadelphia, F. A. Davis, 1963.
13. Gray, H.: Anatomy of the Human Body, 29th ed. Philadelphia, Lea & Febiger, 1973.
14. Haugen, F.P.: The autonomic nervous system and pain. Anesthesiology, *29*:785, 1968.
15. Ischia, S., Luzzan, A., Ischia, A., and Faggion, S.: A new approach to the neurolytic block of the celiac plexus: The transaortic technique. Pain, *16*:333, 1983.
16. Jakobson, S., Fridiksson, H., Hedenstrom, H., and Ivarsson, I.: Effects of intercostal nerve blocks on pulmonary mechanics in healthy men. Acta Anaesthesiol. Scand., *24*:482, 1980.
17. Katz, J.: A survey of anesthetic choice among anesthesiologists. Anesth. Analg. (Cleve.), *52*:373, 1973.
18. Kune, G.A., Cole, R., and Bell, S.: Observations on the relief of pancreatic pain. Med. J. Aust., *2*:789, 1975.
19. Kvalheim, L., and Reiestad, F.: Interpleural catheter in the management of postoperative pain. Anesthesiology, *61*:A231, 1984.
20. Lundy, J.S.: Balanced anesthesia. Minn. Med., *9*:399, 1926.
21. Macintosh, R.R., and Bryce Smith, R.: Local Analgesia: Abdominal Surgery, p. 8. Edinburgh, E & S Livingston, 1953.
22. Moore, D.C.: Pontocaine solutions for regional analgesia other than spinal and epidural block: An analysis of 2500 cases. J.A.M.A., *146*:803, 1951.
23. Moore, D.C., and Bridenbaugh, L.D.: Pneumothorax: Its incidence following intercostal nerve block. J.A.M.A., *174*:842, 1960.
24. Moore, D.C., Bridenbaugh, L.D., Bridenbaugh, P.O., and Thompson, G.E.: Bupivacaine hydrochloride: A summary of investigational use in 3274 cases. Anesth. Analg. (Cleve.), *50*:856, 1971.
25. Moore, D.C., Bridenbaugh, L.D., Thompson, G.E., Balfour,

R.I., *et al.*: Factors determining dosages of amide-type local anesthetic drugs. Anesthesiology, *47*:263, 1977.

26. Moore, D.C.: Intercostal nerve block for postoperative somatic pain following surgery of thorax and upper abdomen. Br. J. Anaesth., *47*:284, 1975.

27. Moore, D.C., Bush, W.H., Scurlock, J.E.: Intercostal nerve block: A roentgenographic anatomic study of technique and absorption in humans. Anesth. Analg. (Cleve.), *59*:815, 1980.

27a. Moore, D.C., Bash, W.H., Burnett, L.L.: Celiac plexus block: A roentgenographic, anatomic study of technique and spread of solution in patients and corpses. Anesth. Analg. (Cleve.), *60*:369, 1981.

28. Moore, D.C., and Scurlock, J.E.: Possible role of epinephrine in prevention or correction of myocardial depression associated with bupivacaine. Anesth. Analg. (Cleve.), *62*:450, 1983.

29. Murphy, D.F.: Continuous intercostal nerve blockade: An anatomical study to elucidate its mode of action. Br. J. Anaesth., *56*:627, 1984.

30. Mushin, W.W.: Bilateral vagal block. Proc. R. Soc. Med., *38*:308, 1945.

31. Nunn, J.F., and Slavin, C.: Posterior intercostal nerve block for pain relief after cholecystectomy. Br. J. Anaesth., *52*:253, 1980.

32. Rawal, N., Sjostrand, U.H., Dahlstrom, B., Nydahl, P.A., *et al.*: Epidural morphine for postoperative pain relief: A comparative study with intramuscular narcotic and intercostal nerve block. Anesth. Analg. (Cleve.), *61*:93, 1982.

33. Ryan, J.R., Adye, B.A., Jolly, P.C., and Mulroy, M.F.: Outpatient inquinal herniorrhaphy with both regional and local anesthesia. Am. J. Surg., *148*:313, 1984.

34. Seddon, S.J.: Intercostal nerve block by jet injection. Anaesthesia, *39*:484, 1984.

35. Singler, R.C.: An improved technique for alcohol neurolysis of the celiac plexus. Anesthesiology, *56*:137, 1982.

36. Thompson, G.E., Artin, R., Bridenbaugh, L.D., and Moore, D.C.: Abdominal pain and alcohol celiac plexus nerve block. Anesth. Analg. (Cleve.), *56*:1, 1977.

37. Thompson, G.E., and Moore, D.C.: Ketamine, diazepam and Innovar: A computerized comparative study. Anesth. Analg. (Cleve.), *50*:458, 1971.

38. Tucker, G.T., Moore, D.C., Bridenbaugh, P.O., Bridenbaugh, L.D., *et al.*: Systemic absorption of mepivacaine in commonly used regional block procedures. Anesthesiology, *37*:277, 1972.

39. Walts, L.F., Forsythe, A.B., and Moore, J.G.: Critique: Occupational disease among operating personnel. Anesthesiology, *42*:608, 1975.

40. Ward, E.M., Rorie, D.K., Nauss, L.A., Bahn, R.C.: The celiac ganglion in man: Normal anatomic variations. Anesth. Analg. (Cleve.), *58*:461, 1978.

section D
HEAD AND NECK

15 SOMATIC BLOCKADE OF HEAD AND NECK

TERENCE M. MURPHY

Regional anesthesia for surgery of the head and neck was used extensively before the introduction of endotracheal intubation. With the widespread use of intubation, however, its popularity waned, and it is now used much less frequently for surgical procedures. Nevertheless, there are still many occasions when it can provide an optimal form of anesthesia, either alone or as a complement to general anesthesia, and it can afford excellent analgesia for postoperative recovery and for chronic pain. Also, local anesthetic blocks have been used in elucidating the mechanisms of voice production.[1]

Because of the very compact anatomy and the close relationship of cranial and cervical nerves to many vital structures, meticulous placement of the needle and small discrete doses of the anesthetic agent are usually required for accurate and safe regional anesthesia in this area. The landmarks for regional anesthesia in the head and neck are relatively constant, easily located, and, for anesthesiologists prepared to acquire the skills necessary in using these techniques,[2-5] predictable, so that satisfactory regional anesthesia can be consistently attained.

The trigeminal nerve and the cervical plexus provide cutaneous sensory innervation to the face, head, and neck. In addition, the glossopharyngeal and vagus nerves supply the pharynx and larynx. This chapter discusses mainly the blocks of these cranial and cervical nerves to provide anesthesia for surgery, endoscopic procedures, and endotracheal anesthesia, as well as the use of such blocks in pain states. I also describe the block of the 11th cranial nerve, the accessory nerve.

The pharmacology of the agents used has considerable effect on regional anesthesia in any region of the body, but probably the greatest reason for failure is incorrect placement of the needle. Correct placement can be ensured only by a thorough understanding of the anatomy of the area in which the needle is inserted. Applied anatomic knowledge is of vital importance for success in regional anesthesia generally, and in regional anesthesia of the head and neck particularly. The anesthesiologist who wishes to become skilled in these techniques would do well to consult references 2–5 and, most important, to familiarize himself with the anatomy[6] by dissecting the cadaver or reviewing prosected specimens whenever possible. Frequent recourse to a skull is advisable when learning how to perform these blocks and even as a means of review just before such procedures.

APPLIED ANATOMY

INNERVATION OF THE FACE

The anatomy and complexity of the nerve supply of the face in the adult is perhaps best understood in light of its development in the embryo, as the face forms around the primitive mouth (the stomodeum). Initially, the stomodeum is surrounded caudally by the mandibular arch (which is supplied by the mandibular nerve), laterally on each side by the maxillary processes (which are supplied by the maxillary division of the trigeminal nerve), and rostrally by the forebrain capsule, from which develops the frontonasal process (which is supplied by the first division of the trigeminal nerve, the ophthalmic nerve). The frontonasal process grows down into the primitive stomodeum from the forebrain capsule; this eventually forms the nose of the mature embryo (Fig. 15-1). The two maxillary processes grow inward from either side and join together below the primitive nose, as shown, and they then form the rostral margin of the primitive mouth. Thus, in the mature face, the forehead, eyebrows, upper eyelids, and nose are supplied by the first ophthalmic division of the trigeminal nerve. The lower eyelid, cheek, and upper lip are supplied by the second division (*i.e.*, the maxillary nerve), and the lower lip, chin, mandibular, and temporal regions are supplied by the third division, mandibular nerve. Because of the disproportionate growth of the cranial cavity in humans, these dermatomal distributions are distorted cranially, with the result that some skin innervated by the cervical plexus is drawn up over the angle of the mandible onto the face and posteriorly over the occipital area and the scalp as far forward as the vertex, as shown in Figure 15-2.

TRIGEMINAL NERVE DISTRIBUTION

The first division of the trigeminal nerve, the ophthalmic (V_1), is primarily distributed to the forehead and nose; the second division, the maxillary (V_2), supplies the upper jaw; and the third division, or mandibular nerve (V_3), supplies the lower jaw (Fig. 15-2).

The gasserian ganglion lies posteromedially in the middle cranial fossa at the junction of its floor and the cavernous sinus. The ganglion invaginates the dura and therefore lies in a dural pouch—Meckel's cave, which contains cerebrospinal fluid (CSF). An injection of local anesthetic or neurolytic agent into the ganglion area can potentially spread to, or accidentally be injected into, this pouch, and therefore into the CSF. This can lead to the spread of analgesia to other adjacent cranial nerves (*e.g.*, abducens, facial) and even total spinal anesthesia. Therefore meticulous aspiration and small (0.25 ml) test doses are mandatory (see Fig. 15-6).

OPHTHALMIC NERVE

In its intracranial course, the trunk of the ophthalmic nerve does not lend itself to regional anesthesia. The intraorbital branches of the nasociliary nerve are blocked by retrobulbar block (see Chap. 17). The intraorbital branches, anterior ethmoidal and infratrochlear, can also be blocked in the orbit (Fig. 15-3).

The terminal divisions in the forehead and nose are suitable for the peripheral nerve blocks of the face (Fig. 15-3).

The mandibular and maxillary divisions can be blocked as they leave the cranial cavity for their respective destinations.

MAXILLARY NERVE

To reach the upper jaw, this nerve leaves the cranial cavity by way of the foramen rotundum and traverses the pterygomaxillary fossa. (This compartment is also referred to as the *pterygopalatine fossa*). This is bounded anteriorly by the maxilla, medially by the palatine bone, and posteriorly by the pterygoid process of the sphenoid bone (see Fig. 15-6). The nerve crosses the fossa anterolaterally to enter the floor of the orbit at the inferior orbital fissure. It can be blocked as it lies in the fossa, producing anesthesia of the upper jaw, the lateral nasal wall, and most of the nasal septum. The superior anterior part of both septum and lateral wall of the nose receive contributions from the anterior ethmoidal branch of the ophthalmic nerve. The entire hard palate is supplied by the maxillary nerve through the sphenopalatine ganglion.

MANDIBULAR NERVE

The mandibular nerve emerges from the cranial cavity through the floor of the middle cranial fossa by way of the foramen ovale to enter the infratemporal fossa. This fossa is a rectangular compartment bounded anteriorly by the posterior wall of the maxilla and posteriorly by the styloid apparatus and carotid sheath. The lateral wall is the ramus and coronoid process of the mandible, and the medial wall is composed anteriorly by the lateral pterygoid plate and posteriorly by the constrictor muscles of the pharynx. It has no floor, but the roof is the floor of the middle cranial fossa in the form of the infratemporal surface of the greater wing of the sphenoid bone. In the infratemporal fossa, the mandibular nerve divides into its terminal branches. Block of the nerve at this site results in anesthesia of the lower jaw, the tongue, and lower teeth; the buccal surface of the cheek; and the skin overlaying the lower jaw, the temporal region, and the anterior superior two thirds

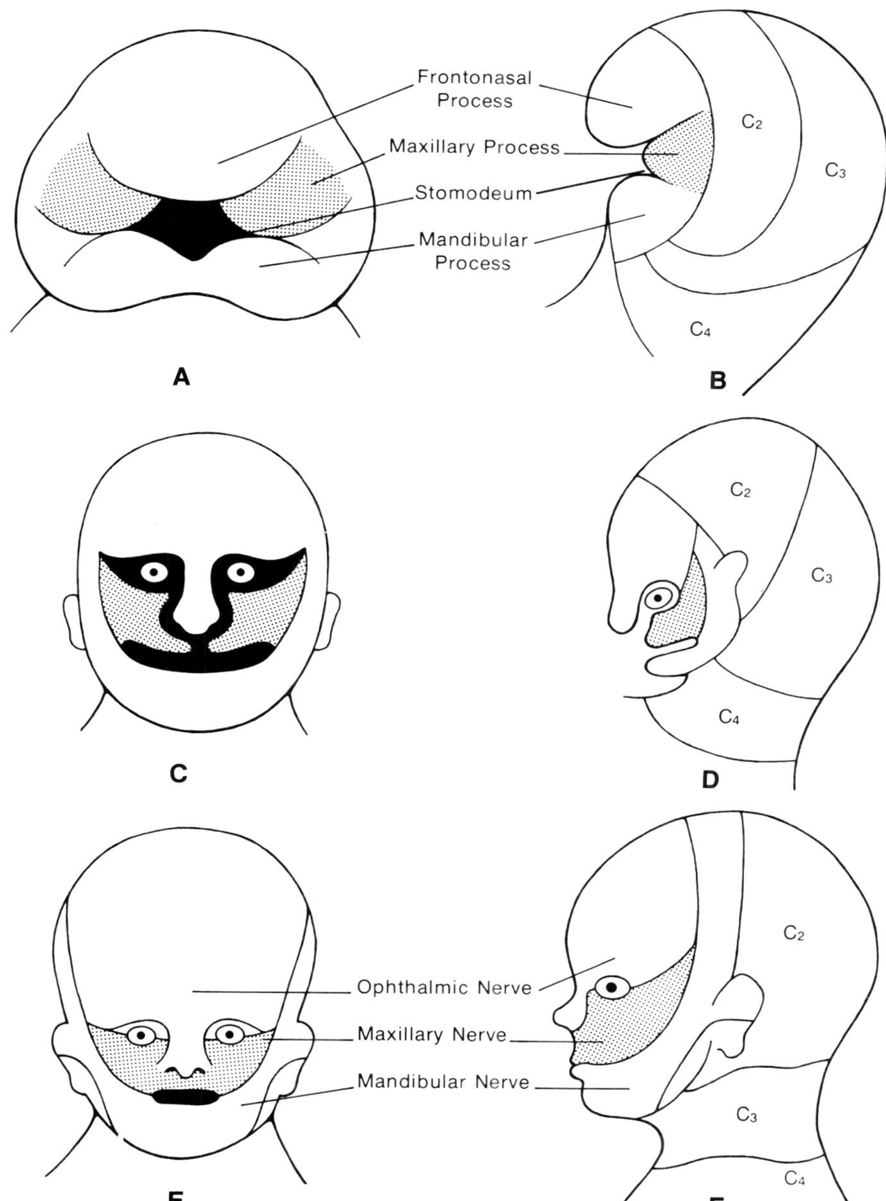

FIG. 15-1. Frontal and lateral views of development of dermatomes of the head and neck. **A, B.** The primitive stomodeum (mouth) is surrounded by the three parts of the developing face. **C, D.** The frontonasal process (supplied by the ophthalmic nerve) grows in from above, the maxillary processes (maxillary nerve) grow in from each side, and the mandibular process (mandibular nerve) forms the caudal margin. **E, F.** The frontonasal process forms the brow, eyebrows, upper eyelid, and nose in the fully developed face. The maxillary process forms both cheeks, lower eyelid, and upper lip. The mandibular process gives rise to the lower lip, the chin, and a strip of skin extending up the side of the face, often to the vertex, including the superior anterior two thirds of the anterior surface of the ear. The cervical plexus derivatives of the second, third, and fourth cervical nerves supply the posterior part of the head and neck from the vertex down. Note in **F** that the skin over the angle of the jaw and the lower part of the auricle on the anterior surface and all of its posterior surface are supplied by cervical plexus dermatomes (C_2).

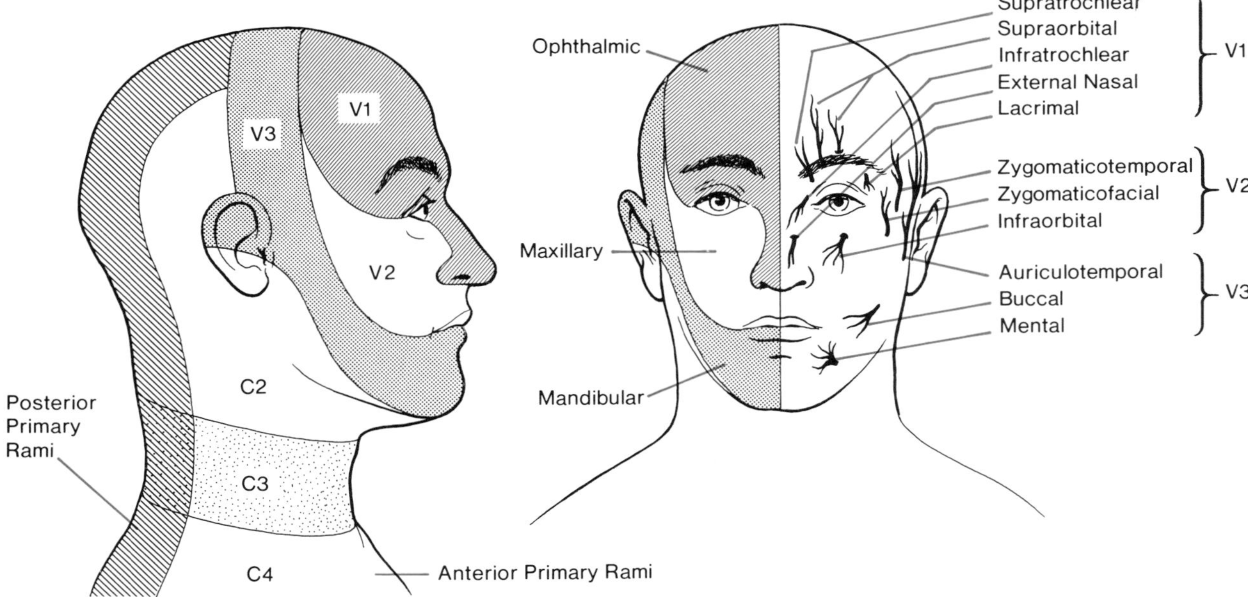

FIG. 15-2. Dermatomes and cutaneous nerves of head, neck, and face. Note that the supraorbital, infraorbital, and mental nerves all lie in the same vertical plane as the pupil, with the eye looking straight forward. The external nasal area is innervated by infratrochlear and external nasal (from anterior ethmoidal *n.*) branches of V1 and the infraorbital branch of V2. The internal nasal cavity is shown in Figure 15-4.

of the surface of the external ear. This nerve can be blocked relatively easily by introducing a needle into the infratemporal fossa through the coronoid notch of the mandible (see Fig. 15-6). It can also be blocked by an intraoral approach (see Chap. 16).

INNERVATION OF EYEBALL AND ORBIT

Innervation of the eye, neural blockade procedures for ocular branches of the trigeminal nerve, and topical analgesia for eye surgery are discussed in Chapter 17.

Local and regional anesthesia lends itself very well to eye surgery, especially in those parts of the world where safe general anesthesia is not readily available. Regional anesthesia is much used also by many ophthalmologists in advanced medial communities for a variety of reasons, including satisfactory analgesia, surgical convenience, and economy. This topic is discussed in more detail in Chapter 17 and for the most part involves blockade of the sensory input to the globe by means of anesthesia of the optic nerve in the posterior part of the orbit, introducing a needle either traditionally along the inferolateral aspects of the orbit or, as has been described more recently, along the superomedial aspect of the orbit.[7] In addition to the retrobulbar anesthesia, these patients also require akinesia, that is, paralysis of the facial and extraocular muscles to prevent compression of the globe during open surgical procedures and to prevent risking extrusion of the globe contents. This is usually achieved by infiltrating the branches of the facial nerve as they cross the zygomatic bone and involves infiltration of a weak local anesthetic solution both lateral and inferior to the margin of the orbit. The facial nerve can also be anesthetized as it crosses the mandibular condyle and can be identified anterior to the ear by asking the patient to open and close his mouth. A needle is inserted through the skin at the point overlying the junction of the superior and middle third of the ramus of the mandible and the nerve is infiltrated by injecting 2 to 3 ml of local anesthetic solution at this point (see Chap. 17).

Although with more ambitious and lengthy ophthalmologic surgical procedures general anesthesia has been used more and more in this subspecialty

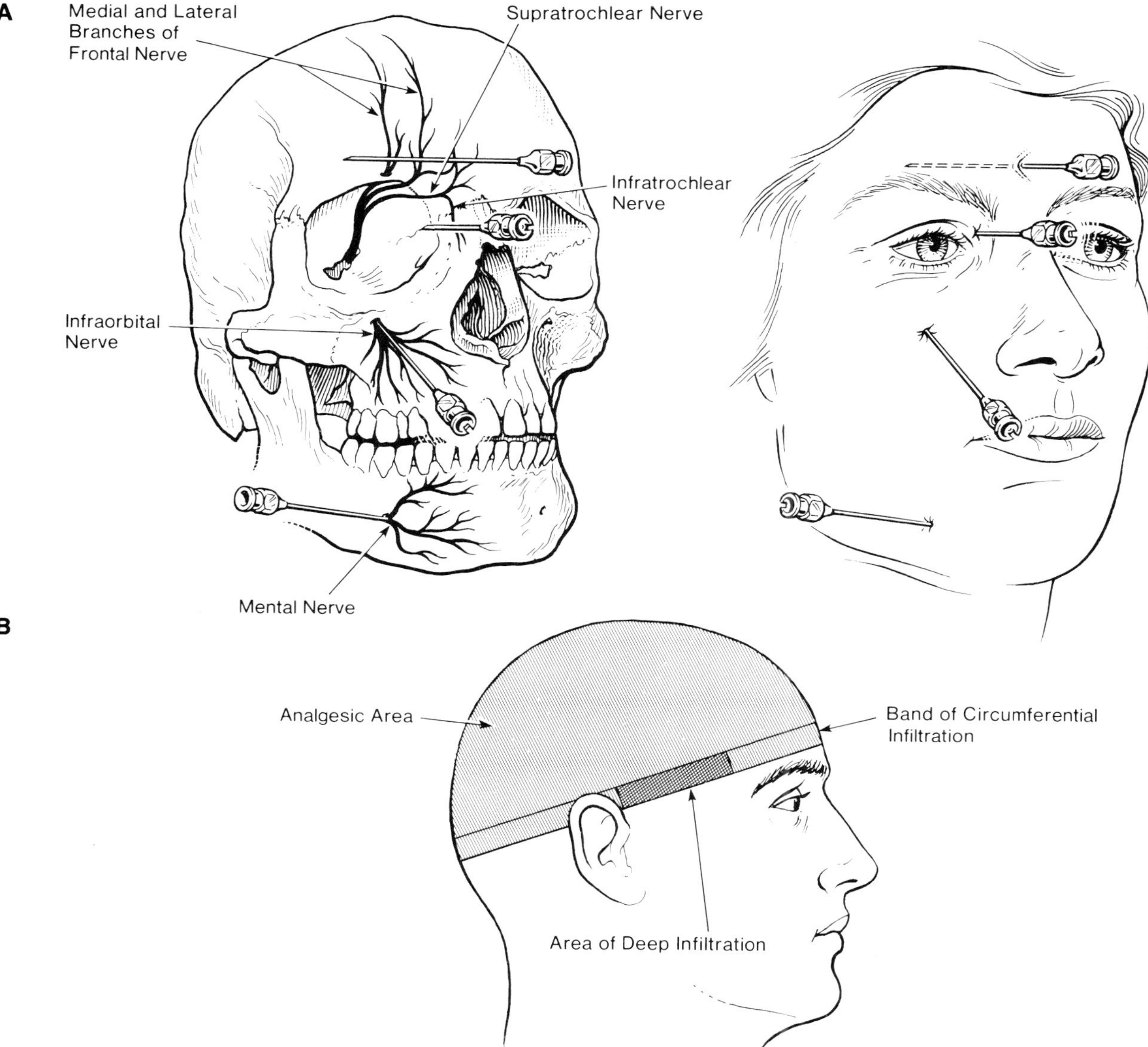

FIG. 15-3. **A.** Nerve block of the superficial branches of the trigeminal nerve. *The supraorbital and supratrochlear* branches of the first division (ophthalmic) can be blocked as they emerge above the orbit. A single needle insertion in the midbrow above the root of the nose can anesthetize the forehead bilaterally by infiltrations on either side through the same insertion. Note that this injection needs to be undertaken above the level of the eyebrow to prevent periorbital hematoma. *The infratrochlear nerve* (and also anterior ethmoidal nerve) is blocked by inserting a needle 1 cm above the inner canthus and just lateral to the medial wall of the orbit. The needle is directed posteriorly and slightly medially to a depth of about 2.5 cm. *The infraorbital nerve* is located one fingerbreadth below the orbital rim in the same vertical position as the pupil with the eye looking forward. To enter the infraorbital foramen, advance the needle cephalad and laterally. It is not necessary, however, to enter the foramen but just to infiltrate the nerve as it emerges at the foramen. *The mental nerve* is anesthetized again in the same vertical line as the pupil; to enter the mental foramen, direct the needle medially as shown in the diagram. The mental foramen lies at a different vertical level in the mandible at different ages (see text). **B.** *Circumferential infiltration of scalp* (see text). Note that infiltration is superficial except in the temporal region where infiltration deep to deep fascia is useful to help prevent movement of the temporalis muscle during surgery. If periosteum will be stimulated, injection must be made deep to deep fascia.

field, local anesthesia still has much to commend it. A recent large review[8] of 10,000 ophthalmological operations identified a subgroup of 288 operations on individuals with previous myocardial infarction who were operated on under regional anesthesia for ophthalmologic surgery, and there was no incidence of reinfarction, suggesting that regional anesthesia (which has been long used in ophthalmologic surgery) may also offer a protective value to patients who have previously had myocardial infarction.

THE NOSE

The external nose requires blockade at three sites: above the inner canthus of the eyelid, at the infraorbital foramen, and at the junction of nasal bone and cartilage (see Fig. 15-3). The nasal cavity is also conveniently blocked at two primary sites: the sphenopalatine ganglion and the point of entry of the anterior ethmoidal nerve at the anterior end of the cribriform plate (Fig. 15-4). Fortunately, both of these sites are high in the nasal cavity in the region known as the *sphenoethmoidal recess.* If the skull is turned upside down, local anesthetic solution instilled by way of the nose pools in this area. Thus both sites of innervation can be blocked simultaneously. The small remaining area on the floor of the nasal cavity innervated by anterior superior alveolar nerve (VII) requires topical local application by holding the nares together after instilling local anesthetic or by direct application (see below).

Innervation of Nasal Sinuses

Maxillary sinus
Maxillary nerve (V_2) and sphenopalatine ganglion
Ethmoidal sinus
Nasociliary nerve (from V_1) by way of anterior and posterior ethmoidal branches
Frontal sinus
Frontal nerve (from V_1)

Thus drainage of the maxillary sinus by an oral approach (Caldwell–Luc) under neural blockade requires maxillary nerve block. Infiltration of the line of the incision over the canine fossa with local anesthetic solution containing epinephrine improves hemostasis. Sometimes the operation of Caldwell–Luc extends to the ethmoidal sinus so that anterior ethmoidal block is also necessary.

CUTANEOUS INNERVATION OF HEAD AND NECK

The cutaneous supply of the head and neck derives from the three divisions of the trigeminal nerve (see below) and from the cervical plexus (see Figs. 15-2; 15-9–15-11).

CERVICAL PLEXUS

The cervical plexus contributes to the nerve supply of both the deep and superficial structures of the neck. The first cervical nerve, C1, is a motor nerve to the muscles of the suboccipital triangle and has no sensory distribution to skin. The skin of the neck is supplied in sequential dermatomal pattern (like the trunk) by the cutaneous branches of C2–C4 by both anterior and posterior primary rami (see Fig. 15-2).

In the neck, all of the cutaneous nerve supply derives from the cervical plexus and can be blocked by a single injection of the superficial cervical plexus at the midpoint of the posterior border of the sternomastoid muscle or by single-injection blockade of the deep cervical plexus (see Figs. 15-11 and 10-7). The latter has the advantage of also blocking the branches of the posterior primary rami if analgesia is required toward the back of the neck; however, it is associated with phrenic nerve palsy.

Blockade of the deep cervical plexus is essentially a paravertebral block in which the needle is inserted and positioned in relation to the transverse processes of the appropriate cervical vertebrae. Because of the obliquity of the transverse processes of the cervical vertebrae, it is important to direct the needle in a caudad fashion. To do otherwise risks entering the spinal canal at this site and thereby, perhaps, producing profound epidural or spinal anesthesia, or even worse—damage to the spinal cord (see Fig. 15-11 and Chap. 10).

Because of the course of the vertebral artery—through the foramina transversaria in each transverse process—it is especially at risk and a potential site for unintentional intravascular injection. Even a very small amount of local anesthetic agent (0.2 ml) injected into this vessel can produce profound toxic effects of convulsions, presumably because of high cerebral blood levels (see Chap. 22).[9]

In the *region of the scalp,* the nerves of supply have long superficial upward courses. Four sensory nerves pass in front of the ear to the scalp (supratrochlear and supraorbital from V_1; zygomaticotemporal from V_2; auriculotemporal from V_3), and four pass behind

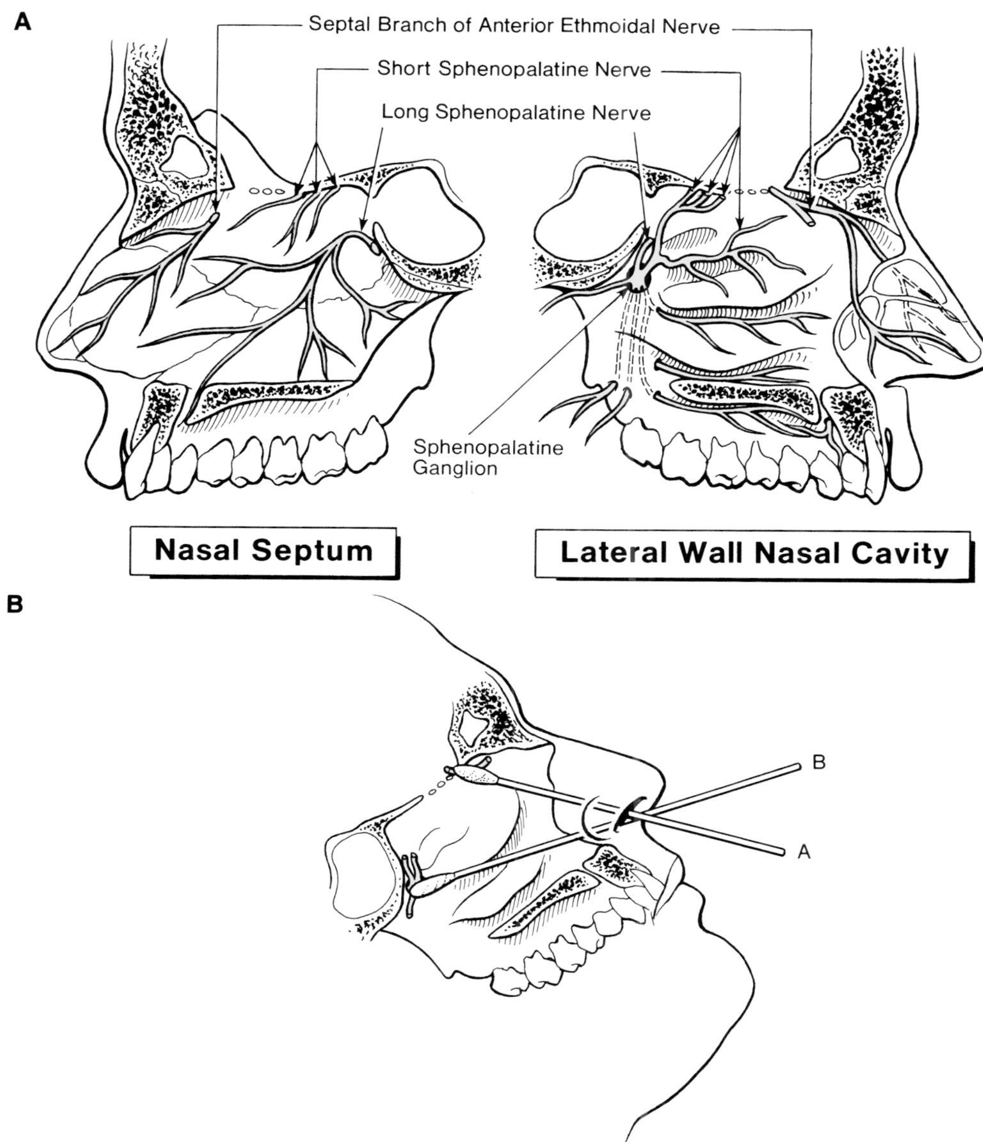

FIG. 15-4. Nerve supply of nasal septum and lateral wall of nasal cavity. Pledgets of cotton wool are soaked in local anesthetic and inserted as shown to contact branches of the anterior ethmoidal nerve **(A)** and the sphenopalatine ganglion and nerves **(B)**. Note pledget A is inserted parallel with the line of the external nose until it reaches the superior extent of the nasal cavity. Pledget B is inserted about 20° to 30° with the horizontal line through the floor of the nose to reach the region of the sphenopalatine foramen.

the ear (great auricular and greater, lesser, and least occipital nerves from cervical plexus). All eight nerves converge toward the vertex of the scalp and are effectively blocked if a band of local anesthetic is infiltrated from the glabella, above the ear to the occiput (Fig. 15-3). Infiltration is made with 0.5% to 1% lidocaine immediately beneath the skin in the subcutaneous tissue. It is useful to inject some solution into the temporalis muscle to prevent undue movement of the muscle during procedures on the scalp. Injection next to the periosteum is required only if bone is to be removed.

In the face, cutaneous branches are short and radiate. Thus, in this area, blockade of individual branches is more satisfactory than "barrage" block. For example, the skin below the eye as far as the upper lip can be anesthetized by infraorbital block (see below).

STYLOID APPARATUS—GLOSSOPHARYNGEAL NERVE

The styloid process is the landmark used in blocking the glossopharyngeal nerve. It is the calcified rostral end of the stylohyoid ligament, and it varies considerably in length from patient to patient. Its tip lies about halfway between the angle of the mandible and the mastoid process and provides a bony landmark when blocks of the glossopharyngeal nerve are planned (see Fig. 15-7). This nerve emerges from the jugular foramen posterior and medial to the styloid process. It exits from the foramen anterior to the 10th and 11th cranial nerves and sweeps down parallel with the posterior border of the styloid process and at a slightly deeper plane. Therefore by "walking" the needle until it just slips off the posterior aspect of the styloid process, the ninth cranial nerve can be blocked (usually along with the 10th and 11th cranial nerves as well). The large vascular conduits of the internal jugular vein and internal carotid artery are very closely related to this nerve at this point, and care must be exercised to avoid injecting into these vessels.

The glossopharyngeal nerve supplies the posterior third of the tongue and the oropharynx from its junction with the nasopharynx at the level of the hard palate. It supplies the pharyngeal surfaces of the soft palate and the epiglottis, the fauces, and the pharyngeal wall as far down as the pharyngoesophageal junction at the level of the cricoid cartilage (C6).

INNERVATION OF THE LARYNX—VAGUS NERVE

The vagus nerve supplies sensation to the larynx. The undersurface of the epiglottis and the laryngeal inlet down to the vocal folds are supplied by the internal laryngeal branch of the vagus. This nerve reaches the larynx by piercing the thyrohyoid membrane, which joins the thyroid to the hyoid cartilages. By blocking its parent nerve (the superior laryngeal branch of the vagus) below the tip of the greater cornu of the hyoid bone, the laryngeal inlet can be rendered insensitive down to the vocal cords. Below the cords, the larynx and trachea are supplied by the recurrent laryngeal branch of the vagus that ascends in the neck in the groove between the trachea and esophagus. Although the nerve can be blocked in this groove (and frequently is as a complication of stellate ganglion block), anesthesia of the trachea is usually effected by spray techniques, either transorally or by percutaneous puncture at the cricothyroid membrane. The recurrent laryngeal nerve also supplies motor function to all the intrinsic muscles of the larynx (except the cricothyroid muscle), and bilateral motor block produces loss of phonation and loss of ability to close the glottis (Fig. 15-8).

INNERVATION OF MOUTH AND PHARYNX

A detailed description of the innervation of teeth and mouth is given in Chapter 17, along with appropriate neural blockade techniques.

INNERVATION OF TONSIL

The tonsil and its surroundings are innervated by the lesser palatine nerve (from V_2), the lingual nerve (from V_3), and the glossopharyngeal nerve by way of the pharyngeal plexus.

Thus it is most practical to denervate the tonsillar fossa by infiltration around the tonsil rather than by blocking individual nerves. This is usually preceded by requesting the patient to suck viscous local anesthetic solutions. Alternatively infiltration can be carried out in association with sedation or light general anesthesia.[10]

TRIGEMINAL NERVE BLOCK

GASSERIAN GANGLION BLOCK

Gasserian ganglion block results in extensive anesthesia of the ipsilateral face over the area shown in Figure 15-2. It was once used extensively for surgery of the head and neck. With the advent of endotracheal intubation and more sophisticated techniques of general anesthesia, however, its appeal as a primary surgical anesthetic declined, but it is still used diagnostically and therapeutically for neuralgias of

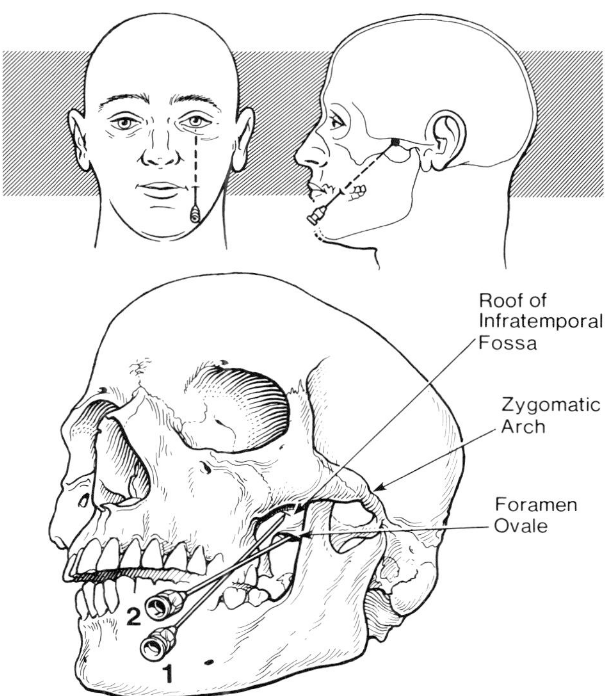

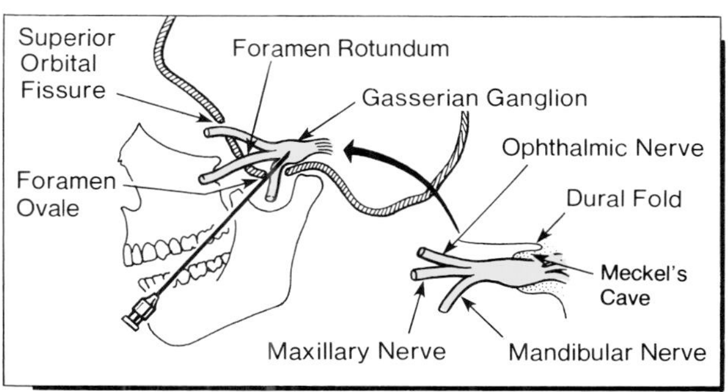

FIG. 15-5. Gasserian ganglion block. **Top Panel.** Note that the needle is inserted in the cheek about 1 cm posterior to the angle of the mouth as shown and directed toward the pupil in the anterior view and the midpoint of the zygoma in the lateral view. In patients with teeth, needle insertion in the cheek is superficial to the teeth of the upper jaw. In edentulous patients this may lie a variable distance between the angle of the mouth and a line midway between upper lip and nose. A palpating finger in the mouth helps to prevent needle penetration into the mouth. **Middle Panel.** As the needle is advanced into the infratemporal fossa, it will usually strike the roof of the infratemporal fossa initially *(1)*; this is the correct depth to seek the foramen ovale. The needle is then directed slightly posteriorly *(2)* to obtain a mandibular nerve *(V3)* paresthesia. **Lower Panel.** The needle can then be advanced through the foramen ovale into the middle cranial fossa where it will be adjacent to the gasserian ganglion as shown. Note the relationships of the dural fold and Meckel's cave containing cerebrospinal fluid. A needle advanced too far through the foramen ovale can enter the Meckel's cave, and subsequent injections could enter the cranial CSF and produce total spinal anesthesia (see text).

the trigeminal system. It has merit as a diagnostic block, a permanent neurolytic block, and as a means of introducing heated probes for the newer technique of thermogangliolysis (see Chaps. 29, 30).[11]

Anatomy

Lying at the apex of the petrous temporal bone at the junction of middle and posterior cranial fossa, the ganglion is situated in a fold of dura mater that forms an invagination around the posterior two thirds of the ganglion. This invagination is in continuity with the CSF and bears the name of Meckel's cave or the cavum trigeminale. It is reached with a needle by traversing the infratemporal fossa and entering the middle cranial fossa by way of the foramen ovale. Medially, the gasserian ganglion is bounded by the cavernous venous sinus, which contains the carotid artery and the third, fourth, and sixth cranial nerves. Superiorly is the inferior surface of the temporal lobe of the brain, and posteriorly the brain stem. Any of these structures might be damaged by the introduction of the needle through the foramen ovale. Also, because the ganglion is partially bathed in CSF, injections into the area might spread into the spinal fluid and hence produce a remote effect on other parts of the central nervous system (CNS) (Fig. 15-5).

Technique

An 8- to 10-cm, 22-gauge needle is required for gasserian ganglion block. The point of introduction of the needle is about one fingerbreadth posterior to the lateral margin of the mouth, next to the medial border of the masseter muscle. In edentulous patients, this landmark may not allow a sufficient angle of approach to the foramen ovale, and therefore a point of insertion more caudad is needed. The direction of the needle is both rostral and medial to a point that coincides with the midpoint of the zygomatic arch from the lateral aspect and the pupil from the anterior view (with the eyes looking straight forward), as in Figure 15-5. It is important to keep a guiding finger in the oral cavity, palpating the cheek to ensure that the needle does not enter the mouth and thereby potentially introduce contaminating bacteria into deeper structures. Such an approach will usually result in impingement of the needle on the roof of the infratemporal fossa (*i.e.*, the base of the skull, which is also the floor of the middle cranial fossa). The needle is then adjusted until it slips through the foramen ovale; usually just before this, a mandibular nerve paresthesia is obtained in the lower jaw or lip. This maneuver is optimally performed under radiographic control, so that the needle and its path through the foramen ovale can be visualized.

Having entered the foramen ovale, the needle should not be advanced more than 1 cm, and usually its advance is guided by the appropriate paresthesia. Initially, there will be a third division mandibular paresthesia, but this can occur while the needle is still in the infratemporal fossa. It is necessary to obtain a second division or first division paresthesia to the upper jaw or frontal area of the face, respectively, to confirm that the needle is, in fact, in the immediate vicinity of the gasserian ganglion. A stimulating device may be used to confirm the position of the needle in patients who are unable to locate the paresthesia accurately. This is, of course, a painful procedure, and it is not inappropriate, perhaps, to administer some intravenous analgesic, for example, 0.05 mg of fentanyl, as a preoperative medication. For diagnostic blocks, however, it is better not to cloud the sensorium with any analgesics in order to obtain a more accurate assessment of the block. Before injection, aspiration tests are, of course, mandatory to ensure that the needle has not entered a blood vessel or, more likely, Meckel's cave with its CSF contents. If these aspiration tests are negative, then the anesthetizing agent, either a local anesthetic (1% lidocaine or the equivalent) or neurolytic agent, is injected in small aliquots (*e.g.*, 0.25 ml at a time) until the desired analgesic effect has been obtained. If injection affords evidence of analgesia in only one of the divisions, then adjustment of the needle can sometimes affect spread to the other divisions in patients in whom the needle is in the same vertical axis as the ganglion. There appear to be some patients, however, in whom the ganglion lies at a more horizontal axis, and in these patients it is sometimes difficult, if not impossible, to obtain a first division paresthesia.

Complications

Depending on the manipulations needed to produce satisfactory block, the patient's face will quite frequently be painful for the following few days, and there is often bruising at the injection site. This usually responds well to treatment with systemic analgesics. Probably the most serious side-effect is injection of local anesthetic or neurolytic agents into the CSF contained within Meckel's cave and its resulting spillover into the circulating CSF of the cranial cavity. In our clinic, injections of as little as 0.25 ml of 1% lidocaine have resulted in unconsciousness and profound paralysis of the ipsilateral cranial nerve system, albeit temporary, but the patient has needed cardiorespiratory support for a brief period (10 minutes). If a hyperbaric solution is used (*e.g.*, 1.5% or 2% lidocaine with 10% dextrose or phenol in glycerine), then the drug that emerges from Meckel's cavity will tend to flow over the free margin of the tentorium cerebelli to affect immediately the 6th, 8th, 9th, 10th, 11th, and 12th cranial nerves and usually consciousness also. With neurolytic agents, there is a potential hazard of spread to these nerves, so that meticulous attention to aspiration tests and perhaps even a test injection of a small dose of local anesthetic is appropriate before the injection of any neurolytic substances. If hypobaric solutions are used (*e.g.*, 1% lidocaine without dextrose, or alcohol), then the flow will tend to be cephalad, involving probably the trochlear and oculomotor nerves initially and almost certainly affecting consciousness to a variable extent.

OPHTHALMIC NERVE BRANCHES: SUPRAORBITAL AND SUPRATROCHLEAR NERVES

Supraorbital and supratrochlear nerve analgesia is a very simple block that can effect excellent analgesia of the forehead and scalp back to the vertex. It is a simple and safe form of anesthesia for minor surgical procedures in this area (*e.g.*, repair of lacerations, removal of cysts). The terminal divisions of the ophthalmic branch of the trigeminal nerve involved are the supraorbital and supratrochlear branches, which emerge from within the orbit. The supraorbital branch, like the infraorbital and mental nerves, lies in the same vertical plane as that of the pupil when the patient is looking straight ahead (see Fig. 15-3). A block of this nerve is best effected above the eyebrow after the nerve has emerged from the orbit through the supraorbital notch. A small dose of 2 to 4 ml of local anesthetic infiltrated between the skin and frontal bone will usually produce satisfactory anesthesia. The other terminal branch that supplies the forehead is the supratrochlear nerve, which emerges from the superomedial angle of the orbit and runs up the forehead parallel to the supraorbital nerve, a fingerbreadth or so medial to it. This nerve is blocked as it emerges above the eyebrow or can be involved by a medial extension of the anesthetic wheal used to block the supraorbital nerve. (Retrobulbar block is described in Chapter 17.)

COMBINED INFRATROCHLEAR AND ANTERIOR ETHMOIDAL NERVE BLOCK

The nasociliary nerve divides into its terminal branches, anterior ethmoidal and infratrochlear nerves, on the medial wall of the orbit 2.5 cm from the orbital margin. Both branches are blocked by inserting a 5-cm, 25-gauge needle 1 cm above the inner canthus. The needle is directed backward and slightly medially to pass just lateral to the inner wall of the orbit and medial to the eyeball and medial rectus muscle (Fig. 15-3). Depth of insertion is 2.5 cm, and at this point 1 ml of 2% lidocaine, or equivalent, is injected as the needle is slowly withdrawn (see Chap. 17). Orbital veins are easily damaged, resulting in proptosis; thus small-gauge needles should be used and repeated insertion avoided. The infratrochlear nerve can be blocked by infiltrating at the superomedial border of the orbit and along its medial wall with 2 to 4 ml of local anesthetic. The external nasal branch of the anterior ethmoidal nerve can also be blocked by infiltration at the junction of nasal bone with cartilage. Anterior ethmoidal and infratrochlear nerve blocks accompanied with an infraorbital nerve block can be very effective when they are performed bilaterally for plastic surgical procedures and reduction operations on the nose.

If the mucous membrane of the nose is likely to be stimulated, as in reduction of fractured nose, then branches of the anterior ethmoidal nerve and sphenopalatine ganglion that supply the septum and lateral wall of the nose should be blocked by topical application of local anesthetic. (see Fig. 15-4).

TOPICAL ANALGESIA OF NASAL CAVITIES

As noted in the description of nerve supply, only two main sites require blockade: the sphenopalatine ganglion and the anterior ethmoidal nerve, both located in the region of the sphenoethmoidal recess (see Fig. 15-4).

Applicators. Macintosh[4] described a technique with 25% cocaine paste applied with nasal probes or applicators. Prior spraying of the nasal cavities with 0.5 ml of 5% cocaine solution on each side provides some shrinking of the mucous membrane and makes the insertion of the applicators more comfortable for the patient. The anesthesiologist then uses a headlight and nasal speculum and gradually applies cocaine paste upward and backward in the nasal cavity. Insertion should initially be close to the septum to avoid injuring the lateral wall. Finally, one applicator is inserted parallel to the anterior border of the nasal cavity until it reaches the anterior end of the cribriform plate at a depth of about 5 cm. A second applicator is inserted at an angle of about 20° to the floor of the nose until bone is felt at a depth of about 6 to 7 cm. The end of the applicator should now lie close to the sphenopalatine foramen. The two applicators are left in place for 10 to 15 minutes, and the patient is asked to breathe through the mouth. Cocaine pastes of 10% are also available and are preferable if bilateral blocks are to be performed. The total dose of solution and paste administered should not exceed 200 mg (*e.g.*, 1 ml of 5% solution [50 mg]; 1.5 ml of 10% paste [150 mg]).

Because of the danger of overdose, some now prefer to use a 10% lidocaine spray for initial anesthesia (20 mg/puff) and then 5% to 10% lidocaine solution up to a maximum dose of 500 mg.

Instillation into sphenoethmoidal recess is unsatisfactory if the mucous membrane is grossly thickened or other abnormalities exist. Also, it requires the patient to lie with his head upside down, which is distressing to many patients.

Technique. The mucous membrane is initially sprayed with local anesthetic solution, as described under Applications. The patient is then placed supine with a pillow under the shoulders and the neck extended so that the skull is upside down. The patient is told to breathe through the mouth. A blunt-nosed 10-cm cannula with a 120° angle at its midpoint is inserted through the nares until the angle lies at the external nares. The cannula is now swiveled, keeping close to the septum, until the end reaches the roof of the nose. Local anesthetic (*e.g.*, 2 ml of 5% cocaine or 2 ml of 10% lidocaine) is injected. The procedure is repeated on the other side. The position is maintained for 10 minutes, and the patient rolls supine, while holding the nares pinched, and lets the solution run out the external nares. Injections into the nasal cavity

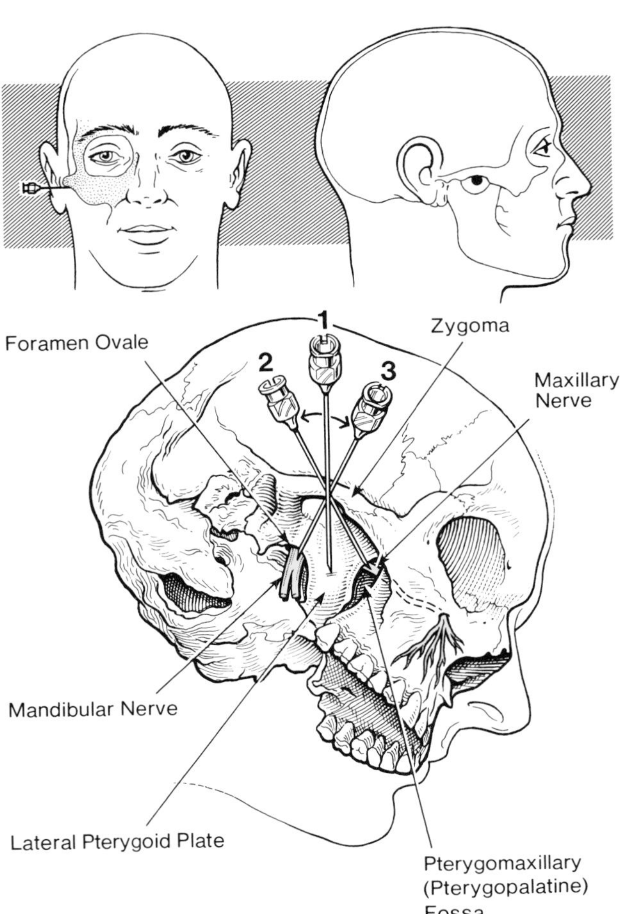

FIG. 15-6. **Upper Panel.** The coronoid notch is located below the midpoint of the zygoma. A finger is placed at this point and the patient asked to open his mouth. The condyle of the mandible should be palpable immediately deep to the fingertip as the mouth opens. The fingertip should then sink into the coronoid notch as the mouth is closed. **Lower Panel.** The maxillary and mandibular nerves are approached by way of the coronoid notch below the midpoint of zygoma. *(1)* The needle passes through the infratemporal fossa to reach the lateral pterygoid plate. Initial direction of the needle should be medial and slightly anterior. *(2)* The needle is then walked anteriorly until it passes into the pterygomaxillary (pterygopalatine) fossa, where the maxillary nerve is blocked. *(3)* The needle is then walked from position *(1)* posteriorly until it passes just posterior to the lateral pterygoid plate to block the mandibular nerve as it emerges from the foramen ovale. The needle point is kept at the same depth as the lateral pterygoid plate to prevent accidental introduction of the needle into the posterior pharynx.

do have significant potential for spread beyond same. Attempts to anesthetize the anterior ethmoidal nerve close to the cribriform plate have resulted in total spinal anesthesia,[12] and it may be that this technique could be performed more safely with the application of anesthetic-soaked pledgets inserted into the nose.

MAXILLARY NERVE

BLOCK OF MAIN TRUNK IN PTERYGOPALATINE FOSSA

As it crosses the pterygopalatine fossa, the maxillary nerve is usually blocked by a lateral approach. The resulting block will produce profound anesthesia of the upper jaw and its teeth on the ipsilateral side of the face (Fig. 15-6).

Technique. The nerve is approached by way of the infratemporal fossa, and the needle is inserted in the skin at a point below the midpoint of the zygomatic arch overlying the coronoid notch of the mandible. Location of the point of needle insertion is aided by asking the patient to open the mouth wide and palpating the condyle of the mandible as it moves anteriorly to the midpoint of the zygoma. When the mouth is closed, the condyle leaves a clear entry path through the coronoid notch. An 8-cm, 22-gauge needle is inserted through the skin and subcutaneous tissues, which contain the parotid gland and possibly some of the rostral portions of the "pes anserinus" branches of the facial nerve destined for the orbicularis oculi muscles. An extensive subcutaneous infiltration of local anesthetic at this site may result in some temporary weakness of these muscles. Having traversed the coronoid notch of the mandible, the needle is directed medially until it reaches the medial wall of the infratemporal fossa, where it will strike the lateral surface of the lateral pterygoid plate, usually at a depth of about 5 cm. The needle is now "walked" anteriorly from the lateral pterygoid plate until it enters the pterygopalatine fossa, where it is advanced a further centimeter into the fossa. Usually, a paresthesia is not obtained or sought, and 5 ml of local anesthetic is injected into this fossa to produce anesthesia of the maxillary nerve. Devogel has reported that the sphenopalatine ganglion can be selectively blocked at this site[14] and used for treatment of refractory headaches. It is almost impossible to block this ganglion selectively without involving the second division of the trigeminal nerve, and this more or less precludes the use of permanent blockade in this area, even if such headaches could conclusively be shown to be relieved by such blockade.

Complications. Because of the highly vascular nature of the contents of this fossa, containing as it does the five terminal branches of the maxillary artery with all their venae comitantes plus the veins that drain the orbit by way of the inferior orbital fissure, a hematoma is frequently a sequel to this block. Such a hematoma can spread into the orbit and produce a profound black eye. The treatment of this is symptomatic, since it usually resolves in several days. Spread of local anesthetic to the optic nerve may occur, producing temporary blindness. The patient should, of course, be forewarned. This approach is not favored for neurolytic blockade because of proximity to the orbit. If maxillary division neurolytic blockade is required, it is common practice to use the approach described under Gasserian Ganglion Block. Alternatively, some favor neurolytic blockade of its infraorbital branch if pain is confined to infraorbital nerve territory.

Alternate Approach by Way of the Orbit. An alternative approach for blocking the maxillary nerve involves traversing the inferolateral borders of the orbit and depositing the local anesthetic in the pterygopalatine fossa superolaterally. A 6-cm, 22-gauge needle is inserted at the junction of the inferior and lateral borders of the orbit and, keeping close to the bone, is advanced for a distance of 4 cm. It will then have entered the inferior orbital fissure, and its tip lies in the pterygopalatine fossa. No attempts are made to seek a paresthesia, and 5 ml of local anesthetic is injected at this site. This approach may also be complicated by hematoma production or spread of local anesthetic to the optic nerve, producing temporary blindness. The eye itself does not encroach directly on the path of the needle in this block, being suspended off the floor of the orbit by the suspending ligament of Lockwood.

Although this is not recommended as a first choice for second division trigeminal block, it is an alternative when local conditions may preclude the conventional approach by the infratemporal fossa.

Alternate Approach by Way of the Infratemporal Fossa. Yet another alternative approach to the maxillary nerve is by way of the anterior aspect of the infratemporal fossa.[4] The needle is introduced anterior to the coronoid process of the mandible at a point below the anterior aspect of the zygomatic arch. This allows a medial approach toward the pupil of the eye, passing posterior to the posterior surface of the maxilla directly into the pterygopalatine fossa. The needle should not be inserted to a depth greater than 5 cm because this approach can lead unchecked into the optic nerve and by way of its foramen into the cranial cavity.[4] Although the bony landmarks for this block are usually constant, sometimes the zygomatic arch is relatively low in position; if this is the case, the second division of the trigeminal can actually be reached in the pterygomandibular fossa by advancing the needle superior to the zygoma.[13] In contrast, the approach by way of the coronoid notch involves an anterior direction so that if the needle is advanced too deeply it will impinge on the posterior surface of the maxillary or palatine bones and thereby be prevented from damaging deeper structures.

BLOCK OF BRANCHES OF MAXILLARY NERVES

Extraoral block of infraorbital nerve is accomplished below the junction of the medial and middle thirds of the lower border of the orbit. This point lies in the same vertical plane as the pupil and the supraorbital and mental foramina (see Fig. 15-3). It is important to appreciate that the infraorbital foramen emerges in a caudad and medial direction, and to enter this foramen it is important to direct a 4-cm, 22- to 25-gauge needle laterally and cephalad. To block the nerve, however, infiltration of 1 to 2 ml of 1% lidocaine or the equivalent at its exit from the foramen is usually all that is needed, and it is not essential to enter the foramen. Block of this nerve will afford satisfactory anesthesia of the skin of the cheek medial to, and only partially including, the nose, which is also supplied by terminal branches of the first division of the trigeminal (*i.e.*, infratrochlear and external nasal nerves). It will provide analgesia of the upper lip to the midline except in patients whose philtrum is derived from first division dermatomes; in them, this middle portion of the upper lip will be supplied by the first division of the trigeminal nerve. This block is useful for superficial surgery in the dermal distribution of the nerve but will not, of course, produce any analgesia of deeper second division structures, such as the teeth, unless the injection is made directly into the canal (see Chap. 16).

The two remaining branches of the maxillary division, zygomaticotemporal and zygomaticofacial, can be anesthetized by infiltration at the sites of emergence from the zygomatic bone, as shown in Figure

15-2. The indications for these are infrequently encountered.

MANDIBULAR NERVE

BLOCK OF MAIN TRUNK IN THE INFRATEMPORAL FOSSA

The approach for blocking the main division of the mandibular nerve in the infratemporal fossa is initially the same as that described for the maxillary nerve, that is, a 6-cm, 22-gauge needle is introduced below the midpoint of the zygomatic arch and passes through the coronoid notch of the mandible, directed medially across the infratemporal fossa until it impinges upon the bony medial wall (*i.e.,* the lateral aspect of the lateral pterygoid plate) (see Fig. 15-6). At this stage, the directions differ from those for a maxillary nerve block. The needle is "walked" posteriorly from the lateral pterygoid plate until a third division paresthesia is obtained. If a paresthesia is not obtained, the needle, once it leaves the posterior aspect of the lateral pterygoid plate, can pierce the attached superior constrictor muscle and enter the pharynx.

Third division block here produces analgesia of the skin over the lower jaw (except at the angle of the mandible), of the superior two thirds of the anterior surface of the auricle, and of a strip of skin that often extends up to the temporal area (see Fig. 15-2). If sufficient concentration of local anesthetic is injected to result in motor blockade (1% lidocaine or equivalent), the muscles of mastication will also be anesthetized, resulting in some incoordination of ipsilateral movements of the jaw. This is well tolerated after temporary blocks but is a long-term complication of permanent blockade. The otic ganglion, lying in such intimate connection posterior to the mandibular division just below the foramen ovale, is inevitably blocked. This nerve supplies secretomotor fibers to the parotid gland, which pursue a peripatetic course from the inferior salivary nucleus, and thus permanent impairment of secretion of this gland is a possible sequel of neurolytic blockade of the mandibular nerve.

Extraoral Block of Mental Nerve. The mental foramen, as mentioned above, lies in the same vertical line as the supraorbital and infraorbital foramen and the pupil, with the pupil in the midposition (see Fig. 15-3). The position of the mental foramen varies with age, being more caudal on the mandibular ramus in youth and much nearer the alveolar margin of the mandible in the edentulous aged person. Although this nerve can be blocked by the intraoral route (see Chap. 16), extraoral blockade can be accomplished. To enter the mental foramen, it is necessary to direct the needle anteriorly and caudad. It is not necessary, however, to enter the foramen, and an infiltration over the midpoint of the mandible in the vertical line is usually sufficient to produce analgesia of the lower lip and chin and is effective anesthesia for operative procedures there.

Auriculotemporal nerve can be blocked as it ascends over the posterior root of the zygoma (see Fig. 15-2) behind the superficial temporal artery, and infiltration of 3 to 5 ml of 1% lidocaine or the equivalent results in anesthesia of the upper two thirds of the temporal fossa.

ALTERNATIVE APPROACHES TO MANDIBULAR NERVE BLOCK

In dental practice where mandibular anesthesia is used for lower jaw procedures, the mandibular nerve is frequently blocked by intraoral approaches that can be accomplished either with an open mouth[16] or even with the jaws closed[17] (see Chap. 16).

GLOSSOPHARYNGEAL NERVE BLOCK

The ninth cranial nerve emerges by way of the jugular foramen in proximity to the vagus and accessory nerves along with the internal jugular vein. It is blocked just below this point, and therefore both temporary and permanent blocks usually involve these other two cranial nerves, all three of which lie in the groove between the internal jugular vein and the internal carotid artery (Fig. 15-7). These two large vascular conduits may well be punctured during attempts to block these nerves at this site, resulting in either intravascular injection or hematoma. Even very small amounts (*e.g.,* 0.25 ml of local anesthetic injected into the carotid artery at this point) can produce quite profound effects of convulsion and loss of consciousness. Therefore, as always, aspiration tests must be meticulous.

The landmarks for this block involve locating the styloid process of the temporal bone. This osseous process represents the calcification of the cephalic end of the stylohyoid ligament. This fibrous band,

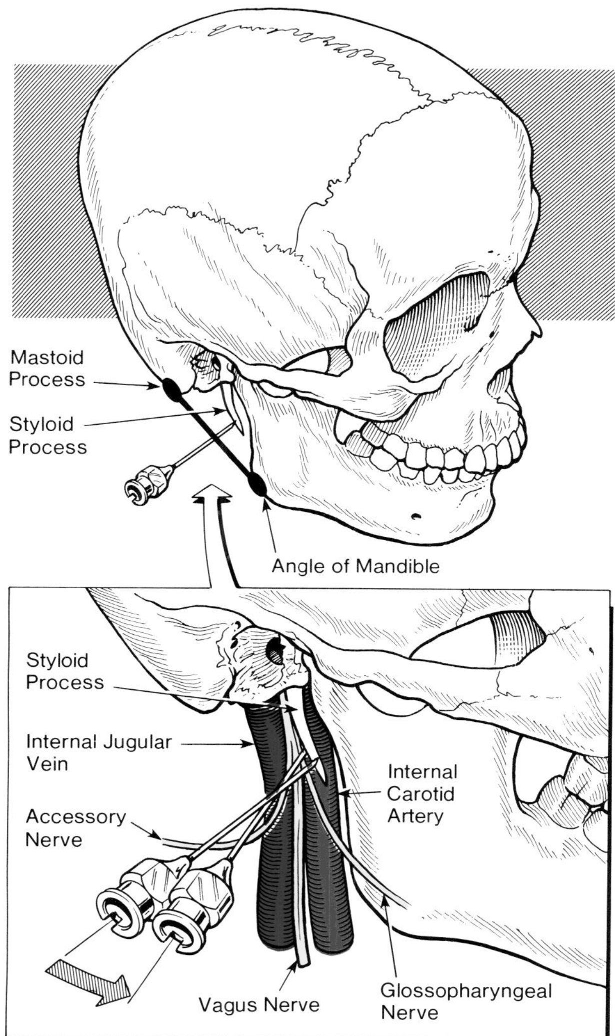

FIG. 15-7. Glossopharyngeal nerve block. **Upper Panel.** The needle is inserted at a point midway between the mastoid process and the angle of the mandible. **Lower Panel.** The needle is inserted at a right angle to the skin. At a depth of 2 to 3 cm the styloid process will be contacted (if present). The needle is then "walked" posteriorly off the styloid process. Local anesthetic deposited at this point will block glossopharyngeal, accessory, and vagus nerves. Note the proximity of the internal carotid artery and the internal jugular vein.

which passes from the base of the skull to the lesser cornu of the hyoid bone, ossifies to a different extent in different patients. Although it is relatively easy to identify in people with a large styloid process, if ossification has been limited then the styloid process sometimes cannot be located with the exploring needle. Sometimes the process may be absent.

TECHNIQUE

A 5-cm, 22-gauge needle is inserted at the midpoint of a line joining the angle of the mandible to the tip of the mastoid process of the occipital bone (Fig. 15-7). The needle is advanced directly medially until it locates the styloid process. In the event that the styloid process is not located, it is inserted to a depth of 3 cm. In patients who have had a radical neck dissection (and therefore are often candidates for this kind of block), the removal of the sternomastoid muscle places the styloid process and its adjacent nerves and vessels at a much more superficial location. In fact, in these patients, the styloid process can often be palpated in the interval between mastoid process and the posterior border of the mandible. The needle will then need to be inserted only 1 to 2 cm. Ideally, the styloid process is located as a bony end point and the needle adjusted posterior to this at the same depth as the process. An injection of 1 to 2 ml of 1% lidocaine or the equivalent will produce anesthesia of the glossopharyngeal, vagus, and accessory nerves. It is not possible at this site to block one of these three nerves selectively.

Glossopharyngeal nerve block is used most frequently for inoperable carcinomas that invade the distribution of the nerve in either the posterior third of the tongue or the pharyngeal areas. Such patients are often quite willing to undergo additional unilateral blockade of the accessory nerve, with resulting weakness of the sternomastoid and trapezius muscles in addition to the numbness of the laryngeal inlet and trachea and paralysis of the ipsilateral vocal cords (with resulting hoarseness).

The injection of neurolytic agents at this site so close to the large vascular carotid and jugular conduits is cause for concern because of the possibility of damage to the walls of these vessels, which might result in slough and necrosis with potentially disastrous sequelae. Such a complication has not, however, yet been reported.

An alternative approach for intraorally blocking the glossopharyngeal nerve has been reported by Cooper.[15] This technique involves injecting local anesthetic into the midpoint of the posterior pillar of the fauces. This appears to offer considerable promise as a means of blocking the glossopharyngeal nerve distribution to the oropharynx and, in combination with laryngeal nerve blocks (see below) and topical anesthesia, provides satisfactory analgesia for endoscopic procedures under regional anesthesia.

VAGUS NERVE BLOCK

The main trunk of the vagus nerve is rarely blocked as a primary procedure (see Fig. 15-7); however, the branches of sensory distribution to the larynx can be blocked simply and efficiently, thereby rendering the laryngeal inlet and adjacent trachea insensitive to pain. This is very useful for intubations performed on conscious patients and other endoscopic procedures. These branches can also be blocked permanently for pain relief in terminal neoplastic disease in the area.

SUPERIOR LARYNGEAL NERVE BLOCK

The superior laryngeal branch of the vagus nerve is easily blocked as it sweeps around the inferior border of the greater cornu of the hyoid bone, which is readily palpable even in the most obese patients. By pressing on the opposite greater cornu of the hyoid bone, the laryngeal structures can be displaced toward the side to be blocked (Fig. 15-8). A small 2.5-cm, 25-gauge needle is usually all that is required. It is "walked" from the inferior border of the greater cornu of the hyoid near its tip, and 3 ml of local anesthetic is infiltrated both superficially and deep to the thyrohyoid membrane. Penetration of this membrane is felt as a slight loss of resistance. The procedure is repeated on the other side. This will produce anesthesia over the inferior aspect of the epiglottis and the laryngeal inlet as far down as the vocal cords. It will also produce motor blockade (if the concentration of lidocaine exceeds 1% or the equivalent for other drugs) of the cricothyroid muscles.

RECURRENT LARYNGEAL NERVE BLOCK

To produce anesthesia below the cords, the simplest and most useful method is transtracheal puncture (Fig. 15-8). Here, a relatively wide-bore needle (*i.e.*, 20- or 22-gauge) is used so that air can be aspirated and rapid injection performed. The needle is introduced in the midline through the cricothyroid membrane. Entry of the needle into the trachea is identified by aspiration of air, and the patient will usually cough slightly at this stage. Rapid injection of 3 to 5 ml of local anesthetic will produce a dramatic cough in all but the most obtunded patients. This spreads the local anesthetic up and down the trachea and yields satisfactory topical anesthesia. It is usually necessary to use a higher concentration for this topical anesthesia than for nerve block. Four percent lidocaine is frequently chosen, although 2% lidocaine will produce adequate blockade but will take a little longer.

The nerve that supplies the wall of the trachea below that of the vocal cords is the recurrent laryngeal nerve. It is possible to block this nerve specifically. (In fact, block of this nerve frequently occurs as a complication of stellate ganglion blocks.)

In the event that blockade of the recurrent laryngeal nerve was ever required (*e.g.*, for a possible neurolytic block for cancers of the vocal cords or below), then the nerve, which lies in the groove between esophagus and trachea, can be blocked at any cervical level below the cricoid cartilage. Attempts at this block would, of course, demand meticulous technique to avoid involvement of brachial plexus with an overly deep insertion of the needle. Block of the auricular branch of the vagus has even been used for resolving bronchial asthma.[18] Block is performed where the nerve exits from the base of the skull between the mastoid process and the external tympanic plate of the temporal bone.

ACCESSORY NERVE (11TH CRANIAL NERVE) BLOCK

There are very few indications to block the accessory nerve. It is useful for trapezius muscle block as an adjunct to interscalene nerve blocks of the brachial plexus for surgery on the shoulder. With interscalene block alone, the patient has adequate analgesia of the operative site, but motor power is maintained in the trapezius muscle. He can, by shrugging his shoulders, inadvertently interfere with the surgical procedure: By blocking the accessory nerve in the posterior triangle of the neck, the trapezius muscle is paralyzed and the surgery often facilitated.

The posterior triangle of the neck is a compartment bounded anteriorly by the posterior border of the sternomastoid muscle, laterally by the anterior border of the trapezius, and inferiorly by the middle third of the clavicle. The accessory nerve traverses this triangle in a very superficial location (Fig. 15-9). It emerges from the substance of the sternomastoid muscle at the junction of the superior and middle thirds of the posterior border of that muscle and proceeds in a downward and lateral course across the

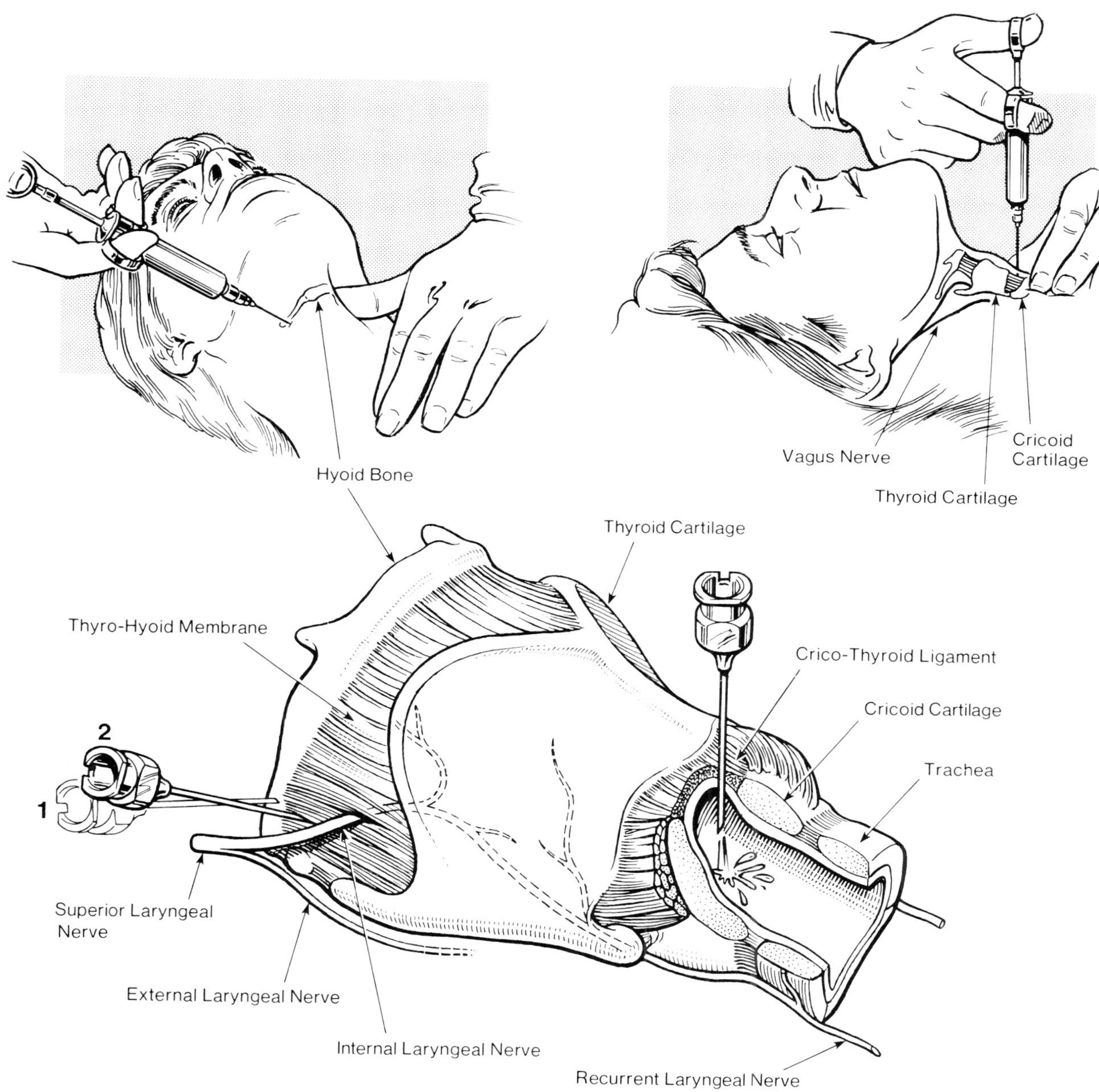

FIG. 15-8. Superior and recurrent laryngeal nerve block. The *superior laryngeal nerve* and its internal and external branches are blocked inferior to the lateral limits of the greater cornu of the hyoid bone. This landmark is brought into prominence by pressing medially on the contralateral cornu of the hyoid bone. *(1)* A needle is inserted onto the greater cornu of the hyoid bone and then walked off the inferior edge of the hyoid *(2)*. Needle depth is not increased beyond the depth of the hyoid to avoid the needle's piercing the larynx. Local anesthetic injected at *(2)* blocks the internal laryngeal nerve and produces anesthesia of the laryngeal inlet, down to the level of the vocal cords. The *recurrent laryngeal nerve* is blocked by introducing a needle through the cricothyroid membrane. Note one hand grasping the cricoid cartilage. The other hand is steadied against the patient's chin. Injection is made after aspirating for air. It is important that the local anesthetic be injected rapidly and the needle immediately removed, since the patient will cough vigorously. Anesthesia is produced over the inferior surface of the vocal cords and the trachea.

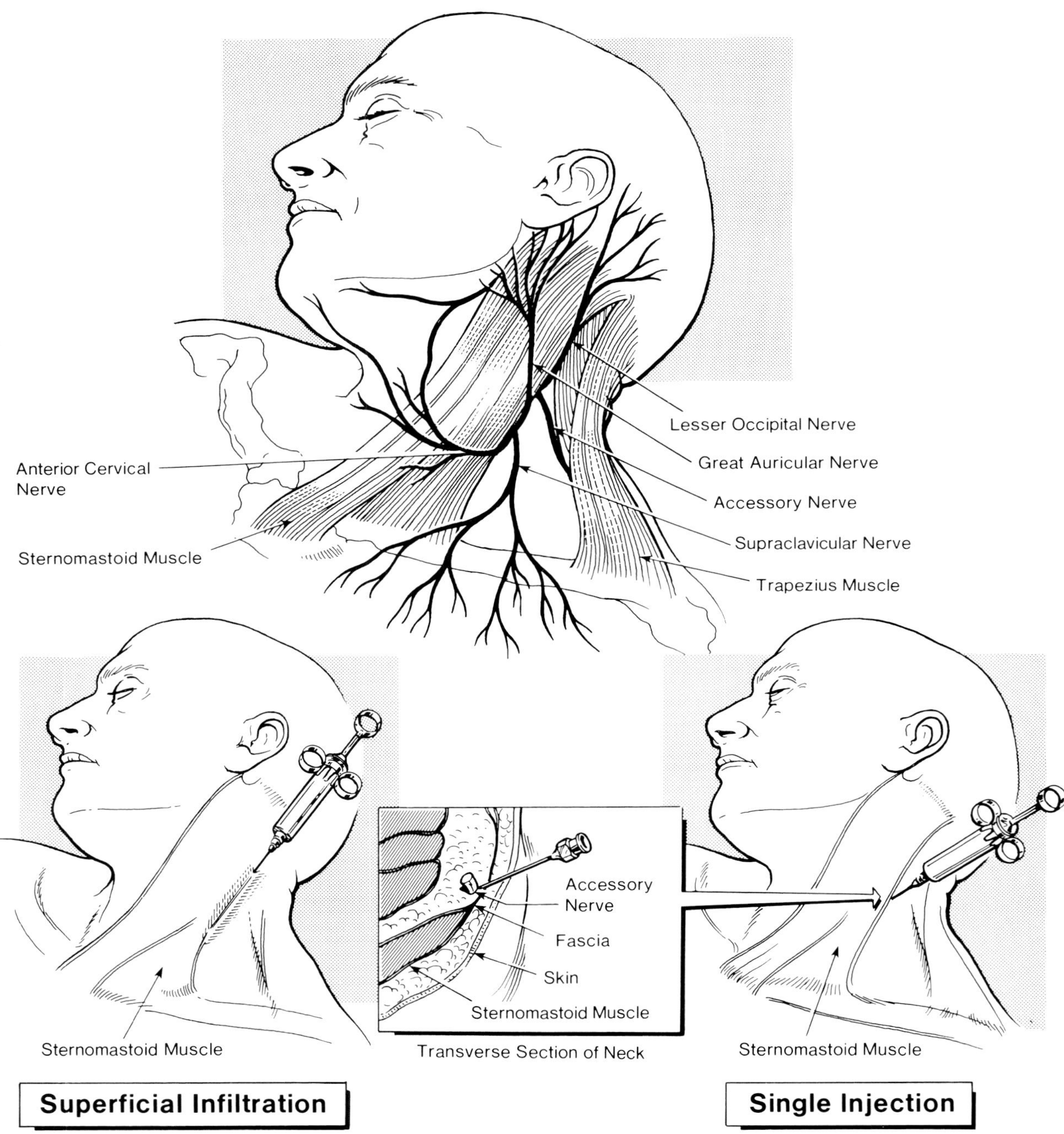

FIG. 15-9. The superficial cervical plexus, which is blocked in the posterior triangle of the neck as it emerges adjacent to the midpoint of the posterior border of the sternomastoid muscle. *Superficial infiltration* is extended along the middle third of the posterior border of the sternomastoid muscle. Note the close relationship of the accessory nerve as it emerges from the posterior border of the sternomastoid muscle at the junction of its middle and upper third, that is, just above the emerging superficial cervical plexus. *Single injection technique for accessory nerve block.* Note that the accessory nerve lies deep to the deep fascia of the neck and that this needs to be pierced as shown in the *"single injection,"* which is sometimes used as an adjunct to produce muscle paralysis of the trapezius muscle in shoulder operations. Successful block of the superficial cervical plexus results in analgesia corresponding to the C2, C3, and C4 dermatomes shown in Figure 15-2.

triangle to enter the trapezius muscle at the junction of the middle and inferior third of its anterior border. Anywhere along this course, it can be successfully blocked. The accessory nerve lies superficial to the prevertebral fascia and therefore is lying deep only to skin, platysma muscle, and deep cervical fascia. Therefore, if a needle is introduced at the junction of the middle and superior thirds of the sternomastoid muscle at its lateral border and an infiltration of 10 ml of local anesthetic is used, block can be accomplished (Fig. 15-9). Accuracy can be increased if a stimulating device is used to locate the nerve. This nerve is not infrequently unintentionally blocked when a superficial cervical plexus block is performed, and *vice versa*.

Ramamurthy[19] has described a technique for blocking this nerve as it lies within the sternomastoid muscle. This is accomplished by infiltrating the substance of the muscle with 10 to 20 ml of local anesthetic below its attachment to the mastoid process. It is used for the therapy of spasms and painful conditions of the sternomastoid muscle itself.

CERVICAL PLEXUS BLOCK

The cervical plexus is formed by loops between the anterior primary rami of the upper four cervical nerves. Its branches are distributed to the prevertebral muscles, strap muscles of the neck, and, of course, the phrenic nerve.

SUPERFICIAL CERVICAL PLEXUS BLOCK

Block at Midpoint of Posterior Border of Sternomastoid. The cervical plexus is distributed to the skin of the anterolateral neck by way of the anterior primary rami of C2–C4. These emerge as four distinct nerves from the posterior border of the sternomastoid at approximately its midpoint, just below the emergence of the accessory nerve. The first branch radiates upward and backward as the lesser occipital nerve to supply part of the posterior surface of the upper part of the ear and skin behind the ear; the second branch runs upward and forward as the great auricular nerve, which supplies skin over the posterior surface of the ear and the anterior lower third of the ear, as well as over the angle of the mandible; the third branch, the anterior cutaneous nerve of the neck, supplies skin from the chin to the suprasternal notch; and the fourth branches, the supraclavicular nerves, supply the skin over the inferior aspect of the neck and the clavicle and down as far as the area overlying the second rib; laterally these supraclavicular nerves supply the skin over the deltoid muscle, and posteriorly as far as the spine of the scapula. All four branches can be blocked by infiltration at the midpoint of the posterior border of the sternomastoid (Fig. 15-9). Lidocaine, 1% (or the equivalent) (5–10 ml) infiltrated at this area produces cutaneous analgesia of the neck from the mandible to the clavicle, both anteriorly and laterally.

BLOCK OF GREATER OCCIPITAL NERVE

The skin over the posterior extensor muscles of the neck and extending up over the occiput as high as the vertex is supplied by the posterior rami of the cervical nerves. Of these, the greater occipital nerve is perhaps the most clinically significant. It is best blocked as it crosses the superior nuchal line, about one third of the way between the external occipital protuberance and the mastoid process (Fig. 15-10). It is located at this site by palpating the occipital artery that lies adjacent to it. Infiltration of 5 ml of 1% lidocaine or the equivalent around the artery will usually effect satisfactory block of this nerve and result in a band of anesthesia from the occiput to the vertex. This block is used along with blocks of the supraorbital, supratrochlear, auriculotemporal, and lesser occipital nerves to render the scalp anesthetic for operative procedures. It is also a useful block in both diagnosis and treatment of occipital "tension" headaches. The mechanism whereby such a block relieves these headaches is often more complex than via the neural blockade *per se* (see Chap. 27.2).

DEEP CERVICAL PLEXUS BLOCK

Deep cervical plexus block is, in effect, a paravertebral nerve block of C2–C4 spinal nerves as they emerge from the foramina in the cervical vertebrae. Each nerve lies in the sulcus in the transverse process of these vertebrae (Fig. 15-11). Three needles were traditionally used, being inserted at the levels of C2, C3, and C4. The sites of insertion are located by reference to a line that joins the tip of the mastoid process with Chassaignac's tubercle of C6, which is readily palpated at the level of the cricoid cartilage. The C2 transverse process is usually located about one fingerbreadth caudad to the mastoid process on this line, and C3 and C4 are at similar intervals caudally on the same line. A horizontal line through the lower

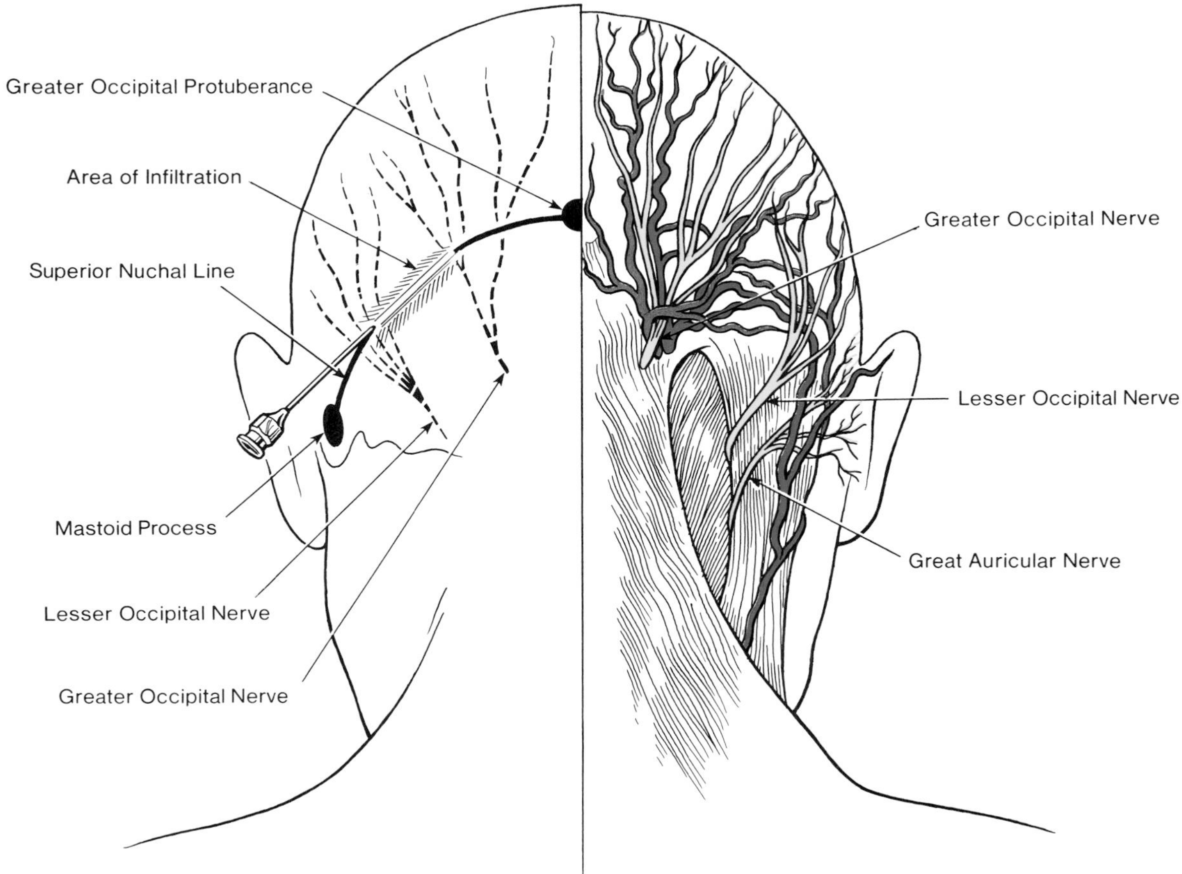

FIG. 15-10. Greater and lesser occipital nerve block. Note the greater and lesser occipital nerve branches crossing the superior nuchal line approximately halfway between the greater occipital protuberance and the mastoid process. Superficial infiltration along this line will produce analgesia of the posterior scalp. The greater occipital nerve can be located by identifying the pulsations of the posterior occipital artery, which crosses the nuchal line in company with the nerve.

border of the ramus of the mandible intersects this line at C4 (Fig. 15-11). Five-centimeter, 22-gauge needles are directed medially and caudally. The reason for the caudad direction is to avoid unintentionally entering the intervertebral foramen and producing a peridural or spinal block. The end point is the bony landmark of the transverse process, and paresthesias are obtained. Injection of 3 or 4 ml of 1% lidocaine or the equivalent on each nerve is usually adequate for anesthesia. Fortunately, the paravertebral space communicates freely in the cervical region, and the anesthetic solution can spread easily to adjacent levels. Deep cervical plexus block can quite often be obtained with injections at just one level with a larger volume, that is, 6 to 8 ml. Cervical plexus block is a frequent sequel to the single-needle interscalene approach that produces brachial plexus block; in fact, if digital pressure is maintained distally in the interscalene groove and the patient is placed in a horizontal or even head-down posture, cervical plexus block can be predictably produced using the same needle insertion technique as for an interscalene brachial plexus block (see Chap. 10).

Deep cervical plexus block is sometimes useful for such procedures as thyroidectomy and tracheostomy under local anesthesia and is also used effectively for carotid endarterectomy or for removal of cervical lymph nodes. A significant complication of the block is due to the proximity of the vertebral artery, because accidental direct intra-arterial injection may produce

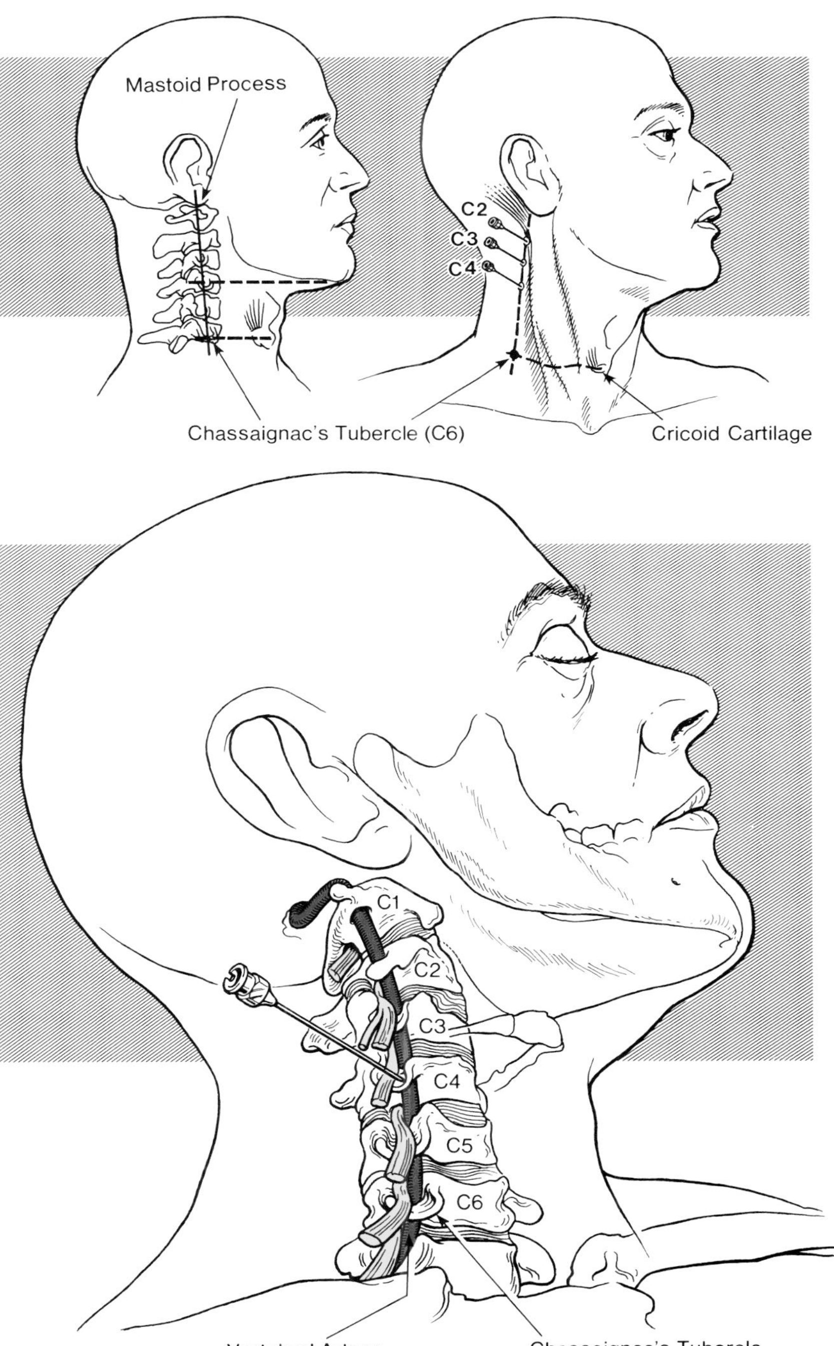

FIG. 15-11. Deep cervical plexus block. A line is drawn from mastoid process to Chassaignac's tubercle (C6). The latter lies on a line extended laterally from the cricoid cartilage. This line lies over the "gutters" in the superior surface of the transverse processes, upon which the cervical nerve roots pass laterally. The *C4 nerve root* is located at the junction of the vertical line and a line horizontally drawn to the lower border of the mandible, with the head in a neutral position. The *C3 and C2 nerve roots* can be located by dividing the distance between the mastoid and horizontal line into thirds (see *right upper panel*). The *C5 nerve root* lies midway between the "C6 line" and the line above. *Individual cervical nerve roots* may be blocked by injecting small volumes of local anesthetics, as shown in the upper right. Single injection block of cervical plexus can be obtained by a technique similar to interscalene brachial plexus block, since the cervical nerve roots are contained in a continuous space between the scalene muscles. A single needle is inserted on the vertical line, at the C4 level, and directed medially and slightly caudad to contact the "gutter" of the transverse process *(lower panel)*. Note that caudad direction is essential to avoid penetration of an intervertebral foramen, with possible injection into epidural space or dural sleeve (and thus direct entry to CSF). Note also the proximity of the vertebral artery passing through the foramina transversaria of the transverse processes.

the profound and very rapid toxic side-effects of convulsions, unconsciousness, and blindness[20]; therefore, aspiration tests are of great importance. Extension of the anesthetic into the epidural or subdural spaces is theoretically possible by either dural sleeves or leakage through intervertebral foramen; thus patients who undergo such procedures must be observed very carefully.

When the block is performed bilaterally, bilateral phrenic nerve block and resultant bilateral diaphragm paralysis is a serious hazard. Because the deep cervical plexus lies deep to the deep cervical fascia, spread to the cervical sympathetic chain should not occur. If, however, infiltration has spread anterior to the prevertebral fascia, the cervical sympathetic chain will be involved, with resultant Horner's syndrome and also spread to the recurrent laryngeal nerve, resulting in hoarseness. Both of these complications in a failed block will indicate that, in fact, the anesthetic has been injected at a site superficial to the deep cervical fascia (Chap. 22).

REGIONAL ANESTHESIA OF THE EAR

The pinnae of the ears are supplied by both cervical plexus and trigeminal nerves. The cervical plexus branches of the great auricular nerve (see Fig. 15-9), and often the lesser occipital (see Fig. 15-10), contribute to the posterior surface of the ear and the lower third of the anterior surface. The superior two thirds of the anterior surface is supplied by the auriculotemporal branch of the mandibular division of the trigeminal (see Fig. 15-2).

The cervical plexus supply to the ear can be anesthetized by infiltration along the posterior aspect of the auricle over the mastoid process where 5 to 8 ml of local anesthetic is infiltrated (see Fig. 15-12). The

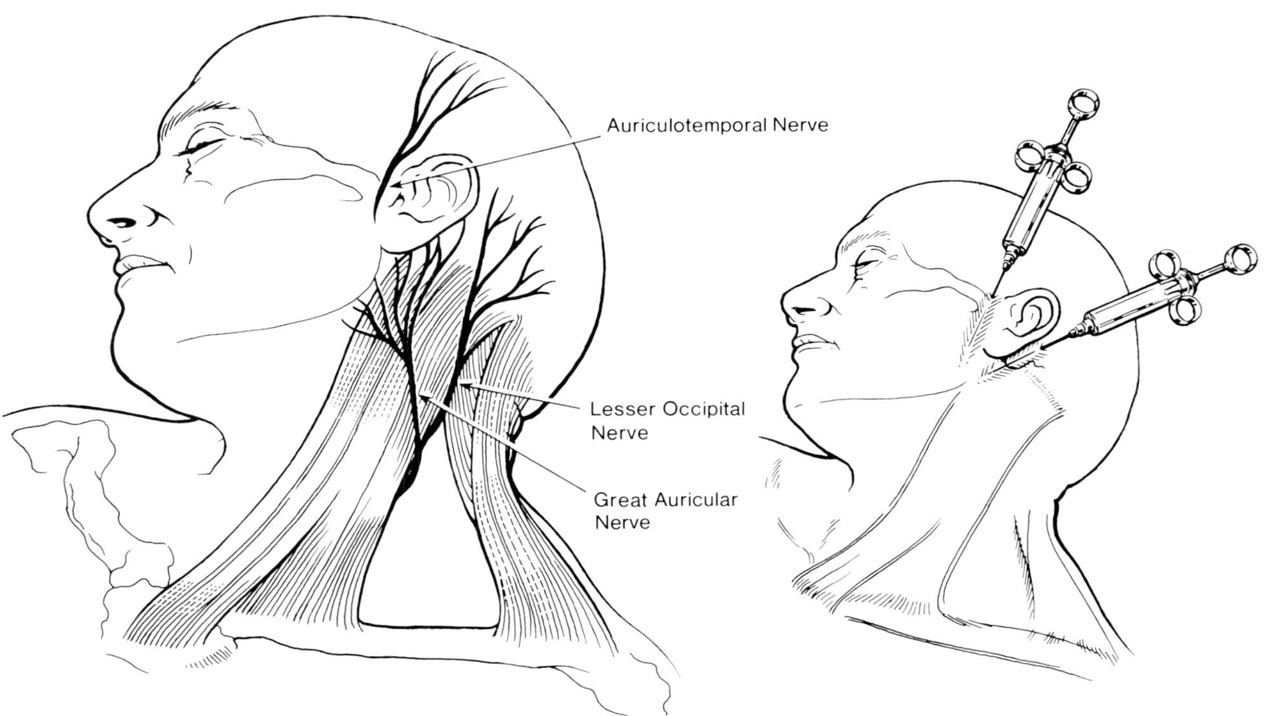

FIG. 15-12. Regional anesthesia of the ear. The *auriculotemporal nerve* (V3) is blocked by infiltration over the posterior aspect of zygoma. The *great auricular nerve* and *lesser occipital nerve* (branches of the cervical plexus) are blocked by infiltration over the mastoid process posterior to the ear.

auriculotemporal contribution to the anterior surface of the ear can be anesthetized by infiltration over the posterior aspect of the zygoma (see Fig. 15-12). A branch of the auriculotemporal nerve supplies the interior of the auditory canal over its superior aspect and is injected at the junction between the bony and cartilaginous parts of the anterior wall of the auditory canal where it can be reached with a 5 to 6 cm needle. Subcutaneous infiltration at the osseous cartilaginous junction is usually done with 2 ml of 1% lidocaine with 1 : 200,000 epinephrine.

The floor of the external auditory canal and the lower part of the tympanum are supplied by a branch of the vagus. This part of the auditory canal can be anesthetized by infiltrating the osseous cartilaginous junction of the external auditory canal over its lower aspect with 2 ml of 1% lidocaine with 1 : 200,000 epinephrine. The tympanum is best anesthetized by direct application of a 4% to 10% lidocaine spray, directing the spray at the roof of the auditory canal and allowing the solution to drain passively over the tympanum rather than directing the spray at the tympanum itself.

CERVICAL EPIDURAL ANESTHESIA

In addition to the discrete regional blocks described for head and neck surgical procedures, it is quite feasible to produce epidural blockade in the cervical region, which can permit extensive head and neck surgery.[21] This might be particularly appropriate because many patients who are candidates for head and neck surgery belong to the older age group and have coexisting chronic obstructive pulmonary and arteriosclerotic cardiovascular disease.

Despite significant preoperative attempts to improve their cardiopulmonary condition, these patients frequently pose significant operative risks. Since the surgical procedures often are very lengthy, the opportunity for administering continuous local anesthetic techniques is enhanced by an epidural catheter (see Chap. 8).

Because of the poor health of many such patients, invasive hemodynamic monitoring may still be required. Resting ventilation after cervical epidural block is similar to that after thoracic epidural block. There might be some statistically significant changes in both carbon dioxide concentration and oxygenation, but Takasaki[22] deemed these to be not clinically significant in a group of surgical patients studied with this technique. It may pose a useful form of analgesia for such patients with compromised cardiorespiratory reserve who have a need for major prolonged head and neck reconstructive surgery.

PRACTICAL APPLICATIONS

Regional anesthesia of the head and neck can be very useful for surgical anesthesia, for the diagnosis and therapy of various pain states, and for postoperative pain relief. This anesthesia is eminently suited for minor plastic and other procedures[30] on superficial structures in select patients (*e.g.*, patients with full stomachs or cardiorespiratory failure). It is well suited for outpatient surgery. It is also very useful as a supplement to light general anesthesia for many of the surgical procedures around the oral cavity, particularly since regional block of the second or third division of the trigeminal nerve with a long-acting local anesthetic agent can afford excellent postoperative analgesia for patients who have had their jaws wired together and since, owing to the threat to the airway, effective doses of narcotics have often been withheld.

Some surgical procedures in the neck lend themselves well to regional anesthesia. Thyroidectomy poses a risk to the recurrent laryngeal nerve, and thus may be performed with an awake, cooperative patient so that the patient's voice can act as an excellent monitor to the integrity of the nerve; however, as noted above, bilateral deep cervical plexus block is required. The patient's state of wakefulness is such a good indication of cerebral perfusion that some vascular surgeons prefer performing their carotid arterial surgery this way. This can be accomplished with deep cervical plexus block.

CAROTID ENDARTERECTOMY

Controversy has existed for some time concerning the relative merits of performing carotid endarterectomy under general or regional anesthesia. This operation poses significant risks to the patient of cerebrovascular ischemia, as a result of interruption of blood flow during the procedure, and poses risks inherent in imposing major anesthetic and surgical stress on patients who usually have significant and serious generalized cardiovascular disease. Although the operation has been traditionally done under general anesthesia with indirect monitors of cerebral function (along with monitoring other bodily functions), there has been a renewed interest displayed in performing this procedure under regional anesthesia, with the patient awake and conscious, allowing direct monitoring of cerebral function by communicating with the patient throughout the procedure, and particularly during the critical stages of clamping of the carotid arteries. Informed opinion is divided as to whether this form of anesthesia provides improved patient care, but there is significant information accumulating in the literature now to suggest it is very worthy of consideration.[23,24]

When the techniques of general as opposed to regional anesthesia have been compared for this operation, regional anesthesia appears to pose advantages with regard to the incidence of postoperative cerebral vascular stroke.[24] Because these patients have systemic cardiovascular disease, myocardial infarction is a risk in these individuals, but in a series of 185 operations for this procedure done under local anesthetic Prough[25] reported no incidence of myocardial infarction. In another comparison between regional and general techniques for carotid endarterectomy, Jopling and co-workers[26] showed that the incidence of both postoperative hypertension and hypotension was lower in the group operated on under regional as opposed to general anesthesia, which may indicate an improved postoperative cardiovascular status.

Controversy still exists in this regard, but with the reports currently available of large series of patients managed successfully under regional anesthesia with awake monitoring, one of the significant objections to regional anesthesia in this technique (*i.e.*, that patients or surgeons could not tolerate same) has been disproved. With appropriate patient (and surgeon) selection, this procedure can be satisfactorily performed under regional anesthesia with a degree of mortality and morbidity that is no worse, and may be even better, than that obtained under general anesthesia. It also appears that the monitoring required for same would be less complicated under regional anesthesia, and since the technique seems to involve less operative and surgical room time[26] it may also have economic advantages.

It is perhaps **in the field of endoscopy** that regional anesthesia of the oral, pharyngeal, and laryngeal compartments has its most frequent application. There are a significant number of instances in anesthesia in which it is desirable to ensure intubation of the trachea before obtunding the patient's normal protective reflexes. This "awake" intubation can be executed admirably with either local anesthetic spray or nerve blocks. Such "awake" intubations are often necessary on patients with an unstable neck, secondary to cervical fracture, and a combination of spray or laryngeal nerve blocks will permit orotracheal or nasotracheal intubation without risking undue flexion or extension movement in the neck, as occurs in routine laryngoscopy. Also, with the patient awake, the integrity of his CNS can be monitored during this maneuver. In cases in which there may be difficulty with intubation, such as facial fractures, intubation under local analgesia does not preclude the use of any alternatives if it fails. Such analgesia also lends itself well to diagnostic endoscopies of the pharnyx, larynx, and even trachea for investigative and biopsy purposes (see also Chap. 16).

For **patients with pain problems** in the head neck, regional analgesia allows elucidation of the pathway of the noxious stimulus (if any), and by an appropriate combination of long- and short-acting local anesthetics, with placebo blocks, it is often possible to predict the effect of nerve section or neurolysis. In patients with cancer of the head and neck, blocks of the trigeminal, glossopharyngeal, laryngeal, or cervical plexus, either alone or in combination, can often afford excellent pain relief (see also Chap. 27).

COMPLICATIONS OF REGIONAL ANESTHESIA OF HEAD AND NECK

Regional anesthesia of the head and neck is an eminently safe procedure; however like all other forms of therapy and intervention a complication rate occurs, and, as with the injection of local anesthetics into other parts of the body, it can be associated with an incidence of syncope, postinjection infection, local tissue trauma, hematoma, and even allergic reactions.[27] Some specific complications are also peculiar to regional anesthetics in this area. These usually involve damage to adjacent structures or spread to the central nervous system by means of direct or vascular spread to produce convulsions or extensive neuraxial anesthesia that requires comprehensive resuscitation.

Accidental injection into one of the vascular conduits carrying blood directly to the brain, for example, carotid or vertebral artery or one of their branches, can produce significant transient losses of consciousness or convulsion, or both, after accidental injection of small (0.5 ml or less) volumes of local anesthetic into the vertebral artery.[9] Total reversible blindness has also been described after similar inadvertent injections of small amounts (1 ml) of local anesthetic accidentally into a vertebral artery.[20] It is also possible for local anesthetic procedures to result in spread of local anesthetic into the neuraxis by means of direct penetration of either the foramina of the skull or the intervertebral foramen in the cervical spine, producing total brain-stem anesthesia.[28]

Infection seems to be a rarely encountered complication of regional anesthesia in the head and neck, which is surprising since many of the injections take place through the mucous membranes of the mouth and oropharynx (which are notorious deposits of microorganisms), possibly because local anesthetics are bacteriostatic and maybe bacteriocidal.[27] There are scant references in the literature of complications, although two surprising cases of atlantoaxial subluxation were deemed to be caused by infection of the anterior transverse ligament following local anesthesia for tonsilectomy.[29]

Systemic toxic reactions to local anesthetic uptake can be produced by applying such agents to mucous membranes in the nose, oropharynx, and larynx, and attention to dose administered is critically important here as in other forms of regional anesthesia. The use of benzocaine and prilocaine has been associated with episodes of methemoglobinemia induced after its application to mucous membranes in the throat and trachea (see Chap. 22).[31–32]

INTRODUCTION TO CLINICAL PRACTICE

Skill in regional anesthesia of this area of the body not only is a challenging and technically satisfying addition to the anesthesiologist's repertoire, but also provides optimal anesthesia for certain kinds of surgical procedures, can provide long-lasting postoperative pain relief, and is important in pain-unit work.

To acquire the required level of expertise, one can begin to learn these techniques on anesthetized patients. Successful blockade then permits reduction, or deletion, of doses of supplemental anesthetics. If long-acting local anesthetics such as bupivacaine or etidocaine are used, the patient receives the benefit of excellent postoperative analgesia in situations in which effective analgesic doses of narcotics are contraindicated (*e.g.*, surgery in proximity to the airway).

Most operations in the head and neck area can be performed under the effects of some of supplementary neural blockade. Only by routine supplementation of light general anesthesia by neural blockade in such cases can the success rate gradually improve. Unless this approach is used, the anesthesiologist will find it difficult to provide an acceptable success rate for patients who have strong indications for head and neck procedures under neural blockade alone. Selection of the appropriate peripheral nerves for blockade can allow very effective and efficient analgesia for a wide range of plastic surgery procedures. Volumes of local anesthetic as small as 1 ml can be used for individual nerves and then supplemented by minimal infiltration of the incision line, which is marked on the skin preoperatively. In one large plastic surgery unit, virtually all major plastic surgery of the face in elderly patients is carried out with peripheral neural blockade.*

REFERENCES

1. Sorensen, D., Hori, Y., and Leonard, R.: Effects of laryngeal topical anesthesia on voice fundamental frequency perturbation. J. Speech Hearing Res., *23*:274–283, 1980.
2. Adriani, J.: Labats Regional Anesthesia: Techniques and Clinical Applications, 3rd ed. Philadelphia, W.B. Saunders, 1967.
3. Bonica, J.J.: The Management of Pain. Philadelphia, Lea & Febiger, 1953.
4. Macintosh, R., and Ostlere, M.: Local Analgesia for Head and Neck. Edinburgh, E. & S. Livingstone, 1967.
5. Moore, D.C.: Regional Block, 4th ed. Springfield, Charles C Thomas, 1975.
6. Last, R.J.: Anatomy: Regional and Applied. Edinburgh, Churchill Livingstone, 1980.
7. Hargrove, J., and Claeys, D.W.: Anesthesia experience in a high volume eye center (abstr.). Reg. Anaesth., *10*:36, 1985.
8. Backer, C.L., Tinker, J.H., Robertson, D.M., and Vlietstra, R.E.: Myocardial reinfarction following local anaesthesia for ophthalmic surgery. Anesth. Analg., *59*:257–261, 1980.
9. Kozody, R., Ready, L.B., Barsa, J.E., et al.: Dose requirement of local anesthetic to produce grand mal seizure during stellate ganglion block. Can. Anaesth. Soc. J., *29*:489, 1982.
10. Boliston, T.A., and Upton, J.J.M.: Infiltration with lignocaine and adrenalin in adult tonsillectomy. J. Laryngol. Otol., *94*:1257–1259, 1980.
11. Loeser, J.D.: What to do about tic douloureux. J.A.M.A., *239*:1153, 1978.
12. Hill, J.N., Gershon, N.I., and Garguiulo, P.O.: Total spinal blockade during local anaesthesia of the nasal passages. Anesthesiology, *59*:144–146, 1983.
13. Priman, J., and Etter, L.E.: Significance of variations of the skull in blocking the maxillary nerve—an anatomical and radiological study. Anesthesiology, *22*:42–48, 1961.
14. Devogel, J.C.: Cluster headache and sphenopalatine block. Acta. Anaesth. Belg., *32*:101–107, 1981.
15. Cooper, M., and Watson, R.L.: An improved regional anaesthetic technique for peroral endoscopy. Anesthesiology, *43*:372–374, 1975.

*Grey, W., Officer Brown Plastic Surgery Unit, Melbourne, Australia: Personal communication.

16. Gow–Gates, G.A., and Watson, J.E.: The Gow–Gates mandibular block: Further understanding. Anesth. Prog., *24*:183–189, 1977.
17. Gustainis, J.F., and Peterson, L.J.: An alternative method of mandibular nerve block. J. Am. Dent. Assoc., *103*:33–36, 1981.
18. Goel, A.C.: Auricular nerve block in bronchial asthma. J. Indian Med. Assoc., *76*:132–134, 1981.
19. Ramamurthy, S., Akkinemi, B., and Winnie, A.P.: A simple method for spinal accessory nerve block. In Abstracts of Scientific Papers—Annual Meeting. Chicago, American Society of Anesthesiologists, 1976.
20. Szeinfeld, M., Laurencio, M., and Pallares, V.S.: Total reversible blindness following stellate ganglion block. Anesth. Analg., *60*:689–690, 1981.
21. Wittich, D.J., Berney, J.J., and Davis, R.K.: Cervical epidural for head and neck surgery. Laryngoscope, *94*:615–619, 1984.
22. Takasaki, M., and Takahashi, T.: Respiratory function during cervical and thoracic extradural analgesia in patients with normal lungs. Br. J. Anaesth., *52*:1271–1275, 1980.
23. Bolisjevac, J.E., and Farha, S.J.: Carotid endarterectomy: Results using regional anaesthesia. Am. Surg., *46*:403–408, 1980.
24. Peitzman, A.B., Webster, M.W., Loubeau, J.M., et al.: Carotid endarterectomy under regional (conductive) anesthesia. Ann. Surg., 196:59–64, 1982.
25. Prough, D.S.,, Schuderi, P.E., Stullken, E., and Davis, C.E.: Myocardial infarction following regional anaesthesia for carotid endarterectomy. Can. Anaesth. Soc. J., *31*:192–196, 1984.
26. Jopling, M.W., deSanctis, C.A., and McDowell, D.E.: Anesthesia for carotid endarterectomy: A comparison of regional and general techniques. Anesthesiology, *59*:217, 1983.
27. Murphy, T.M.: Complications of diagnostic and therapeutic nerve blocks. In Cooperman, L.H., and Orkin, F.K. (eds.): Complications in Anesthesiology. Philadelphia, J.B. Lippincott, 1985.
28. Nique, T.A., and Bennett, C.R.: Inadvertent brainstem anesthesia following extraoral trigeminal V2–V3 blocks. Oral Surg., *51*:468–470, 1981.
29. Sipilia, P., Palva, A., Sorri, M., and Kauko, L.: Atlanto axial subluxation: An unusual complication after local anesthesia for tonsillectomy. Arch. Otolaryngol., *107*:181–182, 1981.
30. Ludwig, B.O.: The role of local anaesthesia in the reduction of long-standing dislocation of the tempero-mandibular joint. Br. J. Oral Surg., *18*:81–85, 1980.
31. Olsen, M.L., and McEvoy, G.K.: Methemoglobinemia induced by local anesthesia. Am. J. Hosp. Pharm., *38*:89–93, 1981.
32. Sandza, J.G., Roberts, R.W., Shaw, T.C., and Connors, J.P.: Symptomatic methemoglobinemia with a commonly used topical anesthetic cetacaine. Ann. Thorac. Surg., *30*:187–190, 1980.

section E
SPECIALIZED APPLICATIONS

16 NEURAL BLOCKADE OF ORAL AND CIRCUMORAL STRUCTURES: INTRAORAL APPROACH

C. RICHARD BENNETT

Local anesthesia of oral and circumoral structures has traditionally been provided by members of the medical profession using *extraoral* techniques. The dental profession, however, relies primarily on *intraoral* techniques to achieve its anesthetic goals. Either approach will usually provide satisfactory results, but there are those occasions in which one method is preferred over the other. The presence of anatomic anomalies, infection, or the nature of an injury, for example, may mitigate for or against a particular technique.

Generally, the extraoral approach is designed to provide anesthesia of a major nerve trunk (*e.g.*, V_2, V_3). The effect of the blockade is to provide anesthesia of a rather wide area of the face, head, or neck. Not infrequently, however, anesthesia of a limited area of the oral cavity is indicated for therapeutic or diagnostic purposes. In these instances the intraoral approach will provide a safe, convenient, and easily mastered alternative to extraoral techniques.

In an attempt to expand the anesthesiologist's armamentarium, this chapter will discuss the most common intraoral techniques used by the dental profession to anesthetize the oral cavity. The techniques themselves are easily mastered and, when administered properly, cause little if any physical discomfort to the patient. The anesthesiologist must also be aware, however, of the existence of tremendous psychological factors associated with manipulations of the oral cavity. Perhaps after performing several intraoral nerve blocks the physician will come to realize the plight of the dentist in dealing with such an anatomically simple yet psychologically involved area as the oral cavity.

To discuss the psychological aspects of the oral cavity, dental phobias, "fear of the dentist," and the like is beyond the scope of this chapter. Suffice it to say that on many occasions in which local anesthesia of the oral cavity (particularly via the intraoral approach) is to be provided, preoperative fear-allaying modalities such as suggestion, hypnosis, or chemically induced sedation must be provided.[2] Management of the apprehensive dental patient may be one of the most challenging problems in the health care delivery field.

PREPARATION

As with all anesthesia, certain requirements must be met before starting the procedure. It will be assumed that the findings of a recent history and physical examination have been reviewed and considered before selecting the anesthetizing technique and drugs that will be used. For the safety of the patient it will also be assumed that the patient's physical condition and ability to tolerate the pending procedure, and the presence of allergies or potentially interfering comedications, have been taken into account.

Special Injection Considerations

Patient Position. The intraoral injections to be described can best be carried out with the patient seated comfortably in the semireclining position (Fig. 16-1). (Most operating and many treatment tables can also be maneuvered into this position.) This position offers at least two advantages over the conventional upright or horizontal position. First, the convenience of the operator is facilitated. All areas of the oral cavity can be visualized easily and access is gained readily. Second, positional support to the patient's cardiovascular and respiratory systems is provided. Not infrequently, the person receiving an intraoral injection will suffer a bout of syncope during the course of anesthetic administration. Perhaps this relates to the psychological aspects that take place upon trespass of the oral cavity.

The semireclining position will not only aid venous return from both the lower extremities and upper torso but also facilitate respiration by relieving the diaphragm of pressure normally applied by the viscera during the horizontal or Trendelenburg position. When using the semireclining position during injections, syncopal episodes are frequently prevented. The incidence of this annoying and often frightening (at least to the patient and surely to dental students) episode has been greatly reduced by the advent of lounge-type contoured dental chairs.

The description of all intraoral injection techniques to be described will rely on anatomic landmarks for their points of reference. This may be in contrast to other textbooks in which an upright or horizontal patient position is assumed. Under those conditions, reference is often made to a syringe positioned perpendicular, parallel, or at an angle to the floor.

Tissue Preparation. Tissue preparation for regional anesthesia at extraoral sites usually involves disinfection of the area with a suitable preparatory solution, draping with sterile towels, and gloving by the operator. It would seem desirable to apply the same principles of "sterile technique" within the oral cavity. In practical terms, however, they are neither necessary nor attainable. Nevertheless, certain basic principles may be applied to minimize the risk of infection and mishap.

Before injection, the hands of the operator should be scrupulously cleansed. Although sterile techniques cannot be adhered to within the oral cavity, it is essential to exercise every precaution to ensure that infection is not introduced into deep structures.

Before inserting a needle into the tissues of the oral cavity, the operator should dry the area with a sterile cotton-tipped applicator stick or a two-by-two gauge sponge. The area should then be scrubbed with a suitable oral antiseptic agent and the antiseptic wiped from the tissue to prevent its introduction into the tissues during needle penetration.

Obviously, the administration of local anesthesia is one of the most frightening aspects of dental care. For this reason it is recommended that tissue penetration be made as painlessly as possible. The application of a topical anesthetic (many flavored brands are available) before tissue penetration aids greatly in reducing discomfort.

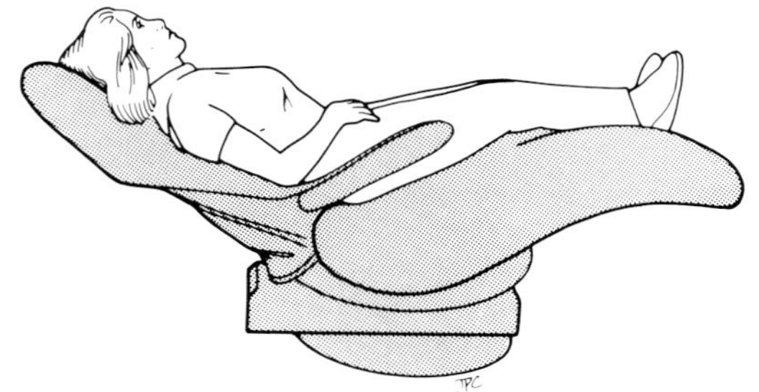

FIG. 16-1. Patient should be placed in semireclining position with legs and thorax slightly elevated.

ARMAMENTARIUM

Although basically similar to the armamentarium used for other types of neural blockade, the equipment used for intraoral anesthesia is sufficiently different and convenient enough to warrant comment. This is not to imply that "standard" equipment cannot or should not be used.

The materials used to obtain intraoral neural blockade may be subdivided as follows:[3]

1. Cartridges containing the anesthetic solution
2. Syringes
3. Needles
4. Auxiliary equipment and supplies

CARTRIDGE

The introduction of the local anesthetic cartridge for dental use was a major step forward because it ensured sterility and uniformity of solution composition. The cartridge is a glass tube sealed at one end by a movable rubber stopper that can be forced into the tube by the plunger of the cartridge-type syringe (Fig. 16-2). The other end of the tube is sealed by an aluminum cap over a rubber diaphragm that is punctured by the cartridge end of the needle (Fig. 16-3). Cartridges are hermetically sealed and contain 1.8 ml of anesthetic solution.

Cartridges are supplied by the manufacturer in either vacuum-packed cans or sealed cartons. After the package containing the cartridges has been opened, it is recommended that cartridges be stored in their original container. Cartridges should not be placed or submerged in any germicide.

Germicides will corrode the metal caps, and the potentially neurolytic germicide agent will eventually seep into the cartridge. The same may be said of the plunger end of the cartridge. In time the germicide will penetrate the rubber stopper if the entire cartridge is submerged.

Problems with Cartridges. Despite care taken in the manufacturing of local anesthetic cartridges, several minor problems may develop:

1. Bubbles. Small bubbles (1 – 2 mm) may be noted within the cartridge. These bubbles are usually nitrogen gas, which has been bubbled into the anesthetic during the manufacturing process to prevent oxygen, which would cause deterioration of the vasoconstrictor, from entering the cartridge. The bubbles are harmless. However, large bubbles in cartridges with or without plungers extended beyond the end of the cartridge (extruded) are caused by freezing. Because the contents may no longer be considered sterile, they should be discarded or returned to the supplier.
2. Extruded plungers. Extruded plungers on cartridges that contain no bubbles usually indicate that the cartridge has been stored in disinfecting solution and that some of the solution has passed through the rubber stopper or diaphragm and contaminated the anesthetic solution. These, too, should be discarded.
3. Corrosion of aluminum cap. Corrosion of the cap is usually caused by immersing the cartridge in chemical disinfecting solutions that contain nitrate antirust materials. Cartridges with corroded caps should not be used.

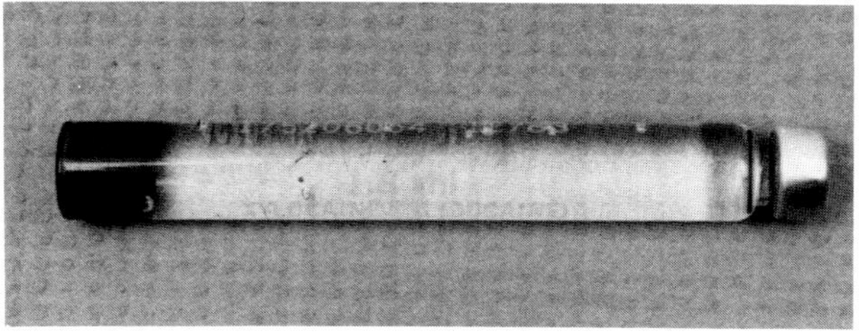

FIG. 16-2. Needle end *(right)* of the cartridge is sealed with a metal cap. A rubber plunger at the other end is used to expel the contents.

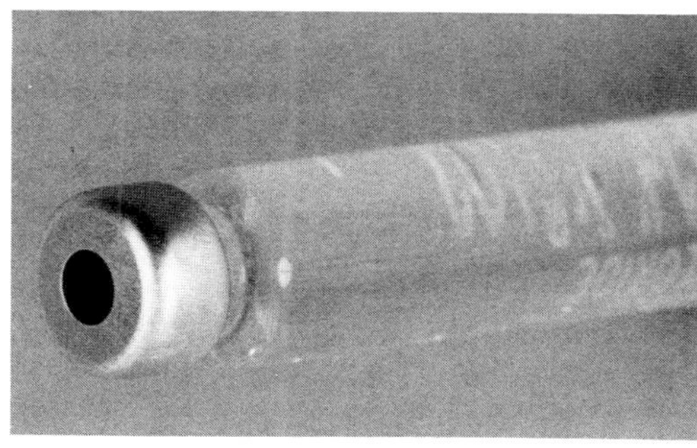

FIG. 16-3. Cartridge with aluminum cap over rubber diaphragm.

SYRINGES

One of the most commonly used syringes for intraoral injections is the side-loading metal cartridge syringe (Fig. 16-4).

Before the needle is attached, the piston of the syringe is retracted and the cartridge inserted, plunger end first into the syringe (Fig. 16-5*A*). Next the piston is pushed forward (not tapped; breakage of the glass cylinder might occur) with moderate pressure until the harpoon on the plunger (Fig. 16-5*B*) is firmly engaged in the rubber stopper. This will allow the stopper to be advanced and withdrawn when aspirating. The needle is then affixed to the threaded end of the syringe provided for this purpose (Fig. 16-5*C*). A few drops of solution are expressed to ensure that the unit is properly assembled and ready for use (Fig. 16-5*D*).

The syringe may be dismantled for cleaning. It may be reassembled and sterilized in the conventional manner.

NEEDLES

Needles for intraoral injection may range from 30 to 25 gauge and from ½ to 1⅝ inches in length.

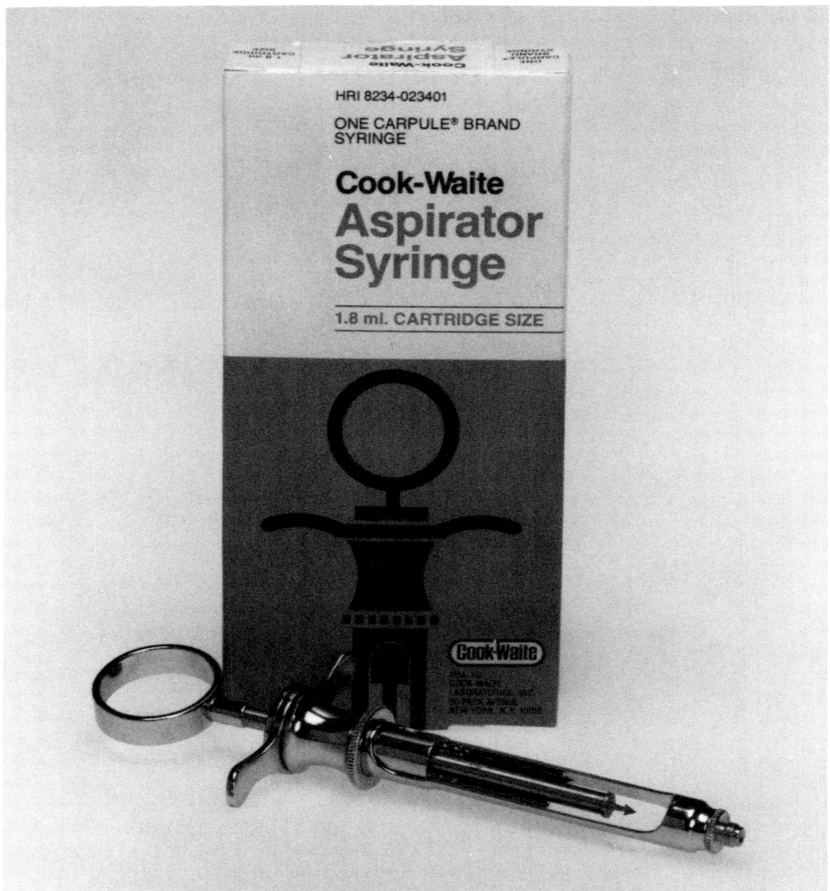

FIG. 16-4. Metal aspirating syringe that can be resterilized. (Courtesy of Cook-Waite Laboratories, Inc.)

A needle that is used in conjunction with dental application is divided into five sections: the bevel, shank, hub, syringe adapter, and syringe end of the needle (Fig. 16-6). The gauge denotes the diameter of the lumen of the shank, while the length is measured from the hub to the point of the bevel.

For deep intraoral injections, the 25-gauge, 1⅝-inch needle is preferred by most practitioners and advocated by most educators. This needle may be painlessly inserted and directed to the desired site with minimal deflection yet is of sufficient gauge to allow reliable aspiration.

As noted above, the "dental needle" is equipped with a pointed extension that protrudes from the syringe adapter toward the barrel of the syringe. Once affixed to the syringe, this end of the needle protrudes through the rubber diaphragm of the cartridge, thus forming a sterile fluid path through which the anesthetic solution may be expressed from the cartridge.

AUXILIARY EQUIPMENT AND SUPPLIES

Because complications and emergencies can occur during the use of regional anesthesia, it is imperative that all necessary equipment and supplies be on hand and readily available for emergency use. An emergency tray containing necessary syringes, needles, and drugs should be within easy reach. In addition, necessary adjuncts to airway maintenance and a manual ventilator should be on hand (see Chap. 6).

Although one may obtain anesthesia within the oral cavity using relatively small doses and volumes of local anesthetic drugs, their administration must not be approached carelessly. The head and neck, after all, constitute a very vascular area of the body. Unintentional intravascular injection or rapid absorption of even relatively small drug doses may precipitate sequellae of major proportion.

In addition, it is estimated that 90% of all medical emergencies occurring in dental offices are psycho-

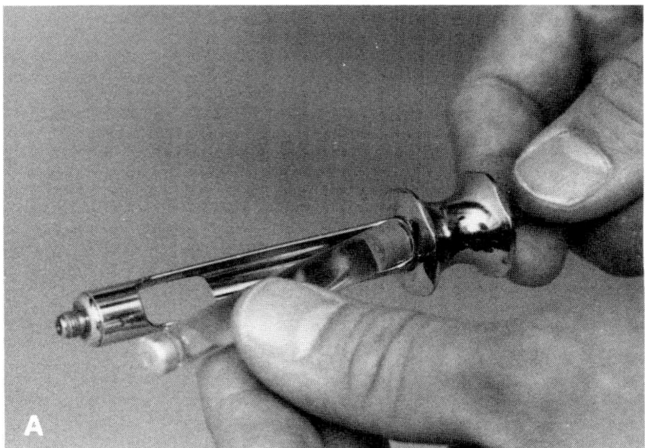

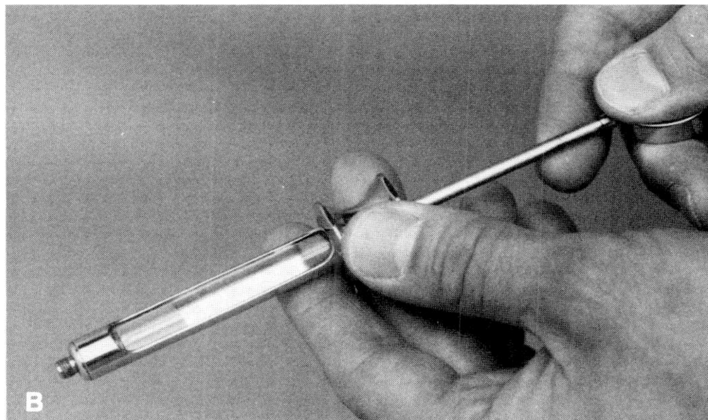

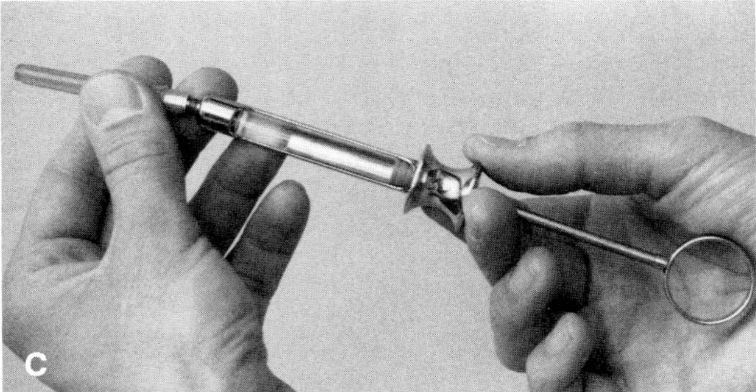

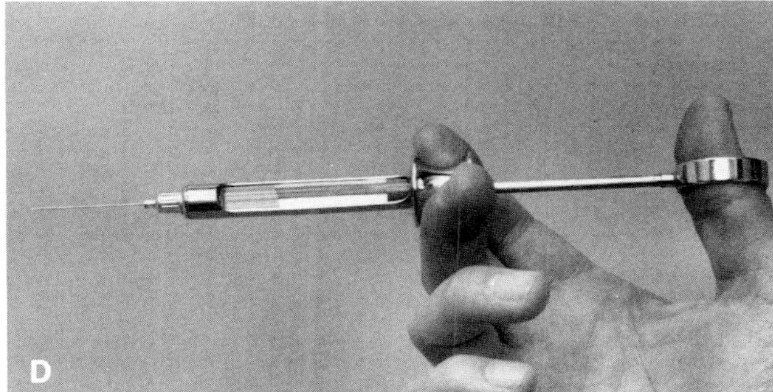

FIG. 16-5. **A.** Plunger is retracted and cartridge inserted into syringe. **B.** Piston pushed forward until harpoon engages plunger. **C.** Needle is affixed to syringe top. **D.** Prepared syringe is ready for use.

logically initiated.[6] They frequently take place in conjunction with, but are not necessarily directly attributable to, the administration of local anesthesia.

Syncope, angina, hyperventilation syndrome, and precipitation of seizure activity in epileptic patients are a few of the reactions reported to have been precipitated by anticipation and fear associated with intraoral neural blockade (see also Chap. 4).[4]

LOCAL ANESTHETIC SOLUTIONS

Although any local anesthetic solution acceptable for neural blockade may be used within the oral cavity, only six agents are currently marketed in cartridge form. Table 16-1 lists these anesthetic agents (by generic and trade names) and the vasoconstrictor that they may contain.

As in other types of neural blockade, the choice of anesthetic agent and vasoconstrictor is based on factors such as physical status, age and weight of the patient, duration required, and the need for hemostasis (see Table 16-2 for representative durations and recommended maximum safe dosages of agents used in dentistry).

In the past, local anesthetic cartridges also contained methylparaben as a germicide/preservative. Because of its documented allergenicity, however, many manufacturers have chosen to delete it from their preparations. To determine whether a particular brand of anesthetic contains methylparaben, one must consult the package insert or take note of the cartridge contents printed on the original container.

Bupivacaine (Marcaine) marketed in dental cartridges contains monothioglycerol and ascorbic acid as antioxidants.[5]

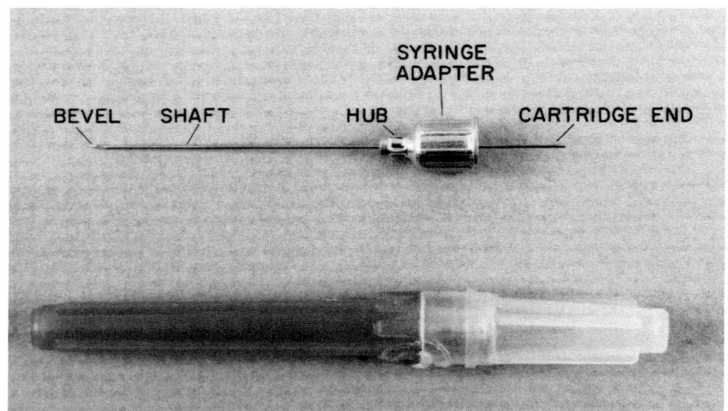

FIG. 16-6. Segments of dental needle.

INTRAORAL INJECTION TECHNIQUES

Anatomy

Innervation of the head and neck is by way of the trigeminal and cervical nerves as depicted in Figure 16-7. More specifically, the trigeminal nerve supplies the face and anterior portions of the scalp by means of its ophthalmic (V_1), maxillary (V_2), and mandibular (V_3) divisions. All areas of the oral cavity are innervated by either V_2 or V_3 (see Chap. 15).

TECHNIQUES OF NEURAL BLOCKADE FOR THE MAXILLARY NERVE AND ITS SUBDIVISIONS

Anatomy of the Maxillary Division (V_2)

The maxillary nerve is entirely sensory (Fig. 16-8). It exits the skull through the foramen rotundum and enters the pterygopalatine fossa, from where it progresses forward into the inferior orbital fissure and passes into the orbital cavity. Here it turns slightly laterally in the infraorbital groove on the orbital surface of the maxilla. As it continues forward it passes through the infraorbital canal and exits onto the front of the maxilla through the infraorbital foramen.

The branches of the maxillary nerve are as follows:

Branches Within the Pterygopalatine Fossa

1. Pharyngeal branch—to mucosa of pharynx
2. Middle and posterior palatine—to tonsil and soft palate
3. Greater palatine—to mucosa of posterior palate
4. Nasopalatine branch—to septal mucosa through incisive canal to the anterior hard palate
5. Posterior and superior lateral nasal branch—to lateral walls of nasal cavity
6. Posterior superior alveolar branch—to second and third maxillary molars as well as palatal and

TABLE 16-1. LOCAL ANESTHETICS IN CARTRIDGE FORM

Generic Name	Trade Name(s)	Vasoconstrictor
Bupivacaine 0.5%	Marcaine	1 : 200,000 epinephrine
Lidocaine 2%	Octocaine	Without vasoconstrictor
	Xylocaine	1 : 50,000 epinephrine
		1 : 100,000 epinephrine
Mepivacaine 3%	Carbocaine	Without vasoconstrictor
Mepivacaine 2%	Carbocaine	1 : 20,000 levonordefrin
Mepivacaine	Isocaine	Without vasoconstrictor
Mepivacaine 3%	Polocaine	Without vasoconstrictor
Prilocaine 4%	Citanest Plain	Without vasoconstrictor
Prilocaine 4%	Citanest Forte	1 : 200,000 epinephrine
Propoxycaine 0.4%*	Ravocaine/	1 : 30,000 levarterenol
Procaine 2%	Novocaine	

*Propoxycaine 0.4% and procaine 2% are combined in the same cartridge. Both compounds are ester-type anesthetic drugs. They are the only esters currently marketed in cartridge form. All other agents are amides.

TABLE 16-2. DURATION AND MAXIMUM SAFE DOSAGE OF AGENTS USED IN DENTISTRY

Drug	Duration Pulpal/ Soft Tissue)	Maximum Dose
Bupivacaine 0.5% 1:200,000 epinephrine	1–2 h/>10 h	1.3 mg/kg 90 mg max
Lidocaine 2% (without vasoconstrictor)	5–10 min/60–120 min	4.4 mg/kg 300 mg max
Lidocaine 2% 1:50,000 epinephrine	60–90 min/3–4 hr	7.0 mg/kg 500 mg max
Lidocaine 2% 1:100,000 epinephrine	60–90 min/3–4 h	7.0 mg/kg 500 mg max
Mepivacaine 3%	20–40 min/2–3 h	6.6 mg/kg 400 mg max
Mepivacaine 2% 1:20,000 levonordefrin	40–60 min/2–4 hr	6.6 mg/kg 400 mg max
Prilocaine plain 4%	10–15 min/2–4 h	7.9 mg/kg 600 mg max
Propoxycaine/ procaine	10–20 min/2–3 h	6.6 mg/kg 400 mg max total ester

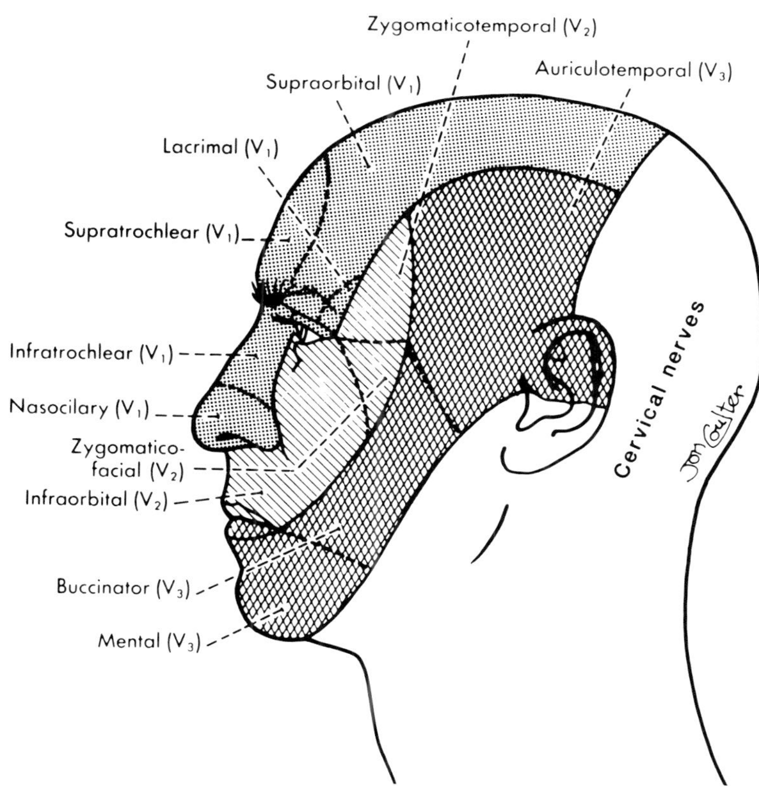

FIG. 16-7. Superficial sensory nerves of the head and neck.

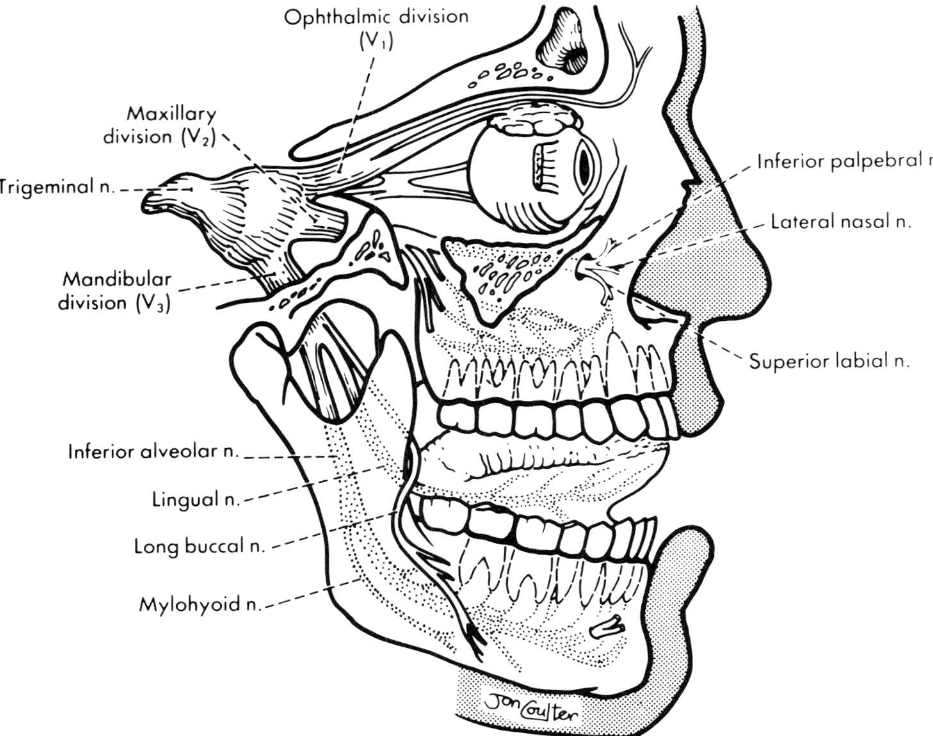

FIG. 16-8. Distribution of the trigeminal nerve.

distobuccal route of first molar, alveolus, and overlying buccal soft tissue. (The mesiobuccal root of the maxillary first molar is innervated by the middle superior alveolar nerve.)

7. Zygomatic branch — to skin of the temple and over the zygomatic bone

At this point the maxillary division becomes known as the infraorbital nerve.

Branches Within the Infraorbital Groove and Canal

1. Middle superior alveolar nerve — to anterior walls of the maxillary sinus, bicuspid teeth, buccal gingiva, and mucosa
2. Anterior superior alveolar nerve — to incisor and cuspid teeth and labial soft tissue

Terminal Branches on the Face

1. Inferior palpebral — to lower eyelid
2. Lateral nasal — to skin of the side of the nose
3. Superior labial — to cheek, skin, and mucosa of the upper lip.

Specific Intraoral Techniques

Local Infiltration. Soft tissues of the oral cavity may be satisfactorily anesthetized with local infiltration.

Technique. A 2.5-cm, 25-gauge needle is inserted beneath the mucous membrane into the connective tissue in the area to be anesthetized, and the solution is infiltrated slowly throughout. Because in many areas of the oral cavity the mucosa is adherent to the underlying periosteum, care must be taken to avoid depositing large volumes of solution. Large volumes may strip the periosteum from the underlying bone or result in pressure-induced soft tissue ischemia. The result will be postinjection pain and, on occasion, tissue slough.

Block of Terminal Branches (Field Block). Terminal branch block is indicated for anesthetizing anterior maxillary teeth or a limited area of the mandible. It is most commonly confined to the maxilla because the porosity of maxillary bone permits diffusion of the anesthetic solution through it. The technique is rarely successful in the mandible because of the density of the cortical plate of the bone. On occasion successful anesthesia of the mandibular anterior teeth may be achieved with this technique, particularly if injections are made on children or adults who have a thin overlying cortical plate. The success of this technique depends on diffusion of the anesthetic solution through the periosteum and underlying bone to come in contact with the nerves therein.

Technique. A 2.5-cm, 25-gauge needle is inserted through the mucous membrane and underlying connective tissue until it contacts the periosteum over the apex of the tooth (or teeth) in question (Fig. 16-9). One milliliter to 2 ml of solution should be injected slowly, allowing about 5 minutes for maximum effect. The maxillary incisors, cuspids, and bicuspids may be anesthetized in this manner. Maxillary molars will require other techniques because their roots are divergent and the overlying bone is rather dense.

Infraorbital Nerve Block (Block of the Anterior and Middle Superior Alveolar Nerves). Infraorbital nerve block is useful for providing anesthesia of the maxillary incisors, cuspids, and bicuspids, including their bony support and surrounding labial soft tissue. The lower eyelid, side of the nose, and upper lip will also be anesthetized.

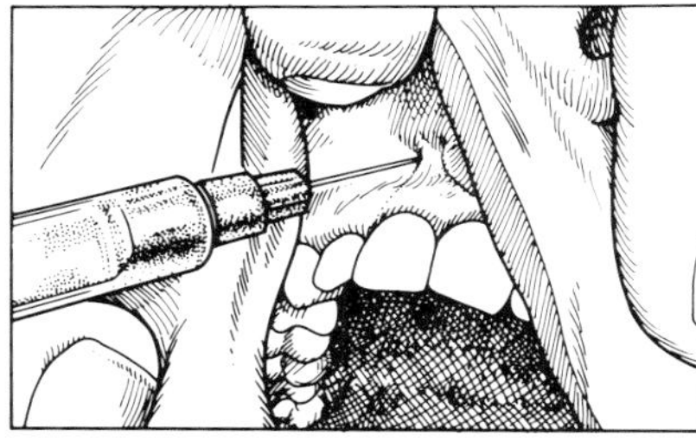

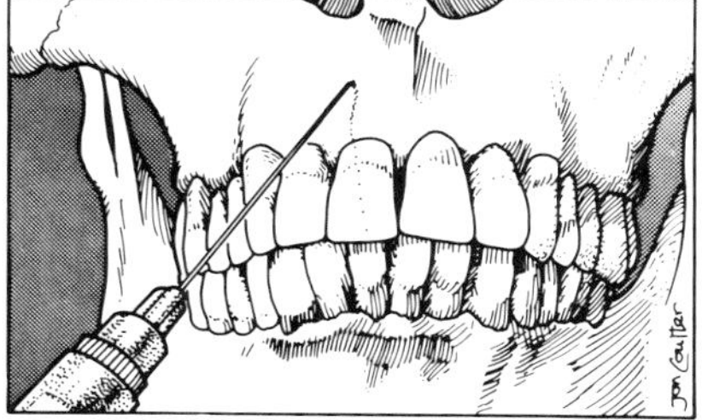

FIG. 16-9. Field block. The needle is inserted through mucous membrane in the area of the tooth or teeth to be anesthetized.

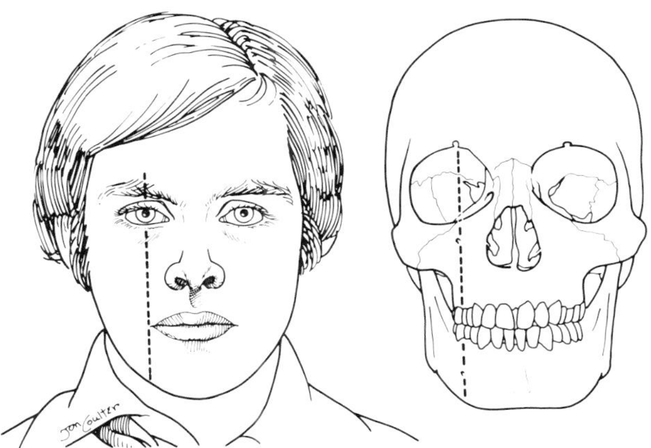

FIG. 16-10. Supraorbital notch, pupil of the eye, infraorbital notch, infraorbital foramen, bicuspid teeth, and mental foramen lie on a straight vertical line.

Technique. The patient is instructed to look directly forward while the operator palpates the supraorbital and infraorbital notches. An imaginary straight line drawn vertically through these landmarks will pass through the pupil of the eye, infraorbital foramen, the bicuspid teeth, and the mental foramen (Fig. 16-10). When the infraorbital notch is located, the palpating finger (or thumb) should follow the vertical line inferiorly about 0.5 cm, at which point a shallow depression will be felt. The infraorbital foramen is located within the depression.

For a block on the right side, the thumb of the operator's left hand is placed over the previously located foramen and the index finger is used to retract the lip (Fig. 16-11). A 4-cm, 25-gauge needle is then inserted along the imaginary vertical line until the foramen is reached. The needle should be inserted a sufficient distance (about 0.5 cm) from the labial plate to bridge the canine fossa. The thumb in place over the foramen should be used to maneuver the needle into position so that it contacts the bone at the entrance to the foramen. The needle should not penetrate soft tissue for more than 2 cm. About 2 ml of solution is deposited.

Tingling and numbness of the lower eyelid, side of the nose, and upper lip will always be produced but is not necessarily an indication of a successful block. In order to anesthetize the anterior and middle superior alveolar nerves that supply the teeth, the solution must enter the infraorbital foramen and flow centrally through the infraorbital canal. Instrumentation

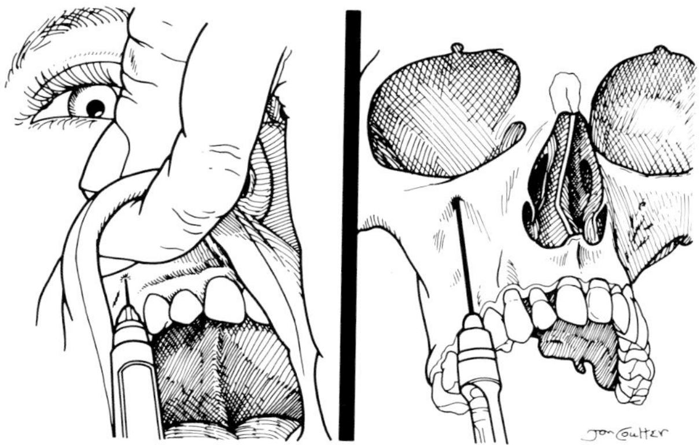

FIG. 16-11. The thumb is maintained in place over the infraorbital foramen.

of the teeth in question will demonstrate success or failure of the block.

Figure 16-12 depicts the anatomic relationships involved when performing the infraorbital nerve block.

Posterior Superior Alveolar Nerve Block. This nerve block provides anesthesia of the third, second, and ⅔ of the first maxillary molar as well as supporting, hard, and buccal soft tissue.

Since the first molar has dual innervation, the posterior superior alveolar nerve block must be coupled with infiltration over the mesiobuccal root to anesthetize it completely.

The posterior superior alveolar nerve arises from the maxillary nerve before it enters the body of the maxilla. It is located distal to the maxillary tuberosity.

Technique. For a block on the right side, the operator places the left forefinger on the buccal surface of the maxillary molars parallel to the occlusal plane. The finger is moved posteriorly until the zygomatic process of the maxilla is reached (Fig. 16-13). At this point the finger is rotated so that the fingernail is adjacent to the alveolar mucosa and its bulbous portion is in contact with the posterior surface of the zygomatic process (Fig. 16-14). The index finger is now pointing in the exact direction the needle is to follow. The insertion is made for a distance of 1.5 to 2 cm, going upward, inward, and backward behind the tuberosity.

To avoid hematoma caused by unintentional trauma to the pterygoid venous plexus, the needle should be kept in contact with the posterior surface of the maxilla throughout the injection. Hematoma caused by a rent in an artery in this area will be rapidly manifest as swelling to the side of the face. Venous hematomas will develop more slowly. Either may produce swelling of surprising proportion. Cold compresses should be applied immediately if a hematoma is suspected.

Maxillary Nerve Block (High Tuberosity Approach). The entire second division of the trigeminal nerve may be anesthetized in a manner almost identical to that described for the posterior superior al-

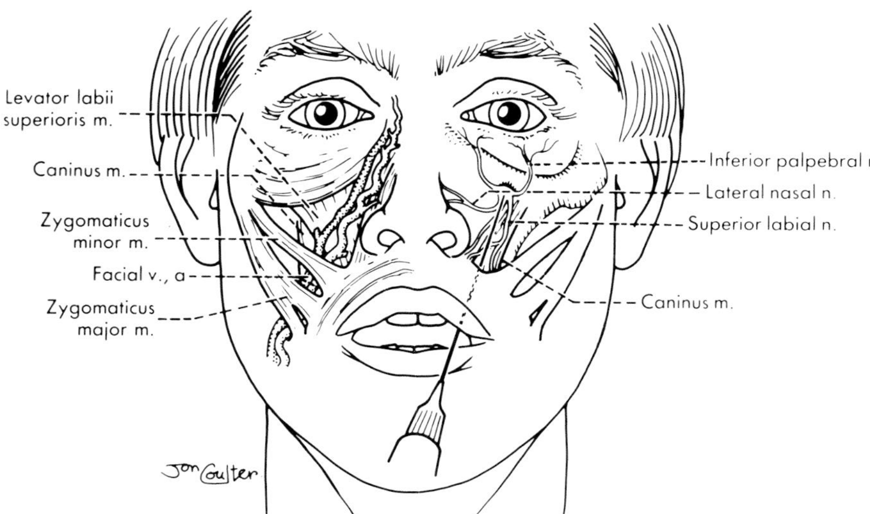

FIG. 16-12. Anatomic relationships relative to the infraorbital nerve block.

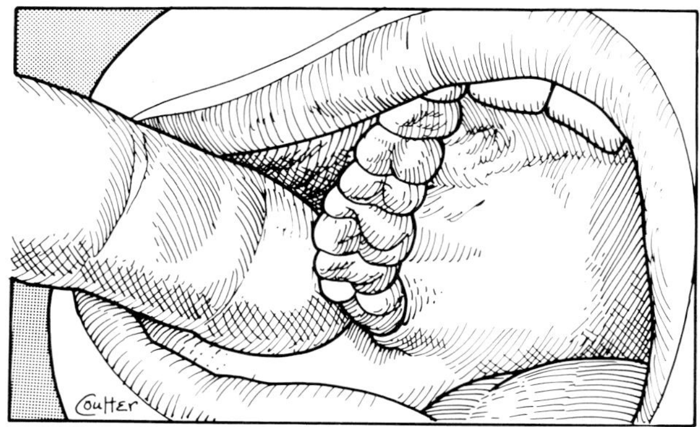

FIG. 16-13. The operator moves the left index finger posteriorly over the buccal surface of the maxillary molars until the zygomtic process of the maxilla is reached.

veolar nerve block. The only difference is that to anesthetize the entire maxillary nerve a 4-cm needle should be inserted to a depth of about 4 cm. The entire contents of the cartridge (1.8–2 ml) should be deposited.

Anesthesia of the three terminal branches as they exit into the face confirms a successful neural blockade of the maxillary nerve.

Nasopalatine Nerve Block. Anesthesia of the nasopalatine nerve will provide palatal hard and soft tissue anesthesia from the bicuspids forward. The procedure for anesthetizing the nasopalatine nerve is relatively simple. Unfortunately, it is also relatively painful.

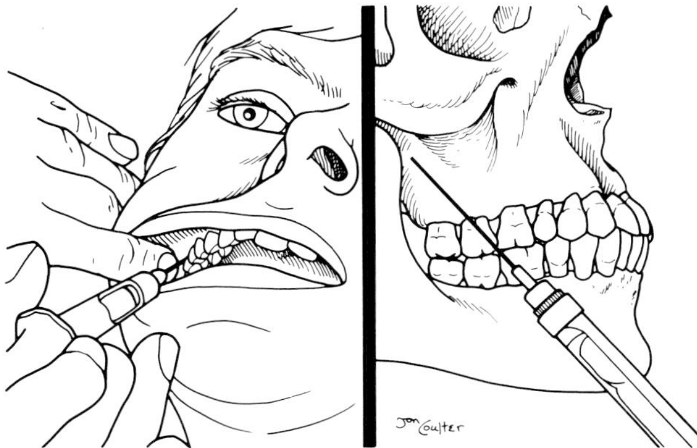

FIG. 16-14. Rotated finger points to path of needle insertion.

Technique. A 2.5-cm, 25-gauge needle is inserted into the incisive papilla just behind the maxillary central incisors (Fig. 16-15). The needle need not be introduced into the nasopalatine canal for successful anesthesia.

Because the soft tissue (particularly submucosal connective tissue) is sparse in this area, only a drop or two of solution can be injected. Care must be taken to avoid injecting too large a quantity of solution lest postinjection pain and tissue slough ensue.

Anterior Palatine Nerve Block. Anesthetizing the anterior palatine nerve results in anesthesia of the posterior hard palate to the midline. This injection too is both relatively simple and painful.

Technique. The anterior palatine nerve emerges into the palate through the greater palatine foramen and courses forward in a groove parallel to the molar teeth. The foramen is situated between the second and third maxillary molars about 1 cm from the teeth toward the midline.

The foramen is approached from the opposite side with a 2.5-cm, 25-gauge needle that is kept as near to a right angle as possible with the curvature of the palatal bone (Fig. 16-16). One-fourth to one-half milliliter is injected. For satisfactory palatal anesthesia, the greater palatine foramen and canal need not be entered.

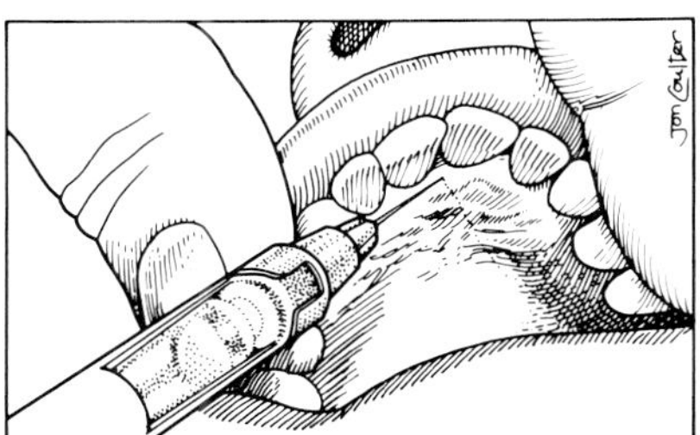

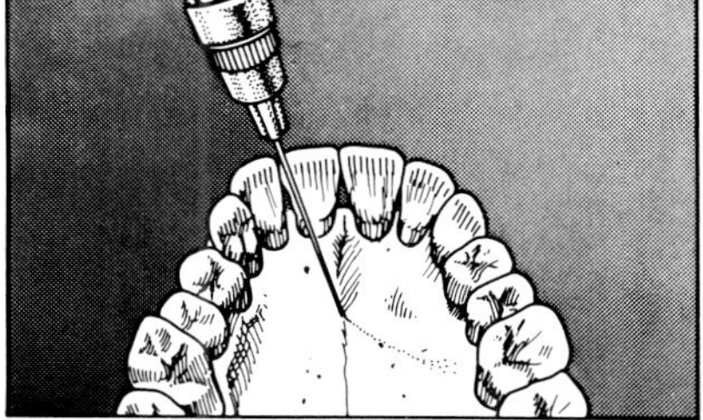

FIG. 16-15. Needle is inserted into the incisive papilla behind the maxillary central incisors.

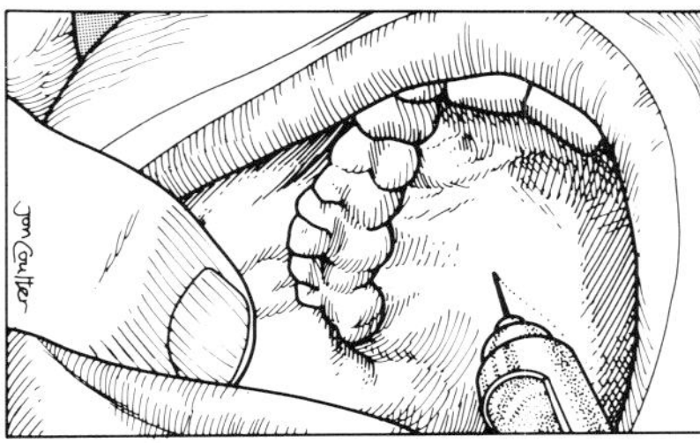

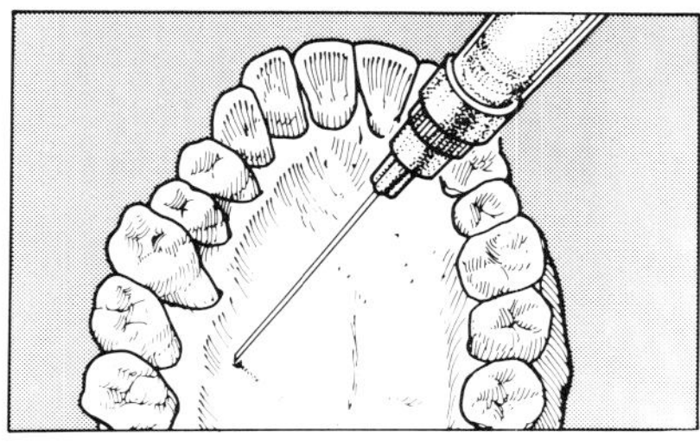

FIG. 16-16. Block of anterior palatine nerve. Needle is inserted from the opposite side, keeping it as near to a right angle as possible with the curvature of the palate.

Maxillary Nerve (Palatal Approach). Using an approach similar to the one described for the anterior palatine nerve block, one may secure anesthesia of the entire distribution of the maxillary nerve. A 4-cm, 25-gauge needle is required.

Once the needle has penetrated the palatal mucosa, the greater palatine foramen is gently probed and the canal entered. The needle is advanced into the canal to a depth not to exceed 4 cm inches. Any resistance encountered should not be overcome with force, but the needle should be withdrawn and again advanced slowly. If continued resistance is met, regardless of how slight, the attempt should be discontinued.

Once resting within the canal at the desired depth, 2 ml of solution is deposited.

TECHNIQUES OF NEURAL BLOCKADE FOR THE MANDIBULAR NERVE AND ITS SUBDIVISIONS

Anatomy of the Mandibular Division (V_3)

The mandibular division of the trigeminal nerve is both sensory and motor. The motor division does not emerge from the gasserian ganglion but joins the sensory branch after it leaves the anteroinferior part of the gasserian ganglion. For a short distance they travel side by side, then form a single trunk to exit the skull through the foramen ovale. From this trunk a motor branch passes to the internal pterygoid and two tensor muscles. The trunk then divides into an anterior and posterior division.

The branches of the anterior division are as follows:

1. External pterygoid nerve—motor
2. Masseter nerve—motor
3. Temporal muscle nerve—motor
4. Long buccal nerve—sensory

The long buccal nerve passes between the two heads of the pterygoid muscle, crosses the anterior border of the ramus at the level of the occlusal plane of the teeth, and supplies the skin and mucous membranes of the cheek and buccal gingiva from the retromolar triangle to the bicuspid teeth.

The branches of the posterior division are as follows:

1. Auriculotemporal nerve—sensory to the parotid gland, temporomandibular joint, external auditory meatus, and scalp in the temporal region.
2. Lingual nerve—sensory to the lingual mucous membranes, anterior two thirds of the tongue, and floor of the mouth. (The chorda tympani nerve from the seventh cranial nerve joins the lingual nerve shortly after its origin and supplies fibers of special sense to taste buds of the anterior two thirds of the tongue.)
3. Inferior alveolar nerve—sensory to the mandibular teeth, body of the mandible, and labial gingiva anterior to the bicuspid teeth. This nerve passes downward on the medial side of the external pterygoid muscle and the medial side of the mandibular ramus. On the medial side of the ramus in the pterygomandibular space it enters the mandibular foramen. It then travels anteriorly within the body of the mandible. In the region of the mental foramen, the inferior alveolar nerve divides into two terminal branches:
   a. Mental nerve—leaves body of the mandible through mental foramen and is sensory to the skin of the chin and lower lip and mucous membrane lining the lower lip.
   b. Incisive nerve—continues anteriorly within the body of the mandible to supply anterior teeth and their supporting hard tissues.

Specific Intraoral Techniques

Classic Inferior Alveolar Nerve Block. This nerve block is used to provide hard tissue anesthesia from the mandible to the midline and labial soft tissue anesthesia from the bicuspid teeth to the midline. For complete anesthesia of the mandible (*e.g.*, for extraction of all teeth), this block must be supplemented with long buccal and lingual nerve blocks.

Technique. The patient is instructed to open the mouth as wide as possible. For a block on the right side the operator palpates the mucobuccal fold in the area of the molar teeth with the left thumb. The thumb is then moved posteriorly until contact is made with the external oblique ridge on the anterior border of the ramus of the mandible. The deepest concavity on the anterior border of the ramus, the coronoid notch, is then identified. The coronoid notch is in a direct line with the lingula, the point at which the inferior alveolar nerve enters the ramus of the mandible (Fig. 16-17).

The palpating thumb is then moved medially onto the internal oblique ridge, the inner "edge" of the ramus. This manuever helps estimate the width of the ramus. The thumb is once again moved to the lateral side of the ramus, retracting soft tissues of the cheek while doing so. At this point the left index finger grasps the posterior border of the mandible from the extraoral approach (Fig. 16-18). In this manner the operator is holding the ramus of the mandible between the thumb and index finger, thus allowing the operator to estimate the anteroposterior width of the ramus.

A syringe with a 4-cm, 25-gauge needle is then inserted parallel to the occlusal plane at a height indicated by the coronoid notch just medial to the internal oblique ridge. The needle should approach the ramus at an angle that is parallel to the inner surface of the ramus (Figure 16-19). Depth of insertion may be determined by estimating when the needle tip has been advanced half the distance between the thumb and index finger. When in proper position for deposition of solution, the needle tip will be close to the inferior alveolar nerve, artery, and vein.

After aspiration, about 2 ml of solution is deposited. Subjective symptoms of anesthesia include tingling and numbness of the lower lip.

Closed-Mouth Approach to Mandibular Nerve Block. On occasion the need arises to anesthetize the mandibular nerve while the teeth are approximated in occlusion (*e.g.*, jaws wired together following mandibular resection). This injection may be invaluable,

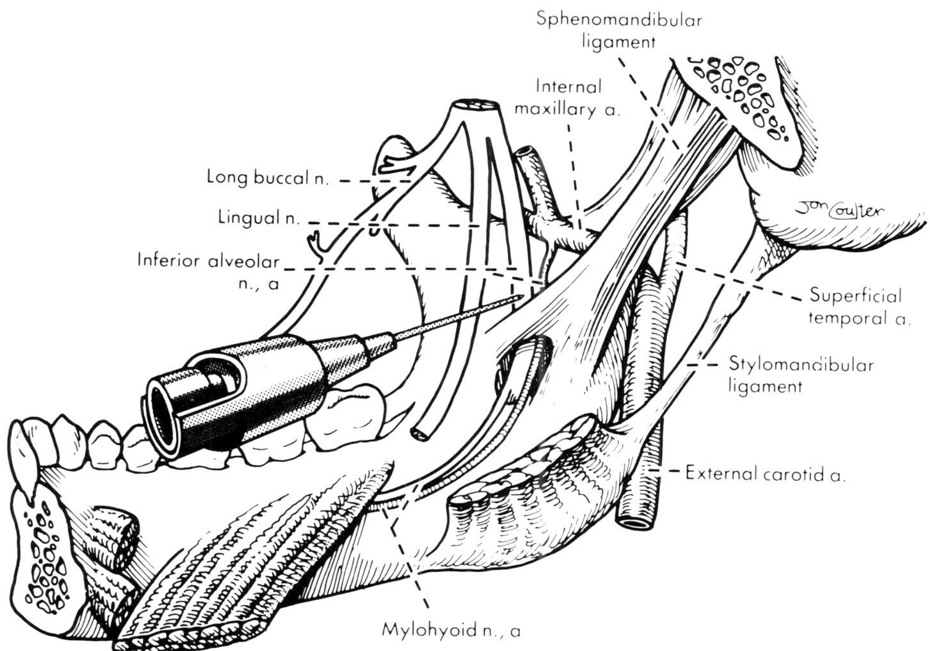

FIG. 16-17. Coronoid notch is in a direct line with the point at which the inferior alveolar nerve enters the ramus of the mandible.

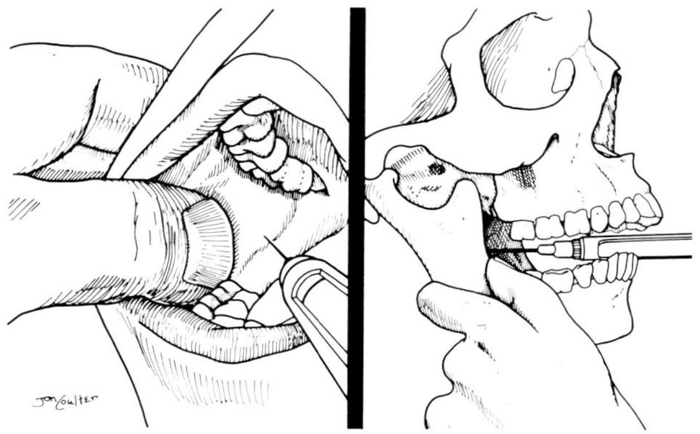

FIG. 16-18. The ramus is grasped between an intraorally placed thumb and an extraorally positioned index finger.

for example, when removing intermaxillary fixation wires.

Since the height of needle insertion and deposition of anesthetic solution is considerably superior to the site for producing inferior alveolar nerve anesthesia, a true mandibular block will be secured[1]; that is to say, the long buccal, inferior alveolar, and lingual nerve distribution will be affected.

Technique. With the teeth in occlusion, the lips are retracted and the needle and syringe are aligned parallel to the occlusal plane at the level of the mucogingival junction of the maxillary molar teeth. The needle penetrates mucosa (Fig. 16-20) just medial to the ramus and is inserted to a depth of about 3 cm. Following negative aspiration, the entire contents of the cartridge are slowly deposited. Successful anesthesia will be confirmed by instrumentation of the mandibular distribution.

Two factors are apt to contribute to failure of this technique. First, the technique relies on a minimum number of bony landmarks for its execution. Depth of needle insertion, in particular, is a nebulous factor. In addition, improper angulation in a superior direction may result in partial or complete anesthesia of the maxilla, particularly if improper medial angulation occurs simultaneously.

Second, because of anatomic restrictions it is impossible to insert the needle parallel to the medial surface of the ramus. In effect, the deeper the needle penetration, the further from the "target" it gets.

Nevertheless, despite its drawbacks, this technique offers a suitable alternative to the classic approach to anesthesia of the mandibule when circumstances dictate its need (see also Chap. 15 and Fig. 15-6).

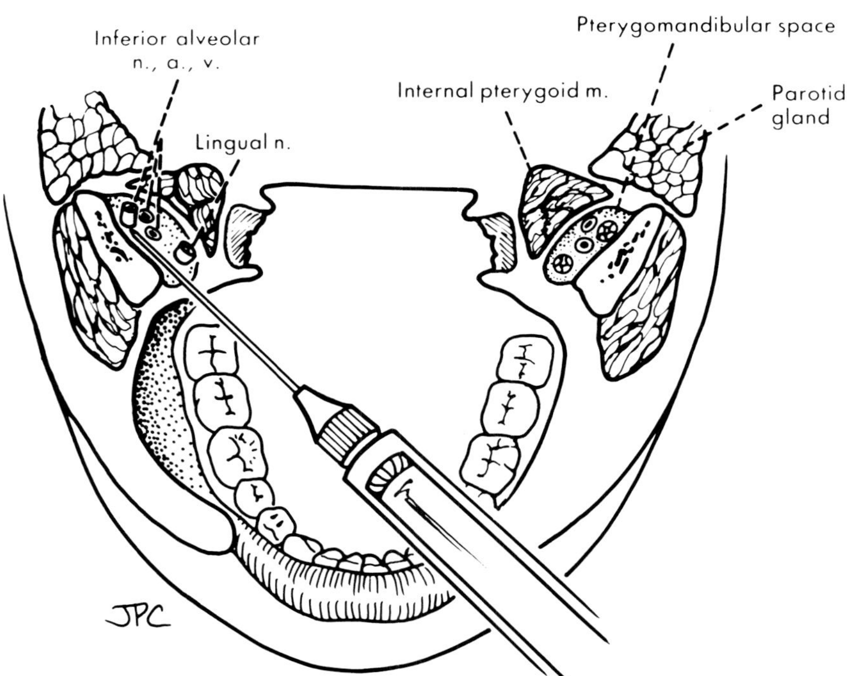

FIG. 16-19. Needle is inserted parallel to the medial surface of the ramus.

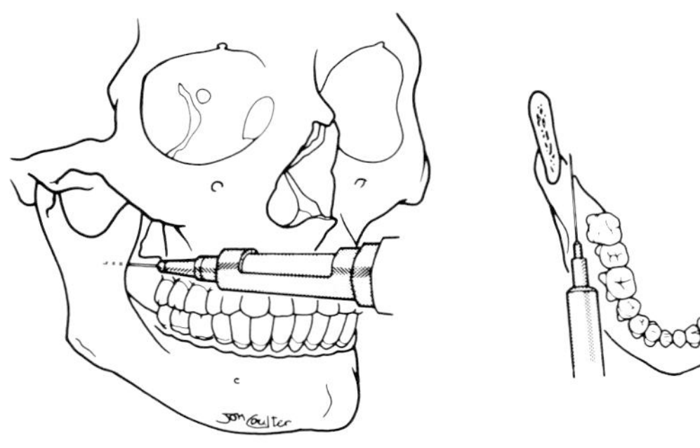

FIG. 16-20. With the teeth in occlusion, the needle is aligned parallel to the occlusal plane and positioned at the level just superior to the maxillary molars.

Lingual Nerve Block. The lingual nerve is close to the inferior alveolar nerve at its point of entry into the ramus of the mandible. For all intents and purposes it is impossible to anesthetize the lingual nerve without simultaneously blocking the inferior alveolar nerve, and *vice versa.* For this reason the injection technique for the lingual nerve block will not be discussed. (At any rate, it is identical to the inferior alveolar nerve block.)

Long Buccal Nerve Block. To provide complete mandibular anesthesia the long buccal nerve block must supplement the inferior alveolar and lingual nerve blocks previously described. The long buccal nerve branches from the mandibular nerve at a point superior to the site for an inferior alveolar nerve block. For this reason a separate injection must be made to provide soft tissue anesthesia adjacent to the molar teeth (see Fig. 16-17).

Technique. The coronoid notch and external oblique ridge are identified in the manner described for the inferior alveolar nerve block. The cheek is retracted and the needle inserted through the soft tissue at the height of the occlusal plane. The needle is directed to the external oblique ridge and inserted until contact is made (Fig. 16-21). One-fourth milliliter to ½ ml of solution is sufficient to anesthetize the long buccal nerve.

Mental Nerve Block. The mental nerve exits the body of the mandible through a foramen (mental foramen) located between the bicuspid teeth near their apices. A block of this nerve provides soft tissue anesthesia of the chin, lower lip, and its underlying mucosa and gingiva.

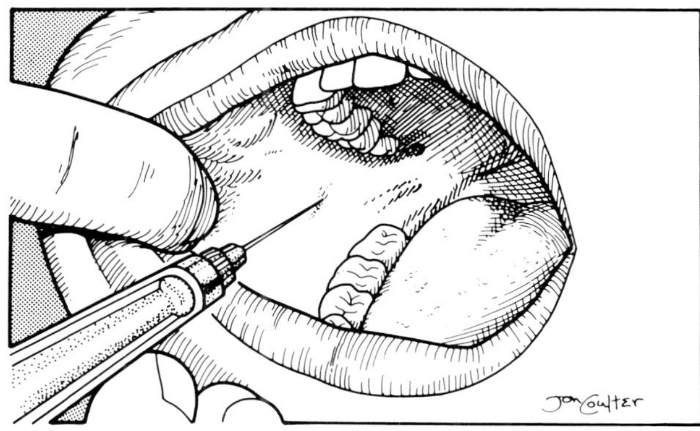

FIG. 16-21. Long buccal nerve block. The needle is inserted through the mucosa and directed toward the external oblique line at the level of the occlusal plane.

Technique. A syringe with 2.5-cm needle attached is inserted through the mucosa and directed to a point approximating the apices of the bicuspid teeth (Fig. 16-22). One-half milliliter to 1 ml of solution is deposited.

Incisive Nerve Block. The incisive nerve is the continuation of the inferior alveolar nerve within the anterior body of the mandible. It supplies the anterior teeth and their supporting hard tissues.

Technique. Access to the incisive nerve is gained through the mental foramen and canal, a structure that opens in a down, forward, and inward direction. For satisfactory anesthesia of the incisive nerve, the

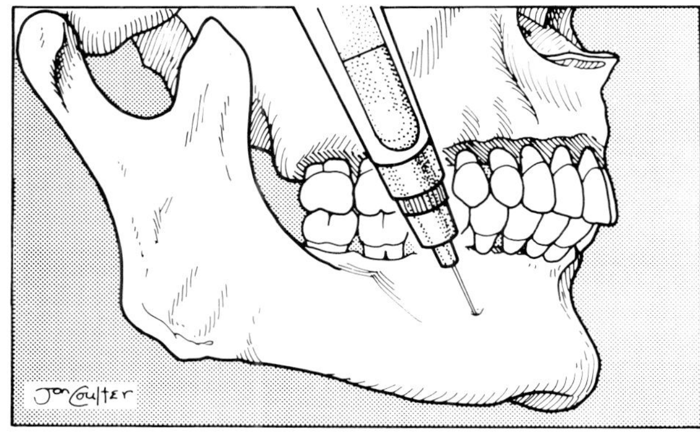

FIG. 16-22. To block the incisive nerve, direct the needle into the mental foramen and canal. The mental nerve will be blocked simultaneously.

mental foramen must be located, gently probed, and then entered by the needle tip. The needle must be directed into the canal at an angle parallel to its long axis.

After deposition of 1/4 to 1/2 ml of solution, anesthesia of the lower anterior teeth and their supporting structures will be produced. Because the mental nerve will be simultaneously anesthetized, anesthesia of the chin and lower lip will ensue.

SUMMARY

Discussed herein are the equipment, supplies, agents, and most common techniques used to provide local anesthesia of selective areas within the oral cavity. Although other techniques or modifications of those presented appear in a number of textbooks, it is hoped that the relatively simple, straightforward methods described will add significantly to the anesthesiologist's armamentarium.

REFERENCES

1. Akinosi, J.O.: A new approach to the mandibular nerve block. J. Oral Surg., *15*:83, 1977.
2. Bennett, C.R.: Conscious-sedation in Dental Practice. ed. 2. St. Louis, C.V. Mosby, 1978.
3. Bennett, C.R.: Monheim's Local Anesthesia and Pain Control in Dental Practice. ed. 7. St. Louis, C.V. Mosby, 1984.
4. Malamed, S.F.: Handbook of Medical Emergencies. ed. 2. St. Louis, C.V. Mosby, 1982.
5. Marcaine Package Insert. New York, Cook–Waite Laboratories, 1985.
6. Monheim, L.M.: Personal correspondence.

17 NEURAL BLOCKADE FOR OPHTHALMOLOGIC SURGERY

MARIANNE E. FEITL
THEODORE KRUPIN

Local anesthesia has been used in ophthalmic surgery for more than 100 years. The requirements and complications of local anesthesia for intraocular and specialized extraocular surgical procedures are unique. The conjunctiva and cornea can be completely anesthetized by topical application of anesthetic agents, and the sensory and motor nervous innervation to the eyeball and the surrounding adnexal tissues by local nerve blocks. A thorough understanding of the mechanism of neural blockade in ophthalmologic surgery depends upon knowledge of the associated anatomy. This chapter outlines the anatomy and techniques necessary to administer successful local anesthesia for ophthalmic surgery.

ANESTHETIC REQUIREMENTS FOR OPHTHALMIC SURGERY

INTRAOCULAR SURGERY

Anesthetic requirements for intraocular surgical procedures include complete akinesia of the extraocular muscles of the eyelid and surrounding face. Incomplete akinesia and subsequent contraction of an extraocular muscle in an eye with an open surgical wound can result in extrusion of intraocular contents. Incomplete akinesia of the eyelid can result in a similar complication secondary to external muscular pressure on the globe.

Satisfactory local anesthesia should provide complete anesthesia of the globe and ocular adnexae. While the duration of the anesthetic should be at least 1½ to 2 hours, longer-acting agents also provide postoperative analgesia.

Normal intraocular pressure is considered to be less than 21 mm Hg. Many surgeons use preoperative hyperosmotic agents to dehydrate the eye (primarily the vitreous) and to lower intraocular pressure. Hyperosmotic agents used before local anesthesia include the following:[4] [a] oral glycerine (1 g/kg) administered 1 hour preoperatively. This agent can cause nausea or vomiting, which may be reduced by prior administration of an antiemetic; [b] oral isosorbide (1 g/kg) given 1 hour before surgery. Isosorbide is not metabolized and results in less nausea than does glycerine; and [c] intravenous mannitol (1 g/kg) administered 15 to 30 minutes before surgery at a rate of 60 drops per minute. Mannitol should be given through a blood filter assembly to remove drug crystals. Many of the barbiturates used for preoperative sedation lower intraocular pressure secondary to a reduction in the rate of aqueous humor formation.[5]

Intraocular pressure should be measured after injection of the local anesthetic agent and before the actual incision into the eye. Incomplete akinesia increases intraocular pressure by mechanical external pressure on the globe. Retrobulbar anesthetic injection does not lower intraocular pressure[24]; however, excessive volume injections into the orbit may increase intraocular pressure secondary to external pressure on the globe. A similar effect results if the injection is complicated by an orbital hemorrhage.

EXTRAOCULAR SURGERY

Requirements for pure sensory or combined sensory/motor blockade vary according to the procedure being performed. Differential sensory blockade can allow surgical correction in the face of an unaltered motor component.

GENERAL VERSUS LOCAL ANESTHESIA

Anesthetic mortality is similar in patients undergoing ophthalmic surgery either under local or general anesthesia.[7] The incidence of operative complications is also similar. Preference between general or local anesthesia prevails in many regions of the United States as well as in different countries.

Cooperation and communication between the anesthesiologist and the surgeon are essential. Individual patient requirements must be satisfied. Preoperative interview and examination are required to determine the patient's physical and mental status and the ability to undergo anesthesia. The patient's medications that could affect anesthesia (*e.g.*, systemic or topical corticosteroids, topical beta-blockers, topical echothiophate) as well as drug allergies must be documented. A history of possible bleeding diathesis should be obtained.

Preoperative preparation of the patient, including explanation of the anesthetic technique, surgical procedure, and postoperative expectations, is a joint venture of the anesthesiologist and ophthalmologist. Anxiety is a common occurrence in patients undergoing eye surgery. This may be a greater problem and therefore requires more patient understanding with local anesthesia.

Continued communication is needed during the surgical procedure. The anesthesiologist should be aware of medications (*e.g.*, epinephrine and acetylcholine [Miochol]) used during the operation and intrasurgical manipulations, in particular tension on extraocular muscles that can result in bradycardia. The ophthalmologist should be informed of the patient's vital signs during the surgery.

LOCAL ANESTHESIA

Local anesthesia results in minimal physiologic alterations during the surgical procedure. Local anesthesia is relatively simple and requires minimal equipment; however, adequate patient monitoring, including electrocardiographic leads, blood pressure monitoring, and an intravenous infusion, is needed. A complete set of resuscitation drugs and equipment are also required. Local anesthesia can provide adequate akinesia and anesthesia as well as postoperative analgesia. Nausea and vomiting are reduced, and less postoperative observation and care of the patient are required.

There are several disadvantages to local anesthesia. It is obviously impossible in children. The patient is awake and it is physically unpleasant to lie still for more than 90 minutes. Complications of local anesthesia include the following:

1. Risk of intravascular injection
2. Risk of oculocardiac reflex
3. Allergy to the anesthetic agent
4. Distortion of the regional anatomy by fluid volume injected or hemorrhage.

Contraindications to local anesthesia include the following;[16]

1. Procedures lasting more than 90 minutes
2. Uncontrolled cough
3. Emotional problems, such as claustrophobia or fear
4. Disorientation or retardation
5. Tremor or convulsive disorders
6. Bleeding or coagulation disorders
7. A perforated globe
8. Deafness (a relative contraindication)

A previous operative complication that may be related to local anesthesia (*e.g.*, blindness secondary to a retrobulbar hemorrhage or to an expulsive hemorrhage) suggests that general anesthesia should be considered for an operation on the remaining eye, if possible.

GENERAL ANESTHESIA

General anesthesia is definitely indicated for most children under the age of 15 years and in trauma patients with a perforating injury to the eyeball. Duration of the operative procedure is not critical, and there is no distortion of the local anatomy. Communication with the patient during surgery is not necessary.

Disadvantages to general anesthesia include the following:

1. Intubation/extubation complications
2. Risk of vomiting or coughing upon awakening

3. Associated physiologic alterations in high-risk patients
4. Surgical field close to the working area of the anesthesiologist
5. Requires additional equipment, personnel, and time

TOPICAL ANESTHESIA

Topical anesthesia is frequently used to eliminate corneal and conjunctival reflexes to obtain ocular measurements. In addition, these agents are used for removal of superficial foreign bodies, for suture removal, and for irrigation of the lacrimal system. Cocaine may be used during dacryocystorhinostomy to provide anesthesia, vasoconstriction, and shrinkage of the nasal mucous membranes.

Although many agents that cause surface anesthesia are available for topical use (Table 17-1), only proparacaine and tetracaine are used widely. All agents have a rapid onset of action, within 30 to 60 seconds, and a duration of action from 10 to 20 minutes.

Ocular or serious systemic reactions to topical anesthetic agents are almost nonexistent with the exception of cocaine. Cocaine penetrates the eye, where it blocks the reuptake of catecholamines at the neuronal level and has a sympathetic potentiating effect. Pupillary dilation occurs. A similar pharmacologic response can occur with systemic absorption of cocaine with resultant hypertensive crisis in patients also taking reserpine, methyldopa, monoamine oxidase inhibitors, or guanethidine. Systemic reactions to cocaine may occur with as little as 20 mg. If intranasal cocaine is used during dacryocystorhinostomy, it is safer to use dilute (5–10%) concentrations. The total dose used should be calculated. Nasal packing rather than a nasal spray of cocaine should be used to control the maximum amount of possible systemic drug absorption.[15]

TABLE 17-1. TOPICAL OPHTHALMOLOGIC ANESTHETIC AGENTS

Agent	Concentration (%)
Proparacaine HCl (Opthaine, Ophthetic)	0.5
Tetracaine HCl (Pontocaine)	0.5
Benoxinate (Dorsacaine)	0.4
Dibucaine HCl (Nupercaine)	0.1
Phenacaine HCl (Holocaine, Tanicaine)	1.0
Piperocaine HCl (Metycaine)	2.0 solution 4.0 ointment
Cocaine	1.0–4.0

All of the topical agents can be toxic to the corneal epithelium with frequent repeated administrations and may delay the healing of corneal epithelial defects by inhibiting cell division and migration.[14] Therefore, they should be used for surgery or diagnostic tests and not for symptomatic relief. Cocaine has the added disadvantage of causing loosening of the epithelium, which can result in large corneal erosions.

ANESTHETIC AGENTS

Agents injected for local anesthesia in ophthalmic surgery (Table 17-2) are basically the same as those used in other peripheral nerve blocks (see Chap. 4). Lidocaine has been the commonly used agent. There is a recent trend, however, toward using the longer-duration agents bupivacaine[8] or etidocaine,[23] which reduce the need for postoperative analgesics and reduce eye movements after surgery. These agents can be used alone or in combination with lidocaine in order to take advantage of the rapid onset of the lidocaine and the long duration of bupivacaine or etidocaine. The longer-duration agents can provide adequate anesthesia for longer and more complicated intraocular procedures.

Epinephrine is frequently added to the injection

TABLE 17-2. LOCAL ANESTHETIC AGENTS USED IN OPHTHALMOLOGY

Agent	Concentration (%)	Maximum Dose (mg)	Onset of Action (min)	Duration of Action
Procaine (Novocaine)	1–4	500	6–8	30–45 min
Mepivacaine (Carbocaine)	1–2	400	3–5	90–120 min
Lidocaine (Xylocaine)	1–2	400	4–6	30–60 min
Prilocaine (Citanest)	1–2	600	3–5	60–90 min
Bupivacaine (Marcaine)	0.25–0.75	175	3–5	4–12 h
Etidocaine (Duranest)	0.5–1	300	3–5	4–6 h

solution for ophthalmologic neural blockade to counteract the vasodilator action of the anesthetic agent. Dilute concentrations of 1:200,000 (1 mg/200 ml) should be used to avoid tissue injury secondary to ischemia. Occasionally, however, epinephrine can result in systemic side-effects and is usually not required with ophthalmic anesthesia. Retrobulbar epinephrine may reduce blood flow to the optic nerve and therefore is best avoided in patients with glaucomatous optic nerve damage.

The enzyme hyaluronidase is frequently added to the anesthetic solution to enhance solution diffusion through the tissues. This action is accomplished by hydrolysis of extracellular hyaluronic acid. For ophthalmic solutions, 7.5 to 15 turbidity reducing units (TRU) per milliliter are used. The addition of hyaluronidase allows a more complete, consistent block with the use of less anesthetic solution, and thus less tissue distortion.

ANATOMY OF THE ORBIT AND THE EYE

A thorough knowledge of the anatomy of the orbit and eye,[13] especially of the nerve supply to the orbital structures, is essential to obtain effective neural blockade. Anatomy related to specific anesthetic blocks is detailed under the description of the regional block.

ORBIT

The bony orbit has the shape of a pear with the stem directed toward the optic canal (Fig. 17-1). The orbit is covered by the outer periosteal layer of the dura mater (periorbita). The orbit is essentially intended as a socket for the eyeball. In addition, it contains the muscles, nerves, and vessels, which are essential for proper functioning of the eye. A number of blood vessels and nerves supplying areas of the face around the orbital aperture pass through the orbit. Important surrounding anatomic associations include the anterior cranial fossa above, the maxillary sinus below, and the nasal cavity and ethmoidal air cells medially. There are nine canals and fissures in the orbit, the most important being the optic foramen, the superior and inferior orbital fissures, and the supraorbital and infraorbital foramina (Fig. 17-2).

EYE

The normal globe is about 24 mm in the anteroposterior diameter. This dimension is increased in myopic

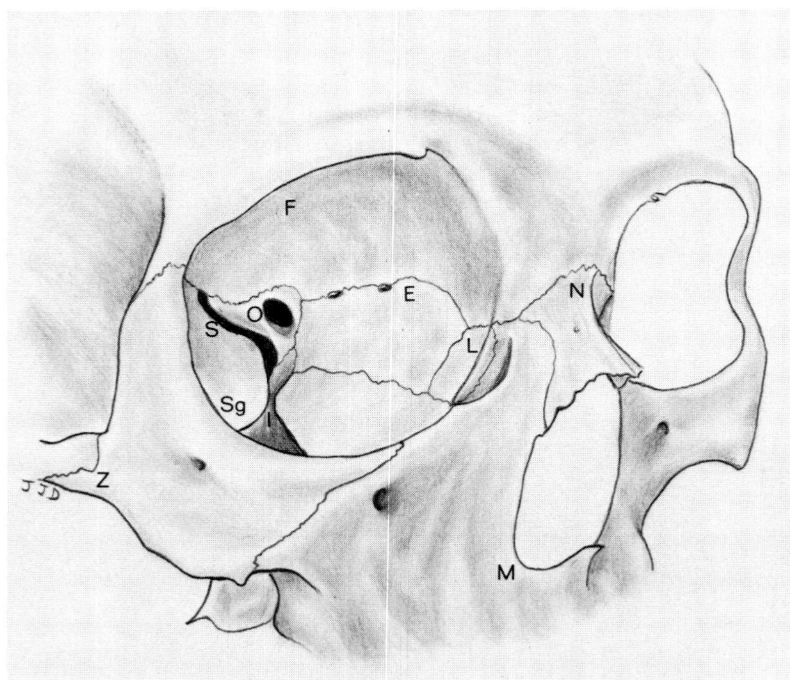

FIG. 17-1. Bony orbit showing the medial wall and floor N, nasal bone; M, maxilla; L, lacrimal bone; E, ethmoid bone; F, frontal bone; O, optic foramen; S, superior orbital fissure; Sg, orbit plate of greater wing of sphenoid; I, inferior orbital fissure; Z, zygomatic bone. (Krupin, T., and Waltman, S.R. [eds.]: Complications in Ophthalmic Surgery. Philadelphia, J. B. Lippincott, 1984.)

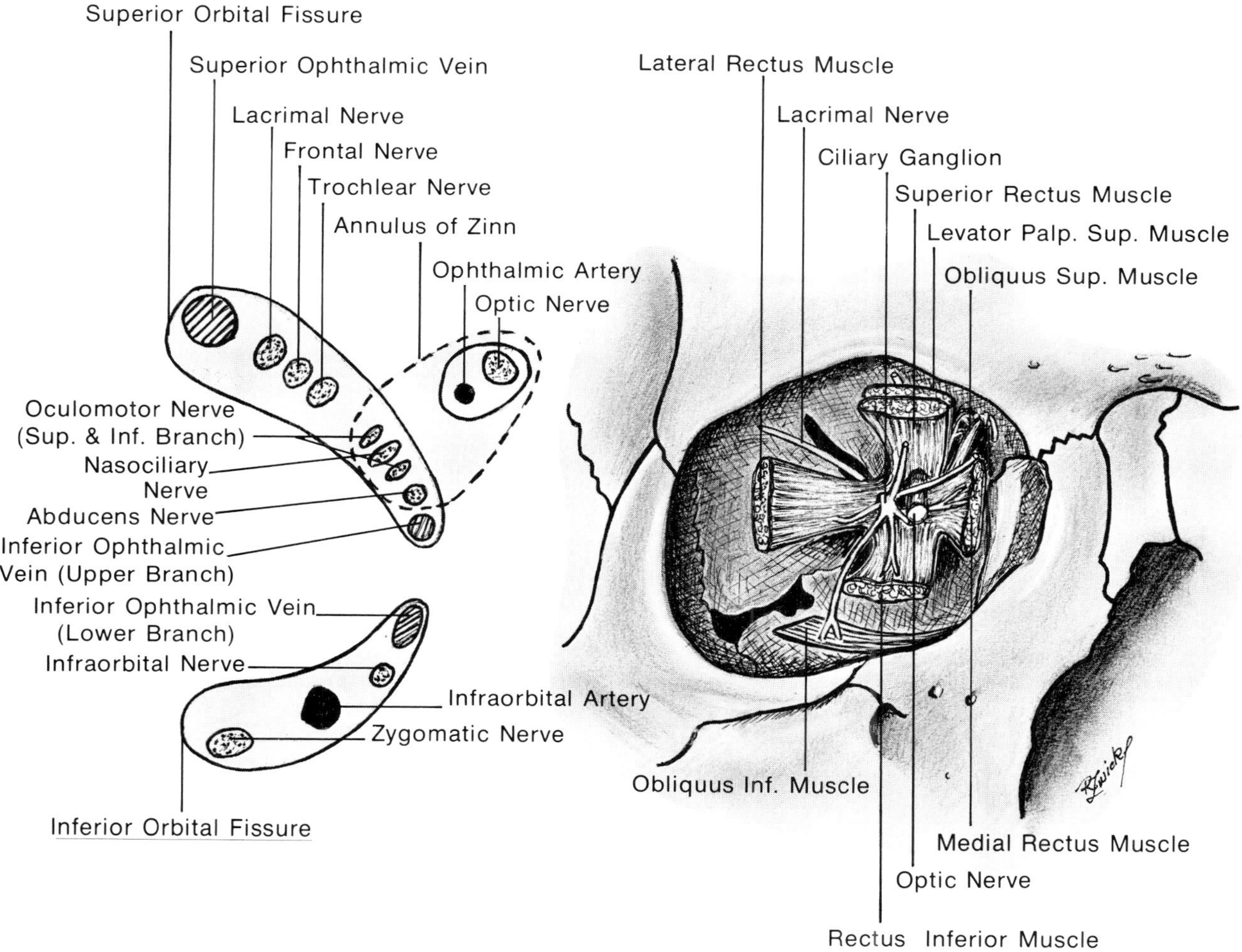

FIG. 17-2. Bony orbit with the superior and inferior orbital fissures and optic canal at the apex of the muscle cone.

(nearsighted) eyes. The eyeball comprises three concentric layers: an outer fibrous layer (the cornea and sclera), a middle vascular layer (the iris, cililary body and choroid), and an inner neural layer (the retina). Intraocular contents consist of the following: aqueous humor in the anterior chamber (space lined by the cornea, iris, and pupil) and in the posterior chamber (space behind the iris and in front of the vitreous), the crystalline lens, and the vitreous humor (space behind the lens and in front of the retina).

The optic nerve (cranial nerve II) pierces the globe just above and 3 mm medial to the posterior pole. The nerve has a diameter of 1.5 mm and an intraorbital length of about 30 mm. The nerve exits the orbit by way of the optic foramen. The traditional upward and inward position of the globe during retrobulbar anesthesia (see below) results in stretching as well as a downward and outward displacement of the optic nerve. This position may place the nerve in a vulnerable position for direct traumatization.[26]

Six extraocular striated muscles control the movements of the globe. The four rectus muscles (superior, medial, inferior, and lateral) originate from a common tendon ring that encircles the optic foramen (annulus of Zinn) with their tendinous insertion 5.5 to 7.5 mm from the limbus of the cornea. The superior oblique muscle originates above and medial to the optic foramen, runs medially to the trochlea, then bends backward to insert on the globe beneath the superior rectus muscle. The inferior oblique muscle originates medially from the periosteum of the lacrimal bone, runs beneath the inferior rectus muscle, and inserts on the posterolateral aspect of the globe. The seventh striated muscle in the orbit is the levator of the upper eye lid, which originates from the periosteum of the apex of the orbit above the superior oblique muscle. The levator runs forward between the roof of the orbit and superior rectus muscle and spreads out into an aponeurosis that inserts into the skin and tarsal plate of the upper eyelid. Cranial nerves III, IV, and VI innervate these striated muscles (Table 17-3).

Innervation of the Eye and Orbital Contents

The sensory supply to the eye and its adnexae is derived from the trigeminal nerve (cranial nerve V).

TABLE 17-3. MOTOR INNERVATION TO OCULAR ADNEXAL MUSCLES

Nerve (Cranial Nerve)	Muscle Innervation
Oculomotor (III)	Superior rectus Medial rectus Inferior rectus Inferior oblique Levator palpebrae superioris
Trochlear (IV)	Superior oblique
Abducens (VI)	Lateral rectus
Facial (VII)	
Upper zygomatic branch	Frontalis Orbicularis oculi upper lid
Lower zygomatic branch	Orbicularis oculi lower lid

This is a mixed nerve that comprises a large sensory part and a small motor part. The sensory portion of the nerve divides at the trigeminal ganglion into three branches: ophthalmic, maxillary, and mandibular (Table 17-4, Figs. 17-3 and 17-4).

The motor supply to the extraocular muscles and levator palpebrae muscle of the upper eyelid is by way of cranial nerves III, IV, and VI (see Table 17-3). The facial nerve (cranial nerve VII) supplies all the muscles of expression, including the orbicularis oculi in the eyelids. The nerve emerges through the stylomastoid foramen, just below the osseus part of the outer ear. The facial nerve then turns forward and enters the parotid gland superficial to the neck of the mandible, where it divides into five branches: temporal, zygomatic, buccal, mandibular, and cervical. The temporal division supplies the upper part of the orbicularis oculi, the corragator supercilii, and the frontalis muscle. The zygomatic branch supplies the lower part of the orbicularis oculi muscle (Fig. 17-5).

The autonomic nervous system supplies the eye through the sympathetic and parasympathetic systems (Table 17-5).

AKINESIA OF THE ORBICULARIS OCULI MUSCLE

Akinesia of the eyelids is essential for all intraocular surgery to prevent squeezing of the lids and expulsion of intraocular contents. Paralysis of the orbicularis oculi muscle may be achieved by either local infiltration of the muscle or proximal infiltration of the branches of the facial nerve that supply it.

TABLE 17-4. TRIGEMINAL (V CRANIAL NERVE) SENSORY INNERVATION OF THE EYE AND ADNEXAL STRUCTURES

Trigeminal Nerve Division	Branch	Sub-branch	Innervation
Ophthalmic	Frontal	Supratrochlear	Skin of lower forehead, skin root of nose, skin and conjunctiva of medial part of upper eyelid
		Supraorbital	Scalp and skin of forehead, skin and conjunctiva of upper eyelid
		Long ciliary	Cornea, iris, ciliary muscle
	Nasociliary	Infratrochlear	Medial upper and lower eyelid, skin and conjunctiva of inner canthus, caruncle, skin root of nose, lacrimal sac
		Long sensory root	Ciliary ganglion (cornea, iris, ciliary body via short ciliary nerves to the ganglion)
		Anterior ethmoid	Tip of nose
	Lacrimal		Outer upper and lower eyelid skin and conjunctiva, lateral canthus, and lacrimal gland
Maxillary	Infraorbital		Entire lower lid, medial and lateral parts of upper and lower lid, lacrimal sac, nasolacrimal duct, upper lip, skin over temple and lateral orbital wall
	Zygomatic		Skin of temporal area and lateral wall of the orbit

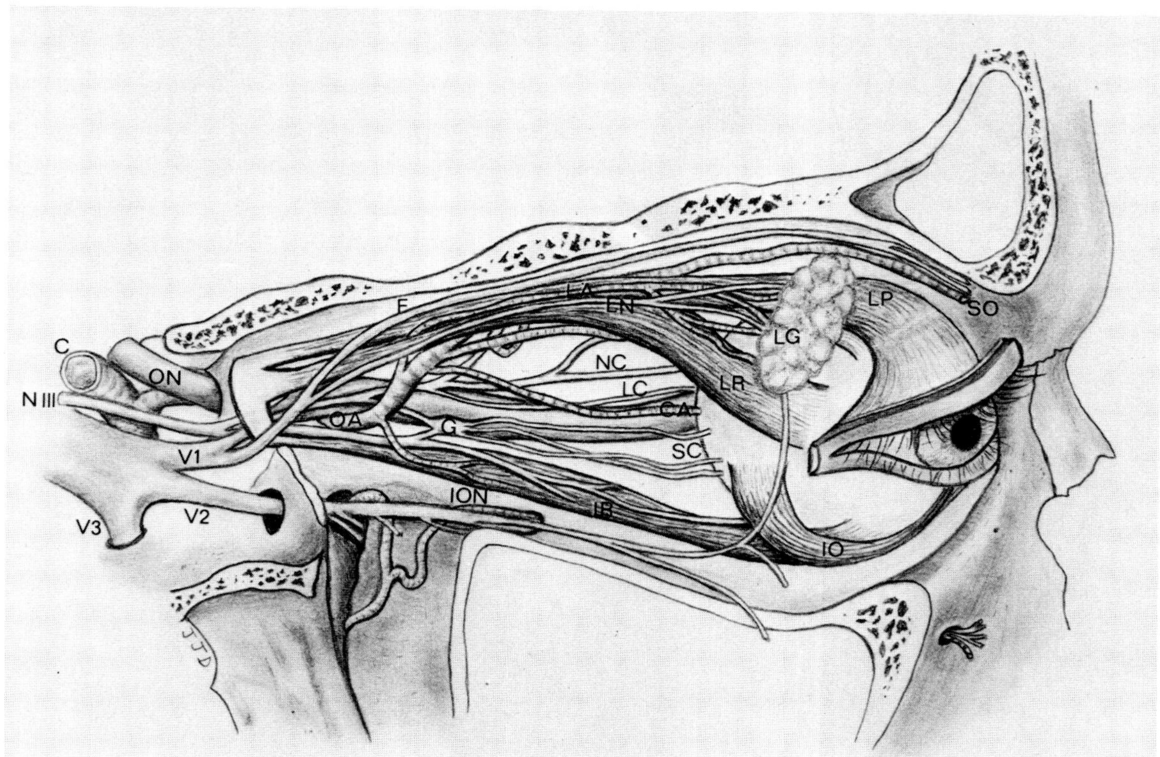

FIG. 17-3. Orbital anatomy as seen from the lateral approach. C, carotid artery; F, frontal nerve; G, ciliary ganglion; IO, inferior oblique muscle; ION, infraorbital neurovascular bundle; IR, inferior rectus muscle; LA, lacrimal artery; LC, long posterior ciliary nerve; LG, lacrimal gland; LN, lacrimal nerve; LP, levator palpebrae superioris; LR, lateral rectus muscle; N III, oculomotor nerve; NC, nasociliary nerve; OA, ophthalmic artery; ON, optic nerve; SC, short posterior ciliary nerve; SO, supraorbital neurovascular bundle; V_1, V_2, and V_3, ophthalmic, maxillary, and mandibular divisions of the trigeminal nerve. (Krupin, T., and Waltman, S.R. (eds.): Complications in Ophthalmic Surgery. Philadelphia, J.B. Lippincott, 1984.)

VAN LINT METHOD

In 1914 van Lint was the first to describe akinesia of the orbicularis oculi for cataract extraction.[27] The classic van Lint technique involves inserting the needle at the lateral orbital rim and making a small intradermal wheal. The needle is then advanced into the deep tissues along the inferolateral orbital margin. As the needle is withdrawn, 2 to 4 ml of anesthetic are injected. The needle is then redirected along the superotemporal orbital margin. Again, anesthetic is injected as the needle is withdrawn. Pressure is then applied to the area to promote diffusion of the anesthetic. This method has the side-effect of producing lid edema. Therefore, the technique has been modified by placing the injections more laterally to block the facial nerve as it crosses the periosteum. The initial injection is made directly on the periosteum of the orbital rim and is followed by inferior and superior injections (Fig. 17-6).

O'BRIEN METHOD

In 1927 O'Brien described a facial nerve block over the mandibular condyle inferior to the posterior zygomatic process.[19] The condyle can be palpated as the patient moves his jaw. The needle is inserted about 1 cm to the level of the periosteum (Fig. 17-7). Anes-

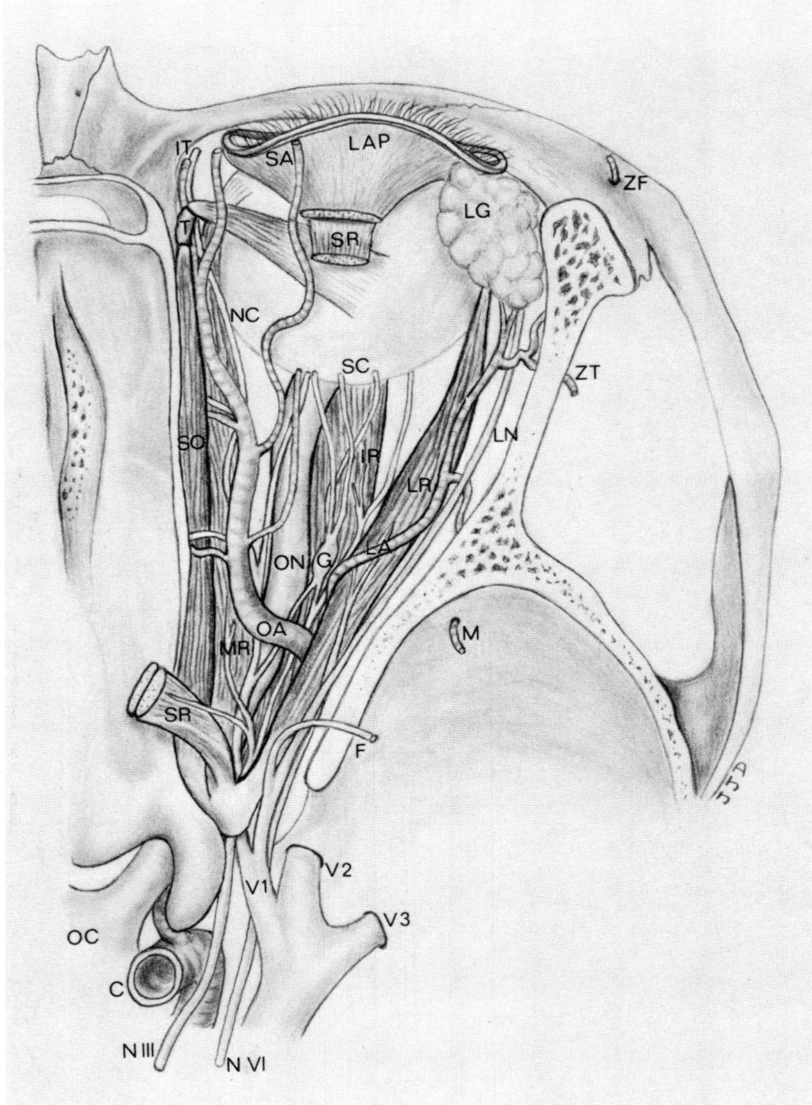

FIG. 17-4. Orbital anatomy as seen from above. C, carotid artery; F, frontal nerve; G, ciliary ganglion; IR, inferior rectus muscle; IT, infratrochlear neurovascular bundle; LA, lacrimal artery; LG, lacrimal gland; LN, lacrimal nerve; LAP, levator aponeurosis; LR, lateral rectus muscle; M, branch of the middle meningeal artery through Hyrtl's canal; MR, medial rectus muscle; NC, nasociliary nerve; N III, oculomotor nerve; N, VI, abducens nerve; OA, ophthalmic artery; OC, optic chiasm; ON, optic nerve; SA, supraorbital artery; SC, short posterior ciliary nerves; SO, superior oblique muscle; SR, superior rectus muscle; T, trochlea; V_1, V_2, and V_3, ophthalmic, maxillary, and mandibular divisions of the trigeminal nerve; ZF, zygomaticofrontal artery; ZT, zygomaticotemporal artery. (Krupin, T., and Waltman, S.R. (eds.): Complications in Ophthalmic Surgery. Philadelphia, J. B. Lippincott, 1984.)

thetic solution (2–3 ml) is injected as the needle is withdrawn. Because of the variable course of the facial nerve, the block may be incomplete. Hence, the following modifications have been recommended: After injecting over the condyle, partially withdraw the needle and redirect it inferiorly along the posterior edge of the ramus of the mandible. Then inject the anesthetic solution while withdrawing the needle. Reposition the needle anteriorly along the zygomatic arch and inject the anesthetic while withdrawing the needle.

ATKINSON METHOD

The Atkinson method involves blocking the branches of the facial nerve to the orbicularis oculi as they cross the zygomatic arch (Fig. 17-8).[2] First, a skin wheal is made at the lower margin of the zygomatic arch below the lateral orbital rim. The needle is then directed superiorly and posteriorly along the zygoma (aimed just lateral to the midpoint between the tragus and lateral orbital rim). Anesthetic (5–10 ml) is injected as the needle is withdrawn.

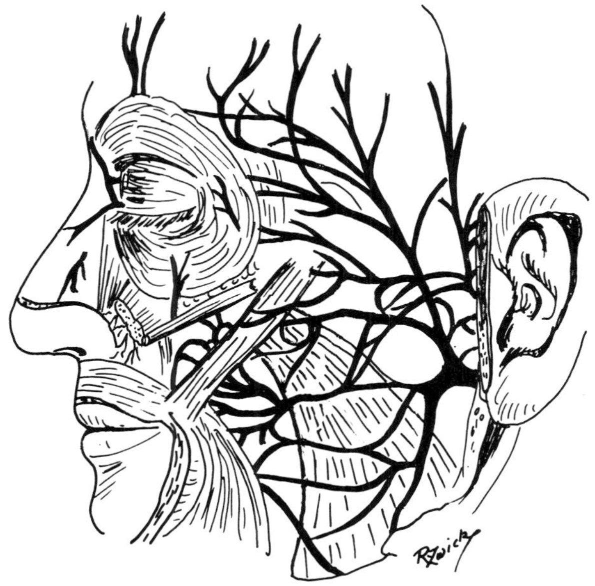

FIG. 17-5. Facial nerve and distribution of its branches.

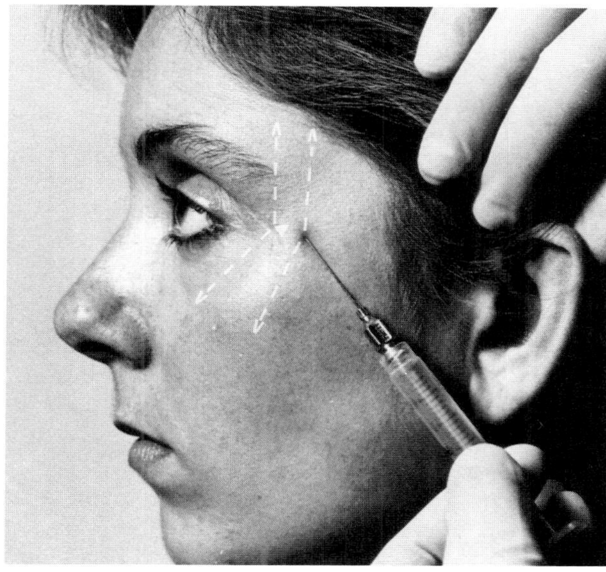

FIG. 17-6. Classic van Lint technique (< - - - -) blocks the facial nerve at the lateral oribital rim. The modified technique (from the needle site) places the injection more lateral to avoid lid edema.

COMBINED METHODS

A number of injection techniques are described that combine the classic with the modified van Lint, O'Brien, and Atkinson methods. Inconsistencies of the different facial nerve blocks relate to individual variability in the course of the nerve after it enters the parotid gland and subsequently divides into the five facial branches.

NADBATH–REHMAN METHOD

Complete akinesia of the muscles innervated by the facial nerve may be achieved with the Nadbath–Rehman block.[18] The main trunk of the facial nerve is blocked at the concavity just below the external auditory meatus between the anterosuperior border of the mastoid process and the posterior border of the mandibular ramus (Fig. 17-9). The site can be identified by palpation and confirmed by having the patient open and close his jaw. A 25-gauge 12-mm needle is inserted into the skin and an intradermal wheal is made. The needle is then advanced its full length perpendicularly into the tissue. The plunger is withdrawn to assure that the needle is not intravascular, and about 3 ml of anesthetic solution is injected as the needle is withdrawn. Gentle massage is applied to the injection site to diffuse the anesthetic. This technique produces complete facial nerve akinesia. The major advantage of this technique is the consistent course of the facial nerve from the stylomastoid foramen to the posteromedial surface of the parotid gland, before branching of the nerve. Akinesia of the lower facial

TABLE 17–5. AUTONOMIC NERVOUS SYSTEM INNERVATION TO THE EYE

System	Source	Nerves	Supply
Sympathetic	Superior cervical ganglion	Long ciliary nerve, (2) short ciliary nerves	Vascular system of choroid, ciliary body, iris (vasoconstrictors); motor impulses to iris dilator muscle
Parasympathetic	Oculomotor nerve (preganglionic fibers) to ciliary ganglion	Short ciliary nerves (postganglionic)	Ciliary body, motor impulse to the iris sphincter muscle and to the ciliary muscle

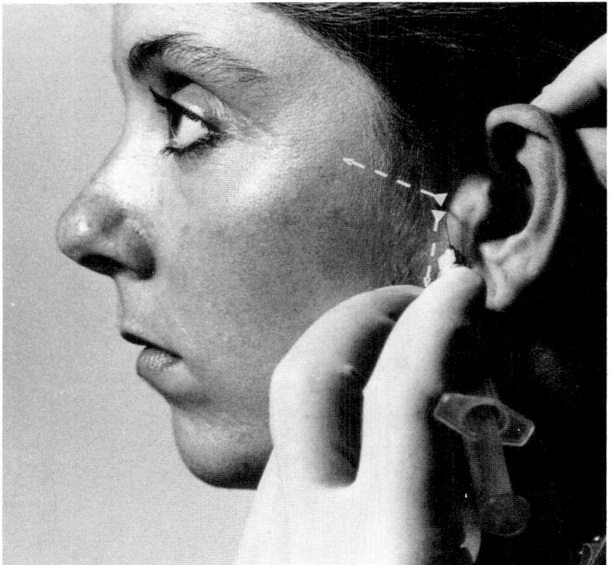

FIG. 17-7. O'Brien technique for facial nerve block. Injection is performed over the mandibular condyle (tip of the needle). A modified technique *(dotted lines)* adds injections along the posterior edge of the mandible and anteriorly along the zygomatic arch.

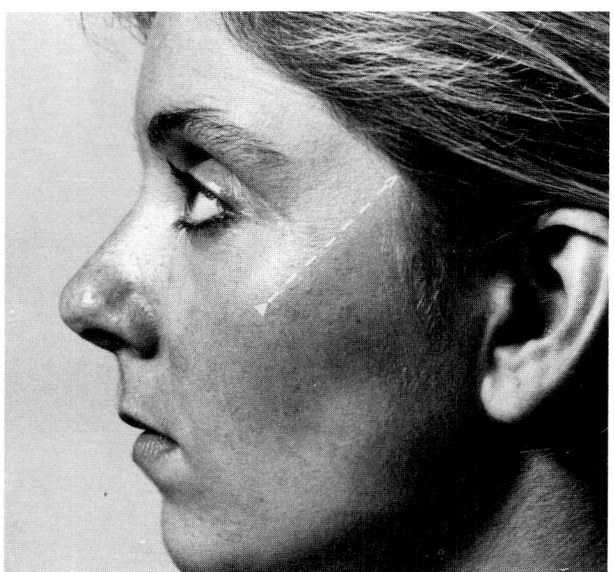

FIG. 17-8. Atkinson method for facial nerve block.

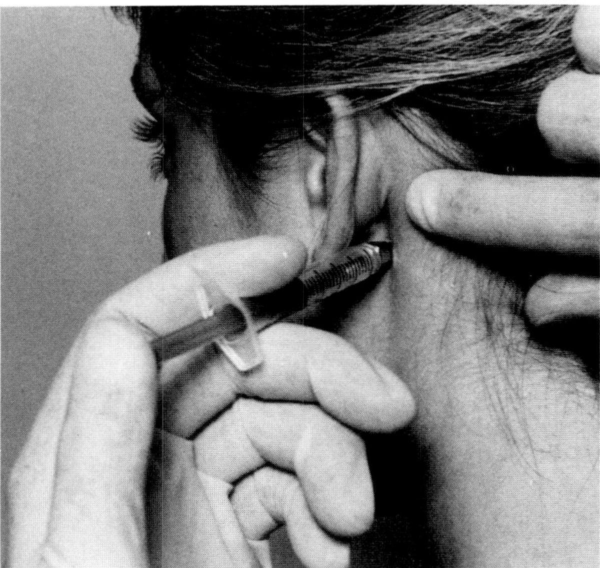

FIG. 17-9. Nadbath–Rehman facial nerve block.

musculature also occurs, but this is not a problem as long as the patient is reassured that the effect is transient.

RETROBULBAR BLOCK

Retrobulbar injection of local anesthetic provides akinesia of the extraocular muscles by blocking cranial nerves III, IV, and VI and anesthesia of the conjunctiva, cornea, and uvea by blocking the ciliary nerves. These effects of retrobulbar anesthesia combined with akinesia of the orbicularis oculi muscle permit intraocular surgery under local anesthesia.

Retrobulbar anesthesia was first described in 1884 when Hermann Knapp used a cocaine injection posterior to the globe to perform an enucleation.[12] Because of serious complications associated with the injection of cocaine, this agent was not commonly used for retrobulbar injection. Retrobulbar injections did not gain widespread use until the later development of procaine. Subsequently, longer-acting agents have been introduced and have become used more frequently owing to their longer duration of action and the postoperative analgesia that they provide.

The administration of the retrobulbar block can be both anxiety producing and painful for the patient.

The use of preoperative medications, such as 25 to 50 mg of hydroxyzine hydrochloride (Vistaril) 1 hour preoperatively may help to reduce the anxiety. In addition, the antiemetic properties of hydroxyzine may help to prevent nausea if an oral hyperosmotic agent is used. A number of techniques have been advocated to lessen the discomfort and awareness of the injection.[16] Intravenous methohexital sodium (Brevital), 15 to 50 mg, or fentanyl (Sublimaze), 0.025 to 0.1 mg, may be given 2 to 4 minutes before the block. Alternatively, 50% to 60% nitrous oxide (*e.g.*, 4 liters/minute nitrous oxide and 3 liters/minute oxygen) may be given by face mask for a few minutes before the retrobulbar and facial nerve blocks. Once the patient feels slightly lightheaded, the injections may be given quickly with little patient discomfort, followed by a few minutes of 100% oxygen to eliminate diffusion hypoxia. This method has few adverse effects when carefully monitered, but nausea, vomiting, and unpleasant dreams may rarely occur. Prior heating of the anesthetic solutions to 40°C on a hot plate may reduce the discomfort associated with injection.[6]

The patient has traditionally been instructed to look upward and nasally during the retrobulbar injection. Atkinson stated that this would place the inferior oblique muscle out of the course of the retrobulbar needle.[3] An additional advantage of this position of the globe is that the patient looks away from the needle and the site of puncture. This position of the globe has been disputed recently in light of a study using CT scanning of a cadaver orbit as the retrobulbar needle is inserted.[26] It was found that in the upward and inward gaze position, the optic nerve, ophthalmic artery and its branches, superior orbital vein, and the posterior pole of the globe rotated into the path of the retrobulbar needle. The chance of perforating the optic nerve is also increased because it is put on stretch in this position. Hence, it has been recommended that the patient be instructed to look in primary gaze (or slightly downward and outward). The choice of a blunted needle (as advocated by Atkinson) also serves to reduce the potential for perforation of orbital vessels or nerves (Fig. 17-10). Patient discomfort with the blunted needle may be diminished by first making an intradermal wheal of local anesthetic at the skin entry site with a sharp 25-gauge needle. This is done just above the inferior orbital rim at the junction of the lateral and middle thirds of the margin (Fig. 17-11). A 3-cm, 23-gauge blunted needle is inserted and directed perpendicular to the skin surface. The bevel of the needle should face the globe to reduce the chance of

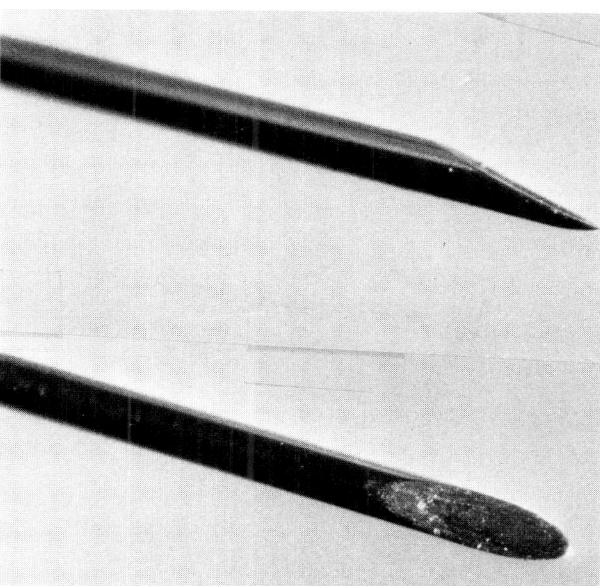

FIG. 17-10. Frontal and lateral views of the Atkinson needle for retrobulbar injection.

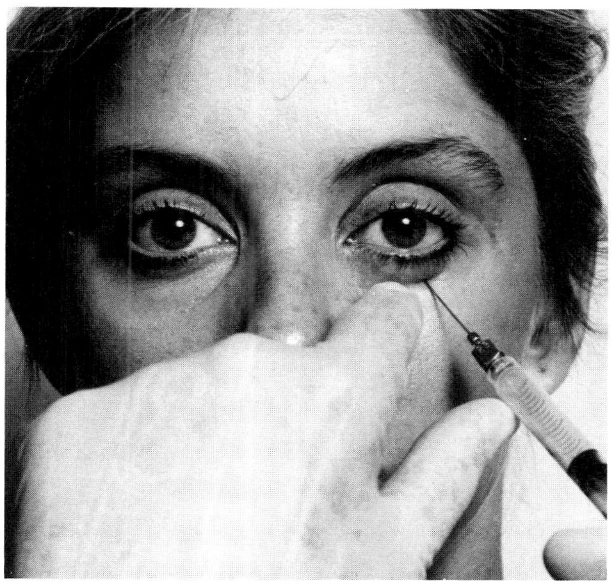

FIG. 17-11. Retrobulbar injection with the eye in primary gaze. The index finger is palpating the orbital rim. The needle is directed slightly below the apex of the orbit (see text).

perforation. Once the needle passes the equator of the globe, it should be directed slightly lower than the orbital apex, toward the inferior part of the superior orbital fissure. After the needle is fully inserted, the syringe should be aspirated before injection to be certain that the needle is not inside a vessel. An adequate retrobulbar block is achieved following injections of 1.5 to 2.0 ml of anesthetic solution in the muscle cone. Many surgeons will inject larger volumes (4.0–5.0 ml) and use hyaluronidase to enhance diffusion through the orbit. These larger volumes may produce additional pressure on the globe and chemosis of the conjunctiva. After the injection, firm intermittent digital pressure is applied for about 5 minutes to help distribute the anesthetic and lower intraocular pressure. If complete akinesia and anesthesia has not been achieved, it may be necessary to perform a supplemental retrobulbar injection or a transconjunctival quadrant block adjacent to the functioning extraocular muscle. The superior oblique muscle, which is outside the annulus of Zinn, will not be paralyzed after a retrobulbar block. Therefore, the eye may intort as the patient is instructed to look down.

Most ophthalmologists perform the retrobulbar injection through the lower eyelid, but a transconjunctival approach may also be used. The lower lid is pulled down and the needle inserted through the inferior cul-de-sac. The direction and technique are otherwise as previously described.

COMPLICATIONS

Retrobulbar injections are associated with both local and systemic complications (Table 17-6). Perforation of the globe can occur during retrobulbar injection despite the use of a blunted retrobulbar needle. This may be a problem particularly in the case of a highly myopic eye, a posterior staphyloma, and after repeated anesthetic injections. The patient has immediate ocular pain and restlessness following unintentional perforation of the globe. Surgery should be postponed and appropriate retinal treatment undertaken.

Retrobulbar hemorrhage is the most common complication seen. Vascular disease may predispose a patient to develop a retrobulbar hemorrhage. It is characterized by increasing proptosis and possibly subconjunctival blood as the hemorrhage extends anteriorly. The patient's intraocular pressure and central retinal artery pulsations should be monitored following a retrobulbar hemorrhage for signs of an impending retinal arterial occlusion. If external pressure on the globe is high enough to result in compression of the retinal arteries, then a deep lateral canthotomy should be performed to decompress the orbit rapidly. When this does not reestablish normal retinal blood flow, an anterior chamber paracentesis should be done to decompress the globe. Failure to treat this complication promptly and sufficiently may result in total loss of vision. An oculocardiac reflex may happen some hours after a retrobulbar hemorrhage as additional blood extravasates. Hence, close monitoring of the patient should be performed for several hours following the hemorrhage. Many retrobulbar hemorrhages are minimal, even subclinical, and on occasion surgery may be continued. There is, however, significant risk of repeat hemorrhage during the surgery with devastating complications. Therefore the more prudent course following a recognized retrobulbar hemorrhage is to postpone surgery until all signs of the hemorrhage have resolved. Surgery can usually be performed 2 to 4 days later, preferably under general anesthesia.

Optic atrophy and permanent loss of vision may occur even in the absence of retrobulbar hemorrhage.[10,11] Postulated mechanisms include direct injury to the nerve, injection into the nerve sheath with compressive ischemia, and intraneural sheath hemorrhage.[10,25] In addition, retinal vascular occlusion has been observed after retrobulbar injection without evidence of a retrobulbar hemorrhage.[11]

Systemic complications associated with retrobul-

TABLE 17-6. COMPLICATIONS OF RETROBULBAR ANESTHESIA

Complication	Signs and Symptoms	Mechanisms
Perforation of the globe	Ocular pain, restlessness, intraocular hemorrhage	Direct trauma (myopic eye, posterior staphyloma, repeated injections)
Retrobulbar hemorrhage	Increasing proptosis, subconjunctival or eyelid ecchymosis, pain, ± increased intraocular pressure	Direct trauma (artery or vein)
Optic nerve	Visual loss, optic disk pallor	Direct injury to nerve or blood vessels, vascular occlusion
CNS	Disorientation, unconsciousness, convulsions, respiratory or cardiac arrest	Excessive total drug injection, injection into sheath and into subarachnoid space, oculocardiac reflex

bar blocks are rare, but potentially serious. These include disorientation, unconsciousness, convulsions, respiratory arrest, and cardiac arrest.[17,21,22] The amount of anesthetic agent given in the retrobulbar block alone is not usually in the toxic range, but the total dose in the retrobulbar and orbicularis blocks may reach dangerously high levels. Unintentional intravascular injection of local anesthetic may precipitate cardiopulmonary arrest or convulsions by means of retrograde flow to the internal carotid artery with subsequent access to midbrain structures. Penetration of the optic nerve dural sheath with diffusion through the cerebrospinal fluid has also been considered as a possible pathway.[9] Prompt recognition and treatment necessitate close monitoring of the patient and the immediate institution of appropriate cardiopulmonary resuscitation (see Chap. 22).

OCULOCARDIAC REFLEX

The oculocardiac reflex is a slowing of the pulse in response to traction on the extraocular muscles or from pressure on the eye. The afferent arc is by way of the trigeminal nerve (ophthalmic division) to the brain stem. Impulses pass through synaptic pathways in the reticular network to the visceral motor nuclei of the vagus nerve, which is the efferent limb of the reflex to the heart. Bradycardia, arrhythmias, and even periods of cardiac asystole may result.[20] A similar reflex, the blepharocardiac reflex, may be elicited by stretching the eyelid muscle during placement of an eyelid retractor.[1]

Children and young adults undergoing eye muscle surgery under general anesthesia are most susceptible to the oculocardiac reflex. Traction on the medial rectus muscle is the most common stimulus, but even retrobulbar injections may cause enough compression to elicit the reflex. Bradycardia persists for 10 to 20 seconds after the muscle traction has been released; however, the reflex may last longer, especially after a retrobulbar injection. All anesthetics produce the reflex with approximately the same frequency. Hypoxemia may increase the occurrence of the reflex.

Premedication with atropine or glycopyrrolate in children and young adults reduces the incidence of the oculocardiac reflex. These agents can also be given intravenously just before surgery. Although retrobulbar block has been advocated for prevention, the block itself may elicit the reflex.

The incidence of the oculocardiac reflex is lower in elderly patients. Prophylactic anticholinergic drugs offer no advantage in this group of patients. Current recommended practice is to keep the patient well ventilated and under constant surveillance on an electrocardiographic monitor. If an arrhythmia develops, surgical manipulation is stopped. Intravenous atropine (0.6 mg) or glycopyrrolate (0.3 mg) is given. Medical attention is given to the cardiac complication and is away from the ocular surgery. If the bradycardia is not treated, hypotension, diaphoresis, and nausea develop, with a myocardial infarction or a cardiac arrest possibly occurring.

The onset of the reflex may be variable. We have observed the oculocardiac reflex immediately after an uncomplicated retrobulbar anesthetic injection and as long as 1 to 1½ hours after uncomplicated retrobulbar anesthesia during the surgical procedure. A retrobulbar hemorrhage can also result in a delayed oculocardiac reflex if bleeding continues with increased pressure on the eye. Adequate cardiac monitoring and an established intravenous pathway are necessary for complete patient care.

SENSORY NERVE BLOCKS

FRONTAL NERVE

The frontal nerve, while still in the orbit, divides into the supraorbital and supratrochlear nerves. A sensory frontal nerve block is very useful in adults undergoing frontalis suspensory surgery for ptosis repair. The block retains motility to the upper eyelid and globe while providing sensory anesthesia to the upper eyelid and eyebrow. A local block can be performed on the frontal nerve within the orbit or on its two branches near the orbit rim.

Frontal Nerve Block

A rigid (22-gauge) 4-cm needle is passed through the center of the eyelid just below the eyebrow and orbital margin. The needle is directed posteriorly in a steplike fashion along the roof of the orbit until the entire 4-cm length of the needle has been passed (Fig. 17-12). This is the location where the frontal and lacrimal nerves enter the orbit. The needle is kept near the roof of the orbit to avoid penetration of the intermuscular septum, which would result in motor anesthesia of the levator and superior rectus muscles and in sensory anesthesia. Not more than 0.5 ml of local anesthetic solution with epinephrine but without hyaluronidase is injected. Complications include penetration of the muscle cone and retrobulbar hemorrhage.

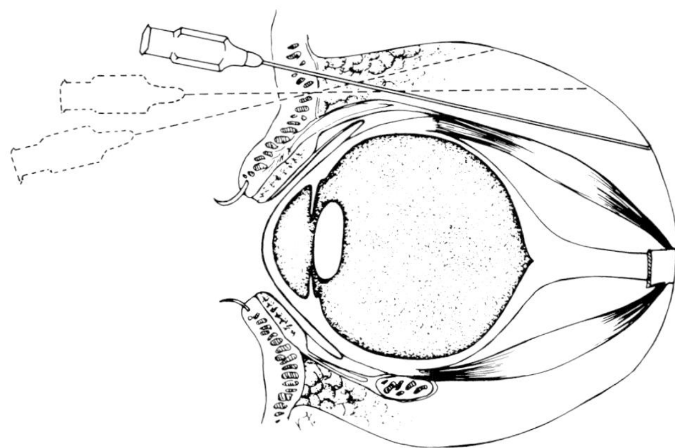

FIG. 17-12. Frontal nerve block. (Krupin, T., and Waltman, S.R. [eds.]: Complications in Ophthalmic Surgery, Philadelphia, J. B. Lippincott, 1984.)

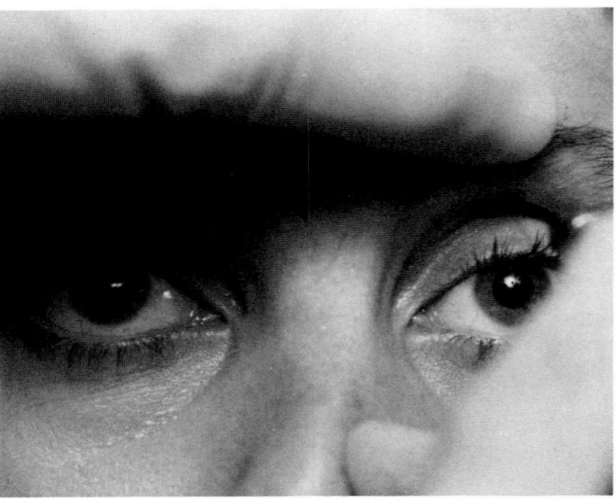

FIG. 17-13. Supraorbital nerve block. The needle is inserted at the supraorbital notch.

Supraorbital Nerve Block

The supraorbital nerve supplies the upper eyelid, the upper conjunctiva, the upper portion of the lacrimal fossa, the upper lacrimal duct, and the supraorbital portion of the forehead. The nerve runs from the superior orbital fissure immediately beneath the periorbita along the orbital roof to emerge from the orbit through the supraorbital foramen or notch. The notch is a separation in the superior orbital rim at the junction of its lateral two thirds and medial one third and is easily palpated. This landmark is on a line with the pupil when the eye is in the primary position. The nerve is blocked by inserting a needle through a skin wheal at the notch and injecting 2 to 3 ml of anesthetic solution (Fig. 17-13). Bleeding can occur from the accompanying supraorbital artery.

Supratrochlear Nerve Block

The supratrochlear nerve supplies the medial part of the upper eyelid, conjunctiva, and forehead. After branching from the frontal nerve, it runs medially to the supraorbital nerve just beneath the periorbita of the orbital roof. The nerve emerges from the orbit between the pulley (trochlea) of the superior oblique muscles and the supraorbital foramen or notch. The supratroclear nerve can be blocked by inserting a needle 1 to 1.5 cm along the superomedial wall, just above the trochlea (Fig. 17-14). One milliliter to 1.5 ml of anesthetic is injected.

NASOCILIARY NERVE

The nasociliary branch of the ophthalmic nerve divides within the orbit into the anterior and posterior ethmoidal nerves and the infratrochlear nerve. The anterior ethmoidal nerve supplies the lateral wall of the nose in the area of the lacrimal fossa and the skin covering the ala nasi. The infratrochlear nerve runs just beneath the periorbita along the medial orbital

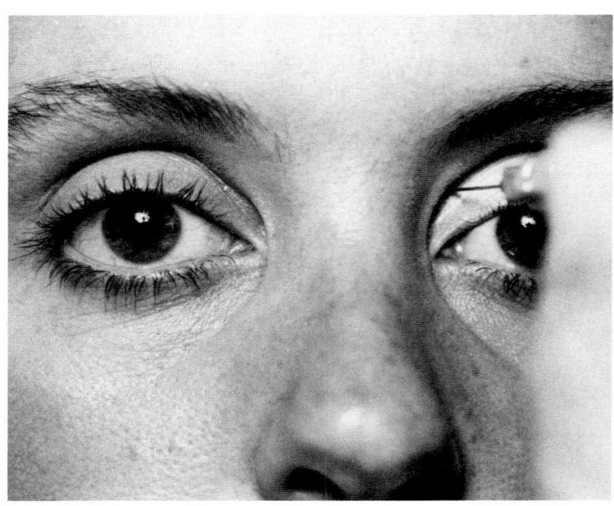

FIG. 17-14. Supratrochlear nerve block.

wall and just above the medial rectus muscle. This nerve innervates the skin of the nose, the skin and the conjunctiva of the inner canthus, and the lacrimal sac. Infiltrative anesthesia of the infratrochlear and infraorbital (see below) nerves is used for surgery on the lacrimal sac (dacryocystorhinostomy).

Infratrochlear Nerve Block

The infratrochlear nerve is blocked by inserting a 25-gauge needle below the trochlea and just above the medial canthal ligament along the medial orbital wall (Fig. 17-15). The needle is inserted to a depth of 2 to 2.5 cm, and 1.5 to 2.0 ml of anesthetic is injected. Introduction of the needle to a depth of 2.5 to 3.5 cm will also anesthetize the anterior ethmoidal nerve.

Terminal branches of the ophthalmic artery and small tributaries of the superior ophthalmic vein can be encountered during an infratrochlear nerve block. Retrobulbar hemorrhage can occur in approximately 2% of blocks. If the hemorrhage is severe, the operation must be postponed.

LACRIMAL NERVE

The lacrimal nerve is located at the superior part of the lateral orbital wall. The nerve supplies the lacrimal gland and the skin and conjunctiva of the lateral part of the upper eyelid. The nerve is anesthetized by introducing a 25-gauge needle through an intradermal wheal in the upper eyelid at the lateral wall of the orbit (Fig. 17-16). The needle is inserted along the lateral wall to a depth of 2.5 cm, and 2 ml of anesthetic solution is injected.

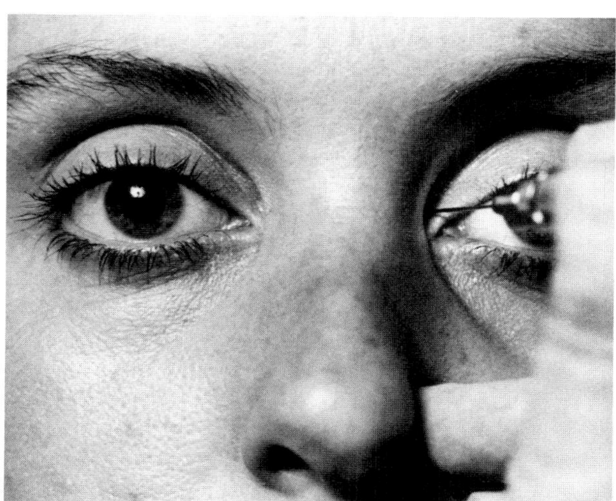

FIG. 17-15. Infratrochlear nerve block.

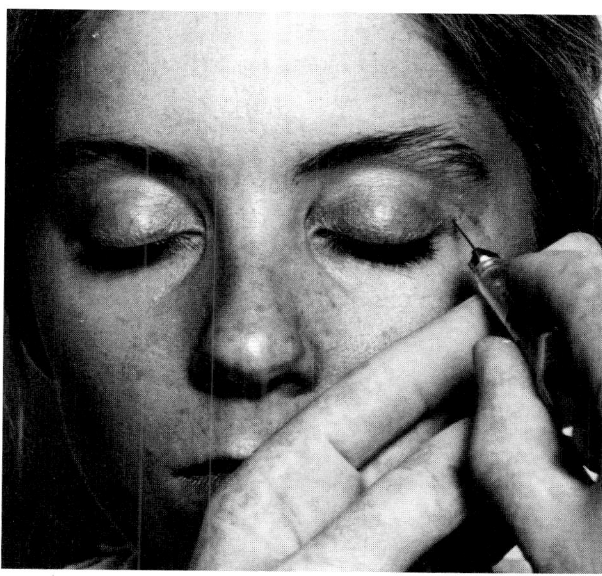

FIG. 17-16. Lacrimal block.

MAXILLARY NERVE

The maxillary nerve, the second division of the trigeminal nerve, runs through the orbit in the infraorbital groove. The nerve divides into the zygomatic and infraorbital nerves.

Zygomatic Nerve Block

The zygomatic nerve innervates the skin of the temporal area and the lateral wall of the orbit. Zygomaticotemporal and zygomaticofacial branches exit through small foramen in the zygomatic bone at the junction of the lateral and inferior orbital rims. Infiltrative anesthesia at these sites will block these nerves.

Infraorbital Nerve Block

The infraorbital nerve within its canal gives off alveolar nerves to the upper teeth, maxillary sinus, and nasal cavity. The infraorbital groove in the central orbital floor becomes bridged-over at its midportion to continue forward as the infraorbital canal. The

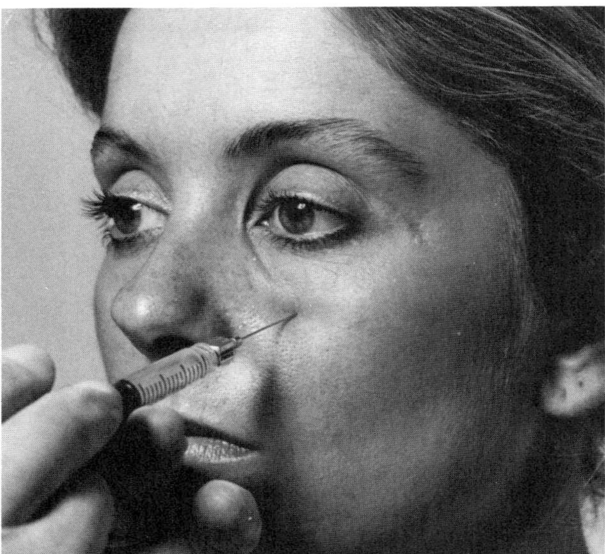

FIG. 17-17. Infraorbital nerve block.

nerve emerges on the face from the infraorbital foramen on the maxilla. The foramen is palpable as a small depression 1.5 cm below the inferior orbital rim. The foramen is on a line with the supraorbital notch and pupil. The nerve supplies the lower eyelid and cheek, inner canthus, and part of the lacrimal sac. Infraorbital combined with infratrochlear nerve block are used for dacryocystorhinostomy.

The infraorbital nerve can be blocked where it enters the canal on the orbital floor. A 2-ml injection of anesthetic is given along the floor, 1.0 to 1.5 cm behind the orbital rim. A block can also be done at the infraorbital foramen. The foramen is palpated on the maxilla, 1.5 cm below the orbital rim on a line with the supraorbital notch and pupil (Fig. 17-17). Anesthetic solution (1.5–2.0 ml) is injected at the external opening of the foramen or just within the canal.

REFERENCES

1. Anderson, R.L.: The blepharocardiac reflex. Arch. Ophthalmol., *96*:1418, 1978.
2. Atkinson, W.S.: Akinesia of the orbicularis, Am. J. Ophthalmol., *36*:1255, 1953.
3. Atkinson, W.S.: The development of ophthalmic anesthesia. Am. J. Ophthalmol., *51*:1, 1961.
4. Becker, B., Kolker, A.E., and Krupin, T.: Hyperosmotic agents. In Leopold, I.H. (ed.): Symposium on Ocular Therapy, Vol. II, pp. 42–53. New York, John Wiley & Sons, 1968.
5. Becker, B., Krupin, T., Podos, S.M.: Phenobarbital and aqueous humor dynamics: Effect in rabbits with intact and transsected optic nerves. Am. J. Ophthalmol., *70*:686, 1970.
6. Bloom, L.H., Scheie, H.G., and Yanoff, M.: The warming of local anesthetic agents to decrease discomfort. Ophthalmic Surg., *15*:603, 1984.
7. Breslin, P.P.: Mortality in Ophthalmic Surgery. Int. Ophthalmol. Clin., *13*:(2): Summer 1975.
8. Chin, G.N., Almquist, H.T.: Bupivacaine and lidocaine retrobulbar anesthesia: A double-blind clinical study. Ophthalmic Surg., *90*:369, 1983.
9. Drysdale, D.B.: Experimental subdural retrobulbar injection of anesthetic. Ann. Ophthalmol., *16*:716, 1984.
10. Ellis, P.P.: Retrobulbar injections. Surv. Ophthalmol., *18*:425, 1974.
11. Klein, M.L., Jampol, L.M., Condon, P.I., Rice, T.A., *et al.*: Central retinal artery occlusion without retrobulbar hemorrhage after retrobulbar anesthesia. Am. J. Ophthalmol., *93*:573, 1982.
12. Knapp, H.: On cocaine and its use in ophthalmic and general surgery. Arch. Ophthalmol., *13*:402, 1884.
13. Last, R.J.: Eugene Wolff's Anatomy of the Eye and Orbit. Philadelphia, W.B. Saunders, 1968.
14. Man, W.G., Wood, R., Senterfit, L., Sigelman, S.: Effect of topical anesthetics on regeneration of the corneal epithelium. Am. J. Ophthalmol., *43*:606, 1957.
15. Meyers, E.F.: Cocaine toxicity during dacryocystorhinostomy. Arch. Ophthalmol., *98*:842, 1980.
16. Meyers, E.F.: Anesthesia. In Krupin, T., Waltman, S.R. (eds.): Complications in Ophthalmic Surgery, 2nd ed., p. 22. Philadelphia, J.B. Lippincott, 1984.
17. Meyers, E.F., Ramirez, R.C., and Boniuk, I.: Grand mal seizures after retrobulbar block. Arch. Ophthalmol., *96*:847, 1978.
18. Nadbath, R.P., and Rehman, I.: Facial nerve block. Am. J. Ophthalmol., *55*:143, 1963.
19. O'Brien, C.S.: Akinesia during cataract extraction. Arch. Ophthalmol., *1*:447, 1929.
20. Pöntinen, P.J.: The importance of the oculocardiac reflex during ocular surgery. Acta. Ophthalmol. (Suppl), *86*:7, 1966.
21. Rosenblatt, R.M., May, D.R., and Barsoumian, K.: Cardiopulmonary arrest after retrobulbar block. Am. J. Ophthalmol., *90*:425, 1980.
22. Smith, J.L.: Retrobulbar bupivacaine can cause respiratory arrest. Ann. Ophthalmol., *14*:1005, 1982.
23. Smith, P.H., and Smith, E.R.: A comparison of etidocaine and lidocaine for retrobulbar anesthesia. Ophthalmic Surg., *14*:569, 1983.
24. Starrels, M., Krupin, T., and Burde, R.M.: Bell's palsy and intraocular pressure. Ann. Ophthalmol., *7*:1067, 1975.
25. Sullivan, K.L., Brown, G.C., Forman, A.R., Sergott, R.C., *et al.*: Retrobulbar anesthesia and retinal vascular obstruction. Ophthalmology, *90*:373, 1983.
26. Unsöld, R., Stanley, J.A., and De Groot, J.: The CT-topography of retrobulbar anesthesia: Anatomic-clinical correlation of complications and suggestions of a modified technique. Albrecht von Graefes Arch. Klin. Ophthalmol., *217*:125, 1981.
27. van Lint, A.: Paralysie palpebrale temporaire provoquee par l'operation de la cataracte. Ann. Ocul., *151*:420, 1914.

18 NEURAL BLOCKADE FOR OBSTETRICS AND GYNECOLOGIC SURGERY

PETER BROWNRIDGE
SHEILA E. COHEN

PART I: NEURAL BLOCKADE FOR OBSTETRICS

If we could induce local anaesthesia without that temporary absence of consciousness which is found in the state of general anaesthesia, many would regard it as a still greater improvement.

James Young Simpson, 1848

Thirty-six years were to lapse before Simpson's wish could become a reality. Simpson, who introduced inhalation analgesia during labor, had been dead 14 years before Koller first demonstrated in 1884 the local anesthetic properties of cocaine. Despite the advantages of neural blockade over inhalation analgesia, its application in obstetric practice was much slower. Subarachnoid block, for example, was first described for vaginal delivery in 1901 by Kreis and caudal analgesia by Cathelin in the same year. Paracervical block was described by Gellert in 1926. Continuous caudal analgesia by way of an indwelling catheter was introduced by Hingson and Edwards in 1942 and continuous lumbar epidural analgesia also by Hingson in 1946.

Neural blockade has a wide application in modern obstetric practice. Several approaches have been described that can provide excellent pain relief during labor and delivery. Because labor pain ranks among the severest forms of pain recorded, having being described as "intolerable" in about one third of women,[217] the ability to provide effective pain relief is desirable enough in its own right. Apart from the relief of suffering, however, neural blockade obtunds certain physiologic changes that are mediated by pain (see also Chap. 5).

Analgesia with neural blockade is achieved without any clouding of consciousness, allowing the mother to remain fully alert throughout labor and delivery and giving her the opportunity to interact with her child immediately after birth. An additional benefit is the ability to provide surgical anesthesia for obstetric emergencies. General anesthesia is hazardous in these circumstances because pregnant patients are particularly prone to regurgitation and pulmonary aspiration. Aspiration pneumonitis and failed intubation are currently the most common causes of maternal death related to anesthesia. Risk is greatest among mothers who have been in labor and those needing emergency anesthesia. Neural blockade is accordingly safer than general anesthesia because the patient's protective reflexes are maintained and intubation is avoided.

For similar reasons, epidural or subarachnoid block is preferred in many centers over general anesthesia for nonurgent cesarean sections. Among the many advantages is that the mother and her partner can see and enjoy the birth of their baby. In the words of Moir,[227] "The delivery of the infant into the arms of a conscious and pain-free mother is one of the most exciting and rewarding moments in medicine." Consumer demand for neural blockade is accordingly high.

Despite the deservedly high current status of regional anesthesia for childbirth, it is not without hazard. Two complications continue to plague neural blockade in obstetric practice. The first of these, systemic toxicity, has caused at least 22 maternal deaths in North America in recent years.[10] In all cases, high concentrations and volumes of bupivacaine had been used, principally for cesarean section but also during labor. Bupivacaine appears to be more cardiotoxic than other local anesthetics; it is likely, however, that rapid injection and inadequate resuscitation accounted for most of these bupivacaine-related maternal deaths. Serious systemic toxicity would probably disappear if local anesthetic agents were always injected slowly and in incremental doses (see Chaps. 3 and 4). The second major complication, a high spinal block, is also largely avoidable, yet it continues to cause maternal deaths. Because both of these complications develop with alarming speed, many centers allow only anesthesiologists to perform epidural anesthesia. Restrictive staffing policies can cause logistical problems, however, and in practice patients with epidural blocks may either suffer periods of inadequate analgesia or be provided with unnecessarily "dense" blockade in order to prolong the duration of analgesia. This practice of "overkill" can be a source of frustration to the mother who is rendered unable to move her legs or feel her contractions and may be unable to bear down effectively during delivery. In an attempt to circumvent these problems, continuous infusion devices have been used or nurse-midwives allowed to administer incremental doses. The latter practice has been approved by the Central Midwives Board in the United Kingdom and other centers in the world subject to certain safeguards. Naturally a high standard of training and supervision is required, and an anesthesiologist should always be readily available to the obstetric unit.

Selective spinal analgesia using opioids has recently found some application in obstetrics, but reports of its efficacy have been conflicting and information remains scanty at this time. Compared with local anesthetics, spinal opioids have not received the same degree of scrutiny or critical evaluation among large obstetric populations. From the reports available to date, however, analgesia is less reliably obtained than with local anesthetic agents and achieved only with doses approaching those used parenterally. Although the absence of motor, sensory, and autonomic block is attractive, spinal opioids can cause somnolence, nausea, vomiting, respiratory depression, and pruritus. The relative merits of opioid drugs versus local anesthetics during labor are discussed more fully later in this chapter.

Experience has shown that the best results are achieved when the anesthesiologist is an integral member of the obstetric team. The anesthesiologist should be experienced and, in addition to technical skills, must have a firm grasp of basic physiologic and pharmacologic principles and an understanding of the medical complications that can arise during pregnancy and childbirth. Every opportunity should be taken to discuss neural blockade in a broad context with both the mother and the rest of the staff, whenever possible allowing the mother to make her own choice regarding analgesia and anesthesia. This implies provision of information that is honest, realistic, and well balanced. Antenatal education classes provide an ideal opportunity for the anesthesiologist to reassure mothers about pharmacologic pain relief. These occasions are also educational for the anesthesiologist because he is made aware of maternal opinions, fears, aspirations, and misconceptions.

PERIPHERAL PAIN PATHWAYS DURING LABOR

The peripheral pain pathways involved during labor were first described by Cleland in 1933[28] and restated more recently by Bonica.[29] It is convenient to discuss separately the pain associated with the first and second stages of labor because these pathways are quite different (Fig. 18-1).

FIRST STAGE OF LABOR

Pain in the first stage of labor primarily results from dilation of the cervix and lower uterine segment and distension of the body of the uterus. The intensity of pain is related to the strength of the contraction and the pressure thus generated. Noxious impulses from the cervix and uterus are transmitted by afferent nerves that accompany sympathetic pathways through, in turn, the pelvic, inferior, middle, and superior hypogastric plexuses; the lumbar sympathetic chain; the white rami of the spinal nerves of T10, T11, T12, and L1; and the posterior roots of these nerves to

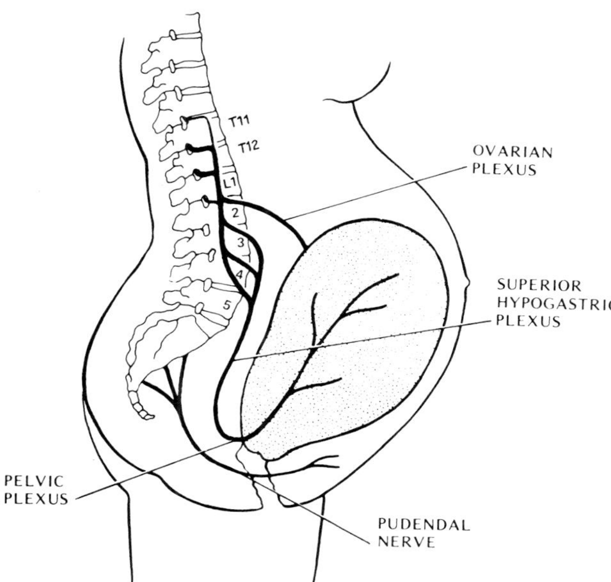

FIG. 18-1. Peripheral pain pathways during labor.

the cord. In early labor only the nerve roots of T11 and T12 are involved, but, as contractions become more intense, segments T10 and L1 also become involved.

Low backache during the first stage of labor is almost certainly referred pain from the *dorsal* rami of T10, to L1, the lateral branches of which descend before becoming superficial and supplying the skin some 10 cm caudal to their spinal origin.[29,333] In addition to the pain of uterine contraction, descent of the fetal head into the pelvis in the latter part of the first stage causes distension of the pelvic structures and pressure on roots of the lumbosacral plexus, producing referred pain by way of segments L2 and below. Thus pain may be felt in the region of L2 low in the back and also in thighs and legs (L2–S1).

SECOND STAGE OF LABOR

Pain produced by stretching of the perineum is transmitted by way of the pudendal nerve. This nerve is derived from the second, third, and fourth sacral nerves and passes posteriorly to the junction of the ischial spine and sacrospinous ligament, and anteriorly to the sacrotuberous ligament. The ischial spine is the bony landmark for pudendal nerve blockade. The analgesia accomplished by a successful pudendal block affects the posterior two thirds of the labia and the rest of the perineal area, including the anus (Fig. 18-2). The anterior third of the labia majora is supplied by the genitofemoral nerve.

APPLIED PHYSIOLOGY

Changes in respiratory, cardiovascular, and gastrointestinal function during pregnancy have particular implications for obstetric neural blockade. Only those relevant to the conduct of regional anesthesia are discussed here.

RESPIRATORY CHANGES

Oxygen consumption increases during pregnancy by about 20% at term and during labor is often doubled.[274,295] This increase during pregnancy is more than adequately compensated for by a 70% rise in alveolar ventilation.[82] Consequently maternal Pa_{CO_2} falls to 30 to 32 mm Hg. During labor further hyperventilation occurs in response to pain,[110] causing considerable hypocarbia and respiratory alkalosis.[294] Minute volumes of 90 liters/minute have been recorded during delivery.[64]

Despite upward displacement of the diaphragm, vital capacity, total lung capacity, and inspiratory reserve volume remain unaltered[320] because an increase in thoracic cage circumference adequately compensates for any diaphragmatic displacement. There is, however, a reduction in expiratory reserve volume and functional residual capacity (FRC).[82] This reduction is sufficient to cause some degree of airway closure in 50% of mothers at term during normal tidal ventilation.[24,292] Obesity, recumbency, and the lithotomy position aggravate this effect further.

There are several clinical implications of these respiratory changes for the anesthesiologist.

1. The increase in pulmonary venous admixture secondary to airway closure may lead to a below-normal Pa_{O_2} in late gestation. Stenger and coworkers,[314] for example, have shown lower maternal Pa_{O_2} values and a wider scatter than in nonpregnant women of the same age.
2. The increased oxygen requirements combined with a diminished FRC mean that hypoxemia occurs very rapidly in the presence of hypoventilation or apnea.[28] It is important to recall that the degree of change in Pa_{O_2} with ventilation follows a series of hyperbolic curves depending on oxygen consumption (Fig. 18-3).[249] Thus, at an oxygen use of 400 ml/minute, Pa_{O_2} shows a rapid decline

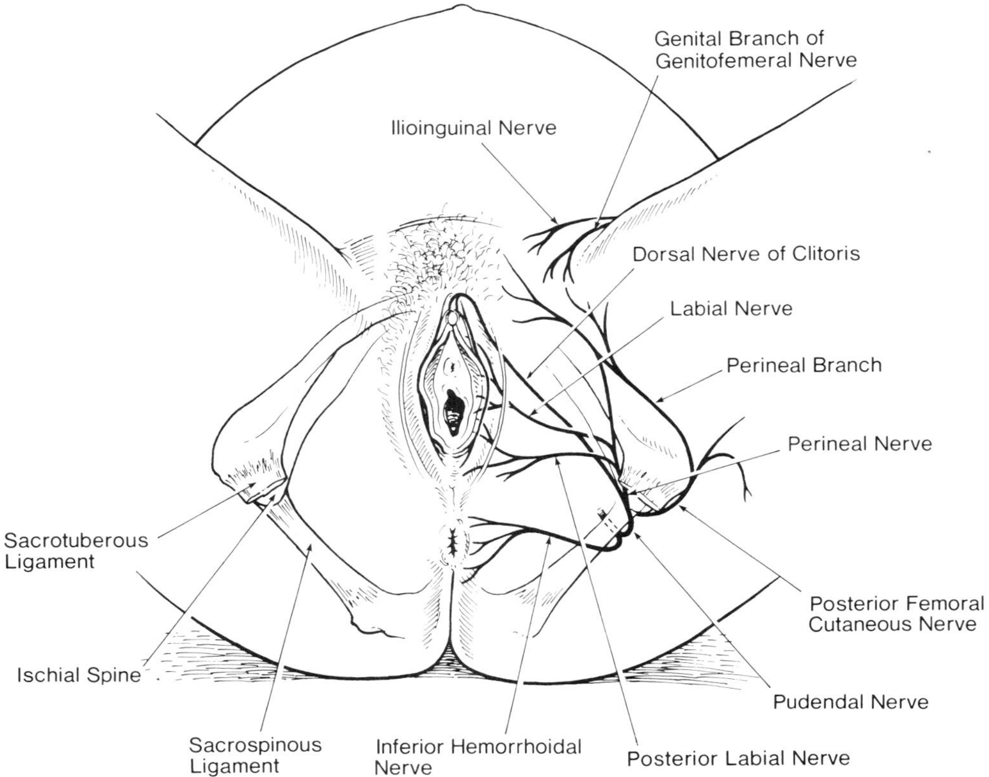

FIG. 18-2. Nerve supply to the perineum.

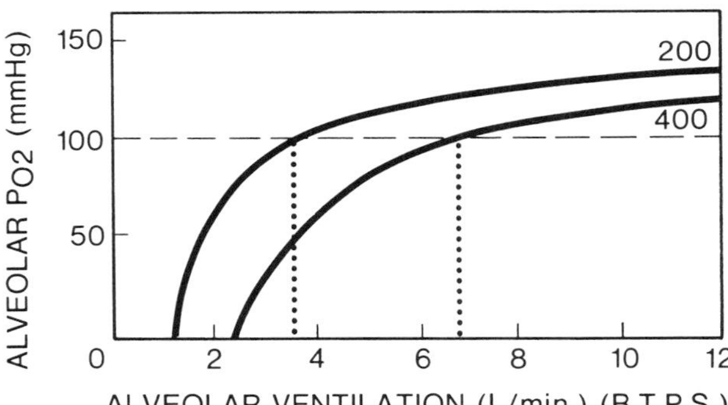

FIG. 18-3. Relationship between alveolar ventilation and alveolar P_{O_2} for values of oxygen consumption of 200 ml/min and 400 ml/min for a patient breathing air at normal barometric pressure. Note the alveolar ventilation required to maintain alveolar P_{O_2} above 100 mm Hg at the higher oxygen consumption in labor. (Modified from Nunn, J.F.: Applied Respiratory Physiology, p. 386. London, Butterworths, 1977.)

once alveolar ventilation falls below approximately 7 liters/minute. For these reasons, if controlled ventilation is required during pregnancy, a higher minute volume is necessary. Preoxygenation is also mandatory before any period of apnea (*e.g.*, at induction of general anesthesia). Further caution is required whenever regional analgesia is performed after parenteral or inhalation analgesia, as the onset of effective pain relief may unmask their depressant effects.

3. Hyperventilation and hypocarbia may reduce perfusion of certain organs. Cerebral blood flow, for example, is extremely sensitive to P_{CO_2} changes, and hypocarbia is associated with dizziness, disorientation, and lightheadedness. Uterine and umbilical artery perfusion also may be reduced in the presence of hypocarbia, thus contributing to the development of fetal acidemia.
4. Respiratory alkalosis can cause paresthesias and even frank tetany secondary to hypocalcemia.

Prolonged acute hypocarbia also results in diminished bicarbonate and buffer base levels that contribute to the development of metabolic acidosis during painful labors (see Figs. 18-6 and 18-8).[259,260]

CARDIOVASCULAR CHANGES

Pregnancy induces a "dynamic circulation." A 30% to 50% increase in both cardiac output and blood volume occurs in conjunction with a fall in peripheral resistance.[186] These changes are such that blood pressure is normally unaltered or slightly reduced. Adequate placental perfusion requires a uterine blood flow of 500 to 700 ml/minute at term.[17] Accordingly, hypotension, myocardial depression, reduced venous return, and hypovolemia should be prevented or quickly remedied. These factors become paramount during cesarean section performed under regional anesthesia: It has been shown, for example, that maternal blood volume expansion improves both uteroplacental and umbilical placental perfusion.[180]

One of the most important (yet easily avoided) causes of decreased venous return, cardiac output, and placental perfusion is aortocaval compression by the gravid uterus. This occurs whenever the mother assumes the supine position (Fig. 18-4). The potentially harmful sequelae of the supine position have been well documented.[25,98,100,176,300,336]

Most mothers are able to "tolerate" the supine position without developing symptoms or hypotension because of an increase in peripheral resistance and heart rate and increased venous return via the epidural and azygos veins.[75] In only 2% to 3% of mothers[148] are the compensatory mechanisms unable to maintain adequate cerebral perfusion, and then the symptoms of the "supine hypotensive syndrome" (pallor, sweating, nausea, and faintness) occur.

Aortocaval compression is of particular importance to the anesthesiologist because major regional and sympathetic blockade diminishes the ability to compensate for a fall in cardiac output and renders supine hypotension inevitable. The supine position must be avoided, therefore, at all times, including delivery in the lithotomy position and during cesar-

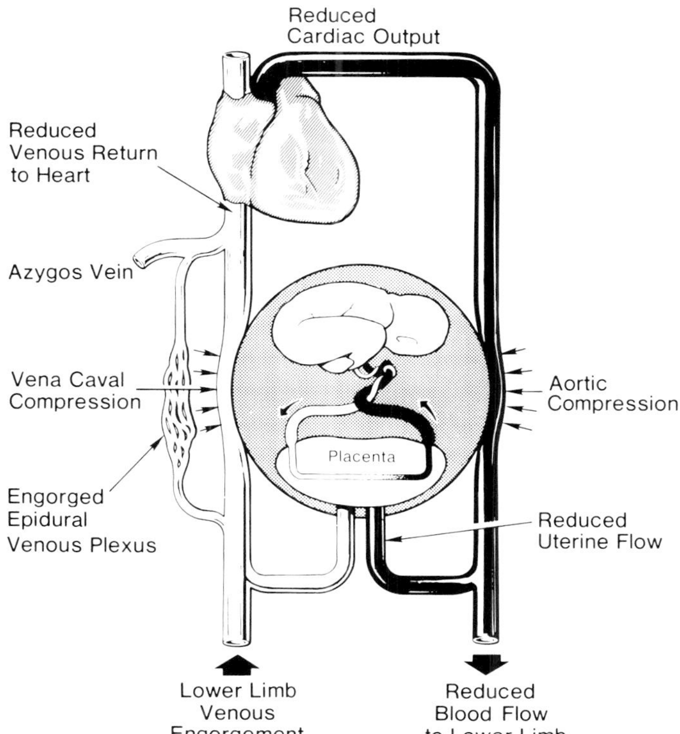

FIG. 18-4. Circulatory effects of aortocaval compression.

ean section.[147,227] In labor the mother should remain on her side, and at cesarean section she should either be suitably tilted or the uterus mechanically displayed laterally (preferably to the left).

Aortocaval compression can jeopardize fetal well-being by reducing uterine blood flow and possibly by interfering with placental venous drainage. Several studies have shown the deleterious effects of the supine posture on neonatal status both in labor[120,151,299] and at cesarean section.[13,79,96,121,327] Changes in fetal heart rate (FHR) are minimal when a lateral-tilt position is maintained during labor.[22,145,152,165,275,299] A further consequence of inferior vena caval compression is an increased venous return by other drainage pathways. In the spinal canal, this leads to engorgement of the epidural venous plexus of Bateson, which in turn diminishes the potential volume of the epidural space. This probably explains why the dose requirements for local anesthetics are reduced in late pregnancy and during labor (Fig. 18-4).[39]

Active bearing-down during delivery can be likened to a series of repeated Valsalva maneuvers. In the presence of central neural blockade, the normal circulatory responses to the Valsalva maneuver are obtunded because peripheral vessels to the lower limbs are unresponsive to sympathetic stimulation. Consequently, a greater fall in blood pressure occurs during active pushing.[335] This may also affect placental perfusion and explain why fetal acidemia develops more rapidly among mothers who push with epidural analgesia than among those who do not (see Fig. 18-8).[258]

Immediately after delivery, maternal blood volume is increased secondary to an autotransfusion of up to 500 ml from the placenta. Hypertension or pulmonary congestion and edema may occur at this time, particularly in those mothers at risk, for example, patients with heart disease and preeclampsia. Pulmonary congestion may also be precipitated after delivery by drugs such as ergometrine and vasopressors, and by drugs that cause fluid retention or circulatory overload, for example, oxytocin and beta-sympathomimetic agents.

Several hematologic changes also occur during pregnancy. Apart from a reduction in hemoglobin level, hematocrit, and blood viscosity[146,236] owing to hemodilution, the most significant are those related to coagulation. The platelet count and fibrinogen levels have doubled by term, whereas other clotting factors increase to a lesser degree.[261] At the same time, fibrinolytic factors decrease with advancing gestation. There is thus an increased risk of thromboembolism associated with pregnancy and childbirth. In many developed countries pulmonary embolism is now the principal cause of maternal death.

In summary, from a teleologic viewpoint, most of the above circulatory changes, that is, increased blood volume, cardiac output, and coagulation, may be seen as providing for increased metabolic demand and as a "protection" against hemorrhage at delivery. The maternal circulation is, however, very susceptible to postural changes, and in the presence of neural blockade aortocaval compression can be life-threatening to both mother and fetus. Attending staff must be alert and ready to treat harmful circulatory changes by measures such as appropriate positioning of the patient, correction of hypovolemia, and, if necessary, using a vasopressor agent intravenously (see below).

UTEROPLACENTAL CIRCULATION AND OXYGEN DELIVERY

Uterine Blood Flow

The uterine circulation can be regarded as a system of low resistance grafted in parallel with other maternal vascular beds.[17] In some respects, it behaves like an arteriovenous shunt. The increase in maternal cardiac output is more than sufficient to supply the uteroplacental circulation (about 500–700 ml/min at term). Blood flow varies directly with perfusion pressure (uterine arterial minus uterine venous pressure) and inversely with uterine vascular resistance. It is important to understand the many factors that can influence these two parameters because fetal homeostasis and survival depend upon adequate placental perfusion.

Uterine perfusion pressure is reduced when systemic hypotension occurs from any cause, including autonomic block and compression of the aorta by the gravid uterus. (Note that the uterine arteries originate at a point distal to the area of aortic compression, that is, at the level of the L4 vertebra; see Fig. 18-4.[25])

Uterine vascular resistance is influenced by both intrinsic and extrinsic factors. Thus uterine arterial vasoconstriction occurs in response to sympathetic stimulation[122] secondary to, for example, pain. The uterine vessels are particularly sensitive to direct-acting alpha-adrenergic drugs,[277] and these agents therefore should be avoided. When a vasopressor is indicated (*e.g.*, to treat hypotension secondary to regional anesthesia), ephedrine is the drug of choice because its effect is predominantly that of a beta-adrenergic agonist. Cardiac output and uterine blood flow consequently improve, as does arterial blood pressure.[278,306]

The addition of epinephrine to local anesthetics in usual clinical concentrations (*i.e.*, <1 : 200,000) has little influence on placental perfusion.[11] Epidural analgesia in labor decreases circulating catecholamines, reduces sympathetic tone, and abolishes hyperventilation; it may thereby improve placental perfusion (see Fig. 18-6). This is considered further in "Physiologic Changes Secondary to Labor Pain" later in this chapter.

Although in the healthy parturient the placental vasculature is maximally dilated, in patients with pregnancy-induced hypertension uterine vascular resistance is increased and placental perfusion impaired. The pathophysiologic mechanisms are complex, but vasospasm is presumed to be an important factor because epidural blockade improves placental blood flow even in the face of moderate falls in systolic blood pressure.[164]

Uterine vascular resistance is influenced *extrinsically* by uterine tone. A uterine contraction reduces uterine flow in proportion to its magnitude when the pressure generated exceeds about 20 mm Hg.[32,185] Attending staff, therefore, must ensure that uterine contractions do not reach an amplitude or frequency sufficient to cause fetal asphyxia. Excessive uterine contractility may be less obvious in the presence of regional blockade. Thus the frequency and strength of contractions must be monitored, either by manual palpation or by intrauterine or abdominal tocodynamometry, preferably in conjunction with continuous monitoring of fetal heart rate.

Oxygen Supply

Oxygen delivery to the fetus depends not only upon placental perfusion but also upon maternal arterial oxygen content. The latter is a product of hemoglobin concentration and saturation. As noted earlier, hemoglobin concentration is lowered during normal pregnancy (the so-called physiologic anemia) and saturation is occasionally reduced in some mothers secondary to an increase in pulmonary venous admixture. During pregnancy there is a significant shift of the oxyhemoglobin dissociation curve to the right compared with the nonpregnant state.[173] This phenomenon is associated with a parallel rise in red cell 2,3 DPG content and signifies an enhanced release of oxygen at a given oxygen tension.[287] In labor, however, extreme hyperventilation and respiratory alkalosis reverse this shift and result in impaired maternal–fetal oxygen transfer.

The fetus is adapted to survive at a much lower arterial oxygen tension than is the adult, umbilical vein Po_2 being about 30 mm Hg. These adaptations include [1] a higher oxygen-carrying capacity (fetal hemoglobin [Hb-F] being 17 g/100 ml); [2] a greater affinity of Hb-F for oxygen: The Hb-F oxygen dissociation curve is shifted well to the left compared with adult Hb (*i.e.*, P50 of 17 mm Hg as opposed to 27 mm Hg); [3] the Bohr effect, which operates on each side of the placental barrier between the maternal and fetal hemoglobins such that oxygen transfer to the fetus is favored at the oxygen tension found in the intervillous space. The Bohr effect accounts for 20% to 40% of oxygen transfer. Oxygen stores in the fetus are, however, very limited, and metabolic acidosis secondary to ischemia is readily incurred whenever oxygen transfer fails to meet oxygen requirements.

Although on breathing air the mother's arterial Hb may be close to full saturation, both maternal and fetal arterial Po_2 are increased significantly when higher oxygen concentrations are inspired. Oxygen therapy should be instituted without hesitation whenever fetal hypoxia is suspected. It should also be administered routinely during cesarean section performed under regional blockade[279] and probably during vaginal delivery. Earlier fears that maternal Pao_2 in excess of 300 mm Hg might cause uterine vasoconstriction and fetal hypoxemia[286] have not been substantiated.[210,279]

GASTROINTESTINAL CHANGES

Acid aspiration is one of the most common causes of maternal death related to anesthesia. The gravid patient is predisposed to this complication, having raised intra-abdominal and intragastric pressures, increased tendency to esophageal reflux, decreased gastric emptying time, and increased gastric acidity. Nausea and vomiting are further exacerbated by labor pain, stress, and the administration of opioids. The importance of the latter was demonstrated by Holdsworth,[141] who found the largest volumes of gastric content among patients who had received meperidine during labor and the smallest in those who had received either epidural or no analgesia. These findings have been supported by Nimmo[247,248] using the acetaminophen absorption test as an indicator of the rate of gastric emptying (Fig. 18-5). Although the risk of regurgitation and pulmonary aspi-

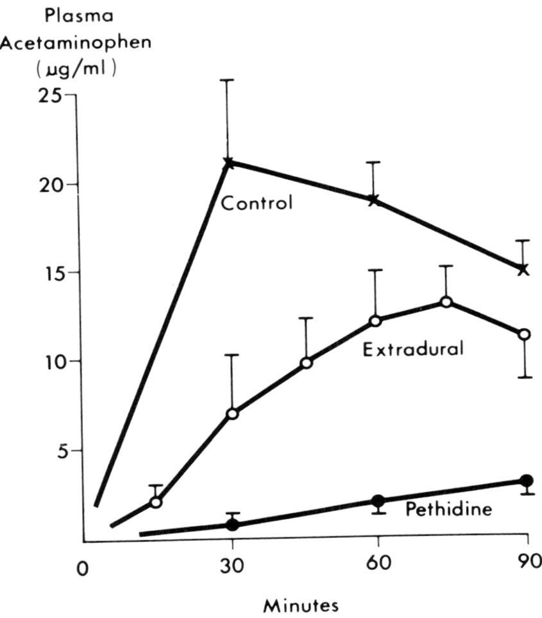

FIG. 18-5. Plasma acetaminophen concentrations (mean ± SD) during labor after 1.5 g of oral acetaminophen. Patients receiving meperidine 150 mg i.m. have a significantly slower acetaminophen absorption than do those receiving no analgesia (control) or epidural bupivacaine. (Nimmo, W.R.: Gastrointestinal function following surgery. Reg. Anaesth., 7:S105, 1982.)

ration is largely associated with general anesthesia, regional blockade is not entirely free from this danger. Aspiration can still occur if consciousness is depressed secondary to, for example, the development of a high spinal block, systemic toxicity, hypovolemia, aortocaval compression, or concurrent medication. Vomiting may also be precipitated by acute hypotension. Ergometrine frequently causes vomiting, especially if given as an intravenous bolus.[228,233] Various prophylactic measures have been suggested to reduce the risk of aspiration, including [a] administration of oral antacids (*e.g.*, 0.3 M sodium citrate) during labor and immediately before surgery; [b] histamine H2-antagonists orally or intravenously; [c] metoclopramide i.v. preoperatively to increase lower esophageal sphinter tone and increase gastric motility; and [d] as a last resort, gastric emptying either by means of an orogastric tube or by inducing emesis with apomorphine. Although these measures have been shown to raise the *p*H or decrease the volume of gastric contents, or both, it is not yet certain whether mortality or serious morbidity is similarly reduced.

PHYSIOLOGIC CHANGES SECONDARY TO PAIN IN LABOR

Several physiologic and biochemical changes occur during labor largely as a result of pain itself; they can be reversed partially or completely by effective regional blockade. These sequelae are summarized in Figure 18-6.

Many of the above effects can be regarded as "stress" responses, similar to those that have been described during surgery (see Chap. 5). Anxiety also may be contributory, yet pain must remain the domi-

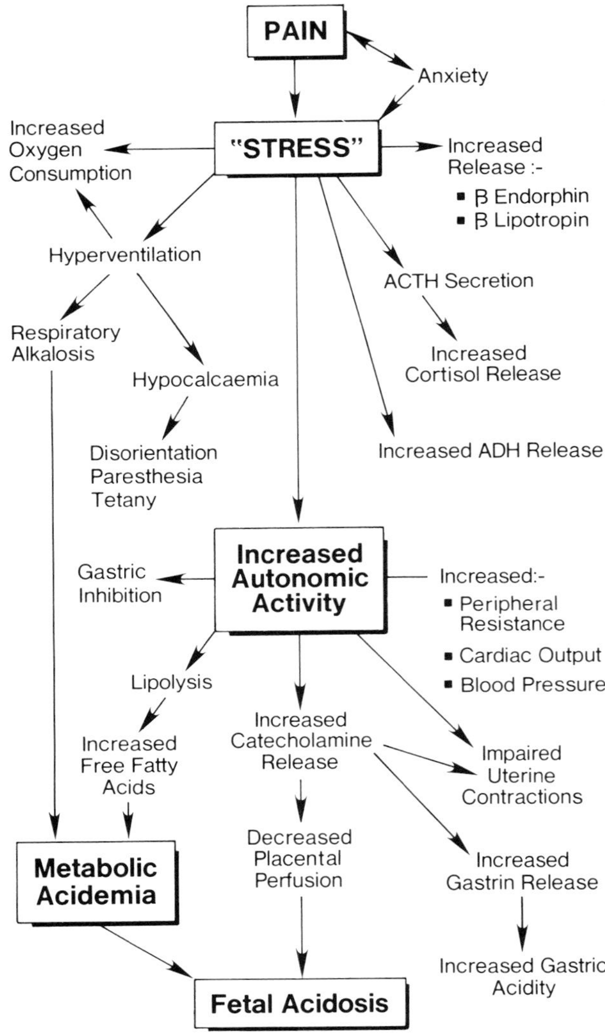

FIG. 18-6. Physiologic changes secondary to pain in labor.

nant factor, since relaxation becomes evident after the onset of good analgesia during labor.

Beta-endorphin, beta-lipotropin, and adrenocorticotropic hormone are derived from a common precursor; all are present in increased amounts during labor.[6,45,106,319] Hormonal secretion from the adrenal cortex similarly increases during labor,[51,53,166,205] whereas thyroid stimulating hormone (TSH) levels remain unchanged.[166] Mothers receiving epidural analgesia have significantly lower circulating levels of beta-endorphin, beta-lipotropin, and corticosteroids, presumably because they are free from pain.[6,45,319] Adrenocortical suppression is related to the extent of neural blockade and the presence of other factors such as physical exertion and emotional stress.[166,205] The clinical significance of the above findings remains conjectural. Although it has been postulated that beta-endorphin release may represent a mechanism for modulation of pain in labor,[118] no change in pain threshold has been demonstrated in humans.[303]

Hyperventilation is prevented when labor is conducted under epidural block[259] and oxygen consumption is similarly reduced.[129,295] Plasma catecholamine levels rise progressively during labor,[104,184] resulting in increased urinary excretion of these substances.[167]

Some of the changes that occur during labor appear to be in response to this increased autonomic activity (Fig. 18-6). The increases in maternal peripheral resistance and blood pressure as labor progresses are examples of this phenomenon because they are reversed by epidural analgesia.

Similarly, inhibition of gastric emptying and of intestinal peristalsis can be explained on this basis.[141] Gastrin release is stimulated during painful labors[133] and results in increased gastric acid secretion. Excessive sympathetic activity is also thought to contribute to a state of incoordinate uterine contractility that can develop during a prolonged labor.[201] In these circumstances epidural analgesia may allow more normal uterine activity and hasten cervical dilation.[232]

Placental perfusion is also probably adversely affected by increased adrenosympathetic activity. For example, a norepinephrine infusion causes uterine vasoconstriction in the pregnant ewe,[290] and uterine blood flow decreases significantly during periods of stress in association with elevated plasma norepinephrine levels (Fig. 18-7).[308]

Whether the circulating catecholamine levels found during normal labor are sufficient to reduce placental perfusion awaits clarification. Epidural analgesia does significantly reduce maternal plasma

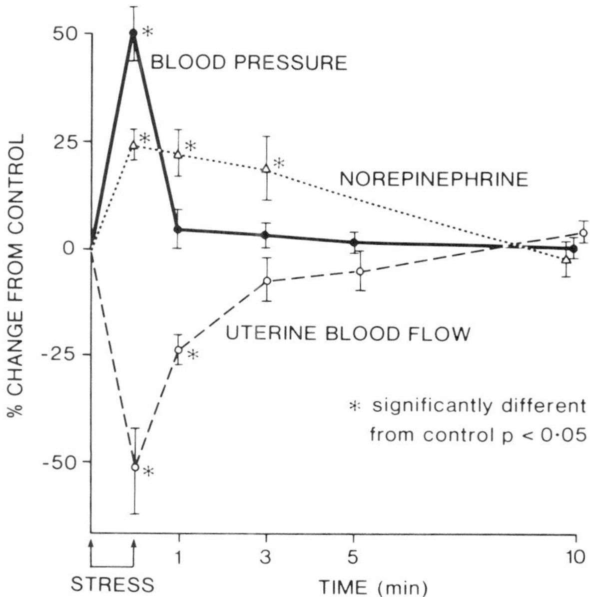

FIG. 18-7. Effects of stress on maternal arterial blood pressure, plasma norepinephrine levels, and uterine blood flow in the pregnant ewe. (Shnider, S.M., *et al.*: Uterine blood flow and plasma norepinephrine changes during maternal stress. Anesthesiology, *50*:524, 1979.)

catecholamine levels during labor,[304] which may account for the improvement in placental perfusion that has been demonstrated following its use in labor.[143,164] The sympathetic blockade and decreased uterine vascular resistance associated with epidural analgesia presumably also contribute to improved perfusion. These effects of neural blockade can be regarded as advantageous to the fetus.

Finally, pain during labor has an influence on acid–base balance. Maternal blood concentrations of free fatty acids and lactate rise to reach a peak at delivery.[166,202,209,259,318] By contrast, when labor is conducted under epidural blockade only minor acid–base changes are observed during the first stage. The most likely explanation for the progressive maternal acidemia that occurs during painful labor is catecholamine-induced lipolytic metabolism, although starvation and a diminished buffering capacity resulting from metabolic compensation for a respiratory alkalosis may also be contributory (Fig. 18-6).

Maternal metabolic acidosis in the second stage of labor is largely related to the degree of exertion during active pushing.[166,260] This occurs irrespective of analgesia and is time dependent. When labor is conducted under epidural analgesia, acidosis is less common among mothers who do not actively push compared with those who do (Fig. 18-8).[260]

The degree of maternal acidosis has implications for patient management because maternal acid–base balance is reflected in the fetus (see Fig. 18-6).[257,258] Although the fetus is less acidotic at the onset of the second stage of labor when regional anesthesia is used (Fig. 18-8), suppression of the bearing-down reflex can lead to a prolonged period of pushing. This not only is unproductive and exhausting for the mother, but also exposes the fetus to increasing acidemia. In the second stage of labor the mother should not be encouraged to push actively until the presenting part has descended as far as the perineum.

APPLIED PHARMACOLOGY

The pharmacology and fetal effects of local anesthetics administered to the mother before delivery have been the subject of several reviews.[89,187,196,224,262,270,277,296,323] It is clear that rapid equilibration occurs between local anesthetic concentrations in the two circulations governed largely by the physiochemical properties of the agents used (see Chap. 3). Certain techniques and agents are more likely to achieve toxic blood levels than others. Direct fetal injection has occurred after attempted paracervical, caudal, and pudendal blocks and even during perineal infiltration.[109] As local anesthetic toxicity is potentially lethal, its recognition and treatment (see Chap. 4) must be well understood by all staff who practice and supervise neural blockade in obstetrics.

RELATIVE MERITS OF LOCAL ANESTHETIC AGENTS IN OBSTETRICS

ESTER-LINKED AGENTS

2-Chloroprocaine has by far the shortest plasma half-life of all local anesthetics. In neonatal blood,

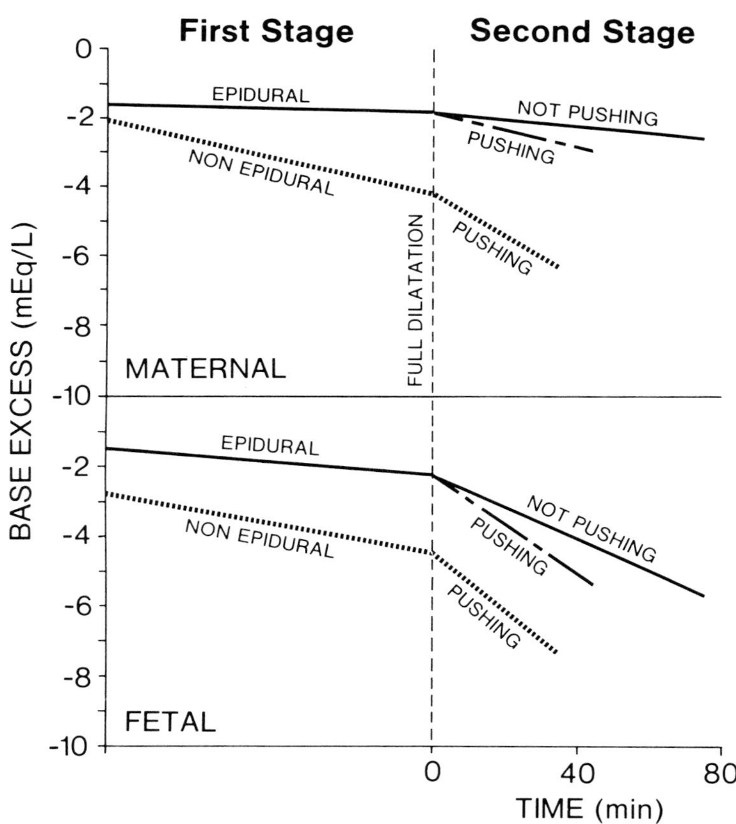

FIG. 18-8. Maternal and fetal acid–base changes during labor, comparing epidural and nonepidural analgesia. During the first stage of labor both maternal and fetal changes are negligible with epidural analgesia. During the second stage, both maternal and fetal acidosis are accelerated owing to active pushing. Although epidural block is associated with a longer duration of the second stage of labor, patients with epidural analgesia demonstrate minimal acidosis at full dilation and a slower *rate* of development of acidosis, especially in the absence of pushing. (Adapted from Pearson and Davies: refs 257–260).

half-life is about 43 seconds, or double the time for adult blood.[107] Fetal blood levels of 2-chloroprocaine following neural blockade are therefore negligible, and it is not surprising that neonatal depression has not been reported following clinical use. Cumulative toxicity does not develop on account of its rapid hydrolysis. For these reasons, it has been recommended for epidural use during labor[139] and for paracervical block.[113] Its shorter duration of action, however, makes 2-chloroprocaine less attractive for continuous epidural analgesia — unless a continuous infusion is used — because more frequent top-up doses are required. Chloroprocaine has, however, been associated with a number of neurologic complications, in most instances after inadvertent intrathecal injection. Although it appears that chloroprocaine itself is no more neurotoxic than other local anesthetics, the combination of a low *p*H in some chloroprocaine formulations and the antioxidant bisulfite could result in neurotoxicity if a large dose was administered intrathecally. This formulation problem is currently being corrected (see Chap. 4).

Tetracaine until recently was the most commonly used intrathecal agent in North America but is not currently available in the United Kingdom or Australasia.

AMIDE-LINKED AGENTS

Unlike ester-linked local anesthetics, the more commonly used amide-linked agents primarily depend on hepatic metabolism before their elimination from the body. Accordingly, the elimination half-life is much longer than that of the esters. Maternal–fetal transfer of the unbound, undissociated form after administration to the mother occurs readily and is dependent upon the maternal blood concentration of free drug. Fetal blood levels therefore represent a balance between the dose administered, the rate of absorption, tissue disposition, metabolism, and excretion. The basic principles of placental transfer and neonatal disposition have been described in Chapter 3; only the clinical implications are discussed here.

The fetal to maternal (F/M) ratio of local anesthetic plasma levels varies widely; prilocaine has a ratio close to unity, whereas lidocaine and mepivacaine have values of 0.5 to 0.7. Bupivacaine and etidocaine, on the other hand, have an F/M ratio of 0.2 to 0.3 (see Fig. 3-32 and Table 3-18). Protein binding in maternal blood may limit the proportion of local anesthetic that is transferable to the fetus;[324] however, the F/M ratio does not indicate the *magnitude* of transfer but rather reflects differences in fetal tissue uptake. Differences in *p*H between maternal and fetal blood also influence local anesthetic uptake by the fetus. Thus in the presence of fetal acidosis, an elevated F/M ratio has been reported with lidocaine,[43,44,240] mepivacaine,[44] and bupivacaine.[269] A decrease in fetal *p*H favors drug ionization and therefore retention within the fetal circulation. Local anesthetic toxicity is also enhanced in the presence of fetal acidosis[240]; thus in the presence of fetal distress, local anesthetics should be administered cautiously.

Although the elimination half-life of lidocaine is greater in the newborn than in the adult because of the larger volume of distribution,[221] metabolic clearance is very similar on a weight-for-weight basis.[108] The plasma half-life of mepivacaine (9 hours) is, however, considerably longer than that of lidocaine (3 hours). Plasma half-life of bupivacaine in the neonate is similar to that in the adult (2 hours).[44]

Toxic effects of local anesthetic agents in the fetus, as in the adult, or neonate are manifested by central nervous and cardiovascular changes. Maternal toxicity has on occasion led to perinatal death[277] after large doses, and fetal cardiotoxicity may have been a contributory factor. More subtle CNS changes have been revealed by neurobehavioral testing of the newborn (see below).

Lidocaine is commonly used in obstetrics for all techniques of neural blockade. Doses may be varied and epinephrine included to provide versatility. Motor block is fairly dense, and development of tachyphylaxis can occur with continuous epidural analgesia.[231] For these reasons bupivacaine has become more popular than lidocaine for labor analgesia, although lidocaine remains the agent of choice in many centers for cesarean section. It is preferable to add epinephrine (1 : 200,000 – 1 : 300,000) to lidocaine in order to limit placental transfer and prolong the duration of analgesia.[3]

Mepivacaine. Placental transfer of mepivacaine is greater, and neonatal metabolism slower, than that of lidocaine.[44] Neonatal neurobehavioral depression has been reported after the epidural administration of mepivacaine, and the potential for frank toxicity makes this agent unattractive for obstetric use.[242]

Prilocaine has the highest F/M ratio, which may indeed exceed unity.[271] Although less toxic than lidocaine, methemoglobinemia has been reported in both mother and neonate.[14] In some instances more than 10% of fetal hemoglobin has been converted, an amount sufficient to produce neonatal cyanosis. These factors outweigh any advantages of prilocaine, except possibly for a single low dose for pudendal block or perineal infiltration, when delivery is imminent.[226]

Bupivacaine is currently the amide agent of choice for epidural analgesia in labor. In concentrations of 0.25% or less, effective analgesia can be provided with minimal motor blockade (see Fig. 4-3). Tachyphylaxis has not been a problem, and the duration of action is convenient for use in labor.

For cesarean section, 0.5% bupivacaine is more popular than lidocaine in some centers. It has been suggested that bupivacaine is relatively more cardiotoxic than other local anesthetic agents, especially in higher concentrations.[10] As discussed in Chapter 4, extreme care should be taken to avoid accidental intravenous injection of large bolus doses of bupivacaine. Precautionary measures include the use of an epinephrine-containing test dose (3 ml of 1 : 200,000 solution) and incremental injections of the total dose.

Etidocaine provides motor blockade out of proportion to its sensory block and therefore is not suitable for epidural analgesia during labor. The rapid onset and good muscle relaxation, however, coupled with a very low F/M ratio, make 1% etidocaine attractive for use in cesarean section.[198]

THE NEUROBEHAVIORAL CONTROVERSY

Frank neonatal local anesthetic toxicity is extremely rare, and Apgar scores and blood gas analyses are usually normal after uncomplicated neural blockade. These tests, however, are useful only in detecting fairly severe depression of vital functions. Neurobehavioral assessments, which more closely scrutinize newborn behavior, have shown that subtle or delayed effects of obstetrical anesthesia can be present even when more gross testing reveals no abnormalities. Neurobehavioral tests examine the neonate's muscle tone and reflex behavior, as well as studying more complex CNS functions such as the ability to change the state of arousal, initiate complex motor acts, and suppress meaningless environmental stimuli. The Early Neonatal Neurobehavioral Scale (ENNS)[297] and the Neurological and Adaptive Capacity Score (NACS)[12] have been extensively used to evaluate the effects of anesthesia on the newborn. Both are simplified versions of the more comprehensive and time-consuming Brazelton Neonatal Behavioral Assessment Scale,[35] differing from each other predominantly in the emphasis placed on the various aspects of neonatal behavior.

Concern regarding the effects of local anesthetics began when Scanlon and his associates compared the neonatal behavioral effects of maternal epidural analgesia with lidocaine and mepivacaine and, in a second study, bupivacaine with that of nonepidural controls.[297,298] Babies whose mothers had received lidocaine or mepivacaine were grouped together and scored less well on the first day of life on tests of muscle strength and tone than did infants whose mothers had received bupivacaine or no anesthesia. The authors described these infants as "floppy but alert" and correlated this finding with the persistence of lidocaine and, to a greater extent, mepivacaine in the newborn.[44] Subsequently, the same group reported that chloroprocaine was similar to bupivacaine in its lack of neurobehavioral depression.[42]

In the United States these findings resulted in the rejection of lidocaine for use in obstetric epidural anesthesia and the widespread adoption of bupivacaine and chloroprocaine. More recently, concerns regarding the potential toxicity of both these agents had led to more critical evaluation of Scanlon's data.[83] One drawback of Scanlon's earliest study is that the epidural group consisted predominantly of patients who had received mepivacaine ($n = 19$), with a much smaller number ($n = 9$) having received lidocaine.[297] This is important because umbilical cord levels of mepivacaine were significantly higher than those of lidocaine.[44] Despite this, patients who received lidocaine and mepivacaine were grouped together for statistical analyses. Another criticism is that the second study was performed at a later date and lacked its own control group, comparisons being made with the nonepidural group of the earlier study. Interpretation of the data is also complicated by the fact that many patients in both the epidural and nonepidural groups received narcotics or barbiturates. Thus it was appropriate to question the validity of the conclusion that bupivacaine was superior to lidocaine; new investigations were clearly necessary.

Abboud and co-workers therefore recently compared neonatal condition following epidural anesthesia with lidocaine, chloroprocaine, and bupivacaine for both vaginal delivery and cesarean section.[4,5] No adverse effects were seen with any agent, and infants in all groups scored equally well on the ENNS. Similarly, Kileff and colleagues[177] found no differences in the ENNS following epidural anesthesia for cesarean section with lidocaine compared with bupivacaine; in fact, infants whose mothers had received lidocaine sucked more vigorously at 24 hours of age. Although one recent study did find that babies performed marginally better on certain aspects of the Brazelton Assessment after chloroprocaine than after lidocaine, these findings were considered to be very subtle and to be significantly less important in influencing neonatal outcome than other perinatal factors.[179]

Neurobehavioral testing also has been performed following systemic medication, as well as other techniques of neural blockade. In general, global depression of the neurobehavioral examination occurs after general anesthesia or administration to the mother of narcotics, barbiturates, or other sedative drugs. The degree and duration of depression is related to the dose to which the newborn has been exposed. Meperidine, in doses as low as 50 mg, has been shown in several studies to produce significant neonatal neurobehavioral depression when administered to the laboring mother.[34,136] As might be expected, subarachnoid block with tetracaine resulted in higher scores on the ENNS than did general anesthesia with either ketamine or thiopental, presumably reflecting the minimal drug exposure involved with spinal anesthesia.[135]

Neurobehavioral testing after paracervical block in which 0.25% bupivacaine was used revealed no difference between the study group and control infants whose mothers had received local infiltration or spinal or pudendal block.[216] In contrast, Nesheim and colleagues[246] reported poorer neurobehavioral scores after paracervical block, also with bupivacaine, than after local infiltration only. This study, however, is difficult to interpret, since paracervical block patients also received significant amounts of lidocaine for pudendal block and local infiltration, and both groups received intravenous sedatives or nitrous oxide. The effects of pudendal block by itself have been studied, comparing outcome after administration of either 0.5% bupivacaine, 15 mepivacaine, or 3% chloroprocaine. In surprising contrast to the findings when similar doses were used for epidural anesthesia, mepivacaine for pudendal block was associated with better performance on the ENNS than were the other agents.[218] Possible explanations for this are the lower neonatal blood concentrations and shorter time from injection to delivery associated with pudendal block.

What are the long-term effects, if any, of abnormal neurobehavioral performance in the early neonatal period? Many studies in which an adverse effect has been attributed to anesthesia are complicated by the inclusion of mothers with abnormalities of pregnancy or delivery. Such problems are likely to affect adversely both newborn behavior and later development. In most of the studies of newborn neurobehavior following neural blockade discussed above, infants were totally normal by the 2nd or 3rd day of life. Ounsted and associates[253,254] prospectively followed 570 children for 4 years after delivery, carefully evaluating neurologic and motor development. No correlation was found between poor outcome and method of pain relief used for delivery, although emergency cesarean section and perinatal asphyxia were strongly associated with abnormal development. In another long-term study of the offspring of healthy mothers with uncomplicated pregnancies, cognitive ability at 5 years of age was not influenced by the method of anesthesia or analgesia used at delivery.[330]

In summary, the neonatal neurobehavioral effects of local anesthetics used for analgesia in childbirth appear to be of minimal significance. It is more important in this respect to avoid maternal hypotension or hypoxia, which could secondarily result in perinatal asphyxia and thereby affect the newborn.

EFFECTS OF LOCAL ANESTHETICS ON THE UTERUS AND UTERINE AND UMBILICAL VESSELS

Clinical studies on the effect of local anesthetics on uterine activity have produced conflicting results. It is unlikely that a direct effect on myometrial contraction will be observed in practice.[270] Isolated human uterine muscle begins to show a significant dose-related depression of contractility with lidocaine, for example, only at levels in excess of 25 μg/ml,[243] a level unlikely to be attained except in the event of gross toxicity or after paracervical block.

Similarly, the actions of local anesthetics on the uterine and umbilical vessels are of dubious clinical significance. *In vitro* studies have demonstrated a vasoconstricting effect of local anesthetics on uterine arteries. With lidocaine, this occurs only at concentrations in excess of 20 μg/ml.[117] In contrast, the umbilical arteries behave differently depending upon the local anesthetic agent. Lidocaine and etidocaine dilate the umbilical vessels, whereas prilocaine and bupivacaine cause vasoconstriction.[325] All these effects have been recorded only at concentrations far exceeding blood levels associated with neural blockade (except possibly with paracervical block).

EFFECTS OF EPINEPHRINE ADDED TO LOCAL ANESTHETICS

The addition of epinephrine to lidocaine and mepivacaine reduces drug absorption, thereby enhancing the spread and quality of neural blockade as well as lowering peak blood levels. With bupivacaine and etidocaine, epinephrine has only marginal effects on the duration of action[67,282] and little effect on reducing peak blood levels.[281]

The action of epinephrine on uterine tone, contractility, and uterine flow remains controversial. Several studies have reported a reduction in uterine activity following epidural blockade and even pudendal block when epinephrine has been added to the local anesthetic.[68,165,211,275,326,348] Other factors, however, such as hypotension and aortocaval compression inhibit contraction,[54] and it is not clear how much epinephrine *per se* contributes to uterine inhibition.

Some investigators have recommended avoidance of epinephrine,[8,262] whereas others consider the addition of 5 μg/ml to be harmless with regard to the progress of labor.[28,226]

Placental blood flow is not significantly altered by the addition of 5 μg of epinephrine to epidural chloroprocaine during labor[11] and therefore is not contraindicated on these grounds.

VASOPRESSOR AGENTS

As mentioned earlier, ephedrine is the most appropriate vasopressor for obstetric purposes. The net effect is to enhance uterine blood flow and restore placental perfusion and maternal arterial blood pressure. Fetal acidosis secondary to hypotension is also arrested and often corrected with epinephrine.[306]

Ephedrine has positive chronotropic activity and is transmitted readily across the placenta. Both maternal and fetal tachycardia, therefore, commonly occur, and increased fetal heart rate variability has also been observed.[343] These effects are dose related, and because they are not associated with fetal acidosis they are regarded as being innocuous.[343]

DRUG INTERACTIONS

Several drugs used in obstetric practice have implications for the patient receiving neural blockade, including oxytocic, hypotensive, and tocolytic agents.

Oxytocic Agents

Oxytocics are commonly given after delivery to improve uterine contractility. Ergometrine (0.25–0.5 mg) and oxytocin (5–10 units) both effectively reduce blood loss,[228,233] although their cardiovascular effects when administered as an intravenous bolus are quite different (Table 18-1).

The vasoconstrictive action of ergometrine can seriously aggravate postpartum hypertension among patients with essential or pregnancy-induced hypertension or pheochromocytoma.[226] Dangerous hypertension can also occur after ergometrine in patients who have already received epinephrine or a vasopressor agent. This may be sufficiently severe to cause a cerebrovascular accident[59] or pulmonary edema.[162]

Nausea, vomiting, and headache are much more common after ergometrine than after oxytocin, and the latter is therefore preferred following delivery or during cesarean section.[223] Despite theoretical concern about hypotension after oxytocin administration in the presence of regional anesthesia,[338] it seldom occurs in practice,[228] especially when the drug is administered as a dilute infusion.[162] Ergometrine should be reserved for intramuscular use (which causes fewer side-effects) except when atonic uterine postpartum hemorrhage fails to respond to oxytocin.

Oxytocin infusions are frequently used in obstetrics for the induction of augmentation of labor; to empty the contents of the uterus in patients with hydatidiform mole; and in midtrimester termination of pregnancy. Even low doses of oxytocin, however, are antidiuretic, and this effect has been demonstrated to occur within 15 minutes of the start of the infusions.[190] When prolonged infusions are given, water intoxication and hyponatremia may develop, resulting in convulsions and loss of consciousness.[9] Hyponatremia must be considered in the differential

TABLE 18–1. SIDE-EFFECTS OF INTRAVENOUS OXYTOCIN VERSUS ERGOMETRINE GIVEN AS A BOLUS DOSE AT DELIVERY

	Oxytocin 5–10 Units	Ergometrine 0.25–0.5 mg
Cardiovascular[162,338]		
Peripheral resistance	↓ (transient)	↑ (prolonged)
Systemic blood pressure	↓ (transient)	↑ (prolonged)
Central venous pressure	↑ (transient)	↑ (prolonged)
Antidiuretic action[190]	Yes	No
Emetic action[223,228,233]	Rare	Common
Headache	Rare	Common

diagnosis, therefore, whenever convulsions occur during labor. The diagnosis should be suspected if the blood sodium concentration is less than 120 to 125 mmol/liter. Water intoxication has usually been associated with oxytocin infusions in excess of 3.5 liters, with 5% dextrose as the vehicle.[105] Careful fluid balance is therefore required, and an isotonic solution is preferred as the vehicle for oxytocin infusions.

Hypotensive Agents

Several drugs are used in the management of pregnancy-induced hypertension, including hydralazine, diazoxide, methyldopa, magnesium sulfate, alpha- and beta-adrenergic antagonists, sodium nitroprusside, and, in some centers, slow-calcium channel blocking agents such as nifedipine. The principles of pharmacologic management of hypertension during pregnancy have been reviewed by Lubbe[197]. Because the blood pressure can be very labile in such patients, regional anesthesia should be applied cautiously and local anesthetics given in small incremental doses.

Tocolytic Agents

Beta-sympathomimetic drugs have been used in the management of premature labor for about 20 years. They act on β_2-receptors on the surface of uterine muscle cells and cause relaxation by inhibiting myosin light-chain phosphorylation (*i.e.*, tocolysis). In therapeutic intravenous infusion doses, unpleasant side-effects are very common and include apprehension, restlessness, skeletal muscle tremor, nausea, tachycardia, and palpitations. Beta-mimetic agents increase heart rate and cardiac output while lowering peripheral vascular resistance.[192] Normally mean blood pressure changes little. These effects accentuate further the hyperdynamic circulatory state that exists in pregnancy, which explains why even with the relatively β_2-selective agents (ritodrine, terbutaline, salbutamol, hexoprenaline, and fenoterol) cardiovascular complications such as myocardial ischemia[346] and pulmonary edema have been reported. Pulmonary edema, in association with β_2-sympathomimetic treatment of premature labor, has been described on 73 occasions and caused 7 deaths.[132] Additional factors that have been incriminated include undiagnosed heart disease, fluid overload, corticosteroid therapy, myocardial depression secondary to general anesthesia, and intravenous ergometrine.

β_2-sympathomimetic agents also produce metabolic changes, including hyperglycemia, hypokalemia, hypocalcemia, and metabolic acidosis secondary to lactate accumulation.[66] These changes are secondary to beta-receptor stimulation of gluconeogenesis and glycogenolysis.

In view of the potentially serious complications of tocolytic therapy, patients require close observation and monitoring in a unit in which resuscitation facilitates exist. Cardiac disease must be excluded and fluid balance, serum glucose, and potassium monitored frequently. It is not entirely clear what the implications are of tocolytic therapy to neural blockade. Epidural blockade may be beneficial in the presence of fluid overload and by reducing endogenous catecholamine release in premature labor.[207] On the other hand, caution must be exercised to avoid further sudden changes in heart rate or peripheral resistance.

TECHNIQUES OF NEURAL BLOCKADE

The blockade techniques commonly used are conveniently divided into two groups: central and peripheral (Fig. 18-9). Descriptions of the applied anatomy and methods for the central techniques are found elsewhere (see Chaps. 7–9). The following peripheral techniques are frequently used in obstetric surgery: local infiltration, pudendal block,, paracervical block.

LOCAL INFILTRATION

Local infiltration is frequently used during a delivery that requires an episiotomy. Subcutaneous infiltration is carried out along the episiotomy incision, followed by deposition of the local anesthetic solution in the ischiorectal fossa in a fan-shaped pattern. Dilute solutions, such as 0.5% lidocaine or 1% chloroprocaine, are usually adequate for infiltration and should be used with epinephrine (1 : 200,000).

After pudendal block, the genitofemoral and ilioinguinal nerves that supply the anterior one third of the labia majora are not blocked. Local bilateral subcutaneous infiltration in this area provides adequate analgesia (see Fig. 18-2). One of the disadvantages of extensive local infiltration is that large volumes of local anesthetic may be necessary. Even infiltration of the perineum with lidocaine prior to episiotomy results in significant transplacental transfer, despite modest doses and a short injection-to-delivery time.[268] The F/M ratio can also be rela-

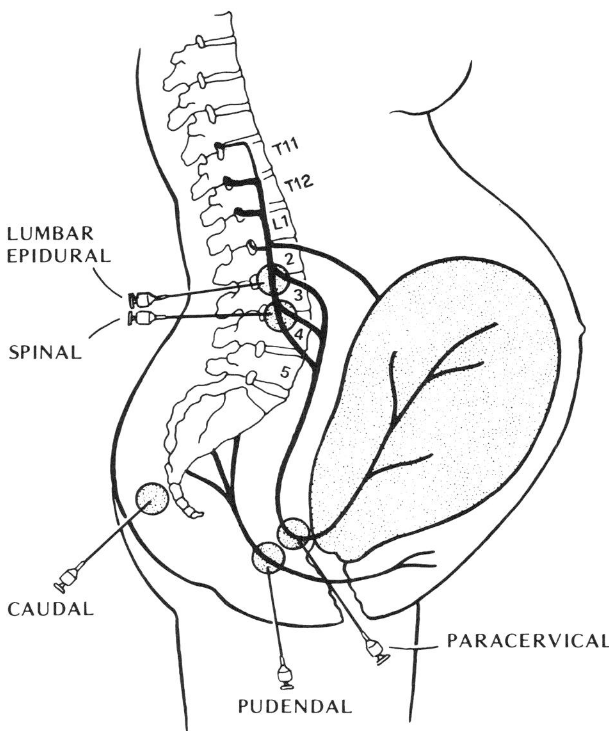

FIG. 18-9. Types of regional blocks that may be used to provide analgesia during obstetric and gynecologic surgery.

tively high (*i.e.*, >1.0) following perineal infiltration and is correlated with the duration of the second stage of labor. This may represent a further example of enhanced local anesthetic transfer in the presence of fetal acidosis (see under *Amide-Linked Agents* earlier in this chapter).

Infiltration analgesia has also been used for cesarean section, but, because large volumes of local anesthetic are required, toxicity is a potential risk. Bonica has described a technique involving separate injections of subcutaneous, intrarectus, parietal peritoneal, visceral peritoneal, and paracervical tissues[28]; however, spinal and epidural block have rendered infiltration methods obsolete except in emergency situations when an anesthesiologist is not immediately available.

PUDENDAL BLOCK

Pudendal nerve block provides analgesia of the lower part of the vagina and perineum to allow an outlet forceps delivery and episiotomy (see Fig. 18-2). Two basic techniques are used in pudendal block: transvaginal and transperineal. The transvaginal technique has a higher success rate, probably owing to its simplicity.[178] In addition, it is less painful for the patient and produces a low incidence of complications. The transperineal pudendal block is now used infrequently and only when the fetal head is fully descended onto the perineum.

TRANSVAGINAL PUDENDAL BLOCK

With the patient in the lithotomy position the ischial spine is palpated vaginally (see Fig. 18-10*a*). A 12- to 14-cm, 20 French gauge needle attached to a 10-ml Luer-Lok syringe filled with local anesthetic solution is guided to the ischial spine through the vaginal wall by the index and middle fingers. The needle is preferably introduced through a needle guide (Iowa Trumpet or Kobak instrument), which limits the penetration of the needle. When the needle is in the sacrospinous ligament, compression of the syringe with local anesthetic solution meets with considerable resistance. As the needle tip passes through the ligament, loss of resistance is felt, and the area should then be infiltrated with local anesthetic solution. This procedure is then repeated on the other side.

TRANSPERINEAL PUDENDAL BLOCK

The transperineal pudendal block requires a skin wheal about 2 to 3 cm posteromedial to the ischial tuberosity. The pudendal needle attached to the syringe as described above is guided to the ischial spine with the index finger usually placed in the vagina, or in the rectum if the fetal head has fully descended to the perineum.

Lidocaine (1%) with epinephrine (1:200,000) is the agent most commonly used for pudendal block. A total volume of 20 to 25 ml should be sufficient to produce the desired block, which usually lasts for 90 to 120 minutes. Chloroprocaine (1.5–2%) can also be used but provides analgesia for only 60 to 90 minutes. Pudendal block produces analgesia in the posterior two thirds of the labia and part of the buttock (see Fig. 18-10*b*). Analgesia of the anterior one third of the labia requires local infiltration as described above. During the deposition of local anesthetic in both approaches, it is mandatory that intravascular injection does not occur; this is assured by frequent aspirations of the syringe.

The success rate of pudendal block is undoubtedly

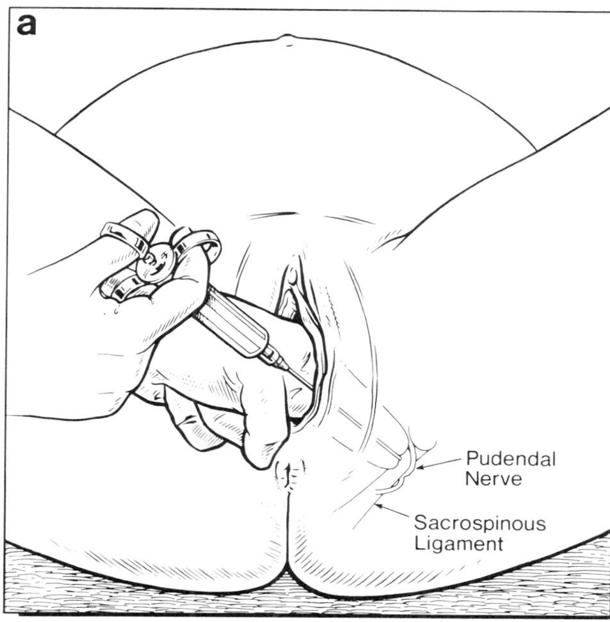

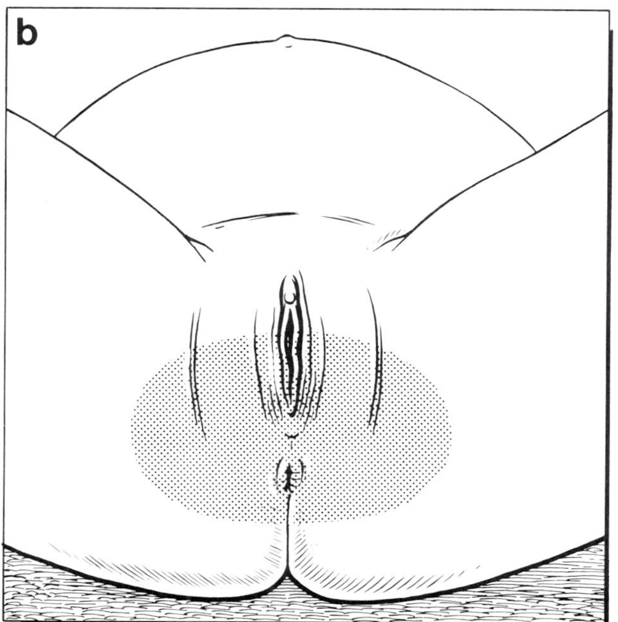

FIG. 18-10. Pudendal block by the transvaginal approach.

related to the experience of the clinician administering it. One study reported a bilateral success rate of 50% with transvaginal blocks and only 25% with transperineal blocks when they were performed by obstetric trainees.[302] Even when successful, the quality of analgesia is limited. In patients undergoing a midcavity or rotational forceps delivery, low subarachnoid or caudal analgesia is far more efficient.[155] Pudendal block should, moreover, be performed only by clinicians who are aware of the symptoms, signs, and treatment of local anesthetic toxicity (see Chap. 4).

PARACERVICAL BLOCK

First described by Gellert in Germany in 1926, paracervical block has been more popular in North America, Scandinavia, and continental Europe than in the United Kingdom.[226] Differing enthusiasm for the technique originally reflected differences in obstetric management. In those countries where paracervical block is popular, the obstetrician is directly involved with management during labor, whereas in the United Kingdom, uncomplicated labor (including analgesia) has traditionally been managed by a midwife.

The technique of paracervical block is relatively simple. To avoid intravascular injection, a 12- to 14-cm French gauge needle is used with a guide (*e.g.*, Iowa Trumpet), so that the needle point can protrude only 5 to 7 mm.[27] The guide, with the needle tip protected, is directed into the lateral fornices between 3 and 4 o'clock, and between 8 and 9 o'clock, by the index and middle fingers, so that the tip of the guide does not depress the vaginal mucosa excessively. An alternative technique uses a short beveled needle with the guide omitted (Fig. 18-11).

Paracervical block provides effective analgesia for the first stage of labor; this is, however, of limited duration (40–90 minutes), and repeated blocks are needed during a long labor. The quality of pain relief is also less reliable than with epidural analgesia. The use of *continuous* paracervical block has not gained acceptance because it is difficult to maintain the tip of the catheter in the correct position. In addition, several cases of paracervical hematoma have been described that developed into a neuropathy of the sacral plexus.[116]

The principal disadvantage of paracervical block is an associated high incidence of fetal arrythmias (particularly bradycardia) that occur within 10 minutes of injection in 5% to 70% of cases and are sometimes accompanied by fetal acidosis and neonatal depression.[16,305] Unexpected fetal death has been reported after paracervical block using mepivacaine and bupivacaine.[244,289] The etiology of the fetal depression is

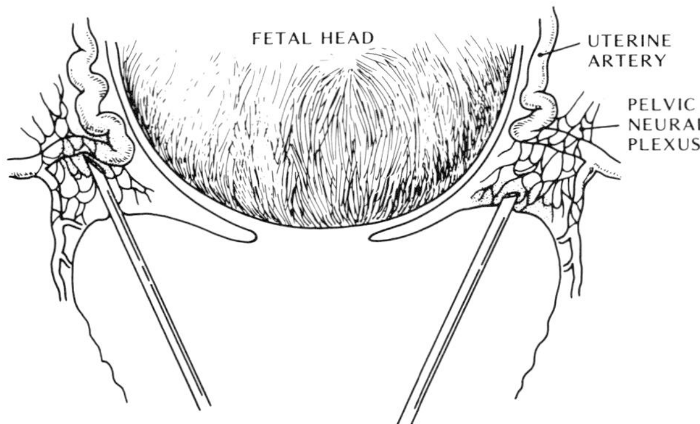

FIG. 18-11. Neurovascular anatomy associated with a paracervical block in obstetrics. The needle in the right fornix is short beveled and shows distribution of the local anesthetic. (Bloom, S.L., *et al.*: Effects of paracervical blocks on the fetus during labor. A prospective study with the use of direct fetal monitoring. Am. J. Obstet. Gynecol., *114*:218, 1972.)

not entirely clear, but three different hypotheses have been proposed:

1. Direct depression of the fetal circulation by local anesthetics has been suggested.[8,16,316] Certainly, absorption from the paracervical area is rapid, with peak maternal and fetal blood levels occurring within 10 minutes,[262] the time at which fetal heart rate (FHR) changes begin to appear; however, bradycardia has occurred even when fetal drug concentrations are low.[193] Freeman and coworkers[114] injected large doses of mepivacaine directly into anencephalic fetuses and found that although myocardial conduction depression invariably ensued, fetal bradycardia occurred only as a preterminal event. The poor correlation that exists between observed FHR changes and fetal local anesthetic concentration therefore makes a direct myocardial mechanism unlikely.
2. Paracervical block may cause uterine arterial vasoconstriction, which in turn leads to decreased placental perfusion, fetal hypoxia, and bradycardia.[62,123] Bradycardia occurs most frequently with bupivacaine and least with chloroprocaine, thereby correlating with the effect of these drugs on uterine arteries. Local anesthetics appear to exert *in vitro* a dose-related *vasoconstrictive* effect on the uterine artery at blood concentrations that occur clinically following paracervical block.[117,123]
3. Fetal hypoxia after paracervical block also may be secondary to an increase in uterine tone[115,241,332] that results from high levels of local anesthetics, although this concept has not been universally accepted.[62,222]
4. Other factors that may be contributory include mechanical distortion of uterine vessels, aortocaval compression, and the addition of epinephrine. The incidence of FHR changes is not significantly altered, however, when epinephrine is added to the local anesthetic.[305,316]

Whatever the mechanism of fetal bradycardia following paracervical block, the incidence appears to be much less following 2-chlorprocaine than with the amide-linked agents.[113,307,317,339] This may be related to the rapid hydrolysis of 2-chloroprocaine by plasma cholinesterase. Only trace levels of 2-chloroprocaine and its principal metabolite (2-chloroaminobenzoic acid) have been detected in the newborn following paracervical block.[267] 2-Chloroprocaine has, however, a short duration of action, and several injections may be required during labor.[267] It is also not available in many countries. Lidocaine 1% is probably the most useful agent for this block.

Paracervical block should in any event be avoided in the presence of prematurity, uteroplacental insufficiency, or fetal distress because the incidence of abnormal FHR changes is significantly higher in the presence of preexisting FHR abnormalities.[183] It is difficult to avoid the conclusion that paracervical block has a very limited role, if any, in modern obstetric practice except when epidural analgesia is either not feasible or unavailable. If it is used, continuous FHR monitoring is mandatory.

LUMBAR EPIDURAL BLOCKADE

ANALGESIA FOR VAGINAL DELIVERY

There is little doubt that the most successful application of epidural analgesia has been during labor. The quality of analgesia is far superior to that which can be achieved by either parenteral or inhalation approaches, and, unlike these methods, the mother remains alert.[283] Epidural analgesia also prevents, or greatly diminishes, most of the physiologic responses to labor pain that have been described earlier in this chapter (see Fig. 18-6). There are considerable benefits, therefore, to both mother and child. Unlike the neural blockade techniques discussed thus far, epidural analgesia usually can be extended to relieve both uterine pain (*i.e.,* T10–T12) and pain related to distension of the lower birth canal (*i.e.*, S2–S4) (see Fig. 18-9), as well as providing analgesia for episiotomy and forceps delivery. A further advantage is the ability to provide continuous pain relief by way of an epidural catheter. Repeat doses can be given as and when required without necessitating further needle injections.

TECHNICAL CONSIDERATIONS

Technical considerations of epidural analgesia are discussed fully in Chapter 8 and in standard obstetric textbooks. Certain difficulties must be appreciated in relation to obstetric practice: The sitting position may be uncomfortable in strong labor; spinal flexion is more difficult to achieve; the patient may be restless; and epidural space pressure is positive during uterine contractions. Meticulous technique is therefore essential if complications such as dural puncture are to be avoided.

DOSE REQUIREMENTS AND SPREAD

Epidural dose requirements are generally accepted to be less during pregnancy,[39] although this has been disputed.[125] An exaggerated spread of local anesthetic may at term be caused by distension of the epidural venous plexus either from vena caval occlusion or secondary to uterine contractions (see Fig. 18-4). Fagraeus and associates[103] have observed facilitated spread of epidural analgesia even in early pregnancy, when mechanical factors related to the gravid uterus are unlikely to be significant. These workers have suggested that increased spread is more likely to be due to a reduction in buffer capacity secondary to respiratory alkalosis than to physical factors.[103] In addition, Datta and colleagues[86] have reported increased sensitivity of isolated nerves during pregnancy, a phenomenon that they attribute to elevated progesterone levels.

Pressure in the epidural space is increased during pregnancy, being higher in the supine than in the lateral position.[220] Epidural space pressure also rises during a uterine contraction,[38] although this effect is lessened after epidural analgesia.[220] Uterine contractions *per se*, however, have little influence on the physical spread of local anesthetic in the epidural space.[309]

Patient posture has minimal effect on the spread of epidural analgesia; similar block is obtained with the mother in the lateral, supine, or sitting position.[219,285] An exception is in the obese patient in whom cephalad spread is limited by the sitting position.[137] Because the supine position leads inevitably to aortocaval compression and sitting occasionally causes symptoms of postural hypotension, the mother should be nursed in the lateral semirecumbent position throughout labor.

MAINTENANCE AND MANAGEMENT

Because bupivacaine causes minimal motor block and is free from neurobehavioral effects, it is commonly regarded as the most suitable agent for epidural analgesia during labor. Various regimens using concentrations ranging from 0.125% to 0.5% (and even 0.0625%[189]) with or without epinephrine have been advocated. Weaker concentrations avoid undesirably dense motor blockade, but analgesia may be inadequate and its duration somewhat limited. Bupivacaine 0.125%, for example, has provided satisfactory analgesia ranging from only 30%[194,313] to 93%[26,322,331,349] of patients; variations in dosage and patient management no doubt explain these differences. The addition of epinephrine (1 : 200,000) improves the quality and duration of analgesia of the weaker concentrations of bupivacaine, but only at the expense of increased motor blockade.[194] Epidural chloroprocaine has also been used during labor, but the duration of action is brief (about 40–50 minutes following 3% chloroprocaine).[56,63] A mixture of chloroprocaine and bupivacaine does not provide any additional advantage over bupivacaine alone.[63] As a result of concern about cardiotoxicity with bupivacaine and neurotoxicity with chloroprocaine, lidocaine has regained popularity in obstetric practice. Although the latter provides a more dense motor block than bupivacaine and is less desirable for routine use, a solution of 1% with epinephrine is helpful to intensify a patchy block or to provide analgesia for a forceps delivery.

Insertion of an epidural catheter early in labor allows the flexibility of the technique to be used to full advantage by tailoring the strength of the blockade to each patient's needs. For example, in most cases 0.125% to 0.25% bupivacaine provides satisfactory analgesia during early labor, and a denser block can be provided later, if necessary, with a more concentrated solution. In the United Kingdom and Australia, top-up doses are often administered by a nurse-midwife trained in the management of epidural block (see Chap. 8) using orders written by the anesthesiologist (Fig. 18-12).

MANAGEMENT OF EPIDURAL ANALGESIA
INSTRUCTIONS

Patient's name .... Date ....

(1) Blood Pressure

B.P. should be taken every 5 mins for 20 mins after top-up

If B.P. falls below .... mmHg Systolic.

(i) turn patient on left side.

(ii) give i.v. infusion of....................

(iii) inform Dr...................

(2) Positioning

Always nurse on side. Use a wedge under the right buttock when patient is in the lithotomy position.

(3) Top-up doses.

* First dose through catheter given at ....(time) by

Dr....................... Agent ....Dose....ml.

*Anaesthetist in charge must be present for first dose through the catheter. Top-up doses may be given in the presence of a qualified midwife. The drug must be

(a) injected through the millipore filter

(b) double checked and

(c) any syringe with unlabelled contents must not be used.

DRUG (Block letters)	Strength	With or Without Adrenaline	Dose in ml	When necessary at intervals of

Signature of Anaesthetist....................

TOP-UP RECORD

TIME	DRUG	STRENGTH	DOSE GIVEN	GIVEN BY	CHECKED BY
1					
2					
3					
4					
5					
6					

Always inform the Anaesthetist if patient requires more analgesia sooner than prescribed for, or if concerned in any way.

FIG. 18-12. Epidural instruction sheet suitable for midwife management of top-up doses.

To ensure continuous analgesia and reduce the demands on medical personnel in centers in which nursing staff are not permitted to administer incremental doses, continuous epidural infusions by means of a mechanical infusion pump have been introduced.[1,102,119,288,315] Other potential advantages include low blood concentrations of local anesthetic and a reduced risk of total spinal block if the catheter becomes positioned in the subarachnoid space. Infusion pumps are not always reliable, however, and adjustments in dosage are often required in order to provide optimal analgesia.[315] It has not been established whether a continuous infusion is, in fact, more effective or safer than intermittent techniques. The same high standards of patient observation and vigilance must be observed with either regimen.

INDICATIONS

The most popular indication for epidural analgesia is the provision of pain relief. A growing number of hospitals are able to offer continuous epidural analgesia at the request of the mother. There are, in addition, certain complications of pregnancy in which epidural analgesia appears to be indicated on therapeutic grounds.

Preeclampsia and Hypertension

Preeclampsia (or pregnancy-induced hypertension) is a potentially serious complication specific to pregnancy that may arise *de novo* or may be superimposed upon an underlying hypertensive disorder. Other causes of hypertension include [a] essential hypertension; [b] renal disease, for example, glomerulonephritis; [c] cardiovascular disease, for example, polyarteritis nodosa and lupus erythematosus; and [d] adrenal disorders, for example, pheochromocytoma and primary aldosteronism. Preeclampsia is rarely manifest before 26 weeks of gestation. Classically the diagnosis is suspected when at least two of the following three conditions arise: hypertension, proteinuria, and edema. Like other hypertensive states, symptoms may be absent until an advanced stage; these include headache, vomiting, epigastric pain, photophobia, and convulsions (eclampsia).

A detailed review of the etiology, pathogenesis, management, and treatment of preeclampsia is beyond the scope of this chapter. It is important to stress, however, that there is widespread vascular dysfunction involving several organs, including the placenta. Preeclampsia is characterized by arterial vasoconstriction and subendothelial intravascular fibrin deposition, especially in the renal glomeruli and spiral arterioles of the placenta.

The increase in systemic blood pressure that occurs in preeclampsia is largely secondary to a rise in peripheral resistance, although cardiac output usually is also increased. The underlying cause of this vasoconstrictive state is unknown; although plasma catecholamine levels are significantly increased in preeclampsia,[2] other factors are likely to be more important. Despite an increase in total body water, the circulatory plasma volume can be contracted by as much as 25%.[273,312] The hematocrit and whole blood viscosity are also raised,[52,134] and these changes further contribute to the increase in peripheral resistance. Both renal and uterine blood flow are decreased, usually in proportion to the severity of the disease.[90] These changes are associated with fibrin deposition and lead to diminished glomerular filtration and intrauterine growth retardation. Liver function may also be abnormal. Plasma colloid oncotic pressure is reduced[23] and may contribute to the development of cerebral or pulmonary edema.[61] These circulatory changes are summarized in Figure 18-13.

Coagulation disorders often exist in preeclampsia, including thrombocytopenia, hypofibrinogenemia, and a prolonged plasma thrombin time.[272] In severe cases, disseminated intravascular coagulation may develop.

Preeclampsia is therefore a complicated disease and, despite a considerable improvement in prognosis over the years, remains one of the major causes of maternal death in developed countries. Cerebral hemorrhage and pulmonary edema are the most common terminal events, although eclampsia and hepatic and renal failure can still occur. The anesthesiologist should play an important role in the management of severe preeclampsia and thus must understand the pathophysiology of the disease. The anesthesiologist must also be familiar with modern obstetric management of preeclampsia because in severe cases the patient is likely to be receiving one or more of several potent drugs that may interact with anesthesia and analgesia. These include sedatives and hypnotics, anticonvulsants, hypotensive agents, diuretics, and, less commonly, heparin and corticosteroids.[197]

When vaginal delivery is planned in preeclampsia, epidural analgesia provides the best method of pain relief while having several additional advantages. Diastolic blood pressure is reduced on average by more than 20%[230] and placental perfusion is either

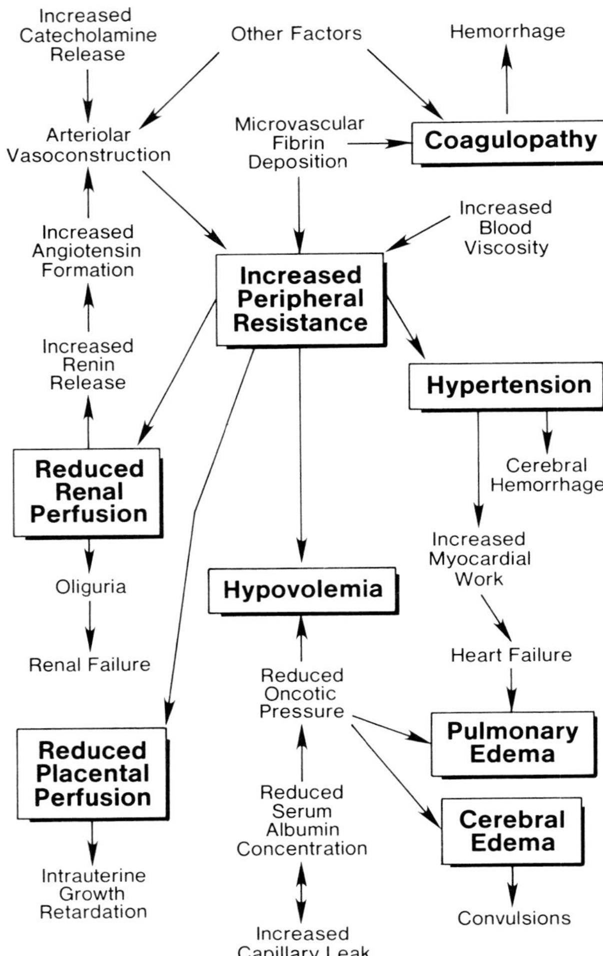

FIG. 18-13. Pathophysiologic changes in preeclampsia (pregnancy-induced hypertension).

unaltered or actually improved (provided that hypovolemia has been corrected and aortocaval compression is avoided).[164] This improvement in uterine blood flow is presumably due to sympathetic blockade. It is likely that renal perfusion is similarly improved, although this has not been confirmed.[159] Other physiologic changes that occur during labor and that are largely secondary to pain or "stress" are also obtunded by epidural analgesia (see Fig. 18-6). Epidural analgesia lowers maternal plasma catecholamine concentrations (which are known to be elevated in preeclampsia) and prevents sudden fluctuations in blood pressure.[2]

Epidural analgesia allows an elective, controlled instrumental delivery to be performed under ideal conditions with perineal relaxation and minimal fetal trauma. There is also less need for maternal sedatives and opioids when epidural analgesia is used. Nevertheless epidural analgesia must not be used in the presence of hypovolemia or significant coagulopathy. Blood volume expansion should precede or accompany the onset of autonomic blockade.

The choice of anesthesia for cesarean section in the presence of hypertension depends on several factors. Epidural analgesia can provide greater stability of systemic and pulmonary artery pressure than can general anesthesia, in which sudden swings in arterial pressure have been recorded, particularly at intubation.[138] Postoperative epidural opioid or local anesthetic analgesia can also contribute to the management of blood pressure following surgery.

Breech Presentation

Formerly regarded as being contraindicated in breech presentations, several studies now have shown that epidural anesthesia is associated with superior conditions for delivery and improved neonatal outcome. Initial fears that it would contribute to morbidity by increasing the breech extraction rate have not been substantiated. Retrospective studies of vaginal breech deliveries comparing epidural analgesia with "conventional" analgesia have found a small prolongation of labor but no increase in the incidence of operative intervention; neonatal condition was actually better in deliveries in which epidural analgesia was used.[33,73,84,92] A prospective study concluded that epidural analgesia did not prolong labor, that breech extraction was reduced, and that the acid–base status of the fetus was better than when labor was conducted with other methods of analgesia.[36] There are several possible explanations for these favorable results. Since the mother is comfortable and cooperative, the progress of labor can be determined by thorough vaginal examinations; the otherwise common urge to push before full dilatation is obtunded; and good perineal relaxation provides optimal conditions for controlled delivery of the fetal head. For these reasons, epidural analgesia can be recommended whenever a vaginal breech delivery is proposed.

Multiple Pregnancy

Until recently, multiple pregnancy was regarded as a contraindication to epidural analgesia on the grounds that a delay in the second stage of labor would lead to more frequent intervention and result in a contracted uterus that would jeopardize the second twin. Mortality and morbidity are greater among second twins and reflect contraction and even separation of the placental bed following delivery of the first infant. Multiple pregnancy is also commonly associated with premature labor and preeclampsia, which contribute further to a higher perinatal mortality. Obstetric intervention may be urgently required to expedite delivery of the second twin.

In the past few years, epidural analgesia for multiple births has been regarded favorably.[74,127,157,161,337] Although most of these studies reported a longer second stage of labor and increased operative intervention compared with other methods of analgesia, neonatal outcome was similar. Moreover, the facility with which obstetric intervention could be performed, without resorting to the induction of urgent general anesthesia, was favorably noted in all these studies. Locked twins have been successfully disimpacted under lumbar epidural blockade.[175]

Incoordinate Uterine Action

Failure to progress during labor in the absence of disproportion is commonly associated with incoordinate uterine activity. Labor is accordingly prolonged, painful, and exhausting for the mother, and the physiologic changes associated with painful labor (see Fig. 18-6) are accentuated with time. Uterine action invariably improves after epidural analgesia and frequently allows labor to progress normally.[201,232]

Maternal Medical Complications

Epidural analgesia is generally recommended for labor in the presence of heart disease and may be a useful adjunct in the prevention of heart failure. Abolition of the physiologic responses to pain (see Fig. 18-6) is beneficial in patients with diminished cardiac reserve. Active bearing-down at delivery represents an additional workload on the heart, and it is not surprising that most maternal deaths caused by heart disease occur at this time. For these reasons, an elective instrumental delivery under epidural analgesia is often preferred. Epidural anesthesia may not be theoretically indicated in patients with aortic stenosis or in those with a right-to-left shunt. Despite theoretical objections, epidural analgesia has been used safely in the presence of Eisenmenger's syndrome.[81]

Epidural analgesia is beneficial in patients with a history of chronic respiratory disease, intracranial surgery, or cerebrovascular accident. Diabetes mellitus is also a relative indication.[226]

Pregnancy superimposed upon severe medical disease, including pregnancy-induced hypertension, can be hazardous and even life-threatening. Such patients should be managed in an environment in which intensive care facilities are accessible. Invasive monitoring may be indicated in order to maintain cardiovascular stability both during delivery and for several hours after.

Fetal Abnormality and Intrauterine Death

It is only reasonable and humane to reduce pain as efficiently as possible in grief-stricken patients. Accordingly, epidural analgesia should be available, although caution is required in patients with coagulopathy.

CONTRAINDICATIONS

With the passage of time, many earlier fears about the safety of epidural analgesia and its influence on the progress of labor have been dispelled. Crawford has proposed that there remain only three absolute contraindications:[75] patient refusal, the presence of a severe coagulation defect, and local or generalized infection. Whether the latter should be an absolute contraindication is controversial. Other relative contraindications are discussed in Chapter 8.

In the past it was feared that by abolishing pain, epidural analgesia might conceal the presence of intra-abdominal hemorrhage or other serious complications, thereby delaying treatment. It is now appreciated that these fears are not well founded and that placental abruption[256] and uterine rupture[328] are still readily recognized under epidural blockade.[75] A trial of labor in the presence of a uterine scar is not, therefore, a contraindication to epidural analgesia; indeed it has even been recommended.[214]

FAILURE OF ANALGESIA

Satisfactory epidural analgesia occurs in 85% to 95% of patients in labor.[26,46,70,71,94,140,145,226,235,276] Ideally, in order to provide pain relief from uterine contractions, local anesthetics should be injected as close as possible to the spinal nerve roots T10–T12 in the posterior midline position of the epidural space. An epidural catheter, although convenient, may on occasion be inserted into a non-midline epidural position or even pass through an intervertebral foramen into the paravertebral space.[329] Analgesia is then likely to be unilateral or incomplete. In this event, which can occur in almost 20% of patients,[46,60,94,140] some readjustment is usually all that is required to achieve satisfactory analgesia. These adjustments include turning the patient to the opposite side and giving a further dose, and partial withdrawal of the catheter or, in the case of persistent unilateral block, reinsertion.

Inadequate perineal analgesia for delivery is a more frequent nuisance, although it usually can be avoided by administering a larger dose of local anesthetic when delivery is imminent.[46,140,142] Some authorities have recommended giving a top-up dose in a sitting position before delivery,[39,94] although this practice has not been validated. Other centers do not aim to achieve perineal analgesia, preferring to supplement with local anesthetic infiltration, a pudendal block, or a caudal block, if required.[170]

EFFECT ON THE COURSE OF LABOR

It is now generally accepted that epidural analgesia does not prolong, and may even shorten, the duration of the first stage of labor.[71,232,266] A transitory decrease in uterine activity has been described,[275,340] but this is of little clinical importance. It is not clear whether the addition of epinephrine has any significant effect on uterine contractions.

The influence of epidural analgesia on the duration of the second stage of labor and on the need for an instrumental delivery remains controversial. Almost all of the case series cited in *Neural Blockade* have demonstrated an increased incidence of forceps delivery or vacuum extraction. This association is, however, complicated by several factors: [a] Epidural analgesia is most commonly used among patients in whom spontaneous delivery is less likely to occur in any case (*e.g.*, fetal malposition, trial of labor; [b] the decision to intervene is determined solely by the attending obstetrician, and there is considerable individual variation in this respect (*e.g.*, in one unit the forceps rate among obstetricians ranged between 10% and 70%[95]; [c] there is still controversy as to when the second stage should be considered to have begun and as to whether a time limit should be set before intervention is indicated. Obviously, all these factors considerably influence the instrumental delivery rate. Despite these difficulties, a *prospective* trial has still shown a fivefold increase in forceps delivery and a threefold increase in malposition among mothers who received epidural analgesia using bupivacaine 0.5%.[149] Although a low cavity forceps delivery is generally regarded as being innocuous to the fetus, a midforceps rotational delivery has been associated with intracranial hemorrhage.[251]

Epidural analgesia may contribute directly to the higher incidence of intervention at delivery if perineal sensation has been abolished and if there has been sufficient loss of pelvic floor muscle tone to interfere with normal rotation of the fetal head. In an attempt to improve the rate of normal delivery, several centers use weaker concentrations of epidural local anesthetics, or a limited "segmental block" for the first stage of labor only.[26,93,145,169,200,212] This practice does increase the likelihood of a spontaneous delivery, but delivery is more likely to be painful. Many patients may, however, prefer to "trade off" some degree of pain for a normal delivery. The final arbiter should be the mother herself.

In conclusion, epidural analgesia does influence management at delivery, and readjustments in policy are often required when the technique is newly introduced. The mother should not be encouraged to push too early, and a longer second stage should be tolerated than in patients without regional blockade. Active intervention is indicated only if signs of fetal distress appear. Such policies have been shown to reduce the instrumental delivery rate considerably.[18,206]

EFFECTS ON FETAL HEART RATE

The reported frequency of FHR abnormalities after epidural analgesia has varied widely. The relatively high incidence documented in early studies was probably related to inadequate intravenous therapy or to aortocaval compression. For example, late decelerations increased fivefold in the supine position[152] or when hypotension occurred.[299] When these factors were avoided, FHR changes related to epidural analgesia were minimal.[165,182,275,349] Abnormalities of FHR are more common during oxytocin infusion,[299] most likely reflecting decreased placental perfusion secondary to uterine contractions.

OTHER EFFECTS

Epidural analgesia prevents, or reverses, most of the pain-mediated physiologic changes summarized in Figure 18-6. In addition, in some circumstances, uterine contractions can become more efficient and placental perfusion improved. These aspects of epidural analgesia can be regarded only as beneficial to the fetus and the neonate. Epidural analgesia also appears to lower the incidence and severity of retinal hemorrhages in the newborn,[203,204] possibly by reducing pelvic floor muscle tone and pressure on the fetal head. It is not known whether *intracranial* hemorrhage is similarly reduced by epidural analgesia.

SIDE-EFFECTS AND COMPLICATIONS

Epidural analgesia is inevitably associated with side-effects. Although minor, these can be a source of frustration and disappointment to the mother. For example, walking is not usually feasible, and the lower limbs may become totally immobile. Awareness of uterine contractions and of a full bladder may be lost and the urge to bear down at delivery abolished altogether. The mother is therefore confined to bed and is more likely to require catheterization, episiotomy, and an instrumental delivery. Although a forceps delivery is generally regarded as atraumatic in experienced hands, it can nevertheless be disappointing for the mother who has anticipated a spontaneous delivery.[239]

Some of the above side-effects can be reduced by using weaker concentrations of local anesthetics, administering them either intermittently or by an infusion device. The mother should be informed about these side-effects and be party to decisions regarding the strength of her neural blockade.

Postural hypotension occasionally results when the mother with an epidural block sits upright, and shivering occurs in up to 50% of mothers.[334] The latter symptom can be reduced by warming both epidural local anesthetics and intravenous fluids to body temperature[215] or by giving epidural meperidine, 25 mg.[49a]

Nonobstetric complications of epidural analgesia (*e.g.*, dural puncture, total spinal, massive epidural, bladder dysfunction, backache, neurologic damage, and epidural hematoma or abscess) are discussed fully in Chapters 7 and 8.

Accidental dural puncture is particularly bothersome in obstetric patients because the incidence of headache is high and, when severe, can be incapacitating.[48,72] An epidural infusion or intermittent bolus injections of saline are the most valuable prophylactic measures in the first 24 hours.[72,311] Failing this, a therapeutic blood patch has proved to be extremely effective[48,72,77,252] provided there is an interval of at least 24 hours[195] and blood is injected directly, rather than by way of an epidural catheter.[252]

Prospective studies have shown that the incidence of backache and bladder dysfunction after epidural analgesia is no different from that which occurs after a pudendal block.[170,229] Neurologic complications also have been extremely rare and invariably attributable to peripheral nerve lesions following instrumental delivery, rather than to epidural analgesia *per se*.[140] A neurologic consultation should nevertheless be sought if paresthesias or prolonged anesthesia occurs in the puerperium.

More serious complications, such as toxicity, total spinal, and unexpected "high epidural" blockade (see Chap. 8), have been reported but are relatively rare in obstetrics. Some are avoidable, and most are readily treatable with high standards of care and supervision. Nevertheless, their occurrence emphasizes the importance of having skilled staff in the labor ward and a physician experienced in resuscitation in close proximity.

ANESTHESIA FOR CESAREAN SECTION

In recent years the incidence of cesarean section has increased steadily, and in many major centers approaches 25% of all deliveries. Regional anesthesia has become increasingly popular during the past decade and is now often preferred to general anesthesia in many centers. The risk of aspiration is lessened and intraoperative blood loss is lower.[225] Early maternal–infant contact is thought by some to encourage the development of strong emotional attachment between the mother and her baby. Early suckling also is important in establishing successful breast-feeding,[293] and this is more likely to occur after epidural cesarean section under regional anesthesia.[50,238]

The advantages of epidural, compared with general, anesthesia extend into the postoperative period: There is less pain, a lower incidence of depression, cough, and pyrexia,[238] and mobility and appetite return more quickly.[50,238] Epidural analgesia can also be maintained in the postoperative period, providing high-quality pain relief without sedation. It is hardly surprising therefore that epidural or spinal anesthesia has become so popular among mothers for this operation.

Cesarean section under epidural block does, however, present certain difficulties for the anesthesiologist. Because premedication is generally avoided, mothers are usually very apprehensive. In addition, if neural blockade should subsequently prove to be inadequate or if unpleasant symptoms such as nausea, vomiting, drowsiness, syncope, dyspnea, or referred retrosternal pain should develop, the patient may become very distressed. Preoperatively the anesthesiologist should establish a good rapport with the patient, and intraoperatively must be prepared to give psychological support and to treat unpleasant symptoms promptly. The confidence of the prospective parents can be enhanced by viewing a film or video of a cesarean section and by meeting other couples who have undergone the operation.

The most commonly used agents are lidocaine (2%), bupivacaine (0.5–0.75%), etidocaine (1.0–1.5%), and chloroprocaine (3%). No clear advantage of one over the other has been demonstrated, and the choice largely seems to depend on regional preference. Chloroprocaine and etidocaine may have a slightly more rapid onset that bupivacaine[99,160,344]; this is a relatively minor advantage but accounts for the higher incidence of hypotension reported with chloroprocaine. The dose requirements are higher for cesarean section than for labor, and it is usually preferable to add epinephrine (1 : 200,000) to reduce systemic absorption (see Chap. 8).

Whichever agent is chosen, neural blockade to T4 provides the best surgical conditions.[69] As is the case with other abdominal surgery, the endocrine stress response is less when cesarean section is performed under epidural than under general anesthesia. Thus maternal (but not fetal) catecholamine release is suppressed,[156] and plasma concentrations of ACTH and cortisol are lower.[191,245] Although many factors influence neonatal outcome, under ideal circumstances there is little difference in acid–base status, Apgar score, time to sustained respiration, or ventilatory pattern after general or regional anesthesia.[21,97,111,112,144,158,255] In the event of a prolonged uterine incision-delivery interval (*e.g.*, greater than 90 seconds), however, neonatal acid–base status deteriorates under general, but not under epidural, anesthesia.[80] Infants presenting by the breech are also in a better clinical condition when delivered under epidural rather than general anesthesia.[80] This beneficial effect of epidural anesthesia may similarly apply in the presence of prematurity, where delay may be experienced in extracting the infant through a poorly formed lower uterine segment. As noted previously, neurobehavioral responses do not appear to be affected after epidural anesthesia with either lidocaine or bupivacaine.[177]

It is vitally important in cesarean section management to ensure cardiovascular stability and immediately correct any hypotension that may develop. Hypotension must be prevented by tilting the patient or mechanically displacing the uterus laterally and by administering an intravenous fluid load of at least 1 and preferably 2 liters of crystalloid before the onset of neural blockade.[188,341] A combination of crystalloid and colloid has also been advocated.[130,280] Dextrose infusions should be avoided, however, since they induce maternal and fetal hyperglycemia, and subsequently neonatal hypoglycemia after delivery.[126,174]

Despite the above measures, hypotension still is not uncommon. Prophylactic intramuscular ephedrine (25–50 mg) has been advocated,[128] but Rolbin and colleagues demonstrated that it was ineffective and that two thirds of patients developed prolonged periods of hypertension after delivery.[284] Ephedrine nevertheless remains the current drug of choice in the treatment of hypotension. Incremental intravenous doses of 5 to 15 mg are usually effective.[85]

Oxygen supplementation during cesarean section improves fetal oxygenation and acid–base status[279] and should be applied routinely. Patient discomfort during surgery may be caused by inadequate neural blockade or visceral stimulation. Suggested remedies include nitrous oxide inhalation,[321] small doses of intravenous ketamine, parenteral or epidural opioids, and sedatives. Sedatives are best avoided, however, because they can cause confusion and amnesia[237] and patient cooperation may be lost. Anesthetic management of cesarean section under regional anesthesia is summarized in Table 18-2.

CAUDAL EPIDURAL ANALGESIA

The caudal approach to the epidural space has become less popular in obstetrics during the past decade. Earlier, several large case series were published reporting high success rates with few complications.[91,101,213,234] A cephalad spread sufficient to provide analgesia in the first stage of labor (*i.e.*, to T10) is more difficult to achieve and requires larger doses than those needed with lumbar epidural analgesia. Also, dense blockade of the sacral nerves tends to occur early in labor with the potential adverse effects discussed earlier. Toxicity is more likely to occur be-

TABLE 18-2. SUMMARY OF REGIONAL ANESTHESIA MANAGEMENT FOR CESAREAN SECTION

1. Preoperative assessment
   Ensure no contraindications to regional anesthesia (*e.g.*, bleeding tendency, hypovolemia, sepsis, or anticipated technical difficulty)
   Discuss procedure with the patient and establish rapport.
   Introduce patient to others on the ward who have recently had a regional CS.
   Whenever feasible, allow patient to choose between regional and general anesthesia
   Prescribe oral antacid preoperatively (*e.g.*, 0.3 M sodium citrate 20 ml)
   Exhort patient to avoid supine position
2. Preanaesthetic preparation
   Check anesthesia and monitoring equipment as for general anesthesia
   Prepare a separate drug tray of labeled syringes containing the following:
   - Ephedrine 30 mg in 6 ml saline
   - Thiopentone 500 mg
   - Suxamethonium 100 mg
   - Atropine 0.6 mg
   - Oxytocin 10 units

   Infuse 1 to 2 liters of dextrose-free electrolyte solution intravenously; 0.5 liters of a colloid solution may be included
3. Management after insertion of epidural or subarachnoid block
   Allow sufficient time for block to become established (T4-S4)
   Establish epidural block with small *incremental* doses
   Ensure left lateral or uterine displacement until delivery
   Monitor ECG, arterial blood pressure, and heart rate
   Provide oxygen supplementation until delivery
   Reassure the patient frequently and treat symptoms promptly
   At delivery, give oxytocin 5 units intravenously
4. Management of symptoms that may arise intraoperatively
   Nausea
   a. Check blood pressure. If hypotensive, treat with ephedrine 5 mg i.v. in increments
   b. Check heart rate. If < 70 treat with atropine 0.3-0.6 mg i.v.
   c. After delivery, treat with antiemetic drug, for example, metaclopromide 10 mg i.v. or droperidol 2.5 mg i.v.

   Pain:
   a. Before delivery, add nitrous oxide by means of face mask (50% in oxygen)
   b. After delivery, treat with i.v. or epidural opioid (*e.g.*, meperidine 25 mg) or alternative such as ketamine 0.2 mg/kg i.v. incrementally

   Shivering/restlessness:
   a. Treat with intravenous or epidural opioid (*e.g.*, meperidine 25 mg)

   Apprehension:
   b. Reassure, nitrous oxide inhalation or intravenous opioid, or both (sedative agents usually contraindicated)

   Respiratory embarrassment/convulsions/panic:
   c. Induce general anesthesia, intubate, and control ventilation

cause of the vascularity of the caudal canal and the large dose of local anesthetic usually employed.

Caudal analgesia is used as part of a two-catheter technique in some centers, although it is doubtful whether this confers great advantage. By itself caudal analgesia can be used for the provision of perineal analgesia when delivery is imminent or an instrumental delivery is planned. Under the latter conditions, many anesthesiologists would prefer to use a low subarachnoid block instead (see Chaps. 7 and 9).

SUBARACHNOID ANALGESIA

ANALGESIA FOR LABOR AND DELIVERY

Subarachnoid blockade has been popular for many years in North America and has a valuable place in obstetrics. The rapid onset, profound degree of blockade, and lack of toxicity due to the low doses required are attractive properties for certain urgent obstetric maneuvers, including operative vaginal delivery, repair of third-degree tear or cervical laceration, and removal of a retained placenta. Low subarachnoid blockade is generally preferable to caudal block or peripheral nerve blocks on these occasions, and it is certainly preferable to the induction of general anesthesia.[49,57,76,226]

All of the standard hyperbaric preparations are suitable (see Chap. 7). In patients undergoing perineal or vaginal surgery or a low instrumental delivery, a sacral (saddle) block is adequate, but for a rotational forceps delivery or placental removal the patient should be so positioned as to ensure a block to T10. It is important to correct any hypovolemia with intravenous fluids before proceeding with subarachnoid block. Hyperbaric lidocaine 25 to 30 mg of a 1.5% or 5% solution in dextrose provides ideal conditions for most obstetric procedures.

ANESTHESIA FOR CESAREAN SECTION

The choice between subarachnoid and epidural block for cesarean section appears to be determined largely by local custom and preference. There have been no prospective studies comparing the two techniques, and yet each has its merits (see Table 18-3).

A major problem with subarachnoid block is difficulty in regulating the upper limit of neural blockade; a level of T8 or less may be unsatisfactory for surgery, and spread above T4 may cause respiratory embarrassment and alarm to the patient. Further, hypotension has been described as occurring in up to 80% of patients despite intravenous fluid preload, uterine displacement, and prophylactic vasopressors.[55,65,291] Systemic hypotension can cause a reduction in perfusion pressure in the uterine vessels and a decrease

TABLE 18-3. RELATIVE MERITS OF SUBARACHNOID VERSUS EPIDURAL ANESTHESIA FOR CESAREAN SECTION

	Subarachnoid	Epidural
Speed of onset	Very rapid	Delayed
Upper limit of block	Variable, unpredictable.	Usually satisfactory to T4
Lower limit of block	Usually satisfactory to S4	Variable, sacral sparing
Density of block	Profound	Variable, agent dependent
Duration of motor block	Agent dependent: may be prolonged	Agent dependent; not usually prolonged
Systemic absorption	Negligible	Substantial; toxicity possible
Hypotension	Common, rapid onset	Variable; gradual onset
Shivering	Rare	Common
Dural puncture headache	Variable, unpredictable	Nil
Provision for postoperative analgesia	Nil	Ideal route for continuous analgesia

in placental blood flow. The degree of fetal acidosis has been associated more with the duration than the severity of hypotension, and a *brief* period of hypotension does not adversely influence Apgar or neurobehavioral scores.[85,208] More recently, it has been shown that a 1500- to 2000-ml infusion, together with early administration of ephedrine, can prevent any reduction in placental perfusion despite a moderate decrease in blood pressure.[163] Thus if precautions are taken and hypotension is treated promptly, there is little difference in neonatal outcome at cesarean section between epidural and subarachnoid anesthesia. The local anesthetic dose requirements, however, are much less with subarachnoid block, and fetal uptake accordingly is negligible.

Management of cesarean section under subarachnoid block is exactly the same as with epidural analgesia. To ensure bilateral blockade, the patient should be tilted to the opposite side after injection. Both epidural and subarachnoid techniques provide satisfactory surgical conditions on most occasions, although a small failure rate exists even in experienced hands. A deliberate combined epidural–subarachnoid approach has therefore been suggested[47,49] that aims to exploit the individual merits of each method.

To some clinicians, postdural puncture headache remains a major objection to subarachnoid block in obstetrics. The incidence has been variously estimated as being between 0 and 30%, and it is generally accepted that obstetric patients are more prone to this complication. Severe headache can be reduced to acceptably low levels by using a fine gauge needle[49,76] and, if persistent, can be readily treated with a blood patch.

SPINAL OPIOIDS IN LABOR

There have been several recent reports on the use of opioids both intrathecally and epidurally during labor. At the time of writing, these reports have included less than 1000 patients overall, and most studies have been uncontrolled. The results and conclusions have not surprisingly been conflicting, and the clinical application of spinal opioids in labor remains controversial (see also Chap. 28).

INTRATHECAL OPIOIDS

Morphine, in doses ranging from 0.5 to 2.0 mg, is the only opioid that has been used intrathecally in labor. Most studies have reported good relief from uterine contraction pain lasting for several hours, but the onset appears to be slow, that is, up to 1 hour after injection.[7,20] At delivery, analgesia is poor, and supplementary pain relief is usually required for instrumental delivery.[7,20,301] Data on the urge to bear down at delivery are incomplete, although some investigators have noted that it was strong; whether this favored spontaneous delivery is not stated.

A major drawback to the use of intrathecal morphine in labor is the high incidence of associated side-effects.[7,20,30,301] These have included pruritus (72–100%), nausea (32–100%), somnolence (43–92%), and urinary retention (12–43%). Although serious respiratory depression did not occur in the studies cited above, the respiratory rate fell to 7/min in one patient 14 hours after injection of morphine 1 mg.[7] It has been suggested that some of these side-effects can be reduced by simultaneous administration of an intravenous naloxone infusion (0.6 mg/h),[40] but this has not been confirmed. A further disadvantage of this technique is the small but still substantial risk of developing a postdural puncture headache, which makes the intrathecal approach much less appealing than the epidural route.

EPIDURAL OPIOIDS

Morphine, meperidine, and fentanyl have all been used epidurally during labor. The results of available studies are summarized below (see also Chap. 28).

Epidural Morphine

There have been nine reports of epidural morphine analgesia during labor, in which doses ranging from 2 to 10 mg were used.[31,78,88,150,154,181,199,250,345] Analgesia has generally been poor, even in the higher dose range, and in many cases was ineffective in relieving uterine contraction pain.[78,154] Like intrathecal morphine, the onset of analgesia, if any, was very slow (up to 1 hour), and supplementary analgesia was invariably needed during delivery. When controlled comparisons were made between epidural morphine and bupivacaine in the studies cited above, the local anesthetic proved to be far superior in providing pain relief.[150,345]

Side-effects such as nausea, vomiting, sedation, and pruritus frequently occur after epidural morphine; in some patients the latter is particularly severe.[181,199] Although respiratory depression has not yet been reported as a complication in labor, the published studies at the time of writing have totaled less than 200 patients. Respiratory depression has been described, however, in other clinical circumstances, and this complication is further compounded by the insidious nature of its onset. The potential for respiratory depression occurring several hours after delivery is a further major disincentive for using epidural morphine in labor.

Epidural Meperidine

Published studies to date have shown that epidural meperidine behaves quite differently from morphine. Thus the onset of analgesia is rapid (within 10 minutes) and is more consistent and reliable than with morphine.[19,131,153,264,265,310] Both the efficacy and duration of analgesia are dose dependent. Meperidine, 25 mg, provides less reliable analgesia than does 0.125% bupivacaine[131] and may have an effective duration of less than 1 hour.[264,310] Increasing the dose to 50 or 100 mg provides analgesia that is equivalent to 0.25% bupivacaine for about 2 hours.[19] Larger doses, however are associated with a higher incidence of side-effects such as nausea, sedation, and pruritus.[19]

The analgesia provided by epidural meperidine, 100 mg, is better than when the same dose is administered by either the intravenous or intramuscular route.[153] The rate of absorption of epidural meperidine into the circulation is of similar order to that which occurs after an intravenous bolus dose;[153] thus repeat doses could lead to fetal accumulation. The addition of epinephrine (1 : 200,000) does not significantly improve the duration or quality of analgesia.[310]

Despite the potential for neonatal depression after epidural meperidine, Apgar scores and neurobehavioral responses were not adversely affected in the reports cited above. The total number of patients studied has, however, been small. From the information available, meperidine seems to be a more suitable agent for epidural administration in labor than does morphine (see Table 18-4). Meperidine also appears to potentiate both the efficacy and the duration of analgesia provided by epidural bupivacaine.[19] It also abolishes shivering that is commonly associated with the latter.[49a]

Epidural Fentanyl

In doses ranging between 0.15 and 0.20 mg, epidural fentany provides effective analgesia from uterine contraction pain within 10 minutes. As with meperidine, the duration of analgesia is about 1.5 to 2.5 hours in early labor and perineal analgesia is poor.[58,347] The incidence of side-effects has varied widely and appears to be partly dose dependent.

The addition of fentanyl, 0.8 mg, to a test dose of bupivacaine provides a more rapid and complete onset of analgesia and significantly prolongs the duration of effect of the local anesthetic.[171,172,347] Such potentiation has been noted only when fentanyl is administered by the epidural rather than the intramuscular route,[172] thereby confirming that the effect is due to a spinal action of the opioid drug.

In summary, the current status and the role of epidural opioid drugs remain controversial. A tentative comparison between the opioids and bupivacaine is shown in Table 18-4.

There are clearly advantages and disadvantages

TABLE 18–4. SCHEMATIC SUMMARY OF EPIDURAL OPIOIDS VERSUS EPIDURAL LOCAL ANESTHETICS IN LABOR

	Hydrophilic Opioid (*e.g.*, morphine 5 mg)	**Lipophilic Opioid (*e.g.*, meperidine 50 mg or fentanyl 50 μg)**	**Low-Dose Local Anesthetic (*e.g.*, bupivacaine 12.5 mg)**	**High-Dose Local Anesthetic (*e.g.*, bupivacaine 50 mg)**
Analgesia				
Onset	30–60 minutes	5–10 minutes	10–20 minutes	5–10 minutes
Duration	Variable, prolonged	1–1.5 hours	1–1.5 hours	1.5–2.5 hours
Quality	Selective	Selective	Moderately selective	Nonselective
First stage of labor	Contraction awareness maintained, but analgesia may be inadequate			Contraction awareness abolished. Analgesia usually complete
At delivery	Urge to bear down retained, but perineal analgesia often inadequate for spontaneous delivery. Unsatisfactory for instrumental delivery			Urge to bear down usually abolished. Instrumental delivery frequently required but perineal analgesia usually satisfactory
Side-effects				
Motor block	Nil	Nil	Slight	Dense
Postural syncope	Nil	Nil	Slight	Not uncommon
Nausea	Common	Not uncommon	Only in presence of hypotension of aortocaval compression.	
Sedation	Not uncommon but variable in degree. Dose dependent.		Only in presence of hypotension of aortocaval compression.	
Pruritus	Common; may be severe	Less common. Not severe	Nil	Nil
Shivering	Nil	Nil	Common	Common
Safety				
Accidental i.v. injection	Innocuous	Innocuous	Systemic toxicity unlikely	Serious toxicity probable
Accidental subarachnoid injection	Severe respiratory depression. Onset may be delayed several hours	Severe respiratory depression of rapid onset probable	Serious degree of somatic blockade unlikely to develop	Life-threatening total spinal block probable

inherent in both classes of drugs administered epidurally during labor. The relative merits of opioid versus local anesthetic agent demand further investigation. A combination of *both* classes of drug in low dosage, either together or sequentially, may provide the best of both worlds in the future (see also Chap. 28).

PART II: GYNECOLOGIC PROCEDURES SUITABLE FOR NEURAL BLOCKADE

DILATATION AND CURETTAGE

Dilatation and curettage is frequently performed in the "day-surgery" setting when the indications are diagnostic or to perform therapeutic abortion. Although some believe that local anesthesia is suitable only for gestations of less than 12 weeks, others have reported use of a combined paracervical–intracervical block for mid-trimester dilatation and extraction.[342] The surgical procedure is preceded by the insertion of laminaria tents on the day before surgery to allow gradual dilatation of the cervix.

Paracervical block is a useful technique for a number of reasons. The technique is relatively easy and contributes significantly to patient safety and early recovery. In addition, only one physician need be involved, and simplified medical facilities can be used. The dangers in this practice, however, should not be underestimated; toxic reactions have led to the death of five women receiving paracervical block for termination of pregnancy in the United States.[124] Full facilities and the necessary resuscitative skills are essential requirements for any physician contemplating its use (see Chap. 4). Because the procedure is short, lidocaine 1% with epinephrine can be used up to a maximum volume of 40 ml (400 mg). Usually, a smaller dose is sufficient. Bupivacaine, 0.5%, also has been used,[342] but its longer duration is probably not necessary for such short procedures. Epinephrine contained in the local anesthetic does not appear to decrease uterine bleeding, although supplementation of the block with intravenous fentanyl in one study was associated with increased blood loss in gestations of greater than 17 weeks.[342]

MAJOR VAGINAL SURGERY

Vaginal surgery can be conveniently separated into two categories, depending upon whether or not the ovarian pedicles are to be stretched or ligated (as in vaginal hysterectomy). These structures have a sensory nerve supply from the T10 level, and therefore regional anesthesia to above that level will be necessary. Any of the centrally acting blocks (caudal or lumbar epidural, subarachnoid) is suitable, provided there are no contraindications to its use. The local anesthetic drugs commonly used for lumbar epidural anesthesia are lidocaine 1.5% to 2%, 18 to 25 ml with epinephrine 1:200,000, or bupivacaine 0.5% to 0.75%. Most major vaginal surgery does not involve the ovarian structures, and therefore caudal analgesia is frequently suitable. Smaller doses of local anesthetic drugs can be used and will provide excellent analgesia for the procedure. Once again, lidocaine 1.5% or bupivacaine 0.5% can be used, depending on the duration of the procedure. Despite adequate analgesia, many patients also require light sedation, for example, with low-dose intravenous infusion techniques as described in Chapter 6.

INTRA-ABDOMINAL PELVIC SURGERY

Many of these operations are eminently suitable for regional block. The duration of the surgical procedure plays an important part in the choice of anesthesia because some reconstructive surgery (tuboplasty), myomectomy) can be inordinately long and result in the patient's becoming restless from remaining in the same position. It is essential to ensure that the height of the block is sufficient, in these patients at least to a level of T8. Of the three blocks previously mentioned, the lumbar epidural is most frequently used, either in a single shot or continuous technique. Regional block is relatively contraindicated for extensive surgery to remove huge uterine or ovarian tumors, partly because the supine hypotensive syndrome can occur but more importantly because the degree of difficulty in excising infiltrating tumors can result in significant blood loss or patient discomfort. Pelvic lymph node dissections, although extensive procedures, frequently benefit from the use of a continuous lumbar epidural technique. The reduction in blood loss and the improved surgical access owing to a small gut make surgery smoother; however, because the length of these procedures is often beyond the tolerance of most patients, it is necessary to supplement the regional block with light general anesthesia (see below).

The types and dosages of drugs used for intra-abdominal pelvic surgery are similar to those used in major vaginal surgery in which traction on the ovarian structures is to be anticipated. The important feature in this situation is muscle relaxation, to achieve which, higher concentrations of lidocaine or bupivacaine are often used. Etidocaine 1%, which produces intense motor blockade, is sometimes useful. Even with blockade to T8, however, some patients experience pain resulting from stimulation of vagal afferents. Thus light general inhalation anesthesia, by means of a face mask, is often administered to supplement the epidural block (see Chap. 8). Equally attractive are newer techniques of low-dose intravenous infusion of narcotic or sedative agents, or both (see Chap. 6). In more extensive procedures in which light general anesthesia is administered, endotracheal intubation is desirable to avoid airway difficulties or hypoxia due to hypoventilation.

The major advantages of regional anesthesia for pelvic surgery are twofold: First, there is a reduction in blood loss with an associated decrease in the surgical time; and, second, the time of recovery from the anesthetic technique is considerably shortened when compared with general anesthesia. Also, there appears to be an earlier return of appetite and improved gut motility when epidural analgesia is continued after operation. Epidural narcotic analgesia can be used and is particularly valuable after cancer surgery. It seems likely that the incidence of deep venous thrombosis also may be reduced after regional anesthesia (see Chap. 8).

POSTPARTUM TUBAL LIGATION

If continuous lumbar or caudal epidural block has been used during labor, it is a simple procedure, postpartum, to administer additional local anesthetic to provide a suitable anesthetic level (T8) for tubal ligation. Lidocaine 1.5% or 2% with epinephrine 1 : 200,000 or chloroprocaine 3% in volumes of 15 to 20 ml is usually adequate. The incision for a postpartum tubal ligation is usually subumbilical and the procedure short. It is important to ensure that cardiovascular stability is present and hydration adequate before administering the dose of local anesthetic because a significant volume of blood frequently is lost during delivery. This is particularly important if a regional block is instituted for the first time postpartum, since the potential for hypotension is high when epidural block is induced in the presence of unrecognized blood loss (see Fig. 18-17). Spinal anesthesia using hyperbaric lidocaine, 50 to 75 mg, also provides excellent anesthesia for tubal ligation. Both epidural and spinal block may be safer than general anesthesia for surgery in the early postpartum period, as the mother is still at risk from aspiration at this time.

LAPAROSCOPY

General anesthesia is most commonly used for laparoscopy because of fears of inadequate ventilation and aspiration during the period of pneumoperitoneum. Both local and epidural anesthesia have, however, been used with success and safety. Zellavos and colleagues[350] reported a series of 1000 outpatient laparoscopic sterilizations using a technique of subumbilical infiltration of the abdominal wall with 2 ml of 1% lidocaine, following which pneumoperitoneum was achieved and each fallopian tube was sprayed by means of the operating laparoscope with 8 ml of the same solution. Penfield[263] used a somewhat more sophisticated technique on 1200 patients, injecting lidocaine directly into the tubes with a 23-gauge needle cannula inserted through the laparoscope. He also administered a paracervical block to permit tolerance of the uterine sound. Both these studies report minimal patient discomfort and an extremely low incidence of complications, none of which was major. They also recommended use of nitrous oxide rather than carbon dioxide as the insufflating gas, since the latter was associated with more patient discomfort. It is important to note that in one study the average operating time was only 8 minutes,[350] emphasizing that surgical expertise is probably an essential component of success with this technique. Diamante and colleagues[87] and Brown and co-workers[41] demonstrated the lack of clinically significant changes in ventilation and blood gases during this procedure, although 2 (of 21) patients became agitated and 2 transiently apneic after sedation in one study.[87] It is vital, therefore, that an anesthesiologist be available, along with adequate resuscitation equipment and surgical facilities, in the event that complications occur.

Epidural anesthesia using lidocaine 1.5% or chloroprocaine 3% also has been performed for laparoscopy[15,37] with only mild shoulder pain and no serious anesthetic or surgical complications. Again, blood gas values were not signigicantly changed during the procedure.[37] For both local and epidural anethesia, the authors claim fewer anesthetic complications (such as cardiac arrhythmias, aspiration, sore throat, and vomiting), reduced costs, and more rapid discharge from the hospital, compared with general anesthesia. With the vast number of outpatient laparoscopies currently being performed for tubal sterilization, and the diagnosis and treatment of infertility, local and regional anesthesia may become more generally accepted.

SUMMARY

Gynecologic surgical procedures are ideally suited for the use of neural blockade. Regional anesthesia frequently reduces the amount of blood loss in the surgical field, and analgesia provided after surgery offers a smooth transition from the operative to the postoperative period. Neurohumoral responses to surgery are reduced, and recovery may be more rapid (see Chaps. 5 and 8).

REFERENCES

1. Abboud, T.K., Afrasiabi, A., Sarkis Daftarian, F., Nagappala, S., *et al.*: Continuous infusion epidural analgesia in parturients receiving bupivacaine, chloroprocaine, or lidocaine—maternal, fetal and neonatal effects. Anesth. Analg., *62*:421, 1983.
2. Abboud, T.K., Artal, R., Sarkis, F., Henrickson, E.H., *et al.*: Sympathoadrenal activity, maternal, fetal, and neonatal responses after epidural anesthesia in the pre-eclamptic patient. Am. J. Obstet. Gynecol., *144*:915, 1982.
3. Abboud, T.K., David, S., Nagappala, S., Costandi, J., *et al.*: Maternal, fetal and neonatal effects of lidocaine with and without epinephrine for epidural anesthesia in obstetrics. Anesth. Analg., *63*:973, 1984.
4. Abboud, T.K., Khoo, S.S., Miller, F., Doan, T., *et al.*: Maternal, fetal and neonatal responses after epidural anesthesia with bupivacaine, 2-chloro-procaine, or lidocaine. Anesth. Analg., *61*:638, 1982.
5. Abboud, T.K., Kim, K.C., Noueihed, R., Kuhnert, B.R., *et al.*: Epidural bupivacaine, chloroprocaine, or lidocaine for cesarean section—maternal and neonatal effects. Anesth. Analg., *62*:914, 1983.
6. Abboud, T.K., Sarkis, F., Hung, T.T., Khoo, S.S., *et al.*: Effects of epidural anesthesia during labor on maternal plasma beta-endorphin levels. Anesthesiology, *59*:1, 1983.
7. Abboud, T.K., Shnider, S.M., Dailey, P.A., Raya, J.A., *et al.*: Intrathecal administration of hyperbaric morphine for the relief of pain in labour. Br. J. Anaesth., *56*:1351, 1984.
8. Abouleish, E.: Pain Control in Obstetrics, pp. 268, 286. Philadelphia, J.B. Lippincott, 1977.
9. Ahmad, A.J., Clark, E.H., Jacobs, H.S.: Water intoxication associated with oxytocin infusion. Postgrad Med, *51*:249, 1975.
10. Albright, G.A.: Cardiac arrest following regional anesthesia with etidocaine or bupivacaine. Anesthesiology, *51*:285, 1979.
11. Albright, G.A., Jouppila, R., Hollmen, A.I., Jouppila, P., *et al.*: Epinephrine does not alter human intervillous blood flow during epidural anesthesia. Anesthesiology, *54*: 131, 1981.
12. Amiel-Tison, C., Barrier, G., Shnider, S.M., Levinson, G., *et al.*: A new neurological and adaptive capacity scoring system for evaluating obstetric medications in full-term newborns. Anesthesiology, *56*:340, 1982.
13. Ansari, I., Wallace, G., Clementson, C.A.B., Mallikarjuneswara, V.R., *et al.*: Tilt caesarian section. J. Obstet. Gynaecol. Br. Commonw., *77*:713, 1970.
14. Arens, J.F., and Carrera, A.E.: Methemoglobin levels following peridural anesthesia with prilocaine for vaginal deliveries. Anesth. Analg., *49*:219, 1970.
15. Aribarg, A.: Epidural analgesia for laparoscopy. J. Obstet. Gynaecol. Br. Commonw., *80*:567, 1973.
16. Asling, J.H., Shnider, S.M., Margolis, A.J., Wilkinson, G.L., *et al.*: Paracervical block anesthesia in obstetrics. II: Etiology of fetal bradycardia following paracervical block anesthesia. Am. J. Obstet. Gynecol., *107*:626, 1970.
17. Assali, N.S., Brinkman, C.R., Nuwayhid, B.: Uteroplacental circulation and respiratory gas exchange. *In:* Gluck, L. (ed.) Modern Perinatal Medicine. p. 67. Chicago, Year Book Medical Publishers, 1974.
18. Bailey, P.W., and Howard, F.A.: Epidural analgesia and forceps delivery: Laying a bogey. Anaesthesia, *38*:282, 1983.
19. Baraka, A., Maktabi, M, Noueihid, R.: Epidural meperidine-bupivacaine for obstetric analgesia. Anesth. Analg., *61*:652, 1982.
20. Baraka, A., Noueihid, R., Hajj, S.: Intrathecal injection of morphine for obstetric analgesia. Anesthesiology, *54*:136, 1981.
21. Belfrage, P., Irestedt, L., Raabe, N., Arner, S.: General anesthesia or lumbar epidural block for cesarean section? Effects on the foetal heart rate. Acta. Anaesthesiol. Scand., *21*:67, 1977.
22. Belfrage, P., Raabe, N., Thalme, B., Berlin, A.: Lumbar epidural analgesia with bupivacaine in labor. Determination of drug concentration and *p*H in fetal scalp blood, and continuous fetal heart rate monitoring. Am. J. Obstet. Gynecol., *121*:360, 1975.
23. Benedetti, T.J., and Carlson, R.W.: Studies of colloid osmotic pressure in pregnancy-induced hypertension. Am. J. Obstet. Gynecol., *135*:308, 1979.
24. Bevan, D.R., Holdcroft, A., Loh L., MacGregor, W.G., *et al.*: Closing volume and pregnancy. Br. Med. J., *1*:13, 1974.
25. Bieniarz, J., Crottogini, J.J., Curuchet, E., Romero-Salinas, G., *et al.*: Aortocaval compression by the uterus in late

human pregnancy. Am. J. Obstet. Gynecol., *100*:203, 1968.
26. Bleyaert, A., Soetens, M., Vaes, L., Van Steenberge, A.L., *et al.*: Bupivacaine 0.125 percent, in obstetric analgesia: Experience in three thousand cases. Anesthesiology, *51*:435, 1979.
27. Bloom, S.L., Horswill, C.W., Curet, L.B.: Effects of paracervical blocks on the fetus during labor. A prospective study with the use of direct fetal monitoring. Am. J. Obstet. Gynecol., *114*:218, 1972.
28. Bonica, J.J.: Principles and Practice of Obstetric Analgesia and Anesthesia, pp. 473, 531. Philadelphia, FA Davis, 1967.
29. Bonica, J.J.: Peripheral mechanisms and pathways of parturition pain. Br. J. Anaesth., *51*:3S, 1979.
30. Bonnardot, J.P., Maillet, M., Colau, J.C., Millot, F., *et al.*: Maternal and fetal concentration of morphine after intrathecal administration during labour. Br. J. Anaesth., *54*:487, 1982.
31. Booker, P.D., Wilkes, R.G., Bryson, T.H.L., Beddard, J.: Obstetric pain relief using epidural morphine. Anaesthesia, *35*:377, 1980.
32. Borell, V., Fernstrom, I., Ohlson, L., Wiquist, N.: Influence of uterine contractions on the uteroplacental flow at term. Am. J. Obstet. Gynecol., *93*:44, 1965.
33. Bowen-Simpkins, P., and Fergusson, I.L.: Lumbar epidural block and the breech presentation. Br. J. Anaesth., *46*:420, 1974.
34. Brackbill, Y., Kane, J., Manniello, R.L., Abramson, D.: Obstetric meperidine usage and assessment of neonatal status. Anesthesiology, *40*:116, 1974.
35. Brazelton, T.B.: Neonatal Behavioural Assessment Scale. Clin. Dev. Med. No. 50. London, Spastics International Medical Publications, William Heinemann Medical Books, 1973.
36. Breeson, A.J., Kovacs, G.T., Pickles, B.G., Hill, J.G.: Extradural analgesia — the preferred method of analgesia for vaginal breech delivery. Br. J. Anaesth., *50*:1227, 1978.
37. Bridenbaugh, L.D., and Soderstrom, R.M.: Lumbar epidural block anesthesia for outpatient laparoscopy. J Reprod Med, *23*:85, 1979.
38. Bromage, P.R.: Continuous lumbar epidural analgesia for obstetrics. Can. Med. Assoc. J., *85*:1136, 1961.
39. Bromage, P.R.: Epidural Analgesia, pp. 141, 548. Philadelphia, W.B. Saunders, 1978.
40. Brookshire, G.L., Shnider, S.M., Abboud, T.K., Kotelko, D.M., *et al.*: Effects of naloxone on the mother and neonate after intrathecal morphine for labor analgesia. [Abstr.] Anesthesiology, *59*:A417, 1983.
41. Brown, D.R., Fishburne, J.I., Robertson, V.O., Hulka, J.V.: Ventilatory and blood gas changes during laparoscopy with local anesthesia. Am. J. Obstet. Gynecol., *124*:741, 1976.
42. Brown, W.U.: Guest discussion. *In* Hodgkinson, R., Marx, G.F., Kim, S.S., *et al.*: Neonatal neurobehavioral tests following vaginal delivery under ketamine, thiopental, and extradural anesthesia. Anesth., Analg., *56*:548, 1977.
43. Brown, W.U., Jr., Bell, G.C., Alper, M.H.: Acidosis, local anesthetics and the newborn. Obstet. Gynecol., *48*:27, 1976.
44. Brown, W.U., Bell, G.C., Lurie, A.O., Weiss, B., *et al.*: Newborn blood levels of lidocaine and mepivacaine in the first postnatal day following maternal epidural anesthesia. Anesthesiology, *42*:698, 1975.
45. Browning, A.J., Butt, W.R., Lynch, S.S., Shakespear, R.A., *et al.*: Maternal and cord plasma concentrations of beta-lipotrophin beta-endorphin and y-lipotrophin at delivery; effect of analgesia. Br. J. Obstet. Gynaecol., *90*:1152, 1983.
46. Brownridge, P.: A three-year survey of an obstetric epidural service with top-up doses administered by midwives. Anaesth. Intens. Care., *10*:298, 1982.
47. Brownridge, P.: Central neural blockade and caesarian section. Part I: Review and case series. Anaesth. Intensive Care, *7*:33, 1979.
48. Brownridge, P.: The management of headache following accidental dural puncture in obstetric patients. Anaesth. Intensive Care, *11*:4, 1983.
49. Brownridge, P.: Spinal anaesthesia revisited. An evaluation of subarachnoid block in obstetrics. Anaesth. Intensive Care, *12*:334, 1984.
49a. Brownridge, P.: Shivering related to epidural blockade in labour, and the influence of epidural pethidine. Anaesth. Intensive Care, *14*:412, 1986.
50. Brownridge, P., and Jefferson, J.: Central neural blockade and caesarian section. II: Patient assessment of the procedure. Anaesth. Intensive Care, *7*:163, 1979.
51. Buchan, P.C.: Emotional stress in childbirth and its modification by variations in obstetric management. Acta Obstet. Gynecol. Scand., *59*:319, 1980.
52. Buchan, P.C.: Pre-eclampsia — a hyperviscosity syndrome. Am. J. Obstet. Gynecol., *142*:111, 1982.
53. Buchan, P.C., Milne, M.K., Browning, M.C.K.: The effect of continuous epidural blockade on plasma 11-hydroxycortico steroid concentrations in labour. J. Obstet. Gynaecol. Br. Commonw., *80*:974, 1973.
54. Caldeyro-Barcia, R.: Effect of position changes on the intensity and frequency of uterine contractions during labor. Am. J. Obstet. Gynecol., *80*:284, 1960.
55. Caritis, S.N., Abouleish, E., Edelstone, D.I., Mueller-Heubach, E.: Fetal acid-base state following spinal or epidural anesthesia for cesarean section. Obstet. Gynecol., *56*:610, 1980.
56. Carlsson, C., Dahlgren, N., Magnusson, J., Hanson, A.: Epidural block with chloroprocaine during labour. Acta. Anaesthesiol. Scand., *24*:469, 1980.
57. Carrie, L.E.S.: Spinal anaesthesia — an alternative route. In Doughty, A. (ed.): Epidural Analgesia in Obstetrics. p. 179. London, Lloyd-Luke, 1980.
58. Carrie, L.E.S., O'Sullivan, G.M., Seegobin, R.: Epidural fentanyl in labour. Anaesthesia, *36*:965, 1981.
59. Casady, G.N., Moore, D.C., Bridenbaugh, L.D.: Post-partum hypertension after use of vasoconstrictor and oxytocic drugs. J.A.M.A., *172*:1011, 1960.
60. Caseby, N.G.: Epidural analgesia for the surgical induction of labour. Br. J. Anaesth., *46*:747, 1974.
61. Chesley, L.: Hypertensive Disorders of Pregnancy. p. 363, New York, Appleton-Century-Crofts, 1978.
62. Cibils, L.A., and Santonja-Lucas, J.J.: Clinical significance of fetal heart rate patterns during labor. III: Effect of para-

cervical block anesthesia. Am. J. Obstet. Gynecol., *130*:73, 1978.

63. Cohen, S.E., and Thurlow, A.: Comparison of a chloroprocaine-bupivacaine mixture with chloroprocaine and bupivacaine used individually for obstetric epidural analgesia. Anesthesiology, *51*:288, 1979.
64. Cole, P.V., and Nainby-Luxmoore, P.C.: Respiratory volumes in labour. Br. Med. J., *1*:1118, 1962.
65. Corke, B.C., Datta, S., Ostheimer, G.W., Weiss, J.B., *et al.*: Spinal anaesthesia for caesarean section. The influence on neonatal outcome. Anaesthesia, *37*:658, 1982.
66. Cotton, D.B., Strassner, H.T., Lipson, L.G., Goldstein, D.A.: The effects of terbutaline on acid base, serum electrolytes, and glucose homeostasis during the management of preterm labor. Am. J. Obstet, Gynecol., *141*:617, 1981.
67. Covino, B.G., and Vassallo, H.G.: Pharmacokinetic Aspects of Local Anesthetic Agents in Local Anesthetics: Mechanism of Action and Clinical Use. p. 103. New York, Grune and Stratton, 1976.
68. Craft, J.B., Jr., Epstein, B.S., Coakley, C.S.: Effect of lidocaine with epinephrine versus lidocaine (plain) on induced labor. Anesth. Analg., *51*:243, 1972.
69. Craft, J.B., Roizen, M.F., Dao, S.D., Edwards, M., *et al.*: A comparison of T4 and T7 dermatomal levels of analgesia for caesarean section using the lumbar epidural technique. Can. Anaesth. Soc. J., *29*:264, 1982.
70. Crawford, J.S.: Lumbar epidural block in labour: A clinical analysis. Br. J. Anaesth., *44*:66, 1972A.
71. Crawford, J.S.: The second thousand epidural blocks in an obstetric hospital practice. Br. J. Anaesth., *44*:1277, 1972B.
72. Crawford, J.S.: The prevention of headache consequent upon dural puncture. Br. J. Anaesth., *44*:598, 1972.
73. Crawford, J.S.: An appraisal of lumbar epidural blockade in patients with a singleton fetus presenting by the breech. J. Obstet. Gynaecol. Br. Commonw., *81*:867, 1974.
74. Crawford, J.S.: An appraisal of lumbar epidural blockade in labour in patients with multiple pregnancy. Br. J. Obstet. Gynaecol., *82*:929, 1975.
75. Crawford, J.S.: Principles and Practice of Obstetric Anaesthesia. 4th ed. Oxford, Blackwell Scientific Publications, 1978.
76. Crawford, J.S.: Experience with spinal analgesia in a British obstetric unit. Br. J. Anaesth., *51*:531, 1979.
77. Crawford, J.S.: Experiences with epidural blood patch. Anaesthesia, *35*:513, 1980.
78. Crawford, J.S.: Experiences with epidural morphine in obstetrics. Anaesthesia, *36*:207, 1981.
79. Crawford, J.S., Burton, M., Davies, P.: Anaesthesia for section: Further refinements of a technique. Br. J. Anaesth., *45*:726, 1973.
80. Crawford, J.S., and Davies, P.: Status of neonates delivered by elective caesarean section. Br. J. Anaesth., *54*:1015, 1982.
81. Crawford, J.S., Mills, W.G., Pentecost, B.L.: Pregnant patient with Eisenmenger's syndrome. Case report. Br. J. Anaesth., *43*:1091, 1971.
82. Cugell, D.W.: Pulmonary function in pregnancy; serial observations in normal women. Am. Rev. Tuberc., *67*:568, 1953.
83. Dailey, P.A., Baysinger, C.L., Levinson, G., Shnider, S.M.: Neurobehavioral testing of the newborn infant. Clinics in Perinatology, *9*:191, 1982.
84. Darby, S., Thornton, C.A., Hunter, D.J.: Extradural analgesia in labour when the breech presents. Br. J. Obstet. Gynaecol., *83*:35, 1976.
85. Datta, S., Alper, M.H., Ostheimer, G.W., Weiss, J.B.: Method of ephedrine administration and nausea and hypotension during spinal anesthesia for cesarean section. Anesthesiology, *56*:68, 1982.
86. Datta, S., Lambert, D.H., Gregus, J., Gissen, A.J., *et al.*: Differential sensitivities of mammalian nerve fibers during pregnancy. Anesth. Analg., *62*:1070, 1983.
87. Diamant, M., Benumof, J.L., Saidman, L.J., Kennedy, J., *et al.*: Laparoscopic sterilization with local anesthesia: Complications and blood-gas changes. Anesth. Analg., *56*:335, 1977.
88. Dick, W., Traub, E., Moller, R.M.: Epidural morphine in obstetric anesthesia. Obstet. Anesth. Digest., *2*:29, 1982.
89. Difazio, C.H.: Metabolism of local anaesthetics in the fetus, newborn and adult. Br. J. Anaesth., *51*:29S, 1979.
90. Dixon, H.G., Browne, J.C.M., Davey, D.A.: Choriodecidual and myometrial blood-flow, Lancet 2:369, 1963.
91. Dogu, T.S.: Continuous caudal analgesia and anesthesia for labor and vaginal delivery. A review of 4071 confinements. Obstet. Gynecol., *33*:92, 1969.
92. Donnai, P., and Nicholas, A.D.: Epidural analgesia. Fetal monitoring and the condition of the baby at birth with breech presentation. Br. J. Obstet. Gynaecol., *82*:360, 1975.
93. Doughty, A.: Selective epidural analgesia and the forceps rate. Br. J. Anaesth., *41*:1058, 1969.
94. Doughty, A.: Lumbar epidural analgesia—the pursuit of perfection. With special reference to midwife participation. Anaesthesia, *30*:741, 1975.
95. Doughty, A.: Epidural analgesia in labour: The past, the present and future. Proc. R. Soc. Med., *71*:879, 1978.
96. Downing, J.W., Coleman, A.J., Mahomedy, M.C., Jeal, D.E., Mahomedy Y.H.: Lateral table tilt for caesarian section. Anaesthesia, *29*:696, 1974.
97. Downing, J.W., Houlton, P.C., Barclay, A.: Extradural analgesia for caesarean section: A comparison with general anaesthesia. Br. J. Anaesth., *51*:367, 1979.
98. Drummond, G.B., Scott, S.E.M., Lees, M.M., Scott, D.B.: Effects of posture on limb blood flow in late pregnancy. Br. Med. J., *4*:587, 1974.
99. Dutton, D.A., Moir, D.D., Howie, H.B., Thorburn, J., Watson, R.: Choice of local anaesthetic for extradural caesarean section—comparison of 0.5% and 0.75% bupivacaine and 1.5% etidocaine. Br. J. Anaesth., *56*:1361, 1984.
100. Eckstein, K.L., and Marx, G.F.: Aortocaval compression and uterine displacement. Anesthesiology, *40*:92, 1974.
101. Epstein, H.M., and Sherline, D.M.: Single-injection caudal anesthesia in obstetrics. Obstet. Gynecol., *33*:496, 1969.
102. Evans, K.R., and Carrie, L.E.S.: Continuous epidural infusion of bupivacaine in labour. Anaesthesia, *34*:310, 1979.
103. Fagraeus, L., Urban, B.J., Bromage, P.R.: Spread of epidural analgesia in early pregnancy. Anesthesiology, *58*:184, 1983.

104. Falconer A.D., and Powles, A.B.: Plasma noradrenaline levels during labour. Anaesthesia, *37*:416, 1982.

105. Feeney, J.G.: Water intoxication and oxytocin. Br. Med. J., *285*:243, 1982.

106. Fettes, I., Fox, J., Kuzniak, S., Shime, J., *et al.*: Plasma levels of immunoreactive beta-endorphin and adrenocorticotropic hormone during labor and delivery. Obstet. Gynecol., *64*:359, 1984.

107. Finster, M., Perel, J.M., Hinsvark, O.N., *et al.*: Pharmacodynamics of 2-chloroprocaine. Fourth Eur. Congr. Anesth., *330*:189, 1974.

108. Finster, M., and Pedersen, J.: Placental transfer and fetal uptake of drugs. Br. J. Anaesth., *51*:25S, 1979.

109. Finster, M., Poppers, P.J., Sinclair, J.C., Morishima, H.O., *et al.*: Accidental intoxication of the fetus with local anesthetic drug during caudal anesthesia. Am. J. Obstet. Gynecol., *92*:922, 1965.

110. Fisher, A., and Prys-Roberts, C.: Maternal pulmonary gas exchange. Anaesthesia, *23*:350, 1968.

111. Fisher, J.T., Mortola, J.P., Smith, B., Fox, G.S., *et al.*: Neonatal pattern of breathing following cesarean section: Epidural versus general anesthesia. Anesthesiology, *59*:385, 1983.

112. Fox, G.S., Smith, J.B., Namba, U., Johnson, R.C.: Anesthesia for cesarean section: Further studies. Am. J. Obstet. Gynecol., *133*:15, 1979.

113. Freeman, D.V., and Arnold, N.I.: Paracervical block with low doses of chloroprocaine—fetal and maternal effects. J.A.M.A., *231*:56, 1975.

114. Freeman, R.K., Gutierrez, N.A., Ray, M.L., Sfovall, D., *et al.*: Fetal cardiac response to paracervical block anesthesia. Am. J. Obstet. Gynecol., *113*:583, 1972.

115. Freeman, R.K., and Schifrin, B.S.: Whither paracervical block? *In:* Advances in Fetal Monitoring and Obstetric Anesthesia. Int. Anesthesiol. Clin., *11*(2):69, 1973.

116. Gaylord, T.G., and Pearson, W.J.: Neuropathy following paracervical block in the obstetric patient. Obstet. Gynecol., *60*:521, 1982.

117. Gibbs, C.P., and Noel, S.C.: Response of arterial segments from gravid human uterus to multiple concentrations of lignocaine. Br. J. Anaesth., *49*:409, 1977.

118. Gintzler, A.R.: Endorphin-mediated increases in pain threshold during pregnancy. Science, *210*:193, 1980.

119. Glover, D.J.: Continuous epidural analgesia in the obstetric patient: A feasibility study using a mechanical infusion pump. Anaesthesia, *32*:499, 1977.

120. Goodlin, R.C.: Importance of the lateral position during labor. Obstet. Gynecol., *37*:698, 1971a.

121. Goodlin, R.C.: Aortocaval compression during cesarean section. Obstet. Gynecol., *37*:702, 1971b.

122. Greiss, F.C., and Gabble, F.L.: Effect of sympathetic nerve stimulation on the uterine vascular bed. Am. J. Obstet. Gynecol., *97*:962, 1967.

123. Greiss, F.C., Still, J.G., Anderson, S.G.: Effects of local anesthetic agent on the uterine vasculature and myometrium. Am. J. Obstet. Gynecol., *124*:889, 1976.

124. Grimes, D.A., and Cates, J.: Deaths from paracervical anesthesia used for first-trimester abortion. N. Engl. J. Med., *295*:1397, 1976.

125. Grundy, E.M., Zamora, A.M., Winnie, A.P.: Comparison of spread of epidural anesthesia in pregnant and nonpregnant women. Anesth. Analg., *57*:544, 1978.

126. Grylack, L.J., Chu, S.S., Scanlon, J.W.: Use of intravenous fluids before cesarean section: Effects on perinatal glucose, insulin and sodium homeostasis. Obstet. Gynecol., *63*:654, 1984.

127. Gullestad, S., and Sagen, N.: Epidural block in twin labour and delivery. Acta. Anaesthesiol. Scand., *21*:504, 1977

128. Gutsche, B.B.: Prophylactic ephedrine preceding spinal analgesia for cesarean section. Anesthesiology, *45*:462, 1976.

129. Hagerdal, M., Morgan, C.W., Sumner, A.E., Gutsche, B.B.: Minute ventilation and oxygen consumption during labor with epidural analgesia. Anesthesiology, *59*:425, 1983.

130. Hallworth, D., Jellicoe, J.A., Wilkes, R.G.: Hypotension during epidural anaesthesia for caesarean section: A comparison of intravenous loading with crystalloid and colloid solutions. Anaesthesia, *37*:53, 1982.

131. Hammonds, W., Bramwell, R.S., Hug, C.C., Najak, Z., *et al.*: A comparison of epidural meperidine and bupivacaine for relief of labor pain. [Abstr.] Anesth. Analg., *61*:187, 1982.

132. Hawker, F.: Pulmonary oedema associated with beta$_2$-sympathomimetic treatment of premature labour. Anaesth. Intensive Care, *12*:143, 1984.

133. Hayes, J.R., Ardill, J., Kennedy, T.L., Shanks, R.G., *et al.*: Stimulation of gastric release by catecholamines. Lancet, *1*: 1972.

134. Hobbs, J.B., Oats, J.N., Palmer, A.A., Long, P.A., *et al.*: Whole blood viscosity in pre-eclampsia. Am. J. Obstet. Gynecol., *142*:288, 1982.

135. Hodgkinson, R., Bhatt, M., Kim, S.S., Grewal, G., *et al.*: Neonatal neuro-behavior tests following cesarean section under general and spinal anesthesia. Am. J. Obstet. Gynecol., *132*:670, 1978.

136. Hodgkinson, R., Bhatt, M., Wang, C.N.: Double-blind comparison of the neuro-behaviour of neonates following the administration of different doses of meperidine to the mother. Can. Anaesth. Soc. J., *25*:405, 1978.

137. Hodgkinson, R., and Husain, F.J.: Obesity, gravity and spread of epidural anesthesia. Anesth. Analg., *60*:421, 1981.

138. Hodgkinson, R., Husain, F.J., Hayashi, R.H.: Systemic and pulmonary blood pressure during caesarean section in parturients with gestational hypertension. Can. Anaesth. Soc. J., *27*:839, 1980.

139. Hodgkinson, R., Marx, G.F., Kim, S.S., Miclat, N.M.: Neonatal neurobehavioural tests following vaginal delivery under ketamine, thiopental and extradural anesthesia. Anesth. Analg., *56*:548, 1977.

140. Holdcroft, A., and Morgan, M.: Maternal complications of obstetric epidural analgesia. Anaesth. Intensive Care, *4*:108, 1976.

141. Holdsworth, J.D.: Relationship between stomach contents and analgesia in labour. Br. J. Anaesth., *50*:1145, 1978.

142. Hollmen, A.: Regional techniques of analgesia in labour. Br. J. Anaesth., *51*:17S, 1979.

143. Hollmen, A.I., Jouppila, R., Jouppila, P., Koivula, A., *et al.*: Effect of extradural analgesia using bupivacaine and 2-chloroprocaine on intervillous blood flow during normal labour. Br. J. Anaesth., *54*:837, 1982.

144. Hollmen, A.I., Jouppila, R., Koivisto, M., Maatta, L., *et al.*: Neurologic activity of infants following anesthesia for cesarean section. Anesthesiology, *48*:350, 1978.

145. Hollmen, A., Jouppila, R., Pihlajaniemi, R., Karvonen, P., *et al.*: Selective lumbar epidural block in labour. A clinical analysis. Acta. Anaesthesiol. Scand., *21*:174, 1977.

146. Holly, R.G.: Anaemia in pregnancy. Obstet. Gynecol., *5*:562, 1955.

147. Holmes, F.: Spinal analgesia and caesarian section—maternal mortality. J. Obstet. Gynaecol. Br. Emp., *64*:229, 1957.

148. Holmes, F.: Incidence of the supine hypotensive syndrome in late pregnancy. J. Obstet. Gynaecol. Br. Emp., *67*:254, 1960.

149. Hoult, I.J., MacLennan, A.H., Carrie, L.E.S.: Lumbar epidural analgesia in labour: Relation to fetal malposition and instrumental delivery. Br. Med. J., *1*:14, 1977.

150. Hughes, S.C., Abboud, T.K., Shnider, S.M., Stefani, S.J., *et al.*: Maternal and neonatal effects of epidural morphine for labour. [Abstr.] Anesth. Analg., *61*:190, 1982.

151. Humphrey, M., Houslow, D., Morgan, S., Wood, C.: The influence of maternal posture at birth on the foetus. J. Obstet. Gynaecol. Br. Commonw., *80*:1074, 1973.

152. Huovinen, K., Kivalo, I., Teramo, K.: Factors influencing the incidence of fetal bradycardia after lumbar epidural block for vaginal labour. Abstract of the Procedures of the 5th European Congress of Perinatal Medicine. Stockholm, Almqvist and Wiksell, 1976.

153. Husemeyer, R.P., Cummings, A.J., Rosonkiewicz, J.R., Davenport, H.T.: A study of pethidine kinetics and analgesia in women in labour following intravenous, intramuscular and epidural administration. Br. J. Clin. Pharmacol., *13*:171, 1982.

154. Husemeyer, R.P., O'Connor, M.C., Davenport, H.T.: Failure of epidural morphine to relieve pain in labour. Anaesthesia, *35*:161, 1980.

155. Hutchins, C.J.: Spinal analgesia for instrumental delivery. A comparison with pudendal nerve block. Anaesthesia, *35*:376, 1980.

156. Irestedt, L., Lagercrantz, H., Hjemdahl, P., Hagnevik, K., *et al.*: Fetal and maternal plasma catecholamine levels at elective cesarean section under general or epidural anesthesia versus vaginal delivery. Am. J. Obstet. Gynecol., *142*:1004, 1982.

157. James, F.M., Crawford, J.S., Davies, P., Naiem, H.: Lumbar epidural analgesia for labor and delivery of twins. Am. J. Obstet. Gynecol., *127*:176, 1976.

158. James, F.M., III, Crawford, J.S., Hopkinson, R., Davies, P., *et al.*: A comparison of general anesthesia and lumbar epidural analgesia for elective cesarean section. Anesth. Analg., *56*:228, 1977.

159. James, F.M., III, and Davies, P.: Maternal and fetal effects of lumbar epidural analgesia for labor and delivery in patients with gestational hypertension. Am. J. Obstet. Gynecol., *126*:195, 1976.

160. James, F.M., III, Dewan, D.M., Floyd, H.M., Wheeler, A.S., *et al.*: Chloroprocaine vs. bupivacaine for lumbar epidural analgesia for elective cesarean section. Anesthesiology, *52*:488, 1980.

161. Jaschevatzky, O.E., Shalit, A., Levy, Y., Grunstein, S.: Epidural analgesia during labour in twin pregnancy. Br. J. Obstet. Gynaecol., *84*:327, 1977.

162. Johnstone, M.: The cardiovascular effects of oxytoxic drugs. Br. J. Anaesth., *44*:826, 1972.

163. Jouppila, P., Jouppila, R., Barinoff, T., Koivula, A.: Placental blood flow during caesarean section performed under subarachnoid blockade. Br. J. Anaesth., *56*:1379, 1984.

164. Jouppila, P., Jouppila, R., Hollmen, A., Koivula, A.: Lumbar epidural analgesia to improve intervillous blood flow during labor in severe pre-eclampsia. Obstet. Gynecol., *59*:158, 1982.

165. Jouppila, P., Jouppila, R., Kaar, K., Merila, M.: Fetal heart rate patterns and uterine activity after segmental epidural analgesia. Br. J. Obstet. Gynaecol., *84*:481, 1977.

166. Jouppila, R., and Hollmen, A.: The effect of segmental epidural analgesia on maternal and foetal acid-base balance, lactate, serum potassium and creatine phosphokinase during labour. Acta. Anaesthesiol. Scand., *20*:259, 1976.

167. Jouppila, R., Hollmen, A., Jouppila, P., Karki, N.: Segmental epidural analgesia and urinary excretion of catecholamines during labour. Acta Anaesthesiol. Scand., *21*:50, 1977.

168. Jouppila, R., Jouppila, P., Hollmen, A., Kuikka, J.: Effect of segmental extradural analgesia on placental blood flow during normal labour. Br. J. Anaesth., *50*:563, 1978.

169. Jouppila, R., Jouppila, P., Karimen, J.M., Hollmen, A.: Segmental epidural analgesia in labour: Related to the progress of labour, fetal malposition and instrumental delivery. Acta Obstet. Gynaecol., Scand., *58*:135, 1979.

170. Jouppila, R., Pihlajaniemi, R., Hollmen, A., Jouppila, P.: Segmental epidural analgesia and post partum sequelae. Ann. Chir., Gynaecol. Fenn., *67*:85, 1978.

171. Justins, D.M., Francis, D., Houlton, P.G., Reynolds, F.: A controlled trial of extradural fentanyl in labour. Br. J. Anaesth., *54*:409, 1982.

172. Justins, D.M., Knott, C., Luthman, J., Reynolds, F.: Epidural versus intramuscular fentanyl: Analgesia and pharmacokinetics in labour. Anaesthesia, *38*:937, 1983.

173. Kambam, J.R., Handte, R.E., Brown, W.R., Smith, B.E.: Effect of pregnancy on oxygen dissociation. [Abstr.] Anesthesiology, *59*:A395, 1983.

174. Kenepp, N.B., Kumar, S., Shelley, W.C., Stanley, C.A., *et al.*: Fetal and neonatal hazards of maternal hydration with 5% dextrose before caesarean section. Lancet, *1*:1150, 1982.

175. Kenney, A., Koh, L.S., Pole, Y.L.: A case of locked twins managed under lumbar epidural analgesia. Anaesthesia, *33*:32, 1978.

176. Kerr, M.G., Scott, D.B., Samuel, E.: Studies of the inferior vena cava in late pregnancy. Br. Med. J., *1*:532, 1964.

177. Kileff, M.E., James, F.M., III, Dewan, D.M., Floyd, H.M.: Neonatal neurobehavioral responses after epidural anesthesia for cesarean section using lidocaine and bupivacaine. Anesth. Analg., *63*:413, 1984.

178. Kobak, A.S., Evans, E.F., Johnson, G.R.: Transvaginal pudendal block. Am. J. Obstet. Gynecol., *71*:981, 1956.

179. Kuhnert, B.R., Harrison, M.J., Linn, P.L., Kuhnert, P.M.: Effects of maternal epidural anesthesia on neonatal behavior. Anesth. Analg., *63*:301, 1984.
180. Lah, F., Giles, W.R., Trudinger, B.J.: Epidural anaesthesia for caesarean section and its effect on maternal uterine and fetal umbilical placental arterial blood flow velocity-time waveform. [Abstr.] Can. Anaesth. Soc. J., *32*:S76, 1985.
181. Lassner, J., Barrier, G., Talafre, M.L., Durupty, D.: Failure of extradural morphine to provide adequate pain relief in labour. [Abstr.] Br. J. Anaesth., *53*:112P, 1981.
182. Lavin, J.P., Samuels, S.V., Miodovnik, M., Holroyde, J., *et al.*: The effects of bupivacaine and chloroprocaine as local anesthetics for epidural anesthesia on fetal heart rate monitoring parameters. Am. J. Obstet. Gynecol., *141*:717, 1981.
183. LeFevre, M.L.: Fetal heart rate pattern and post paracervical fetal bradycardia. Obstet. Gynecol., *64*:343, 1984.
184. Lederman, R.P., McCann, D.S., Work, B., Huber, M.J.: Endogenous plasma epinephrine and norepinephrine in last-trimester pregnancy and labor. Am. J. Obstet. Gynecol., *129*:5, 1977.
185. Lees, M.H., Hill, J.D., Ochsner, A.J., Thomas, C.L., Novy, M.J.: Maternal placental and myometrial blood flow of the rhesus monkey during uterine contractions. Am. J. Obstet. Gynecol., *110*:68, 1971.
186. Lees, M.M., Scott, D.B., Kerr, M.G.: Haemodynamic changes associated with labour. J. Obstet. Gynaecol. Br. Commonw., *77*:29, 1970.
187. Levinson, G., and Shnider, S.M.: Placental transfer of local anesthetics. Clinical Implications. *In* Marx, G.F. (ed.): Parturition and Perinatology. p. 173. Philadelphia, Williams and Wilkins, 1973.
188. Lewis, M., Thomas, P., Wilkes, R.G.: Hypotension during epidural analgesia for caesarean section. Anaesthesia, *38*:250, 1983.
189. Li, D.F., Rees, G.A.D., Rosen, M.: Continuous extradural infusion of 0.0625% or 0.125% bupivacaine for pain relief in primigravid labour. Br. J. Anaesth., *57*:264, 1985.
190. Liggins, G.C.: Antidiuretic effects of oxytocin, morphine and pethidine in pregnancy and labour. Aust. N.Z. J. Obstet. Gynaecol., *3*:81, 1963.
191. Lindahl, S., Norden, N., Nybell-Lindahl, G., Westgren, M.: Endocrine stress response during general and epidural anaesthesia for elective caesarean sections. Acta. Anaesthesiol. Scand., *27*:50, 1983.
192. Lipshitz, J.: Beta adrenergic agonists. Seminars in Perinatology, *5*:252, 1981.
193. Liston, W.A., Adjepon-Yamoah K.K., Scott, D.B.: Foetal and maternal lignocaine levels after paracervical block. Br. J. Anaesth., *45*:750, 1973.
194. Littlewood, D.G., Buckley, P., Covino, B.G., Scott, D.B., *et al.*: Comparative study of various local anaesthetic solutions in extradural block in labour. Br. J. Anaesth., *51*:47S, 1979.
195. Loeser, E.A., Hill, G.E., Bennett, G.M., Sederberg, J.H.: Time vs. success rate for epidural blood patch. Anesthesiology, *49*:147, 1978.
196. Lofstrom, B.: Aspects of the pharmacology of local anaesthetic agents. Br. J. Anaesth., *43*:194, 1970.
197. Lubbe, W.F.: Hypertension in pregnancy. Pathophysiology and management. Drugs., *28*:170, 1984.
198. Lund, P.C., Cwik, J.C., Gannon, R.T., Vassallo, H.G.: Etidocaine for caesarean section — effects on mother and baby. Br. J. Anaesth., *49*:457, 1977.
199. Magora, F., Olshwang, D., Eimerl, J., Shorr, J., *et al.*: Observations on extradural morphine analgesia in various pain conditions. Br. J. Anaesth., *52*:247, 1980.
200. Maltau, J.M., and Andersen, H.T.: Continuous epidural anaesthesia with a low frequency of instrumental deliveries. Acta. Obstet. Gynecol. Scand., *54*:401, 1975.
201. Maltau, J.M., and Andersen, H.T.: Epidural anaesthesia as an alternative to caesarean section in the treatment of prolonged, exhaustive labour. Acta. Anaesthesiol. Scand., *19*:349, 1975.
202. Maltau, J.M., Andersen, H.T., Skrede, S.: Obstetrical analgesia assessed by free fatty acid mobilisation. Acta. Anaesthesiol. Scand., *19*:245, 1975.
203. Maltau, J.M., and Egge, K.: Epidural analgesia and perinatal retinal haemorrhages. Acta. Anaesthesiol. Scand., *24*:99, 1980.
204. Maltau, J.M., Egge, K., Moe, N.: Retinal hemorrhages in the preterm neonate. A prospective randomised study comparing the occurrence of hemorrhages after spontaneous versus forceps delivery. Acta. Obstet. Gynecol. Scand., *63*:219, 1984.
205. Maltau, J.M., Eielson, O.V., Stokke, K.T.: Effects of stress during labor on the concentration of cortisol and estriol in maternal plasma. Am. J. Obstet. Gynecol., *134*:681, 1979.
206. Maresh, M., Choong, K.-H., Beard, R.W.: Delayed pushing with lumbar epidural analgesia in labour. Br. J. Obstet. Gynaecol., *90*:623, 1983.
207. Marks, R.J., and DeChazol, R.C.S.: Ritodrine-induced pulmonary oedema in labour. Anaesthesia, *39*:1012, 1984.
208. Marx, G.F., Cosmi, E.V., Wollman, S.B.: Biochemical status and clinical condition of mother and infant at cesarean section. Anesth. Analg., *48*:986, 1969.
209. Marx, G.F., and Greene, N.M.: Maternal lactate, pyruvate and excess lactate production during labour and delivery. Am. J. Obstet. Gynecol., *90*:786, 1964.
210. Marx, G.F., Mateo, C.V.: Effects of different oxygen concentrations during general anaesthesia for elective caesarian section. Can. Anaesth. Soc. J., *18*:587, 1971.
211. Matadial, L., Cibils, L.A.: The effect of epidural anesthesia on uterine activity and blood pressure. Am. J. Obstet. Gynecol., *125*:846, 1976.
212. Matouskova, A., Dottori, O., Forssman, L., Victorin, L.: An improved method of epidural analgesia with reduced instrumental delivery rate. Acta. Obstet. Gynecol. Scand., *54*:231, 1975.
213. Meehan, F.P.: Continuous caudal analgesia in obstetrics. Proc. R. Soc. Med., *62*:185, 1969.
214. Meehan, F.P., Moolgaoker, A.S., Stallworthy, J.: Vaginal delivery under caudal analgesia after caesarean section and other major uterine surgery. Br. Med. J., *2*:740, 1972.
215. Mehta, P., Theriot, E., Mehrotra, D., Patel, K., *et al.*: Shivering following epidural anesthesia in obstetrics. Reg. Anesth., *9*:83, 1984.

216. Meis, P.J., Reisner, L.S., Payne, T.F., Hobel, C.J.: Bupivacaine paracervical block: Effects on the fetus and neonate. Obstet. Gynecol., *52*:545, 1978.

217. Melzack, R.: The myth of painless childbirth. Pain, *19*:321, 1984.

218. Merkow, A.J., McGuiness, G.A., Erenberg, A., Kennedy, R.L.: The neonatal neuro-behavioral effects of bupivacaine, mepivacaine, and 2-chloroprocaine used for pudendal block. Anesthesiology, *52*:309, 1980.

219. Merry, A.F., Cross, J.A., Mayadeo, S.V., Wild, C.J.: Posture and spread of extradural analgesia in labour. Br. J. Anaesth., *55*:303, 1983.

220. Messih, M.N.A.: Epidural space pressures during pregnancy. Anaesthesia, *36*:775, 1981.

221. Mihaly, G.W., Moore, R.G., Thomas, J., Triggs, E.J., *et al*: The pharmacokinetics of anilide-local anaesthetics in neonates. I: Lignocaine. Eur. J. Clin. Pharmacol., *13*:143, 1978.

222. Miller, F.C., Quesnel, G., Petrie, R.H., Paul, R.H., *et al.*: The effects of paracervical block on uterine activity and beat-to-beat variability of the fetal heart rate. Am. J. Obstet. Gynecol., *130*:284, 1978.

223. Milne, M.K., and Murray Lawson, J.I.: Epidural analgesia for caesarian section. Br. J. Anaesth., *45*:1206, 1973.

224. Mirkin, B.L.: Perinatal pharmacology, placental transfer, fetal localization and neonatal disposition of drugs. Anesthesiology, *43*:156, 1975.

225. Moir, D.D.: Anaesthesia for caesarian section: An evaluation of a method using low concentrations of halothane and 50 percent oxygen. Br. J. Anaesth., *42*:136, 1970.

226. Moir, D.D.: Obstetric Anaesthesia and Analgesia. London, Bailliere Tindall, 1976.

227. Moir, D.D.: Extradural analgesia for caesarian section. Br. J. Anaesth., *51*:79, 1979.

228. Moir, D.D., Amoa A.B.: Ergometrine or oxytocin: Blood loss and side effects at spontaneous vertex delivery. Br. J. Anaesth., *51*:113, 1979.

229. Moir, D.D., Davidson, S.: Postpartum complications of forceps delivery performed under epidural and pudendal nerve block. Br. J. Anaesth., *44*:1197, 1972.

230. Moir, D.D., Victor–Rodrigues, L., Willocks, J.: Epidural analgesia during labour in patients with pre-eclampsia. J. Obstet. Gynaecol. Br. Commonw., *79*:465, 1972.

231. Moir, D.D., Willocks, J.: Epidural analgesia in British obstetrics. Br. J. Anaesth., *40*:129, 1968.

232. Moir, D.D., Willocks, J.: Management of inco-ordinate intrauterine action under continuous epidural analgesia. Br. Med. J., *3*:396, 1967.

233. Moodie, J.E., Moir, D.D.: Ergometrine, oxytocin and extradural analgesia. Br. J. Anaesth., *48*:571, 1976.

234. Moore, D.C., Bridenbaugh, L.L., Bridenbaugh, P.O., Tucker, G.T.: Caudal and epidural blocks with bupivacaine for childbirth. Report of 657 parturients. Obstet. Gynecol., *37*:667, 1971.

235. Moore, J., Murnaghan, G.A., Lewis, M.A.: A clinical evaluation of the maternal effects of lumbar extradural analgesia for labour. Anaesthesia, *29*:537, 1974.

236. Mor, A., Yang, W., Schwarz, A., Jones, W.C.: Platelet counts in pregnancy and labor, a comparative study. Obstet. Gynecol., *16*:338, 1960.

237. Morgan, B.M., Aulakh, J.M., Barker, J.P., Goroszeniuk, T., *et al.*: Anaesthesia for caesarean section—a medical audit of junior anaesthetic staff practice. Br. J. Anaesth., *55*:885, 1983.

238. Morgan, B.M., Aulakh, J.M., Barker, J.P., Reginald, P.W., *et al.*: Anaesthetic morbidity following caesarean section under epidural or general anaesthesia. Lancet, *1*:328, 1984.

239. Morgan, B.M., Bulpitt, C.J., Clifton, P., Lewis, P.J.: Analgesia and satisfaction in childbirth (The Queen Charlotte's 1000 mother survey). Lancet, *2*:808, 1982.

240. Morishima, H.O., and Covino, B.G.: Toxicity and distribution of lidocaine in nonasphyxiated and asphyxiated baboon fetuses. Anesthesiology, *54*:182, 1981.

241. Morishima, H.O., Covino, B.G., Yeh, M.-N., Stark, R.I., *et al.*: Bradycardia in the fetal baboon following paracervical block anesthesia. Am. J. Obstet. Gynecol., *140*:775, 1981.

242. Morishima, H.O., Daniel, S.S., Finster, M., Poppers, P.J., *et al.*: Transmission of mepivacaine hydrochloride across the human placenta. Anesthesiology, *27*:147, 1966.

243. Munson, E.S., Embro, W.J.: Lidocaine, monoethylglycinexylidide, and isolated human uterine muscle. Anesthesiology, *48*:183, 1978.

244. Murphy, P.J., Wright, J.D., Fitzgerald, T.B.: Assessment of paracervical nerve block anaesthesia during labour. Br. Med. J., *1*:526, 1970.

245. Namba, Y., Smith, J.B., Fox, G.S., Challis, J.R.G.: Plasma cortisol concentrations during caesarean section. Br. J. Anaesth., *52*:1027, 1980.

246. Nesheim, B.I., Lindbaek, E., Storm–Mathisen, I., Jenssen, H.: Neuro-behavioural response of infants after paracervical block during labour. Acta. Obstet. Gynecol., Scand., *58*:41, 1979.

247. Nimmo, W.S.: Gastrointestinal function following surgery. Reg. Anesth., *7*:S105, 1982.

248. Nimmo, W.S., Wilson, J., Prescott, L.F.: Narcotic analgesics and delayed gastric emptying during labour. Lancet, *1*:890, 1975.

249. Nunn, J.F.: Applied Respiratory Physiology, p. 386, 2nd ed. Butterworths, London, 1977.

250. Nybell—Lindahl, G., Carlsson, C., Ingemarsson, I., Westgren, M., *et al.*: Maternal and fetal concentrations of morphine after epidural administration during labor. Am. J. Obstet. Gynecol., *139*:20, 1981.

251. O'Driscoll, K., Meagher, D., MacDonald, D., Geoghegan, F.: Traumatic intracranial haemorrhage in first born infants and delivery with obstetric forceps. Br. J. Obstet. Gynaecol., *88*:577, 1981.

252. Ostheimer, G.W.: Prophylactic epidural blood patch. Reg. Anesth., *4*:17, 1979.

253. Ounsted, M.: Pain relief during childbirth and development at 4 years. J. R. Soc. Med., *74*:629, 1981.

254. Ounsted, M., Scott, A., Moar, V.: Delivery and development: To what extent can one associate cause and effect? J. R. Soc. Med., *73*:786, 1980.

255. Palahniuk, R.J., Scatliff, J., Biehl, D., Wiebe, H., *et al.*: Maternal and neonatal effects of methoxyflurane, nitrous oxide

and lumbar epidural anaesthesia for caesarean section. Can. Anaesth. Soc. J., *24*:586, 1977.

256. Paterson, M.E.L.: The aetiology and outcome of abruptio placentae. Acta Obstet. Gynecol. Scand., *58*:31, 1979.
257. Pearson, J.F., and Davies, P.: The effect of continuous lumbar epidural analgesia upon fetal acid-base status during the first stage of labour. J. Obstet. Gynaecol. Br. Commonw., *81*:971, 1974a.
258. Pearson, J.F., and Davies, P.: The effect of continuous lumbar epidural analgesia upon fetal acid-base status during the second stage of labour. J. Obstet. Gynaecol. Br. Commonw., *81*:975, 1974b.
259. Pearson, J.F., and Davies, P.: The effect of continuous lumbar epidural analgesia on the acid-base status of maternal arterial blood during the first stage of labour. J. Obstet. Gynaecol. Br. Commonw., *80*:218, 1973a.
260. Pearson, J.F., and Davies, P.: The effect of continuous lumbar epidural analgesia on maternal acid-base balance and arterial lactate concentration during the second stage of labour. J. Obstet. Gynaecol., Br. Commonw., *80*:225, 1973b.
261. Pechet, L., Alexander, B.: Increased clotting factors in pregnancy. N. Engl. J. Med., *265*:1093, 1961.
262. Pedersen, H., Morishima, H.O., Finster, M.: Uptake and effect of local anesthetics in mother and fetus. Int. Anesthesiol. Clin., *16*:4, 73, 1978.
263. Penfield, A.J.: Laparoscopic sterilization under local anesthesia — 1200 cases. Obstet. Gynecol., *49*:725, 1976.
264. Perris, B.W.: Epidural epthidine in labour. A study of dose requirements. Anaesthesia, *35*:380, 1980.
265. Perris, B.W., and Malins, A.F.: Pain relief in labour using epidural pethidine with adrenaline. Anaesthesia, *36*:631, 1981.
266. Phillips, J.C., Hochberg, C.J., Petrakis, J.K., Van Winkle, J.D.: Epidural analgesia and its effects on the "normal" progress of labor. Am. J. Obstet. Gynecol., *129*:316, 1977.
267. Philipson, E.H., Kuhnert, B.R., Syracuse, C.B., Reese, A.L.P., *et al.*: Intrapartum paracervical block anesthesia with 2-chloroprocaine. Am. J. Obstet. Gynecol., *146*:16, 1983.
268. Philipson, E.H., Kuhnert, B.R., Syracuse, C.B.: Maternal, fetal, and neonatal lidocaine levels following local perineal infiltration. Am. J. Obstet. Gynecol., *149*:403, 1984.
269. Pickering, B., Biehl, D., Meatherall, R.: The effect of foetal acidosis on bupivacaine levels in utero. Can. Anaesth. Soc. J., *28*:544, 1981.
270. Poppers, P.J.: Evaluation of local anaesthetic agents for regional anaesthesia in obstetrics. Br. J. Anaesth., *47*:322, 1975.
271. Poppers, P.J., and Finster, M.: Use of prilocaine hydrochloride for epidural analgesia in obstetrics. Anesthesiology, *29*:1134, 1968.
272. Pritchard, J.A., Cunningham, F.G., Mason, R.A.: Coagulation changes in eclampsia: Their frequency and pathogenesis. Am. J. Obstet. Gynecol., *124*:855, 1976.
273. Pritchard, J.A., and Stone, S.R.: Clinical and laboratory observations in eclampsia. Am. J. Obstet. Gynecol., *99*:754, 1967.
274. Prowse, C.M., Gaensler, E.A.: Respiratory and acid-base changes during pregnancy. Anesthesiology, *26*:381, 1965.
275. Raabe, N., Belfrage, P.: Epidural analgesia in labour. IV: Influence on uterine activity and fetal heart rate. Acta Obstet. Gynecol. Scand., *55*:305, 1976.
276. Raabe, N., Belfrage, P.: Lumbar epidural analgesia in labour. A clinical analysis. Acta Obstet. Gynecol. Scand., *55*:125, 1976.
277. Ralston, D.H., Shnider, S.M.: The fetal and neonatal effects of regional anesthesia in obstetrics. Anesthesiology, *48*:34, 1978.
278. Ralston, D.H., Shnider, S.M., De Lorimer, A.A.: Effects of equipotent ephedrine, metaraminol, mephentermine and methoxamine on uterine blood flow in the pregnant ewe. Anesthesiology, *40*:354, 1974.
279. Ramanthan, S., Gandhi, S., Arismendy, J., Chalon, J., *et al.*: Oxygen transfer from mother to fetus during cesarean section under epidural anesthesia. Anesth. Analg., *61*:576, 1982.
280. Ramanathan, S., Masih, A., Rock, I., Chalon, J., Turndorf, H.: Maternal and fetal effects of prophylactic hydration with crystalloids or colloids before epidural anesthesia. Anesth. Analg., *62*:673, 1983.
281. Reynolds, F., Hargrove, R.I., Wyman, J.B.: Maternal and foetal plasma concentrations of bupivacaine after epidural block. Br. J. Anaesth., *45*:1049, 1973.
282. Reynolds, F., and Taylor, G.: Plasma concentrations of bupivacaine during continuous epidural analgesia in labour: The effect of adrenaline. Br. J. Anaesth., *43*:436, 1971.
283. Robinson, J.O., Rosen, M., Evans, J.M., Revill, S.I., *et al.*: Maternal opinion about analgesia for labour. A controlled trial between epidural block and intramuscular pethidine combined with inhalation. Anaesthesia, *35*:1173, 1980.
284. Rolbin, S.H., Cole, A.F.D., Hew, E.M., Pollard, A., *et al.*: Prophylactic intramuscular ephedrine before epidural anaesthesia for caesarean section: Efficacy and actions on the foetus and newborn. Can. Anaesth. Soc., J., *29*:148, 1982.
285. Rolbin, S.H., Cole, A.F.D., Hew, E.M., Virgint, S.: Effect of lateral position and volume on the spread of epidural anaesthesia in the parturient. Can. Anaesth. Soc. J., *28*:431, 1981.
286. Rorke, M.J., Davey, D.A., Du Toit, H.F.: Foetal oxygenation during cesarean section. Anaesthesia, *23*:585, 1968.
287. Rorth, M., and Bille Brahe, N.E.: 2,3 Diphosphoglycerate and creatinine in the red cell membrane during pregnancy. Scand. J. Clin. Lab. Invest., *28*:271, 1971.
288. Rosenblatt, R., Wright, R., Denson, D., Raj, P.: Continuous epidural infusions for obstetric analgesia. Reg. Anesth., *8*:10, 1983.
289. Rosefsky, J.B., and Petersiel, M.E.: Perinatal deaths associated with mepivacaine paracervical block anesthesia in labor. N. Engl. J. Med., *278*:530, 1968.
290. Rosenfeld, C.R., and West, J.: Circulating response to systemic infusion of norephinephrine in the pregnant ewe. Am. J. Obstet. Gynecol., *127*:376, 1977.
291. Russell, I.F.: Spinal anaesthesia for caesarean section: The use of 0.5% bupivacaine. Br. J. Anaesth., *55*:309, 1983.
292. Russell, I.F., and Chambers, W.A.: Closing volume in normal pregnancy. Br. J. Anaesth., *53*:1043, 1981.
293. Salariya, E.M., Easton, P.M., Cater, J.I.: Duration of breast

feeding after early initiation of frequent feeding. Lancet, *2*:1141, 1978.

294. Saling, E., and Ligdas, P.: The effect on the foetus of maternal hyperventilation during labour. J. Obstet. Gynaecol. Br. Commonw., *76*:877, 1969.

295. Sangoul, F., Fox, G.S., Houle, G.L.: Effect of regional analgesia on maternal oxygen consumption during the first stage of labor. Am. J. Obstet. Gynecol., *121*:1080, 1975.

296. Scanlon, J.W., and Alper, M.H.: Perinatal pharmacology and evaluation of the newborn. Int. Anesthesiol. Clin., *11*:163, 1973.

297. Scanlon, J.W., Brown, W.U., Weiss, J.B., Alper, M.H.: Neurobehavioral responses of newborn infants after maternal epidural anesthesia. Anesthesiology, *40*:121, 1974.

298. Scanlon, J.W., Ostheimer, G.W., Lurie, A.O., Brown, W.U., *et al.*: Neurobehavioral responses and drug concentrations in newborns after maternal epidural anesthesia with bupivacaine. Anesthesiology, *45*:400, 1976.

299. Schifrin, B.S.: Fetal heart rate patterns following epidural anaesthesia and oxytocin infusion during labour. J. Obstet. Gynaecol. Br. Commonw., *79*:332, 1972.

300. Scott, D.B., Kerr, M.G.: Inferior vena caval pressure in late pregnancy. J. Obstet. Gynaecol., Br. Commonw., *70*:1044, 1963.

301. Scott, P.V., Bowen, F.E., Cartwright, P., Rao, B.C.M., *et al.*: Intrathecal morphine as sole analgesic during labour. Br. Med. J., *2*:351, 1980.

302. Scudamore, J.H., and Yates, M.J.: Pudendal block—A misnomer? Lancet, *1*:23, 1966.

303. Sengupta, P., and Nielsen, M.: The effect of labour and epidural analgesia on pain threshold. Anaesthesia, *39*:982, 1984.

304. Shnider, S.M., Abboud, T.K., Artal, R., Henrikson, E.H., *et al.*: Maternal catecholamines decrease during labor after lumbar epidural anesthesia. Am. J. Obstet. Gynecol., *147*:13, 1983.

305. Shnider, S.M., Asling, J.H., Hall, J.W., Margolis, A.J.: Paracervical block anesthesia in obstetrics. I: Fetal complications and neonatal morbidity. Am. J. Obstet. Gynecol., *107*:619, 1970.

306. Shnider, S.M., DeLorimer, A.A., Hall, J.W., Chapler, F.K., *et al.*: Vasopressors in obstetrics. I: correction of fetal acidosis with ephedrine during spinal hypotension. Am. J. Obstet. Gynecol., *102*:911, 1968.

307. Shnider, S.M., and Gildea, J.: Paracervical block anesthesia in obstetrics. Am. J. Obstet. Gynecol., *116*:320, 1973.

308. Shnider, S.M., Wright, R.G., Levinson, G., Roizen, M.F., *et al.*: Uterine blood flow and plasma norepinephrine changes during maternal stress. Anesthesiology, *50*:524, 1979.

309. Sivakumeran, C., Ramanathan, S., Chalon, J., Turndorf, H.: Uterine contractions and the spread of local anesthetics in the epidural space. Anesth. Analg., *61*:127, 1982.

310. Skjoldebrand, A., Garle, M., Gustafsson, L.L., Johansson, H., *et al.*: Extradural pethidine with and without adrenaline durine labour: Wide variation in effect. Br. J. Anaesth., *54*:415, 1982.

311. Smith, B.E.: Prophylaxis of epidural "wet tap" headache. Anesthesiology, *51*:S304, 1979.

312. Soffronoff, E.C., Kauffman, B.M., Connaughton, J.F.: Intravascular volume determinations and fetal outcome in hypertensive disease of pregnancy. Am. J. Obstet. Gynecol., *127*:4, 1977.

313. Stainthorp, S.F., Bradshaw, E.G., Challen, P.D., Tobias, M.A.: 0.125% bupivacaine for obstetric analgesia? Anaesthesia, *33*:3, 1978.

314. Stenger, V., Eitsman, D., Anderson, T., DePadua, C., *et al.*: Observations on placental exchange of the respiratory gases in pregnant women at cesarean section. Am. J. Obstet. Gynecol., *88*:45, 1964.

315. Taylor, H.J.C.: Clinical experience with continuous epidural infusion of bupivacaine at 6 ml per hour in obstetrics. Can. Anaesth. Soc. J., *30*:277, 1983.

316. Teramo, K.: Effects of obstetrical paracervical blockade on the fetus. Acta. Obstet. Gynecol. Scand., *50*[*Suppl.*]:16, 1971.

317. Teramo, K., and Widholm, O.: Studies of the effect of anesthetics on the foetus. Part I: The effect of paracervical block with mepivacaine upon foetal acid-base values. Acta. Obstet. Gynecol. Scand., *46*[*Suppl.*]:1, 1967.

318. Thalme, B., Belfrage, P., Raabe, N.: Lumbar epidural analgesia in labour: I. Acid-base balance and clinical condition of mother, fetus and newborn child. Acta. Obstet. Gynecol. Scand., *53*:27, 1974.

319. Thomas, T.H., Fletcher, J.E., Hill, R.G.: Influence of medication, pain and progress in labour on plasma beta-endorphin-like immunoreactivity. Br. J. Anaesth., *54*:401, 1982.

320. Thomson, K.J., and Cohen, N.E.: Vital capacity observations in normal pregnant women. Surg. Gynecol. Obstet., *66*:591, 1938.

321. Thorburn, J., and Moir, D.D.: Epidural analgesia for elective caesarean section—technique and its assessment. Anaesthesia, *35*:3, 1980.

322. Thorburn, J., and Moir, D.D.: Extradural analgesia: The influence of volume and concentration of bupivacaine on the mode of delivery, analgesic efficacy and motor block. Br. J. Anaesth., *53*:933, 1981.

323. Tucker, G.T.: Plasma binding and disposition of local anesthetics. Int. Anesthesiol. Clin., *13*:33, 1975.

324. Tucker, G.T., Boyes, R.N., Bridenbaugh, P.O., Moore, D.C.: Binding of anilide-type local anesthetics in human plasma II: Implications in vivo with special reference to transplantal distribution. Anesthesiology, *33*:304, 1970.

325. Tuvemo, T., and Willdeck-Lund, G.: Smooth muscle effects of lidocaine, prilocaine, bupivacaine and etidocaine on the human umbilical artery. Acta. Anesthesiol. Scand., *26*:104, 1982.

326. Tyack, A.J., Parsons, R.J., Millar, D.R., Nicholas, A.D.: Uterine activity and plasma bupivacaine levels after caudal epidural and analgesia. J. Obstet. Gynaecol. Br. Commonw., *80*:896, 1973.

327. Ueland, K., Gills, R., Hansen, J.M.: Maternal cardiovascular dynamics. I: Cesarian section under subarachnoid block anesthesia. Am. J. Obstet. Gynecol., *100*:42, 1968.

328. Uppington, J.: Epidural analgesia and previous caesarean section. Anaesthesia, *38*:336, 1983.

329. Usubiaga, J.E., Reis, A., Usubiaga, L.E.: Epidural misplace-

ment of catheters and mechanisms of unilateral blockade. Anesthesiology, *32*:158, 1970.

330. Van den Berg, B.J., Levinson, G., Shnider, S.M., Hughes, S.C., *et al.*: Evaluation of long-term effects of obstetrics medication on clinical development. p. 52. Abstracts of the Society for Obstetric Anesthesia and Perinatology, Boston, 1980.

331. Vanderick, G., Geerinckx, K., Van Steenberge, A.L., De Muylder, E.: Bupivacaine 0.125% in epidural block analgesia during childbirth: Clinical evaluation. Br. J. Anaesth., *46*:338, 1974.

332. Vasicka, A., Robertazzi, R., Raji, M., Scheffs, J., *et al.*: Fetal bradycardia after paracervical block. Obstet. Gynecol., *38*:500, 1971.

333. Warwick, R., Williams, P.L. (eds.): Dorsal rami of the spinal nerves. *In:* Grays Anatomy. ed. 35. p. 1032. Norwich, Longman, 1973.

334. Waters, H.R., Rosen, N., Perkins, D.H.: Extradural blockade with bupivacaine. Anaesthesia, *25*:184, 1970.

335. Weaver, J.B., Pearson, J.F., Rosen, M.: Response to a Valsalva manoeuvre before and after epidural block. Anaesthesia, *32*:148, 1977.

336. Weaver, J.B., Pearson, J.F., Rosen, M.: The effect of posture and epidural block upon limb blood flow and radial artery pressure in term pregnant women. Br. J. Obstet. Gynaecol., *82*:844, 1975.

337. Weeks, A.R., Cheridjian, V.E., Mwanje, D.K.: Lumbar epidural analgesia in labour in twin pregnancy. Br. Med. J., *2*:730, 1977.

338. Weis, F.R., Markello, R., Mo, B., Bochiechio, P.: Cardiovascular effects of oxytocin. Obstet. Gynecol., *46*:211, 1975.

339. Weiss, R.R., Halevy, S., Almonte, K.O., Gundersen, K., *et al.*: Comparison of lidocaine and 2-chloroprocaine ini paracervical block: Clinical effects and drug concentration in mother and child. Anesth. Analg., *62*:168, 1983.

340. Willdeck-Lund, G., Lindmark, G., Nilsson, B.A.: Effect of segmental epidural analgesia upon the uterine activity with special reference to the use of different local anaesthetic agents. Acta. Anaesthesiol. Scand., *23*:519, 1979.

341. Wollman, S.B., and Marx, G.F.: Acute hydration for prevention of hypotension of spinal anesthesia in parturients. Anesthesiology, *29*:374, 1968.

342. Woodward, G.: Intraoperative blood loss in midtrimester dilatation and extraction. Obstet. Gynecol., *62*:69, 1983.

343. Wright, R.G., Shnider, S.M., Levinson, G., Rolbin, S.H., *et al.*: The effect of maternal administration of ephedrine on fetal heart rate and variability. Obstet. Gynecol., *57*:734, 1981.

344. Writer, W.D.R., Dewan, D.M., James, F.M., III: Three percent 2-chloroprocaine for cesarean section: Appraisal of a standardised dose technique. Can. Anaesth. Soc., *31*:559, 1984.

345. Writer, W.D.R., James, F.M., III, Scott-Wheeler, Z.: Double-blind comparison of morphine and bupivacaine for continuous epidural analgesia in labor. Anesthesiology, *45*:215, 1981.

346. Ying, Y.-K., and Tejani, N.A.: Angina pectoris as a complication of ritodrine hydrochloride therapy in premature labor. Obstet. Gynecol., *60*:385, 1982.

347. Youngstrom, P., Eastwood, D., Patel, H., Bhatia, R., *et al.*: Epidural fentanyl and bupivacaine in labor: Double-blind study. [Abstr.] Anesthesiology, *61*:A414, 1984.

348. Zador, G., Lindmark, G., Nilsson, B.A.: Pudendal block in normal vaginal deliveries: Clinical efficacy, lidocaine concentrations in maternal and fetal blood, fetal and maternal acid-base values and influence of uterine activity. Acta Obstet. Gynecol. Scand., *34*[*Suppl.*]:51, 1974.

349. Zador, G., and Nilsson, B.A.: Low dose intermittent epidural anaesthesia in labour: Influence on labour and fetal acid-base status. Acta Obstet. Gynecol. Scand., *34*[*Suppl.*]:17, 1974.

350. Zellavos, H., Shah, Y., Moody, L.: Outpatient laparoscopy with local anesthesia. Int. J. Gynaecol. Obstet., *17*:379, 1980.

19 NEURAL BLOCKADE FOR PLASTIC SURGERY

LORNE ELTHERINGTON
ROBERT CHASE

A decorous silence ought to be observed. It may be humane and salutatory, however, for one of the attending physicians or surgeons to speak occasionally to the patient; to comfort him under his sufferings; and to give him assurance if consistent with truth, that the operation goes well, and promises a speedy and successful termination.

Thomas Percival, M.D., 1803

Socioeconomic changes in medicine and health care and the advent of new pharmacologic agents for conduction anesthesia and sedation have stimulated a sharp increment in the number of surgical outpatient centers (surgicenters) and the frequency of office surgery. An increasing percentage of plastic and reconstructive operations are being performed on outpatients often outside the hospital setting and frequently without the help of an anesthesiologist. Plastic surgeons are likely to be expert in the anatomy of innervation patterns of body regions where they habitually operate. Such surgeons may be technically adept in performing local nerve blocks for operations they perform. Technical expertise and anatomic knowledge in and of themselves are obviously insufficient to assure safety and feasibility of the situation in which the surgeon is responsible for both the anesthesia and some of the more extensive procedures that currently are being performed in this way.

A surgeon cannot simultaneously monitor a patient pharmacologically rendered semiconscious or unconscious and attend to the details of the surgical procedure itself. This is particularly true when the patient's face is draped out of the operative field. It seems fitting to discuss some of the indications, contraindications, pitfalls, and risks of local anesthesia and sedation, as well as monitoring and the local anesthetic techniques most useful to plastic and reconstructive surgeons.

Preoperative, intraoperative, and postoperative management of the patient is described in detail because it is the key to the successful use of neural blockade for plastic surgery.[25,50] *It is also the key to the safe use of neural blockade.*

GENERAL PRINCIPLES

1. No more anesthesia should be used than the minimum necessary to perform the operation and give the patient postoperative comfort.
2. No anesthesia should be used before taking a careful history and performing a physical evaluation, *if indicated by history.*
3. Patients must be protected and educated so as not to cause secondary injuries simply because a part is anesthetized or paralyzed.
4. A safe level of consciousness or arousability must be constantly maintained during operations under local anesthesia and sedation.
5. Safe, titrated dosages of pharmacologic agents for each specific patient must be understood by the surgeon using the agent.
6. Interactions of drugs being used or contemplated must be known.
7. No agents should be administered unless proper

equipment is available for resuscitation and the surgical team is trained and prepared to deal with adverse reactions.
8. The surgeon should never operate alone or without help immediately available to him and the patient.
9. Establishing good rapport with the patient is an important part of anesthesia care.
10. Monitoring equipment and a functional intravenous line are mandatory requirements for significant procedures under local anesthesia.
11. The surgeon must be assured of a fail-safe mechanism to be certain that the agent he is using is the one that he thinks he is using.
12. Waiting patiently by the clock for the full local anesthetic effect is the best way to avoid fear owing to pain at the start of the operation and continuing concern of the patient throughout the operation.
13. The individual who administers local anesthetic agents and monitors the patient must be well aware of premonitory signs and symptoms of overdose and reaction to the agent, vasoactive additives, and preservatives found in the standard preparations.
14. The secondary gain achieved by using local anesthesia with vasoconstrictors is a clean operative field free of excessive bleeding. A surgeon who habitually uses local anesthetic agents with vasoconstrictors must constantly be aware of the dangers of such agents around end arteries, such as those to toes, fingers, and the penis. He must also be cognizant of the dangers of the systemic effect of such agents in patients with hypertension, coronary insufficiency, and cerebrovascular insufficiency and other diseases associated with increased sensitivity to vasoconstrictors.
15. Operating room decorum on the part of all present should be of the highest order. Percival's admonition (see introductory quote) remains timely now, a lifetime after he wrote it.

PREOPERATIVE EVALUATION

In Chapter 6 Bridenbaugh describes a traditional preoperative evaluation of patients scheduled for surgery under regional or local anesthesia with an anesthesiologist in attendance. He suggests, quite appropriately, that the aim is to evaluate the patients as candidates for general anesthesia before they may be considered as appropriate candidates for regional anesthesia.

This "classic" preoperative evaluation by the anesthesiologist needs modification when a plastic surgeon is evaluating an asymptomatic patient who is to have elective low blood loss surgery under local or regional anesthesia administered by the surgeon. In this case the surgeon needs to look for and optimize conditions that may change surgical outcome. Unfortunately, this process often consists of an expensive, time-consuming, and often not helpful physical and, especially, laboratory examination.

To place this evaluative process in perspective, it is necessary to first list rational goals of preoperative evaluation for the plastic surgeon and second, describe how "best" to achieve these goals.

Goals of Preoperative Evaluation

1. To be sure the patient is in an optimum physiologic and psychological condition to undergo regional or local anesthesia and plastic surgery.
2. If this is not the case, to treat or obtain medical consultation that will lead to treatment designed to optimize the patient's health before surgery. This consultation is not designed to obtain "clearance" for surgery, but to obtain assurance that the patient is in the best physical and psychological condition for the proposed surgery.
3. To make the surgical team aware of and prepared to manage any preexisting or potential problems that might arise during the perioperative period.
4. To plan safe and effective pharmacologic management of the patient.
5. To establish a rational perioperative management plan that will allow the safest, most pleasant, and most efficient recovery of patients to their preoperative state or better.

Traditional Preoperative Evaluation

A number of authors[69,72] have provided convincing arguments as to why the usual preoperative evaluation by anesthesiologists and surgeons needs major modification to include reliance on well-documented risk-benefit and cost-benefit data.

Others[38,92] have demanded that more emphasis be placed on the preoperative emotional state of patients, beginning when surgery is first scheduled and continuing through the perioperative and recovery periods. Failure to determine and treat preoperative fear and anxiety may result in technically perfect anesthetic and surgical management complicated by a prolonged, stormy recovery period and a dissatisfied patient. This patient will probably neither return to nor recommend the surgeon to others.

Usual preoperative evaluation involves a "routine" history and physical examination, followed by (or often even preceded by) "routine" laboratory testing, which may include chest x-ray, electrocardiogram, CBC, electrolyte panel, urinalysis, and coagulation measurements. This commonly used preparation makes little sense in, for example, an asymptomatic 50-year-old plastic surgery patient scheduled for rhinoplasty under local anesthesia. Most preoperative testing is a result of irrational habits that provide little useful information, at great cost to the patient and health care system.

Rather than ask which laboratory tests are necessary for asymptomatic plastic surgery patients when minor blood loss is expected, one could rationally ask whether *any* tests are necessary?

Robbins and Mushlin[69] and Roizen[72] have provided excellent arguments for considering the following preoperative laboratory testing in the type of healthy, asymptomatic patients mentioned earlier.

No tests in healthy men under age 40.
A hematocrit in healthy women under age 40, and a test for pregnancy if they are at risk.
Men and women between 40 and 60 years of age would require an ECG, BUN, and blood glucose, plus a hematocrit for women.
Over age 60, all patients would have hematocrit, BUN, blood sugar, ECG, and chest x-ray.

Note that urinalysis is not suggested in any of the above patient groups.

These ideas could be modified even further to include serum creatinine as a better measure of renal function than BUN, or perhaps better, to question at all the testing of renal function in any asymptomatic patient. These suggestions will be met with great skepticism by many surgeons, anesthesiologists, nurses, and hospital administrators. The skeptics should at least read the papers by authors cited above before they close their minds on the subject and merely follow tradition.

The obvious, but often not appreciated necessity to allow rational and cost-effective laboratory testing is a comprehensive search for symptoms (*i.e.*, the history). A comprehensive medical and psychological history could best be started as a detailed questionnaire given to the patient when first seen by the plastic surgeon. For example, the checklist suggested by de Bass[14] could be modified and expanded. The answers to the questionnaire would be used by a nurse to question the patient further. Any deviations from "normal" would assist the surgeon to provide an appropriate, individualized physical examination and laboratory investigation.

A routine physical examination, like anything "routine," does not recognize patients' individuality in terms of prior health and the potential perioperative difficulties they might encounter. The truly asymptomatic patient, as determined by a comprehensive history, does not require a physical examination, except for perhaps baseline pulse and blood pressure obtained at each visit. To rationally analyze the suggestions above, it is necessary to ask the following question: What conditions could possibly be found by a routine preoperative physical examination that would influence anesthetic and surgical outcome and would not be suggested by a comprehensive history?

Black adds further emphasis to this point when he states,[5]

> "In developed countries at least, it is quite rare to find diagnostic physical signs in patients who are truly free from all symptoms.[5]

Using data provided by Robbins and Mushlin,[69] it is estimated that diagnosis of one hepatitis case in 1000 asymptomatic surgical patients, by measuring SGOT in every patient, would cost approximately $36,000. The diagnosis of interstitial lung disease in the same group of patients would cost $500,000 per case and, incredibly, to find an asymptomatic bleeding disorder in the same group could cost the health care system more than $1 million! Unfortunately, little thought is given to the cost of preoperative testing because "everybody does it." Surely this is an unacceptable reason in a time of rapidly escalating health care costs and demands by government and other third party payment groups that physicians reduce costs. Applying the ideas above could save millions of dollars per year without sacrificing health care standards.

Such an approach relies heavily on a comprehensive medical and psychological history. Any abnormalities revealed by the history require appropriate physical examination and laboratory tests. The combination of *no* or sloppy history taking and this approach would fail to gain any benefit because of missing important and potentially costly medical problems.

PREOPERATIVE PREPARATION

Psychological

Reports from the 1970s[6] reveal a strong association between preoperative neuroticism and postoperative pain intensity. They also show that vital capacity is significantly impaired in proportion to patients' pain complaints. Neuroticism has also been related to long-term prognosis after gastric ulcer surgery.[48] Because neuroticism is a good measure of predisposition to anxiety, these and other studies help to document that patients with elevated preoperative anxiety experience more postoperative pain and resultant morbidity than do patients with low anxiety. In fact, it has been suggested[64] that the well-recognized and yet unexplained great variations in postoperative pain complaints may simply reflect differences in the preoperative personality characteristics of patients. These characteristics continue through the perioperative and recovery periods, so it should come as no surprise that long-term patient recovery could be adversely affected.[20,38,53,92] Recent studies indicated that anxiety state correlates well with postoperative pain—regardless of anxiety trait (see Chap. 25).[65]

Of considerable interest to plastic surgeons, as regards preoperative anxiety, is the finding[88] that a Multiple-Affect Adjective Check List could reproducibly measure preoperative anxiety. Lorazepam, a benzodiazepine, anxiolytic drug, effectively reduced preoperative anxiety, while papaveretum, a mixture of narcotic analgesics, not only did not lower anxiety, but also resulted in significantly greater depression in patients before surgery. This finding fits well with the observations of Jaffe[37] that many pain-free patients become dysphoric after receiving narcotics, rather than developing the euphoria or lack of emotional change experienced by patients in pain.

One means of reducing perioperative anxiety is by providing extensive preoperative counseling and information.[10,92] The information should include a thorough explanation of the whole perioperative period, including the sequence of events to be expected after entering the surgical facility. Patients should know who they will meet, what will be done; where and when they will change clothes; injections or pills to expect as well as feelings to expect from medication; what questions will be asked; and where they will wait before entering the operating room. They should also be told what activity, and especially what noise level, to expect around them. The information regarding noise becomes even more significant when one realizes that noise in an operating room is frequently greater than that found on an automotive freeway and approximates the 90 db measured in a household kitchen when a food blender is running.[73] This so-called Third Pollution, following that of air and vision, may easily add to the preoperative and intraoperative anxiety already present in most patients.

Further detailed information, often neglected but of major importance, is what will happen after patients enter the operating room. They need to be told about monitoring devices, injections, medication-induced bodily feelings, the amount of "undress," and initial coldness to expect. Further counseling must stress that repeated questioning during surgery regarding how they feel does not mean that something is wrong, but is used as a most important monitor of their physical and psychological well-being. Patients should be encouraged to tell the surgical team of any "bad feelings" they may be having at any time. Heavy reliance on central nervous system depressant drugs will eliminate this most important monitor.

Finally, patients need to be told the details regarding postoperative care, including the amount of pain to expect and how it will be treated, what will be done for nausea and vomiting, what bandages to expect, and what monitoring will be done. Telling patients what criteria will be used to determine their suitability for discharge is also important.

Patients may be unusually concerned about their recovery at home. They need information and reassurance concerning how much pain to expect and how it will be treated, or, preferably, prevented. They should be encouraged to call a designated member of the surgical team if they have any questions at home concerning their recovery, especially what is normal and abnormal in terms of bodily feelings and appearance.

Much, if not all, of this information could be provided to the patient in written form once they are scheduled for surgery, so as to allow time for them to read the material several times and ask questions if they do not completely understand the information. This approach would also fulfill most legal requirements for informed consent.

The primary goal of providing patients with such detailed information concerning the perioperative and recovery periods is to reduce anxiety and provide patients with a feeling of self-control from knowing what to expect. They will thus have less tendency to develop unrealistic expectations of what will happen and have greater overall satisfaction with the whole experience.[46] It has been shown[81] that loss of control results in patients becoming angry, and dissatisfied postoperatively with resultant increased anxiety and pain (see Chap. 25).

Pharmacologic

Not only does anxiety result in more postoperative pain, but it may also result in several other unpleasant symptoms during the perioperative period, including paresthesias, tremor, shakiness, dizziness, palpitations, giddiness, feeling cold, nervousness, dyspnea, chest pain, blurred vision, chills, weakness, lump in the throat, smothering feelings, headache, faintness, irritability, nausea, and choking.[66]

The autonomic nervous system (ANS) signs and symptoms of anxiety — tachycardia, palpitations, tremor, and hypertension — may be effectively blocked by beta-adrenergic receptor blocking drugs. For example, propranolol in a dose of 20 to 40 mg four times per day, or even a single oral dose of 40 mg 1 hour before surgery, will not only block the ANS manifestations of anxiety, but also sometimes reduce unpleasant psychological components, such as feelings of doom.[35,80] Even 5 mg of intravenous propranolol, given slowly in 1-mg increments just before surgery, can reduce the ANS stimulation that may be causing serious hypertension in an otherwise normotensive patient. This type of unexpected hypertension just before plastic surgery is not uncommon and usually leads to case cancellation and an expensive, nonrevealing cardiovascular evaluation. Beta-blockade by agents with a β_2-action should be avoided in asthmatics.

The signs and symptoms of anxiety unrelated to ANS activation, such as sweating, tachypnea, and dyspnea, will usually not be affected by propranolol-like drugs. Attenuation of these feelings requires the use of other pharmacologic anxiolytics. The benzodiazepine class of sedative-hypnotic "tranquilizing" drugs, as represented by diazepam, are the most rational anxiolytic agents to use. These drugs have been widely used for premedication and anxiolysis and differ from one another mainly in their clearance from the body, as represented by their terminal half-lives. For example, the half-life of diazepam, that amount of time it takes to reduce the diazepam blood concentration to 50% of its initial value, varies from 9 to 53 hours.[3] On the other hand, oxazepam is a short-acting benzodiazepine metabolite of diazepam with a half-life of 10 to 14 hours (see Chap. 6).[3]

Older drugs used for anxiolysis include the barbiturates; sedative antihistamines like hydroxyzine; phenothiazine and butyrophenone tranquilizers chlorpromazine and droperidol; sedative narcotics like morphine; and miscellaneous sedative-hypnotics exemplified by chloral hydrate.

Benzodiazepines are rational, safe, and effective anxiolytics for premedication because they can be effective at doses that cause little sedation.[18] Most sedating drugs, with the notable exception of narcotics and droperidol, possess anxiolytic properties. The problem with these "other drugs" is that the dose–response relationship for anxiety relief closely parallels that for sedation, that is, anxiolysis occurs in proportion to sedation. This relationship is notably absent with droperidol. It has been shown to produce excellent sedation when given to patients preoperatively but no anxiolysis.[21] Likewise, as mentioned previously in this chapter, it has been reported[88] that the sedating properties of narcotics may be associated with dysphoria in pain-free patients as well as dizziness, sweating, dry mouth, nausea and vomiting, weakness, syncope, mood change, mental clouding, and tachycardia.[78] It is interesting that many of these signs and symptoms are the same as those found preoperatively in non-premedicated anxious patients. This potential toxicity should be considered when using narcotic premedication in pain-free plastic surgery patients. Gravenstein gives the following warning[28]:

> "Whenever a physician prescribes a narcotic preoperatively (even a short acting one) he assumes special responsibilities to protect the patient before, during and after the operation against such effects as orthostatic hypotension, respiratory depression, and postoperative pulmonary complications as well as nausea and vomiting."

Although this warning was directed to anesthesiologists contemplating the use of narcotics before general anesthesia, it has perhaps even greater importance to the plastic surgeon operating "alone."

At one time[19] it was thought that oral absorption of diazepam was "better" than that after intramuscular administration. Many anesthesiologists and surgeons still think this is true. However, it was well demonstrated, in 1975,[41] that injection of diazepam into the deltoid muscle achieved more rapid and higher blood levels than did the oral route of administration. Since then it has been shown convincingly[29] that blood flow to the injection site is the rate-limiting factor for absorption of intramuscular drugs, with the deltoid > vastus lateralis > gluteus in terms of blood flow and absorption. Despite these findings, we believe that oral administration of benzodiazepine drugs is the safest, most rational and effective means of providing the only pharmacologic premedication, other than perhaps for propranolol-like drugs, necessary to produce anxiety-free patients. A recent study[67] has shown that only 10 ml of water is necessary, in most patients, for a rapid passage of diazepam through the stomach and into the small intestine. However, the authors recommend that 50 ml of water taken in the sitting position will guarantee rapid oral absorption in virtually all patients.

These considerations point out the irrationality and "traditionalism" of giving multiple preoperative drugs such as barbiturates, narcotics, tranquilizers, anticholinergics, and antihistamines, usually by the unpredictable intramuscular route, only 1 hour before local or even general anesthesia in pain-free patients. If the *only* goal of preoperative medication is the attenuation of perioperative anxiety, anxiolytic benzodiazepines should be started at least the night before and perhaps even several days before surgery. For example, two studies[24,51] revealed that starting chlordiazepoxide orally, a few days before surgery resulted in patients for cardiac and general surgery who were truly "tranquilized" and anxiety-free on the morning of surgery.

However, "nothing is for free," especially where drugs are concerned. An editorial by Hollister[32] claimed that chronically anxious patients taking chlordiazepoxide over a 90-day period had ten times more traffic accidents than predicted for a normal population. Whether this result was due to the drug alone or would also be found in a nontreated group of chronically anxious patients is not clear. "Chronic" anxiolytic premedication needs to be considered in terms of risk-benefit, and patients must be warned regarding potential dangers, such as driving.

The following "idealized" preoperative treatment plan is an example of what is meant by rational, safe, and effective premedication for plastic surgery patients.

1. Diazepam in an oral dose of 10 to 20 mg, beginning at least the night before surgery, but in very anxious patients preferably a few days before surgery. One half the chosen dose, assuming it was effective in providing excellent sleep, would be given orally on the day of surgery after the patient is admitted to the surgical unit. If signs or symptoms of ANS stimulation are present, propranolol, 40 mg orally, could be given at this time at least 1 hour before surgery. If signs and symptoms of anxiety should still be present when the patient is stabilized in the operating room but before surgery, intravenous diazepam or propranolol (for hypertension) could be slowly titrated to provide optimum individualized anxiolysis. If beta blockade is used, intravenous atropine or, better, glycopyrrolate may be needed if heart rate decreases excessively.
2. Rather than intravenous diazepam, which, because of the presence of an irritating solvent, is painful when injected, a new water-soluble, nonirritating benzodiazepine could be used in the operating room. This new agent, midazolam (Versed), is said to produce more anterograde amnesia than does diazepam, is shorter lasting, and in doses of 0.07 mg/kg produces excellent sedation and anxiolysis for gastroscopy.[7] A smaller titrated dose should provide excellent anxiolysis as an adjunct to preoperative, oral diazepam.
3. In the postoperative recovery period, which will be considered later in this chapter, a benzodiazepine could be continued nightly for sleep until the patient has truly returned to "normal." The decision to use this approach must be evaluated for each patient, but there is no question that control of postoperative anxiety will lead to a marked reduction, or even elimination, of the need for postoperative analgesia. Two interesting studies[8,16] show that diazepam or chlordiazepoxide *alone* provide good postoperative analgesia.

In the preceding treatment plan, diazepam is recommended as the anxiolytic drug of choice because of its long half-life. This fact allows the agent to be given as a single bedtime dose. The major side-effect, sedation, will allow sleep, while residual anxiolytic action usually continues throughout the next day. A possible disadvantage of diazepam is its unpredictable oral bioavailability and variable half-life. Because of this, some patients may require day-time dosing with diazepam to achieve adequate long-term anxiety relief, for example, 20 mg at night and 5 mg two to three times per day.

In healthy young people a 20-mg oral dose the night before surgery should be effective and well tolerated. Older patients require less drug; a 10-mg tablet may suffice. They will also tolerate chloral hydrate well in a dose of 1 to 2 g, with half the bed-time amount repeated orally the morning of surgery. However, if there is any doubt as to an older patient's need for sedative drugs, do not give them. Follow Roberts' admonition[71] when giving any drugs to older patients:

> "The straw which breaks the camel's back may be very small when the camel is nearing the end of its journey."

In summary, rational psychological and pharmacologic preparation of the asymptomatic plastic surgery patient, for low blood loss procedures under local anesthetic administered by the surgeon, should concern itself *only* with the prevention or reduction of anxiety. This is best achieved by the surgical team providing empathetic counseling and detailed information. Further anxiolysis, if required, may be achieved pharmacologically by the use of benzodiazepines or beta-adrenergic blocking drugs in selected patients.

CHOICE OF LOCAL ANESTHETIC AND ROUTE OF ADMINISTRATION

This topic is discussed under Preoperative Evaluation earlier in this chapter, and the reader is referred to Chapters 3 and 4 for detailed information.

INTRAOPERATIVE CONSIDERATIONS

ANALGESIA

Operating analgesia should be established and maintained by the careful and rational use of local anesthetics. Before local anesthesia, most plastic surgeons provide intravenous analgesia to reduce the discomfort of injection.

In this context, Farr shows great insight into this problem when he states, quite emphatically[22]:

> He who cannot do an operation painlessly under local anesthesia alone should not hide behind the veil of a preliminary narcotic. Some surgeons who have had difficulty in establishing good local anesthesia have found in this preliminary medication a panacea for all their "local" troubles, so to speak, and have with the aid of huge and possibly dangerous doses of those preliminary drugs, been able to perform painless operations. It is a mistake to class this work as local anesthesia. As a matter of fact the use of the local anesthetic in these cases plays only a minor part, and without the aid of this preliminary medication the operation could not be done under local anesthesia provided by the technic employed.

A good example of what Farr means is illustrated by the following irrational and potentially dangerous technique[85]: intramuscular premedication with secobarbital 100 mg, promazine 25 mg, Pantopon 20 mg, followed 2 hours later by up to 20 mg of intravenous diazepam, 75 mg of intravenous ketamine, and local anesthesia with 0.5% lidocaine containing epinephrine, 5 μg/ml. Another 50 mg of intravenous ketamine may be used 30 minutes later. There is considerable "tranquility" produced by this technique, but at what price? In fact, Cullen[12] questioned the risk of any premedication designed to depress the central nervous system. Imagine what he would have said regarding the above scheme!

Patients receiving such medications are not only tranquil, but in a condition of general anesthesia as well, at least part of the time. According to the author, however, the patients are not receiving general anesthesia, but are "completely asleep and not responsive to voice command." Although this technique works and has apparently been safe in the hands of one plastic surgeon, it is *not* recommended. The same author has claimed[86] that anesthesiologists disagree with his "analgesic" technique because of "anxieties raised by many anesthesiologists when others perform procedures they feel are in their domain." This anxiety is certainly not universal among anesthesiologists.[26,61] However, *analgesic* doses of ketamine for the purpose of pain-free local anesthetic injection is a totally different concept than using larger doses of ketamine as part of what can only be described as a "balanced" technique of general anesthesia, even though the surgeon describes the technique[86] as one that "borders on general anesthesia." That border is too close for the comfort of most anesthesiologists and, more important, for patient safety.

A number of other schemes for facilitating painful local anesthetic injection have been suggested.[9,13,49] A major shortcoming of most methods has to do with the rather indiscriminate and often dangerous use of intravenous narcotic analgesics that can produce significant respiratory depression not diagnosed by the surgical team, as well as other toxicities mentioned earlier.[37,78] Of even greater potential consequence to the patient is undetected respiratory depression (elevation of Pa_{CO_2}) combined with hypoxemia. Reports[34,50] from plastic surgeons routinely using narcotic drugs provide ample evidence of potential hypoxemia and the need for supplemental oxygen to prevent its occurrence.

As mentioned previously, narcotics are poor anxiolytics, only fair sedatives, and therefore *not* recommended for premedication. The surgeon should be providing analgesia during surgery by local anesthetics. Therefore, the only possible rationale for narcotic use is in the few minutes required to reduce the pain from injection of the local anesthetic. In most cases the surgeon requires only 5 to 10 minutes for this injection. For this purpose it makes no sense to inject a long-acting, long-onset narcotic such as morphine or meperidine. Rather, rapid-onset, short-acting fentanyl could be slowly administered, as suggested by some authors.[42,76] Unfortunately, satisfactory analgesia for skin injection is not guaranteed and significant undetected respiratory depression may occur later in the case.

There are a number of safer and more easily controlled analgesia choices, than narcotics, to achieve a short pain-free injection period. Ketamine in low intravenous doses of 0.5 mg/kg, given slowly over 1 minute, will reliably provide a 5- to 10-minute pain-free interval in an apparently unconscious patient who will, however, take a deep breath when instructed to do so. Elderly patients require only 10 to

20 mg of ketamine intravenously. This period is one of *analgesia,* not general anesthesia. Some plastic surgeons use as much as 1 mg/kg of intravenous ketamine to achieve a longer period of more profound analgesia for local anesthetic injection. Some of these patients will in fact be "under" general anesthesia for this short period. Any central nervous system (CNS) depressant drug given before the ketamine will add to the amount of CNS depression elicited by ketamine. This fact provides even more reason to avoid premedication with narcotics and other CNS depressants, except the benziodiazepines, that demonstrate dose–response relationships separating anxiolysis and CNS depression.

Many surgeons precede ketamine injection by approximately 5 minutes with a small intravenous dose of diazepam, 2.5 to 5 mg, or midazolam, 1 to 2 mg. This may reduce the blood pressure stimulation often produced by ketamine as well as the incidence of "ketamine dreaming." However, it has been shown[13] that with low-dose ketamine "bad dreams" seldom occur and may not be affected by diazepam given before or after the ketamine. Other evidence[54] suggests that dreams are reduced. It is interesting that adverse ketamine reactions have been prevented by *psychological* pretreatment.[77]

More important than bad dreams is the well-documented[11] diazepam protection of ketamine-induced tachycardia and hypertension. Other benzodiazepines, including oxazepam, lorazepam, and flunitrazepam, would also likely be protective. Of even more interest is the claim[11] by these authors that oxygen inhalation also attenuates cardiovascular stimulation by ketamine. Although the benzodiazepines will obviously add to the CNS depression produced by ketamine, this risk is more than justified by the benefits of cardiovascular stabilization and perhaps dream reduction.

It is now recognized[4] that ketamine sedation may be nonspecifically antagonized by physostigmine, while leaving the analgesia unaltered. If this finding is upheld with further investigation, it would make low-dose ketamine analgesia as a prelude to local anesthetic injection even safer than it is now.

Another way[63] to provide ketamine analgesia is by continuous intravenous infusion rather than by bolus injection. Volunteers were infused with ketamine to provide "satisfactory" analgesia, sedation, and amnesia in 50% of the patients. This was accomplished with a bolus of 1 mg/kg, followed by 1 mg/kg/h (approximately 14 μg/kg/min). With this technique one must be cautious to inject the bolus of 1 mg/kg slowly over 2 minutes so as to avoid possible apnea.

Some plastic surgeons have advised the liberal use of narcotics before, during, and after surgery because, after all, narcotic toxicity can be readily reversed by naloxone. This "antidote mentality" is dangerous. As previously mentioned,[34,50] it is possible to have significant hypoventilation and hypoxemia secondarily to narcotic-induced respiratory depression without it being apparent to the patient or the surgical team. Obviously, then, the best narcotic antagonist is of no value unless narcotic toxicity can be diagnosed before it causes complications. Naloxone antagonism of long-acting morphine and meperidine depression is much shorter than the respiratory depression itself. Thus patients may appear adequately reversed but unexpectedly "re-narcotize" with the attendent patient risk, while the surgical team is lulled into a false sense of patient safety. Moreover, naloxone antagonism of narcotics, unless skillfully managed, may result in nausea, vomiting, hypertension, restlessness, and dysphoria.

There are other safer and more effective analgesic methods than narcotics. Two authors[23,61] reported the use of nitrous oxide as a safe, effective analgesic for use in minor painful procedures, such as local anesthetic infiltration. This may be administered by way of a dental-type nose mask that allows gas scavenging and prevents operating room contamination. The technique is also advocated by dentists.[70] The mask and tubing may be sterilized and placed in a sterile surgical field. After the use of nitrous oxide in oxygen during injection of the local anesthetic, oxygen only could be maintained throughout the case. This is especially important if the patient has received, or will receive, a narcotic injection. Nitrous oxide, in most circumstances, is best administered by anesthesia personnel or others trained in its use.

Hypnosis has been successfully used[83] by plastic surgeons in place of drugs for producing anxiolysis and analgesia before local anesthetic injection. In fact, hypnosis has even been used as a substitute for local anesthesia for cosmetic surgery.[73] Experts in hypnosis claim[83] that after 3 to 4 days of training, plastic surgeons should be able to use hypnotic techniques to reduce pain and anxiety as an adjunct to local anesthesia and even for removal of superficial skin lesions without drugs.

Other drug-free analgesic techniques have also been used[70] and include the following:

Acupuncture analgesia with needles either manually twirled or electrically stimulated by an acupuncture machine.

Audioanalgesia during which the patient wears

earphones and controls the volume of the "white sound." This may be the original patient-controlled analgesia now so popular for providing narcotic analgesia.[90]

Electrical analgesia, introduced by the Russians to provide pain relief during dental surgery. The same technique could possibly be modified and used as a form of transcutaneous electrical nerve stimulation (TENS), to elicit skin analgesia before local anesthetic injection. The method would also provide analgesia under patient control, which appears to be important in any problem involving pain therapy.

Finally, all plastic surgeons realize that superb surgical technique is a prerequisite for surgical success. Many have forgotten, however, that superb local anesthetic injection techniques can make this procedure readily acceptable by most patients *without the supplemental use of analgesic drugs.* A recent report[1] looked at the influences of rate and depth of injection and temperature of local anesthetic solution as determinants of injection discomfort. They found that the rate and depth of local anesthetic injection were important in minimizing injection pain. There was no difference in the duration of skin anesthesia with subcutaneous versus intradermal injection. Intradermal placement of local anesthetic resulted in a more rapid onset of anesthesia at the expense of more pain on injection. Further, they advocated the use of a 30-gauge needle and subcutaneous injection to produce excellent skin anesthesia in 5 to 6 minutes.

Intradermal saline containing 0.9% benzol alcohol has also been recommended as a rapid, painless method for obtaining good skin anesthesia lasting approximately 3 minutes.[82] The mixture comes ready-mixed from the manufacturer as bacteriostatic saline in a multidose bottle. This finding was first reported in a 1976 paper[91] that compared a number of compounds used for intradermal anesthesia, including saline, saline with benzol alcohol, lidocaine 0.5% plain and with 0.1% methylparaben, lidocaine 1%, and procaine 1%.

One of the most interesting descriptions[43] of local anesthetic injection technique appears in the translation of a Russian text. The authors describe local infiltration according to A. V. Vishnevsky ("the Russian method"), in which the anesthetic solution is advanced under pressure, "along the sheaths and fascial slits of the human body." They refer to this as the "method of creeping infiltrate." It uses 0.25% procaine with epinephrine and tissue layer by layer infiltration along the incision line. They claim that the injection is painless and allows immediate incision for virtually any type of surgery.

States, Robert Farr, a Minneapolis general surgeon, writing in 1923[22]:

> It is possible to make a complete infiltration of a given field without any painful sensation except in the production of the first wheal, provided the injection is made of the proper cadence and the necessary precautions are taken."

Using the saline-containing benzyl alcohol skin wheal referred to above[82] would conceivebly make the infiltration pain free. After the skin wheal Farr then proceeded to slowly and gently infiltrate subcutaneous local anesthesia up to within a centimeter of the needle hub. At this point, and critical to the success of his pain-free technique, he depressed the skin just ahead of the needle point, and thus created a second intradermal skin wheal from below the skin instead of through the epidermis from above. He proceeded by withdrawing the needle and reinserting it through the intradermal area of anesthesia (Fig. 19-1). This intradermal wheal, made from injecting the dermis by a subcutaneous approach, was immediately anesthetic and allowed the surgeon to quickly proceed with further infiltration. In contrast, it may take 5 to 6 minutes for subcutaneous infiltration to produce surgical anesthesia.

MONITORING AND OTHER MEASURES

All patients undergoing surgery with local anesthesia should have an intravenous line established, either with a heparin-lock or, preferably, connected to an infusing physiological solution. If the patient has been fasting overnight, the solution should contain 5% glucose so as to replace liver glycogen that has diminished during the overnight "starvation." The theoretical other advantage of plain 5% glucose is that it provides free water to allow the urinary excretion of fixed acids and other cellular metabolites that have accumulated in plasma during the fasting period, as well as replacing hypotonic, insensible fluid losses.

One could certainly make a case for "visual monitoring" without an intravenous line in a patient having "lump and bump" plastic surgery, in which the only drug used is a small amount of local anesthetic (*e.g.*, less than 1.5 mg/kg of lidocaine). The only possible toxicity from this type of procedure would be a rare allergic reaction or vasovagal bradycardia and possibly syncope, owing to psychic stimulation caused by the injection itself. When there is any

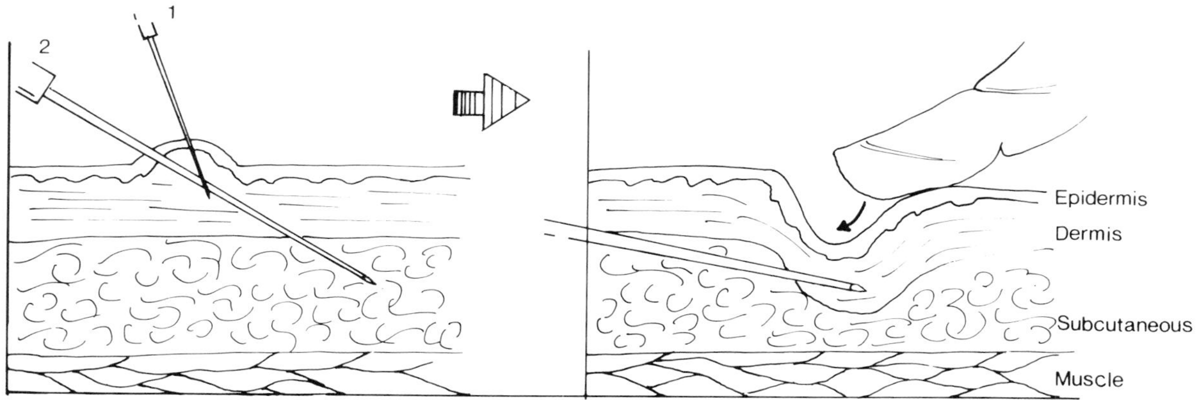

FIG. 19-1. **Left.** Skin wheal and subcutaneous infiltration. **Right.** Intradermal wheal produced painlessly via the subcutaneous space.

doubt as to whether or not an intravenous cannula should be inserted, insert one.

It is unacceptable to use a metal, butterfly-type intravenous needle. These devices become easily dislodged or pierce the vein, often at a time of maximum need, when an emergency occurs. A small 20- or 22-gauge plastic cannula, securely taped, is well tolerated by patients. However, it is often just as easy and as well tolerated by the patient to insert an 18-gauge or larger cannula. The larger the cannula, the more rapidly drugs and fluids can be infused if needed in an emergency. A small amount of nitroglycerin ointment (Nitrobid) may be rubbed over the hand to produce venous dilatation and facilitate cannulation.

Monitoring of plastic surgery patients should be dictated by the patient's health, degree of expected pharmacologic and surgical intervention, and, most important, being prepared to treat any major problem, even cardiopulmonary arrest. Hence the suggestion for large intravenous cannula. This caution may appear to be excessive for asymptomatic healthy patients. However, it has been shown[2] that in healthy asymptomatic patients receiving *general anesthesia,* there is a higher percentage of more serious respiratory mishaps than occur in the sicker surgical population. The same situation may be true in healthy patients under local anesthesia. For example, it has been shown[42] that "conscious sedation" using diazepam, fentanyl, and methohexital led to significant hypercarbia and, more important, hypoxemia in conscious patients who were able to respond to verbal commands. Their respiratory rates were above 12 per minute and their "clinical appearance" did not indicate that 36% of the patients had significant respiratory depression. Supplemental oxygen with a nasal mask at 6 liters per minute totally prevented the hypoxemia in the face of significant respiratory depression (a mean transcutaneous Pco_2 rise of 9 mm Hg).

It follows therefore that in the absence of respiratory function monitoring (pulse oximetry, end-tidal CO_2, or transcutaneous O_2 and CO_2), respiratory depressant drugs should be accompanied by supplemental oxygen. It has been pointed out[45] that when the surgeon is responsible for doing the operation, providing the anesthetic, and monitoring the patient, "trouble may occur." Adequate monitoring, training, and, when necessary, the use of anesthesia personnel can usually prevent this unwanted trouble.

With this in mind, the first step in monitoring, even before intravenous placement, is "all personnel in the outpatient surgery unit should be trained and certified in cardiopulmonary resuscitation (CPR) techniques. Further, at least the physicians in the unit should be trained and certified in advanced CPR techniques." This statement,[26] by a well-known plastic surgeon with considerable expertise in the potential dangers of surgeon-administered local anesthesia, underlines the fact that even sophisticated and invasive monitoring is useless unless the people doing the monitoring can interpret the signals and are trained to successfully treat significant deviations from normal.

The best monitor of a plastic surgery patient under local anesthesia is frequent communication with the patient.[26,45] Of secondary importance are mechanical, electrical, noninvasive monitors that produce reliable and useful information regarding the patient's physiologic state during surgery and recovery.

Blood Pressure Monitoring

Systemic blood pressure is usually measured in patients, but even this apparently simple procedure may be poorly done. For example, the American Heart Association publishes "Recommendations for Human Blood Pressure Determination by Sphygmomanometers."[39] These recommendations include cuff size being more than 40% and less than 70% of arm circumference and the cuff length covering at least 60% of the upper arm.

Automated blood pressure recording with easily seen digital readings can be taken at set time intervals and may be used in place of manual measurements. The sophisticated, but expensive units can be obtained with serial printout of systolic, mean, and diastolic blood pressure, and pulse. It has been demonstrated[74] that inexpensive instruments designed for home use are also reliable.

Surgeons, and even anesthesiologists, tend to be quite complacent when blood pressure is normal during general anesthesia, and perhaps even more so when patients are awake during surgery. However, it has been well documented that blood pressure is really an insensitive and crude monitor of cardiovascular function. Nickerson suggested that[60] "our reason for measuring blood pressure is not so much its importance as the ease with which it can be measured." A patient may have low cardiac output (CO) and high systemic vascular resistance (SVR) with subsequent low tissue oxygen delivery in the face of "normal" blood pressure.[93] It is obvious, then, that marked drug-induced, potentially harmful cardiovascular changes can take place to which the patient may adjust, and thus present with normal blood pressure.

Monitoring of Oxygenation

Even invasive monitoring with measurement of CO and calculation of SVR may not really tell what is happening as regards the prime function of the cardiovascular system to deliver adequate oxygen to tissues. For example, either decreased oxygen content of arterial blood or increase in tissue oxygen demand over supply may be reflected by a "normal" CO.

It is now possible to easily monitor, noninvasively, the hemoglobin oxygen saturation of arterial blood by pulse oximetry.[94] This may prove to be the overall "best" noninvasive objective monitor of patients during surgery under regional/local anesthesia. Quite simply, pulse oximetry provides a frequent digital display of hemoglobin saturation in arterial blood, using spectrophotoelectric oximetric techniques. A fall in saturation below 98% in a healthy awake patient, breathing room air, must be due to hypoxemia. The severity of hypoxemia, as measured by oximetry, has been correlated with the Pao_2 of arterial blood.[40] Slight, moderate, and profound hypoxemia would be represented by Pao_2's of 50 to 70 mm Hg, 35 to 50 mm Hg, and <35 mm Hg, respectively. Arterial blood oxygen saturations, Sao_2, correlating with the Pao_2s are slight hypoxemia 85% to 95%, moderate hypoxemia 65% to 85%, and profound hypoxemia <65% saturation. A simple approximation for calculation of oxygen tension from hemoglobin saturation <90% is $P_ao_2 = S_ao_2 - 30$.

Knill suggests[40] that pulse or ear oximetry is too expensive to be routinely used during anesthesia. We suggest that oximetry as a noninvasive monitor of arterial blood oxygenation is too important *not* to be used during anesthesia, especially by a surgical team operating without an anesthesiologist or an anesthetist. Because the cardiovascular and respiratory systems have, as a major function, the oxygenation of tissues, any monitoring device that noninvasively measures a major index of this function, such as arterial hemoglobin oxygen saturation, is worth using.

Electrocardiogram

An electrocardiogram (ECG) should be used in every case where blood pressure recording is done. One outstanding monitor of significantly diminished myocardial perfusion and oxygenation in the awake patient is the presence of angina pectoris. Again, this fact points out the necessity for having an awake, communicative patient. A single-lead ECG, commonly lead II, will only provide information regarding cardiac rhythm. An optional printout attachment to the ECG monitor is helpful to accurately diagnose rhythm disturbances. However, this single ECG lead is not adequate to diagnose myocardial ischemia. Even the use of a more appropriate V4, V5, or modified precordial lead may miss the presence of significant myocardial ischemia owing to the regional nature of this phenomenon. No single precordial lead will detect ischemia in all patients. To be sure that the patient is not having myocardial ischemia, in the absence of complaints of angina, requires a 12-lead ECG. Hence, for operative monitoring, the plastic surgeon should use a single V5 lead so as to evaluate cardiac rhythm disturbances as well as *possibly* see evidence of myocardial ischemia in the anterior myocardium.

Supplemental Oxygen

If respiratory depressant drugs are used, then an absolute necessity for care of these patients during and after surgery is supplemental oxygen. This can easily be supplied by way of inexpensive, sterilized nasal prongs, even for patients having operations around the face. As mentioned previously, mild to moderate hypoventilation and hypercarbia is usually not a serious problem unless hypoxemia occurs. Supplemental oxygen, along with pulse oximetry monitoring, can help to guarantee that hypoxia does not occur.

USE OF VASOCONSTRICTORS

Vasoconstrictor drugs are universally used by plastic surgeons as part of local anesthetic infiltration to provide hemostasis,[31] reduce systemic absorption, and extend the duration of anesthesia. For example, plain 0.5% lidocaine, a frequently used local anesthetic, provides approximately 75 minutes of skin anesthesia (range of 30–90 minutes). Adding 5 μg/ml of epinephrine (1:200,000) results in anesthesia from 60 to 300 minutes with a mean of 200 minutes. However, there are some disadvantages to the use of epinephrine in combination with local anesthetics. Lidocaine solution containing epinephrine has been reported[89] to produce more injection pain than plain lidocaine. The use of subcutaneous epinephrine, in a rat model, has also been shown[56] to markedly reduce tissue oxygenation and increase carbon dioxide proportional to its concentration. It is not known whether or not this tissue ischemia results in any serious human toxicity, such as tissue necrosis. Excellent hemostasis can be obtained[30] with an epinephrine concentration of less than 2.5 μg/ml (1:400,000).*

An important reason for using vasoconstrictors with any local anesthetic solution is reduction of vascular absorption, and resultant decreased blood levels of the drug. Unfortunately, most studies evaluating the hemostatic efficacy of epinephrine do not correlate this property with the amount of systemic local anesthetic absorption. For example, a recent report[9] describing a "new system" of infiltration anesthesia used an epinephrine concentration of 0.6 μg/ml (1:1,666,666) combined with 0.26% lidocaine. They used up to 382 ml of this solution that contained 993 mg of lidocaine and "only" 299 μg of epinephrine. Although "effective" vasoconstriction and anesthesia were claimed, no information was reported on blood levels of lidocaine and possible contribution of systemically absorbed lidocaine to complications the authors reported, such as excitement, nausea, dizziness, and hypertension. The same study did show the incidence of ventricular arrhythmias in hypertensives increased with increasing doses of epinephrine, as well as the degree of tachycardia, palpitations, and excitement.

Another important aspect of vasoconstrictor use not appreciated by all plastic surgeons is the difference in effectiveness between local anesthetic-vasoconstrictor solutions *premixed* by the manufacturer and containing the antioxidant sodium metabisulfite, and solutions *freshly mixed* in the operating room immediately before use. Auto-oxidation of epinephrine to ineffective pink adrenochromes in manufactured solutions is prevented by adding the metabisulfite, which lowers, for example, lidocaine *p*H from greater than 6 to less than 4.5. This more acidic solution, while reducing oxidation, results in more of the lidocaine existing in an ionized form (as the cation). This solution requires greater alkaline buffering in tissue to produce the lipid-soluble moiety that is able to penetrate neuronal lipid membranes and produce anesthesia. Clinically, the onset and intensity of local anesthesia, and even the duration, may be adversely influenced. Adding epinephrine to the local anesthetic just before use provides a more alkaline solution and a simple step method, if mixing instructions are always referred to by both nurse and surgeon so as to eliminate mixing mistakes (see also Chaps. 3 and 4).

Habit, tradition, and usage have made epinephrine the vasoconstrictor of choice for mixing with local anesthetics. If pharmacologists were asked today to pick a rational vasoconstrictor for adding to local anesthetics, epinephrine would probably not be the first choice. The drug has a number of adverse cardiovascular actions, including cardio-acceleration and vasodilatation, especially in skeletal muscle, owing to stimulation of beta-adrenergic receptors, and vasoconstriction owing to alpha-adrenergic receptor activation with "larger doses." Absorption of epinephrine from injection sites, or accidental intravenous injection, may produce, in the patient, fear, anxiety, tenseness, restlessness, throbbing headache, tremor, weakness, dizziness, pallor, respiratory distress, and palpitations.[36] More rational agents that elicit only

*A solution of epinephrine 1 mg in 1 ml is a 1:1000 solution that contains 1000 μg; the maximum safe dose is 200 μg (0.2 ml of the 1:1000 solution). Thus a 5 μg/ml solution is 1:200,000, and 40 ml of this is a maximum safe dose. If large volumes are needed, 1:400,000 dilution may be used.

vasoconstriction include norepinephrine, felypressin, ornipressin, and phenylephrine (see also Chap. 4).

Norepinephrine has been used with local anesthetics in concentrations of 12.5 to 40 μg/ml (1 : 25,000 to 1 : 80,000). Because norepinephrine is a pure alpha-adrenergic receptor agonist in all vascular beds, it is more dependable than epinephrine as a "tissue tourniquet." Its use has not become popular based largely on tissue-irritating properties, supposedly greater than those of epinephrine. This information derives mainly from unfortunate accidents in which large intravenous doses of norepinephrine were infused and infiltrated into surrounding tissues producing extensive tissue necrosis, in patients treated for shock, with pre-existing vasoconstriction. Dilute norepinephrine solutions containing local anesthetics have been successfully used to provide hemostasis, extend local anesthetic duration, and minimize systemic absorption. Untoward effects of norepinephrine are said to be qualitatively the same as those produced by epinephrine but considerably less intense.[36] Most common are anxiety, respiratory distress, headache, and reflex cardiac slowing.

Perhaps the most rational vasoconstrictor, at least in theory, is felypressin, a synthetic posterior pituitary hormone that has been shown to be effective in a concentration of 0.03 U/ml (1 : 2,000,000) without increasing tissue metabolism as seen with sympathomimetic amines, thus reducing the potenial of local tissue damage. Ornipressin 1 IU/ml has also been shown to be effective in plastic surgery with minimal cardiac effects.

Levonordefrin (Neo-cobefrin) is used as a vasoconstrictor in dentistry, in a concentration of 50 μg/ml. It has more stability than epinephrine and norepinephrine but in the high concentrations used, possesses similar toxicity. More dilute concentrations may be suitable for use in plastic surgery.

Phenylephrine, a direct-acting sympathomimetic amine producing alpha-adrenergic receptor stimulation only, has been used in local anesthetic solutions. Concentrations of 500 μg/ml (1 : 2000) provide subcutaneous vasoconstriction that lasts more than twice as long as that produced by epinephrine.[36] It also produces much less subjective toxicity than does epinephrine. It would be worthwhile to use much greater dilutions of phenylephrine and to measure local anesthetic duration, systemic absorption, and resulting hemostasis.

Despite these suggestions, it is apparent that epinephrine will continue to be the vasoconstrictor of choice for mixing with local anesthetic solutions unless a drug company decides to manufacture and test other agents for efficacy, safety, and cost, when compared with epinephrine as the "golden standard."

POSTOPERATIVE CARE

The following comment typifies the inadequacy of modern postoperative pain management: "The most common treatment for postoperative pain remains a standard intramuscular dose of an opiate administered at the discretion of a nurse, on demand by a patient whose pain tolerance has been exceeded."[87] The same authors go on to remind us that despite revolutionary changes in anesthesia over the past century, we are still practicing 19th-century medicine in the use of postoperative analgesics.

The recovery period after local anesthesia should not be considered a separate part of the patient's care. As discussed earlier, preoperative psychological and pharmacologic preparation can markedly influence a patient's postoperative state. Therefore, postoperative analgesia should begin preoperatively and continue during and after surgery. Less postoperative anxiety means less postoperative pain and other discomforting feelings.

Rather than make a senseless transition between operative and postoperative analgesia (which often happens with general anesthesia), it is important to consider the patient's postoperative analgesic needs in choosing the appropriate local anesthetic agent and technique for surgery. For example, a surgical procedure planned to last for 3 hours or less could easily be accomplished with 0.5% lidocaine freshly mixed with 5 μg/ml of epinephrine. This would provide approximately 3 hours of surgical anesthesia and probably at least another hour of analgesia to allow a smooth postoperative transition from surgical facility to home without the need for supplemental analgesia. In fact, for most infiltration procedures, 0.25% bupivacaine is as effective as 1% lidocaine and the onset of anesthesia is thought to be the same.[75] Duration of action, using this low concentration, mixed with epinephrine, may be more than 7 hours (range of 6.5 – 7.5 hours). Provided intravascular injection of high concentrations (0.5% and 0.75%) is avoided, the risk of bupivacaine toxicity can be minimized (see Chap. 4). The recommended single, safe infiltration dosage of bupivacaine mixed with epinephrine is 200 mg. This means that 80 ml of the 0.25% concentration may be safely infiltrated at one time, in healthy patients.

Long-lasting local anesthesia can also be obtained

with a 0.5% lidocaine-epinephrine mixture to which 1 mg/ml of tetracaine (Pontocaine) is added to a maximum total tetracaine dose of 1 mg/kg. Some physicians have attempted to mix the rapid-onset, short-duration amide chloroprocaine (Nesacaine) with the slow-onset, long-duration amide bupivacaine (Marcaine). Because of the low *p*H of the resultant mixture, the block is of shorter duration than that produced by bupivacaine alone and often is unpredictable in onset (see Chap. 4).

It has been suggested[15] that mixtures of local anesthetics are no more toxic than the drugs in the mixture. This means that, for example, if the maximum, single recommended dose of lidocaine with epinephrine is 500 mg and the maximum for tetracaine plus epinephrine is 200 mg, a mixture of the two local anesthetics to provide rapid onset and long duration of local anesthesia (4 to 6 hours and longer) should contain no more than 250 mg of lidocaine and 100 mg of tetracaine. This allows the use of 100 ml of the solution.[59] This analgesia should last throughout the immediate postoperative period and allow oral analgesia to be commenced before discharge.

After entering the recovery room, the patient could take an oral loading dose of an appropriate analgesic, prescribed by the surgeon and brought to the surgical facility by the patient the morning of surgery. If the oral dose were given immediately on stabilization in the recovery room, any toxicity from the drug should be apparent before discharge from the facility.

What oral analgesics are rational, safe, and effective in the immediate postoperative period? Usual postoperative analgesia is provided by intramuscular injection of meperidine, often combined with promethazine. As stressed earlier in this chapter, intramuscular drug administration makes little sense *at any time* when considering healthy patients for plastic surgery. In fact, the same statement could easily be made concerning the use of intramuscular analgesics in *any patient* able to take oral medication.

Patients with mild to moderate pain postoperatively may get effective analgesia from aspirin or other nonsteroidal anti-inflammatory drugs (NSAIDs) given in large doses on a time-contingent (not prn) basis. For example, aspirin 1300 mg is administered to start, followed by 650 mg every 4 hours with meals or a large glass of fluid. Of some interest is the report[58] that shows 650 mg of aspirin is a superior analgesic to ten commonly used oral analgesics, including narcotics. Other investigators showed[44] that it takes 2 or more hours to achieve maximum blood salicylate level after a dose of plain aspirin. In contrast, sodium salicylate, in a glass of warm water, results in maximum blood salicylate levels in 30 minutes, and is less prone to cause gastrointestinal irritation or bleeding.[44]

Longer-lasting and more expensive NSAIDs can also be used:

Diflunisal (Dolobid), 1 g initial dose and 500 mg b.i.d., or even t.i.d.
Piroxicam (Feldene), 40 mg initial dose and 20 mg daily
Sulindac (Clinoril), 400 mg initial dose up to 200 mg b.i.d.
Ibuprofen (Motrin), 1600 mg initial dose and up to 3200 mg per day

Many other NSAIDs are available and could be substituted for the above according to cost, convenience, efficacy, and patient tolerance.

If the pain is not significantly reduced by NSAIDs, the addition of 60 to 120 mg of codeine is valuable to provide added pain relief mediated by a different mechanism. Adequate doses of codeine, given at least every 6 hours to begin with, are necessary to serve this purpose. A rational drug combination in this case (even though fixed-dose drug mixtures are usually not advised) might be aspirin 325 mg and codeine 60 mg (sold as ASA #4) two tablets orally with a large glass of fluid every 6 hours. If analgesia evaluation, done in the first 8 hours after surgery as it should be, reveals good analgesia for less than 6 hours, the timing should be changed to every 4 hours. If analgesia lasts for the necessary period of time but is not intense enough, the dosage could be increased to three tablets.

If NSAIDs are not indicated because of a history of ulcers or concern for postoperative bleeding, then acetaminophen (Tylenol) can be given in place of a NSAID in the same dosage and interval as aspirin. Codeine, 60 mg, is also available as a mixture (acetaminophen #4) under several trade names. Some plastic surgeons prefer acetaminophen to NSAIDs because of concern about subcutaneous hematoma formation.

The analgesic regimen described assumes that anxiolytic therapy continues during the postoperative and recovery period. For example, diazepam in a sleep dose usually provides antianxiety action throughout the next day. It also assumes that the patient has no nausea or vomiting and is able to tolerate oral fluids.

To treat moderate to severe postoperative pain, or to use as a substitute when codeine is not tolerated because of nausea and vomiting, oral morphine has much to recommend it. Many plastic surgeons may be shocked by this idea until they realize that codeine is really weak morphine. That is, approximately 10% of the codeine absorbed from the stomach is converted to morphine and it is this morphine "metabolite" that produces most of the analgesia attributed to codeine.[37] This being the case, why not give morphine itself rather than a precursor?

Oral morphine demonstrates extensive first-pass liver metabolism, that is, it takes approximately 40 to 60 mg of oral morphine to provide the same amount of analgesia as that obtained from 10 mg of intramuscular morphine. It takes approximately 160 mg of codeine to achieve the same analgesic effect.[27] For patients expected to have moderate to severe postoperative pain, the following regimen may be started in the recovery room: oral morphine 40 to 60 mg every 4 hours together with an NSAID or acetaminophen in adequate dose. A new long-acting oral morphine preparation (Morphine Contin) may be given in a 30 or 60 mg dose every 12 hours. This regimen should be evaluated during the first 8 hours and modified as necessary.

Meperidine is not recommended for oral use, even though it can produce effective analgesia in 300- to 400-mg doses (equivalent to 100 mg intramuscularly). The drug is not as anxiolytic as morphine and, even more important, its major metabolite, normeperidine, has been associated with CNS toxicity.[27]

A number of other oral narcotic analgesics have been used to treat postoperative pain. For example, oxycodone (sold as Percodan when combined with aspirin and Percocet when combined with acetaminophen), hydromorphone (Dilaudid), and weak narcotic agonist antagonist drugs, such as pentazocine (Talwin), are common alternative agents. These drugs are not recommended as being equally effective or as well tolerated as the drugs described above.

NAUSEA AND VOMITING

In addition to bradycardia, nausea and vomiting (N/V) may occur as part of a vasovagal response. This stressful event can usually be successfully treated using intravenous glycopyrrolate, 0.4 mg. Atropine, 0.8 mg, may also be used, but because it is a tertiary amine, it enters the brain and may produce CNS effects. The use of an ionized quaternary amine, such as glycopyrrolate, which does not cross the blood–brain barrier, is more rational.

The most common cause of postoperative N/V in patients recovering from local anesthesia is the preoperative and intraoperative use of narcotics.[68] These agents all cause direct stimulation of the brainstem, chemoreceptor, trigger zone and have been shown to cause nausea in 40% and vomiting in 16% of ambulatory patients. This suggests a vestibular component to the N/V.[37] It is interesting that morphine, and presumably other narcotics, depress the vomiting center when used chronically. Vomiting, if it does occur, usually happens only after the first dose, and as long as plasma levels are maintained, nausea and vomiting should not occur as a result of subsequent doses.[37] Unfortunately, this is not always the case.

A Scottish plastic surgery group studied N/V after general anesthesia. They stated in their introductory comments that avoidance of narcotic premedication was a major factor in reducing postoperative vomiting. They went on to strongly support the view that the indiscriminate use of antiemetic drugs was undesirable because many of them delay recovery from anesthesia. The phenothiazine group of agents also produced a high incidence of postural hypotension.[84] The authors also studied nausea and vomiting in patients who had received both a narcotic and an antiemetic phenothiazine before general anesthesia. Their data suggest that children, females, and patients having ear surgery were most apt to vomit postoperatively. Men over 40 seldom vomited, irrespective of the operative procedure.

In some plastic surgery patients, postoperative vomiting is not only a nuisance, but also a serious danger. Such patients are those who have had skin grafts or flaps, or who have had intraoral and nasal surgery, where bleeding spells failure. Vomiting can markedly increase venous pressure in the head and neck, which may result in significant bleeding and consequent hematoma formation. With plastic surgery patients who have intraoral or nasal surgery, it is especially important to prevent blood from entering the stomach, where it can act as a potent emetic. Such swallowed blood and resultant vomiting tends to create more bleeding.[62] It appears reasonable that if narcotics are extensively used preoperatively or intraoperatively with patients in whom postoperative vomiting is a hazard, a prophylactic antiemetic drug needs to be administered. These statements should make one realize that giving potentially toxic drugs, such as phenothiazines, to help reduce a toxic effect of a narcotic whose use is probably not indicated makes little sense.

One group showed recently[52] that N/V after narcotics could be markedly decreased by giving naloxone (Narcan) 0.4 mg intravenously and 0.4 mg subcutaneously early in the postoperative period. However, if the narcotic was providing analgesia for the patient, this analgesic effect would be rapidly and dramatically reversed by these doses of naloxone. This reversal might then cause hypertension, resulting in bleeding and hematoma—a consequence worse than the vomiting that the naloxone was used to prevent. Although these last two reports concern patients having general anesthesia, the results and concepts are applicable to plastic surgery patients receiving local or regional anesthesia.

The following are suggestions to prevent or treat postoperative nausea and vomiting fully realizing that drugs effective prophylactically against vomiting may be of no value once active vomiting starts.

Avoid narcotics completely.

Prophylaxis against postoperative nausea and vomiting is not dependable, but the following drugs or techniques are suggested:

Preoperative, posthypnotic suggestion.

Postoperative perphenazine (Trilafon) or prochlorperizine (Compazine) 5 mg, intramuscularly. These representative phenothiazine drugs may, however, cause postural hypotension and extrapyramidal side-effects, such as restlessness. The restlessness may last for 24 hours after a single dose of perphenazine. Paradoxical as it sounds, restlessness may be treated by another phenothiazine, promethazine (Phenergan), in a dose of 10 to 25 mg, intravenously.* One must always remember that a prime cause of restlessness is cerebral hypoxia. This possible cause must be discounted before giving sedative drugs.

Preoperative, prophylactic droperidol 1.25 mg intravenously and 1.25 mg intramuscularly. This butyrophenone will produce a long duration of sedation and, possibly, adverse postural hypotension.

Glycopyrrolate, 0.4 mg intravenously (only for vomiting after bradycardia). Expect a dry mouth and tachycardia if glycopyrrolate is used.

Haloperidol (Haldol) in a dose of 2 mg intravenously is another butyrophenone with a rapid onset of action like droperidol but with a short (3-hour) duration.[55] It may be an effective antiemetic and can also be given orally.

Transdermal scopolamine is an option that awaits assessment.[79]

If nausea is the complaint and the occurrence of vomiting will not be dangerous to the patient, an effective and relatively harmless treatment is to give the patient a sweet carbonated drink to induce vomiting. Once vomiting occurs, the nausea usually passes and the patient feels much better. Using drugs to treat nausea is often not successful, and this should be tried only when subsequent vomiting would be dangerous to the patient.

HYPERTENSION

Once postoperative hypertension becomes manifest, it is often difficult to treat. When hypertension does occur, the etiology must be assumed to be hypoxemia unless proved otherwise. Administration of oxygen should be the first therapeutic choice. An elevated blood pressure often occurs in asymptomatic, normotensive women who have had a meloplasty. In this group of patients especially, hypertension-induced bleeding and subsequent hematoma formation can set the stage for serious complications. Pain and anxiety may also be major causes of postoperative hypertension. Treatment should be initiated by sitting the patient straight up and making sure she is warm. Fentanyl in 25-μg doses, given over 1 minute every 5 minutes, or 15 mg of alphaprodine administered in the same manner, are reasonable choices for rapid-onset, short-acting pain relief. If it is practical or possible to reinject the wound with local anesthetic, this is a good alternative for pain relief. For example, local anesthetics may be injected into breast drains after augmentation mammoplasty to provide excellent postoperative analgesia.

Anxiety-induced stimulation of the ANS, with resulting tachycardia and hypertension, can be treated by slowly injecting propranolol, 0.5 mg intravenously, together with hydralazine 5 mg.[55] This combination may be repeated safely in 10 minutes. If more than two doses of hydralazine and propranolol are required, consideration should be given to obtaining a medical consultation.

If hypertension occurs in a patient with normal or lowered heart rate, a full bladder should be considered as a possible cause. If it is not, then nitroglycerin paste could be used on the forearm (approximately 1 inch [2.5 cm]). If this application is successful in reducing the hypertension, it may be continued as necessary. Sublingual and chewable isosorbide dinitrate, 10 mg, may provide 2 to 3 hours of hypertension control.[57] Likewise, Labetalol, a combined alpha- and beta-adrenergic receptor antagonist in an i.v. dose of 5 to 10 mg, may provide several hours of hypertension control. Postural hypotension may occur with

*In older age-group patients, and rarely in younger patients, a parkinsonian type of extrapyramidal syndrome may develop with any phenothiazine. This requires urgent treatment with cogentin.

these drugs and patients need to be made aware of this possibility.

Chlorpromazine is a blood pressure-lowering agent widely used by plastic surgeons.[26] In repeated intravenous doses of 1 to 2 mg it may be effective in treating intraoperative and postoperative hypertension. The drug has some significant drawbacks, however. They include [1] unpredictable efficacy with too much or too little effect on blood pressure in any given patient; [2] sometimes significant, long-lasting sedation, dysphoria, and postural hypotension will occur; [3] the drug has other pharmacologic actions, including direct and indirect CNS effect on the heart and blood vessels.

The more specific antihypertensive drugs are recommended over chlorpromazine-like agents because they have more specific, tritratable, and evanescent cardiovascular effects. The emergence of calcium channel blocking drugs raises further blood pressure control options yet to be evaluated in the setting described above.

HYPOTENSION

Postoperative hypotension can occur without apparent cause in otherwise healthy patients. As mentioned in the section on monitoring, changing to a larger blood pressure cuff or using a different automatic blood pressure device may mislead the observer into misdiagnosing "hypotension." The intraoperative blood pressure cuff should be left applied to the patient for recovery room use. A manual blood pressure taken by the recovery room nurse will diminish the risk of such misdiagnosis. If the hypotension should be "real," the first step is to lower the head and raise the legs while administering oxygen by mask and rapid intravenous fluids.

Tachycardia associated with the hypotension suggests hypovolemia, best corrected by the position change mentioned above and rapid volume infusion. A seriously low blood pressure, that is, more than 50% below average intraoperative levels, should be immediately treated with ephedrine, 12.5 mg intravenously, every 5 minutes while fluid is infusing. If a bradycardia exists along with the hypotension, a bolus of intravenous glycopyrrolate, 0.4 mg, should be given rather than ephedrine. This dosage can be repeated every 10 minutes until the pulse returns to the normal range. Failure of glycopyrrolate to reverse the hypotension should then be followed with the ephedrine therapy.

Cardiac arrhythmia is a possible but infrequent cause of hypotension during early recovery. This should be readily apparent on the ECG monitor.

Narcotics, coupled with upright posture, are a common cause of hypotension because of narcotic-induced increase in venous capacitance. The supine or head-down position should readily reverse hypotension from this etiology.

Very fit athletes who engage in endurance sports, such as long-distance running and cycling, are often chronically hypovolemic and prone to exhibit hypotension from narcotics, minor blood loss, and phenothiazines. Such patients should have a large intravenous cannula placed preoperatively and receive at least 1 liter of balanced salt solution before entering the operating room. Hypotension should be expected and prepared for in this unusually "healthy" patient group who would not normally be expected to have problems with plastic surgery under local anesthesia.

RESTLESSNESS

This behavior in the operating room or recovery room could represent hypoxemia, and the patient needs to be placed on oxygen as the first step in therapy. Other causes of restlessness can be a full bladder, pain, anxiety, prior use of phenothiazine drugs, and prior use of atropine and other potentially dysphoric drugs, such as narcotics and droperidol. After oxygenation and reassurance the patient should be closely observed to determine whether or not signs or symptoms are progressing. If the restlessness persists in spite of oxygenation (checked by blood gases or pulse oximetry, or both) and reassurance, a small dose of intravenous benzodiazepine, for example, 1 mg of midazolam, may be helpful. Tachycardia coupled with restlessness suggests ANS activation. This may require intravenous propranolol for successful resolution.

VOIDING DIFFICULTIES

A full bladder not only is uncomfortable for the patient, but also can produce significant bradycardia and hypotension. The recovery room environment may make patients unable to void. Rather than persist with encouragement and sounds of running water, it is better to do a single straight catheterization. If sterile technique is strictly adhered to, the risk of infection from bladder catheterization is small in healthy patients.

SPECIFIC REGIONAL NERVE BLOCKS FOR OPERATIVE PROCEDURES, AND RELATED ANESTHESIA

Most of the regional nerve blocks and local anesthetic techniques are described in other chapters in this text. Many plastic surgery procedures are amenable to the use of spinal, epidural, or caudal blocks (see Chaps. 7 through 9).

Procedures in the *arms or legs* can use the large number of single-shot or continuous techniques described in Chapters 10 through 12. It is worth noting that the role of sympathetic blocks in maintaining blood supply to flaps, pedicles, and plastic reconstruction requires investigation (see Chap. 13).

Thoracic and abdominal region plastic surgery may use a number of peripheral nerve blocks, described in Chapter 14. Some of these techniques, such as rectus sheath block and iliac crest block, are being "rediscovered."

Perhaps the highest volume of plastic surgery under neural blockade uses techniques described in the *head-neck, eye, and oral cavity* region (see Chaps. 15 through 17). The reader should compare some of the alternative approaches with blocks in the vicinity of the mouth, described separately in Chapters 15 and 16. *Pediatric patients* have received too little consideration with respect to the use of neural blockade for plastic surgery. A surprising number of techniques are described in Chapter 21, as well as the selection and management of patients.

A sobering note should be added. Anyone performing neural blockade should be familiar with the physiology, pharmacology, and toxicology of these drugs (see Chaps. 2 through 4). They should also understand the neurologic complications (see Chap. 22) and the basis of the rare neuropathology (see Chap. 29.1) that may occur.

Some blocks and techniques of particular interest to the plastic surgeon[17,47] will be discussed in this chapter. These include local anesthesia infiltration techniques suitable for head and neck surgery, breast augmentation, tissue expansion, lipectomy and liposuction, and regional anesthetic nerve blocks suitable for plastic surgery of the genitalia.

BLEPHAROPLASTY, MELOPLASTY, AND MENTOPLASTY

Local anesthesia with a vasoconstrictor is preferred to general anesthesia in combination with local anesthesia for procedures on the aging face because there is a significant reduction in bleeding. In addition, this method facilitates the ease of positioning and draping and provides greater mobility of the head for surgical dissection. By combining local infiltration with nerve blocks, less agent is used and less tissue distention is noted. In meloplasty, 1% lidocaine (Xylocaine) with epinephrine is used in the infraorbital (see Fig. 15-3), mandibular (see Fig. 15-6), and superficial cervical plexus blocks (see Figs. 15-9, 15-11). The major local infiltration (0.5%) is administered along the lines of the incision. Each case varies significantly, as does the distribution of the local infiltration and dissection. For example, more local anesthetic is used in the mastoid area and in the upper neck above the sternocleidomastoid muscle level, since the skin is inherently associated with the overlying fascial tissue. Total quantity of local anesthetic used varies somewhat; however, usually not more than 500 mg of lidocaine with 1:400,000 epinephrine is used during the entire procedure, which may last up to 4 hours. The anesthetic is instilled into the area of dissection approximately 20 to 30 minutes before surgery.

Another benefit of nerve blocks plus infiltrative anesthesia is that the motor branches of the facial nerve can be stimulated and isolated for identification during the procedure itself, whereas during muscle-relaxant/general anesthesia techniques, responses of facial muscles may be abolished by the combined effects of neuromuscular blockade and general anesthesia.

Techniques

As shown in Figure 15-3, the foramen of exit for the supraorbital, infraorbital, and mental nerves passes through a vertical line located just medial to the pupil in adults, but which bisects the pupil in children.

Infraorbital Block. The infraorbital foramen is located in line with the pupil, below the bony orbital margin (see Fig. 15-3). Approximately 2 ml of local anesthetic agent are infiltrated in and around the infraorbital foramen.

Mandibular Block, by Way of the Mandibular Notch. The puncture site is below the zygomatic arch in the middle of the mandibular notch (see Fig. 15-6).

The needle is directed perpendicular to the skin to a depth of about 4 cm. The mandibular nerve is found just posterior to the lateral pterygoid plate (see Fig. 15-6). Four milliliters of 1% lidocaine is used. Chapter 15 should also be consulted for a more detailed account of the anatomy of this technique.

Superficial Cervical Plexus Block. Four milliliters of agent is instilled into the central area of the posterior margin of the sternocleidomastoid muscle (see Fig. 15-9). The distribution of the agent is both subcutaneous and subfascial (see Chap. 15).

RHINOPLASTY

Technique

Ten to 20 minutes before surgery, cotton applicators moistened with 2 ml of 10% cocaine or 4% lidocaine are applied transnasally to the area of the nasociliary nerve and the sphenopalatine ganglion (Fig. 19-2). While this topical anesthetic is taking effect, the local agent can be injected, to block in turn (1) nasal branches of the supraorbital nerve; (2) external branch of the anterior ethmoidal nerve; (3) nasal branches of the infraorbital nerve (see also Fig. 15-3). Approximately 6 to 10 ml of 2% lidocaine with epinephrine, 1 : 200,000 is administered, using the least volume possible. The agent is injected slowly through a No. 27 hypodermic needle 4 cm in length. The rate of distention of the tissue appears to be directly related to the amount of pain incurred with the injection. Starting the injection in the glabellar area at the junction of the nose and forehead, the dorsum is infiltrated (see Fig. 19-2). Next, the infraorbital block is completed (see Fig. 15-3). Finally, the nasal spine is infiltrated for completion of the block (Fig. 19-2). The cotton applicators are then replaced with 2.5 cm nasal packing that has been soaked in 1 to 2 ml of 4% cocaine. The packing is used primarily to prevent blood from dripping into the nasopharyngeal area, but the local anesthetic effect is also important (see also Figs. 15-3 and 15-4).

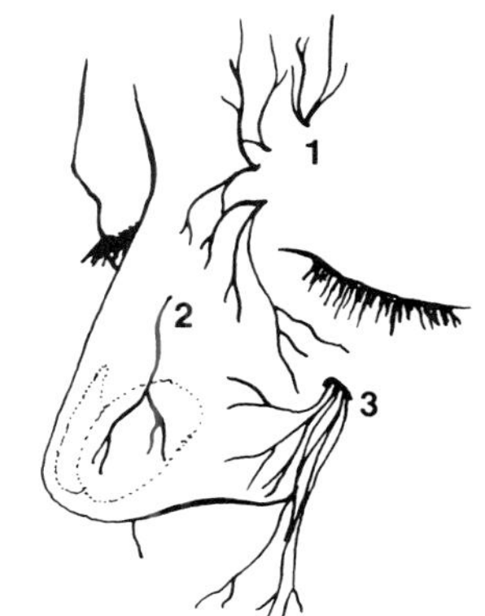

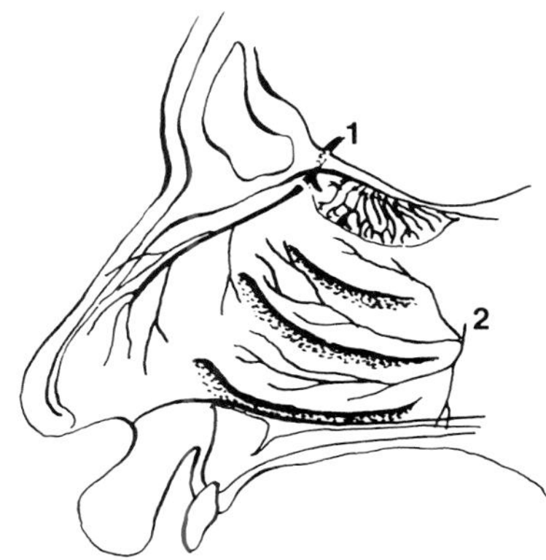

FIG. 19-2. Innervation of the nose as applied to rhinoplasty. **Top.** Nasal branches of the supraorbital nerve *(1)*, external branch of the anterior ethmoid nerve *(2)*, and nasal branches of the infraorbital nerve *(3)*. **Bottom.** Anterior ethmoidal nerve *(1)* and sphenopalatine ganglion area *(2)*.

"EAR BLOCK"

This is useful for plastic surgery on the ear. The technique is shown in Figure 15-12.

LOCAL ANESTHESIA FOR BREAST SURGERY

The skin of the infraclavicular region of the anterior chest wall receives sensory innervation from supraclavicular nerves C_3 and C_4 as primary branches from the cervical plexus. These nerves supply some sensibility as low as the third rib on the chest wall (see Figs. 8-35 and 15-2). There is some crossover innervation from the first three intercostal nerves. Most of the rest of the sensory innervation to the anterior chest wall is supplied by the intercostal nerves 3 through 7 (see Chap. 14). There are, however, afferent components in the nerves to the muscles of the anterior chest wall, such as the pectoralis major. Discomfort may occur with retraction and pulling of this muscle pedicle unless anesthesia is supplied to the pectoral nerves.

Nerve Block Anesthesia

The supraclavicular nerves are effectively blocked by subcutaneous infiltration in a linear area just below the clavicle, crossing the anterior axillary fold into the skin of the axilla. With the arm fully abducted, intercostal nerves 3 through 7 may be blocked by palpating the ribs in the axilla anterior to the anterior border of the latissimus dorsi (Fig. 19-3A). Skin wheals are raised at each intercostal space, using dilute anesthetic agent. Each intercostal nerve, 3 through 7, is blocked by palpation of the inferior portion of the rib with the needle. The needle is walked inferiorly to the rib margin. At the inferior margin of the rib the needle is advanced enough to penetrate the intercostal muscle fascia but not the pleura (see Chap. 14 and Fig. 14-3). Five milliliters of anesthetic agent is deposited at this point. Additional anesthetic solution is injected just beneath the pectoralis muscle pedicle to avoid discomfort when the muscle is retracted or pulled on. It is often necessary to supplement such blocks with a circular field block of anesthetic agent subcutaneously along the lateral sternal border to anesthetize the anterior branch of the intercostals in the event that one or more may not be completely anesthetized at the lateral intercostal site (Fig. 19-3B). These nerve blocks are particularly useful in diminishing postoperative discomfort, thus avoiding the need for narcotics with the cascade of events, including nausea and vomiting, that often follow the use of such agents. The intercostal blocks, therefore, are often done using long-acting anesthetics such as 0.5% bupivacaine, whereas the local subcutaneous infiltration is done using a dilute lidocaine solution. Such solution is safer and of longer duration if it is combined with dilute epinephrine as well. An example of such an agent might be 0.25% lidocaine with 1 : 300,000 epinephrine. In this way a substantial volume of anesthetic solution (up to 160 ml) may be given safely to an adult patient. As the volume of local anesthetic agent increases, concomitantly the total dosage increases. The patient obviously needs to be monitored carefully for increased pulse rate or other evidence of anesthetic agent toxicity. Oftentimes augmentation mammoplasty is done through axillary incisions and a drain is inserted for a short-time postoperatively. It may be helpful to inject 10 ml of 0.25% bupivacaine into the drain for prophylaxis against postoperative discomfort. This, together with the bupivacaine intercostal blocks, results in patient comfort after surgery and diminished need for systemic analgesia.

As an alternative, a "field block" may be used as a sole anesthetic. Local anesthetic is injected in the retromammary space over the entire breast area (Fig. 19-3B). However, this technique is far inferior to that described above.

The above techniques are suitable for *simple mastectomy* or *augmentation* mammoplasty.

Radical mastectomy may be performed with epidural block at C7–T1 interspace. This has been reported to be associated with decreased blood loss compared to general anesthesia.[80a] A regional block may also be performed as described by Labat:[43a] (1) supraclavicular brachial plexus block; (2) intercostal block of the 4th, 5th, 6th, 7th, and 8th intercostal nerves; (3) infiltration subcutaneously in the axilla; (4) infiltration subcutaneously below the clavicle, then down the midsternal region to the xiphisternum, then laterally to the midaxillary line. Even when dilute local anesthetic is used for (2) through (4) above, the dose is likely to be high. Thus epinephrine is used, and injections are made slowly.

BLOCK ANESTHESIA FOR GENITAL PLASTIC SURGERY

Saddle-block spinal anesthesia is frequently chosen if conduction anesthesia is desired for perineal and genital surgery (see Chap. 7). Nerve block anesthesia is a safe alternative when used with skill and attention to anatomic detail.

The key nerve to the region is the pudendal nerve, which may be blocked quite effectively in the perineal area. If the pudendal nerve is blocked at the terminal end of the pudendal canal (Alcock's canal), additional injection should be made to block the long posterior scrotal/labial nerve over the ischial tuberosity (see Chap. 18 and Fig. 18-10).

Sensory nerve branches of the ilioinguinal, iliohypogastric, and genitofemoral nerves come down to the perineal and genital areas from above and anteriorly. Blocking the ilioinguinal and iliohypogastric nerves close to the anterior superior iliac spine and the genitofemoral branches in the pubic area at the external inguinal ring will complete the block of sensibility from the perineum and external genitalia (see Chap. 14 and Fig. 14-12).

Supplemental use of dilute lidocaine with epinephrine 1 : 300,000 in the pubic region may be particularly useful for hemostasis during surgery.

Pudendal Nerve Block

Effective block of the branches of the pudendal nerve that emerge from Alcock's canal to the perineum can

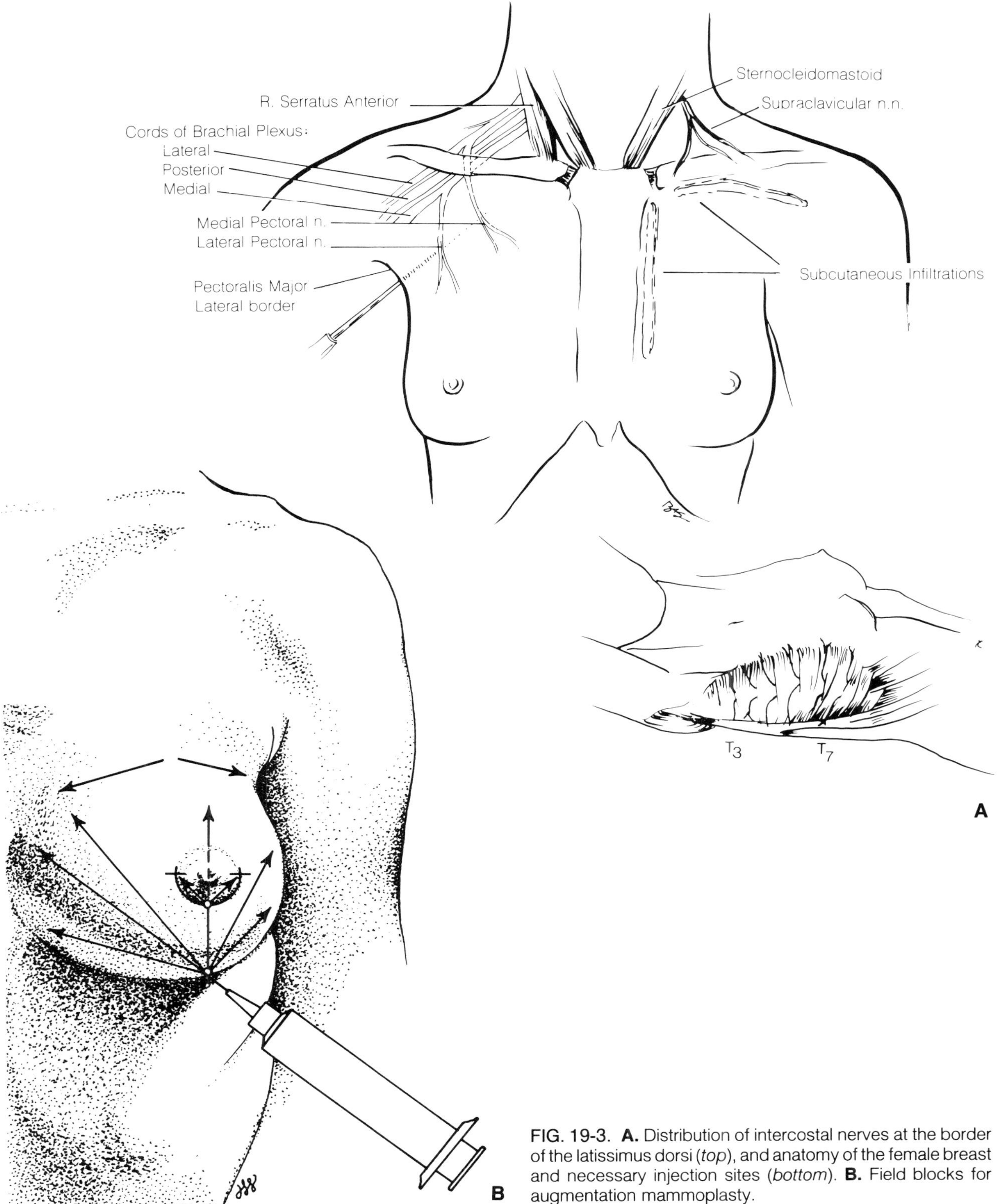

FIG. 19-3. **A.** Distribution of intercostal nerves at the border of the latissimus dorsi (*top*), and anatomy of the female breast and necessary injection sites (*bottom*). **B.** Field blocks for augmentation mammoplasty.

be accomplished regularly with a little practice and attention to anatomic landmarks (Fig. 19-4A).

The patient is placed in a slightly exaggerated lithotomy position. After raising a skin wheal between the easily palpable ischial tuberosity and anus just anterior to the palpable perineal border of the gluteus maximus, a needle is passed just deep to the fascia and the injection is made (Fig. 19-4B). This will not block the long posterior scrotal/labial branch of the pudendal nerve. It may be blocked by depositing local anesthetic just superficial and lateral to the ischial tuberosity. The tuberosity may be palpated with the needle tip and by walking the needle tip to the lateral surface of the ischial tuberosity; injection can

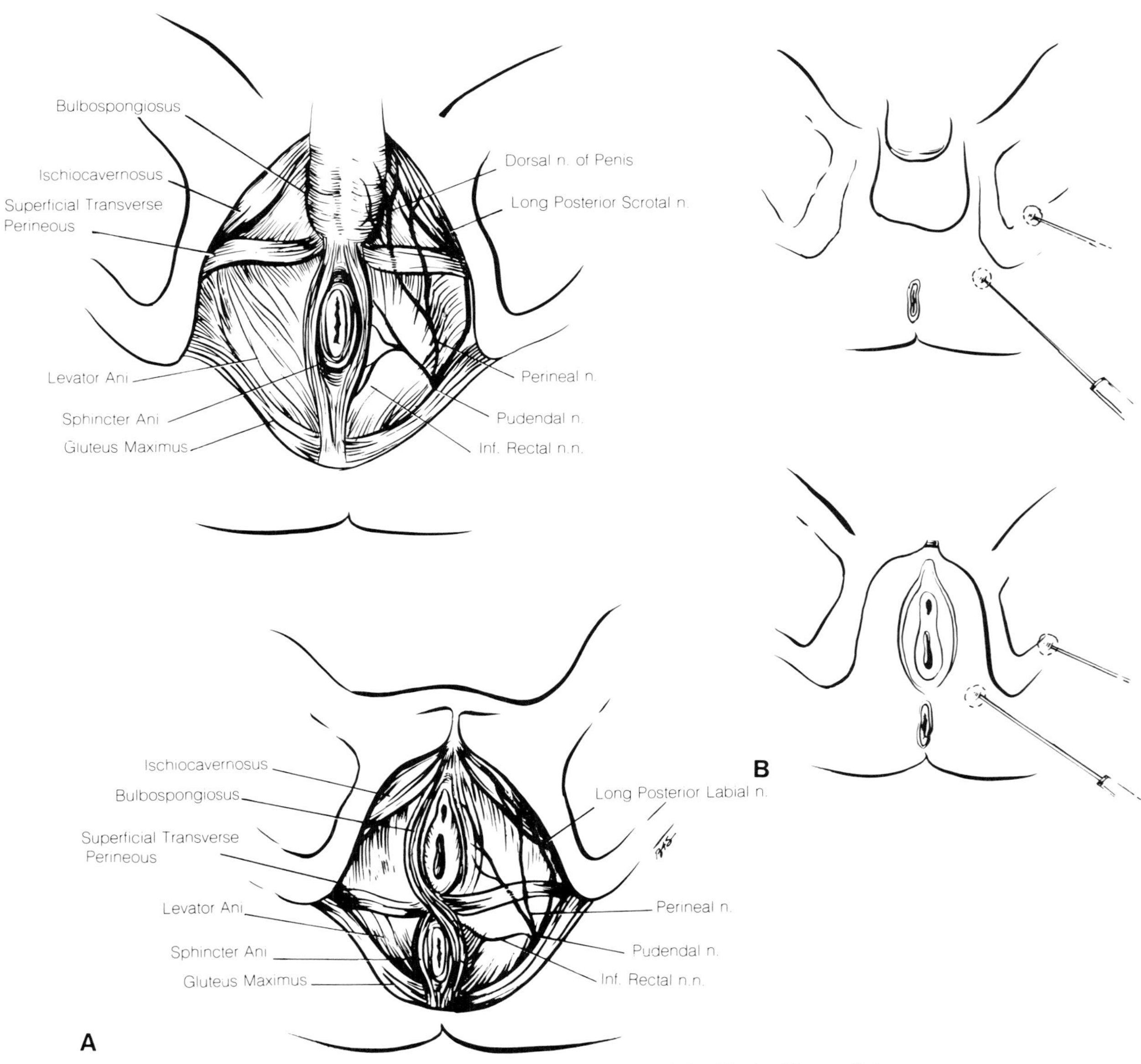

FIG. 19-4. **A.** Anatomy of the male and female perineum illustrating nerves to be blocked for genital surgery. **B.** Sites for needle insertion.

be made at the point of passage of the long posterior scrotal/labial nerve to the perineum (see also Fig. 18-10).

The whole pudendal nerve, including the scrotal/labial branch, may be blocked more proximally in the pudendal canal of Alcock. A clear understanding of anatomic relationships is as important in performing a successful pudendal block as it is in any nerve block procedure in the body. The nerve lies close to the sciatic nerve as both pass out of the pelvis just below the piriformis muscle through the greater sciatic foramen. The pudendal nerve then courses in through the lesser sciatic foramen just below the spine of the ischium to enter the pudendal canal. With the finger in the vagina or rectum, one readily can palpate the ischial spine. With the palpating finger in place, one may insert a needle through the skin wheal between the prominent ischial tuberosity and the rectum. The needle may be guided to the ischial spine and to the palpable attached sacrospinous ligament. Injection should be made by either passing the needle through the ligament or passing it just inferior to the spine and ligament. A sense of decreased resistance occurs after the recognizable resistance that is created by passing the needle through the ligament. The point at which the decreased resistance is felt is the proper point for injection to block the trunk of the pudendal nerve. Truncal blocks done bilaterally at this level give effective anesthesia when supplemented by blocks of the ilioinguinal, iliohypogastric, and terminal branches of the genitofemoral nerves (see Fig. 14-12).

Ilioinguinal Nerve Block

The ilioinguinal nerve, which has origins from T_{12} and, more particularly, L_1, is readily blocked as it passes close to the prominent anterior superior iliac spine (see Fig. 14-12). It lies deep to the fascia of the external oblique muscle and emerges with the spermatic cord through the external inguinal ring to continue to the penoscrotal area in the male or the labial area in the female. Although there is variability in the distance above and medial to the anterior superior iliac spine that the nerve courses, it quite regularly lies in the areolar layer of fascia just deep to the thick fascia of the external oblique muscle. Thus an injection about 2 or 3 cm medial and superior to the anterior superior spine, after palpable penetration of the definable external oblique fascia, will block the nerve, particularly if the area injected is expanded in this layer medially toward the umbilicus (Fig. 19-5). This medial spread will also block the iliohypogastric nerve, which lends sensibility to the pubic skin (see Chap. 14 and Fig. 14-12 and Chap. 21, Fig. 21-17).

The Genitofemoral Nerve

The genitofemoral nerve contributes some sensory nerve supply to the genital area as is suggested by its name. It can be blocked effectively as it enters the area by injection of the local anesthetic solution using the pubic spine as a landmark (Fig. 19-5). The nerve branches pass with the spermatic cord structures in the male and the counterpart round ligament extension in the female. Thus an injection at the location of the external inguinal ring just lateral to the pubic spine infiltrating the tissue surrounding the cord structure is sufficient to block the genitofemoral contribution to sensibility in the region (see Chap. 14).

PENILE BLOCK FOR CIRCUMCISION

Circumcision is generally performed for cosmetic reasons, usually as an elective procedure. Surprisingly, general anesthesia is commonly used for this operation, whereas all that is required is 5 ml of local anesthetic. The size of the operative procedure and the relative risks of the two anesthetic techniques bring into question the routine use of general anesthesia for circumcision. Certainly the procedure has psychological overtones; however, adequate preoperative explanation and appropriate premedication can almost always alleviate such problems. Even if light general anesthesia is used in young children, the additional benefits of penile block are reduced reflex activity during the procedure and the possibility of prolonged postoperative pain relief. The alternative technique of single-shot caudal block is described in Chapter 9 for adults and Chapter 21 for pediatric patients (see Fig. 21-18).

Technique

The dorsal nerves of the penis may be blocked at the base of the penis by two separate injections of 1 ml of 1% lidocaine by way of a 26- or 27-gauge needle inserted at the 10:30 o'clock and 1:30 o'clock positions on the penis; it is necessary for the needle to pierce the deep fascia, but great care should be taken that the needle does not lie in a blood vessel (see Fig. 21-18).

If the injection is made close to the pubic bone, the dorsal nerve is blocked before its posterior branches pass toward the undersurface of the penis. If the posterior branches are not blocked, the frenulum and undersurface of the penis will not be anesthetized,

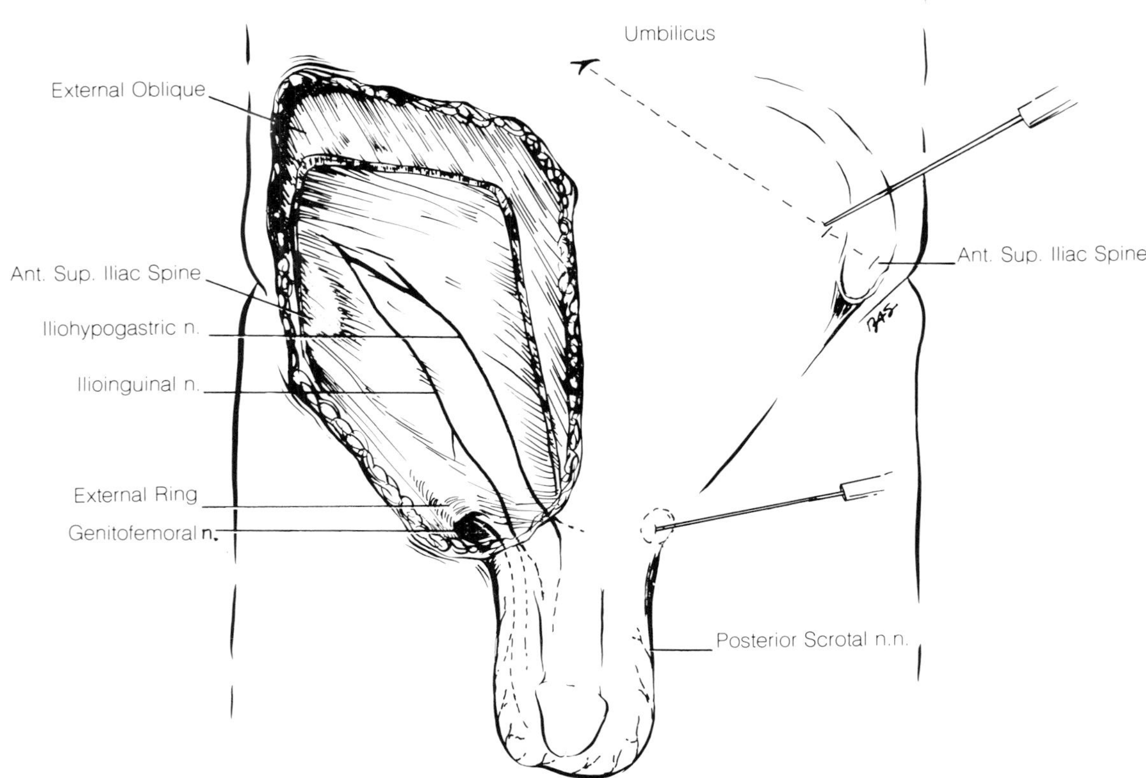

FIG. 19-5. Anatomy and needle insertion sites for anesthesia of the ilioinguinal and genitofemoral nerves.

and a separate injection will be required along the lateral surface of the penis.

If postoperative analgesia is required, 0.25% to 0.5% bupivacaine is used. Circumferential infiltration at the base of the penis is avoided and vasoconstrictors are not used for fear of causing ischemia. Also, great care should be taken not to use large needles, which may cause hematomas.

PLASTIC SURGERY OF THE ARM AND HAND

Brachial Plexus Block. The axillary technique of brachial plexus block is well suited to plastic surgical operations on the arm or hand (Fig. 10-7). This neural blockade technique is described in detail in Chapter 10. It should be stressed that it is a major plexus block requiring local anesthetic at doses close to toxic so that the knowledge, skill, and equipment to deal with local anesthetic toxicity is a prerequisite to its use (see Chap. 4).

Peripheral Nerve Blocks at the Elbow and Wrist. As described in Chapter 10, there is seldom any advantage in blocking the radial and median nerves at the elbow rather than at the wrist, where blockade is easily accomplished by the plastic surgeon after draping and skin preparation. Sometimes it is desirable to produce sensory blockade without significant motor blockade so that movement can be evaluated during tendon repair surgery. Experience has shown that motor block is difficult to avoid if adequate sensory block is achieved by axillary brachial block. In this situation individual branches of peripheral nerves can be blocked at the wrist, leaving long flexors intact. If the duration of the operation is kept brief and the patient is adequately premedicated, patients will tolerate the required arm tourniquet (see Chap. 10, Figs. 10-9 to 10-15).

Digital nerve block is perhaps one of the most useful techniques for minor plastic surgery on the digits. The various approaches are described in Chapter 10, Figure 10-16.

PLASTIC SURGERY ON THE LEG

A considerable improvement in efficacy of nerve blocks in the leg has resulted from use of nerve stimulators. Blocks at the level of pelvis, knee, ankle, and toes are described in Chapter 11.

Skin Graft with Infiltration or Nerve Block. Many skin grafting procedures are performed under general anesthesia in order to provide analgesia for the donor site on the thigh. Many years ago Hamilton Brailey described a simple procedure for obtaining skin from the thigh under the cover of a circumscribed "fence" of local anesthesia. The area of the thigh from which the graft is to be taken is marked as a rectangular area by an indelible marking pen or merely as an extra rectangle of preparation solution. This rectangular fence is then thoroughly infiltrated with 0.5% lidocaine or 0.25% bupivacaine. The latter is preferable because donor sites are often quite painful postoperatively. It is important that the area of infiltration is marked beforehand and that the graft be taken only from within this area. Alternatively, the technique of lateral femoral cutaneous nerve block extends the anesthetized area available for graft donation. This techniqus is described in Chapter 11 and Figure 11-8.

Procedures on the Foot with Ankle Block. Neural blockade of the individual nerves at the ankle is an easy technique that provides excellent operating conditions for foot surgery and superb postoperative analgesia. These techniques are described in Chapter 11 and Figure 11-11.

LIPOSUCTION

Patients having this procedure frequently wish to have fat removed from multiple areas (*e.g.*, thighs, abdomen). Thus the use of field blocks would involve a large dose of local anesthetic, even using a dilute solution. In this situation, an epidural block offers an attractive alternative to general anesthesia.

For more limited areas, such as one or both thighs, lateral femoral cutaneous nerve blocks and other nerve blocks of the thigh may be used (see Chap.11). It is also possible to use a"fence" of local anesthetic infiltrated around the entire area to receive liposuction.

ACUTE POST-TRAUMATIC PROCEDURES

A wide range of neural blockade techniques are applicable to repair of soft tissue trauma in various regions of the body. Particular mention should be made of the following:

For major lacerations of the scalp, circumferential infiltration above the level of the ears provides complete analgesia of the entire scalp (see Chap. 15 and Fig. 15-3).

For superficial injuries in the region of the eye, a combination of topical and nerve block techniques is often useful (see Chap. 17).

Repair of lacerations in the mouth, lips, and surrounding region lends itself to a considerable range of nerve block and infiltration techniques, which are common knowledge to dentists and oral surgeons but are too infrequently used by others. These techniques are described in Chapter 16.

A number of the alternative techniques for nerve block in head/neck, mouth, and eye are suitable for plastic surgery. These are described in detail in Chapters 15, 16, and 17.

In particular inferior mental nerve block deserves more frequent use; block of this nerve with 5 ml of local anesthetic provides anesthesia of one half of the lower jaw and its overlying mucous membrane, including the lower lip (see Fig. 16-18).

REFERENCES

1. Arndt, K.A., Burton, C., and Noe, J.M.: Minimizing the pain of local anesthesia. Plast. Reconstr. Surg., *72*:676, 1983.
2. Aukburg, S.J.: Monitor selection—a physician's perspective. Int. Anesth. Res. Soc. Rev. Course Lectures. p. 17. 1985.
3. Avery, G.S. (ed.): Principles and Practice of Clinical Pharmacology and Therapeutics. Sydney, ADIS Press, 1976.
4. Balmer, H.G.R., and Wyte, S.R.: Antagonism of ketamine with physostigmine. Br. J. Anaesth., *49*:510, 1977.
5. Black, D.A.K.: The present status of presymptomatic screening. Proc. R. Soc. Med., *59*:1223, 1966.
6. Boyle, P., and Parbrook, G.D.: The interrelation of personality and post operative factors. Br. J. Anaesth., *49*:259, 1977.
7. Brophy, T., Dundee, J.W., Hazelwood, V., Kaware, P., Varghese, A., and Ward, M.: Midazolam, a water soluble benzodiazepine, for gastroscopy. Anesth. Intens. Care, *10*:344, 1982.
8. Bruce, I.S.: *In* Knight, P.F., and Burgess, C.G. (eds.): Postoperative Use of Diazepam, p. 89. Bristol, Wright, 1968.
9. Buffington, C.W., Buchler, P.K., Glauber, D.T., Hornbein, T.F., and Hamacher, E.N.: A new system of infiltration anes-

thesia and sedation for plastic surgery. Plast. Reconstr. Surg., *74*:671, 1984.
10. Cassileth, B.R., Zupkis, R.V., Sutton-Smith, K., and March, V.: Why are goals imperfectly realized? N. Engl. J. Med., *302*:896, 1980.
11. Cremonesi, E., and Bairao, G.S.: Farmacologia da ketamina: Mecanismo da hipertensa arterial. Rev. Hosp. Clin. Fac. Med. (Sao Paulo), *28*:3, 1973.
12. Cullen, S.C.: What price tranquillization? Anesthesiology, *20*:697, 1959.
13. Cunningham, B.L., and McKinney, P.: Patient acceptance of dissociative anesthetics. Plast. Reconstr. Surg., *72*:22, 1983.
14. de Bass, F.W.J.: A preanesthesia screening system. Anaesthesia, *27*:217, 1972.
15. de Jong, R.H., and Bonica, J.D.: Mixtures of local anesthetics are no more toxic than the parent drugs. Anesthesiology, *54*:177, 1981.
16. Derrick, W.S., Wette, R., and Hill, D.B.: Librium in the recovery room. Anesth. Analg. (Cleve.), *46*:171, 1967.
17. Dicker, R.L., and Syracuse, U.K.: Local anesthesia in facial plastic surgery. Otolaryngology, *86*:461, 1978.
18. Dundee, J.W., and Haslett, W.H.K.: The benzodiazepines—A review of their actions and uses relative to anesthetic practice. Br. J. Anaesth., *42*:217, 1970.
19. Dundee, J.W., Gample, J.A.S., and Assaf, R.A.E.: Influence of the model of administration of the action of diazepam (Valium). IV European Congress of Anaesthesiology, September 5–11, Madrid. Excerpta Medica, *330*:194, 1974.
20. Egbert, L.D., Battit, G.E., Welch, C.E., and Bartlett, M.K.: Reduction of postoperative pain by encouragement and instruction of patients. A study of doctor–patient rapport. N. Engl. J. Med., *270*:823, 1964.
21. Ellis, F.R., and Wilson, J.: An assessment of droperidol as a premedicant. Br. J. Anaesth., *44*:1288, 1972.
22. Farr, R.E.: Practical local anesthesia and Its Surgical Technic. London, Henry Kimpton, 1923.
23. Flomenbaum, N.: Self-administered nitrous oxide: An adjunct analgesic. J. Am. Coll. Emerg. Phys., *8*:95, 1979.
24. Gibbs, L., Svigals, R.E., and Riklan, M.: A double-blind study of chlordiazepoxide as a preanesthetic agent in cardiac surgery. Anesth. Analg. (Cleve.), *50*:17, 1971.
25. Goin, J.M., and Goin, M. Kroft.: Local anesthesia, intravenous sedation, and intraoperative psychological reactions. *In* Goin, J.M., and Goin, M. Kroft (eds.): Changing the Body: Psychological Effects of Plastic Surgery. Baltimore, Williams & Wilkins, 1981.
26. Gordon, H.L.: Drugs for outpatient surgery. *In* Regnault, P., and Daniel, R.K. (eds.): Plastic Surgery: Principles and Techniques. Boston, Little, Brown, 1984.
27. Gourlay, G.K., and Cousins, M.J.: Strong analgesics in severe pain. Drugs, *28*:79, 1984.
28. Gravenstein, J.S.: Preanesthetic medication. Pharmacol. Phys., *3*:1, 1969.
29. Greenblatt, D.J., and Koch, Weser, J.: Intramuscular injection of drugs. N. Engl. J. Med., *295*:542, 1976.
30. Grubb, W.C.: A concentration of 1:500,000 epinephrine in a local anesthetic solution is sufficient to provide excellent hemostasis. Plast. Reconstr. Surg., *63*:834, 1979.
31. Hirshowitz, B., and Eliachar, I.: Effective haemostasis with local anesthesia in nasal surgery. Br. J. Plast. Surg., *25*:335, 1972.
32. Hollister, L.E.: Tranquillity—at a price. Clin. Pharm. Exp. Ther., *6*:417, 1965.
33. Houle, G.: Practical considerations in regional anaesthesia. Can. Anaesth. Soc. J., *32*:547, 1985.
34. Huang, T.T., Rejaie, I., and Lewis, S.R.: Relative hypoxemia during rhytidoplasty. Plast. Reconstr. Surg., *58*:32, 1976.
35. Imhof, P.R., Blatter, K., Fuccella, L.M., and Turri, M.: Beta-blockade and emotional tachycardia, radiotelemetric investigations in ski jumpers. J. Appl. Physiol., *27*:366, 1969.
36. Innes, I.R., and Nickerson, M.: Drugs acting on postganglionic adrenergic nerve endings and structures innervated by them. (sympathomimetic drugs) *In* Goodman, L.S., and Gilman, A. (eds.): The Pharmacological Basis of Therapeutics, 4th ed., pp. 478. New York, Macmillan, 1970.
37. Jaffe, J.H.: Narcotic analgesics. *In* Goodman, L.S., and Gilman, A. (eds.): The Pharmacological Basis of Therapeutics, 4th ed., pp. 237. New York, Macmillan, 1970.
38. Johnson, M., and Carpenter, L.: Relationship between preoperative anxiety and postoperative state. Psychol. Med., *10*:361, 1980.
39. Kirkendall, W.N., Feinleib, M., Freis, E.D., and Mark, A.L.: Recommendations for human blood pressure determination by sphygmomanometers. Circulation, *62*:1145A, 1980.
40. Knill, R.L.: Evaluation of arterial oxygenation during anaesthesia. Can. Anaesth. Soc. J., *32*:516, 1985.
41. Korttila, K., and Linnoila, M.: Absorption and sedative effects of diazepam after oral administration and intramuscular administration into the vastus lateralis muscle and deltoid muscle. Br. J. Anaesth., *47*:857, 1975.
42. Kraut, R.A.: Continuous transcutaneous O_2 and CO_2 monitoring during conscious sedation for oral surgery. J. Oral Maxillofac. Surg., *42*:489, 1985.
43. Kuzin, M.I., and Kharnas, S.Sh.: Local Anesthesia. p. 116. Moscow, Mir Publishers, 1983.
43a. Labat, G.: Operations on the Thorax. In Regional Anesthesia: Its Technique and Clinical Application, pp 339–347. Philadelphia, W.B. Saunders, 1922.
44. Leonards, J.R.: Are all aspirins alike? Aust. N.Z. J. Med., *6*:8, 1976.
45. Levin, N.: Monitoring the patient under local anesthesia. *In* Courtiss, E.H. (ed.): Anesthetic Surgery Trouble: How to Avoid It and How to Treat It. p. 25. St. Louis, C.V. Mosby, 1978.
46. Ley, P.: Satisfactory compliance and communication. Br. J. Clin. Psychol., *21*:241, 1982.
47. Lynch, S.: Anesthesia. *In* Rees, T.D. (ed.): Anesthetic Plastic Surgery. Philadelphia, W.B. Saunders, 1980.
48. McColl, I., Drinkwater, J.E., Hulme-Moir, I., and Donnan, S.B.: Prediction of success or failure of gastric surgery. Br. J. Surg., *58*:768, 1971.
49. McDowell, A.J., and Whitlaw, D.R.: Reversible titration deep sedation for major office surgery. Plast. Reconstr. Surg., *59*:21, 1977.
50. McNabb, T.G., and Goldwyn, R.M.: Blood gas and hemodynamic effects of sedatives and analgesics when used as a

supplement to local anesthesia in plastic surgery. Plast. Reconstr. Surg., *58*:37, 1976.

51. McNaught, Inglis, J., and Barrow, M.E.H.: Premedication—a reassessment. Proc. R. Soc. Med., *58*:29, 1965.
52. Magnusson, J.: Narcotic antagonism by naloxone. Few side effects after a short procedure? Anaesthesia, *38*:103, 1983,
53. Martinez-Urrutia, A.: Anxiety and pain in surgical patients. J. Consult. Clin. Psychol., *43*:437, 1975.
54. Mattila, M., Carni, H.M., Nummi, S.E., et al.: Effect of diazepam on emergence from ketamine anesthesia: A double-blind study. Anaesthetist, *28*:20, 1979.
55. Miller, E.D., Jr.: Perioperative hypertension. Can. Anaesth. Soc. J., *32*:542, 1985.
56. Miller, S.H., Buck, M.M., Woodward, W.R., and Dermuth, R.J.: Alterations in local blood flow, tissue gas tension by epinephrine. Plast. Reconstr. Surg., *73*:797, 1984.
57. Mintz, G.S..: Newer applications of organic nitrate vasodilator therapy. Drug Ther., December 5, 1976.
58. Moertel, C.G.: Relief of pain with oral medications. Aust. NZ. J. Med., *6*:1, 1979.
59. Moore, D.C., Bridenbaugh, L.D., Bridenbaugh, P.O., Thompson, G.E., and Tucker, G.T.: Does compounding of local anesthetic agents increase their toxicity in humans? Anesth. Analg., *51*:579, 1972.
60. Nickerson, M.: Drug therapy of shock. *In* Bock, K.D. (ed.): Shock, Pathogenesis and Therapy. Heidelberg, Springer-Verlag, 1962.
61. Obi, L.J.: Oranges, lemons and persimmons—the ketamine question. Plast. Reconstr. Surg., *4*:527, 1980.
62. Palazzo, M.G.A., and Strunin, L.: Anaesthesia and emesis. II. Prevention and management. Can. Anaesth. Soc. J., *31*:407, 1984.
63. Pandit, S.K.: Low dose intravenous infusion technique with ketamine. Anaesthesia, *35*:669, 1980.
64. Parkhouse, J., Lambrechts, W., and Simpson, B.R.: The incidence of postoperative pain. Br. J. Anaesth., *33*:345, 1961.
65. Peck, C.L.: Psychological factors in acute pain management. *In* Cousins, M.J., and Phillips, G.D. (eds.): Acute Pain Management, pp 251-274. New York, Churchill Livingstone, 1984.
66. Pitts, F.N., and Allen, R.E.: Beta-adrenergic blockade in the treatment of anxiety. *In* Mathew, R.J. (ed.): The Biology of Anxiety. p. 134. New York, Brunnel-Mazel, 1982.
67. Richards, D.G., McPherson, J.J., Evans, K.T., and Rosen, M.: Effect of volume of water taken with diazepam tablets on absorption. Br. J. Anaesth., *58*:41, 1986.
68. Riding, J.E.: Post-operative vomiting. Proc. R. Soc. Med., *53*:671, 1960.
69. Robbins, J.A., and Mushlin, A.I.: Preoperative evaluation of the healthy patient. Med. Clin. North Am., *63*;1145, 1969.
70. Roberts, D.H., and Sowray, J.H.: Local Analgesia in Dentistry. Bristol, John Wright & Sons, 1979.
71. Roberts, M.T.S.: Anesthesia for the geriatric patient. Drugs, *11*:200, 1976.
72. Roizen, M.F.: Routine preoperative evaluation. *In* Miller, R.D. (ed.): Anesthesia. p. 3. New York, Churchill Livingstone, 1981.
73. Scott, D.L., and Holbrook, L.A.: Hypnotic psychotherapy and cosmetic surgery. Br. J. Plast. Surg., *34*:478, 1981.
74. Scott, W.A.C.: Haemodynamic monitoring: Measurement of systemic blood pressure. Can. Anaesth. Soc. J., *32*:294, 1985.
75. Seow, L.T., Lips, F.J., Cousins, M.J., and Mather, L.E.: Lidocaine and bupivacaine mixtures for epidural blockade. Anesthesiology, *56*:177, 1982.
76. Simmons, R.L.: The office surgical suite: Pros and cons. Otolaryngol. Clin. North Am., *13*:391, 1980.
77. Sklar, G.S., Zukin, S.R., and Reilly, T.A.: Adverse reactions to ketamine anesthesia. Abolition by a psychological technique. Anaesthesia, *36*:183, 1981.
78. Small, E.W.: Preoperative sedation in dentistry. Dent. Clin. North Am., *3*:1, 1969.
79. Snyder, G.B.: Transdermal scopolamine. Plast. Reconstr. Surg., *74*:729, 1985.
80. Taggart, P., Carruthers M., and Somerville, W.: Electrocardiogram, plasma catecholamines and lipids, and their modification by oxprenolol when speaking before an audience. Lancet, *2*:341, 1973.

80a. Takeshima, R., Dohi, S.: Cervical epidural anesthesia and surgical blood loss in radical mastectomy. Reg. Anaesth., *11*:171, 1986.

81. Taylor, J.E.: Hospital patient behavior: Reactance, helplessness or control? J. Soc. Issues, *35*:156, 1979.
82. Thomas, D.V.: Pain of skin infiltration with local anesthetics. Anesth. Intens. Care, *13*:101, 1984.
83. Tucker, K.R., and Virnelli, F.R.: The use of hypnosis as a tool in plastic surgery. Plast. Reconstr. Surg., *76*:140, 1985.
84. Vance, J.P., Neill, R.S., and Norris, W.: The incidence of and aetiology of post-operative nausea and vomiting in a plastic surgery unit. Br. J. Plast. Surg., *26*:336, 1973.
85. Vinnik, C.A.: An intravenous dissociation technique for outpatient plastic surgery. Tranquility in the office surgical facility. Plast. Reconstr. Surg., *67*:799, 1981.
86. Vinnik, C.A.: Letter to the Editor. Plast. Reconstr. Surg., *69*:1028, 1982.
87. Wallace, P.G.M., and Norris, W.: The management of postoperative pain. Br. J. Anaesth., *47*:113, 1975.
88. Wassenaar, W., Lancee, W.J., Galloon, S., and Gale, G.D.: The measurement of anxiety in the pre-surgical patient. Br. J. Anaesth., *49*:605, 1977.
89. Weimer, R.D.: Epinephrine pain with local anesthesia. Plast. Reconstr. Surg., *73*:997, 1984.
90. Weisbrod, R.L.: Audio analgesia revisited. Anaesthesia Prog., *16*:8,1969.
91. Wightman, M.A., and Vaughan, R.W.: Comparison of compounds used for intradermal anesthesia. Anesthesiology, *45*:687, 1976.
92. Wilson, J.F.: Behavioral preparation for surgery: Benefit or harm? J. Behav. Med., *4*:79, 1981.
93. Wynands, J.E.: Haemodynamic monitoring: Cardiovascular system function. Can. Anaesth. Soc. J., *32*:288, 1985.
94. Yelderman, M., and New, W., Jr.: Evaluation of pulse oximetry. Anesthesiology, *59*:349, 1983.

20 NEURAL BLOCKADE FOR OUTPATIENTS

L. DONALD BRIDENBAUGH

Although many medical centers, particularly in the United States, will perform 30% to 40% of surgical procedures on an outpatient basis, either in special ambulatory care centers, emergency rooms, or physicians' offices, it is important that anesthesiologists keep a proper perspective when selecting regional anesthesia as the anesthetic technique. The efficacy of the technique as applied to the usual circumstances for inpatients should be foremost in the anesthetic selection and the fact that the surgery is being done on an outpatient basis used as a final consideration. Compared to a fully equipped operating room, the outpatient clinic, emergency room, or private office is often rather primitive, and local infiltration may be the only logical anesthetic choice. Specific peripheral nerve blocks would be appropriate and have a definite advantage if the physician was capable of performing them. Unfortunately, because of the apparent simplicity of the method and the equipment required, many physicians working in these areas do not even have available resuscitation equipment or personnel who can use that equipment should a complication occur. This practice should never be condoned. The same equipment and personnel necessary for a similar procedure on an inpatient should always be available for procedures performed on the outpatient.

Regional block with its selective local action and simple equipment can offer an excellent anesthetic choice in an outpatient facility. However, the techniques are not universally appropriate, and proper selection of patients, procedures, and surgeons is essential for success of the method.

PATIENT SELECTION

Although patients considered eligible for outpatient surgery are usually suitable candidates for almost any type of anesthesia, the use of a neural block technique requires more patient acceptance, cooperation, and understanding than is needed for a general anesthetic. An extremely apprehensive or reluctant patient is likely to require sufficient supplemental sedation so as to negate the relative advantage of the block technique. Cooperation and understanding by the patient are necessary if an operation is to be performed solely under local anesthesia. He must be willing to undergo surgery while awake and submit to the slight discomfort of the application of the regional block. As compensation, the advantage of somewhat less rigid rules on fasting and probably less need for preoperative laboratory tests is obtained. In addition, the hazards of unconsciousness during general anesthesia, some of the sequelae such as nausea, vomiting, aspiration, or the physiologic upsets are avoided.

Without regard to the anesthetic technique to be used, some important general principles or requirements have evolved as experience with outpatient surgery has become more commonplace.

Most outpatients will be of physical status ASA I or II, which will allow them to be safely dismissed to their home, and many institutions will limit procedures only to ASA physical status I or II patients. However, an indication for a regional block anesthetic may be the poor-risk patient (ASA physical status III or IV). If the surgical procedure *per se* does not require hospitalization, there is no reason that it cannot be performed under neural blockade anesthesia on an outpatient basis no matter what the patient's physical status. If the medical condition is stable and the surgical procedure does not change the medical problems that the patient was managing at home before surgery, then certainly he can continue to be managed at home after the surgery and recovery from anesthesia.

Patients will usually accept the decision to use local anesthesia, but a few are terrified by the thought of being awake during the procedure. It may be wise to reject these patients as candidates for regional block because, apart from upsetting the patient, it is highly likely that the technique will prove to be a failure. How often this kind of patient is met will vary according to national and local tradition and, most important, local reputation. In countries where anesthesiology is not a specialty in its own right, local analgesia has been used extensively and with great skill to avoid the complications that follow poorly conducted general anesthesia. Conversely, in some countries, general anesthesia has been administered by specialists, only a few of whom have bothered to learn regional blocks.

To encourage the most extensive use of regional anesthesia, the public must be educated. Because patients learn quickly from the experience of others, the best way to introduce regional anesthesia as an accepted procedure is to make certain that no patient is forced to submit to a painful operation because of an inadequate regional block.

Small children cannot be expected to cooperate and should not be treated under local anesthesia without appropriate supplemental sedation. The age at which children can tolerate local anesthesia will vary individually and with the ability of the physician to gain the confidence of the child.

Some patients with anatomic abnormalities or who are very obese may produce technical difficulties in performing the blocks. Discretion is the better part of valor. Perhaps these patients should be rejected as candidates for a regional block procedure.

SURGEON AND ANESTHETIST

Skill and patience are the primary requirements for physicians involved in the surgical procedure to be performed on outpatients under neural blockade anesthesia. The surgeon must be supportive of regional techniques, both in preoperative discussion with the patient and during intraoperative management of the procedure. The surgeon must occasionally be willing to wait a few minutes for the block to "set up." He must also conduct the surgery gently, realizing that the patient may perceive pressure as pain. Surgeons who are convinced of the advantages of nerve block anesthetics in providing greater alertness, less risk, and earlier recovery for their patients are willing to tolerate occasional inconveniences and may even suggest regional analgesia to their patients.

The anesthesiologist must also demonstrate skill and patience. Skill can be acquired and maintained only if the physician is sufficiently interested in regional blocks to undergo a period of training that involves considerable practice. Even for an expert, a successful block will not be obtained in all cases, and the beginner must certainly expect a number of failures. Thus it is recommended that the necessary experience be acquired by performing regional blocks as supplementary analgesia in patients for whom general anesthesia is part of the inpatient routine. The anatomy of landmarks can be learned from a textbook, but experience can be gained only by repeated administration. Patience is mandatory because a block may take as long as 30 minutes to perform and become completely effective. No surgery must ever be performed until the effect of the block has been tested.

SELECTION OF TECHNIQUE

Because the morbidity of surgery and anesthesia increases with time, it has been advised that outpatient procedures be restricted to those of less than 2 hours' duration. However, a peripheral nerve block with a long-acting local anesthetic drug frequently negates this problem and allows prolonged procedures such as plastics or orthopedics to be performed on an outpatient basis.

Many physicians using local anesthesia in their offices or emergency centers frequently ignore the inpatient concerns for n.p.o. status or the necessity for an appropriate physical workup or laboratory work. This again is not to be condoned. Surgical or anesthetic complications can and do occur in simple procedures under local anesthesia. Individuals practicing on an outpatient basis must be prepared to treat and legally defend any complication. (Treatment of reactions to local anesthetic drugs is discussed in Chapter 4).

The preparation and supervision of the patient for an outpatient procedure should include a written record that contains a short history with special attention given to previous experiences with local anesthetic drugs. If a reaction to a local anesthetic drug has occurred, its nature must be explored.

Most patients are more nervous than they will admit, and the attitude of the medical personnel is of enormous psychological importance in relieving this anxiety. Some patients will benefit from a pharmacologic sedative; however, this may lead to lack of cooperation, and the result is a patient who requires prolonged supervision and may be unfit to go home. Although rapport, gentleness, and skill in performing the block usually make premedication unnecessary, preoperative sedation for regional anesthesia may be appropriate. Midazolam 1 to 2 mg, or diazepam, 2.5 to 10 mg, is an effective anxiolytic that may be useful if given orally with sips of water. Administered intravenously, immediately before performing the block, diazepam may cause painful irritation to the vein. This, plus its amnesic effect, can limit its usefulness. The short-acting narcotic fentanyl, in 50 to 100 μg doses, is ideal for outpatient use because it attenuates patient discomfort associated with the performance of the blocks or eliciting of a paresthesia but does not abolish patient cooperation. We have not seen clinically significant respiratory depression with these doses. Currently some of the ambulatory care centers are testing the use of beta-blocking drugs, for example, 10 to 20 mg of propranolol, as "premedication" for relieving the anxiety associated with nerve block techniques (see Chap. 6).

Patients scheduled in advance for minor surgery under neural blockade should still be advised to have only a light meal or take nothing by mouth no later than 4 hours before the procedure. Although all patients treated for emergencies are, on principle, assumed to have a full stomach, if regional block can be used, there is no reason to subject them to the ordeal of manipulations with the stomach tube. Some of the patients who come to the emergency room will be under the influence of alcohol, which in itself is no contraindication to regional block. The decision for a regional block is solely a matter of the patient's desire, and ability to cooperate.

Ideally, all patients should have vital signs measured and recorded from the moment the block is started. But since local infiltration and peripheral neural blockade normally will not interfere with the physical or mental condition of a patient, under certain circumstances it may be permissible to observe only the following basic requirements:

1. A patient must never be left alone.
2. Regular verbal contact with the patient must be maintained to ensure consciousness and comfort.
3. Whether every patient receiving a nerve block should have an intravenous needle in place as well as oscilloscopic monitoring of the heart is a matter of physician judgment and would depend on the amount of local anesthetic drugs, the site injected, technique, and the patient's physical status.
4. Pulse and blood pressure should be measured and recorded before starting the block and then as clinically indicated.
5. Resuscitation equipment and knowledgeable, helpful personnel must be available to treat a complication in the event that it does occur.

LOCAL ANESTHETIC DRUGS

In choosing the appropriate anesthetic drug for outpatient regional nerve block anesthesia, duration of action is the primary criterion. Procaine and 2-chloroprocaine are the briefest in action, but these ester-linked compounds are associated with potential allergenic sensitivity. Procaine is adequate for local infiltration but in standard concentrations (0.5–2.0%) may produce unreliable peridural anesthesia. 2-Chloroprocaine is contraindicated for intravenous regional block because of possible resultant phlebitis.[3] Neurologic damage on accidental subarachnoid injection of 2-chloroprocaine has been reported.[9] Therefore, although their short duration of action is desirable, the usefulness of these local anesthetic esters may be limited.

The intermediate-acting amide anesthetics lidocaine, mepivacaine, and prilocaine appear to be safer and more reliable in the usual clinical doses and do not unduly prolong recovery if epinephrine is not administered concomitantly. The risk of undesirably rapid systemic absorption must be considered when deleting the customary 1:200,000 concentration of epinephrine from local anesthetic solutions. Doses of prilocaine in excess of 500 mg are best avoided because of ensuing methemoglobinemia.[4] For peridural anesthesia, 2% lidocaine, 2% prilocaine, and 1.5% mepivacaine are useful, whereas lower concentrations are more appropriate for peripheral nerve blockade. Bupivacaine, tetracaine, and etidocaine generally have little use in outpatient surgery because of their long duration of action; however, as previously mentioned, they can be very useful in providing prolonged postoperative analgesia when used for wound infiltration or arm blocks. The local anesthetic drugs are discussed in detail in Chapter 4. No matter which drug is chosen, one basic principle is imperative and generally accepted: Only the smallest volume of the local anesthetic drug in a solution of the lowest possible concentration that will give the desired effect should be used.

NEURAL BLOCKADE TECHNIQUES

The specific details and diagrams for performing the various nerve blocks are found in other chapters in *Neural Blockade* and should be referred to by individuals unfamiliar with a certain technique.

Of the block techniques suitable for outpatient application, local infiltration of the site of surgery is the safest and simplest. Intracutaneous and subcutaneous infiltration with a suitable dilute concentration (0.5% or 1%) of an intermediate-acting anesthetic drug is sufficient for removal of superficial scars or lesions. An expansion of this technique is the "field block" by subcutaneous infiltration blocking of nerves that supply a particular area. This is most commonly used for hernia blocks, penile blocks for circumcisions, or breast blocks for excision of breast lumps. This procedure is usually performed by the surgeon and provides good postoperative analgesia as well as good operative anesthesia. The addition of epinephrine can be helpful in obtaining hemostasis, although it is not indicated in procedures on the digits or penis.

For the anesthesiologist, the simplest and most reliable anesthesia is the intravenous regional technique usually ascribed to August Bier. It is suitable for most superficial surgical procedures on extremities that take less than 90 minutes to perform (the limiting factor being tourniquet time). The major hazard of this technique is the accidental or premature release of the tourniquet or inadequate tourniquet pressure with resulting excessive blood levels of the local anesthetic drug. Close monitoring is essential, and two-stage release of the tourniquet is required if tourniquet time is less than 40 minutes. It is recommended that the tourniquet pressure be at least 100 mm Hg above the patient's normal systolic pressure if leakage of the local anesthetic drug under the tourniquet into the systemic circulation is to be prevented.[5]

This technique is obviously unsuitable when a tourniquet is contraindicated, as in amputations or vascular access procedures. It is useful for excision of neuromas, release of carpal tunnel compression, and other orthopedic and general procedures (see Chap. 12).

If more profound, deep anesthesia of the upper extremity is required, regional block of the brachial plexus is favored. The plexus can be approached in the interscalene groove, as it crosses the first rib, or in the axilla. Each technique has its advantages and proponents. The supraclavicular and interscalene approaches are usually avoided in outpatients because of the small but disabling incidence of pneumothorax. The axillary approach provides good anesthesia to the forearm, as long as care is taken to block the musculocutaneous nerve by infiltration.

The main problem of the axillary block for outpatient surgery is that it may take 15 to 20 minutes to achieve surgical levels of anesthesia. The major hazard of this technique is unintentional intravascular injection. The details for performing these techniques are all described in Chapter 10.

Unilateral or bilateral intercostal nerve blocks are ideally suited for surgical procedures of the abdomen and chest wall. This procedure does involve a small risk of pneumothorax but does not limit ambulation or function and does not create the sympathetic blockade seen with central (peridural or spinal) blocks. Early ambulation and discharge make this a particularly effective choice for outpatients.

In the leg, any combination of sciatic, femoral, lateral femoral cutaneous, and obturator nerve blocks is possible for lengthy and involved procedures. These blocks are particularly appropriate anesthesia for fractures and dislocations of the ankle or distal leg. Use of regional anesthesia for surgery on the foot, recently reviewed and described by McCutcheon and Schurman,[6,11] is especially valuable for procedures on the sole of the foot such as cuts, foreign bodies, and plantar warts because this is a very sensitive area but tough and difficult to infiltrate locally. Posterior tibial nerve block at the ankle is one of the most rewarding and easy to perform. It is preferable to perform the posterior tibial block on patients in the prone position so that they cannot kick away from the needle when parasthesias are elicited; also, the sural nerve can conveniently be blocked at the same time by a wheal from the lateral border of the Achilles tendon to the lateral malleolus. It is usually easier to perform surgery on the sole of the foot with the patient in the prone position.

A midcalf tourniquet, if properly applied, is well tolerated by most patients for at least 30 minutes; this is essential for the removal of foreign bodies from the sole of the foot.

A femoral nerve block yields almost total analgesia to the patient with a fractured shaft of the femur, so that it may be of value for pain relief while the patient is awaiting more definitive therapy in an emergency room.[1] A lateral femoral cutaneous nerve block frequently is the technique of choice for obtaining analgesia for taking the skin for minor skin grafts.

Although spinal anesthesia and epidural anesthesia may negate some of the advantages of a regional technique, that is, early ambulation, lack of general physiologic effects, and minimal potential complications, they are the simplest and most reliable of the regional techniques. Spinal (subarachnoid block) using 50 to 75 mg of 5% lidocaine diluted with CSF or a standard 6 to 10 mg tetracaine without epinephrine can provide from 30 to 60 minutes of rapid and dense perineal, leg, or lower abdominal anesthesia. A major limitation of spinal anesthesia has been the incidence of postlumbar puncture headache, which approaches 10% overall in outpatients but can be reduced to less than 1% by the use of a 25- or 26-gauge spinal needle and by restricting the technique to older patients. We have found that if a headache does occur, treatment with epidural blood patch on an outpatient basis is effective in remedying this complication without the need for a hospital admission.

In younger patients or in those in whom the potential for headache is unacceptably high or the patient's resistance to the technique, epidural anesthesia is a suitable alternative. Both caudal and lumbar epidural anesthesia are more difficult technically and slightly less reliable than subarachnoid block but have worked very successfully in our experience for perineal, lower extremity orthopedic, and gynecologic procedures. Lumbar epidural anesthesia is particularly effective for gynecologic laparoscopic procedures. This requires a modern Trendelenburg position to keep the nitrous oxide pneumoperitoneum in the pelvis, thereby reducing the incidence of shoulder pain caused by a diaphragmatic irritation. Although patients perceive difficulty with deep inspiration in this situation, no problem with clinical insufficiency has been demonstrated.[2]

Another application of epidural anesthesia is in the repair of inguinal or femoral hernias.[10] The surgeon may delay the onset of postoperative pain by supplementing the short-acting epidural anesthetic with wound infiltration with a long-acting local anesthetic drug, for example, 0.25% bupivacaine or 0.5% etidocaine at the end of surgery. This technique is preferable to reliance on a "hernia block" since the latter involves femoral nerve anesthesia, which may be prolonged and limit ambulation. Patients who have adequate surgical anesthesia with a combination of epidural and local infiltration may be discharged comfortably to their homes before postoperative pain begins.[12]

This discussion has covered only some of the commonly used techniques of regional anesthesia in outpatient surgery. In addition, there are multitudes of specialized blocks, such as the supraorbital or infraorbital nerve blocks, scalp blocks for procedures on the face, ear, and tongue, which are difficult to anesthetize locally, and superficial cervical plexus blocks for head and neck procedures. Many diagnostic and therapeutic nerve blocks for pain can be adapted for use in outpatients. The specific techniques for performing any of the individual nerve blocks are detailed in other sections of *Neural Blockade.* The use of regional anesthesia in outpatients is limited only by the imagination and ability of the anesthesiologists and the surgeons involved.

POSTOPERATIVE RECOVERY

Before discharge, the patient should recover sufficiently from anesthesia to approach his preoperative physical and mental status. This does not imply full recovery, particularly if a neural blockade technique has been used because the block will likely still be effective. If the patient is properly instructed, however, he can usually be sent home during this period. The risk of a delayed toxic reaction after 30 minutes decreases rapidly and is very remote after 1 hour. Careful instruction must be given in order to avoid injury, and the patient must be provided with an appropriate sling or protection for the numb extremity or anesthetized area. Those who have received epidural or spinal block must have full recovery of motor function before discharge. If all sensory anesthesia has regressed, particularly with a full return of perineal sensation, then sympathetic blockade and orthostatic hypotension should not be a problem on ambulation.[8] Because most of the patients who have had regional block anesthesia have had minimal premedication or sedation, they spend a shorter time in the postoperative recovery unit than those having general anesthesia. Studies conducted in an ambulatory surgery unit comparing the recovery time and complications of general anesthesia and the various local anesthetic drugs available for epidural anesthesia when used for outpatient laparoscopies demonstrated a significant advantage for this type of anesthesia in our surgery.[2,7]

When the effects of the neural blockade wear off, the patient may need an analgesic, which should be prescribed as part of the postoperative care. It is well worth stressing that a very effective analgesic for operations on extremities is provided by elevation and immobilization. If narcotics are demanded urgently by a patient in the immediate postoperative period, the possibility of a complication should be considered because minor surgical procedures normally will not be followed by severe pain. The requirements for postoperative analgesics will depend on the nature of the surgery and the needs of the patient. It does not depend on whether the patient has undergone surgery as an outpatient or an inpatient.

There are several approaches to the problem of postoperative pain. For example, as mentioned, a field block or local infiltration of the wound at the termination of surgery can be accomplished with a long-acting local anesthetic drug, which will allow a fairly long postoperative period of analgesia while the patient is recovering. This is especially effective in pediatric patients. Research is being done today on the use of transcutaneous nerve stimulators to reduce the amount of postoperative pain and thereby reduce the need for medication. Fentanyl can be effective for short-term pain. Most pain can be alleviated by aspirin, percocet, or mild oral analgesics.

In most institutions in which procedures are being performed on outpatients, patients are provided with a form that warns of possible sequelae, a brief instruction sheet on preoperative care, appointments with the responsible physician, and advice about food or drink. The form emphasizes the need for patients to be accompanied by a responsible adult, not only to and from the surgical center, but at home for the first 24 hours. Any other relevant information can also be given at that time. A similar instruction sheet is given to the patient on discharge from the outpatient facility.

SUMMARY

At present, about one third of the surgical procedures in the United States are either being performed or could be performed on an outpatient basis. The principles of anesthetic management for outpatients are the same as those for inpatients, bearing in mind that most of the procedures will be short, the surgical procedure itself should not necessitate postoperative hospitalization, and the operating facilities may be limited—all making neural blockade an excellent anesthetic choice. The customary modifications that have been made for anesthetic management of the outpatient under neural blockade include [1] the selection of patients, surgeons, and anesthetists qualified and motivated toward nerve block anesthesia; [2] written preoperative instructions and information to all patients because of the short period available for evaluation amd rapport; [3] little or no preanesthetic medication; [4] use of regional block anesthetic techniques wherever possible, including the infiltration of the wound with a long-acting local anesthetic drug to decrease the need for postoperative narcotics; [5] written postoperative instructions and a method for telephone or return follow-up on discharge; and [6] no limitation as to the ASA physical status of the patients or the techniques of anesthesia.

If the above considerations are followed, the use of neural blockade in outpatients will be a most satisfying experience.

REFERENCES

1. Berry, F.R.: Analgesia in patients with fractured shaft of femur. Anaesthesia, *32*:576, 1977.
2. Bridenbaugh, L.D., and Soderstrom, R.M.: Lumbar epidural block anesthesia for outpatient laparoscopy. J. Reprod. Med., *23*:85, 1979.
3. Harris, W.H.: Choice of anesthetic agents for intravenous regional anesthesia. Acta Anaesthesiol. Scand., *36*(Suppl.):47, 1969.
4. Hjelm, M., and Holmdahl, M.H.: Clinical chemistry of prilocaine and clinical evaluation of methaemoglobinaemia induced by this agent. Acta Anaesthesiol. Scand., *16*(Suppl.):161, 1965.
5. Lawes, E.G., Johnson, T., Pritchard, P., and Robbins, P.: Venous pressures during simulated Bier's block. Anaesthesia, *39*:149, 1984.
6. McCutcheon, R.: Regional anesthesia of the foot. Can. Anaesth Soc. J., *12*:465, 1965.
7. Mulroy, M.F., and Bridenbaugh, L.D.: Regional anesthetic techniques for outpatient surgery. Int. Anesthesiol. Clin., *20*:71, 1982.
8. Pflug, A.E., Aasheim, G.M., and Fosler, C.: Sequence of return of neurological function and criteria for safe ambulation following subarachnoid block. Can. Anaesth. Soc. J., *25*(2):133, 1978.
9. Ravendran, R.S., *et al.*: Prolonged neural blockade following regional analgesia with 2-chloroprocaine. Anesth. Analg. (Cleve.), *59*:447, 1980.
10. Ryan, J.A., Adye, B.A., Jolly, P.C., and Mulroy, M.F.: Outpatient inguinal herniorrhaphy with both regional and local anesthesia. Am. J. Surg., *1948*(3):313, 1984.
11. Schurman, D.J.: Ankle block anesthesia for foot surgery. Anesthesiology, *44*:348, 1976.
12. Thompson, G.E.: Celiac plexus, intercostal, and minor peripheral blockade. In Cousins, M.J., and Bridenbaugh, P.O. (eds.): Neural Blockade in Clinical Anesthesia and Management of Pain, pp. 384–404. Philadelphia, J. B. Lippincott, 1980.

21 NEURAL BLOCKADE FOR PEDIATRIC SURGERY

T. C. KESTER BROWN
OTTO SCHULTE-STEINBERG

Local anesthesia has been used in pediatric surgery since at least 1900 when Bainbridge reported on spinal anesthesia in children.[7] Reports on the use of regional and local nerve block techniques in children were sporadic until relatively recently. A number of factors have led to the rapid increase in interest in regional anesthesia in children during the past 10 to 15 years, including the advent of newer long-acting local anesthetics, an increasing awareness of the inadequacies of the methods used for postoperative analgesia, and the toxicity problems with some of the inhalational agents. Additional factors in the neonate include the relative sensitivity to *d*-tubocurarine and problems with airway maintenance and ventilation in the newborn by anesthesiologists not experienced in this field. Although over 1000 spinal anesthetics were given to children in Montreal between 1940 and 1947[62] and its use had been reported in Toronto in 1933[54] and in England in 1934,[31] the current wave of interest in regional anesthesia seems to have stemmed from the increasing use of caudal anesthesia, particularly for circumcision.[42,64,105]

GENERAL CONSIDERATIONS

Children vary in size, and aspects of their anatomy change as they grow. The dura and spinal cord reach lower levels in the spinal canal in infants.[30,43,44] The epidural space is shallower and the epidural fat differs so that spread of local anesthetic is more even in young children (Table 21-1).[106] Ligaments and fasciae are thinner and therefore easier to penetrate. It may be more difficult in infants to feel fascial planes and aponeuroses with the needle tip because there is less resistance. A short beveled needle is particularly useful in this age group, but also in older children, because it helps the anesthesiologist feel the loss of resistance as fascia or aponeurosis is penetrated. This is important in techniques such as femoral or ilioinguinal nerve blocks where accurate depth location depends on feeling the loss of resistance.[16]

In small children the nerves are thinner, allowing easier diffusion of the local anesthetic solution and a more rapid onset of action. In neonates, myelination of nerves is also incomplete. These factors allow adequate block to be achieved with lower concentrations of local anesthetic.

The vascular response to regional anesthesia is less marked in children, and hypotension is uncommon even after fairly extensive regional block.[27]

Some peripheral nerve blocks can be done in conscious older children, but generally children do not like needles and can be frightened in the strange operating theater environment so that blocks are often done under deep sedation or light general anesthesia. Emotional trauma is thus avoided, and the following benefits of regional anesthesia can be obtained.

1. The block provides analgesia intraoperatively and postoperatively, thereby reducing the amount of general anesthetic required. The patient awakens

TABLE 21-1. ANATOMIC DIFFERENCES OF IMPORTANCE IN SPINAL AND EPIDURAL ANESTHESIA IN CHILDREN AND ADULTS

Anatomic Variable	Neonate	Infant	Small Child	Older Child	Adult
Position of lower end of spinal cord	L3		L1 at 12 months		L1
Position of lower end of dural sac	S4		S2		S2
CSF/kg	4 ml	4 ml	3 ml	2 ml	2 ml
Condition of epidural fat	Loose	Loose	Loose	± loose	Firmly packed

more rapidly and is free of pain and tranquil in the recovery room.

2. The neural blockade suppresses undesirable reflexes such as laryngospasm during circumcision and perianal procedures.
3. Muscle relaxation can be obtained with etidocaine (0.75 – 1.0%) or with higher concentrations (0.5%) of bupivacaine, both of which block motor nerve fibers.
4. Neural blockade can minimize the "stress response" to surgery, resulting in more rapid recovery and shorter hospital stay (see Chap. 5).[12,81]
5. Neural blockade facilitates immobilization of a limb after nerve or tendon repair or skin grafting.
6. Postoperative vomiting is less after regional anesthesia than when opiates are used for analgesia and earlier resumption of oral fluid intake is possible.[20,86]
7. Bleeding during surgery may be reduced and the risk of further bleeding and dislodgement of dressings in the recovery room lessened.

The advantages of regional anesthesia in adults also apply in children. The anesthesiologist should be familiar with the technique and aware of the differences between adults and children before embarking on nerve blocks in young patients. There should also be a justifiable advantage to the patient before a block is used, especially when it is done in conjunction with a light general anesthetic. Neural blockade should be done only when adequate equipment is available to induce and maintain general anesthesia in case toxic reactions such as convulsions occur or the block is inadequate (see Chaps. 4 and 6 for more detail).

DOSAGE OF LOCAL ANESTHETICS IN CHILDREN

The recommendations for safer maximal dosage in children are scaled-down doses for weight based on maximum adult doses for a 70-kg person. Although the maximum dose can be defined as that which produces no toxic effects, a number of factors make this definition difficult. First, during general anesthesia, signs of toxicity, including convulsions, may be masked. Second, the blood levels achieved by any route of administration may vary even though the dose and technique of administration is standardized. Third, the blood levels at which toxic signs occur are not clearly defined in humans for all the local anesthetics, and they may be lower in very young children because the blood – brain barrier is immature. If accidental intravascular injection occurs even with normally safe doses, toxic effects may occur.

Table 21-2 outlines the generally accepted doses per kilogram for children. Although these may seem conservative and may have been exceeded by some anesthesiologists, they are a guide for safe practice. When the volume and concentration needed for a block have been determined, the dose should be calculated to ensure that it is in the safe range (1 ml of 1% = 10 mg). If it is too high, either the concentration or the volume may be reduced. For example, if the maximum dose of lidocaine without epinephrine for a 12-kg child is 60 mg, this may be given as 3 ml of 2%, 4 ml of 1.5%, or 6 ml of 1% solution.

In general, satisfactory nerve block can be produced by lower concentrations in children than in adults because the nerves are smaller and their connective tissue sheaths are thinner, so that diffusion of the local anesthetic into them is easier.

PLASMA CONCENTRATIONS

Many factors influence the plasma concentration in children, and most will be similar to those discussed for adults in Chapter 3. Volume of distribution is reported to be greater and clearance more rapid in children than in adults.[85a]

1. Peak arterial plasma levels are higher than peak venous levels initially, but shortly after the peak has been reached the levels approximate each other (Fig. 21-1).[33]

TABLE 21-2. LOCAL ANESTHETIC AGENTS AND DOSES IN CHILDREN

Agent	Topical Use: Concentration (%)	Topical Use: Dose (mg/kg)*	Injection: Plain Solution Dose (mg/kg)*	Injection: Dose with Epinephrine (mg/kg)*
Lidocaine	2–10	3†	5	7
Mepivacaine		5	5	7
Prilocaine			5–7 (Dose not to exceed 600 mg; single dose only)	7–9
Chloroprocaine and procaine			7	10
Bupivacaine			2	2
Etidocaine			3	3–4
Dibucaine	0.2–0.5	1	2 (Subarachnoid use only)	2
Cocaine	3–10	2		
Amethocaine (tetracaine)	0.5–2	1	1.5 (Subarachnoid use only)	1.5

*These doses are the same on a milligram per kilogram basis as in adults and are based on measurements of plasma levels after safe clinical use, compared to toxic plasma levels.

†This low dose is preferable below the age of 3 years since plasma levels following topical use at this age are relatively higher than those for older children.[35]

2. Route of administration: Eyres and colleagues, using 4 mg/kg lidocaine, showed that peak plasma levels were lowest with subcutaneous administration in the groin, slightly higher but well within safe levels with caudal, and highest with topical tracheal spray (Fig. 21-2).[35] Higher plasma levels were obtained with 3 mg/kg bupivacaine in children over 5 years when given by lumbar epidural than by caudal injection (Fig. 21-3), but the levels with younger children were lower by the lumbar route.[35] Although initial studies showed that younger children developed higher plasma levels with topical tracheal lignocaine (see Fig. 21-1),[35] further studies on 99 children[33,37] showed a wide variation in peak plasma levels, with the mean peak plasma levels rising from 5.2 μg/ml in the under-1 year group to only 5.9 μg/ml in children over 5 years. Four children had levels over 10 μg/ml, but none had convulsions because they were all anesthetized (Table 21-3). The mean times until peak plasma levels were reached were shorter in the younger age groups. Rothstein and associates studied intercostal nerve block with bupivacaine 0.5% in children aged 3 months to 16 years. Three different dosages of bupivacaine resulted in the following blood concentrations: 2 mg/kg, 0.77 ± 0.53 μg/ml; 3 mg/kg, 1.37 ± 0.23 μg/ml; and 4 mg/kg, 1.87 ± 0.53 μg/ml. Absorption seemed more rapid than in adults, and the results indicated a maximum safe dose in children of 3 mg/kg.[85a]

3. Age: The peak plasma levels varied with age with some but not all routes of administration. With lumbar epidural the levels were higher in children over 3 years of age.[36] In some studies peak plasma levels were reached earlier in younger children, probably because of their higher cardiac output and more rapid circulation,[33] but it was also noted

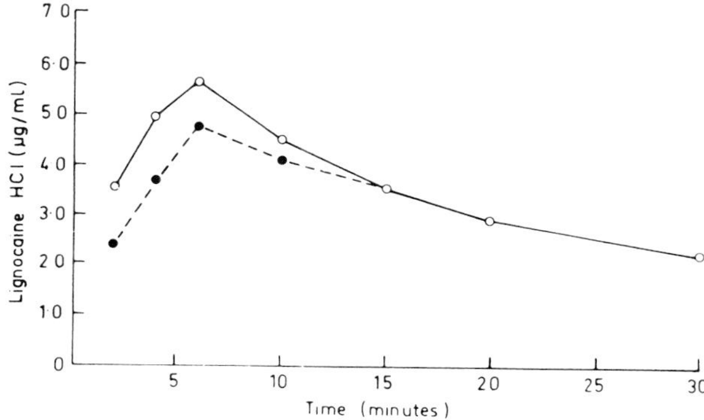

FIG. 21-1. Mean plasma lidocaine concentrations against time for 12 patients having simultaneous arterial and venous sampling. ○——○, mean arterial plasma levels; ●---●, mean venous plasma levels. (Eyres, R.L., *et al.*: Anaesth. Intens. Care, *11*:23, 1983.)

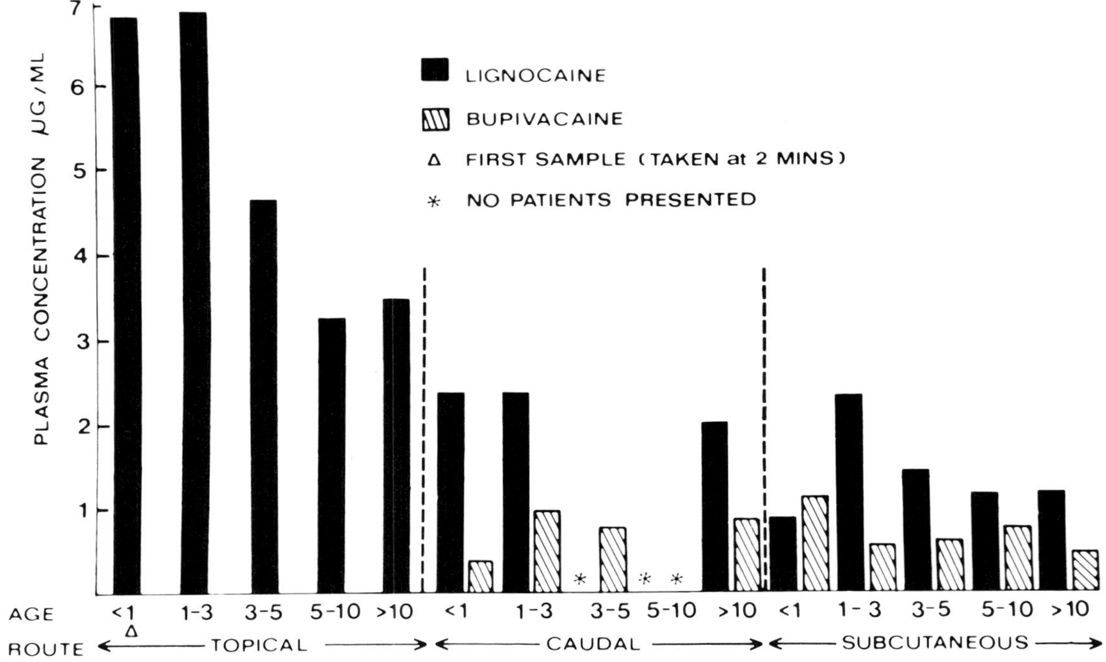

FIG. 21-2. Summary of mean plasma concentrations for different ages and routes of administration. Lignocaine (lidocaine), 4 mg/kg; bupivacaine, 2 mg/kg. (Eyres, R.L., *et al.*: Anaesth. Intens. Care, *6*:247, 1978.)

that high levels tended to be reached more quickly.

A litter of puppies studied several times during the first 4 months of life were given lidocaine, 4 mg/kg by tracheal spray; results showed that a peak plasma level was highest in younger puppies (Fig. 21-4).[48]

4. Local anesthetic and dosage: Studies comparing plasma concentrations of different local anesthetics given in the same dose by the same route are lacking. The mean peak plasma levels of lidocaine after 4 mg/kg by caudal injection (2.4 µg/ml) are relatively greater than after bupivacaine 2 mg/kg (0.8 µg/ml) and 3 mg/kg (1.3 µg/ml) (see Figs. 21-2, 21-3).[34,35]
5. Physiologic and pharmacologic factors: Lidocaine has been shown to be less protein bound in children than in adults.[106] Many enzyme systems are not fully developed at birth, and those responsible for the metabolism of mepivacaine are deficient.[29] Enzyme activity increases with development, particularly during the neonatal period.[13] This is accompanied by more rapid metabolism as the activity of the enzymes involved matures.
6. Elimination: A study in which an intravenous infusion of lidocaine 4 mg/kg over 60 seconds was repeated several times in a litter of puppies during the first 4 months of life showed that elimination was slower at the youngest ages (Fig. 21-5).[47] Elimination is also slower under halothane anesthesia than thiopentone, nitrous oxide, and relaxant anesthesia, probably because of decreased liver blood flow and suppression of liver metabolism under halothane anesthesia.[8,47,87]

TOXICITY

The manifestations of local anesthetic toxicity and their management are discussed in Chapters 2–4. The signs in children are similar to those in adults (see Fig. 4-14) but may be suppressed by general anesthesia, during which the threshold for convulsions may be approximately doubled while the earlier symptoms cannot be recognized. Reports of blood levels during convulsions in children are rare, particularly when the patient is anesthetized. One 12-year-old had an arterial level of 7.5 µg/ml during a convulsion following bupivacaine given by lumbar epidural.[38]

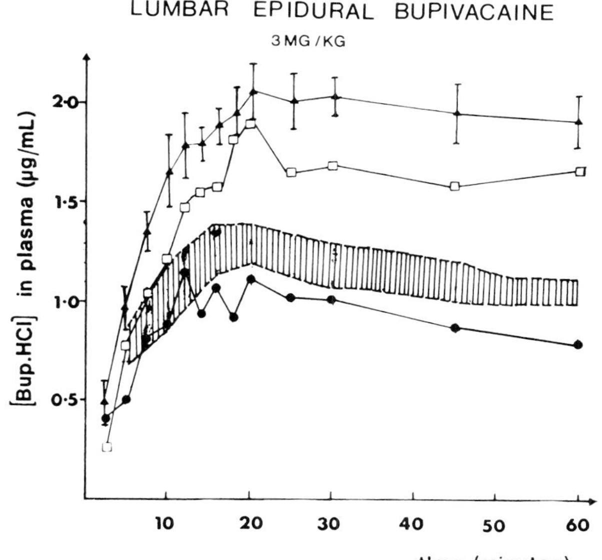

FIG. 21-3. Mean plasma bupivacaine levels following 3 mg/kg administered by the lumbar route in three age groups: ● 1–3 years, n = 5; □ 3–5 years, n = 5; ▲ older than 5 years, n = 6. The mean plasma concentrations for the same dose in these age groups after caudal anesthesia fell in the shaded area.[33] (Eyres, R.L., *et al.*: Plasma bupivacaine levels following lumbar epidural anaesthesia in children. Anaesth. Intens. Care, *14*:131, 1986.)

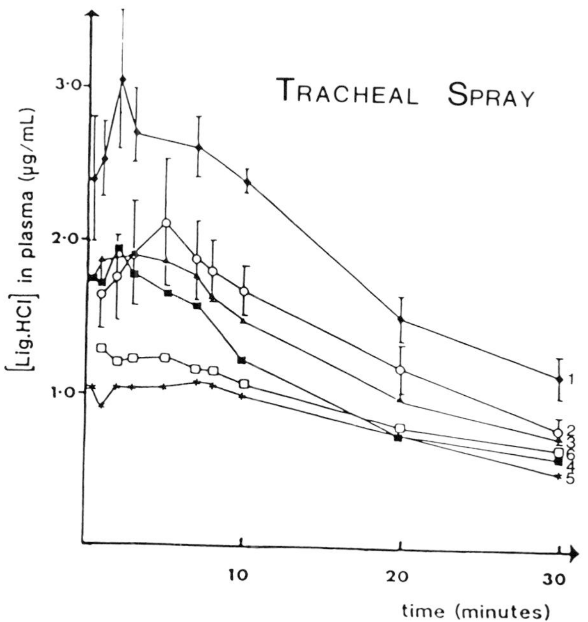

FIG. 21-4. Changes in plasma lidocaine levels with age in puppies under 4 months old following midtracheal spray of 4 mg/kg. The same seven puppies from one litter were used throughout. 1, 20 days; 2, 20–30 days; 3, 40–50 days; 4, 50–64 days; 5, 65–89 days; 6, 90–110 days. (Hastings, C.L., et al.: The influence of age on plasma lignocaine levels following tracheal spray in young dogs. Anaesth. Intens. Care, *13*:392, 1985.)

Another problem in assessing toxic levels and doses is circadian rhythm, which has been shown in mice to affect toxicity.[68]

The causes of toxic reactions in children are the same as those in adults: intravascular injection or overdosage. Other reactions include reaction to vasoconstrictor or, in conscious patients, vasovagal reactions. Hypotension associated with sympathetic block during spinal or epidural anesthesia is less likely in children than in adults.[27] Anaphylaxis, if it occurs with pure local anesthetics, is very rare.

The management of toxicity is discussed in Chapter 4. It is desirable to have intravenous access before inserting the block, especially if the child is fat, has constricted veins due to apprehension, or if, for any reason, access to a vein is likely to be difficult. Should convulsions occur, assisted ventilation with oxygen is of prime importance to prevent hypoxia, hypercarbia, and acidosis. If an anticonvulsant is needed, thiopentone is often at hand or diazepam may be used, but it should be remembered that these drugs will increase the central depression caused by the local anesthetic.

Cardiotoxicity with cardiac arrest has occurred in a small child after etidocaine administration. The arrest

TABLE 21-3. OBSERVATIONS AFTER TRACHEAL LIDOCAINE SPRAY (4 mg/kg) IN CHILDREN

Age (yr)	Number of Children	Mean Peak Plasma Level	Highest Peak Plasma Level	Percentage Over 7 µg/ml	Mean Time to Peak in Minutes
1	13	5.2	10.1	23	6.1
1–3	21	5.7	7.2	10	6.5
3–5	23	5.8	10.1	13	7.9
5+	42	5.9	10.3	19	10.8

(Eyres, R.L., et al.: Plasma lignocaine concentrations following topical analgesia. Anaesth. Intens. Care [In Press])

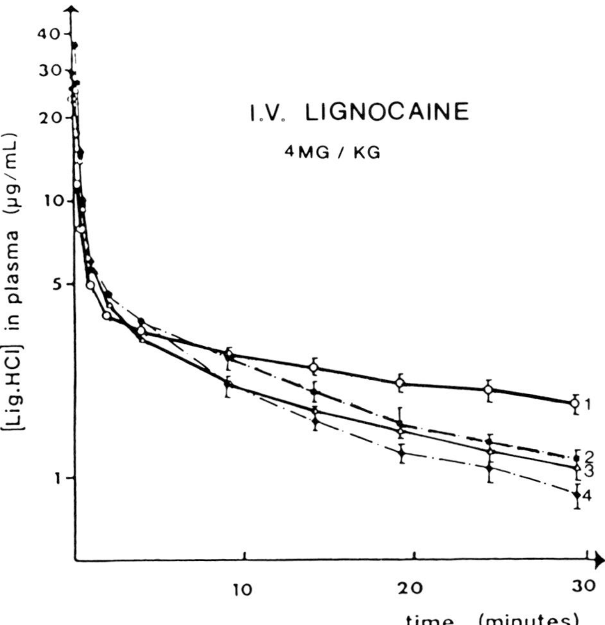

FIG. 21-5. Mean plasma levels following 4 mg/kg of lidocaine administered intravenously over 60 seconds in a litter of eight puppies at intervals during the first 6 months of life. 1, 8 ± 5 days; 2, 43 ± 6 days; 3, 94 ± 6 days; 4, 185 ± 5 days. (Hastings, C.L., et al.: The influence of age on plasma lignocaine levels following tracheal spray in young dogs. Anaesth. Intens. Care, *13*:392, 1985.)

may occur several minutes after the injection has been completed (see Chap. 4).

NEURAL BLOCKADE WITHOUT GENERAL ANESTHESIA

Most children do not like needles or injections. Small children who are frightened are unlikely to keep still unless well sedated. Thus local anesthetic techniques alone are not usually used in children under about age 7 years except for very minor procedures. An exception may be the use of local anesthesia to reduce the stress of circumcision in the newborn.[108] After that age a cooperative child who has had the procedure explained may tolerate local infiltration or a nerve block for suturing lacerations, an intravenous arm block, or axillary brachial plexus block for reduction of a fracture or minor procedures on the arm. Usually adequate sedation beforehand or the presence of a reassuring parent, or both, facilitates the procedure.

When the child has pain from, for instance, a fractured femur, the insertion of a block to relieve the pain may be of less concern to the patient than the painful fracture. A skilled, sympathetic assistant and continued reassurance are necessary. Those undertaking the procedure must remember that the patient is awake, and they must behave appropriately.

When a child requires an emergency procedure, such as a fracture reduction or suturing a laceration, preoperative sedation is usually helpful. If an appropriate choice is made, local anesthesia is usually well tolerated. The combination of an analgesic such as morphine or papaveretum, if there is pain, an amnesic such as hyoscine, or a tranquilizer such as diazepam or lorazepam, which also have amnesic properties, will usually produce reasonable sedation. Alternatively, particularly for elective procedures, neuroleptanalgesia with droperidol or a benzodiazepine and fentanyl can produce satisfactory conditions (Table 21-4). New methods of giving sedatives, opioids, and local anesthetics transdermally will be of great benefit to local anesthetic techniques in the conscious child (see Chap. 32).

If it has been proposed to use a nerve stimulator, the child will need to be well sedated, preferably with a combination including an analgesic drug. A nerve stimulator may permit the use of neural blockade in an anxious child, since motor responses can be obtained without causing discomfort if sedation is adequate (see Chap. 6).

COMBINED LOCAL AND GENERAL ANESTHESIA

In children, local or regional anesthesia is often combined with light general anesthesia, but there must be justifiable advantages to the child. Such potential advantages are summarized above. In addition, both general anesthesia and diazepam suppress CNS toxicity caused by local anesthetics.[112]

The same preoperative assessment, premedication, preparation, and checking of the anesthetic equipment should be carried out as for general anesthesia. Anesthesia is induced, and when intravenous access has been assured and monitoring equipment attached, the patient is positioned for the block. A competent assistant is required to maintain the airway and ventilation while the block is performed. The patient can be monitored with a precordial stethoscope, which provides information about heart rate, rhythm, intensity of heart sounds, and respiration. The decision to intubate should be based on the usual criteria, such as a full stomach, upper abdominal surgery, or the need to maintain adequate ventilation. If

TABLE 21-4. PREMEDICATION IN CHILDREN

Drug	Dose (mg/kg)	Route	Time Preoperative (h)	Main Actions and Comments
Chloral hydrate	50	Oral	¾–1	Sedative, good for young children, some preparations have unpleasant taste.
Diazepam	0.3–0.4	Oral	½–2	Tranquilizer, amnesic, better for older children.
Trimeprazine	3	Oral	2	Prolonged postoperative sleep, patient often agitated if roused.
Morphine	0.2	i.m.	1¼	Analgesic, euphoric, sedative, increased nausea and vomiting.
Papaveretum (omnopon)	0.4	i.m.	1¼	Analgesic, euphoric, sedative, increased nausea and vomiting.
Meperidine (pethidine)	1	i.m.	1	Analgesic, less calming than morphine and papaveretum, better than above two agents in asthmatic patients.
Hyoscine	0.008	i.m.	1¼	(With papaveretum) Antisialagogue, amnesic, antiemetic.
Atropine	0.01	i.m.		Blocks vagal reflexes and dries secretions.

indicated, the patient should be intubated before the block is begun. The local anesthetic can be drawn up after the skin has been prepared; this gives more time for the antiseptic solution to act and greatly decreases the risk of accidentally exchanging the local anesthetic syringe with one containing another drug such as thiopentone.

Blocks that do not require paresthesias are ideal for use with general anesthesia, but where paresthesias are usually sought a nerve stimulator can be used to locate the nerve.

Basal anesthesia during the operation can be maintained with nitrous oxide, oxygen, and, if necessary, low concentrations of an inhalational agent such as halothane; with intravenous supplements such as diazepam; or with ketamine, which can be given intramuscularly or intravenously. When ketamine is used, it is advisable to give diazepam for premedication or intravenously to minimize undesirable psychic effects.

SPECIFIC BLOCKS AND THEIR USE IN CHILDREN

Any of the techniques for regional or nerve blocks described elsewhere in *Neural Blockade* can be used in children provided the anesthesiologist bears in mind the principles already discussed in relation to anatomic and physiologic differences related to the patient's size. The techniques described in other chapters can be consulted before proceeding with the block. Various blocks will now be discussed with particular reference to their use in children.

CENTRAL NEURAL BLOCKADE

History

Spinal subarachnoid block in infants and children was developed by Gray as early as 1909.[45] There were a number of reports in the 1930s and 1940s, particularly from Canada, where it was used even for intrathoracic operations.[32,54,58,61,62,83,98] With the advent of better methods of general anesthesia, spinal anesthesia lost popularity in the 1950s, and with the current widespread use of epidural, particularly caudal, anesthesia in children, recent reports of spinal anesthesia are sparse.[1,72]

An early publication on caudal anesthesia by Campbell[30] appeared in 1933. In 1962 Spiegel[101] and more recently many others[5,24,25,42,55,64,66,102] have reported its use. Epidural block in children was first reported in 1936 by Sievers[97] and later by Schneider in 1951.[91] Ruston perfected the technique and introduced the continuous method.[88-90] In 1971 Russian authors reported the use of thoracic epidural block for postoperative analgesia after thoracic surgery in children.[53]

Anatomy and Physiology

It is important to remember that the spinal cord and dural sac reach a lower level in infants. The tip of the spinal cord is at L3 at birth and by 1 year it is at its final position at L1. The position of the lower end of the dural sac is independent of the spinal cord and is usually at the level of S2. The spinal cord occasionally reaches S1 and the dural sac as low as S4 (see Table 21-1).[30] The low dural sac accounts for the occasional dural puncture reported during caudal anesthesia.

The cardiovascular effects of spinal and epidural block in children are reported by several authors with extensive experience to be less marked than in adults.[9,27,36,42,63,72,77,78,84,88] Melman reported no hypotension in 200 cases,[36] and Ruston's cases of spinal anesthesia also failed to show the decrease in blood pressure seen in adults. Children have an active sympathetic nervous system, which compensates rapidly for minor falls in blood pressure.[63] Buckley and colleagues have shown differing rates of postnatal maturation of the cardiovascular responses to catecholamines in piglets, but the variation is greatest in the first few weeks of life.[19]

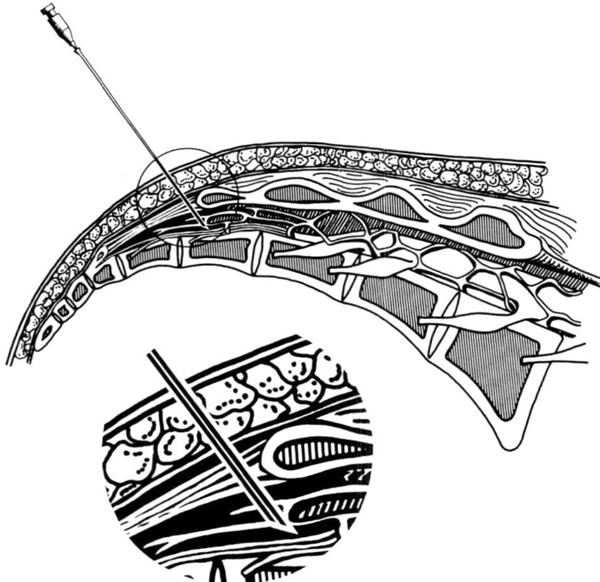

FIG. 21-6. Caudal epidural blockade in the child. Anatomic view of the needle path, which is directed at an angle of 65° to 70° and passes almost at a right angle through the sacrococcygeal ligament. The enlarged view *(inset)* shows the needle passing into the caudal epidural space, which offers no resistance to the advancing needle until it reaches the anterior table of the sacrum.

CAUDAL EPIDURAL ANESTHESIA

Caudal epidural anesthesia is much more widely used than lumbar epidural or spinal anesthesia in children, probably because the block is easy to do and because of its applicability to several of the common pediatric operations such as circumcision, hypospadias repair, and inguinal hernia repair. It is also useful as an adjunct for rectosigmoidectomy, other perineal and perianal procedures, and operations on the lower extremities.

The caudal injection is done with the child lying on the side with the knees drawn up, the upper knee being flexed more than the lower. If general anesthesia is used, a competent assistant must maintain the airway. The sacral hiatus is palpated between the sacral cornua, and the skin is cleansed with antiseptic. The needle is inserted at an angle between 60° and 90° to the skin (Fig. 21-6). If a short beveled needle is used, the loss of resistance is felt more easily as the sacrococcygeal membrane is penetrated. After aspirating to ensure there is no blood or cerebrospinal fluid, the local anesthetic is injected. Some anesthesiologists advance the needle upward into the canal before injecting. This ensures that the needle tip is in the canal, which is much shallower in children, but it may increase the risk of dural puncture, especially in infants. There is no advantage in inserting the needle any further than 2 to 3 mm past the sacrococcygeal membrane. If the needle is halted at this point, it will be less likely to puncture the dura. It is possible to insert an epidural catheter through a large cannula or a needle in the sacral hiatus in children if prolonged block is wanted or as an alternative to lumbar epidural injection. The catheter can usually be passed up to the lower lumbar region. In children under 3 years of age, even higher levels may be reached.[95] The catheter should never be forced if an obstruction is felt because it could puncture a blood vessel or loop back on itself.

The epidural fat in infants and small children has a gelatinous spongy appearance with spaces between the lobules so that there is an easier spread of local anesthetic solution than in adults, in whom the fat lobules are more densely packed and interrupted by fibrous strands.

The height of a block achieved by caudal injection depends on the volume of local anesthetic used. In one study,[14] 0.5 ml/kg of contrast medium injected at autopsy spread consistently to at least L2 and sometimes to T10–T11 (Figs. 21-7, 21-8). Similar studies by Schulte–Steinberg using contrast medium mixed with the local anesthetic showed that the anesthesia produced extended about five segments higher than the radiopaque contrast when tested by pinprick.[94,95] In another study,[34] 3 mg/kg of bupivacaine 0.25% produced analgesia up to the midthoracic region.

Dosage has been shown to increase linearly with age from 4 to 18 years for lumbar epidural anesthesia (Fig. 21-9). For caudal anesthesia in children, Schulte–Steinberg demonstrated a strong correlation between dose of lidocaine (1%), mepivacaine (1%), and bupivacaine (0.25%) and age, weight, and height. The correlation was highest with age (correlation coefficient 0.94). The dose ascertained by loss of sensation to pinprick was 0.1 ml per segment per year of age (±0.2 ml) (Fig. 21-10).[92–95] From the study of a large series of children, Busoni has developed a dose related to age and the level required for mepivacaine with 1:400,000 epinephrine (Fig. 21-11).[20] In children under 8 years of age, his doses are higher than Schulte–Steinberg's because he used the more intense stimulus of pinching with fingernails (carried by A-fiber) as opposed to the weaker pain stimulus of pinprick (carried by C-fibers). For example, a 3-year-old child given 5 ml of 1% mepivacaine by the caudal route was anesthetic to pinprick for 18 segments (0.09 ml/segment/year) compared with 12 segments that were insensitive to pinching (0.14 ml/segment/year).

Because the main purpose of using caudal anesthesia is to provide analgesia and not motor blockade, a dilute solution (0.25–0.35%) of bupivacaine is adequate and avoids overdosage if larger volumes are used for extension of blocks to high segmental levels.

Whatever method is used to determine the dose, the total mg/kg dosage should always be checked to ensure that it is below the recommended safe level.

In order to ensure an adequate block, enough time must be allowed before surgery for the local anesthetic to act. This may be 15 to 20 minutes with bupi-

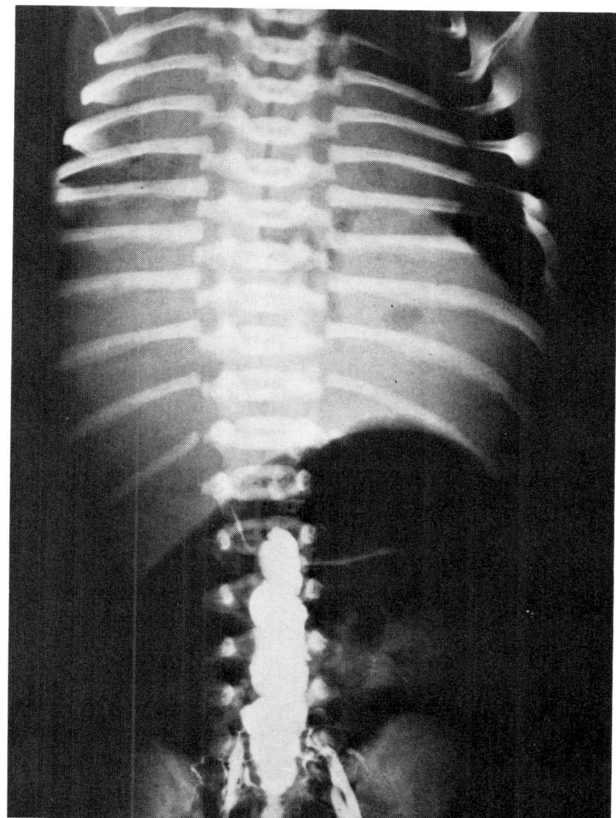

FIG. 21-7. Radiograph shows the spread of 2 ml radiopaque material injected into the sacral hiatus of a stillborn baby. Note the spread to L1 and the escape from intervertebral foramina following the course of the nerves.

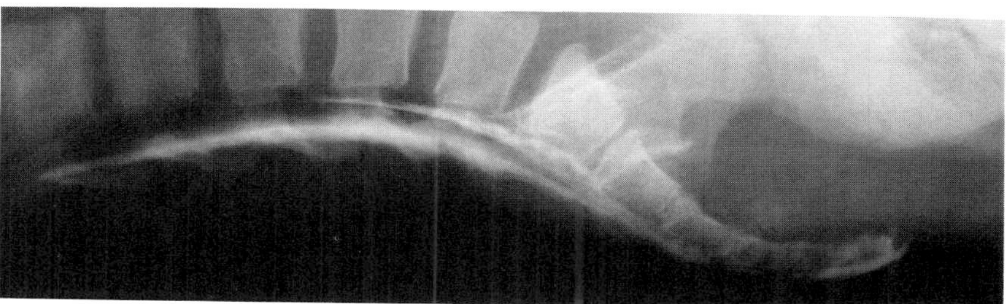

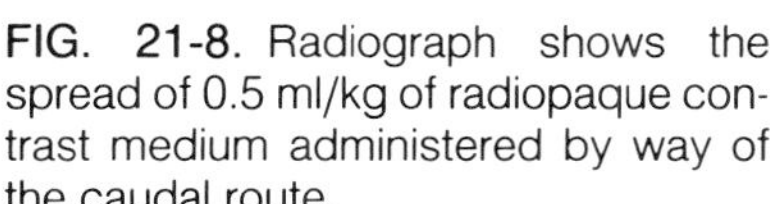

FIG. 21-8. Radiograph shows the spread of 0.5 ml/kg of radiopaque contrast medium administered by way of the caudal route.

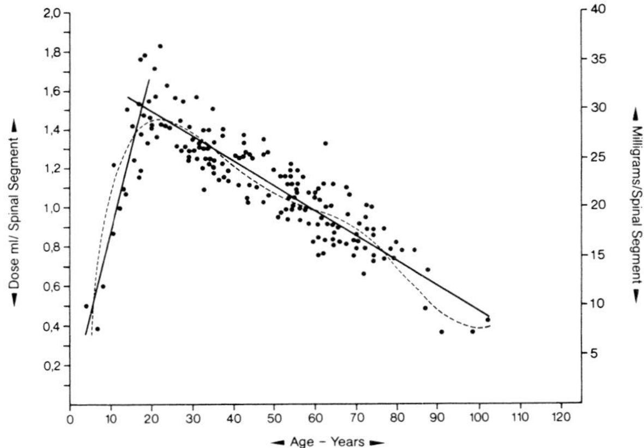

FIG. 21-9. Lumbar epidural block. Segmental dose requirements are related to age (between 4 and 102 years). Computer-fitted linear (——) and curvilinear (- - -) lines have been drawn through the data points. Four children under the age of 12 years were included. Note the linear increase in dose requirements to age 20 and then the linear decrease as age increases. (Bromage, P.R.: Aging and epidural dose requirements. Segmental spread and predictability of epidural analgesia in youth and extreme age. Br. J. Anaesth., *41*:1016, 1969.)

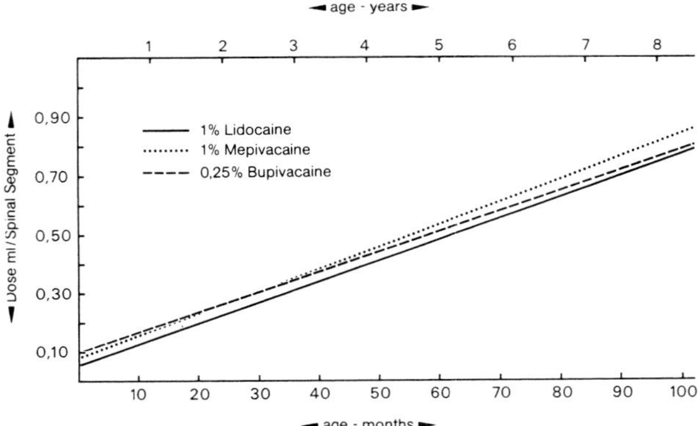

FIG. 21-10. Caudal epidural blockade in children. Segmental dose requirements of lidocaine, bupivacaine, and mepivacaine are related to age.

vacaine, although in children the onset of block tends to be quicker.

The advantages of caudal anesthesia are that it provides good intraoperative and postoperative analgesia, provides reduced bleeding, prevents erection, and prevents the reflex laryngeal spasm commonly seen when circumcision is performed with halothane anesthesia alone. It is easily administered in children.

Dural puncture is a rare hazard. If not recognized, it may result in a total spinal anesthetic. At the Royal Children's Hospital, Melbourne, there have been 3 cases of dural puncture in 18 years (in about 5000 cases): Two had a normal sacral hiatus, and 1 had incomplete sacral laminae. Fortuna reported 2 cases in 156 patients.[42] The potential for it to occur is increased by passing the needle up the sacral canal or by the presence of incomplete lower sacral laminae so that the hiatus is located at a higher level. It can be recognized by free flow of CSF from the needle if one of adequate size is used (21-gauge), or by careful aspiration.

Intravascular injections leading to toxic manifestations such as convulsions and possibly cardiovascular depression may result from accidental intravenous or interosseous injection. The latter is more likely in young infants when a sharp needle is used and it penetrates the body of the vertebra anteriorly or the lamina posteriorly.

The administration of a small test dose of local anesthetic with epinephrine will cause tachycardia and hypertension if the injection is intravascular. Recognition of this will avoid toxic doses being given. If convulsions, hypotension, or arrhythmias occur, the child should be hyperventilated with oxygen.

If there is free flow of blood from the needle or the appearance of blood on aspiration, the needle may be repositioned. Saline followed by a test dose of local anesthetic with epinephrine can then be injected. If tachycardia does not develop, the injection of local anesthetic can be completed. On rare occasions, rapid vascular absorption can occur despite watching for blood and aspirating.

Intrapelvic injection is possible but unlikely with experienced anesthesiologists.[14]

EPIDURAL BLOCKADE

Compared with caudal, the lumbar epidural approach is much less commonly used in children, probably because of uncertainty about the depth of the epidural space in the growing child; fear of

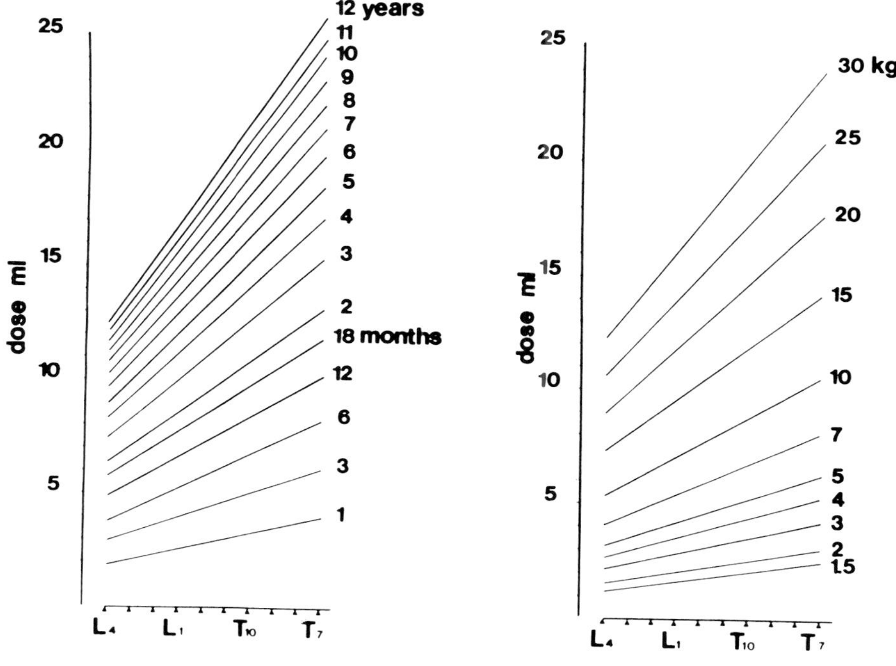

FIG. 21-11. Graph used to calculate the caudal dose of 1% mepivacaine according to age or weight and the desired extent of the block. (Busoni, P., and Andreucetti, T.: The spread of caudal anaesthesia in children: A mathematical model. Anaesth. Intens. Care 14:140, 1986)

dural puncture owing to the epidural space being narrower in children; and because most procedures where it might be used are done under general anesthesia with muscle relaxation. Epidural anesthesia should therefore be used only in situations in which it offers distinct advantages.

The depth of the epidural space from the skin increases as the child grows. It is about 1 mm/kg in children who are not obese.[36] The ligamentum flavum is softer and thinner than in adults, allowing easier passage of the needle, thus facilitating identification of the epidural space using a syringe filled with normal saline. The space is narrower, but the injections of saline as it is entered will push the dura away from the needle. This technique is particularly useful if a catheter is to be inserted.[71] Epidural anesthesia has been used to a limited extent via both the lumbar and thoracic routes in children, but its use should be restricted to those who are already expert with the technique in adults.

Dosages of local anesthetics are similar to those used for caudal anesthesia.[20,92–95] Eyres has reported using 3 mg/kg in children by the lumbar route, although doses of this magnitude are not always needed.[36] A 0.1 ml/year/segment has been used for thoracic epidurals in children by Isakob and colleagues.[53] Infusion of 4 to 6 mg/kg/day has been used as a satisfactory alternative to intermittent doses for postoperative pain relief.[71]

Epidural opiates can be used, as in adults, for pain therapy or postoperative analgesia in children. Morphine, 1 to 2 mg in 5 ml of normal saline, has been used successfully in children 3 to 11 years of age.[96] Children with metastases and increasing pain may need steadily increasing doses.[59] As in adults, care must be taken to monitor respiration in the event that delayed respiratory depression occurs (see Chap. 28).

Dural puncture occurs occasionally even with experienced anesthesiologists, but, provided that it is recognized, the serious consequences of total spinal anesthesia (hypotension and respiratory arrest) can be avoided.

Accidental intravascular injection is an uncommon complication. Intravascular injection may be recognized by the rapid onset of tachycardia and hypertension following a small test dose if epinephrine is added to the local anesthetic.

Other complications such as hematoma, infection, and their consequences are the same in children as in adults (see Chap. 22).

SPINAL SUBARACHNOID ANESTHESIA

Provided one is familiar with the technique of lumbar puncture in children and knows the appropriate doses (Table 21-5), spinal anesthesia can be performed in children. It must be remembered that the spinal cord reaches L3 in infants and lumbar puncture should therefore be performed at a lower level in this age group. Although this form of anesthesia was widely used during the earlier part of the century, reports of its use in recent years have been sporadic. Improved general anesthesia and the increased use of caudal epidural anesthesia probably account for this change. The principles of spinal anesthesia, including the use of posture to control spread, are the same as in adults (see Chap. 7).

The dose per kilogram of local anesthetic is greater in children under 3 years of age and gradually decreases thereafter. Abajian and co-workers used 0.25 mg/kg of 1% tetracaine in infants under 1 year of age with an equivalent volume of 10% dextrose. If a prolonged procedure was anticipated, 0.02 ml of 1 : 1000 epinephrine was added.[1] The reason given for the larger dose in infants is that CSF volume in babies is at least twice that in adults (2 ml/kg). Figures vary from 4 ml/kg[23] to 40 to 60 ml in babies.[67] There is also considerable variation quoted in anesthesia and physiology literature for the percentage of CSF in the spinal canal. Because the doses needed in infants are relatively greater, it is possible that their spinal CSF volume:body weight ratio is greater than in adults.

UPPER LIMB BLOCKS

BRACHIAL PLEXUS BLOCKADE

Brachial plexus block was first described in children by Farr in 1920.[40] Since 1941, more reports have appeared.[26,65,69,80,99]

The **axillary** approach in children was described by Accardo and Adriani in 1949.[2] This approach is preferable in children if the arm can be abducted and externally rotated because of its safety and ease of performance (Table 21-6). The technique is the same as that used in adults (see Chap. 10). It must be remembered that the plexus lies at a more superficial level in children and that inappropriately deep injection is the most common cause of failed block. When paresthesias or muscle contraction in response to a nerve stimulator (first described in children by Aisenberg[3,4]) are obtained, the local anesthetic can be injected. Continued compression of the artery and adduction of the arm aid spread of the solution upward and increase the probability of blocking the musculocutaneous nerve, which has a high origin. The intercostobrachial nerve can be blocked by a skin wheal as the needle is withdrawn.

Supraclavicular brachial plexus block, although less commonly used, can be done successfully in children.[61] The anatomy can be more easily recognized

TABLE 21-5. RECOMMENDED DOSAGES FOR SPINAL ANESTHESIA IN CHILDREN

Agent	Expected Duration of Anesthesia (min)	Dose
Lidocaine, 5% in 8% glucose	45	2 mg/kg (3 years of age), decreasing doses down to 1 mg/kg (3–10 years)
Tetracaine, 1% plus 10% glucose	45–90	1 mg per year of age; below 3 years, 0.2 mg/kg
Dibucaine 0.5% in 6% glucose	100–160	0.2 mg/kg
Tetracaine, 1% plus 10% glucose that contains 2 mg phenylephrine in 1 ml	100–200	0.2 mg/kg 1 mg per year of age; below 3 years, 0.2 mg/kg

Data from Gouveia[43] and Berkowitz and Green.[9]

TABLE 21-6. AXILLARY BRACHIAL PLEXUS BLOCK VOLUMES EQUIPOTENT TO 1% PRILOCAINE*

Age (yr)	Volume† (ml)
1-3	6-9
4-6	9-11
7-9	14-20
10-12	21-25
13-15	28-35

*Alternatively, a volume of 0.6 to 0.7 ml/kg may be used as a guide.
†To avoid toxic levels, it is important to calculate the dosage on a milligram per kilogram basis and to reduce the volume accordingly.
Data from Eriksson.[31]

by palpation than in adults. The interscalene groove and subclavian artery can be easily felt.

The Kuhlenkampf method in which the first rib is used as a landmark is less satisfactory in children than is Fortin's method using a short fine (25-26-gauge) needle, which will be described here.[41] It does not require contacting the first rib, and pneumothorax is a less likely complication.

The brachial plexus is brought toward the surface by placing a rolled towel lengthwise between the shoulders along the spine with the child lying supine with his head turned away from the side to be blocked. By pushing the shoulders back on to the table, the first rib is elevated, carrying the brachial plexus and subclavian artery closer to the skin. The site of injection is 1 cm above the midpoint of the clavicle, just lateral to the subclavian artery. The position is confirmed if the first rib can be felt (see Chap. 10).

The anesthesiologist stands at the head of the table.[61] behind the shoulder, inserts the short fine needle, and walks it posteriorly until paresthesias are obtained. If the child is anesthetized, muscle twitching in the hand or forearm in response to a nerve stimulator will indicate that the nerves have been touched. If the rib is hit, the needle is too deep. When paresthesias are elicited, all the local anesthetic is injected, since it will be in the perivascular sheath surrounding the plexus. The main hazard is pneumothorax if the needle is too medial and deep and passes the first rib.

The **interscalene** approach to the brachial plexus was introduced by Winnie.[109] A technique not depending on paraesthesias that is also used in adults has been described by Miranda.[72] The needle is introduced at the level of the cricoid cartilage at the apex of the triangle formed by the scalenus anterior and medius muscles. The needle is directed downward at a 45° angle toward the midline in the interscalene groove. It is advanced until loss of resistance is felt as it penetrates the fibrous sheath of perivascular space. One milliliter or 2 ml of local anesthetic are injected, and the syringe is disconnected. If a few drops of fluid run back from the needle, it is in the correct plane. This occurs because the local anesthetic produces a positive pressure in the potential space. Paresthesias are not essential but can be obtained in the conscious child if desired. The remainder of the local anesthetic is then injected (see Chap. 10).

The potential complications of this approach are vertebral artery injection leading to convulsions, injection of a dural cuff leading to total spinal anesthesia and phrenic nerve or recurrent laryngeal nerve block.

Various dosage schedules have been devised for arm blocks in children.[31,49,75,109] Table 21-7 outlines a simplified summary of these. Alternatively, 0.6 to 0.7 mg/kg of 1% prilocaine or lignocaine can be used. The total dose should be calculated to ensure that it is below the toxic dose.

Intravenous regional anesthesia, originally described by Bier[10] and reintroduced by Holmes (see Chap. 12),[51] can be used in cooperative children usually over about 7 years of age, although its use has been reported in a child of 3 years. They usually need some preliminary sedation or light general anesthesia. The presence of a parent, especially for emergency outpatient procedures such as fracture reduction, is helpful.

A butterfly needle or cannula is inserted in the hand. The arm is then exsanguinated by gravity if the patient is conscious. The arterial supply can be occluded before the upper tourniquet cuff is inflated to aid exsanguination. The tourniquet pressures should be 180 to 240 mm Hg for the upper limb and 350 to

TABLE 21-7. SIMPLIFIED DOSAGE FOR ARM PLEXUS BLOCKS

Age (yr)	Formula to Determine Volume (ml)	Concentration of Lidocaine and Mepivacaine (%)	Concentration of Bupivacaine (%)
0-4	$\frac{\text{Height (cm)}}{12}$	0.7-0.8	0.2
5-8	$\frac{\text{Height (cm)}}{10}$	0.8-0.9	0.25
9-16	$\frac{\text{Height (cm)}}{7}$	0.9-1	0.25

Data based on dosages suggested by Winnie[110] and Lanze (personal communication).

500 mm Hg for the leg. The dose is 3 mg/kg of 0.5% lidocaine or prilocaine. This is a volume of 0.6 ml/kg. After 5 to 7 minutes, the lower cuff is inflated and the upper one released. Mean peak plasma levels of 1.95 μg/ml with a maximum of 2.8 μg/ml have been measured when the cuff was released after 20 minutes.[39] High levels while the cuff is inflated may result from leakage under the cuff or through bone.[83] Inadequate cuff inflation or use of defective tourniquets may lead to toxicity (see Chap. 12).[85] This technique has been used successfully for emergency reduction of fractures.[22,39,107]

PERIPHERAL BLOCKS

The radial, ulnar, and median nerves can easily be blocked at the wrist. Only small volumes (about 0.5–1 ml each) are needed, injected through a fine-bore needle. Details are provided in Chapter 10.

LOWER LIMB BLOCKS

Caudal, epidural, or spinal anesthesia can be used for lower limb surgery, but several of the more specific nerve blocks have a place in the management of children. These lower limb blocks are discussed in Chapter 11; this discussion will consider only some specific anatomic points and clinical uses.

The nerves are smaller, the tissue barriers are thinner, and penetration by the local anesthetic of even the larger nerves is more rapid, so that smaller doses will produce adequate block. Dosage should be related to the size of the child compared with an adult and be correspondingly reduced. It is always wise in pediatric anesthesia to check that the milligram per kilogram dosage is within the recommended safe limits.

SCIATIC NERVE BLOCK

Sciatic nerve block can be used for much lower limb surgery but is particularly useful in the early management of leg trauma and fractures, especially of the tibia and fibula. There are several approaches: The posterior one with the patient lying prone or on the side is probably the most commonly used (see Chap. 11); the lithotomy approach, where the nerve lies midway between the greater trochanter and the ischial tuberosity, is relatively easy, but the anterior one will be more useful with fractures if turning the patient is going to cause further discomfort. The needle is inserted until it contacts the femur and is then redirected past the lesser trochanter. The key to finding the right depth is feeling loss of resistance as the fascia posterior to adductor magnus is penetrated.[70] The nerve lies just medial to the lesser trochanter and just deep to this fascia (Fig. 21-12). Its position can be confirmed by the use of a nerve stimulator (see Chap. 11).

FEMORAL NERVE BLOCK

Femoral nerve block is easy to perform provided one uses a short beveled needle and understands the anatomy. The nerve is located just lateral to the femoral artery but is deep to both fascia lata and fascia iliaca, which can both be located by the loss of resistance or the sound of a "pop" as they are penetrated. The artery is deep only to fascia lata and superficial to fascia iliaca (Fig. 21-13). The nerve can be blocked adequately by a single injection just lateral to the artery provided two fascial planes are penetrated.[55] To obtain a lumbar plexus block, including the lateral femoral cutaneous and obturator nerves, as described by Winnie, the same approach is used employing a larger volume of local anesthetic and putting pressure just below the site of injection so that the solution tracks upward in the fascial canal to the lumbar nerve roots.[110] Fanwise injection of the femoral nerve is inappropriate if the anatomy is clearly understood.

The femoral nerve block can be used to anesthetize parts of the leg not blocked by the sciatic, tibial, or common peroneal nerves. It is particularly useful in the early management of fractured femoral shaft in children so that transport, x-rays, and manipulation can be carried out without discomfort. It relieves muscle spasm around the fracture and provides immediate analgesia. It is also a useful block when a split thickness skin graft is being taken from the front of the thigh.

LATERAL CUTANEOUS NERVE OF THIGH BLOCK

Several methods have been described for blocking the lateral cutaneous nerve of the thigh. The most reliable landmark is the anterior superior iliac spine. The nerve emerges in a fascial canal immediately medial to it to pass just below the lateral attachment of the inguinal ligament (Fig. 21-14). If a needle is inserted vertically just medial to the anterior superior

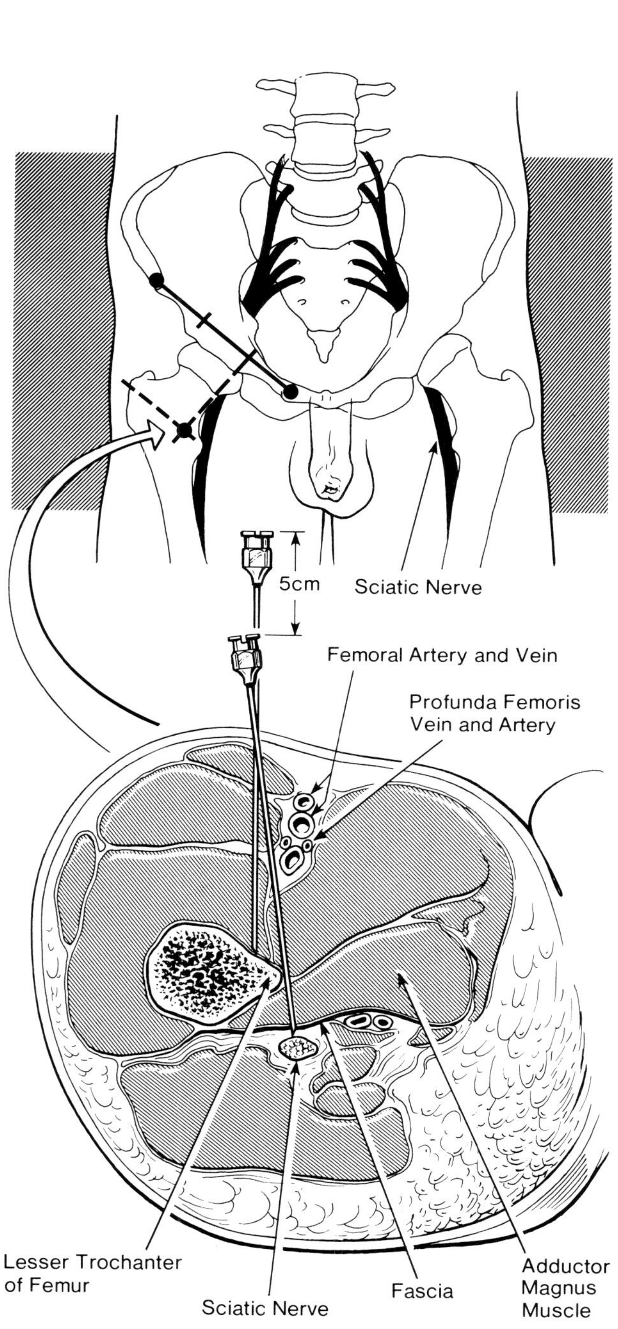

FIG. 21-12. Anterior approach to sciatic nerve block (see text). Cross-section of the leg at the level of the lesser trochanter to show the relationship between the sciatic nerve and the femur, and the fascia separating it from adductor magnus.

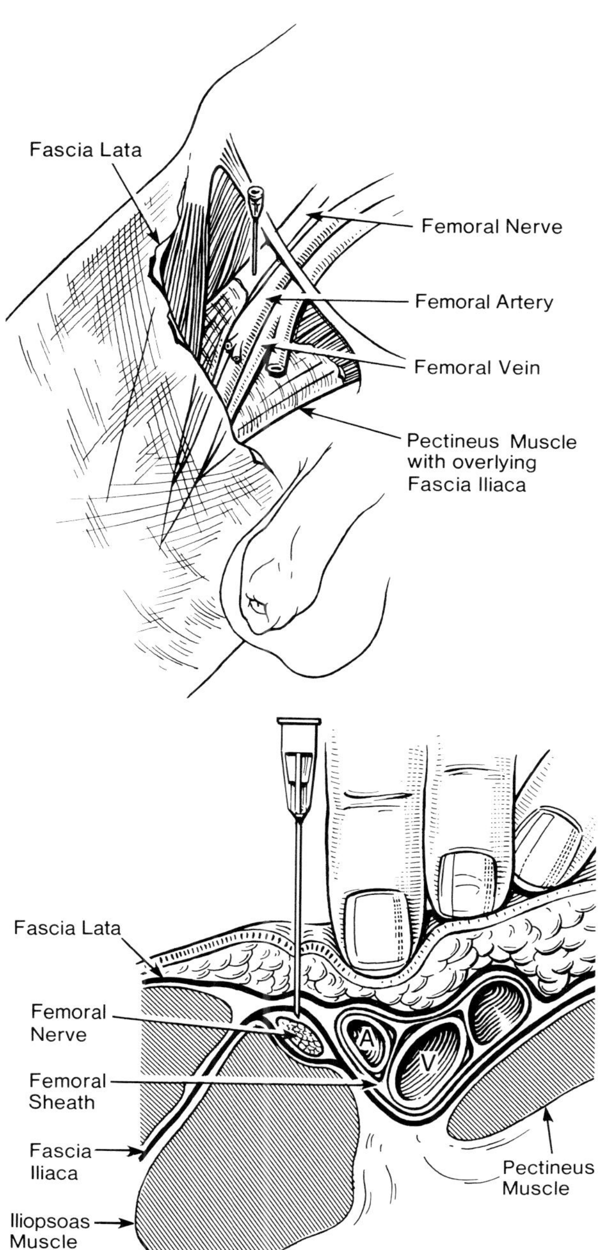

FIG. 21-13. Femoral nerve block (see text). The femoral nerve lies in a canal immediately lateral to the femoral artery just below the inguinal ligament. It lies deep to fascia lata and fascia iliaca. Loss of resistance can be felt twice when a short beveled needle is inserted through these two layers. The femoral artery and vein lie deep to fascia lata but superficial to fascia iliaca. (Khoo, S.T., and Brown, T.C.K.: Anaesth. Intens. Care, *11*:40, 1983.)

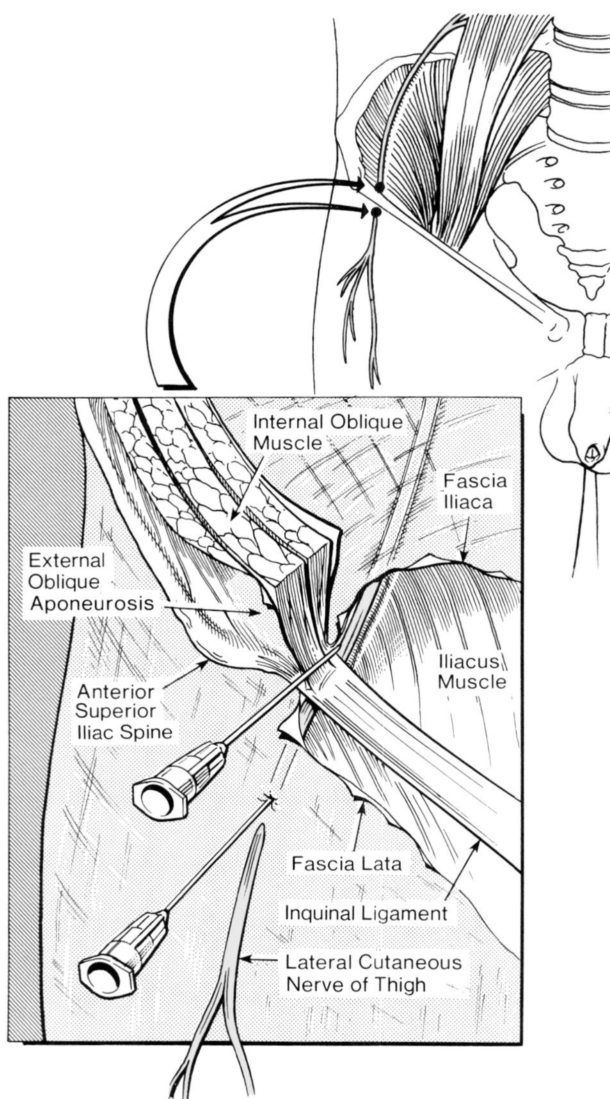

FIG. 21-14. Lateral cutaneous nerve block (see text). The lateral cutaneous nerve of the thigh passes inferiorly on iliacus muscle covered by iliacus fascia. Just medial to the anterior superior iliac spine it turns anteriorly to pass just below the inguinal ligament and runs deep to the fascia lata until it emerges subcutaneously. The lateral cutaneous nerve can be blocked [1] just medial to the anterior superior iliac spine, when loss of resistance is felt on passing through the external oblique aponeurosis and on emerging through the internal oblique muscle or [2] 1 to 2 cm below the anterior superior iliac spine by injecting deep to fascia lata.

iliac spine, a loss of resistance will be felt as the needle passes through external oblique aponeurosis. It is difficult to inject while the needle passes through internal oblique muscle. A second loss of resistance is felt as it emerges and enters the fascial canal containing the nerve. The local anesthetic is then injected.[18]

POSTERIOR CUTANEOUS NERVE OF THIGH BLOCK

The posterior cutaneous nerve of the thigh lies close to the sciatic nerve as it emerges from the sciatic foramen. It then lies medial to it and often divides before it reaches the level of the gluteal fold, where the branches emerge below the lower border of gluteus maximus. At this point a perineal branch passes medially, a few small branches pass up to supply part of the buttock, and others continue down to supply the posterior aspect of the thigh. A needle is inserted into or immediately below the gluteal fold one quarter of the distance from the ischial tuberosity to the greater trochanter. A loss of resistance can be felt twice as it passes through the superficial fascia and a much thicker and more fibrous deep fascia and enters the space just below and medial to the gluteus maximus where the branches of the posterior cutaneous nerve lie. Injection of about 0.25 ml/kg of local anesthetic at this point will bathe the nerves in the underlying space. This block is particularly useful when donor skin graft is cut from the back of the thigh (Fig. 21-15).[52]

TIBIAL NERVE BLOCK

Tibial nerve block can be performed with the patient prone by inserting a short beveled needle just lateral to the midpoint of a line drawn from the apex of the popliteal fossa and the midpoint of a line drawn between the femoral condyles (Fig. 21-16). Loss of resistance is felt as the fascia covering the popliteal fossa is penetrated. The nerve lies about 0.5 cm deep to this and is contained in a neural sheath. It can be located accurately with a nerve stimulator.[56]

Although this nerve can be blocked to provide surgical anesthesia of the part of the leg and foot supplied, this block has proved most useful in pediatrics to relax the calf muscles in those with spastic disorders or extensor muscle spasms following head injury. After the block the ankle can be manipulated and splinted with plasters. One or several manipulations may be necessary to obtain the correct position of the feet for standing. Initially the child will require support, but the postural reflexes return and eventually the child may be able to stand and walk much more quickly than with less active management.[54]

COMMON PERONEAL NERVE BLOCK

The common peroneal nerve leaves the tibial nerve at the apex of the popliteal fossa and runs laterally just medial to the biceps femoris muscle and deep to the popliteal fascia. It can be blocked at the point shown in Figure 21-16. It should not be blocked as it passes around the neck of the fibula, since neuralgia is more likely to occur.

Tibial, common peroneal, and femoral (or saphenous) nerve blocks can be used for operations below the knee. The saphenous nerve does not have a specific landmark and is blocked by infiltration just posterior to the medial border of the tibia in the vicinity of the long saphenous vein just below the knee.

Blocks around the ankle can be used for removal of plantar warts or foreign bodies in the foot or to provide analgesia, particularly postoperatively, following removal of ingrowing toenails, bunions, and the like (see Chap. 11).

ABDOMINAL AND THORACIC NERVE BLOCKS

ILIOINGUINAL NERVE BLOCK

Ilioinguinal nerve block is now in common use in children having inguinal hernia repair. It is useful for the provision of operative and postoperative analgesia, particularly when no opiate analgesia has been given (see also Chap. 14).

The block is performed by inserting a short beveled needle just below and 0.5 to 2 cm medial to the anterior superior iliac spine (the distance depending on the size of the child) until loss of resistance is felt as the needle penetrates the external oblique aponeurosis. The ilioinguinal nerve emerges through the internal oblique muscle around this point (Fig. 21-17). The injection of 0.25 mg/kg of 0.5% bupivacaine will spread between the muscle and aponeurosis and bathe the nerve. An alternative technique is described in Chapter 14.

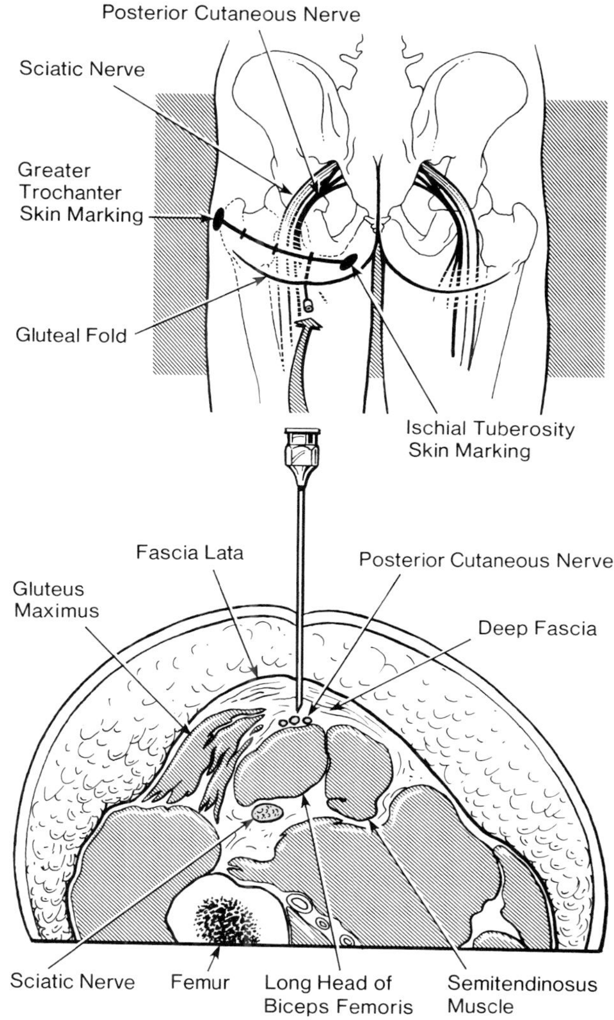

FIG. 21-15. Posterior cutaneous nerve block (see text). The posterior cutaneous nerve can be blocked where the branches emerge below the lower border of gluteus maximus muscle, medial to the sciatic nerve, and deep to both the superficial and the thick fibrous deep fascia. The needle is inserted through the gluteal fold at a point level with one fourth of the distance from the ischial tuberosity to the greater trochanter.

DORSAL NERVE OF PENIS BLOCK

Block of the **dorsal nerve of penis** is becoming more widely used for circumcision and in many centers is preferred to caudal anesthesia because it does not

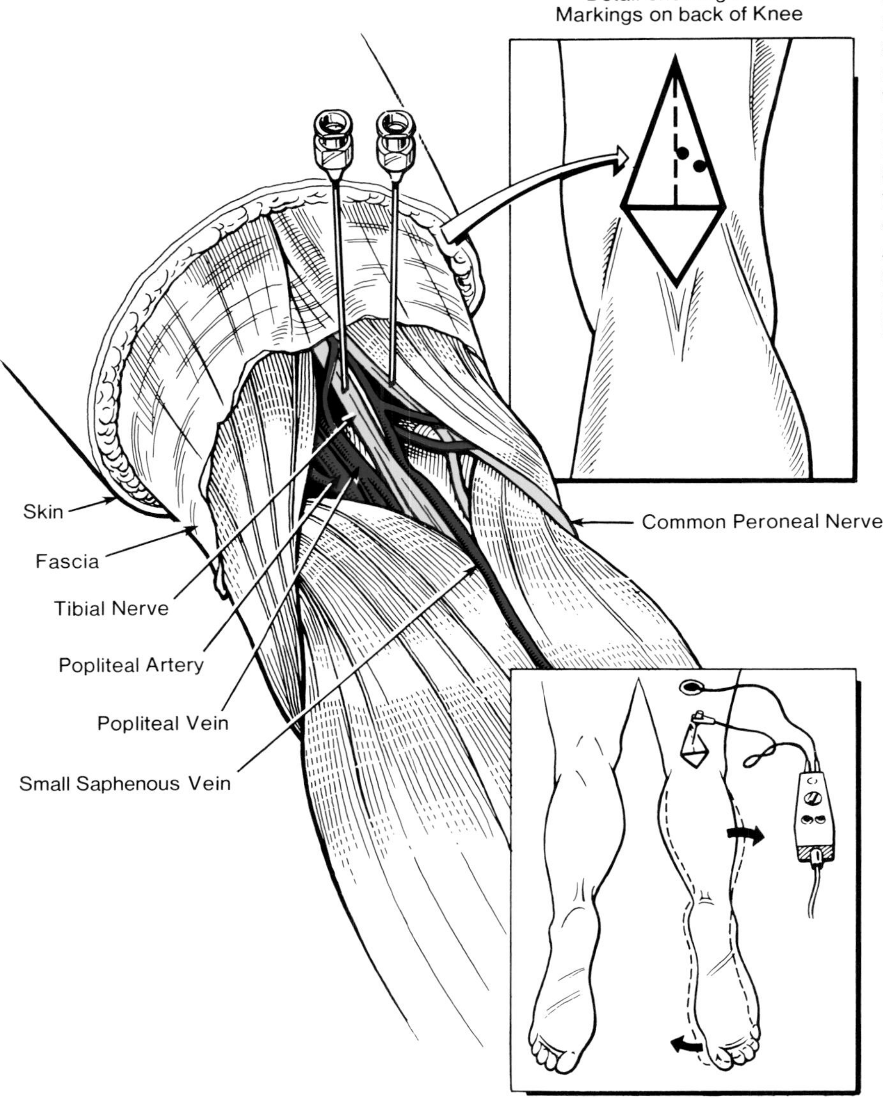

FIG. 21-16. Tibial and common perineal nerve block (see text). The tibial and common peroneal (lateral popliteal) nerves diverge in the popliteal fossa, which is bounded by biceps femoris muscle laterally and semimembranosus muscle medially. They can be blocked as they pass through the triangle formed by these muscles and a line drawn between the femoral condyles. As the needle is inserted, a loss of resistance should be felt as the needle penetrates the fascia overlying the popliteal fossa.

affect the lower limbs and urinary retention is less likely.[16,111]

It is important to remember that the nerves are bilateral. They emerge from under the pubis near the symphysis and pass forward on the surface of the crura of the penis as these converge. At this part of their course they lie on the deep aspect of a triangle bounded superiorly by Buck's fascia, posteriorly by the symphysis pubis, and inferiorly by the crura and their continuation, the corpora cavernosa. This space is divided vertically by the suspensory ligament of the penis which divides over the crura. The nerves lie on the crura deep to the suspensory ligament (Fig. 21-18).

To block the dorsal nerves, the needle is inserted to the symphysis pubis, then withdrawn and advanced just below it until loss of resistance is felt as Buck's fascia is penetrated. Buck's fascia is attached to the anterior border of the symphysis pubis and crosses to the base of the penis. In infants, where the fascia is thin, detection of its penetration is facilitated by the use of a short beveled needle. If Buck's fascia is not located, it will usually have been penetrated if the needle has been advanced 5 mm deep to the anteroinferior border of the symphysis. Once the needle is in the triangular space, the local anesthetic can be injected. A single injection is used in the technique described by Bacon[6]; an alternative is to inject on each side of the midline. Successful block depends on diffusion of local anesthetic through the suspensory ligament, unless the needle enters the triangular space containing the nerves (Fig. 21-18).

A third approach is to inject superficially under the skin, around the base of the penis where the two dorsal nerves are in proximity and lie subcutaneously. Care must be taken at this point to avoid the accompanying blood vessels.

Postoperative analgesia for circumcision has also been provided by the application of local anesthetic ointment to the operative site.[103] Although the pain is greatest soon after the operation, the ointment can be reapplied or the dorsal nerve blocks can be repeated.

A dose of 1 ml per 3 years (minimum 1 ml) of 0.5% bupivacaine is injected after aspiration to ensure a vessel has not been penetrated.

Epinephrine must *never* be used because ischemia

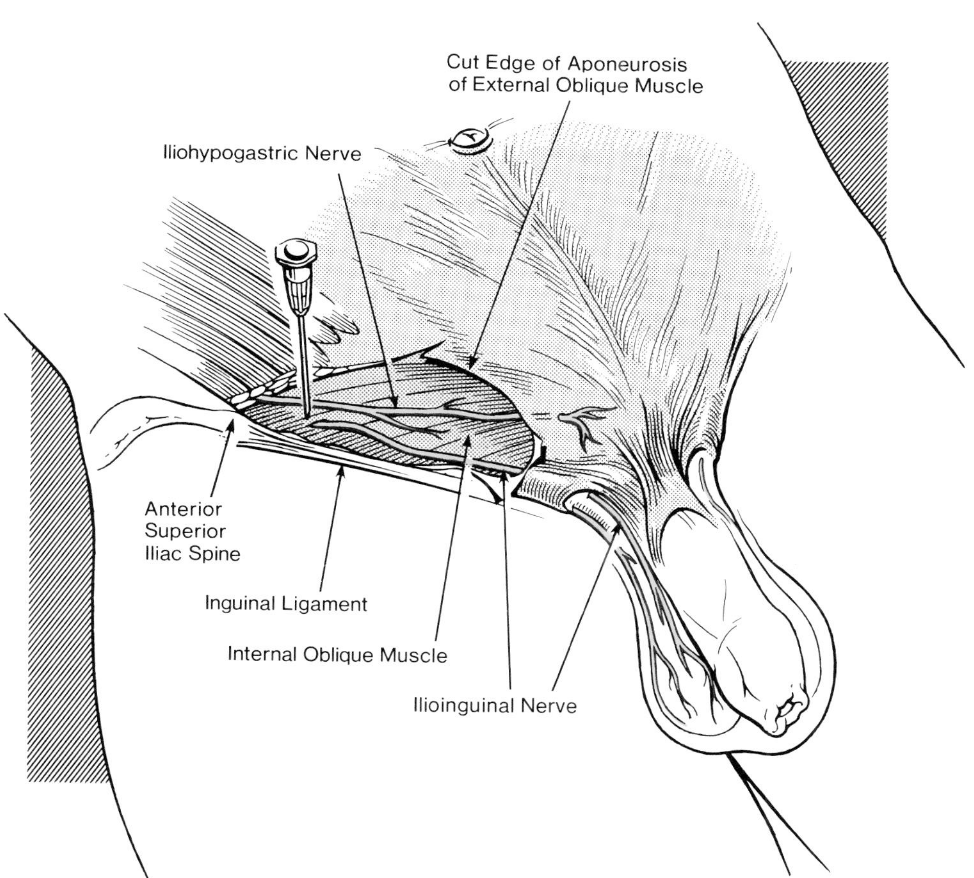

FIG. 21-17. Ilioinguinal and iliohypogastric nerve block (see text). The ilioinguinal nerve emerges through the internal oblique muscle about 1 to 2 cm medial to the anterior superior iliac spine. It lies deep to the external oblique aponeurosis, which can be felt when a short beveled needle is passed through it.

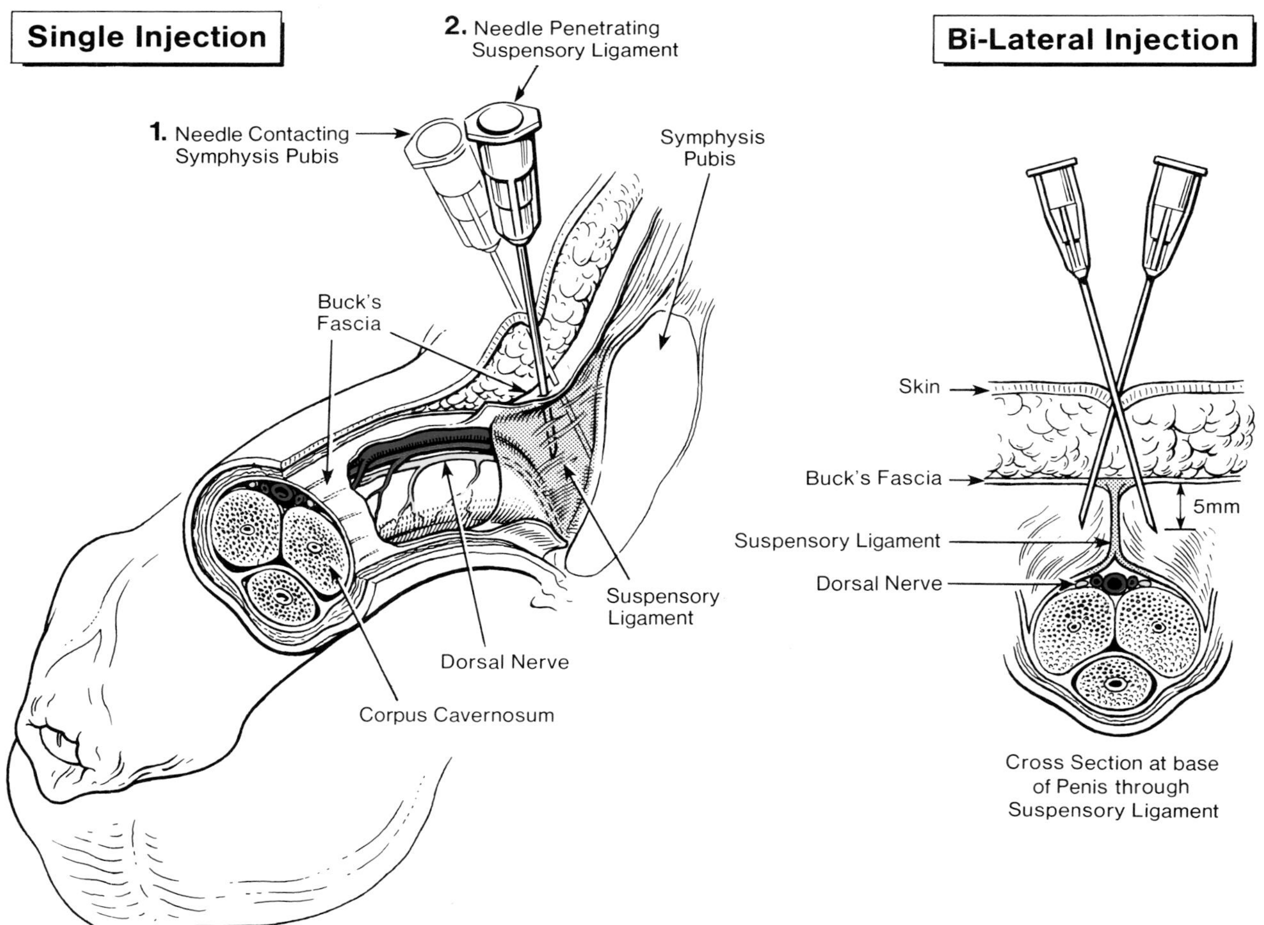

FIG. 21-18. Dorsal nerve of penis block (see text). The dorsal nerves of the penis, derived from the pudendal nerve, run anteriorly below the pubis on the corpora cavernosa. They are most commonly blocked as they traverse the triangular space bounded by the pubic symphysis, the corpora cavernosa, and Buck's fascia. In the transverse section the nerves lie deep to the suspensory ligament of the penis, at which point it splits to surround the penis. **Left.** Lateral view. **Right.** Cross-section. The needle must penetrate Buck's fascia. The injection is then made on either side of the suspensory ligament: through a single midline insertion or through bilateral insertions.

may result. Other potential complications are hematoma and intravascular injection.

INTERCOSTAL NERVE BLOCK

Intercostal nerve blocks are very useful for thoracic or upper abdominal surgery and for the provision of postoperative analgesia if a long-acting local anesthetic is used. They also provide pain relief following chest trauma. They should be performed at the angle of the rib or just posteriorly where there is an innermost intercostal muscle lying deep to the space containing the nerve and vessels. The needle with the syringe attached should be held in the hand resting on the back so that the depth of the needle is not affected by patient movement (see Chap. 14 and Fig. 14-3). The needle is inserted over the rib and "walked" down until it advances below the rib margin. A grating is often felt as it passes through the external and internal intercostal muscles — about 1 to 2 mm in a child. After aspirating to ensure that a vessel has not been punctured, the local anesthetic is injected. Some authors recommend a single large volume injection so that the local anesthetic runs posteriorly. Beyond the insertion of the innermost intercostal muscle, the solution can spread extrapleurally to adjacent intercostal spaces.[74] Alternatively small volumes can be injected into a number of intercostal spaces. Because the diaphragm is relatively more important for respiration in infants than the intercostal muscles, bilateral blocks are well tolerated for an upper abdominal incision that crosses the midline.

PARAVERTEBRAL BLOCK

Paravertebral block is rarely used in children. It might be indicated when an incision or fracture is posterior to the angle of the rib. It must be remembered that the paravertebral space angles deeply from the intercostal space to the spinal canal. The hazards of this block in children are that the space is smaller, making epidural block and the possibility of puncturing a dural cuff and producing spinal anesthesia more likely. The technique is described in Chapter 14.

LUMBAR SYMPATHETIC BLOCK

Lumbar sympathetic block is very occasionally performed in children, mainly for the treatment of reflex sympathetic dystrophy associated with pain in the foot or leg. If this condition is not recognized and allowed to continue in children, osteoporosis and growth retardation of the long bones can occur. Catch-up growth has been reported after a curative block.[28] Reflex sympathetic dystrophy requiring sympathetic block may respond to one block or require repeated local anesthetic blocks. Occasionally, if the condition is longstanding, a more permanent block with phenol will be required (see Chap. 13).

UPPER LIMB SYMPATHETIC BLOCK

Sympathetic block of the upper limb is usually achieved by blocking the fibers carried in the brachial plexus. Stellate ganglion block has been reported for the successful treatment of an ischemic arm in a neonate (Lagade), but this block is rarely used in children. An alternative is the use of an intravenous guanethidine block (see Chaps. 12 and 13).[46]

HEAD AND NECK

Blocks of branches of the cranial nerves supplying the face and scalp can be used with deep sedation or with general anesthesia. They have the benefits of providing postoperative analgesia and preventing restlessness and movement of skin grafts (see Chap. 15).

TOPICAL ANESTHESIA TO THE AIRWAYS

Lidocaine is commonly used topically for laryngoscopy, bronchoscopy, and bronchography in children. These procedures are most commonly done under general anesthesia with the patient either breathing spontaneously with an inhalational agent such as halothane or with controlled ventilation using a relaxant and one of several ventilating techniques described.[15] Local anesthesia reduces the reactivity of the airways.

The local anesthetic can be applied by a spray, through a catheter, or nebulized. Using a 2-ml syringe and a Cass needle with four side holes and an end hole (Fig. 21-19) allows an easily measured volume of known concentration to be applied.[23] For bronchography, a pediatric Y-piece such as that made by Portex is useful because a catheter can be inserted through it to administer the local anesthetic, and then the radiopaque dye. It can also be used for oxygen and suction. This arrangement allows unimpeded spontaneous or controlled ventilation.[17]

Pelton and colleagues showed that blood levels following 3 mg/kg of lidocaine reached 3.2 μg/ml.[79] Eyres and associates found that after 4 mg/kg the mean peak plasma level was about 5.5 μg/ml, although levels up to 10 μg/ml were reached in occasional patients.[37] No toxic manifestations were seen at these levels in children under anesthesia. Lidocaine 2% in the tracheobronchial tree suppresses the cough reflex for about 20 to 30 minutes. There is evidence that the duration of action of topical lidocaine increases when higher concentrations are used.[82]

Bronchoscopy and bronchography can be carried out in older children under sedation alone, but the procedure is unpleasant for the patient. The techniques are the same as those used for adults (see Chap. 16).

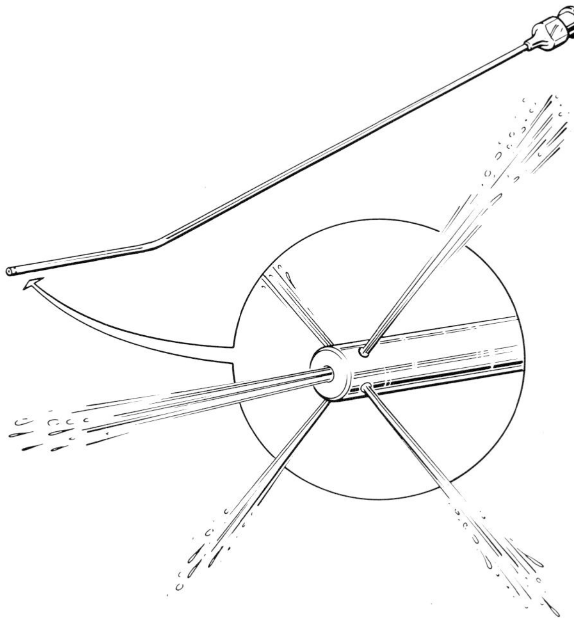

FIG. 21-19. Cass-Waldie needle has a terminal opening and four side holes so that the local anesthetic sprays laterally and distally from the needle.

MINOR INFILTRATION AND TOPICAL TECHNIQUES

Adequate prior sedation allows many minor procedures, such as suture of a small laceration, to be performed with local anesthesia. Attempts to carry out such procedures without adequate premedication are very likely to result in a highly distressed child who will then require general anesthesia.

REFERENCES

1. Abajian, J.C., Mellish, R.W.P., Browne, A.F., Perkins, F.M., *et al.*: Spinal anesthesia for surgery in the high risk infant. Anesth. Analg., *63*:359, 1984.
2. Accardo, N.J., and Adriani, J.: Brachial plexus block: A simplified technique using the axillary route. South. Med. J., *42*:920, 1949.
3. Aizenberg, V.L.: The technique of regional anesthesia of the extremities in combination with nitrous oxide general anesthesia in children. Vestn. Khir., *108*(5):88, 1972.
4. Aizenberg, V.L., and Moisenko, O.L.: Regional anesthesia of the upper extremity in combination with nitrous oxide analgesia in children. Khirurgiia (Mosk.), *48*:26, 1972.
5. Armitage, E.N.: Caudal block in children. Anaesthesia, *34*:396, 1979.
6. Bacon, A.K.: An alternative block for post circumcision analgesia. Anaesth. Intens. Care, *5*:63, 1977.
7. Bainbridge, W.B.: Analgesia in children by spinal injection with a report of a new method of sterilization of the injection fluid. Med. Record, *58*:937, 1900.
8. Bentley, J.B., Class, S., and Gandolfi, J.: The influence of halothane on lidocaine pharmacokinetics in man. Anesthesiology, *59*:A246, 1983.
9. Berkowitz, S., and Greene, B.A. Spinal anesthesia in children: Report based on 350 patients under 13 years of age. Anesthesiology, *12*:376, 1977.
10. Bier, A.: Ueber einen neuen Weg Lokalanasthesie an den Gliedmassen zu erzeugen. Verh. Dtsch. Ges. Chir., *37*(2):204, 1908.
11. Bromage, P.R.: Aging and epidural dose requirements: Segmental spread and predictability of epidural analgesia in youth and extreme age. Br. J. Anaesth., *41*:1016, 1969.
12. Bromage, P.R., Shibata, R.R., and Willoughby, H.W.: Influence of prolonged epidural blockade on blood sugar and cortisol responses to operations upon the upper part of the abdomen and thorax. Surg. Gynecol. Obstet., *132*:1057, 1971.
13. Brown, T.C.K., and Fisk, G.C.: Anaesthesia for Children, p. 26. Oxford, Blackwell, 1979.
14. Brown, T.C.K., and Fisk, G.C.: Anaesthesia for Children, p. 258. Oxford, Blackwell, 1979.
15. Brown, T.C.K., and Fisk, G.C.: Anaesthesia for Children, p. 205. Oxford, Blackwell, 1979.
16. Brown, T.C.K.: Local and regional anaesthesia in children. Anaesthesia, *40*:407, 1985.
17. Brown, T.C.K.: Uses of the Portex Y piece in paediatric anaesthesia. Anaesth. Intens. Care, *3*:215, 1985.
18. Brown, T.C.K., and Dickens, D.R.V.: Another approach to lateral cutaneous nerve of thigh block. Anaesth. Intensive Care, *14*:126, 1986.
19. Buckley, N.M., Gootman, P.M., Yellin, E.L., and Brazeau, P.: Age related cardiovascular effects of catecholamines in anaesthetized piglets. Circ. Res., *45*:282, 1979.
20. Busoni, P., and Andreucetti, T.: The spread of caudal anaesthesia in children: a mathematical model. Anaes. Intens. Care *14*:140, 1986.
21. Campbell, M.F.: Caudal anesthesia in children. Am. J. Urol., *30*:245, 1933.
22. Carrell, E.D., and Eyring, E.J.: Intravenous regional anesthesia for childhood fractures. J. Trauma, *11*:301, 1971.
23. Cass, N.M., Waldie, L.A.: A robust, reliable throat spray. Br. J. Anaesth., *36*:61, 1964.
24. Castanos, C.C., Rollano, J., and Beltran, J.J.: Anestesia peridural sacra em criancas. Rev. Bras. Anest., *20*:348, 1970.
25. Davenport, H.T.: Paediatric Anaesthesia, p. 97. London, Heinemann Medical Books, 1967.
26. De Pablo, J.S., and Diez-Mallo, J.: Experiences with 3000 cases of brachial plexus blocks: Its dangers: Report of a fatal case. Ann. Surg., *128*:956, 1948.
27. Dohi, S., Naito, H., and Takahashi, T.: Age related changes in blood pressure and duration of motor block in spinal anaesthesia. Anesthesiology, *50*:319, 1979.

28. Doolan, L.A., and Brown, T.C.K.: Reflex sympathetic dystrophy in a child. Anaesth. Intens. Care, *12*:70, 1984.
29. Eather, K.F.: Regional anesthesia for infants and children. Int. Anesthesiol. Clin., *13*:19, 1975.
30. Elze, C.: Centrales Nervensystem. In Braus, H. (ed.): Anatomie des Menschen. Berlin, Springer-Verlag, 1932.
31. Eriksson, E.: Axillary brachial plexus anaesthesia in children with Citanest. Acta Anaesthesiol. Scand., *16*:291, 1965.
32. Etherington-Wilson, W.: Spinal anaesthesia in the very young and further observations. Proc. R. Soc. Med., *388*:109, 1944.
33. Eyres, R.L., Bishop, W., Oppenheim, R.C., and Brown, T.C.K.: Plasma lignocaine concentrations following topical laryngeal application. Anaesth. Intens. Care, *11*: 23, 1983.
34. Eyres, R.L., Bishop, W., Oppenheim, R.C., and Brown, T.C.K.: Plasma bupivacaine concentrations in children during caudal epidural anaesthesia. Anaesth. Intens. Care, *11*:20, 1983.
35. Eyres, R.L., Kidd, J., Oppenheim, R.C., and Brown, T.C.K.: Local anaesthetic plasma levels in children. Anaesth. Intens. Care, *6*:243, 1978.
36. Eyres, R.L., Hastings, C., Brown, T.C.K., and Oppenheim, R.C.: Plasma bupivacaine concentrations following lumbar epidural anaesthesia in children. Anaesth. Intens. Care, *14*:131, 1986.
37. Eyres, R.L., Hastings, C.: Personal communication.
38. Eyres, R.L., Brown, T.C.K., and Hastings, C.: Plasma level of bupivacaine during convulsions. Anaesth. Intens. Care, *11*:385, 1983.
39. Eyres, R.L.: Personal communication.
40. Farr, R.E.: Local anesthesia in infancy and childhood. Arch. Pediatr., *37*:381, 1920.
41. Fortin, G., and Tremblay, L.: The short-needle technique in brachial plexus block. Can Anaesth. Soc. J., *6*:32, 1959.
42. Fortuna, A.: Caudal analgesia: A simple and safe technique in paediatric surgery. Br. J. Anaesth., *39*:165, 1967.
43. Gouveia, M.A.: Raquianestesia para pacientes pediatricos. Rev. Bras. Anest., *4*:503, 1970.
44. Gray's Anatomy of the Human Body, 29th ed., p. 792. Philadelphia, Lea & Febiger, 1973.
45. Gray, T.: Study of spinal anaesthesia in infants and children. Lancet, *25*:9, 1909; *10*:10, 1909; and *10*:6, 1910.
46. Hannington-Kiff, J.G.: Intravenous regional sympathetic block with guanethidine. Lancet, *1*:1019, 1974.
47. Hastings, C., Brown, T.C.K., Eyres, R.L., and Oppenheim, R.C.: The influence of age on lignocaine pharmacokinetics in young puppies. Anaesth. Intens. Care, *14*:135, 1986.
48. Hastings, C., Brown, T.C.K., Eyres, R.L., and Oppenheim, R.C.: The influence of age on plasma lignocaine levels following tracheal spray in young dogs. Anaesth. Intens. Care, *13*:392, 1985.
49. Hempel, V., and Baur, K.F.: Regionalanaesthesie fuer Schulter, Arm und Hand. Munich, Urban and Schwarzenberg, 1982.
50. Holland, A.J.C., Davies, K.H., and Wallace, D.H.: Sympathetic blockade of isolated limbs by intravenous guanethidine. Can. Soc. Anaesth. J., *24*:597, 1977.
51. Holmes, C. McK.: Intravenous regional anaesthesia. Lancet, *1*:245, 1963.
52. Hughes, P.J., and Brown, T.C.K.: Posterior cutaneous nerve of thigh block. Anaesth. Intensive Care (In Press).
53. Isakob, Y.F., Geraskin, B.L., and Koshevnikov, V.A.: Long term peridural anesthesia after operations on the organs of the chest in children. Grudn. Chir., *13*:104, 1971.
54. Junkin, C.L.: Spinal anesthesia in children. Can. Med. Assoc. J., *28*:51, 1933.
55. Kay, B.: Caudal block for postoperative pain relief in children. Anaesthesia, *29*:610, 1974.
56. Kempthorne, P.M., and Brown, T.C.K.: Nerve blocks around the knee in children. Anaesth. Intens. Care, *12*:14, 1984.
57. Khoo, S.T., and Brown, T.C.K.: Femoral nerve block—the anatomical basis for a single injection technique. Anaesth. Intens. Care, *11*:40, 1983.
58. Koster, H.: Spinal anesthesia in head and neck surgery. Am. J. Surg., *5*:554, 1928.
59. Kuhn, K.: Postoperative Schmerzbekaempfung mittels periduraler Opiat Analgesie bei Kindern. In Kuhn, K. (ed.): Regional Anaesthesie im Kindesalter, p. 31. Berlin, Springer-Verlag.
60. Lagade, M.R.G., and Poppers, P.J.: Stellate ganglion block: A therapeutic modality for arterial insufficiency of the arm in premature infants. Anesthesiology, *61*:203, 1984.
61. Leak, W.D., Winchell, S.W.: Regional anesthesia in pediatric patients—Review of clinical experience. Reg. Anaesth., *7*:64, 1982.
62. Leigh, M.D.: Spinal anaesthesia in infants and children. Int. Anesthesiol. Clin., *1*:825, 1963.
63. Leigh, M.D., and Belton, M.K.: Pediatric Anesthesia, 2nd ed. New York, Macmillan, 1960.
64. Lourey, C.J., and McDonald, I.H.: Caudal anaesthesia in infants and children. Anaesth. Intens. Care, *1*:547, 1973.
65. Lundy, J.S., Tuphy, E.B., Adams, R.C., and Mousel, C.H.: Clinical use of local and intravenous anesthetic agents: General anesthesia from the standpoint of hepatic function. Proc. Staff Meetings Mayo Clin., *16*:73, 1941.
66. Lunn, J.N.: Postoperative analgesia after circumcision. Anaesthesia, *34*:552, 1979.
67. Lups, S., and Haan, A.M.F.H.: The cerebrospinal fluid. Amsterdam, Elsevier, 1964.
68. Lutsch, E.F., and Morris, R.W.: Circadian periodicity in susceptibility to lidocaine hydrochloride. Science, *156*:100, 1967.
69. Macintosh, R.R., and Mushin, W.W.: Local anaesthesia: Brachial Plexus. Oxford, Blackwell, 1944.
70. McNicol, L.R.: Sciatic nerve block by the anterior approach for postoperative pain relief in paediatric practice. Anaesthesia, *40*:410, 1985.
71. Meigner, M., Souron, R., and Le Neel, J.C.: Postoperative dorsal epidural analgesia in the child with respiratory disabilities. Anesthesiology, *59*:473, 1983.
72. Melman, E., Pennelas, J., and Maruffo, J.: Regional anesthesia in children. Anesth. Analg. (Cleve.), *54*:387, 1975.
73. Miranda, D.R.: Continuous brachial plexus block. Acta Anaesthesiol. Belg., *4*:323, 1977.

74. Murphy, D.F.: Continuous intercostal nerve blockade: An anatomical study to elucidate its mode of action. Br. J. Anaesth., *52*:253, 1980.
75. Niesel, H.C., Rodrigues, P., and Wilsmann, I.: Regional Anaesthesie der oberen Extremitaet bei Kindern. Anaesthetist, *23*:1788, 1974.
76. Nunn, J.F., and Slavin, G.: Posterior intercostal nerve block for pain relief after cholecystectomy. Br. J. Anaesth., *52*:2523, 1980.
77. Parnes, D.I., and Gordeyev, V.I.: Some indices of external respiration in the postoperative peridural blockade in children. Vestn. Khir., *105*:66, 1970.
78. Parnes, D.I., *et al.*: Hemodynamics and respiration in the postoperative peridural blockade in children. Vestn. Khir., *106*:110, 1971.
79. Pelton, D.A., Daly, M., Cooper, P.D., and Conn, A.W.: Plasma lidocaine concentrations following topical aerosol application to the trachea and bronchi. Can. Anaesth. Soc. J., *17*:350, 1970.
80. Pitkin, G.P.: Conduction anesthesia: Clinical studies of George P. Pitkin. In Southwerth, J.L., and Hingson, R. (eds.), 387. Philadelphia, J.B. Lippincott, 1946.
81. Reinauer, H., and Hollman, S. Der Einfluss der Narkoseart auf den Gehalt an Adeninnucleotiden Lactat and Pyruvat in Herz, Leber und Milz der Ratte. Anaesthesist, *15*:327, 1966.
82. Robinson, E.P., Rex, M.A.E., and Brown, T.C.K.: A comparison of different concentrations of lignocaine hydrocloride used for topical anaesthesia of the larynx of the cat. Anaesth. Intens. Care, *13*:137, 1985.
83. Robson, C.H.: Anesthesia in children. Am. J. Surg., *34*:468, 1936.
84. Rodrigues, L.A.: Anestesia peridural no pacienta pediatrico. Rev. Bras. Anest., *14*:116, 1964.
85. Rosenberg, P.H., Kalso, E.A., Tuominen, M.K., and Linden, H.B.: Acute bupivacaine toxicity as a result of venous leakage under the tourniquet cuff during a Bier block. Anesthesiology, *58*:95, 1983.
85a. Rothstein P., Arthur, G.R., Feldman, H.S., Kopf, G.S., *et al.*: Bupivacaine for intercostal nerve blocks in children: Blood concentrations and pharmacokinetics. Anesth. Analg., *65*:625, 1986.
86. Rowley, M.P., and Brown, T.C.K.: Postoperative vomiting in children. Anaesth. Intens. Care, *10*:309, 1982.
87. Runciman, W.B., Mather, L.E., Ilsley, A.H., Carapetis, R.J., *et al.*: A sheep preparation for studying interactions between blood flow and drug disposition: III. Effects of general and spinal anaesthesia on regional blood blow and oxygen tensions. Br. J. Anaesth., *56*:1247, 1984.
88. Ruston, F.G.: Epidural anaesthesia in infants and children. Can. Anaesth. Soc. J., *1*:37, 1954.
89. Ruston, F.G.: Epidural anesthesia in paediatric surgery: Present status at the Hamilton General Hospital. Can. Anaesth. Soc. J., *11*:12, 1964.
90. Schettler, D.: Untersuchungen der Ventilation der Atemmechanik, der Blutgase und des Saeure-Basen-Haushaltes bei Saeuglingen mit Lippen-, Kiefer-, Gaumenspalten vor, waehrend und nach der Operation. Dusseldorf, Habil Schr, 1970.
91. Schneider Kinderklinik, Leipzig: Peridural Anaesthesie im Kindesalter. Z. Urol. Chir., *76*:704, 1951.
92. Schulte-Steinberg, O.: Die Caudalanaesthesie im Kindersalter unter besonderer Berucksichtigung der Frage der Ausbreitung und des Wirkungsortes von Localanaesthetika im Kindlichwn Epiduralraum. In Wust, H.J., Schulte-Steinberg, O. (eds.): Epidural Anaesthesie bei Kindern und Alteren Patieuten. Berlin, Springer-Verlag, 1983.
93. Schulte-Steinberg, O., and Rahlfs, V.W.: Caudal anaesthesia in children and spread of 1 per cent lignocaine: A statistical study. Br. J. Anaesth., *42*:1093, 1970.
94. Schulte-Steinberg, O.: Caudal Anaesthesie bei Kindern und die Ausbreitung von 0.25% iger Bupivacaine Loesung. Anaesthetist, *21*:94, 1972.
95. Schulte-Steinberg, O.: Zum gegenwaartigen Stand der kaudalen Epiduralanaesthesie in Kindersalter. Anaesthesiol. u. Reanimat., *6*:323, 1981.
96. Schapiro, L.A., Jedeikin, R.J., Shalev, D., and Hoffman, S.: Epidural morphine analgesia in children. Anesthesiology, *61*:210, 1984.
97. Sievers, R.: Peridural Anaesthesie zur Cystoscopie beim Kind. Arch. Klin. Chir., *185*:359, 1936.
98. Slater, H.M., and Stephen, C.R.: Hypobaric pontocaine spinal anaesthesia in children. Anesthesiology, *11*:709, 1950.
99. Small, G.A.: Brachial plexus block anesthesia in children. J.A.M.A., *147*:1648, 1951.
100. Smith, R.M.: Anesthesia for infants and children, 3rd ed. St. Louis, C.V. Mosby, 1968.
101. Spiegel, P.: Caudal anesthesia in pediatric surgery: A preliminary report. Anesth. Analg. (Cleve.), *41*:218, 1962.
102. Spiegel, P.: Anestesia peridural sacra em pacientes pediatros Panorama Atual. Rev. Bras. Anest., *26*:566, 1976.
103. Thara Tree-traken, Pirayavaropron, S.: Personal communication.
104. Touloukian, R.J., Ulugmeister, M., Pickett, L.K., and Hehre, F.W.: Anaesthesie for neonatal, anoperineal and rectal operations. Anaesth. Analg., *50*:565, 1971.
105. Tretjakoff, D.: Das epidurale Fettgewebe. Z. Anat., *79*:100, 1926.
106. Tucker, G.L., and Mather, L.E.: Pharmacokinetics of local anaesthetic agents. Br. J. Anaesth., *47*:213, 1975.
107. Turner, P.L., Batten, J.B., Hjorth, D., Ross, E.R.S., *et al.*: Intravenous regional anaesthesia for the treatment of upper limb injuries in childhood. Aust. N.Z. J. Surg., *56*:153, 1986.
108. Williamson, P.S., Williamson, M.L.: Physiologic stress reduction by a local anesthetic during newborn circumcision. Pediatrics, *71*:36–40, 1983.
109. Winnie, A.P.: Interscalene brachial plexus block. Anesth. Analg. (Cleve.), *49*:455, 1970.
110. Winnie, A.P., Ramamurthy, S.R., and Durrany, Z.: The inguinal perivascular technique of lumbar plexus anesthesia: The "3-in-1 block". Anesth. Analg. (Cleve.), *52*:989, 1973.
111. Yeoman, P.M., Cooke, R., and Hain, W.R.: Penile block for circumcision? Anaesthesia, *38*:862, 1983.
112. Yoshikawa, K., Mima, T., and Egawa, J.: Blood level of marcaine. (LAC-43) in axillary plexus blocks, intercostal nerve blocks and epidural anaesthesia. Acta Anaesthesiol. Scand., *12*:1, 1968.

section F

COMPLICATIONS OF NEURAL BLOCKADE

22 COMPLICATIONS OF LOCAL ANESTHETIC NEURAL BLOCKADE

PHILLIP O. BRIDENBAUGH

It is often difficult for the anesthetist to be objective when discussing complications of any kind. The word itself has a negative connotation and is frequently used to imply fault, failure, or even negligence. Although elements of such may be present in many complications, there is virtually nothing in life, medicine, anesthesia, or neural blockade that is totally without risk of complication—cause not withstanding. The safest approach to a discussion of complications of local anesthetic neural blockade, therefore, is to have a clear understanding of what the complications of a given procedure might be and be prepared to prevent or diagnose and treat them appropriately.

Unfortunately, many unsuccessful procedures or poor results are automatically attributed to "complications." This may preserve the anesthetist's reputation but, unfortunately, tends to reflect poorly on the procedure instead. Stated differently, is there really a high complication rate to neural blockade, or is it "just a low success rate" in many hands?

Many times normal responses to neural blockade are called complications, for example, hypotension with high spinal anesthesia. One must differentiate, therefore, between normal "side-effects" and true complications. *Webster's Dictionary* defines a complication as "a difficult factor or issue, often appearing unexpectedly and changing existing plans, methods or attitudes." Clearly, hypotension with a high spinal block may be sudden, but it should not *usually* be unexpected. Conversely, *Webster's* defines a side-effect as "a secondary and usually adverse effect." Certainly much of what occurs with neural blockade is physiologic side-effect as opposed to unexpected complications.

CAUSES OF COMPLICATIONS

One classic way of discussing the complications of a given entity is by cause. For neural blockade, therefore, one might discuss complications owing to equipment, drugs, and, perhaps, human error. Such an approach makes it more difficult to anticipate the complications and side-effects of new or different techniques. A more systematic approach is to discuss causes as something common to all neural blockade techniques and then proceed to their logical classification.

If, as defined, side-effects were anticipated and therefore prevented, the resultant complications would also be avoided. The causes of these "unanticipated side-effects" can be categorized into three general areas: All may be referred to as "errors in judgment" as they relate to [1] technique, [2] drugs, and [3] management of the patient.

TECHNIQUE

Errors in judgment related to technique are concerned with selecting the nerve block technique (if in fact one is appropriate) to best fit the needs of the patient and the surgeon and the abilities of the anesthetist. This is often the precursor, but quite different from actual technical errors in performing the block.

Clearly, abstinence is the best way to avoid complications, but, if one is carefully selective in the application of nerve block procedures, the inverse ratio of high success with few complications will prevail. Anesthetists are taught, however, that regional anesthesia is the anesthesia of choice for poor risk and trauma patients. The morbidity and the mortality associated with regional anesthesia often occur in the poor selection for the poor-risk or emergency patient, for example, the morbidly obese, belligerent patient and the full stomach hypovolemic patient, who may require a nerve block that the anesthetist has seldom done. Even if the technique is suited to the patient, it may not be suited to the abilities of the anesthetist.

DRUGS

A successfully accomplished technique puts the needle next to the nerves to be blocked. The successful nerve block comes in the selection of the correct local anesthetic agent or, more frequently, the right concentration or volume. Poor judgment leads to a partial block (inadequate concentration or volume) or one that wears off before the surgery finishes (wrong drug). All too frequently, patients were selected for a nerve block because of a relative contraindication to general anesthesia, that is, a full stomach or difficult intubation. The risk of complications secondary to an inadequate block in this circumstance is clearly greater. The opposite error in drug selection is that of excess volume or concentration, or both, leading to toxicity or prolonged neural blockade. The use of 0.75% bupivacaine, for example, for an arm block in an outpatient will subject the patient to many hours of a vasodilated, useless extremity or the risk of a grand mal seizure from drug overdose 30 minutes after completing the block.

PATIENT MANAGEMENT

The end result of any nerve block, no matter how successfully administered, is dependent upon how well the patient's total anesthetic experience is managed. Clearly, the successful management of the patient can become extremely difficult and complex if there have been preceding errors in judgment relating to just the neural blockade portion of the patient's anesthetic care.

Most patients require some measure of supplemental sedation, amnesia, or analgesia, or all three in order to be psychologically satisfied with their anesthetic experience. Inappropriate selection of drugs, such as the dissociative agents, can convert a responsible and cooperative patient into a restless, belligerent, or even unmanageable and disoriented patient who must then receive a full general anesthetic.

Conversely, overdose of the sedative or hypnotic agents may result in loss of consciousness, airway obstruction, and hypotension and require resuscitative intubation and ventilation. Technicians may be skilled at doing perfect nerve blocks, but trained anesthetists must learn how to select and manage patients in whom a regional anesthetic technique will be an important adjunct to their total successful anesthetic management.

CLASSIFICATION OF COMPLICATIONS AND SIDE-EFFECTS

In discussing the complications of a major area of medical practice, such as neural blockade, there is a tendency to provide an outline or structure that will cover all the complications of all the procedures. The most thorough, repetitive, and tedious approach is to make a list of all reported or theoretical complications for each of the nerve block techniques. Other authors have approached the discussion by etiology, that is, complications owing to equipment, to drugs, and to human error. There are, however, many complications for which we do not know the cause. Further, such an approach does not allow one to predict what complications might occur with new techniques.

The approach here is to suggest that there is an anatomic and therefore physiologic commonality for the nerve block techniques that allows one to predict which complications might occur and the magnitude and frequency of such complications. Because most of the nerves to be blocked are surrounded by major blood vessels and lie in proximity to major body organs (*i.e.*, lung, liver, kidney), it seems reasonable to classify complications into three major systemic groups: [1] vascular complications, [2] respiratory complications, and [3] neurologic complications. A fourth miscellaneous group will collect those complications or side-effects not having a relationship to the other three systems.

VASCULAR COMPLICATIONS AND SIDE-EFFECTS

At nearly every site of the body where neural blockade is accomplished, the nerves to be blocked are surrounded by arteries and veins forming the neurovascular bundle. Naturally, the larger or more proximal the nerve, the greater is the likelihood that the surrounding vessels are also large. There has been a tendency in the past to consider all vascular complications as unintentional intravenous injections of local anesthetics in sufficient volume or dose to precipitate a grand mal seizure. Less frequent, but just as important, are complications from intra-arterial injections and hematoma formation.

Arterial

The deceptive difference between intravenous and intra-arterial complications comes as a result of our failure to realize that although all venous blood empties into the heart and goes through the lungs before going to the target organ (*i.e.,* the brain), the injection of drugs into the internal carotid or vertebral arteries goes directly to the brain. Therefore, a very small dose of local anesthetic will result in CNS toxicity. All other arterial injections just feed into the venous circulation and will behave similarly to intravenous injections. The potential for this complication occurring was noted by Moore in his textbook *Stellate Ganglion Block* in 1954.[46] Since that time, isolated case reports have appeared in the literature, usually after stellate ganglion block. If one reflects on the anatomy of the vertebral and internal carotid arterial system (Fig. 22-1), however, it is apparent that a similar complication may result from any practitioner inserting needles into the neck of his patient. Certainly, interscalene block, cervical plexus block, vagal nerve block, and, perhaps, even local infiltration for insertion of central lines are but a few of the techniques that could result in intra-arterial-induced local anesthesia seizures.

Korevaar and co-workers[37] stressed the small doses required to precipitate toxicity by comparing the actual doses of seven previous case reports with their estimated toxic dose. The minimum toxic dose injected into a vertebral or internal carotid artery as a bolus can be estimated by accepting that 15% of the cardiac output that goes to the brain is equally divided among the four arteries supplying the brain. Therefore, 15% of the minimum intravenous toxic dose divided by four will be the estimated bolus toxic dose intra-arterially (Table 22-1).

Convulsions are not the only complication of bolus injection into the internal carotid or vertebral artery: Total blindness, aphasia, hemiparesis, and unconsciousness of a transient and completely recoverable nature have also been reported.[62,66] It is equally probable that local anesthetic injections around the head

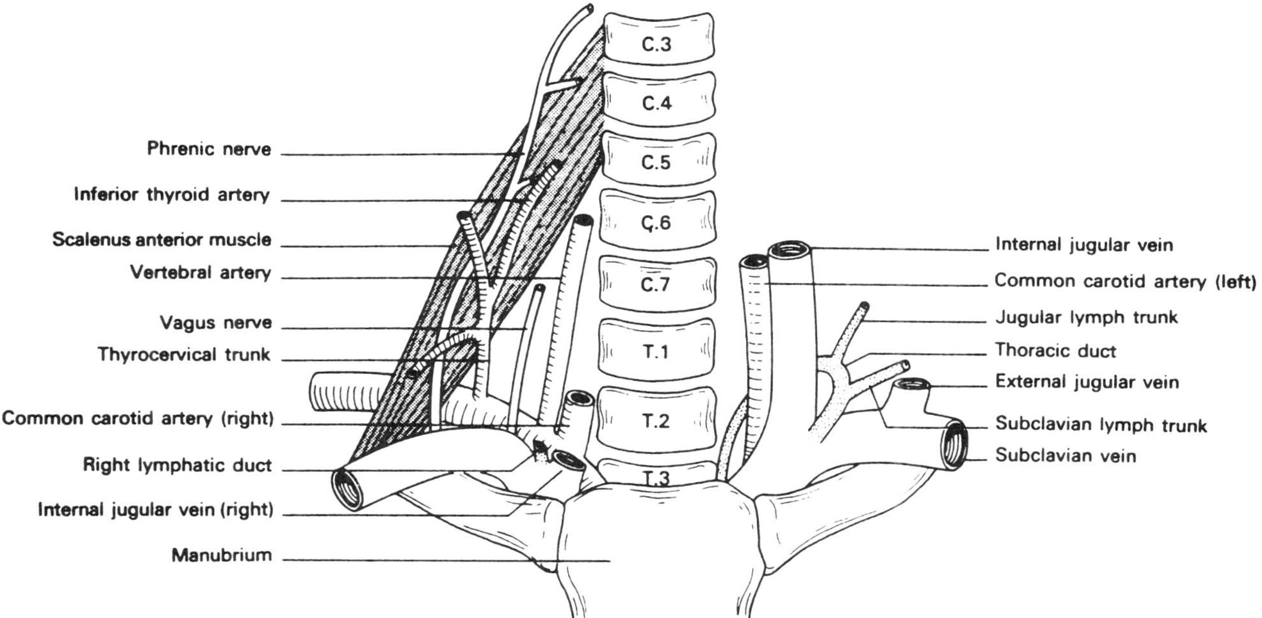

FIG. 22-1. Relationship of carotid and vertebral arteries to neural structures of the neck. (Thompson, J.S.: Core Textbook of Anatomy, p. 228. Philadelphia, J. B. Lippincott, 1977.)

TABLE 22-1. ANESTHETIC AGENTS AND TOXIC DOSES*

Local Anesthetic Agent	Minimum Toxic Intravenous Dose (mg/kg)	Estimated Intra-Arterial Toxic Dose* (mg)	Reported Toxic Doses (mg)
Procaine	19.2	43.2	100
Tetracaine	2.5	5.6	2.5
Lidocaine	6.4	14.4	10
			16
			90
Bupivacaine	1.6	3.6	32.5
			7.5

*Estimated for injection into a vertebral or internal carotid artery for a 60-kg subject.

(Korevaar, W.C., Burney, R.G., and Moore, P.A.: Convulsions during stellate ganglion block: a case report. Anesth. Analg., *58*:330, 1979.)

and neck may enter small arteries and, by retrograde flow, pass into the cerebral circulation. Tomlin, in a review of death in outpatient dental anesthesia, commented on the case of a 22-year-old woman who, after receiving an inferior dental nerve block with 1.5 ml of 2% lignocaine with 1:80,000 norepinephrine, lost consciousness, paled, convulsed, had a cardiac arrest, and died.[70] In an effort to demonstrate retrograde flow by bolus injection into small arteries, Aldrete[2] performed lingual artery lidocaine injections in baboons and measured lidocaine levels in the internal carotid artery. Six seconds after lingual artery injection, the lidocaine levels in the internal carotid artery were 28 μg/ml. Injection of microspheres further illustrated retrograde flow.

Injections made into brachial and femoral arteries also demonstrated retrograde flow into the internal carotid system. This study, along with clinical reports, suggests that ophthalmologists, dentists, otorhinolaryngologists, and other surgeons injecting local anesthetics around the head and neck should aspirate gently and repeatedly and inject slowly if they wish to avoid such complications.

Intravenous

As previously noted, most clinicians from the time they were taught how to do a venipuncture were taught that inviolate dictum, "Aspirate before you inject." The humorous but irrational extreme of this dictum is observing people painfully insert a needle subcutaneously and faithfully aspirate before making a skin wheal with a local anesthetic agent. The scientific world anxiously awaits the first report of a toxic reaction secondary to intravascular injection of a skin wheal.

Although direct intravenous injections are much more likely than intra-arterial, the safety from seizure comes in the larger volumes or doses required for such a complication. A cautious anesthetist and a conscious patient can *usually* detect the prodroma of CNS toxicity before frank seizures occur (see Chap. 4). Certainly, unintentional intravenous injection is possible with all of the regional block techniques, with the remote exception of subarachnoid block. In point of fact, as one listens to anesthesia colleagues or reads the literature on CNS and cardiovascular toxicity of local anesthetics, it becomes apparent that most of these unintentional intravenous injections result from injections through an indwelling epidural catheter. Many novices to the use of indwelling epidural or caudal catheters are unaware of the gentleness with which aspiration must be accomplished if blood (or CSF) is to be aspirated at all—let alone the full length of the catheter to the aspirating syringe. It is common that the negative pressures exerted at the tip of the catheter by a strong anesthetist on the proximal end of a 20-ml syringe will instantly collapse vein or dura and nothing will be returned, only to result in complications when too much local anesthetic is injected too quickly. A moderate practice suggests use of a small test dose of local anesthetic containing 1:200,000 epinephrine with appropriate cardiovascular monitors followed by slow injection of 5-ml increments of local anesthetic to reach the final preselected total dose (see Chap. 4).

Another more subtle form of intravenous toxicity has come to light over the past few years as reported by the practitioners of intravenous regional anesthesia (see Chap. 12). Heath,[30] in a letter to the editors of *Anesthesiology*, drew attention to the fact that from 1979 to early 1983, "seven patients have died in the United Kingdom as a result of Bier blocks in which bupivacaine was used." The role of bupivacaine in those fatalities is not the issue here (see Chaps. 4 and 12). Other factors that contribute to such complications relate to the fact, first, that many practitioners other than trained anesthetists are performing Bier blocks, even in offices and outpatient facilities where neither equipment nor trained personnel are available to treat seizures or perform resuscitation.[25] Death and, much more commonly, CNS toxicity from intravenous regional anesthesia may result from errors of technique or drug dosage along with failure of resuscitation. Disasters have certainly resulted from tourniquet failure, illustrating the point that tourniquet equipment should be well maintained and checked frequently for maintenance of accurately displayed pressures.[58] It has now become apparent, however, that the injected solution can "leak" beneath a correctly inflated cuff. Subsequent to a patient having seizures and cardiovascular collapse with intravenous regional anesthesia despite an accurate tourniquet pressure of 120 mm Hg over systolic (180/300 mm Hg), Rosenberg and colleagues[59] performed phlebographic studies in three patients and three volunteers. In four of the six subjects, contrast medium leakage was seen proximal to the tourniquet. To study further the problem of leakage under the tourniquet, Lawes and colleagues[39] measured the pressures generated in the venous system of the arm during injection of a simulated intravenous regional anesthetic. Should the recommended tourniquet pressure of 50 mm Hg over systolic be adhered to, three of four subjects would have sustained periods of venous pressure in excess of tourniquet pressure, thus allowing leakage of injected solution under the cuff and into the systemic circulation. Even with the tourniquet inflated to 250 mm Hg, one of four subjects would still have had leakage under the cuff. These situations of high venous pressure are more likely to occur if the injection is made rapidly or into a proximal vein, if the volume injected is large, or if the extremity is inadequately exsanguinated.[28] The effect of speed of injection and method of exsanguination was studied by Duggan and associates.[17] They noted that venous pressures were dependent upon the methods of exsanguination, with highest pressures occurring when no exsanguination was done and lowest with exsanguination by Esmarch bandage, regardless of the rate of injection. The slow rate of injection always produced significantly lower peak pressures than did the faster rate at all degrees of exsanguination (Table 22-2). The severity of the clinical response depends on the dose and concentration of local anesthetic being injected, which is able to gain access to the systemic circulation. One should not, however, overlook the obvious: that sudden or early tourniquet release, or both, are still the most common cause(s) of CNS or cardiovascular complications associated with intravenous regional anesthesia.

Hematoma

Only in the past decade or so has the practitioner of neural blockade become concerned about the risks of hematoma formation coincident with or subsequent to his block. The major concern with hematoma formation is not if it will occur, but where. Hematoma after most peripheral nerve blocks is uncommon and usually of little consequence. The major awareness of this potential complication focuses on the subarachnoid and epidural spaces (see Chaps. 7, 8) and in retrobulbar block (see Chap. 17), where diagnosis is more difficult, treatment complicated, and complications serious. After the early enthusiastic reports[33] on the use of low-dose heparin to prevent deep vein thrombosis, the major question has become, "When it is, or is it, safe to use spinal or epidural anesthesia in patients receiving low-dose heparin therapy?"

Initially there was hope that if the heparin dose remained below an agreed upon level, regional anesthesia would be safe; however, Cooke and coworkers[11] measured blood heparin levels in ten consecutive patients who received 5000 units of heparin before elective hip operations and found a wide variation in dose response (Fig. 22-2). Anticoagulation activity does not, however, always parallel heparin blood levels. For that reason, it is believed that accepted tests for anticoagulation should be performed and be in an acceptable range before doing a block.

Because heparin inhibits multiple clotting factors, several coagulation assays are altered. The whole blood clotting time has been the standard test for many years; however, it lacks precision, must be per-

TABLE 22-2. EFFECT OF RATE OF INJECTION AND PREINJECTION EXSANGUINATION ON MEAN PEAK VENOUS PRESSURES

Rate of Injection	Preinjection Exsanguination	Mean Peak Venous Pressures (mm Hg ± SD)	Range
0.833 ml^{-1}	Nil	213.33 ± 48.34	280-150
	Elevation	161.67 ± 44.80	230-105
	Elevation and Esmarch	105.83 ± 25.38	130-70
0.42 ml^{-1}	Nil	151.67 ± 47.40	210-90
	Elevation	95.00 ± 26.83	130-60
	Elevation and Esmarch	70.83 ± 21.31	100-50

(Duggan, J., McKeown, D.W., and Scott, D.B.: Venous pressures generated during IV regional anaesthesia [IVRA]. Br. J. Anaesth., *55*:1158P, 1983.)

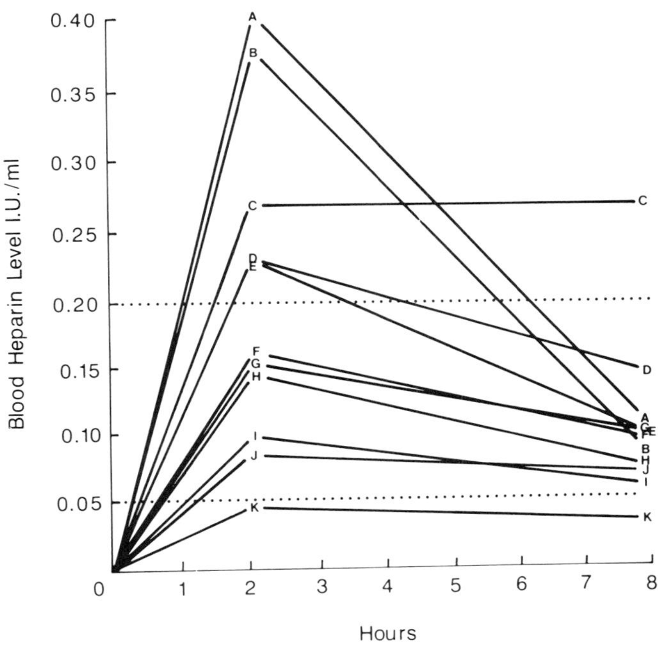

FIG. 22-2. Blood heparin levels following subcutaneous injection of 5000 units of heparin in ten consecutive patients. (Cooke, E.D.: Monitoring during low dose heparin prophylaxis. N. Engl. J. Med., *294*:1066, 1976.)

formed at the bedside, and may require up to 45 minutes for completion at therapeutic levels of heparin. The activated partial thromboplastin time (APTT) is more reproducible, has a more rapid endpoint, is sensitive to low doses of heparin, and can be performed at a convenient time in a central laboratory. The activated coagulation time (ACT) is also a sensitive test with reproducible results, has a short endpoint, and can be automated. It must be remembered that low doses of heparin may have little or no effect on coagulation tests. In a double-blind study comparing 5000 units of heparin against saline administered subcutaneously every 12 hours, no significant differences in parameters of coagulation or fibrinolysis were noted between the two groups.[31]

The risk of subarachnoid or epidural hematoma cannot be predicted. For the past century, mainly case reports have been published about these complications, and with a variety of causes. In the recent past, two larger series of continuous epidural and spinal anesthesia for vascular surgery in anticoagulated patients have been reported. Rao and El-Etr[53] reported on 3164 patients receiving continuous epidural and on 847 receiving continuous subarachnoid anesthesia for lower extremity vascular surgery over a 6-year period (1973–1978). All of their patients received heparin anticoagulation to twice baseline activated clotting time levels approximately 1 hour after insertion of the anesthetic catheter. There was no incidence of peridural or subarachnoid hematoma. Similarly, Odoom and Sih reported on 1000 lumbar epidural blocks in 950 patients undergoing vascular surgery during a 3-year period between 1977 and 1980.[50] A significant difference in this series from that of Rao was that all of these patients were receiving preoperative oral anticoagulation therapy. No side-effects were observed in any patient that could be related to hemorrhage or hematoma formation in the epidural space. Two additional smaller series of 187 and 40 patients, respectively, were reported on the use of epidural for surgery[3] and for intrathecal morphine[43] to 40 cardiac surgical patients 50 minutes before heparinization. Neither group had any evidence of neurologic sequelae (see also Chap. 8).

Having noted what little evidence is available relating to incidence of such complications does not dismiss the possibility that hematomas may occur and for a variety of reasons, not all related to low-dose heparin. Scott and associates[61] reported two cases of acute, *spontaneous* spinal hematoma and noted that about 100 additional cases had been reported since the original report by Hughling Jackson in 1869. The hematoma is not considered spontaneous if it is associated with a bleeding disorder, trauma, or other causes. Hematoma may also occur secondary to full anticoagulation therapy. Harik and colleagues[27] reported the second case of complete spontaneous recovery from subarachnoid hemorrhage of more than 100 cases found in the literature at that time. Similarly, lumbar puncture or needle trauma into the subarachnoid or epidural space may result in hematoma. Rengarchy[57] and Greensite[26] reported such cases and noted very few similar cases in the literature. It comes as no surprise, then, that there are several reports of hematoma after the combination of patients receiving spinal or epidural anesthesia and who had been, were, or subsequently were anticoagulated.[15,73] Anesthetists should bear in mind that heparin or, for that matter, standard anticoagulants are not the only medications that might predispose to subarachnoid or epidural hematomas. Locke and colleagues[40] reported a case of spontaneous acute spinal epidural hematoma unassociated with trauma, conventional anticoagulant therapy, coagulopathy, or vascular abnormalities. They attributed the etiology to two doses of aspirin, two tablets each.

Conversely, however, Benzon[6] prospectively studied 100 consecutive patients on low, intermediate, and high doses of aspirin for less than 1 week, less than 1 month, and greater than 1 month. The average bleeding time and the incidence of prolonged bleeding time were not significantly different in any of the groups. Benzon performed 246 epidural and spinal blocks on 87 patients (8 who had bleeding times prolonged to 10.5 minutes) without any signs or symptoms of epidural hematoma.

Still unresolved is the question of when it is safe to use spinal and epidural anesthesia in the face of altered coagulation. Clearly, hard and fast rules are impossible and inappropriate; however, there seems to be some common ground for caution that has been expressed in the aforementioned reports. First, of course, is an awareness by the anesthetist of what medications the patient is taking and their effect on coagulation. If there is any evidence that the patient has received such drugs in the past *or will receive such drugs* intraoperatively, then appropriate coagulation studies should be accomplished. Acceptable deviations from the norm become very individualized and matters of local practice. Patients considered not suitable for continuous epidural or spinal by some authors[50,53] include those with preexisting neurologic disease, blood dyscrasias, aspirin therapy of long duration, infection at the puncture site, and preoperative full heparin therapy.

Equally as important as proper patient selection and careful anesthetic technique is the requirement for constant intraoperative and postoperative monitoring of neurologic stability. Many authors stress that failure to make an early diagnosis of hematoma, or diagnosis not followed by immediate decompression, will likely result in little or incomplete neurologic improvement. The real risk in using these techniques is less in the occurrence than in the failure to diagnose and treat accurately and quickly. It has been suggested that patients should be monitored daily in the hospital after removal of the epidural or spinal catheter.[50] Whenever the patients return to outpatient clinics, they should undergo appropriate neurologic examination. Finally, but most importantly, the presence of a severe or prolonged backache with or without neurologic signs, local tenderness, fever, or leukocytosis is an indication for early spinal x-ray and myelography. Any clinical or radiologic evidence of cord compression should be followed by an immediate laminectomy and decompression, since complete recovery becomes less likely as surgery time is delayed (see Table 22-3 for other signs and symptoms of epidural and spinal hematoma).

More devastating, and fortunately very rare, are intracranial hematomas after subarachnoid puncture for either diagnostic or anesthetic purposes, especially in patients without preexisting intracranial disease. Newrick and Read[48] noted 12 such patients in five previous reports in the literature and discussed two additional cases of theirs. The case report of Erola and associates[21] noted herniation of the uncus rather than hemorrhage. Although rare, the presumed pathophysiology is similar and carries a clear clinical implication.

The brain is suspended in cerebrospinal fluid with the additional support of vessels and venous sinuses

TABLE 22-3. SIGNS AND SYMPTOMS OF SPINAL AND EPIDURAL HEMATOMA

Local and radiating pain at site of hematoma
Headache or stiff neck, or both, with subarachnoid hematoma
Bilateral numbness and weakness (paraparesis/quadriparesis)
Loss of bowel and bladder sphincter function
Decreased or lost reflexes distal to lesion
Blood stained CSF after lumbar puncture
Defect on myelography

(see Fig. 22-5). When the amount of cerebrospinal fluid is decreased by spinal tap or leakage through the needle hole in the dura, the brain tends to sag, especially when the patient is upright. The downward traction on pain-sensitive cerebral vessels is assumed to produce the clinical situation of "postlumbar puncture headache." If allowed to persist untreated, the most serious consequences of cerebrospinal fluid leak with further sagging of the brain is rupture of small cerebral vessels resulting in subdural hematoma. The time-interval from the dural puncture to serious neurologic symptoms has been from a few days to 4 months. If not evacuated, these hematomas have been fatal. Similar to the spinal and epidural hematomas, even when evacuated, recovery has been nil to incomplete in most cases.

The clinical implication in this rare but devastating complication is the presenting feature of typical postlumbar puncture headache (discussed later in this chapter). It would seem that early and aggressive treatment of this early but minor complication would prevent these hemorrhages and should become part of our practice. There seems to be no benefit in delayed symptomatic, prolonged, and ineffective treatment of these headaches. Early neurologic examination and follow-up are essential.

RESPIRATORY COMPLICATIONS AND SIDE-EFFECTS

Clinical impressions about the respiratory complications of neural blockade are, unfortunately, too simplistic and misinformed. Most practitioners believe that as long as they avoid doing supraclavicular brachial plexus blocks or intercostal nerve blocks, which "everyone knows have a high incidence of pneumothorax," they will have no respiratory complications to worry about. In point of fact, the incidence of pneumothorax is much less than they expect, and there are other problems they need to consider.

Excluding *central* respiratory depression, there are two primary mechanisms whereby neural blockade may produce respiratory complications: [1] interference with the neuromuscular mechanics of ventilation; and [2] interference with the thoracic volume of the lungs. Practically speaking, the first complication arises from blockade of the cervical nerve roots or phrenic nerves that are the motor nerves to the diaphragm or, in isolated cases, abolition of the motor power to the abdominal and intercostal muscles of respiration. The second complication of thoracic volume comes through pneumothorax, hemothorax, or hydrothorax, all of which serve to reduce functional lung volume. The true incidence of these complications is difficult to determine. The patient with normal pulmonary function can easily tolerate loss of his respiratory muscles if his diaphragm is intact or, conversely, loss of unilateral diaphragmatic function if the other muscles are intact. It is the respiratory cripple subjected to these side-effects of neural blockade who has a problem. This illustrates the difference between a side-effect and a complication. High spinal, epidural, and intercostal nerve blocks will functionally block those muscles of respiration, a physiologic side-effect that is not a complication until applied to the wrong patient or not diagnosed and treated properly. A few prospective studies do, however, give us some idea of the variation of the occurrence of these problems.

Interference with Mechanics of Respiration

Many thousands of nerve blocks (intercostal, thoracic epidural) have been done for relief of postoperative and traumatic pain. There is also significant evidence in the literature that this form of analgesia is less depressing to ventilation than either narcotics or no treatment at all; however, there are reports that blockade of the nerves to the muscles of respiration in elderly patients and in patients who have chronic obstructive pulmonary disease may be harmful. Engberg[20] compared narcotics with unilateral and bilateral intercostal nerve blocks for pain relief after subcostal and midline incisions. Whereas the use of unilateral intercostal blocks had a positive effect on pulmonary function, the bilateral intercostal blockade in elderly patients was suspected of contributing to postoperative pulmonary complications. More recently, there have been two similar case reports[10,12] of elderly patients who received intercostal nerve blocks immediately after operation and who were pain free with apparently adequate ventilation, but in less than 50 minutes both required reintubation and ventilation owing to inadequate ability to sustain themselves with spontaneous ventilation. Neither patient had pneumothorax or any other new radiographic evidence of pulmonary complications. Thus it appears that intercostal block should be used with caution in this very select group of patients. Clearly, a select number of unilateral nerves blocked with weaker (nonmotor blocking) concentrations of local anesthetic solutions would still be preferred therapy over no pain relief or high-dose narcotics.

Since the earliest days of neural blockade, there has been an awareness of the importance of the diaphragm to good ventilation, and therefore to the potential respiratory complications that might arise from blockade of its motor nerve supply—the phrenic nerves. The difficulty for the clinician is in trying to predict either the incidence or the magnitude of this risk. Labat[1] states in his early book *Regional Anesthesia* that "*bilateral* blocking of the cervical plexus is not attended by any appreciable or dangerous functional disturbances due to block of the phrenic nerves. The paresis (of the diaphragms)—caused by a bilateral cervical plexus block—is apparently insufficient to interfere with ventilation. Perhaps the intercostal muscles compensate for the decreased diaphragmatic activity." Similar statements have been made by other authors regarding the seriousness of this complication, especially unilateral diaphragmatic paralysis; however, most do caution against doing nerve blocks that might result in bilateral involvement. It is even more difficult to arrive at an incidence of this complication, since the incidence clearly varies with technique, method of diagnosis, concentration of local anesthetic solution, and skill of the anesthetist. More important is an awareness of the anatomy of the cervical nerve roots and phrenic nerves above the clavicle so that appropriate precautions may be taken whenever any practitioner injects local anesthetic solutions into the neck for whatever reason.

The phrenic nerve (C3,4,5) is the most important branch of the cervical plexus. In addition to providing motor innervation to the diaphragm, it transmits proprioceptive sensory fibers from the central part of the diaphragm. In addition, it supplies filaments to pleura and pericardium. The principal component of the nerve is derived from the anterior primary ramus of C4, but contributions are provided by C3 and C5. The three roots join at the lateral border of the scalenus anterior muscle when the full constituted nerve passes downward and medially across the face of the muscle covered by a very thin prevertebral fascia and then over the subclavian artery and behind the vein to enter the thorax (Fig. 22-3). After encountering a

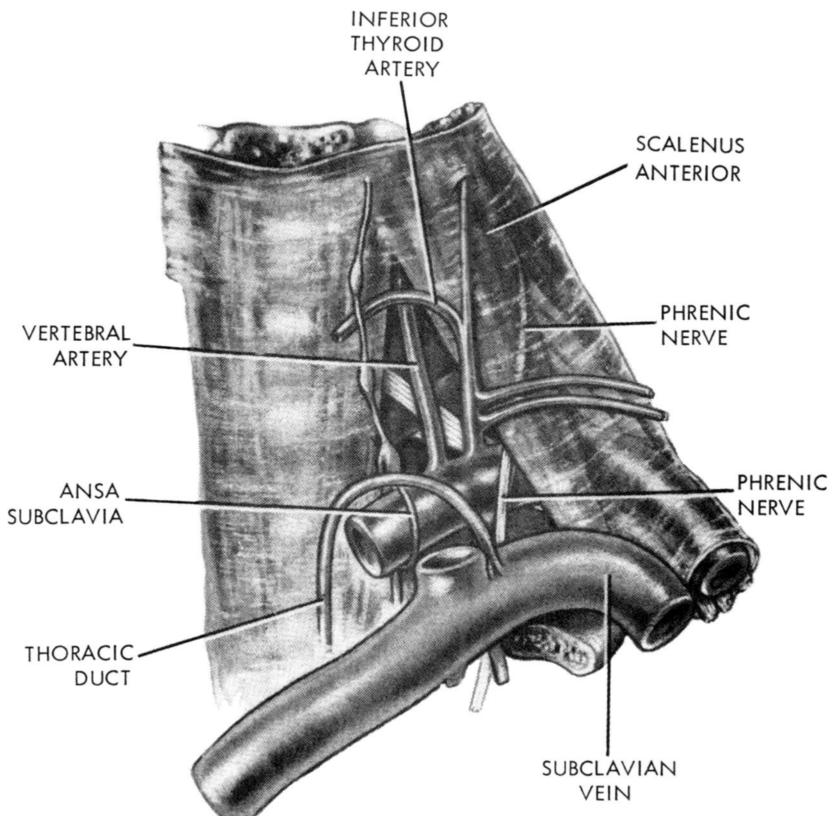

FIG. 22-3. Relationship between the phrenic nerve and the scalene muscles and subclavian vessels. (Last, R.J.: Anatomy: Regional and Applied, p. 376. New York, Churchill Livingstone, 1978.)

case of respiratory failure caused by phrenic nerve block secondary to brachial plexus block, Knoblanche[36] studied 15 select patients having supraclavicular brachial plexus block with x-ray examination of the diaphragm 3 hours after successful block. Ten of the 15 patients (67%) demonstrated diaphragmatic paralysis, and 5 had Horner's syndrome. Thirty milliliters of 0.5% bupivacaine was the solution used.

Virtually any nerve block or local anesthetic infiltration with significant volumes in the area of the cervical nerve roots or scalenus muscles could result in blockade of the phrenic nerve, including deep cervical plexus block, interscalene brachial plexus block, supraclavicular brachial plexus block, stellate ganglion block, and probably even superficial cervical plexus block if not carefully done. Just as in the case of intercostal nerve block, if respiratory compromise from a paralyzed diaphragm could be a risk to a given patient, then bilateral blocks should not be done; if unilateral paralysis is deemed risky, then abstinence or dilute (nonmotor blocking) concentrations and small volumes of local anesthetic solutions should be used.

Interference with Thoracic Volume

The vast majority of these types of complications are, obviously, pneumothoraces caused by needle puncture of the pleural surface. Although this has most often been identified with supraclavicular brachial plexus block and intercostal nerve block, it may also occur with stellate ganglion block, interscalene plexus block, deep cervical plexus block, subclavian plexus block, and paravertebral thoracic nerve blocks (somatic and sympathetic). Just as was true with phrenic nerve block, true incidence of pneumothorax with any technique is unknown. Most of the reports in the literature varied widely from author to author and are now decades old (Table 22-4). More recent reports account for the unusual complications that also interfere with lung and thoracic volume. As an added complication of regional blocks in the face of anticoagulation, a case of hemopneumothorax following subclavian perivascular brachial plexus block has been reported by Mani and colleagues[47] in a patient who received heparin therapy intraoperatively and postoperatively. The patient became dyspneic and complained of chest pain on the third postoperative day; x-ray film showed massive hemopneumothorax. About 1700 ml of blood-stained fluid was aspirated. Although spontaneous hemothorax has been reported with anticoagulant therapy, the presence of an associated 10% pneumothorax on the same side as the brachial block suggests needle trauma to the lung. A reminder of the additional risks of performing neural blockade on the left side of the neck came from the report of Thompson and coworkers.[67] One day after unsuccessful attempts at left stellate ganglion block, the patient returned to the hospital complaining of dyspnea and chest pain. X-ray film revealed a left pneumothorax with a fluid level. Two aspirations over 1 hour's time produced 1375 ml of milky fluid reported to be chyle. Although all physicians are cautioned about injury to the thoracic duct in the left neck, it is a rare *clinical* complication. It is important for anesthetists to realize that iatrogenic trauma to the thoracic duct is not unique to neural blockade but has been reported as a complication of subclavian vein catheterization in the placement of hyperalimentation lines.[69] Further illustrating the fact that other than nerve blocking needles may result in air or fluid in the chest is the report of Ghani and Berry[24] of *right* hydrothorax after left external jugular vein catheterization for fluid infusion.

Two important clinical considerations must be kept in mind regarding needle puncture of the lung without regard to fault. If any of the patient's care after such trauma involves positive intrapleural pressure (*e.g.*, endotracheal anesthesia or ventilation), then one must be alert to the possibility of a tension pneumothorax. Such an occurrence could result in a crisis intraoperatively if not recognized early and treated properly. Less serious, but of no small consequence, is the fact that even intermittent positive pressure breathing from respiratory therapy may convert a small asymptomatic pneumothorax into a large and clinically significant one requiring chest tube drainage.

The role of chest x-ray, empiric or when clinically indicated, in the diagnosis of pneumothorax is variable according to personal or specialty practice standards. Appropos to the previous reports on central

TABLE 22-4. REPORTED INCIDENCE OF PNEUMOTHORAX AFTER VARIOUS NERVE BLOCKS

Nerve Block	Incidence (%)
Supraclavicular brachial plexus block	0.6–2
Stellate ganglion block	
Anterior approach	0.25
Anterolateral approach	0.5–8
Posterior approach	3–13
Thoracic paravertebral (somatic) block	0–6
Thoracic paravertebral (sympathetic) block	1.4–7.9

venous line placement is the recommendation by those authors that all central lines be x-rayed to verify correct placement. Pneumothorax, depending upon the magnitude of the pleural trauma, may not appear on x-ray film for 6 to 12 hours. Therefore, routine chest x-rays in the recovery room may not be helpful. If one accepts the philosophy that most clinically significant pneumothoraces are symptomatic and that there is an incidence of less than 5%, then there is little justification for empiric chest x-rays as opposed to individual clinical indications.

Treatment or management of pneumothorax is also variable and often determined by a consultant surgeon rather than an anesthetist. Moore[47] recommends that pneumothorax of approximately 20% or less will likely resolve spontaneously and therefore require no treatment. Anything over 20% should be aspirated. Those only slightly larger and asymptomatic may be aspirated with a needle; the larger and symptomatic ones likely will require chest tube and suction drainage. Periodic follow-up x-rays should be taken to ensure that there has been no recurrence of pneumothorax post-therapy.

NEUROLOGIC COMPLICATIONS AND SIDE-EFFECTS

The area of neurologic complications is clearly the one of most notoriety and misinformation of all the complications of neural blockade. There are the rare but often disastrous complications to the spinal cord and surrounding structures, and the more frequent complications of headache and peripheral nerve disturbances. Despite the incidence of these serious and often permanent complications being severalfold less than the mortality with general anesthesia, they remain as a daily reminder to all and therefore have a more negative impact on the respective nerve block techniques than mortality has on general anesthesia techniques. Equally important in maintaining a global perspective on all the complications of anesthesia and surgery is the continued necessity of determining that all neurologic sequelae are not necessarily due to the neural blockade technique. Nicholson and McAlpin[49] quote two large surgical series of 50,000 and 30,000 patients, respectively. Seventy-two patients in the former series and 31 patients in the latter developed postoperative neural complications, usually peripheral nerve and usually related to positioning of the patient.

Delayed Systemic Toxicity

At first glance, it may seem unusual to separate *acute* (intravascular) systemic toxicity (previously discussed in this chapter) from delayed (absorption) systemic toxicity. The acute problem, however, clearly results as a complication of unintentional vascular injection, whereas delayed systemic toxicity is really a neurologic consequence of relative overdose of local anesthetic agent. Most anesthetists memorize a single maximum allowable dose of each local anesthetic agent on a milligram per body weight basis and are quite unaware of all the technical, physiologic, pharmacologic, and pathologic variables that might predispose a patient to toxicity at "normal" doses (see Chap. 4). Less appreciated than toxicity from single injection overdose is the very delayed CNS toxicity that may result from toxic blood levels achieved through cumulative overdose (see Chap. 3). The potential for more serious or even fatal complications from this type of CNS toxicity is a result of the very late insidious onset of the convulsions and the very long time they may persist. Whereas the direct intravascular injection of a local anesthetic agent will precipitate an immediate *but* very transient convulsion, the CNS toxicity secondary to relative overdose (single or cumulative) may not occur for 20 minutes to several hours. This also means that the patient having the immediate seizure will likely be attended by the practitioner administering the block, who presumably has the equipment and ability to provide appropriate resuscitation. With the delayed onset of toxicity, patients may have been moved to nontreatment areas, and most likely the administering practitioner has left to attend to other anesthetic duties, resulting in an unattended patient vulnerable to a prolonged seizure. All patients who have received a single large dose or who are receiving intermittent doses of local anesthetics must be attended by trained personnel in areas where such complications may be treated quickly and appropriately. Such occurrences after intermittent dose local anesthetics are most likely to occur in obstetric or postoperative pain patients. Thorburn and Moir[68] reported two patients who had bupivacaine epidural analgesia for labor followed by cesarean section, and who manifested seizure activity after 10 hours (357.5 mg) and 9 hours (356.25 mg), respectively. Similar situations may result in surgical anesthesia in which a major nerve block is missed and repeated by another anesthetist using full doses of local anesthetic; if still unsatisfactory, the surgeon infiltrates even more "local" and the patient convulses. Although *neural* absorption of local anesthetic cannot be guaranteed, the *vascular* bed is ubiquitous and virtually guarantees that every milligram of administered local anesthetic will contribute to a higher blood level.

An obvious preventive measure to this "total dose —high blood level" problem would be the monitoring of plasma levels of the local anesthetics. The seizure level of these agents has been studied extensively (see Chaps. 3 and 4), and the ability to measure blood levels is clinically possible. Unfortunately, the precise seizure level for a given patient is not predictable nor constant; in addition to body weight, it depends on site of injection, presence of vasoconstrictors, lipid solubility, pKa and protein binding of the injected drug, *p*H of the patient's blood, and the patient's cardiac, renal, and hepatic function. Hasselstrom and Mogensen[29] reported a toxic reaction to bupivacaine in a patient whose plasma bupivacaine level was 1.1 μg/ml. The accepted toxic threshold for bupivacaine is in the range of 4 μg/ml or greater. It seems, therefore, that plasma level monitoring by itself will not prevent all toxic reactions. On the other hand, monitored levels approaching 4 μg/ml or greater should alert the clinician to take corrective action.

COMPLICATIONS IN SUBARACHNOID AND EPIDURAL SPACES

Before discussing the major permanent complications, I must comment on the clinical syndromes known as "total spinal" anesthesia. Most anesthetists realize that if large volumes or doses of local anesthetic are unintentionally injected into the subarachnoid space the patient will become apneic, unresponsive, and usually hypotensive and require immediate supportive therapy. Usually after a period of time commensurate with the duration of action of the injected drug, the spinal anesthetic regresses and the patient recovers. The element of concern to the clinician, however, is the fact that uneventful recovery does not always occur. Reasons for this are not all known, but failure to recognize and treat properly certainly provides a setting for serious, irreversible complications. The unintentional subarachnoid injection during placement of an epidural or caudal anesthetic is usually recognized. Unfortunately, there are many other situations in neural blockade in which local anesthetics may be placed into the subarachnoid or epidural space and not be recognized.

These unexpected complications usually result from paravertebral nerve block techniques such as deep cervical plexus block, interscalene block, stellate ganglion block, intercostal nerve block, infraclavicular nerve block, thoracic and lumbar somatic and sympathetic nerve blocks, and celiac ganglion block. Recently, Hill and co-workers[32] reported a case of total spinal blockade during local anesthesia of the nose by the surgeon. Had not the patient failed to answer a question, the surgical drapes covering her comatose apneic state would not have been removed, and a fatality may have resulted. Similar unexpected spinal or segmental epidural anesthetics have resulted from intrathoracic intercostal nerve block by surgeons before closing.[23] The risk of failure to suspect, diagnose, and treat these complications of surgically induced neural blockade is probably greater than if the anesthetist performing the block is sensitized to its possible complications. Not surprising, then, is the occurrence of epidural[38] and total spinal[60] anesthesia after interscalene arm block. Finally, in discussing the unsuspected onset of neurologic (or vascular) complications, one needs to keep in mind that epidural catheters may migrate into blood vessels or subarachnoid space, resulting in toxic reaction or total spinal from what had previously been a functional epidural anesthetic.[51]

An unfortunate and severe complication to unintentional subarachnoid injection was reported in the United States after the use of 2-chloroprocaine for epidural anesthesia. Unlike the traditional circumstances just noted in that the patient made a complete recovery as soon as the local anesthetic wore off, a few patients developed serious neurologic sequelae (see Chap. 4).[54,56] Of interest is that the resulting neuropathology varied from just prolonged motor and sensory effect to cauda equina syndrome to adhesive arachnoiditis. In an effort to gain a true perspective on the serious neurologic complications after spinal and epidural, Kane[34] did an extensive literature search on this topic. His review serves to illustrate an important fact all physicians must keep in mind. The multiple case reports of various complications that abound in the literature draw our attention to the *kinds* of complications that may occur. Reviews such as this or those of Usubiaga[72] and Dawkins,[14] to name only a few, indicate the frequency and varied circumstances under which these might occur. Kane's review found three patients with permanent paralysis or paresis in a series of 50,000 epidural anesthetics (Table 22-5); in 65,000 spinal anesthetics, one permanent paralysis occurred (Table 22-6). Usubiaga studied more than 750,000 epidural anesthetics and concluded an incidence of 1 neurologic complication per 11,000 anesthetics. Of 32,718 cases reviewed, Daw-

TABLE 22-5. SURVEY REPORTS OF EPIDURAL ANESTHESIA

Reference*	Number of Patients	Anesthetics	Procedures	Neurologic Sequelae
Bleyaert (3)	3,000	Bupivacaine, 0.125%, 1:800,000 epinephrine	Obstetric	None
Moore (4)	11,080	Bupivacaine, 0.25%, 0.5%, or 0.75%, with or without epinephrine'	Surgical, obstetric, diagnostic	None
Holdcroft (5)	1,000	Bupivacaine, 0.5%, or lidocaine, 1.5% (32 patients)	Obstetric	1 foot drop; 1 paresthesia of thigh
Moore (6)	7,286	Lidocaine + tetracaine with epinephrine in 6,270 patients; various agents in remaining cases	Surgical, obstetric	1 bilateral paralysis of quadriceps muscles
Lund (7)	10,000	Lidocaine, 2% (8,000 patients); chloroprocaine, 3% (700 patients); hexylcaine, 2% (200 patients)	Surgical, obstetric, diagnostic	1 paresis of 1 leg (subarachnoid hexylcaine); 4 paresthesias of thigh; 1 persistent numbness; 3 bladder or rectal incontinence
Eisen (8)	9,532	Lidocaine	Obstetric	16 paresthesias; 9 numbness of thigh; 1 paraplegia (1 of 5,091 surgical cases)
Bonica (9)	3,885	Various; mostly lidocaine	Surgical, obstetric, diagnostic	1 hypalgesia of trunk, weakness of leg (subarachnoid lidocaine); 1 paresthesias, numbness weakness of leg

*Refers to references listed within Kane's original article (see citation below).
(Kane, R.E.: Neurologic deficits following epidural or spinal anesthesia. Anesth. Analg., *60*:151, 1981.)

TABLE 22-6. SURVEY REPORTS OF SPINAL ANESTHESIA

Reference*	Number of Patients	Anesthetics	Procedure	Neurologic Sequelae
Kortum (23)	2,592	Bupivacaine, 0.5%	Surgical	1 lumbar plexus injury
Bergman (24)	10,000	Lidocaine, mepivacaine, bupivacaine	Various	None
Phillips (25)	10,440	Lidocaine	Obstetric, surgical	8 persistent peripheral neuropathy
Moore (26)	11,574	Tetracaine, dibucaine: with epinephrine or phenylephrine in 8,852	Surgical, obstetric	1 persistent muscular weakness of legs, impotence
Sadov (27)	20,000	Tetracaine, procaine, dibucaine	Various	1 paraplegia due to spinal tumor; 3 meningitis
Dripps (28); Vandam (29–31)	10,098	Tetracaine, procaine, dibucaine: with epinephrine in 2,000		No major neurologic sequelae; 2 foot drop; 1 leg weakness (trauma); 12 exacerbation of previous neurologic disease
Brown (32)	600	Tetracaine	Surgical	2 peroneal paresis, unilateral

*Refers to references listed within Kane's original article (see citation below).
(Kane, R.E.: Neurologic deficits following epidural or spinal anesthesia. Anesth. Analg., *60*:152, 1981.)

kins reported an incidence of transient neurologic lesions of 0.1% and permanent lesions of 0.02%.

The kinds of neurologic sequelae causing permanent disturbances and their etiology are not always precise because only surgical or autopsy examination will provide tissue diagnosis. Paralysis or paresis may be due to cord ischemia or infarct secondary to hematoma or anterior spinal artery occlusion. This may be caused by severe hypotension of any etiology and not just spinal or epidural anesthesia. Direct injury to the spinal cord, roots, and their coverings may be traumatic or chemical. Chemical contaminants such as detergents, preservatives, and neurolytics act as irritants and may induce meningeal or arachnoid inflammatory responses. Excessive doses or concentrations of local anesthetics and vasoconstrictors have also been incriminated in this process. Previously undiagnosed spinal tumors, or other spinal abnormalities, may be "revealed" at the time of spinal or epidural anesthesia (see Chap. 8).

Another complication of spinal and epidural anesthesia that seems to be recurring in the literature is that of subdural injection of local anesthetic solutions.[41,52] The subdural space consists of a potential space between the dura and the arachnoid. Unlike the epidural space, the subdural space extends intracranially (Fig. 22-4). It contains a minute quantity of serous fluid to moisten the opposing membranes. It does not communicate directly with the subarachnoid space but extends laterally over the nerve roots and ganglia. The subdural space is wider in the cervical region than elsewhere and also adjacent to the nerve roots, which is where the unintentional entry by epidural needle or catheter is likely to occur.[44] The clinical manifestations of this complication are variable, having been described as both fast and slow in

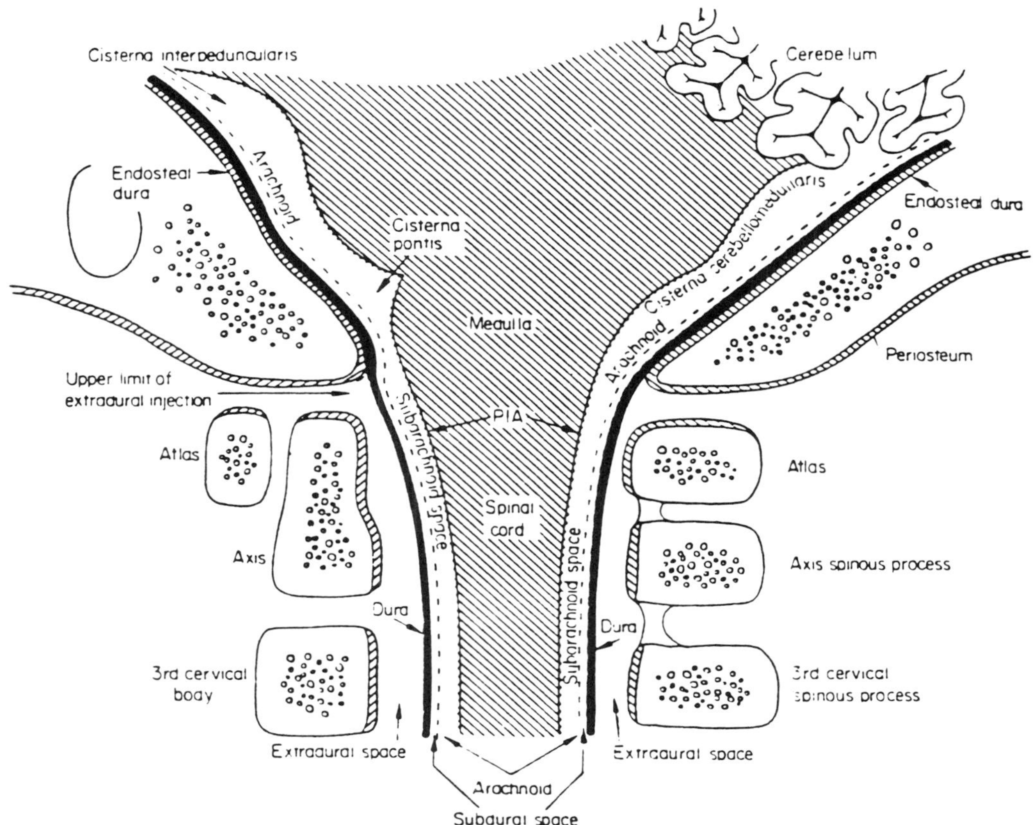

FIG. 22-4. Diagrammatic representation of the layers covering the spinal cord to show the site of the cervical subdural space and its extension into the cranial cavity. (Mehta, M., and Maher, R.: Injection into the extra arachnoid subdural space. Anaesthesia, *32*:762, 1977.)

onset. All are characterized by inordinantly high levels of sensory anesthesia with very low doses or volumes of local anesthesia. Symptoms may be unilateral or bilateral, but in every case the reactions of the patients required immediate support or resuscitation of cardiovascular or respiratory function, or both, for a duration of 1 hour to several hours. Contrary to the expressed rationalizations of clinicians, it is not a silent repository to which all missed spinals and epidurals may be attributed (see Chap. 7).

Infection

Bacterial infection is a possible risk of all neural blockade, but, like hematoma, it is of greatest concern if it occurs around the spinal cord and its coverings or spaces. Microorganisms may be transmitted by syringes, catheters, and needles. They may come from the anesthetist or from the patient with a septic process of the skin, tissue, or blood. The most common site for infection is skin and subcutaneous tissue in patients on chronic pain therapy with indwelling catheters left in place for days to weeks. The serious neural infections of abscess, meningitis, and arachnoiditis are quite rare. Usubiaga[72] reported on seven cases and noted that most reports came in earlier years. More recently, Kilpatrick and Gingis[35] reported 17 cases of meningitis after spinal anesthesia over a 5-year period in a Cairo, Egypt, ward treating 1429 meningitis patients. Only 10 of the 17 had positive CSF cultures: Eight were *Pseudomonas aeruginosa,* 1 was *Staphylococcus aureus,* and 1 was *Streptococcus mitis.* These organisms were *not* cultured from the other patients who had not had spinal anesthesia. They concluded that meningitis in patients after recent spinal anesthesia commonly is due to unusual or nosocomial organisms and recommended aggressive, meticulous bacteriologic evaluation and early treatment. Beaudoin and Klein[5] reported a patient who developed back pain following five spinal anesthetics and who was found, 4 weeks after the last spinal, to have a large epidural abscess. CSF examination was sterile and normal except for elevated protein content (0.9 g/liter). They presumed infection of a hematoma but could not determine whether the source of contamination was blood-borne or external. These reports serve as a warning to the practitioner who initiates epidural or spinal anesthesia in the face of a local or systemic infection. Although fever, by itself, may be of many causes other than bacteremia, and therefore may not mitigate against such anesthetics, extreme caution and thought should be used when doing these blocks in septic patients.

Headache

The most minor, but also the most common, complication of spinal anesthesia, and perhaps epidural anesthesia, is postdural puncture headache. It is important to the image of spinal anesthesia that the age-old term "spinal headache" be discarded in favor of "postdural puncture headache" because this specific syndrome more frequently occurs subsequent to dural puncture for myelogram, diagnostic neurologic studies, and even unintentional dural puncture secondary to epidural anesthesia (see Chap. 7). Despite the significant progress in preventing or treating some complications of neural blockade, little has changed in the prevention and treatment of postdural puncture headaches over the past 2 decades. Most authors writing on the topic still quote authors and series dating back 3 to 4 decades. Two prospective studies of this complication were recently reported. Driessen and colleagues[16] studied 613 patients in whom a total of 783 spinal anesthetics had been performed. Subjective complaints (13%) were more common among the female patients. Twenty-three patients (2.9%) developed a typical postspinal headache. A later study by Eckstein and associates[19] of 1009 patients compared the 22-gauge and 25-gauge Quincke tip spinal needle with a 22-gauge Whitacre tip needle. The smaller needle caused only one half as many headaches as the larger needles. There was no difference between the 22-gauge Quincke tip and the 22-gauge Whitacre tip. The overall incidence of headache was about 5%. Interestingly, and contrary to common belief, the highest frequency of headaches was reported in female patients in the 5th decade. An increase with younger age patients was *not* noted. Definite bloody taps were associated with significantly higher rates. Although nearly all series report a higher incidence of postlumbar puncture headaches in obstetric patients receiving spinal anesthesia, the reasons are not clear. Ravindran and co-workers[55] studied the effect of "bearing-down" at the time of delivery in 100 patients and compared them with studies in 100 patients having outlet forceps delivery. They found no difference in the incidence of headache in the two groups (9% versus 10%).* Little new has been added

*Brownridge reported on a series of obstetric patients with accidental dural puncture associated with epidural block. He also proposed a management plan.[9a]

to the therapeutic regime, with conservative treatment and autologous epidural blood patch still being the favored treatment (see Chap. 7). Early diagnosis and treatment are essential because, as noted earlier in this chapter, there are case reports of intracerebral hematomas in patients with prolonged, untreated postpuncture headaches, presumably from significant losses of CSF. A summary of proposed factors in postdural puncture headache is shown in Figure 22-5.

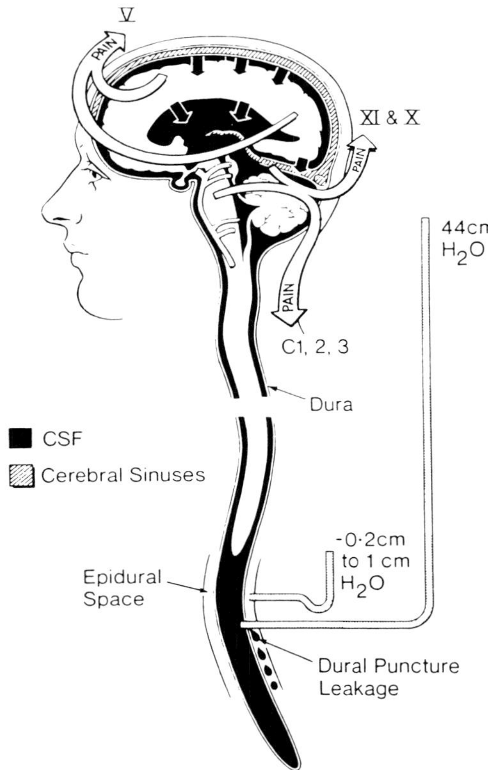

FIG. 22-5. Pathophysiology of dural puncture headache. Barometric figures are those to be expected in the subarachnoid and epidural spaces in the upright position at the site of lumbar puncture. The pressure differential favors CSF leakage. Note that CSF pressure is approximately atmospheric at the base of the brain. CSF leakage leads to descent of the brain in the upright position *(dark arrows)* on pain-sensitive intracranial vessels and the tentorium. Pain is referred *(open arrows)* above the tentorium via the trigeminal nerve *(V)* to the frontal region, and below the tentorium via the glossopharyngeal and vagal nerves *(IX, X)* to the occiput and via the upper cervical nerves *(C1, 2, 3)* to the neck and shoulders. (Brownridge, P.: The management of headache following accidental dural puncture in obstetric patients. Anaesth. Intensive Care, *11*:9, 1983.)

COMPLICATIONS OF PERIPHERAL NERVE BLOCKS

Less dramatic, but equally important, as the complications of the spinal cord, its coverings, and spaces are the complications related to the peripheral nerves. Many advocates of regional anesthesia stress the need for paresthesias as an integral part of the nerve block technique to ensure successful anesthesia. Conversely, critics of the "paresthesia" approach to neural blockade have been equally vocal about the damage that could, theoretically, result from repeated needle trauma to the nerves. Clinical reports by many authors of thousands of peripheral nerve blocks of all types made this criticism seem more theoretical than real. Reports by Selander and colleagues,[65] however, provide sufficient evidence to cause anesthetists to reexamine the risks of eliciting paresthesias during nerve blocks. They studied the frequency of nerve lesions after axillary plexus block performed with nerve location either by paresthesias or by axillary artery pulsation. Their study included 290 patients in the paresthesia group and 243 in the arterial group. It should be noted, however, that paresthesias were still elicited in 40% of patients in the arterial group. Postanesthetic nerve lesions were seen in 8 patients in the paresthesia group and in only 2 in the arterial group. All patients had received 1% mepivacaine containing 1 : 200,000 epinephrine. Symptoms varied from light dysesthesias lasting a few weeks to severe dysesthesias with aching and paresis lasting more than 1 year (Table 22-7). The presumed etiology of these nerve complications was either direct nerve trauma from the needle or drug induced from direct intraneural injection. To elucidate these differences, the same group[64] studied the effects of intrafascicular or topical application of bupivacaine on isolated rabbit sciatic nerve. Whereas the topical application of saline, bupivacaine, and bupivacaine plus epinephrine to the nerve caused no detectable nerve injury, the intrafascicular injections resulted in

TABLE 22-7. NUMBER OF PATIENTS WITH SYMPTOMS OF POSTANESTHETIC NERVE LESION

	Number of Patients	Nerve Lesion	
		Patients	%
Paresthesia group	290	8	2.8
Artery group	243	2	0.8
Total	533	10	1.9

(Selander, D., Edshage, S., Wolff, T.: Paresthesiae or no paresthesiae? Acta Anesthesiol. Scand., *23*:29, 1979.)

axonal degeneration and damaged blood nerve barrier.

Axonal degeneration was the same after physiologic saline as after plain bupivacaine in low concentrations. It did increase, however, with increasing concentrations of bupivacaine and with the epinephrine-containing solutions (Table 22-8). They concluded that intraneural injections should be avoided, and, whenever possible, nonepinephrine containing solutions should be used. Earlier work by Selander[63] using the same sciatic nerve preparation studied the effect of the angle of the needle bevel on nerve injury. One needle was the conventional sharp-pointed needle (14° bevel) and the other, a very blunt-tipped (45° bevel) needle. Their results showed that whereas the sharp needle tended to cut the nerve fiber in both the parallel and horizontal approaches, the 45° short-bevel needle tended to push the nerve fiber away and, therefore, produced less axonal damage (see Table 6-2). The clinical importance of these studies is to stress not only that each variable — drug, needle, and epinephrine — may by itself cause axonal damage, but combined in the form of an intraneural injection of a significant volume of solution will likely cause serious problems. Barutell and colleagues[4] reported the case of a 49-year-old woman who received 8 ml of 1% prilocaine for interscalene brachial plexus block. "The patient suffered a sharp paresthesia — when the needle was inserted, and, at the same time, a brisk jerk of the hand occurred. Neither spinal fluid nor blood escaped. The paresthesia became worse when the injection of the local anaesthetic began, but in spite of this, injection was continued. . . . When 8 ml had been injected, the patient suddenly became hoarse — loss of consciousness and respiratory failure followed." The day after operation, the patient had a paralyis of the extensor muscles of her fingers and of the flexor and intrinsic muscles of the hand. These deficits never recovered. This case is extremely important in illustrating the dictum that one should never continue injecting local anesthesia if a patient complains of severe pain. Retraction or movement of the needle 1 to 2 mm will ensure that it is not intraneural, and such complications should be avoided.

Because most of the complications to peripheral nerves manifest in the postoperative period, it is essential that patients be followed by the anesthetist in the prolonged postoperative period through close communication with the primary surgeon. Winchell[74] reported on 854 consecutive patients receiving upper arm block for upper extremity surgery who were evaluated on their first and second postoperative visits to the surgeon for evidence of neuropathy. They found three patients with unequivocal evidence of nerve damage, for an incidence of 0.36%. It is equally important that possible causes other than a given nerve block technique be included in the etiologic diagnoses. All patients, but especially trauma patients, should have neurologic examination results noted on their chart. In addition to anesthetic causes, faulty positioning of the patient and surgical trauma may result in damage to peripheral nerves. Nicholson and McAlpine,[49] in writing about neural injuries associated with surgical positions and operations, quote series of 50,000 and 30,000 patients, respectively. Seventy-two patients in the first series developed postoperative nerve complications believed to be related to the period during which the patient was anesthetized. Brachial plexus palsy was the most common injury occurring in 23 of 28 patients who had undergone open heart surgery. Other nerves involved included peroneal, radial, ulnar, median, and sciatic. In the study of 30,000 patients (1940–1945), 31 patients had paresis of one or more nerves during the postoperative period — 26 in the upper extremity and 5 in the lower (all common peroneal nerve).

Three cases of femoral neuropathy as a complication of lithotomy position under spinal anesthesia reported by Tondare and co-workers[71] illustrate one of the most troublesome areas for the diagnosis of postsurgical complications. These authors reported on three patients who sustained unilateral peripheral femoral neuropathy of 4 to 8 weeks' duration after vaginal hysterectomy operations in the lithotomy position lasting 2 to 2½ hours. They attributed the complication to the extreme abduction of the thighs with external rotation at the hip causing ischemia of

TABLE 22-8. AXONAL DEGENERATION AFTER INTRAFASCICULAR INJECTION OF 0.05 ML

Agent	Concentration (mg/ml)	Axonal Degeneration*		
		0 → +	++	+++
Physiologic saline		11	4	1
Bupivacaine	5	10	6	–
Bupivacaine	10	4	7	5
Bupivacaine with epinephrine, 5 μg/ml	5	–	11	5

*Degrees of axonal degeneration: 0 → +: none or insignificant; ++: significant but <50% of axons; +++: ≥50% of axons.

(Selander, D., Brattsand, R., Lundborg, G., Nordborg, C., et al.: Local anesthetics: Importance of mode of application, concentration and adrenaline for the appearance of nerve lesions. Acta Anesthesiol. Scand., *23*:129, 1979.)

the femoral nerve as it is kinked beneath the tough inguinal ligament. All too often, if a patient has had spinal or epidural anesthesia, the surgical and nursing staff will suggest to the patient that the complications are a result of anesthesia. The anesthetist who makes careful postoperative rounds can become aware of these latent complications and solicit appropriate neurologic consultations. Most unilateral peripheral nerve problems will not be a result of spinal, caudal, or epidural anesthesia but from some more peripheral cause.

One of the proposed explanations for peripheral nerve injury has been that smaller nerves, especially when they lie over bone or in restricted fascial compartments, are more vulnerable to ischemia or traumatic injury (*e.g.*, pressure), or both. Some practitioners have discouraged block of nerves at the knee (see Chap. 11) and digits for that very reason. Nerves in tight places also will not slide away as easily from the advancing block needle and are therefore more vulnerable to intraneural injection. Born[7] recently reported a series of 49 patients receiving 0.5% bupivacaine for wrist and metacarpal nerve blocks. Seven patients developed hyperesthesia in the blocked nerve distribution lasting from 1 week to 4 months. Relatively large total volumes of solution were used, and three patients had 1 : 200,000 epinephrine added to their solutions. This then reinforces the admonition of teachers of regional block, that is, when blocking small nerves, use small volumes of weak concentrations of local anesthetic solutions *without* epinephrine. In addition, extreme caution should be used to avoid nerve trauma or intraneural injections.

MISCELLANEOUS COMPLICATIONS OF NEURAL BLOCKADE

Although the manifestations of the complications to be noted herein will likely be neurologic or vascular, they arise from a variety of causes in the performance of neural blockade and tend to be discrete entities; they thus are grouped together in a miscellaneous category to include such diverse topics as allergy, methemoglobinemia, backache, and equipment failure.

Allergy to Local Anesthetics

Many patients, and all too often their physicians and dentists, believe themselves "allergic" to a local anesthetic (see Chap. 4) and subject themselves to a life of inconvenience or therapeutic confusion everytime they require a procedure done under "local." In point of fact, although allergic reactions to the ester family of local anesthetics are known to occur, they are *not* common. Even more relevant in today's practice of infiltration and regional neural blockade using amide types of local anesthetics is the fact that clinically manifest allergic reactions in this group of drugs are extremely rare. Brown and colleagues[8] reported on a patient who presented with a history "years ago" of a reaction to lignocaine. They skin tested, uneventfully, with 0.2 ml of 0.5% prilocaine, but when they skin tested with 0.2 ml of 0.5% bupivacaine the patient immediately developed a tight chest, rash, and visual disturbances. Immunologic studies showed a decrease in plasma complement C4 concentration, which they thought indicated the reaction was immunologically mediated. Soon thereafter, Fischer and Pennington[22] reported on a patient who had a very positive history for lidocaine and prilocaine allergy in whom they performed a variety of dilutional intradermal tests. The tests confirmed her clinical sensitivity and suggested no allergy to bupivacaine, which she subsequently received without untoward effect (Table 22-9). They emphasize that skin tests for one group of local anesthetics give no information about the other and that both should be tested.

Methemoglobinemia

An increased level of methemoglobin has been a recognized complication of receiving the local anesthetic agent prilocaine since its introduction in the early 1960s (see Chaps. 3 and 4). Although as little as 1.52% may cause visible cyanosis, it is of little consequence. The formation of methemoglobin is dose re-

TABLE 22-9. INTRADERMAL TESTING IN A PATIENT AFTER SEVERE ANAPHYLACTOID REACTIONS TO LOCAL ANESTHETIC

	Dilution			
Drug	**1:10,000**	**1:1,000**	**1:100**	**1:10**
1% procaine	NT*	NT	–	0.8†
1% xylocaine	14/40	14/40	NT	NT
1% mepivacaine	0/0	0/0	0/0	0/0
1% bupivacaine	0/0	0/0	0/0	0/0
0.5% amethocaine	5/15	12/28	NT	NT
1% prilocaine	10/45	15/45	NT	NT

*NT = not tested.
†Expressed as weal size over flare size (mm).
(Fisher, M., Pennington, J.C.: Allergy to local anaesthesia. Br. J. Anaesth., *54*:893, 1982.)

lated, with doses of >8 mg/kg for peripheral nerve blocks required to produce symptoms. This phenomenon is still of importance to clinicians as the drug becomes more commonly used for intravenous regional anesthesia and infiltration. Duncan and Kobrinsky[18] reported extremely high levels of methemoglobin in a neonate receiving 7.5 mg of 4% prilocaine for surgical infiltration of a palate repair.

This serves to indicate that different patients may metabolize the drug differently and that should cyanosis occur in any patient who has received prilocaine, a methemoglobin determination should be obtained. The cyanosis of methemoglobinemia has a late onset — a few hours after injection — and therefore may be missed as the causative factor when diagnosed by recovery room nurses and surgical staff.

Backache

Pain of any kind is a subjective complaint the cause of which may be as obscure as its symptoms. Headache and backache are two such relatively frequent pain problems, usually associated with spinal, epidural, and paravertebral neural blockade. Since headache of neural blockade origin is a more specific syndrome attributed to postdural puncture, it is discussed in detail in Chapter 7. Backache, however, may also follow surgery under general anesthesia. An early study evaluated patients who received either spinal or general anesthesia and found no significant difference in incidence of backache between the two techniques.[9] It is generally accepted that most commonly backache occurs after procedures in which there is flattening of the normal lumbar curve owing to relaxation of the paraspinous muscles (with either muscle relaxants or local anesthetics), allowing stretch of the joint capsules and spinous ligaments. Such an effect is exaggerated if the patient is further manipulated, as might occur during the lithotomy position. Regional anesthesia has likely been unfairly incriminated as the cause of this problem for two reasons: First, there is a high use of regional anesthesia for surgical procedures employing the lithotomy position (*e.g.*, urology, obstetrics, and gynecology); and second, there is the natural "cause and effect" reaction of many patients who reason that "I received a needle puncture in my back (especially if traumatically done) and developed pain in my back after surgery; therefore, the needle must have caused the back pain." Moir and Davidson[45] compared 50 patients receiving pudendal nerve block for vaginal delivery with 50 patients who received epidural analgesia and noted 32% incidence of backache in the pudendal group and 22% in the epidural group. Crawford,[13] in analyzing 923 lumbar epidural blocks for labor, noted that 45% of his patients complained of backache on one or more of the first 6 postnatal days. In 32% of the total series, backache began on the day after delivery. He believed that in most patients, there was no evidence that it was related to the epidural block.

The importance of discussing this relatively benign complication is not to encourage practitioners to further deny that nerve block techniques may cause such a problem; rather, it is extremely important that the patients undergoing these procedures be informed preanesthetically that backache may occur as a result of the procedure (surgery, anesthesia, *and* position) but that it is usually transient and can be successfully treated with analgesics.

Faulty Equipment and Technique

Clearly these are not complications but rather the cause of some relatively minor complications. Perhaps the most notable is that of the "sheared catheter." The majority of reports indicate the cause of this complication is attempts by the operator to withdraw the epidural catheter back into a needle, with the sharp edge of the needle shearing the catheter (Fig. 22-6). Occasionally, catheters that have been in the patient for some time will break off at the skin surface. Despite the universal dictum "Never pull a catheter back through a needle," these complications still occur. There is, however, increasing agreement among practitioners of epidural anesthesia that if a catheter is sheared or broken off in the epidural space, it does not necessarily have to be surgically removed even if it is impossible to remove it any other way. Most of the current catheters are made of inert materials and not likely to cause tissue reaction or injury to vessels and organs. The patient should be informed of the occurrence and be given the recommendation that it be left in place unless it subsequently becomes a problem.

Earlier authors cautioned about broken needles and the damage that might occur. Recommendations for removal of broken needles still prevail, since they might migrate from the site of entry and lead to more serious complications. A minor, but often unappreciated, complication of the current long-beveled disposable needles used for neural blockade is their predisposition to "spur" upon striking a bony surface. The result, when examined closely (Fig. 22-7), is a

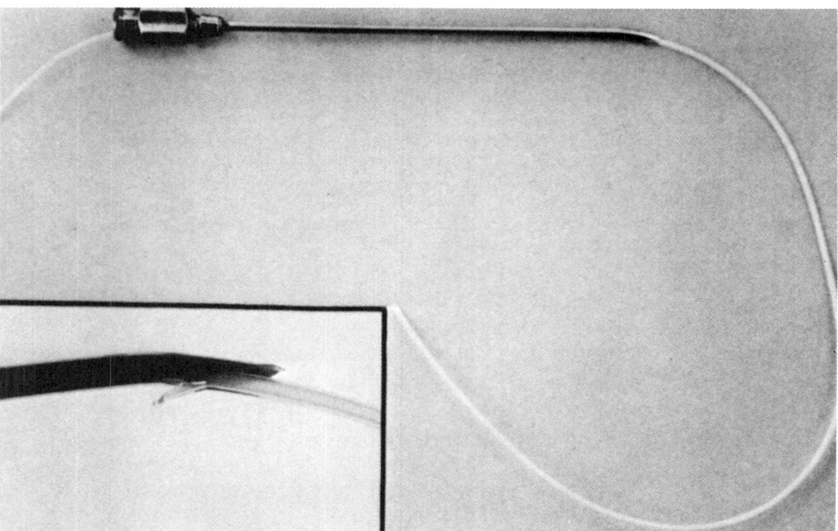

FIG. 22-6. A needle "shearing off" a catheter.

needle tip resembling a small fish hook. Clearly, such a needle tip passing in and out of nerves, arteries, and veins could cause significant damage. It is important, therefore, that such needles be tested frequently by passing the tip over gauze or cotton and be discarded for a new one at the first indication of spur formation.

PROPHYLAXIS OR TREATMENT OF COMPLICATIONS

It was suggested at the beginning of this chapter that many of the complications of neural blockade were a result of errors in judgment, related to choice of patient, technique, drug, concentration, volume, supplementation with sedation, and so forth. Prophylaxis comes in avoiding, whenever possible, situations that could lead to an increased risk of complications. Of prime importance, therefore, is a careful and thorough preanesthetic evaluation of the patient to be anesthetized, with special attention given to features of the preselected regional block technique, for example, altered anatomy, coagulopathies, altered blood volume, and any restrictions to supplementation or resuscitation.

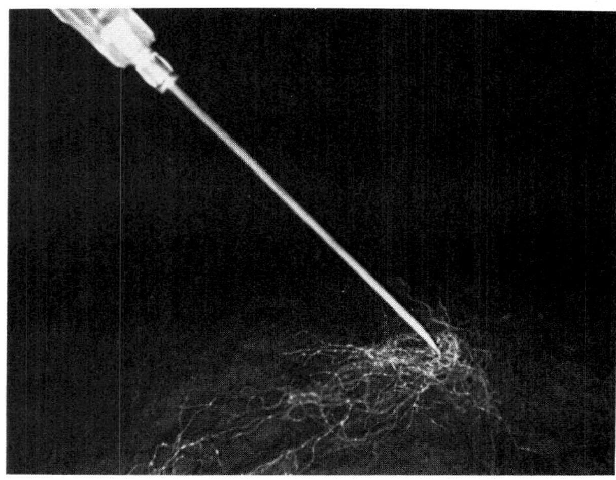

FIG. 22-7. Needle with barb or "fish hook."

Equally important in the preanesthetic evaluation is a discussion with the patient of the proposed technique, its benefits, and significant risks necessary to provide a legitimate informed consent. This discussion should be in sufficient detail that the patient understands, in advance, his role in cooperating with the administration of the anesthetic and how he will be managed intraoperatively (see Chap. 6). Many complications incur the potential for medicolegal problems through patient–physician misunderstanding or lack of rapport.

Perhaps most important in preventing complications is insurance of adequate and functional equipment not only for performance of the anesthetic but also for resuscitation, the latter being extremely important for nerve blocks performed in offices and outpatient settings. Unfortunately, centers or practitioners who perform regional blocks infrequently will attempt to assemble a disarray of obsolete needles and syringes on an "as needed" basis and then wonder at their high incidence of failures and complications. *Everyone* who undertakes the practice of neural blockade, no matter how minor, should be trained in cardiopulmonary resuscitation and have immediate access to the essential equipment and supplies. Incurring complications can be avoidable; failure to diagnose and treat those complications appropriately may be negligence.

Although many of the complications discussed herein will occur almost immediately or within the anesthetic period, others, such as neuropathies, headache, and pneumothorax, occur some days later in the postsurgical period. It is important, therefore, that all patients undergoing neural blockade be visited a sufficient number of times postanesthetically so that the documented record will show evidence of the anesthetist's awareness of any complications that may occur. Most postanesthesia complications are erroneously attributed to an anesthetic cause by other physicians and nurses in the absence of adequate anesthesia follow-up during the postsurgical period. Early diagnosis, consultation with appropriate specialists, and early initiation of corrective therapy are medicolegal and professional responsibilities of all anesthetists. This, coupled with good patient rapport and record-keeping, will ensure the maximum beneficial outcome from any postregional anesthetic complication.

REFERENCES

1. Adriani, J.: Labat's Regional Anesthesia. 3rd ed. p. 192. Philadelphia, W.B. Saunders, 1967.
2. Aldrete, J.A., Romo-salas, F., Arora, S., Wilson, R., *et al.*: Reverse arterial blood flow as a pathway for central nervous system toxic responses following injection of local anesthetics. Anesth. Analg., *57*:428, 1978.
3. Allemann, B.H., Gerber, H., Gruber, U.F.: Spinal conduction anesthesia in the face of subcutaneously administered heparin-dihydro ergot for thromboembolism prophylaxis. Anaesthetist *32*:80, 1983.
4. Barutell, C., Vidal, F., Raich, M., Montero, A.: A neurological complication following interscalene brachial plexus block. Anaesthesia, *35*:365–367, 1980.
5. Beaudoin, M.G., and Klein, L.: Epidural abscess following multiple spinal anaesthetics. Anaesth Intensive Care, *12*:163, 1984.
6. Benzon, H.T., Brunner, E.A., Vaisrub, N.: Bleeding time and nerve blocks after aspirin. Reg. Anesth., *9*:86, 1984.
7. Born, G.: Neuropathy after bupivacaine wrist and metacarpal nerve blocks. J. Hand. Surg., *9A*:109, 1984.
8. Brown, D.T., Beamish, D., Wildsmith, J.A.W.: Allergic reaction to an amide local anaesthetic. Br. J. Anaesth., *53*:435, 1981.
9. Brown, E.M., Elman, D.S.: Postoperative backache. Anesth. Analg., *40*:683, 1961.

9a. Brownridge, P.: The Management of Headache Following Accidental Dural Puncture in Obstetric Patients. Anaesth. Intensive Care, *11*:4, 1983.

10. Casey, W.F.: Respiratory failure following intercostal nerve blockade. Anaesthesia, *39*:351, 1984.
11. Cooke, E.D.: Monitoring during low dose heparin prophylaxis. N. Engl. J. Med., *294*:1066, 1976.
12. Cory, P.C., and Mulroy, M.F.: Postoperative respiratory failure following intercostal block. Anesthesiology, *54*:418, 1981.
13. Crawford, J.S.: Lumbar epidural block in labor: A clinical analysis. Br. J. Anaesth., *44*:66, 1972.
14. Dawkins, C.J.M.: An analysis of the complications of extradural and caudal block. Anesthesia, *24*:554, 1969.
15. DeAngelis, J.: Hazards of subdural and epidural anesthesia during anticoagulant therapy: A case report and review. Anesth. Analg., *51*:676, 1972.
16. Driessen, A., Mauer, W., Fricke, M., Kossmann, B., Schleinzer, W.: Prospective studies on the pathologic mechanism of post spinal headache in a select group of patients. Anaesthetist, *29*:38, 1980.
17. Duggan, J., McKeown, D.W., Scott, D.B.: Venous pressures generated during IV regional anaesthesia (IVRA). Br. J. Anaesth., *55*:1158P, 1983.
18. Duncan, P., and Kobrmsky, N.: Prilocaine induced methemoglobinemia in a newborn infant. Anesthesiology, *59*:75, 1983.
19. Eckstein, K.L., Rogacev, Z., Vincente–Eckstein, A., Grahovac, A.: Prospective comparative study of postspinal headache in young patients (less than 51 years). Reg. Anesth., *5*:57, 1982.
20. Engberg, G.: Relief of postoperative pain with intercostal blockade compared with the use of narcotic drugs. Acta. Anaesthesiol. Scand., *70(Suppl)*:1136, 1978.
21. Erola, M., Kaukinen, L., Kaukinen, S.: Fatal brain lesion following spinal anaesthesia. Acta. Anaesthesiol. Scand., *25*:115, 1981.
22. Fisher, M., and Pennington, J.C.: Allergy to local anaesthesia. Br. J. Anaesth., *54*:893, 1982.
23. Gallo, J.A., Lebowitz, P.W., Battit, G.E., Bruner, J.M.R.: Complications of intercostal nerve blocks performed under direct

vision during thoracotomy. J. Thorac. Cardiovasc. Surg., *86*:628, 1983.

24. Ghani, G.A., and Berry, A.J.: Right hydrothorax after left external jugular vein catheterization. Anesthesiology, *58*:93, 1983.
25. Gould, J.E., Casey, W.F., Reynolds, F.: Bupivacaine intravenous anaesthesia and resuscitation (Letters). Anaesthesia, *39*:612, 1984.
26. Greensite, F.S., and Katz, J.: Spinal subdural hematoma associated with attempted epidural anesthesia and subsequent continuous spinal anesthesia. Anesth. Analg., *59*:72, 1980.
27. Harik, S.I., Raichle, M.E., Reis, D.J.: Spontaneously remitting spinal epidural hematoma in a patient on anticoagulants. N. Engl. J. Med., *284*:1355, 1971.
28. Hassan, E.K., Hutton, P., Black, A.M.S.: Dangers of cubital fossa injections for Bier's blockade. Br. J. Anaesth., *55*:1158P, 1983.
29. Hasselstrom, L.J., and Mogensen, T.: Toxic reaction of bupivacaine at low plasma concentration. Anesthesiology, *61*:99, 1984.
30. Heath, M.L.: Bupivacaine toxicity and Bier blocks (Letter). Anesthesiology, *59*:480, 1983.
31. Heglund, P.O., and Blomback, M.: The effect of prophylaxis with low dose heparin on blood coagulation parameters. Thromb. Haemost., *41*:337, 1979.
32. Hill, J.N., Gershon, N.I., Gargiulo, P.O.: Total spinal blockade during local anesthesia of the nasal passages. Anesthesiology, *59*:144, 1983.
33. Kakkar, V.V., Corrigan, T., Fossard, D.P.: Prevention of fatal postoperative pulmonary embolism by low doses of heparin. Lancet, *2*:45, 1976.
34. Kane, R.E.: Neurologic deficits following epidural or spinal anesthesia. Anesth. Analg., *60*:150, 1981.
35. Kilpatrick, M.E., and Girgis, N.I.: Meningitis: A complication of spinal anesthesia. Anesth. Analg., *62*(5):513, 1983.
36. Knoblanche, G.E.: The incidence and aetiology of phrenic nerve blockade associated with supraclavicular brachial plexus block. Anaesth. Intensive Care, *7*:346, 1979.
37. Korevaar, W., Burney, R.G., Moore, P.A.: Convulsions during stellate ganglion block: A case report. Anesth. Analg., *58*:329, 1979.
38. Kumar, A., Battit, G.F., Fraese, A.B., Long, M.C.: Bilateral cervical and thoracic epidural blockade complicating interscalene brachial plexus block. Anesthesiology, *35*:650, 1971.
39. Lawes, E.G., Johnson, T., Pritchard, P., Robbins, P.: Venous pressures during simulated Bier's block. Anaesthesia, *39*:147, 1984.
40. Locke, G.E., Giorgio, A.J., Biggers, S.L.: Acute spinal epidural hematoma secondary to aspirin-induced prolonged bleeding. Surg. Neurol., *5*:292, 1976.
41. Manchanda, V.N., Murad, S.H.N., Shilyansky, G., Mehringer, M.: Unusual clinical course of accidental subdural local anesthetic injection. Anesth. Analg., *62*:1124, 1983.
42. Mani, M., Ramamurthy, N., Rao, T.L.K., Winnie, A.P., *et al.*: An unusual complication of brachial plexus block and heparin therapy. Anesthesiology, *48*:213, 1978.
43. Mathews, E.T., and Abrams, L.D.: Intrathecal morphine in open heart surgery. Lancet, *2*:543, 1980.
44. Mehta, M., and Maher, R.: Injection into the extra-arachnoid subdural space. Anaesthesia, *32*:760, 1977.
45. Moir, D.D., and Davidson, S.: Postpartum complications of forceps delivery performed under epidural and pudendal nerve block. Br. J. Anaesth., *44*:1197, 1972.
46. Moore, D.C.: Stellate Ganglion Block. p. 110. Springfield, Illinois, Charles C. Thomas, 1954.
47. Moore, D.C.: Regional Block. 4th ed. p. 240. Springfield, Illinois, Charles C. Thomas, 1965.
48. Newrick, P., and Read, P.: Subdural haematoma as a complication of spinal anesthetic. Br. Med. J., *285*:341, 1982.
49. Nicholson, M.J., and McAlpine, F.S.: Neural injuries associated with surgical positions and operations. *In* Martin, J.T.: Positioning in Anesthesia and Surgery. pp. 193–224. Philadelphia, W.B. Saunders, 1978.
50. Odoom, J.A., and Sih, I.L.: Epidural analgesia and anticoagulant therapy. Experience with one-thousand cases of continuous epidurals. Anaesthesia, *38*:254, 1983.
51. Park, R.: A migrating epidural cannula. (Letter) Anaesthesia, *39*:289, 1984.
52. Pearson, R.M.G.: A rare complication of extradural analgesia. Anaesthesia, *39*:460, 1984.
53. Rao, T.K.L., and El-Etr, A.A.: Anticoagulation following placement of epidural and subarachnoid catheters. Anesthesiology, *55*:618, 1981.
54. Ravindran, R.S., Bond, V.K., Tasch, M.D., Gupta, C.D., *et al.*: Prolonged neural blockade following regional analgesia with 2-chloroprocaine. Anesth. Analg., *59*:447, 1980.
55. Ravindran, R.S., Viegas, O.J., Tasch, M.D., Cline, R.P., *et al.*: Bearing down at the time of delivery and the incidence of spinal headache in parturients. Anesth. Analg., *60*:524, 1981.
56. Reisner, L.S., Hochman, B.N., Plumer, M.H.: Persistent neurologic deficit and adhesive arachnoiditis following intrathecal 2-chloroprocaine injection. Anesth. Analg., *59*: 452, 1980.
57. Rengarchy, S.S., and Murphy, D.: Subarachnoid hematoma following lumbar puncture causing compression of the caudal equina. J. Neurosurg., *41*:252, 1974.
58. Reynolds, F.: Bupivacaine and intravenous regional anaesthesia (Editorial). Anaesthesia, *39*:105, 1984.
59. Rosenberg, P.H., Kalso, E.A., Tuominen, M.K., Linden, H.B.: Acute bupivacaine toxicity as a result of venous leakage under the tourniquet cuff during Bier block. Anesthesiology, *58*:95, 1984.
60. Ross, S., and Scarborough, C.D.: Total spinal anesthesia following brachial plexus block. Anesthesiology, *39*:458, 1973.
61. Scott, D.B., Quisling, R.G., Miller, C.A.: Spinal epidural hematoma. J.A.M.A., *235*:513, 1976.
62. Scott, D.L., Ghia, J.N., Teeple, E.: Aphasia and hemiparesis following stellate ganglion block. Anesth. Analg., *62*:1038, 1983.
63. Selander, D., Dhuner, K.S., Lundberg, G.: Peripheral nerve injury due to injection needles used for regional anesthesia. Acta. Anaesthesiol. Scand., *21*:182, 1977.
64. Selander, D., Brattsand, R., Lundborg, G., Nordborg, C., *et al.*: Local anesthetics: Importance of mode of application, concentration and adrenaline for the appearance of nerve lesions. Acta Anaesthesiol. Scand., *23*:127, 1979.

65. Selander, D., Edshage, S., Wolff, T.: Paresthesiae or no paresthesiae? Acta Anaesthesiol. Scand., *23*:27, 1979.
66. Szienfeld, M., Laurencio, M., Pallares, V.S.: Total reversible blindness following stellate ganglion block. Anesthesiol. Analg., *60*:689, 1981.
67. Thompson, K.J., Melding, P., Hatangdi, V.S.: Pneumochylothorax: A rare complication of stellate ganglion block. Anesthesiology, *55*:589, 1981.
68. Thorburn, J., Moir, D.D.: Bupivacaine toxicity in association with extradural analgesia for caesarean section. Br. J. Anaesth., *56*:551, 1984.
69. Thurer, R.J.: Chylothorax: A complication of subclavian vein catheterization and parenteral hyperalimentation. J. Thorac. Cardiovasc. Surg., *71*:465, 1976.
70. Tomlin, P.J.: Death in outpatient dental anesthetic practice. Anaesthesia, *29*:551, 1974.
71. Tondare, A.S., Nadkarn, A.V., Sathe, C.H., Dave, V.B.: Femoral neuropathy: A complication of lithotomy position under spinal anesthesia. Can. Anaesth. Soc. J., *30*:84, 1983.
72. Usbiaga, J.E.: Neurological complications following epidural anesthesia. Int. Anesthesiol. Clin., *13*:1, 1975.
73. Varkey, G.P., and Brindle, G.F.: Peridural anaesthesia and anticoagulant therapy. Can. Anaesth. Soc. J., *21*:106, 1974.
74. Winchell, S.W., and Wolfe, R.: The incidence of neuropathy following upper extremity nerve blocks. Reg. Anesth., *10*:12, 1985.

23 COMPLICATIONS OF NEUROLYTIC NEURAL BLOCKADE

MARK SWERDLOW

GENERAL CONSIDERATIONS

The performance of neurolytic neural blockade entails the general hazards described in Chapter 22, but, in addition, the introduction of irritating sclerosing substances involves risks that are generally longer lasting and more serious than those caused by local anesthetics. This is especially so if the neurolytic agent unintentionally overspills the intended site or is unknowingly injected into an unseen hazard (*e.g.*, dural cuff).

Because the dose of neurolytic agent injected is much smaller than that in the corresponding local anesthetic block, complications that result from overflow or spread are less likely. If, however, the neurolytic solution impinges upon a neighboring structure, the effects will be longer lasting and destructive; thus, for example, overflow onto the brachial plexus while chemical stellate block is being performed may yield protracted sensory and motor loss in the arm. The prolonged duration of action of the agents must particularly be borne in mind when chemical nerve block is contemplated in patients with existing physical disabilities, especially neurologic or respiratory. In such patients, an unexpected complication caused by injection of local anesthetic might result in temporary difficulties and embarrassment, but the same accident produced by a neurolytic drug could prove serious. Thus, in a case reported by Peyton and his colleagues, paresis due to a spinal cord lesion was precipitated into complete paralysis by a subarachnoid injection of alcohol.[98] Similarly, unintentional chemical phrenic nerve block could be dangerous in a patient with existing respiratory difficulty.

With regard to the effect of neurolytic agents on nerve tissue itself, Sunderland has stated that the neural damage sustained by injection of sclerosing substances varies in severity from rapidly reversible changes that cause only transient loss of function to permanent constrictive scarring in and about the nerve, sufficient to prevent recovery in the affected fibers.[111]

The effects of alcohol and of phenol on nerve tissue have been found to be histologically almost identical.[79] The extent and severity of damage are influenced by such factors as the internal structure of the nerve at the site of injection, the amount of material injected, and its sclerosing properties. A further important risk is vascular damage caused by the neurolytic agent, especially damage to the vascular supply of the central nervous system (CNS).[112] Phenol has been stated to have an even greater affinity for vascular tissue than for brain (see also Chap. 29.1).[92]

In light of the dangers of chemical neurolysis, it is clear that with peripheral nerve blocks a preliminary injection of a test dose (1 – 2 ml) of local anesthetic is usually advisable, especially when there is doubt about which nerve is involved and whether blocking it will provide effective pain relief. Such prognostic blocking has the added advantage that it may provide the patient with a chance to evaluate possible side-effects. This is not always the case because the path taken by the needle in a subsequent neurolytic injection might not be identical, and a blood vessel, dural cuff, or pleura involved on the first occasion would not necessarily be involved during the subsequent neurolytic injection and, of course, *vice versa.*

Following neurolytic block, a day or two should be allowed to elapse before the degree of depletion of nerve function that has resulted is determined. After phenol, this depletion may not be as serious as appeared at first, perhaps because of the biphasic effect of the agent.[89] Thus, for example, phenol injected into the cisterna has been reported to have produced quadriplegia that "lasted for 30 minutes in full intensity, then gradually cleared."[130]

If a neurolytic solution does cause persistent unwanted nerve block, the nerve will regenerate in time (except for the optic nerve), and treatment should be aimed at relieving pain, preventing disuse atrophy, and reassuring the patient. To reduce the anxiety that the occurrence of a complication may cause the patient (and the anesthesiologist!) and to avoid legal action, it is well to explain the procedure and likely complications to the patient and to have a "consent" form signed *before* beginning treatment. Needless to say, if complications do occur, appropriate specialists should be consulted so that recovery and rehabilitation are as complete and expeditious as possible.

Table 23-1 shows details of 25 cases in which neurolytic block was followed by legal action; all but one of these patients were suffering from noncancer pain.

Legal action may be brought on a number of grounds,[116] namely that

1. Complications were caused by the injection;
2. The patient did not consent to the procedure;
3. The procedure was carried out inexpertly;
4. The wrong procedure was performed; or
5. Treatment of the complication(s) was inadequate.

Injection of neurolytic solutions is sometimes followed by pain at the site of injection that lasts a few days and is presumably due to local tissue irritation. Persistence of the pain suggests a possible complication such as a slough or sterile abscess formation. Chemical neurolysis may also be followed by a troublesome neuritis, especially after alcohol.

Petrillo and colleagues,[97] who performed tibial nerve block with 5% aqueous phenol in 30 hemiplegic patients for the treatment of spasticity, reported the development of a burning sensation and paresthesia in the sensory distribution of the tibial nerve. The dysesthesia was moderate in 5 patients and severe in 3; it started 5 days to 3 weeks after the block and lasted 1 to 8 weeks. Katz and his colleagues[55] had a case in which paresthesia persisted longer than 2 months after ulnar nerve block with phenol. If this is of moderate degree, it should be treated with appropriate analgesics; in more severe cases of neuralgia a somatic nerve block plus sympathetic block may be indicated, and occasionally the help of a neurosurgeon may be required. Reports of the incidence of paresthesias after phenol block range from 14.7%[59] to 30%.[13]

Swelling, cellulitis, and sloughing of tissues have been reported in perineural tissues; May found that alcohol caused severe adhesions as well as neurolysis.[72] When the needle is being withdrawn after neurolytic block, there is a risk that some of the chemical will be left in the track of the needle with troublesome sequelae. It is advisable, therefore, to inject a little saline or local anesthetic as the needle is being removed. There is a special risk when a chemical is being injected at a superficial site (*e.g.*, intercostal block, neurolytic block for coccydinia); the dose at such sites should be minimal and the needle flushed out with the saline during withdrawal. I had one patient with sloughing of a small area of skin over the coccyx after injection of 1 ml of 10% phenol and a similar complication after intercostal phenol block (Fig. 23-1). Complete healing eventually occurred in both patients.

Intravascular injection should be avoided by aspirating repeatedly during injection of alcohol, phenol, or other neurolytic agents. Intravascular injection of 10% phenol causes "severe tinnitus and flushing within a few seconds but recovery is rapid and complete."[100] Phenol stimulates the CNS, causing muscle tremors and eventually convulsions.[6,31] Absorption of large amounts of phenol, however, will depress consciousness and blood pressure and cause renal damage.[35] Accidental intravascular injection of absolute alcohol results in effects that are "entirely pleasurable and will require no specific therapy"[17]; however, intravenous alcohol may sometimes cause thrombosis of the vessel.

Another neurolytic agent is ammonium sulphate. It was considered by Stewart and colleagues[109] to produce sensory blockade without motor block, although Davies and his colleagues[26] describe a case of foot drop after the application of 15% ammonium chloride solution to the peroneal nerve. It has been claimed that neuritis does not follow the injection of ammonium salts.[77,129]

Neurolytic chemical agents are used for a more restricted and defined range of nerve blocks than are local anesthetics, and this reflects, in part, the risks

TABLE 23-1. CASE DETAILS

Techniques	Number of Cases	Complication(s)	Disposition	Comments
Intrathecal neurolysis	1	Sensation and bladder impaired	Settled out of court	Technique unwise in young man with benign condition
	1	Paresis and bladder impaired	Settled out of court	Injection unwise
	1	Paresis and impaired sensation	Judgment for the doctor	Valid informed consent
	1	Paresis, sensory and bladder impairment	Judgment for the patient	Use of 10% phenol unwise
	1	Paresis, sensory and bladder impairment	Judgment for the patient	Use of phenol and volume (3 ml) criticized
	1	Sensory and bladder impairment	Judgment for the doctor	
	1	Paresis, sensory impairment	Judgment for the patient	
	1	Paresis	Pending	
	1	Paraparesis, double incontinence	Settled out of court £25,000 + costs	Use of phenol unjustifiable in nonmalignant case and dose (3 ml) excessive
	1	Right paresis + anesthesia perineum	Settled out of court £18,680 damages	Use of phenol unwise in nonmalignant young case
	1	Right paresis + double incontinence	Pending	
Lumbar sympathetic block (neurolytic)	1	Paresis, bladder impaired	Pending	? Accidental intrathecal block
	1	Paresis	Proceeding	
	1	Paresis	Judgment for the doctor	
	1	Ureter damaged; → nephrectomy performed	Settled out of court	Procedure indefensible
Lumbar sympathetic block, phenol in almond oil	1	Unilateral paralysis of leg	Plaintiff awarded £33,000 damages	Accidental intrathecal injection
Phenol block, lower sacral nerves	1	Sensory and bladder impairment	Pending	
Procaine injection, scalenus anterior	1	Pneumothorax	Judgment for the doctor	
Alcohol, perineal block	1	Sloughing perineal skin	Pending	
Phenol caudal block	1	Bladder function impaired	Judgment for the doctor	
Lesser occipital nerve block with absolute alcohol + 1% lidocaine	1	Dysphagia and hoarseness	Pending	
Splanchnic block (neurolytic)	1	Paraplegia	Pending	
Subarachnoid hypertonic saline	1	Bowel and bladder impairment, impotence, and paraparesis	Case proceeding	
Subarachnoid barbotage	2	Permanent paraplegia	Cases proceeding	

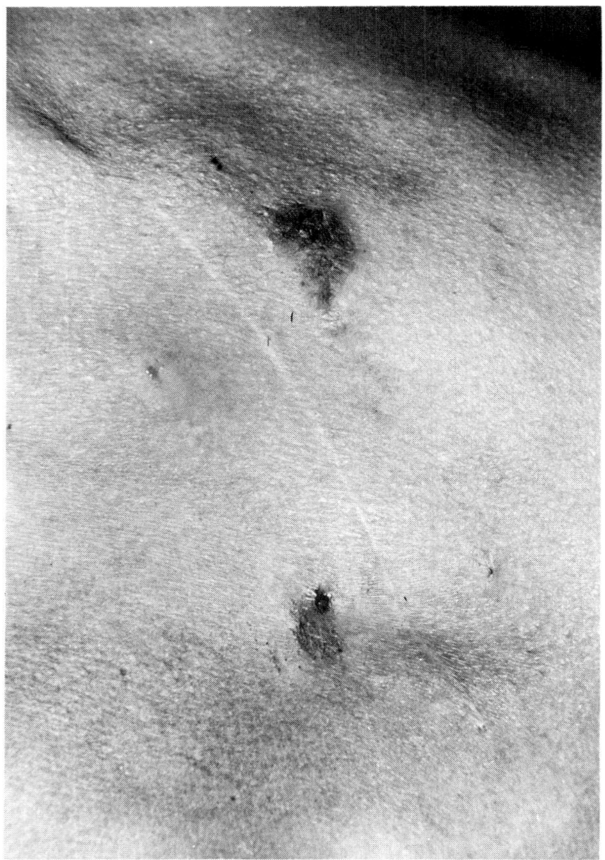

FIG. 23-1. Sloughing of a small area of skin over the chest after intercostal phenol block.

involved. Because of these risks, thermogangliolysis or neurosurgery rather than chemical neurolysis may be advised for specific nerves (*e.g.*, trigeminal ganglion, thoracic sympathetic ganglia).

SUBARACHNOID CHEMICAL BLOCK

Intrathecal neurolysis is undoubtedly a most valuable means of providing relief for intractable pain. The accessibility of the spinal nerve roots within the theca to injected fluids is, however, a mixed blessing because motor, sensory, and autonomic nerves may unintentionally be involved by the injected chemical (see Chap. 29.1). The complications that result are usually only temporary, but, as will be seen later, sometimes persist and give rise to difficulties in patient management.

It is difficult to make any valid comparison among reported differences in incidence of the various complications because of the great individual variation in the patients treated. Most patients who undergo intrathecal neurolysis are suffering from pain caused by malignant disease, and a number of factors may affect the incidence of complications. There are considerable interpatient differences in the size and position of the primary or secondary tumor that causes the pain and also in whether or not the patient has had radiotherapy. Further, many of the patients already have some degree of sensory, motor, or autonomic impairment in the painful region of the body before the injection is given.[49,113] It is therefore difficult to conduct a comparative study of the potential for complications of different intrathecal neurolytic agents other than to encompass a very large number of patients in the hope, thereby, of eliminating these variables. A further difficulty in assessing reported results is that the degree and duration of the complications are not always described.

The incidence of complications depends to a great extent on which part of the cord is being blocked and how many nerve roots are involved. Thus, paresis will be in evidence only when the cervicothoracic or lumbar cord is blocked, and bladder or rectal sequelae are very unlikely after subarachnoid blocks solely at the thoracic level. I had one patient, however, who developed bladder paralysis after phenol block at T11 following three previous uncomplicated blocks at lower spinal levels and a second patient who developed bladder paresis after phenol block at T7.[114] The second patient had previously received extensive radiotherapy to the lower thoracic spine. On the other hand, Tank, Dohn, and Gardner, who administered 37 intrathecal alcohol blocks for intractable sacral plexus pain, reported that half their patients suffered transient loss of bladder control and three had permanent loss, and Papo and Visca noted 5 permanent and 10 temporary interruptions of bladder function after phenol saddle block in 39 patients.[94,118] Finally, injection in the cervical part of the subarachnoid space entails the risk of respiratory arrest.[45,112] These cases stress the danger of an excessive dose of a neurolytic agent.

Capuzzo and his colleagues[15] have recently described an unusual complication following subarachnoid phenol injection. A needle was introduced in the L1–L2 space and 1.5 ml of contrast medium was injected and found to move caudally. The table was given some headdown tilt, and 0.7 ml of 10% phenol was injected. Six hours later there was evidence of cranial nerve involvement; the patient gradually recovered after 48 hours. Vesical and anal sphincter control, however, were absent until death 2 months later.

The incidence of complications must, of course, be considered in relation to the quality of results obtained. A new agent or method that gives rise to an increased incidence of complications might be acceptable if it provided longer and more complete pain relief—it would certainly not be welcomed if it did not! These facts should be remembered in considering the following incidence of reported complications.

I have analyzed the complications that occurred in 300 patients who had received a total of 453 intrathecal injections at the Regional Pain Relief Centre, Hope Hospital (University of Manchester School of Medicine). All the patients, as detailed in Table 23-2, had been followed for at least 3 months or until death (if this occurred earlier).

TABLE 23-2. ANALYSIS OF AGENT INJECTED IN SWERDLOW'S SERIES OF 300 PATIENTS GIVEN INTRATHECAL INJECTIONS

Drugs Administered	Number of Patients
Phenol, 5% or 7% in glycerine	145
Chlorocresol, 1:50 or 1:40 in glycerine	138
Phenol and chlorocresol	17
Total	300

Table 23-3 lists the complications that lasted for not more than 3 days. Of the 300 patients,

48 had one or more complications that persisted more than 3 days; 21 of these patients had received more than one intrathecal injection.
28 had one or more complications that persisted more than 1 week.
19 had one or more complications that persisted more than 2 weeks.
10 had one or more complications that persisted more than 1 month.

Table 23-4 cites patients who had one or more complications that persisted for more than a week.

Nathan reported a 12% incidence of sphincter disorder following intrathecal phenol.[87] Bonica found that vesical paralysis, rectal dysfunction, or limb paralysis occurred in 25% of patients after subarachnoid neurolytic injection.[5] It has been claimed that phenol in iophendylate (Pantopaque) has a less injurious effect on bladder innervation, but Pantopaque may introduce complications of its own.[47,118] Interference with bladder function will necessitate the use of an indwelling catheter, while timely doses of carbachol may be both prognostic and therapeutic. The data provided by other publications on phenol are summarized in Table 23-5.[71,73,94,110,128]

With regard to the sequelae of *alcohol* injection, Derrick performed 485 intrathecal alcohol blocks in

TABLE 23-3. COMPLICATIONS THAT LASTED 72 HOURS OR FEWER

	Number of Patients							
Drugs Administered	**Bladder Paresis**	**Bowel Paresis**	**Muscle Paresis**	**Headache**	**Paresthesia**	**Numbness**	**Hyper-esthesia**	**Others**
Phenol	7			5		7		Nausea
Chlorocresol	4		7	4	1	13	2	Backache, nausea (2)
Phenol and chlorocresol	2	2			1	2		Backache Involuntary movements of contralateral leg
Total	13	2	7	9	2	22	2	6

TABLE 23-4. COMPLICATIONS THAT LASTED LONGER THAN 7 DAYS

	Number of Patients					
Drugs Administered	**Bladder Paresis**	**Bowel Paresis**	**Muscle Paresis**	**Headache**	**Paresthesia**	**Numbness**
Phenol	8	1	3		1	4
Chlorocresol	11	1	7	1	1	5
Phenol and chlorocresol	3	1		1		1
Total	22	3	10	2	2	10

TABLE 23-5. REPORTED COMPLICATIONS OF INTRATHECAL PHENOL

Authors	Total Number of Patients	Number of Patients					
		Bladder Paralysis	Bowel Paralysis	Headache	Paresis	Dysesthesia	Loss of Proprioception
Papo and Visca (1979)[95]	290	16			25		
Stovner and Endresen (1972)[110]	151	6	2	14	10	3	
Mark and colleagues (1962)[71]	30				4	4	4
White and Sweet (1969)[128]	26	2			6	2	
Mehta (1973; phenol or chlorocresol)[73]	55	8		2	10	27	
Nathan (1972)[88]	62	11	9		11		
Litshitz et al[63]	90	20	3	5	23		

322 patients, 18 of whom developed muscle weakness or bladder disturbance, two with permanent paralysis of both legs.[28] Hay[42] details the results of 407 alcohol injections in 252 patients. Two patients developed temporary urinary incontinence—one with paraparesis, and one with lasting urinary incontinence and paralysis of the left leg. There were two other cases of limb paralysis, and four patients had temporary marked proprioceptive loss.

Hand has reported the use of subarachnoid ammonium sulphate in 50 patients.[41] Transient complications were nausea, retching, and headache, whereas paresthesias or a burning sensation occurred in 30.4% of patients (especially when 500 mg was given) and lasted 2 to 14 days. Judovich and his colleagues[53] reported a number of patients with bowel and bladder involvement following a subarachnoid injection of ammonium salts, and they advocated reducing the dose of ammonium sulphate to 200 mg. The dangers of intrathecal ammonium salts were further illustrated by Guttman and Pardee,[38] who described two cases of paraparesis owing to spinal cord level syndrome following ammonium sulphate injection.

In view of the pain-riddled state of many of the patients who receive intrathecal neurolytics and the new sensations that the patient experiences immediately after the procedure, it is somewhat problematic whether subarachnoid alcohol sometimes causes alcohol neuritis. In one such possible case, Katz has suggested that the neuritis may have been caused by spilling of alcohol into the epidural space during the intrathecal injection.[54]

Meningismus is a rare complication of subarachnoid alcohol block.[10] Three days to 4 days after the injection, the patient exhibits headache, neck rigidity, and pain over the vertebral column; the CSF pressure is found to be raised. Treatment consists of bed rest, removal of CSF, and administration of appropriate analgesics. It has been suggested that the relatively scanty subarachnoid space in the cervical part of the spine could predispose a patient to a meningeal reaction there.[105]

Cauda equina lesion may, on occasion, be a sequel of intrathecal injection of alcohol, although the reported cases date from before the introduction of the autoclave.[104,123] Posterior spinal artery thrombosis has been reported after intrathecal injection of phenol; the syndrome appeared on the 2nd day and had practically cleared up a week later.[48] Anterior spinal artery thrombosis is also a risk.

Totoki and co-workers[122] reported a disastrous case of anterior spinal artery occlusion after cervical subarachnoid injection of 0.3 ml of 10% phenol in glycerine. A further case was described by Churcher,[21] whose patient developed permanent paraparesis following intrathecal injection of 0.4 ml of 5% phenol in glycerine. It was thought that surgery and radiotherapy had already impaired the blood supply to the spinal cord and the phenol acted as the "ultimate insult."

Subarachnoid Hypertonic Saline. A number and variety of complications have been reported following intrathecal administration of hypertonic saline. Lucas and his colleagues have reviewed the adverse reactions encountered by a number of workers in a total of 2105 patients.[66] Complications of some degree occurred in 10.59% of the patients; in 1.03% there was "significant morbidity." Two patients treated by this method died as a result of myocardial infarction. It has been shown that during saline injection, sinus tachycardia or ventricular ectopic beats may be exhibited and that when the injection is administered intracisternally, sinus bradycardia may occur.[67] Hammermeister and Reichenbach suggested that intrathecal saline may excite a sympathetic discharge that could cause myocardial damage.[40] It would therefore appear inadvisable to use this method in patients who suffer from cardiovascular or hypertensive disease.

Ventafridda and Spreafico have reported localized paresis lasting for many hours and paresthesias that sometimes persisted for weeks.[125] Transient hemiplegia has also been reported to follow subarachnoid hypertonic saline injection, and Thompson recorded the case of a patient who developed pulmonary edema that responded to treatment with diuretics.[93,119] Hitchcock has stated that after cisternal injection of hypertonic saline, one patient developed pain in the ear and vestibular disturbances that persisted for some weeks.[44] Finally, persisting loss of sphincter control with sacral anesthesia has occurred in two patients who had "presumptive evidence of gross arteriosclerosis in the blood supply to the roots of the cauda equina."[12]

EXTRADURAL ANALGESIA

In theory, the extradural route should have advantages for the production of chemical neurolysis; there are, however, relatively few reports on the results of this procedure.[14] Grunwald[37] has reported on the use of extradural 6% to 10% aqueous phenol in 221 patients with cancer pain. Urinary incontinence occurred in 57 patients and lasted longer than 2 weeks in 17 of them. There was bowel incontinence in 21 patients and muscular weakness in 14: These complications persisted longer than 2 weeks in 8 and 3 patients, respectively.

Bromage[14] reported on 55 epidural neurolytic injections. One patient exhibited temporary weakness of arm and intercostal muscles after a thoracic level block with alcohol, and one patient had a short-lasting slight paraparesis after an alcohol lumbar block. Two patients had transient urinary retention after sacral epidural block, one with alcohol and one with phenol.

Epidural injection of alcohol may be followed by distressing neuritis. Colpitt and associates[22] reported the occurrence of uncomfortable dysesthesia of 24 to 48 hours' duration in two of their patients given 7% phenol epidurally. Hypertonic saline administered epidurally has resulted in permanent paraplegia.[124]

PERIPHERAL NERVE BLOCKS

BLOCKS OF THE HEAD AND NECK

Trigeminal Nerve

Gasserian Ganglion Block. Because of the anatomic situation of the ganglion, gasserian ganglion chemical block may be followed by a number of different complications, many of which are of serious import; indeed, Stender reports a 0.9% fatality rate after alcohol blocks for trigeminal neuralgia.[108] The risks of diffusion of alcohol can be so serious that boiling water has been suggested as a safer means of destroying the ganglionic cells, although new radiofrequency techniques now appear the best choice (see Chaps. 15 and 30).[50] Another technique that appears to have advantages on the grounds of safety is the injection of small volumes of glycerol as advocated by Hakanson.[39]

Puncture of veins in the subtemporal region can cause hemorrhage, which spreads in the temporal fossa and cheek and should be controlled by firm pressure. Care, gentleness, experience, and a careful study of the anatomy all help, to some extent, to decrease the incidence of complications, as, it is hoped, will more recent techniques.[91] In particular, in performing gasserian ganglion block the greatest care should be taken to avoid accidental movement of the needle tip once accurate placement has been assured; the dosage must be precisely checked, and the injection should be slow and controlled.

Some patients find the resulting anesthesia of the face a great disability, but they can be reassured that some sensation will return. A number of side-effects, which are usually neither grave nor lasting, may follow shortly after the injection of alcohol. Thus, block of the paratrigeminal sympathetic fibers produces Horner's syndrome, which gradually diminishes, whereas involvement of the motor fibers of the trigeminal nerve will interfere with mastication.[25] The parasympathetic fibers of the third cranial nerve may be affected, giving rise to mydriasis with an irregular oval pupil that does not react to light. Block of the oculomotor nerve itself causes strabismus and diplopia, which usually fade in a few days. The abducens nerve is not uncommonly affected, and Ruge and colleagues have reported two cases of permanent lateral rectus palsy.[103] It has been suggested that the patient should be requested to move the eyes during the injection and that if signs of incipient muscle weakness become apparent, the injection should be discontinued.[91]

Involvement of other nearby nerves may be more serious. Thus diffusion of solution to the eighth nerve causes loss of hearing, whereas involvement of the cochlear-vestibular nerve results in dizziness (aggravated by postural changes), nausea, vomiting, and nystagmus; the vestibular effects are usually short lasting. Spread of alcohol may also occur in the space around the posterior root of the facial nerve; the facial muscles on the blocked side are paralyzed and the eye will not close. Prolonged inability to close the eyelid may result in corneal ulcer or keratitis. The facial weakness may prove to be temporary or permanent.[86,103] Corneal ulcers or keratitis may follow gasserian ganglion block because the nerve to the cornea travels through the ganglion. The corneal reflex is obtunded, which exposes the eye to trauma. Worse, because of paralysis of the greater superficial petrosal nerve, there is a lack of tear formation, and this may well encourage conjunctivitis. If the ganglion has been blocked with chemical, therefore, long-term protection must be provided for the eye. In one reported series, keratitis occurred in 28 of 64 patients.[99] Cervical sympathectomy has been advocated in the treatment of keratitis.[29]

Table 23-6 shows the incidence of complications in two large reported series.

The later results of destruction of the ganglion can, according to Thurel, be divided into trophic disturbances and anesthesia dolorosa, and herpes simplex of the lips and delayed facial paralysis.[121] Trophic disturbances include mucous erosions in the mouth, nasal ulceration, keratitis, and facial "algae." These may result from trauma in an anesthetic area in the presence of diminished tissue resistance from neuromotor disturbances. Bactericidal ointments and the wearing of gloves at night are useful therapeutic measures. Anesthesia dolorosa and paresthesia in the numb area may follow gasserian ganglion alcohol injection; Sperling and Stender reported that 10 of 85 patients given ganglion block suffered later from burning pain in the blocked area, and Ramb found similar complications in 4 of 46 patients.[99,107] The use of a "drop-by-drop" method with positioning of the patient's head during injection has produced a diminution in the incidence of these complications. Jefferson's method of injecting the ganglion with 5% phenol in glycerine (with the patient in a sitting position) appears to control even better the spread of the neurotoxic agent; of 50 patients reported by Jefferson, none developed either corneal ulceration or anesthesia dolorosa.[51]

Overflow onto the optic nerve may occur if the needle is directed incorrectly during gasserian ganglion block or supraorbital or infraorbital nerve block. Chemical block of the optic nerve yields partial or total blindness, which may persist.[81,99] Overflow onto the glossopharyngeal nerve may also occur,[43] resulting in dysphagia. Another complication that has been reported after gasserian ganglion block is osteomyelitis of the mandible.[103]

According to Labat, alcohol frequently causes an inflammatory reaction, producing adhesions in the tissues around the ganglion—this may later render surgery difficult.[61] Labat considered that neurolytic agents should never be used in the retrobulbar area (*e.g.*, ophthalmic nerve, ethmoidal nerve block) because of the proximity of the optic, trochlear, and oculomotor nerves.[61] Henderson[43] abandoned injection of the maxillary nerve in the pterygopalatine fossa because of the proximity of the optic nerve and the risk of causing blindness.

Supraorbital Nerve Block. The dose of neurolytic solution injected should not exceed 0.5 ml because of the risk of diffusion into the orbit. If injected too

TABLE 23-6. COMPLICATIONS OF ALCOHOL GASSERIAN GANGLION BLOCK

Complication	Miles[76] (130 injections)	Henderson[43] (196 injections)
Oculomotor palsy (temporary)	4	6
Abducens palsy (temporary)	–	2
Glossopharyngeal palsy (temporary)	–	1
Corneal anesthesia	20	69
Permanent anesthesia of cheek and nose	?	66
Nasal ulceration	2	12
Blindness	–	1
Corneal ulceration	2	?
Trigeminal motor weakness	1	–

superficially, it may cause sloughing of superficial tissues and skin overlying the nerve.

Maxillary Division Trigeminal Nerve. Neurolytic solutions must be used with caution when they are given extraorally. Not more than 1 ml of solution should be injected because excess may pass through the inferior orbital fissure into the orbit and damage the optic and oculomotor nerves, producing visual difficulties and even blindness. Alcohol block (or indeed surgical section) of the maxillary nerve at the foramen rotundum or of the infraorbital nerve can be followed by ulceration and sloughing of the cheek and ala of the nose or of the soft or hard palate (Fig. 23-2). I had one patient in whom a small area of ulceration occurred on the cheek following infraorbital block with 10% aqueous phenol, and a similar accident was reported by Churcher.[20] Churcher[21] has more recently had a further case in which infraorbital nerve block with 0.28 ml of absolute alcohol caused rapid development of ischemic necrosis of the mucosa and cartilage of the palate, resulting in a large hole over half the roof of the mouth on the ipsilateral side. It was thought that the alcohol precipitated intense vasospasm in the area supplied by the maxillary artery. Such damage usually occurs in the area innervated by the infraorbital nerve, but Moore reported a case of a patient in whom sloughing occurred in the posterior part of the superior ridge of the maxilla.[68,81,96] With ulceration of the cheek, stellate ganglion block may be helpful by improving the circulation.

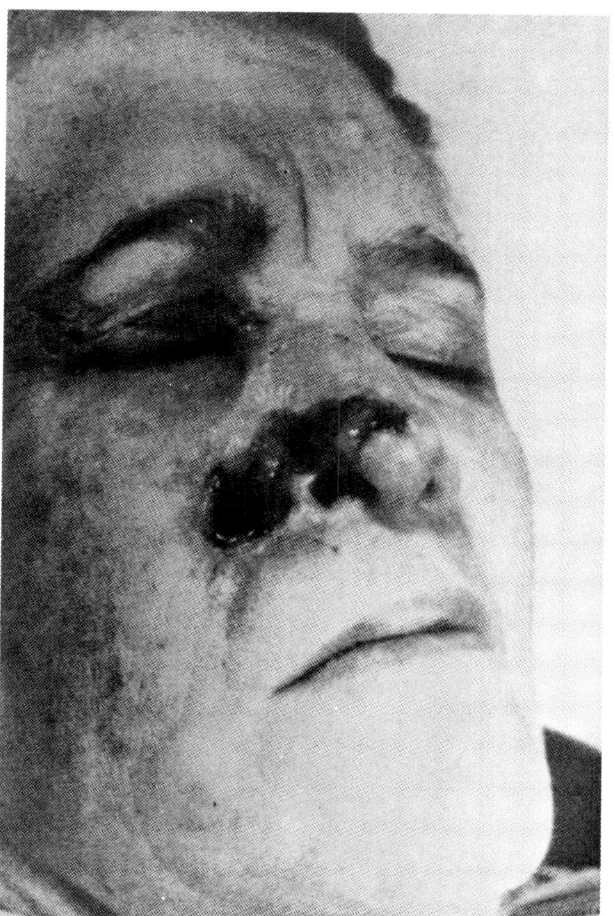

FIG. 23-2. Ulceration and sloughing of the cheek and ala of the nose after alcohol block of the maxillary nerve. (Macomber, D.W.: Plas. Reconstr. Surg., *11*:337, 1953.)

Mandibular Nerve Block. As it emerges from the foramen ovale, the mandibular nerve contains motor as well as sensory fibers. Consequently, neurolytic block may result in paresis or paralysis of the muscles of mastication on the affected side, and the mandible may deviate from the midline. If a neurolytic solution is used, not more than 1 to 2 ml should be injected lest some solution pass upward and affect the gasserian ganglion. White and Sweet reported one case of a patient who developed permanent anesthesia dolorosa following alcohol block of the third division of the trigeminal nerve at the forearm ovale.[128] When trigeminal branch block is being performed by way of the mandibular notch, the facial nerve may also be involved. Finally, a fatality caused by injury to the carotid artery in the cavernous sinus has been reported.[46]

Facial Nerve. Neurolytic agents should be used with the greatest caution in the facial nerve because they may cause permanent paralysis of facial muscles.

Glossopharyngeal nerve may be blocked near the stylomastoid process, but the vagus, accessory, and hypoglossal nerves are in proximity and are at risk if neurolytic agents are injected. Montgomery and Cousins have recommended that glossopharyngeal nerve block always be carried out under radiographic control.[80] Glossopharyngeal block causes dysphagia from paralysis of pharyngeal muscles, and it is recommended that unilateral block only should be performed.[1] Further, neurolytic solutions may cause sloughing and fibrosis in surrounding tissues, and, in particular, the carotid artery and internal jugular vein may be involved with erosion or thrombosis. Facial nerve block may also follow chemical glossopharyngeal block distal to the jugular foramen.[54] Despite these hazards, surgery of the nerve often is not preferable to neurolytic block, since patients who are candidates for this procedure have terminal diseases or have severe systemic contraindications to surgery.

Cervical Nerve. Block of the cervical nerves should be performed with great care to avoid the risk of accidental intrathecal or intravascular injection. In addition, introducing the needle too deeply into the neck may result in involvement of the esophagus or of the spinal accessory nerve, causing paresis of the trapezius. Overflow onto the cervical sympathetic nerve will lead to Horner's syndrome; the patient may complain of ptosis or of nasal congestion.

Brachial Plexus. The use of neurolytic agents is not advised for the brachial plexus because of the risk of paresis or paralysis of muscles of the upper limb and the danger of erosion or thrombosis of blood vessels.

Stellate Ganglion. Chemical block of the stellate ganglion carries the risks of prolonged Horner's syndrome and of possible involvement of the brachial plexus or of the recurrent laryngeal nerve. Recurrent laryngeal nerve block causes hoarseness and some difficulty in swallowing, but both are temporary and require no more than the reassurance of the patient and a warning to take great care with eating and drinking. In addition to these risks, the solution may spread paravertebrally, which in a case reported by Superville–Sovak and colleagues gave rise to extensive extraspinal lesions and spinal cord infarction.[112]

Parastellate injections may reach the subarachnoid space, especially in the presence of enlarged or damaged dural root sleeves.[58] Intrathecal extension of a stellate injection is often heralded by severe headache and may cause respiratory arrest.[2]

CHEMICAL ABLATION OF THE PITUITARY

The destruction of the pituitary gland by alcohol injected through a needle inserted by the nasal, transphenoidal route[85] has now been widely adopted for the relief of cancer pain. The procedure may cause, or be followed by, a number of troublesome sequelae. Some of these are consequences of the absence of the pituitary gland, whereas others are complications owing to the actual injection procedure (see Chap. 29.2).

HORMONAL MORBIDITY

Diabetes insipidus is perhaps the most common sequel. It is a danger only if there is abnormal electrolyte balance or dehydration. It can usually be controlled by inhalation of desmopressin or if this is ineffective, by the use of injections of diuretic hormone (Pitressin). Takeda and co-workers[117] believe that excessive urinary excretion can be prevented by use of indomethacin suppositories. Indomethacin reduces polyuria by suppressing renal prostaglandin E_2, which interferes with inactivation of ADH and does not disturb the diurnal pattern of urinary excretion in polyuria. Lloyd and his colleagues[65] claim that the incidence of diabetes insipidus can be reduced by injecting the alcohol only into the anterior part of the gland, but Lipton[64] was unable to confirm this. Corticosteroid deficiency requires administration of steroids. Hypothyroidism necessitates thyroxin replacement in long-surviving patients.[65,69] Hypothermia, hyperphagia, hypoadrenalism, and lowering of libido are other sequelae. Corssen and associates[23] believe that determination of cortisol and prolactin levels may reliably show whether the patient requires hormone substitution therapy.

COMPLICATIONS

Death occurred in 2 of Ventafridda and De Conno's 96 patients[126] and in 8 of the 122 patients reported by Miles,[75] who stresses that it is important to assess the condition of the patient and to be sure that he can withstand the operation. The most common complication is CSF rhinorrhea; it usually stops in a day or two. According to Madrid,[69] rhinorrhea can be prevented by the use of a nasal tube with a double cuff rather than gauze packing. To prevent leakage of CSF, Katz and Levin[56] now inject 0.5 ml of alpha-ethylcyanoacrylate as the needle is being withdrawn from the sella. If bleeding through the needle should occur during the procedure, the needle should be occluded until bleeding has stopped and adenosis postponed.[23]

Two of Miles' patients showed evidence of hypothalamic injury—progressive impairment of consciousness level, in one associated with hemiparesis.[75] In each case autopsy confirmed extensive infarction of the pituitary stalk and suggested infarction of the hypothalamus with separation of the ependyma. Autopsy in five of Madrid's cases[69] showed complete necrosis of the anterior lobe with no evidence of damage to hypothalamic nuclei.

Neurologic complications. The incidence of neurologic complications is shown in Table 23-7. Involvement of the second or third cranial nerve can result from alcohol diffusing up from the pituitary gland; pupillary response to light should be carefully observed throughout the operation.

Corssen and associates[23] believe that the carotid arteries and extraocular nerves can be avoided by keeping the needle close to the midline during the procedure; however, Newfield and colleagues[90] point out that keeping the needle close to the midline will not always avoid trauma to important structures. Although the cavernous sinuses are located laterally, there are intercavernous connections within the sella that pass anterior, posterior, and inferior to the gland. The location of these sinuses across the midline increases the risk of intraoperative bleeding and provides a port of entry for venous air embolism during transphenoidal adenolysis. Newfield and colleagues recently reported three cases of air embolism in patients undergoing transphenoidal hypophysectomy in the semisitting position.

If visual defects occur, cisternal puncture should be performed and prednisolone or hydrocortisone injected.[64,117] Takeda and co-workers[117] had a case in which hemianopsia was immediately relieved by cisternal puncture with removal of 10 ml of CSF and instillation of prednisolone into the cisterna. Takeda and colleagues[117] consider that by fluoroscopic observation of the spread of neurolytic solution, ophthalmologic complications can be avoided; they advocate a phenol–metrizamide solution. If the injected solution is seen to be spreading in an undesirable direction, suction of the syringe will withdraw some of the solution.

Takeda believes that insufficient alcohol can result in incomplete pain relief but that an excess amount of neurolytic agent increases the danger of damage to the optic chiasma. He considers that the optimal dose of alcohol is 1.8 to 2.4 ml.

Meningitis is a risk, especially if CSF rhinorrhea occurs. Prophylactic sulfonamide may be given; should meningitis occur, it should be treated with antibiotics. Lipton[64] reported a case of empyema of the sphenoid that gave rise to meningitis. He recommended that the sphenoid sinus be aspirated during cannulation.

INTERCOSTAL NEUROLYSIS

Injection of neurolytic agents onto intercostal nerves can be followed by distressing neuritis, especially if

TABLE 23-7. COMPLICATIONS OF CHEMICAL ABLATION OF THE PITUITARY

Study	Number of Patients	Complications and Incidence	Comment
Visual field defects			
Takeda et al[117]	102	10	
Miles[75]	122	2	Some permanent deficiency
Ventafridda and De Conno[126]	96		
Katz and Levin[56,57]	27	2	Temporary
Lloyd et al[65]	35	1	
Ocular nerve palsy			
Corssen et al[23]	24	1	14 days
Madrid[69]	329	7	Permanent in two cases
Katz and Levin[56,57]	27	5	Two permanent, slight
Ventafridda and De Conno[126]	96	32	
Takeda et al[117]	102	3	10 days' duration
CSF rhinorrhea			
Katz and Levin[56,57]	27	3	
Madrid[69]	329	2	Several days
Takeda et al[117]	102	1	
Lloyd et al[65]	35	2	
Miles[75]	122	10–20%	>6 weeks in 1 patient
Ventafridda and De Conno[126]	96	14	
Meningitis			
Madrid[69]	329	1	
Takeda et al[117]	102	2	
Miles[75]	122	2	

alcohol is used. Another danger is of subcutaneous and cutaneous tissue sloughing.

If solutions of local anesthetic in oil or glycol are used, particularly in generous quantity, there is a risk of pleural irritation and effusion and nerve damage.[83]

PARAVERTEBRAL SYMPATHETIC BLOCK

Because of the anatomic position of the sympathetic chain, there is a genuine risk of the needle's entering the aorta, the vena cava, or the theca. Klopfer[60] believes that the technique can be made safer by introducing the needle with the patient in the semiprone position "so that the point of insertion of the needle lies vertically over the point of desired placement of neurolytic solution." Subarachnoid injection is a very serious hazard; the first complaint may be dyspnea or paralysis of the arms or legs, and there is also a sharp fall in blood pressure.[17] It is important to remember that the dural cuff extends out of the intervertebral foramen, and it may accidentally (and perhaps unwittingly) be punctured while paravertebral nerve block is being performed; if a neurolytic solution is being injected, troublesome neurologic sequelae may well result. Smith and associates[106] reported a case of permanent paraparesis following sympathetic block at right L3–L4 levels. Autopsy suggested that some of the aqueous phenol injected must have entered the theca.

Fraser and colleagues[33] described three instances of ureteric injury during chemical sympathectomy, one of which necessitated a nephrectomy. Churcher[21] also reported a case of ureteric damage requiring nephrectomy. He considers that either the needle itself damaged the ureter or the phenol injected caused thrombosis in the branch of the ovarian artery supplying the ureter.

Rose,[101] who has performed 2500 lumbar sympathetic blocks with phenol, reported the following major complications: In 3 patients there were permanent paresthesias in the L1–L2 dermatomes; 3 patients had permanent weakness of one nerve root in the leg, and 1 patient developed persistent weakness of the whole leg. One patient developed motor and sensory defects in the lower limbs 12 hours after the sympathetic block, and a paraparesis ensued that was considered to be due to thrombosis of the venous plexus to the cauda equina. The condition gradually improved over the next 2 years. There were also two cases of damage to a ureter with ulceration and leakage of urine, in one of which there was a urinary fistula in the loin. This emphasizes the added safety provided by radiographic confirmation of needle position.

Backache is a common sequel of lumbar paravertebral block and usually clears up in 24 to 48 hours. Less common and more troublesome is spillover of neurolytic agent onto intercostal nerves or onto paravertebral somatic nerves, in particular the genitofemoral and lumboinguinal nerves; this may cause motor or sensory loss.

Figure 23-3 shows how phenol spreads in the psoas sheath. Paravertebral spillover is usually the result of not having the needle point advanced far enough, but it may also be caused by drug spilling as the needle is withdrawn past the nerve. Because of the risk of adventitious neuritis, many workers prefer to use phenol rather than alcohol.[27,70] Reid and colleagues reported the complications encountered in 1666 injections of 6.7% aqueous phenol onto the lumbar sympathetic chain. They found that 9% of injections produced neuritis in the groin or the medial aspect of the thigh and occasionally the outer side of the thigh. Pain may be accompanied by hyperesthesia or numbness; the numbness may outlast the pain, which rarely persists more than 6 to 8 weeks although Miles and Rothman had one patient in whom

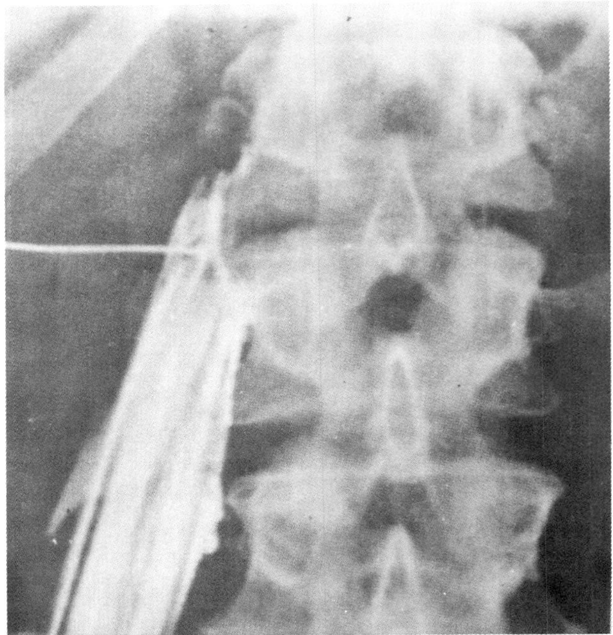

FIG. 23-3. Spread of phenol in the psoas sheath. (Feldman, S.A., and Yeung, M.L.: Treatment of intermittent claudication. Lumbar paravertebral somatic block with phenol. Anaesthesia, *30*:174, 1975.)

neuritic pains in the thighs lasted more than 4 months.[74] Boas[9] considers that this postsympathectomy dysesthesia is a deafferentation-type neuralgia and postulates that the loss of sympathetic afferent input may cause referred pain in a somatic distribution. Cherry[18] has stated that postsympathectomy genitofemoral neuralgia occurs in 7% to 20% of cases and generally lasts up to 5 weeks; however, deposit of phenol in the psoas muscle can result in permanent neuralgia of L1 or L2.

The use of radiopaque solution and x-ray screening, if available, can be of great value in safe and accurate needle placement. Careful monitoring of the direction of spread of the neurolytic solution can forewarn about deposit in a dangerous place (*e.g.*, dural cuff) or tracking in an undesirable direction. X-ray monitoring, however, does not guarantee safety, and it is still important to be attentive and careful during neurolytic injections.

Encroachment of the needle and injection into the abdomen are occasionally the cause of troublesome complications. Feldman and Yeung have reported one patient who developed transient abdominal pain and slight tenderness, possibly owing to extraperitoneal spread of phenol.[30] Puncture of the kidney sometimes occurs and is recognized by a pendulum swing of the needle or by the escape of urine through the needle. Injury of the kidney may produce hematuria, renal colic, or dysuria, but in most cases the symptoms are transient and full recovery results. Bilateral lumbar sympathetic block causes loss of ejaculation; impotence does not occur and the patient may not be sterile. Baxter and O'Kafo[3] reported the case of a patient who developed failure of ejaculation after bilateral phenol lumbar sympathectomy; the condition persisted for 5 weeks. It was considered that there may have been complete failure of the ejaculatory mechanism caused by block of sympathetic innervation or that there was retrograde ejaculation into the bladder caused by failure of bladder neck closure.

Pneumothorax is a not infrequent complication of upper thoracic block and has been reported after high lumbar sympathetic block. Hemoptysis has occurred on a few occasions without sequelae.[100] After paravertebral block of the highest sympathetic ganglia with alcohol, White has reported the case of a patient with severe pleuritic pain that he considered to be due to alcohol leaking into the pleural cavity.[35] Molitch and Wilson reported a case of temporary Brown–Sequard paralysis following paravertebral injection of alcohol beneath the first rib for anginal pain.[78] The chemical may reach the spinal cord by way of an extended dural cuff of the perineural space or because of a misdirected needle. Intercostal neuritis, perhaps with hyperesthesia of the chest wall and medial aspects of the arm, is a not uncommon complication of paravertebral sympathetic block in the thoracic segments; it usually clears in a month or two.

Beddard has advised against the performance of lumbar sympathetic block in patients who receive anticoagulant treatment because this may "spread the necrosive action of the phenol"; he has reported the case of a patient in whom "the greater part of the psoas muscle was found gangrenous at autopsy."[4]

Thoracic paravertebral sympathetic block with alcohol can be followed by pleuritic pain and also by intercostal neuralgia.[32] Finneson[32] had a similar case with permanent paraplegia, Brown–Sequard paralysis following the inadvertent intrathecal injection of alcohol during a thoracic paravertebral block.

CELIAC PLEXUS BLOCK

The anatomic position of the celiac plexus renders it susceptible to many hazards from nerve block,[115] although Moore[82] considers that complications other than back pain and hypotension are due to incorrect performance of the block (see Chap. 14). Certainly the use of x-ray control and the addition of contrast medium to the neurolytic solution are to be strongly recommended to ensure that the needle is correctly placed and to monitor the spread of the neurolytic solution. Computed tomography, if available, can give even more precise and useful information.[84] Celiac block, being retroperitoneal, has no fixed route of spread, and the solution will tend to diffuse along paths of least resistance. For example, pleuritic pain can occur if the neurolytic solution spreads to involve the lower edge of the pleura,[8] and Thompson and his colleagues[120] reported a case where, following celiac block with the patient lying on his side, spread of alcohol solution to the nerve roots of the lumbar plexus gave partial unilateral leg paralysis. The dangers are accentuated by the relatively large volume of alcohol commonly injected.

Accidental subarachnoid puncture is a risk that must be borne in mind: Moore[82] has encountered it 18 times in 3000 celiac plexus blocks. If neurolytic solution is inadvertently injected intrathecally, the results can, of course, be serious. Leung and his colleagues[62] reported one case in which after celiac plexus block with alcohol, the patient suffered weakness of the left lower limb and loss of anal and bladder sphincter function, necessitating suprapubic cystostomy.

Intravascular injection and pneumothorax are ever-present possibilities, as is the risk of hemorrhage. The dangers are accentuated by the relatively large volume of alcohol commonly injected. Spinal or paraspinal pain at the level of injection is not uncommon; it may be severe and last 24 to 48 hours and may be due to spilling of alcohol in the track of the needle. Spill of alcohol onto the first lumbar (somatic) nerve can give rise to neuritis,[52,70] which can be persistent.

Increased bowel motility and more frequent bowel motion are common during the first few days after the block but gradually revert to normal. Temporary urinary difficulty can also occur.[7]

Hematuria can result from puncture of a kidney, particularly if the path of the needle is too far lateral.[82] One of Leung's patients had hematuria for 2 days after the block.[62] Puncture of the aorta or vena cava should be avoided by careful aspiration test and by the use of a fine needle. Much of the celiac plexus lies in front of the aorta, but the needle should be kept close to the vertebra (*i.e.*, behind the aorta), for the volume of solution is adequate to spread and envelope the whole plexus.[82]

Hypotension commonly follows celiac plexus block; it results from interruption of vasoconstrictor fibers in the viscera and omentum. An intravenous infusion immediately should be available, and ephedrine should be ready for i.v. administration, if necessary. Younger patients can compensate by constriction of unaffected vessels, but, in the elderly and in arteriosclerotic patients, postural hypotension may require bed rest and the use of an abdominal binder and elastic stockings for a few days. It is important in such patients to monitor pulse and blood pressure and to ensure circulatory stability while sitting before allowing the patients to stand and then before allowing them to walk. It has been suggested that preliminary local anesthetic block be performed and, if an exaggerated hypotensive response results, alcohol block should not be given.[36]

Two cases of paraplegia have been reported following celiac plexus block with 6% aqueous phenol. In one, vascular ischemia of the cord was thought to be the cause, although the possibility of injection of phenol into a dural cuff in the paravertebral region was not ruled out.[34] In the other, some of the phenol was thought to have entered the subarachnoid space.[106] Cherry and Lamberty[19] have recently reported a case in which, despite the use of x-ray control, celiac plexus block was followed by paraparesis, areflexia, and partial sensory loss, attributed to anterior spinal artery syndrome.

Failure of ejaculation is another possible complication; it was noted in two of Black and Dwyer's patients owing to interruption of the central connections of the hypogastric plexus.[7]

MISCELLANEOUS COMPLICATIONS

Finally, a word must be said about the unintentional and unwitting injection of neurolytic agents during the course of nerve blocks. In the days of sterilization of instruments and needles in antiseptic solutions, the occurrence of neurologic damage from contamination by such solutions was not uncommon. Currently, despite the general use of aseptic methods of sterilization, such complications still occur occasionally; when performing nerve blocks, it behooves the operator to be ever watchful against the possibility of accidental neurolytic contaminants. The following recent cases are salutory:

1. A patient receiving obstetric epidural anesthesia had a catheter placed epidurally after accidental lumbar puncture. Delivery was carried out under epidural anesthesia, and 1½ hours later 40 ml of 0.9% saline (containing 1.5%-[benzyl] alcohol preservative) was injected. Thirty hours later the patient had severe flaccid paraparesis that largely disappeared over the next 2 years and that was due to damage to the motor and sensory roots of the cauda equina.[24]
2. A patient was rendered permanently quadriplegic because an epidural "top-up" dose contained or was contaminated by paraldehyde.[116]
3. Fortunately of a less serious nature, 2.5% thiopentone was mistakenly administered for an intended caudal epidural anesthesia. The patient had difficulty with micturition for 3 days, but there were no other sequelae.[16]

REFERENCES

1. Adriani, J. (ed.): Labat's Regional Anesthesia, 3rd ed. Philadelphia, W.B. Saunders, 1967.
2. Adriani, J., Parmley, J., and Ochsner, A.: Fatalities and complications after attempts at stellate ganglion block. Surgery, 32:615, 1952.
3. Baxter, A.D., and O'Kafo, B.A.: Ejaculatory failure after chemical sympathectomy. Anesth. Analg., *63*:770–771, 1984.

4. Beddard, J.R.J.: Twenty years of clinical nerve blocking. Br. J. Anaesth., *30*:367, 1958.
5. Bell, S.N., Cole, R., and Roberts–Thomson, I.C.: Coeliac plexus block for control of pain in chronic pancreatitis. Br. Med. J., 281:1604, 1980.
6. Benzon, H.T.: Convulsions secondary to intravascular phenol; a hazard of celiac plexus block. Anesth. Analg., *58*:150–151, 1979.
7. Black, A.C., Dwyer, B.: Coeliac plexus block. Anaesth. Intensive Care, *1*:315, 1973.
8. Boas, R.A.: Sympathetic blocks in clinical practice. In Stanton–Hicks, M.D. (ed.): Int. Anesthesiol. Clin., *16*(4): 1978.
9. Boas, R.A.: The sympathetic nervous system and pain relief. In Swerdlow, M. (ed.): Relief of Intractable Pain, 3rd ed. Amsterdam, Elsevier, 1983.
10. Bonica, J.J.: Management of Pain. Philadelphia, Lea & Febiger, 1953.
11. Bonica, J.J.: Diagnostic and therapeutic blocks: A reappraisal based on 15 years' experience. Anesth. Analg. (Cleve.), *37*:58, 1958.
12. Booth, A.E.: Intrathecal hypertonic saline. Proc. R. Soc. Med., *67*:772, 1974.
13. Brattstrom, M., Moritz, U., and Svantesson, G.: Electromyographic studies of peripheral nerve block with phenol. Scand. J. Rehabil. Med., *2*:17–22, 1970.
14. Bromage, P.R.: Epidural Analgesia. Philadelphia, W.B. Saunders, 1978.
15. Capuzzo, M., Gritti, G., and Vassalli, A.: Anomala diffusione di fenolo in un caso di neurolisi subarachnoidea. Algos., *1*:58, 1984.
16. Cay, D.L.: Accidental epidural thiopentone. Anaesth. Intensive Care, *12*:61–63, 1984.
17. Challenger, J.: Sympathetic nervous system blocking. In Swerdlow, M. (ed.): Relief of Intractable Pain. Amsterdam, Excerpta Medica, 1974.
18. Cherry, D.A.: Chemical lumbar sympathectomy. Curr. Concepts in Pain, *2*:12–15, 1984.
19. Cherry, D.A., and Lamberty, J.: Paraplegia following coeliac plexus block. Anaes. Intensive Care, *12*:59–72, 1984.
20. Churcher, M.: Peripheral nerve blocks. In Swerdlow, M. (ed.): Relief of Intractable Pain. 3rd ed. Amsterdam, Elsevier, 1983.
21. Churcher, M.: Personal communication, 1984.
22. Colpitt, M.R., Levy, B.A., and Lawrence, M.: Treatment of cancer related pain with phenol epidural block. Abstracts of 2nd World Congress on Pain, p. 147, 1978.
23. Corssen, G., Holcomb, M.C., Moustapha, I., Langford, K., *et al.*: Alcohol induced adenolysis of the pituitary gland; a new approach to control of intractable cancer pain. Anesth. Analg., *56*:414–421, 1977.
24. Craig, D.B., and Habib, G.G.: Flaccid paraparesis following obstetrical epidural anesthesia. Possible role of *benzyl alcohol.* Anesth. Analg., *56*:219–221, 1977.
25. Crimeni, R.: Clinical experience with mepivacaine and alcohol in neuralgia of the trigeminal nerve. Acta Anaesthesiol. Scand., *24*[*Suppl.*]:173, 1966.
26. Davies, J.I., Steward, P.B., and Fink, P.: Prolonged sensory block using ammonium salts. Anesthesiology, *28*:244, 1967.
27. Dekrey, J.A., Schroeder, C.F., and Buechel, D.R.: Selective chemical sympathectomy. Anesth. Analg. (Cleve.), *47*:633, 1968.
28. Derrick, W.S.: Subarachnoid alcohol block for the control of intractable pain. Acta Anaesthesiol. Scand., *24*[*Suppl.*]:167, 1966.
29. Dott, N.H.: Facial pain. Proc. R. Soc. Med., *44*:1034, 1951.
30. Feldman, S.A., and Yeung, M.L.: Treatment of intermittent claudication. Lumbar paravertebral somatic block with phenol. Anaesthesia, *30*:174, 1975.
31. Felsenthal, G.: Pharmacology of phenol in peripheral nerve blocks; a review. Arch. Phys. Med. Rehabil., *55*:1, 1974.
32. Finneson, B.E.: Diagnosis and management of pain syndromes, 2nd ed., pp. 239–240. Philadelphia, W.B. Saunders, 1969.
33. Fraser, I., Windle, R., Smart, J.G., and Barrie, W.W.: Ureteric injury following chemical sympathectomy. Br. J. Surg., *71*:349, 1984.
34. Galizia, E.J., and Lahiri, S.K.: Paraplegia following coeliac plexus block with phenol. Br. J. Anaesth., *46*:539, 1974.
35. Goodman, L.S., and Gilman, A.: A Pharmacological Basis of Therapeutics, 4th ed. London, Macmillan, 1970.
36. Gorbitz, C., and Leavens, M.E.: Alcohol block of the celiac plexus for control of upper abdominal pain caused by cancer and pancreatitis. J. Neurosurg., *34*:575, 1971.
37. Grunwald, I.: Neurolise com fenol: Uso da via peridural no tratamento da dor de cancer. Rev. Bras. Anestes., *26*(4):628–633, 1976.
38. Guttman, S.A., and Pardee, I.: Spinal cord level syndrome following intrathecal ammonium sulphate and procaine hydrochloride. A case report with autopsy findings. Anesthesiology, *5*:347–353, 1944.
39. Hakanson, S.: Retrogasserian glycerol injection as a treatment of tic douloureux. In Bonica, J.J., Lindblom, U., and Iggo, A. (eds.). Res. Ther., *5*:927–933, 1983.
40. Hammermeister, K.E., and Reichenbach, D.D.: QRS changes, pulmonary edema, and myocardial necrosis associated with subarachnoid hemorrhage. Am. Heart J., *78*:94, 1969.
41. Hand, L.V.: Subarachnoid ammonium sulfate therapy for intractable pain. Anesthesiology, *5*:354, 1944.
42. Hay, R.C.: Subarachnoid alcohol block in the control of intractable pain. Anesth. Analg., *41*:12–16, 1962.
43. Henderson, W.R.: Trigeminal neuralgia: The pain and its treatment. Br. Med. J., *1*:7–15, 1967.
44. Hitchcock, E.: Osmotic neurolysis for intractable facial pain. Lancet, *1*:434, 1969.
45. Holland, A.J.C., and Yousseff, M.: A complication of subarachnoid phenol blockade. Anaesthesia, *34*:260, 1979.
46. Horowitz, N.H., and Rizzoli, H.V.: Postoperative Complications in Neurosurgical Practice, p. 666. Baltimore, Williams & Wilkins, 1967.
47. Howland, W.J., Curry, J.L., and Butler, A.K.: Pantopaque arachnoiditis; experimental study of blood as a potentiating agent. Radiology, *80*:489, 1963.

48. Hughes, J.T.: Thrombosis of the posterior spinal arteries. Neurology (Minneap.), *20*:659, 1970.
49. Ischia, S., Luzzani, A., Ischia, A., Magon, F., *et al.*: Subarachnoid neurolytic block (L5–S1) and unilateral percutaneous cervical cordotomy in the treatment of pain secondary to pelvic malignant disease. Pain, *20*:139–49, 1984.
50. Jaeger, R.: The results of injecting hot water into the gasserian ganglion for the relief of tic douloureux. J. Neurosurg., *16*:656, 1957.
51. Jefferson, A.: Trigeminal neuralgia: Trigeminal root and ganglion injections using phenol in glycerin. In Knighton, R.S., and Dumke, P.R. (eds.): Pain, p. 365. Boston, Little, Brown, 1966.
52. Jones, R.R.: Technic for injection of splanchnic nerves with alcohol. Anesth. Analg. (Cleve.), *36*:75, 1957.
53. Judovich, B.D., Bates, W., and Bishop, K.: Intraspinal ammonium salts for the intractable pain of malignancy. Anesthesiology, *5*:341–346, 1944.
54. Katz, J.: Pain theory and management. In Scurr, C.B., and Feldman, S. (eds.): Scientific Foundations of Anaesthesia, p. 226. London, Heinmann, 1970.
55. Katz, J., Knott, L.W., and Feldman, D.J.: Peripheral nerve injections with phenol in the management of spastic patients. Arch. Phys. Med. Rehabil., *48*:97–99, 1967.
56. Katz, J., and Levin, A.B.: Treatment of diffuse metastatic cancer pain by installation of alcohol into the sella turcica. Anesthesiology, *46*:115–121, 1977.
57. Katz, J., and Levin, A.B.: Long-term follow-up study of chemical hypophysectomy and additional cases. Anesthesiology, *51*:167–169, 1979.
58. Keim, H.A.: Cord paralysis following injection into traumatic cervical meningocele. Complication of stellate ganglion block. N.Y. State J. Med., *70*:2115, 1970.
59. Khalili, A.A., and Betts, H.B.: Peripheral nerve block with phenol in the management of spasticity. J.A.M.A., *200*(13):103–105, 1967.
60. Klopfer, G.T.: Neurolytic lumbar sympathetic blockade: A modified technique. Anaesth. Intensive Care, *11*:43–46, 1983.
61. Labat, G.: Regional anesthesia technique and clinical applications. In Adriani, J. (ed.): Labat's Regional Anesthesia, 3rd ed. Philadelphia, 1967.
62. Leung, J.W.C., Bowen-Wright, M., Aveling, W., Shorvon, P.J., *et al.*: Coeliac plexus block for pancreatitis. Br. J. Surg., *70*:730–732, 1983.
63. Lifshitz, S., Debacker, L.J., and Buchsbaum, H.J.: Subarachnoid phenol block for pain relief in gynaecologic malignancy. Obstet. Gynecol., *48*:316–320, 1976.
64. Lipton, S.: Percutaneous cervical cordotomy and pituitary injection of alcohol. In Swerdlow, M. (ed.): Relief of Intractable Pain, 3rd ed. Amsterdam, Elsevier, 1983.
65. Lloyd, J.W., Rawlinson, W.A.L., and Evans, P.J.D.: Selective hypophysectomy for metastatic pain. Br. J. Anaesth., *53*:1129–1133, 1981.
66. Lucas, J.T., Ducker, T.B., and Perot, P.L.: Adverse reactions to intrathecal saline injection for control of pain. J. Neurosurg., *42*:557, 1975.
67. McKean, M.C., and Hitchcock, E.: Electro-cardiographic changes after intrathecal hypertonic saline solution. Lancet, *2*:1083, 1968.
68. Macomber, D.W.: Necrosis of the nose and cheek, secondary to treatment of trigeminal neuralgia. Plast. Reconstr. Surg., *11*:337, 1953.
69. Madrid, J. Chemical Hypophysectomy. Adv. Pain Res. Ther., *2*:381–391, 1979.
70. Mandl, F.: Aqueous solution of phenol as substitute for alcohol in sympathetic block. J. Int. Coll. Surg., *13*:566, 1950.
71. Mark, V.H., White, J.C., Zervas, N.T., Ervin, F.R., *et al.*: Intrathecal use of phenol for the relief of chronic severe pain. N. Engl. J. Med., *267*:589, 1962.
72. May, O.: The functional and histological effects of intraneural and intraganglionic injections of alcohol. Br. Med. J., *2*:465, 1912.
73. Mehta, M.: Intractable Pain. London, W.B. Saunders, 1973.
74. Miles, E., and Rothman, J.S.: Experiences with the use of 10% aqueous phenol for chemical sympathectomy. Preliminary report. Am. J. Surg., *87*:830, 1954.
75. Miles, J.: Chemical hypophysectomy. In Bonica, J.J., and Ventafridda, V. (eds.): Advances in Pain Research and Therapy, Vol. 2. New York, Raven Press, 1979.
76. Miles, J.: Trigeminal neuralgia. In Lipton, S. (ed.): Persistent Pain, Vol. 2. London, Academic Press, 1980.
77. Miller, R.D., Johnston, R.R., and Hosobuchi, Y.: Treatment of intercostal neuralgia with 10% ammonium sulfate. J. Thorac. Cardiovasc. Surg., *69*:476–478, 1975.
78. Molitch, M., and Wilson, G.: Brown-Sequard paralysis following a paravertebral alcohol injection for angina pectoris. J.A.M.A., *97*:247, 1931.
79. Moller, J.E., Helweg-Larson, J., and Jacobsen, E.: Histopathological lesions in the sciatic nerve of the rat following perineural application of phenol and alcohol solutions. Dan. Med. Bull., *16*:116–119, 1969.
80. Montgomery, W., and Cousins, M.J.: Aspects of management of chronic pain illustrated by ninth nerve block. Br. J. Anaesth., *44*:383, 1972.
81. Moore, D.C.: Epidural anaesthesia. *In* Complications of Regional Anaesthesia. Springfield, Il., Charles C Thomas, 1965.
82. Moore, D.C.: Celiac (splanchnic) plexus block with alcohol. Adv. Pain Res. Ther., 2:357–371, 1979.
83. Moore, D.C., and Bridenbaugh, L.D.: Intercostal nerve block in 4,333 patients: Indications, technique and complications. Anesth. Analg. (Cleve.), *41*:1, 1962.
84. Moore, D.C., Bush, W.H., and Burnett, L.L.: Celiac plexus block: A roentgenographic study of technique and spread of solution in patients and corpses. Anesth. Analg., *60*:369–379, 1981.
85. Moricca, G.: The management of cancer pain. *In* Progress in Anaesthesiology, pp. 266–270. Amsterdam, Excerpta Medica, 1968.
86. Mousel, L.H.: Treatment of intractable pain of the head and neck. Anesth. Analg. (Cleve.), *46*:705, 1967.
87. Nathan, P.W.: Control of pain. Ann. R. Coll. Surg. Engl., *41*:82, 1967.
88. Nathan, P.W. Pain in cancer; comparison of results of cordo-

tomy and chemical rhizotomy. In Pusek, I., and Kune, Z. (eds.): Present limits of neurosurgery. Amsterdam, Excerpta Medica, 1972.

89. Nathan, P.W., and Sears, T.A.: Effects of phenol on nervous conduction. J. Physiol., *150*:565, 1960.
90. Newfield, P., Maroon, J.C., and Albin, M.S.: Pituitary adenolysis. Anesth. Analg., *56*:879, 1977.
91. Northfield, D.W.C.: The Surgery of the Central Nervous System. Oxford, Blackwell, 1973.
92. Nour-Eldin, F.: Preliminary report: Uptake of phenol by vascular and brain tissue. Microvasc. Res., *2*:224, 1970.
93. O'Higgins, J.W., Padfield, A., and Clapp, H.: Possible complication of hypothermic-saline subarachnoid injection. Lancet, *1*:567, 1970.
94. Papo, I., and Visca, A.: Phenol rhizotomy in the treatment of cancer pain. Anesth. Analg. (Cleve.), *53*:99, 1974.
95. Papo, I., and Visca, A.: Phenol subarachnoid rhizotomy for the treatment of cancer pain. A personal account of 290 cases. Adv. Pain Res. Ther., *2*:339–346, 1979.
96. Peet, M.M.: Major trigeminal neuralgia post-op. complications. Lewis's Practice of Surgery, *12*:48, 1954.
97. Petrillo, C.R., Chu, D.S., and Davis, S.W.: Phenol block of the tibial nerve in the hemiplegic patient. Orthopedics, *3*:871–874, 1980.
98. Peyton, W.T., Semansky, E.J., and Baker, A.B.: Subarachnoid injection of alcohol for relief of intractable pain with discussion of cord changes found at autopsy. Am. J. Cancer, *30*:709, 1937.
99. Ramb, H.: Die Alkoholinjektion ins Ganglion Gasseri bei der Trigeminusneuralgie. Dtsch. Med. Wochenschr., *74*:826, 1949.
100. Reid, W., Watt, J.K., and Gray, T.G.: Phenol injection of sympathetic chain. Br. J. Surg., *47*:45, 1970.
101. Rose, S.S.: Personal communication, 1984.
102. Rovenstine, E.A., and Papper, E.M.: Glossopharyngeal nerve block. Am. J. Surg., *75*:713, 1948.
103. Ruge, D., Brochner, R., and Davis, L.: A study of the treatment of 637 patients with trigeminal neuralgia. J. Neurosurg., *15*:528, 1958.
104. Sloane, P.: Syndrome referrable to the cauda equina following the intraspinal injection of alcohol for the relief of pain. Arch. Neurol. Psychiatr., *34*:1120, 1935.
105. Smith, M.C.: Histological findings following intrathecal injections of phenol solutions for relief of pain. Br. J. Anaesth., *36*:387, 1964.
106. Smith, R.C., Davidson, N.McD., and Ruckley, C.V.: Hazard of chemical sympathectomy. Br. Med. J., *1*:552, 1978.
107. Sperling, E., and Stender, A.: Tic Douloureux and Gesichtsschmerz (Therapeutische und Pathogenetische Betrachtungen). Dtsch. Zahn. Mund. Kieferheilkd., *173*:161, 1955.
108. Stender, A.: Excerpta Medica International Congress Series. Washington D.C., *36*, 1961.
109. Stewart, W., Hughes, J., and Judovich, B.D.: Ammonium chloride in the relief of pain. Am. J. Physiol., *129*:475, 1940.
110. Stovner, J., and Endresen, R.: Intrathecal phenol for cancer pain. Acta Anaesthesiol. Scand., *16*:17, 1972.
111. Sunderland, S.: Nerves and Nerve Injuries. Edinburgh, E. & S. Livingstone, 1978.
112. Superville-Sovak, B., Rasminsky, M., and Finlayson, M.H.: Complications of phenol neurolysis. Arch. Neurol., *32*:226, 1975.
113. Swerdlow, M.: 4 year's pain clinic experience. Anaesthesia, *22*:568, 1967.
114. Swerdlow, M.: Intrathecal and Extradural Block. *In* Relief of Intractable Pain, 2nd ed. Amsterdam, Excerpta Medica, 1978.
115. Swerdlow, M.: Peripheral nerve blocking in the relief of pain. *In* Lipton, S. (ed.): Persistent Pain. London, Academic Press, 1977.
116. Swerdlow, M.: Medicolegal aspects of complications following pain relieving block. Pain, *13*:321–331, 1982.
117. Takeda, F., Fujii, T., Uki, J., Fuse, Y., *et al.*: Cancer pain relief and tumour regression by means of pituitary neuroadenolysis and surgical hypophysectomy. Neurol. Medico-Chirurgia Tokyo, *23*:41–49, 1983.
118. Tank, T.M., Dohn, D.F., and Gardner, W.J.: Intrathecal injections of alcohol or phenol for relief of intractable pain. Cleve. Clin. Q., *30*:111, 1963.
119. Thompson, G.E.: Pulmonary edema complicating intrathecal hypertonic saline injection for intractable pain. Anesthesiology, *35*:425, 1971.
120. Thompson, G.E., Moore, D.C., Bridenbaugh, L.D., and Artin, R.Y.: Abdominal pain and alcohol celiac plexus nerve block. Anesth. Analg., *56*:1–5, 1977.
121. Thurel, R.: Alcoolisation du ganglion de gasser. Complications tardives troubles trophiques et sympathalgies. Rev. Neurol., *104*:334, 1961.
122. Totoki, T., Kato, T., Nomoto, Y., Kurakazu, M., *et al.*: Anterior spinal artery syndrome—a complication of cervical intrathecal phenol injection. Pain, *6*:99, 1979.
123. Tureen, L.L., and Gitt, J.J.: Cauda equina syndrome following subarachnoid injection of alcohol. J.A.M.A., *106*:18, 1936.
124. Usubiaga, J.E.: Neurological complications following epidural anesthesia. Boston, Little, Brown, 1975.
125. Ventafridda, V., and Spreafico, R.: Subarachnoid saline perfusion. Adv. Neurol., *4*:477, 1974.
126. Ventafridda, V., and De Conno, F.: Moricca's operation at the National Cancer Institute of Milan. In Ischia, S., Lipton, S., and Maffezzoli, G.F. (eds.): Pain Treatment. Verona, Cortina Internat., 1983.
127. White, J.C.: Technique of paravertebral alcohol injection. Surg. Gynecol. Obstet., *71*:334, 1940.
128. White, J.C., and Sweet, W.H.: Pain and Neurosurgeon. Springfield, Il., Charles C Thomas, 1969.
129. Wright, B.D.: Treatment of intractable coccygodynia by transsacral ammonium chloride injection. Anesth. Analg., *50*:519, 1971.
130. Wilkinson, H.A., Mark, V.H., and White, J.C.: Further experiences with intrathecal phenol for the relief of pain. J. Chronic Dis., *17*:1055, 1964.

part three

NEURAL BLOCKADE IN THE MANAGEMENT OF PAIN

24.1 INTRODUCTION TO ACUTE AND CHRONIC PAIN: IMPLICATIONS FOR NEURAL BLOCKADE

MICHAEL J. COUSINS

PAST DEFICIENCIES AND NEW INITIATIVES

Since the publication of the first edition of *Neural Blockade in Clinical Anesthesia and Management of Pain*, there have been significant initiatives aimed at improving the treatment of all types of pain.

Cancer Pain

The World Health Organization (WHO) is collaborating with the International Association for the Study of Pain (IASP) in a program aimed at effective treatment of cancer pain throughout the world by the year 2000.[20] This program includes an "analgesic ladder" (Table 24-1) as a guideline to oral drug therapy for cancer pain; a text on cancer pain for distribution throughout the world; educational activities in many countries; initiatives with governments and other agencies to help implement effective treatment of cancer pain, which, in some countries, requires that oral opioid drugs be made available as a vital ingredient of treatment. Several studies confirm that carefully titrated oral opioid therapy results in good pain control, without escalation of dosage, in many patients.[8,9] Also, evaluations of the relative role of various modalities for cancer pain treatment have begun.[8,21] This information will be of great importance to the rational use of the neural blockade techniques described in this text. In a major study from the Milan Cancer Centre, a high percentage of patients obtained pain relief with oral opioid and/or "co-analgesic" drugs.[21] Neural blockade techniques were reported to be effective in some patients who were not effectively treated with drug therapy, and in some patients they allowed reestablishment of oral drug therapy at a lower dose. Some patients ceased oral drug therapy, for variable periods of time, after neural blockade. A substantial number of patients, however, continued to need carefully controlled oral opioid and "co-analgesic" drugs, as well as drugs for treatment of other symptoms, such as nausea and vomiting, constipation, and pruritus.[21] In the hospice setting, subcutaneous opioid infusion is reported to be useful; objective evaluation is not yet available. As in other forms of pain, neural blockade should be used as part of an overall treatment strategy and in the setting of good collaboration with the appropriate specialties.[2,3,7,8]

The incidence of cancer pain is generally agreed to be approximately 40% of patients with cancer and 60% to 80% of patients with terminal cancer.[2,3,8,20] Contrary to anecdote, pain can and does occur early in the course of cancer and requires effective treatment.[2] Inadequacies in the treatment of cancer pain have been documented throughout the world, varying from 30% to 80% of patients with unrelieved pain in the developed world.[2,20] In the underdeveloped world less than 10% of patients obtain relief of severe pain.[20] These are the reasons that WHO identified cancer pain as a major world health problem.[20] National and state governments in the United States, Canada, Europe, the United Kingdom, New Zealand, Australia, and other countries have now begun to respond by forming committees of their health and medical research bodies to recommend measures that need to be taken. Vigorous programs of education, research, and clinical care have

TABLE 24-1. ANALGESIC LADDER IN CANCER PAIN

Step 1:	Paracetamol, aspirin or other NSAIDs ± adjuvants* (co-analgesics)
Step 2:	Codeine, dextropropoxyphene (or ? oxycodone) ± NSAID ± adjuvants*
Step 3:	Morphine, methadone, ± NSAID ± adjuvants*

Paracetamol = acetaminophen; NSAIDs = nonsteroidal anti-inflammatory drugs.
*Psychotropics (anxiolytics, antidepressants) anticonvulsants, steroids, etc.

begun in some parts of the world. This impetus needs to be maintained in order to reach the goal of the year 2000 set by the IASP and WHO.

Chronic Noncancer Pain

The community, governments, and the medical profession have begun to recognize chronic pain as a major community, medical, and financial problem. Bonica's estimate of the costs in the United States of $50 billion annually has been supported by report of similar costs (on a population basis) in Australia of $5 billion annually.[10] More rational and humane attitudes toward occupationally related pain syndromes have made insurance companies, employers, and the general public more aware that large savings can be made in the financial costs and unnecessary human suffering incurred in patients with chronic pain. Ignorant dogma about "compensation neurosis" has been replaced by clear data showing that pain in patients with compensation claims responds to treatment equally as well as pain in patients without claims—provided appropriate treatment is given (see Chap. 25).[14]

The complex interaction of psychological and physical factors in chronic pain has been recognized by the establishment of multidisciplinary "pain clinics" in many countries (see Chap. 31). Such clinics can function effectively only if they have appropriate physical facilities, the required range of health professionals, and adequate funding (see Chap. 31). It is in such a setting that the use of neural blockade is likely to be most effective and safest. Those involved in the use of neural blockade must play a part in obtaining or maintaining the financial support required. Such support is clearly justified by the savings that can be made in areas such as occupationally related pain syndromes. Other savings can be made with neural blockade techniques that permit same-day treatment of large numbers of patients. For example, Cousins and associates reported a saving of more than 2800 inpatient bed days* in about 400 patients treated for rest pain with neurolytic, rather than surgical, sympathectomy (see Chap. 13).[6] Many other neural blockade treatments can be carried out on a day-patient basis if a dedicated pain unit facility and staff are available (see Chaps. 27.2, 27.3, 28, 29.2, 30, 31, and 32). Also, adjunctive treatments such as physical therapy, and psychological therapy can best take advantage of neural blockade in a pain clinic setting. In the absence of such a setting, *ad hoc* arrangements can still be made, using operating theaters, recovery rooms, day wards, and so on. However, such arrangements are logistically difficult and should be replaced by dedicated space and staff when this becomes feasible.

*In the United States this would be a saving of $1,400,000.

Acute Pain

Recognition of acute pain as a major problem has been unacceptably slow, in view of repeated documentation of inadequacies of treatment of such pain (see references 1 and 5). In a study of acute pain of various causes, Marks and Sacher[12] reported that three quarters of the patients who received narcotics for severe pain continued to experience pain. These findings have been confirmed in adults by Cohen[4] and in children by Mather and Mackie.[13]

It is likely that all forms of acute pain are poorly managed: postoperative, post-trauma, acute medical diseases (*e.g.*, pancreatitis, myocardial infarction),[1,5] obstetric pain[1] (see Fig. 25-5). The effective relief of labor pain with epidural block in more than 95% of patients gives hope that other types of acute pain can also be relieved (see Chap. 18). This does not imply that neural blockade is "the answer" to acute pain—it is one of the answers. A wide range of pharmacological, physical, and psychological treatments are now available, or under investigation, for acute pain.[1,5] (see Chaps. 25, 26, 28, and 32). Improved understanding of peripheral and central mechanisms of pain offers new treatment options (see Chap. 24.2). Pain treatment techniques will depend, for their effective use, on overcoming financial, administrative, and logistical hurdles.[5] Funding is needed for staff (nursing, medical, and other, *e.g.*, psychology, physical therapy), equipment, and perhaps space. There is discussion of the value of an "open ward" plan for stabilization of pain therapy for the first 24 to 48 hours in those patients who do not require the intensive care unit setting (see Chap. 28). Protocols and nursing procedures need to be developed (see Figs. 26-8, 9) to monitor and manage the various options, such as intravenous infusion of opioids, patient-controlled analgesic therapy, epidural local anesthetic or opioid (see Chaps. 8, 18, 26, and 28). Educational programs need to be developed and implemented for nursing, medical, and other staff. Much of this depends on a close collaboration between medical, nursing, and administrative staff. The regimens chosen for each institution must be appropriate to the resources and range of expertise in that setting. A powerful aid to improving acute pain treatment would be the use of a "pain control audit." In some hospitals, pain is now charted, along with temperature and pulse, and orders for treatment are based on pain score obtained with visual analogue scale or other techniques (see Figs. 25-3, 4) described in Chapter 25. Audit of the efficacy of pain control becomes feasible if a record of this type is a routine part of the medical record. Acute pain in children is a special case requiring urgent attention. This is because of fallacious dogma that children suffer less pain than do adults.[13] Techniques developed in adults can be applied in children (see Chap. 21); however, problems in implementation need to be overcome.

In addition to humanitarian reasons for improving acute pain treatment, there is now convincing evidence that unrelieved acute pain may result in harmful physiological effects[1,5] (see Chaps. 5, 8, 18, and 26) and psychological effects (see Chap. 25). These adverse effects may result in significant morbidity, and even mortality.

PAIN: A PHYSICAL AND PSYCHOLOGICAL EXPERIENCE

The IASP defines pain as "an unpleasant sensory and emotional experience associated with actual or potential tissue damage, or described in terms of such damage."[15]

Sensory mechanisms of pain are described in Chapter 24.2 and psychological aspects, in Chapter 25; however, they are intricately intertwined. The neurologic and pharmacological information in Chapter 24.2 provides some of the "wiring" and "neurochemical mediators" for the powerful influences of psychological factors on the pain experience (see also Figs. 25-1, 2).

At a peripheral level there are now known to be highly complex neural, humoral, and biochemical influences on the sensitivity of pain receptors.[22] An introductory and simplified version is shown in Figure 24-1; however, full details are given in Chapter 24.2.

Visceral pain is now better understood: convergence of visceral and somatic afferents has been proven and this helps to explain referred pain. Also, important viscerosomatic reflexes have been identified (see Fig. 24-2). Temporary relief of visceral pain by blockade of the somatic referred area poses potential problems of interpretation of "diagnostic" local anesthetic nerve blocks (see Chap. 27.1). Experimental evidence for these important mechanisms is given in Chapter 24.2.

Central mechanisms are now known to be complex.[17] The introductory scheme shown in Figure 24-3 emphasizes that afferent input may ascend by way of many alternative pathways (*e.g.*, spinothalamic, spinoreticular), that afferent input may activate descending modulation, and that descending modulation may have powerful inhibitory influences on pain transmission at many levels (see also Fig. 28-4). Central mechanisms are described in detail in Chapter 24.2. It is worth bearing in mind that clear definition of spinal inhibitory mechanisms led rapidly to a new method of neural blockade, spinal opioids (see Chap. 28). There are undoubtedly many other treatments that will arise from mechanisms described in Chapter 24.2.

The assessment of pain and its treatment is difficult and influenced by psychological as well as physical and other aspects of pain. The importance of these factors cannot be overemphasized. One example is the variation in placebo response in proportion to the potency of "active" drug used, even in double-blind studies (see Chap. 25). Neural blockade techniques have potentially powerful placebo effects.

DIFFERENT CATEGORIES OF PAIN

Noordenbos[16] has given a helpful description of the various situations in which pain arises*:

"**Pain caused by external events** (special senses excepted) has the following features: [a] It always involves the skin. [b] The pain is of short duration, except when tissue injury is the result. [c] Localization, identification, or verification of its cause by the subject is usually possible. [d] Withdrawal is possible (if prevented, we are dealing with torture). [e] The nervous system is intact; conduction is not interfered with; modulating factors are fully operative. This category includes the majority of methods of experimentally produced pain and represents the conditioning mechanism that teaches the individual to avoid injury. It also includes the clinical sensory examination that ascertains whether this function is intact.

Pain Caused by Internal Events. Receptors are activated whatever their nature or the mechanism of

*Reproduced with permission from Noordenbos, W.: Prologue: *In* Wall, P.D., and Melzack, R. (eds.): Textbook of Pain. Edinburgh, Churchill Livingstone, 1984.

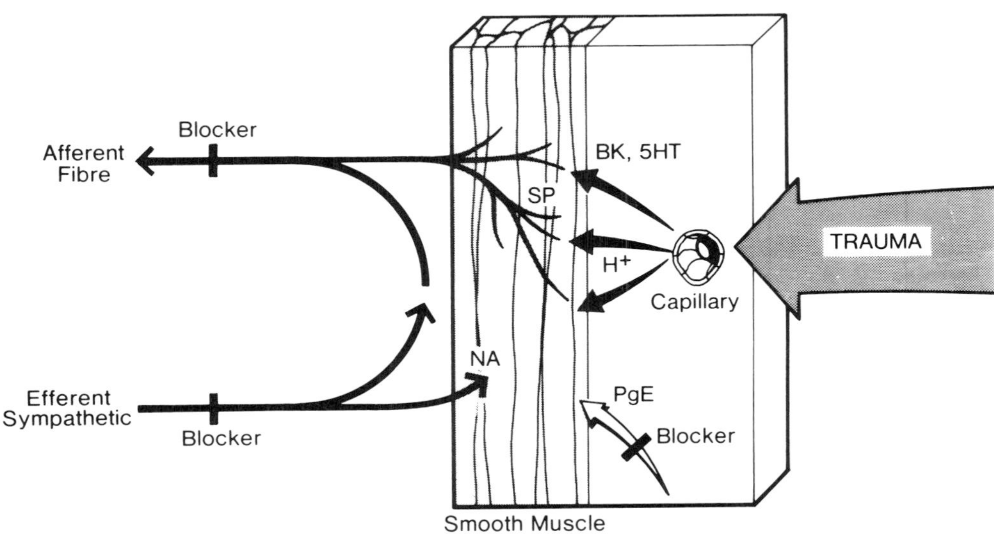

FIG. 24-1. Simplified schema of peripheral pain receptors and modification of their activity. *Increased responsiveness of receptors* results from release of bradykinin *(BK)*, 5-hydroxytryptamine *(5HT)*, and histamine (not shown) and a number of other algesic substances (see Chap. 24.2). Local changes in hydrogen ion concentration (acidosis) and microcirculatory changes (ischemia) may also increase receptor sensitivity. Prostaglandin E *(PgE)* increases the algesic effects of BK, 5HT, and other algesic substances but is not algesic itself. Local release of substance P *(SP)* results in local vascular changes and release of algesic substances. Increased sympathetic activity increases receptor sensitivity by means of norepinephrine (noradrenaline, *NA*) release and possibly by means of local circulatory changes. Increased pain may cause reflex increases in sympathetic activity, thus setting up a repetitive cycle. *Decreased receptor sensitivity* results from local injection of local anesthetics, and perhaps steroids, near receptors; depletion of substance P by injection of capsaicin; and administration of cyclo-oxygenase inhibitors that decrease synthesis of prostaglandins (see also Chap. 13). Sympathetic blockade may also decrease receptor sensitivity, if performed in a patient with increased sympathetic tone. (*Reproduced from* Cousins, M.J., Phillips, G.D. (eds.): Acute Pain Management. London, Churchill Livingstone, 1986.)

this activation may be. An afferent pattern is set up that is perceived as pain. This group has the following features: [a] The skin is usually not involved, except when directly injured or in referred pain. [b] The pain is of longer duration. It lasts until the source is ascertained and, if possible, adequately treated. [c] Localization and identification of the source by the patient is often impossible. [d] Withdrawal is not possible, or only partially so (*i.e.*, not moving an injured joint). [e] The nervous system is intact: the focus or pathologic process is peripheral to the receptors. Conduction is normal; modulating factors are operative.

This group may be subdivided according to which type of tissue is involved—ectodermal, mesodermal, or endodermal—each having its own particular type of afferent innervation.

This group also includes pain caused by physiologic events, such as labor pains.

Pain associated with lesions of the nervous system, especially the afferent system, has the following characteristics: [a] The skin is often involved, which makes correct identification of external events difficult, if not impossible. [b] Localization of the source may be faulty. [c] The pain is prolonged; it may last for years, or even a lifetime. [d] Withdrawal is impossible. [e] The nervous system is not intact. Conduction is faulty; modulating mechanisms have become disrupted. In such cases the lesion is proximal to the receptors. It may involve peripheral nerves, the spinal cord, or higher levels. It may be localized or of a systemic nature.

This group represents the real problems, the Puzzles of Pain (postherpetic neuralgia, causalgia, phantom limb pain, plexus avulsions, thalamic syndrome). The pain may be of a more general nature, as in polyneuropathies.

None of the above; the pain is associated with psychological, social, or environmental factors."

In each of these categories, cognitive and emotional aspects have to be taken into account, although the emphasis will differ markedly, depending on how the pain arises.

Another approach that overlaps, to a degree, is to categorize pain on the basis of the *predominant* part of the nervous system that is responsible for the pain. This is somewhat artificial, since it can be argued that "all" of the nervous system is almost invariably active or involved in any pain. However, the diagnosis and treatment may be helped by this approach, with the proviso that it is remembered that this only identifies which aspect is predominant.

Pain of Predominantly "Peripheral" Origin (*i.e.*, peripheral to dorsal horn). This has also been termed *nociceptive* pain. It could include, for example, acute postoperative pain and chronic back pain caused by nerve root compression. It would also include post-thoracotomy neuralgic pain and trigeminal neuralgia

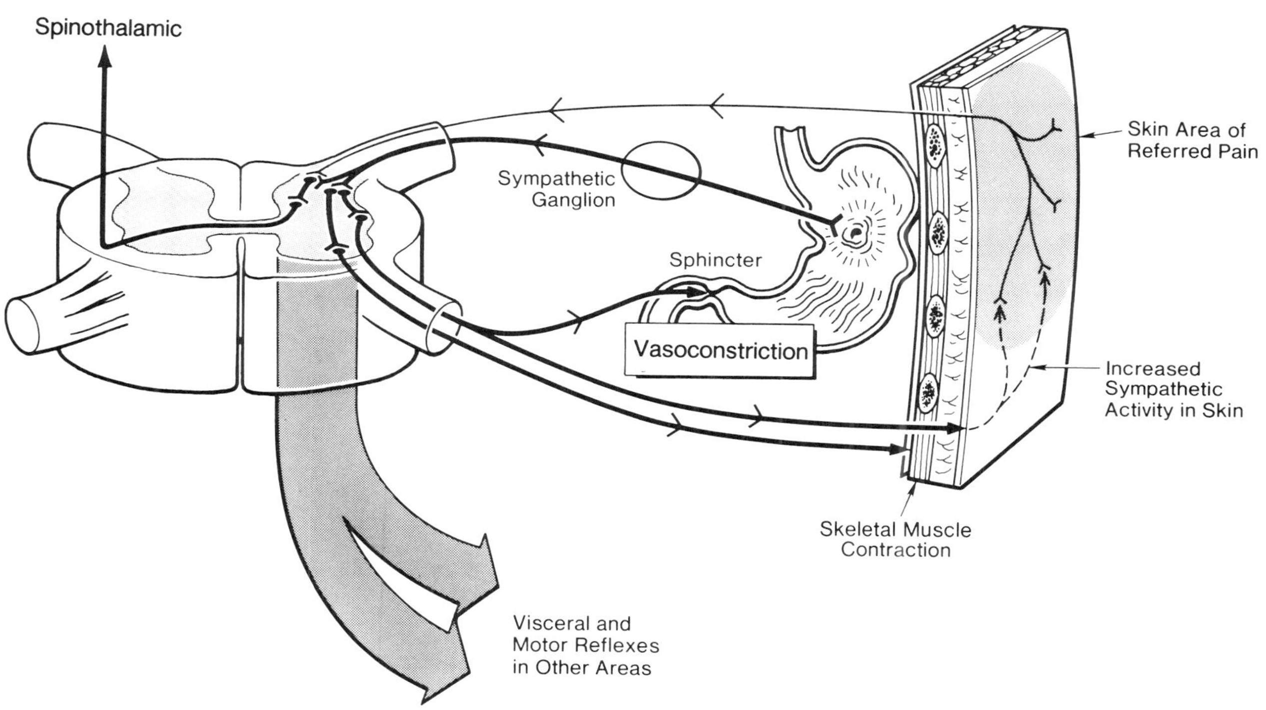

FIG. 24-2. Visceral pain: convergence of visceral and somatic nociceptive afferents. Visceral sympathetic afferents converge on the same dorsal horn neuron as do somatic nociceptive afferents. Visceral noxious stimuli are then conveyed, together with somatic noxious stimuli, by means of the spinothalamic pathways to the brain. *Note the following: 1.* Referred pain is felt in the cutaneous area corresponding to the dorsal horn neurons upon which visceral afferents converge. This is accompanied by allodynia and hyperalgesia in this skin area. *2.* Reflex somatic motor activity results in muscle spasm, which may stimulate parietal peritoneum and initiate somatic noxious input to dorsal horn. *3.* Reflex sympathetic efferent activity may result in spasm of sphincters of viscera over a wide area, causing pain remote from the original stimulus. *4.* Reflex sympathetic efferent activity may result in visceral ischemia and further noxious stimulation. Also, visceral nociceptors may be sensitized by norepinephrine release and microcirculatory changes (see also Fig. 24-1). *5.* Increased sympathetic activity may influence cutaneous nociceptors (see Fig. 24-1), which may be at least partly responsible for referred pain. *6.* Peripheral visceral afferents branch considerably, causing much overlap in the territory of individual dorsal roots. Only a small number of visceral afferent fibers converge on dorsal horn neurons compared with somatic nociceptor fibers. Also, visceral afferents converge on the dorsal horn over a wide number of segments. Thus dull, vague visceral pain is very poorly localized. This is often called "deep visceral pain."

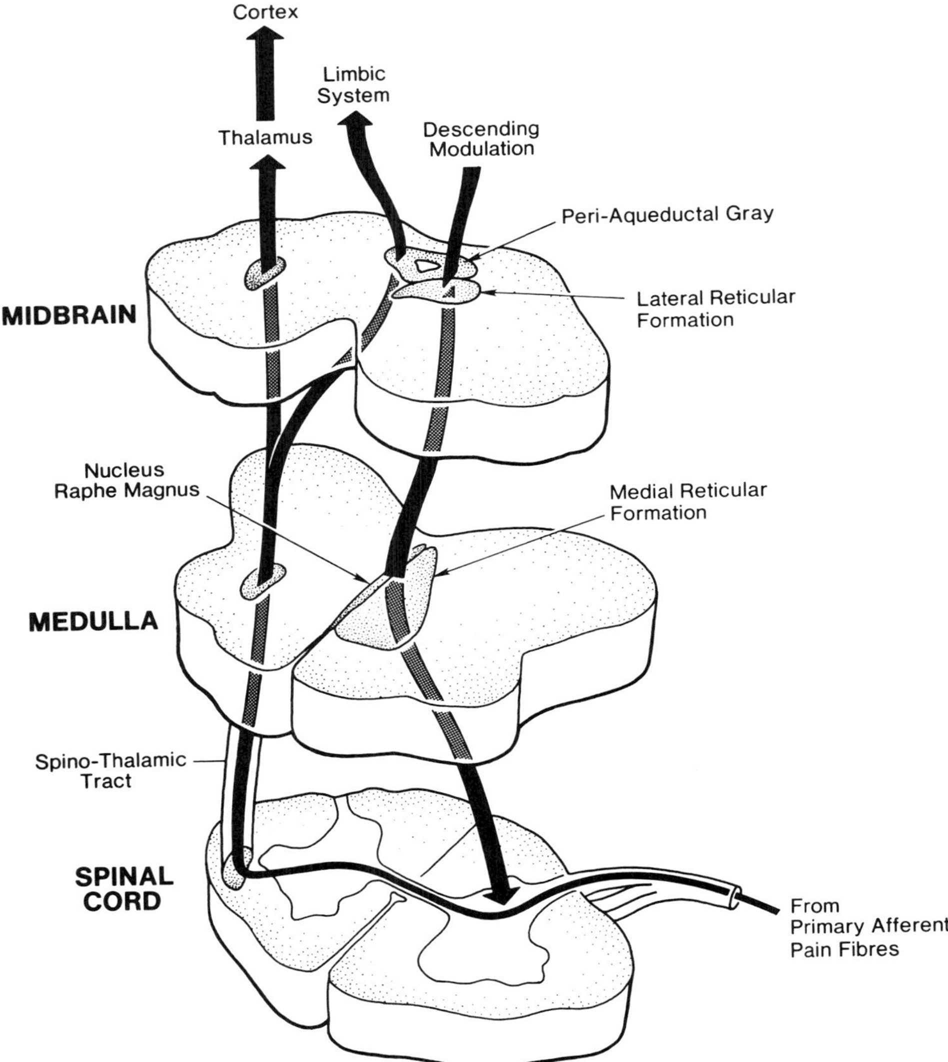

FIG. 24-3. Simplified schema of modulation of pain at spinal cord, medulla, and midbrain. Note initial modulation in dorsal horn of spinal cord and descending modulation by means of the periaqueductal gray matter, in the medial and lateral reticular formation, and in the nucleus raphe magnus. Descending inhibitory tracts in the dorsolateral funiculus then impinge on dorsal horn and release several inhibitory neurotransmitters. Note that the main afferent pain pathway ascends by means of the thalamus to the cerebral cortex, probably to produce the physical aspects of pain (oligosynaptic pathway). Other afferent pathways, however, such as spinoreticular, are important (polysynaptic pathways). An offshoot relays to the limbic system, probably resulting in the emotional aspects of pain. There are also afferent pathway influences on descending modulation (negative feedback) and cortical influences that may modulate pain at brain-stem level (see Chap. 24.2 for details). (Reproduced from Cousins, M.J., Phillips, G.D. (eds.): Acute Pain Management. London, Churchill Livingstone, 1986.)

of reasonably short duration. However, if such pain persists, it progressively develops a *central* component,[11] as do many other syndromes that begin as a peripheral problem (*e.g.*, reflex sympathetic dystrophy).[24]

Pain of Predominantly Neurogenic Origin. This includes lesions or disturbances anywhere in the nervous system.[17] Spinal lesions include traumatic paraplegia and deafferentation owing to surgery. Brain lesions include stroke, tumors, and trauma. *Central pain* was previously limited to the so-called thalamic syndrome, owing to selective thalamic lesions. It is now recognized that lesions or disturbances in many parts of the brain may cause pain (see Appendix B). One view holds that loss of afferent input results in decreased drive of descending inhibition, and thus loss of normal pain modulation. This has been termed *deafferentation pain* (see Chap. 30). However, there are other theories of central pain, and it is possible that different mechanisms may operate in different types of central pain.[17]

The term **neurogenic pain** is also used to describe pain caused by lesions in the peripheral nervous system. It includes such disorders as peripheral nerve injuries, peripheral neuropathies,[18] causalgia, and reflex sympathetic dystrophy. Although such problems may begin at "peripheral" levels, they rapidly develop all the hallmarks of central pain.

Pain of Predominantly Psychological Origin (psychogenic pain). This does not exclude a *contribution* from physical factors.

ETIOLOGY AND FEATURES OF ACUTE AND CHRONIC PAIN

Acute and chronic pain may arise from cutaneous, deep somatic or visceral structures. Careful mapping of the principal superficial dermatomes is important for effective use of neural blockade techniques. Dermatomes are shown in Figure 8-35. Visceral pain is much more vaguely localized than somatic pain and has other unique features (Table 24-2); its relief requires blockade of visceral nociceptive fibers that travel to the spinal cord by way of the sympathetic chain (see Fig. 13-1). The viscera and their spinal cord segments associated with their visceral nociceptor afferents are shown in Table 24-3. Visceral pain is "referred" to the body surface areas, as shown in Figure 24-4. It should be noted that there is considerable overlap for the various organs. Thus it is not surprising that there is a substantial error rate in the diagnosis of visceral pain. Also, there are important viscerosomatic and somaticovisceral reflexes that may make diagnosis and treatment difficult (Fig. 24-2). Pain pathways for gynecologic pain have been poorly understood; they are shown in Figure 24-5.

Features of Acute Pain

There are important differences between most types of acute pain and chronic pain.[19] In acute pain the nervous system is usually intact; the pain is caused by trauma, surgery, acute "medical" conditions, or a physiologic process (*e.g.*, labor). Facial grimaces and

TABLE 24-2. VISCERAL PAIN COMPARED WITH SOMATIC PAIN

	Somatic	Visceral
Site	Well localized	Poorly localized
Radiation	May follow distribution of somatic nerve	Diffuse
Character	Sharp and definite	Dull and vague (may be colicky, cramping, squeezing, etc.)
Relation to stimulus	Hurts where the stimulus is; associated with external factors	May be "referred" to another area; associated with internal factors
Time relations	Often constant (sometimes periodic)	Often periodic and builds to peaks (sometimes constant)
Associated symptoms	Nausea usually only with deep somatic pain owing to bone involvement	Often nausea, vomiting, sickening feeling

TABLE 24–3. VISCERA AND THEIR SEGMENTAL NOCICEPTIVE NERVE SUPPLY

Viscus	Spinal Segments of Visceral Nociceptive Afferents*
Heart	T1–T5
Lungs	T2–T4
Esophagus	T5–T6
Stomach	T6–T10
Liver and gallbladder	T6–T10
Pancreas and spleen	T6–T10
Small intestine	T9–T10
Large intestine	T11–T12
Kidney and ureter	T10–L2
Adrenal glands	T8–L1
Testis, ovary	T10–T11
Urinary bladder	T11–L2
Prostate gland	T11–L1
Uterus	T10–L1

*These travel with sympathetic fibers and pass by way of sympathetic ganglia to the spinal cord. However, they are *not* sympathetic (efferent) fibers. They are best referred to as visceral nociceptive afferents. *Note:* Parasympathetic afferent fibers may be important in upper abdominal pain (vagal fibers, celiac plexus).

signs of increased autonomic activity and other potentially harmful effects may be evident: for example, hypertension, tachycardia, vasoconstriction, sweating, increased rate and decreased depth of respiration, skeletal muscle spasm (see Fig. 26-1), increased gastrointestinal secretions, decreased intestinal motility and increased sphincter tone, urinary retention, venous stasis and potential for thrombosis, and possible pulmonary embolism; anxiety, confusion and delirium (see Chaps. 5 and 26). Also, the pain usually ceases when the wound heals or the medical condition improves. Patients are usually aware that the pain will improve as they recover, and thus an end is in sight. This may not be so if patients are ill-prepared and poorly informed (see Chap. 25).

Some severe and prolonged acute pain may progressively become more like chronic pain (see below). Some patients with chronic pain may have superimposed acute pain (*e.g.*, when they require further surgery or develop a bone fracture owing to metastatic cancer).[8] Such patients may not have an intact ner-

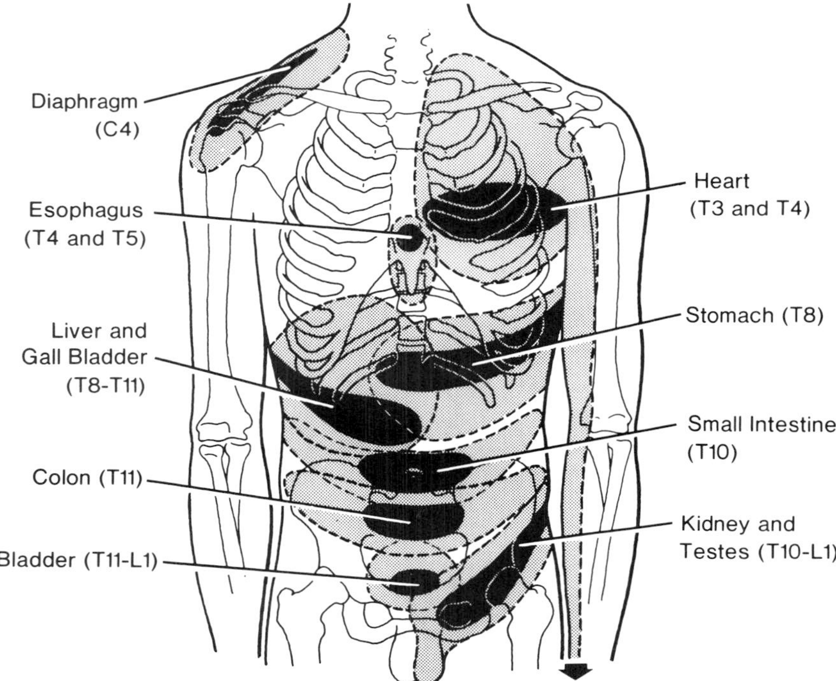

FIG. 24-4. Viscerotomes. Approximate superficial areas to which visceral pain is referred, with related dermatomes in brackets. The dark areas are those most commonly associated with pain in each viscus. The gray areas indicate approximately the larger area that may be associated with pain in that viscus. (Reproduced with permission from Cousins, M.J.: Visceral pain. In Andersson, S., Bond, M., Mehta, M., and Swerdlow, M. [eds.]: Chronic Non-Cancer Pain: Assessment and Practical Management. Lancaster, MTP Press, 1987.)

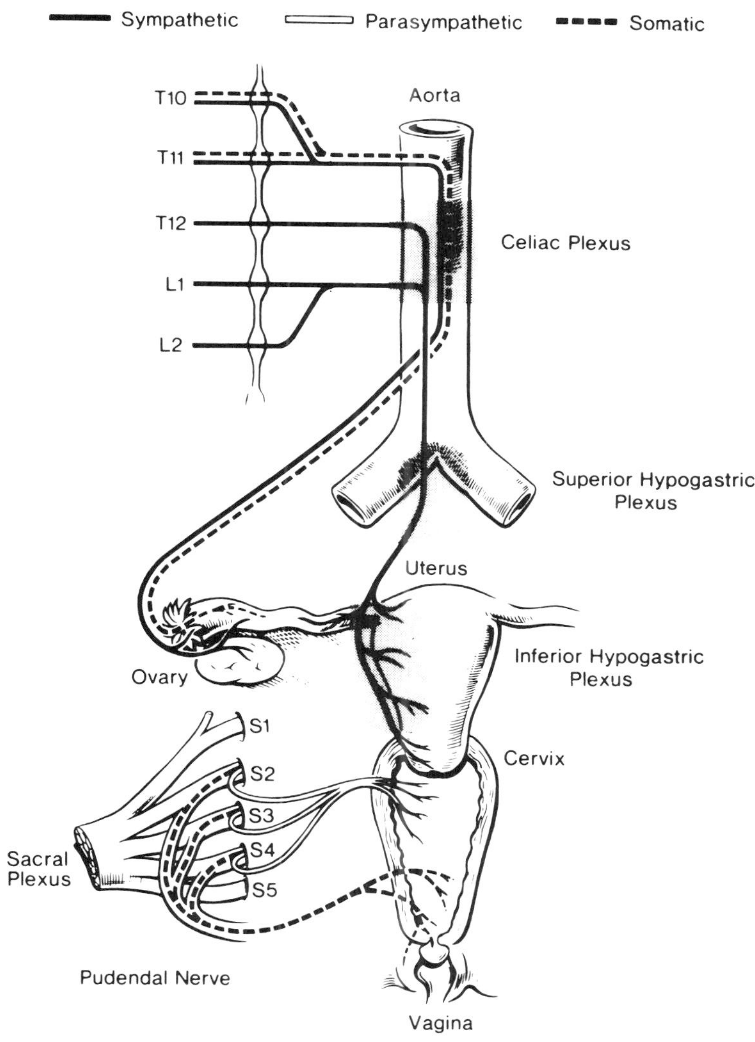

FIG. 24-5. Pain pathways in gynecologic pain. Somatic afferents from lower vagina are also shown. (Reproduced with permission from Cousins, M.J., Wilson, P.R.: Gynecologic pain. In Coppleson, M. [ed.]: Gynecologic Oncology. Edinburgh, Churchill Livingstone, 1981.)

vous system and may have marked preexisting psychological problems, opioid tolerance, and other problems.

Extensive somatic *and* sympathetic blockade may be required to relieve acute pain associated with some types of major surgery. For example, the following may be required for pain after thoracoabdominal esophagogastrectomy with cervical anastomosis: *C3–C4 and T2–T12 sensory nerves* (somatic structures in neck, thorax, and abdomen); *cervicothoracic sympathetic chain and celiac plexus* (intrathoracic and abdominal viscera); *C3, C4 phrenic nerve sensory afferents* (pain from incision in central diaphragm referred to shoulder tip).

Segmental and suprasegmental reflex responses to acute pain result in muscle spasm, immobility, vasospasm, and other adverse effects, as described above (see Chaps. 5 and 26). This may intensify the pain by way of various vicious cycles (see Fig. 24-2), which include increased sensitivity of peripheral nociceptors (Fig. 24-1; see Chap. 24.2). Acute pain that is unrelieved results in anxiety and sleeplessness, which in turn increase pain (see Chap. 26). Also anxiety and a feeling of helplessness, before as well as after surgery, increase pain (see Fig. 26-2). Their prevention and relief are valuable adjuncts to other treatments. Psychological journals contain much of relevance to acute pain (see Chap. 26). After major surgery, or severe trauma, or painful medical conditions (*e.g.*, pancreatitis), acute pain may persist for more than 10 days.[1] In such situations the pain and its sequelae become similar to chronic pain. It is not uncommon for such patients to show anger, depression, and other characteristics of chronic pain[1,5] (see Chap. 25). Thus one should be wary of drawing too sharp a distinction between acute and chronic pain: as acute pain persists, more emphasis may need to be placed on psychological *in addition to* physical and pharmacologic approaches to treatment.

Features of Chronic Pain

It has been arbitrarily agreed that chronic pain is that pain which persists "past the time of healing" or for more than about 3 months.[15] However, sometimes severe acute pain may become essentially chronic after only approximately 10 to 14 days (see above). Chronic pain progressively leads to limitation of physical, mental, and social activities, with accompanying anger, depression, and family and socioeconomic disruption. It seems that sympathoadrenal responses "habituate" or become exhausted in chronic pain and then vegetative responses emerge: sleep disturbance, irritability, loss of appetite for food and sex, decreased motor activity, mental depression (see Chap. 25). The facial expression of patients with chronic pain may be subdued, sad, or even "sleepy," owing to excessive medication. This may give the impression that pain cannot be present. Patients with chronic pain are often exhausted from lack of sleep and from extreme demands on their mental and physical resources. Severe psychoneurosis and other psychological disturbances may result from severe unrelieved chronic pain. These may be rapidly and completely reversed on relief of the pain. Treatment must address these components of chronic pain syndromes (see Chap. 25). Outstanding progress in understanding neurologic mechanisms of pain has helped greatly in treatment of chronic pain (see Chaps. 24.2 and 25).

CLASSIFICATION OF CHRONIC PAIN

Diagnosis and treatment of chronic pain has been greatly helped by the development of a "Classification of Chronic Pain: Description of Chronic Pain Syndromes and Definitions of Pain Terms."[15] This monumental task was taken on by the Subcommittee on Taxonomy of the IASP, headed by Professor Harold Merskey. Its publication in *Pain* represents a landmark in the history of pain diagnosis and treatment. It will aid treatment by greatly improving the recognition of various chronic pain syndromes. It will also encourage the use of a universal "language" of pain, and thus permit precise reporting and the gathering of vital statistical and epidemiological information about chronic pain. The Definitions of Pain Terms are reproduced in their entirety as Appendix A. It should be stressed that the definition of pain is equally applicable to acute and chronic pain. The Description of Chronic Pain Syndromes is reproduced in part as Appendix B with the kind permission of Professor Harold Merskey (Chairman, Taxonomy Subcommittee, IASP), Professor Patrick Wall (Editor, *Pain*), and the publishers of *Pain*, Elsevier Science Publishers. The scheme for coding is given in detail and then some complete examples of classifications and descriptions of pain syndromes are given. This is followed by a complete listing of all chronic pain syndromes that are described in the IASP Classification. Those that are common or potentially amenable to diagnosis or treatment with neural blockade are reproduced in full. The reader is strongly encouraged to consult the full classification for the full range of descriptions.[15]

Several points pertinent to neural blockade can be made.

1. The scheme for coding encourages precise description of region of body, system involved, temporal characteristics of pain, intensity, time since onset, and etiology. This helps to identify pain syndromes that are known to be responsive to neural blockade and pinpoints anatomic regions involved.
2. The classification refers first to *generalized* syndromes (*e.g.*, peripheral neuropathy) that may have important underlying medical diseases (*e.g.*, amyloid, diabetes). Some of these may be amenable to treatment of the disease as a means of pain treatment and are frequently, but not invariably, unresponsive to neural blockade. Some may require a good knowledge of the disease process in order to effectively *and safely* treat the pain. *Regionalized* pain syndromes are then described and some of these are amenable to neural blockade.
3. The use of neural blockade is appropriate and effective only in some of these many syndromes (see Chaps. 27.2, 27.3, 28, 29.2, 30, 31). Those using neural blockade should be familiar with all of the syndromes in the classification and with the treat-

ments other than neural blockade that are effective for some syndromes. In particular, it should be recognized that there are many well-described pain syndromes of predominant psychological etiology. However, in some of these, neural blockade may be useful as an *adjunct* to psychological measures (see Chaps. 27.2 and 31).

4. The classification and coding system can be used to obtain precise information about the efficacy of neural blockade in many pain syndromes in which it has as yet not been *objectively* evaluated.

Chronic Pain Syndromes in Cancer Patients

Treatment of cancer pain has been helped by clear descriptions of major categories of pain problems that commonly occur in cancer patients and etiologic factors in cancer pain[2,3,8] (Tables 24-4 through 24-8).

TABLE 24-4. TYPES OF PAIN IN PATIENTS WITH CANCER

I. Patients with acute cancer-related pain
   a. Associated with the diagnosis of cancer
   b. Associated with cancer therapy (surgery, chemotherapy, or radiation)
II. Patients with chronic cancer-related pain
   a. Associated with cancer progression
   b. Associated with cancer therapy (surgery, chemotherapy, or radiation)
III. Patients with preexisting chronic pain and cancer-related pain
IV. Patients with a history of drug addiction and cancer-related pain
   a. Actively involved in illicit drug use
   b. In methadone maintenance programs
   c. With a history of drug abuse
V. Dying patients with cancer-related pain

Incidence of different types of pain is approximately as follows: Directly caused by cancer (78%); caused by treatment (19%); indirectly related or unrelated to cancer (3%). However, many patients have multiple pains (*e.g.*, a high percentage [30% to 40%] of patients have myofascial syndromes) *in addition* to cancer-related pain. (Data from Foley, K.M.: The treatment of cancer pain. *N. Engl. J. Med., 313:*84, 1985.)

TABLE 24-5. PAIN SYNDROMES IN PATIENTS WITH CANCER: PAIN DIRECTLY CAUSED BY CANCER* (PRIMARY OR METASTATIC)

Mechanism	Common Sites and Characteristics of Pain
Infiltration of bone by tumor	Dull, constant aching; ± muscle spasm
Base of skull (jugular foramen, clivus, sphenoid sinus)	Early onset pain in occiput, vertex, frontal areas, respectively
Vertebral body (subluxation atlas, metastases C7–T1, L1 sacral)	Early onset pain in neck and skull, neck and shoulders, midback, lower back, and coccyx, respectively ± neurologic deficit
Metastatic fracture close to nerves	Acute onset pain + muscle spasm
Infiltration or compression of nerve tissue by tumor	
Peripheral nerve (± peripheral and perivascular lymphangitis)	Burning constant pain in area of peripheral sensory loss ± dysesthesia and hyperalgesia ± signs of sympathetic over-activity. See neuropathy definition.
Plexus, *e.g.*, lumbar	Radicular pain to anterior thigh and groin (L1–L3) or to leg and foot (L4–S2)
e.g., sacral	Dull aching midline perianal pain + sacral sensory loss and fecal and urinary incontinence.
e.g., brachial	Radicular pain in shoulder and arm ± Horner's syndrome (superior pulmonary sulcus or Pancoast syndrome)
Meningeal carcinomatosis	Constant headache ± neck stiffness or low back and buttock pain
Epidural spinal cord compression (± vertebral body infiltration)	Severe neck and back pain locally over involved vertebra, or radicular pain
Obstruction of hollow viscus *e.g.*, gut, genitourinary tract)	Poorly localized, dull, sickening pain, typical visceral pain
Occlusion of arteries and veins by tumor	Ischemic pain like rest pain (skin) or claudication (muscle) or pain ± venous engorgement
Stretching of periosteum or fascia, in tissues with tight investment, by tumefaction	Severe localized pain (*e.g.*, periosteum) *or* typical visceral pain (*e.g.*, ovary)
Inflammation owing to necrosis and infection of tumors (±superficial ulceration)	Severe localized pain (*e.g.*, perineum), visceral pain (*e.g.*, cervix)
Soft tissue infiltration	Localized pain; unsightly and foul-smelling if ulcerated
Raised intracranial pressure	Severe constant headache, behavioral changes, confusion, etc.

*A subcategory can be defined as *Pain related to the cancer: e.g.*, muscle spasm, constipation, bedsores, lymphedema, candidiasis, herpetic and postherpetic neuralgia, deep venous thrombosis, pulmonary embolism.

TABLE 24–6. PAIN SYNDROMES IN PATIENTS WITH CANCER: PAIN ASSOCIATED WITH CANCER THERAPY

Mechanism	Common Sites and Characteristics of Pain
Following surgery	
Acute postoperative pain	Wound or referred pain; back or other sites (owing to posture during surgery)
Nerve trauma	Neuralgic pain in area of peripheral nerve or spinal nerve
Entrapment of nerves in scar tissue	Superficial wound scar hypersensitivity of area supplied by scarred nerves (*e.g.*, perineum)
Amputation of limb or other area (*e.g.*, breast)	Localized stump pain (neuroma) *or* phantom pain referred to absent region
Following radiotherapy	
Acute lesions or inflammation of nerves or plexuses	Pain associated with motor and sensory loss.
Radiation fibrosis of nerves or plexuses	*e.g.*, brachial plexus, lumbar plexus distribution; diffuse limb pain, 6 months to many years after radiation ± lymphedema and local skin changes ± sensory loss ± motor loss (difficult to distinguish from tumor recurrence)
Myelopathy of spinal cord	Brown-Sèquard syndrome (ipsilateral sensory and contralateral motor loss) with pain at level of spinal cord damage or referred pain
Peripheral nerve tumors owing to radiation	Painful enlarging mass in area of radiation along line of peripheral nerve or plexus
Following chemotherapy	
Vinca alkaloid (vincristine > vinblastine)-induced peripheral neuropathy	Burning pain in hands and feet associated with symmetrical polyneuropathy
Steroid pseudorheumatism owing to slow as well as rapid withdrawal of steroid treatment	Diffuse joint and muscle pain with associated tenderness to palpation but no inflammatory signs Pain resolves when steroid reinstituted.
Aseptic necrosis of bone (femoral or humoral head) with chronic steroid therapy	Pain in knee, leg, or shoulder with limitation of movement; bone scan changes delayed after pain onset
Postherpetic neuralgia, following herpes zoster infection in area of tumor or area of radiotherapy with onset during chemotherapy	Continuous burning pain in area of sensory loss *or* Painful dysesthesias *or* Intermittent, shocklike pain

TABLE 24–7. PAIN SYNDROMES IN PATIENTS WITH CANCER: PAIN UNRELATED TO CANCER OR CANCER THERAPY

Mechanism	Common Sites and Characteristics of Pain
Neuropathy (*e.g.*, diabetic)	Burning pain in hands, feet
Degenerative disk disease	Back pain ± radicular pain
Rheumatoid arthritis	Joint pain, on movement
Diffuse osteoporosis	Back pain, limb pain (may be like causalgia)
Posture abnormalities after surgery	Back pain and muscle spasm ± radicular pain
Myofascial syndromes owing to anxiety	Local pain in muscle with muscle spasm ± referred pain; trigger areas in muscle
Headache	Typical migraine or tension type

TABLE 24-8. PAIN SYNDROMES IN PATIENTS WITH CANCER: PAIN EXACERBATED OR ENTIRELY CAUSED BY PSYCHOLOGICAL FACTORS

Psychological Factor	Possible Causes
Anxiety	Sleeplessness
	Fear of death; loss of dignity (loss of self-control)
	Fear of surgical mutilation; uncontrollable pain
	Fear of the future; loss of social position and work
	Confused understanding of disease owing to poor communication
	Family and financial problems
Depression	Sleeplessness
	Loss of physical abilities
	Sense of helplessness
	Disfigurement
	Loss of valued social position; financial problems
Anger	Frustration with therapeutic failures
	Resentment of sickness
	Irritability caused by pain and general discomfort

A vicious cycle usually develops:

ANXIETY
SLEEPLESSNESS ← PAIN → ANGER
DEPRESSION

It will be clear that neural blockade offers an effective means of treatment of only some of these syndromes. Failure to assess *and reassess* cancer pain in the light of these potential etiologies will result in poor results from use of neural blockade. It should be remembered that central pain, including deafferentiation pain, can occur in patients with cancer.[23] This is not responsive, on a continued basis, to neural blockade, except sometimes to stimulation techniques (see Chap. 30). Precise description of the origin *and pattern* of cancer pain is important. For example, it has been reported that intermittent visceral pain responds poorly to spinal opioids (see Chap. 28).

REFERENCES

1. Bonica, J.J.: Biology, pathophysiology and treatment of acute pain. *In* Lipton, S., and Miles, J. (eds.): Persistent Pain, vol. 5. pp. 1–32. Orlando, Grune & Stratton, 1985.
2. Bonica, J.J.: Treatment of cancer pain: Current status and future needs. *In* Fields, H.L., *et al.* (eds.): Advances in Pain Research and Therapy, vol. 9. pp. 589–616.. New York, Raven Press, 1985.
3. Bonica, J.J., and Ventafridda, V.: Pain of advanced cancer. *In* Fields, H.L., *et al.* (eds.): Advances in Pain Research and Therapy, vol. 2. New York, Raven Press, 1979.
4. Cohen, F.L.: Postsurgical pain relief: Patient's status and nurses' medication choices. Pain, *9*:265, 1980.
5. Cousins, M.J., and Phillips, G.D.: Acute Pain Management. *In* Clinics in Critical Care Medicine. Edinburgh, Churchill Livingstone, 1986.
6. Cousins, M.J., Reeve, T.S., Glynn, C.J., Walsh, J.A., and Cherry, D.A.: Neurolytic lumbar sympathetic blockade: Duration of denervation and relief of rest pain. Anaesth. Intensive Care, *7*:121, 1979.
7. Foley, K.M.: Pharmacologic approaches to cancer pain management. *In* Fields, H.L., *et al.* (eds.): Advances in Pain Research and Therapy, vol. 9. pp. 629–653. New York, Raven Press, 1985.
8. Foley, K.M.: The treatment of cancer pain. N. Engl. J. Med., *313*:84, 1985.
9. Gourlay, G.K., Cherry, D.A., and Cousins, M.J.: A comparative study of the efficacy and pharmacokinetics of oral methadone and morphine in the treatment of severe pain in patients with cancer. Pain, 25:297, 1986.
10. Gross, P.: Cost of chronic pain in Australia. Abstracts of Scientific Meeting of Australian Pain Society, Melbourne, 1986.
11. Loeser, J.D.: Tic douloureux and atypical facial pain. *In* Wall, P.D., and Melzack, R. (eds.): Textbook of Pain. pp. 426–434, Edinburgh, Churchill Livingstone, 1984.

12. Marks, R.M., and Sacher, E.J.: Undertreatment of medical patients with narcotic analgesics. Ann. Intern. Med., *78*:173, 1973.
13. Mather, L.E., and Mackie, J.: The incidence of postoperative pain in children. Pain, *15*:271, 1983.
14. Mendelsson, G.: Compensation, pain complaints, and psychological disturbances. Pain, *20*:169, 1984.
15. Merskey, H. (ed.): Classification of chronic pain. Description of chronic pain syndromes and definitions of pain terms. Pain, *3*[*Suppl.*]:1, 1986.
16. Noordenbos, W.: Prologue. *In* Wall, P.D., and Melzack, R. (eds.): Textbook of Pain. Edinburgh, Churchill Livingstone, 1984.
17. Pagni, C.A.: Central pain due to spinal cord and brain stem damage. *In* Wall, P.D., and Melzack, R. (eds.): Textbook of Pain. pp. 481–495. Edinburgh, Churchill Livingstone, 1984.
18. Scadding, J.W.: Peripheral neuropathies. *In* Wall, P.D., and Melzack, R. (eds.): Textbook of Pain. pp. 413–425. Edinburgh, Churchill Livingstone, 1984.
19. Sternbach, R.A.: Acute versus chronic pain. *In* Wall, P.D., and Melzack,, R. (eds.): Textbook of Pain. pp. 173–177. Edinburgh, Churchill Livingstone, 1984.
20. Sternsward, J.: Cancer pain relief: An important global public health issue. *In* Fields, H.L.,, *et al.* (eds.): Advances in Pain Research and Therapy. pp. 555–558. New York, Raven Press, 1985.
21. Ventafridda, V., Tamburini, M., and DeConno, F.: Comprehensive treatment in cancer pain. *In* Fields, H.L., *et al.* (eds.): Advances in Pain Research and Therapy. pp. 617–628. New York, Raven Press, 1985.
22. Wall, P.D.: Introduction. *In* Wall, P.D., and Melzack, R. (eds.): Textbook of Pain. pp. 1–16. Edinburgh, Churchill Livingstone, 1984.
23. Wall, P.D.: Cancer pain: Neurogenic mechanisms. *In* Fields, H.L., *et al.* (eds.): Advances in Pain Research and Therapy, vol. 9. pp. 575–587. New York, Raven Press, 1985.
24. Wynnparry, C.B., and Withrington, R.W.: The management of painful peripheral nerve disorders. *In* Wall, P.D., and Melzack, R. (eds.): Textbook of Pain. pp. 395–401. Edinburgh, Churchill Livingstone, 1984.

APPENDIX A: TAXONOMY OF PAIN*

PAIN

An unpleasant sensory and emotional experience associated with actual or potential tissue damage, or described in terms of such damage.

Note: Pain is always subjective. Each individual learns the application of the word through experiences related to injury in early life. Biologists recognize that stimuli that cause pain are liable to damage tissue. Accordingly, pain is the experience that we associate with actual or potential tissue damage. It is unquestionably a sensation in a part or parts of the body, but it is also always unpleasant, and therefore an emotional experience as well. Experiences that resemble pain (*e.g.*, pricking) but are not unpleasant should not be called pain. Unpleasant abnormal experiences (dysesthesias) may also be pain but are not necessarily so because, subjectively, they may not have the usual sensory qualities of pain.

Many people report pain in the absence of tissue damage or any likely pathophysiologic cause; usually this happens for psychological reasons. There is no way to distinguish their experience from that due to tissue damage if we take the subjective report. If they regard their experience as pain and if they report it in the same ways as pain caused by tissue damage, it should be accepted as pain. This definition avoids tying pain to the stimulus. Activity induced in the nociceptor and nociceptive pathways by a noxious stimulus is not pain, which is always a psychological state, even though we may well appreciate that pain most often has a proximate physical cause.

ALLODYNIA

Pain due to a stimulus that does not normally provoke pain.

Note†: This was first introduced as a term intended to refer to the situation in which otherwise normal tissues, which may have abnormal innervation or may be referral sites for other loci, give rise to pain on stimulation by nonnoxious means. "Allo" means "other" in Greek and is a common prefix for medical conditions that diverge from the expected. "Odynia" is derived from the Greek word *odune* or *odyne*, which is used in "pleurodynia" and "coccydynia," and is similar in meaning to the root from which words with -alga or -algesia in them are derived. Allodynia was suggested after discussions with Professor Paul Potter of the Department of the History of Medicine and Science at The University of Western Ontario.

See also the notes on hyperalgesia and hyperpathia.

*Reprinted with permission from Pain, 3[Suppl.]:216–221, 1986. The "Taxonomy of Pain" (Appendix A) is reprinted in full. Note that the "Classification of Chronic Pain and Description of Chronic Pain Syndromes" (Appendix B) is greatly abridged. The reader is advised to consult the full version in **Pain,** 3(Suppl.):217, 1986.

†Abridged. See full note in Pain, 3[Suppl.]:217, 1986.

ANALGESIA

Absence of pain in response to stimulation that would normally be painful.

Note: As with allodynia, the stimulus is defined by its usual subjective effects.

ANESTHESIA DOLOROSA

Pain in an area or region that is anesthetic.

CAUSALGIA

A syndrome of sustained burning pain, allodynia, and hyperpathia after a traumatic nerve lesion, often combined with vasomotor and sudomotor dysfunction and later trophic changes.

CENTRAL PAIN

Pain associated with a lesion of the central nervous system.

DYSESTHESIA

An unpleasant abnormal sensation, whether spontaneous or evoked.

Note: Compare with pain and with paresthesia. Special cases of dysesthesia include hyperalgesia and allodynia. A dysesthesia should always be unpleasant and a paresthesia should not be unpleasant, although it is recognized that the borderline may present some difficulties when it comes to deciding whether a sensation is pleasant or unpleasant. It should always be specified whether the sensations are spontaneous or evoked.

HYPERALGESIA

An increased response to a stimulus that is normally painful.

Note: The changes here relate to two matters. One is the avoidance of the word noxious in the definition because of difficulties in its use. The second is the inclusion of some features of allodynia in the definition of hyperalgesia. Many cases of hyperalgesia have features of allodynia. The term allodynia should be preferred when there is not an increased response to a stimulus that normally provokes pain. However, when there is also a response of increased pain to a stimulus that normally is painful, hyperalgesia is the appropriate word. It should also be recognized that with allodynia, the stimulus and the response are in different modes, whereas with hyperalgesia they are in the same mode.

See also notes on allodynia and hyperpathia.

HYPERESTHESIA

Increased sensitivity to stimulation, excluding the special senses.

Note: The stimulus and locus should be specified. Hyperesthesia may refer to various modes of cutaneous sensibility, including touch and thermal sensation without pain, as well as to pain. The word is used to indicate both diminished threshold to any stimulus and an increased response to stimuli that are normally recognized.

Allodynia is suggested for pain after stimulation that is not normally painful. Hyperesthesia includes both allodynia and hyperalgesia, but the more specific terms should be used whenever they are applicable.

HYPERPATHIA

A painful syndrome, characterized by increased reaction to a stimulus, especially a repetitive stimulus, as well as an increased threshold.

Note: It may occur with hyperesthesia, hyperalgesia, or dysesthesia. Faulty identification and localization of the stimulus, delay, radiating sensation, and aftersensation may be present, and the pain is often explosive. The change in this note is the inclusion of hyperalgesia explicitly, whereas previously it was implied, since hyperesthesia was mentioned and hyperalgesia is a special case of hyperesthesia.

The implications of some of the above definitions may be summarized for convenience as follows:

Allodynia	Lowered threshold	Stimulus and response mode differ
Hyperalgesia	Increased response	Stimulus and response mode are the same
Hyperpathia	Raised threshold; increased response	Stimulus and response mode may be the same or different
Hypoalgesia	Raised threshold; lowered response	Stimulus and response mode are the same

The essentials of the definitions do not have to be symmetrical, and are not symmetrical at present. Lowered threshold may occur with hyperalgesia but is not required. Also, there is no category for lowered threshold and lowered response—if it ever occurs.

HYPOALGESIA

Diminished pain in response to normally painful stimulus.

Note: Hypoalgesia was formerly defined as diminished sensitivity to noxious stimulation, making it a particular case of hypoesthesia. However, it now refers only to the occurrence of relatively less pain in response to stimulation that produces pain. Hypoesthesia covers the case of diminished sensitivity to stimulation that is normally painful.

HYPOESTHESIA

Decreased sensitivity to stimulation, excluding the special senses.

Note: Stimulation and locus to be specified.

NEURALGIA

Pain in the distribution of a nerve or nerves.

Note: Common usage, especially in Europe, often implies a paroxysmal quality, but neuralgia should not be reserved for paroxysmal pains.

NEURITIS

Inflammation of a nerve or nerves.

Note: Not to be used unless inflammation is thought to be present.

NEUROPATHY

A disturbance of function or pathological change in a nerve; in one nerve, mononeuropathy; in several nerves, mononeuropathy multiplex; if diffuse and bilateral, polyneuropathy.

Note: Neuritis is a special case of neuropathy and is now reserved for inflammatory processes affecting nerves. Neuropathy is not intended to cover cases like neurapraxia, neurotmesis, or section of a nerve.

NOCICEPTOR

A receptor preferentially sensitive to a noxious stimulus or to a stimulus that would become noxious if prolonged.

Note: Avoid use of terms like pain receptor or pain pathway.

NOXIOUS STIMULUS

A noxious stimulus is one that is damaging to normal tissues.

Note: Although the definition of a noxious stimulus has been retained, the term is not used in this list to define other terms.

PAIN TOLERANCE LEVEL

The greatest level of pain that a subject is prepared to tolerate.

Note: As with pain threshold, the pain tolerance level is the subjective experience of the individual. The stimuli that are normally measured in relation to its production are the pain tolerance level stimuli and not the level itself. Thus the same argument applies to pain tolerance level as to pain threshold, and it is not defined in terms of the external stimulation as such.

PAIN THRESHOLD

The least experience of pain that a subject can recognize.

Note: Traditionally the threshold has been defined as the least stimulus intensity at which a subject perceives pain. Properly defined, the threshold is really the experience of the patient, whereas the intensity measured is an external event. It has been common usage for most pain research workers to define the threshold in terms of the stimulus, and that should be avoided. However, the threshold stimulus can be recognized as such and measured. In psychophysics, thresholds are defined as the level at which 50% of stimuli are recognized. In that case the pain threshold would be the level at which 50% of stimuli would be recognized as painful. The stimulus is not pain and cannot be a measure of pain.

PARESTHESIA

An abnormal sensation, whether spontaneous or evoked.

Note: Compare with dysesthesia. After much discussion it has been agreed to recommend that paresthesia be used to describe an abnormal sensation that is not unpleasant, whereas dysesthesia be used preferentially for an abnormal sensation considered to be unpleasant. The use of one term (paresthesia) to indicate spontaneous sensations and the other to refer to evoked sensations is not favored. There is a sense in which, since paresthesia refers to abnormal sensations in general, it might include dysesthesia, but the reverse is not true. Dysesthesia does not include all abnormal sensations, but only those that are unpleasant.

APPENDIX B: CLASSIFICATION OF CHRONIC PAIN AND DESCRIPTION OF CHRONIC PAIN SYNDROMES*

SCHEME FOR CODING CHRONIC PAIN DIAGNOSES

All diagnoses may need to be preceded by a special number or letter chosen arbitrarily and not otherwise used in the International Classification of Diseases (ICD) (*e.g.*, P or Y). Such a letter would identify the fact that this is a pain classification. Give priority to the main site of the pain.

Axis I: Regions

Record main site first, Record two important regions separately. If there is more than one site of pain, separate coding will be necessary. More than three major sites can be coded, optionally, as shown.

Head, face, and mouth	000
Cervical region	100
Upper shoulder and upper limbs	200
Thoracic region	300
Abdominal region	400
Lower back, lumbar spine, sacrum, and coccyx	500
Lower limbs	600
Pelvic region	700
Anal, perineal, and genital regions	800
More than three major sites	900

Axis II: Systems

Nervous system (central, peripheral, and autonomic) and special senses; physical disturbance or disfunction	00
†Nervous system (psychological and social)	10
Respiratory and cardiovascular systems	20
Musculoskeletal system and connective tissue	30
Cutaneous and subcutaneous and associated glands (breast, apocrine, etc.)	40
Gastrointestinal system	50
Genitourinary system	60
Other organs or viscera (*e.g.*, thyroid, lymphatic, hemopoietic)	70
More than one system	80

Note: The system is coded whose abnormal functioning produces the pain (*e.g.*, claudication = vascular). Similarly, the nervous system is to be coded only when a pathological disturbance in it produces pain. Thus pain from a pancreatic carcinoma = gastrointestinal; pain from a metastatic deposit affecting bones = musculoskeletal.

Axis III: Temporal Characteristics of Pain: Pattern of Occurrence

Not recorded, not applicable, or not known	0
Single episode, limited duration (*e.g.*, ruptured aneurysm, sprained ankle)	1
Continuous or nearly continuous, nonfluctuating (*e.g.*, low back pain, some cases)	2
Continuous or nearly continuous, fluctuating severity (*e.g.*, ruptured intervertebral disk)	3
Recurring, irregularly (*e.g.*, headache, mixed type)	4
Recurring, regularly (*e.g.*, premenstrual pain)	5
Paroxysmal (*e.g.*, tic douloureux)	6
Sustained with superimposed paroxysms	7
Other combinations	8
None of the above	9

Axis IV: Patient's Statement of Intensity: Time Since Onset of Pain*

Not recorded, not applicable, or not known		.0
Mild	—1 month or less	.1
	1 month to 6 months	.2
	more than 6 months	.3
Medium	—1 month or less	.4
	1 month to 6 months	.5
	more than 6 months	.6
Severe	—1 month or less	.7
	1 month to 6 months	.8
	more than 6 months	.9

Axis V: Etiology

Genetic or congenital disorders (*e.g.*, congenital dislocation)	.00
Trauma, operation, burns	.01
Infective, parasitic	.02
Inflammatory (no known infective agent), immune reactions	.03
Neoplasm	.04

*Reprinted with permission from Pain, 3[Suppl.]:10–214, 1986.
†To be coded for psychiatric illness without any relevant lesion.

*Decide the time at which pain is recognized retrospectively as having started even though the pain may occur intermittently. Grade for intensity in relation to the level of current pain problem.

Toxic, metabolic (*e.g.*, alcoholic neuropathy, anoxia, vascular, nutritional, endocrine), radiation	.05
†Degenerative, mechanical	.06
‡Dysfunctional (including psychophysiologic)	.07
Unknown or other	.08
Psychological origin (*e.g.*, conversion hysteria, depressive hallucination). *Note:* No physical cause should be held to be present nor any pathophysiologic mechanism	.09

Some examples:

Mild prostherpetic neuralgia of T5 or T6 6 months' duration	302.22b or 303.22b
Severe tension headache More than 6 months' duration	033.97b
Moderately severe mechanical low back pain More than 6 months' duration	533.68b
Severe primary dysmenorrhea Duration not recorded	765.07b

PAIN SYNDROMES, DESCRIPTIONS, AND CODES

GROUP 1 RELATIVELY GENERALIZED SYNDROMES

PERIPHERAL NEUROPATHY (I-1)

Definition. Constant or intermittent burning, aching, or lancinating limb pains caused by generalized or focal diseases of peripheral nerves.

Site. Usually distal (especially the feet) with burning pain, but often more proximal and deep with aching. Focal with mononeuropathies, in the territory of the affected nerve (*e.g.*, meralgia paresthetica).

System. Peripheral nervous system.

Main Features.

Prevalence. Common in neuropathies of diabetes, amyloid, alcoholism, polyarteritis, Guillain-Barré syndrome, neuralgic amyotrophy, Fabry's disease.

†*E.g.*, biliary colic, lumbar puncture headache would be mechanical.

‡*E.g.*, migraine, irritable bowel syndrome, tension headache. *Note:* Include syndromes in which a pathophysiologic alteration is recognized. Emotional causes may or may not be present.

Age of Onset. Variable, usually after second decade.

Quality. (a) Burning, superficial distal pain often with dysesthesia, constant. May be in the territory of a single affected nerve; (b) deep aching, especially nocturnal, constant; and (c) sharp lancinating "tabetic" pains, especially in legs, intermittent.

Associated Symptoms. Sensory loss, especially to pinprick and temperature; sometimes weakness and muscle atrophy (especially in neuralgic amyotrophy); sometimes reflex loss; sometimes signs of loss of sympathetic function, smooth, fine skin, hair loss.

Laboratory Findings. (a) Features of the primary disease (*e.g.*, diabetes) and (b) features of neuropathy: reduced or absent sensory potentials, slowing of motor and sensory conduction velocities, electromyographic evidence of muscle denervation.

Usual Course. Distal burning and deep aching pains are often long lasting and the disease processes are relatively unresponsive to therapy. Pain resolves spontaneously in weeks or months in self-limited conditions such as Guillain-Barré syndrome or neuralgic amyotrophy.

Complications. Drug abuse, depression.

Social and Physical Disabilities. Decreased mobility.

Pathology. Nerve fiber damage, usually axonal degeneration. Pain especially occurs with small fiber damage (sensory fibers). Nerve biopsy may reveal the above, plus features of the specific disease process (*e.g.*, amyloid).

Summary of Essential Features and Diagnostic Criteria. Chronic distal burning or deep aching pain with signs of sensory loss with or without muscle weakness, atrophy, and reflex loss.

Differential Diagnosis. Spinal cord disease, muscle disease.

Code.

Arms: 203.X2a (infective), 203.X3a (inflammatory or immune reactions), 203.X5a (toxic, metabolic, etc.), 203.X8a (unknown or other).

Legs: 603.X2a, 603.X3a, 603.X5a, 603.X8a.

References. Thomas, P.K.: Pain in peripheral neuropathy: Clinical and morphological aspects. *In* Ochoa, J., and Culp,

W. (eds.): Abnormal Nerves and Muscles as Impulse Generators. New York, Oxford University Press, 1982. Asburn, A.K., and Fields, H.L.: Pain due to peripheral nerve damage: An hypothesis. Neurology, *34*:1587, 1984.

STUMP PAIN (I-2)

Definition. Pain at the site of an extremity amputation.

Site. Upper or lower extremity at the region of amputation. Pain is not referred to the absent body part, but is perceived in the stump itself, usually in region of transected nerve(s).

System. Peripheral nervous system; perhaps central nervous system.

Main Features. Sharp, often jabbing pain in stump, usually aggravated by pressure on or infection in the stump. Pain often elicited by tapping over neuroma in transected nerve(s).

Associated Symptoms. Refusal to use prosthesis.

Signs. Pain elicited by percussion over stump neuromata.

Laboratory Findings. None.

Usual Course. Develops several weeks to months after amputation; persists indefinitely if untreated.

Relief. (a) Alter prosthesis to avoid pressure on neuromata; (b) resect neuromata so that they no longer lie in pressure areas; and (c) use neurosurgical procedures, such as rhizotomy and ganglionectomy, or spinal cord or peripheral nerve stimulation in properly selected patients.

Complications. Refusal to use prosthesis.

Social and Physical Disabilities. Severe pain can preclude normal daily activities; failure to use prosthesis can add to functional limitations.

Pathology. Neuroma at site of nerve transection.

Essential Features. Pain in stump.

Differential Diagnosis. Phantom limb pain, radiculopathy.

Code. 203.X1a, 603.X1a.

PHANTOM PAIN (I-3)

Definition. Pain referred to a surgically removed limb or portion thereof.

Site. In the absent body part.

System. Central nervous system.

Main Features. Follows amputation; may commence at time of amputation or months to years later. Varies greatly in severity from person to person. Reports of prevalence vary from <1% to >50% of amputees. Believed to be more common if loss of limb occurs later in life, in limbs than in breast amputation, in the breast before the menopause rather than after it, and particularly if pain was present before the part was lost. Pain may be continuous, often with intermittent exacerbations. Usually cramping, aching, burning; may have superimposed shocklike components. Seems to be less likely if the initial amputation is treated actively and a prosthesis is promptly used. Phantom limb pain is almost always associated with distorted image of lost part.

Associated Symptoms. Aggravated by stress, systemic disease, poor stump health.

Signs. Loss of body part.

Usual Course. Complaints persist indefinitely, frequently with gradual amelioration over years.

Relief. No therapeutic regimen has more than a 30% long-term efficacy. TENS, anticonvulsants, antidepressants, or phenothiazines may be helpful. Sometimes sympathectomy or surgical procedures on spinal cord and brain, including stimulation, are helpful.

Social and Physical Disabilities. May preclude gainful employment or normal daily activities.

Pathology. Related to deafferentation of neurons and their spontaneous and evoked hyperexcitability.

Essential Features. Pain in an absent body part.

Differential Diagnosis. Stump pain.

Code. 203.X7a (arms), 603.X7a (legs).

CAUSALGIA (I-4)

Definition. Burning pain, allodynia, and hyperpathia, usually in the hand or foot, after partial injury of a nerve or one of its major branches.

Site. In the region of the limb innervated by the damaged nerve.

Main Features. Onset usually immediately after partial nerve injury or may be delayed for months. Causalgia of the radial nerve is uncommon. The nerves most frequently involved are the median, the sciatic and tibial, and the ulnar. Spontaneous pain. Pain described as constant, burning; exacerbated by light touch, stress, temperature change or movement of involved limb, visual and auditory stimuli (*e.g.*, a sudden sound or bright light), emotional disturbances.

Associated Symptoms. Atrophy of skin appendages, secondary atrophic changes in bones, joints, and muscles. Cool, red, clammy skin with excessive sweating. Sensory and motor loss in structure innervated by damaged portion of nerve.

Signs. Cool, red, clammy, sweaty skin with atrophy of skin appendages and deep structures in painful area.

Laboratory Findings. Galvanic skin responses and plethysmography reveal signs of sympathetic nervous system hyperactivity. Roentgenograms may show atrophy of bone.

Usual Course. If untreated, the majority of patients will have symptoms that persist indefinitely; spontaneous remission occurs.

Relief. In early stages of causalgia (first few months) sympathetic blockade plus vigorous physical therapy usually provides transient relief; repeated blocks usually lead to long-term relief. When a series of sympathetic blocks does not provide long-term relief, sympathectomy is indicated. Long-term persistence of symptoms reduces the likelihood of successful therapy.

Social and Physical Disabilities. Disuse atrophy of involved limb; complete disruption of normal daily activities by severe pain. Risk of suicide, drug abuse if untreated.

Pathology. Partial injury to major peripheral nerve; actual cause of pain is unknown. Peripheral, central, and sympathetic mechanisms involved in an unexplained way.

Essential Features. Burning pain and cutaneous hypersensitivity with signs of sympathetic hyperactivity in portion of limb innervated by partially injured nerve.

Differential Diagnosis. None

Code. 207.91 (arm), 607.91 (leg).

REFLEX SYMPATHETIC DYSTROPHY (I-5)

Definition. Continuous pain in a portion of an extremity after trauma that may include fracture but does not involve a major nerve, associated with sympathetic hyperactivity.

Site. Usually the distal extremity adjacent to a traumatized area.

System. Peripheral nervous system; possibly the central nervous system.

Main Features. The pain follows trauma (usually mild), not associated with significant nerve injury; the pain is described as burning and continuous and exacerbated by movement, cutaneous stimulation, or stress. Onset usually weeks after injury.

Associated Symptoms. Initially there is vasodilatation with increasing temperature, hyperhidrosis, and edema. Hyperhidrosis and reduced sympathetic activity also occur. Atrophy of skin appendages, cool, red clammy skin are variably present. Disuse atrophy of deep structures may progress to Sudeck's atrophy of bone. Aggravated by use of body part, relieved by immobilization. Sometimes follows a herniated intervertebral disk, spinal anesthesia, poliomyelitis, severe iliofemoral thrombosis, or cardiac infarction. This may appear as the shoulder-hand syndrome. Later vasospastic symptoms become prominent with persistent coldness of the affected extremity, pallor and cyanosis, Raynaud's phenomenon, atrophy of the skin and nails and loss of hair, atrophy of soft tissues and stiffness of joints. Without therapy these symptoms may persist. It is not necessary for one patient to exhibit all symptoms together. An additional limb or limbs may be affected as well.

Signs. Variable; there may be florid sympathetic hyperactivity.

Laboratory Findings. In advanced cases, roentgenograms may show atrophy of bone.

Usual Course. Persists indefinitely if untreated; small incidence of spontaneous remission.

Relief. Sympathetic block and physical therapy; sympathectomy if long-term results not achieved with repeated blocks; may respond in early phases to high doses of corticosteroids (*e.g.*, prednisone 50 mg daily).

Complications. Disuse atrophy of involved limb; suicide and drug abuse if untreated; sometimes spreads to contralateral limb.

Social and Physical Disability. Depression, inability to perform daily activities.

Pathology. Unknown.

Essential Features. Burning pain in distal extremity, usually after minor injury without nerve damage.

Differential Diagnosis. Unrecognized local pathology (fracture, strain, sprain). Causalgia, post-traumatic vasospasm or thrombosis.

Code. 203.91b (arms), 603.91b (legs).

CENTRAL PAIN (INCLUDING THALAMIC AND PSEUDOTHALAMIC PAIN) (I-6)

Definition. Diffuse unilateral pain, often burning with allodynia, hypoesthesia, hypoalgesia, hyperpathia, dysesthesiae, and neurologic signs of damage to structures that supply the affected region.

Site. Usually one half of the whole body, contralateral to a cerebral lesion; seldom the face and/or the head alone (more often one lower limb alone); sometimes the upper extremity, with or without the head; most often by far the entire contralateral half of the body or the upper and lower extremities together. In some cases the face on one side and limb(s) on the opposite side (as with bulbar) lesions).

System. Central nervous system.

Main Features. Onset is most often after age 40 in groups subject to cardiovascular disease. Pain most often appears within a few weeks to 2 years later. The pain is spontaneous, continuous, burning, stabbing, and often aching. It varies from mild to intolerable in different cases and is localized to the skin, muscle, or bone in the majority of patients. Usually constant and persistent by day, the pain is subject to exacerbations that may occur for no apparent reason or be evoked by normally nonnoxious stimuli, such as light touch, heat, cold, movements, TENS. It can be made worse by auditory or visual stimuli (*e.g.*, sudden sound or light) and by visceral activity (*e.g.*, micturition) and is often exacerbated by anxiety and emotional arousal.

Associated Symptoms and Signs. There may be various neurologic symptoms and signs, especially those typical of hemiparesis. Most often there are motor impairments and sensory deficits in the affected areas. Light touch is impaired. Allodynia and hyperpathia are almost always found and dysesthesias often occur either spontaneously or otherwise. Vasomotor and sudomotor atrophic changes are often present. Anxiety and depression commonly occur with the syndrome.

Laboratory Findings. Computed tomography scan may indicate a relevant lesion in the thalamus or elsewhere, especially the cerebral peduncles.

Usual Course. Persists indefinitely in most cases. In some, may show signs of diminution.

Relief. May be relieved by centrally active medications, such as phenothiazines and tricyclic antidepressants. Stabbing element often appears to be helped by carbamazepine or diphenyl hydantoin.

Complications. Depression, suicide.

Social and Physical Disabilities. Work impairment.

Pathology. Thalamic lesions caused by any pathological process that damages the ventral posterolateral nucleus. More than 80% of cases are due to cerebrovascular hemorrhage or occlusion. May be complication of surgery, neoplasm, trauma, multiple sclerosis. Lesions in cerebral peduncles, pons and medulla, and juxtathalamic areas may produce similar syndrome owing to comparable causes, but pain is ipsilateral in the face and contralateral to the lesion elsewhere. Within these areas the following types of cause are particularly likely to produce pain: occlusion of posteroinferior cerebellar artery; occlusion of posterior cerebral artery or of its branches to the brain stem; hematobulbia or syringobulbia; neoplasm; multiple sclerosis; trauma; and stereotaxic surgical lesions. Facial pain may also be due to bulbar lesions. Occasional cases of localized cerebral lesions producing central pain have also been reported.

Diagnostic Criteria. Spontaneous pain with allodynia, hypoesthesia, hypoalgesia, and hyperpathia with evidence of damage to the thalamus or structures or the central nervous system that supply the affected region.

Differential Diagnosis. If pain involves all of one half of body, differentiation from hysteria may be required. Pain localized to the head alone, or one limb alone, may require differentiation from other neurologic disorders. Pain from spinal lesions is not included.

Code. X03.X5c, or X03.X1c, X03.X2c, X03.X4c, X03.X8c; 003.X5c when affecting head and face; code additional entries for other areas.

SYNDROME OF SYRINGOMYELIA (I-7)

Definition. Aching or burning pain usually in a limb, commonly with muscle wasting caused by tubular cavitation gradually developing in the spinal cord.

Code. 007.X0 (face), 207.X0 (arm), 607.X0 (leg).

POLYMYALGIA RHEUMATICA (I-8)

Definition. Diffuse aching, and usually stiffness, in neck, hip girdle, or shoulder girdle, usually associated with a markedly raised sedimentation rate, sometimes associated with giant cell vasculitis, and promptly responsive to steroids.

System. Musculoskeletal.

Code. X32.X3a

FIBROSITIS OR DIFFUSE MYOFASCIAL PAIN SYNDROME (I-9)

(Nonarticular rheumatism, fibromyalgia)

Definition. Diffuse, aching musculoskeletal pain associated with multiple discrete predictable tender points and stiffness.

Site. Multiple anatomic areas.

System. Musculoskeletal (ligaments and tendons).

Main Features.

Epidemiology. Primary fibrositis, without important associated disease is uncommon compared with secondary diffuse fibrositis. It usually occurs in the 3rd to 4th decade. The sex ratio is five females to one male (5 : 1).

Pain. Widespread aching, of more than 3 months' duration, poorly circumscribed and perceived as deep, usually referred to muscle or bony prominences. Although pain in the trunk and proximal girdle is aching, distal limb pain is often perceived as associated with swelling, numbness, or stiffness. Day-to-day fluctuation in pain intensity and shifting from one area to another is characteristic, although the pain is usually continuous.

Stiffness is perceived as an increased resistance to joint movement, particularly toward the end of the range of movement. It is worse in the mornings. Both the pain and the stiffness are maximal within the broad sclerotomic and myotomic areas of reference of the lower segments of the cervical and lumbar spine. Chronic exhaustion is often marked in the morning and associated with feeling unrefreshed after rest or sleep.

Tender Points. Synonym: trigger points (TP). Discrete local areas of deep tenderness involving a variety of otherwise normal tissues are a pathognomonic feature, provided that at least 12 are present. The tender points usually lie within an area of taut muscle fibers ("taut bands") or over origins and insertions (entheses). The patient is usually unaware of the existence of these points. Palpation of them may be associated with a "jump sign," in which the patients move or cry out with minimal pressure at these points. The pressure may cause pain at a different site (area of reference), usually reproducing the pain complained of by the patient. The predictable location of these tender points and their multiplicity are essential features of the syndrome.

Associated Symptoms.

Skinfold Tenderness and Reactive Hyperemia. Rolling of the skin and subcutaneous tissue of the upper scapula region between the examiner's thumb and index finger characteristically elicits tenderness and reactive hyperemia, particularly in the general regions of deep tenderness. The distal limbs and lumbar region usually are devoid of this phenomenon of reactive hyperemia.

Autonomic Phenomena. Although a variety of autonomic phenomena are described as associated features, only reactive hyperemia or erythema is common.

Aggravating and Relieving Factors. Cold, damp weather, interrupted sleep, fatigue, mental stress, and under exercise or overexercise accentuate the widespread aching and stiffness. Local heat, massage, warm dry weather, moderate activity and exercise,and relief from stress, such as vacations, give temporary symptomatic relief.

Chronic muscle overloads may occur in settings that demand repetitive or sustained contractions, poor posture or work habits, and stress that is manifested by increased muscle tension. Chronic overload is also related to skeletal asymmetry or disproportion, dental malocclusion, ergonomically inappropriate furniture, and prolonged constrictive pressure or immobility. Trigger point sensitivity is positively correlated with a sedentary life-style; and myofascial pain with associated headache, neck pain, or low back pain is common among persons reporting many hours of TV viewing.

There may also be indirect routes of TP activation, including visceral disease (myocardial infarctions, peptic ulcer, cholelithiasis, renal colic), nerve compression, disk disease, arthritic joint involvement, and neuropathy.

Signs. See also tender points. Widespread tenderness over the trapezius muscles at the midpoint of the upper fold as well as at the second costochondral junctions is found.

Further tender points occur 1 to 2 cm distal to the lateral epicondyle; at the origin of the supraspinatus tendons, the interspinous ligaments of L4–S1, the upper outer quadrants of buttocks, and the medial fat pads of the knees.

Relief. Relief may be provided by reassurance and explanation about the nature of the illness and possible mechanism of pain, by symptomatic treatment with heat or massage, and by encouraging moderate activity. Low-dose amitriptyline may help.

Pathology. No consistent specific or nonspecific pathological feature has been demonstrated in the tissues. Thermography may demonstrate patterns of skin thermal radiation correlated with tender points.

Some authors imply an association between chronic cervical and lumbar strain and the frequent occurrence of tender points and areas of aching that are found in the broad sclerotomal and myotomal reference areas of the lower cervical and lumbar segments. It is in these motion segments that degenerative changes maximally occur.

Etiology. Unknown. One view holds that physical or mental stress or fatigue exacerbate a pathophysiologic dysfunction. Another view suggests that this syndrome represents epiphenomena and that the basic problem is altered behavior of the lower cervical and lumbar motion segments where postural stress and mobility requirements are high.

Experimental reproduction of the diffuse fibrositis syndrome was obtained in some healthy university students by means of deprivation of slow-wave non-REM sleep.

Diagnostic Criteria.

Primary Diffuse Fibrositis Syndrome. (1) Widespread aching of more than 3 months' duration; (2) skinroll tenderness over the upper scapular region; (3) disturbed sleep, with morning fatigue and stiffness; (4) demonstrated bilateral tender points in at least six areas, midpoint of upper fold of trapezius; superolateral aspect of 2nd costochondral junction; anterior aspect of interspinous spaces of C4–6; lateral epicondyle within proximal muscle belly of the long finger extensor; interspinous ligament region of L4–S1; upper outer buttock over gluteus medius; medial knee fat pad, overlying medial collateral ligament, proximal to joint line; and (5) absence of laboratory evidence of inflammation or muscle damage.

Note: Criteria 1, 4, and 5 are essential to establish a diagnosis of primary diffuse fibrositis syndrome. Criteria 1 and 4 only are needed for a diagnosis of secondary diffuse fibrositis syndrome.

Code. X33.X8a.

References. Cyriax, J.: Textbook of Orthopaedic Medicine, vol. 1. Fam, A.G., and Smythe, H.A.: Musculoskeletal chest wall pain. Can. Med. Assoc. J., *133*:379, 1985. Hier, D.B., and Spector, R.H.: Neuropsychiatric disorders. *In* Samuels, M.A. (ed.): Manual of Neurologic Therapeutics, 3rd ed. Boston, Little, Brown, 1985. Kellgren, J.H.: Observations on referred pain from muscle. Clin. Sci., *3*:175, 1938. Ochoa, J., and Torebjörk, H.E.: Pain from skin and muscle. Pain, *1*[Suppl.]:88, 1981. Reynolds, M.D.: The development of the concept of fibrositis. J. Hist. Med. Allied Sci., *38*:5, 1983. Simons, D.G.: Myofascial pain syndrome. *In* Basmajian, J., and Kirby, R.L., (eds.): Medical Rehabilitation, pp. 209–214.

NOTE: SPECIFIC MYOFASCIAL PAIN SYNDROMES

Synonyms: Fibrositis (syndrome), myalgia, muscular rheumatism, nonarticular rheumatism.

Specific myofascial syndromes may occur in any voluntary muscle with referred pain, local and referred tenderness, and a tense shortened muscle. The pain has the same qualities as that of the diffuse syndromes. Passive stretch or strong voluntary contraction in the shortened position of the muscle is painful. Satellite tender points may develop within the area of pain reference of the initial trigger point. Other phenomena resemble those of the diffuse syndromes. Diagnosis depends on the demonstration of a trigger point (tender point) and reproduction of the pain by maneuvers that place stress on proximal structures or nerve roots. This suggests that the syndrome is an epiphenomenon secondary to proximal pathology such as nerve root irritation. Relief may be obtained by stretch and spray techniques, tender point compression, or tender point injection, including the use of "dry" needling.

Some individual syndromes are described here (*e.g.*, sternocleidomastoid and trapezius). Others may be coded as required according to individual muscles that are identified as being a site of trouble.

RHEUMATOID ARTHRITIS (I-10)

Definition. Aching, burning joint pain caused by systemic inflammatory disease affecting all synovial joints, muscle, ligaments, and tendons in accordance with diagnostic criteria below.

Site. Symmetrical involvement of small and large joints.

System. Musculoskeletal system and connective tissue.

Main Features. Diffuse aching, burning pain in joints, usually moderately severe; usually intermittent with exacerbations and remissions. The condition affects about 1% of the population and is more common in women. Diagnostic criteria of the American Rheumatism Association describe and further define the illness. They are as follows: (1) morning stiffness; (2) pain on motion or tenderness at one joint or more; (3) swelling of one joint; (4) swelling of at least one other joint; and (5) symmetrical joint swelling.

All of the above have to be of at least 6 weeks' duration. Further criteria include (6) subcutaneous nodules; (7) typical radiographic changes; (8) positive test for rheumatoid factor in the serum; (9) a poor response in the mucin clot test in the synovial fluid; (10) synovial histopathology consistent with rheumatoid arthritis; and (11) characteristic nodule pathology.

Classic rheumatoid arthritis requires seven criteria to be diagnosed. Definite rheumatoid arthritis may be diagnosed on five criteria and probable rheumatoid arthritis on three criteria.

Associated Symptoms. Morning stiffness usually greater than half an hour's duration; chronic fatigue. Inflammation may affect eyes, heart, lungs.

Signs. Tenderness, swelling, loss of range of motion of joints, ligaments, tendons. Chronic destruction and joint deformity are common.

Laboratory Findings. Anemia, raised ESR (sedimentation rate), rheumatoid factor in the serum in the majority of cases.

Relief. Usually good relief of pain and stiffness can be obtained with nonsteroidal anti-inflammatory drugs, but some patients require therapy with gold or other agents.

Pathology. Chronic inflammatory process of synovium, ligaments, or tendons. There may be systemic vasculitis.

Essential Features. Aching, burning joint pain with characteristic pathology.

Differential Diagnosis. Systemic lupus erythematosus, palindromic rheumatism, mixed connective tissue disease, psoriatic arthropathy, calcium pyrophosphate deposition disease, seronegative spondyloarthropathies, hemochromatosis (rarely).

Code. X34.X3a.

OSTEOARTHRITIS (I-11)

Definition. Deep, aching pain caused by a "degenerative" process in a single joint or multiple joints, as either a primary phenomenon or secondary to other disease.

Site. Joints most commonly involved are distal and proximal interphalangeal joints of the hands, the carpometacarpal thumb joint, the knees, the hips, and cervical and lumbar spines. Many joints or only a few joints may be affected, (*e.g.*, at C5 or L5, the hip or knee); proximal joints may be involved alone or only distal interphalangeal joints.

System. Musculoskeletal.

Main Features. There is deep, aching pain that may be severe as the disease progresses. The pain is felt at the joint or joints involved but may be referred to adjacent muscle groups. Usually the pain increases in proportion to the amount of use of the joint. As the disease progresses, there is pain at rest and later nocturnal pain. The pain tends to become more continuous as the severity of the process increases. Stiffness occurs after protracted periods of inactivity and in the morning but lasts for less than half an hour as a rule.

There is a discrepancy between radiologic prevalence and clinical complaints. Radiologic evidence of osteoarthritis occurs in 80% of individuals over 55 years of age. Only about 25% of those with radiographic changes report symptoms. The incidence increases with age. There is a greater prevalence relatively in men under the age of 45 compared with women, and in women over the age of 45 compared with men.

Code. X38.X6a.

CALCIUM PYROPHOSPHATE DEPOSITION DISEASE* (CPPD) (I-12)

Definition. Attacks of aching, sharp and throbbing pain with acute or chronic recurrent inflammation of a joint caused by calcium pyrophosphate crystals.

Code. X38.X0 or X38.X5a.

GOUT (I-13)

Definition. Paroxysmal attacks of aching, sharp or throbbing pain, usually severe and owing to inflammation of a joint caused by monosodium urate crystals.

**Editor's note:* Only major features of pain syndromes are reproduced in Appendix B from here onward. The reader should consult Pain, 3(Suppl.):25–213, 1986 for full details.

Code. X38.X5b.

HEMOPHILIAC ARTHROPATHY (I-14)

Definition. Bouts of acute, constant, nagging, burning, bursting, and incapacitating pain or chronic, aching, nagging, gnawing, and grating pain occurring in patients with congenital blood coagulation factor deficiencies and secondary to hemarthrosis.

Code. X34.X0a.

PAIN OF PSYCHOLOGICAL ORIGIN: MUSCLE TENSION PAIN (I-16)

Definition. Virtually continuous pain in any part of the body owing to sustained muscle contraction and provoked by emotional causes or by persistent overuse of particular muscles.

Code. X33.X7b. *Note:* (b) coding used to allow the (a) coding to be employed if an acute syndrome needs to be specified.

PAIN OF PSYCHOLOGICAL ORIGIN: DELUSIONAL OR HALLUCINATORY PAIN (I-16)

Definition. Pain of psychological origin and attributed by the patient to a specific delusional cause.

Code. X1X.X9a. X = to be completed individually according to circumstances in each case.

PAIN OF PSYCHOLOGICAL ORIGIN: HYSTERICAL OR HYPOCHONDRIACAL (I-16)

Definition. Pain specifically attributable to the thought processes, emotional state, or personality of the patient in the absence of an organic or delusional cause or tension mechanism.

Code. X1X.X9b.

A NOTE ON FACTITIOUS ILLNESS AND MALINGERING (I-17)

Factitious illness is of concern to psychiatrists because both it and malingering are frequently associated with personality disorder. Physicians in any discipline may encounter the problem in differential diagnosis. No coding is given for pain in these circumstances because it will be either induced by physical change or counterfeit. In the first instance it can be coded under the appropriate physical heading. In the second case the complaint of pain does not represent the presence of pain. The code for factitious illness and malingering in the International Classification of Diseases may be used, viz: -V65.2

RELATIVELY LOCALIZED SYNDROMES

GROUP II: NEURALGIAS OF THE HEAD AND FACE

TRIGEMINAL NEURALGIA (TIC DOULOUREUX) (II-1)

Definition. Sudden severe brief stabbing recurrent pains in the distribution of one or more branches of the 5th cranial nerve.

Site. Strictly limited to the distribution of the 5th nerve. Usually involves one branch; may involve two. More common on the right side.

System. Nervous system.

Main Features.

Prevalence. Relatively uncommon. Incidence: men 2.7, women 5.0/100,000/annum in U.S.A.

Age of Onset. After fourth decade, with peak onset fifth and sixth decades; earlier onset does occur but is extremely uncommon before age 30.

Sex Ratio. Women affected more commonly than men in ratio of approximately 3 : 2.

Quality. Sharp, agonizing electric shocklike stabs of pain felt superficially in the skin or buccal mucosa, triggered by light mechanical contact from a more or less restricted site (trigger point or trigger zone) usually of brief duration—seconds—with repetition in bursts for several seconds to a minute or two, followed by a refractory period of 30 seconds or so up to a few minutes.

Time Pattern. Episodes may occur at intervals of several or many times daily or, in rare instances, succeed one another almost continuously. Periodicity is characteristic, with episodes occurring as described for a few weeks to a month or two, followed by pain-free interval of months or years and then recurrence of another bout.

Intensity. Extremely severe, probably one of the most intense of all acute pains.

Usual Duration. As described above.

Associated Symptoms. Occasionally a mild flush may be noted during episodes. Precipitated by mechanical stimuli, as noted, but contrary to earlier reports no seasonal predominance. No particular aggravating factors; some relief obtained by firm pressure as with the hands around but not touching the trigger point.

Signs and Laboratory Findings. In true trigeminal neuralgia, apart from the trigger point, neurologic examination is negative. In symptomatic trigeminal neuralgia, areas of hypoesthesia on the face or absence of the corneal reflex may occur; if sensory deficit is detected, a lesion is probably responsible.

Usual Course. Recurrent bouts over periods of years interspersed with more or less prolonged asymptomatic phases.

Complications. None.

Social and Physical Disability. Only as related to the pain episodes.

Pathology. When present always involves the peripheral trigeminal (primary afferent) neuron. Impingement on root by vascular loops, etc. appears to be most common cause. Demyelination and hypermyelination on electron microscopy.

Summary of Essential Features and Diagnostic Criteria. Sudden, transient, intense bouts of superficially located pain, strictly confined to the distribution of one or more divisions of the trigeminal nerve, usually precipitated by light mechanical activation of a trigger point or area. No sensory or reflex deficit detectable by routine neurologic testing.

Differential Diagnosis. Must be differentiated from symptomatic trigeminal neuralgia, owing to a small tumor such as an epidermoid or small meningioma involving either the root or the ganglion. Sensory and/or reflex deficit in the face may be detected in a significant proportion of such cases. Differential diagnosis between trigeminal neuralgia of mandibular division and glossopharyngeal neuralgia may, in rare instances, be difficult.

Code. 006.X8a.

SECONDARY NEURALGIA (TRIGEMINAL) FROM CENTRAL NERVOUS SYSTEM LESIONS (II-2)

Definition. Sudden severe brief stabbing recurrent pains in the distribution of one or more branches of the fifth cranial nerve, attributable to a recognized lesion, such as tumor or aneurysm.

Code. 006.X4 (tumor) or 006.X0 (aneurysm).

SECONDARY TRIGEMINAL NEURALGIA FROM FACIAL TRAUMA (II-3)

Definition. Chronic throbbing or burning pain with paroxysmal exacerbations in the distribution of a peripheral trigeminal nerve subsequent to injury.

Code. 006.X1.

ACUTE HERPES ZOSTER (TRIGEMINAL) (II-4)

Definition. Pain associated with acute herpetic lesions in the distribution of a branch or branches of the 5th cranial nerve.

Code. 002.X2a.

POSTHERPETIC NEURALGIA (TRIGEMINAL) (II-5)

Definition. Chronic pain with skin changes in the distribution of one or more roots of the 5th cranial nerve subsequent to acute herpes zoster.

Site. Face. Usually distribution of first (ophthalmic) division.

System. Trigeminal nerve.

Main Features.

Prevalence. Relatively infrequent.

Age of Onset. Sixth and later decades.

Sex Ratio. More common in males.

Quality. Burning, tearing, itching dysesthesia and crawling dysesthesias in skin of affected area. Exacerbated by mechanical contact.

Time Pattern. Constantly present with exacerbations. May last for years but spontaneous subsidence is not uncommon.

Intensity. Usually moderate, but constancy and intractability, in many instances, contribute to intolerable nature of complaint.

Usual Duration. Months to years.

Associated Symptoms. Depression, irritability.

Signs and Laboratory Findings. Cutaneous scarring, loss of normal pigmentation in area of earlier herpetic eruption. Hypoesthesia to touch, hypoalgesia, hyperesthesia to touch and hyperpathia may occur.

Usual Course. Chronic, intractable; may last for years. Some cases "burn out" spontaneously.

Complications. None.

Social and Physical Disability. Severe impairment of most or all social activities because of constant pain. Suicide occasionally.

Pathology. Loss of many large fibers in affected sensory nerve. Chronic inflammatory changes in trigeminal ganglion and demyelination in root entry zone.

Summary of Essential Features and Diagnostic Criteria. Chronic burning, dysesthesias, paresthesias, and intractable cutaneous pain in distribution of the ophthalmic division of the trigeminal associated with cutaneous scarring and history of herpetic eruption in an elderly patient.

Differential Diagnosis. The syndrome is usually characteristic. Other conditions (*e.g.*, metastatic carcinoma) under treatment may promote its occurrence.

Code. 003.X2b.

GENICULATE NEURALGIA (7TH CRANIAL NERVE): RAMSAY HUNT SYNDROME (II-6)

Definition. Severe lancinating pains felt deeply in external auditory canal subsequent to an attack of acute herpes zoster.

Code. 006.X2.

GLOSSOPHARYNGEAL NEURALGIA (9TH CRANIAL NERVE) (II-7)

Definition. Sudden, severe, brief stabbing recurrent pains in the distribution of the glossopharyngeal nerve.

Code. 006.X8b.

NEURALGIA OF THE SUPERIOR LARYNGEAL NERVE (VAGUS NERVE NEURALGIA) (II-8)

Definition. Paroxysms of unilateral lancinating pain radiating from the side of the thyroid cartilage or pyriform sinus, to the angle of the jaw and occasionally to the ear.

Code. 006.X8c.

OCCIPITAL NEURALGIA (II-9)

Definition. Pain, usually deep and aching, in the distribution of the 2nd cervical dorsal root.

Site. Suboccipital area, unilateral in the 2nd cervical root distribution from occiput to vertex. May radiate still further forward, see below.

System. Nervous.

Main Features.

Prevalence. Quite common; no epidemiological data; most often follows acceleration/deceleration injuries.

Age off Onset. From second decade to old age. More common in 3rd to 5th decades.

Sex Ratio. Women more frequently affected, but statistical data lacking.

Quality. Deep, aching, pressure pain in suboccipital area, sometimes stabbing also. Unilateral usually; may radiate toward vertex or to fronto-orbital area and/or face.

Time Pattern. Irregular, usually worse later in day.

Intensity. From moderate to severe.

Associated Symptoms. Hyperesthesia of scalp. A variety of symptoms such as vertigo, tinnitus, tears, etc. have been described in some cases, but probably these are transitional forms to cluster headache. Nerve block may give effective relief.

Signs and Laboratory Findings. Diminished sensation to pinprick in area of C2 and tenderness of great occipital nerve may be found.

Usual Course. Chronic, recurrent episodes. May cease spontaneously on occasion.

Complications. None.

Social and Physical Disability. Only as related to pain episodes.

Pathology. Unknown. Perhaps related to increased muscle activity in cervical muscles. May be secondary to trauma, including flexion-extension (whiplash) injury.

Summary of Essential Features and Diagnostic Criteria. Intermittent episodes of deep, aching, and sometimes stabbing pain in suboccipital area on one side. Marked tendency to chronicity. Often associated with tender posterior cervical muscles. Can be bilateral.

Differential Diagnosis. Cluster headaches, posterior fossa and high cervical tumor, herniated cervical disk, uncomplicated flexion-extension injury. Metastatic neoplasm at the base of the skull.

Code. 004.X8 or 004.X1 if subsequent to trauma.

References. Behrman, S.: Brit. Med. J., *286*:1312, 1983.

GROUP III: CRANIOFACIAL PAIN OF MUSCULOSKELETAL ORIGIN

ACUTE TENSION HEADACHE (III-1)*

Definition. Acute, continuous unilateral or diffuse head pain related to anxiety, depression, or emotional tension.

Code. 034.X7a.

TENSION HEADACHE: CHRONIC FORM (SCALP MUSCLE CONTRACTION HEADACHE) (III-2)

Definition. Virtually continuous head pain, usually symmetrical, associated with muscle tension, anxiety, and "depression." Exacerbations with increased pounding headache, nausea, and vomiting are typical; usually responds to measures for treatment of anxiety and depression, including particularly antidepressant medication.

Code. 033.X7b.

*Note: all greatly abbreviated. See Pain, 3(Suppl.):217, 1986.

TEMPOROMANDIBULAR PAIN AND DYSFUNCTION SYNDROME (III-3)

(also called myofascial pain dysfunction syndrome)

Definition. Aching in the muscles of mastication plus, in some cases, an occasional brief severe pain on chewing, possibly leading to restricted jaw movement.

Summary of Essential Features and Diagnostic Criteria. Muscle tenderness; temporomandibular joint clicking; mandibular dysfunction; high psychophysiologic stress response. Dull ache with severe exacerbations. Frequently long standing. Associated with trismus, clicking, locking of the joint, and bruxism. Related to adverse life events. Association with malocclusion unproven.

Code. 034.X8a.

References. Feinmann, C., Harris, M., and Cawley, R.M.: Psychogenic facial pain. Presentation and treatment. Brit. Med. J., *288*:436, 1984.

OSTEOARTHRITIS OF THE TEMPOROMANDIBULAR JOINT (III-4)

Definition. Degenerative change, possibly leading to the masticatory dysfunction syndrome and associated pain.

Code. 033.X6.

RHEUMATOID ARTHRITIS OF THE TEMPOROMANDIBULAR JOINT (III-5)

Definition. Part of the systemic disorder of rheumatoid arthritis with granulation tissue proliferating onto the articular surface.

Code. 032.X3b.

GROUP IV: LESIONS OF THE EAR, NOSE, AND ORAL CAVITY

MAXILLARY SINUSITIS (IV-1)

Definition. Constant burning pain with zygomatic and dental tenderness from inflammation of the maxillary sinus.

Code. 031.X2a.

ODONTALGIA: TOOTHACHE 1. OWING TO DENTINO-ENAMEL DEFECTS (IV-2)

Definition. Short-lasting, diffuse orofacial pain owing to dentino-enamel defects and evoked by local stimuli.

Code. 034.X2b.

ODONTALGIA: TOOTHACHE 2. PULPITIS (IV-3)

Definition. Orofacial pain owing to pulpal inflammation, often evoked by local stimuli.

Code. 031.X2c.

ODONTALGIA: TOOTHACHE 3. PERIAPICAL PERIODONTITIS AND ABSCESS (IV-4)

Definition. Orofacial pain owing to the causes named and having a graduated response to local stimulation.

Code. 031.X2d.

ODONTALGIA: TOOTHACHE 4. TOOTH PAIN NOT ASSOCIATED WITH LESIONS (ATYPICAL ODONTALGIA) (IV-5)

Definition. Severe throbbing pain in the tooth without major pathology.

Code. 034.X8b.

GLOSSODYNIA AND SORE MOUTH (ALSO KNOWN AS BURNING TONGUE OR ORAL DYSESTHESIA) (IV-6)

Definition. Burning pain in the tongue from any cause.

Code. 041.X5 (if known) or 041.X8 (alternative).

CRACKED TOOTH SYNDROME (IV-7)

Definition. Brief, sharp pain in a tooth, often not understood until a piece fractures off the tooth.

Code. 034.X1.

DRY SOCKET (IV-8)

Definition. Unilateral pain in the jaw, usually lower, usually associated with additional tenderness owing to submandibular lymphadenitis after dental extraction and caused by a localized osteitis.

Code. 031.X1.

GROUP V: PRIMARY HEADACHE SYNDROMES*

CLASSIC MIGRAINE (V-1)

Definition. Unilateral, throbbing head pain often with a prodromal state and usually preceded by an aura that is usually visual; nausea, vomiting, and photophobia often accompany the pain.

Code. 004.X7a.

COMMON MIGRAINE (V-2)

Common migraine has the same characteristics as classic migraine with the following differences.

Definition. Unilateral, throbbing head pain often with a prodromal state but without a distinct aura, usually accompanied by nausea, vomiting, and photophobia.

Code. 004.X7b.

MIGRAINE VARIANTS (V-3)

Hemiplegic migraine, migraine accompagnée, basilar migraine, ophthalmoplegic migraine, retinal migraine.

Code. 004.X7c for all except migraine cervicale.

CAROTIDYNIA (V-4)

Definition. A form of migraine in which the pain occurs in the distribution of the external carotid artery, thus being experienced in the head, face, and neck.

Code. 004.X7d.

MIXED HEADACHE (V-5)

Mixed headache probably refers, in most cases, either to migraine with interparoxysmal headache or to chronic ten-

*Abbreviated. See Pain, 3(Suppl.):217, 1986.

sion headache as described above. The term should therefore be avoided when possible.

Code. 003.X7b.

CLUSTER HEADACHE (V-6)

Definition. Unilateral pain principally in the ocular, frontal, and temporal areas recurring in separate bouts with daily attacks for several months, usually with rhinorrhea or lacrimation.

Code. 004.X8a.

CHRONIC PAROXYSMAL HEMICRANIA (CHRONIC STAGE) (V-7)

Definition. Multiple daily attacks of pain usually in females and principally in ocular, frontal, and temporal areas by day and night, usually with lacrimation and nasal stuffiness and/or rhinorrhea, with absolute relief from indomethacin.

Code. 006.X8c.

CHRONIC CLUSTER HEADACHE (V-8)

The features of chronic cluster headache are the same as those for cluster headache with the following differences.

Definition. Bouts of unilateral pain usually in males, principally in the ocular, frontal, and temporal areas occurring at least twice a week for more than one year.

Relief. The same measures are effective as for cluster headache, but lithium carbonate tends to work relatively better for chronic cluster headache.

Code. 004.X8b.

CLUSTER-TIC SYNDROME (V-9)

Definition. The association of the features of cluster headache and tic douloureux (trigeminal neuralgia), whether the two entities occur concurrently or separated in time in the same individual.

Code. 006.X8d.

POST-TRAUMATIC HEADACHE (V-10)

Definition. Continuous, or nearly continuous, diffusely distributed head pain associated with personality changes involving irritability, loss of concentration ability, dizziness, visual accommodation problems, change in tolerance to ethyl alcohol, loss of libido and depression, and with or without post-traumatic stress disorder and with or without post-traumatic migraine, after head injury.

Code. 002.X1.

References. Tyler, G.S., McNeely, H.E., and Dick, M.L.: Treatment of post-traumatic headache with amitriptyline. Headache. *20*:213, 1980.

GROUP VI: PAIN OF PSYCHOLOGICAL ORIGIN IN THE HEAD AND FACE

DELUSIONAL OR HALLUCINATORY PAIN (VI-1)

Code. 01X.X9a.

HYSTERICAL OR HYPOCHONDRIACAL PAIN (VI-2)

Code. 01X.X9b.

GROUP VII: SUBOCCIPITAL AND CERVICAL MUSCULOSKELETAL DISORDERS

MYOFASCIAL SYNDROME: CERVICAL SPRAIN OR CERVICAL HYPEREXTENSION INJURY (VII-1)

("Whiplash")

Definition. Dull, aching pain, in back of head or neck or both in an area of reference from one or more muscles of the occiput and neck and with a trigger point usually outside the painful area from hyperextension injury.

Site. Back of head or neck or both, with spread in area of the affected muscle (*e.g.*, trapezius). Particularly common just medial to the right or left inferior scapula pole.

System. Musculoskeletal.

Associated Symptoms. The pain is aggravated by motion of the cervical spine, tension, sitting, reading; relieved by mild analgesics, cervical collar, heat; more prolonged symptoms helped by cervical traction, biofeedback. Sometimes there is dizziness and tinnitus. Pain may shift to the axilla, arm, or anterior upper chest, or inferior scapula pole.

Signs and Laboratory Findings. Limited motion of cervical spine, especially toward flexion and rotation. Tenderness to palpation in trapezius and posterior cervical spine (diffuse). Muscle spasm and trigger points in one or more muscles of occiput or neck. Prolonged or repetitive use of the shoulder girdle muscles (*e.g.*, carrying dishes or washing them may induce radiation of pain into the upper extremity). Push/pull activities (*e.g.*, vacuum cleaning) may aggravate pain also.

Laboratory findings normal.

X-rays. Normal, although loss of usual cervical lordosis common; lateral flexion/extension views may reveal motion at one or two segments as opposed to all.

Usual Course. Gradual complete recovery over a 1 to 3-month period. The emphasis is on regaining a normal range of motion concurrently with symptomatic treatment. If the initial symptoms are severe, or premorbid personality disorder exists, the symptoms may persist or even increase. In a group of patients they persist longer than 3 years, even independently of litigation.

Complications. Reactive depression, unemployment. Role changes may occur.

Social and Physical Disability. Significant stress may be experienced by the patient or family if endurance at work is decreased and social and financial problems follow.

Pathology. Unknown; may represent injury to ligamentous tissue and/or skeletal muscle.

Summary of Essential Features and Diagnostic Criteria. Posterior/cervical/upper trapezius—mild/moderate pain precipitated by a traumatic event. Differential diagnosis primarily one of excluding disk herniation or cervical fracture.

Differential Diagnosis. Degenerative disk; brachial neuritis; cervical disk herniation; pancoast tumor; cervical fracture; infection.

Codes. 133.X1, 233.X1.

References. MacNab, I.: The whiplash syndrome. Clin. Neurosurg., *20*:232, 1973. Mendelson, G.: Not "cured by a verdict." Effect of legal settlement on compensation claimants. Med. J. Aust., 2:132, 1982. Merskey, H.: Psychiatry and the cervical sprain syndrome. Can. Med. Assoc. J., *130*:1119, 1984.

MYOFASCIAL SYNDROME: STERNOCLEIDOMASTOID MUSCLE (VII-2)

Definition. Continuous aching pain sometimes with autonomic phenomena that may arise from hyperactive trigger points (TP) in either the sternal or clavicular division of the muscle. Each will produce a different pattern of referred phenomena.

System. Musculoskeletal.

Site. Sternocleidomastoid muscle.

Main Features. Pain is usually described as dull and aching. The associated symptoms vary in intensity from mild to disabling but generally persist over a period of weeks to months, more intense at times of stress or seeming to recur without a known precipitating cause. Sternocleidomastoid TPs are the most commonly overlooked source of multiple symptoms.

Sternal Division. (1) Trigger points (TP) in the lower third may refer continuous, dull, aching pain to the upper portion of the sternum so that a paroxysmal dry cough will be produced; (2) trigger points in the middle level refer pain across the cheek into the maxilla, over the supraorbital ridge, deep into the orbit, sometimes into the external auditory canal. Along the inner margin TP will refer pain to the pharynx and back of tongue (during the act of swallowing), creating a sore throat, and to the tip of the chin; and (3) trigger points in the upper third refer pain to the occipital ridge behind but not close to the ear, and the vertex of the head along with surrounding scalp tenderness.

Clavicular Division. (1) Trigger points located in the middle level refer pain to the frontal forehead area, which, when severe, crosses the midline and becomes bilateral; and (2) trigger points located in the upper level refer pain ipsilaterally deep into the ear and posterior auricular zone. Occasionally there may be poorly localized pain ipsilaterally in the cheek and molars.

Associated Symptoms.

Sternal Division. Autonomic phenomena are experienced in the ipsilateral eye and nose. Eye symptoms may include increased lacrimation; conjunctival reddening secondary to vascular engorgement; apparent ptosis owing to spasm of the orbicularis oculi muscle such that to look upward the head must be tilted backward; visual disturbances such as blurred vision and dimming of perceived light intensity. Nasal symptoms consist of coryza and maxillary sinus congestion. Decreased hearing may also occur on the ipsilateral side of the affected muscle.

Clavicular Division. Autonomic phenomena are experienced as localized sweating and vasoconstriction in the frontal forehead area.

Proprioceptive disturbances may be numerous and can be more disabling themselves than the referred pain. Possible symptoms include, among others,, postural dizziness, motion sickness, disequilibrium (sudden falling when bending/stooping and ataxia), occasional vertigo (on either sudden rotations of the head or after sustained periods wherein the head has been tilted to one side), and, in severe cases, syncope. Nausea and vomiting may also occur. These changes create a state wherein there are exaggerated postural responses (*e.g.*, while looking downward the patient falls forward and while looking up the patient falls backward). Alone or together these disturbances may interfere with daily functions.

Satellite Trigger Points. Satellite TP are usually found in such nearby muscles as scaleni, levator scapulae, trapezius, and splenius cervicis. In the zone of referred pain, satellite TP may occur in the following muscles: masseter, temporalis, orbicularis oculi, and frontalis.

Physical Examination. Examination should reveal palpable band(s), area(s) of deep tenderness, and a local twitch response. Marked limitation of rotation and flexion may occur.

Pathology. See myofascial pain syndrome, I-9.

Etiology. SCM trigger points may be activated through mechanical overload in situations where there are protracted periods of neck extension (*e.g.*, overhead work, sports overuse, and accidental injury [whiplash]). Other potential acute precipitants include sleeping on two pillows, whereby the neck is flexed, reading in bed with a light placed to one side, cocking the head to avoid glare or improve hearing, compression from a tight collar or necktie.

Chronic stress can result from the following: postural stress owing to deformity or an injury that acts to restrict upper extremity movement. The former may arise from either a short leg or small hemipelvis. The latter would result in awkward compensatory neck positioning. Other sources of chronic overload may arise through paradoxical breathing or chronic cough, which would then strain the accessory muscles of respiration.

Differential Diagnosis. Vascular headache, trigeminal neuralgia, Horner's syndrome, congenital torticollis, and other neurologic disease; Ménière's disease, other vestibular disease; nonvestibular sources of dizziness (*e.g.*, internal carotid artery stenosis, hypertension, intracranial tumor/aneurysm, drug side-effects, excess ear wax impinging on the temporomandibular joint; and conversion hysteria.

Code. 132.X7a, 232.X7a.

MYOFASCIAL SYNDROME: TRAPEZIUS MUSCLE (VII-3)

Definition. Dull, aching, continuous pain arising from hypersensitive trigger points (TP) in the upper, middle, or lower portions of the trapezius muscle.

Site. Trapezius muscle.

System. Musculoskeletal.

Main Features. Continuous, dull aching or burning pain with myofascial trigger points in the affected area, often bilateral but more on one side. There are seven potential sites for their development throughout the length of the muscle. There are potentially two TP in each of the upper, middle, and lower portions of the muscle. A seventh is also possible, although seldom present in the middle portion of the muscle.

Upper Trapezius. Trigger points (TP) refer pain unilaterally upward along the posterolateral aspect of the neck to the mastoid process and the posteroinferior area behind the ear. When intense, the pain can extend cross to the other side of the head, where it concentrates in the temple area. From there, it may travel to the back of the orbit, the angle of the jaw, the lower molar teeth, and the pinna of the ear. Complaints may include any of the following: posterolateral neck pain, temporal headache, a stiff neck, and intolerance to heavy clothing.

Middle Trapezius. TP here cause local pain or referred pain in the posterior cervical region and the top of the acromion process.

Lower Trapezius. TP here cause local pain and refer pain to the following areas: the high cervical region of the paraspinal muscles, adjacent mastoid area, the acromion, and the suprascapular region. In addition, the pain may be referred to the medial border of the scapula.

Associated Symptoms.

Entrapments. (1) Greater occipital nerve: Tautness of the trapezius muscle can create a shearing stress that may contribute, but alone be insufficient, to entrap the greater occipital nerve; and (2) spinal accessory nerve: If this is entrapped by sternocleidomastoid muscle fibers, the trapezius muscle will appear weakened on examination.

Satellite Trigger Points. These may develop in temporalis and occipitalis muscles.

Signs.

Standing Posture. The patient may develop an abnormal stance wherein there is bilateral shoulder elevation with a slight tilting of the head toward the more affected side.

Seated Posture. The patient will usually sit with arms crossed and chin cradled.

Behavior. The patient may rub the muscle in an attempt to reduce the pain as he may also move his head about in an attempt to stretch out the muscle and thereby reduce the pain.

Pathology. See myofascial pain syndrome (I-9).

Etiology. The antigravity function may be overlooked by any activity that requires the trapezius to carry the weight of the homolateral arm for an extended period. A few such examples would be telephoning, sitting without adequate armrest support, holding the forearms up to reach a high typewriter. Chronic overloads may appear as a cumulative stress from any of the following: clothing and accessories (narrow brassiere straps, shoulder bags, backpacks); activities that involve prolonged periods of shoulder elevation (long telephone calls, playing of the violin); and holding the head far to one side in a fixed position for an extended period. Cervical radiculopathies can, as part of their sequelae, result in the development of TP in the upper trapezius muscle.

Middle Trapezius. This part of the muscle may become overloaded when the arm is held up and forward for extended periods. An example of this would be the driving of a car with both hands held gripping the top of the steering wheel, creating a round-shouldered posture.

Lower Trapezius. This can be overloaded through long periods of bending and reaching forward. An example of such an activity would be sitting with the chin supported by the hand, with the elbow resting on the chest, because of inadequate armrest support.

Code. 132.X7b, 232.X7b.

STYLOHYOID PROCESS SYNDROME (EAGLE'S SYNDROME) (VII-4)

Definition. Pain after trauma in the region of a calcified stylohyoid ligament.

Code. 036.X6.

GROUP VIII: VISCERAL PAIN IN THE NECK

CARCINOMA OF THYROID (VIII-1)

Definition. Pain in the thyroid gland, aggravated by palpation and associated with an adherent neoplastic mass.

Code. 172.X4.

CARCINOMA OF LARYNX (VIII-2)

Definition. An aching soreness in the throat, aggravated by swallowing with hoarseness and dysphagia.

Code. 122.X4.

TUBERCULOSIS OF LARYNX (VIII-3)

Definition. A painful irritation in the throat on air flow during breathing, coughing, and swallowing owing to tuberculosis lesions.

Code. 123.X2.

GROUP IX: PAIN OF NEUROLOGIC ORIGIN IN NECK, SHOULDER, AND UPPER EXTREMITY

PROLAPSED DISK (IX-1)

Definition. Pain in the distribution of a dermatome owing to a prolapsed intervertebral disk.

Essential Features. Segmental pain aggravated by coughing, sneezing, and neck movements and relieved by neck traction. Sensory deficit and diminished deep tendon reflexes at appropriate levels.

Differential Diagnosis. Osteoarthritic changes, fracture, abscess, intraspinal, vertebral, and superior pulmonary sulcus tumors, traumatic avulsion of nerve root and brachial plexus lesions, syringomyelia, herpes zoster, tuberculosis, syphilis, and transverse myelitis.

Code. 203.X6a (arm). *Note:* Because of similar codings with other syndromes, a, b, or c is used in the sixth digit place to distinguish them from each other.

OSTEOPHYTE: CERVICAL SPONDYLOSIS (IX-2)

Definition. Pain in the distribution of a dermatome owing to protrusion of a vertebral bony spur.

Code. 203.X6b.

INTRA-SPINAL TUMOR (IX-3)

Definition. Neck pain or dermatomal pain or both, associated with intraspinal tumor, aggravated by traction, coughing, or sneezing.

Code. 202.X4a.

FRACTURE OR COLLAPSE OF CERVICAL VERTEBRAE (IX-4)

Definition. Neck pain and dermatomal pain, or both, associated with fracture.

Code. 203.X1b.

EPIDURAL ABSCESS (IX-5)

Definition. Pain at site of infection, exacerbated by movement, with consequent spasm of erector spinae muscles and root pains after 2 to 3 days owing to abscess.

Code. 202.X2a.

VERTEBRAL TUMOR (IX-6)

Definition. Neck pain and tenderness followed by radiculalgia owing to primary or metastatic tumor.

Code. 202.X4b.

HERPES ZOSTER: ACUTE (IX-7)

Definition. Pain associated with acute herpetic lesions in a dermatomal distribution.

Code. 203.X2a.

POSTHERPETIC NEURALGIA (IX-8)

Definition. Chronic pain with skin changes in a dermatomal distribution after acute herpes zoster.

Code. 203.X2b.

SYPHILIS: TABES DORSALIS AND HYPERTROPHIC PACHYMENINGITIS (IX-9)

Diagnostic Criteria. Lightning pains plus neurologic diagnosis of tabes dorsalis.

Code. 206.X2 or 207.X2 if associated with root pain.

MENINGITIS AND ARACHNOIDITIS (IX-10)

Acute infectious meningitis will, rarely, produce radicular pain. Occasionally it will progress to arachnoiditis involving one or more spinal segments, causing root pain in the upper limb. More frequently the arachnoiditis is relatively diffuse with widespread and bilateral symptoms.

Definition. Continuous increasing pain, usually associated with a bandlike constricting sensation and owing to local infection and scar tissue formation.

Code. 203.X2c, 203.X4, if caused by neoplasm.

TRAUMATIC AVULSION OF NERVE ROOTS (IX-11)

Definition. Pain in one or more root distributions from traumatic avulsion.

Code. 203.X1b.

SUPERIOR PULMONARY SULCUS SYNDROME (PANCOAST TUMOR) (IX-12)

Definition. Progressively intense pain in the shoulder and ulnar side of the arm associated with sensory and motor deficits and Horner's syndrome owing to neoplasm.

Code. 102.X6a.

Reference. Bonica, J.J., Ventafridda, V., and Pagni, C.A. (eds.): Management of Superior Pulmonary Sulcus Syndrome (Pancoast Syndrome) (Advances in Pain Research and Therapy, vol. 4). New York, Raven Press, 1982.

THORACIC OUTLET SYNDROME (IX-13)

(Includes Scalenus Anticus Syndrome, Cervical Rib Syndrome)

Definition. Pain in the root of the neck or shoulder radiating to the arm most often down the ulnar aspect. Caused by compression of the brachial plexus by an hypertrophied or abnormal scalenus anticus muscle, or a cervical rib or malformed first thoracic rib (cf. IX-14).

Summary of Essential Features and Diagnostic Criteria. Patients with scalenus anticus syndrome suffer from compression of the brachial plexus by an hypertrophied or abnormal scalenus anticus muscle. They characteristically develop pain and paresthesias in the upper extremities with activity and are relieved by rest. Adson's sign is positive. Electromyographic studies indicate delayed conduction time across the thoracic outlet.

Code. 133.X6, 233.X6.

CERVICAL RIB OR MALFORMED FIRST THORACIC RIB (IX-14)

It is impossible to differentiate the scalenus anticus syndrome from cervical or malformed first thoracic rib, except by x-ray. The presentations are identical. The diagnosis and differential diagnoses are the same. The only variation from the scalenus anticus syndrome is the finding of the abnormal or deformed rib on x-ray. The code is the same and the reference for this syndrome is the same.

PAIN OF SKELETAL METASTATIC DISEASE OF THE ARM OR SHOULDER GIRDLE (IX-15)

Definition. Dull aching pain in the shoulder girdle or upper extremity owing to tumor infiltration of bone.

Code. 233.X4.

GROUP X: LESIONS OF THE BRACHIAL PLEXUS

TUMORS OF THE BRACHIAL PLEXUS (X-1)

Definition. Progressive aching, burning pain with paresthesias and sensory and motor impairment in the distribution of a branch or branches of the brachial plexus owing to tumor.

Summary of Essential Features and Diagnostic Criteria. The tumors are associated with slowly progressive pain and paresthesias, and subsequently severe sensory loss and motor loss. The diagnostic criteria are the increasing aching, burning pain, its distribution in the brachial plexus, the associated paresthesias, motor and sensory loss, and the presence of a mass by palpation and on x-ray or CT scan.

Code. 102.X6b, 202.X6b.

CHEMICAL IRRITATION OF THE BRACHIAL PLEXUS (X-2)

Definition. Continuous burning pain occasionally accompanied by severe paroxysms, in the distribution of the brachial plexus or one of its branches, with sensory-motion deficits owing to effects of local injection of chemical irritants.

Code. 102.X5, 202.X5.

TRAUMATIC AVULSION OF THE BRACHIAL PLEXUS (X-3)

Definition. Pain, most often burning or crushing with superadded paroxysms, after avulsion lesions of the brachial plexus.

Summary of Essential Features and Diagnostic Criteria. The pain in avulsion lesions of the brachial plexus is almost invariably described as severe burning and crushing pain, constant, and often with paroxysms of sharp, shooting pains that last for seconds and vary in frequency from several times an hour to several times a week. So characteristic is the pain of an avulsion lesion that it is virtually diagnostic of an avulsion of one or more roots. Traction lesions of the brachial plexus that involve the nerve roots distal to the posterior roots ganglion are seldom, if ever, associated with pain. Sometimes in regeneration spontaneously, or after nerve grafts for rupture of nerve roots, distal to the intervertebral foramen, a causalgic type of pain develops, but this is highly characteristic of causalgia and cannot be confused with avulsion or deafferentation pain.

Code. 203.X1c.

Reference. Wynn Parry, C.B.: Pain in avulsion lesions of the brachial plexus. Pain, *9*:41, 1980.

PAINFUL ARMS AND MOVING FINGERS (X-5)

See XXX-7.

Reference. Verhagen, W.I.M., Horstink, M.W.I.M., and Notermans, S.L.H.: Painful arm and moving fingers. J. Neurol. Neurosurg. Psychiatry, *48*:384, 1985.

GROUP XI: PAIN IN THE SHOULDER, ARM, AND HAND

BICIPITAL TENDINITIS (XI-1)

Definition. Severe pain with acute onset owing to inflammation of the longhead biceps tendon.

Essential Features. Acute pain in the anterior shoulder, aggravated by forced supination of the flexed forearm.

Code. 231.X3.

SUBACROMIAL BURSITIS (SUBDELTOID BURSITIS, SUPRASPINATUS TENDINITIS) (XI-2)

Definition. Aching pain in the shoulder owing to inflammation of subacromial bursa.

Essential Features. Aching pain in shoulder with inflammation of the subacromial bursa and exacerbation on movement, as well as tenderness over the insertion of the supraspinatus tendon.

Code. 238.X3.

ROTATOR CUFF TEAR—PARTIAL OR COMPLETE (XI-3)

Definition. Acute severe aching pain owing to traumatic rupture of supraspinatus tendon.

Code. 231.X1.

LATERAL EPICONDYLITIS (TENNIS ELBOW) (XI-4)

Definition. Pain in the lateral epicondylar region of the elbow owing to strain or partial tear of the extensor tendon of the wrist.

Code. 235.X1a.

MEDIAL EPICONDYLITIS ("GOLFER'S ELBOW") (XI-5)

Definition. Pain in the medial epicondylar region of the elbow.

Code. 235.X1b.

DEQUERVAIN'S TENOSYNOVITIS (XI-6)

Definition. Severe aching and shooting pain owing to stenosing tenosynovitis of abductor pollicis longus or extensor pollicis brevis.

Essential Features. Severe aching and shooting pain in the radial portion of the wrist related to movement.

Code. 233.X3.

OSTEOARTHRITIS OF THE HANDS (XI-7)

Definition. Chronic aching pain in the fingers with degenerative changes of distal and proximal phalangeal joints of the hands.

Code. 238.X6b.

CARPAL TUNNEL SYNDROME (XI-8)

Definition. Stinging, burning, or aching pain in the hand, often nocturnal, owing to entrapment of the median nerves in the carpal tunnel.

Summary of Essential Features and Diagnostic Criteria. Episodic paresthetic nocturnal pain in the hand with electrophysiologic evidence of delayed conduction in the median nerve across the wrist.

Code. 204.X6.

PAIN OF PSYCHOLOGICAL ORIGIN IN THE SHOULDER AND ARM (XI-9)

Code. 233.X7b (tension: arm), 21X.X9a (delusional: arms), 21X.X9b (conversion: arms).

GROUP XII: VASCULAR DISEASE OF THE LIMBS

RAYNAUD'S DISEASE (XII-1)

Definition. Episodic attacks of aching, burning pain associated with vasoconstriction of the arteries of the extremities in response to cold or emotional stimuli.

Site. Predominantly in the hands, unilateral initially, later bilateral. Rarely lower limbs and exposed areas of face.

System. Cardiovascular.

Main Features.

Prevalence. Raynaud's phenomena can occur in 5% of normal females as secondary to connective tissue disease. Raynaud's disease is uncommon, with a female-male ratio of 5:1, onset most common between puberty and age 40. Exacerbations during emotional stress and possibly at time of menses.

Start. Evoked by cold, nervousness, and other stimuli, which vary among patients. A typical attack occurs in three phases. Initially the digits become ashen white and then turn blue as the capillaries dilate and fill with slowly flowing deoxygenated blood. Finally the arterioles relax and the attack comes to an end with a flushing of the diseased parts.

Quality. Initially the pain is deep and aching and varies from mild to severe, changing to severe burning dysesthesias in the phase of reactive hyperemia.

Occurrence. Recurring irregularly with changes in environmental temperature and emotional status.

Intensity. Variable from mild to severe, depending on the temperature and other stimuli.

Duration. Minutes to hours. Sometimes may last for days if painful ischemic skin ulcers develop.

Associated Symptoms and Signs. Numbness or hypoesthesia is present. Progressive spasm of the vessels leads to atrophy of the tip, giving the finger a tapered appearance. The nail becomes brittle and paronychia is common. Advanced cases may develop focal areas of necrosis at the fingertip, occasionally preceded by cutaneous calcification. These areas are extremely painful and tender to palpation. Anxiety and other signs of sympathetic overactivity, such as increased sweating in the limbs and piloerection, develop.

Relief. Temporary relief from sympathetic block occurs and occasional prolonged relief from sympathectomy in the early phases. Calcium channel blocking agents may help.

Pathology. The cause of "cold sensitivity" is unknown. Abnormalities in sympathetic activity have not been proved. However, local application of cold is necessary to elicit the response of Raynaud's syndrome and the threshold for triggering the response is lowered by any factor that increases sympathetic outflow or circulating catecholamines.

Essential Features. Color changes of digits, excited by cold or emotions, involving both upper extremities and absence of specific disease.

Differential Diagnosis. Raynaud's disease, which has no other known cause, and Raynaud's phenomenon, which is a response occurring in other illnesses, should be distinguished. The following other diseases should be recognized: collagen vascular diseases: scleroderma, rheumatoid arteritis, systemic lupus erythematosus, dermatomyositis, periarteritis nodosa; other vascular diseases: thromboangiitis obliterans, thrombotic or embolic occlusion, arteriosclerosis obliterans, syphilitic arteritis; trauma: vibration (air-hammer disease, etc.), percussion (digital—pianist, typist, etc.), palmar (hypothenar hammer syndrome); neurovascular syndromes: thoracic outlet syndromes, spondylitis, causalgia; central and peripheral nervous disorders (rarely): syringomyelia, poliomyelitis, ruptured cervical disk, progressive muscular atrophy; cold injury: frostbite, nonfreezing cold injury, (pernio, immersion foot), cold sensitivity syndrome; lack of suspension stability of blood: cold agglutinins, cryoglobulinemia, cryofibrinogenemia, polycythemia vera; intoxication: ergot, arsenic, heavy metals (lead), nicotine and tobacco.

Code. 224.X7a Raynaud's disease, 224.XXb Raynaud's phenomenon, 624.X7a (legs), 624.XXb (legs), 024.X7a (face), 024.XXb (face). Note: When the legs are affected, codes are altered to provide a 6 in the first digit. When the face is affected, codes are altered to provide a 0 in the first digit.

RAYNAUD'S PHENOMENON (XII-2)

Definition. Attacks like those of Raynaud's disease but related to one or more other disease processes.

Usual Course. In accordance with the underlying disease.

Pathology. Systemic and vascular diseases such as collagen disease, arteriosclerosis obliterans, nerve injuries, occupational trauma, for example, in chain saw operators, painists, and pneumatic hammer operators, may all contribute to the development of Raynaud's phenomenon.

Code. 224.XXb Raynaud's phenomenon, 624.XXb (legs), 024.XXb (face). Note: When the legs are affected, codes are altered to provide a 6 in the first digit. When the face is affected, codes are altered to provide a 0 in the first digit.

FROSTBITE AND COLD INJURY (XII-3)

Definition. Severe burning pain in digits or exposed areas of face owing to cold injury.

Essential Features. Exposure to cold below 0°C, followed by tissue injury a variable period after exposure.

Code. 222.X1a (arms), 622.X1a (legs).

ERYTHEMA PERNIO (CHILBLAINS) (XII-4)

Definition. Pain and itching in areas of extremities after exposure to cold and wet environment above 0°C and associated with pigmented or purpuric skin lesions.

Code. 225.X1 (arms), 625.X1 (legs).

ACROCYANOSIS (XII-5)

Definition. Persistent blueness and coldness of hands and feet, sometimes with aching pain.

Code. 222.X1b (arms), 622.X1b (legs).

LIVEDO RETICULARIS (XII-6)

Definition. Common, possibly, vasospastic disorder in women under the age of 40; associated with persistent aching in the skin of the arms, itching of circular and reticular lesions that have a mottled cyanotic appearance.

Code. 222.68a (arms), 622.68a (legs).

GROUP XIII: COLLAGEN DISEASE OF THE LIMBS

SCLERODERMA (XIII-1)

Definition. Intermittent vasospasm often with soreness, stiffness, or swelling of peripheral joints of the fingers and toes owing to collagen disease of the skin, particularly affecting the limbs.

Code. 226.X5 (arms), 626.X5 (legs).

ERGOTISM (XIII-2)

Definition. Burning pain in the extremities, identical to Raynaud's phenomenon, associated also with systemic symptoms attributable to excessive ergot intake.

Code. 281.X5 (upper limbs), 681.X5 (lower limbs).

GROUP XIV: VASODILATING FUNCTIONAL DISEASE OF THE LIMBS

ERYTHROMELALGIA (XIV-1)

Definition. Episodic burning pain in the extremities accompanied by bright red discoloration in response to increased environmental temperature.

Code. 224.X8b (hands), 624.X8b (legs). *Note:* Add code for secondary cases according to etiology.

THROMBOANGIITIS OBLITERANS (XIV-2)

Definition. Pain in the fingers or hands or small digits of the feet, usually in males who smoke; associated with ulceration of fingertips and margins of nails; related initially to segmental inflammation of walls of medium and small arteries and veins.

Code. 224.X3b (arms), 624.X3b (legs).

CHRONIC VENOUS INSUFFICIENCY (XIV-3)

Definition. Dull, aching pain in limbs, especially legs, characterized by abnormally dilated or tortuous veins.

Essential Features. Signs of venous insufficiency. Deep venous thrombosis in history.

Code. 222.X4 (neoplasm), 222.X6 (arms), 622.X4 (legs, neoplasm), 622.X6 (legs).

References. Juergens, J.L., et al.: Peripheral Vascular Diseases, 5th ed. Philadelphia, W.B. Saunders, 1980.

GROUP XV: ARTERIAL INSUFFICIENCY IN THE LIMBS

INTERMITTENT CLAUDICATION (XV-1) AND REST PAIN (XV-2)

Definition. Intermittent cramping pain in a muscular area produced by exercise and relieved by rest (XV-1) or constant pain in an extremity associated with hypoesthesia and/or dysesthesia and areas of skin ulceration or gangrene (XV-2).

Relief. Relief may be provided by sympathectomy for rest pain; claudication is less often relieved by this technique.

Code. 224.X8c (arms) intermittent claudication, 624.X8c (legs), 222.X8b (arms) Rest pain, 622.X8b (legs).

GROUP XVI: PAIN OF PSYCHOLOGICAL ORIGIN IN THE LIMBS (XVI-1)

General Descriptions
See section I-16

Pain in the limbs of psychological origin is seldom considered to be caused by muscle tension. Delusional or conversion pain in these (and other) locations may be more common on the left. Recurrent or chronic limb pain owing to inappropriate use of muscle groups whether or not for psychological reasons may be quite common.

Code. 233.X7b (tension: upper limb), 633.X7b (tension: lower limb); 21X.X9a (delusional: upper limb); 61X.X9a (delusional: lower limb), 21X.X9b (conversion: upper limb), 61X.X9b (conversion: lower limb).

References. Merskey, H., and Watson, G.D.: The lateralization of pain. Pain, *7*:271, 1979. Hall, W., and Clarke, I.M.C.: Pain and laterality in a British pain clinic sample. Pain, *14*:63, 1982.

GROUP XVII: CHEST PAIN

POSTINFECTIOUS AND SEGMENTAL PERIPHERAL NEURALGIA (XVII-3)

Definition. Paroxysmal pain in the distribution of an intercostal nerve commonly associated with cutaneous tenderness in the affected dermatome.

Code. 306.X2 postinfectious, 306.X8 unknown, 306.X1 or 303.X1a (post-traumatic).

ANGINA PECTORIS (XVII-4)

Definition. Pain, usually constricting, and a heavy feeling in the chest, related to ischemia of the myocardium without myocardial necrosis.

Summary of Essential Features and Diagnostic Criteria. Crushing retrosternal chest pain brought on by stress (physical or psychological) and relieved by rest and nitroglycerin, with ST depression on ECG but no evidence of infarction on sequential ECGs and cardiac enzymes.

Code. 324.X6, 224.X6 if mostly in the arms.

MYOCARDIAL INFARCTION (XVII-5)

Definition. Pain, usually crushing, from myocardial necrosis secondary to ischemia.

Summary of Essential Features and Diagnostic Criteria. Crushing retrosternal chest pain with myocardial necrosis as evidenced by ECG and enzyme changes.

Code. 321.X6 221.X6 if in the arms.

PERICARDITIS (XVII-6)

Definition. Pain, often sharp, arising from inflammation of the pericardium.

Summary of Essential Features and Diagnostic Criteria. Sharp retrosternal pain aggravated by breathing and relieved by leaning forward, with auscultation revealing a friction rub, ECG showing ST elevation or T wave inversion and echocardiogram showing an echo-free pericardial space.

Code. 323.X2 known infection, 323.X3 unknown infective cause, 323.X1 trauma, 323.X4 neoplasm, 323.X5 toxic.

ANEURYSM OF THE AORTA (XVII-7)

Definition. Pain from an abnormal widening of the aorta.

Main Features. Deep, diffuse, central chest pain is associated with large aneurysms. If dissection occurs, sudden and severe pain occurs, maximal at onset.

Summary of Essential Features and Diagnostic Criteria. An uncommon cause of chronic chest pain with a wide superior mediastinum on chest x-ray. A dramatic cause of excruciating acute pain with importance because of medical and surgical therapies available.

Code. 322.X6 (chronic aneurysm).

DISEASES OF THE DIAPHRAGM (XVII-8)

Definition. Pain from the diaphragm related to irritation of the diaphragmatic nerves by a disease process above the diaphragm, in the diaphragm (uncommon), or below the diaphragm.

Summary of Essential Features and Diagnostic Criteria. Abdominal pain in epigastrium with radiation to central chest, posterior midthorax, and shoulder tip(s), with evidence of space-occupying lesions above or below the diaphragm.

Code. 423.X2 infection: chest or pulmonary source, 423.X4 neoplasm: chest or pulmonary source, 433.X2 musculoskeletal, 453.X2 infection: gastrointestinal source, 453.X4a neoplasm: gastrointestinal source, 453.X6 cholelithiasis.

FRACTURE OR COLLAPSE OF THORACIC VERTEBRAE (XVII-9)

Definition. Thoracic pain or dermatomal pain or both associated with fracture of a vertebra.

Code. 303.X1b.

SLIPPING RIB SYNDROME (XVII-10)

(also known as Clicking Rib Syndrome and Rib Tip Syndrome)

Definition. Chronic pain at the costal margin that may mimic visceral pain.

Summary of Essential Features and Diagnostic Criteria. A fairly common condition that should be considered in any patient complaining of upper abdominal pain. The diagnosis is clinical and should be made only when the patient's symptoms are *exactly reproduced* by manipulation of the appropriate rib or ribs. An intercostal nerve block with local anesthetic may produce confirmatory evidence when the clinical findings are equivocal.

Code. 333.X6.

References. Copeland, G.P., Machin, D.G., and Shennan, J.M.: Surgical treatment of the slipping rib syndrome. Brit. J. Surg., *71*:522, 1984.

POSTMASTECTOMY PAIN: ACUTE AND SUBACUTE (XVII-11)

Definition. Acute and semiacute pain after extensive breast surgery, either radical mastectomy or modified radical mastectomy.

Main Features. *Burning pain* in the axilla and upper lateral chest and medial aspect of the arm, owing to complete transection or neurapraxia of the intercostobrachial nerve. Sometimes worse on light touch to the skin. *Intercostobrachial nerve pain* with paresthesias or anesthesia occurs after this type of surgery and lasts for up to 3 months but seldom persists and is not usually a problem. *Incisional pain* is minimal after breast surgery because of the hypoesthesia that develops after the flaps are mobilized.

Associated Symptoms. Dysesthesia in the distribution of the intercostobrachial nerve. Sometimes allodynia or other evidence of partial innervation is found.

Code. 303.X1c.

POSTMASTECTOMY PAIN: CHRONIC NONMALIGNANT (XVII-12)

Definition. Chronic pain beginning immediately or soon after mastectomy in a nonanatomic area on the anterior thorax.

Summary of Essential Findings and Diagnostic Criteria. Intractable pain, onset postoperatively, in anterior hemithorax, present more than 1 month, with superficial local sensitivity to touch, and nonanatomic neurologic findings. Poor motivation to flexion of the arms against resistance. More common on the nondominant side.

Differential Diagnosis. Herpes zoster, local infection, radiation necrosis in ribs, incisional neuralgia (intercostobrachial nerve syndrome of acute and subacute postmastectomy pain), and neuromata.

Code. 303.X9.

LATE POSTMASTECTOMY PAIN OR REGIONAL CARCINOMA (XVII-13)

Definition. Shooting, jabbing, or burning pain commencing more than 3 years after the initial treatment for cancer of the breast and caused by local metastases.

Summary of Essential Findings and Diagnostic Criteria. Chronic pain of cutaneous, visceral, skeletal, or neurogenic pattern arising more than 3 years after the initial diagnosis of cancer of the breast, associated with classic signs of lymphadenopathy, neurologic findings, weight loss, and anemia. Neurogenic pain of radiation or brachial plexus infiltration is commonly refractory to narcotics.

Code. 307.X4.

POST-THORACOTOMY PAIN SYNDROME (XVII-14)

Definition. Pain that recurs or persists along a thoracotomy scar at least 2 months after the surgical procedure.

Site. Chest wall.

Systems. Skeletal and nervous system.

Main Features. Pain after thoracotomy is characterized by an aching sensation in the distribution of the incision. It usually resolves in the 2 months after the surgery. Pain that persists beyond this time or recurs may have a burning dysesthetic component. There may also be a pleuritic component to the pain. Movements of the ipsilateral shoulder make the pain worse.

Signs and Laboratory Findings. There is usually tenderness, sensory loss, and absence of sweating along the thoracotomy scar. Auscultation of the chest may reveal decreased breath sounds owing to underlying lung consolidation or a malignant pleural effusion. A specific trigger point with dramatic pain relief after local anesthetic injection suggests that the pain is benign in nature and caused by the formation of a traumatic neuroma. A CT scan through the chest is the diagnostic procedure of choice to establish the presence or absence of recurrent tumor.

Usual Course. If the pain is due to traumatic neuromata, it usually declines in months to years and can be relieved by antidepressant-type medications and anticonvulsants. If the pain is due to tumor recurrence, some relief may be obtained by an intercostal nerve block or radiation therapy.

Summary of Essential Features and Diagnostic Criteria. Persistent or recurrent pain in the distribution of the thoracotomy scar in patients with lung cancer is commonly associated with tumor recurrence. CT scan of the chest is the diagnostic procedure of choice to demonstrate this recurrence.

Differential Diagnosis. Epidural disease and tumor in the perivertebral region can also produce intercostal pain if there is recurrent disease after thoracotomy.

Code. 303.X1d (neuroma), 333.X4 (metastasis).

GROUP XVIII: CHEST PAIN OF PSYCHOLOGICAL ORIGIN

MUSCLE TENSION PAIN (XVIII-1)

Definition. Virtually continuous pain in the thorax, owing to sustained muscle contraction and related to emotional causes.

Code. 333.X7b.

DELUSIONAL PAIN (XVIII-2)

See the general description of delusional pain (I-16). Perhaps more frequent in the precordial region.

Code. 31X.X9a.

CONVERSION PAIN (XVIII-3)

See the description of conversion pain in general (I-16). Most frequent in precordium; may be associated with tachycardia and fear or conviction of heart disease being present. Often mimics angina, but without adequate evidence of organic disease.

Code. 31X.X9b.

GROUP XIX: CHEST PAIN: REFERRED FROM ABDOMEN OR GASTROINTESTINAL TRACT

SUBPHRENIC ABSCESS (XIX-1)

Definition. Pain, often referred to the shoulder, from a collection of pus under the diaphragm.

Summary of Essential Features and Diagnostic Criteria. Chronic illness often after abdominal surgery with fever and abdominal pain, often with shoulder tip radiation.

Code. 353.X2 (thorax), 453.X2 (abdomen).

HERNIATED ABDOMINAL ORGANS (XIX-2)

Definition. Pain related to the protrusion of an abdominal organ through the normal containing walls of the abdomen.

Summary of Essential Features and Diagnostic Criteria. Epigastric discomfort and esophageal reflux are key symptoms with radiographic or endoscopic evidence of extra-abdominal organs.

Code. 355.X6 thoracic pain, 455.X6 abdominal pain.

ESOPHAGEAL MOTILITY DISORDERS (XIX-3)

Definition. Attacks of severe pain, usually retrosternal and midline, owing to a diffuse disorder of the esophageal musculature with severe attacks of spasm and/or failure of relaxation of the cardiac sphincter.

Summary of Essential Features and Diagnostic Criteria. This syndrome consists of short attacks of acute severe retrosternal pain that may be relieved by nitrites, with or without dysphagia. The diagnosis is made with a combination of barium swallow appearances and disordered esophageal motility and normal mucosal appearances on esophagoscopy.

Differential Diagnosis. Pericarditis, pulmonary embolism, angina pectoris, dissecting aneurysm, tertiary esophageal contractions in the elderly, and carcinoma of the esophagus.

Code. 356.X7.

ESOPHAGITIS (XIX-4)

Definition. Pain caused by inflammation of the esophageal mucosa.

Summary of Essential Features and Diagnostic Criteria. Burning retrosternal pain from esophageal inflammation.

Code. 355.X2 monilial, 355.X3a peptic.

REFLUX ESOPHAGITIS WITH PEPTIC ULCERATION (XIX-5)

Definition. Retrosternal burning chest pain owing to acid reflux causing inflammation and ulceration.

Summary of Essential Features and Diagnostic Criteria. Esophagitis with nonmalignant ulceration presents with retrosternal pain, especially on bending or lying down, or on drinking hot or cold fluids or acidic foods. The diagnosis is made on the history, esophagoscopy, and esophageal motility studies.

Code. 355.X3b.

CARCINOMA OF ESOPHAGUS (XIX-6)

Definition. Pain caused by malignant disease of the esophagus resulting from malignant transformation of either the squamous epithelium of the upper esophagus or the mucosa of the lower esophagus.

Site. Retrosternal pain, extending sometimes to the back.

Summary of Essential Features and Diagnostic Criteria. Presents with dysphagia with pain as a late feature. Diagnosed by barium swallow and esophagoscopy with biopsy or cytology.

Code. 354.X4.

GROUP XX: ABDOMINAL PAIN OF NEUROLOGIC ORIGIN

SEGMENTAL OR INTERCOSTAL NEURALGIA (XX-3)

See description of these conditions in thoracic section. Characteristics as for thoracic pain of similar etiology.

Code. 406.X2 postinfectious, 406.X8 unknown, 406.X1 or 403.X1 post-traumatic.

TWELFTH RIB SYNDROME (XX-4)

Definition. Chronic pain in the loin, sometimes with acute exacerbations and radiation to the groin.

Summary of Essential Features and Diagnostic Criteria. Loin pain, either intermittent or continuous and sometimes with radiation to the groin. Frequently misdiagnosed as pain of renal origin. Diagnosis is clinical and depends on exactly reproducing the patient's pain by palpation of the rib. Confirmatory evidence can often be obtained by using local anesthetic to block the appropriate intercostal nerve, but a negative test would not necessarily exclude the syndrome.

Differential Diagnosis. Renal or ureteric pathology, spinal problems, pulmonary pathology.

Code. 433.X6a.

Reference. Machin, D.G., and Shennan, J.M.: Twelfth rib syndrome; a differential diagnosis of loin pain. Brit. Med. J., *287*:586, 1983.

ABDOMINAL CUTANEOUS NERVE ENTRAPMENT SYNDROME (XX-5)

Definition. Segmental pain in the abdominal wall owing to cutaneous nerve entrapment in its muscular layers, commonly at the outer border of the rectus sheath or by involvement in postoperative scar tissue.

Differential Diagnosis. Serious intra-abdominal pathology, such as acute appendicitis, is normally not so prolonged over weeks or months. The pain of appendicitis is present even when the abdomen is relaxed and usually is association with other well-known physical signs. Entrapment neuropathy may require distinction from other causes of segmental pain (see intercostal neuralgia). Pain of psychological origin, especially in young women, is another diagnostic alternative.

Code. 433.X6b.

GROUP XXI: ABDOMINAL PAIN OF VISCERAL ORIGIN

CARDIAC FAILURE (XXI-1)

Definition. Dull aching pain from congestive failure.

Essential Factors. Dull aching right upper quadrant and epigastric pain with a large tender liver and elevated liver enzymes in association with other findings of heart failure.

Differential Diagnosis. Hepatitis and diseases of the gallbladder.

Code. 452.X6.

GALLBLADDER DISEASE (XXI-2)

Definition. Pain caused by an inflammatory disorder of the gallbladder usually associated with gallstones.

Summary of Essential Features and Diagnostic Criteria. Acute right upper quadrant pain, dyspepsia to fatty foods. Diagnosis by ultrasound or cholecystogram.

Code. 456.X6.

POSTCHOLECYSTECTOMY SYNDROME (XXI-3)

Definition. Right upper quadrant pain in patients after cholecystectomy.

Summary of Essential Features and Diagnostic Criteria. Right upper quadrant pain in a patient after cholecystectomy with no obvious cause. Endoscopic retrograde cholangiography often reproduces the pain.

Differential Diagnosis. Retained bile duct stone, hepatic flexure syndrome.

Code. 457.X1.

CHRONIC GASTRIC ULCER (XXI-4)

Definition. Attacks of periodic upper abdominal pain owing to ulceration of the gastric mucosa.

Summary of Essential Features and Diagnostic Criteria. Chronic gastric ulcer is a syndrome of periodic diffuse postprandial, upper abdominal pain relieved by antacids. The diagnosis is made by endoscopy or barium contrast radiology.

Code. 455.X3a.

CHRONIC DUODENAL ULCER (XXI-5)

Definition. Attacks of periodic epigastric pain owing to ulceration of the first part of the duodenal mucosa.

Summary of Essential Features and Diagnostic Criteria. Chronic duodenal ulcer is a syndrome of periodic, highly localized, upper epigastric pain relieved by antacids. The diagnosis is made by endoscopy or barium contrast radiology.

Code. 455.X3b.

CARCINOMA OF THE STOMACH (XXI-6)

Definition. Constant upper abdominal pain owing to neoplasm of the stomach.

Summary of Essential Features and Diagnostic Criteria. Indefinite onset of anorexia, weight loss, and fatigue in an elderly patient with vague upper abdominal discomfort developing into constant upper abdominal pain associated with anemia. The overall prognosis depends on the stage of the tumor at the time of diagnosis, early resectable tumors having an excellent prognosis.

Code. 453.X4b.

CARCINOMA OF PANCREAS (XXI-7)

Definition. Chronic constant abdominal pain or discomfort owing to neoplasia anywhere within the pancreatic gland.

Summary of Essential Features and Diagnostic Criteria. Indefinite onset of anorexia, weight loss, and fatigue in an elderly patient with vague central abdominal discomfort eventually turning to severe constant pain with or without obstructive jaundice. The overall prognosis even with modern imaging techniques is poor.

Code. 453.X4c.

CHRONIC MESENTERIC ISCHEMIA (XXI-8)

Definition. Intermittent central abdominal pain or discomfort related to ischemia of the large or small intestine.

Summary of Essential Features and Diagnostic Criteria. Mesenteric ischemia may result in central abdominal pain, associated with ingestion of meals. When this becomes severe, weight loss results and sudden small bowel infarction may occur.

Code. 455.X5.

CROHN'S DISEASE (XXI-9)

Definition. Pain caused by chronic granulomatous disease of the gastrointestinal tract.

Main Features. Becoming increasingly common in young adults but can occur at any age; males and females affected equally; pain usually caused by obstruction in the distal ileum with colicky central abdominal pain in bouts; or localized inflammation (abscess formation) may cause a constant severe pain. Both pains will persist until treated.

Essential Features. Pain caused by a chronic inflammatory granulomatous condition of the GI tract resulting in narrowing of the ileum and inflammatory "skip" lesions of the colon.

Code. 456.X3 (colicky pain), 452.X3 (sustained pain).

CHRONIC CONSTIPATION (XXI-10)

Definition. Abdominal pain, usually dull, caused by chronic alteration in bowel habit resulting in fewer bowel movements and diminished mean daily fecal output.

Summary of Essential Features and Diagnostic Criteria. Abdominal pain, usually dull, sometimes exacerbated by eating owing to chronic constipation, which is largely a disorder of Western civilization and increases with age. The diagnosis is made from the history and physical examination.

Code. 453.X7a.

IRRITABLE BOWEL SYNDROME (XXI-11)

Definition. Chronic abdominal pain of no apparent cause associated with alteration of bowel habit.

Essential Features. Usually there is a long history of constant abdominal pain and tenderness in young women; associated with alteration in bowel habit and no abnormal investigations.

Code. 453.X7b.

DIVERTICULAR DISEASE OF THE COLON (XXI-12)

Definition. Pain, usually dull, arising in relation to multiple small sac-like projections from the lumen of the colon through the muscular wall and beyond the serosal surface.

Summary of Essential Features and Diagnostic Criteria. A common chronic condition of the elderly resulting in constipation, colonic distension and sometimes abdominal pain. The diagnosis is made by identification of diverticuli on barium enema.

Code. 454.X6.

CARCINOMA OF THE COLON (XXI-13)

Definition. Pain caused by malignant neoplasm of the large bowel.

Summary of Essential Features and Diagnostic Criteria. One of the most common cancers in the Western world manifesting either as iron deficiency anemia, rectal bleeding, or an alteration in bowel habit, sometimes with abdominal or perineal pain. Diagnosed by endoscopy or barium enema.

Differential Diagnosis. Benign polyps and strictures, diverticular disease, ischemic colitis.

Code. 452.X4

GROUP XXII: ABDOMINAL PAIN SYNDROMES OF GENERALIZED DISEASES

FAMILIAL MEDITERRANEAN FEVER (XXII-1)

Definition. Disease of unknown cause predominant in those of Mediterranean stock, notably Sephardic Jews, Armenians, and Arabs. Classic features are periodic acute self-limiting febrile episodes with peritonitis, pleuritis, synovitis, and/or erythema resembling erysipelas.

Code. 434.X0b or 334.X0b.

ABDOMINAL MIGRAINE (XXII-2)

Definition. Characterized by recurrent attacks of abdominal pain and/or vomiting occurring in association with typical migraine or as a replacement or migraine equivalent.

Code. 404.X7.

PORPHYRIA—HEPATIC PORPHYRIAS

INTERMITTENT ACUTE PORPHYRIA (XXII-3)

Definition. Inherited disturbance of porphyrin metabolism *not* associated with photosensitivity, with attacks of abdominal pain as a constant feature, and sometimes variable hypertension, peripheral and central neuropathy (mainly motor), or psychosis.

Laboratory Findings. X-rays often show areas of intestinal distention proximal to areas of spasm. Hyponatremia may be severe. Porphobilinogen and ALA (delta-amino-levulinic acid) in urine.

Code. 404.X5a.

HEREDITARY COPROPORPHYRIA (XXII-4)

Definition. An inherited disturbance of porphyrin metabolism characterized by attacks of abdominal pain, occasional photosensitivity, neurologic and mental disturbance (see Intermittent Acute Porphyria).

Pathology. Owing to probable partial block in conversion of coproporphyrin III to protoporphyrinogen IX. Coproporphyrinogen oxidase activity decreased, probably mainly in liver.

Code. 404.X5b.

VARIEGATE PORPHYRIA (V.P.) (XXII-5)

(South African genetic porphyria or protocoproporphyria hereditaria)

Definition. An uncommon hereditary disorder of porphyria metabolism characterized by acute attacks of *abdominal pain,* neuropsychiatric manifestations, *and* photocutaneous lesions.

Laboratory Findings. Excretion of large amounts of protoporphyrin and coproporphyrin in feces. Urinary porphyrin precursors only modestly increased or normal, except during acute attacks. Dehydration may lead to azotemia and hyponatremia is common.

Code. 404.X5c.

GROUP XXIII: ABDOMINAL PAIN OF PSYCHOLOGICAL ORIGIN

MUSCLE TENSION PAIN (XXIII-1)

Uncommon. See General description (I-16-1 and III-1, -2).

Code. 433.X7b.

DELUSIONAL OR HALLUCINATORY PAIN (XXIII-2)

See general description (I-16-2).

Code. 41X.X9a.

CONVERSION PAIN (XXIII-2)

See general description (I-16-3).

Abdominal pain of psychological origin occurs as the Couvade syndrome in men during their wives' pregnancies. This may be manifest as pains of discomfort, or at the time of labor, seldom in developed societies, as an episode of pains resembling contractions.

Code. 41X.X9b.

ABDOMINAL PAIN—VISCERAL PAIN REFERRED TO THE ABDOMEN

Pericarditis—See XVII-4.

Diaphragmatic Hernia—See XIX-2.

GROUP XXIV: DISEASES OF UTERUS, OVARIES, AND ADNEXA

MITTELSCHMERZ (XXIV-1)

Definition. Mittelschmerz, also called midcycle pain, occurs as recurrent pain episodes at the time of ovulation.

Code. 765.X7a.

Reference. Renaer, M.: Midcycle pain. *In* Renaer, M. (ed.): Chronic Pelvic Pain. pp. 65–68. Berlin, New York, Springer-Verlag, 1981.

SECONDARY DYSMENORRHEA (XXIV-2)

Definition. Dysmenorrhea is called secondary if a structural anomaly is found that is probably responsible for the pain or when the pain seems to have a psychological origin.

Code. 765.X6a (endometriosis), 765.X4 (adenomyosis or fibrosis), 765.X0 (congenital obstruction), 765.X6b (acquired obstruction), 765.X9a (psychological tension), 765.X9b (psychological, delusional), 765.X9c (psychological, conversion).

PRIMARY DYSMENORRHEA (XXIV-3)

Note: *Endometritis* does not cause pain neither acute or chronic.

Definition. Dysmenorrhea, or painful menstruation, refers to episodes of pelvic pain whose duration is limited to the period of menstrual blood flow, or which start 1 or, at the earliest, 2 days before and stop 1 or, at the latest, 2 days after the blood flow. In primary dysmenorrhea there is no structural lesion.

Code. 765.X7b.

ENDOMETRIOSIS (XXIV-4)

Definition. Lower abdominal pain caused by foci of ectopic endometrium located outside the uterus (endometriosis externa of endometriosis).

Code. 764.X6.

POSTERIOR PARAMETRITIS (XXIV-5)

Definition. Pain with low-grade infection of parametrial tissues, especially the posterior parametrium. Synonyms: pelvic lymphangitis, chronic parametrial cellulitis.

Code. 733.X2.

Reference. Renaer, M.: Chronic Pelvic Pain in Women. Berlin, Springer-Verlag, 1981.

TUBERCULOUS SALPINGITIS (XXIV-6)

Definition. Pelvic pain caused by tuberculosis salpingitis.

Code. 763.X2.

RETROVERSION OF THE UTERUS (XXIV-7)

Definition. Lower abdominal pain caused by a retroverted uterus.

Code. 765.X7c.

Reference. Renaer, M.: Pain in gynecologic practice. III. The symptomatology of uterine retroversion and, in particular, pain in uterine retroversion (Dutch). Verhand. Koninkl. Acad. voor Gen. van België, *17*:433, 1955.

OVARIAN PAIN (XXIV-8)

Definition. Lower abdominal pain caused by an ovarian lesion.

Recurrent Painful Functional Ovarian Cysts. Main Features. Lower abdominal pain owing to recurrent painful functional cysts is sometimes, although rarely, seen in young women. It is called by some "painful ovarian dystrophy." Diagnostic Criteria. If the condition is very painful, laparoscopy may be indicated in order to ascertain the cause of the pain; the cystic fluid may then be aspirated and submitted to cytologic examination. If the result of this examination is compatible with a functional cyst, it is recommended to treat it conservatively by means of oral contraceptives. There is a good chance that the cyst and the pain will disappear, whereas surgical exploration with wedge resection of the ovary is likely to be followed by a recurrence of the cyst and of the painful episode.

Code. 764.X7a.

Ovarian Remnant Syndrome. Pain caused by ovarian remnants after operation. Main Features. When a bilateral oophorectomy has been performed in conditions that make it difficult to be sure that all ovarian tissue is removed (*e.g.*, when the ovaries were embeded in endometriotic scar tissue or were surrounded by dense adhesions), active rests of ovarian tissue may cause a painful condition called the "ovarian remnant syndrome." Diagnostic Criteria. An ovarian remnant will be suspected when the patient presents evidence of estrogen secretion that persists after a short course of corticoids prescribed to suppress adrenal androstenedione secretion and its peripheral conversion to estrone. Treatment will consist of meticlous excision of the residual ovarian tissue.

Code. 764.X7b.

References. Stone, S.C., and Schwartz, W.J.: A syndrome characterized by recurrent symptomatic functional ovarian cysts in young women. Am. J. Obstet. Gynecol., *134*:310, 1979. Symmonds, R.E., and Pettit, P.D.N.: Ovarian remnant syndrome. Obstet Gynecol., *54*:174, 1979.

CHRONIC PELVIC PAIN WITHOUT OBVIOUS PATHOLOGY (XXIV-9)

Definition. Chronic or recurrent pelvic pain that has apparently a gynecologic origin but for which no definite lesion or cause is found.

Main Features. Chronic pelvic pain without obvious pathology is the name given recently to a syndrome that has been known and described for more than a century under many names, some of them being parametropathia spastica, pelvic congestion and fibrosis, pelipathia vegetativa, pelvic sympathetic syndrome. *Prevalence.* This syndrome is rather uncommon. Until 30 years ago, it was considered rather common, but the diagnosis should be considered only under the following conditions: (1) if the patient's symptoms are not due to a gynecologic cause; (2) if the pain has characteristics of a gynecological pain; and (3) if the syndrome is not due to one of the acknowledged causes of gynecological pain which supposes that the patient underwent a laparoscopy.

It has become clear that formerly many chronic painful conditions have erroneously been classified under the above heading.

Code. 763.X8. See also I-16.

References. Renaer, M., Jijs, P., Van Assche, A., and Vertommen, H.: Chronic pelvic pain without obvious pathology: Personal observations and a review of the problem. Eur. J. Obstet. Gynaecol. Reproductive Biol., *10*:415, 1980.

GROUP XXV: PAIN IN THE RECTUM, PERINEUM, AND EXTERNAL GENITALIA

NEURALGIA OF ILIOHYPOGASTRIC, ILIOINGUINAL, OR GENITOFEMORAL NERVES (XXV-1)

Definition. Burning or lancinating or other pain syndrome owing to injury of the respective nerve, usually after surgical intervention in the hypogastric or inguinal region.

Main Features. The pain can occur immediately after the operation but not infrequently occurs after months or years. Sometimes there is no history of operation or trauma. The pain is burning or lancinating and radiates to the area supplied by the sensory nerve. For the iliohypogastric nerve, the pain radiates to the midline above the pubis but also laterally to the hip region. For the ilioinguinal and the genitofemoral nerve, the pain radiates from the groin into the anterior part of the labia major (or the scrotum and the root of the penis) and on the inside or the anterior surfaces of the thigh, sometimes down to the knee.

Usually the pain is continuously present, but it can be intensified by forcible stretching of the hip joint, by coughing, sneezing, sexual intercourse, or general tension in the abdominal muscles. The patient frequently adopts a posture that eases discomfort, with a slight flexure of the hip and a slight forward inclination of the trunk.

Differential Diagnosis. Inguinal and femoral hernia; lymphadenopathy; periostitis of pubic tubercle.

Code. 407.X7b, 407.X1 testicular pain.

TUMOR INFILTRATION OF THE SACRUM AND SACRAL NERVES (XXV-2)

Definition. Dull aching sacral pain accompanied by burning or throbbing pain in the rectum and perineum.

Summary of Essential Features and Diagnostic Criteria. The essential features are dull aching sacral pain with burning or throbbing perineal pain. There is usually sacral sensory loss and sphincter incontinence. A CT scan of the pelvis may show sacral erosion and a presacral soft tissue mass.

Code. 702.X4 nerve infiltration. 732.X4 musculoskeletal deposits.

RECTAL, PERINEAL, AND GENITAL PAIN OF PSYCHOLOGICAL ORIGIN (XXV-3)

About 10% of psychiatric patients with pain have rectal, perineal, or genital pain. This is usually mentioned as a secondary site of pain. Only about 2% report pain in these parts as the primary site. When that happens the rectal pain is usually associated with severe depressive or schizophrenic illness but may also be associated with conversion symptoms. It occurs in a few patients. For the general description, see I-16.

Conversion pain in these patients is usually accompanied by pains elsewhere. See also I-16.

Code. 81X.9a delusional, 81X.9b conversion.

GROUP XXVI: BACKACHE AND PAIN OF NEUROLOGIC ORIGIN IN TRUNK AND BACK

Prolapsed Intervertebral Disk (XXVI-1) See (XXVII-9)	502.X1c
Acute Herpes Zoster (XXVI-2)	303.X2a chest
	403.X2a abdomen
	503.X2a low back
	603.X2a leg
Postherpetic Neuralgia (XXVI-3)	303.X2b chest
	403.X2b abdomen
	503.X2b low back
	603.X2b leg
Intraspinal Tumor (XXVI-4)	302.X4a thorax
	402.X4a abdomen
	502.X4a low back
Fracture of Lumbar Vertebrae (XXVI-5) (See Section XXVII)	
Collapse of Lumbar Vertebrae (XXVI-6)	503.X1a trauma
	503.X4a neoplasm
	503.X5a metabolic
Epidural Abscess (XXVI-7)	302.X2a thorax
	402.X2a abdomen
	502.X2a low back

VERTEBRAL TUMOR (XXVI-8)

Definition. Pain in the midback or low back region, often with a radicular component, owing to tumor infiltration of the vertebral body and the epidural space.

Summary of Essential Features and Diagnostic Criteria. Metastases to the lumbosacral spine produce local and radicular pain, which can progress to paraplegia, sensory loss, and sphincter disturbance if untreated. The pain is usually worsened by lying and sitting and alleviated by standing or walking. One or more of the following studies may show the level of involvement—plain films, bone scan, and myelography.

Differential Diagnosis. The differential diagnosis includes benign disease such as disk herniation and other malignant conditions, such as meningeal carcinomatosis and tumor infiltration of the lumbosacral plexus.

Code. 303.X4 nerve involvement: thorax, 333.X4 musculoskeletal involvement: thorax, 403.X4 nerve involvement:

abdomen, 433.X4 musculoskeletal involvement: abdomen, 503.X4b nerve involvement: low back, 533.X4 musculoskeletal metastasis: low back.

MENINGEAL CARCINOMATOSIS (XXVI-11)

Definition. Dull aching pain in the lower back or buttocks with radiation into the legs on a radicular basis. There are usually more signs than symptoms, indicating involvement of multiple levels of the neuraxis.

Summary of Essential Features and Diagnostic Criteria. The essential features are low back pain with a radicular component and evidence of involvement of multiple levels of the neuraxis. The CSF is almost always abnormal and CSF cytology may be positive.

Differential Diagnosis. It is important to exclude a chronic meningeal infection such as fungal meningitis. Metastatic epidural disease can be ruled out by performing a myelogram.

Code. 502.X4c (low back), 302.X4c (thorax) 402.X4c (abdomen).

TUMOR INFILTRATION OF THE LUMBOSACRAL PLEXUS (XXVI-12)

Definition. Progressively intense pain in the low back or hip with radiation into the lower extremity.

Summary of Essential Features and Diagnostic Criteria. Low back and hip pain radiating into the leg is followed in weeks to months by progressive numbness, paresthesias, weakness, and leg edema. The physical findings indicate that more than one nerve root is involved. CT scan of the abdomen and pelvis is the study of choice.

Differential Diagnosis. Myelography and CSF analysis should rule out epidural and meningeal metastatic disease, respectively. Other entities to consider are radiation fibrosis, lumbosacral neuritis, and disk disease.

Code. 502.X4d.

GROUP XXVII: BACK PAIN OF MUSCULOSKELETAL ORIGIN

OSTEOPHYTE (XXVII-1)

Definition. Pain in the distribution of a dermatome owing to encroachment on a foramen by a bony spur.

Differential Diagnosis. Ruptured lumbar disk, fracture, abscess, intraspinal tumor, causes of nonradicular paralysis involving the lumbar plexus (*e.g.*, diabetic neuropathy), vascular lesions of the iliac arteries and their branches and stenosis of the lumbar canal.

Code. 533.X6a.

LUMBAR SPONDYLOLYSIS (XXVII-2)

Definition. Lumbar spondylolysis is an acquired bony defect in the pars interarticularis and is not necessarily painful.

Summary of Essential Features and Diagnostic Criteria. Lumbar spondylolysis occurs commonly in the second decade of life and is associated with low back discomfort. Some patients have radiculopathy as a result of neural compression secondary to exuberant bone formation. The diagnosis is generally made from roentgenograms of the lumbosacral spine. A bone scan is also helpful in the assessment and diagnosis of patients.

Differential Diagnosis. Lumbar spondylolysis as a cause of significant back pain should be a diagnosis of exclusion, since many patients do not have long-term symptoms. Spondylolisthesis, the dislocation of one vertebral body on its neighbor, occurs in a small fraction of the patients with bilateral spondylolysis. Spondylolisthesis can lead to deep aching lumbosacral pain and radicular pain if nerve roots are compressed.

Code. 531.X1a.

SPINAL STENOSIS (XXVII-3)

Definition. Chronic pain usually experienced in the buttocks and legs, at times extremely severe, usually deep and aching with "heaviness" and "numbness" in the leg, from buttock to foot secondary to compression of the cauda equina, of multiple etiology, common but often missed.

Code. 533.X6b (back), 633.X6 (legs).

SACRALIZATION OR LUMBARIZATION (TRANSITIONAL VERTEBRA) (XXVII-4)

Definition. Approximately 5% to 6% of patients have radiographic evidence for transitional lumbar vertebra representing either lumbarization of S1 or sacralization of L5.

This condition may be either unilateral or bilateral. The syndrome usually represents a failure of segmentation involving the development of the lumbosacral junction region.

Summary of Essential Features and Diagnostic Criteria. This anomaly can be recognized on roentgenograms. No specific clinical features have been observed. No neurologic deficits occur.

Code. 530.X0.

ABNORMAL ARTICULAR FACETS (FACET TROPISM) (XXVII-5)

Definition. Facet tropism is a developmental or acquired condition in which the lumbar articular facets are in different planes. Specifically, one facet joint is in a coronal plane, whereas the contralateral facet joint is in the sagittal plane. Thus, *in vivo* stress and strain patterns are altered by this developmental anomaly.

Summary of Essential Features and Diagnostic Criteria. Facet tropism represents a developmental alteration in the anatomy of the lumbar facet joints typified by one joint being in the sagittal plane while the other is in a coronal plane. Patients have minimal symptoms, and disability as a direct result of this variation is uncommon.

Code. 530.X6.

ACUTE LOW BACK STRAIN (XXVII-6)

(Acute mechanical backache, lumbosacral strain, acute ligamentous strain, acute discogenic backache)

Definition. Acute dull aching, cramping or knifelike back pain caused by minimal trauma or to precipitate movement with sudden loading of a motion segment.

Summary of Essential Features and Diagnostic Criteria. Onset of symptoms immediately after minor trauma or brief unexpected high-magnitude forces; local muscle spasm and tenderness; symptoms usually resolve. Recurrences likely.

Differential Diagnosis. Herniated nucleus pulposus (especially "midline" at L3–4, L4–5, or L5–S1), degenerative arthritis of lumbar spine, congenital abnormalities of spine, retroperitoneal pathology, disk-space infection.

Code. 531.X8 or 531.X1b.

RECURRENT LOW BACK STRAIN (XXVII-7)

(Postural backache, recurrent mechanical backache)

Definition. Mild or moderately severe dull aching or burning back pain correlated with prolonged posture of sitting or standing or repetitive awkward movements or postures.

Essential Features. Recurring pain exacerbated by specific activities, particularly those activities associated with repetitive loading or prolonged loading with hyperextension of a motion segment.

Code. 532.X7b.

TRAUMA, ACUTE (XXVII-8)

Definition. Pain in low back, usually severe, associated with fractures or dislocation of spine and disruption of joints, ligaments, tendons, from major trauma (usually motor vehicle accident or fall of greater than 6 feet [1.85 m]).

Differential Diagnosis. Injury to retroperitoneal structures.

Code. 531.X1c.

CHRONIC MECHANICAL LOW BACK PAIN (XXVII-9)

Definition. Continuous dull aching or burning pain in the low back associated with motion segment failure and made worse by specific activities. Duration beyond 6 months and associated with significant impairment of activities of daily living and/or work activities.

Code. 533.X1 mechanical instability.

ANKYLOSING SPONDYLITIS (XXVII-12)

Definition. Aching low back pain and stiffness of gradual development owing to chronic inflammatory change of unknown origin.

Radiographic Findings. Bilateral symmetrical sacroiliitis; syndesmophytes of lumbar thoracic spines.

Essential Features. Chronic aching lumbar pain and stiffness with "gelling" and with characteristic x-ray changes as described.

Code. 533.X8b.

QUADRATUS LUMBORUM SYNDROME (XXVII-14)

Definition. Dull aching pain arising from either the deep or the superficial fibers of the quadratus lumborum muscle.

Code. 532.X7c.

GLUTEAL SYNDROMES (XXVII-14)

Definition. Aching myofascial pain arising from trigger points located in one of the three gluteal muscles.

Code. 533.X7c.

Editor's note: Pyriformis muscle spasm may produce a syndrome of pain in buttock and thigh, occasionally with "sciatica." Marked spasm of pyriformis is detectable on palpation.

GROUP XXVIII: BACK PAIN OF VISCERAL ORIGIN

CARCINOMA OF THE RECTUM (XXVIII-1)

Code. 753.X4 (pelvic pain), 853.X4 (perineal pain).
See also XVII, XXI, XXIV, and XXV.

GROUP XXIX: LOW BACK PAIN OF PSYCHOLOGICAL ORIGIN

Code. 533.X7b (tension), 51X.X9a (delusional), 51X.X9b (conversion).

GROUP XXX: LOCAL SYNDROMES IN THE LEG OR FOOT—PAIN OF NEUROLOGIC ORIGIN

LATERAL FEMORAL CUTANEOUS NEUROPATHY (MERALGIA PARAESTHETICA) (XXX-1)

Definition. Hypoesthesia and painful dysesthesia in the distribution of the lateral femoral cutaneous nerve.

Code. 602.X1a.

OBTURATOR NEURALGIA (XXX-2)

Definition. Pain in the distribution of the obturator nerve.

Essential Features. Pain in groin and medial thigh; with time the development of sensory and motor changes in obturator nerve distribution.

Differential Diagnosis. Tumor or inflammation involving L2–4 roots, psoas muscle, pelvic side wall. Hip arthropathy.

Code. 602.X6a (obturator hernia), 602.X1b (surgery), 602.X2a (inflammation), 602.X4a (neoplasm).

FEMORAL NEURALGIA (XXX-3)

Definition. Pain in the distribution of the femoral nerve.

Essential Features. Pain, weakness, and sensory loss in the distribution of the femoral nerve or its branches.

Code. 602.X2b (inflammation), 602.X4b (neoplasm), 602.X6b (arthropathy).

SCIATICA NEURALGIA (XXX-4)

Definition. Pain in the distribution of the sciatic nerve owing to pathology of the nerve itself.

Main Features. Continuous or lancinating pain or both, referred to the region innervated by the damaged portion of the nerve; exacerbated by manipulation or palpation of the involved segment of the sciatic nerve.

Code. 602.X1c.

INTERDIGITAL NEURALGIA OF THE FOOT (MORTON'S METATARSALGIA) (XXX-5)

Definition. Pain in the metatarsal region.

Essential Features. Pain in region of metatarsal heads exacerbated by weight-bearing.

Code. 603.X1b.

PAINFUL LEGS AND MOVING TOES (XXX-7)

Definition. Deep pain, often gnawing, twisting, or aching in an extremity, with involuntary movements of the extremity, especially the digits.

Code. 602.X8 (legs), 202.X8 (arms) (See X-5 for reference).

References. Nathan, P.W.: Painful legs and moving toes: Evidence on the site of the lesion. J. Neurol. Neurosurg. Psychiatry, *41*:934, 1978. Montagna, P., Cirignotta, F., Sacquegna, T., Martinelli, P., Ambrosetta, G., and Lugaresi, E.: Painful legs and moving toes: Associated with polyneuropathy. J. Neurol. Neurosurg. Psychiatry, *46*:399, 1983.

METASTATIC DISEASE (XXX-8)

Definition. Pain in the hip joint and thigh region owing to tumor infiltration of bone.

Summary of Essential Features and Diagnostic Criteria. The essential features for disease in the hip joint are severe pain in the groin with radiation into the buttock and down the medial thigh. There is usually tenderness in the groin and increased pain on internal and external rotation. Plain films and bone scan may be positive.

Differential Diagnosis. The differential diagnosis includes upper lumbar plexopathy, avascular necrosis of the femoral head, and septic arthritis and radiation fibrosis of the hip joint.

Code. 633.X4.

GROUP XXXI: PAIN SYNDROMES OF HIP AND THIGH OF MUSCULOSKELETAL ORIGIN

ISCHIAL BURSITIS (XXXI-1)

Definition. Severe, sharp, or aching syndrome arising from inflammatory lesion of ischial bursa.

Essential Features. Recurring pain in ischial region aggravated by sitting or lying, relieved by injection.

Differential Diagnosis. Acute sciatica, spondyloarthropathies, prostatitis.

Code. 533.X3.

TROCHANTERIC BURSITIS (XXXI-2)

Definition. Aching or burning pain in the high lateral part of the thigh and in the buttock caused by inflammation of the trochanteric bursa.

Essential Features. Local pain aggravated by climbing stairs, extension of the back from flexion with knees straight.

Code. 634.X3b.

OSTEOARTHRITIS OF THE HIP (XXXI-3)

Definition. Pain caused by primary or secondary degenerative process involving the hip joint.

Main Features. As for osteoarthritis. Often felt deep in the groin, sometimes buttock or thigh, reproduced on passive or active movement of hip joint through a range of motion. As disease progresses, range of motion declines. Other features as for osteoarthritis (I-11).

Code. 638.X6b.

GROUP XXXII: MUSCULOSKELETAL SYNDROMES OF THE LEG

OSTEOARTHRITIS OF THE KNEE (XXXII-2)

Definition. Pain caused by a degenerative process of one or more of the three compartments of the knee joint.

Main Features. As for osteoarthritis but localized to the knee. Epidemiology, aggravating and relieving features, signs, usual course, physical disability, pathology, and differential diagnosis as for osteoarthritis (I-11).

Code. 638.X6c.

NIGHT CRAMPS (XXXII-3)

Definition. Painful nocturnal cramps in the calves.

Code. 634.X8.

PLANTAR FASCIITIS (XXXII-4)

Definition. Pain in the foot caused by inflammation of the plantar aponeurosis.

Code. 633.X3.

Editor's note: The reader is reminded that many of the above have been abbreviated and the full descriptions should be consulted in Pain, 3(Suppl.):217, 1986.

24.2 NEUROLOGIC MECHANISMS OF PAIN

TONY L. YAKSH

From a teleological standpoint, certain classes of unconditioned stimuli that interact with visceral, somatic or muscular receptor systems give rise to a complex syndrome of behavior in the unanesthetized organism that we refer to as pain. This syndrome is frequently characterized by vocalization or efforts to escape. Moreover, when such stimuli are provided repetitively, the organism, when given the opportunity, will go to great lengths to avoid this input. This led Sherrington to suggest that "stimuli become adequate as excitants of pain when they are of such intensity as threatens damage to the skin."[565] To generalize on this phenomenon, we note that other unconditioned stimuli, such as electrical stimuli, that do not produce evident damage will, however, produce the same behavioral syndrome. We would thus conclude that these stimuli have activated portions of the circuitry that mimics the input produced by the stimulus that physically damages the organism. Similarly, displacement of a joint beyond its normal range of motion, reversible ischemia of cardiac muscle, or gall bladder sphincter contractions, although not necessarily leading to acute and immediate damage, produce similar response syndromes (*e.g.*, vocalization, guarding), which suggests that the organism is responding to the input provided by that stimulus in a fashion similar to that of the tissue-damaging stimulus. The substrate by which these classes of information gain access to the central nervous system will be one of the principal subjects of this chapter.

The behavior of the organism in context thus provides corollaries as to the pain characteristics of the stimulus. In contrast, although a particular stimulus may indeed give rise to a "pain" response, it is not necessarily true that that physiologic stimulus will be an absolutely reliable predictor of the pain behavior it will evoke. Thus the response may be uncoupled from the stimulus by the context of the stimulus situation. Well-known exceptions occur during emotionally pervasive circumstances such as men injured in battle and athletes with traumatic injury in which no pain is expressed. The apparent disruption of this linkage between stimulus and response, however, does not occur because of a random association between the stimulus and the evoked behavior, but from the very properties of the system that we have chosen to investigate. The appreciation of the complex relation between stimulus and response indeed represents one of the major advances in conceptualization of the pain response that has occurred in the past 15 to 20 years. It is now apparent that one cannot consider the afferent limb through which "pain" information travels (*e.g.*, the pain pathway) without considering the systems that modulate at every level that very transmission (see Fig. 24-3).

NOCICEPTIVE PROCESSING: ROSTRALLY PROJECTING SUBSTRATES

In the following sections are discussed the substrates through which information generated by high-intensity stimuli gains access to higher centers. Anatomically the substrates may be broadly considered in terms of the primary afferents, the spinal cord, the brain stem (medulla, mesencephalon, diencephalon), and the cortex. In each case, one must consider the presumptive evidence associating activity in elements of that substrate with the afferent and efferent connections of that substrate and the behavioral sequelae that might be predicted secondary to the physiologic manipulations (lesion, stimulation) of that substrate.

PRIMARY AFFERENT SYSTEMS

In the following sections are addressed the anatomic, physiologic, and pharmacologic characteristics of afferents as they appear to relate to nociceptive transmission.

Myelinated and Unmyelinated Afferents

Afferent fibers can be broadly classified according to whether they are myelinated or unmyelinated. Large diameter peripheral afferents enveloped in Schwann cell sheets range in diameter from about 6 to 14 μm in human cutaneous nerve. Nonmyelinated fibers range in diameter from 0.2 to 2.0 μm and, although not possessing the Schwann cell investment, are commonly co-located in proximity with other small fibers within a common Schwann cell sheath. Myelinated to unmyelinated fiber ratios in cutaneous nerves are about 1 : 3 to 1 : 5 in humans.[184,481] Thus while the largest of myelinated fibers represent the largest area in a cross-section of nerve, numerically they likely constitute a relatively small proportion of the afferent pathways. The peripheral terminals of these axons ramify extensively in the subcutaneous layer, sending collaterals into the dermis. In this process some fibers lose their Schwann cell investment and become nonmyelinated. Conduction velocities of myelinated fibers thus decrease and approach that of unmyelinated fibers when measured near their site of termination (see also Table 2-1 and Figs. 2-1–2-4).[307]

Afferent axons in the skin ramify profusely,[112] losing their perineural sheath. Large diameter fibers, commonly excited by low-intensity mechanical stimuli, may develop specialized terminals with distinctly organized encapsulations constructed of non-neuronal elements.[61,89,659] The vast majority of nerve terminals, and certainly those deriving from unmyelinated fibers, however, show little evidence of specialization.[659] Unmyelinated terminals show extensive branching in a horizontal layer in the superficial dermis, and several axon branches may be invested by a single Schwann cell. Axon collaterals enter the epidermal layer with the basement membrane of the nerve terminal becoming contiguous with that of the epidermis. Unmyelinated fiber terminals are directed toward the stratum corneum and, there, lie between the juxtaposed epidermal cells.[111,130] Similar reorganization is observed in different target tissues such as the cornea (see Fig. 24-6). In tooth pulp, both myelinated and unmyelinated fibers appear to lose their Schwann cell sheath in the dentinal tubules.[16]

Free nerve endings commonly display agranular vesicles and numerous mitochondria (see Fig. 24-6).[111,299,592–594] As will be discussed in the comments on the peripheral pharmacology of afferents, these vesicle populations provide the substrate for the release of locally active agents at the *distal* terminals of the sensory axon.

It appears likely that certain "free" nerve endings are characteristically sensitive to physical stimuli that evoke pain behavior: [1] Activation of small diameter myelinated and unmyelinated fibers is associated with tissue damage (see below), and most small diameter fibers apparently end in unencapsulated terminals; [2] electrical, mechanical, thermal, or chemical stimuli, when applied to certain structures such as the cornea or the tooth pulp, which possess no encapsulated endings, will evoke a pain report.[15,16,128,405,477]

Primary Afferent Neuron Morphology

Primary sensory neurons are pseudounipolar with the soma located in the dorsal root ganglion (DRG) or, for the fifth nerve, in the trigeminal ganglion. The DRG may be divided into two categories:[21] large, lightly staining cells (type A) that give rise to large diameter myelinated fibers, and small darkly staining cells (type B) from which derive the small diameter myelinated or unmyelinated primary afferent axons.[690] Morphologically, type A and type B neurons have been differentiated on the basis of structural components such as relative content of granular and smooth endoplasmic reticulum and of ribosomes and neural filaments and microtubules, Golgi apparatus, and lysosomal bodies (*c.f.* Ref. 414). Histochemical differences also exist. Fluoride-resistant acid phosphatase,[141,152,379,380,382] cholinesterase,[336,337] and a number of peptides appear to be preferentially located in type B cells (see below).

Because axon terminals do not possess ribosomes with which to manufacture peptides and proteins, such materials are synthesized in the soma[175] and transported to the distal terminals of the neuron by means of an energy-dependent axon transport system.[482,483] Differences have not been observed between myelinated and unmyelinated fibers in the velocity or character of axon transport,[94,484] and the ability to conduct an action potential does not depend

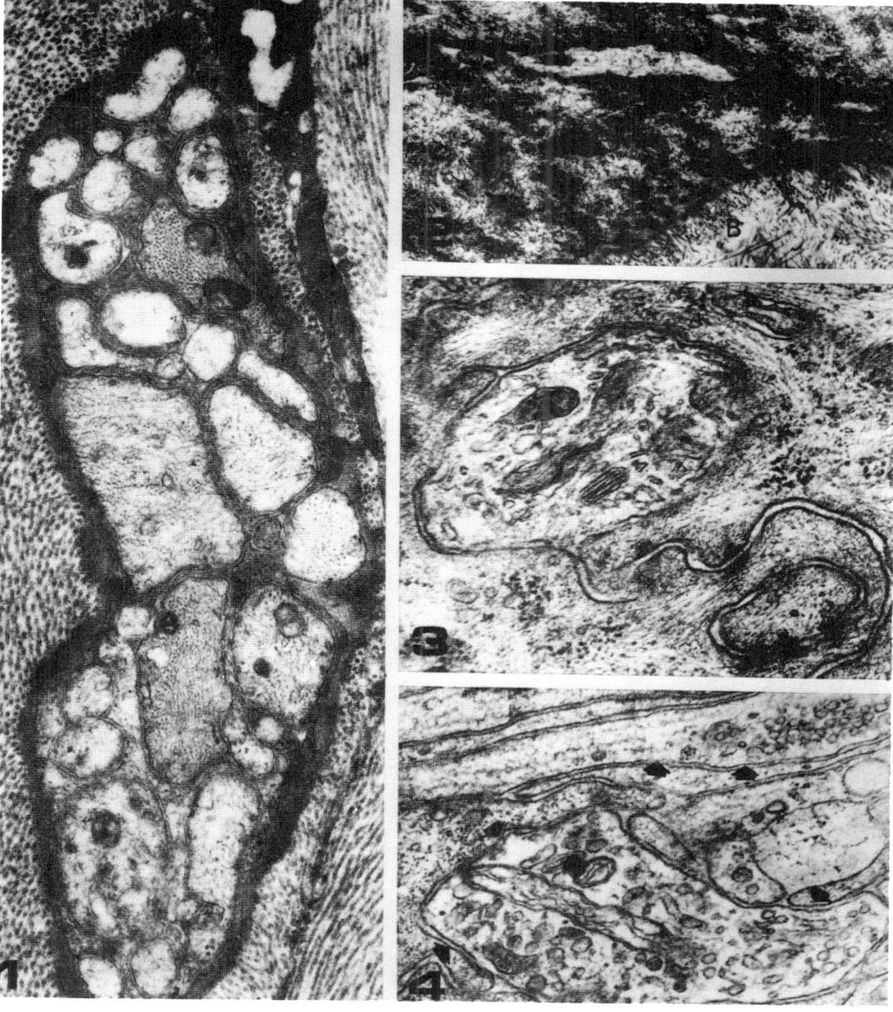

FIG. 24-6. *1.* A nerve trunk in the stroma of the rat cornea. Glutaraldehyde-OsO_4 fixation. (Original magnification ×32,500) *2.* An axon *(arrow)* penetrating between two basal epithelial cells. B, Bowman's layer. Glutaraldehyde-OsO_4 fixation. (Original magnification ×22,000). *3.* An intraepithelial axon profile containing mitochondria and agranular vesicles of varying shapes and sizes. Glutaraldehyde-OsO_4 fixation. (Original magnification ×59,100). *4.* Two intraepithelial axons *(arrows)* containing agranular vesicles. Glutaraldehyde-OsO_4 fixation. (Original magnification ×19,000) (Tervo, T., et al.: Pain, *6*:57–70, 1979.)

on the viability of axon transport systems. Changes, however, in the transport of materials to the distal terminals appear to play several important roles in the maintenance of the axon. With the blockade of axon transport (as with certain neuropathy-inducing agents such as colchicine or vinblastine), trophic changes in axon structure result.[381] Moreover, the likely role of certain peptides in primary afferent neurotransmission and the inability of nerve terminals to synthesize peptides argue for the importance of such a transport system.

Correlation of Behavior and Sensory Afferent Activity

Direct Activation of Axons. Zotterman,[703] using multiple unit recording, observed that high-intensity electrical stimulation in the periphery activated rapidly and slowly conducting fibers. Based on conduction velocity of cutaneous sensory nerves, fibers were subsequently designated as A-beta (30–100 m/sec) and A-delta (4–30 m/sec). The C component was those fibers conducting at less than 2.5 m/sec.[227] This classic definition is shown in the recording presented in Figure 24-7). Based on dissection, muscle afferents in the cat have been divided into the following groups on the basis of axon diameter: group I, greater than 12 μm; group II, 6 to 12 μm; group III, 1 to 6 μm; and group IV, less than 1 μm.[425] Given the close relationship between axon diameter in myelinated/unmyelinated axons and conduction velocities, the following relationships are normally accepted: group I, no homologue; group II, A-alpha/beta; group III, A-delta; and group IV, C.

Electrical stimulation that produced synchronous volleys in high-threshold cutaneous afferents (and therefore slowly conducting and small diameter) evoked massive sympathetic discharges and pseudoaffective responses even in lightly anesthetized animals,[703] suggesting that the activation was associated with a noxious stimulus. In humans, stimulation that evoked only fast conducting volleys in cutaneous nerve gave rise to sensations of tickling or light pressure, whereas stimulation that evoked fast and slow components resulted in pain.[144,597] High-intensity stimulation applied during selective blockade of large diameter fibers by anoxia, leaving A-delta/C fibers active, produces a short lasting pain of a pricking nature. The sensation appears similar to that often reported as "first" pain. Activation limited to more slowly conducting fiber populations (C or group IV) has given rise to dull, diffusely localized sensations that were likened to burning or so-called second pain.[272,596-600,620]

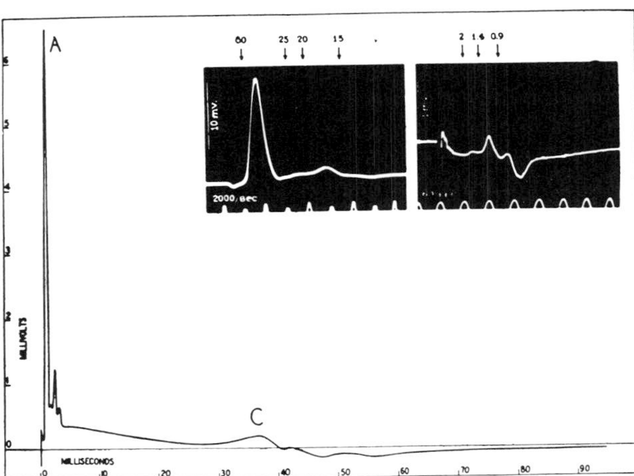

FIG. 24-7. Scale drawing of complete compound action potential of mammalian saphenous nerve. **Left Inset.** Recording of A fiber components. **Right Inset.** Recording of C fiber components. Numbers above arrows give maximal conduction rates (m/sec) of each component. (Patton, H.D.: In Ruch, T.C., and Patton, H.D. [eds]: Physiology and Biophysics, pp. 73–94. Philadelphia, W.B. Saunders, 1965.)

Afferent Activity Evoked by Stimuli Associated with Behavioral Signs of Pain. Although electrical activation of gross fiber populations may produce pain, it does not necessarily follow when a high-intensity somatic stimulus is applied that specific afferent populations are activated, or that their specific activation is uniquely correlated with pain sensations. Using single unit recording in human nerve fascicles *in situ*, it has been shown that stimuli that produce sensations of light touch or vibration are accompanied by the activation of rapidly conducting afferents.[325,373-375] Needle pricks associated with verbal reports of marked discomfort evoked rapid firing in C cutaneous afferents (0.5–1.5 m/sec). Chemical (acetic acid or intradermal histamine) or thermal stimuli that produce reports of pain or itch activate populations of slowly conducting fibers.[596,598-601,620] An example of such recording and a modality definition of peripheral sensory afferents conducting at a C-fiber velocity are shown in Figure 24-8. Such investigations have provided a number of insights: [1] Activation of only a few C fibers appears not to be sufficient to evoke a pain report[601,619]; and [2] although the activation of fibers conducting at velocities corresponding to A-delta and C fibers is a prerequisite for evoking somatic pain in humans, activity in all slowly conducting fibers is not uniquely associated with a pain event. Populations of slowly conducting afferents communicate information on warmth, cooling, or muscle pressure,[89,306] stimulus conditions that are not normally aversive. This heterogeneity is emphasized in Table 24-9, where the classes of afferents (as defined by conduction velocity) are correlated with the categories of "natural" stimuli that result in their excitation; and [3] electrical or mechanical stimulation sufficient to activate a slowly conducting component of a compound action potential and evoke a pain event will also evoke activity in rapidly conducting afferent fibers. Although the above observations indicate that the pain report may be obtained in the absence of large fibers, they cannot absolutely exclude them from a role in characterizing the pain event. Thus a prolonged intense mechanical stimuli will give rise to an initial burst of activity in low threshold afferents which, unlike the small diameter fibers, is not sustained. Willer and associates[650] observed that high-frequency stimulation of sural nerve at an intensity at which the electrical stimulus was just sufficient to generate a rapidly

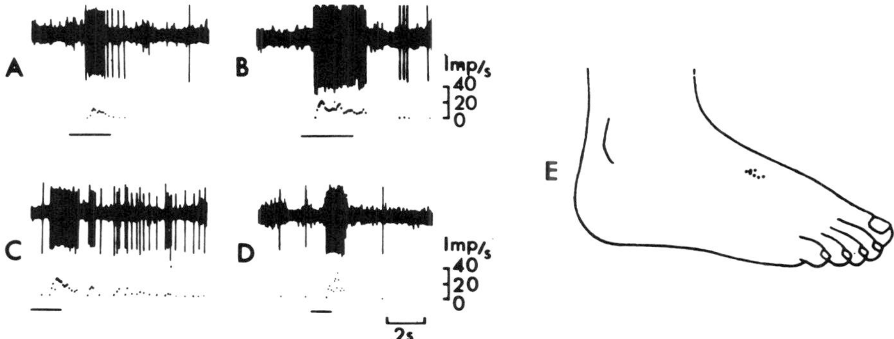

FIG. 24-8. Activity in afferent C unit (conduction velocity 0.64 m/sec) recorded in peroneal nerve at knee level. Various stimuli applied to receptive field on dorsum of big toe are indicated by bars under recordings. **A.** Sustained pressure with Frey hair, 2 g. Sensation: itch after about 2 seconds. **B.** Needle penetration through skin. Sensation: pricking and delayed pain. **C.** Touching skin with nettle leaf. Sensation: pain followed by itch. **D.** Touching skin with glowing match. Sensation: pricking followed by burning pain. **E.** Example of receptive field of C unit, recording being made from superficial peroneal nerve. Field measured 0.6 cm by 1.7 cm and consisted of seven receptive maxima *(dots)* surrounded by unresponsive areas. (Hagbarth, K.E.: Mayo Clin. Proc., *54*:353–365, 1979.)

TABLE 24–9. SUMMARY OF SENSORY AFFERENTS AND THEIR CHARACTERISTICS

Receptor Type	Effective Stimulus	Background Activity	Range of Conduction Velocity (m/sec)	Selected References
Cutaneous mechanoreceptors				
Type I	Identation of dome	0	30–90	374, 502
Type II	Skin deformation	+	30–70	374, 502
C mechanoreceptor	Skin indentation	0	<1	47
Meissner's corpuscle and Krause's end-bulb	Skin indentation	0	40–80	373, 591
Pacinian corpuscle	Vibration	0	50–80	373, 502
Cutaneous nociceptors				
A-delta mechanical	Damage	0	5–60	228, 502
C mechanical	Damage	0	<1	49, 228
A-delta heat	Noxious heat or mechanical damage	0	4–40	228, 307
C polymodal	Noxious heat; mechanical; algesic agents	0	<1	36, 150, 620
Warm	Increased temperature	+		
Muscle nociceptors				
Group III	Pressure; damage	+/0	60–90	494
Group IV	Pressure; damage	+/0	<2.5	219
Group III	Pressure; damage	+/0	60–90	494
Group IV	Pressure; damage	+/0	<2.5	219
Joint nociceptors				
A-delta	Extreme bending		<30	134
Visceral mechanoreceptors				
Intestine	Distension, tension on mesentery or blood vessels (intestine)	+/0	<1–30	48, 137, 456
Bladder	Distension or contraction	+/0	<2–20	137, 660
Visceral nociceptors				
	Intense mechanical, thermal, and chemical stimuli	+/0		137

conducting volley (A-alpha) was adequate to provoke reports of pricking pain. Finally, in Fabry's disease, small diameter fibers are damaged, the largest fibers remain functional, but pain sensations remain.[183,184,490]

Sensory Afferents Excited by Natural Stimuli

Table 24-9 presents a summary of the classes of afferents that are activated by various physical stimuli capable of evoking pain behavior. In the following section, characteristics of these afferents as a function of their respective innervated organ are discussed.

Cutaneous Stimuli. *Mechanosensitive Afferents.* High-threshold mechanoreceptive fibers responding only at pressure sufficient to produce tissue damage innervating glabrous tissue and conducting the range of A-delta fibers (15–25 m/sec) have been identified.[36,88,89,228,502] These afferents tend to respond with a rate of discharge proportional to the magnitude of the pressure applied. Receptive fields for these mechanoreceptors are large in the trunk (1–8 cm^2) and smaller on the face (1–2 cm^2). While on the limbs, distal receptive fields tend to be smaller than proximal fields. Mechanoreceptors conducting at C fiber velocities have been shown with thresholds requiring Von Frey hair stimuli greater than 2 g and with receptive fields ranging from small (5 mm^2) to strips covering several square centimeters. These fibers discharge with a frequency that is monotonically proportional to the stimulus intensity.[49,228]

Thermoreceptive Afferents. Warm receptors have been observed that respond to temperature increments of less than 1°C within the range of 30°C to 40°C with small peripheral receptive fields (less than 0.5 mm in diameter).[305] These fibers have also been shown to respond to thermal stimuli of noxious intensity with an increasing frequency of discharge. High-intensity stimulation within the range of 47° to 51°C evokes a transient high-frequency discharge. These response characteristics are to be differentiated from those reported for the mechanical–thermal receptive units (see below) in that the response rate commonly is all or none in character.[176,177,276,277] Certain afferent cutaneous fibers that respond to decreases in temperature on the order of less than 1°C (*i.e.*, "cold" receptors) may show a paradoxical response to heat. As skin temperature has risen to 45° to 52° C, the fiber's rate of discharge has also increased.[171,178,275,400]

Mechano–Thermoreceptive Nociceptive Afferents. Afferents have been reported that respond to high-intensity mechanical and thermal stimulation, conduct within an A-delta range (10–40 m/sec) and exhibit a positively accelerating monotonic stimulus response function.[35,89] Activation threshold may lie between 40° and 60°C, and a maximum response is commonly observed at 45° to 53°C.[176,177,228,307] Receptive fields for these units are small (less than 5 mm^2) and frequently occur as several spots, suggesting extensive collateralization of the terminals. These afferents may mediate the "first" pain of heat, for example, the pricking sensation reported immediately after the application of a strong thermal stimulus.[519]

Polymodal C Fiber Afferents. A major portion of C fiber afferents that respond to nociceptive stimuli are "polymodal" in character. These fibers may constitute 80% to 90% of the primate nociceptive C fiber population.[38] These axons are activated equally well by several classes of stimuli, including mechanical (greater than 1 g), thermal (45–53°C), and frequently by chemical stimuli applied to the characteristically small (<3 mm^2) receptive field. The response to such ongoing stimuli is a sustained, vigorous discharge the frequency of which is monotonically related to stimuli intensity.[38,39,49,393]

Recordings in humans from single afferents conducting in the range of 0.5 to 2.0 m/sec have been made from sensory nerves innervating nonglabrous skin. These fibers are activated by strong mechanical stimuli (Von Frey hairs of 0.7–13 g; needle pricks; and local compression) and produce an ongoing discharge that adapts slowly in the presence of the sustained stimulus.[596,598,599,601,620] An example of one such unit is presented in Figure 24-8. Such units are not spontaneously active at temperatures up to about 40°C, but temperatures in excess of 45°C evoke activity in an increasing number of units.[596,601,619] Local application of acid, histamine, or potassium chloride evoke a prolonged discharge.[596,601,619] Receptive fields of polymodal C afferents tend to be larger in humans (1 mm^2–1 cm^2) but frequently may also display several sites, suggesting extensive collateralization.[596,600,601,620] These slowly conducting fibers, presumably unmyelinated in character, show clear signs of fatigue and failure of conduction upon repeated high-frequency electrical stimulation.[598,599]

Skeletal Muscle. It has been reported[577] that, excluding the stretch receptors, the principal sensory innervation of the skeletal muscle derives from free nerve endings in fascia and the adventitia of blood vessels that arise from myelinated and nonmyelinated fibers. High-threshold groups III and IV mechanoreceptors in muscle activated by intense contraction have been reported.[304,391] Intense thermal stimuli applied to muscle belly evokes monotonically increasing activity in these afferents.[280] Hypertonic solutions of sodium chloride[494] and close intra-arterial injections of a number of algogenic agents (histamine, bradykinin, and serotonin) evokes significant activity in groups III and IV afferents.[212,219,450] The terminals are, however, not functionally homogeneous. At least three groups of afferents have been identified: [1] activated by algogenic agents but not by muscle activity; [2] activated by muscle activity but not by algogenic agents; and [3] activated by both sustained muscle activity and algogenic agents.[377] The sensitivity to chemical agents makes it likely that these nociceptive groups III and IV afferents are activated by agents that are released locally during muscle contraction. Extracellular potassium levels double (5–15 mM) during isometric testing in cat.[284] Failure of nominal concentrations of phosphate and lactate to alter group IV afferents activity suggests that metabolic by-products alone do not constitute a source of muscle pain.[377] The apparent ability of prostaglandins to sensitize algogenic receptors to otherwise inactive concentrations of chemical stimulants in cardiac muscle (see below), and the likelihood of their release during intense skeletal muscle contraction, could be of significance in the activation of groups III and IV skeletal muscle afferents by metabolic by-products.

Cardiac Muscle. Occlusion of the coronary artery leading to ischemia of ventricular muscle produces pain in humans[56,640] and pseudoaffective response in animals.[584] Sensory afferents in the inferior cardiac nerve projecting to the T1–T5 segments of the spinal cord mediate the transmission of such information.[213,215,420,641] Recording single units from the T2–T3 rama communicans reveals that during coronary occlusions, activity in A-delta/C afferents increases.[81,82,611] The cardiac afferents are activated by moderate- to high-intensity mechanical stimulation,[82,429,610] noxious heating,[476] and several algogenic agents.[87,476,612] The stimulus for angina may be the release from ischemic muscle of humoral factors that sensitize or activate cardiac afferents. Serotonin and histamine stimulate cardiac afferent fibers,[173,475,476] and blood levels of bradykinin in the coronary sinus after occlusion are sufficient to evoke pseudoaffective responses when administered in dogs.[251,369,578,611] In an interesting series of experiments, Staszewska–Barcak and co-workers[578] observed [1] reflex cardiovascular changes suggestive of angina discomfort following the topical application of several algogenic agents to the wall of the left ventricle; and [2] that temporary occlusion of the coronary artery supplying the area of the ventricle under study sensitizes the heart to the algogenic effects of bradykinin. Importantly, coapplication of prostaglandins ($PGE_1 > PGE_2 > PGF_{2\alpha}$) with bradykinin has significantly potentiated the algogenic effects of bradykinin. Pretreatment with a prostaglandin synthesis inhibitor reduced the algogenic effects of bradykinin and the sensitizing effects of prior ischemia. The potentiation of bradykinin's algogenic effects by exogenous prostaglandins was evident for as long as 60 minutes and could not be attenuated by indomethacin. These observations are consistent with the observation that prostaglandins are formed and released in heart muscle following hypoxia or ischemia.[10,55,637] Thus angina could speculatively result, in part, from the neurohumoral activation of afferent terminals by the joint release of both prostaglandins and bradykinin.

Teeth. Innervation of the teeth occurs both intradentally (within the tooth) and periodontally (within the surrounding connective tissue). Free nerve endings are found within the pulp and the surrounding blood vessels. Fibers that originate in afferent plexi adjacent to the inner dentinal surface pass through the odontoblasts to the dentinal tubules that run parallel to the odontoblast processes.[218,486] In tooth pulp, the unmyelinated fibers are ensheathed by Schwann cells and interlace with the odontoblast somata. Tooth pulp afferents consist of fibers having diameters and apparent conduction velocities in the A-delta and C fiber range.[18,164,246,694] The periodontal afferents travel through the maxillary and mandibular branches of the trigeminal nerve to terminate within collagen fibers of the alveolar ligament with specializations similar to the Meissner corpuscle.

Transdentinal electrical stimulation produces sharp pain of brief duration[128] that gives rise to jaw opening and closing reflexes and attempts to escape.[618,626,627] In shock titration paradigms, primates maintain the current intensity of dental stimulation at or immediately above that intensity which, in a single escape paradigm, will support escape behavior.[485] These observations correspond to studies in humans suggesting that the difference between a perceivable threshold stimulus (prepain) and a stimulus sufficient to evoke a pain report is small.[15,16] Conversely, activity in intradentinal sensory nerves has been shown to correlate closely with the sensation of pain.[188] Pressure, touch, or tooth movement is likely mediated by afferents from the periodontal and gingival structures in which the tooth is embedded.[70,508]

Thermal stimulation of teeth has been reported to evoke neuronal activity in dental nerves.[222,437] In cats, frequency of discharge of dental afferents rose when the dentin temperature was elevated from 34°C to 37°C within a 10-second period.[559] Slow heating of the cat tooth surface to 47°C failed to elicit such activity.[3] Repeated intense thermal stimulation of the tooth (60°C), however, did evoke a persistent afferent discharge. Pretreatment, but not posttreatment with prostaglandin synthesis inhibitors, reduced the discharge associated with repetitive heating.[4] The generation of cyclooxygenase products may therefore sensitize nerve endings to stimuli originating in the local pulpal environment.

Because nerve endings do not penetrate to the enamel dentin interface, the effective stimulus in tooth sensations has been proposed to be the distortion of odontoblasts or alterations in hydraulic flow produced by changes in temperature.[69] Inflammation or edema associated with thermal damage as described above, or direct pressure, could increase pulpal volume and deform the mechanically sensitive nerve terminals that lie between the odontoblasts. That changes in pulpal pressure can evoke activity in tooth afferents is supported by the observations that [1] bursts of 1 to 4 spikes occur in synchrony with the systolic pulse and [2] pulpal pressure change as much as 5 mm Hg with the systolic pulse pressure in the normal tooth.[51,559] Presumably, where inflammation has occurred, such changes may be augmented because of the increased pulpal volume in a restricted space.

Synovial Joints. Cutaneous afferents and branches of adjacent muscle afferents innervate the joints.[226] Intense deformation or inflammation-induced expansion within the joint will evoke activity in the group III (A-delta) fibers.[132–134] Urate crystals,[2,85,208] carrageenin,[453,617] and endotoxin[279] injected into the synovial joint evokes an acute local inflammation, whereas the intradermal injection of killed bacteria suspended in Freund's adjuvant results in a chronic polyarthritis.[242] A marked sensitivity to stimulation of the affected limbs is observed in animals so treated. Joint pain associated with gout-induced arthritis in humans likely results from urate crystal deposition.[442] Altered sensitivity to mechanical stimulation may be mediated by the generation of chemical intermediaries such as prostaglandins. The ability of cyclooxygenase or phospholipase A inhibitors to reduce the sensitivity associated with the inflamed joints and to reduce the inflammation is consistent with this hypothesis.[85,617] Other inhibitors of cyclooxygenase such as paracetamol are effective against joint pain but exert no effect on arthritic swelling.[663]

Visceral Organs. Although manipulation of a number of visceral organs such as liver, kidney, and spleen does not appear to give rise to reports of pain, internal body organs clearly become symptomatic in the presence of mechanical distortion and particularly during inflammation (as discussed above for cardiac muscle). Although the characteristics of the sensing element that gives rise to these sensations are not generally known, stimulation of visceral afferents or mechanical distortion in animal models clearly gives rise to pain-associated autonomic reflex activity or verbal reports of pain, or both, in humans. The characteristic of the effective stimuli suggests the existence of both chemoreceptive and mechanoreceptive systems. Thus severe pain may occur secondary to the strong contraction of smooth muscle, that is, as secondary to the obstruction of the hollow viscus, or in the presence of biliary or uretric distension. Chemosensitivity also appears to be a not uncommon phenomenon in visceral afferents that give rise to pain-associated behaviors. Thus lung nociceptors would appear likely to be responsible for pain secondary to pulmonary congestion, and atelectasis. In addition, as noted above, injection of bradykinin into the cardiac circulation results in powerful pseudoaffective responses and may be responsible for the pain associated with an ischemic myocardium.[214]

Abnormal Origins of Activity in Peripheral Afferents. Commonly, orthodromic discharge of a peripheral afferent originates at the distal terminals secondary to generator potentials induced by the appropriate peripheral stimulus. Pressure briskly applied midaxon evokes only a transient neural activity (see Fig. 24-9).[298,634] Acute nerve compression in humans may be reported as transiently painful, if perceived at all.[185,342] Simple slow distortion of midaxon regions, however, is ineffective in generating neural activity.[1,240,243,333,634] Thus chronic pressure alone, such as that generated by benign tumors, is often not reported as painful.[342] Mechanical insensitivity of the midaxon region is, however, altered after nerve injury. Upon severance of a nerve there is a shower of activity that disappears. With time, the cut end reseals and a neuroma develops. Systematic studies in animal models have shown that this neu-

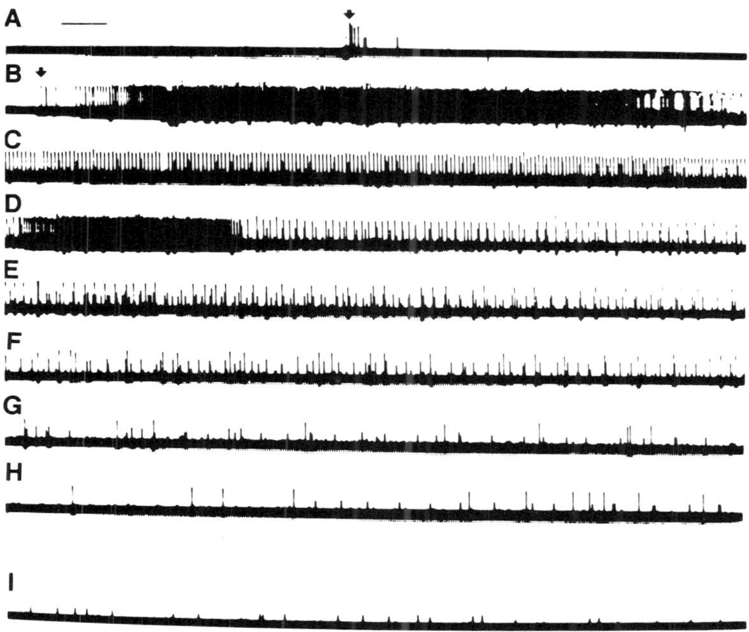

FIG. 24-9. Effects of dorsal root ganglion (DRG) compression. Multiple unit recording from a small filament of dorsal root. **A.** For contrast, the response of the units to dorsal root compression. **B–H.** Response in same filament to maintained DRG compression. Each line represents the first 3 seconds of successive 1-minute intervals. **I.** The first 3 seconds of activity sampled 25 minutes after initiation of DRG compression, showing persistent A-delta activity. Time bar, 200 msec. Compression begins at the arrow in *B* and is maintained throughout the recording. (Howe, J.F., et al.: Pain, *3*:25–41, 1977.)

roma frequently gives rise to ongoing orthodromic activity in the nerve. The activity occurs within fibers having conduction velocities, suggestive of small diameter myelinated fibers.[631] Small distortions of the cut region now produce long periods (30 seconds) of repetitive discharge. These observations suggested that the local injury had transformed that region of the axon and endowed it with properties of excitability similar to those of the terminal region. Ectopic foci such as these have been suggested to be the source of the abnormal sensations that occur after amputation.[101,174] Neurotomy in several species, including mice, rats, cats, and rabbits,[33,168,631] gives rise to autonomy of the denervated region that may result from the abnormal discharges generated by the neuroma formed. The self-mutilation, when and if it does develop, apparently is not due to the anesthetic state: [1] Mutilation begins only after several days[633]; [2] guanethidine, which suppresses the ectopic discharges associated with neuromas in mice, suppresses the autotomy in neurectomized rats and mice[633]; and [3] selective spinal tractotomies abolish the autonomy.[33] It should be noted that neurectomies produce marked transganglionic changes in the chemistry of the dorsal horn. Thus section of the peripheral nerve results in a loss of fluoride-resistant acid phosphatase and substance P in the dorsal horn.[323,379,380,383] The role these subtle changes play in the phenomenon of autonomy has yet to be assessed.

Dorsal root ganglion cells are apparent exceptions to the above discussion of nonterminal spike generation. As shown in Figure 24-9, slow, minor distortion of the dorsal root ganglion evokes repetitive firing that lasts minutes. Similar distortion of the dorsal roots was not as effective.[298] That this stimulation evoked a pain event is evidenced by the fact that acute injury to the dorsal root ganglion evokes immediate tachycardia and mass flexion reflexes in the lightly anesthetized animal. These observations support the suggestion that the radicular pain of sciatica might be associated with such a focal distortion of the dorsal root ganglion and not the root or nerve proper.

Patients suffering from tic douloureux are often reported to have an artery or a small tumor or plaque impinging upon the trigeminal root.[315,347,348] Although such mechanical stimulation may not account for the unique sensory barrage associated with tic episodes, the mechanical sensitivity of the dorsal root may provide a background upon which a mechanical stimulus, such as that provided by the adjacent artery, might alter innocuous sensory input and thus generate the pain event.[29,97–99,297]

SPINAL TERMINALS OF PRIMARY AFFERENTS

Dorsal Root Entry Zone

As the dorsal root approaches the spinal cord, small myelinated and unmyelinated fibers tend to aggregate in the lateral aspect of the dorsal root, and larger myelinated fibers aggregate medially (see Fig. 24-10).[354,416,530,531,574] Entering the spinal cord, the primary afferents bifurcate into rostrally and caudally projecting branches. Large fibers proceed along the dorsal columns for varying distances; many terminate in the spinal gray.[102,580] Large diameter afferent collaterals exit from the dorsal column axis perpendicularly and pursue a ballistic trajectory, coursing deeply into the gray matter before turning dorsally to terminate in the upper portions of the gray matter.[95] The smaller caliber fibers project rostrally and caudally one or two segments into the medial portion of the tract of Lissauer. Small diameter fibers enter the dorsal gray matter directly and terminate dorsally, as will be discussed. Both large and small diameter fibers give rise to collaterals that distribute ventrally in the spinal gray matter (see Fig. 28-2).

Although the preponderance of afferents terminate ipsilaterally, there is evidence that a small proportion of the afferents also terminate contralaterally.[17,416,417,524,533] These fibers travel dorsal to the central canal to terminate in laminae III and IV of the contralateral dorsal horn, forming a longitudinally oriented plexus one to two segments in length.[154] These contralateral projections occur most commonly at the cervical and sacral levels of the spinal cord, although crossing fibers have been described in lumbar cord.[416,417]

Early work demonstrated the behavioral significance of the medial to lateral distribution of the large and small primary afferents by making discrete lesions in the dorsal root entry zone.[531] Lateral cuts, presumably severing the smaller caliber myelinated fiber population, produced significant blockade of the pseudoaffective response of the animal to strong, otherwise aversive, stimuli on the side where the lesions were made. Such section also likely produced local infarcts of the adjacent dorsal gray matter.[271] Discrete surgical lesions directed at the dorsal horn through the dorsal root entry zone have been shown to alleviate pain, particularly that associated with root avulsions.[467,468]

The principal portion of the sensory afferents enters the spinal cord through the dorsal root entry zone, consistent with the "law" of Bell and Magendie. A significant number of unmyelinated afferent fibers that arise from dorsal root ganglion cells, however, also exist within the ventral roots.[25,136,137,139,140] After the injection of horseradish peroxidase into the spinal gray matter of cats with previously sectioned dorsal roots, reaction products appeared in small dorsal root ganglion cells. Failure to label large dorsal

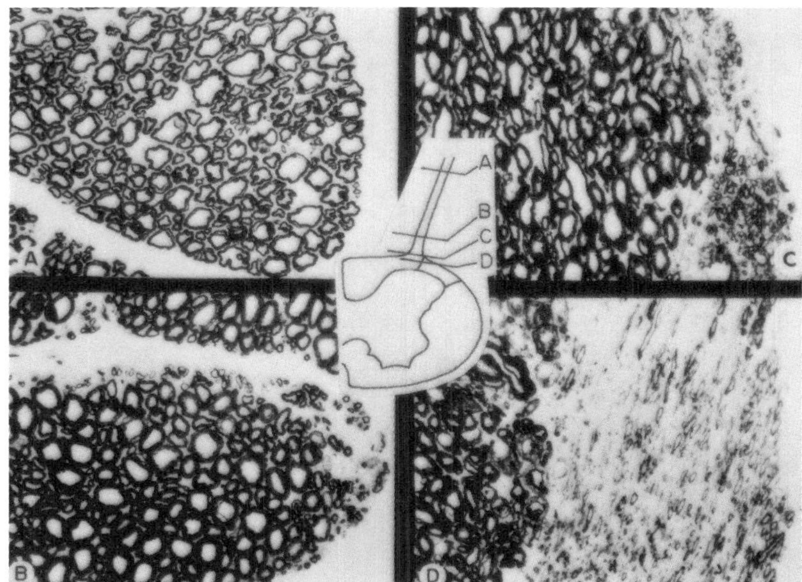

FIG. 24-10. Distribution of large and small fibers in the L7 dorsal root of the cat at selected intervals. **A.** At 5 mm from the root entry zone (REZ) there is no evidence of segregation. **B.** At approximately 1 mm from the REZ the small fibers are arranged in a peripheral ring. **C.** Just before entering the REZ, the great majority of small fibers are located in the lateral aspect of the rootlet. **D.** The small fibers have merged with the tract of Lissauer. (Kerr, F.W.L.: Mayo Clin. Proc., *50*:685–690, 1975.)

root ganglion neurons is consistent with the observation that the ventral root afferents are largely unmyelinated.[441] Similar results have been reported by Yamamoto and colleagues.[685] The relevance of the ventral root afferents in pain transmission remains to be fully described. This alternate pathway may account for the failure of dorsal rhizotomies to reliably relieve pain.[491] The origin of dorsal and ventral root afferents in dorsal root ganglion neurons would suggest that ganglionectomy would be superior to rhizotomy if afferent input is to be abolished.[492]

Afferent Terminals in Dorsal Horn

The concept that the spinal gray matter of the adult spinal cord may be organized according to a distinctive lamination of cell bodies and terminal regions has been used fruitfully to delimit the anatomy of the spinal gray matter (see Fig. 24-11).[534,535]

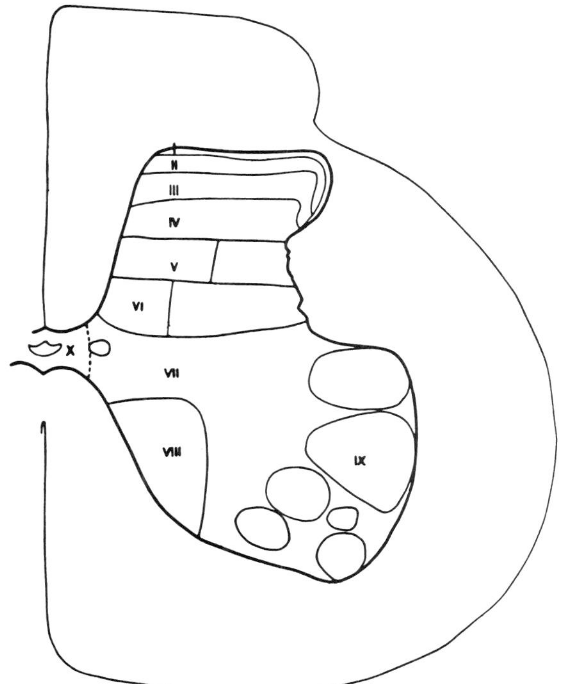

FIG. 24-11. Schematic drawing of the lamination of the ventral cell column of the 7th lumbar spinal cord segment in the full-grown cat. Lamina VIII occupies only the medial part of the ventral horn, lamina IX with its large motor nuclei has swung laterally and dorsally, and lamina VII extends between them both deeply into the horn. (Rexed, B.: J. Comp. Neurol., *96*:415–495, 1952.)

Retrograde transport of horseradish peroxidase to the distal cut ends of primary afferent fibers after medial section of the dorsal root revealed that horseradish peroxidase reaction product was located primarily in the dorsalmost laminae of the spinal gray matter. Terminals from smaller myelinated fibers were located in the marginal zone, the ventral portion of lamina II, and throughout lamina III.[416] Fine caliber unmyelinated fibers largely terminated throughout lamina II. In contrast, the large caliber fibers passing in the medial portion of the root entry zone terminated largely in the nucleus proprius and in more ventral regions of the dorsal gray matter. These larger fibers made few direct contacts with neurons of the substantia gelatinosa and marginal layer. Similar results were obtained in studies in which the distribution of functionally defined afferents was examined after intra-axonal application of horseradish peroxidase.[417] Intermediate-to-fine diameter cutaneous nociceptive mechanoreceptors terminated largely in the marginal zone. Terminals of low threshold mechanoreceptors activated by D-hair-type (down hair) receptors were distributed in the dorsal portion of laminae IV and V as well as in the ventral portions of the substantia gelatinosa. These comments are summarized schematically in Figure 24-12).

PHARMACOLOGY OF PRIMARY AFFERENTS

Central (Spinal) Terminals

The synapse made by primary afferents with neurons of the spinal cord represents the first-order link between the periphery and the central nervous system. Electrophysiologic studies have provided substantial evidence that conducted potentials interact with the second-order neuron by an excitatory synapse. No evidence of a classic monosynaptic inhibitory influence by primary afferents has been presented.[294] These considerations, along with morphologic evidence such as synaptic vesicles, end-plate specializations, and synaptic clefts, are consistent with the premise that the primary afferent exerts its effect on the second-order neuron by the release of excitatory neurotransmitters.

Considerable efforts have been directed at establishing the identity of neuroactive substances in the primary afferent. Several criteria are classically accepted as minimum requirements in the establishment of the correspondence between the endoge-

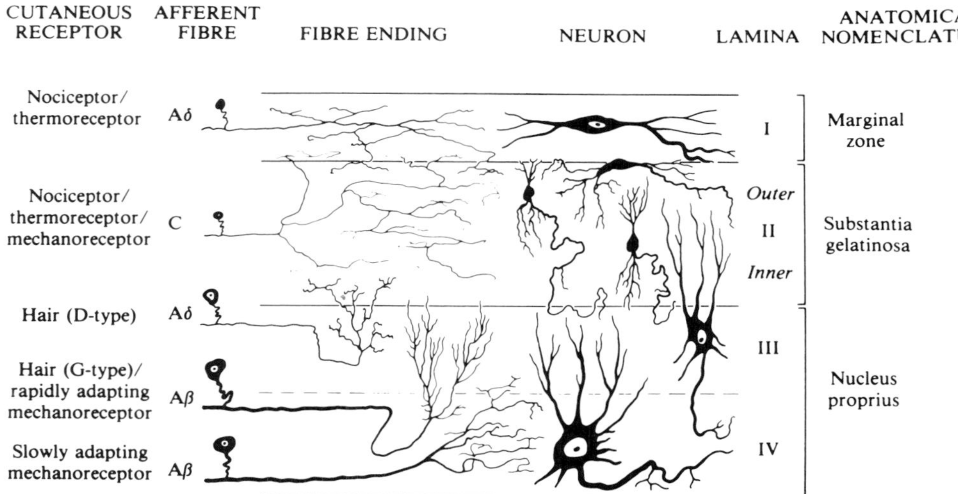

FIG. 24-12. Schematic diagram of the neuronal organization of, and afferent input to, the superficial dorsal horn. The diagram represents an imaginary transverse section of the dorsal horn and illustrates the afferent fiber endings and neuronal elements present in the first four laminae of the dorsal horn. To the left of the diagram the types of afferent fiber and relevant receptor groups associated with them are listed. Fiber endings in the dorsal horn are schematized diagrams taken from published morphologic studies. Neurons in the diagram represent standard types of neuron in the superficial dorsal horn. The following types have been illustrated *(from top to bottom):* a marginal cell, an SG limiting cell, two SG central cells, and two neurons of the nucleus proprius, the most superficial of which has dendrites penetrating lamina II. Indicated at the right of the diagram are the laminar division of the superficial dorsal horn and corresponding anatomic nomenclature. (Cervero, F., and Iggo, A.: Brain, *103*:717–772, 1980.)

nous material and a given substance: [1] The material must be found in the terminals of the afferent population in question (and it or its precursor in the respective dorsal root ganglion cell); [2] the material must be present in a fraction that is released when the appropriate afferents undergo depolarization; [3] the postsynaptic effects of the exogenously applied materials must mimic the effects that result when the endogenous afferent systems are physiologically activated; and [4] those physiologic effects that result from the actions of the endogenously released and exogenously administered agents must possess an identical pharmacology (*i.e.,* the characteristics of the receptor acted upon by the endogenous and exogenous agents must be indistinguishable).

Localization of Putative Afferent Neurotransmitters. Currently, excitatory amino acids such as aspartate and glutamate[157] and a number of peptides including substance P (sP), vasoactive intestinal peptide (VIP), somatostatin, a VIP homologue (PHI), cholecystokinin (CCK), angiotensin II, bombesin, and related peptides have been observed to possess the following characteristics: [1] They have been found in the dorsal horn of the spinal cord (where most primary afferent terminals are found); [2] the levels in dorsal horn are reduced by rhizotomy or ganglionectomy, or both; and [3] the peptides have been shown to exist within subpopulations of small dorsal root ganglion cells (type-B cells of Anders) (see Table 24-10). This latter observation is of particular importance because it is thought to be small afferents arising from the type-B cells that are perhaps relevant to pain transmission (see also Fig. 28-4).

Immunohistochemical studies directed at the dorsal horn have revealed discriminable differences in the discrete distribution of the several peptides in the dorsal laminae. sP is predominantly located in Rexed lamina I and the outer layer of II; VIP is principally found in lamina I, whereas somatostatin is found in the outer layer of II. Fluoride-resistant acid phosphatase, found in small ganglion cells separate from

TABLE 24-10 SUMMARY OF EVIDENCE SUGGESTING THE PRESENCE OF CERTAIN PEPTIDES IN SPINAL PRIMARY AFFERENT TERMINALS

Peptide	Dorsal Horn > Ventral Horn		DRG/Roots	Effect of Rhizotomy on Dorsal Horn Levels
	Immunohistochemistry/ RIA-Bioassay			
sP	Yes (1)	Yes (2)	+ (1)	(3)
Somatostatin	Yes (4)	Yes (2)	+ (4)	(5)
VIP	Yes (6)	Yes (7)	+ (8)	(7)
PHI	–	Yes (9)	Yes (9)	–
Cholecystokinin	Yes (10)	Yes (7)	+ (10)	(7)
Angiotension II	Yes (11)	–	Yes (11)	–
Bombesin	Yes (12)	–	Yes (13)	–

(1) 287; (2) 225; (3) 589; (4) 285; (5) Micevych, P.E., and Yaksh, T.L.: Unpublished observations; (6) 339; (7) 678; (8) 428; (9) Yaksh, T.L., Michener, S., and Go, V.L.W.: Unpublished observations; (10) 159; (11) 286; (12) 495; (13) 496.

those containing sP or somatostatin,[463] is distributed primarily in the inner layer of lamina II in regions distinct from those that sP, VIP, or somatostatin project.[464]

Additionally, a decrease in sP levels in the dorsal horn after ventral rhizotomies has been reported in cats.[665] These observations are consistent with findings discussed previously that unmyelinated afferent fibers course in the ventral roots.

Ability of Putative Afferent Neurotransmitters to Be Released. Important considerations are whether the materials present in afferent terminals exist within a releasable fraction and whether the axons from which they derive are relevant to pain transmission. From spinal cord slices, sP and somatostatin levels in the extracellular fluid have been shown to be elevated in a Ca^{++}-dependent fashion by depolarization.[5,322,493,550,564] *In vivo* studies using a spinal superfusion model[680] have demonstrated the release of materials from primary afferents, including sP,[396,676] VIP, and CCK.[54,673] With these peptides, release was produced by stimulation that activated A-delta/C but not A-beta afferents. The release of sP from spinal cord has been shown to be antagonized by the local application of mu and delta but not kappa opioid agonists and by α_2-agonists.[671] These observations are consistent with the presence of opioid and alpha-adrenergic receptors on primary afferent terminals and the effects of opiates and adrenergic agonists on afferent terminals.[317,549,670,702]

Postsynaptic Actions. Glutamate and aspartate applied onto dorsal horn neurons result in a powerful reversible depolarization with rapid onset accompanied by an increase in membrane conductance (see, for example, Ref. 698). Examination of the subclasses of neurons excited by glutamate or aspartate reveals no functional selectivity. Thus motor horn cells and dorsal horn neurons excited by A-beta, A-delta, and C fibers show a characteristic excitatory response to glutamate administration.[46,698]

Iontophoretic application onto the dorsal horn of several peptides found in primary afferents has been shown to produce excitatory effects. The focal administration of sP onto spinal neurons results in a slow progressive depolarization of the cell.[273,462,699]

Substance P will excite cells that are naturally activated by noxious radiant heat,[273] strong mechanical stimuli,[528] and the intra-arterial injection of bradykinin[509,664] and facilitate the response of cells activated by noxious cutaneous stimuli. Other agents such as glutamate, CCK, and VIP appear somewhat less selective, since they have been shown to produce excitatory and facilitatory effects on neurons that respond to a wide variety of innocuous stimuli (see above). Thus, there appears to be a significant correlation between the ability of sP to evoke a progressive depolarization in a dorsal horn neuron and the existence of an afferent drive from small fibers (see, however, Ref. 509).

VIP and CCK have similarly been shown to evoke excitation of dorsal horn neurons.[318,319] Somatostatin has been shown to produce an inhibition of the activity of dorsal horn neurons after iontophoretic administration.[528] This finding is somewhat surprising because a monosynaptic inhibition by primary afferents on second-order neurons has not been described, but reflects the fact that these agents may exist in several systems, not in primary afferents alone.

It is likely that some populations of afferents, particularly those of small diameter, may have more than one material in their terminals that can be released. Electron microscopy has long indicated the presence of several morphologically distinct vesicle populations in primary afferent terminals, notably those that are dense core and now thought to contain peptides and smaller clear vesicles that may contain amino acids (see Ref. 446). Intracellular recording in rat spinal cord slices has revealed that repetitive stimulation of the dorsal roots results in an initial burst of monosynaptically driven spikes followed by a prolonged slow hypopolarization.[615] The slow depolarization of dorsal horn neurons evoked by afferent stimulation or focally applied sP (but not VIP) was blocked by coadministration of a putative sP receptor antagonist, such as D-Pro^2-D-Try^{7,9}-sP, or by the prior administration of capsaicin, a neurotoxin that results in the depletion of afferent stores of sP and CCK, destroys small afferents marked by the cytosol enzyme fluoride-resistant acid phosphatase, but has no effect on large diameter afferents (see Ref. 671). The early depolarization was unaffected by these manipulations. These observations suggest that for this particular neuronal population in neonatal rat spinal cord, afferent stimulation results in two events: a delayed depolarization likely mediated by a population of sP-containing terminals and an immediate depolarization mediated by a second neuroactive agent, perhaps an excitatory amino acid (see Ref. 311).

Role of Neurotransmitters in Pain Transmission. In view of the above data, one may tentatively hypothesize that sP may play some role in pain transmission. *In vivo*, intrathecal, or systemic capsaicin has been shown to produce a reduction in the response to thermal and chemical stimuli,[670] and this treatment will produce powerful depleting effects on the levels of sP, somatostatin, and FRAP in primary afferent terminals (see above).

The direct application of sP into the dorsal horn of the spinal cord results in mild scratching behavior,[301] but this effect is translated into a profound increase in behavioral signs of irritation when the peptide is coadministered with the excitatory amino acid glutamate.[671] The potentiating effects are reduced when this is coadministered with low doses of putative sP receptor antagonists. Importantly, the direct spinal administration of sP antagonists results in a significant increase in the nociceptive threshold, but this effect is associated with significant changes in motor function.[6,671]

Peripheral Terminals

A common result of a high-intensity thermal or mechanical stimulus is tissue damage and is termed by Lewis[412] as the "triple response": a flush at the site of the stimulus accompanied by a flare resulting from widespread arterial dilation and a local edema secondary to increased vascular permeability. This state of inflammation is often accompanied by a local decrease in the magnitude of the stimulus required to elicit a pain response, that is, a primary hyperalgesia,[52,661] referred to by Lewis[412] as "nocifensor tenderness." The region of primary hypersensitivity is often surrounded by a much larger region of secondary hypersensitivity.[412] Evidence that these phenomena were mediated by a peripheral mechanism derives from the following observations: [1] Antidromic electrical activation of sensory afferent fibers produces hypersensitivity and flare in the skin region innervated by the nerve; and [2] blockade of the nerve central to the site of antidromic stimulation does not block the hypersensitivity evoked by such nerve stimulation.[410] Because the antidromic volley evokes a primary hyperalgesia and vasodilation in the absence of sympathetic innervation and the required stimulation intensities evoke discharges in C fibers, it appears likely that the effects are mediated by unmyelinated somatic afferents.[124,282,410]

Lewis[410] presciently suggested that primary hypersensitivity was due to the release of algogenic agents from damaged tissue and from nerve terminals in the skin by means of an axon reflex activated by the proximate tissue damage. In this case, it is suggested that action potentials evoked in the terminals of a sensory fiber which are in the damaged regions travel not only back to the spinal cord, but also antidromically into the surrounding vascular bed by means of axon collaterals. This is associated with the release of a vasodilator agent that increases blood flow (thereby producing the flare), increases vascular permeability (producing edema), and, as a result of either a direct effect or a subsequent release of an intermediate agent, activates or facilitates the activation of peripheral sensory afferent terminals (hypersensitivity).

The local release of chemical intermediates as suggested above may also explain the occurrence of continued sensation after the primary stimulus (*e.g.*, thermal or mechanical) has been removed. Thus mild heat damage to the receptive fields has been shown to produce significant increases in the excitability of polymodal nociceptors (C fibers, see below)[38,49,503] and high threshold mechanoreceptors.[206] As noted above, the paradoxical discharges of cold receptors to noxious heat also display sensitization.[178] A chemical intermediary with a prolonged half-life that alters the environs of the adjacent nerve terminals and facilitates their activity could explain the accompanying hypersensitivity.

Endogenous agents that may mediate these effects can be categorized according to their presumed origin: tissue (serotonin; histamine; potassium; members of the arachidonic acid cascade), plasma (kinins), or nerve terminals (substance P; sP). This listing is meant only to be representative and is neither inclusive nor exclusive (see Refs. 122, 700).

Histamine (granules of mast cells, basophils, and platelets[245]) and serotonin (mast cells and platelets[195]) are released by mechanical trauma, heat, radiation, and certain by-products of tissue damage, most notably neutrophil lysosomal materials, certain immunologic processes, thrombin, collagen, and epinephrine, as well as by lipid acids of the arachidonic acid cascade, such as the leukotryines, and the prostaglandins.[338,457,583,616]

Prostanoids are synthesized upon the release of cell-membrane-derived arachidonic acid by the activation of phospholipase A.[546] Various agents, including norepinephrine and dopamine, stimulate synthesis of cellular phospholipids by releasing nonesterified free fatty acid precursors.[211,436] Membrane-bound enzymes lipoxygenase,[478] or cyclooxygenase[545] act on these substrates to synthesize the leukotrienes and the prostanoids. Agents such as acetylsalicylic acid and indomethacin inhibit cyclooxygenase[210,573,621] and prevent the synthesis of these agents.

Bradykinin is synthesized by the cascade that is triggered when the factor XII is activated by agents such as kallikrein and trypsin. In the course of the cascade even more kallikrein is produced; this is converted to bradykinin by the enzyme timenogenase.[125,138] This factor is released by noxious insult.[538,658]

Agents directly relevant to nociception that are released from tissue in response to injury may activate small diameter afferent fibers and evoke pain when applied locally. Serotonin, histamine, acetylcholine, bradykinin, and potassium have all been shown to excite primary afferents. Close intra-arterial injection of serotonin excites populations of cutaneous mechanoreceptive and high-threshold afferents.[35,36] Similar administration of histamine was shown to excite populations of C fiber/group IV cutaneous mechanoreceptors and nociceptors sensitive to thermal and mechanical stimuli, but not myelinated (presumably non-noxious) mechanoreceptive afferents.[209,212] Administration of 48/80, which releases histamine from mast cells, activated small diameter fiber nociceptors.[49] A variety of agents (acetylcholine, potassium, histamine, serotonin, bradykinin) injected into the ear of a rabbit isolated from the body except for its nerve supply evoked a reflex depressor response indicative of the activation of small diameter cutaneous nociceptive afferents.[331]

Direct application of histamine, SRSA, or bradykinin onto a blister base induced by cantharidin or the direct injection of these agents into the skin induced a significant pain response in humans.[26,191,340] In dogs, the intra-arterial but not the intravenous injection of serotonin, histamine, and bradykinin induced pseudoaffective responses (barking, efforts to escape, pupil dilatation), the most potent agent being bradykinin (see also Fig. 24-1).[251]

Prostaglandins injected alone evoked little pain response except in high doses.[151,198,295] Although these prostanoids commonly have little evocative effect, they readily facilitate the pseudoaffective and autonomic responses produced by intra-arterial administration of bradykinin in dogs and rabbits.[198,331] Intradermal injections of PGE_1 augmented the pain evoked by [1] peripheral injections of bradykinin and histamine[196]; [2] the writhing response evoked by intraperitoneal phenylbenzoguinone[142,312]; [3] the response to pressure in the inflamed rat's paw[197,609]; and [4] the dog's inflammed knee joint.[453] Perfusion of the receptive field of a thermal nociceptive afferent with PGE_2 did not alter its resting discharge. PGE_2 did, however, produce a dose-dependent increase in the discharge rate of the fiber in response to a stimulus.[266] Similarly, the simultaneous administration of PGE_1 and bradykinin, each in a dose that by itself was ineffective, together produced significant activity in afferent fibers.[123] That some or all of bradykinin's algogenic effects may be mediated or potentiated by prostaglandins is suggested by nociceptive response to the kinin being blocked by prior treatment with a cyclooxygenase inhibitor.[198,407,453]

If the prostaglandins produce their sensitizing effects by a common biochemical mechanism in the different species and several organ systems, a common order of potency for the several lipidic acids should be observed. Where examined, the following rank order has, in fact, been observed: $PGE_1 > PGE_2 > PGF_{2\alpha} \geq PGF_{2\beta} \geq PGA_1 = PGB_2 = PGI_2 = 0$.[198,331,453,609,622]

Given prostaglandins' presumed role in the sensitizing effects of injury, it is thus important to note that [1] in damaged skin there is a significant elevation in prostanoid levels that is blocked by cyclooxygenase inhibition[244,259,651]; and [2] local intra-arterial bradykinin will enhance the formation and release of prostaglandins.[330,332,408,443]

Substance P, an undecapeptide, is located in small diameter unmyelinated primary afferent neurons, as well as in peripheral terminals in the skin,[224,287,288] cortical blood vessels,[438,459] tooth pulp,[487] and eye.[53] Nearly four times as much sP is transported toward the peripheral as the central terminals.[73] Stimulation of the trigeminal nerve has been shown to release sP from tooth pulp,[75] which, like exogenously administered sP, evokes an increase in local blood flow and capillary permeability. The effects of either manipulation are reversed by putative sP antagonists.[148,540] These observations appear to reflect mechanisms that may be quite common. The sP in plexi surrounding cerebral vessels and that originates in the trigeminal ganglion may be released and occasion the vascular syndrome of migraine.[459]

It should be stressed that *antidromic* nerve activity in dorsal roots secondary to afferent input in an adjacent root is readily demonstrated and is commonly seen in the early phases of primary afferent depolarization.[31,186,187] The ability of visceral and somatic afferent terminals to mutually produce primary afferent depolarization and dorsal root reflexes in the other has been described.[560,561] Thus, given that visceral and autonomic terminals possess stores of sP that are associated with primary afferents (see Ref. 153), one might propose that somatic input directly interacts with autonomic/visceral systems, and *vice versa*. The relevance of such systems to various somatovisceral reflexes is clear (see Fig. 24-2).

With regard to cutaneous terminals, sP has been shown not to be algogenic when administered peripherally[406] and will not activate peripheral nociceptive afferents.[390] Antidromic nerve stimulation, as noted above, will produce flare and sensitization in the region of skin innervated by the stimulated sensory nerve. As exogenously administered, sP has been shown to induce plasma extravasation in both normal and denervated skin,[406] and, because other peptides such as VIP do not produce such extravasation,[224] sP appears a likely mediator for the neurogenically evoked increase in capillary wall permeability. The release of a kinin in skin following antidromic activation of the dorsal root has been shown.[127] Administration of capsaicin will deplete sP content in skin,[224] which is accompanied by a loss of the ability of peripheral nerve stimulation to produce extravasation.[314,587] This supports the idea that the antidromically induced changes in vascular permeability may be mediated through the release of this peptide. Importantly, topical treatment with capsaicinoids also attenuates the pseudoaffective pain response of animals or humans to otherwise algogenic chemical stimuli applied in that region.[313,586]

The pharmacology of the peripheral neurotransmitter terminals has only just begun to be examined, but it is likely that since the activity of central terminals is governed by selected receptor populations, so might be the peripheral terminals. Thus the characteristics of the effects of neurotoxins (such as capsaicin) after topical application to the skin or to the cord are identical.[324] Opiate binding sites are known to be transported peripherally in afferents,[695] and the release of sP from tooth pulp has been shown to be antagonized by morphine, suggesting that these binding sites in the distant terminals are coupled.[76] Given the presence of other primary afferent terminal receptors, for example, GABA and α_2-adrenergic, the possibility of a complicated peripheral pharmacology cannot be dismissed. These observations together thus suggest that the primary afferent neurotransmitter systems may play a pervasive role far beyond their coding of afferent information by also influencing peripheral vascular and autonomic systems, a perhaps not unexpected consequence of a reasonable interpretation of Dale's Principle.[158]

NOCICEPTIVE ELEMENTS IN SPINAL CORD

The differential distribution in the Rexed lamina[534] of terminals associated with fibers that are activated by specific noxious stimuli is consistent with the existence of populations of second-order neurons relevant to the rostrad transmission of nociceptive information (see Fig. 24-12).

Marginal Zone (Lamina I)

The superficial layer of the dorsal horn comprises classes of large neurons oriented transversely across the cap of the dorsal gray matter. Some cells project to the thalamus by means of contralateral ascending pathways[354,398,522,603,604,655]; others project intrasegmentally and intersegmentally along the dorsal and dorsolateral white matter.[93,551,585]

The dendritic plexus of these neurons extends up to several hundred micra along both the transverse and longitudinal axes of the cord, although the dendritic tree is largely confined to the marginal layer.[95,235] As displayed schematically in Figure

24-12) afferent terminals tend to synapse distally in the dendritic tree whereas nonafferent terminals tend to be proximal on the cell body.[352,354]

Lamina I neurons may be divided physiologically into three groups: [1] neurons activated by fibers having A-delta/C fiber conduction velocities that respond to intense mechanical stimulation; [2] neurons activated by innocuous skin cooling with afferents having a conduction velocity akin to those of an A-delta fiber; and [3] a small percentage of neurons activated by C fiber polymodal afferents.[117,131,394,395,522,656] Although initial observations suggested that these neurons of lamina I were specifically sensitive to intense stimuli, a significant proportion of these cells also possess wide dynamic range, that is, a response frequency proportional to the intensity of the stimulus.[117] Importantly, those neurons responding to A-delta and C fiber input can also be activated by group III and group IV muscle afferents, indicating a convergence of muscle and cutaneous input.

Substantia Gelatinosa (Laminae II and III)

The clear band of neural tissue lying ventral to the marginal layer and dorsal to a region of coarser texture known as the nucleus proprius was given the name substantia gelatinosa by Rolando.[539] The substantia gelatinosa, defined by gross observation in unfixed or semifixed tissue, corresponds to the laminae II and III of Rexed. The question as to whether only lamina II[236,416,417,527,534] or laminae II and III[354] constitute the substantia gelatinosa is one of nomenclature and is resolved by definition of the precise area under study.[114]

Lamina II is divided into an outer and inner layer. The former is characterized by small, densely packed cells and a neuropil made complex by the presence of a larger number of dendrites. The latter zone is similar but has a less coarse texture owing to the relative paucity of terminals.[416,527] The principal cell type in lamina II is the stalk cell, with cone-shaped dendritic trees arborizing through lamina II into III and axons branching into lamina I.[236,551] The terminals of A-delta afferents that project to this lamina are a likely source of the numerous axodendritic contacts observed in this region.[141,182,234,352,526,639]

Lamina III contains fewer neurons and a less dense neuropil than does lamina II. In addition, the islet neuron[233,238] (Golgi type II) appears in high concentration, in contrast to the stalk cells that occur predominantly in the outer layer of lamina II.

A detailed review of this complex region has been published.[115]

A significant proportion of the substantia gelatinosa neurons receive A-delta/C fiber input.[118,392,394,418,632] Neurons located in lamina II (the outer portion of the substantia gelatinosa) tend to be excited by activation of thermal receptive or mechanical nociceptive afferents.[418]

Neurons retrogradely labeled with horseradish peroxidase and activated by nociceptive input display dendritic branching in the outer layer of the substantia gelatinosa, whereas neurons activated by innocuous mechanical stimuli have dendritic trees in the inner layer of the substantia gelatinosa.[417] Receptive fields of gelatinosa neurons responsive to peripheral stimuli are small (less than 2 cm^2).

The properties of gelatinosa neurons are not well examined, but several interesting characteristics have emerged. First, unlike those cells lying more deeply (see below), neurons of the substantia gelatinosa commonly exhibit prolonged periods of excitation and inhibition after afferent activation.[278,632] Second, islet and stalked cells constitute several classes of functionally distinct cells, with variable degrees of background activity and in which afferent input will drive complex "on/off" responses. Significantly, those cells inhibited by non-noxious stimuli were excited by noxious input, whereas cells inhibited by noxious input were excited by non-noxious input.[114,119] Such profiles suggest that the activity of substantia gelatinosa neurons is governed by a convergence of large and small fiber input acting either directly on these neurons or by inhibitory interneurons.

Nucleus Proprius (Laminae IV and V)

Lamina IV, as defined by Rexed, is composed of a broad layer of relatively large neurons (10 to 15 μm in diameter) that endows this region with its characteristic morphology. The dendritic tree of these neurons transversely and dorsally spreads into laminae II and III. The neuropil is characterized by axodendritic and axoaxonic synapses[351,526] originating from [1] afferent input of the large diameter fibers that contact the apical portion of the dendritic tree[525] and [2] local axonal plexi derived from intrinsic fibers.[354]

Lamina V, located along the neck of the dorsal horn, displays a dendritic organization that does not differ from that of neurons in lamina IV. Neurons in both lamina IV and V project to the ventrobasal thalamus and mesencephalon[229,360,602,603,604] and the lateral cervical nucleus,[80,116] and provide propriospinal projections within the spinal cord in various species (see below).

Cells in the nucleus proprius may be broadly classed as those that respond to A-beta input and those that respond to A-beta, A-delta, and C and are referred to as wide dynamic range neurons.[448] The latter class responded to transient brush and touch but showed no elevation in activity with prolonged pinch; these cells are often referred to as lamina IV neurons because of the early studies that localized them in that region.[630] In the latter classes of cells, light innocuous touch evokes activity that increases as the intensity of pressure or pinch is increased. Thermal stimuli applied to the receptive field will similarly evoke a rate of discharge that is proportional to temperature; some units show an exponential increase in discharge rate at temperatures above 45°C.[401,402,518,520] Repetitive electrical stimulation at 0.5 to 1 Hz of C fiber input onto a wide dynamic range neuron produces a gradual increase in the frequency discharge until the neuron is in a state of virtually continuous discharge. This is referred to as "windup."[448] The possibility that this repetitive activity derived from C fiber input may occur secondary to the release of sP has been previously noted.

Although these WDR neurons are commonly referred to as lamina V neurons, precise assignment of cells to given functional class cannot be made on the basis of absolute depth within the dorsal gray matter.[84]

Receptive fields for wide dynamic range neurons are more extensive than those of the primary afferent neurons that impinge upon them, indicating convergence of afferent input onto the dendritic tree. As with marginal neurons (and the primary afferents), receptive field size decreases as one moves distally on the extremities.[83,86,117] Although somatotopically convergent input is the rule for wide dynamic range neurons and the activity of such neurons can be highly influenced by input from several adjacent spinal cord segments, these neurons are activated most effectively by input arriving from the dermatome in which they lie.[521,628] Importantly, many of the early investigations were carried out in decerebrate or decerebrate/spinal animals to avoid the use of anesthetics. In experiments using intact anesthetized preparations, receptive fields, sometimes including the whole body, have been found in addition to the more restricted ones observed when the spinal cord has been transected. Moreover, the magnitude of the receptive field is under an ongoing modulation by intrinsic systems that can increase and decrease the size of the field complex (see below).

Wide dynamic range neurons commonly demonstrate organ convergence as well as somatic convergence. Thus neurons in the n. proprius have been observed that are activated by [1] stimulation of sympathetic afferents and by coronary artery occlusion, as well as by noxious pinches applied within the dermatomes that coincided with the segmental location of those cells (T1–T5)[215]; [2] stimulation of the splanchnic nerve and A-beta/A-delta cutaneous input[265,512,560,561]; [3] distension of hollow viscera (bladder, small intestine, and gallbladder)[636]; [4] injection of bradykinin into the mesenteric artery and cutaneous input[249]; and [5] close intra-arterial administration of bradykinin or the injection of hypertonic saline into muscle/tendon or group III afferent stimulation from the gastrocnemius[216,512] and cutaneous input field. Correlation of those areas of the skin (forepaw, hind paw, hind leg, abdomen, thorax) where stimulation would evoke activity in neurons known to be activated by distension of the gallbladder or the urinary bladder revealed that about one third of the units examined responded to stimulation of both the gallbladder and various cutaneous regions with the highest percentage associated with the thorax and perineum.[203] Progressive bladder distension activated cells in widespread dermatomal regions, but most effectively activated neurons responsive to cutaneous stimuli applied to the abdomen. These results indicate that the phenomenon of referred visceral pain likely has its substrate in viscerosomatic and musculosomatic convergence onto dorsal horn neurons.[542]

Central Canal (Lamina X)

Although the central canal is a parvicellular region, recent studies have demonstrated that branches of small lightly myelinated fibers were observed to enter the region.[416] Transport studies have further demonstrated that a significant proportion of these neurons projected both ipsilaterally and contralaterally in the ventrolateral tract into the bulbar reticular formation. Recent studies have demonstrated that cells in this region possess properties similar to those of the marginal cells noted above. Thus cells have been observed that respond primarily to high-threshold temperature and noxious pinch with small receptive fields.[291,293,465]

ASCENDING SPINAL TRACTS

Ventral Funicular Systems

Unilateral and ventrolateral tractotomies elevate the threshold for visceral and somatic pain reports on the side contralateral to the lesion.[398,576,623,625,643] Conversely, stimulation of the ventrolateral tracts in awake subjects undergoing percutaneous cordotomies has resulted in reports of contralateral warmth and pain.[440,643] The analgesia is characterized by a loss or reduction in the response to thermal (heat and cold), mechanical (pinprick), itch,[645] and deep somatic (Achilles tendon) stimuli. Midline myelotomies that destroy fibers crossing the midline at the levels of the cut produce bilateral pain deficits.[283,554] These observations jointly suggest that the relevant pathways for nociception are predominantly crossed. It should be stressed that midline myelotomies are not identical with ventrolateral cordotomies. As summarized by Vierck and colleagues,[623] after midline myelotomy there tends to be [1] an increased incidence of paresthesias; [2] no decrease in the magnitude of evoked cutaneous pain; [3] preserved dull – sharp discrimination; and [4] enduring losses of deep pain.

The rostrad transmission of nociceptive information, however, is not unique to the ventrolateral funiculus (VLF). This is evidenced by [1] the anomalous recovery of pain 3 months to 1 year after cordotomy; [2] the persistence of contralateral pain sensations after a unilateral lesion (suggestive of bilateral projections); and [3] the ability of high-intensity stimulation to produce a "break through" of pain resembling the diffuse, burning pain of C fiber activation.[644]

Origin. Localization of the cells of origin of this system have been made by [1] examining chromatolytic reaction after spinal section, [2] antidromic activation of spinal neurons by brain-stem electrodes, and [3] labeling of spinal neurons with horseradish peroxidase injected into probable terminal regions of axons projecting in the VLF.

Retrograde chromatolytic reactions were observed early in neurons of the marginal zone and of the deeper laminae (IV and V) of the dorsal horn of patients with clinically effective lesions of the VLF.[398] Chromatolytic cell bodies lying more deeply in the ventral horn were also found after ventrolateral cordotomy.

Injection of horseradish peroxidase into the lateral thalamic nuclei or into the spinothalamic tract itself resulted in labeled neurons in the marginal zone, the substantia gelatinosa,[655] and laminae IV and V.[602] Stimulating electrodes placed in the contralateral VLF at cervical or mesodiencephalic levels will antidromically activate neurons in the marginal zone, the substantia gelatinosa, and laminae IV and V, as well as in laminae VII and VIII in the cat.[8,9,170,229,522,603] Fibers in the ventral funiculi are myelinated with diameters of 1 to 11 μm.[422] Application of the Hursh factor for myelinated fibers estimates conduction velocities that closely correspond to those reported for these fibers by several laboratories (18 – 58 m/sec in cats[170]; 7 – 74 m/sec in primates[656]).

Organization. Fibers traveling rostrad in this tract originate in the dorsal horn and cross in the dorsal commissure at levels up to two segments from the point of origin.[398,645,655] White and associates[642] noted a rostral displacement of the analgesic dermatomes after a ventrolateral cordotomy and suggested that before crossing, these axons may remain medial for one or two segments. A somatotopic arrangement within the VLF has been described such that the fibers arising from the more caudal segments are located laterally, whereas those entering from the more rostral segments lie medially and ventrally in the funiculi.[303]

Although it has been suggested that there may also be an anatomically defined organization by modality in the ventrolateral tract, for example, pain and touch, single unit recording studies in primates have failed to document such modality segregation (see Ref. 653).

Rostral Terminals. Because spinofugal tracts do not appear to show major or reliable differences with regard to their point of origin within the spinal gray matter (see below), the tracts projecting rostrally within the VLF are commonly considered according to the brain regions in which they terminate. Long tract systems that may be relevant to the rostrad transmission include the spinoreticular, spinomesencephalic, and spinothalamic tracts. The first two have often been referred to as the paleospinothalamic system, and the last as the neospinothalamic system by virtue of the increasing size of the diencephalic projections in phylogenetically advanced species.[444] It should be remembered, however, that up to half of the fibers in the VLF in humans (which are not destined for the cerebellum) terminate caudal to the rostral aspect of the inferior olive.[66]

Spinoreticular Fibers. Spinoreticular axons terminate both ipsilaterally and contralaterally to their site of origin in the spinal cord.[204,696] Entering the medulla, the fibers aggregate laterally, and collaterals of these fibers terminate in the more medially situated brain-stem reticular nuclei (the n. reticularis gigantocellularis, the n. reticularis paragigantocellularis, the n. reticularis pontis caudalis, and the n. subceruleus[64,355,445,541,696]). Terminals have also been reported in the n. raphe magnus and pallidus,[71,74,445] making both somatic and dendritic contacts.[638]

Stimulating electrodes in the reticular formation antidromically activate neurons in laminae V through VIII.[200,204,409] Discrete injections of horseradish peroxidase into the n. reticularis gigantocellularis and the magnocellular part of the lateral reticular nucleus have labeled neurons situated throughout the contralateral spinal cord in laminae IV, V, and VIII and in the ipsilateral laminae IV and V.[360,365] Lamina I neurons have not been identified as an origin of spinoreticular fibers in the above cited studies. This suggests that marginal zone neurons, some reportedly specifically nociceptive in function, do not contribute a significant projection into the medial medullary region. It is important to remember that although many of the projects to the bulbar reticular formation are ipsilateral, a small contingent of fibers may cross at the medullary level. Degeneration in this bulbar region after extensive midline myelotomies has not been observed.[362] Consistent with these anatomic observations, response latencies of neurons in the n. reticulogigantocellularis to stimulation of the ipsilateral hind paw in cat were shorter in 60% of the units examined.[67] Using stimulating electrodes placed at several brain-stem levels, it has been shown in cats that axons projecting no further than the brain-stem reticular formation do exist and possess cell bodies located throughout the n. proprius of the dorsal horn, as well as laminae VI–IX.[200] This suggests that spinoreticular terminals do not represent only the collaterals of fibers in transit to more rostrad sites. Retrograde transport studies have, however, demonstrated that some spinofugal axons do indeed project to both the brain stem and thalamus.[366,367]

With regard to electrophysiologic properties, spinoreticular neurons have been shown to possess receptive fields that may be restricted cutaneous, restricted deep, or complex extensive. Although the receptive fields are predominantly ipsilateral excitatory, bilateral fields and fields with inhibitory components have also been observed. A high proportion of spinoreticular neurons have wide dynamic range response characteristics.[200]

Spinomesencephalic Fibers. Fibers originate from neurons located in the spinal gray matter in regions similar to those reported for spinoreticular fibers. Two spinomesencephalic tracts have been reported. The largest tract crosses within the spinal cord; the lesser tract ascends ipsilaterally and crosses in the tegmentum at the level of the intertectal commissure.[445,696] Degenerating terminals following lesions of the ventrolateral cord have been observed in the midbrain reticular formation, for example, the nucleus cuneiformis, the inferior and superior colliculi, and the periaqueductal gray matter of several species.[24,63,64,355,445,696] In contrast to the spinoreticular projections, midline myelotomies produce extensive signs of degeneration in the mesencephalon.[362] Using retrograde labeling, cells of origin have been demonstrated in laminae I and V.[423,449]

Physiologic properties of identified spinomesencephalic neurons have not been examined extensively. Uniformly shorter response latencies of these neurons in the mesencephalon have been reported for contralateral as compared with ipsilateral somatic stimulation, suggesting a largely crossed afferent input.[11,41,68] A population of these cells displays a significant response to noxious stimuli.[687]

Spinothalamic Fibers. The cells of origin of this tract, the most extensively studied of the spinal projection systems, are as in previously discussed ventrolateral tract systems not limited to the dorsal gray matter. Figure 24-13 presents a summary of the position of cells in three species located by retrograde transport or antidromic activation. The existence of cell systems lying in the dorsal gray matter is expected, but the density around the neck of the proprius and the central canal emphasizes the possible role of this deep system in nociceptive transmission.[465] The tract ascends predominantly in the contralateral ventral quadrant. Crossed fibers predominate, but it is clear that uncrossed fibers represent a significant component of the spinothalamic population. Retrogradely labeled neurons following unilateral injection of horseradish peroxidase into the thalamus of the monkey revealed that about 25% of the projections from the sacral cord were ipsilateral.[655] The spinothalamic system ascends in the medulla, dorsolaterally to the pyramid, and inferiorly to the olivary nucleus. In the rostral mesencephalon, fibers are located ventromedially to the inferior colliculus. The spinothalamic fibers differentiate into a lateral and medial component in the posterior portions of the thalamus: The medial component passes through the internal medullary lamina to terminate in the n. parafascicularis and intralaminar and paralaminar nuclei.[445,454,696] The majority of fibers pass laterally

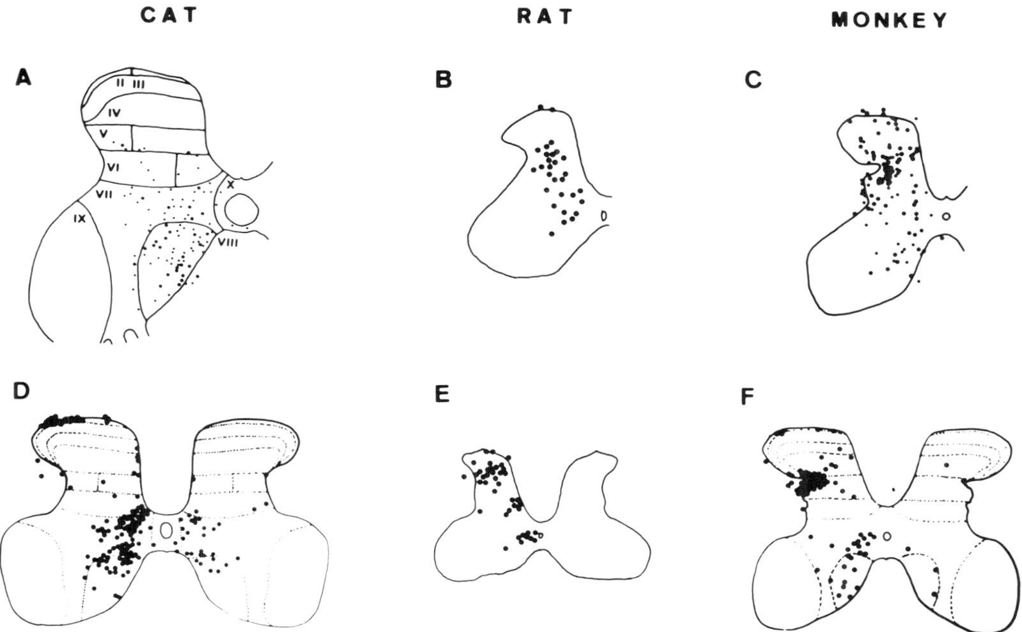

FIG. 24-13. **A–C.** Recording sites from which antidromic action potentials can be recorded from spinothalamic tract cells in the lumbosacral enlargement of the cat, rat, and monkey following stimulation in the contralateral thalamus. **D–F.** Location of spinothalamic tract cells labeled retrogradely following injection of horseradish peroxidase into the thalamus in cat, rat, and monkey. (Willis, W.D.: In Yaksh, T.L. [eds.]: Spinal Afferent Processing. New York, Plenum Press, 1986.)

through the external medullary lamina to terminate in small clusters scattered throughout the n. ventralis posterolateralis, the medial aspects of the posterior n. complex, and the intralaminar nuclei.[44,60,149,355,445,507] In primates, thalamic stimulation evokes antidromic activation of neurons located dorsally in the lateral aspect of the nucleus proprius and in the marginal zone.[8,603,656] With horseradish peroxidase studies, neurons in lamina I project uniquely to the region lying between the rostral, ventrolateral, and caudal ventrolateral thalamic nuclei. Spinothalamic neurons lying in laminae IV and V terminate in the posterior nuclei of the thalamus, whereas neurons in laminae VII and VIII are generally labeled after injections of horseradish peroxidase into the intralaminar thalamic nuclei.[104,230,602]

Giesler and colleagues[230a] have demonstrated a principal subdivision in primate spinothalamic projections. A significant proportion of the neurons projecting laterally in the thalamus (ventral posterior lateral complex) also projected to the medial (central lateral nucleus or dorsal medial nucleus) portion. In contrast, a second population of neurons projected only to the medial thalamus.

At least four classes of spinothalamic neurons may be tentatively identified: [1] Narrow dynamic range neurons that respond only to innocuous tactile stimuli (laminae IV and V); [2] neurons situated deep that are responsive to proprioceptive input (laminae IV and V); [3] wide dynamic range neurons that respond in a frequency-dependent fashion to stimuli of increasing intensity, receive convergent input from cutaneous, visceral, and muscle sources, respond to thermal and chemical stimuli in the noxious range, and display a sustained discharge to pressure but a rapid adaptation to light tactile input (lamina V); and [4] neurons that respond uniquely to high-intensity noxious stimuli. These high-threshold units display a slowly adapting response to noxious cutaneous mechanical and thermal stimuli. Lamina I neurons having such properties have been observed.[131,216,217,264,392,394,656] In the studies noted above,[230a] neurons that project to both the medial and the lateral thalamus have displayed a significant proportion of wide dynamic-range-type cells. In contrast, medially projecting cells have been largely characterized as high-threshold-selective.

With regard to receptive fields, antidromic activation of spinothalamic neurons with electrodes placed in both the medial thalamus and lateral thalamus has revealed three types of spinothalamic neurons: [1] those that project only to the lateral thalamus; [2] those that project only to the medial thalamus; and [3] those that project to both the medial *and* the lateral thalamus. Receptive field properties of those neurons that project to the lateral thalamus are conventional (small fields with larger surrounding regions that require more intense stimulation for activation of the neuron), and many neurons have inhibitory fields extending over broad body areas. Neurons projecting to the medial thalamus display large, often whole body receptive fields, although the contralateral field often is most effective in activating the cell. These neurons display discharge patterns that last beyond the stimulus. Severing the cord reduces the receptive field to that observed for spinal animals and abolishes the poststimulus discharge. Thus somatic stimuli gaining access to supraspinal centers can readdress spinal projection neurons in what appears to be a spino(contralateral)-bulbo (crossed)-spinal (ipsilateral) feedback circuit (see Ref. 652).

Dorsal Funicular Systems

Transections of the dorsal quadrant of the spinal cord in the cat produce significant increases in the nociceptive threshold.[343] Severance of the dorsal columns or the spinocervical tract, or both, may account for this elevation. In primates and humans, lesions of the dorsolateral quadrant have been reported to produce a hyperalgesia.[471,624] Although large diameter afferent fibers, sensitive to light touch and vibration, terminate in the dorsal column nuclei after ascending in the dorsal columns, many nonprimary afferent fibers originating in lamina V ascend in the dorsal column as well.[543,544] These fibers respond to tactile and to noxious mechanical and thermal stimuli.[22] Dorsal column lesions in humans[145] do not alter pain threshold, and stimulation of the dorsal columns in humans often gives rise to sensations of vibration, not of pain.[469] In primates, a slight decrease in pain reactivity has been observed.[624] As noted, a postsynaptic pathway originating from lamina V neurons in the dorsal horn has been shown. The role of this system is not known.

Axons of spinocervical neurons project ipsilaterally in the dorsolateral quadrant of the spinal cord to terminate in the lateral cervical nucleus.[80,86] These neurons lie predominantly in the nucleus proprius (laminae III and IV).[80,86] Several types of spinocervical neurons have been identified, and they appear to be activated by tactile (hair movement, pressure), noxious thermal (40 – 53 °C), and noxious mechanical (pinch) stimuli[77,78,79,116] and close intra-arterial injection of algogenic agents.[376]

The spinocervical tract has been well described in cats,[455] but its presence is much reduced in lower primates[253,254,473] and is practically nonexistent in humans.[605]

Intersegmental Systems

The ability of ventrolateral cordotomies to alter pain illustrates the important role of long tracts in the rostral transmission of nociceptive information. For reasons stated above, the existence of alternate spinal pathways appears certain. Early studies showed that alternating hemisections will abolish neither the behavioral nor the autonomic responses to strong stimuli.[32,72,372] These observations suggest that systems that project for short distances ipsilaterally may contribute to the rostrad transmission of nociceptive information. Kerr[350,357] proposed that selective destruction of the dorsal gray matter, for example, spinonucleolysis, might prove to be a possible method of pain management in light of the relevance of nonfunicular pathways traveling in the spinal gray matter. Subsequent work by Nashold and coworkers.[467] and Schvarcz[555,556] revealed that such lesions could produce significant and prolonged pain relief associated with nerve avulsions and other chronic, otherwise intractable, somatosensory pain syndromes. These procedures, using focal electrolytic lesions, strive to leave the superficial funicular pathways intact. These results offer support for the proposed relevance in pain transmission of systems traveling within the dorsal gray matter. Alternately, the recent role of cell systems in lamina X and the likelihood of local systems traveling in the dorsal columns indicates the possibility that midline myelotomies may not only act by the severance of crossing fibers, but also do damage to relevant midline systems. Early studies[161] suggested that visceral pain was dependent upon the central core (see Ref. 623). Several segmental pathways that may be relevant to the rostrad transmission of nociceptive information include the Lissauer tract, the dorsolateral propriospinal system, and the dorsal intracornual tract.

The tract of Lissauer is divided into medial and lateral components. The medial portion of the tract consists largely of collaterals of the unmyelinated or lightly myelinated primary afferent fibers that travel several segments rostrally and caudally before entering the dorsal horn gray matter.[354,529,530,585] The lateral tract lies in the dorsolateral funiculus immediately lateral to the dorsal root entry zone and consists of myelinated or small myelinated fibers deriving from neurons in the substantia gelatinosa and marginal layers.[585] These fibers may travel only a few millimeters in either direction before disappearing into the dorsal horn.[118,354,632,635] Although the medial and lateral components of Lissauer's tract can be separated at the dorsal root entry zone, they merge at the cervical level and cannot be easily differentiated (*c.f.* Ref. 635).

Lesions of the dorsolateral quadrant that destroy Lissauer's tract have been reported to elevate the nociceptive threshold[302,343] and enlarge the dermatomal fields associated with a given segment of the spinal cord. Tractotomies of the medial Lissauer tract in primates exert the opposite effect and result in shrinkage of the dermatome associated with a given spinal cord root.[166]

The ipsilateral projections of the dorsolateral propriospinal system travel lateral to the axis of the nucleus proprius and contain axons originating from neurons of the substantia gelatinosa and marginal zone.[95] The role of many marginal neurons in pain transmission and the possibility that these neurons may project in this pathway suggest that a certain proportion of nociceptive information may be transmitted by means of the dorsolateral propriospinal tract.

The dorsal intracornual tract consists of small diameter fibers coursing longitudinally through the medial regions of the nucleus proprius. Because rhizotomies do not reduce the number of these fibers, it appears they arise from intrinsic neurons.[354]

Despite corollary evidence suggesting that intrasegmental systems may transmit nociceptive information, the role of these pathways in pain transmission remains speculative. The results of a ventrolateral cordotomy clearly indicate the importance of crossed pathways; the segmental pathways are largely ipsilaterally organized. Yet there is evidence that some primary afferent neurons do terminate contralaterally (see above) and interneurons do cross the midline along the longitudinal axis of the cord as evidenced by the existence of crossed reflexes. Crossing fibers may serve to transmit the ipsilateral message to a contralateral projection. The existence of segmental spinal systems might explain the recurrence of pain 3 to 12 months after ventrolateral cordotomy and, particularly, the "breakthrough" mediated by small fibers that occurs when high-intensity stimuli are applied (see above and Ref. 623).

Consideration of Special Sensory Systems

In the preceding section, specific interest was directed at general systems whereby sensory information enters the central nervous system. Although the essential characteristics of the afferent input are reasonably uniform across the sensory systems, two systems have special complexities that render them of particular interest: These are the trigeminal system and the systems whereby visceral information enters the central nervous system.

Trigeminal System. The essential characteristics of afferent input through the trigeminal system are similar to those to the spinal cord. Certain morphologic and functional considerations, however, make it worth noting this system separately.

Trigeminal Input. The face, head, and buccal regions are innervated by the ophthalmic, mandibular, and maxillary divisions of the trigeminal nerve, the cell bodies of which are located in the ganglion of the 5th nerve (gasserian). The afferents are organized somatotopically in the sensory root in a medial to lateral fashion: The mandibular nerve branch is posterolaterally positioned, the ophthalmic branch anteromedially located, and the maxillary branch situated in an intermediate position.[34,160,349] The more rostral the peripheral terminal fields, the more ventrally and laterally situated are the cell bodies in the ganglia.[34,363]

As in the spinal cord, a large proportion of the afferent input enters through the sensory root (the portio major), but sensory fibers might also enter by way of the portio minor or the efferent outflow of the trigeminal system. Because visceral efferent fibers are not thought to course in the portio minor, the observation that about 20% of the axons are unmyelinated suggests a situation analogous to that studied in greater detail in the lumbar and sacral cord.[692] The continued presence of these afferent fibers may be a possible reason for the preservation of tactile sensitivity and of various pathologic facial pains following trigeminal nerve rhizotomy.[167,316]

Brain Stem Organization. The trigeminal sensory nucleus is divided into the main sensory and the more caudally located spinal nucleus (extending as far caudally as the cervical spinal cord). The spinal nucleus is further divided into three subdivisions: the n. oralis, n. interpolaris, and n. caudalis (rostral–caudal presentation).[489] The central processes of the trigeminal afferent neurons enter the brain stem at the level of the pons to terminate in these nuclei.[135] The somatotopic arrangement of the three branches of the trigeminal nerve observed within the ganglion is maintained in the descending trigeminal tract and in the main sensory[349,388] and the spinal[349,518] nuclei.

Large diameter afferents bifurcate within the brain stem, giving rise to ascending and descending branches that terminate in the main sensory and spinal nuclei, respectively.[27,95] Horseradish peroxidase injected into axons of physiologically identified afferents of vibrissae has confirmed the bifurcation of these afferents and their coinnervation of the main sensory and spinal nuclei.[269] A population of large diameter afferents also exists that does not bifurcate but descends in the spinal tract to innervate the entire rostrocaudal extent of the spinal nucleus, a course similar to that followed by smaller diameter myelinated and unmyelinated fibers.

Physiologic studies have supported the anatomic evidence for widespread termination of trigeminal afferents within the several nuclear subdivisions.

Neurons responsive to tactile stimuli (subserved by activity in large diameter afferents) are not localized to any one nucleus. Neurons of the n. oralis,[361,368] the n. interpolaris,[361] the n. caudalis,[361,389,461,518] and neurons within the main sensory nucleus[361,368,389] are activated by the application of tactile stimuli (light touch, hair movement, brush) to their receptive fields. Neurons responsive to thermal or noxious stimuli have been reported in the n. caudalis.[169,460,461,517,518,688] Significantly, trigeminal neurons may be driven by input from spinal afferent collateral and other cranial nerves. Thus stimulation as far caudally as the C2 root will produce an excitatory drive of neurons receiving trigeminal input.[345,353,364] Kerr[346] pointed to the likelihood that unusual pain syndromes such as are seen in atypical facial neuralgias might reflect these collateral projections.

The role of the n. caudalis in pain has been emphasized on the basis that trigeminal tractotomy at the level of the medullary obex relieves ipsilateral facial pain with preservation of touch.[570,645] The nociceptive responses of neurons situated in the n. caudalis reveal two populations of neurons that are remarkably similar to those reported in the spinal cord.[518] One population located in the marginal rim of the n. caudalis (corresponding to lamina I of the spinal cord[237]) has been termed "nociceptive specific." The receptive fields of these neurons are predominantly ipsilateral and small in size.[460,461,517,518,688] The second population of nociceptive neurons is "wide dynamic range" and is situated ventrally in the magnocellular portion of the n. caudalis. These neurons receive convergent input from large diameter afferents being activated by stimulation of low-threshold rapidly conducting fibers, as well as by light touch, hair movement, and vibration.[461,517,518]

After the injection of horseradish peroxidase into the ventrobasal thalamus of the rat, retrogradely labeled neurons are found throughout the entire trigeminal sensory complex, with the possible exception of the n. oralis of the spinal nucleus.[90,221] These trigeminothalamic projections are predominantly contralateral, although a small ipsilateral projection from the main sensory nucleus has been described.[90,221] Neurons in the n. caudalis responsive to noxious or innocuous stimuli, or both, project to the ventroposterior thalamus[518] and to the adjacent reticular formation.[595] Neurons of the n. caudalis also project within the trigeminal tract to the more rostral sensory nuclei.[239,300,581,595] This intranuclear projection may serve to modulate the activity of neurons in the more rostral trigeminal sensory nuclei and may explain why neurons responsive to noxious stimuli are not localized to the n. caudalis.[368] Neurons of the main sensory nucleus and n. oralis are activated by electrical stimulation of the n. caudalis,[368] and activation of n. caudalis neurons by topical application of strychnine potentiates the response of main sensory and n. oralis neurons to both noxious and innocuous stimuli. Conversely, cold block of the n. caudalis decreases the responses of neurons in the n. oralis and main sensory nucleus to peripheral stimuli.[247] Consistent with these observations, electrical stimulation or strychnine on the n. caudalis has been reported to hyperpolarize the preterminal endings of primary afferent neurons in the n. oralis.[558] The application of strychnine to the n. caudalis potentiates the hyperpolarization induced by dental pulp stimulation of primary afferent terminals located in the rostral sensory nuclei.[693] Thus neurons of the n. caudalis may hyperpolarize primary afferent terminals synapsing on neurons in the more rostral sensory trigeminal nuclei. Behavioral evidence for such a facilitatory action of n. caudalis neurons on afferent impulse transmission in the n. oralis and main sensory nucleus has been obtained in the cat. Thus, after application of strychnine to the n. caudalis, strong pseudoaffective responses to stroking of the fur have occurred.[370]

Clinical observations on patients with syringomyelia progressing to syringobulbia are not, however, in agreement with the proposed role of ipsilateral projections within trigeminal nuclei in pain. Because this lesion normally does not involve the trigeminal nuclei, the loss of pain coincident with the rostral progression of thermalgesia into the facial region in an onion-skin distribution cannot be attributed to severance of rostrocaudal projections within the trigeminal nuclei. Rather, such observations would suggest that fibers decussating within the brain stem have been interrupted (Kerr, F.W.L.: Personal observation).

Visceral Afferent Organization. Innervation of the visceral organs derives from sensory afferents the cell bodies of which are in the dorsal root ganglia, and the fibers of which travel with sympathetic and parasympathetic axons. It has been estimated that the visceral afferents account for about 10% of the fibers that run in the dorsal roots. Yet these visceral afferents serve an organ surface area equivalent to about 25% of the body surface,[523] which suggests that visceral sensitivity will be poorly localized.

To understand visceral pain, one must recognize that these afferents appear to converge onto dorsal horn systems, which receive cutaneous input. Figure 24-14 displays systematic studies by Fields and colleagues[203] that show the convergence of gallbladder and urinary bladder stimulation as a function of the somatic receptive field of dorsal horn neurons. Thus it is not surprising that certain visceral pains are localized predominantly with certain dermatomal segments. Such segments correspond with the cutaneous innervation of that particular spinal segment. With regard to thoracic input, therefore, sensory information from thoracic viscera will serve to activate sensory afferents traveling with sympathetic fibers that terminate in cord segments T1–T4. Similarly, sensory input that results in activity in visceral sympathetic afferents will enter the spinal cord at segments T5–T12/L1, traveling via the splanchnic nerves through the celiac plexus (see Fig. 24-2).

These afferents enter the dorsal horn of the spinal cord to terminate in the dorsal gray matter. At this point convergence with somatic afferent input onto common postsynaptic neurons occurs. As noted in previous sections, both spinoreticular and spinothalamic projecting neurons showed such viscerosomatic and muscular somatic convergence as a common property. Such neurons will respond not only to noxious events, that is, cardiac ischemia or smooth muscle spasm, but also to more benign input such as distension of the bladder (see above).

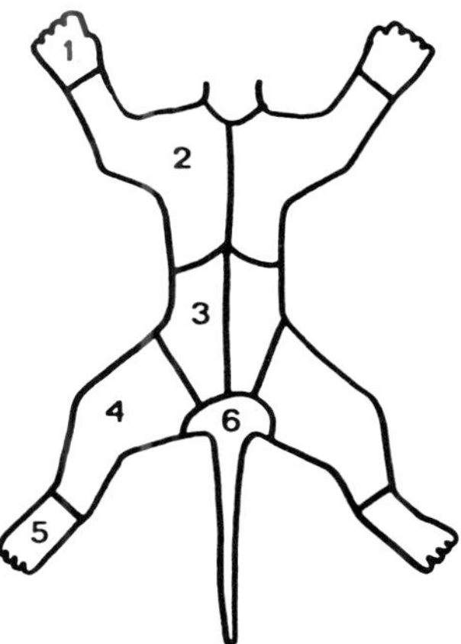

FIG. 24-14. Partitioning of cat's body surface for principal cutaneous receptive fields of spinal neurons. Percentage of cells by region that responds to somatic stimulation and also to gall bladder or urinary bladder stimulation (/) is 1: 40/18; 2: 56/11; 3: 38/44; 4: 33/31; 5: 35/28; 6: 43/25. (Adapted from Fields, H.L., *et al.*: J. Neurophysiol., *33*:827–837, 1970.)

SUPRASPINAL ELEMENTS IN NOCICEPTIVE TRANSMISSION

Supraspinal nuclear groups participating in the processing of pain-relevant information have been tentatively identified on the basis of their connectivity and their response to a peripheral stimulus adequate to evoke pain behavior. The accessibility of the pathways that project in the VLF has facilitated extensive investigations of the supraspinal connections of these pathways. As noted earlier, there are essentially three major sites of termination: the medulla, the mesencephalon, and the diencephalon.

Medullary Reticular Formation

Given the spinopetal projections and the reticulothalamic projections from the medullary reticular neurons to the intralaminar and ventrobasal nuclei of the thalamus, the medullary reticular formation has been suggested as a "relay" station for the rostrad transmission of nociceptive information. Retrogradely labeled neurons have been localized to neurons in the medullary reticular formation following the injection of horseradish peroxidase into the thalamus.[360] Medullary reticular neurons are activated antidromically by stimulation in the thalamus[431]; conversely, stimulation of the medullary reticular formation has been reported to activate thalamic neurons.[67,341,431]

Physiologic studies support the anatomic evidence that medullary reticular neurons receive peripheral input by means of spinal systems that travel in the VLF. Neurons of the lateral reticular nucleus,[11] the n. gigantocellularis,[106,250,404,498,499] the n. raphe magnus and applidus,[19] and the n. locus coeruleus[113] are activated by noxious or innocuous stimuli, or both, applied to their peripheral receptive fields. These receptive fields, both ipsilateral and contralateral, are large, often including an entire limb or extending over the entire body.[11,19,42,106] Because the spinoreticular fibers that project to these regions do not commonly display such broad receptive fields and project predominantly ipsilaterally (see above), the existence of extensive receptive fields suggests supraspinal convergence. Many of these neurons that are responsive to somatic input are also activated by auditory and visual stimuli.[67]

A significant proportion of neurons of the various medullary reticular nuclei behave as spinal wide dynamic range neurons.[19,106,113,498] Neurons of the n. gigantocellularis are most effectively activated following electrical stimulation of nerves sufficient to evoke afferent volleys in A-delta and C fibers; volleys in larger diameter A fibers are ineffective or less so.[106,241,404,499] Intra-arterial injection of algogenic agents such as bradykinin[250] or intense stimulation of the splanchnic nerve will alter the discharge of n. gigantocellularis neurons.[515] Although the number of neurons responding to muscle afferents is small, the most effective input has arisen from group II and III fibers.[419,513]

Several lines of evidence may be marshaled to correlate neural activity in the n. gigantocellularis with pain behavior in unanesthetized animals.[107,108,109,341]

1. In unanesthetized cats, as the intensity of an electrical stimulus applied to the radial nerve is elevated (through chronically implanted electrodes), so too is the discharge frequency of single neurons of the n. gigantocellularis. The stimulus intensity that evokes escape behavior is also the minimum intensity that produces a maximum discharge rate in that neuron.
2. The discharge frequency of thalamic neurons has been correlated with the intensity of stimuli delivered to the n. gigantocellularis and the escape threshold in awake animals.
3. Stimulation of the gigantocellularis may be used to evoke learned escape behavior in rats and cats. Additionally, such stimuli can serve as an unconditioned stimulus in pavlovian conditioning paradigms. In unanesthetized animals, the activity of n. gigantocellularis neurons covarys with the intensity of somatic stimulation, and stimuli applied to the n. gigantocellularis will drive thalamic neurons, evoke escape behavior, and support pavlovian conditioning.
4. Lesions of the n. gigantocellularis have been shown to attenuate the response to otherwise aversive stimuli in the absence of any significant signs of motor impairment.[258,498]

Several cautionary notes should be considered in these and other studies in which the behavioral effects of stimulating and lesioning of supraspinal systems are used to examine the involvement of a given structure in a pain event. Electrical stimulation or lesions of nuclei also affect fibers of passage and so may inhibit or activate ascending or descending pathways relevant to the pain event. Thus stimulation of spinothalamic fibers could produce a direct drive of thalamic substrates in a manner independent of the system within the nuclei being stimulated. Within the brain stem, particularly the n. gigantocellularis, there is a preponderance of connections with autonomic nuclei and sensations related to gastric secretion, nausea, or tachycardia that are likely stimulated by activation of efferent/autonomic pathways. These syndromes might be unpleasant, and such sensations themselves might underlie the "aversive" characteristics of local stimulation. It is thus possible that the role played by these nuclei is not related to the "conscious" perception of a pain event, but rather they could serve as the mediators of the autonomic sequelae evoked by high-intensity somatic stimulation.

Mesencephalic Reticular Formation and Central Gray Matter

These regions receive crossed/uncrossed projections from spinomesencephalic neurons. Neurons of the central gray project rostrally to terminate in the midline and intralaminar nuclei of the thalamus and the caudal hypothalamus.[65,129,261,431,537] Of particular interest are the massive projections that connect the central gray matter with the subadjacent tegmentum.[261]

Units in the mesencephalic central gray matter and in the adjacent mesencephalic reticular formation are differentially responsive to innocuous and noxious cutaneous and electrical stimuli,[30,37,143,189,691] with units phasically excited by innocuous mechanical stimulation but responding to noxious stimuli (such as pinching or heating) with sustained discharges. There is a close correlation between the high-frequency discharge of these neurons evoked by noxious natural stimulation and the ability of electrical C fiber activation to drive the unit.[37,143,189] As in other brain-stem regions, few, if any, neurons in this region are uniquely nociceptive. Thus cells that appear to be activated only by noxious tail pinch can be driven weakly by electrical stimulation of the coccygeal nerve at intensities that evoke only a fast conducting (A-beta) volley.[189] Thus experiments that examine only "natural" input may fail to observe the presence of weak but clearly present connections.

Neurons of the mesencephalic reticular formation display a high degree of convergence with bilateral receptive fields that may include the entire body.[30,41,189,691] There is little evidence for a specific somatotopic organization of input to these regions, although there may be a distribution.[248,415]

Stimulation of the mesencephalic central gray matter and adjacent mesencephalic reticular formation evoke signs of intense discomfort in the cat as characterized by flattening of the ears, vocalization, pupil dilatation, and attempts to escape. In humans, autonomic responses are elicited along with reports of dysphoria.[165,371,470,572,575]

Although electrolytic lesions of the central gray/mesencephalic reticular nuclei have been reported to alter nociceptive responsiveness,[257,446] a significant portion of the literature suggests little, if any, effect after either lesion or reversible blockade.[50,162,413,683]

Observations that activation of these several areas has an aversive consequence are consistent with the known projections of these nuclei to the medial and intralaminar nuclei of the thalamus. Yet the failure of lesions to elevate the pain threshold indicates that this region is not essential. It might be argued that lesions failed to affect a sufficient volume of tissue and that total destruction of this complex region would, however, leave the animal moribund. Willis' observation that electrical stimulation of the mesencephalic reticular formation would excite *spinothalamic cells* suggests that pathways either originating in, or passing through, the mesencephalon may exert an excitatory effect on the activity of spinothalamic neurons otherwise evoked by noxious peripheral stimuli (see Ref. 652). Such a situation might explain why stimulation in the mesencephalon would be aversive while lesions would fail to block the rostrad transmission of information via the diffuse spinothalamic and mesencephalic system and so not alter the pain threshold.

Diencephalon

Several nuclear groups of the thalamus primarily receive projections from the spinal cord thought to be associated with the transmission of somatic information evoked by noxious stimuli: the posterior nuclear complex, the ventrobasal complex, and the medial intralaminar nuclear complex. (For further comments, see previous section on ventrolateral tract projections.)

Posterior Nuclear Complex

The posterior nuclear area comprises the suprageniculate limitans and a heterogeneous region of ill-defined cell groups extending rostrally in the medial geniculate toward the caudal pole of the ventromedial group.[92] Input into this region is primarily contributed by the spinothalamic system[58,60,355,427] and lemniscal input from the dorsal column nuclei and the spinocervical tract.[57] Projections arising from the posterior complex are several in number, but of principal interest are the projections to the posterior portion of the somatosensory area (I–II) of the cortex.[92,329]

Populations of neurons in the posterior nuclear complex respond to noxious stimuli.[105,344,506,510] These neurons display large bilateral receptive fields. A number of the neurons resemble the wide dynamic range neurons in the spinal cord (discharge frequency proportional to the intensity of the applied stimulus). Electrical activation of A-delta afferents from tooth pulp, presumably noxious in nature, also evokes activity in neurons of the posterior thalamic complex.[566] Although these investigations clearly suggest the existence of neurons in the posterior complex that can be activated by nociceptive input, other investigations have failed to observe as large a population of neurons responsive to noxious input.[43,156,480]

Lesions of monkey posterior nuclear complex reduce responsiveness of animals to maximum mechanical stimuli,[557] but the literature is generally inconclusive concerning the effects of such lesions in humans; at best, the effects are transient.[268]

Ventrobasal Complex

The ventrobasal complex (n. ventralis posterior and n. ventralis lateralis) is situated in the ventrolateral quadrant of the thalamus. Neurons of this region project in a somatotopic manner to SI and SII of the somatosensory cortex. The projection to SI is greater than that to SII. The SII receives no independent input, but appears rather innervated by collaterals of the projection to SI.[220,327,328,432,548,648]

The ventrobasal nuclei have classically been thought to receive primarily lemniscal input[511] from the dorsal column nuclei.[59,427] The spinothalamic tract is a minor source of input.[60,445,646] After sectioning of the dorsal columns that spare the VLF, only a small number of neurons in the ventrobasal region are activated by either noxious or non-noxious peripheral stimuli.[504]

Most neurons in the ventrobasal complex are responsive to innocuous tactile or thermal stimuli or to joint movement.[91,267,387,511,514] The number of neurons responsive to noxious stimuli is much smaller, about 6% to 10% of the sample.[267,479,566] In the ventroposterolateral axis, large populations of neurons responsive to noxious input have been identified.[110,292,378]

Lesions in the ventrobasal complex in a variety of species alter somatosensory discrimination. White and Sweet[645] noted in humans that such lesions produce transient analgesia. Similar findings have been reported in cats.[231] Stimulation of the ventrobasal complex in humans commonly produces non-noxious paresthesias and tingling.[590]

Medial and Intralaminar Nuclei

The intralaminar nuclear complex forms a shell around the lateral aspect of the nucleus medialis dorsalis and comprises five nuclear groups: the n. paracentralis, n. centralis medialis, n. centromedian, n. centralis lateralis, and n. parafasicularis. Input to these nuclei is contributed primarily by the spinothalamic tract[58,60,427,445] and the n. reticularis gigantocellularis. These reticulothalamic projections are thought to be a major source of input to the intralaminar complex.[67,430,501] The intralaminar thalamic complex projects diffusely to wide areas of the cerebral cortex, including the frontal, parietal, and limbic regions.[326]

Populations of neurons in the medial and intralaminar nuclei respond to noxious stimuli and encode the stimulus intensity in the duration and frequency of patterned discharges.[192] A proportion of neurons in these regions respond exclusively to innocuous stimuli or respond to both innocuous and noxious stimuli.[7,23,105,172,500,504,614] Consistent with these observations, volleys in A-delta and C fibers produced by electrical stimulation of peripheral nerves evoke activity in neurons of the medial and intralaminar nuclei.[172,309] The receptive fields of neurons in these regions are large, often bilateral with little evidence for a somatotopic organization of input.[7,172,500,614] Neurons of the medial and intralaminar nuclei receive convergent input from skin, joints, and muscle.[7,172] In humans, neurons in the centromedian–parafascicular region that possess large receptive fields, occasionally including the contralateral half and ipsilateral upper half of the body, are found that are responsive to noxious stimuli.[310] Two classes of neurons have been described: those activated with a short latency to response and those activated with a long latency. The former category of neurons is found predominantly in the basomedial portions of the parafascicular nucleus, and the latter group is localized to the dorsal centromedian and parafascicular regions.

The analyses strongly implicate intralaminar nuclei, particularly the centromedian–parafascicular region, in nociception. Lesion studies conducted in rats, cats, and monkeys have, however, failed to report an alteration in the animals' response to noxious stimuli following large lesions.[163,205,684] Such lesions have, however, produced increases in nociceptive threshold as assessed by tooth pulp stimulation in cats[335,452] and operant response to shock in primates.[435,607] In addition, a significant relief of intractable pain arising from neoplastic disease has been reported following lesions of the medial thalamus.[547,582,613] The centromedian–parafascicular–medialis dorsalis complex appears to be a critical determinant of effectiveness. Conversely, electrical stimulation of these nuclei has commonly elicited sensations of burning pain experienced contralaterally.[547]

Cortex

The somatosensory areas (SI/SII) receive input indirectly from the three major spinal systems through which ascending sensory and noxious information may travel.[61] Investigations have focused attention on the importance of the SII area in the reception and perception of pain information. This area of cortex may be divided into an anterior and a posterior region.[647] The anterior region is thought to receive input primarily from the ventrobasal thalamic nuclei,[220,327,328,548] and neurons in this region are activated by light tactile stimuli. Input to this region is somatotopically arranged; receptive fields correspond with precise symmetrical sites on both sides of the body.[647]

Posterior SII receives input largely from the posterior thalamic complex.[92,329] Neurons in this region possess receptive fields that encompass large asymmetrical areas of the body.[647] These neurons are polysensory, and a number respond to high-intensity mechanical stimuli.[103,647] The responsive properties of these neurons resemble those reported for neurons in the posterior thalamic nuclei.[504,510] Neurons in the posterior thalamic complex are antidromically activated by stimulation of posterior SII,[155] and nociresponsive neurons could still be observed in the cortex of cats having lesions of the dorsal funiculus,[20] suggesting that input eventually arriving at the cortex could, in fact, travel over the ventrolateral quadrants. Berkley and Palmer[45] have observed that bilateral destruction of that area to which the posterior thalamic nuclei project produces an increase in the nociceptive threshold.

NOCICEPTIVE PROCESSING: MODULATORY SUBSTRATES

As noted in the introductory paragraph of this chapter, the consideration of ascending pathways through which pain-related information travels may be thought of not only in terms of the elements through which the information travels, but also as to the systems that modulate transmission at each level of the synapse. For the sake of discussion, however, we shall consider five basic divisions: [1] intrinsic spinal systems; [2] brain-stem–spinal projection systems; [3] intrinsic brain-stem systems; [4] brain-stem ascending systems; and [5] suprathalamic systems.

INTRINSIC SPINAL SYSTEMS

Presynaptic and Postsynaptic Inhibitory Systems in Spinal Cord

Dorsal root potentials (DRP) related to primary afferent depolarization are associated with a reduction in the amount of primary afferent transmitter release by an incoming impulse[553] and are thus associated with a reduction of the efficiency of transmission to the first synaptic link. Stimulation of the dorsal columns, which mimics the activation of large diameter primary afferent collaterals, inhibits discharge of dorsal horn interneuron nociceptors.[36,281] These results fulfilled one prediction of the gate control theory originally proposed by Melzack and Wall[447] and led to the clinical use of dorsal column stimulation for the relief of pain,[472,563] although the procedure has not been uniformly successful. The neuronal pathways that mediate the mechanisms of inhibition of the cord are not well understood. Primary afferent depolarization has been suggested to originate within the substantia gelatinosa.[629] Stimulation of the lateral Lissauer tract (a presumed outflow of gelatinosa neurons) resulted in the development of segmental DRPs and a concurrent inhibition of the polysynaptic ventral root reflex, as well as the discharge of lamina V neurons evoked by noxious stimulation.[635,681] As indicated, substantia gelatinosa neurons are activated by primary afferent input, and it is conceivable that presynaptic inhibitory effects of afferent input are mediated by such circuitry.

Postsynaptic effects are also well described. Systematic studies have suggested that these inhibitory effects are mediated by an interneuron.[46,294]

Pharmacology of Intrinsic Spinal Systems

Considerable insight into the systems that may modulate sensory transmission, particularly that relevant to pain processing, has been shed by studies on the characteristic neurotransmitter systems that interact with cord function. Classically, the inhibitory amino acids (gamma-aminobutyric acid) and glycine have been thought to mediate the classically observed presynaptic and postsynaptic inhibitions, respectively.[223] These agents, however, do not appear to possess any particular specificity with regard to classes of sensory input.

More recently, it has become clear that the pharmacology of the dorsal horn with regard to modulatory influences is considerably more complex, and several possible controlling systems have been identified (see Table 24-11). Most interesting with regard to intrinsic circuitry has been the growing appreciation of the role of endorphinergic systems in spinal function. Several lines of evidence may be briefly considered: [1] Opiates administered systemically will produce an inhibition of nociceptive reflexes in spinal transected animals[649]; [2] the iontophoretic administration of opiates into the dorsal horn will produce a significant inhibition of the discharge of nociceptive neurons[96,179,180,697]; [3] systemically administered opiates in decerebrate spinal animals will produce a relatively selective suppression at low doses of A-delta/C-fiber-evoked activity in dorsal horn neurons and a reduction in the size of the neuronal receptive field.[334,402,662,666]; [4] the release of putative neurotransmitters from primary afferents such as substance P has been demonstrated to be inhibited by locally administered opiate receptor agonists (see Fig. 24-15)[322,672,676]; and [5] the intrathecal administration of opioid agonists will produce a powerful analgesia in all species thus far examined (see also Fig. 28-3).

Importantly, with few exceptions, the pharmacology of the above electrophysiologic, biochemical, and behavioral events is identical, suggesting that the characteristics of the receptors acted upon by the exogenously administered opiates are the same.[147,667,677] Multiple discrete populations of opioid receptors have been identified, notably mu, delta, kappa, sigma, and epsilon (see Refs. 668, 669). Systematic studies have clearly demonstrated that mu, delta, and kappa receptor systems in spinal cord are able to alter significantly the response to noxious stimulation after the intrathecal administration of the appropriate ligand.[552,677] Opioid binding studies have indicated the presence of opiate binding sites on primary afferent terminals.[202,399,474] The presence of these receptors and the powerful effects of exogenously administered opiates on spinal nociceptive functioning lead to the question of what are the *endogenous* systems that normally act on these receptors and what normally activates those systems. Several populations of endorphins have been identified, including those deriving from the pre/pro hormones of proopiomelanocortin, pre/pro-enkephalin, and pre/pro-dynorphin (see Refs. 668, 669). Products of the latter two populations such as met and leu enkephalin, and various extended peptides such as Phe^7-Arg^6-Met^5-enkephalin and extended chains of leu-enkephalin (yielding dynorphins), have been identified in dorsal horn neurons. Importantly, these several classes of opioids have been shown to possess a differential receptor preference (see Refs. 668, 669).

Evidence that these endogenous systems may play an ongoing role in certain aspects of modulating sensory transmission is presented in an extensive literature, which suggests that decreasing opiate tone in spinal transected animals by the injection of opiate antagonists will increase the amplitude of ventral root reflexes and the discharge rate of nociceptive neurons,[40,207,274] although these findings are controversial (see Ref. 181). Other lines of investigation have demonstrated that enkephalin and various radioreceptor assayable endorphins are released from spinal cord in animal models by high- but not low-intensity stimulation; by the C fiber stimulation with the excitotoxin capsaicin; and by noxious pinch and

TABLE 24-11. SUMMARY OF EFFECTS OF INTRATHECALLY ADMINISTERED AGONISTS FOR DIFFERENT RECEPTOR POPULATIONS ON SPINAL (TAIL FLICK), SUPRASPINALLY ORGANIZED THERMAL (HOT PLATE), AND CHEMICAL (WRITHING) NOCICEPTIVE RESPONSE

				Antinociceptive Effects		
Neurotransmitter Systems	**Proposed Receptor**	**Endogenous Ligand**	**Exogenous Ligand**	**Tail Flick**	**Hot Plate**	**Writhing**
Opioid*	mu	β-endorphin; met/leu enkephalin	Morphine	+	+	+
	delta	Met/leu enkephalin	DADL	+	+	0
	kappa	Dynorphin	U50488H	0	0	+
Adrenergic†	α_1	Norepinephrine	Methoxamine	+?	+	+?
	α_2	Norepinephrine	Clonidine	+	+	+
	beta	Epinephrine	Isoproterenol	0	0	0
Serotonergic‡	5-HT	Serotonin	Serotonin	+	+	+
Gabaergic§	1	GABA	Baclofen	+	+	+
	2	GABA	Muscimol	0?	0?	0?
Neurotensin‖	–	Neurotensin	Neurotensin	+	+	?
Cholinergic¶	Muscarinic	Acetylcholine	Oxotremorine	+	+	+

(?) Motor effects at antinociceptive doses. *552,668,669. †532,670. ‡682. §657; Yaksh and Harty, unpublished observations. ‖674. ¶678.

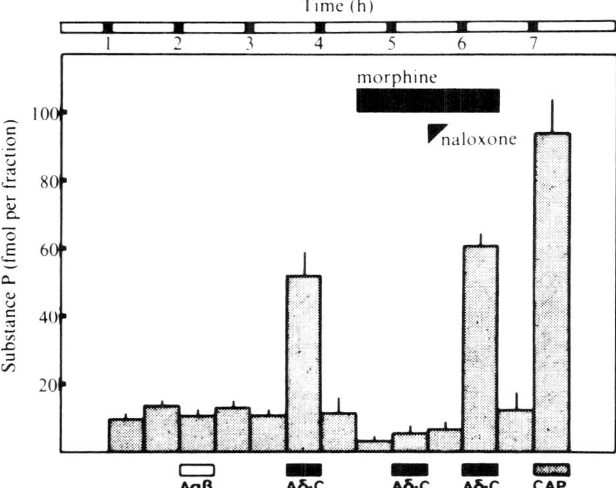

FIG. 24-15. Release of substance P from superfused cat spinal cord in response to sciatic nerve stimulation and capsaicin. Cats were anaesthetized with chloralose-urethane (100 mg/kg) and prepared with a tracheal tube and jugular and carotid catheters. An incision was made in the cisterna magna and the perfusion cannula inserted after retraction of the arachnoid layer. The perfusion cannula consisted of a length of polyethylene PE-90 (1.0 mm outer diameter) tubing through which was passed a length of polyethylene PE-10 tubing. The PE-10 served as inflow cannula, whereas the PE-90 was used as collection cannula. Both cannulae were inserted through the retracted incision in the cisterna membrane 37 to 40 cm down the spinal cord (upper sacral region), and the PE-90 cannula was then retracted 10 cm. Perfusion was therefore localized to the upper sacral and lumbar spinal cord. The position of the inflow and outflow cannulae was determined by x-ray films after infusion of radiopaque dye. The sciatic nerve was exposed and prepared for stimulation and recording of the compound action potential. Stimulation of the nerve was performed with rectangular pulses (3–4 V, 0.05 msec, 50 Hz for activation of A-alpha and A-beta fibers and 40–50 V, 0.05 msec, 50 Hz for recruitment of A-delta and C fibers). Superfusate in all experiments consisted of NaCl, 151.1 mM; KCl, 2.6 mM; $MgSO_4$, 0.9 mM; $CaCl_2$, 1.3 mM; $NaHCO_3$, 21.0 mM; K_2HPO_4, 2.5 mM, gassed with 95% O_2 and 5% CO_2 before perfusion. Perfusion samples (3 ml) were collected into glacial acetic acid (final concentration of 2 N) and immediately frozen and lyophilized. Samples were reconstituted in 1.0-ml assay buffer, neutralized, and aliquots of each fraction were used to determine the content of substance P, by radioimmunoassay, using antibody R6P with a sensitivity of 1.5 fmol per assay tube. Serial dilutions of synthetic substance P and immunoreactivity in superfusate samples and produced parallel dilution curves. Each value is the mean ± SEM from four separate experiments. (Yaksh, T.L., et al.: Nature, *286*:155–156, 1980.)

the application of acetic acid.[120,675,679] Since the afferent-evoked release of methionine enkephalin-like immunoreactivity is not abolished in spinal blocked animals, at least one spinal enkephalin releasing terminal system would appear to be locally organized.[675]

BRAIN-STEM–SPINAL PROJECTION SYSTEMS

Classic work by Hagbarth and Kerr[256] demonstrated the ability of descending long tract systems to modulate spinal-evoked activity. Takagi and colleagues[588] early pointed to a possible role of descending systems in mediating the effects of morphine. It has long been known that activation of the pathways originating in the brain stem and descending to the spinal cord can inhibit activity evoked in flexor reflex afferents.[193,194,289] Virtually every pathway carrying nociceptive information, including the spinoreticular[290] and spinothalamic,[654] has been shown to be under modulatory control of pathways that originate supraspinally. The classic observations that microinjections of morphine into the brain stem could inhibit spinal reflex activity,[606] and the subsequent demonstration that stimulation in the mesencephalon and medulla will inhibit the discharge of neurons in the spinal cord and trigeminal nucleus[199,201,426,562,654,689] evoked by nociceptive stimulation, emphasized the likely role of spinopetal systems in controlling spinal processing. In unanesthetized animals, such stimulation has been shown to alter the response to noxious stimuli and inhibit reflex function.[439,488]

The mechanism of this descending inhibition has been a subject of considerable investigation during the past 10 years, and it is increasingly apparent that a significant proportion of this modulation is mediated by the activation of descending monaminergic pathways. Evidence for this may be briefly summarized as follows: [1] Electrical stimulation or microinjections of opiates at brain-stem sites such as the periaqueductal gray or the nucleus gigantocellularis will inhibit nociceptive reflexes, and this effect is antagonized by the intrathecal administration of serotonergic or noradrenergic antagonists, or both[100,262,666]; [2] microinjections of morphine or focal stimulation in the medulla or periaqueductal gray that alter nociceptive thresholds are associated with an increased release of serotonin or norepinephrine in the spinal cord[263,680]; and [3] the spinal application of adrenergic or serotonergic agonists either by iontophoresis or by intrathecal administration in the unanesthetized animal will significantly antagonize the A-delta/C-fiber-evoked activity in dorsal horn neurons and is associated with significant analgesia, respectively.[270,532,682] Studies examining the characteristics of the systems from which these materials are released in spinal cord have demonstrated that high- but not low-intensity stimulation of afferent input (sciatic nerve) produces a significant stimulus-related increase in the release of both serotonin and norepinephrine from spinal cord.[608] Importantly, spinal transections inhibit this effect, indicating that the release is mediated by a spinobulbospinal loop. Significantly, stimulation of regions remote from the lumbar spinal cord region from which the release has been measured (infraorbital branch of the trigeminal nerve) also produces release of serotonin and norepinephrine in the lumbar spinal cord region. This suggests that these particular descending systems, the activity of which is manifested by serotonin and norepinephrine release, are globally activated by afferent input. This is in marked contrast to the enkephalin-evoked release from the spinal cord, where such distal stimulation has failed to have any influence on spinal release (see also Fig. 28-4).[608,675]

Although the principal interest thus far has focused largely on spinopetal aminergic pathways, other neurotransmitter systems have been shown to project to the spinal cord, including dopamine,[62,571] substance P,[62] thyrotropin-releasing hormone,[62] and cholecystokinin.[434] The complexity of this system is emphasized further by the fact that a number of these agents may be co-contained, such as substance P and serotonin[126] and enkephalin and serotonin.[232] The role of these several systems has yet to be ascertained, but clearly they provide additional substrates whereby brain-stem systems may interact with spinal cord sensorimotor processing.

BRAIN-STEM SUBSTRATES

Although most work examining the effects of brain-stem manipulations on nociceptive responsiveness has focused on projections to the spinal cord, significant evidence suggests that supraspinal, brain-stem–brain-stem, modulatory influences are being exerted by various systems. Thus the nucleus gigantocellularis, as discussed previously, may represent an important supraspinal link in systems through which nociceptive information may travel *en route* to higher centers. It has been demonstrated that mesencephalic stimulation will inhibit the discharge of neurons in the nucleus gigantocellularis in response to peripheral stimulation.[458]

Thus, although brain-stem manipulations that inhibit spinal reflex functions (such as the tail flick) may indeed alter the rostral transmission of information relevant to pain behavior, it is likely that this is not the only method whereby these supraspinal systems modulate the ascending pain message. Intrathecal administration of aminergic antagonists, therefore, will produce a significant reversal of the effects of these descending systems on spinal reflex function but has a subtotal effect on the supraspinally mediated aspects of the behavior.[100,320,321] This suggests that these supraspinal systems may act at several levels to modulate the animal's processing of nociceptive information (see Figs. 25-1, 25-2).

ROSTRALLY PROJECTING BRAIN-STEM SYSTEMS

Several lines of evidence have recently begun to emphasize the role of descending systems in the modulation of the organism's response to noxious stimulus. Current evidence indicates that there are significant projections from the mesencephalic central gray matter into the vicinity of the medial thalamus.[260,433,505] Stimulation in the periaqueductal gray matter has been demonstrated to produce a significant inhibition of the response of these medial thalamic neurons.[13,308] The neurotransmitter mediator of this is not known, although ascending serotonergic projections from the raphe have been well described and the iontophoretic administration of serotonin will reduce the firing of these thalamic neurons.[12,28] Importantly, stimulation of the dorsal raphe will produce similar effects on the firing of parafasicular neurons.[13] These observations are of particular interest in view of the clinical reports that brain-stem stimulation can produce significant changes in the patient's response in various chronic pain conditions. Although it has been suggested that this is due to the activation of *descending* pathways, such stimulation rarely has any effect on spinal reflex function, even in those limited cases in which analgesia has been reported and documented (see, for example, Refs. 252, 296, 451, 536).

SUPRATHALAMIC SUBSTRATE SYSTEMS

Early studies have demonstrated that stimulation of the caudate nucleus produces significant interaction of the medial thalamic and interlaminar nuclei and that this interaction is largely inhibitory in character.[384,386,397] Electrical stimulation of the caudate nucleus in primates has been reported to reduce the affective response to strong cutaneous stimulation.[385,421]

Corticospinal systems have long been known to have a significant effect on spinal afferent transmission. Thus electrical stimulation of the sensory cortex has been reported to affect afferent transmission and reflex pathways.[14,256,424] More recently, it has been demonstrated that the stimulation of the somatosensory S1 region of the cortex can result in a significant reduction in the response of spinothalamic neurons to C fiber activity evoked by high-intensity thermal mechanical stimuli.[686]

In summary, it is apparent that afferent input itself undergoes significant modulation at all levels of transmission. In the limited studies that have been done thus far, it is clear that the modulation may certainly occur in a reflex fashion. Thus the release of enkephalins from the spinal cord can be evoked in a spinal transected animal by the afferent message. Similarly, the descending noradrenergic/serotonergic system is activated by what appear to be obligatory reflex actions. The fact that the release of serotonin, norepinephrine, and enkephalin from the lumbar cord is associated with a significant decrease in the rostrad transmission of nociceptive information when these agents are applied to the spinal cord clearly suggests that activity in small diameter afferents may reflexly activate modulatory circuits, creating the possibility of an automodulation of the sensory message (see also Fig. 28-4).

Whether these endogenous systems defined in certain animal models are relevant to pain processing in the unanesthetized preparation in man is not certain. There is, however, ample evidence that certain somatic and visceral input will significantly alter the organism's response to otherwise aversive stimuli, and that these effects may be mediated by these intrinsic systems. Thus vaginal probing in rats will evoke a significant increase in the nociceptive threshold, and this effect is antagonized by intrathecal amine antagonists.[579] Sjölund and colleagues noted that levels of endorphin were increased after somatic stimulation, which was observed to produce change in pain threshold in patients.[567–569] Some evidence has indeed been generated to suggest that certain cases of congenital insensitivity to pain, which is naloxone reversible, may be associated with altered characteristics of cerebrospinal fluid endorphins.[121]

ROLE OF ENDOGENOUS MODULATORY SYSTEMS

Although there are systems that serve to modulate sensory transmission related to pain processing, it should not be concluded that this modulation serves that purpose in a global sense as an "antipain" system. Such systems likely serve other more subtle functions.

Modality Selectivity. A significant proportion of the cells in spinal cord are wide dynamic range in character. The descending pathways originating in the brain stem that modulate wide dynamic range neuron activity are commonly thought to inhibit the response to A-delta/C fibers, leaving A-beta responses intact. Although one may consider this as an antinociceptive mechanism, from the point of view of the nervous system, it is likely that these effects are related to the production of a modality-specific neuron that responds only to A-beta fibers. It is significant that stimulation of the somatosensory cortex has been demonstrated under certain stimulus conditions to produce a selective inhibition of A-beta activity, leaving unaffected the prolonged stimulation generated by C fiber input.[146] Such pyramidal input would therefore produce a modality-specific neuron shown to respond to A-delta/C fiber input.

Gain Control. Examination of stimulus response curves for afferents of dorsal horn neurons in response to afferent stimulation has demonstrated that various manipulations, including the local action of opiates[666] and brain-stem stimulation (see Ref. 701), can result in a change in threshold or a significant reduction in the slope of the stimulus response curve, or both. Although currently not well studied, it appears that different modulatory substrates may interact with sensory processing in various ways to alter the response characteristics of high-order spinal neurons.

Given that the systems that produce such modulation are themselves activated by input into the nervous system, it appears that this organization can provide for a variable gain or threshold control. Given the vast amount of information available for transmission, and the theoretically limited capacity of spinal transmission systems, such a mechanism would permit the system to be as sensitive as possible under normal circumstances. As intensity or amount of sensory information in the system increases, the system must increasingly reject some of the information in favor of other aspects of the environment. Thus the modulatory circuitry would serve as a gain-tuning device designed to accentuate different types of input. Under these conceptions, the vast majority of so-called wide dynamic neurons in spinal cord would represent broad-band tuning devices the messages of which are rendered modality specific by the particular modulatory circuit that has been activated.

Given this variability, it is reasonable to conclude that some elements of the system may exist that are not subject to the gain control; otherwise there would be no bench mark to permit the system to assess the extent of the ongoing modulation. One might speculate that certain inputs that respond only to nociceptive (marginal cells) or innocuous (lamina IV cells) stimulation might serve in that capacity. It is significant that in the case of morphine, sharp or first pain (such as the pain of incision) is rarely abated.

Excitatory Effects. All modulation need not be inhibitory. Iontophoretically applied serotonin on certain dorsal horn neurons has been shown to be excitatory (see Ref. 270). It is intriguing to speculate that the broad receptive fields reported in spinothalamic neurons and examined in nontransected animals may in fact reflect such an activation of a descending excitatory system. Thus descending pathways may serve to facilitate transmission and alter the characteristics of the receptive field.

CONCLUDING COMMENTS

In the preceding sections, an outline has been provided of systems that potentially serve as substrates through which information initiated by high-intensity stimuli may gain access to various regions within the nervous system. The likelihood that "pain-relevant" information passes along a diversity of pathways is clear even at the level of the spinal cord. Upon reaching the second-order neuron, the most apparent characteristic is that of polymodal convergence. At supraspinal levels the issue becomes predictably even more complex. The "meaning" of activity evoked in a given system by such stimulation depends on what function that system serves, for example, autonomic reflexes, somatomotor organization or sensory processing. It is thus not surprising in view of the global system response evoked by noxious stimuli that small fiber afferent input will have pervasive influences on systems throughout the nervous system. Yet when we speak of pain we are commonly referring to those systems that are central to the issues of motivation (*e.g.*, escape). We do not routinely escape an unconditioned somatic stimulus because our heart beats rapidly and our mouth becomes dry; rather these are sequelae of the systems to which that somatic input, activating small afferents, has access.

The observation that these afferent processing systems are powerfully influenced by modulatory substrates may imply the presence of an antipain system, but more likely it reflects a focusing mechanism for attention to allow a cursory screening of the tremendous amount of somatic information entering the spinal cord, which, because of limited channel capacity, cannot reach supraspinal structures but which can be summoned to consciousness instantaneously (*e.g.*, consider your right big toe and its associated condition—a subject that now leaps instantly to mind). As such, these modulatory systems provide the substrate whereby one may account for the anomalies considered in the introductory paragraphs of this chapter, for example, the discontinuities between stimulus and response.

It appears likely, however, that the question of modulating systems may be the tip of a more profound issue in understanding pain: the question of how pain is coded. At an elemental level, one may present a line-labeled hypothesis in which activity, yes or no, "means" tissue damage. For these, nociceptive specific neurons such as those described in the marginal layer would appear to be an element. More complexly, there are gradations of pain, and it can be hypothesized that the intensity is frequency coded. The wide dynamic range neurons could provide such information.[516] Such systems generally imply that pain is the reliable product of frequency-coded information traveling in certain pathways (see Refs. 192, 516). The issue of convergence, however, prevents the wholesale acceptance of this specificity analysis. As noted, most spinal and brain-stem neurons are polymodal, potentially responding to noxious and non-noxious stimuli and different afferent systems, for example, light touch, hair cells, high-threshold mechanical distension. The ability to detect the difference and to not perceive, under normal circumstances, light touch as painful clearly suggests that the information is interpreted on the basis of the physiologic context of the message. Such coding considerations are, in part, elements in such coding systems as those proposed by Melzack and Wall,[447] Kerr,[356,358,359] and, more recently, the DNIC circuitry formulated by LeBars and colleagues.[403] In a sense, all of these paradigms seek to have the meaning of the sensory message be a function of the context of the stimulus environment. The presence of powerful modulating circuits in the unanesthetized and intact organism reflects mechanisms that can produce a modality-coded element in the system and represents a way in which the stimulus environment can accentuate or, perhaps, as in the case of transcutaneous stimulation, blur the message generated by information arriving over specific classes of primary afferents. The present state of our understanding is just beginning to provide an appreciation of the physiology and pharmacology of the substrate that can account for the complexity of the pain experience.

REFERENCES

1. Adrian, E.D.: The effects of injury on mammalian nerve fibers. Proc. R. Soc. B, *106*:596–618, 1930.
2. Agudelo, C.A., Schumauser, H.R., Phelps, P.: Effect of exercise on urate crystal–induced inflammation in canine joints. Arthritis Rheum., *15*:609–616, 1972.
3. Ahlberg, K.F.: Dose–dependent inhibition of sensory nerve activity in the feline dental pulp by anti–inflammatory drugs. Acta Physiol. Scand., *102*:434–440, 1978.
4. Ahlberg, K.F.: Influence of local noxious heat stimulation on sensory nerve activity in the feline dental pulp. Acta Physiol. Scand., *103*:71–80, 1978.
5. Akagi, H., Otsuka, M., Yanagisawa, M.: Identification by high–performance liquid chromatography of immunoreactive substance P released from isolated rat spinal cord. Neurosci. Lett., *20*:259–263, 1980.
6. Akerman, B., Rosell, S., Folkers, K.: Intrathecal (D–Pro^2, D–Trp^{7,9})–SP elicits hypoalgesia and motor blockade in the rat and antagonizes noxious responses induced by substance P. Acta Physiol. Scand., *114*:631–633, 1982.
7. Albe–Fessard, D., Kruger, L.: Duality of unit discharges from cat centrum medianum in response to natural and electrical stimulation. J. Neurophysiol., *25*:3–20, 1962.
8. Albe–Fessard, D., Levante, A., Lamour, Y.: Origin of spinothalamic tract in monkeys. Brain Res., *65*:503–509, 1974.
9. Albe–Fessard, D., Levante, A., Lamour, Y.: Origin of spinothalamic and spinoreticular pathways in cats and monkeys. Adv. Neurol., *4*:157–166, 1974.
10. Alexander, R.W., Kent, K.M., Pisano, J.J., Keiser, H.R., *et al.*: Regulation of canine coronary blood flow by endogenous synthesized prostaglandins. Circulation, *48(Suppl.* IV):107, 1973.
11. Amassian, V.E., Waller, H.J.: Spatiotemporal patterns of activity in individual reticular neurones. *In* Jasper, H.H., Proctor, L.D., Knighton, R.S., Noshay, W.C., (eds.): Reticular Formation of the Brain, pp. 69–108. Boston, Little, Brown & Co., 1958.
12. Andersen, E., Dafny, N.: Microiontophoretically applied 5–HT reduces responses to noxious stimuli in the thalamus. Brain Res., *241*:176–178, 1982.
13. Andersen, E., Dafny, N.: Dorsal raphe stimulation reduces responses of parafasicular neurons to noxious stimulation. Pain, *15*:323–331, 1983.
14. Andersen, P., Eccles, J.C., Sears, T.A.: Cortically evoked depolarization of primary afferent fibers in the spinal cord. J. Neurophysiol., *27*:63–77, 1964.
15. Anderson, D.J., Curwen, M.P., Howard, L.V.: The sensitivity of human dentin. J. Dent. Res., *37*:669–677, 1958.
16. Anderson, D.J., Hannam, A.G., Matthews, B.: Sensory mechanisms in mammalian teeth and their supporting structures. Physiol. Rev., *50*:171–195, 1970.
17. Anderson, F.D.: Distribution of dorsal root fibers in the cat spinal cord. Anat. Rec., *136*:154–155, 1960.
18. Anderson, K.V., Perl, G.S.: Conduction velocities in afferent fibers from feline tooth pulp. Exp. Neurol., *43*:281–283, 1974.
19. Anderson, S.D., Basbaum, A.I., Fields, H.L.: Response of medullary raphe neurons to peripheral stimulation and to systemic opiates. Brain Res., *123*:363–368, 1977.
20. Andersson, S.A.: Projection of different spinal pathways to the second somatic sensory area in cat. Acta Physiol. Scand., *56(Suppl.* 194):1–74, 1962.
21. Andres, K.H.: Untersuchungen uber den Feinbau von Spinalganglien. Z. Zellforsch., *55*:1–48, 1961.
22. Angaut–Petit, D.: The dorsal column system: II. Functional properties and bulbar relay of the postsynaptic fibers of the cat's fasciculus gracilis. Exp. Brain Res., *22*:471–493, 1975.
23. Angel, A.: The effect of peripheral stimulation on units located in the thalamic reticular nuclei. J. Physiol. (Lond.), *171*:42–60, 1964.
24. Antonetty, C.M., Webster, K.E.: The organization of the spinotectal projection. An experimental study in the rat. J. Comp. Neurol., *163*:449–466, 1975.
25. Applebaum, M.L., Clifton, G.L., Coggeshall, R.E., Coulter, J.D., *et al.*: Unmyelinated fibres in the sacral 3 and caudal 1 ventral roots of the cat. J. Physiol. (Lond.), *256*:557–572, 1976.
26. Armstrong, D., Dry, R., Keele, C.A., Markham, J.W.: Observations on chemical excitants of cutaneous pain in man. J. Physiol (Lond.), *120*:326–351, 1953.
27. Astrom, K.E.: On the central course of afferent fibers in the trigeminal, facial, glossopharyngeal, and vagal nerves and their nuclei in the mouse. Acta Physiol. Scand., *29(Suppl.* 106):209–230, 1953.
28. Azmitia, E.C.: The serotonin–producing neurons of the midbrain–medial and dorsal raphe nuclei. *In* Eversen, L.I., et al. (eds.): Handbook of Psychopharmacology, vol. 9, pp. 233–314, New York, Plenum Press, 1981.
29. Baker, G.S., Kerr, F.W.L.: Structural changes in the trigeminal system following compression procedures. J. Neurosurg., *20*:181–184, 1963.
30. Barnes, K.L.: A quantitative investigation of somatosensory coding in single cells of the cat mesencephalic reticular formation. Exp. Neurol., *50*:180–193, 1976.
31. Barron, D.H., Matthews, B.H.C.: Dorsal root reflexes. J. Physiol. (Lond.), *94*:26P–27P, 1939.
32. Basbaum, A.I.: Conduction of the effects of noxious stimulation by short-fiber multisynaptic systems of the spinal cord in the rat. Exp. Neurol., *40*:699–716, 1973.
33. Basbaum, A.I.: Effects of central lesions on disorders pro-

duced by multiple dorsal rhizotomy in rats. Exp. Neurol., *42*:490–501, 1974.

34. Beaudreau, D.E., Jerge, C.R.: Somatotopic representation in the gasserian ganglion of tactile peripheral fields in the cat. Arch. Oral. Biol., *13*:247–256, 1968.
35. Beck, P.W., Handwerker, H.O.: Bradykinin and serotonin effects on various types of cutaneous nerve fibers. Pflugers Arch., *374*:209–222, 1974.
36. Beck, P.W., Handwerker, H.O., Zimmerman, M.: Nervous outflow from the cat's foot during noxious radiant heat stimulation. Brain Res., *67*:373–386, 1974.
37. Becker, D.P., Gluck, H., Nulsen, F.E., Jane, J.A.: An inquiry into the neurophysiological basis for pain. J. Neurosurg., *30*:1–13, 1969.
38. Beitel, R.E., Dubner, R.: Response of unmyelinated (C) polymodal nociceptors to thermal stimuli applied to monkey's face. J. Neurophysiol., *39*:1160–1175, 1976.
39. Beitel, R.E., Dubner, R.: Fatigue and adaptation in unmyelinated (C) polymodal nociceptors to mechanical and thermal stimuli applied to the monkey face. Brain Res., *112*:402–406, 1976.
40. Bell, J.A., Martin, W.R.: The effect of narcotic antagonists naloxone, naltrexone and nalorphine on spinal cord C–fibers reflexes evoked by electrical stimulation or radiant heat. Eur. J. Pharmacol., *42*:147–154, 1977.
41. Bell, C., Sierra, G., Buendia, N., Segundo, J.P.: Sensory properties of neurons in the mesencephalic reticular formation. J. Neurophysiol., *27*:961–987, 1964.
42. Benjamin, R.M.: Single neurons in the rat medulla responsive to nociceptive stimulation. Brain Res., *24*:525–529, 1970.
43. Berkley, K.J.: Response properties of cells in ventrobasal and posterior group nuclei of the cat. J. Neurophysiol., *36*:940–952, 1973.
44. Berkley, K.J.: Spatial relationships between the terminations of somatic sensory and motor pathways in the rostral brainstem of cats and monkeys. I. Ascending somatic sensory inputs to lateral diencephalon. J. Comp. Neurol., *193*:283–317, 1980.
45. Berkley, K.J., Palmer, R.: Somatosensory cortical involvement in response to noxious stimulation in the cat. Exp. Brain Res., *20*:363–374, 1974.
46. Besson, J.M., Catchlove, R.F.H., Feltz, P., Le Bars, D.: Further evidence for postsynaptic inhibitions on lamina V dorsal horn interneurons. Brain Res., *66*:531–536, 1974.
47. Bessou, P., Burgess, P.R., Perl, E.R., Taylor, C.B.: Dynamic properties of mechanoreceptors with unmyelinated (C) fibers. J. Neurophysiol., *34*:116–131, 1971.
48. Bessou, P., Perl, E.R.: A movement receptor of the small intestine. J. Physiol., *182*:404–426, 1966.
49. Bessou, P., Perl, E.R.: Response of cutaneous sensory units with unmyelinated fibers to noxious stimuli. J. Neurophysiol., *32*:1025–1043, 1969.
50. Beven, T., Pert, A.: The effect of midbrain and diencephalic lesions on nociception and morphine induced antinociception in the rat. Fed. Proc., *34*:713, 1975.
51. Beveridge, E.E., Brown, A.: The measurement of human dental intrapulpal pressure and its response to clinical variables. Oral Surg., *19*:655–668, 1965.
52. Bilisaly, F.N., Goodell, H., Wolff, H.G.: Vasodilatation, lowered pain threshold, and increased tissue vulnerability. Effects dependent upon peripheral nerve function. Arch. Intern. Med., *94*:759–773, 1954.
53. Bill, A., Stjernschantz, J., Mandahl, A., *et al.*: Substance P: Release on trigeminal nerve stimulation, effects in the eye. Acta Physiol. Scand., *106*:371–373, 1979.
54. Blank, M.A., Anard, P., Lumb, B.M., Morrison, J., *et al.*: Release of vasoactive intestinal polypeptide–like immunoreactivity (VIP) from cat urinary bladder and sacral spinal cord during pelvic nerve stimulation. Dig. Dis. Sci., *27*:11S, 1984.
55. Block, A.R., Feinberg, H., Herbaczynska–Cedra, K., Vane, J.R.: Anoxia–induced release of prostaglandins in rabbit isolated hearts. Circ. Res., *36*:34–42, 1975.
56. Blumgart, H.L., Schlesinger, M.J., Davis, D.: Studies on the relation of the clinical manifestations of angina pectoris, coronary thrombosis and myocardial infarction to the pathological findings, with particular reference to the significance of the collateral circulation. Am. Heart J., *19*:1–91, 1940.
57. Boivie, J.: The termination of the cervicothalamic tract in the cat. An experimental study with silver impregnation methods. Brain Res., *19*:333–360, 1970.
58. Boivie, J.: The termination of the spinothalamic tract in the cat. An experimental study with silver impregnation methods. Exp. Brain. Res., *12*:331–353, 1971.
59. Boivie, J.: Anatomical observations on the dorsal column nuclei and the cytoarchitecture of some somatosensory thalamic nuclei. J. Comp. Neurol., *178*:17–48, 1978.
60. Boivie, J.: An anatomical reinvestigation of the termination of the spinothalamic tract in the monkey. J. Comp. Neurol., *186*:343–370, 1979.
61. Boivie, J., Perl, E.R.: Neural substrates of somatic sensation. *In* Hunt, C.C. (ed.): MTP International Review of Science, Physiology Series One, vol. 3, pp. 303–411. Baltimore, University Press, 1975.
62. Bowker, R.M., Westlund, K.N., Sullivan, M.C., Wilber, J.F., *et al.*: Descending serotonergic, peptidergic and cholinergic pathways from the raphe nuclei: A multiple transmitter complex. Brain Res., *288*:33–48, 1983.
63. Bowsher, D.: Termination of the central pathway in man: The conscious appreciation of pain. Brain, *80*:606–622, 1957.
64. Bowsher, D.: The sub–diencephalic distribution of fibres from the anterolateral quadrant of the spinal cord in man. Mschr. Psychiatr. Neurol., *143*:75–99, 1962.
65. Bowsher, D.: Diencephalic projections from the midbrain reticular formation. Brain Res., *95*:211–220, 1975.
66. Bowsher, D.: Role of the reticular formation in responses to noxious stimulation. Pain, *2*:361–378, 1976.
67. Bowsher, D., Mallart, A., Petit, D., Albe–Fessard, D.: A bulbar relay to the centromedian. J. Neurophysiol., *31*:288–300, 1968.
68. Bowsher, D., Petit, D.: Place and modality analysis in nu-

cleus of posterior commissure. J. Physiol. (Lond.), *206*:663–675, 1970.

69. Brännstrom, M., Astrom, A.: The hydrodynamics of the dentine; its possible relationship to dentinal pain. Int. Dent. J., *22*:219–227, 1972.
70. Brashear, A.D.: The innervation of the teeth. An analysis of nerve fiber components of the pulp and peridental tissues and their probable significance. J. Comp. Neurol., *64*:169–185, 1936.
71. Breazile, J.E., Kitchell, R.L.: Ventrolateral spinal cord afferents to the brain stem in the domestic pig. J. Comp. Neurol., *133*:363–372, 1968.
72. Breazile, J.E., Kitchell, R.L.: A study of fiber systems within the spinal cord of the domestic pig that subserve pain. J. Comp. Neurol., *133*:373–382, 1968.
73. Brimijoin, S., Lundberg, J.M., Brodin, E., *et al.*: Axonal transport of substance P in the vagus and sciatic nerves of the guinea pig. Brain Res., *191*:443–457, 1980.
74. Brodal, A., Walberg, F., Taber, E.: The raphe nuclei of the brain stem in the cat. II. Afferent connections. J. Comp. Neurol., *114*:261–279, 1960.
75. Brodin, E., Gazelius, B., Olgart, L., Nilsson, G.: Tissue concentration and release of substance P–like immunoreactivity in the dental pulp. Acta Physiol. Scand., *111*:141–149, 1981.
76. Brodin, E., Gazelius, B., Panopoulos, P., Olgart, L.: Morphine inhibits substance P release from peripheral sensory nerve endings. Acta Physiol. Scand., *117*:567–570, 1983.
77. Brown, A.G.: Organization in the Spinal Cord. New York, Springer–Verlag, 1981.
78. Brown, A.G.: Ascending and long spinal pathway: Dorsal columns, spinocervical tract and spinothalamic tract. *In*: Iggo, A. (ed.) Handbook of Sensory Physiology, vol. II, pp. 315–338, New York, Springer–Verlag, 1973.
79. Brown, A.G., Franz, D.N.: Responses of spinocervical tract neurons to natural stimulation of identified cutaneous receptors. Exp. Brain Res., *7*:231–249, 1969.
80. Brown, A.G., Fyffe, R.E.W., Noble, R., Rose, P.K., *et al.*: The density, distribution and topographical organization of spinocervical tract neurones in the cat. J. Physiol. (Lond.), *300*:409–428, 1980.
81. Brown, A.M.: Excitation in afferent cardiac sympathetic nerve fibers during myocardial ischemia. J. Physiol. (Lond.), *190*:35–53, 1967.
82. Brown, A.M., Malliani, A.: Spinal sympathetic reflexes initiated by coronary receptors. J. Physiol. (Lond.), *212*:685–705, 1971.
83. Brown, P.B., Fuchs, J.L.: Somatotopic representation of hindlimb skin in cat dorsal horn. J. Neurophysiol., *28*:1–9, 1975.
84. Brown, P.B., Fuchs, J.L., Tapper, D.N.: Parametric studies of dorsal horn neurons responding to tactile stimulation. J. Neurophysiol., *28*:19–25, 1975.
85. Brune,K., Walz, D., Bucher, K.: The avian microcrystal arthritis. I. Simultaneous recording of nociception and temperature effect in the inflamed joint. Agents Actions 4:21–26, 1974.
86. Bryan, R.N., Trevino, D.L., Coulter, J.D., Willis, W.D.: Location and somatotopic organization of the cells of origin of the spinocervical tract. Exp. Brain Res., *17*:177–189, 1973.
87. Burch, G.E., DePasquale, N.P.: Bradykinin. Am. Heart J., *65*:116–123, 1963.
88. Burgess, P.R., Perl, E.R.: Myelinated afferent fibers responding specifically to noxious stimulation of the skin. J. Physiol. (Lond.), *190*:541–562, 1967.
89. Burgess, P.R., Perl, E.R.: Cutaneous mechanoreceptors and nociceptors. *In* Iggo, A. (ed.): Handbook of Sensory Physiology, Vol. II, pp. 29–78. New York, Springer–Verlag, 1973.
90. Burton, H., Craig, A.D., Jr.: Distribution of trigeminothalamic projection cells in cat and monkey. Brain Res., *161*:515–521, 1976.
91. Burton, H., Forbes, D.J., Benjamin, R.M.: Thalamic neurons responsive to temperature changes of glabrous hand and foot skin in squirrel monkey. Brain Res., *24*:179–190, 1970.
92. Burton, H., Jones, E.G.: The posterior thalamic region and its cortical projection in new world and old world monkeys. J. Comp. Neurol. *168*:249–302, 1976.
93. Burton, H., Loewy, A.D.: Descending projections from the marginal cell layer and other regions of the monkey spinal cord. Brain Res., *116*:485–491, 1976.
94. Byers, M.R., Fink, B.R., Kennedy, R.D., Middaugh, M.E., *et al.*: Effects of lidocaine on axonal morphology, microtubules, and rapid transport in rabbit vagus nerve *in vitro*. J. Neurobiol. 4:125–143, 1973.
95. Cajal, S.R., y: Histologie du Systeme Nerveux de l' Hommes et des Vertebres. Madrid, Instituto Ramon y Cajal, 1952 reprint, 1909.
96. Calvillo, O., Henry, J.L., Neuman, R.S.: Actions of narcotic analgesics and antagonists on spinal units responding to natural stimulation in the cat. Can. J. Physiol. Pharmacol. *51*:652–663, 1979.
97. Calvin, W.H.: Some design features of axons and how neuralgias may defeat them. *In* Bonica, J.J., Liebeskind, J.C., Albe–Fessard, D. (eds.): Advances in Pain Research and Therapy, vol. 3, pp. 297–309. New York, Raven Press, 1979.
98. Calvin, W.H., Howe, J.F., Loeser, J.D.: Ectopic repetitive firing in focally demyelinated axons and some implications for trigeminal neuralgia. *In* Anderson, D., Matthews, B. (eds.): Pain in the Trigeminal Region, pp. 125–136. Amsterdam, Elsevier/North Holland, 1977.
99. Calvin, W.H., Loeser, J.D., Howe, J.F.: A neurophysiological theory for the pain mechanism of tic douloureux. Pain, *3*:147–154, 1977.
100. Camarata, P.J., Yaksh, T.L.: Characterization of the spinal adrenergic receptors mediating the spinal effects produced by the microinjection of morphine into the periaqueductal gray. Brain Res., *336*:133–142, 1985.
101. Carlen, P.L., Wall, P.D., Nadvorna, H., Steinbach, T.: Phantom limbs and related phenomena in recent traumatic amputations. Neurology, *28*:211–217, 1978.
102. Carpenter, M.D., Stein, B.M., Shriver, J.E.: Central projections of spinal dorsal roots in the monkey. II. Lower thoracic,

lumbosacral and coccygeal dorsal roots. Am. J. Anat., *123*:75–118, 1968.

103. Carreras, M., Andersson, S.A.: Functional properties of neurons of the anterior ectosylvian gyrus of the cat. J. Neurophysiol., *26*:100–126, 1963.

104. Carstens, E., Trevino, D.L.: Laminar origins of spinothalamic projections in the cat as determined by the retrograde transport of horseradish peroxidase. J. Comp. Neurol. *182*:151–166, 1978.

105. Casey, K.L.: Unit analysis of nociceptive mechanisms in the thalamus of the awake squirrel monkey. J. Neurophysiol., *29*:727–750, 1966.

106. Casey, K.L.: Somatic stimuli, spinal pathways, and size of cutaneous fibers influencing unit activity in the medial medullary reticular formation. Exp. Neurol., *25*:35–56, 1969.

107. Casey, K.L.: Responses of bulboreticular units to somatic stimuli eliciting escape behavior in the cat. Int. J. Neurosci., *2*:15–28, 1971.

108. Casey, K.L.: Escape elicited by bulboreticular stimulation in the cat. Int. J. Neurosci., *2*:29–34, 1971.

109. Casey, K.L., Keene, J.J.: Unit analysis of the effects of motivating stimuli in the awake animal: Pain and self stimulation. *In* Phillips, M.I. (ed.): Brain Unit Activity During Behavior, pp. 115–129. Springfield, IL, Charles C Thomas, 1973.

110. Casey, K.L., Morrow, T.J.: Ventral posterior thalamic neurons differentially responsive to noxious stimulation of the awake monkey. Science, *221*:675–677, 1983.

111. Cauna, N.: Fine structure of the receptor organ and its probable functional significance. *In* de Reuck, A.V.S., Knight, J. (eds.): Touch, Heat and Pain, pp. 117–127. CIBA Symposium. London, Churchill, 1966.

112. Cauna, N.: The fine morphology of the sensory receptor organs in the auricle of the rat. J. Comp. Neurol. *136*:81–98, 1969.

113. Cedarbaum, J.M., Aghajanian, G.K.: Activation of locus coeruleus neurons by peripheral stimuli: modulation by a collateral inhibitory mechanism. Life Sci., *23*:1383–1392, 1978.

114. Cervero, F.: Dorsal horn neurons and their sensory inputs. *In* Yaksh, T.L. (ed.): Spinal Afferent Processing, pp. 197–216. New York, Plenum Press, 1986.

115. Cervero, F., Iggo, A.: The substantia gelatinosa of the spinal cord. A critical review. Brain, *103*:717–772, 1980.

116. Cervero, F., Iggo, A., Molony, V.: Responses of spinocervical tract neurones to noxious stimulation of the skin. J. Physiol. (Lond.), *267*:537–558, 1977.

117. Cervero, F., Iggo, A., Ogawa, H.: Nociceptor–driven dorsal horn neurones in the lumbar spinal cord of the cat. Pain, *2*:5–24, 1976.

118. Cervero, F., Molony, V., Iggo, A.: Extra– and intracellular recordings from neurones in the substantia gelatinosa. Brain Res., *136*:565–569, 1977.

119. Cervero, F., Molony, V., Iggo, A.: Supraspinal linkage of substantia gelatinosa neurones: Effects of descending impulses. Brain Res., *175*:351–355, 1979.

120. Cesselin, F., Oliveras, J.L., Bourgoin, S., Sierralta, F., *et al.*: Increased levels of met–enkephalin–like material in the CSF of anaesthetized cats after tooth pulp stimulation. Brain Res., *237*:325–338, 1982.

121. Cesselin, F., Bourgoin, S., Artaud, F., Hamon, M.: Basic and regulatory mechanisms of *in vitro* release of met–enkephalin from the dorsal zone of the rat spinal cord. J. Neurochem., *43*:763–773, 1984.

122. Chahl, L.A.: Pain induced by inflammatory mediators. *In* Beers, R.F., Jr., Bassett, E.G. (eds.): Mechanisms of Pain and Analgesic Compounds, pp. 273–284, New York, Raven Press, 1979.

123. Chahl, L.A., Iggo, A.: The effects of bradykinin and prostaglandin E_1 on rat cutaneous afferent nerve activity. Br. J. Pharmacol., *59*:343–374, 1977.

124. Chahl, L.A., Ladd, R.J.: Local oedema and general excitation of cutaneous sensory receptors produced by electrical stimulation of the saphenous nerve in the rat. Pain, *2*:25–34, 1976.

125. Chan, J.V.C., Burrowes, C.E., Movat, H.Z.: Surface activation of factor XII (Hageman factor)–critical role of high molecular weight kininogen and another potentiator. Agents Actions, *8*:65–72, 1978.

126. Chan–Palay, V.: Combined immunocytochemistry and autoradiography after *in vivo* injections of monoclonal antibody to substance P and ^{3}H–serotonin. Anat. Embryol., *156*:241–255, 1979

127. Chapman, L.F., Ramos, A.O., Goodell, H., Wolff, H.G.: Neurohumoral features of afferent fibers in man. Arch. Neurol., *4*:617–650, 1961.

128. Chatrain, G.E., Canfield, R.C., Knauss, T.A., Lettich, E.: Cerebral responses to electrical tooth pulp stimulation in man: An objective correlate of acute experimental pain. Neurology, *25*:745–757, 1975.

129. Chi, C.C.: An experimental silver study of the ascending projections of the central gray substance and adjacent tegmentum in the rat with observation in the cat. J. Comp. Neurol., *139*:259–272, 1970.

130. Chouchkov, C.N.: On the fine structure of free nerve endings in human digital skin, oral cavity and rectum. Z. Mikrosk. Anat. Forsch. *86*:273–288, 1972.

131. Christensen, B.N., Perl, E.R.: Spinal neurons specifically excited by noxious or thermal stimuli: marginal zones of the dorsal horn. J. Neurophysiol., *33*:293–307, 1970.

132. Clark, F.J.: Central projection of sensory fibers from the cat knee joint. J. Neurobiol., *3*:101–110, 1972.

133. Clark, F.J.: Information signaled by sensory fibers in medial articular nerve. J. Neurophysiol., *38*:1464–1472, 1975.

134. Clark, F.J., Burgess, P.R.: Slowly adapting receptors in cat knee joint: Can they signal joint angle? J. Neurophysiol., *38*:1448–1463, 1975.

135. Clarke, W.B., Bowsher, D.: Terminal distribution of primary afferent trigeminal fibers in the rat. Exp. Neurol., *6*:372–383, 1962.

137. Clifton, G.L., Vance, W.H., Applebaum, M.L., Coggeshall, R.E., *et al.*: Responses of unmyelinated afferents in the mammalian ventral root. Brain Res., *82*:163–167, 1974.

136. Clifton, G.L., Coggeshall, R.E., Vance, W.H., Willis, W.D.: Receptive fields of unmyelinated ventral root afferent fibers in the cat. J. Physiol. (Lond.), *256*:573–600, 1976.

138. Cochrane, C.G.: The Hageman factor pathways of kinin formation, clotting and fibrinolysis. *In* Beers, R.F., Bassett, E.G. (eds.): The Role of Immunological Factors in Infectious, Allergic and Autoimmune Processes, pp. 237–245. New York, Raven Press, 1976.

139. Coggeshall, R.E., Applebaum, M.L., Fazen, M., Stubbs, T.B., *et al.*: Unmyelinated axons in human ventral roots, a possible explanation for the failure of dorsal rhizotomy to relieve pain. Brain, *98*:157–166, 1975.

140. Coggeshall, R.E., Coulter, J.D., Willis, W.D., Jr.: Unmyelinated axons in the ventral roots of the cat lumbosacral enlargement. J. Comp. Neurol., *158*:39–58, 1974.

141. Coimbra, A., Sodre–Borges, B.P., Magalheas, M.M.: The substantia gelatinosa Rolandi of the rat. Fine structure cytochemistry (acid phosphatase) and changes after dorsal root section. J. Neurocytol., *3*:199–217, 1974.

142. Collier, J.G., Karim, S.M.M., Robinson, B., Somers, K.: Action of prostaglandins A_2, B_1, E_2, F_2 on superficial hand veins of man. Br. J. Pharmacol., *44*:374P–375P, 1972.

143. Collins, W.F., Randt, C.T.: Midbrain evoked responses relating to peripheral unmyelinated or "C" fibers in cat. J. Neurophysiol., *23*:47–53, 1960.

144. Collins, W.F., Nulsen, F.E., Randt, C.T.: Relation of peripheral nerve fiber size and sensation in man. Arch. Neurol., *3*:381–385, 1960.

145. Cook, A.W., Browder, E.: Function of posterior columns in man. Arch. Neurol., *12*:72–79, 1965.

146. Coulter, J.D., Foreman, R.D., Beall, J.E., Willis, W.D.: Cerebral cortical modulation of primate spinothalamic neurons. *In* Bonica, J.J., Albe–Fessard, D. (eds.): Advances in Pain Research and Therapy, vol. 1, pp. 271–277. New York, Raven Press, 1976.

147. Cousins, M.J., Mather, L.E.: Intrathecal and epidural administration of opioids. Anesthesiology, *61*:276–310, 1984.

148. Couture, R., Cuello, A.C.: Substance P antagonists and the antidromic stimulation of peripheral sensory branches of the trigeminal nerve. *In*: Substance P, pp. 192–193, Dublin, 1983.

149. Craig, A.D., Burton, H.: Spinal and medullary lamina I projection to nucleus submedius in medial thalamus: A possible pain center. J. Neurophysiol., *45*:443–466, 1981.

150. Croze, S., Duclaux, R., Kenshalo, D.R.: The thermal sensitivity of the polymodal nociceptors in the monkey. J. Physiol., *263*:539–562, 1976.

151. Crunkchorn, P., Willis, A.L.: Cutaneous reactions to intradermal prostaglandins. Br. J. Pharmacol., *41*:49–56, 1971.

152. Csillik, B., Knyihar, E.: Biodynamic plasticity in the Rolando substance. In Progress in Neurobiology, vol. 10, pp. 203–230. Oxford, Pergamon Press, Ltd., 1978.

153. Cuello, A.C., Priestley, J.V., Matthews, M.R.: Localization of substance P in neuronal pathways. *In* Ciba Foundation Symposium 91, Substance P in the Nervous System, pp. 55–83. London, Pitman, 1982.

154. Culberson, J.L., Haines, D.E., Kimmel, D.L., Brown, P.B.: Contralateral projection of primary afferent fibers to mammalian spinal cord. Exp. Neurol., *64*:83–97, 1979.

155. Curry, M.J.: The effects of stimulating the somatic sensory cortex on single neurones in the posterior group (PO) of the cat. Brain Res., *44*:463–481, 1972.

156. Curry, M.J.: The exteroceptive properties of neurones in the somatic part of the posterior group (PO). Brain Res., *44*:439–462, 1972.

157. Curtis, D.R., Johnston, G.A.R.: Amino acid transmitters in the mammalian central nervous system. Rev. Physiol. Biochem., Pharmacol., *69*:98–188, 1974.

158. Dale, H.H.: Pharmacology and nerve endings. Proc. R. Soc. Med., *28*:319–332, 1935.

159. Dalsgaard, C.J., Vincent, S.R., Hökfelt, T., *et al.*: Coexistence of cholecystokinin–and substance P–like peptides in neurons of the dorsal root ganglia of the rat. Neurosci. Lett., *33*:159–163, 1982.

160. Darian–Smith, I., Mutton, P., Proctor, R.: Functional organization of tactile cutaneous afferents within the semilunar ganglion and tri–trigeminal spinal tract in the cat. J. Neurophysiol., *28*:682–694, 1965.

161. Davis, L.E., Hart, J.T., Crain, R.C.: The pathway for visceral afferent impulses within the spinal cord. II. Experimental dilatation of the biliary ducts. Surg. Gynecol. Obstet., *48*:647–651, 1929.

162. Deakin, J.F.W., Dostrovsky, J.O.: Involvement of the periaqueductal grey matter and spinal 5–hydroxytryptaminergic pathways in morphine analgesia. Effects of lesions and 5–hydroxytryptamine. Br. J. Pharmacol., *63*:159–165, 1978.

163. Delacour, J., Borst, A.: Failure to find homology in rat, cat and monkey for functions of a subcortical structure in avoidance conditioning. J. Comp. Physiol. Psychol., *80*:458–468, 1972.

164. Delange, A., Hannam, A., Matthews, B.: The diameters and conduction velocities of fibers in the terminal branches of the inferior dental nerve. Arch. Oral Biol., *14*:513–520, 1969.

165. Delgado, J.M.R., Rosvald, H.E., Looney, E.: Evoking conditioned fear by electrical stimulation of subcortical structures in the monkey brain. J. Comp. Physiol. Psychol., *49*:373–380, 1956.

166. Denny–Brown, D., Kirk, E.J., Yanagisawa, N.: The tract of Lissauer in relation to sensory transmission in the dorsal horn of the spinal cord in the Macaque monkey. J. Comp. Neurol., *151*:175–200, 1973.

167. Denny–Brown, D., Yanagisawa, N.: The function of the descending root of the fifth nerve. Brain, *96*:783–814, 1973.

168. Devor, M., Schonfeld, D., Seltzer, Z., Wall, P.D.: Two modes of cutaneous reinnervation following peripheral nerve injury. J. Comp. Neurol., *185*:211–220, 1979.

169. Dickenson, A.H., Hellon, R.F., Taylor, D.L.M.: Facial thermal input to the trigeminal spinal nucleus of rabbits and rats. J. Comp. Neurol., *185*:203–210, 1979.

170. Dilly, P.N., Wall, P.D., Webster, K.E.: Cells of origin of the spinothalamic tract in the cat and rat. Exp. Neurol., *21*:550–562, 1968.

171. Dodt, E., Zotterman, Y.: The discharge of specific cold fibers at high temperatures. Acta Physiol. Scand., *26*:358–365, 1952.

172. Dong, W.K., Ryu, H., Wagman, I.H.: Nociceptive responses of neurons in medial thalamus and their relationship to spinothalamic pathways. J. Neurophysiol., *41*:1592–1613, 1978.

173. Douglas, W.W., Ritchie, J.M.: Non–medullated fibers in the saphenous nerve which signal touch. J. Physiol. (Lond.), *139*:385–399, 1957.

174. Doupe, J., Cullen, C.H., Chance, G.Q.: Post–traumatic pain and the causalgic syndrome. J. Neurol. Neurosurg. Psychiatry, *7*:33–48, 1944.

175. Droz, B.: Renewal of synaptic proteins. Brain Res., *62*:383–394, 1973.

176. Dubner, R., Beitel, R.E.: Neural correlates of escape behavior in rhesus monkey to noxious heat applied to the face. *In* Bonica, J.J., Albe–Fessard, D. (eds.): Advances in Pain Research and Therapy, vol. 1, pp. 155–160. New York, Raven Press, 1976.

177. Dubner, R., Gobel, S., Price, D.D.: Peripheral and central trigeminal "pain" pathways. *In* Bonica, J.J., Albe–Fessard, D., (eds.): Advances in pain Research and Therapy, vol. 1, pp. 137–147, New York, Raven Press, 1976.

178. Dubner, R., Sumino, R., Wood, W.I.: A peripheral "cold" fiber population responsive to innocuous and noxious thermal stimuli applied to the monkey's face. J. Neurophysiol., *38*:1373–1389, 1975.

179. Duggan, A.W., Hall, J.G., Headley, P.M.: Suppression of transmission of nociceptive impulses by morphine: Selective effects of morphine administered in the region of the substantia gelatinosa. Br. J. Pharmacol, *61*:65–76, 1977.

180. Duggan, A.W., Johnson, S.M., Morton, C.R.: Differing distributions of receptors for morphine and Met^5–enkephalinamide in the dorsal horn of the cat. Brain Res., *229*:379–387, 1981.

181. Duggan, A.W., North, R.A.: Electrophysiology of opioids. Pharmacol. Rev., *35*:219–281, 1984.

182. Duncan, D., Morales, R.: Relative numbers of several types of synaptic connections in the substantia gelatinosa of the cat spinal cord. J. Comp. Neurol., *182*:601–610, 1978.

183. Dyck, P.J.: Detection thresholds of cutaneous sensations in health and disease in man. *In* Yaksh, T.L. (ed.): Spinal Afferent Processing, pp. 345–362. New York, Plenum Press, 1986.

184. Dyck, P.J., Lambert, E.H., Nicholas, P.C.: Quantitative measurement of sensation related to compound action potential and number and sizes of myelinated and unmyelinated fibres of the sural nerve in health, Friedreich's ataxia, hereditary sensory neuropathy, and tabes dorsalis. *In* Cobb, W.A. (ed.): Handbook of Electroencephalography and Clinical Neurophysiology, vol. 9, pp. 83–118. Amsterdam, Elsevier, North–Holland, 1971.

185. Dyson, C., Brindley, G.S.: Strength–duration curves for the production of cutaneous pain by electrical stimuli. Clin. Sci., *30*:237–241, 1966.

186. Eccles, J.C., Eccles, R.M., Magni, F.: Central inhibitory action attributable to presynaptic depolarization produced by muscle afferent volleys. J. Physiol. (Lond.), *159*:147–166, 1961.

187. Eccles, J.C., Kostyuk, P.G., Schmidt, R.F.: Central pathways responsible for depolarization of primary afferent fibers. J. Physiol. (Lond.), *161*:237–257, 1962.

188. Edwall, L., Olgart, L.: A new technique for recording of intradental sensory nerve activity in man. Pain, *3*:121–125, 1977.

189. Eickhoff, R., Handwerker, H.O., McQueen, D.S., Schick, E.: Noxious and tactile input to medial structures of midbrain and pons in the rat. Pain, *5*:99–113, 1978.

190. Eisenman, J., Landgren, S., Novin, D.: Functional organization in the main sensory trigeminal nucleus and in the rostral sub–division of the nucleus of the spinal trigeminal tract in the cat. Acta Physiol. Scand., *59*:(*Suppl.* 214):1–44, 1963.

191. Elliot, D.E., Horton, E.W., Lewis, G.P.: Actions of pure bradykinin. J. Physiol. (Lond.) *153*:473–480, 1960,

192. Emmers, R.: Pain: A Spike–Interval Coded Message in the Brain. New York, Raven Press, 1981.

193. Engberg, I., Lundberg, A., Ryall, R.W.: Reticulospinal inhibition of transmission in reflex pathways. J. Physiol. (Lond.), *194*:201–223, 1968.

194. Engberg, I., Lundberg, A., Ryall, R.W.: Reticulospinal inhibition of interneurones. J. Physiol. (Lond.), *194*:225–236, 1968.

195. Essman, W.B.: Serotonin distribution in tissues and fluids. *In* Essman, W.B. (ed.): Availability, Localization and Disposition, vol. I. Serotonin in Health and Disease, pp. 15–178. New York, Spectrum Publications, 1968.

196. Ferreira, S.H.: Prostaglandins, aspirin–like drugs and analgesia. Nature New Biol., *240*:200–203, 1972.

197. Ferreira, S.H., Lorenzetti, B.B., Correa, F.M.A.: Central and peripheral antialgesic action of aspirin–like drugs. Eur. J. Pharmacol., *53*:39–48, 1978.

198. Ferreira, S.H., Moncada S, Vane, J.R.: Prostaglandins and the mechanism of analgesia produced by aspirin–like drugs. Br. J. Pharmacol., *49*:86–97, 1973.

199. Fields, H.L., Anderson, S.D.: Evidence that raphe–spinal neurons mediate opiate and midbrain stimulation–produced analgesias. Pain, *5*:333–349, 1978.

200. Fields, H.L., Basbaum, A.I., Clanton, C.H., Anderson, S.D.: Nucleus raphe magnus inhibition of spinal cord dorsal horn neurons. Brain Res., *126*:441–453, 1977.

201. Fields, H.L., Clanton, C.H., Anderson, S.D.: Somatosensory properties of spinorecticular neurons in the cat. Brain Res., *120*:49–66, 1977.

202. Fields, H.L., Emson, P.C., Leigh, B.K., *et al.*: Multiple opiate receptor sites on primary afferent fibres. Nature, *284*:351–353, 1980.

203. Fields, H.L., Partridge, L.D., Winter, D.L.: Somatic and visceral receptive field properties of fibers in ventral quadrant white matter of the cat spinal cord. J. Neurophysiol., *33*:827–837, 1970.

204. Fields, H.L., Wagner, G.M., Anderson, S.D.: Some properties of spinal neurons projecting to the medial brain–stem reticular formation. Exp. Neurol., *47*:118–134, 1975.

205. Finger, S., Frommer, D.: Effects of cortical and thalamic lesions on temperature discrimination and responsiveness to foot shock in the rat. Brain Res., *24*:69–89, 1970.

206. Fitzgerald, M., Lynn, B.: The sensitization of high threshold mechanoreceptors with myelinated axons by repeated heating. J. Physiol. (Lond.), *265*:549–563, 1977.

207. Fitzgerald, M., Woolf, C.J.: The stereospecific effect of naloxone on rat dorsal horn neurones: Inhibition in superficial laminae and excitation in deeper laminae. Pain, *9*:293–306, 1980.

208. Fitzgerald, T.J., Williams, B., Uyeki, E.M.: Effects of antimitotic and antiinflammatory agents on sodium urate-induced pain swelling in mice. Pharmacology, *6*:265–273, 1971.

209. Fjallbrant, N., Iggo, A.: The effect of histamine, 5-hydroxytryptamine and acetylcholine on cutaneous afferent fibers. J. Physiol. (Lond.), *156*:578–590, 1961.

210. Flower, R.J.: Drugs which inhibit prostaglandin biosynthesis. Pharmacol., Rev., *26*:33–67, 1974.

211. Flower, R.J.: Steroidal anti-inflammatory drugs as inhibitors of phospholipase A_2. *In* Galli, C., Galli, G., Porcellati, G. (eds.): Advances in Prostaglandin Thromboxane Research, vol. 3, pp. 105–112. New York, Raven Press, 1978.

212. Fock, S., Mense, S.: Excitatory effects of 5-hydroxytryptamine, histamine and potassium ions on muscular group IV afferent units: A comparison with bradykinin. Brain Res., *105*:459–469, 1976.

213. Foreman, R.D.: Viscerosomatic convergence onto spinal neurons responding to afferent fibers located in the inferior cardiac nerve. Brain Res., *137*:164–168, 1977.

214. Foreman, R.D.: Spinal substrates of visceral pain. *In* Yaksh, T.L. (ed.): Spinal Afferent Processing, pp. 217–242. New York, Plenum Press, 1986.

215. Foreman, R.D., Ohata, C.A., Gerhart, K.D.: Neural mechanisms underlying cardiac pain. *In* Schwartz, P.J., Brown, A.M., Malliani, A., Zanchetti, A. (eds.): Neural Mechanisms in Cardiac Arrhythmias, pp. 191–207. New York, Raven Press, 1978.

216. Foreman, R.D., Schmidt, R.F., Willis, W.D.: Convergence of muscle and cutaneous input onto primate spinothalamic tract neurons. Brain Res., *124*:555–560, 1977.

217. Foreman, R.D., Schmidt, R.F., Willis, W.D.: Effect of mechanical and chemical stimulation of fine muscle afferents upon primate spinothalamic tract cells. J. Physiol. (Lond.), *286*:215–231, 1979.

218. Frank, R.M.: Ultrastructural relationship between the odontoblast, its process and the nerve fiber. *In* Symins, N.D.J. (ed.): Dentine and Pulp: Their Structure and Relations, pp. 115–145. Livingstone, 1968.

219. Franz, M., Mense, S.: Muscle receptors with group IV afferent fibres responding to application of bradykinin. Brain Res., *92*:369–383, 1975.

220. Friedman, D.P., Jones, E.G.: Focal projection of electrophysiologically defined groupings of thalamic cells on the monkey somatic sensory complex. Brain Res., *191*:249–252, 1980.

221. Fukushima, T., Kerr, F.W.L.: Organization of trigeminothalamic tracts and other thalamic afferent systems of the brainstem in the rat: Presence of gelatinosa neurons with thalamic connections. J. Comp. Neurol., *183*;169–184, 1979.

222. Funakoshi, M., Zotterman, Y.: A study in the excitation of dental pulp nerve fibres. *In* Anderson, D.J. (ed.): Sensory Mechanisms in Dentine, pp. 60–72. Oxford, Pergamon, 1963.

223. Game, C.J.A., Lodge, D.: The pharmacology of the inhibition of dorsal horn neurones by impulses in myelinated cutaneous afferents in the cat. Exp. Brain Res., *23*:75–84, 1975.

224. Gamse, R., Holzer, P., Lembeck, F.: Decrease of substance P in primary afferent neurones and impairment of neurogenic plasma extravasation by capsaicin. Br. J. Pharmacol., *68*:207–213, 1980.

225. Gamse, R., Leeman, S., Holzer, P., Lembeck, F.: Differential effects of capsaicin on the content of somatostatin, substance P, and neurotensin in the nervous system of the rat. Naunyn-Schmiedeberg's Arch. Pharmacol., *317*:140–148, 1981.

226. Gardner, E.: The distribution and termination of nerves in the knee joint of the cat. J. Comp. Neurol., *80*:11–32, 1944.

227. Gasser, H.S.: Unmedulated fibers originating in dorsal root ganglia. J. Gen. Physiol., *33*:651–690, 1950.

228. Georgopoulos, A.P.: Functional properties of primary afferent units probably related to pain mechanisms in primate glaborous skin. J. Neurophysiol., *39*:71–83, 1976.

229. Giesler, G.J., Menetrey, D., Guilbaud, G., Besson, J.M.: Lumbar cord neurons at the origin of the spinothalamic tract in the rat. Brain Res., *118*:320–324, 1976.

230. Giesler, G.J., Jr., Menetrey, D., Basbaum, A.I.: Differential origins of spinothalamic tract projections to medial and lateral thalamus in the rat. J. Comp. Neurol., *184*:107–126, 1979.

230a. Giesler, G.J., Jr., Yezierski, R.P., Gerhart, K.D., Willis, W.D.: Spinothalamic tract neurons that project to medial and/or lateral thalamic nuclei: Evidence for a physiologically novel population of spinal cord neurons. J. Neurophysiol., *46*:1285–1308, 1981.

231. Glassman, R.D., Forgus, M.W., Goodman, J.E., Glassman, H.N.: Somesthetic effects of damage to cat's ventrobasal complex, medial lemniscus or posterior group. Exp. Neurol., *48*:460–492, 1975.

232. Glazer, E.J., Steinbusch, H., Verhofstad, A., Basbaum, A.I.: Serotonin neurons in nucleus raphe dorsalis and paragigantocellularis of the cat contain enkephalin. J. Physiol. (Paris) *77*:241–245, 1981.

233. Gobel, S.: Golgi studies of the substantia gelatinosa neurons in the spinal trigeminal nucleus. J. Comp. Neurol., *162*:397–415, 1975.

234. Gobel, S.: Dendroaxonic synapses in the substantia gelatinosa trigeminal nucleus of the cat. J. Comp. Neurol., *167*:165–176, 1976.

235. Gobel, S.: Golgi studies of the neurons in layer I of the dorsal horn of the medulla (trigeminal nucleus caudalis). J. Comp. Neurol., *180*:375–393, 1978.

236. Gobel, S.: Golgi studies of the neurons in layer II of the dorsal horn of the medulla (trigeminal nucleus caudalis). J. Comp. Neurol., *180*:395–414, 1978.

237. Gobel, S., Falls, W.M., Hockfield, S.: The division of the dorsal and ventral horns of the mammalian caudal medulla into eight layers using anatomical criteria. *In* Anderson, D.J., Matthews, B. (eds.): Pain in the Trigeminal Region, pp. 443–453, Amsterdam, Elsevier/North-Holland, 1977.

238. Gobel, S., Hockfield, S.: An anatomical analysis of the synaptic circuitry of layers I, II and III of trigeminal nucleus caudalis in the cat. *In* Anderson, D.J., Matthews, B. (eds.): Pain in the Trigeminal Region, pp. 203–211. Amsterdam, Elsevier/North–Holland, 1977.

239. Gobel, S., Purvis, M.B.: Anatomical studies of the organization of the spinal V nucleus: The deep bundles and the spinal V tract. Brain Res., *48*:27–44, 1972.

240. Goldman, D.E.: Responses of nerve fibers to mechanical forces. *In* Iggo, A. (ed.): Handbook of Sensory Physiology, vol. 1, pp. 340–344. New York, Springer, 1971.

241. Goldman, P.L., Collins, W.F., Taub, A., Fitzmartin, J.: Evoked bulbar reticular unit activity following delta fiber stimulation of peripheral somatosensory nerve in cat. Exp. Neurol., *37*:597–606, 1972.

242. Gouret, C., Mocquet, G., Raynaud, G.: Use of Freund's adjuvant arthritis test in anti–inflammatory drug screening in the rat: Value of animal selection and preparation at the breeding center. Lab. Anim. Sci., *26*:281–287, 1976.

243. Gray, J.A.B.: Effects of stretch on single myelinated nerve fibres. J. Physiol. (Lond.), *124*:84–98, 1954.

244. Greaves, M.W., Sodergaard, J., McDonald–Gibson, W.: Recovery of prostaglandins in human cutaneous inflammation. Br. Med. J., *2*:258–260, 1971.

245. Green, J.P., Johnson, C.L., Weinstein, H.: Histamine as a neurotransmitter. *In* Lipton, M.A., DiMascio, A., Killam, K.F. (eds.): Psychopharmacology: A Generation of Progress, pp. 319–332. New York, Raven Press, 1978.

246. Greenwood, L.F., Horiuchi, H., Matthews, B.: Electrophysiological evidence on the types of nerve fibers excited by electrical stimulation of teeth with a pulp tester. Arch. Oral Biol., *17*:701–709, 1972.

247. Greenwood, L.F., Sessle, B.J.: Inputs to trigeminal brain stem neurones from facial, oral, tooth pulp and pharyngolaryngeal tissues: II. Role of trigeminal nucleus caudalis in modulating responses to innocuous and noxious stimuli. Brain Res., *117*:227–238, 1976.

248. Groves, P.M., Miller, S.W., Parker, M.V., Rebec, G.V.: Organization of sensory modality in the reticular formation of the rat. Brain Res., *54*:207–224, 1973.

249. Guilbaud, G., Benelli, G., Besson, J.M.: Responses of thoracic dorsal horn interneurons to cutaneous stimulation and to the administration of algogenic substances into the mesenteric artery in the spinal cat. Brain Res., *124*:437–448, 1977.

250. Guilbaud, G., Besson, J.M., Oliveras, J.L., Wyon–Maillard, M.C.: Modifications of the firing rate of bulbar reticular units (nucleus gigantocellularis) after intra–arterial injection of bradykinin into the limbs. Brain Res., *63*:131–140, 1973.

251. Guzman, F., Braun, C., Lim, R.K.S.: Visceral pain and the pseudaffective response to intra–arterial injection of bradykinin and other algesic agents. Arch. Int. Pharmacodyn Ther., *136*:353–384, 1962.

252. Gybels, J.M.: Electrical stimulation of the central gray for pain relief in humans: A critical review. *In* Bonica, J.J., *et al.* (eds.): Advances in Pain Research and Therapy, vol. 3, pp. 499–509, New York, Raven Press, 1979.

253. Ha, H., Kitai, S.T., Morin, F.: The lateral cervical nucleus of the raccoon. Exp. Neurol., *11*:441–450, 1965.

254. Ha, H., Liu, C.N.: Organization of the spino–cervico–thalamic system. J. Comp. Neurol., *127*:445–470, 1966.

255. Hagbarth, K.E.: Exteroceptive, propioceptive, and sympathetic activity recorded with microelectrodes from human peripheral nerves. Mayo Clin. Proc., *54*:353–365, 1979.

256. Hagbarth, K.E., Kerr, D.I.B.: Central influences on spinal afferent conduction. J. Neurophysiol., *17*:295–307, 1954.

257. Halpern, M.: Effects of midbrain central gray matter lesions on escape–avoidance behavior in rats. Physiol. Behav., *3*:171–178, 1968.

258. Halpern, B.P., Halverson, J.D.: Modification of escape from noxious stimuli after bulbar reticular formation lesions. Behav. Biol., *11*:215–229, 1974.

259. Hamberg, M., Jonsson, C.E.: Increased synthesis of prostaglandins in the guinea pig following scalding injury. Acta Physiol. Scand., *87*:240–245, 1973.

260. Hamilton, B.L.: Projections of the nuclei of the periaqueductal grey matter of the cat. J. Comp. Neurol., *152*:45–58, 1973.

261. Hamilton, B.L., Skultety, M.: Efferent connections of the periaqueductal gray matter in the cat. J. Comp. Neurol., *139*:105–114, 1970.

262. Hammond, D.L., Yaksh, T.L.: Antagonism of stimulation–produced antinociception by intrathecal administration of methysergide or phentolamine. Brain Res., *298*:329–337, 1984.

263. Hammond, D.L., Tyce, G.M., Yaksh, T.L.: Efflux of 5–hydroxytryptamine and noradrenaline into spinal cord superfusates during stimulation of the rat medulla. J. Physiol., *359*:151–162, 1985.

264. Hancock, M.B., Foreman, R.D., Willis, W.D.: Convergence of visceral and cutaneous input onto spinothalamic tract cells in the thoracic spinal cord of the cat. Exp. Neurol., *47*:240–248, 1975.

265. Hancock, M.B., Rigamonti, D.D., Bryan, R.N.: Convergence in the lumbar spinal cord of pathways activated by splanchnic nerve and hind limb cutaneous nerve stimulation. Exp. Neurol., *38*:337–348, 1973.

266. Handwerker, H.O.: Influences of algogenic substances and prostaglandins on the discharges of unmyelinated cutaneous nerve fibers identified as nociceptors. *In* Bonica, J.J., Albe–Fessard, D. (eds.): Advances in Pain Research and Therapy, vol. 1, pp. 41–45. New York, Raven Press, 1976.

267. Harris, F.A.: Wide–field neurons in somatosensory thalamus of domestic cats under barbiturate anesthesia. Exp. Neurol., *68*:27–49, 1980.

268. Hassler, R.: Die Zentralen Systeme des Schmerzes. Acta Neurochir (wien), *8*:353–423, 1960.

269. Hayashi, H.: Distribution of vibrissae afferent fiber collaterals in the trigeminal nuclei as revealed by intra–axonal injection of horseradish peroxidase. Brain Res., *183*:442–446, 1980.

270. Headley, P.M., Duggan, A.W., Griersmith, B.T.: Selective reduction by noradrenaline and 5–hydroxytryptamine of nociceptive responses of cat dorsal horn neurones. Brain Res., *145*:185–189, 1978.

271. Heimer, L., Wall, P.D.: The dorsal root distribution to the substantia gelatinosa of the rat with a note on distribution in the cat. Exp. Brain Res., *6*:89–99, 1968.

272. Heinbecker, P., Bishop, G.H., O'Leary, J.: Pain and touch fibers in peripheral nerves. Arch. Neurol. Psychiatr. (Chic.), *29*:771–789, 1933.
273. Henry, J.L.: Effects of substances P on functionally identified units in cat spinal cord. Brain Res., *114*:439–451, 1976.
274. Henry, J.L.: Naloxone excites nociceptive units in the lumbar dorsal horn of the spinal cat. Neuroscience, *4*:1485–1491, 1979.
275. Hensel, H.: Cutaneous thermoreceptors. *In* Iggo, A. (ed.): Handbook of Sensory Physiology, vol. 2, pp. 79–110. New York, Springer–Verlag, 1973.
276. Hensel, H., Huopaniemi, T.: Static and dynamic properties of warm fibres in the intraorbital nerve. Pflugers Arch., *309*:1–10, 1969.
277. Hensel, H., Iggo, A.: Analysis of cutaneous warm and cold fibres in primates. Pflugers Arch., *329*:1–8, 1971.
278. Hentall, I.: A novel class of unit in the substantia gelatinosa of the spinal cat. Exp. Neurol., *57*:792–806, 1977.
279. Herman, A.C., Moncada, S.: Release of prostaglandins and incapacitation after injection of endotoxin in the knee joint of the dog. Br. J. Pharmacol., *53*:465P, 1975.
280. Hertel, H.C., Howaldt, B., Mense, S.: Responses of group IV and group III muscle afferents to thermal stimuli. Brain Res., *113*:201–205, 1976.
281. Hillman, P., Wall, P.D.: Inhibitory and excitatory factors influencing the receptive fields of lamina 5 spinal cord cells. Exp. Brain Res., *9*:284–306, 1969.
282. Hinsey, J.C., Gasser, H.S.: The components of the dorsal root mediating vasodilatation and the Sherrington contracture. Am. J. Physiol., *92*:679–689, 1930.
283. Hitchcock, E.: Stereotaxic cervical myelotomy. J. Neurol. Neurosurg. Psychiatr., *33*:224–230, 1970.
284. Hnik, P., Holas, M., Krekvle, I., Kriz, N., *et al.*: Work induced potassium changes in skeletal muscle and effluent venous blood assessed by liquid ion–exchanger microelectrodes. Pflugers Arch., *362*:85–94, 1976.
285. Hökfelt, T., Elde, R., Johansson, O., Luft, R., *et al.*: Immunohistochemical evidence for separate populations of somatostatin-containing and substance P–containing primary afferent neurons in the rat. Neuroscience, *1*:131–136, 1976.
286. Hökfelt, T., Johansson, O., Ljungdahl, A., *et al.*: Peptidergic neurones. Nature, *284*:515–521, 1980.
287. Hökfelt, T., Kellerth, J.O., Nilsson, G., Pernow, B.: Experimental immunohistochemical studies on the localization and distribution of substance P in cat primary sensory neurones. Brain Res., *100*:235–252, 1975.
288. Hökfelt, T., Kellerth, J.O., Nilsson, G., Pernow, B.: Substance P: Localization in the central nervous system and in some primary sensory neurons. Science, *190*:889–890, 1975.
289. Holmqvist, B., Lundberg, A.: On the organization of the supraspinal inhibitory control of interneurones of various spinal reflex arcs. Arch. Ital. Biol., *97*:340–356, 1959.
290. Holmqvist, B., Lundberg, A., Oscarsson, O.: Supraspinal inhibitory control of transmission to three ascending spinal pathways influenced by the flexion reflex afferents. Arch. Ital. Biol., *98*:60–80, 1960.
291. Honda, C.N.: Convergence of visceral and somatic afferent conversions onto neurons near the central canal in the sacral spinal cord of the cat. J. Neurophysiol., *53*:1059–1078, 1985.
292. Honda, C.N., Mense, S., Perl, E.R.: Neurons in ventrobasal region of cat thalamus selectivity responsive to noxious mechanical stimuli. J. Neurophysiol., *49*:662–673, 1983.
293. Honda, C., Perl, E.R.: Functional and morphological features of neurons in the midline region of the caudal spinal cord of the cat. Brain Res., *340*:285–295, 1985.
294. Hongo, T., Jankowska, E., Lundberg, A.: Post–synaptic excitation and inhibition from primary efferents in neurones of the spinocervical tract. J. Physiol., *199*:569–592, 1968.
295. Horton, E.W.: Action of prostaglandin E_1 on tissues which respond to bradykinin. Nature, *200*:892–893, 1963.
296. Hosobuchi, Y.: The current status of analgesic brain stimulation. Acta Neurochirur., *30(Suppl.)*:219–227, 1980.
297. Howe, J.F., Calvin, W.H., Loeser, J.D.: Impulses reflected from dorsal root ganglia and from focal nerve injuries. Brain Res., *116*:139–144, 1976.
298. Howe, J.F., Loeser, J.D., Calvin, W.H.: Mechanosensitivity of dorsal root ganglia and chronically injured axons: A physiological basis for the radicular pain of nerve root compression. Pain, *3*:25–41, 1977.
299. Hoyes, A.D., Barber, P.: Ultrastructure of the corneal nerves in the rat. Cell. Tiss. Res., *172*:133–144, 1976.
300. Hu, J.W., Sessle, B.J.: Trigeminal nociceptive and nonociceptive neurons: Brain stem intranuclear projections and modulation by orofacial, periaqueductal gray and nucleus raphe magnus stimuli. Brain Res., *170*:547–552, 1979.
301. Hylden, J.L.K., Wilcox, G.L.: Intrathecal substance P elicits a caudally-directed biting and scratching behavior in mice. Brain Res., *217*:212–215, 1981.
302. Hyndman, O.R.: Lissauer's tract section. A contribution to chordotomy for the relief of pain (preliminary report). J. Int. Coll. Surgeons, *5*:394–400, 1942.
303. Hyndman, O.R., Van Epps, C.: Possibility of differential section of the spinothalamic tract. Arch. Surg., *38*:1036–1053, 1939.
304. Iggo, A.: Nonmyelinated afferent fibers from mammalian skeletal muscle. J. Physiol. (Lond.), *155*:52–53P, 1961.
305. Iggo, A.: Cutaneous thermoreceptors in primates and subprimates. J. Physiol. (Lond.), *200*:403–430, 1969.
306. Iggo, A., Kornhuber, H.H.: A quantitative study of C–mechanoreceptors in hairy skin of the cat. J. Physiol. (Lond.), *271*:549–565, 1977.
307. Iggo, A., Ogawa, H.: Primate cutaneous thermal nociceptors.J. Physiol. (Lond.), *216*:77P, 1971.
308. Ishida, Y., Kitano, K.: Raphe induced inhibition of intralaminar thalamic unitary activities and its blockade by para–chlorophenylalanine in cats. Naunyn–Schmiedebergs Arch. Pharmacol., *301*:1–4, 1977.
309. Ishijima, B., Sano, K.: Responses of specific and nonspecific thalamic nuclei to the selective A and C fiber stimulation and their interactions in cat's brain. Neurol. Med. Chir., *11*:84–100, 1971.
310. Ishijima, B., Yoshimasu, N., Fukushima, T., Hori, T., *et al.*: Nociceptive neurons in the human thalamus. Confin. Neurol., *37*:99–106, 1975.
311. Jahr, C.E., Jessell, T.: Amino acid neurotransmission in dor-

sal horn spinal cord cell monolayer cultures. J. Neurosci., in press, 1985.

312. James, G.W.L., Church, M.K.: Hyperalgesia after treatment of mice with prostaglandins and arachidonic acid and its antagonism by antiinflammatory—analgesic compounds. Arzneimittelforsch., *28*:804–807, 1978.
313. Jancso, N.: Desensitization with capsaicin as a tool for studying the function of pain receptors. *In* Lim, R.K.: Pharmacology of Pain: Proceedings, vol. 9, pp. 33–55. Oxford, Pergamon Press, 1968.
314. Jancso, N., Jancso–Gabor, A., Szolcsanyi, J.: Direct evidence for neurogenic inflammation and its prevention by denervation and by pretreatment with capsaicin. Br. J. Pharmacol. Chemother., *31*:138–151, 1967.
315. Jannetta, P.J.: Microsurgical approach to the trigeminal nerve for tic douloureux. Prog. Neurol. Surg., *7*:180–200, 1976.
316. Jannetta, P.J., Rand, R.W.: Transtentorial retrogasserian rhizotomy in trigeminal neuralgia. In Rand, R.W. (ed.): Microsurgery, pp. 156–169. St. Louis, C.V. Mosby, 1969.
317. Jeftinija, S., Miletic, V., Randic, M.: Cholecystokinin octapeptide excites dorsal horn neurons both in vivo and in vitro. Brain Res., *213*:231–236, 1981.
318. Jeftinija, S., Semba, K., Randic, M.: Norepinephrine reduces excitability of single cutaneous primary afferent C–fibers in the cat spinal cord. Brain Res., *219*:456–463, 1981.
319. Jeftinija, S., Murase, K., Nedeljkov, V., Randic, M.: Vasoactive intestinal polypeptide excites mammalian dorsal horn neurons both *in vivo* and *in vitro.* Brain Res., *243*:158–164, 1982.
320. Jensen, T.S., Yaksh, T.L.: I. Comparison of antinociceptive action of morphine in the periaqueductal gray, medial and paramedial medulla in rat. Brain Res., *363*:99–113, 1986.
321. Jensen, T.S., Yaksh, T.L.: II. Examination of spinal monoamine receptors through which brain stem opiate sensitive systems act in the rat. Brain Res., *363*:114–127, 1986.
322. Jessell, T., Iversen, L.L.: Opiate analgesics inhibit substance P release from rat trigeminal nucleus. Nature, 549–551, 1977.
323. Jessell, T., Tsunoo, A., Kanazawa, I., Otsuka, M.: Substance P: Depletion in the dorsal horn of rat spinal cord after section of the peripheral processes of primary sensory neurons. Brain Res., *168*:247–259, 1979.
324. Jhamandas, K., Yaksh, T.L., Harty, G., Szolcsanyi, J., *et al.*: Action of intrathecal capsaicin and its structural analogues on the content and release of spinal substance P: Selectivity of action and relationship to analgesia. Brain Res., *306*:215–225, 1984.
325. Johansson, R.S.: Tactile sensibility in the human hand: Receptive field characteristics of mechanoreceptor units in the glabrous skin area. J. Physiol. (Lond.), *281*:101–123, 1978.
326. Jones, E.G., Leavitt, R.Y.: Axonal transport and the demonstration of non-specific projections to the cerebral cortex and striatum from thalamic intralaminar nuclei in the rat, cat and monkey. J. Comp. Neurol., *154*:349–378, 1974.
327. Jones, E.G., Powell, T.P.S.: The cortical projection of the ventroposterior nucleus of the thalamus in the cat. Brain Res., *13*:298–318, 1969.
328. Jones, E.G., Powell, T.P.S.: Connexions of the somatic sensory cortex of the rhesus monkey. III. Thalamic connexions. Brain, *93*:37–56, 1970.
329. Jones, E.G., Powell, T.P.S.: An analysis of the posterior group of thalamic nuclei on the basis of its afferent connections. J. Comp. Neurol., *143*:185–216, 1971.
330. Juan, H.: Mechanism of action of bradykinin–induced release of prostaglandin E. Naunyn–Schmiedebergs Arch. Pharmacol., *300*:77–85, 1977.
331. Juan, H., Lembeck, F.: Action of peptides and other algesic agents on paravascular pain receptors of the isolated perfused rabbit ear. Naunyn–Schmiedebergs Arch. Pharmacol., *283*:151–164, 1974.
332. Juan, H., Lembeck, F.: Release of prostaglandins from the isolated perfused rabbit ear by bradykinin and acetylcholine. Agents Actions, *6*:642–645, 1976.
333. Julian, F.J., Goldman, D.D.: The effects of mechanical stimulation on some electrical properties of axons. J. Gen. Physiol., *46*:297–313, 1962.
334. Jurna, I., Grossmann, W.: The effect of the activity evoked in ventrolateral tract axons of the cat spinal cord. Exp. Brain Res., *24*:473–484, 1976.
335. Kaelber, W.W., Mitchell, C.L., Yarmat, A.J., Afifi, A.K., *et al.*: Centrum medianum–parafasicularis lesions and reactivity to noxious and non-noxious stimuli. Exp. Neurol., *46*:282–290, 1975.
336. Kalina, M., Bubis, J.J.: Ultrastructural localization of acetylcholine esterase in neurons of rat trigeminal ganglia. Experientia, *25*:388–387, 1967.
337. Kalina, M., Wolman, M.: Correlative histochemical and morphological study on the maturation of sensory ganglion cells in the rat. Histochemie, *22*:100–108, 1970.
338. Kaliner, M., Austen, K.F.: Immunological release of chemical mediators from human tissues. Ann. Rev. Pharmacol., *15*:177–189, 1975.
339. Kawatani, M., Lowe, I.P., Nadelhaft, I., Morgan, C., *et al.*: Vasoactive intestinal polypeptide in visceral afferent pathways to the sacral spinal cord of the cat. Neurosci. Lett., *42*:311–316, 1983.
340. Keele, C.A., Armstrong, D.: Substances producing pain and itch. *In* Barcroft, H., Davson, H., Paton, W.D.M. (eds.): Monographs of the Physiological Society, vol. 12, pp. 1–374. London, Edward Arnold, 1964.
341. Keene, J.J., Casey, K.L.: Rewarding and aversive brain stimulation: Opposite effects on medial thalamic units. Physiol. Behav., *10*:283–287, 1973.
342. Kelly, M.: Is pain due to pressure on nerves? Spinal tumors and the intervertebral dic. Neurology (Minneap.), *6*:32–36, 1956.
343. Kennard, M.A.: The course of ascending fibers in the spinal cord of the cat essential to the recognition of painful stimuli. J. Comp. Neurol., *100*:511–524, 1954.
344. Kenshalo, D.R., Jr., Giesler, G.J., Leonard, R.B., Willis, W.D.: Responses of neurons in primate ventral posterior lateral nucleus to noxious stimuli. J. Neurophysiol., *43*:1594–1614, 1980.
345. Kerr, F.W.L.: A mechanism to account for frontal headache in cases of posterior–fossa tumors. J. Neurosurg., *18*:605–609, 1961.
346. Kerr, F.W.L.: Atypical facial neuralgias, their mechanism as

inferred from anatomic and physiologic data. Mayo Clin. Proc., *36*:254–260, 1961.

347. Kerr, F.W.L.: Trigeminal neuralgia, pathogenesis and description of a possible etiology for the cryptogenic variety. Trans. Am. Neurol. Assoc., *87*:118–120, 1962.

348. Kerr, F.W.L.: The etiology of trigeminal neuralgia. Arch. Neurol., *8*:15–25, 1963.

349. Kerr, F.W.L.: The divisional organization of afferent fibres of the trigeminal nerve. Brain, *86*:721–732, 1963.

350. Kerr, F.W.L.: Spinal V nucleolysis and intractable craniofacial pain. Surg. Forum, *17*:419–421, 1966.

351. Kerr, F.W.L.: The fine structure of subnucleus caudalis of the trigeminal nerve. Brain Res., *23*:129–145, 1970.

352. Kerr, F.W.L.: The organization of primary afferents in the subnucleus caudalis of the trigeminal: A light and electron microscopic study of degeneration. Brain Res., *23*:147–165, 1970.

353. Kerr, F.W.L.: Central relationships of trigeminal and cervical primary afferents in the spinal cord and medulla. Brain Res., *43*:561–572, 1972.

354. Kerr, F.W.L.: Neuroanatomical substrates of nociception in the spinal cord. Pain, *1*:325–356, 1975.

355. Kerr, F.W.L.: The ventral spinothalamic tract and other ascending systems of the ventral funiculus of the spinal cord. J. Comp. Neurol., *159*:335–356, 1975.

356. Kerr, F.W.L.: Pain: a central inhibitory balance theory. Mayo Clin. Proc., *50*:685–690, 1975.

357. Kerr, F.W.L.: Segmental circuitry and ascending pathways of the nociceptive system. *In* Beers, R.F., Jr., Bassett, E.G. (eds.): Mechanisms of Pain and Analgesic Compounds, pp. 113–141. New York, Raven Press, 1979.

358. Kerr, F.W.L.: Segmental circuitry and spinal cord nociceptive mechanisms. *In* Bonica, J.J., Albe–Fessard, D. (eds.): Advances in Pain Research and Therapy, vol. 1, pp. 75–89. New York, Raven Press, 1976.

359. Kerr, F.W.L.: Craniofacial neuralgias. *In* Bonica, J.J., Liebeskind, J.C., Albe–Fessard, D. (eds.): Advances in Pain Research and Therapy, vol. 1, pp. 283–295, New York, Raven Press, 1979.

360. Kerr, F.W.L., Fukushima, T.F.: New observations on the nociceptive pathways in the central nervous system. *In* Bonica, J.J. (ed.): Pain, pp. 47–61. New York, Raven Press, 1980.

361. Kerr, F.W.L., Kruger, L., Schwassmann, H.O., Stern, R.: Somatotopic organization of mechanoreceptor units in the trigeminal complex of the macaque. J. Comp. Neurol., *34*:127–144, 1968.

362. Kerr, F.W.L., Lippman, H.H.: The primate spinothalamic tract as demonstrated by anterolateral cordotomy and commissural myelotomy. Adv. In Neurol., *4*:147–156, 1974.

363. Kerr, F.W.L., Lysak, W.R.: Somatotopic organization of trigeminal ganglion neurones. Archiv. Neurol., *11*:593–602, 1964.

364. Kerr, F.W.L., Olafson, R.A.: Trigeminal and cervical volleys, convergence on single units in the spinal gray at C–1 and C–2. Arch. Neurol., *5*:171–178, 1961.

365. Kevetter, G.A., Haber, L.H., Yezierski, R.P., Chung, J.M., *et al.*: Cells of origin of the spinoreticular tract in the monkey. J. Comp. Neurol., *207*:61–74, 1982.

366. Kevetter, G.A., Willis, W.D.: Spinothalamic cells in the rat lumbar cord with collaterals to the medullary reticular formation. Brain Res., *238*:181–185, 1982.

367. Kevetter, G.A., Willis, W.D.: Collaterals of spinothalamic cells in the rat. J. Comp. Neurol., *215*:453–464, 1983.

368. Khayyat, G.F., Yu, Y.J., King, R.B.: Response patterns to noxious and non–noxious stimuli in rostral trigeminal relay nuclei. Brain Res., *97*:47–60, 1975.

369. Kimura, E., Hashimoto, K., Furukawa, S., Hayakawa, H.: Changes in bradykinin level in coronary sinus blood after the experimental occlusion of a coronary artery. Am. Heart J., *85*:635–647, 1973.

370. King, R.B., Barnett, J.C.: Studies of trigeminal nerve potentials. Over reaction to tactile facial stimulation in acute laboratory preparations. J. Neurosurg., *14*:617–627, 1957.

371. Kiser, R.S., Lebovitz, R.M., German, D.C.: Anatomic and pharmacologic differences between two types of aversive midbrain stimulation. Brain Res., *155*:331–342, 1978.

372. Kletzin, M., Spiegel, E.A.: Spinal conduction by chains of short neurons. Fed. Proc., *11*:83–84, 1952.

373. Knibestöl, M.: Stimulus–response functions of rapidly adapting mechanoreceptors in the human glabrous skin area. J. Physiol. (Lond.), *232*:427–52, 1973.

374. Knibestöl, M.: Stimulus–response functions of slowly adapting mechanoreceptors in the human glabrous skin area. J. Physiol. (Lond.), *245*:63–80, 1975.

375. Knibestöl, M., Vallbo, A.B.: Single unit analysis of mechanoreceptor activity from the human glabrous skin. Acta Physiol. Scand., *80*:178–195, 1970.

376. Kniffki, K.D., Mense, S., Schmidt, R.F.: Activation of neurones of the spinocervical tract by painful stimulation of skeletal muscle. Proc. Int. Union Physiol. Sci., *13*:393, 1977.

377. Kniffki, K.D., Mense, S., Schmidt, R.E.: Responses of group IV afferent units from skeletal muscle to stretch, contraction and chemical stimulation. Exp. Brain Res., *31*:511–522, 1978.

378. Kniffki, K.D., Mizumura, K.: Responses of neurons in VPL and VPL–VL region of the cat to algesic stimulation of muscle and tendon. J. Neurophysiol., *49*:649–661, 1983.

379. Knyihar, E., Csillik, B.: Effect of peripheral axotomy on the fine structure and histochemistry of the Rolando substances: Degenerative atrophy of central processes of pseudounipolar cells. Exp. Brain Res., *26*:73–87, 1976.

380. Knyihar, E., Csillik, B.: Representation of cutaneous afferents by fluoride-resistant acid phosphatase (FRAP)–active terminals in the rat substantia gelatinosa Rolandi. Acta Neurol. Scand., *53*:217–225, 1976.

381. Knyihar–Csillik, E., Csillik, B.: FRAP: Histochemistry of the primary nociceptive neuron. Progr. Histochem. Cytochem., *14*:1–137, 1981.

382. Knyihar, E., Gerebtzoff, M.A.: Extra–lysosomal localization of acid phosphatase in the spinal cord of the rat. Exp. Brain Res., *18*:383–395, 1973.

383. Knyihar, E., Laszlo, I., Tornyos, S.: Fine structure and fluoride–resistant acid phosphatase activity of electron dense sinusoid terminals in the substantia gelatinosa Rolandi of the rat after dorsal root transection. Exp. Brain Res., *19*:529–544, 1974.

384. Krauthamer, G.M., Albe–Fessard, D.: Inhibition of nonspe-

cific sensory activities following striopallidal and capsular stimulation. J. Neurophysiol., *28*:100–124, 1965.

385. Krauthamer, G., Dalsass, M.: Differential synaptic modulation of polysensory neurons of the intralaminar thalamus by medial and lateral caudate nucleus and substantia nigra. Brain Res., *154*:137–143, 1978.

386. Krauthamer, G., Feltz, P., Albe–Fessard, D.: Neurons of the medial diencephalon. II. Excitation of central origin. J. Neurophysiol., *30*:81–97, 1967.

387. Kruger, L., Albe–Fessard, D.: Distribution of responses to somatic afferent stimuli in the diencephalon of the cat under chloralose anesthesia. Exp. Neurol., *2*:442–467, 1960.

388. Kruger, L., Michel, F.: A morphological and somatotopic analysis of single unit activity in the trigeminal sensory complex of the cat. Exp. Neurol., *5*:139–156, 1962.

389. Kruger, L., Michel, F.: Reinterpretation of the representation of pain based on physiological excitation of single neurons in the trigeminal sensory complex. Exp. Neurol., *5*:157–178, 1962.

390. Kumazawa, T., Mizumura, K.: The polymodal receptors in the testis of dog. Brain Res., *136*:553–558, 1977.

391. Kumazawa, T., Mizumura, K.: Thin–fibre receptors responding to mechanical, chemical, and thermal stimulation in the skeletal muscle of the dog. J. Physiol. (Lond.), *273*:179–194, 1977.

392. Kumazawa, T., Perl, E.R.: Differential excitation of dorsal horn and subsantia gelatinosa marginal neurons by primary afferent units with fine (A–delta and C) fibers. *In*: Zotterman, Y. (ed.): Sensory Functions of the Skin in Primates, with Special Reference to Man, pp. 67–88. New York, Pergamon, 1976.

393. Kumazawa, T., Perl, E.R.: Primate cutaneous sensory units with unmyelinated (C) afferent fibers. J. Neurophysiol., *40*:1325–1338, 1977.

394. Kumazawa, T., Perl, E.R.: Excitation of marginal and substantia gelatinosa neurons in the primate spinal cord: Indications of their place in dorsal horn functional organization. J. Comp. Neurol., *177*:417–434, 1978.

395. Kumazawa, T., Perl, E.R., Burgess, P.R., Whitehorn, D.: Ascending projections from marginal zone (lamina I) neurons of the spinal dorsal horn. J. Comp. Neurol., *162*:1–12, 1975.

396. Kuraishi, Y., Hirota, N., Sugimoto, M., Satoh, M., *et al.*: Effects of morphine on noxious stimuli–induced release of substance P from rabbit dorsal horn *in vivo.* Life Sci., *33*:693–696, 1983.

397. Kuromi, H., Satoh, M., Takagi, H.: Effects of morphine and methotrimeprazine (levomepromazine) on the caudate–induced inhibition of the thalamic somatosensory evoked potential. Eur. J. Pharmacol., *24*:317–320, 1973.

398. Kuru, M.: Sensory Paths in the Spinal Cord and Brain Stem of Man. Tokyo, Sogensya, 1949.

399. LaMotte, C., Pert, C.B., Snyder, S.H.: Opiate receptor binding in primate spinal cord: Distribution and changes after dorsal root section. Brain Res., *112*:407–412, 1976.

400. LaMotte, R.H., Campbell, J.N.: Comparison of responses of warm and nociceptive C–fiber afferents in monkey with human judgments of thermal pain. J. Neurophysiol., *41*:509–528, 1978.

401. Le Bars, D., Dickenson, A.H., Besson, J.M., Villanueva, L.: Aspects of sensory processing through convergent neurons. In Yaksh, T.L. (ed.): Spinal Afferent Processing, pp. 467–504. New York, Plenum Press, 1986.

402. Le Bars, D., Guilbaud, G., Jurna, I., Besson, J.M.: Differential effects of morphine on responses of dorsal horn lamina V type cells elicited by A and C fibre stimulation in the spinal cat. Brain Res., *115*:518–524, 1976.

403. Le Bars, D., Menetrey, D., Consieller, C., Besson, J.M.: Depressive effects of morphine upon lamina V cells activities in the dorsal horn of the spinal cat. Brain Res., *93*:261–277, 1975.

404. LeBlanc, H.J., Gatipon, G.B.: Medial bulboreticular response to peripherally applied noxious stimuli. Exp. Neurol., *42*:264–273, 1974.

405. Lele, P.P., Weddell, G.: The relationship between neurohistology and corneal sensibility. Brain, *79*:119–154, 1956.

406. Lembeck, F., Gamse, R., Juan, H.: Substance P and sensory nerve endings. *In* von Euler, U.S., Pernow, B. (eds.): Substance P, pp. 169–181. New York, Raven Press, 1977.

407. Lembeck, F., Juan, H.: Interaction of prostaglandins and indomethacin with algesic substances. Naunyn-Schmiedebergs Arch. Pharmacol., *285*:301–313, 1974.

408. Lembeck, F., Popper, H., Juan, H.: Release of prostaglandins by bradykinin as an intrinsic mechanism of its algesic effect. Naunyn–Schmiedeberg's Arch. Pharmacol., *294*:69–73, 1976.

409. Levante, A., Albe–Fessard, D.: Localisation dans les couches VII and VIII de Resed de cellules d'origine d'un faisceau spinoreticulaire croise. G. R. Acad. Sci. D., *274*:3007–3010, 1972.

410. Lewis, T.: Experiments relating to cutaneous hyperalgesia and its spread through somatic nerves. Clin. Sci., *2*:373–423, 1936.

411. Lewis, T.: The nacifensor system of nerves and its reactions. Br. Med. J., *1*:431–435, 1937.

412. Lewis, T.: Pain. New York, MacMillian, 1942.

413. Lewis, V.A., Gebhart, G.F.: Evaluation of the periaqueductal central gray (PAG) as a morphine–specific locus of action and examination of morphine-induced and stimulation–produed analgesia at coincident PAG loci. Brain Res., *124*:283–303, 1977.

414. Lieberman, A.R.: Sensory ganglia. *In* Landon, D.N. (ed.): The Peripheral Nerve, pp. 188–278. London, Chapman & Hall, 1976.

415. Liebeskind, J.C., Mayer, D.J.: Somatosensory evoked responses in the mesencephalic central gray matter of the rat. Brain Res., *27*:133–151, 1971.

416. Light, A.R., Perl, E.R.: Re–examination of the dorsal root projection to the spinal dorsal horn including observations on the differential termination of coarse and fine fibers. J. Comp. Neurol., *186*:117–132, 1979.

417. Light, A.R., Perl, E.R.: Spinal termination of functionally identified primary afferent neurons with slowly conducting myelinated fibers. J. Comp. Neurol., *186*:133–150, 1979.

418. Light, A.R., Trevino, D.L., Perl, E.R.: Morphological features of functionally defined neurons in the marginal zone and substantia gelatinosa of the spinal dorsal horn. J. Comp. Neurol., *186*:151–172, 1979.

419. Limansikyi, Y.P.: Response of neurones of the medullary reticular formation to afferent impulses from cutaneous and muscle nerves. Fiziol. Zh., *11*:151–153, 1965.

420. Lindgren, I., Olivecrona, H.: Surgical treatment of angina pectoris. J. Neurosurg., *4*:19–39, 1947.

421. Lineberry, C., Vierck, C.: Attenuation of pain reactivity by caudate nucleus stimulation in monkeys. Brain Res., *98*:110–134, 1975.

422. Lippman, H.H., Kerr, F.W.L.: Light and electron microscopic study of crossed ascending pathways in the anterolateral funiculus in monkey. Brain Res., *40*:496–499, 1972.

423. Liu, R.P.C.: Laminar origins of spinal projection neurons to periaqueductal gray of the rat. Brain Res., *264*:118–122, 1983.

424. Lloyd, D.P.C.: The spinal mechanism of the pyramidal system in cats. J. Neurophysiol., *4*:525–546, 1941.

425. Lloyd, D.P.C.: Neuron patterns controlling transmission of ipsilateral hind limb reflexes in cat. J. Neurophysiol., *6*:293–315, 1943.

426. Lovick, T.A., Wolstencroft, J.H.: Inhibitory effects of nucleus raphe magnus on neuronal responses in the spinal trigeminal nucleus to nociceptive compared with non–nociceptive inputs. Pain, *7*:135–145, 1979.

427. Lund, R.D., Webster, K.E.: Thalamic afferents from the spinal cord and trigeminal nuclei. An experimental anatomical study in the rat. J. Comp. Neurol., *130*:313–328, 1967.

428. Lundberg, J.M., Hökfelt, T., Nilsson, G., Terenius, L., *et al.*: Peptide neurons in the vagus splanchnic and sciatic nerves. Acta Physiol. Scand., *104*:499–501, 1978.

429. Malliani, A., Recordati, G., Schwartz, P.J.: Nervous activity of afferent cardiac sympathetic fibres with atrial and ventricular endings. J. Physiol. (Lond.), *229*:457–469, 1973.

430. Mancia, M., Broggi, G., Margnelli, M.: Brain stem reticular effects on intralaminar thalamic neurons in the cat. Brain Res., *25*:638–641, 1971.

431. Mancia, M., Marginelli, M., Mariotti, M., *et al.*: Brainstem-thalamus reciprocal influences in the cat. Brain Res., *69*:297–314, 1974.

432. Manson, J.: The somatosensory cortical projection of single nerve cells in the thalamus of the cat. Brain Res., *12*:489–492, 1969.

433. Mantyh, P.W.: Connections of midbrain periaqueductal gray in the monkey. I. Ascending efferent projection. J. Neurophysiol., *49*:567–581, 1983.

434. Mantyh, P.W., Hunt, S.P.: Evidence for cholecystokinin–like immunoreactive neurons in the rat medulla oblongata which project to the spinal cord. Brain Res., *291*:49–54, 1984.

435. Marburg, D.J.: The effect on reaction to painful stimuli of lesions in the centromedian nucleus in the thalamus of the monkey. Int. J. Neurosci., *5*:153–158, 1973.

436. Marcus, A.J.: The role of lipids in platelet function with particular reference to the arachidonic acid pathway. J. Lipid Res., *19*:793–826, 1978.

437. Matthews, B.: The response of pulpal nerves to thermal stimulation of dentine. J. Dent. Res., *46*:1279, 1967.

438. Mayberg, M., Langer, R.S., Zervas, N.T., Moskowitz, M.A.: Perivascular meningeal projections from cat trigeminal ganglia: Possible pathway for vascular headaches in man. Science, *213*:228–230, 1981.

439. Mayer, D.J., Liebeskind, J.C.: Pain reduction by focal electrical stimulation of the brain: An anatomical and behavioral analysis. Brain Res., *68*:73–93, 1974.

440. Mayer, D.J., Price, D.D., Becker, D.P.: Neurophysiological characterization of the anterolateral spinal cord neurons contributing to pain perception in man. Pain, *1*:51–58, 1975.

441. Maynard, C.W., Leonard, R.B., Coulter, J.D., Coggeshall, R.E.: Central connections of ventral root afferents as demonstrated by the HRP method. J. Comp. Neurol., *172*:601–608, 1977.

442. McCarty, D.J., Gatter, R.A., Brill, J.M., Hogan, J.M.: Crystal deposition disease—sodium urate (gout) and calcium pyrophosphate (chondrocalcinosis, pseudogout). J.A.M.A., *193*:129–132, 1965.

443. McGiff, J.C., Terragno, N.A., Malik, K.U., Lonigro, A.J.: Release of a prostaglandins E–like substance from canine kidney by bradykinin. Circ. Res., *31*:36–43, 1972.

444. Mehler, W.R.: Some neurological species differences—a posteriori. Ann. N. Y. Acad. Sci., *167*:89–114, 1969.

445. Mehler, W.R., Feferman, M.E., Nauta, W.J.H.: Ascending axon degeneration following anterolateral cordotomy. An experimental study in the monkey. Brain, *83*:718–750, 1960.

446. Melzack, R., Stotler, W.A., Livingston, W.K.: Effects of discrete brainstem lesions in cats on perception of noxious stimulation. J. Neurophysiol., *21*:353–367, 1958.

447. Melzack, R., Wall, P.D.: Pain mechanisms: A new theory. Science, *150*:971–980, 1965.

448. Mendell, L.M.: Physiological properties of unmyelinated fiber projection to the spinal cord. Exp. Neurol., *16*:316–332, 1966.

449. Menetrey, D., Chaouch, A., Binder, D., Besson, J.M.: The origin of the spinomesencephalic tract in the rat: An anatomical study using the retrograde transport of horseradish peroxidase. J. Comp. Neurol., *206*:193–207, 1982.

450. Mense, S., Schmidt, R.F.: Activation of group IV afferent units from muscle by algesic agents. Brain Res., *72*:305–310, 1974.

451. Meyerson, B.A., Boethius, J., Carlsson, A.M.: Alleviation of malignant pain by electrical stimulation in the periventricular–periaqueductal region: Pain relief as related to stimulation sites. *In* Bonica, J.J., Albe–Fessard D. (eds.): Advances in Pain Research and Therapy, vol. 3, pp. 525–533. New York, Raven Press, 1979.

452. Mitchell, C., Kaelber, W.: Effect of medial thalamic lesions on responses elicited by tooth pulp stimulation. Am. J. Physiol., *210*:263–269, 1966.

453. Moncada, S., Ferreira, S.H., Vane, J.R.: Inhibition of prostaglandin biosynthesis as the mechanism of analgesia of aspirin–like drugs in the dog knee joint. Eur. J. Pharmacol., *31*:250–260, 1975.

454. Morin, F.: A new spinal pathway for cutaneous impulses. Am. J. Physiol., *183*:245–252, 1955.

455. Morin, F., Schwartz, H.G., O'Leary, J.L.: Experimental study

of the spinothalamic and related tracts. Arch. Psychol. Neurol. Scand., *26*:371–396, 1951.

456. Morrison, J.F.B.: The afferent innervation of the gastrointestinal tract. *In* Brooks, F.P., Evers, P.W., (eds.): Nerves and the Gut, pp. 297–322. Slack, Thorofare, N. J., 1977.

457. Morrison, D.C., Henson, P.M.: Release of mediators from mast cells and basophils induced by different stimuli. *In* Bach, M.K. (ed.): Immediate Hypersensitivity: Modern Concepts and Developments, pp. 431–502. New York, Marcel Dekker, 1978.

458. Morrow, T.J., Casey, K.L.: Analgesia produced by mesencephalic stimulation: Effect on bulboreticular neurons. *In* Bonica, J.J., Albe–Fessard, D. (eds.): Advances in Pain Research and Therapy, vol. 1, pp. 503–510. New York, Raven Press, 1976.

459. Moskowitz, M.A., Reinhard, J.F., Jr., Romero, J., *et al.*: Neurotransmitters and the fifth cranial nerve: Is there a relation to the headache phase of migraine? The Lancet, *1*:883–885, 1979.

460. Mosso, J.A., Kruger, L.: Spinal trigeminal neurons excited by noxious and thermal stimuli. Brain Res., *38*:206–210, 1972.

461. Mosso, J.A., Kruger, L.: Receptor categories represented in spinal trigeminal nucleus caudalis. J. Neurophysiol. *36*:472–488, 1973.

462. Murase, K., Randic, M.: Actions of substance P on rat spinal dorsal horn neurones. J. Physiol., *346*:203–217, 1984.

463. Nagy, J.I., Hunt, S.P.: Fluoride–resistant acid phosphatase–containing neurones in dorsal root ganglia are separate from those containing substance P or somatostatin. Neuroscience, *7*:89–97, 1982.

464. Nagy, J.I., Hunt, S.P.: The termination of primary afferents within the rat dorsal horn—evidence for rearrangement following capsaicin treatment. J. Comp. Neurol., *218*:145–158, 1983.

465. Nahin, R.L., Madsen, A.M., Giesler, G.J.: Anatomical and physiological studies of the grey matter surrounding the spinal cord and central canal. J. Comp. Neurol., *220*:321–335, 1983.

466. Narotzky, R.A., Kerr, F.W.L.: Marginal neurons of the spinal cord: types, afferent synaptology and functional considerations. Brain Res., *139*:1–20, 1978.

467. Nashold, B., Urban, B., Zorub, D.S.: Phantom pain relief by focal destruction of the substantia gelatinosa of Rolando. *In* Bonica, J.J., Albe–Fessard, G. (eds.): Advances in Pain Research and Therapy, vol. 1, pp. 959–963. New York, Raven Press, 1976.

468. Nashold, B.J., Ostdahl, R.H.: Dorsal root entry zone lesions for pain relief. J. Neurosurg., *51*:59–69, 1979.

469. Nashold, B.S., Jr., Friedman, N.: Dorsal column stimulation for control of pain. Preliminary report on 30 patients. J. Neurosurg., *36*:590–597, 1972.

470. Nashold, B.S., Jr., Wilson, W.P., Slaughter, D.: Sensation evoked by stimulation in the hindbrain of man. J. Neurosurg., *30*:14–24, 1969.

471. Nathan, P.W., Smith, M.C.: Some tracts of the anterior and lateral columns of the spinal cord. *In* Knighton, R.S., Dumke, P.R., (eds.): Pain, pp. 47–57. Little, Brown & Co., Boston, 1966.

472. Nielson, K.P., Adams, J.E., Hosobuchi, Y.: Phantom limb pain. Treatment with dorsal column stimulation. J. Neurosurg., *42*:301–307, 1975.

473. Nijensohn, D.E., Kerr, F.W.L.: The ascending projections of the dorsolateral funiculus of the spinal cord in the primate. J. Comp. Neurol., *161*:459–470, 1975.

474. Ninkovic, M., Hunt, S.P., Kelly, J.S.: Effects of dorsal rhizotomy on the autoradiographic distribution of opiate and neurotensin receptors and neurotensin–like immunoreactivity within the rat spinal cord. Brain Res., *230*:111–119, 1981.

475. Nishi, K.: The action of 5–hydroxytryptamine on chemoreceptor discharges of the cat's carotid body. Br. J. Pharmacol., *55*:27–40, 1975.

476. Nishi, K., Sakanashi, M., Takenaka, F.: Activation of afferent cardiac sympathetic nerve fibers of the cat by pain producing substances and by noxious heat. Pflugers Arch., *372*:53–61, 1977.

477. Noyes, F.B., Thomas, N.G.: Dental Histology and Embryology, pp. 142–143. Philadelphia, Lea & Febiger, 1938.

478. Nugteren, D.H.: Arachidonate lipoxygenase. *In* Silver, M., Smith, B.J., Kocsis (eds.): Prostaglandins in Hematology, pp. 11–25. New York, Spectrum Publications, 1977.

479. Nyquist, J.K.: Somatosensory properties of neurons of thalamic nucleus ventralis lateralis. Exp. Neurol., *48*:123–135, 1975.

480. Nyquist, J.K., Greenhoot, J.H.: Unit analysis of nonspecific thalamic responses to high–intensity cutaneous input in the cat. Exp. Neurol., *42*:609–622, 1974.

481. Ochoa, J., Mair, W.G.: The normal sural nerve in man. I. Ultrastructure and numbers of fibers and cells. Acta Neuropathol. (Berl.), *13*:127–216, 1967.

482. Ochs, S.: Energy metabolism and supply of nerve by axoplasmic transport. Fed. Proc., *33*:1049–1057, 1974.

483. Ochs, S., Hollingsworth, D.: Dependence of fast axoplasmic transport in nerve on oxidative metabolism. J. Neurochem., *18*:107–114, 1971.

484. Ochs, S., Jersild, R.A., Jr.: Fast axoplasmic transport in unmyelinated nerve fibers shown by electron microscopic radioautography. J. Neurobiol., *5*:373–377, 1974.

485. Oleson, T.D., Kirkpatrick, D.B., Goodman, S.J.: Elevation of pain threshold to tooth shock by brain stimulation in primates. Brain Res., *194*:79–95, 1980.

486. Olgart, L.: Local mechanisms in dental pain. *In* Beers, R.F., Bassett, E.G. (eds.): Mechanisms of Pain and Analgesic Compounds, pp. 285–294. New York, Raven Press, 1979.

487. Olgart, L., Hökfelt, T., Nilsson, G., Pernow, B.: Localization of substance P-like immunoreactivity in nerves in the tooth pulp. Pain, *4*:153–159, 1977.

488. Oliveras, J.L., Redjemi, G., Guilbaud, G., Besson, J.M.: Analgesia induced by electrical stimulation of the inferior centralis nucleus of the raphe in the cat. Pain, *1*:139–145, 1975.

489. Olszewski, J.: On the anatomical and functional organization of the spinal trigeminal nucleus. J. Comp. Neurol., *92*:401–413, 1950.

490. Onishi, A., Dyck, P.J.: Loss of small peripheral sensory neurons in Fabry's disease. Arch. Neurol., *31*:120–127, 1974.

491. Onofrio, B.M., Campa, H.K.: Evaluation of rhizotomy: Review of 12 years' experience. J. Neurosurg., *36*:751–755, 1972.

492. Osgood, C.P., Dujovny, M., Faille, R., Abassy, M.: Microsurgical ganglionectomy for chronic pain syndromes. J. Neurosurg., *45*:113–115, 1976.

493. Otsuka, M., Konishi, S.: Release of substances P–like immunoreactivity from isolated spinal cord of newborn rat. Nature, *264*:83–84, 1976.

494. Paintal, A.S.: Functional analysis of group III afferent fibres of mammalian muscles. J. Physiol. (Lond.), *152*:250–270, 1960.

495. Panula, P., Yang, H.Y., Costa, E.: Neurohumoral localization of bombesin–like immunoreactivity in the CNS of the rat. Regul. Pept., *4*:275–283, 1982.

496. Panula, P., Hadjiconstantinou, M., Yang, H.Y., Costa, E.: Immunohistochemical localization of bombesin, substance P and gastrin–releasing peptide in primary sensory neurons. J. Neurosci., *3*:2021–2029, 1983.

497. Patton, H.D.: Special properties of nerve trunks and tracts. *In* Ruch, T.C., Patton, H.D. (eds.): Physiology and Biophysics, pp. 73–94. Philadelphia, W.B. Saunders, 1965.

498. Pearl, G.S., Anderson, K.V.: Effects of nociceptive and innocuous stimuli on the firing patterns of single neurons in the feline nucleus reticularis gigantocellularis. *In* Bonica, J.J., Albe–Fessard, D. (eds.): Advances in Pain Research and Therapy, vol. 1, pp. 259–265, New York, Raven Press, 1976.

499. Pearl, G.S., Anderson, K.V.: Response patterns of cells in the feline caudal nucleus reticularis gigantocellularis after noxious trigeminal and spinal stimulation. Exp. Neurol., *58*:231–241, 1978.

500. Pearl, G.S., Anderson, K.V.: Response of cells in feline nucleus centrum medianum to tooth pulp stimulation. Brain Res. Bull., *5*:41–45, 1980.

501. Pearl, G.S., Anderson, K.V.: Interactions between nucleus centrum medianum and gigantocellularis nociceptive neurons. Brain Res. Bull., *5*:203–206, 1980.

502. Perl, E.R.: Myelinated afferent fibers innervating the primate skin and their response to noxious stimuli. J. Physiol. (Lond.), *197*:593–615, 1968.

503. Perl, E.R.: Sensitization of nociceptors and its relation to sensation. *In* Bonica, J.J., Albe–Fessard, D. (eds.): Advances in Pain Research and Therapy, vol. 1, pp. 17–28. New York, Raven Press, 1976.

504. Perl, E.R., Whitlock, D.C.: Somatic stimuli exciting spinothalamic projections to thalamic neurons in cat and monkey. Exp. Neurol., *3*:256–296, 1961.

505. Peschanski, M., Besson, J.M.: Diencephalic connections of the raphe nuclei of the rat brainstem: An anatomical study with reference to the somatosensory system. J. Comp. Neurol., *224*:509–534, 1984.

506. Peschanski, M., Guilbaud, D., Gautron, M.: Posterior intralaminar region in rat: Neuronal responses to noxious and nonnoxious cutaneous stimuli. Exp. Neurol., *72*:226–238, 1981.

507. Peschanski, M., Mantyh, P.W., Besson, J.M.: Spinal afferents to the ventrobasal thalamic complex in the rat: An anatomical study using wheatgerm agglutinin conjugated to horseradish peroxidase. Brain Res., *278:240–244, 1983.*

508. Pfaffman, C.: Afferent impulses from the teeth due to pressure and noxious stimulation. J. Physiol. (Lond.), *97*:207–219, 1939.

509. Piercey, M.F., Einspahr, F.J., Dobry, P.G.K., *et al.*: Morphine does not antagonize the substance P mediated excitation of dorsal horn neurons. Brain Res., *186*:421–434, 1980.

510. Poggio, G.F., Mountcastle, V.B.: A study of the functional contributions of the lemniscal and spinothalamic systems to somatic sensibility. Bull. Johns Hopk. Hosp., *106*:266–316, 1960.

511. Poggio, G.F., Mountcastle, V.B.: The functional properties of ventrobasal thalamic neurons studied in unanesthetized monkeys. J. Neurophysiol., *26*:775–806, 1963.

512. Pomeranz, B., Wall, P.D., Weber, W.V.: Cord cells responding to fine myelinated afferents from viscera, muscle, and skin. J. Physiol. (Lond.), *199*:511–532, 1968.

513. Pomepiano, O., Swett, J.E.: Actions of graded cutaneous and muscular afferent volleys on brain stem units in the decrebrate, cerebellectomized cat. Arch. Ital. Biol., *101*:552–583, 1963.

514. Poulos, D.A., Benjamin, R.M.: Response of thalamic neurons to thermal stimulation of the tongue. J. Neurophysiol., *31*:28–43, 1968.

515. Preobrazhenskii, N.N., Limanskyi, Y.P.: Activation of bulbar reticular neurones by visceral afferents. Neirofiziol. (Kiev), *1*:177–185, 1969.

516. Price, D.D.: The question of how the dorsal horn encodes sensory information. *In* Yaksh, T.L. (ed.): Spinal Afferent Processing, pp. 445–466. New York, Plenum Press, 1986.

517. Price, D.D., Dubner, R., Hayes, R., *et al.*: Trigemino–thalamic and spinothalamic neurons that subserve sensory discrimination aspects of pain. *In* Anderson, D.J., Matthew, B. (ed.): Pain in the Trigeminal Region, pp.225–232. Amsterdam, Elsevier/North Holland, 1977.

518. Price, D.D., Dubner, R., Hu, J.W.: Trigeminothalamic neurons in nucleus caudalis responsive to tactile, thermal, and nociceptive stimulation of monkey's face. J. Neurophysiol, *39*:936–953, 1976.

519. Price, D.D., Hu, J.W., Dubner, R., Gracely, R.: Peripheral suppression of first pain and central summation of second pain evoked by noxious heat pulses. Pain, *3*:57–68, 1977.

520. Price, D.D., Hull, C.D., Buchwald, N.A.: Intracellular responses of dorsal horn cells to cutaneous and sural nerve A and C fiber stimuli. Exp. Neurol., *33*:291–309, 1971.

521. Price, D.D., Mayer, D.J.: Physiological laminar organization of the dorsal horn of M. mulatta. Brain Res., *79*:321–325, 1974.

522. Price, D.D., Mayer, D.J.: Neurophysiological characterization of the anterolateral quadrant neurons subserving pain in M. mulatta. Pain, *1*:59–72, 1975.

523. Procacci, P., and Zoppi, M.: Pathophysiology and clinical aspects of visceral and referred pain. *In* Bonica, J., Lindblom, U., and Iggo, A. (eds.): Advances in Pain Research and Therapy, vol. 5, pp. 647–658. New York, Raven Press, 1983.

524. Proshansky, E., Egger, M.D.: Dendritic spread of dorsal horn neurons in cats. Exp. Brain Res., *28*:153–166, 1977.

525. Ralston, H.J.: The organization of the substantia gelatinosa Rolandi in the cat lumbosacral spinal cord. Z. Zellforsch., *67*:1–23, 1965.

526. Ralston, H.J.: Dorsal root projection to dorsal horn neurons in the cat spinal cord. J. Comp. Neurol., *132*:303–330, 1968.

527. Ralston, H.J.: The fine structure of laminae I, II and III of the macaque spinal cord. J. Comp. Neurol., *184*:619–642, 1979.

528. Randic, M., Miletic, V.: Effect of substance P on cat dorsal horn neurons activated by noxious stimuli. Brain Res., *128*:164–169, 1977.

529. Ranson, S.W.: The course within the spinal cord of the non–medullated fibers of the dorsal roots: A study of Lissauer's tract in the cat. J. Comp. Neurol., *23*:259–281, 1913.

530. Ranson, S.W.: An experimental study of Lissauer's tract and the dorsal roots. J. Comp. Neurol., *24*:531–545, 1914.

531. Ranson, S.W., Billingsly, P.R.: The conduction of painful afferent impulses in the spinal nerves. Am. J. Physiol., *40*:571–584, 1916.

532. Reddy, S.V.R., Maderdrut, J.L., Yaksh, T.L.: Spinal cord pharmacology of adrenergic agonist–mediated antinociception. J. Pharmacol. Exp. Ther., *213*:525–533, 1980.

533. Rethelyi, M., Trevino, D.L., Perl, E.R.: Distribution of primary afferent fibers within the sacrococcygeal dorsal horn: An autoradiographic study. J. Comp. Neurol., *185*:603–622, 1979.

534. Rexed, B.: The cytoarchitectonic organization of the spinal cord in the cat. J. Comp. Neurol., *96*:415–495, 1952.

535. Rexed, B.: A cytoarchitectonic atlas of the spinal cord in the cat. J. Comp. Neurol., *100*:297–380, 1954.

536. Richardson, D.E., Akil, H.: Pain reduction by electrical brain stimulation in man. J. Neurosurg., *47*:178–183, 1977.

537. Robertson, R.T., Lynch, G.S., Thompson, R.F.: Diencephalic distributions of ascending reticular systems. Brain Res., *55*:309–322, 1973.

538. Roca e Silva, M., Antonio, A.: Release of bradykinin and the mechanism of production of a thermic edema (45°C) in the rat's paw. Med. Exp. (Basel), *3*:371, 1960.

539. Rolando, L.: Richerche anatomie sulla struttura del midollo spinal, pp. 1–118. Torino, Dalla Stamperia Reale, 1824.

540. Rosell, S., Olgart, L., Gazelius, B., Panopoulos, P., *et al.*: Inhibition of antidromic and substance P–induced vasodilatation by a substance P–antagonist. Acta Physiol. Scand., *111*:381–382, 1981.

541. Rossi, G.F., Brodal, A.: Terminal distribution of spinoreticular fibers in the cat. Arch. Neurol. Psychiatr., *78*:439–453, 1957.

542. Ruch, T.C.: Pathophysiology of pain. *In* Ruch, T.C., Patton, H.D., Woodbury, J.W., Towe, A.L. (eds.): Neurophysiology, pp. 350–368. Philadelphia, W.B. Saunders, 1961.

543. Rustioni, A.: Nonprimary afferents to the nucleus gracilis from the lumbar cord of the cat. Brain Res., *51*:81–95, 1973.

544. Rustioni, A.: Nonprimary afferents to the cuneate nucleus in the brachial dorsal funiculus of the cat. Brain Res., *75*:247–259, 1974.

545. Samuelsson, B.: Biosynthesis of prostaglandins. Fed. Proc., *31*:1442–1460, 1972.

546. Samuelsson, B., Goldyne, M., Granstrom, E., Hamberg, M., *et al.*: Prostaglandins and thromboxanes. *Ann. Rev. Biochem.*, *47*:997–1029, 1978.

547. Sano, K., Yoshioka, M., Ogashiwa, M., Ishijima, B., *et al.*: Thalamotominotomy. Confin. Neurol., *27*:63–66, 1966.

548. Saporta, S., Kruger, L.: The organization of projections to selected points of somatosensory cortex from the cat ventrobasal complex. Brain Res., *178*:275–295, 1979.

549. Sastry, B.R.: Potentiation of presynaptic inhibition of nociceptive pathways as a mechanism for analgesia. Can. J. Physiol. Pharmacol., *58*:97–100, 1980.

550. Sawynok, J., Kato, N., Havlicek, V., Labella, F.S.: Lack of effect of baclofen on substance P and somatostatin release from the spinal cord *in vitro*. Naunyn-Schmiedebergs Arch. Pharmacol., *319*:78–81, 1982.

551. Scheibel, M.E., Scheibel, A.B.: Terminal axonal patterns in the cat spinal cord. II. The dorsal horn. Brain Res., *9*:32–58, 1968.

552. Schmauss, C., Yaksh, T.L.: *In vivo* studies on spinal opiate receptor systems mediating antinociception. II. Pharmacological profiles suggesting a differential association of mu, delta and kappa receptors with visceral chemical and cutaneous thermal stimuli in the rat. J. Pharmacol. Exp. Ther., *228*:1–12, 1983.

553. Schmidt, R.F.: Presynaptic inhibition in the vertebrate central nervous system. Ergebn. Physiol., *63*:21–101, 1971.

554. Schvarcz, J.R.: Spinal cord stereotactic surgery. *In* Sano, K., Ishii, S., LeVay, D. (eds.): Recent Progress in Neurological Surgery, pp. 234–241. New York, Elsevier, 1974.

555. Schvarcz, J.R.: Post–herpetic craniofacial dyaesthesiae. Their management by stereotaxic trigeminal nucleotomy. Acta Neurochir. (Wien). *38*:65–72, 1977.

556. Schvarcz, J.R.: Stereotaxic spinal trigeminal nucleotomy for dysesthetic facial pain. *In* Bonica, J.J., Liebeskind, J.C., Albe–Fessard, D. (eds.): Advances in Pain Research and Therapy, vol. 3, pp. 331–336, New York, Raven Press, 1979.

557. Schwartzman, R.J.: Thalamic sensory nuclear ablations in trained monkeys. Arch. Neurol., *23*:419–429, 1970.

558. Scibetta, C.J., King, R.B.: Hyperpolarizing influence of trigeminal nucleus caudalis on primary afferent preterminals in trigeminal nucleus oralis. J. Neurophysiol., *32*:229–238, 1969.

559. Scott, D., Jr., Maziarz, R.: What is the most unique form of stimulus to evoke dental pain: *In* Bonica, J.J. and Albe–Fessard, D. (eds.): Advances in Pain Research and Therapy, vol. 1, pp. 205–213, New York, Raven Press, 1976.

560. Selzer, M., Spencer, W.A.: Convergence of visceral and cutaneous afferent pathways in the lumbar spinal cord. Brain Res., *14*:331–348, 1969.

561. Selzer, M., Spencer, W.A.: Interactions between visceral and cutaneous afferents in the spinal cord: Reciprocal primary afferent fibre depolarization. Brain Res., *14*:349–366, 1969.

562. Sessle, B.J., Dubner, R., Greenwood, L.F., Lucier, G.E.: Descending influences of periaqueductal gray matter and somatosensory cerebral cortex on neurones in trigeminal brain stem nuclei. Can. J. Physiol. Pharmacol., *54*:66–69, 1975.

563. Shealy, C.N., Mortimer, J.T., Hagfors, N.R.: Dorsal column electroanalgesia. J. Neurosurg., *32*:560–564, 1970.

564. Sheppard, M., Kronheim, S., Adams, C., Pimstone, B.: Immunoreactive somatostatin release from rat spinal cord *in vitro*. Neurosci. Lett., *15*:65–70, 1979.

565. Sherrington, C.: The Integrative Action of the Nervous System, p. 228. New Haven, Yale University Press, 1947.

566. Shigenaga, Y., Matano, S., Okada, K., Sohai, A.: The effects of tooth pulp stimulations in the thalamus and hypothalamus of the rat. Brain Res., *63*:402–407, 1973.

567. Sjölund, B., Eriksson, M.: Electroacupuncture and endogenous morphins. Lancet, *2*:1085, 1976.

568. Sjölund, B., Eriksson, M.: The influence of naloxone and analgesia produced by peripheral conditioning stimulation. Brain Res., *173*:275–302, 1979.

569. Sjölund, B., Terenius, L., Eriksson, M.: Increased cerebrospinal fluid levels of endorphins after electroacupuncture. Acta Physiol. Scand., *100*:382–384, 1977.

570. Sjöqvist, O.: Studies on pain conduction of the trigeminal nerve. Acta Psychiat. Neurol. Scand., *17(Suppl.)*:1–139, 1938.

571. Skagerberg, G., Bjorklund, A., Lindvall, O., Schmidt, R.H.: Origin and termination of the diencephalo-spinal dopamine system in the rat. Brain Res. Bull., *9*:237–244, 1982.

572. Skultety, F.M.: Stimulation of periaqueductal gray and hypothalamus. Arch. Neurol., *8*:608–620, 1963.

573. Smith, J.B., Willis, A.L.: Aspirin selectively inhibits prostaglandin production in human platelets. Nature, *231*:235–236, 1971.

574. Snyder, R.: The organization of the dorsal root entry zone in cats and monkeys. J. Comp. Neurol., *174*:47–70, 1977.

575. Spiegel, E.A., Keltzkin, M., Szekely, E.G.: Pain reactions upon stimulation of the tectum mesencephali. J. Neuropathol. Exp. Neurol., *13*:212–220, 1954.

576. Spiller, W.G., Martin, E.: The treatment of persistent pain of organic origin in the lower part of the body by division of the anterolateral column of the spinal cord. J.A.M.A., *58*:1489–1490, 1912.

577. Stacey, M.J.: Free nerve endings in skeletal muscle of the cat. J. Anat., *105*:231–254, 1969.

578. Staszewska-Barczak, J., Ferreira, S.H., Vane, J.R.: An excitatory nociceptive cardiac reflex elicited by bradykinin and potentiated by prostaglandins and myocardial ischaemia. Cardiovasc. Res., *10*:314–327, 1976.

579. Steinman, J.L., Komisaurak, B.R., Tyce, G.M., Yaksh, T.L.: Spinal cord monoamines mediate the antinociceptive effects of vaginal stimulation in rats. Pain, *16*:155–166, 1983.

580. Sterling, P., Kuypers, H.G.J.M.: Anatomical organization of the brachial spinal cord of the cat. I. The distribution of dorsal root fibers. Brain Res., *4*:1–15, 1967.

581. Stewart, W., King, R.B.: Fiber projections from the n. caudalis of the spinal trigeminal nucleus. J. Comp. Neurol., *121*:271–286, 1963.

582. Sugita, K., Mutsuga, N., Takaoka, Y., Doi, T.: Results of stereotaxic thalamotomy for pain. Confin. Neurol., *34*:265–274, 1972.

583. Sullivan, T.J., Parker, C.W.: Possible role of arachidonic acid and its metabolites in mediator release from rat mast cells. J. Immunol., *122*:431–436, 1979.

584. Sutton, D.C., Lueth, H.C.: Experimental production of pain on excitation of the heart and great vessels. Arch. Intern. Med., *45*:827–867, 1930.

585. Szentagothai, J.: Neuronal and synaptic arrangement in the substantia gelatinosa Rolandi. J. Comp. Neurol., *122*:219–239, 1964.

586. Szolcsanyi, J.: A pharmacological approach to elucidation of the role of different nerve fibres and receptor endings in mediation of pain. J. Physiol. (Paris), *73*:251–259, 1977.

587. Szolcsanyi, J., Jancso-Gabor, A., Joo, F.: Functional and fine structural characteristics of the sensory neurone blocking effect of capsaicin. Naunyn-Schmiedebergs Arch. Pharmacol., *287*:157–168, 1975.

588. Takagi, H., Matsumura, M., Yanai, A., Ogui, K.: The effect of analgesics on the spinal reflex activity of the cat. Jpn. J. Pharmacol., *4*:176–187, 1955.

589. Takahashi, T., Otsuka, M.: Regional distribution of substance P in the spinal cord and nerve roots of the cat and the effect of dorsal root section. Brain Res., *87*:1–11, 1975.

590. Talairach, J., Hecaen, M., David, M., Recherches sur la coagulation therapeuthique des structures sous-carticates chez l'homme. Rev. Neurol., *81*:4–24, 1949.

591. Talbot, W.H., Darian-Smith, I., Kornhuber, H.H., Mountcastle, V.B.: The sens of flutter-vibration: Comparison of the human capacity with response patterns of mechanoreceptive afferents from the monkey hand. J. Neurophysiol., *31*:301–334, 1968.

592. Tervo, T., Palkama, A.: Innervation of the rabbit cornea. A histochemical and electron-microscopic study. Acta. Anat., *102*:164–175, 1978.

593. Tervo, T., Palkama, A.: Ultrastructure of the corneal nerves after fixation with potassium permanganate. Anat. Rec., *190*:851–860, 1978.

594. Tervo, T., Joo, F., Huikuri, K.T., Toth, I., *et al.*: Fine structure of sensory nerves in the rat cornea: An experimental nerve degeneration study. Pain, *6*:57–70, 1979.

595. Tiwari, R.K., King, R.B.: Fiber projections from trigeminal nucleus caudalis in primate (squirrel monkey and baboon). J. Comp. Neurol., *158*:191–206, 1974.

596. Torebjork, H.E.: Afferent C units responding to mechanical, thermal and chemical stimuli in human non-glabrous skin. Acta Physiol. Scand., *92*:374–390, 1974.

597. Torebjork, H.E., Hallin, R.G.: Perceptual changes accompanying controlled preferential blocking of A and C fibre responses in intact human skin nerves. Exp. Brain Res., *16*:321–332, 1973.

598. Torebjork, H.E., Hallin, R.G.: Responses in human A and C fibres to repeated electrical intradermal stimulation. J. Neurol. Neurosurg. Psychiatry, *37*:653–664, 1974.

599. Torebjork, H.E., Hallin, R.G.: Excitation failure in thin nerve fiber structures and accompanying hypalgesia during repetitive electric skin stimulation. *In* Bonica, J.J. (ed.): Advances in Neurology, vol. 4, pp. 733–735. New York, Raven Press, 1974.

600. Torebjork, H.E., Hallin, R.G.: Identification of afferent C units in intact human skin nerves. Brain Res., *67*:387–403, 1974.

601. Torebjork, H.E., Hallin, R.G.: Skin receptors supplied by unmyelinated (C) fibres in man. *In* Zotterman, Y. (ed.): Sensory Function of the Skin in Primates, pp. 475–487. Oxford, Pergamon, 1976.

602. Trevino, D.L., Carstens, E.: Confirmation of the location of spinothalamic neurons in the cat and monkey by the retrograde transport of horseradish peroxidase. Brain Res., *98*:177–182, 1975.

603. Trevino, D., Coulter, J.D., Willis, W.D.: Location of cells of origin of spinothalamic tract in lumbar enlargement of the monkey. J. Neurophysiol., *36*:750–761, 1973.

604. Trevino, D.L., Maunz, R.A., Bryan, R.N., Willis, W.D.: Location of cells of origin of the spinothalamic tract in the lumbar enlargement of cat. Exp. Neurol., *34*:64–77, 1972.

605. Truex, R.C., Taylor, M.J., Smythe, M.Q., Gildenberg, P.L.: The lateral cervical nucleus of cat, dog and man. J. Comp. Neurol., *139*:93–104, 1970.

606. Tsou, K., Jang, C.S.: Studies on the site of analgesic action of morphine by intracerebral microinjection. Sci. Sin., *13*:1099–1109, 1964.

607. Tsutsumi, H., Mark, V.H.: Experimental local thalamic application of xylocaine through silicone rubber chemode. J. Neurosurg., *38*:743–747, 1973.

608. Tyce, G.M., Yaksh, T.L.: Monoamine release from cat spinal cord by somatic stimuli: An intrinsic modulatory system. J. Physiol. (Lond.), *314*:513–529, 1981.

609. Tyers, M.B., Haywood, H.: Effect of prostaglandins on peripheral nociceptors in acute inflammation. Agents Actions, *6*:(*Suppl.*)65–78, 1979.

610. Uchida, Y., Kamisaka, K., Ueda, H.: Experimental studies on anginal pain: Mode of excitation of afferent cardiac sympathetic nerve fibers. Jpn. Circulation J., *35*:147–161, 1971.

611. Uchida, Y., Murao, S.: Excitation of afferent cardiac sympathetic nerve fibers during coronary occlusion. Am. J. Physiol., *226*:1094–1099, 1974.

612. Uchida, Y., Murao, S.: Bradykinin–induced excitation of afferent cardiac sympathetic nerve fibers. Jpn. Heart J., *15*:84–91, 1974.

613. Urabe, M., Tsubokawa, T.: Stereotaxic thalamotomy for the relief of intractable pain. Tohoku J. Exp. Med., *85*:286–300, 1965.

614. Urabe, M., Tsubokawa, T., Watanabe, Y.: Alteration of activity of single neurons in the nucleus centrum medianum following stimulation of the peripheral nerve and application of noxious stimuli. Jpn. J. Physiol., *16*:421–435, 1966.

615. Urban, L., Randic, M.: Slow excitatory transmission in rat dorsal horn: Possible mediation by peptides. Brain Res., *290*:336–341, 1984.

616. Uvnas, B.: The mechanism of histamine release from mast cell. *In* Rocha e Silva, M. (ed.): Handbuch der Experimentallelen Pharmacologie, vol. 18, (part 2), pp. 75–92. New York, Springer–Verlag, 1978.

617. Van Arman, C.G., Carlson, R.P., Risley, E.A., *et al.*: Inhibitor effects of indomethacin, aspirin and certain other drugs on inflammations induced in rat and dog by carrageenan, sodium urate and ellagic acid. J. Pharmacol. Exp. Ther., *175*:459–468, 1970.

618. Van Hassel, H.J., Biedenback, M.A., Brown, A.C.: Cortical potentials evoked by tooth pulp stimulation in rhesus monkeys. Arch. Oral Biol., *17*:1059–1066, 1972.

619. Van Hees, J.: Human C fiber input during painful and nonpainful skin stimulation with radiant heat. *In* Bonica, J.J., and Albe–Fessard, D. (eds.): Advances in Pain Research and Therapy, vol. 1, pp. 35–40. New York, Raven Press, 1976.

620. Van Hees, J., Gybels, J.M.: Pain related to single afferent C fibers from human skin. Brain Res., *48*:397–400, 1972.

621. Vane, J.R.: Inhibition of prostaglandins synthesis as a mechanism of action for aspirin–like drugs, Nature, New Biol., *291*:23–25, 1971.

622. Vane, J.R.: The mode of action of aspirin and similar compounds. J. Allergy Clin. Immunol., *58*:691–712, 1976.

623. Vierck, C.J., Jr., Greenspan, J.D., Ritz, L.A., Yeomans, D.C.: The spinal pathways contributing to the ascending conduction and the descending modulation of pain sensations and reactions. *In* Yaksh, T.L. (ed.): Spinal Afferent Processing, pp. 275–329. New York, Plenum Press, 1986.

624. Vierck, C.J., Jr., Hamilton, D.M., Thornby, J.I.: Pain reactivity of monkeys after lesions to the dorsal and lateral columns of the spinal cord. Exp. Brain Res., *13*:140–158, 1971.

625. Voris, H.C.: Variations in the spinothalamic tract in man. J. Neurosurg., *14*:55–60, 1957.

626. Vyklicky, L., Keller, O.: Central projection of tooth pulp primary afferents in the cat. Acta Neurobiol. Exp., *33*:803–809, 1973.

627. Vyklicky, L., Keller, O., Brozek, G., Butkhuzi, S.M.: Cortical potentials evoked by stimulation of tooth pulp afferents in the cats. Brain Res., *41*:211–213, 1972.

628. Wagman, I.H., Price, D.D.: Response of dorsal horn cells of Macaca mulatta to cutaneous and sural nerve A and C fiber stimuli. J. Neurophysiol., *32*:803–817, 1969.

629. Wall, P.D.: The origin of a spinal cord slow potential. J. Physiol. (Lond.), *164*:508–526, 1962.

630. Wall, P.D.: The laminar organization of dorsal horn and effects of descending impulses. J. Physiol. (Lond.), *188*:403–423, 1967.

631. Wall, P.D., Gutnick, M.: Ongoing activity in peripheral nerves: The physiology and pharmacology of impulses originating from a neuroma. Exp. Neurol., *43*:580–593, 1974.

632. Wall, P.D., Merrill, E.G., Yaksh, T.L.: Responses of single units in laminae II and III of cat spinal cord. Brain Res., *160*:245–261, 1979.

633. Wall, P.D., Scadding, J.W., Tomkiewicz, M.M.: The production and prevention of experimental anaesthesia dolorosa. Pain, *6*:175–182, 1979.

634. Wall, P.D., Wasman, S., Basbaum, A.I.: Ongoing activity in peripheral nerve: Injury discharge. Exp. Neurol., *45*:576–589, 1974.

635. Wall, P.D., Yaksh, T.L.: The effect of Lissauer tract stimulation on activity in dorsal and ventral roots. Exp. Neurol., *60*:570–583, 1978.

636. Weber, W.V.: Some actions and interactions of visceral and somatic afferents in the thoracic spinal cord. *In* Kornhuber, J.J. (ed.): The Somatosensory System, Thieme Ed, pp. 227–238, Publishing Sciences Group, Acton, MA, 1975.

637. Wennmalm, A., Chanh, P.H., Junstad, M.: Hypoxia causes prostaglandin release from perfused rabbit hearts. Acta Physiol. Scand., *91*:133–135, 1974.

638. Westman, J., Bowsher, D.: Ultrastructural observations on the degeneration of spinal afferents to the nucleus medullae oblongatae centralis (pars caudalis) of the cat. Brain Res., *26*:395–398, 1971.

639. Westrum, L.E., Black, R.C.: Fine structural aspects of the

synaptic organization of the spinal trigeminal nucleus (pars interpolaris) of the cat. Brain Res., *25*:265–288, 1971.

640. White, J.C., Bland, E.F.: The surgical relief of severe angina pectoris: Methods employed and end results in 83 patients. Medicine (Baltimore), *27*:1–42, 1948.
641. White, J.C., Garrey, W.E., Atkins, J.A.: Cardiac innervation: Experimental and clinical studies. Arch. Surg., *26*:765–786, 1933.
642. White, J.C., Richardson, E.P., Sweet, W.H.: Upper thoracic cordotomy for relief of pain: Postmortem correlation of spinal incision with analgesic levels in 18 cases. Ann. Surg., *144*:407–420, 1956.
643. White, J.C., Sweet, W.H., Hawkins, R., Nilges, R.G.: Anterolateral cordotomy: Results, complications and causes of failure. Brain, *73*:346–367, 1950.
644. White, J.C., Sweet, W.H.: Pain, Its Mechanisms and Neurosurgical Control. Springfield, IL. Charles C Thomas, 1955.
645. White, J.C., Sweet, W.H.: Pain and the Neurosurgeon. Springfield, IL. Charles C Thomas, 1969.
646. Whitlock, D.G., Perl, E.R.: Thalamic projections of spinothalamic pathways in monkeys. Exp. Neurol., *3*:240–255, 1961.
647. Whitsel, B.L., Petrucelli, L.M., Werner, G.: Symmetry and connectively in the map of the body surface in somatosensory area II of primates. J. Neurophysiol., *32*:170–183, 1969.
648. Whitsel, B.L., Rustioni, A., Dreyer, D.A., Loe, P.R., *et al.*: Thalamic projections to S 1 in Macaque monkeys. J. Comp. Neurol., *178*:385, 1978.
649. Wikler, A.: Sites and mechanisms of action of morphine and related drugs in the central nervous system. Pharmacol. Rev., *2*:435–506, 1950.
650. Willer, J.C., Boureaux, F., Albe-Fessard, D.: Role of large diameter cutaneous afferents in transmission of nociceptive messages: Electrophysiological study in man. Brain Res., *152*:385–364, 1978.
651. Willis, A.L.: Release of histamine, kinin and prostaglandin during carrageenin-induced inflammation in the rat. *In* Montegazza, P., Horton, E.W. (eds.): Prostaglandins, Peptides and Amines, pp. 31–38. Academic Press, London, 1969.
652. Willis, W.D.: Ascending somatosensory systems. *In* Yaksh, T.L. (ed.): Spinal Afferent Processing, pp. 243–274. New York, Plenum Press, 1986.
653. Willis, W.D., Coggeshall, R.E.: Sensory Mechanisms of the Spinal Cord. New York, Plenum Press, 1978.
654. Willis, W.D., Haber, L.H., Martin, R.F.: Inhibition of spinothalamic tract cells and interneurons by brainstem stimulation in the monkey. J. Neurophysiol., *40*:968–981, 1977.
655. Willis, W.D., Kenshalo, D.R., Jr., Leonard, R.B.: The cells of origin of the primate spinothalamic tract. J. Comp. Neurol., *188*:543–574, 1979.
656. Willis, W.D., Trevino, D.L., Coulter, J.D., Maunz, R.A.: Responses of primate spinothalamic tract neurons to natural stimulation of hindlimb. J. Neurophysiol., *37*:358–372, 1974.
657. Wilson, P.R., Yaksh, T.L.: Baclofen is antinociceptive in the spinal intrathecal space of animals. Eur. J. Pharmacol., *51*:323–330, 1978.
658. Winkelmann, R.K.: Kinins from human skin. *In* Kenshalo, D.R. (ed.): The Skin Senses, chap. 25, pp. 499–511. Charles C Thomas, 1968.
659. Winkelmann, R.K.: Sensory receptors of the skin. In Yaksh, T.L. (ed.): Spinal Afferent Processing, pp. 19–57. New York, Plenum Press, 1986.
660. Winter, D.L.: Receptor characteristics and conduction velocities in bladder afferents. J. Psychiatr. Res., *8*:225–235, 1971.
661. Wolff, H.G., (Dalessio, D.J., rev.): Wolff's Headache and Other Head Pain, 3rd ed. reviewed by D.J. Dalessio, New York, Oxford University Press, 1972.
662. Woolf, C.J., Fitzgerald, M.: Lamina-specific alteration of C-fibre evoked activity by morphine in the dorsal horn of the rat spinal cord. Neurosci. Lett., *25*:37–41, 1981.
663. Woodbury, D.M., Fingl, E.: Analgesic antipyretics, anti-inflammatory agents, and drugs employed in the therapy of gout., *In* Goodman, L.S., Gilman, E.A. (eds.): The Pharmacological Basis of Therapeutics, 5th ed., pp. 325–358. New York, MacMillan, 1975.
664. Wright, D.M., Roberts, M.H.T.: Responses of spinal neurones to a substance P analogue, noxious pinch and bradykinin. Eur. J. Pharmacol., *64*:165–167, 1980.
665. Yaksh, T.L.: Neuropharmacology of the spinal cord reaction to noxious inputs. Proc. Int. Union Physiol. Sci., *14*:283, 1980.
666. Yaksh, T.L.: Inhibition by etorphine of the discharge of dorsal horn neurons: Effects upon the neuronal response to both high- and low-threshold sensory input in the decerebrate spinal cat. Exp. Neurol., *60*:23–40, 1978.
667. Yaksh, T.L.: Spinal opiate analgesia: Characteristics and principles of action. Pain, *11*:293–346, 1981.
668. Yaksh, T.L.: Multiple opioid receptor systems in brain and spinal cord: Part 1. Eur. J. Anaesthesiol., *1*:171–199, 1984.
669. Yaksh, T.L.: Multiple opioid receptor systems in brain and spinal cord. Part 2. Eur. J. Anaesthesiol., *1*:201–243, 1984.
670. Yaksh, T.L.: Pharmacology of spinal adrenergic systems which modulate spinal nociceptive processing. Pharmacol. Biochem. Behav., *22*:845–858, 1985.
671. Yaksh, T.L.: The central pharmacology of primary afferents with emphasis on the disposition and role of primary afferent substance P., *In* Yaksh, T.L. (eds.): Spinal Afferent Processing, pp. 165–195. New York, Plenum Press, 1986.
672. Yaksh, T.L.: The effects of intrathecally administered opoid and adrenergic agents on spinal function. *In* Yaksh, T.L. (ed.): Spinal Afferent Processing, pp. 505–539. New York, Plenum Press, 1986.
673. Yaksh, T.L., Abay, E.O., Go, V.L.W.: Studies on the location and release of cholecystokinin and vasoactive intestinal peptide in rat and cat spinal cord. Brain Res., *242*:279–290, 1982.
674. Yaksh, T.L., Dirksen, R., Harty, G.J.: Antinociceptive effects of intrathecally injected cholinomimetic drugs in the rat and cat. Eur. J. Pharmacol., *117*:81–85, 1985.
675. Yaksh, T.L., Elde, R.P.: Factors governing the release of methionine-enkephalin-like immunoreactivity from the mesencephalon and spinal cord of the cat *in vivo*. J. Neurophysiol., *46*:1056–1075, 1981.
676. Yaksh, T.L., Jessell, T.M., Gamse, R., Mudge, A.W., *et al.*:

Intrathecal morphine inhibits subsance P release from mammalian spinal cord *in vivo*. Nature, *286*:155–156, 1980.

677. Yaksh, T.L., Noueihed, R.: The physiology and pharmacology of spinal opiates. Annu. Rev. Pharmacol., Toxicol., *25*:433–462, 1985.

678. Yaksh, T.L., Schmauss, C., Micevych, P.E., Abay, E.O., *et al.*: Pharmacological studies on the application, disposition and release of neurotensin in the spinal cord. Annu. NY Acad. Sci., *400*:228–243, 1982.

679. Yaksh, T.L., Terenius, L., Nyberg, F., Jhamandas, K., *et al.*: Studies on the release by somatic stimulation from rat and cat spinal cord of active materials which displace dihydromorphine in an opiate–binding assay. Brain Res., *268*:119–128, 1983.

680. Yaksh, T.L., Tyce, G.M.: Resting and K^+ evoked release of serotonin and norepinephrine *in vivo* from the cat and rat spinal cord. Brain Res., *192*:133–146, 1980.

681. Yaksh, T.L., Wall, P.D.: Activation of a local spinal inhibitory system by focal stimulation of the lateral Lissauer tract in cats. Fed. Proc., *37*:398, 1978.

682. Yaksh, T.L., Wilson, P.R.: Spinal serotonin terminal system mediates antinociception. J. Pharmacol. Exp. Ther., *208*:446–453, 1979.

683. Yaksh, T.L., Yeung, J.C., Rudy, T.A.: Systematic mapping of the central gray medial thalamic axis of the rat: evidence for a somatotopic distribution of morphine sensitive sites within the periaqueductal gray (abstr.). Neuroscience, *1*:283, 1975.

684. Yaksh, T.L., Yeung, J.C., Rudy, T.A.: Medial thalamic lesions in the rat: Effects on nociceptive threshold and morphine antinociception. Neuropharmacology, *16*:107–114, 1977.

685. Yamamoto, T., Takahashi, K., Satomi, H., Ise, H.: Origins of primary afferent fibers in the spinal ventral roots in the cat as demonstrated by the horseradish peroxidase method. Brain Res., *126*:350–354, 1977.

686. Yezierski, R.P., Gerhart, K.D., Schrock, B.J., Willis, W.D.: A further examination of effects of cortical stimulation on primate spinothalamic tract cells. J. Neurophysiol., *49*:424–441, 1983.

687. Yezierski, R.P., Schwartz, R.H.: Receptive field properties of spinomesencephalic tract (SMT) cells (Abstr.) Pain, (*Suppl.*)*2*:184, 1984.

688. Yokota, T.: Excitation of units in marginal rim of trigeminal subnucleus caudalis excited by tooth pulp stimulation. Brain Res. *95*:154–158, 1975.

689. Yokota, T., Hashimoto, S.: Periaqueductal gray and tooth pulp afferent interaction on units in caudal medulla oblongata. Brain Res., *117*:508–512, 1976.

690. Yoshida, S., Matsuda, Y.: Studies on sensory neurons of the mouse with intracellular–recording and horseradish peroxidase–injection techniques. J. Neurophysiol., *42*:1134–1145, 1979.

691. Young, D.W., Gottschaldt, R.M.: Neurons in the rostral mesencephalic reticular formation of the cat responding specifically to noxious mechanical stimulation. Exp. Neurol., *51*:628–636, 1976.

692. Young, R.F.: Unmyelinated fibers in the trigeminal motor root. Possible relationship to the results of trigeminal rhizotomy. J. Neurosurg., *49*:538–543, 1978.

693. Young, R.F., King, R.B.: Excitability changes in trigeminal primary afferent fibers in response to noxious and nonnoxious stimuli. J. Neurophysiol., *35*:87–95, 1972.

694. Young, R.F., King, R.B.: Fiber spectrum of the trigeminal sensory root of the baboon determined by electron microscopy. J. Neurosurg., *38*:65–72, 1973.

695. Young, W.S., Wamsley, J.K., Zarbin, M.A., Kuhar, M.J.: Opioid receptors undergo axonal flow. Science, *210*:76–78, 1980.

696. Zemlan, F.P., Leonard,C.M., Kow, L.M., Pfaff, D.W.: Ascending tracts of the lateral columns of the rat spinal cord: A study using the silver impregnation and horseradish peroxidase techniques. Exp. Neurol., *62*:298–334, 1978.

697. Zieglgänsberger, W., Bayerl, H.: The mechanisms of inhibition of neuronal activity by opiates in the spinal cord of the cat. Brain Res., *115*:111–128, 1976.

698. Zieglgänsberger, W., Puil, E.A.: Actions of glutamic acid on spinal neurons. Exp. Brain Res., *17*:35–49, 1973.

699. Zieglgänsberger, W., Tulloch, I.F.: Effects of substance P on neurones in the dorsal horn of the spinal cord of the cat. Brain Res., *166*:273–282, 1979.

700. Zimmerman, M.: Neurophysiology of nociception. *In* Porter, R. (ed.): Int. Rev. Physiol., Neurophysiol. II, Vol. 10, pp. 179–221. Baltimore, University Park Press, 1976.

701. Zimmerman, M.: Encoding in dorsal horn interneurons receiving noxious and non–noxious afferents. J. Physiol. (Paris), *73*:221–232, 1977.

702. Zimmerman, M., Carstens, E., Schreiber, H., Gilly, H.: Excitability changes at intraspinal terminals of afferent C– and A–fibers produced by midbrain stimulation and iontophoretic application of transmitters in cat. Soc. Neurosci. Abstr., *9*:254, 1983.

703. Zotterman, Y.: Touch, pain, and tickling: An electrophysiological investigation on cutaneous sensory nerves. J. Physiol. (Lond.), *95*:1–28, 1939.

25 PSYCHOLOGICAL ASPECTS OF PAIN: IMPLICATIONS FOR NEURAL BLOCKADE

RONALD MELZACK

Pain is a personal, subjective experience influenced by cultural learning, the meaning of the situation, attention, and other psychological variables. Pain processes do not begin with the stimulation of receptors. Rather, injury or disease produces neural signals that enter an active nervous system that (in the adult organism) is the substrate of past experience, culture, anxiety, and so forth. These brain processes actively participate in the selection, abstraction, and synthesis of information from the total sensory input. Pain, then, is not simply the end product of a linear sensory transmission system; rather, it is a dynamic process that involves continuous interactions among complex ascending and descending systems.

PSYCHOLOGICAL CONTRIBUTIONS TO PAIN

When compared with vision or hearing, the perception of pain seems simple, urgent, and primitive. We expect the nerve signals evoked by injury to "get through," unless we are unconscious or anesthetized. But experiments and clinical observations show that pain is much more variable and modifiable than many people have believed in the past. Pain differs from person to person, culture to culture. Stimuli that produce intolerable pain in one person may be tolerated without a whimper by another. Pain perception, then, cannot be defined simply in terms of particular kinds of stimuli. Rather, it is a highly personal experience that depends in part on psychological factors that are unique to each individual.[40]

CULTURAL DETERMINANTS

It is often asserted that variations in pain experience from person to person are due to different "pain thresholds"; however, there are several thresholds related to pain, and it is important to distinguish among them. Typically, thresholds are measured by applying a stimulus such as electric shock or radiant heat to a small area of skin and gradually increasing the intensity. Four thresholds can be measured by this technique: [1] sensation threshold (or lower threshold)—the lowest stimulus value at which a sensation such as tingling or warmth is first reported; [2] pain perception threshold—the lowest stimulus value at which the person reports that the stimulation feels painful; [3] pain tolerance (or upper threshold)—the lowest stimulus level at which the subject withdraws or asks to have the stimulation stopped; and [4] encouraged pain tolerance—the same as #3, but the person is encouraged to tolerate higher levels of stimulation.

There is now evidence that all people, regardless of cultural background, have a uniform *sensation threshold.* Sternbach and Tursky[49] made careful measurements of sensation threshold, using electric shock as the stimulus, in American-born women belonging to four different ethnic groups: Italian, Jewish, Irish, and Old American. They found no differences among the groups in the level of shock that was first reported as producing a detectable sensation. The sensory conducting apparatus, in other words, appears to be essentially similar in all people so that a given critical level of input always elicits a sensation.

Cultural background, however, has a powerful effect on the *pain perception threshold*. For example, levels of radiant heat that are reported as painful by people of Mediterranean origin (such as Italians and Jews) are described merely as warmth by Northern Europeans.[17] Similarly, Nepalese porters on a climbing expedition are much more stoical than the Occidental visitors for whom they work: Even though both groups are equally sensitive to changes in electric shock, the Nepalese porters require much higher intensities before they call them painful.[8]

The most striking effect of cultural background, however, is on *pain tolerance levels*. Sternbach and Tursky[49] report that the levels at which subjects refuse to tolerate electric shock, even when they are encouraged by the experimenters, depend in part on the ethnic origin of the subject. Women of Italian descent tolerate less shock than women of Old American or Jewish origin. In a similar experiment[25] in which Jewish and Protestant women served as subjects, the Jewish, but not the Protestant, women increased their tolerance level after they were told that their religious group tolerated pain more poorly than others.

These differences in pain tolerance reflect different ethnic attitudes toward pain. Zborowski[54] found that Old Americans have an accepting, matter-of-fact attitude toward pain and pain expression. They tend to withdraw when the pain is intense, and cry out or moan only when they are alone. Jews and Italians, on the other hand, tend to be vociferous in their complaints and openly seek support and sympathy. The underlying attitudes of the two groups, however, appear to be different. Jews tend to be concerned about the meaning and implications of the pain, whereas Italians usually express a desire for immediate pain relief.

PAST EXPERIENCE

The evidence that pain is influenced by cultural factors leads naturally to an examination of the role of early experience in adult behavior related to pain. It is commonly accepted that children are deeply influenced by the attitudes of their parents toward pain. Some families make a great fuss about ordinary cuts and bruises, whereas others tend to show little sympathy toward even fairly serious injuries. There is reason to believe, on the basis of everyday observations, that attitudes toward pain acquired early in life are carried into adulthood. These observations have been confirmed experimentally in dogs[36] and monkeys.[27] In both studies, young animals were raised in cages that protected them from the usual injuries encountered in normal development. At maturity, these animals exhibited abnormally little response to injurious stimuli. The monkeys, for example, when released into a normal environment, often engaged in suicidal attacks against older and stronger monkeys. They also viciously bit their own limbs. These acts of self-destruction by the monkeys "have on occasion resulted in broken bones and torn skin and blood vessels. After being repaired, many of these animals fail to profit from their experiences, continuing to bite themselves and to attack larger animals who inflict new wounds. . . ."[27]

MEANING OF THE PAIN-PRODUCING SITUATION

There is considerable evidence to show that people attach variable meaning to pain-producing situations and that the meaning greatly influences the degree and quality of pain they feel. Beecher[2] observed that soldiers wounded in battle rarely complained of pain, whereas civilians with similar surgical wounds usually claimed that they were in severe pain. Beecher[2] concluded the following from his study:

> The common belief that wounds are inevitably associated with pain, and that the more extensive the wound the worse the pain, was not supported by observations made as carefully as possible in the combat zone. . . . The data state in numerical terms what is known to all thoughtful clinical observers: there is no simple direct relationship between the wound *per se* and the pain experienced. The pain is in very large part determined by other factors, and of great importance here is the significance of the wound. . . . In the wounded soldier [the response to injury] was relief, thankfulness at his escape alive from the battlefield, even euphoria; to the civilian, his major surgery was a depressing, calamitous event.

A similar study[7] of Israeli soldiers with traumatic amputations after the Yom Kippur War provided similar observations. Most of the wounded men spoke of their initial injury as painless and used neutral terms such as "bang," "thump," or "blow" to describe their first sensation. They often volunteered their surprise that the injury did not hurt.

Melzack, Wall, and Ty[41] recently examined the features of acute pain in patients at an emergency clinic. Patients who had severe, life-threatening injuries or who were agitated, drunk, or "in shock" were excluded from the study. Of 138 patients who were alert, rational, and coherent, 51 (37%) stated that they did not feel pain at the time of injury. The majority of these patients reported onset of pain within an hour of injury, although the delays were as long as 9 hours or more in some patients. The predominant emotions of the patients were embarrassment at appearing careless or worry about loss of wages.

The occurrence of delays in pain onset was related to the nature of the injury. Of 46 patients whose injuries were limited to skin (lacerations, cuts, abrasions, burns) 53% had a pain-free period. Of 86 patients with deep-tissue injuries (fractures, sprains, bruises, amputation of a finger, stabs and crushes), 28% had a pain-free period. The results indicate that the relation between injury and pain is highly variable and complex.

ATTENTION, ANXIETY, AND DISTRACTION

If a person's attention is focused on a potentially painful experience, he will tend to perceive pain more intensely than he would normally. Hall and Stride[16] found that the simple appearance of the word "pain" in a set of instructions made anxious subjects more likely to report a given level of electric shock as painful; the same level of shock was rarely reported to be painful when the word was absent from the instructions. Thus the mere anticipation of pain is sufficient to raise the level of anxiety and thereby the intensity of perceived pain. Similarly, Hill, Kornetsky, Flanary, and Wikler[19,20] have shown that if anxiety is dispelled (by reassuring the subject that he has control over the pain-producing stimulus), a given level of electric shock or burning heat is perceived as significantly less painful than the same stimulus under conditions of high anxiety.

In contrast to the effects of attention on pain, it is well known that distraction of attention away from pain can diminish or abolish it. Distraction of attention may partly explain why boxers, football players, and other athletes sometimes sustain severe injuries during the excitement of the sport without being aware that they have been hurt.

Distraction of attention, however, is usually effective only when the pain is steady or rises slowly in intensity.[42] If radiant heat is focused on the skin, for example, the pain may rise so suddenly and sharply that subjects are unable to control it by distraction. But when the pain rises slowly, people may use various stratagems to distract their attention from it. They often find that the pain actually levels off or decreases *before* it reaches the anticipated intolerable level. Distraction stratagems are used effectively by some people to control pain produced by dental drilling and extraction.[15]

FEELINGS OF CONTROL OVER PAIN

It is now apparent that the severity of postsurgical pain is significantly reduced when patients are taught how to cope with their pain. Patients who were scheduled to undergo major surgery to remove the gall bladder, uterus, or portions of the digestive tract were given detailed information about the pain they would feel after the operation and how they could best cope with it. They were told where they would feel pain, how severe it could be, how long it could last, and that such pain is normal after an operation. They were also shown how to relax by using breathing and relaxation stratagems. Finally, they were told that total relaxation is difficult to achieve and that they should request medication if they were uncomfortable. The results showed that patients who received these instructions reported significantly less pain, asked for many fewer medications during recovery, and spent less time in hospital than a similar group of patients who received no instructions.[12]

It was originally thought that the information alone is sufficient psychological preparation to reduce the uncertainty and anxiety associated with major surgery. It is evident, however, that knowledge, in this case, may only increase the anxiety because of the certain expectation of pain and various discomforts. The essential ingredient is providing the patient with skills to cope with the pain and anxiety —at the very least, to provide the patient with a sense of control. Recent studies have shown that simply giving patients information about their pain tends to make them focus on the discomforting aspects of the experience, and their pain is magnified rather than reduced; however, when the patients are taught skills to cope with their pain, such as relaxation or distraction strategies, the pain is less severe.[26] Other studies have shown that the amount of postsurgical pain is directly proportional to the amount of anxiety perceived by the patient.[28] Achieving a sense of control, then, appears to diminish both anxiety and pain.

SUGGESTION AND PLACEBOS

The influence of suggestion on the intensity of perceived pain is clearly demonstrated by studies of the effectiveness of placebos. Clinical investigators[2] have found that severe pain, such as postsurgical pain, can be relieved in some patients by giving them a placebo (usually some nonanalgesic substance such as a sugar or salt solution) in place of morphine or other analgesic drugs. About 35% of the patients report marked relief of pain after being given a placebo. This is a strikingly high proportion because morphine, even in large doses, relieves severe pain in only about 75% of patients.

A surprising recent discovery about placebos is that their effectiveness is always about 50% of that of the drug with which it is being compared, even in double-blind experiments[13]; that is, if the drug is a mild analgesic such as aspirin, then the pain relief produced by the placebo is half that of the aspirin. If it is a powerful drug such as morphine, the placebo has greater pain-relieving properties, again about 50% of that of morphine. This indicates that even though the "double-blind" is maintained, the therapist's enthusiasm is conveyed to the patient.

There are large individual differences in susceptibility to placebos, and studies have been done to determine some of the factors involved.[13] These studies have revealed that placebos are more effective for severe pain than for mild pain and are more effective when the patients are under great stress and anxiety than when they are not. McGlashan and coworkers[29] have shown that placebo-induced analgesia is not significantly related to suggestibility, hypnotic susceptibility, or anxiety induced specifically by pain or the therapeutic situation (which is known as "state-anxiety"); however, placebo effects occur more powerfully in people who have chronic generalized anxiety (personality "trait-anxiety").

There are other fascinating factors in the placebo response. Two placebo capsules, for example, are more effective than one capsule, and large capsules are better than small ones. A placebo is more effective when injected than when given by mouth and is more potent when accompanied by strong suggestion that a powerful analgesic has been given. In short, the greater the implicit and explicit suggestion that pain will be relieved, the greater is the relief obtained by the patient. Unfortunately, however, patients tend to get less and less relief from repeated administration of placebos.

HYPNOSIS

The manipulation of attention together with strong suggestion is part of the phenomenon of hypnosis. The hypnotic state eludes precise definition. Loosely speaking, hypnosis is a trance state in which the subject's attention is focused intensely on the hypnotist while attention to other stimuli is markedly diminished. After people are hypnotized they can, with appropriate suggestion, be cut or burned yet report that they did not feel pain.[17] They may say that they felt a sharp tactile sensation or strong heat, but they maintain that the sensations never welled up into pain. Evidently a small percentage of people can be hypnotized deeply enough to undergo major surgery entirely without anesthesia. For a larger number of people, hypnosis reduced the amount of pain-killing drug required to produce successful analgesia.

Despite the long history of hypnotism, which goes back hundreds of years under different names such as animal magnetism and mesmerism, very little is known about its mechanisms. Still worse, most of its major features are highly controversial. For example, there is a vigorous debate on the nature of hypnosis: Is it a special state of consciousness known as a "trance state," or is it merely a trait of responsiveness to strong suggestion? There is no resolution yet to this question.[46]

Nevertheless, anyone who has observed the behavior of people who have been hypnotized realizes that this is an especially interesting phenomenon. Under hypnosis, people sustain pain, during demonstrations or experiments, at levels at which they would normally cry out and withdraw. Major surgery on every part of the body has been carried out on hypnotized patients. Countless articles describe these procedures, and there are reports that hypnosis is effective in relieving severe clinical pains, such as phantom limb pain. Although excellent studies of hypnotic analgesia have been carried out with experimentally induced pains,[18] there are as yet no convincing studies, using the necessary control groups, of clinical pain. The evidence thus far is observational or "anecdotal."

It is known, however, that not all people can be hypnotized. About 30% of people can reach a state of deep hypnosis, 30% reach a moderate state, and another 30% achieve a drowsy-light state. About 10% of people are not susceptible at all. These figures resemble the proportions of placebo reactors and nonreactors. There is, however, strong evidence that the lack of responsiveness to pain in hypnotized subjects is more than a placebo effect. An elegantly designed experiment[29] has shown that pain perception threshold and pain tolerance level are strikingly increased during hypnosis but that only the pain perception threshold is raised after administration of a placebo. In fact, this study demonstrated that the hypnotic procedure itself has not only a placebo effect, but also an additional effect that raises pain threshold and tolerance still further.

PSYCHOGENIC PAIN

Because psychological factors play such a powerful role in pain, several clinical pain syndromes have been labeled as "psychogenic," with the implication that the primary cause of the pain is psychological; that is, the person is presumed to be in pain because he needs or wants it.

It is clear that we must recognize the psychological contribution to pain, but we must also maintain a balanced view of it. Psychological factors contribute to pain, and pain may be helped by using psychological approaches. But there are also physical contributions. This does not deny the existence of patients who need their pain and whose lives derive meaning from it. Such patients complain of terrible pain yet discontinue certain types of therapy because of minor unpleasantness, such as an injection or the taste of a particular drug. Even when psychological factors appear to play a major role, there is often tissue damage that can also be treated. In such cases, the physical symptoms as well as the psychological symptoms require treatment.

Perhaps the most convincing evidence that chronic pain is usually the cause rather than the result of neurotic symptoms derives from studies of patients who are eventually relieved of their pain. Typically, these patients, while they are suffering chronic pain, show evidence of psychological disturbance on the Minnesota Multiphasic Personality Inventory (MMPI). In particular, they have elevated scores on the scales for hysteria, depression, and hypochondriasis; however, these patients usually show significant decreases in MMPI indices of psychological disturbance when their pain is abolished by successful surgery. The results, the authors conclude, "support the hypothesis that the neuroticism associated with chronic pain is the result of it, and may be reversible when the pain is reduced or abolished."[48]

It is evident from this study that it is unreasonable to ascribe chronic pain to neurotic symptoms. Although psychological processes contribute to pain, they are only part of the activity in a complex nervous system. All too often, the diagnosis of neurosis as the cause of pain hides our profound ignorance of many aspects of pain mechanisms.

THE GATE CONTROL THEORY OF PAIN

The traditional specificity theory of pain, which is still widely taught, proposes that pain is a specific sensation and that the intensity of pain is proportional to the extent of tissue damage. The theory implies a fixed, straight-through transmission system from somatic pain receptors to a pain center in the brain. The evidence just reviewed, however, shows that pain not only is a function of injury, but also is influenced by psychological variables.

In 1965, Melzack and Wall[39] proposed the gate control theory of pain. Basically, the theory proposes that neural mechanisms in the dorsal horns of the spinal cord act like a gate that can increase or decrease the flow of nerve impulses from peripheral fibers to the spinal cord cells that project to the brain. Somatic input is therefore subjected to the modulating influence of the gate *before* it evokes pain perception and response. The theory suggests that large-fiber inputs tend to close the gate whereas small-fiber inputs generally open it, and that the gate is also profoundly influenced by descending influences from the brain. It further proposes that the sensory input is modulated at successive synapses throughout its projection from the spinal cord to the brain areas responsible for pain experience and response. Pain occurs when the number of nerve impulses that arrives at these areas exceeds a critical level.

Melzack and Wall[40] have recently assessed the present-day status of the gate-control theory in light of new physiologic research. Despite considerable controversy and conflicting evidence, the concept of gating (or input modulation) is stronger than ever. A slightly revised model of the gate control theory has recently been presented (Fig. 25-1).[40]

DIMENSIONS OF PAIN EXPERIENCE

Research on pain, since the beginning of this century, has been dominated by the concept that pain is purely a sensory experience. Yet pain also has a distinctly unpleasant, affective quality. It becomes overwhelming, demands immediate attention, and disrupts ongoing behavior and thought. It motivates or drives the organism into activity aimed at stopping the pain as quickly as possible. To consider only the sensory features of pain and ignore its motivational-affective properties is to look at only part of the problem. Even the concept of pain as a perception, with full recognition of past experience, attention, and

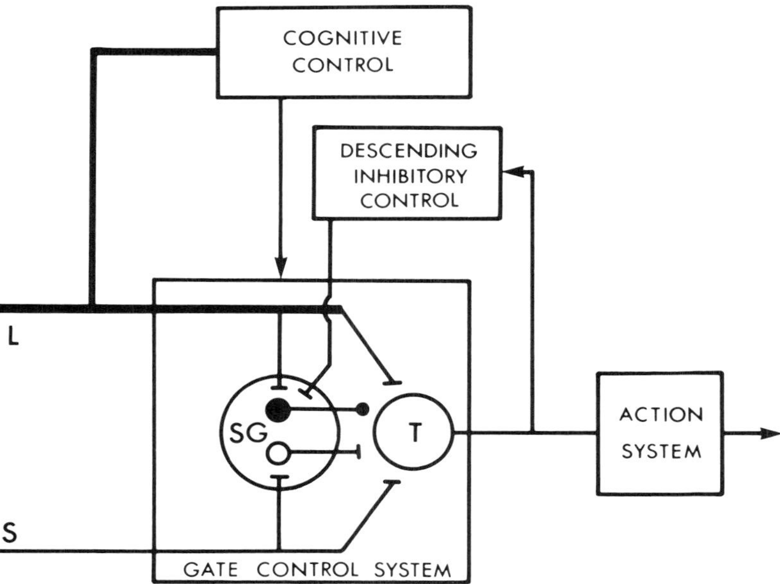

FIG. 25-1. The gate-control theory: Mark II. The new model includes excitatory *(white circle)* and inhibitory *(black circle)* links from the substantia gelatinosa *(SG)* to the transmission *(T)* cells, as well as descending inhibitory control from brain-stem systems. The round knob at the end of the inhibitory link implies that its action may be presynaptic, postsynaptic, or both. All connections are excitatory, except the inhibitory link from SG to T cell.

other cognitive influences, still neglects the crucial motivational dimension.

These considerations led Melzack and Casey[32] to suggest that there are three major psychological dimensions of pain: sensory-discriminative, motivational-affective, and cognitive-evaluation. They proposed that they are subserved by physiologically specialized systems in the brain (Fig. 25-2):

1. The sensory-discriminative dimension of pain is influenced primarily by the rapidly conducting spinal systems.
2. The powerful motivational drive and unpleasant affect characteristic of pain are subserved by activities in reticular and limbic structures that are influenced primarily by the slowly conducting spinal systems.
3. Neocortical or higher central nervous system processes, such as evaluation of the input in terms of past experience, exert control over activity in both the discriminative and motivational systems.

It is assumed that these three categories of activity interact with one another to provide *perceptual information* on the location, magnitude, and spatiotemporal properties of the noxious stimuli, *motivational tendency* toward escape or attack, *cognitive information* based on past experience, and probability of outcome of different response strategies. All three forms of activity could then influence motor mechanisms responsible for the complex pattern of overt responses that characterize pain.

MEASUREMENT OF PAIN

PSYCHOPHYSICAL APPROACHES

Until recently, the methods used for pain measurement treated pain as though it were a single, unique quality that varied only in intensity.[2] The most common of these methods is the use of words such as "mild," "moderate," and "severe," and subjects (or patients) are asked to choose the word that best describes the intensity of their pain. Another method consists of a five-point scale that ranges from 1 (mild pain) to 5 (unbearable pain), and subjects are asked to choose the most appropriate number. In this way, some quantitative measure of pain is obtained. Still another method is the use of fractions; subjects who have received injections of analgesic drugs such as morphine are asked whether their pain is a third or a half of what it was before the injection. Yet another method is the "visual analogue scale."[45] The patient or subject is presented with a line 10 cm long and is told that one end represents no pain and the other represents the worst pain imaginable. He is then

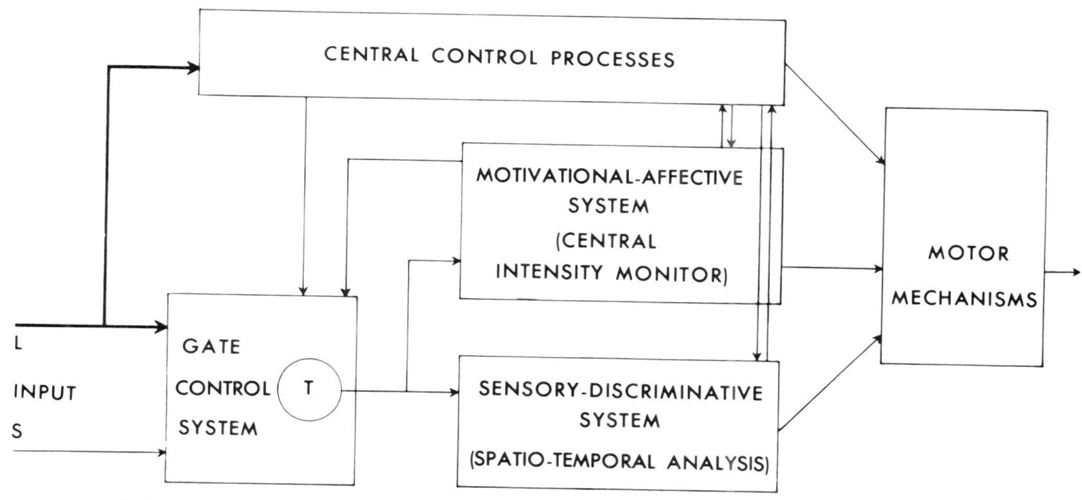

FIG. 25-2. Conceptual model of the sensory, motivational, and central control determinants of pain. The output of the T cells of the gate-control system projects to the sensory-discriminative system (via neospinothalamic fibers) and the motivational-affective system (via the paramedial ascending system). The central control trigger is represented by a line running from the larger fiber system to central control processes; these, in turn, project back to the gate-control system and to the sensory-discriminative and motivational-affective systems. All three systems interact with one another and project to the motor system.

asked to make a mark on the line that represents the intensity of his pain. A ruler is then used to get a numerical measure of pain intensity such as 7 cm, or units, of pain intensity. These simple methods have all been used effectively in hospital clinics and have provided valuable information about pain and analgesia.

All of these methods specify only intensity. It is now clear, however, that the word "pain" refers to an endless variety of qualities that are categorized under a single linguistic label, not to a specific, single sensation that varies only in intensity. Each pain has unique qualities. The pain of a toothache is obviously different from that of a pinprick, just as the pain of a coronary occlusion is uniquely different from that of a broken leg.

THE MCGILL PAIN QUESTIONNAIRE

Melzack and Torgerson[38] have made a start toward specifying the qualities of pain. In the first part of their study, subjects were asked to classify 102 words, obtained from the clinical literature relating to pain, into smaller groups that describe different aspects of the experience of pain. On the basis of the data, the words are categorized into 3 major classes and 16 subclasses. The classes are [1] words that describe the *sensory qualities* of the experience in terms of temporal, spatial, pressure, thermal, and other properties; [2] words that describe *affective qualities,* in terms of tension, fear, and autonomic properties that are part of the pain experience; and [3] *evaluative* words that describe the subjective overall intensity of the total pain experience. Each subclass, which was given a descriptive label, consists of a group of words that were considered by most subjects to be qualitatively similar.

The second part of the study was an attempt to determine the pain intensities implied by the words within each subclass. Groups of doctors, patients, and students were asked to assign an intensity value to each word, using a numerical scale ranging from least (or mild) pain to worst (or excruciating) pain. When this was done, it was apparent that several words within each subclass had the same relative intensity relationships in all three sets. For example, in the spatial subclass, "shooting" was found to represent more pain than "flashing," which in turn implied more pain than "jumping." Although the precise intensity values differed for the three groups, all three agreed on the positions of the words relative to each other.

Because of the high degree of agreement on the intensity relationships among pain descriptors by subjects who have different cultural, socioeconomic, and educational backgrounds, it has been possible to develop a questionnaire (Fig. 25-3) for use as a measuring instrument in studies of clinical pain.[30,31]

One of the most exciting features of the McGill Pain Questionnaire is its potential value as a diagnostic technique.[11] The questionnaire was administered to 95 patients suffering from one of eight known pain syndromes: postherpetic neuralgia, phantom limb pain, metastatic carcinoma, toothache, degenerative disk disease, rheumatoid arthritis or osteoarthritis, labor pain, and menstrual pain. A multiple group discriminant analysis revealed that each type of pain is characterized by a distinctive constellation of verbal descriptors. Further, when the descriptor set for each patient was classified by the computer program into one of the eight diagnostic categories, a correct classification was made in 77% of cases. It is evident, then, that there are appreciable and quantifiable differences in the way various types of pain are described, and that patients with the same disease or pain syndrome tend to use remarkably similar words to communicate what they feel.

ACUTE AND CHRONIC PAIN

The time-course of pain is profoundly important in determining its psychological effects on an organism. Acute pain, which is usually associated with a well-defined cause (such as a burned finger or a ruptured appendix), normally has a characteristic time-course and vanishes after healing has occurred. The pain usually has a rapid onset—the *phasic* component—and then a subsequent *tonic* component that persists for variable periods of time.[9] Chronic pain states such as low back pain, the neuralgias, or phantom limb pain may begin as acute pain and pass through both the phasic and tonic phases. The tonic pain, however, may persist long after the injury has healed. It is then labeled as "chronic pain" and appears to involve neural mechanisms that are far more complex than those of acute pain. The pain not only persists but also may spread to adjacent or more distant body areas. It is resistant to surgical control, and its prolonged time-course is characteristically associated with high levels of anxiety and depression.[6]

One of the major advances in the field of pain in recent years has been the recognition that chronic, persistent pain is a medical entity that differs from acute pain in many respects. Chronic pain, which persists after all possible healing has occurred or at least long after pain can serve any useful function, is no longer simply a symptom of injury or disease. It becomes a pain *syndrome*—a medical problem in its own right that requires urgent attention. Chronic pain becomes debilitating and often produces severe depression. Most important for diagnosis, treatment, and prognosis is the recognition that treatments that are normally effective for most kinds of acute pain are not necessarily effective for chronic pain. Pain, which is normally associated with the search for treatment and optimal conditions for recovery, now becomes intractable. Patients are beset with a sense of helplessness, hopelessness, and meaninglessness. The pain becomes evil; it is intolerable and serves no useful function. We are especially indebted to Bonica[5,6] for the recognition of chronic pain as a distinct medical entity that requires special investigation and treatment; chronic, intractable pain presents a special challenge to the physician or health professional.

Recently we have learned to recognize that chronic pain rarely has a single cause but is instead the result of multiple, interacting causes. A variety of subtle physical and psychological factors interact and contribute to chronic pain.[34,40]

THE RATIONALE OF PAIN CONTROL

The specificity theory of pain, with its concept of a fixed one-to-one relationship between stimulus and sensation, has given rise to the expectation, in patient and physician alike, that a given form of therapy, in the hands of *all* doctors, should work for *all* patients and for *all* pains. No such therapy has yet been found, and the complexity and diversity of pain and of patients' and doctors' personalities suggest that it never will. Nevertheless, the idea of the ultimate panacea of total pain relief for *everyone* pervades our Western culture. The patient who visits a clinic and is told that he must learn to live with his pain usually concludes that the physician is incompetent, and therefore visits doctor after doctor in search of the all-encompassing, perfect pain-control method. The patients with the thick dossiers (the "crocks") may, possibly, have deep-seated psychological problems, but they are also a product of our Western all-or-nothing, pill-popping ethos, which promises instant, total pain relief—if not now, then tomorrow.

Medical practitioners must also accept a portion of the blame for this occurrence, and their training in specificity concepts underlies it: one pain, one cause; eliminate the cause by an operation or a drug and the

McGill Pain Questionnaire

Patient's Name ______ Date ______ Time ______ am/pm

PRI: S ______ (1-10) A ______ (11-15) E ______ (16) M ______ (17-20) PRI(T) ______ (1-20) PPI ______

1 FLICKERING, QUIVERING, PULSING, THROBBING, BEATING, POUNDING
2 JUMPING, FLASHING, SHOOTING
3 PRICKING, BORING, DRILLING, STABBING, LANCINATING
4 SHARP, CUTTING, LACERATING
5 PINCHING, PRESSING, GNAWING, CRAMPING, CRUSHING
6 TUGGING, PULLING, WRENCHING
7 HOT, BURNING, SCALDING, SEARING
8 TINGLING, ITCHY, SMARTING, STINGING
9 DULL, SORE, HURTING, ACHING, HEAVY
10 TENDER, TAUT, RASPING, SPLITTING
11 TIRING, EXHAUSTING
12 SICKENING, SUFFOCATING
13 FEARFUL, FRIGHTFUL, TERRIFYING
14 PUNISHING, GRUELLING, CRUEL, VICIOUS, KILLING
15 WRETCHED, BLINDING
16 ANNOYING, TROUBLESOME, MISERABLE, INTENSE, UNBEARABLE
17 SPREADING, RADIATING, PENETRATING, PIERCING
18 TIGHT, NUMB, DRAWING, SQUEEZING, TEARING
19 COOL, COLD, FREEZING
20 NAGGING, NAUSEATING, AGONIZING, DREADFUL, TORTURING

PPI
0 NO PAIN
1 MILD
2 DISCOMFORTING
3 DISTRESSING
4 HORRIBLE
5 EXCRUCIATING

BRIEF	RHYTHMIC	CONTINUOUS
MOMENTARY	PERIODIC	STEADY
TRANSIENT	INTERMITTENT	CONSTANT

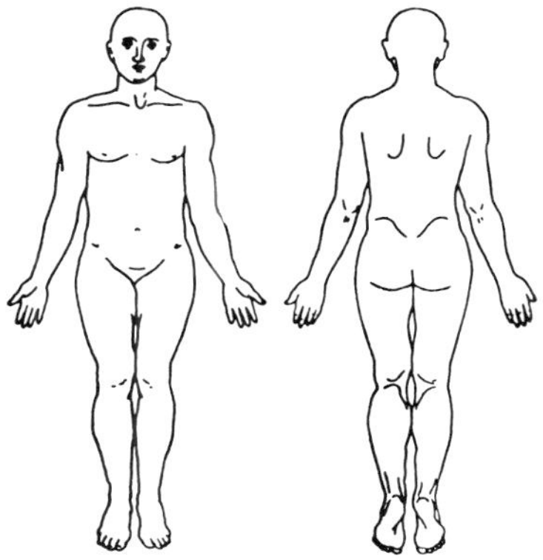

E = EXTERNAL
I = INTERNAL

COMMENTS:

FIG. 25-3. McGill Pain Questionnaire, adapted for a study of narcotic drugs. Descriptors fall into four major groups: sensory, 1 to 10; affective, 11 to 15; evaluative, 16; and miscellaneous, 17 to 20. The rank value for each descriptor is based on its position in the word set. The sum of the rank values is the "pain rating index" *(PRI)*. The "present pain intensity" *(PPI)* is based on a scale of 0 to 5.

pain should vanish. This works often enough for acute pain.

Chronic pain, however, which generally has multiple determinants, is an entirely different story. Treatment may sometimes enhance rather than diminish pain, which may lead to further treatment that may make the patient even worse. We have all seen patients crippled with back pain who have undergone several disk operations, rhizotomies, and cordotomies and who are finally turned over to the psychiatrist. The so-called pain tract was cut, not once but several times, and if the patients are still in pain they are, by definition in terms of specificity theory, malingerers or neurotics. Small wonder that by this time the patients are depressed, resentful, anxious, and attentive to their pain and nothing else. It is a fundamental fact in the field of pain that some patients will suffer pain for the rest of their lives. In such cases, the most effective therapy may be to teach them to live with their pain, to carry on productive lives despite it.

WORKER'S COMPENSATION AND PAIN

Patients who receive worker's compensation or are awaiting litigation after an accident have long been regarded as neurotics or malingerers who are exaggerating their pain for financial gain. There is, however, a growing body of evidence that patients who receive worker's compensation are no different from patients who do not. In particular, a recent study[43] found no differences between compensated and noncompensated patients based on pain scores obtained with the McGill Pain Questionnaire (MPQ). A subsequent study of 145 patients suffering low-back and musculoskeletal pain also revealed that compensated and noncompensated patients had virtually identical sensory and total pain scores and pain descriptor patterns.[33] They were also similar on the MMPI pain triad (depression, hysteria, hypochondriasis) and on several other personal variables that were examined. The only differences were small but significantly lower affective scores in the low-back group and lower evaluative scores in the musculoskeletal group. These results suggest that the financial security provided by compensation decreases anxiety, which is reflected in the lower affective or evaluative ratings but not in the sensory or total MPQ scores. Compensated patients, contrary to traditional opinion, appear not to differ from people who do not receive compensation. Accidents that produce injury and pain should be considered as potentially psychologically traumatic as well as conducive to the development of subtle physiologic changes such as trigger points. Patients on compensation or awaiting litigation deserve the same concern and compassion as all other patients who suffer chronic pain. It is prejudice, not evidence, that underlies the old idea of "the compensation neurotic" and adds insult to the patient's injury.

PSYCHOLOGICAL CONTROL OF PAIN

Many psychological approaches are known to produce some measure of pain relief, including [1] the use of operant conditioning to diminish the frequency of pain-related behavior patterns; [2] teaching patients to utilize feedback of electroencephalographic or other indices of physiologic activity to develop a state of mind that allows them to cope with pain; [3] hypnotic suggestion techniques; [4] the use of stratagems to distract attention or change the meaning of the pain; [5] social modeling techniques; and [6] psychotherapeutic or pharmacologic techniques to relieve depression. All of these approaches have value for the treatment of pain in some patients at least. They may not abolish pain entirely but may decrease some kinds of pain from unbearable to bearable levels for variable periods of time.

OPERANT-CONDITIONING TECHNIQUES

Operant-conditioning methods are based on observations that complex patterns of behavior can be modified by the manipulation of rewards and punishments. Fordyce[14] assumes that pain consists of "behaviors" that have been reinforced or rewarded, and the way to abolish "pain behaviors" is to stop all such rewards. Fordyce[14] has provided a thorough description of his procedures to retrain the patient who suffers chronic pain. The patient enters the hospital for a prolonged period (an average of 8 weeks), and all the usual "crutches" are removed. Pain behaviors such as complaint are ignored. All physical activity is rewarded with smiles and praise. During this period, medication is reduced to the barest minimum ("detoxification"). After the operant procedure, Fordyce reports, the patients are more active, complain less, take fewer drugs, work, and generally lead more normal lives.

There have not, however, been any controlled studies that compare Fordyce's operant technique to other therapeutic methods. Even without controlled data, the results are not impressive. In a study of a treatment program essentially like Fordyce's, Anderson and colleagues[1] found that 74% of the patients who completed the program reported "leading normal lives without drugs" when they were contacted 6 months to 7 years after discharge; however, the patients constituted a highly selected group so that they were hardly "typical" patients with chronic pain. Only 60 of 130 patients (46%) referred to the program were accepted for treatment. Only 37 (29%) chose to enter, and 3 of these dropped out before the program had been completed. As Turk and Genest[52] point out, "when Anderson *et al.* report that 74% of the patients treated were 'leading normal lives,' they are actually speaking of only 26 (19%) of the original patients screened over a 7-year period." It may be added that few conclusions can be drawn from a follow-up study that ranges from 4 months to 7 years without knowing how many patients were interviewed at each year after treatment.

BIOFEEDBACK

The most enthusiastic claims for biofeedback were related to alpha-brainwave activity.[23] Some practitioners of yoga or transcendental meditation can produce large amounts of alpha-brainwaves at will and simultaneously report feeling no pain when stuck with pins. Many observers, including writers for the mass media, quickly concluded that, by simply learning to increase alpha-output, sufferers could banish pain. Given these suggestive data, as well as the massive advertising campaign by "mind-control experts" who claimed they could teach people to abolish all kinds of clinical pain with only a few easy biofeedback lessons, Melzack and Perry[35] carried out a study to test the claims. Their patients were in continuous pain of known physical origin. Although the patients learned to produce significant increases in the amount of alpha-rhythm in their brainwaves, they did not experience greater reductions in pain than those reductions that occurred in "placebo" baseline sessions. In these sessions, given before the alpha-training, the patients were allowed to relax in a comfortable reclining chair, were distracted from their pain by being given a thorough description of the training procedures they would receive later, and were given strong anxiety-relieving assurances that the biofeedback would diminish their pain. This placebo condition, then, was just as effective as the elegant, extremely expensive electronic biofeedback equipment and procedure.

This conclusion is now supported by an impressive amount of research. Three major reviews of the literature on biofeedback have recently appeared. One of them[47] asks in its title, "Are the machines really necessary?" Two of them deal specifically with biofeedback for pain problems,[22,53] and one of them reviews 100 papers that were published in the 1970s. Turk and associates[53] conclude the following:

> The biofeedback literature for the regulation of pain is reviewed and found wanting on both conceptual and methodological grounds. In particular, studies on the use of biofeedback for the treatment of tension and migraine headaches and chronic pain indicate that biofeedback was not found to be superior to less expensive, less instrument-oriented treatments such as relaxation and coping skills training.

The biofeedback procedure *does* add something important to psychological therapy for pain.[35] It is a useful vehicle for distraction of attention, for relaxation, suggestion, and for providing the patient with a sense of control over his pain. Under certain conditions, and for particular patients, it may provide a valuable additional contribution for pain control.

HYPNOSIS

The number of people who can undergo major surgery solely with hypnotic analgesia is very small. There is no reason to doubt the reports that hypnosis can be used effectively to control a wide variety of pain problems such as labor pain, phantom limb pain, cancer pain, and headache.[18] But these studies generally consist of a small number of individual cases, and it is not known what proportion of patients suffering these pains can be helped by hypnosis, how long the effects last, or whether a placebo treatment would work equally well.

RELAXATION

Benson and his colleagues[3] have proposed that the "relaxation response" is the basis of all meditative practices. Relaxation, they suggest, induces the subjective experience of well-being that is often referred to as an "altered state of consciousness." In contrast to Jacobson's method of "progressive relaxation," in which people are taught to relax individual muscle groups in progression throughout a therapy session, Benson and co-workers[3] have developed a simple technique to induce general relaxation based on a variety of historical religious practices. Their instructions for this noncultic technique have been shown to produce striking physiologic changes characteristic of deep relaxation, such as decreased metabolism and lower blood pressure and respiration rate. The procedure has also been shown to produce significant reductions in chronic pain.[4]

COGNITIVE COPING SKILLS

Everyone, beginning at an early age, learns to cope with pain by using various strategies. In recent years, psychologists have devised a large number of ingenious methods that employ different kinds of strategies or coping mechanisms.[51] The following is a partial list of the strategies.

Imaginative Inattention. The patient is trained to ignore the pain by evoking imagery that is incompatible with pain. For example, the patient is instructed to imagine himself at the beach, at a party, or in the country, depending on the image he can conjure up most vividly.

Imaginative Transformation of Pain. The patient is instructed to interpret the subjective experience in terms other than "pain" (*e.g.*, transforming it into tingling or other purely sensory qualities) or to minimize the experience as trivial or unreal.

Imaginative Transformation of Context. The patient is trained to acknowledge the pain but to transform the setting or context. For example, a patient with a sprained arm may picture himself as a fighter pilot who has been shot in the arm while being chased by an enemy plane.

Attention-Diversion to External Events. The patient focuses attention on environmental objects and may count ceiling tiles or concentrate on the weave of a piece of clothing.

Attention-Diversion to Internal Events. The patient focuses attention on self-generated thoughts such as mental arithmetic or composing a limerick.

Somatization. The patient is trained to focus attention on the painful area but in a detached manner. For example, the patient may analyze the pain sensations as if preparing to write a magazine article about them.

Two recent studies indicate that coping-strategy techniques are effective for clinical pain. The first[21] investigated the effects of pleasant imagery guided by a tape on dental pain. The results showed that patients who used this strategy had significantly less discomfort than did a control group that received no treatment instructions and, more importantly, than did a second control group instructed in "neutral" imagery—that is, imagining numbers on a poster. The second study[44] examined patients who suffered severe pain owing to amputation, rheumatoid arthritis, fractures, and other diseases or injuries. The results showed that patients who were trained in the coping strategy of imaginative transformation (or reinterpretation) of the pain had significantly less pain than did patients who were taught two other strategies: diverting attention from the pain, or concentrating on the pain (somatization). It is apparent, then, that particular procedures are effective for some patients and for some kinds of pain. The approach is promising and may become more effective when patients' personalities are taken into account. For example, some people are less capable than others of generating imagery, and some people have a greater desire to cope personally with their pain than do others, who may be more passive and prefer to have other people take full responsibility for its alleviation.[51]

PREPARED CHILDBIRTH TRAINING

The most famous of all psychological approaches to the control of pain is prepared childbirth training. Labor pain is one of the severest forms of pain, and several procedures have been developed to teach pregnant women how to cope with their pain when they are in labor. One of the methods, developed by Grantly Dick-Read,[10] is known as "childbirth without fear." More recently, Fernand Lamaze[24] developed a program for "painless childbirth" that is widely known as "Lamaze training." Basically, these techniques include [1] providing detailed information on pregnancy and labor to the mother-to-be so that she knows what to expect, and therefore experiences less anxiety; [2] relaxation training so that the woman can try to relax and calm herself when uterine contractions begin to increase in frequency, duration, and intensity; [3] coping strategies to distract attention from pain; and [4] breathing exercises that are useful to enhance relaxation and distract attention.

Women in labor are subject to intense fears and anxieties related to their ability to bear the pain, to the possibility of medical complications, and to the baby's health. Prepared childbirth training, which is designed to reduce fear, anxiety, and tension, should therefore also decrease pain. A recent study[37] demonstrates that it does, but the effects are not as great as people generally believe. Several factors are significant predictors of labor pain. Primiparas generally have *less* pain if they [1] belong to higher socioeconomic status groups, [2] do not have a history of menstrual difficulties, and [3] practiced the procedures they learned in prepared childbirth training. Labor pain in multiparas is influenced by the same factors, but it is especially important that the women believe that they have been adequately prepared for labor.[37]

Figure 25-4 shows the average pain scores (Pain Rating Index of the McGill Pain Questionnaire) of primiparas who received prepared childbirth training (PCT) and those who did not. The results for individual PCT instructors are also shown. PCT, in all cases, consisted of a series of classes that included instruction in obstetrical physiology, breathing exercises, and relaxation techniques. Clearly, there is considerable variability among different instructors' groups in the scores obtained during labor. Discussions held with some of the women suggested that this is partly due to differences in the instructors' enthusiasm about PCT.

Figure 25-4 shows that PCT produces a significant decrease in total pain scores when compared with the scores of women who did not receive any training. Moreover, PCT does not only diminish the affective

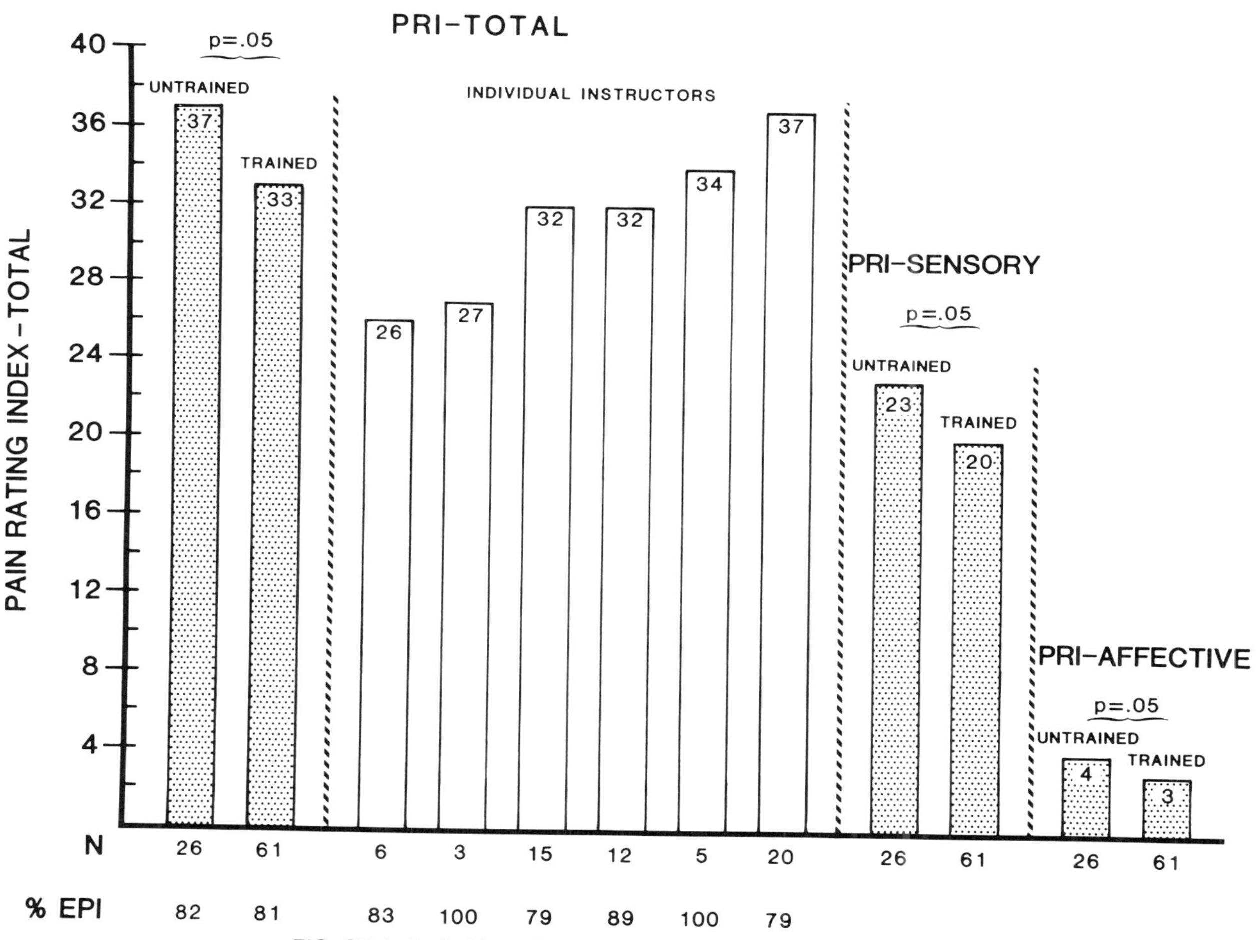

FIG. 25-4. **Left:** Mean PRI scores obtained by untrained and trained primiparas.[37] **Center:** The average PRI scores of trained women categorized by individual prepared-training instructors. **Right:** Mean PRI scores for the sensory and affective descriptor sets of the MPQ. The percentages of women who received an epidural block are indicated at the bottom.

dimension of pain, but also produces a significant decrease in the sensory dimension. A striking feature of Figure 25-4, however, is that the average scores of women who received PCT are still very high. Instructor 1, for example, was clearly the most effective of all; yet the mean total pain scores of her patients are at about the same level as the average totals recorded for outpatients with chronic back pain and cancer (Fig. 25-5). Most significant is the fact that although this instructor strongly encouraged her patients to forgo epidural spinal blocks, five of the six women specifically requested an epidural block during the late stages of labor.

These observations should be interpreted in a positive sense.[37] The fact that the current training procedures have statistically significant effects on pain is encouraging and indicates that psychological preparation is valuable. The additional fact that the average pain reduction is relatively small means that there is a need for further development of these procedures.

INTERACTING DETERMINANTS OF PAIN

There is no longer any doubt about being able to reduce many kinds of clinical pain by different psychological therapies. It is important to keep in mind, however, that these therapies rarely abolish pain entirely and are not equally effective for everyone. There are no perfect therapies of any kind. We have learned, as a result of literally hundreds of experiments, that there is a limit to the effectiveness of any

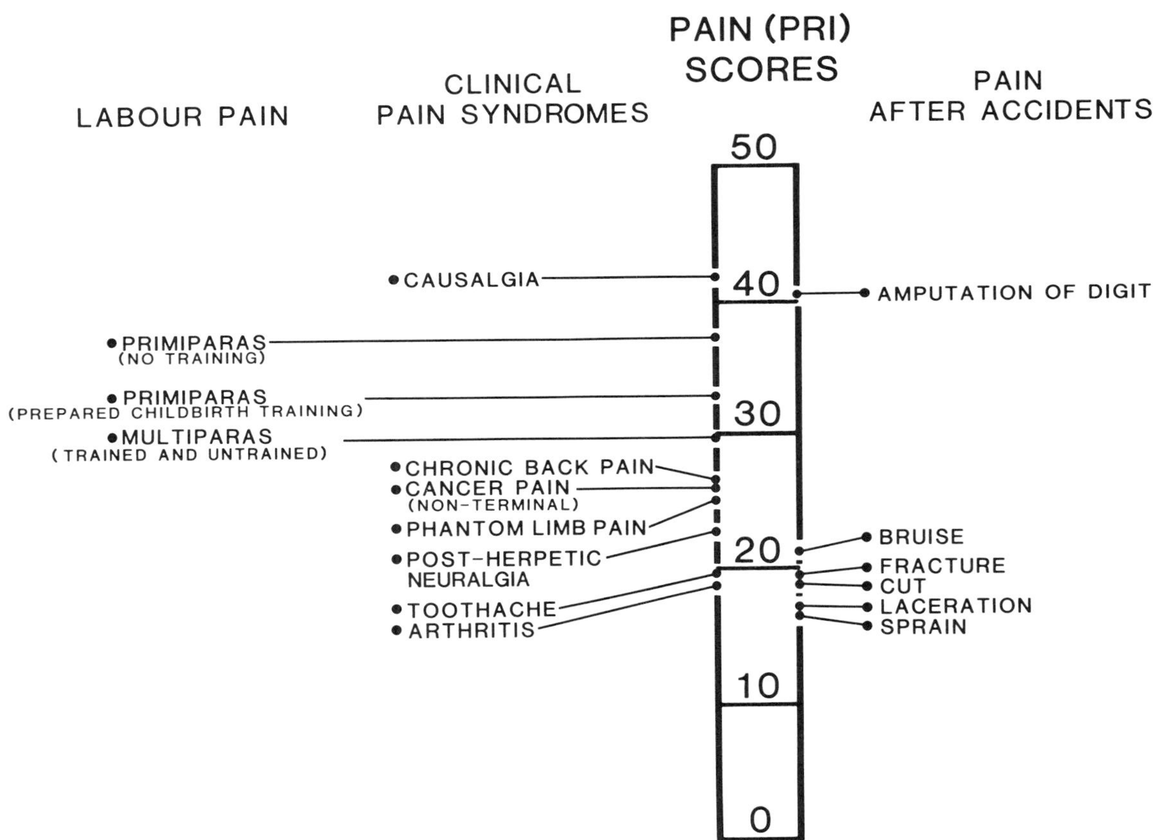

FIG. 25-5. Comparison of pain scores, using the McGill Pain Questionnaire, obtained from women during labor[37] and from patients in a general hospital pain clinic[30] and an emergency department.[41] The pain score for causalgic pain is reported by Tahmoush.[50]

given therapy, but, happily, the effects of two or more therapies given in combination are cumulative. Two therapies, each with slight effects that do not reach statistical significance, may produce significant reductions in pain when given together.[35,42] For this reason, *multiple convergent therapy* increasingly is becoming the standard psychological approach to pain problems. Biofeedback, hypnosis, and stress-inoculation training may each produce small effects. Two of the procedures together may have a large, significant effect; however, multiple convergent therapy does not refer only to psychological approaches. A psychological method may be used in combination with anesthetic blocks, analgesic or antidepressant drugs, or sensory modulation procedures.

The data indicate that multiple convergent therapy using several psychological procedures is effective because each kind of therapy may have its predominant effect on a different mechanism. Relaxation, for example, may reduce muscle tension and generally reduce activity in the sympathetic nervous system. Hypnosis, however, may have its predominant effect by activating control processes that modulate the input as it is transmitted through the brain. Procedures that involve the diversion of attention (so that even spinal reflexes may fail to occur) may, conceivably, activate the descending systems of the brain stem so that inputs are modulated at spinal levels. It is evident, then, that different psychological approaches can have powerful effects on pain. There are, however, limitations to the procedures, and it is important to recognize them. By doing so, we set the stage for new approaches, or the use of old approaches in different combinations. The field is young and growing rapidly. It holds great promise as an approach by itself or together with the powerful yet simple methods of sensory modulation that we are also just beginning to understand.

REFERENCES

1. Anderson, T.P., Cole, T.M., Gullickson, G., Hudgens, A., *et al.*: Behavior modification of chronic pain: A treatment program by a multidisciplinary team. J. Clin. Orthop., *129*:96, 1977.
2. Beecher, H.K.: Measurement of Subjective Responses. New York, Oxford University Press, 1959.
3. Benson, H., Kotch, J.B., Crassweller, K.D., and Greenwood, M.: Historical and clinical considerations of the relaxation response. American Scientist, *65*:441, 1977.
4. Benson, H., Pomeranz, B., and Katz, I.: The relaxation response and pain. *In* Wall, P.D., and Melzack, R. (eds.): Textbook of Pain. Edinburgh, Churchill Livingstone, 1984.
5. Bonica, J.J.: The Management of Pain. Philadelphia, Lea & Febiger, 1953.
6. Bonica, J.J.: Organization and function of a pain clinic, *In* Bonica, J.J. (ed.): Advances in Neurology. vol. 4. New York, Raven Press, 1974.
7. Carlen, P.L., Wall, P.D., Nadvorna, H., and Steinbach, T.: Phantom limbs and related phenomena in recent traumatic amputations. Neurology, *28*:211, 1978.
8. Clark, W.C., and Clark, S.B.: Pain responses in Nepalese porters. Science, *209*:410, 1980.
9. Dennis, S.G., and Melzack, R.: Pain-signalling systems in the dorsal and ventral spinal cord. Pain, *4*:97, 1977.
10. Dick-Read, G.: Childbirth without Fear. New York, Harper & Row, 1944.
11. Dubuisson, D., and Melzack, R.: Classification of clinical pain descriptions by multiple group discriminant analysis. Exp. Neurol., *51*:480, 1976.
12. Egbert, L.D., Battit, G.E., Welch, C.D., and Bartlett, M.K.: Reduction of post-operative pain by encouragement and instruction of patients. N. Engl. J. Med., *270*:825, 1964.
13. Evans, F.J.: The placebo response in pain reduction. *In* Bonica, J.J. (ed.): Advances in Neurology. vol. 4. New York, Raven Press, 1974.
14. Fordyce, W.E.: Behavioral Methods for Chronic Pain and Illness. St. Louis, MO, C.V. Mosby, 1976.
15. Gardner, W.J., and Licklider, J.C.R.: Auditory analgesia in dental operations. J. Am. Dent. Assn., *59*:1144, 1959.
16. Hall, K.R.L., and Stride, E.: The varying response to pain in psychiatric disorders: A study in abnormal psychology. Br. J. Med. Psychol., *27*:48, 1954.
17. Hardy, J.D., Wolff, H.G., and Goodell, H.: Pain Sensations and Reactions. Baltimore, Williams & Wilkins, 1952.
18. Hilgard, E.R., and Hilgard, J.: Hypnosis in the Relief of Pain. Los Altos, CA, Kaufmann, 1975.
19. Hill, H.E., Kornetsky, C.H., Flanary, H.G., and Wikler, A.: Effects of anxiety and morphine on discrimination of intensities of painful stimuli. J. Clin. Invest., *31*:473, 1952a.
20. Hill, H.E., Kornetsky, C.H., Flanary, H.G., and Wikler, A.: Studies of anxiety associated with anticipation of pain. I. Effects of morphine. Arch. Neurol. Psychiat., *67*:612, 1952b.
21. Horan, J.J., Layng, F.C., and Pursell, C.H.: Preliminary study of effects of "in vivo" emotive imagery in dental discomfort. Percept. Motor Skills, *42*:105, 1976.
22. Jessup, B.A., Newfield, R.W.J., and Merskey, H.: Biofeedback therapy for headache and other pain: An evaluative review. Pain, *7*:225, 1979.
23. Kamiya, J.: Conscious control of brainwaves. Psychology Today, *1*:56, 1968.
24. Lamaze, F.: Painless Childbirth: Psychoprophylactic Method. Chicago, Regnery, 1970.
25. Lambert, W.E., Libman, E., and Poser, E.G.: Effect of increased salience of membership group on pain tolerance. J. Pers., *28*:350, 1960.
26. Langer, E., Janis, I.L., and Wolfer, J.A.: Reduction of psychological stress in surgical patients. J. Exp. Soc. Psychol., *11*:155, 1975.
27. Lichstein, L., and Sackett, G.P.: Reactions by differentially

raised Rhesus monkeys to noxious stimulation. Dev. Psychobiol., *4*:339, 1971.

28. Martinez–Urrutia, A.: Anxiety and pain in surgical patients. J. Consult. Clin. Psychol., *43*:437, 1975.
29. McGlashan, T.H., Evans, F.J., and Orne, M.T.: The nature of hypnotic analgesia and placebo response to experimental pain. Psychosom. Med., *31*:227, 1969.
30. Melzack, R.: The McGill Pain Questionnaire: Major properties and scoring methods. Pain, *1*:277, 1975.
31. Melzack, R.: Pain Measurement and Assessment. New York, Raven Press, 1984.
32. Melzack, R., and Casey, K.L.: Sensory, motivational, and central control determinants of pain: A new conceptual model. *In* Kenshalo, D. (ed.): The Skin Senses. Springfield, IL, Charles C. Thomas, 1968.
33. Melzack, R., Katz, J. and Jeans, M.E.: The role of compensation in chronic pain: Analysis using a new method of scoring the McGill Pain Questionnaire. Pain, *23*:101, 1985.
34. Melzack, R., and Loeser, J.D.: Phantom body pain in paraplegics: Evidence for a central "pattern generating mechanism" for pain. Pain, *4*:195, 1978.
35. Melzack, R., and Perry, C.: Self-regulation of pain: The use of alpha-feedback and hypnotic training for the control of chronic pain. Exp. Neurol., *46*:452, 1975.
36. Melzack, R., and Scott, T.H.: The effects of early experience on the response to pain. J. Comp. Physiol. Psychol., *50*:155, 1957.
37. Melzack, R., Taenzer, P., Feldman, P., and Kinch, R.A.: Labour is still painful after prepared childbirth training. Can. Med. Assoc. J., *125*:357, 1981.
38. Melzack, R., and Torgerson, W.S.: On the language of pain. Anesthesiology, *34*:50, 1962.
39. Melzack, R., and and Wall, P.D.: Pain Mechanism: A new theory. Science, *150*:971, 1965.
40. Melzack R., and Wall, P.D.: The Challenge of Pain. New York, Basic Books, 1982.
41. Melzack, R., Wall, P.D., and Ty, T.C.: Acute pain in an emergency clinic: Latency of onset and descriptor patterns. Pain, *14*:33, 1982.
42. Melzack, R., Weisz, A.Z., and Sprague, L.T.: Stratagems for controlling pain: Contributions of auditory stimulation and suggestion. Exp. Neurol., *8*:239, 1963.
43. Mendelson, G.: Compensation, pain complaints, and psychological disturbance. Pain, *20*:169, 1984.
44. Rybstein–Blinchik, E.: Effects of different cognitive stratagies on chronic pain experience. J. Behav. Med., *2*:93, 1979.
45. Scott, J., and Huskisson, E.C.: Graphic representation of pain. Pain, *2*:175, 1979.
45. Sheehan, P.W., and Perry, C.W.: Methodologies of Hypnosis: A Critical Appraisal of Contemporary Paradigms of Hypnosis. Hillsdale, NJ, Erlbaum Associates, 1976.
47. Silver, B.V., and Blanchard, E.G.: Biofeedback and relaxation training in the treatment of psychophysical disorders: Or, are the machines really necessary? J. Behav. Med., *1*:217, 1978.
48. Sternbach, R.A., and Timmermans, G.: Personality changes associated with reduction of pain. Pain, *1*:177, 1975.
49. Sternbach, R.A., and Tursky, B.: Ethnic differences among housewives in psychophysical and skin potential responses to electric shock. Psychophysiology, *1*:73, 1965.
50. Tahmoush, A.J.: Causalgia: Redefinition as a clinical pain syndrome. Pain, *10*:187, 1981.
51. Tan, S.-Y.: Cognitive and cognitive-behavioral methods for pain control: A selective review. Pain, *12*:201, 1982.
52. Turk, D.C., and Genest, M.: Regulation of pain: The application of cognitive and behavioral techniques for prevention and remediation. In Kendall, P.C., and Hollon, S.D. (eds.): Cognitive-Behavioral Interventions: Theory, Research and Procedures. New York, Academic Press, 1979.
53. Turk, D.C., Meichenbaum, D.H., and Berman, W.H.: Application of biofeedback for the regulation of pain: A critical review. Psychol. Bull., *86*:1322, 1979.
54. Zborowski, M.: Cultural components in responses to pain. J. Soc. Issues, *8*:16, 1952.

26 ACUTE PAIN MANAGEMENT

D. BRUCE SCOTT

Acute pain in most cases is a valuable physiologic reaction to an acute pathologic event. In the case of a bony fracture the pain prevents excessive movement, identifies the bone concerned, and helps immobilize the affected parts. Pain caused by stones in the kidney, ureter, bladder, or gallbladder again identifies the underlying cause. Ischemic pain such as angina or claudication warns the patient to rest.

When the acute pain continues, however, its physiologic benefit is less easy to discern. In what way does continuing toothache or earache help the sufferer? Clearly once a definitive diagnosis has been made, relieving the pain will be an important part, albeit noncurative, of the patient's treatment. On the other hand, the definitive treatment of the condition frequently will quickly relieve the pain, for example, reducing a dislocation or evacuating an abscess. When this cannot be done, some form of analgesia will be needed.

The choice of analgesia in such cases will be between analgesic drugs and regional anesthesia. The former have the great advantage that they are simple to prescribe and administer and they can be used in many conditions in which regional anesthesia could not be used, for example, the toothache and earache mentioned above. The place for regional anesthesia is limited but nevertheless should be considered in some situations, particularly if systemic analgesics have proved ineffective.

Blockade of sensory nerves subserving an area of the body involved in acute pain can produce total relief for that pain, but ways and means have to be found to prolong the nerve block for the duration of the pain, since most local anesthetic drugs have a relatively short-lived effect.

Acute pain should be treated only if a definitive diagnosis has been made and the resultant analgesia will not affect clinical assessments with regard to the diagnosis and progress of the underlying cause. The most common cause of acute pain is trauma, and in this respect the anesthesiologist will be most concerned with the alleviation of postoperative pain. In most other cases of traumatic pain, the anesthesiologist will usually be called only to anesthetize the patient while the necessary surgery is carried out. There are instances, however, in which the continuing pain from trauma, after its initial treatment, can be relieved with a local anesthetic technique much to the patient's benefit (Fig. 26-1).

There are, in addition, a limited number of conditions in which neural blockade can be used to treat pain. Because of its importance, postoperative pain will be considered separately in this chapter. Other forms of acute pain amenable to neural blockade will be divided into those mediated by somatic sensory nerves and those by autonomic sensory nerves.

ACUTE PAIN INVOLVING SOMATIC SENSORY NERVES

TRAUMATIC PAIN

Like postoperative pain, the pain of fractures and other traumatic conditions often poses considerable problems in providing continuous adequate analgesia. This is especially so in the case of those bony fractures that are difficult to immobilize. Thus a parenteral opioid may produce considerable relief to a patient with a fractured shaft of the femur, but any movement involving the thigh will still cause great distress. In such cases a femoral nerve block will not

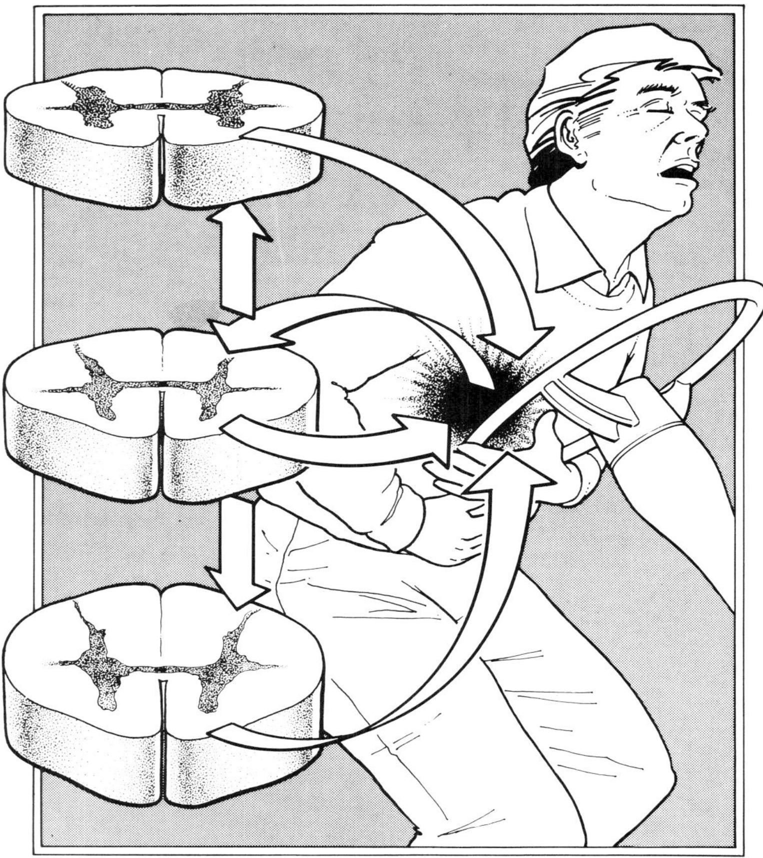

FIG. 26-1. Acute pain and trauma. Muscle "splinting" may result in severe compromise of respiratory function and may serve a protective role until intra-abdominal and intrathoracic trauma have been diagnosed. As soon as this is accomplished, however, pain must be relieved. (Reproduced with permission from Cousins, M.J., and Phillips, G.D. (eds.): Acute Pain Management. In Clinics in Critical Care Medicine. Edinburgh, Churchill Livingstone, 1986.)

TABLE 26-1. ACUTE PAIN INVOLVING SOMATIC SENSORY NERVES

Condition	Regional Technique	Drug and Administration
Fractured femur	Femoral nerve block	10 ml 0.5% bupivacaine intermittently via indwelling cannula
Fractured humerus	Brachial plexus block, interscalene or supraclavicular	30 ml 0.25% bupivacaine intermittently via indwelling cannula
Fractured ribs (up to four in number)	Intercostal nerve block just posterior to fracture	2–4 ml 0.5% bupivacaine for each nerve, intermittently. Because of subpleural spread, it may suffice to inject one intercostal space with 10 to 20 ml 0.5% bupivacaine
Fractured ribs, multiple	Thoracic epidural	4–6 ml 0.5% bupivacaine followed by 0.125%, 10 ml/hr continuously through epidural cannula. Adjust according to need
Supraspinatus tendon hematoma	Local infiltration	2–5 ml 0.25% bupivacaine
Poisonous bite	Local infiltration	5–10 ml 0.25% bupivacaine

only relieve the pain completely but will allow the painless reduction of the fracture and the setting up of traction (see Chap. 11).[4] Fracture of the shaft of the humerus is almost impossible to immobilize unless the patient is upright. If perforce the supine position has to be used, for example, during ventilator treatment of multiple fractured ribs, the pain can become intolerable since the shoulder tends to move with respiration. A continuous brachial plexus block is very efficacious in such cases (see Chap. 10). A fracture of even a single rib is a most painful event, and excellent relief can be obtained by intercostal nerve block. Underlying pulmonary disease can make treatment with opioids hazardous because of the inability of the patient to cough. Multiple fractured ribs can give rise to severe respiratory problems, and positive pressure respiration has proved life saving. In recent years, however, total relief of the pain with continuous thoracic epidural block has avoided the respiratory problems in many cases (see Chap. 8).[17,20,21]

Plaster casts must be used cautiously in the treatment of fractures, since pain is a major warning sign of ischemia owing to compression by the plaster. Fortunately the immobilization of a fracture within a plaster cast confers, of itself, considerable analgesia.

NONTRAUMATIC PAIN

Most nontraumatic pain involving somatic sensory nerves is due to infection and is unsuitable for treatment with regional anesthesia. Acute back pain or sciatica is often caused by sudden movement or exertion, but the amount of pain is disproportionate to the degree of trauma. Patients are almost always treated with bed rest and analgesics. If the pain persists, however, and the diagnosis is clear, treatment with an epidural or facetal block might be considered (see Chap. 27).

Supraspinatous tendon hematoma often has an acute onset and is extremely painful. Simple local infiltration of local anesthetic with or without steroid induces rapid effective relief (see Chap. 27).

Local infiltration is very useful but seldom considered in the treatment of a painful bite from a poisonous insect or animal. Scorpion bites are extremely painful; the pain can be relieved rapidly and completely by local infiltration. If the bite is life threatening, for example, snake bite, relief of the pain will not remove the need to watch the patient closely and to give appropriate antivenom therapy.

ACUTE PAIN INVOLVING AUTONOMIC NERVES

The most common cause of acute pain subserved by autonomic nerves is that associated with uterine contractions. The relief of pain in labor is discussed in Chapter 18.

There remain a few conditions that are extremely painful and in which regional anesthesia can be effective. Stones within the upper urinary tract are a good example, especially when conservative treatment has been decided on and permanent relief will occur only when the stone reaches the bladder. If satisfactory analgesia cannot be obtained with opioids, continuous epidural block or lumbar sympathetic block can be considered (see Chaps. 8, 13).[5,35,59]

Acute pancreatitis has been treated with epidural,[10,48] celiac plexus,[11] or splanchnic nerve block.[37] It is vitally important, however, to have established the diagnosis, preferably by laparotomy, before relieving the pain in this way. The pancreas is supplied by the greater splanchnic nerves deriving fibers from T7, T8, and T9. An epidural block covering these segments will relieve the pain of pancreatitis and improve respiratory function. In addition, it prevents splanchnic vasoconstriction and may relax the sphincter of Oddi (see Chaps. 8, 13).

Herpes zoster in its acute stage is often not referred to an anesthesiologist, but a sympathetic block, for example, stellate ganglion block, can relieve the pain and may prevent the onset of chronic herpetic pain (see Chap. 13).

POSTOPERATIVE PAIN

One of the more obvious benefits of regional anesthesia is the degree of analgesia it provides in the immediate postoperative period. Clearly, a technique that can be used for the surgical procedure is going to give near-perfect analgesia, provided the nerve block outlasts the duration of surgery.

It seems an obvious step, therefore, to try to achieve prolongation of the effect into the hours or days following the operation. Such prolongation is not difficult to achieve, yet it is seldom used except by enthusiasts or in intensive care units where sufficient staff to continue the nerve block and monitor its effects are available. Thus, although there is no lack of knowledge as to how regional analgesia could be used, the practical difficulties of managing patients in a standard surgical ward seem to be insurmountable in many centers.

TABLE 26-2. ACUTE PAIN INVOLVING AUTONOMIC SENSORY NERVES

Condition	Regional Technique	Drug and Administration
Stone in upper urinary tract	Epidural	0.25–0.5% bupivacaine 5–10 ml intermittently or continuous infusion of 10–15 ml/hr of 0.125%
Acute pancreatitis	Celiac plexus	20–40 ml of 0.25% bupivacaine intermittently using indwelling catheter inserted under x-ray control
	Splanchnic nerve block (bilateral)	5–10 ml of 0.25% bupivacaine for each side. Catheters inserted under x-ray control and injections made intermittently
	Thoracic epidural block	Catheter inserted at intervertebral space between T10–T11 or T11–T12. 5–8 ml 0.5% bupivacaine intermittently or continuous infusion 0.125% 10–15 ml/hr
Acute herpes zoster involving head and neck	Stellate ganglion block	5–10 ml 0.25% bupivacaine intermittently through indwelling cannula

In this, of course, it does not differ much from the more widespread use of systemic opioids, which are seldom given in an optimal way and are not individually tailored to the patient's need. It is not surprising, therefore, that postoperative pain relief is a largely unsolved medical problem and has driven most anesthesiologists to a state of therapeutic nihilism exemplified by the prescription of intramuscular opioids p.r.n.

Much more could be done with regional anesthesia without undue risk to the patient if only the anesthesiologist would contemplate the possibility. This chapter will describe several techniques that can be used for postoperative pain relief but will exclude intraspinal opioids, which are discussed in Chapter 28.

GENERAL PRINCIPLES

Although most operations can be performed under regional anesthesia, which should therefore be able to obtund all pain from the operative site, it is idle to think that 100% analgesia can be achieved in 100% of patients using regional anesthesia alone. Postoperative pain does not arise only in the wound but is often multifactorial.[12a] Wound pain, when it is unrelieved, concentrates the patient's mind so that little else worries him. Remove that pain, and many and varied are the other discomforts which then appear and, if unrelieved, become intolerable. Thus a patient with a totally analgesic abdominal wound may be made extremely uncomfortable by visceral pain, shoulder pain owing to diaphragmatic irritation, nasogastric tubes, and even intravenous drips. All these discomforts become less bearable if long periods of insomnia must also be endured (Fig. 26-2); because none are of themselves very painful, they are easily relieved by modest doses of parenteral analgesics, which would seldom relieve the pain of the wound. Morphine, 10 mg intramuscularly (even p.r.n.), now becomes a highly effective prescription and, by having sedative properties, allows the patient to sleep, with little risk of respiratory depression.

Having performed a nerve block that has totally relieved the wound pain, it is disappointing when the patient still complains bitterly, and it is understandable that one becomes disenchanted with the method. The anesthesiologist should therefore not expect a regional anesthetic technique to be the sole method of relieving postoperative pain. Although it may be achieved in some patients, it is no more illogical to give parenteral drugs in addition than it is to give similar agents during surgery performed under regional anesthesia.

Patients frequently (and understandably) have a different perception of analgesia from that of the medical and nursing staff, particularly with regard to the time-course of the pain. The anesthesiologist who achieves good analgesia for 16 hours out of the first 24 postoperatively will believe that he has done a good, even a superb, job. The patient who has had severe pain for four periods of 2 hours is unlikely to agree. It is therefore preferable to speak about pain prevention rather than analgesia, and methods that do not have painful gaps between reapplication are much the best. Thus a steady-state of therapeutic effect should be the goal, so that peaks and troughs are avoided.

Regional anesthesia for postoperative pain should in the main be concentrated on the operative wound site. Blockade of nerves for prolonged periods has to be done with care, and the fewer nerves blocked the better. Thus, although the best operating conditions for a lower abdominal operation may be achieved by blocking the T5–S5 spinal nerves, postoperatively the block should ideally be confined to the T9–T12 nerves. Widespread nerve block will have profound effects on autonomic and motor function, which will contribute little to postoperative analgesia. Hypotension and inability to move the lower limbs or micturate are obvious disadvantages and should be avoided. Autonomic block, however, has advantages in blocking the surgical stress reactions,[29] increasing blood flow to the lower limbs,[39] and improving gastrointestinal motility.[44]

The benefits of relieving pain after operation are by no means confined to humanitarian considerations.

Regional anesthesia has many advantages over general anesthesia, but often these advantages cease when the nerve block wears off. For example, the surgical stress response can be greatly modified by regional anesthesia, but the response will develop whenever pain appears.[30] Thus a significant reduction in surgical stress will be apparent only when the regional anesthesia is continued well into the postoperative period (see Chap. 5). Protection against deep venous thrombosis to the lower limbs, by increasing the blood flow, will depend on the duration of the sympathetic blockade in those limbs. Gastrointestinal function is severely depressed by opioid drugs,[43] and if the amount of these agents can be reduced or their effects opposed by sympathetic blockade, so much the better. Thus to obtain these kinds of advantages, the regional analgesia must be continued for at least 24 hours and sometimes longer.

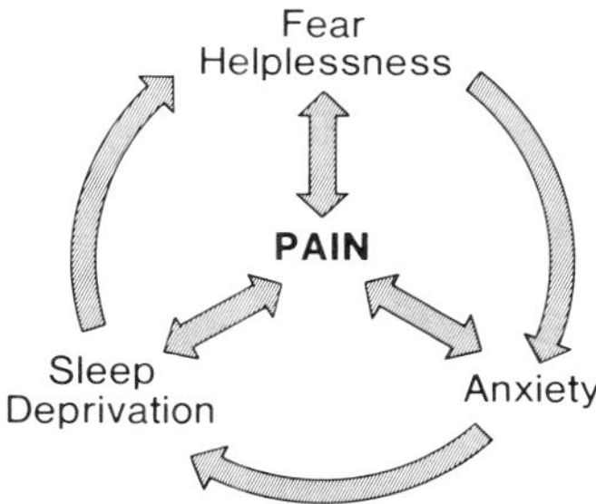

FIG. 26-2. Vicious cycle of pain, anxiety, sleep deprivation. Relief of pain helps reduce anxiety and sleeplessness; however, it is necessary to use appropriate psychological and pharmacologic measures aimed specifically at anxiety and sleeplessness. If pain remains unrelieved for days, anger and depression also begin to add to the vicious cycle as patients become demoralized and lose confidence in the ability (and motivation) of their medical attendants to relieve their pain. (Reproduced with permission from Cousins, M.J., and Phillips, G.D. (eds.): Acute Pain Management: In Clinics in Critical Care Medicine. Edinburgh, Churchill Livingstone, 1986.)

TECHNIQUES

Using regional anesthetic techniques for postoperative pain relief does not, by any means, always involve the more major forms of nerve blockade. Many minor operations, for example, removal of a toenail or anal stretch, can be very painful, although the pain is of relatively short duration. In these, excellent analgesia can be achieved by using a local anesthetic method for the operation itself, relying on the duration of the block to outlast the potential painful period. In this, the use of long-acting drugs is recommended. The duration of a nerve block is directly related to the dose of local anesthetic,[5] and if postoperative pain relief is a prime objective, then solutions of higher concentration of long-acting local anesthetic agents are indicated provided there are no implications regarding toxicity or inappropriate motor blockade. Thus a digital ring block using plain 0.75% bupivacaine, although a much greater concentration than is required for surgery, would give many hours of analgesia.

In children it is common practice to combine a regional technique with general anesthesia (see Chap. 21). The ability of the regional anesthesia to allow recovery of consciousness with the child remaining free of pain is a major advantage.

Even when the anesthesia does not involve a regional technique, excellent analgesia can be obtained by injecting local anesthetic at the end of surgery while the patient is still unconscious. Thus intercostal blocks can provide many hours of useful analgesia after a cholecystectomy performed under general anesthesia.[46]

The techniques that can be used will be divided into infiltration, minor, major, and central nerve blocks.

Local Infiltration

Infiltration of local anesthetic into a surgical wound can produce analgesia at the operative site lasting several hours,[50,51] particularly if epinephrine is added. With day case surgery being used more frequently for operations such as inguinal hernia or varicose vein ligation, patients may be made much more comfortable by local infiltration of the areas to be incised, even if general anesthesia is being used. Plastic surgery is particularly suitable for this approach (see Chap. 19).

In more major surgery, there has been renewed interest in repeated irrigation of wounds with local anesthetic solutions.[73] For this a multihole catheter is left in place under the skin and the muscle layers of the incision, and injections of local anesthetic, for example, bupivacaine 0.125%, are made intermittently. Good analgesia of the wound is claimed, but the method should be augmented by parenteral opioids. It is of interest that normal saline irrigated in the same way also appears to have an analgesic effect.[34]

It has been suggested that bupivacine used for intravenous regional anesthesia (Bier's block), which is a form of infiltration, could give a useful period of postoperative analgesia. The dose required for this, however, was prohibitively high and cannot be recommended (see Chap. 12).

TABLE 26-3. METHODS OF NEURAL BLOCKADE IN POSTOPERATIVE PAIN: LOCAL INFILTRATION OF SURGICAL WOUNDS

Method	Drug and Dose
Single injection into wound	Bupivacaine 10–20 ml 0.5% at end of surgery
Continuous irrigation	Bupivacaine 10–20 ml 0.125% twice daily through catheter

Minor Nerve Blocks

Many small nerves not only are anatomically easy to block, but also remain blocked for many hours with standard doses of local anesthetic.

Digital nerve blocks of fingers and toes are easily performed by ring blocks at the proximal end of the digit. Removal of a toenail is a very painful procedure, the pain lasting a substantial time afterward. Often a ring block is not considered if the surgeon requests a tourniquet proximal to the foot, and general anesthesia is given instead. If a ring block were performed as well, the amount of general anesthetic would be greatly reduced, and several hours of postoperative analgesia would also be provided.

Wrist blocks, although simple to do, are also infrequently used because a tourniquet on the upper arm is often required. Personal preference will decide whether the operation is performed under Bier's block, brachial plexus block, or general anesthesia. Nevertheless, in many patients, the additional blockade of the terminal parts of the median, radial, and ulnar nerves at the wrist will give significant analgesia following hand surgery (see Chap. 10).

Ankle blocks are in a similar category. The saphenous, deep and superficial peroneal, sural, and plantar nerves are all readily available for blockade, which will decrease the requirement for general anesthesia and provide several hours of increased patient comfort (see Chap. 11).[63]

The iliohypogastric and ilioinguinal nerves can be blocked as they run forward in proximity to the anterior superior iliac spine and the inguinal ligament. The injection of local anesthetic in this area will render an inguinal hernia wound analgesic for several hours. The terminal branches of the genitofemoral nerve can also be blocked by direct infiltration of the spermatic cord. In outpatient surgery, the patient can be transported home pain free at the completion of surgery, and this will greatly assist in patient management (see Chaps. 14 and 21).

The dorsal nerve of the penis is a branch of the pudendal nerve and supplies most of the shaft and glans of the penis. It can be blocked on each side of the superior portion of the penis at the pubic bone, allowing the painless performance of circumcision and providing postoperative pain relief (see Chap. 21).

TABLE 26-4. METHODS OF NEURAL BLOCKADE IN POSTOPERATIVE PAIN: MINOR NERVE BLOCKS

Method	Indications	Drug and Dose
Digital ring block	Ingrowing toenail. Operations on fingers or toes	Bupivacaine (plain) 2-3 ml 0.5%
Wrist block	Operations on hand not affected by prolonged anesthesia, *e.g.*, Dupuytren's contracture	Bupivacaine 6-10 ml 0.5%
Ankle block	Foot operations	Bupivacaine 10-15 ml 0.5%
Iliohypogastric and ilioinguinal nerve block	Hernia repair	Bupivacaine 5-8 ml 0.5%
Dorsal nerve of the penis blockade	Circumcision	Bupivacaine 4-6 ml 0.5%

Major Nerve Blocks

The blockade of several nerves or a major nerve plexus will produce widespread analgesia that can be used postoperatively. The greater the number of nerves involved, the larger is the amount of associated dysfunction, and this should be weighed against the advantages of the analgesia. For example, a prolonged brachial plexus block will produce a painless but paralyzed upper limb. If the surgery is confined to the hand, it might be more appropriate to perform a wrist block for analgesia at the end of surgery.

Brachial plexus blockade can be indefinitely extended postoperatively by the simple method of leaving a plastic cannula within the neurovascular sheath of the plexus. A needle and cannula as used for intravenous infusions are ideal for performing a brachial plexus block. If paresthesia is being sought to identify correct placement, the withdrawal of the needle leaving the blunt plastic cannula *in situ* will largely obviate the possibility of direct injection into a nerve. If a nerve stimulator is being used, it is again ideal since only the needle tip is uninsulated. Having withdrawn the needle, the anesthesiologist can firmly tape the cannula in place and make injections of local anesthetic at will (see Chaps. 10, 27.2).

The block will usually cause paralysis of the whole limb, which must be well supported with a sling to avoid swelling of the hand. Other potentially undesirable side-effects are Horner's syndrome caused by stellate ganglion blockade and phrenic nerve block.

Femoral nerve block is a relatively simple procedure and produces analgesia of the shaft of the femur.[4] Patients who require traction or who have undergone surgery for a shaft fracture will benefit from such a block. Again, if it is necessary, a cannula can be left in place for repeated injection (see Chaps. 11, 21).

Intercostal nerve block of the appropriate nerves can give very gratifying pain relief, especially after abdominal surgery. It is usually recommended that intercostal nerves be blocked close to the angle of the rib,[15] thus requiring the patient's back to be accessible for the injections. Recent studies, have shown, however, that injections into the intercostal space travel several centimeters in either direction from the needle tip.[41,45] Perfectly good blocks are thus obtainable in the midaxillary line and with much less disturbance to the patient. Likewise the use of large volumes of local anesthetic are generally unnecessary, 2 ml of 0.75% or 0.5% bupivacaine with epinephrine 1:200,000 for each nerve blocked being sufficient (see Chap. 14).

For abdominal surgery, the best results are obtained with a unilateral Kocher's incision, as used for cholecystectomy. This requires the blockade of the 7th to 11th intercostal nerves (and sometimes the 6th) on the right side.

Midline incisions will, of course, require bilateral intercostal blocks, and the results are not as impressive as those with a unilateral incision. For upper abdominal operations the 6th to 10th nerves should be blocked, and for lower abdominal incisions, the 8th to the 12th (more accurately the subcostal nerve) should be blocked. An appendectomy wound would require blockade of the 8th to 12th nerves on the right side only. Good results have been reported after flank incisions[14,45] by blocking T9-T12.

As mentioned above, intercostal block for postoperative pain is a good choice even if general anesthesia has been used for the operation. Much pain could

TABLE 26-5. METHODS OF NEURAL BLOCKADE IN POSTOPERATIVE PAIN: MAJOR NERVE BLOCKS

Method	Indications	Drug and Dose
Brachial plexus block	Operations on upper limb not affected by prolonged action	Bupivacaine 30–40 ml 0.25%
Femoral nerve block	Fractured shaft of femur	Bupivacaine 10 ml 0.5%
Intercostal nerve block	Abdominal surgery	Bupivacaine 2–3 ml 0.5% for each nerve
	Thoracic surgery	Cryoanalgesia

be prevented if anesthesiologists would consider spending only a few minutes at the end of surgery to perform this very simple block. The analgesia, of course, will only last as long as the block, and many find the repetition of the multiple nerve blocks rather daunting; however, if bupivacaine has been used in the higher concentration range, many hours of analgesia are obtainable. Even if the blocks are repeated, the actual discomfort to the patient (especially if he can remain recumbent) is minimal in relation to the relief obtained.

For thoracic operations, the situation is much more problematic. Thoracotomy wounds involve not only the intercostal space through which entry to the thorax is obtained, but also the muscles of the shoulder girdle. In addition, the parietal pleura will be involved, especially when large intercostal drains have been inserted. Although good results have been claimed, the amount of analgesia that is likely to accrue from intercostal blocks with local anesthetic drugs is relatively small. The best results have been obtained with cryoanalgesia,[28,47] the nerves being frozen under direct vision by the surgeon. Even then the analgesia is not outstanding until the drains are removed. Epidural block would appear to be the only regional anesthetic technique likely to succeed in this problem.[23]

The only complication of any import with intercostal block is pneumothorax. Provided the anesthesiologist keeps his needle tip in proximity to the rib, there is little danger that the pleura will be pierced. That possibility should, however, be remembered, and, if confirmed by radiography, a chest drain may have to be inserted (see Chap. 22).

In recent years there has been discussion that local anesthetic injected into a single intercostal space may spread subpleurally and affect several adjacent intercostal nerves. Anatomic evidence for and against this has been reported.[41,46] A clinical report has claimed, however, that a single intercostal injection of 20 ml of 0.5% bupivacaine at T9 is at least as effective as multiple intercostal nerve blocks, giving good analgesia to 87.5% of patients undergoing cholecystectomy.[32] Because only one injection site is used, a catheter may be left in place for repeated injections.

An even more novel method is the intrapleural injection of local anesthetic.[55] The pleural space is entered at the angle of a rib below the lower border of the lung using a standard epidural needle and catheter. Twenty milliliters of 0.5% bupivacaine is said to give several hours of unilateral analgesia, presumably by transpleural absorption of the local anesthetic into the intercostal nerves. The method has been used after both cholecystectomy and thoracotomy operations. The risk of pneumothorax is apparently very small, but time and further studies will quantify the risk/benefit of the procedure.

Central Nerve Blocks

For major abdominal and thoracic surgery, central nerve blocks offer the easiest method of producing widespread analgesia; however, they are also associated with a greater degree of autonomic block, which can have a profound physiologic effect on the patient. Thus a balance must be found between effective pain relief and possible danger. Autonomic dysfunction will affect cardiovascular control, gastrointestinal function, and micturition. The sympathetic outflow derives from the T1–L2 spinal segments, whereas the sacral parasympathetic nerves are from S1–S4. The cranial parasympathetic nerves are not involved, and the vagus nerve in particular will remain unblocked.

During surgery performed under epidural or spinal anesthesia, a widespread blockade of all modalities of nerve function, sensory, motor, and autonomic, is well tolerated (and even desirable) provided that the patient is adequately monitored by an experienced anesthesiologist. For postoperative pain relief this kind of supervision is not usually available. It is

TABLE 26-6. METHODS OF NEURAL BLOCKADE IN POSTOPERATIVE PAIN: CENTRAL NERVE BLOCKS

Method	Indications	Drug and Dose
Thoracic epidural block	Upper abdominal and thoracic operations	Bupivacaine intermittent injections 4-6 ml 0.5%. Continuous infusions 8-10 ml/hr of 0.1-0.125%
Lumbar epidural block	Lower abdominal, hip surgery, knee surgery	Bupivacaine intermittent injections 4-8 ml 0.5%. Continuous infusions 10-20 ml/hr of 0.1-0.125%
Cervical epidural block	Mastectomy	Bupivacaine 5-8 ml 0.25%
Spinal block	Hip and knee surgery	Bupivacaine 1-1.5 ml 0.5% plain

therefore necessary to restrict the nerve block to provide analgesia of the wound, leaving motor and autonomic function as unaffected as possible.

Catheter techniques, both epidural and spinal, offer the most convenient and practical methods of prolonged central nerve blockade. To achieve analgesia of the minimum number of spinal segments, the catheter tip ideally should be at the center of the required band of anesthesia, for example, T8 for upper abdominal incisions, T11 for lower abdominal, and L2 for hip surgery.

In attempting these very restricted levels of analgesia postoperatively, particularly with epidural blocks, there are two practical difficulties to overcome:

1. Small volumes of local anesthetic solutions do not always spread equally in the epidural space, and unilateral block is not uncommon.
2. Small volumes necessitate small doses, restricting the useful duration of effect. Thus an epidural injection of 10 ml of 0.5% bupivacaine gives pain relief for 1½ to 2 hours but involves several segments beyond the area of the required block. Five milliliters of the same solution, although restricted to the appropriate segments, will last only ¾ to 1 hour, that is, pain will appear as soon as regression begins to occur. If small bolus injections are used, they must be given frequently, for instance, hourly, and this requires some form of automatic injection pump, which is not readily available commercially.

The most practical way to achieve a restricted block is to use a continuous infusion of local anesthetic.[12a] The concentration and volume used are of great import. With a bupivacaine infusion of 0.5% solution at 5 ml/hr, too few segments may be blocked. Better results are obtained with 0.125% at 15 ml/hr or 0.1% at 20 ml/hr. The infusion rates can be varied up or down depending on the extent of the nerve block. When using dilute solutions, it is necessary initially to achieve a solid block with 0.5% solution. The 0.1% and 0.125% solutions can maintain a block but cannot achieve one or restore one that has worn off. If at any time the block regresses and pain reappears, it is necessary to top up with a small volume (5-8 ml) of the 0.5% solution.

In general, bupivacaine is the best drug to use because of its sparing effects on motor nerve fibers.

Unilateral block is probably the most common cause of failure and can be corrected only by topping up with 0.5% bupivacaine. It frequently helps if the catheter is withdrawn a centimeter or so before topping up to allow the injected solution to take another path and be distributed more evenly.

Lumbar epidural blockade at the L2-L3 or L3-L4 intervertebral space can produce excellent postoperative analgesia of the lower limbs and has been widely used with good results in hip replacements.[39] If the blockade can be restricted to an upper limit of T10 or T11, there is little or no risk of developing severe hypotension. The sympathetic innervation to the lower limbs derives from L1 and L2 and the reduction in vascular tone, and increased blood flow produced by nerve blockade considerably reduces the incidence of deep venous thrombosis and pulmonary embolus. This increase in lower limb blood flow is also of great value in major vascular surgery.[13]

For lower abdominal operations the catheter should be inserted between T11-T12 or T12-L1. The epidural space in this area is more superficial than in the midlumbar region but is easily identifiable. The catheter should not be inserted more than 2 to 3 cm and must be firmly fixed to the back with adhesive plaster. If the patient is topped up with 8 to 10 ml of 0.5% bupivacaine at the end of surgery, a continuous infusion of 15 ml/hr of 0.125% solution will maintain a blockade between T8 and L1 indefinitely in most patients. Motor paralysis is minimal after the motor effects of the 0.5% top-up dose have worn off. It is important to check the level of block occasionally and adjust the infusion rate appropriately.

Upper abdominal surgery requires a midthoracic catheter since the T6–T11 spinal nerves are the target nerves. Thus the epidural space should be entered between T7–T8, T8–T9, or T9–T10. This is a little more difficult than farther down, and the epidural needle must be considerably angled (see Chap. 8). Because of narrowing of the epidural space in this area, smaller volumes are usually required, for example, a top-up of 4 to 6 ml of 0.5% bupivacaine followed by 6 to 10 ml/hr of 0.125% solution.

Thoracic blocks can also be used for thoracic operations and are now popular for treating chest injuries.[17,20,21] The catheter site will depend on the nerves that need to be blocked. Again small doses will usually suffice, as with upper abdominal operations.

Cervical epidural blocks are seldom used either for surgery or for postoperative pain but can be highly effective in operations of the chest wall such as mastectomy.

Continuous spinal blockade, although used only rarely, is nevertheless gaining popularity in the management of elderly patients undergoing hip surgery. The advantages claimed are the reproducibility of the block[74] and the greatly reduced dosage as compared with epidural blockade. Catheter migration is not, of course, to be feared. Spinal puncture should be performed at the L3–L4 or L4–L5 interspaces and a catheter inserted 2 to 3 cm. Five milligrams to 7.5 mg of isobaric bupivacaine or tetracaine will usually suffice and can be repeated with appropriate adjustments as indicated by the extent of the block obtained. The block is usually maintained by top-up injections, continuous infusions not having been reported. The size of the needle required can be a problem (although spinal headache is surprisingly infrequent in this elderly age group), but fine catheters designed for use in pediatric epidural block are now becoming available. Obviously very strict aseptic precautions must be taken, and the blocks should be terminated after 24 to 36 hours to allow active movement of the legs.

PHYSIOLOGIC CHANGES ASSOCIATED WITH PROLONGED CENTRAL NERVE BLOCKS

Epidural and spinal blockade will affect all modalities of nerve function and lead to changes, sometimes profound, in the patient's physiology. Autonomic blockade of the sympathetic and pelvic parasympathetic nerves is most important, although loss of somatic sensory and motor function is not without effect.

The physiologic changes produced by central nerve block are described in detail in Chapter 8. Most studies of these changes have, however, been obtained from subjects not in pain, for example, patients about to undergo operative procedures or volunteers. Patients in pain in the postoperative period are somewhat different in that

1. The pain itself may produce a greater or smaller degree of sympathetic activity.
2. Hypovolemia may be present.
3. If a general anesthetic has been given, there will be a lack of vasomotor control for some hours in many cases.
4. The patient's general condition may be less than ideal.
5. Pain may be interfering with normal respiratory function.
6. Gastrointestinal function will be abnormal due to either opioid administration or operations on the gastrointestinal tract.

CARDIOVASCULAR EFFECTS

Central Hemodynamics

In a study of patients undergoing cholecystectomy in whom postoperative analgesia was achieved with a continuous epidural block (using an epidural infusion of 0.4% lidocaine), cardiac output was increased by 44% compared to preoperative measurements.[66] Heart rate was increased only by 12%, whereas mean arterial pressure was decreased by 11%. Allowing the epidural block to wear off the day after surgery caused an increase in both heart rate (10%) and arterial pressure (22%) without any substantial effect on cardiac output. Thus ventricular work and myocardial oxygen consumption increased considerably (Fig. 26-3).

A high degree of sympathetic activity in the postoperative period is often seen after coronary artery,

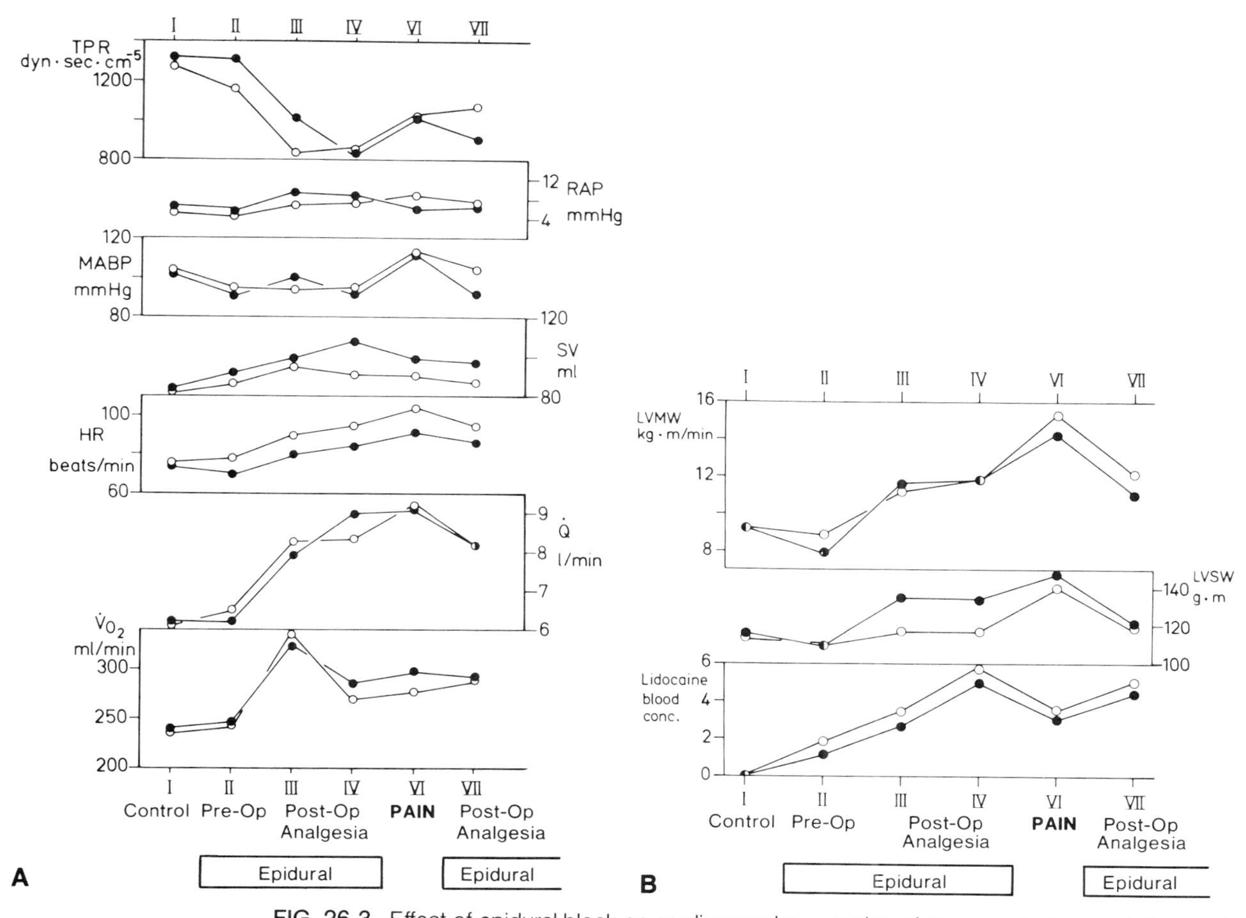

FIG. 26-3. Effect of epidural block on cardiovascular sequelae of severe pain. I, period of control CVS measurements; II, 30 minutes after epidural injection of 2% lidocaine either in the lumbar region, 15 ml *(open circles),* or the thoracic region, 8 ml *(closed circles);* III, 1 hour after cholecystectomy analgesia maintained with 0.4% lidocaine drip; IV, on the morning after surgery, after 17 hours of continuous pain relief by epidural; V, (not shown) pain returning, when epidural drip ceased for 30 to 60 minutes; VI, 60 to 90 minutes after epidural drip ceased, severe pain present; VII, 90 minutes after pain relief reestablished by epidural drip. **A.** Changes in total peripheral resistance (TPR); right atrial pressure (RAP); stroke volume (SV); heart rate (HR); cardiac output (Q); oxygen uptake (VO_2). **B.** Changes in left ventricular minute work (LVMW); left ventricular stroke work (LVSW) and lidocaine venous blood concentrations. *Note*: Pain is associated with increased TPR, MABP, HR, and CO, as well as with increased LVMW and LVSW. Pain relief by the thoracic epidural route restored all these variables to levels near those before the emergence of pain. Open circles = lumbar epidural; closed circles = thoracic epidural. (Reproduced with permission from Sjogren, S., Wright, B.: Circulatory changes during continuous epidural blockade. Acta Anaesthesiol. Scand. *16:*5–25, 1972.)

aortic, and vascular surgery. The consequent tachycardia and hypertension are likely to have deleterious effects, particularly in patients with coronary insufficiency. A central nerve block can restore more normal function by reducing sympathetic tone and blocking the sympathetic tone to the adrenal medulla. By instituting an epidural block in the upper thoracic segments after coronary artery surgery, arterial pressure decreased from 156/89 mm Hg to 105/60 mm Hg.[27] Because the cardiac output was also decreased by

15% (although still remaining within normal limits), there was a considerable decrease in myocardial oxygen consumption.

Similar advantageous effects of epidural block were seen in a study of patients all of whom had had a myocardial infarct within 3 months of undergoing major abdominal surgery.[56] Compared to neuroleptanesthesia, epidural block plus light general anesthesia did not increase myocardial oxygen consumption, and there were fewer incidents of ischemic ECG changes and arrhythmias.

After aortic surgery, arterial pressure was maintained at a significantly lower level (133 mm Hg systolic versus 155 mm Hg) when a continuous epidural block was used for postoperative pain compared to opioid infusion.[33]

An important consideration after major vascular surgery is the maintenance of blood flow through an arterial graft. Surgeons are apprehensive that any reduction in arterial pressure will reduce flow and encourage clotting within the graft; however, provided the decrease in pressure is not excessive, the flow through the graft will be increased considerably by epidural block owing to the lowered arterial resistance in the lower limbs.[13]

Hypotension is the most common effect of central blockade and must be regarded with respect, although its dangers are often greatly exaggerated. It can occur as a result of a reduction in cardiac output or peripheral resistance, or both. Hypotension resulting from vasodilatation, and unaccompanied by a significant fall in cardiac output, is relatively benign and is a common event in normal sleep. Hypotension occurring suddenly as a result of sympathetic blockade in a hypovolemic patient, however, is quite another matter. Vasovagal fainting also causes a dramatic decrease in arterial pressure but is almost always self-reversing, and the correct diagnosis (usually confirmed by the presence of marked bradycardia) is of great import (see Chap. 8).

Central nerve blocks reduce arterial pressure primarily by sympathetic blockade, which must be widespread enough to overcome any compensatory vasoconstriction in unblocked segments.[6] Thus hypotension is much more common in thoracic than in lumbar blocks. Moreover, if the sympathetic supply to the heart (T1 – T5) is affected, the heart may not be able to adjust to the changes in pressure. However, because upper thoracic blocks are rarely required for postoperative analgesia, this complication would occur only in an unexpected high block. Even so, in the absence of hypovolemia, any fall in cardiac output is commensurate with the heart rate reduction, stroke volume being unchanged.[38,49]

Widespread reduction in venous tone leads to a decrease in central venous pressure, although venous return remains within normal limits. The patient will, however, be sensitive to postural changes in the head-up position.

Thus hypotension occurring during the postoperative period may be due to

1. Sympathetic blockade alone. This will seldom cause a decrease in arterial pressure of more than 10% to 20%.
2. Hypovolemia such as unsuspected postoperative bleeding. Significant operative blood loss should have been replaced with appropriate amounts of blood or colloid during surgery; however, minor degrees of hypovolemia, which would have little effect in a normal patient, may precipitate a significant degree of hypotension in the presence of sympathetic blockade.[7]
3. Posture. Sympathectomized patients tolerate the head-up posture poorly. Even low blocks affecting only the lower limbs (L1 – L2) can cause pooling of 1 to 2 liters of blood. The sitting-up posture for postoperative patients is very popular with surgeons and nurses, but its benefits, if any, in the early postoperative period are minimal. Pooling of blood is the result of gravity and cannot occur with the patient lying supine or with his head slightly down.
4. Vasovagal fainting. This may result from changes in the sympathetic/parasympathetic balance brought on by the sympathetic blockade. It can also be triggered by mild hypotension or sudden changes in posture. In general, although dramatic at the time, particularly if accompanied by transient unconsciousness or temporary cardiac arrest, or both, it is self-limiting provided that the patient is not maintained in the head-up position. Treatment should be by posture (head down and legs raised) and by modest doses of vasopressor (ephedrine, 10 – 15 mg i.v.) if hypotension persists. Atropine is seldom effective.
5. Cardiovascular instability in the early postoperative period. This is probably the most common cause of hypotension in the first few hours after surgery and is not confined to patients receiving regional anesthesia. It is due to a lack of vasomotor control and can almost always be prevented by a prophylactic vasopressor given intramuscularly. Although usually quite benign if the patient is left

supine or head down, it can be treated with intravenous fluids or a vasopressor, or both.

Organ Blood Flow

Heart. Because both the oxygen supply and the demand of the myocardium are directly proportional to afterload, ischemia does not occur in normal hearts even with a very low arterial pressure. This may not be the case, however, in the presence of coronary artery disease because ECG evidence of myocardial ischemia has been seen at systolic pressures of 75 mm Hg.[9] The rate of decrease in arterial pressure is of import,[24] as is the heart rate. With a slow heart rate, diastole is prolonged, allowing adequate coronary perfusion. Although anesthesiologists and surgeons are impressed by, and often over-react to, hypotension, they should be more concerned by hypertension accompanied by tachycardia.[53] This combination, not infrequent after general anesthesia, is very uncommon during spinal or epidural block. Hypertension and tachycardia both cause a considerable increase in myocardial oxygen demand.

Brain. Cerebral blood flow is susceptible to rapid changes in arterial pressure and to posture. In the supine or head-down position, only a very low pressure would cause significant reductions in blood flow in conscious patients.

Lower limb blood flow is increased by sympathetic blockade even though arterial pressure may fall.[39] This increased flow is mostly to skin; muscle blood flow may actually decrease (Fig. 26-4). Nevertheless the entire flow must leave the lower limbs through

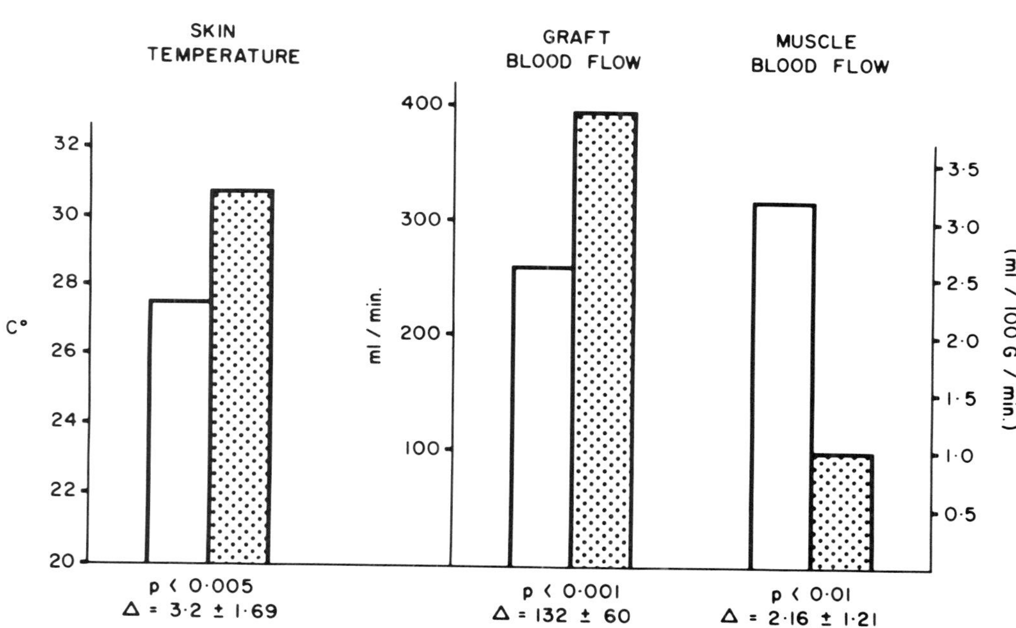

FIG. 26-4. Epidural block and blood flow in vascular surgical patients. Blood flow in femoral artery (electromagnetic flow meter) is increased, as is skin blood flow (skin temperature); however, muscle blood flow (^{133}Xe clearance) is reduced. Measurements were taken at the completion of vascular surgery, before epidural block, and then after epidural block. (Reproduced with permission from Cousins, M.J., and Wright, C.J.: Graft, muscle, skin blood flow after epidural block in vascular surgical procedures. Surg. Gynecol. Obstet., *133*:59, 1971.)

the femoral and iliac veins where the most dangerous thrombi are formed. Increasing the blood flow through these major veins has been the rationale for the early ambulation of postoperative patients. Nevertheless the very temporary increase in flow caused by muscular activity, undertaken for a few minutes at a time, should be compared with the sustained increase of about 100% seen with epidural block.[8] This has been shown to be of more than theoretical interest. Hip replacements have a high incidence of deep venous thrombosis, and continuous epidural analgesia for 24 hours postoperatively has produced a significant decrease in thrombus formation (particularly in the larger veins) and pulmonary embolism.[39] Thus only 13% developed thrombi in the popliteal and femoral veins, compared to 67% given opioid analgesia instead. The figures for pulmonary embolus (as detected by lung scan) were 10 and 33%, respectively.

It might be thought that relief of pain *per se* would increase lower limb blood flow by reducing sympathetic tone. This did not prove to be the case when epidural analgesia was compared with optimal analgesia using intravenous diamorphine, the latter having no effect on blood flow (Figs. 26-5, 26-6).[8]

Apart from the effects of neural blockade on blood flow, local anesthetics themselves have both a fibrinolytic and an antithrombotic effect,[40] along with a reduced incidence of leukocyte infiltration of damaged vein epithelium (see Chap. 5).[70]

Gastrointestinal Tract and Liver. Splanchnic and hepatic blood flow have been shown to increase in postoperative patients given a splanchnic block,[77] probably owing to vasodilation resulting from sympathetic block and an increase in gastrointestinal activity.

In dogs, spinal anesthesia has been shown to in-

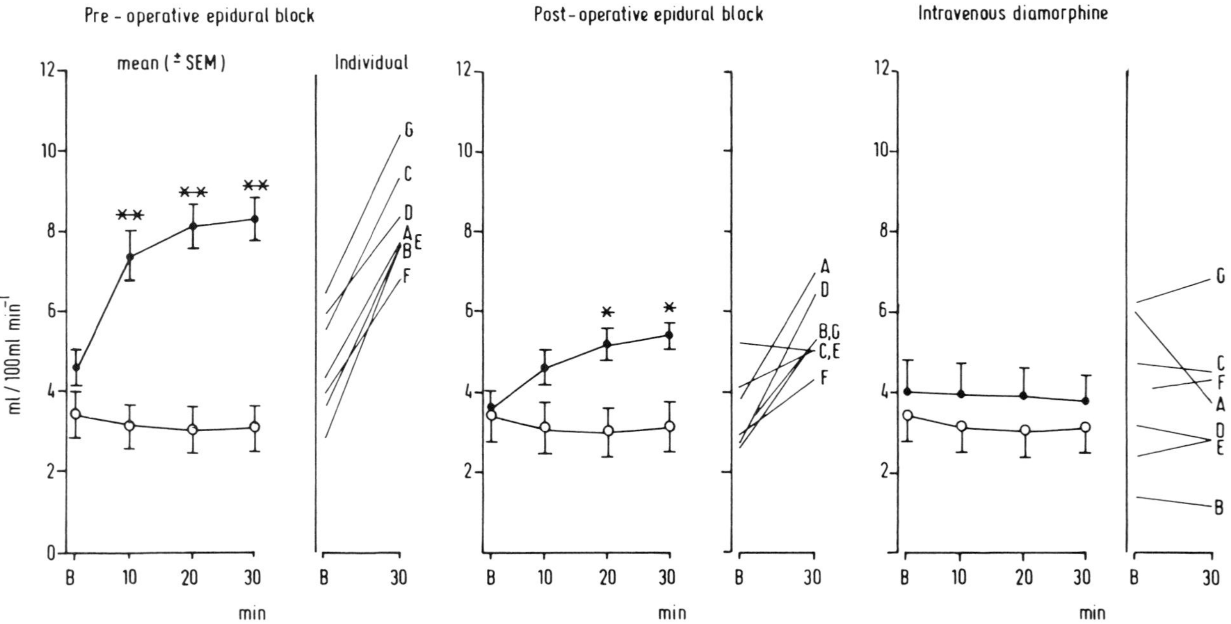

FIG. 26-5. Calf arterial flow was measured using venous occlusion plethysmography immediately before and on the day after lower abdominal surgery in seven patients. Ten milliliters of 0.5% bupivacaine was injected at the T11–T12 intervertebral space for the epidural block (EDB). Intravenous diamorphine was given until the patients were completely free of pain (mean dose 8.6 mg). EDB blockade was followed by an increase in leg blood flow, whereas i.v. diamorphine was not. Relief of pain *per se* does not result in the increased leg blood flow that follows EDB and that may be responsible for the reduced incidence of postoperative thromboembolism. ● = treatment measurements; O = control measurements; B = before injection; *$p < 0.05$; **$p < 0.01$. (Reproduced with permission from Bowler, G.M.R., Lamont, M.C., and Scott, D.B.: Effect of postoperative analgesia with extradural bupivacaine or intravenous diamorphine on calf blood flow. Br. J. Anaesth. [In Press].)

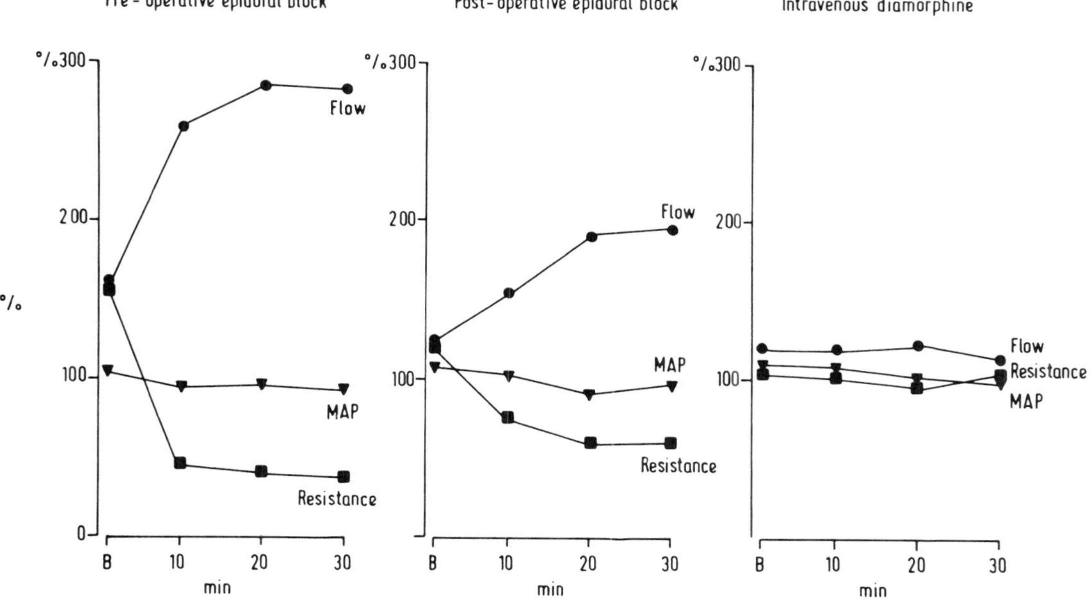

FIG. 26-6. Calf blood flow, mean arterial pressure (MAP), and derived arterial resistance in seven patients given epidural block using 10 ml of 0.5% bupivacaine at the T11–12 interspace before surgery and 24 hours after surgery. When pain reappeared after regression of block, i.v. diamorphine was given until complete analgesia was obtained, and the calf flow measurements were repeated. Preoperatively calf flow increased by 123% and postoperatively by 68% in response to epidural bupivacaine. (The control value 100% was measured either 24 hours before surgery or 8 days after surgery.) Intravenous diamorphine had no effect on calf blood flow. (Reproduced with permission from Bowler, G.M.R. Lamont, M.C., and Scott, D.B.: Effect of post-operative analgesia with extradural bupivacaine or intravenous diamorphine on calf blood flow. Br. J. Anaesth. [In Press].)

crease colonic blood flow by 22%[1]; this may be related to the lower incidence of colonic anastomosis dehiscence seen in patients receiving neural blockade instead of general anesthesia.[2]

Kidneys. High epidural block has been shown to cause a reduction in renal blood flow in normal volunteers[31] but not in sheep given a spinal block.[61] There are no data available from postoperative patients.

RESPIRATORY EFFECTS

Surgery, particularly thoracic and abdominal, has marked effects on respiration owing to alterations in the action of the muscles of respiration. Although quiet respiration may be little affected, the ability to take deep breaths or cough is considerably limited (Fig. 26-7). In these circumstances a central block may have two opposed actions: On the one hand by relieving pain, muscular movement may improve; on the other hand, motor blockade may reduce the activity of the intercostal and abdominal muscles and make effective coughing more difficult.

Almost all studies of the effect of epidural and spinal block below T4 on normal subjects not in pain indicate that lung volumes and blood gases are little changed. Higher blocks can, however, lead to a reduction in the expiratory reserve volume.[19]

Because there is a sympathetic nerve supply to the bronchi, sympathetic blockade might be thought to cause bronchoconstriction, but several studies have failed to show this.[67,71,75] There are isolated reports, however, of asthmatic patients suffering an acute attack of bronchospasm during epidural blocks, although several other factors, such as drug sensitivity, are often present.

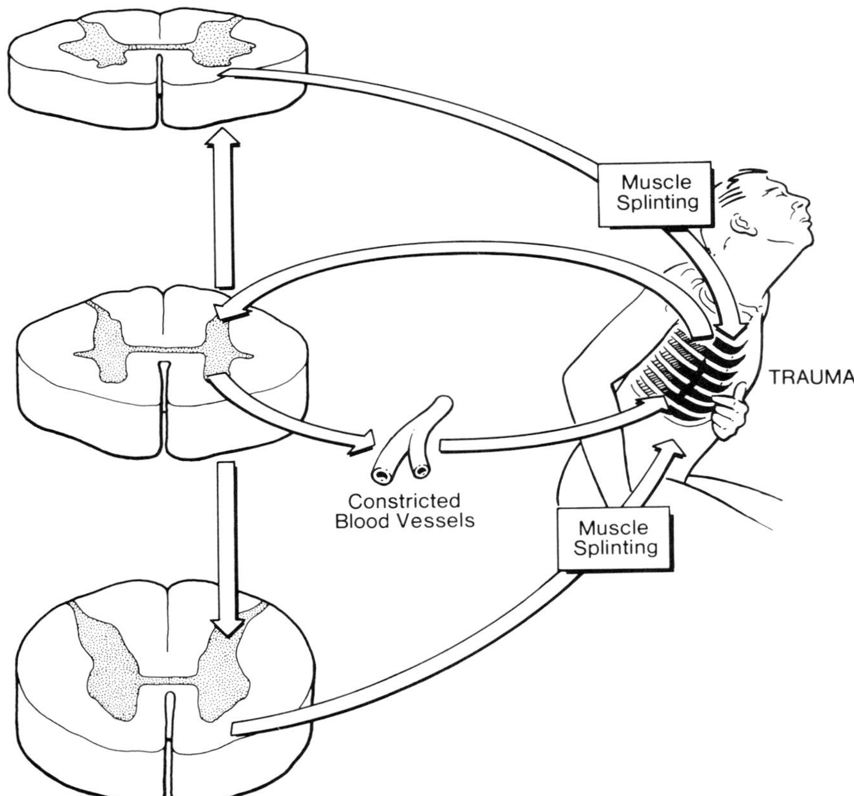

FIG. 26-7. Some effects of postoperative pain. Surgery or trauma may result in a vicious cycle of pain – muscle spasm – increased sympathetic activity and other adverse reflex changes. Note that interneuronal activity increases several segments above and below the pain stimulus. This may result in widespread increases in motor and sympathetic activity. Increased motor activity results in muscle spasm, causing further stimulus at the site of pain stimulus and more pain. Increased sympathetic activity releases norepinephrine, which sensitizes pain receptors. Also local microcirculatory vasospasm results in changes in local *p*H and release of algesic substances, further increasing pain. These vicious cycles can be broken by peripheral (intercostal) or epidural neural blockade.

After abdominal and thoracic surgery, there is a large reduction both in vital capacity (VC) and in functional reserve capacity (FRC). VC decreases by about 60% after upper abdominal surgery, whereas FRC decreases by around 20%.[75] The patients breathe small tidal volumes rapidly and are unwilling either to take deep breaths or to cough.

VC can be returned toward normal by epidural block, but invariably there remains a considerable deficit of about 30% to 40%.[67,75] Epidural blockade has a variable effect on FRC, some studies showing an increase[75] and others no change,[18] depending on whether the operation was in the upper or lower abdomen. In chronic airways disease, however, epidural block is more effective in increasing VC than it is in normal patients.[65]

Postoperative hypoxemia almost always occurs for some days after abdominal or thoracic surgery, and even when a fully effective epidural block is obtained there is little improvement seen in the short term[18,42,52,68] despite some increase in VC and FRC. However, the duration of hypoxemia is shorter and the incidence of chest infection lower when epidural blockade is used postoperatively rather than opioids.[69] This is probably due to the greater ability to cough and remove secretions. Beneficial effects of epidural block on respiratory function, when compared to more standard methods of pain relief with intramuscular opioids, have been demonstrated after upper abdominal surgery,[52,69] transvesical prostactectomy,[58] and hip replacement.[52,76]

Perhaps more important are the beneficial effects in patients with chronic lung disease with copious secretions. In these patients, epidural block may be lifesaving.[64,69] The only alternative in many patients lies in postoperative ventilator treatment, which is likely to be very prolonged.

GASTROINTESTINAL TRACT

The effects of sympathetic blockade on the blood supply to the gut have been mentioned above. There are, in addition, important effects on gut motility. Thus sympathetic blockade in the presence of an unaffected vagus nerve will increase the motility of the stomach, small intestine, and the proximal part of the large bowel. If, as is commonly the case, the epidural block affects the sacral nerves, there will be a parasympathetic block to the distal colon. Thus food transit time to the colon will be decreased, but defecation may be delayed.

Conversely, opioids have a marked inhibitory effect on the motility of the gastrointestinal tract, especially with regard to gastric emptying.[43] The use of epidural block in the postoperative period is associated with much less impairment of gastric emptying than is the case with intramuscular opioids.[44] Decreased gut motility can lead to abdominal distension and ileus, which will have deleterious effects on lung function and intestinal anastomoses.[3]

URINARY BLADDER

Parasympathetic block results from involvement of the S2, S3, and S4 spinal segments and will cause urinary retention. If the block extends to the lower thoracic segments, the discomfort of a full bladder will not be appreciated by the patient and gross overdistension may occur. It is therefore necessary to monitor urine output and catheterize the patient, if necessary.

METABOLIC AND HORMONAL EFFECTS

The trauma of surgery causes a variety of bodily changes — metabolic, hormonal, and immunologic — known as the "surgical stress response," which is fully described elsewhere (see Chap. 5). By blocking afferent impulses to, and autonomic efferent impulses from, the central nervous system during and after surgery, many of these changes can be considerably modified or abolished.[29]

The body's reaction to severe trauma is to mobilize substrate and to enter a catabolic phase. Thus there develops a state of negative nitrogen balance, with increases in plasma glucose, amino acids, and free fatty acid. These are mediated through changes in functions of the pituitary and adrenal glands and the pancreas, leading to increased secretion of cortisol, epinephrine, aldosterone, and antidiuretic hormone (see Chap. 5).

Although regional anesthesia during operation greatly modifies the stress response, especially after lower abdominal and lower limb surgery, the response will nevertheless be provoked by postoperative pain once the anesthesia wears off.[22,62] Only by prolonging the block well into the postoperative period for 24 to 48 hours can a substantial reduction be achieved.

Immunologic changes are also seen with a decrease in lymphocytes and an increase in granulocytes; both of these changes are again modified by regional anesthesia.[57]

Although the exact significance of reducing surgical stress has not yet been defined, there is a strong clinical impression that the postoperative well-being of patients, which is associated with regional anesthesia, is causally connected.

PHARMACOLOGIC EFFECTS OF LOCAL ANESTHETIC DRUGS

Given over a prolonged period, local anesthetics must perforce be given in large doses, and quite high plasma levels of bupivacaine have been recorded after 48 hours of continuous epidural injection.[60] Toxic effects are usually not seen, however, unless too fast an infusion is given by accident (see Chap. 4). An epidural infusion rate of more than 25 mg/hr is seldom required, and 30 mg/hr should be considered the upper limit.

The pharmacologic effects of nontoxic concentrations of bupivacaine, particularly on cardiovascular function, are described elsewhere (see Chap. 4) but have little, if any, clinically significant implications in treating postoperative pain.

MANAGEMENT OF POSTOPERATIVE EPIDURAL BLOCKADE

1. Insert an epidural catheter at or near the middle of the required band of analgesia and protect it with a bacterial filter. It must be firmly fixed to the patient's back by adhesive strapping.
2. Ensure that an effective block is still present at the end of surgery and, if necessary, inject a top-up dose of 0.5% bupivacaine, 4 to 6 ml for upper abdominal or lower limb surgery and 8 to 10 ml for lower abdominal surgery.
3. Start an infusion of dilute bupivacaine, 0.125% or 0.1%. A dose of 15 ml/hr will usually suffice, although 6 to 10 ml can be used in upper abdominal and thoracic operations. A roller pump is

ideal because it is unaffected by the resistance of the catheter.

4. Prepare a reservoir of drug sufficient to last 24 hours, and use a pediatric drip set to avoid accidental overdose. A set with a 30-ml measuring chamber is ideal. It must be refilled every 2 to 3 hours from the reservoir but allows accurate monitoring of the infusion rate. Not more than 30 ml can be given before an incorrect infusion rate is diagnosed.
5. An injection of ephedrine, 30 mg i.m., at the end of surgery will largely eliminate hypotension.
6. When handed into the care of the nursing staff, the patient must be monitored with regard to arterial pressure, heart rate, and rate of infusion. In addition, it is helpful if the height of block can be checked by pinprick and the patient's ability to move the legs noted. The effectiveness of the analgesia should also be occasionally recorded. A special chart for the nursing staff is of inestimable value, reminding them of the observations to be made and containing the written orders of the anesthesiologist (Figs. 26-8, 26-9).
7. Should hypotension occur, there should be a written protocol for the nursing staff (on the special form) instructing them to raise the foot of the bed and infuse electrolyte solution rapidly intravenously, for example, 250 ml of Hartmann's solution in 10 to 15 minutes. If hypotension persists, they should call for medical help and, in the interim, give ephedrine 30 mg i.m. What level of arterial pressure is deemed "hypotension" is a matter of opinion. I consider a systolic pressure of 80 mm Hg or more to be satisfactory and well tolerated if the patient remains supine. If hypotension does not respond to the above simple measures, a source of postoperative bleeding should be sought.
8. The patient should remain horizontal (unless hypotension occurs), although turning (to prevent pressure sores) should be done every 2 hours.
9. If the patient complains of discomfort from the wound, a top-up dose of 0.5% solution should be given by the medical staff.
10. If the patient complains of discomfort despite a painless wound (*e.g.*, owing to a nasogastric tube or to referred pain in the abdomen or shoulder), the nursing staff should be encouraged to give intramuscular opioid in conventional doses. This will not only relieve the discomfort, but also encourage sleep. Since the worst of the postoperative pain is alleviated by the epidural block, any other pain is likely to be mild and easily relieved by opioid.
11. If urinary retention occurs, it will be necessary to institute continuous bladder drainage. The danger of infection must be considered but is probably slight in comparison with the advantages of successful epidural analgesia.
12. Active physiotherapy should be given the day after surgery before the block wears off.

Provided the anesthesiologist is prepared to look after these patients and the nursing staff has received adequate instruction, there is no reason why patients cannot receive this form of analgesia in an ordinary surgical or gynecologic ward. There are clear advantages in this respect in the "Nightingale" ward with many beds. Single rooms pose considerable difficulties for the proper monitoring and care of this type of analgesia.

ADVANTAGES OF POSTOPERATIVE REGIONAL ANESTHESIA

The alternative to regional analgesia postoperatively is opioid given intramuscularly, intravenously, or intraspinally.

Intramuscular Opioid. Opioid given intramuscularly has several drawbacks that are both inherent and a result of the way it is applied. All too frequently conventional doses are quite ineffective, and there is a great reluctance on the part of the nursing staff to increase the dose or give injections frequently. Nausea and vomiting are common, and gastrointestinal motility is greatly reduced. The only advantages are simplicity and relative freedom from life-threatening complications. The widely shared view that postoperative pain is still a major problem is testimony to its inadequacy.

Regional blockade, particularly when prolonged, is far more effective in relieving pain.

Intravenous Opioid. There is now considerable interest in using the intravenous route for administering opioid drugs. This may be done as an initial bolus and continued either with intermittent small boluses controlled by the patient (PCA) or as a continuous infusion.[72] It has many attractions over the i.m. route. The patient can be given the appropriate amount of drug to relieve the pain, and the troughs and peaks of effectiveness are largely avoided.

It is as well to consider what is being achieved. The opioid is being used to depress brain function to the point at which severe pain is not appreciated as such. Thus analgesia must be accompanied in some pa-

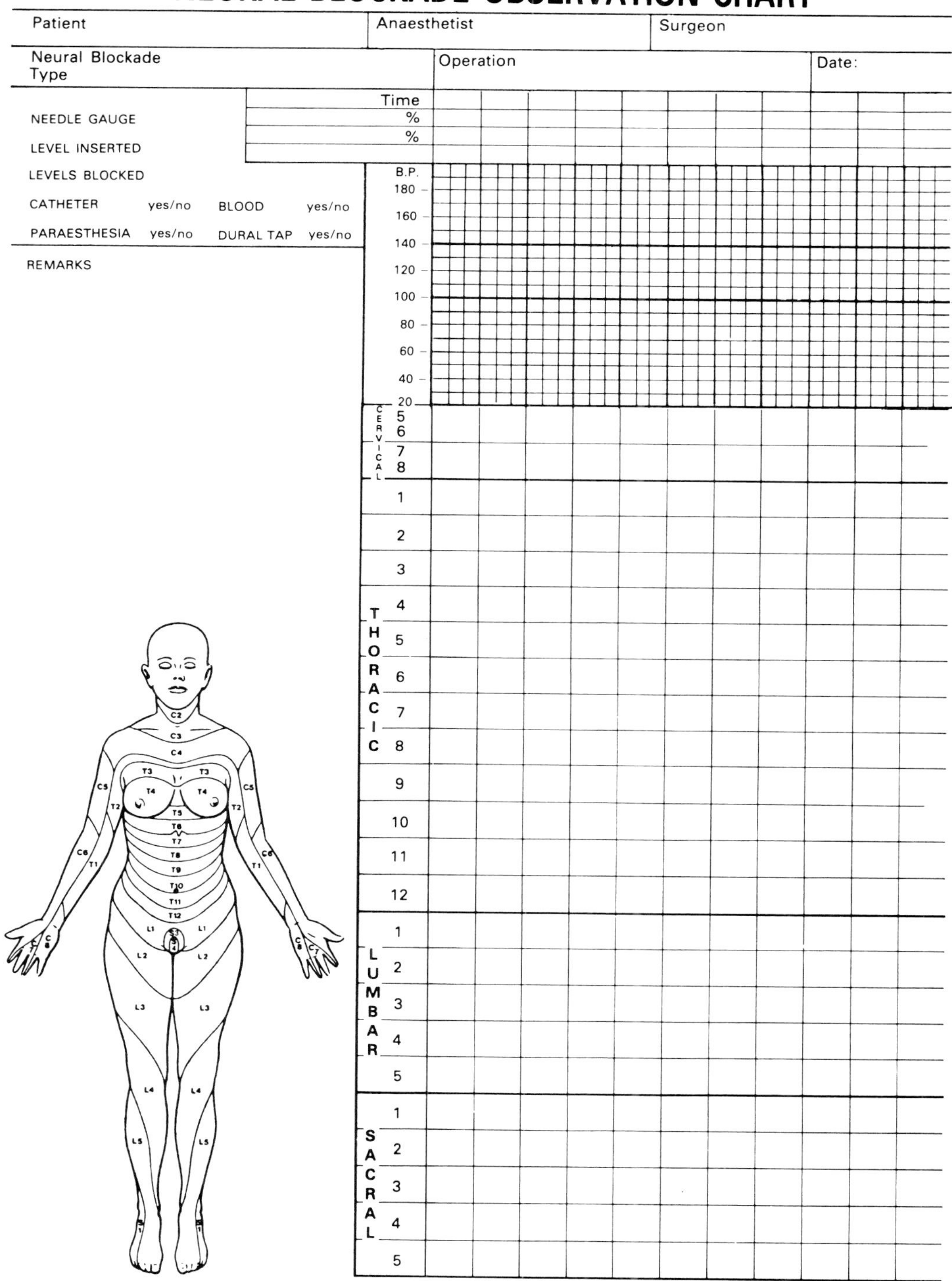

NEURAL BLOCKADE OBSERVATION CHART

MR 114

Patient	Anaesthetist	Surgeon

Neural Blockade Type	Operation	Date:

NEEDLE GAUGE

LEVEL INSERTED

LEVELS BLOCKED

CATHETER yes/no BLOOD yes/no

PARAESTHESIA yes/no DURAL TAP yes/no

REMARKS

Time

%

%

B.P.

180

160

140

120

100

80

60

40

20

CERVICAL 5 6 7 8

THORACIC 1 2 3 4 5 6 7 8 9 10 11 12

LUMBAR 1 2 3 4 5

SACRAL 1 2 3 4 5

FIG. 26-8. Charting of epidural analgesia. Details of insertion of epidural catheter should be clearly recorded and available to the staff managing prolonged epidural block. Also, cardiovascular parameters and level of block should be charted.

FLINDERS MEDICAL CENTRE

INFUSION CHART
(Sage Pump)

PUMP No.:

Ward	
Unit No.	
Surname	
Other Names	
D.O.B./Sex	
Address	

DOCTOR'S ORDERS Date: / /

__________mgm ______________________________(drug) in __________mls solution

To run at__________mls/hour Setting:_______

Doctor's signature:_____________________________

Time	30 min. check	Amt left (mls)	Amt given (mls)	Setting	RN signature	Time	30 min. check	Amt left (mls)	Amt given (mls)	Setting	RN signature

PROBLEMS
(refer Nursing Procedures Manual pp 82A-D)

____

____

____

____

Time Changed	R.N. Signatures

FIG. 26-9. Chart for recording observations on infusion pump for epidural local anesthetic. Note that amount ordered and amount actually infused are checked at set time-intervals.

tients, at least, by marked CNS depression, with somnolence and respiratory depression. Because of this and the difficulty of monitoring respiration, there is a temptation not to use fully effective analgesic doses. The patient with some pain is unlikely to suffer severe respiratory depression.

Regional block is usually much more effective and achieves analgesia without central nervous system depression. It may be argued that it replaces respiratory depression with hypotension, but the latter is much easier to detect before serious consequences arise.

Intraspinal Opioid. Opioid given intraspinally is discussed in Chapter 28. Although frequently impressive in the degree of analgesia it provides, it is not infrequently quite unsuccessful. Certainly serious respiratory depression has been observed many times, and again the problem of respiratory monitoring is apparent. Minor side-effects, particularly itching, nausea, and urinary retention are common. Prolonged analgesia is obtained only with morphine. If the more lipid-soluble drugs are used, they must be given frequently or infused continuously.

Two of the main advantages of regional analgesia are prevention of deep venous thrombosis and reduction in surgical stress. Neither of these is shared by intraspinal opiates, since they do not cause sympathetic blockade or have any effect on the surgical stress reaction even when analgesia is optimal.[12,25,26]

Combined Epidural Anesthetic and Opioid. Local anesthetics and opioids have quite different effects on the transmission and interpretation of nociceptive impulses. There is recent evidence, however, that these differing effects may be additive or even synergistic. One problem of continuous epidural block is the development of tachyphylaxis. Whether it is a true tachyphylaxis or not is debatable, but in any event it is quite common for an epidural block to regress several spinal segments over a period of hours despite maintenance of a constant rate of infusion. It has now been shown that this regression can be halted and indeed reversed by giving intravenous opioid without altering the infusion of local anesthetic.[36] If the main contribution of opioids in this effect is at the spinal cord level, either in the substantia gelatinosa of the dorsal horn or, possibly, the inhibitory descending pathways, then it would be logical to combine local anesthetic with opioids for infusion into the epidural space. Moreover, it should be possible to reduce significantly the dose of opioid and reduce the possibility of central depression. In a double-blind study comparing the epidural infusion of bupivacaine (0.1% at 3–4 ml/hr), or morphine (0.3–0.4 mg/hr), or both (with a saline control group and a nonepidural group), the combination was statistically superior to the other groups.[16] Even better results might have been obtained with a higher dose of bupivacaine. A combination of bupivacaine and meperidine has also proved effective.[54] This line of approach offers clear theoretical advantages and should be pursued with well-designed trials.

CONCLUSION

I am convinced that continuous epidural block offers the most effective form of postoperative analgesia and that it can be performed safely in most surgical units without recourse to intensive care units or prolonged stay in recovery wards. The best results, however, are obtained when epidural block is backed by the intelligent use of opioids when necessary. Whether the opioids are better given conventionally or intraspinally has yet to be decided

REFERENCES

1. Aitkenhead, A.R., Gilmour, D.G., Hothersall, A.P., and Leadingham, I.M.: Effects of subarachnoid nerve block and arterial P_{CO_2} on colon blood flow in the dog. Br. J. Anaesth., *52*:634P, 1980.
2. Aitkenhead, A.R., Wishart, H.Y., Peebles-Brown, D.A.: High spinal nerve block for large bowel anastomosis. Br. J. Anaesth., *50*:177, 1978.
3. Aitkenhead, A.R.: Anaesthesia and bowel surgery. Br. J. Anaesth., *56*:95, 1984.
4. Berry, F.R.: Analgesia in patients with fractured shaft of femur. Anaesthesia, *32*:576, 1977.
5. Bonica, J.J.: The management of pain with special emphasis on the use of analgesic block in diagnosis, prognosis and treatment. pp. 1404–5. Philadelphia, Lea & Febiger, 1953.
6. Bonica, J.J., Berges, P.U., Morikawa, J.: Circulatory effects of peridural block. I: Effects of level of analgesia and dose of lidocaine. Anesthesiology, *33*:619, 1970.
7. Bonica, J.J., Kennedy, W.F., Akamatsu, T.J., and Gerbershagen, H.U.: Circulatory effects of peridural block. III. Effects of acute blood loss. Anesthesiology, *36*:219, 1972.
8. Bowler, J.R., Lamont, M., and Scott, D.B.: Effect of extradural blockade on lower limb blood flow. Br. J. Anaesth. [in press].
9. Bromage, P.R.: Epidural Analgesia. pp. 376–377. Philadelphia, W.B. Saunders, 1978.
10. Browne, R.A., and Ashworth, E.J.: The use of epidural block in acute pancreatitis: A report of eight cases. Can. Anaesth. Soc. J., *16*:416, 1969.
11. Carron, H., Korbon, G.A., and Rowlingson, J.C.: Regional Anesthesia. p. 138. Orlando, FL, Grune & Stratton, 1984.

12. Christensen, P., Brandt, M.R., Rem, J., and Kehlet, H.: Influence of extradural morphine on the adrenocortical and hyperglycaemic response to surgery. Br. J. Anaesth., *54*:24, 1982.
12a. Cousins, M.J., Phillips, G.D.: Acute Pain Management in Clinics in Critical Care Medicine. Edinburgh, Churchill Livingstone, 1986.
13. Cousins, M.J., and Wright, C.J.: Graft, muscle, skin blood flow after epidural block in vascular surgical procedures. Surg. Gynec. Obstet., *133*:59, 1971.
14. Crawford, E.D., and Skinner, D.G.: Intercostal nerve block with thoracoabdominal and flank incisions. Urology, *19*:25, 1982.
15. Crawford, R.D., and Thompson, G.E.: Intercostal block. In Cousins, M.J., and Phillips, G.D. (eds.): Acute Pain Management. ed. 1. p. 239. New York, Churchill Livingstone, 1986.
16. Cullen, M.L., Staren, E.D. El-Ganzouri, A., Logas, W.G., *et al.*: Continuous epidural infusion for analgesia after major abdominal operations: A randomized, prospective double-blind study. Surgery, *98*:718, 1985.
17. Dittmann, M., Steenblock, U., Kranzlin, M., and Wolff, G.: Epidural analgesia or mechanical ventilation for multiple rib fractures? Intensive Care Med., *8*:89, 1982.
18. Drummond, G.B., and Littlewood, D.G.: Respiratory effects of extradural analgesia after lower abdominal surgery. Br. J. Anaesth., *49*:999, 1977.
19. Freund, F.B., Bonica, J.J., Ward, R.J., Akamatsu, T.J., *et al.*: Ventilatory reserve and the level of motor block during high spinal and epidural anesthesia. Anesthesiology, *28*:834, 1967.
20. Gibbons, J., James, O., and Quail, A.: Management of 130 cases of chest injury with respiratory failure. Br. J. Anaesth., *45*:1130, 1973a.
21. Gibbons, J., James, O., and Quail, A.: Relief of pain in chest injury. Br. J. Anaesth., *45*:1136, 1973b.
22. Gordon,N.H., Scott, D.B., and Percy-Robb, I.W.: Modification of plasma corticosteroids during and after surgery by epidural blockade. Br. Med. J., *1*:581, 1973.
23. Griffiths, D.P.G., Diamond, A.W., Cameron, J.D.: Postoperative extradural analgesia following thoracic surgery. A feasibility study. Br. J. Anaesth., *47*:48, 1975.
24. Hackel, D.B., Sancretta, S.M., and Kleinerman, J.: Effect of hypotension due to spinal anesthesia on coronary blood flow and myocardial metabolism. Circulation, *13*:92, 1956.
25. Hakanson, E., Rutberg, H., Jorfeldt, L., and Martensson, J.: Effects of the extradural administration of morphine or bupivacaine on the metabolic response to upper abdominal surgery. Br. J. Anaesth., *57*:394, 1985.
26. Hjortso, N-C., Christensen, N.J., Andersen, T., and Kehlet, H.: Effects of extradural administration of local anaesthetic agents and morphine on the urinary excretion of cortisol, catecholamines and nitrogen following abdominal surgery. Br. J. Anaesth., *57*:400, 1985.
27. Hoar, P.F., Hickey, R.F., and Ullyot, D.J.: Systemic hypertension following myocardial revascularization. A method of treatment using epidural anesthesia. J. Thorac. Cardiovasc. Surg.: *71*:859, 1976.
28. Katz, J., Nelson, W., Forest, R., and Bruce, D.L.: Cryoanalgesia for post-thoracotomy pain. Lancet, *1*:512, 1980.
29. Kehlet, H.: The modifying effect of general and regional anesthesia on the endocrine-metabolic response to surgery. Reg. Anaesth., *7*[*Suppl*]:S38, 1982.
30. Kehlet, H.: The endocrine-metabolic response to postoperative pain. Acta Anaesthesiol. Scand., *74*[*Suppl*]:173, 1982.
31. Kennedy, W.F., Sawyer, T.K., Gerbershagen, H.U., Cutler, R.E., *et al.*: Systemic cardiovascular and renal hemodynamic alterations during peridural anesthesia in normal man. Anesthesiology, *31*:414, 1969.
32. Kirno, K., and Lindell, K.: Intercostal nerve blockade. Br. J. Anaesth., *58*:246, 1986.
33. Kumar, B., and Hibbert, G.R.: Control of hypertension during aortic surgery using lumbar extradural blockade. Br. J. Anaesth., *56*:797P, 1984.
34. Levack, I.: Personal communication, 1986.
35. Lloyd, J.W., and Carrie, L.E.S.: A method of treating renal colic. Proc. R. Soc. Med., *58*:634, 1965.
36. Lund, C., Mogensen, T., Hjortso, N., and Kehlet, H.: Systemic morphine enhances spread of sensory analgesia during postoperative epidural bupivacaine infusion. Lancet, 2:1156, 1985.
37. Marion, P.: Sur le traitement des pancreatites aigues par les infiltrations splanchniques. Lyon Chir., *40*:315, 1945.
38. McLean, A.P.H., Mulligan, G.W., Otton, P., and MacLean, L.D.: Hemodynamic alterations associated with epidural anesthesia. Surgery, *62*:79, 1967.
39. Modig, J., Borg, T., Karlstrom, G., Maripuu, E., *et al.*: Thromboembolism after total hip replacement: Role of epidural and general anesthesia. Anesthesia & Analgesia, *62*:174, 1983.
40. Modig, J., Borg, T., Bagge, L., and Haldeen, T.: Role of extradural and of general anaesthesia in fibrinolysis and coagulation after total hip replacement. Br. J. Anaesth., *55*:625, 1983.
41. Moore, D.C.: Intercostal nerve block: Spread of India ink injected to the rib's costal groove. Br. J. Anaesth., *53*:325, 1981.
42. Muneyuki, M., Ueda, Y., Urabe, N., Takeshita, H., *et al.*: Postoperative pain relief and respiratory function in man. Anesthesiology, *29*:304, 1968.
43. Nimmo, W.S., Heading, R.C., Wilson, J., Tothill, P., *et al.*: Inhibition of gastric emptying and drug absorption by narcotic analgesics. Br. J. Clin. Pharmacol., 2:509, 1975.
44. Nimmo, W.S., Littlewood, D.G., Scott, D.B., and Prescott, L.F.: Gastric emptying following hysterectomy with extradural analgesia. Br. J. Anaesth., *50*:559, 1978.
45. Noller, D.W., Gillenwater, J.Y., Howards, S.S., and Vaughan, E.D.: Intercostal nerve block with flank incision. J. Urol., *117*:759, 1977.
46. Nunn, J.F., and Slavin, G.: Posterior intercostal nerve block for pain relief after cholecystectomy: Anatomical basis and efficacy. Br. J. Anaesth., *52*:253, 1980.
47. Orr, I.A., Keenan, D.J.M., Dundee, J.W., Patterson, C.C., *et al.*: Post thoracotomy pain relief: Combined use of cryoprobe and morphine infusion techniques. Ann. R. Coll. Surg. Engl., *65*:366, 1983.
48. Orr, R.B., and Warren, K.W.: Continuous epidural analgesia in acute pancreatitis. Lahey Clin. Bull., *6*:204, 1950.
49. Otton, P.E., and Wilson, E.J.: The cardiocirculatory effects of upper thoracic epidural analgesia. Can. Anaesth. Soc. J., *13*:541, 1966.

50. Owen, H., Galloway, D.J., and Mitchell, K.G.: Analgesia by wound infiltration after surgical excision of benign breast lumps. Ann. R. Coll. Surg. Engl., *67*:114, 1985.
51. Patel, J.M., Lanzufame, R.J., Williams, J.S., and Mullen, B.V., *et al.*: The effect of the incisional infiltration of bupivacaine hydrochloride upon pulmonary functions, atelectasis and narcotic need following elective cholecystecomy. Surg. Gynecol. Obstet., *157*:338, 1983.
52. Pflug, A.E., Murphy, T.M., Butler, S.H., and Tucker, G.T.: The effects of postoperative peridural analgesia on pulmonary therapy and pulmonary complications. Anesthesiology, *41*:8, 1974.
53. Prys-Roberts, C., Meloche, R., and Foex, P.: Studies of anaesthesia in relation to hypertension. Br. J. Anaesth., *43*:122, 1971.
54. Raj, P.P., Knarr, D., Vigdorth, E., Gregg, R., *et al.*: Comparative study of continuous epidural infusions versus systemic analgesics for postoperative pain. Anesthesiology, *63*:A238, 1985.
55. Reiestad, F., and Stromskag, K.E.: Intrapleural catheter in the management of postoperative pain—a preliminary report. Reg. Anaesth., *11*:89, 1986.
56. Reiz, S., Balfors, E., Sorensen, M.B., Haggmark, S., *et al.*: Coronary hemodynamic effects of general anesthesia and surgery: Modification by epidural analgesia in patients with ischemic heart disease. Reg. Anaesth., *7*:S8, 1982.
57. Rem, J., and Brandt, M.R., Kehlet, H.: Prevention of postoperative lymphopenia and granulocytosis by epidural analgesia. Lancet, *1*:283, 1980.
58. Renck, H.: The elderly patient after anaesthesia and surgery; with special regard to certain respiratory, circulatory, metabolic and muscular functions. Acta Anaesthesiol. Scand., *34*[*Suppl.*]:5, 1969.
59. Romagnoli, A., and Batra, M.S.: Continuous epidural block in the treatment of impacted ureteric stones. Can. Med. Assoc. J., *109*:968, 1973.
60. Ross, R.A., Clarke, J.E., and Armitage, E.N.: Postoperative pain prevention by continuous epidural infusion. Anaesthesia, *35*:663, 1980.
61. Runciman, W.B., Mather, L.E., Isley, A.H., Carapetis, R.J., *et al.*: A sheep preparation for studying interactions between blood flow and drug disposition. III. Effect of general and spinal anaesthesia on regional blood flow. Br. J. Anaesth., *56*:1247, 1984.
62. Sandberg, A.A., Eik-Nes, K., Samuels, L.T., and Tyler, F.H.: The effects of surgery on the blood levels and metabolism of 17-hydroxycorticosteroids in man. J. Clin. Invest., *33*:1507, 1954.
63. Sharrock, N.E., Waller, J.F., and Fierro, L.E.: Midtarsal block for surgery of the forefoot. Br. J. Anaesth., *58*:37, 1986.
64. Shuman, P.L., and Peters, R.M.: Epidural anesthesia following thoracotomy in patients with chronic obstructive airway disease. J. Thorac. Cardiovasc. Surg., *71*:82, 1976.
65. Simpson, B.R., Parkhouse, J., Marshall, R., and Lambrechts, W.: Extradural analgesia and the prevention of postoperative respiratory complications. Br. J. Anaesth., *33*:628, 1961.
66. Sjogren, J., and Wright, B.: Circulatory changes during continuous epidural blockade. Acta Anaesthesiol. Scand. *46*[*Suppl.*]:5, 1972.
67. Sjogren, J., Wright, B.: Respiratory changes during continuous epidural blockade. Acta. Anaesthesiol. Scand. *46*[*Suppl.*]:27, 1972.
68. Spence, A.A., and Smith, G.: Postoperative analgesia and lung function: A comparison of morphine with extradural block. Br. J. Anaesth., *43*:144, 1971.
69. Spence, A.A., and Logan, D.A.: Respiratory effects of extradural nerve block in the postoperative period. Br. J. Anaesth., *47*:281, 1975.
70. Stewart, G.J.: Antithrombotic activity of local anesthetics in several canine models. Reg. Anaesth. *7*[*Suppl.*]:S89, 1982.
71. Takasaki, M., and Takahashi, T.: Respiratory function during cervical and thoracic extradural analgesia in patients with normal lungs. Br. J. Anaesth., *52*:1271, 1980.
72. Tamsen, A.: Comparison of patient-controlled analgesia with constant infusion and intermittent intramuscular regimes. In Harmer, M., Rosen, M., and Vickers, M.D. (eds.): Patient-controlled analgesia. p. 111. Oxford, Blackwell Scientific Publications. 1985.
73. Thomas, D.F.M., Lambert, W.G., and Lloyd-Williams, K.: The direct perfusion of surgical wounds with local anaesthetic solutions: An approach to postoperative pain. Ann. R. Coll. Surg. Engl., *65*:226, 1983.
74. Underwood, R.J.: Experiences with continuous spinal anesthesia in physical status group IV patients. Anaesth. Analg. (Cleve.), *47*:18, 1968.
75. Wahba, W.M., Craig, D.B., Don, H.F., and Becklake, M.R.: The cardiorespiratory effects of thoracic epidural anaesthesia. Can. Anaesth. Soc. J., *19*:8, 1972.
76. Wahba, W.M., Don, H.F., and Craig, D.B.: Postoperative epidural analgesia: Effects on lung volumes. Can. Anaesth. Soc. J., *22*:519, 1975.
77. Wiklund, L.: Postoperative hepatic blood flow and its relation to systemic circulation and blood gases during splanchnic blockade and fentanyl analgesia. Acta Anaesthesiol. Scand., *58*[*Suppl.*]:5, 1975.

27.1 DIAGNOSTIC NEURAL BLOCKADE

ROBERT A. BOAS
MICHAEL J. COUSINS

Evaluation of patients who are in chronic pain is as difficult a challenge as any other in medical practice —[1,9,10,22,25,27] so difficult, in fact, that some patients may proceed through a full specialist workup with nothing more than "low back pain" or "chest pain" as their eventual label. Sometimes this is the sole diagnosis preceding therapy. In patients with chronic pain, it is essential to have skilled examination and comprehensive history before attempting to assign any provisional diagnosis. Depending on the problem, it may be necessary to have further specialized evaluation, for example, a gynecologist to evaluate a patient with pelvic pain. Psychological evaluation is important and should be performed independently by a trained psychologist, including the use of objective testing (see Chap. 25). All of the above information should be discussed in a pain clinic conference (see Chap. 31), where a differential diagnosis and treatment plan will be formulated. It is essential to use precisely defined terminology ("pain terms") and to assign the patient's problems to pain syndromes that are now classified and coded (see Appendices A and B, Chap. 24.1). Thus, for example, "headache" would not be an acceptable diagnosis and would be replaced by coded diagnoses such as classic migraine or cluster headache (see Appendix B, Chap. 24.1). The importance of such precision mainly lies in avoiding the use of diagnostic and therapeutic measures that may be unnecessary, or even undesirable, in some conditions.[1] This requires a broad knowledge of medicine and of human behavior.[25,27] No individual specialty, particularly anesthesiology, provides such knowledge during training. Most medical specialties are deficient in emphasizing psychological aspects, particularly in the context of chronic pain. This highlights the importance of the multimodal approach to both diagnosis and treatment of chronic pain in adults[1,9,10] and children.[22]

The temptation that befalls some who work without the help of psychologists in their patient workup is to seek nonorganic and behavioral interpretations from the results of nerve blocks. What nerve blocks cannot do is offer any contribution to the presence or absence of psychological aberrations in the pattern of pain behavior. Specialized psychologists in the field of pain, and purpose-designed psychological tests, offer remarkably precise and efficient methods for deriving this information. For anesthesiologists to seek psychological diagnoses from the interpretation of nerve blocks is an arrogance evolved from ignorance. Such practice should not be countenanced. Nor do diagnostic nerve blocks provide accurate prognoses for the outcome of permanent ablative procedures, the experience reported by Tasker[23] being one of 100 consecutive surgical failures after positive responses to diagnostic blocks (see Chap. 30). Similarly, the results of diagnostic paravertebral blocks were shown by Loeser to have no correlation with the outcome of dorsal rhizotomy.[18] All who have gained experience in long-term patient care can attest to such errors made from well-intentioned but misinterpreted blocks of years past. The aim of this chapter is to outline the scope of diagnostic nerve blocking procedures in a multidisciplinary pain clinic setting and to provide guidelines for their interpretation, so as to avoid the many pitfalls that might otherwise arise from inappropriate use.

APPLICATIONS AND SCOPE OF DIAGNOSTIC BLOCKS

The aim of diagnostic nerve block techniques is to help in determining or differentiating the site, organ, or pathway by which a presumed nociceptive input mediates pain. Practically speaking, this almost involves a separation of the "pain" from the individual, as if the patient were dissociated from the disease process, the very issue that causes some of the concerns already cited. Clearly, diagnostic blocks are only part of the evaluation process, giving clues as to the nociceptive component of painful disease (see also Chap. 31). In general terms, this can be accomplished at six functional levels (as shown in Fig. 27-1) using either anatomic or pharmacologic distinctions to identify specific structures, nerves, or processes involved in pain generation. When this information is combined with a detailed physical and psychological workup, it may be possible to provide accurate detail as to one or more aspects of a patient's pain, as is shown in Table 27-1. Such an approach is equally applicable in both adults[9,10] and children[22] who suffer from either noncancer pain or cancer pain.[21]

Anatomic Localization of Pain Source

Direct injection of low-concentration local anesthetic solutions into superficial sites of pain or tenderness can readily elicit the precise tissue source of pain and offer a definitive diagnosis. Frequent examples are those of nerve entrapments from trauma, local disease, or postsurgical scar entrapment.[3] Trigger points and soft-tissue sites of pain can also be readily identified, even in patients with cancer pain,[21] and may provide an opportunity for concurrent therapy (see Chap. 27.2). Similarly, the ability to direct needles to deep-sited joint structures allows the localization of pain to tissues within or around the joint itself or to adjacent structures mimicking articular pain. Low back pain is a good example of a syndrome complex that can be defined more precisely by such methods. Injections conducted with radiographic control give such precision of needle and anesthetic solution placement that it is possible to distinguish whether pain is arising from a facet joint (see Chap. 27.3), from nerve root damage/foraminal stenosis,[14] or from ligamentous or soft-tissue muscle sites. This is one of the most valuable and underused applications

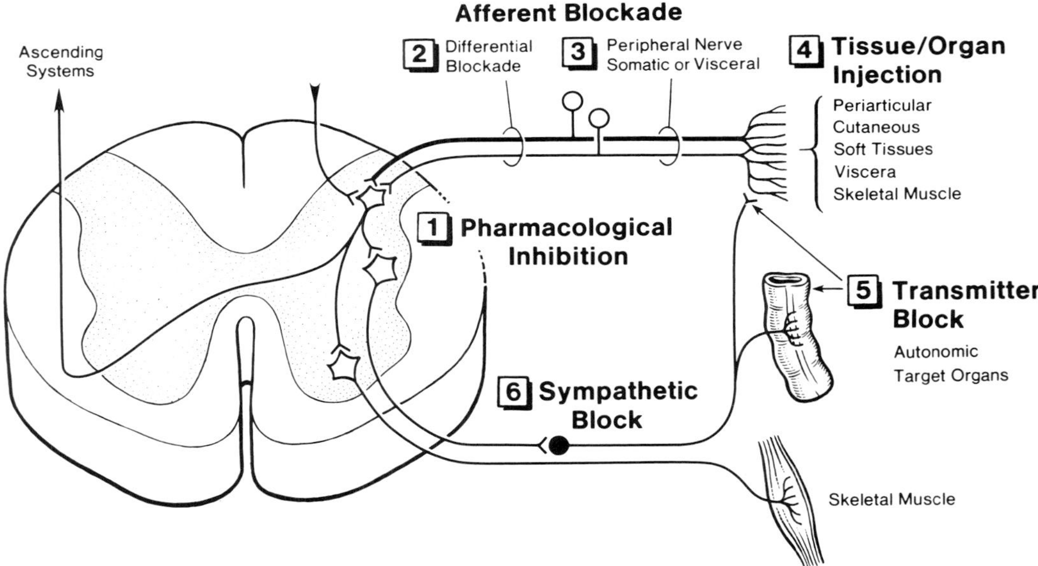

FIG. 27-1. Peripheral nociceptive pathways and sites for diagnostic neural blockade. Both pharmacologic (*e.g.*, spinal opioid versus local anesthetic) and anatomic (*e.g.*, spinal nerve versus peripheral nerve) approaches are used to identify specific structures, nerves, or processes involved in pain generation.

of all the diagnostic block techniques. Even when radiologic abnormality is absent, other than for reduction in size of intervertebral disk space, the resolution of back pain after injections into a facet joint is virtually diagnostic for early-stage degenerative pains that arise at these posterior elements of the spinal vertebrae (see Figs. 27-24 through 27-30). Another example is radiographic-controlled injection of local anesthetic containing contrast medium into the temporomandibular joint. This diagnostic block is helpful in diagnosis of pain in the jaw region.[16]

TABLE 27-1. SCOPE OF DIAGNOSTIC BLOCKS

1. Anatomically localize and delineate pain source.
2. Determine visceral or somatic origin of thoraco-abdominal pain.
3. Separate "sympathetic" from "somatic" etiology of peripheral pain.
4. Help identify syndromes of referred pain.
5. Establish segmental levels of nociceptive input.
6. Determine by somatic block (*e.g.*, brachial plexus) the role of pain and muscle spasm or bone/tendon/joint capsule fixed deformity in conditions such as reflex sympathetic dystrophy.
7. Assist in diagnosis of central pain.

Visceral Versus Somatic Pain

Sometimes trunk pain involving the chest, abdomen, or pelvis can provide diagnostic difficulties. Some cases may undergo extensive investigation, or even surgery, before proceeding to a pain clinic referral. In many such cases the body wall, rather than the visceral structures, is an overlooked focus of pain. Rib cartilages, nerve, or soft tissues provide sites at which diagnostic injections can readily and often dramatically relieve pain. Posthoractomy, postcholecystectomy, or inguinal herniorrhaphy repair pains caused by nerve entrapment, neuroma, and deafferentation, or combinations of these, can be aided diagnostically on this basis.

Another frequently encountered presentation is that of the abdominal cutaneous nerve entrapment syndrome,[3] mimicking severe abdominal pain. Placement of local anesthetic solution at the deep layer of the rectus sheath to produce loss of pain and tenderness is the diagnostic confirmation for this disorder (see Fig. 14-11).

Epigastric pain or poorly defined lower chest pains can be separated as to somatic or visceral origin by the use of intercostal nerve blocks (see Fig. 14-3) to provide trunk anesthesia, or with celiac plexus or splanchnic blocks (see Figs. 14-6 through 14-8), to identify visceral pain sources (see Chap. 14). For most cases, it is usually sufficient to exclude body-wall pain in order to ascribe a visceral source, especially if a disease has already been identified. At other times, when no focus can be identified in terms of disease or afferent nerve source, it may be acceptable to use diagnostic epidural blocks, graded in concentration and with progressive rostral spread, to ascertain the anatomic level and possible nature of pain input[26] (see below). In some instances, full somatic block and visceral block to levels of T4 provide no relief. In such cases pain must be ascribed to supraspinal processes. However, no decision can be made about physical or psychological cause of this supraspinal pain. It should be noted that interpretation of a single somatic or visceral block is difficult because of the convergence of somatic and visceral nociceptive fibers on the same dorsal horn neuron (see Fig. 24-2). Thus it is preferable to carry out both somatic and visceral blocks and to note efficacy and duration of analgesia (see below).

Sympathetic Versus Somatic Origin of Peripheral Pain

Sympathetic fiber activity produces or contributes to pain by means of sensitization of peripheral pain receptors, local ischemia, and reflex changes depicted in Figure 24-1. History, physical examination, and investigations (*e.g.*, radiography) helps point to conditions in which sympathetic fiber (efferent) activity may be the cause of, or contribute to, pain (*e.g.*, reflex sympathetic dystrophy, Raynaud's disease or phenomenon, vascular insufficiency; see Appendix B, Chap. 24.1). It should be emphasized that careful medical investigation may make diagnostic neural blockade unnecessary. For example, the differential diagnosis of Raynaud's phenomenon is extensive, and for some of these diseases the diagnostic and therapeutic procedures used do not involve nerve blocks (see Chap. 24.1, Appendix B, X11—1 and 2).

Diagnostic sympathetic nerve blocks should be carried out at anatomic sites where sympathetic fibers are separate from somatic fibers: cervicothoracic sympathetic chain, splanchnic nerves, celiac plexus, and lumbar sympathetic chain (see Chaps. 13 and 14). Objective documentation of the efficacy of sympathetic block should be obtained (*e.g.*, skin conductance response; see Chap. 13) independent of evaluation of pain relief (*e.g.*, visual analogue scale; see below and Chap. 25). Changes in skin temperature and blood flow may also be documented (see Chap. 13). A useful technique in this aspect is thermography,[13,20,24] which may produce a qualitative "picture" of areas of ischemia and their change or otherwise after sympathetic block (Fig. 27-2). Color photographs taken before and at various stages during treatment also help to document results of diagnostic and therapeutic nerve blocks (Fig. 27-3). Radiographs of both hands or feet should also be taken to document any osteoporosis (Fig. 27-4).

Intravenous regional sympathetic block (see Chap. 12) is an alternative to blocking the sympathetic chain for diagnosis of pain in the limbs. Patients usually find it more acceptable than, for example, cervicothoracic sympathetic block. However, if a series of diagnostic blocks are to be performed in a patient with lower limb pain, it may be equally acceptable to place a catheter near the lumbar sympathetic chain and leave it *in situ* (see Chaps. 13 and 27.2). This permits either prolonged sympathetic block or use of different local anesthetic drugs to produce different durations of sympathetic block. Intravenous regional sympathetic blocks with guanethidine have a duration of sympathetic block of approximately 2 to 3 days. It is useful to carry out at least two diagnostic blocks to determine whether pain has improved. In patients with arteriopathy, it may be preferable to use slow intra-arterial infusion of guanethidine, since inflation of a cuff above arterial pressure for 10 minutes may produce ischemia that does not recover (see Chap. 13).

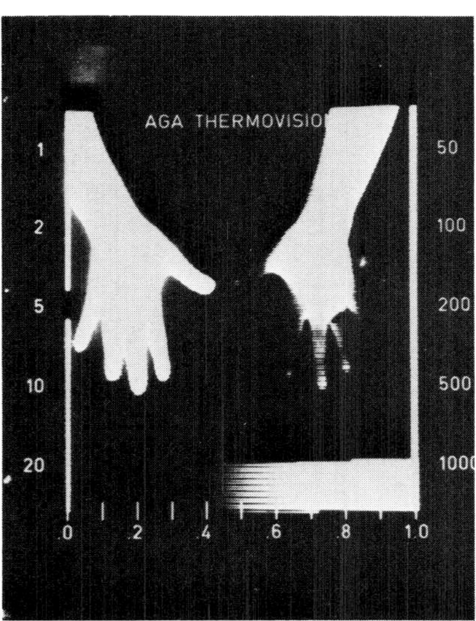

AFFECTED HAND(LEFT)

FIG. 27-2. Thermogram of the hands of a patient with clinical symptoms and signs suggestive of reflex sympathetic dystrophy. Thermography revealed reduced blood flow and temperature in the left hand (dark areas), indicating increased sympathetic activity. Right hand temperature was 29.1°C and left hand was 26.5°C. After diagnostic left stellate ganglion block, the thermogram of the left hand was the same as that of the right hand. *Note:* Thermograms can also be obtained *in color* with equipment of varying degrees of complexity and cost. The advantage of color lies in a clearer depiction of areas of reduced blood flow and decreased skin temperature.

If the results of diagnostic block are favorable, a series of therapeutic blocks may be performed. In arterial disease, it may be necessary to carry out only a few therapeutic blocks each time an "acute on chronic" episode occurs (*e.g.*, during winter). There is no way to know beforehand whether a patient with severe arterial disease will benefit from sympathetic block. Thus the first sympathetic block may be both diagnostic and therapeutic. The use of such blocks in arteriopathies such as scleroderma may relieve pain and improve skin nutrition in patients who have no other hope of relief. Thus a diagnostic block is worthwhile (see Chap. 13). In patients with painful peripheral nerve disorders, Wynn–Parry and colleagues recommend a series of five or six sympathetic blocks over 2 weeks, combined with mobilization physiotherapy.[29] They have found that patients in whom hyperpathia (see Chap. 24.1, Appendix A) is a prominent feature usually respond to diagnostic intravenous guanethidine blocks and subsequently benefit from a course of blocks. Patients in whom paresthesias predominate seem to respond best to transcutaneous electrical nerve stimulation.[29]

Pain caused by somatic factors in the limbs may have diagnosis helped by somatic nerve blocks, but it is difficult to produce somatic blocks without some degree of sympathetic block. Thus it is often best to carry out sympathetic block before somatic blocks. Injection of trigger points (see Chap. 27.2), painful scars, neuromas, and other localized disease may result in a relatively pure somatic block. An example is the differentiation of stump pain (which may respond to local infiltration but not to sympathetic block) from causalgia (which may respond to sympathetic block but usually not to somatic block, except for brief poorly reproduced periods). Somatic nerve block of individual branches of nerves may also produce relatively pure somatic block. An example is block of the lateral femoral cutaneous nerve (see Fig. 11-8) in the diagnosis of meralgia paresthetica (see Chap. 24.1, Appendix B). Block of sensory as well as motor fibers may be necessary in pain syndromes in

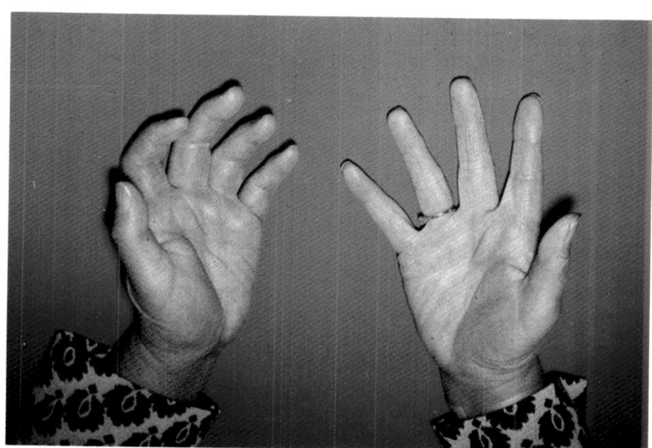

FIG. 27-3. Patient with reflex sympathetic dystrophy in the left hand (left side of figure). Note the venous congestion and mottled areas of pink-blue color and some areas of pallor in the fingers. Note also the flexed position of the fingers; this was unchanged after attempts at active or passive movement. Diagnostic intravenous regional sympathetic block with guanethidine (Ismelin) reversed the swelling, congestion, and color changes but had no effect on range of movement in the fingers. Diagnostic brachial plexus block revealed that limitation of movement was due to pain and muscle spasm, since the fingers could be passively moved through a full range at each joint.

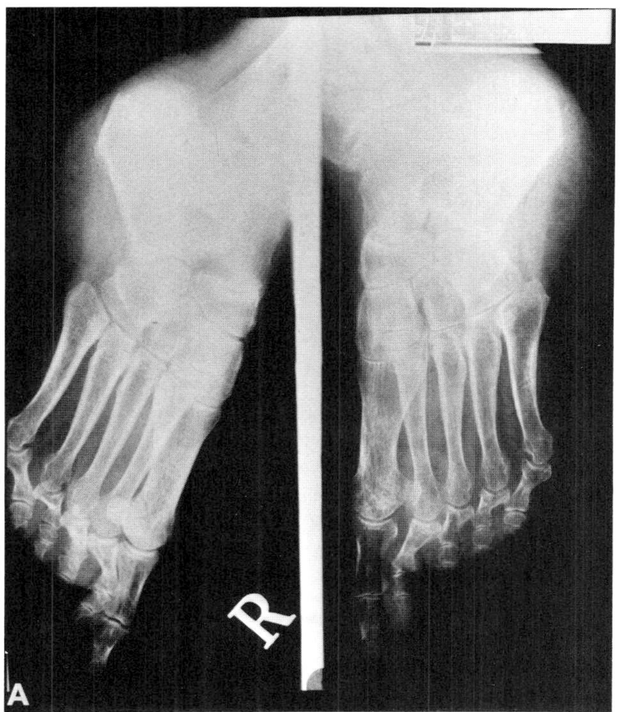

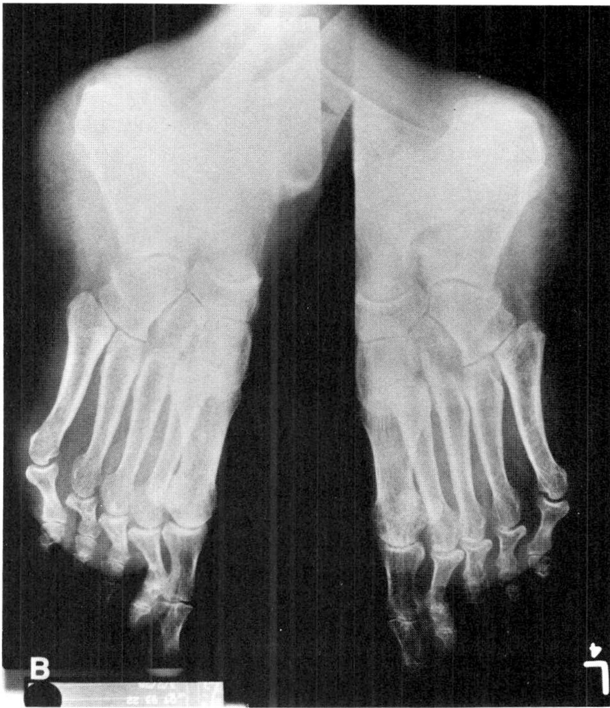

FIG. 27-4. Simultaneous radiographs of both feet of a patient suspected of having reflex sympathetic dystrophy in the left lower limb. **A.** Before treatment, osteoporosis is seen in the affected left foot. (Note the right foot is marked with a large R.) Osteoporosis can be identified by great reduction in calcification in the cortex of all toes and by some areas in the more central regions that appear as dark areas of almost total loss of calcium. **B.** Three months after treatment that included lumbar sympathetic neurolytic block, there is considerable resolution of osteoporosis. Note that the affected left foot is marked with an inverted L.

which muscle spasm is a major component of the syndrome. An example is abdominal cutaneous nerve entrapment syndrome (see Chap. 27.2). Blockade of the appropriate intercostal nerve at the level of the rectus sheath (see Fig. 14-11) relieves pain and muscle spasm.

"Differential" somatic blockade is a more contentious approach to diagnosis of a somatic versus sympathetic etiology of pain. A catheter may be placed in the site of the brachial or lumbosacral plexus (see Chap. 27.2) in the epidural or subarachnoid space. Local anesthetic solutions of increasing concentration are then injected to block sympathetic, sensory, and then motor fibers. Alternatively, a maximum clinical dose and concentration of solution is injected, and effects on pain are observed as the block wears off. Both approaches assume that there will be clear-cut phases of [a] motor, sensory, and sympathetic block; [b] sensory and sympathetic block; [c] sympathetic block alone; [d] no block. Unfortunately, this seems not to be reliable (see below) from the point of view of the "differential" nature of the nerve block. Also, there will be carry-over effects from the earlier, more intense block.

Referred Versus Focal Pain

Pain may be referred from viscera to the skin surface or deeper integumental structures (see Chap. 24.1 and Figs. 24-2 and 24-4). It is less well known that pain from deep somatic structures may be referred to other somatic regions and may even produce reflex changes in viscera. For example, pain caused by zygapophyseal joint (facet joint) disease may be referred to other regions of the back or to the limbs. Blockade of the facet joint or of the medial branch of the dorsal root of the spinal nerves helps to diagnose facet joint disease (see Chap. 27.3). In comparison, some back pain may be due to local soft-tissue, ligamentous, or muscle pathology. Local infiltration into "trigger" areas may relieve such pain (*i.e.*, by injection in the painful area). Discogenic back pain may be referred to the back and limbs and may require blockade of one or more nerve roots (see Fig. 14-10) to achieve pain relief. However, such nerve root blocks are seldom discrete blocks of an individual nerve root, since local anesthetic may diffuse into dural root sleeves and then into cerebrospinal fluid (CSF). Epidural block is seldom useful in providing a precise diagnosis of focal versus referred back pain because it may relieve both types of pain. Sometimes blocking the entire referred area relieves pain in the area of pain focus; this may complicate diagnosis (see Fig. 24-2).

Establishing Segmental Levels of Nociceptive Input

Diagnosis of somatic or visceral pain may be aided by determining which spinal segments are associated with the pain. This then gives a clue to the likely structure(s) involved. A summary of the spinal segments associated with pain in various viscera is given in Figures 24-4 and 24-5 and in Table 24-3.

Somatic pain may be elucidated by progressively blocking somatic nerve roots or intercostal nerves (see Chap. 14). If the pain is bilateral, this must be done on both sides. An alternative is to place an epidural catheter close to the center of the putative segmental area of the pain. Small doses of local anesthetic are then given, and the band of segmental anesthesia is gradually increased until the pain is relieved. Inevitably, some degree of sympathetic block may occur. Thus it is preferable to be sure that the pain is of somatic origin before using an epidural segmental block.

For visceral pain, segmental epidural blockade can be used as described above. In this case, dilute local anesthetic is used in increasing doses (*e.g.*, 0.5% lidocaine). Again, there is the problem that some sensory block may occur; thus it is preferable to have first established that the pain is of visceral origin by blockade of visceral nociceptive fibers (*e.g.*, at celiac plexus and other sites; see Figs. 14-6 through 14-8). An example would be placement of an epidural catheter at T10–T11 for suspected pain of the uterus or ovary. Injection of a small dose to block T10–11 in a female may relieve pain and point to the ovary as the source of pain (see Fig. 24-5). If a large area of segmental block is required (*e.g.*, T10–L1), then the uterus is a more likely source. On the other hand, if blockade of T11–T12 segments relieves pain, the urinary bladder may be the source of pain (see Table 24-3). Even with careful testing for loss of pinprick sensation, it is difficult to be certain that only T10–T11 segments are blocked. It need only be recalled that labor pain is often relieved by epidural block when there is no evidence of loss of cutaneous sensation.

Blockade at the level of autonomic plexus will give only general information. However, this may be a useful starting point. For example, pain in the region of the lower chest/upper abdomen may be difficult to elucidate because of overlap of referred areas from thoracic and abdominal viscera (see Fig. 24-4). Thus blockade of cervicothoracic ganglia (T1–T5) by way of the "stellate" approach may relieve pain and point to heart (T1–T5), lungs (T2–T4), or esophagus (T5–T6) as the source of pain. More precise blockade of thoracic ganglia could then be considered, if necessary. On the other hand, relief of pain with celiac plexus blockade would indicate that pain was arising from upper abdominal viscera, such as stomach (T6–T10), liver, and gallbladder (T6–T10). This approach can be used only for broad information about segmental levels.

A more precise approach is to block individual sympathetic ganglia bilaterally. Thus, for ovarian pain, T10 and T11 ganglia would be blocked on both sides. The precision of this approach can be increased by using local anesthetic mixed with radiographic contrast medium (*e.g.*, Angiographin) and injecting small doses under image-intensifier control (see Figs. 13-25 through 13-31).

Although such an approach was used by Bonica[8] to help elucidate the spinal segments associated with labor pain, it seems to have been infrequently used in diagnosis of chronic visceral pain.

In summary, somatic segmental levels of nociceptive input are best established by blockade of somatic nerve roots (see Fig. 14-10) or intercostal nerves (see Fig. 14-3). Visceral segmental levels are most precisely determined by blockade of sympathetic ganglia (see Figs. 13-25 and 14-6 through 14-8).

Central Pain

The term "central pain" refers to pain arising from the spinal cord or the brain. It includes thalamic syndrome, deafferentation syndrome, and other causes of lesions or disturbances in modulation of nociception in the central nervous system (CNS) (see Chap. 24.1, Appendix B). It was originally believed that local anesthetic blocks would not relieve central pain. However, it has been reported that brief periods of relief of central pain may follow afferent as well as efferent neural blockade of the painful region involved in central pain.[15,19] This may be due to an effect of altered neural traffic on the disturbed neural activity ("turbulence") in the CNS or perhaps to absorbed local anesthetic.[28] However, the effect is short-lived and does *not* predict long-lasting pain relief with a permanent nerve block or neural lesion. An important clue to central pain is failure to achieve pain relief with opioid drugs by any route. Neurogenic pain, owing to nerve lesion or neuropathy, may be relieved by intravenous infusion of local anesthetic[7] (see Chap. 27.2). One approach to diagnosis of central versus more peripheral mechanisms in pain is the "diagnostic epidural opioid block"[11] (see below). This aims to identify pain arising at or peripheral to the dorsal horn, which may respond to epidural opioid. However, certain types of "peripheral pain" may not be relieved (*e.g.*, intermittent deep somatic or visceral pain[4]; see Chap. 28). In a further approach, there are some reports that central pain may be relieved by intravenous barbiturate as a "diagnostic test." However, it appears to be necessary to give doses of, for example, thiopental, which are little different from anesthetizing doses. The test is of no proven clinical usefulness.

Psychogenic Pain

Psychogenic pain refers to pain that is predominantly, but not exclusively, caused by psychological factors (see Chap. 24.1). As discussed earlier, the results of diagnostic nerve blocks should *not* be used to make such a diagnosis. Independent psychological or psychiatric assessment, or both, should be the basis of such a diagnosis. However, the results of all evaluations by pain unit members can help in reaching such a diagnosis.[9,10,22,25,27]

TECHNIQUES OF DIAGNOSTIC NEURAL BLOCKADE

Infiltration Techniques

Infiltration techniques are perhaps some of the most reliable and least controversial because of their unequivocal site of action and effects. Trigger point or "tender point" (TP) injection produces rapid and complete relief of pain, muscle spasm, (see Figs. 27-6 and 27-7), and other symptoms associated with the many and varied myofascial syndromes (see Chap. 24.1, Appendix B, 1-9, VII-1, VII-2, VII-3). The technique of trigger-point injection is described in Chapter 27.2 and shown in Figure 27-18.

Local infiltration techniques include subcutaneous infiltration of local anesthetic to determine whether pain is arising superficially, as in postsurgical scar entrapment of cutaneous nerves.

Patients with local areas of pain, such as suspected nerve entrapment neuromas, may have the cause of pain determined by careful infiltration of the region. If pain relief is obtained, further benefit can be derived from repeated blocks at 1- to 3-month intervals, with local anesthetic and steroid. The membrane-stabilizing action of the steroid extends the period of quiescence in the damaged nerve.[12] Prolongation of pain relief tends to confirm the diagnosis and offers a therapeutic option.

Peripheral Nerve Blocks and Spinal Somatic Nerve Blocks

Blockade of individual peripheral nerves (see Chaps. 10, 11, 14) and cranial nerves (see Chaps. 15, 16, 17) may be useful in confirming that pain has a significant peripheral nociceptive component. However, it should be remembered that central pain may be relieved for a short time with peripheral blockade. Also, absorbed local anesthetic may produce central effects.[6] Thus minimal doses of drug should be administered and local anesthetics of different duration used and effects observed. Some of the pain syndromes amenable to treatment with peripheral blockade are described in Chapter 27.2.

Accuracy of needle placement is essential to ensure effective blockade with minimal doses of local anesthetic (see below). This requires a sound knowledge of the anatomic basis of each nerve block (see Chaps. 7 through 21). The use of radiologic techniques also may be helpful for some blocks, such as maxillary and mandibular block, paravertebral somatic nerve block, obturator nerve block (see Chaps. 11, 14, 15), and blocks of the medial branch of dorsal rami (see Chap. 27.3). Some blocks lend themselves to injection of local anesthetic mixed with contrast medium (*e.g.*, paravertebral somatic nerve block). In others, contrast medium may be injected first to check accuracy of placement (*e.g.*, spinal facet block; see Chap. 27.3 and Figs. 27-24, 27-26, 27-29, and 27-30).

Block of peripheral nerves that are located in regions less amenable to radiographic control may be facilitated by use of a peripheral nerve stimulator (see Chap. 6).

Other aids used to confirm nerve block of the intended region include skin temperature measurements, laser Doppler flowmetry, infrared thermography, and liquid crystal thermography (see below). These aids rely on the fact that blockade of a spinal nerve or peripheral nerve results in vasodilation in the area of distribution of that nerve. However, it is necessary to compare the same area on the contralateral side, since some preexisting conditions produce changes in skin blood flow and temperature. For example, it is reported that in spinal nerve root irritation, there is sympathetic hyperactivity along the affected dermatome, producing a decrease in temperature in that area.[20,24] After nerve block, the temperature may be increased only to a "normal" level, which is the same as that on the opposite side.

Diagnostic Plexus Blockade

Local anesthetic blockade of a major plexus such as the brachial plexus produces profound sensory, motor, and sympathetic block in a limb. This may be used to investigate pain and limitation of movement associated, for example, with reflex sympathetic dystrophy (see Fig. 27-3). Initial examination of such patients may reveal limited movement at all joints in the limb. It may be impossible to determine the relative contribution of capsulitis of the joint, tendon sheath fibrosis, and fixed bone deformity, compared with pain and muscle spasm. Under plexus blockade, pain and muscle spasm are absent and passive movement may reveal a full range of movement. Residual restriction of movement is due to other factors mentioned earlier (see Fig. 27-5). Sometimes chronic muscle spasm has resulted in muscle shortening. A skilled physical therapist can gently and gradually stretch such muscles to regain normal length, sometimes during several separate plexus blocks. Violent attempts to "break adhesions" are usually counterproductive and may result in hematoma formation and increased pain and sympathetic activity. The value of diagnostic plexus blocks lies in providing information about the cause of restricted movement, pointing to the possible value of further plexus blocks to aid mobilization and demonstrating to the patient the improvement that may be obtained.

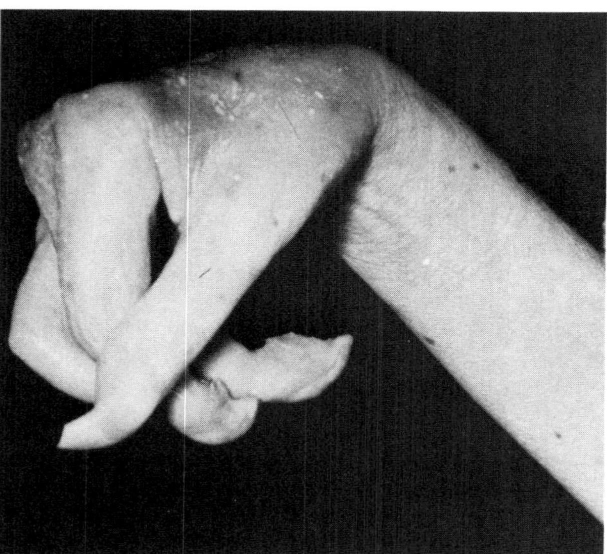

FIG. 27-5. Hand of patient with fixed deformity caused by reflex sympathetic dystrophy, which followed amputation of an infected finger. Diagnostic brachial plexus block provided temporary pain relief but revealed that the range of movement in the hand and wrist could not be increased because of tendon sheath fibrosis, contractures, and bony deformity. At this stage, the condition had been present for 15 years and remained unresponsive to all treatments attempted.

"Differential" Intrathecal and Epidural Neural Blockade

As discussed in Chapters 2 and 3, the classic concepts of "differential" blockade have recently come into question. The reader should consult this discussion, which makes it clear that there is no way to be certain of producing a "pure" block of sympathetic, sensory, or motor fibers. It was originally thought that fiber size was the predominant factor governing sensitivity to local anesthetics. Subsequent studies have drawn attention to other factors, such as frequency-dependent conduction block (see Chap. 2), spinal cord long tract blockade (see Chap. 8), and the direct effect of absorbed local anesthetics on spinal neurons.[28] These studies make the concept of "differential" neural blockade[2,26] increasingly contentious and cast considerable doubt on the interpretation of such blocks. Absorption into the vascular system of substantial amounts of local anesthetic occurs with epidural block and all major nerve blocks. Recent studies of systemic administration of local anesthetics have reported a selective depression of C-afferent fiber-evoked activity in the spinal cord.[28] These data imply that injection of significant amounts of local anesthetic anywhere in the body could result in widespread effects on spinal antinociceptive mechanisms, regardless of the area or modality of peripheral axonal blockade.

Thus interpretation of the results of diagnostic spinal blockade, by whatever technique, must be considered as dubious if conclusions are to be made on the basis of differing nerve fiber blockade and the presence or absence of pain. However, the use of spinal injection of local anesthetics to determine the segmental level from which pain is derived or transmitted can be accomplished by producing ascending spinal blockade with dose increments to achieve rising segmental anesthesia. In theory, this may be best achieved by subarachnoid injection because of the use of much smaller doses of local anesthetic and thus less drug absorbed into the vasculature to produce the effects described above. In the future, development of very fine subarachnoid catheters may make this approach more attractive because incremental doses can be given and patients can carry out movements that may usually provoke pain.*

Differential epidural block[26] was advocated in an attempt to overcome some limitations of differential spinal subarachnoid block. Use of an epidural catheter allowed better patient movement and associated testing for pain, while providing for repeated tests if some responses were equivocal. Avoidance of headache, especially in young patients, was a further advantage. Despite these considerations, diagnostic "differential" epidural local anesthetic blockade carries the same limitations of interpretation as spinal subarachnoid block, and the technique must be considered as one of limited value.

What positive information can be derived from spinal subarachnoid or epidural diagnostic local anesthetic blockade?

1. The segmental level of nociceptive input may be established.
2. Continuation of pain in or below an area fully blocked suggests pain of a higher central focus. Additional issues relating to interpretation pitfalls are discussed under "Evaluation of Block."

Diagnostic Epidural Opioid Blockade. This technique is based on the assumption that epidural opioids block nociceptive input at the level of the dorsal horn, leaving sensory, sympathetic, and motor function unchanged and without giving the patient "cues" that blockade has occurred.[11] Relief of pain would point to a nociceptive focus either in the dorsal horn or peripheral to the dorsal horn. Failure of pain relief would point to more central pain (see Table 27-2). However, there are two problems with this technique: [1] Some types of pain may not be abolished by spinal opioids, for example, intermittent deep somatic and visceral pain[4] (see Chap. 28); and [2] opioid drugs migrate in CSF to the brain and are absorbed into the vasculature (see Chap. 28); this may produce "cues" to the patient and may also exert a significant analgesic effect at the level of the brain.

To resolve these problems, the following are needed: [1] blood and CSF pharmacokinetic studies after epidural, and intrathecal,* opioids used for diagnostic purposes (*e.g.*, fentanyl, Table 27-2); [2] simultaneous documentation of pharmacodynamic effects; and [3] statistical analysis of the reliability of diagnostic opioid blockade in predicting the etiology of pain syndromes that are precisely documented. In cancer pain, it certainly seems worthwhile using a trial of opioid by means of a percutaneous catheter before implanting an expensive "portal" or pump system (see Chap. 28).

Diagnostic Epidural Stimulation. In "deafferentation" pain syndromes, in some cases, transcutaneous nerve stimulation (TCNS) produces good pain relief but is impractical for long-term use. In other cases, TCNS is ineffective or only partly effective. In all these situations, a trial of epidural stimulation may be considered. This is highly preferable to implanting such devices as a "last-resort" maneuver. The stimulating electrodes are placed by means of an epidural needle under an image intensifier and positioned percutaneously. Stimulation is then carried out for 1 to 2 days on a trial basis, and careful records of pain relief, opioid requirements, and activity are kept. Unfortunately, there are no objective data of specific pain syndromes evaluated with "trial" stimulation and then followed up after definitive implantation of an epidural stimulator (see Chap. 30).

Differential Brachial Plexus or Lumbosacral Plexus Block. It is possible to place a catheter next to either of these plexuses (see Chaps. 10 and 11). In theory, placebo, sympathetic block, sensory block,

TABLE 27-2. DIAGNOSTIC EPIDURAL OPIOID BLOCKADE

1. 10 ml of 0.9% saline without preservative (epidural) (placebo)
2. 10 ml of 0.9% saline without preservative (epidural) (placebo)
3. 10-ml solution of fentanyl 100 μg (epidural)
4. Naloxone 0.4 mg (intravenous)
5. Lidocaine 2% 20 ml (epidural)

A visual analogue scale is used to record pain relief. The pattern of response is suggested as being useful.

*A 32-gauge × 36-inch polyamide microcatheter has been developed (Encapsulon, FX Medical, West Eatontown, New Jersey). It can be inserted through a 26-gauge spinal needle. This equipment may prove useful for diagnostic spinal local anesthetic and also opioid blockade.

and then motor block could be produced by saline, 40 ml of 0.25% lidocaine, 40 ml of 0.5% lidocaine, and 40 ml of 1% lidocaine, respectively. However, the same problems arise as with differential epidural block. In the arm and the leg, it is preferable to carry out a sympathetic block at the cervicothoracic level (arm) and lumbar sympathetic chain (leg). Then, on a separate occasion, somatic blocks can be performed.

Sympathetic Chain Blockade. This represents the most discrete method of determining whether pain is predominantly of sympathetic origin. The following techniques are described in Chapter 13: cervicothoracic ("stellate") sympathetic block, splanchnic nerve block, thoracic sympathetic ganglion block, celiac plexus block, and lumbar sympathetic ganglion block.

For the upper limb, it is necessary to block at least T1–T4 and preferably T1–T6 ganglia. Thus 15 ml of 1% lidocaine is required (see Figs. 13-19 and 13-20). If pain relief does not occur with sympathetic blockade, then a brachial plexus block is performed with 40 ml of 1% lidocaine with epinephrine 1 : 200,000. This should not be done sooner than 1 to 2 hours after the sympathetic block, to avoid cumulative toxicity.

For the lower limb, needles are inserted at L2 or L3, as shown in Figure 13-25, and 10 ml of 0.5% lidocaine is injected. Independent assessment of pain relief, sympathetic function, and blood flow is carried out. The results may help to determine whether a neurolytic block is likely to be helpful (see Fig. 13-7).

If pain is not relieved by sympathetic block, then somatic block is performed using sciatic, femoral, lateral femoral cutaneous, and obturator block (see Chap. 11).

Intrathoracic pain may be diagnosed using thoracic paravertebral (see Fig. 13-21) or "stellate ganglion level" (see Fig. 13-19) block. The former carries a greater risk of pneumothorax than the latter. Both may result in severe bradycardia if carried out bilaterally.

Intra-abdominal pain may be diagnosed using splanchnic or celiac plexus block (see Figs. 14-6 through 14-8).

Intrapelvic pain may be diagnosed using blockade of lumbar sympathetic ganglia bilaterally (see Figs. 13-22 and 25).

Intravenous Regional Blockade. Intravenous regional blockade with local anesthetic may be a convenient method of determining whether pain arises from a peripheral focus in the upper or lower limb (see Chap. 12). Pain relief can be assessed only while the cuff is inflated, since generalized effects will be produced as soon as local anesthetic is released into the circulation. However, there may also be some escape of local anesthetic under the cuff and by way of intraosseus blood flow, even when the cuff is inflated (see Chap. 12).

Intravenous regional sympathetic block (see Chaps. 12 and 13) may be used as a diagnostic test for causalgia, reflex sympathetic dystrophy, and other conditions with increased sympathetic activity. However, sympathetic block does *not* invariably relieve pain in such conditions; it seems more effective when hyperpathia is present than when paresthesias are predominant. Thus a positive response helps to confirm the diagnosis of sympathetic overactivity, whereas a negative result must be interpreted with caution. Some authors advise that solutions for diagnostic intravenous sympathetic blocks should not contain local anesthetic, since it is important to determine whether the sympathetic block relieves pain.[29]

Intravenous Infusion of Local Anesthetic. Interest has been rekindled in the use of intravenous lidocaine[7,28] and 2-chloroprocaine to treat central pain states. Before a series of infusions is initiated, the results of a "diagnostic" infusion should be carefully documented. The currently recommended dose and rate of infusion are given in Chapter 27.2.

A future application may be the use of intravenous infusion of local anesthetic to separate the effects of neural blockade from those of absorbed local anesthetic. For example, blood concentration of local anesthetic could be measured in each patient during the neural blockade procedure. On a separate occasion, local anesthetic would be infused to produce similar blood concentrations. The effects of both procedures on pain could be compared. A degree of pain relief with intravenous infusion similar to that obtained with nerve block suggests a central pain.

The mechanism of pain relief with intravenous local anesthetic is uncertain. Possibilities include [1] interference with central processing of pain, perhaps by membrane stabilization of central neurons; [2] suppression of "turbulent" neuronal activity at level of spinal cord or brain; and [3] a possible action on a spinal receptor mediating antinociception.[28]

PROCEDURAL REQUIREMENTS AND METHODS OF EVALUATION OF DIAGNOSTIC NERVE BLOCK

Physical Examination and History-Taking

It is highly desirable that a careful history be taken of both physical and psychosocial aspects of the pain[1,9,10,25,27] (see Chaps. 24.1 and 31). Psychological tests such as the Minnesota Multiphasic Personality Inventory and the illness behavior questionnaire are used (see Chap. 25). Also, any family and social problems should be explored.[1] The following aspects of the pain should be sought: onset and duration, site(s), character (intermittent, constant, or episodic), intensity, radiation, factors increasing or decreasing pain, symptoms associated with the pain; effect of pain on sleep; medications taken for pain, sleep, anxiety, depression, if any; effect of pain on patient's behavior, social life, work, sexual activity; effect on family; activities prevented by pain; patient's occupation, and response of other workers to the pain; existence of financial problems; and possibility of pending litigation or financial compensation.[1,9,10,25,27]

Physical examination should include careful neurologic examination and, if necessary, diagnostic tests such as x-rays, electromyography, myelography, and computed tomography scan. It should be remembered that there may be several pain sites, each with a different cause. If the physical and psychological evaluation is thorough, it is often possible to assign the patient to a well-recognized chronic pain syndrome (see Chap. 24.1, Appendix B). Such assignment may clarify whether diagnostic neural blockade is desirable or necessary. It may be sobering for those accustomed to using nerve blocks empirically to read the descriptions of pain syndromes with largely psychological bases and with other etiologies that permit diagnosis without neural blockade.

The myth that patients with pending litigation should not be considered for diagnostic neural blockade, or be actively treated, has been exploded. Patients undergoing litigation respond as well to treatment as do those not undergoing litigation (see Chap. 25). Nevertheless, litigation can make some patients anxious and depressed, and this should be taken into account when they are prepared for diagnostic neural blockade.

Patient Preparation

Patients should fast and be prepared as for any nerve block (see Chap. 6). Patients with chronic pain require careful explanation of the block procedure and considerable reassurance. Although the explanation is first given by the physician, it is usually the nursing staff of the unit that answers the patients' questions and ensures that they have the correct information. It is important that patients understand they are to undergo a *diagnostic* test that may or may not relieve their pain. Otherwise, they may feel "cheated" if definitive pain relief does not occur (see also Chap. 31).

Block Room Facilities

Full resuscitative equipment should be available in an appropriate setting for neural blockade (see Chap. 6). Adequate assistance is essential. Image intensifiers, nerve stimulators, thermography, and other equipment (see Chaps. 6 and 13) help greatly in performing the block and documenting its effects (see also Chap. 31).

Objective Tests of Function Before and After Blockade

Patients may be asked to keep a diary of activity (*e.g.*, time in bed, time "up," time working, time walking) for several weeks before presenting to the clinic. Immediately before blockade, baseline measurements of sensory, motor, and sympathetic function may be made (see Chaps. 8 and 13). The help of a physical therapist may be invaluable to document range of joint movement and other indices of physical activity. These measurements are repeated after the block.

Pain Measurement

A "pain diary" may be kept by patients before they are seen at the clinic. This should include a record of medications. The visual analogue scale is a useful method of documenting pain before and after block (see Chap. 25). The scales should be filled out without reference to previously marked scales. It is important that patients undergoing diagnostic neural blockade are free from analgesic and sedative drugs. Also, there should be a significant level of pain before blockade; otherwise, the block should be postponed.

Examination of painful area will reveal before-and-after differences in tenderness, sensory change, and reflex responses in addition to those affected by the conduction block itself.

Procedural Requirements

As with any regional procedure, the critical factor in determining whether the desired block will be attained is the site of final solution dispersion. How one begins or reaches this point is not of concern, but in principle the use of radiologic control with contrast medium-containing solutions is advocated as a graphic measure of correct technique. The ultimate test lies in the use of adequate and appropriate testing after local anesthetic injection to affirm the adequacy or otherwise of the conduction block (see Chap. 31).

Objective Evidence of Specific Block. Neurologic changes consequent to and consistent with the intended block should always be confirmed. Sensory and motor loss and deep tendon reflexes are commonly used for somatic pain, but abolition of twitch responses to nerve stimulation is helpful in difficult situations. Sympathetic block is confirmed by vasodilation (see Fig. 13-6), loss of sweating, temperature rise (see Fig. 13-7), evidence of a Horner's syndrome (see Fig. 13-19) for cervical sympathetic or postural hypotension, and increased gut motility with visceral block.

Time-Course of Response. As much information is gained from the duration of response as from the nature of the response. If subjective relief is considerably less than the duration of block, a nonspecific effect is surmised. No clinical deductions can be made, the reaction being other than pharmacologically induced analgesia. However, when block duration and analgesia are in parallel, almost certainly the effect is specific and caused by local somatic disease. Extended pain relief generally indicates an element of reflex activity, either muscle spasm or sympathetic overactivity, as part of the presentation.

Interpretation Pitfalls

Without doubt, the most difficult aspect of regional block use in pain diagnoses is in the interpretation of the clinical findings produced. Two general categories of misinterpretation are presented in this context.

False Positives. These arise when pain reduction is inferred as being a specific consequence of the block, when in fact the pain reduction is due to some action other than that intended or supposed. There are at least four possibilities.

Placebo Response. In the context of diagnostic blocks, a placebo response is one that reduces or abolishes pain by means other than the pharmacologic conduction block by the anesthetic used.[5,6,17] It occurs in approximately 30% of all procedures and indicates nothing more than an individual's capacity to develop such a response (see Chap. 25). Whatever mechanism is involved in its generation, this response conveys no significance as to diagnosis. Recognition of placebo versus specific analgesia is difficult, but in general a placebo effect is less complete, of less duration, and less reproducible with successive use (see Chap. 25). Examination reveals an inconsistency between subjective report and objective findings.

Unreliable Patient Report of Effects of Block. Diagnostic local anesthetic blocks inevitably suffer from the problem that the patient experiences an area of loss of sensation (sensory block) or a feeling of warmth (sympathetic block) that will act as a "cue." Some patients respond to that change in sensation by stating it as a genuinely perceived reduction in pain. Others may deceitfully report pain relief, since they believe that such a report may provide access to further medication, attention, or other desired gains.

Effects of Local Anesthetic Absorbed into the Circulation. It is clear that lidocaine and probably other local anesthetics may act as analgesics when absorbed into vasculature[7,28] (see above). Thus pain relief may be due to absorbed drug rather than to the nerve block. This is more likely if large doses of local anesthetic are used in highly vascular areas.

Effects of Peripheral Block on Central Processing. A nonspecific reduction in afferent input to the nervous system may result in temporary relief of central pain.[19,22] This does not imply that the pain focus lies peripheral to the nerve block but rather that normal peripheral input is activating a low-threshold central neuronal pool.

False Negatives. These incorrect deductions arise when a block does not relieve the pain, inferring that the site or nerve is not involved in the pain process.

Incomplete Block or Alternative Pain Pathways. All the nerve fibers may not be completely blocked, or alternative pathways may continue to provide nociceptive input from the same site or structure. In some patients, anatomic variants may be responsible for apparent failure. Joint structures in particular have multiple innervation.

If confirmatory testing for a successful block is undertaken, missed nerves or partial block will be identified. Sometimes a particular nerve may not be amenable to test, so techniques such as identification by means of twitch responses with a nerve stimulator or radiographic control of drug placement using contrast solutions will aid in ensuring high rates of successful block. Suprascapular block and segmental facet block (see Chap. 27.3) are examples of these approaches. It is equally important in making confirmatory tests that these techniques be applied to the correct level. For instance, a Horner's syndrome does not necessarily indicate successful sympathetic block to the arm after a stellate ganglion injection. The affected limb must show increased warmth, increased blood flow, loss of sweating, and loss of psychogalvanic reflex to provide proof of interruption of arm as opposed to cervical sympathetics (see Chap. 13).

Referred Pains. Facet joint disease may produce referred pain that does not precisely correspond with the segment associated with that facet (see Chap. 27.3). Thus somatic nerve root block at the level of the referred pain may not result in pain relief, whereas blockade of the diseased facet joint or medial branch of dorsal ramus at this level would relieve the pain. Another example is sacroiliac disease, which may produce pain referred to the back of the thigh and leg. Sciatic nerve block may not relieve this pain, whereas local injection into the sacroiliac joint would produce positive results. On the other hand, pain from facets at the L4 – L5 level may be referred to the sacroiliac area. Block at the sacroiliac level may have no effect, whereas block of L4 – L5 facet joints would relieve the pain.

Unreliable Patient Reports of Effects of Block. Some patients whose pain is relieved by diagnostic block may nevertheless fail to report pain relief because they wish the doctor to be seen to "fail" or they believe that this is their most effective route to the treatment, drugs, attention, and so forth that they desire. Psychological evaluation usually reveals serious personality disorder in such patients.

Testing at Inappropriate Time. Patients with little pain before the block may report little change after the block; thus diagnostic block should be postponed until the patient is again experiencing sustained pain. Testing too early, before complete onset of block, or too late, after the block has regressed, will result in a false negative. Some patients hold on to the idea that if the nerve block is successful, it should relieve the pain immediately and permanently. No amount of instruction about its temporary nature will change their minds.

Prognostic Blocks

As mentioned earlier, it was formerly a common practice to carry out a local anesthetic block of an appropriate peripheral nerve, nerve root, or other neural pathway before making a permanent surgical or neurolytic lesion to relieve pain. In a sense, such blocks were both "diagnostic" and "prognostic." However, all of the limitations that apply to the diagnostic use also apply to a purported prognostic application. The results obtained with a local anesthetic block are not always entirely "prognostic" of the results obtained with a neurolytic solution or with a surgical or other destructive technique. This is particularly so when a single local anesthetic block of rather short duration is carried out. It is possible that better "prognosis" could be obtained if catheter techniques were used to produce a longer-lasting block. As noted earlier, a single local anesthetic injection may predict rather poorly the intensity of pain relief and side-effects obtained with a permanent procedure.[18,23] This is hardly surprising when one considers that the spread of local anesthetic agents into neural structures and other surrounding structures may be quite different from the spread of the neurolytic solution or from the lesion produced by the surgical or other destructive measures. Also, a patient experiencing an area of sensory loss for a short period of time may not be at all disturbed by this. In contrast, it has now become clear that sensory loss extending over many days, weeks, and then years may become extremely disturbing to patients and may result in a "deafferentation syndrome."[23] Another frequent consequence of permanent neuroablative techniques is that they all may lead to subsequent fibrosis and possible scar entrapment of remaining fibers. Thus a patient's report of no discomfort from an anesthetic area after a nerve block cannot be interpreted with confidence as a prediction that such a patient will experience no discomfort when that area is denervated on a permanent basis.

CONCLUSION

Diagnostic and prognostic nerve blocks can provide useful information as part of a multidisciplinary management of chronic pain. They should be performed only by those skilled in neural blockade. Objective evidence of completeness of blockade should always be documented independently of measurements of effects of blockade, such as increased blood flow, and assessment of pain relief. It is desirable to use catheter technique and to randomize placebo solutions with local anesthetics of different duration. The use of an independent observer to document results improves reliability. Precise documentation and coding (see Chap. 24.1) of the pain syndrome under investigation will permit future assessment of the usefulness of diagnostic neural blockade in various chronic pain syndromes.

REFERENCES

1. Abram, S.E., Anderson, R.A., and Maitra-D'Cruze, A.M.: Factors predicting short-term outcome of nerve blocks in the management of chronic pain. Pain, *10*:323, 1981.
2. Ahlgren, E.W., *et al.*: Diagnosis of pain with a graduated spinal block technique. JAMA, *195*:813, 1966.
3. Applegate, W.V.: Abdominal cutaneous nerve entrapment syndrome. Surgery, *71*:118, 1972.
4. Arner, S., and Arner, B.: Differential effects of epidural morphine in the treatment of cancer related pain. Acta Anaesthesiol. Scand., *29*:32, 1985.
5. Beecher, H.K.: The powerful placebo. JAMA, *159*:1602, 1955.
6. Benson, H., and Epstein, M.D.: The placebo effect. A neglected asset in the care of patients. JAMA, *232*:1225, 1975.
7. Boas, R.A., Covino, B.G., and Shahwarian, A.: Analgesic response to IV lignocaine. Br. J. Anaesh., *54*:501, 1982.
8. Bonica, J.J.: Current role of nerve blocks in the diagnosis and therapy of pain. *In* Bonica, J.J. (ed.): Advances in Neurology, vol. 4, p. 445. New York, Raven Press, 1974.
9. Brena, S.F.: Nerve blocks and chronic pain states: An update. I. Basic Considerations. II. Clinical Indications. Postgrad. Med., *78*:62, 1985.
10. Catchlove, R.F.: Integrated management of chronic pain. Can. Anaesth. Soc. J., *33*:S13, 1986.
11. Cherry, D.A., Gourlay, G.K., McLachlan, M., and Cousins, M.J.: Diagnostic epidural opioid blockade and chronic pain. Pain, *21*:143, 1985.
12. Devor, M., Govrin-Lippmann, R., and Raber, P.: Corticosteroids suppress ectopic neural discharge originating in experimental neuromas. Pain, *22*:127, 1985.
13. Diaz, P.M.: Use of liquid crystal thermography to evaluate sympathetic blocks. Anesthesiology, *44*:443, 1976.
14. Hoppenstein, R.: A new approach to the failed, failed back syndrome. Spine, *5*:371, 1980.
15. Kibler, R.F., and Nathan, P.W.: Relief of pain and paresthesiae by nerve blocks distal to a lesion. J. Neurol. Neurosurg. Psychiatry, *23*:91, 1960.
16. Klineberg, I., and Lillie, J.: Regional nerve block of the temporomandibular joint capsule: A technique for clinical research and differential diagnosis. J. Dent. Res., *59*:1930, 1980.
17. Laska, E., and Sunshine, A.: Anticipation of analgesia—A placebo effect. Headache, *13*:1, 1973.
18. Loeser, J.D.: Dorsal rhizotomy for the relief of chronic pain. J. Neurosurg., *36*:745, 1972.
19. Loh, L., Nathan, P.W., and Schott, G.: Pain due to lesions of the central nervous system removed by sympathetic block. Br. Med. J., *282*:1026, 1981.
20. Pochaczevsky, R., Wexler, C.E., Meyers, P.H., *et al.*: Liquid crystal thermography of the spine and extremities; its value in the diagnosis of spinal root syndromes. J. Neurosurg., *56*:386, 1982.
21. Porges, P.: Local anesthetics in the treatment of cancer pain. Recent Results Cancer Res., *89*:127, 1984.
22. Schechter, N.L.: Pain and pain control in children. Curr. Probl. Pediatr., *15*:1, 1985.
23. Tasker, R.: Deafferentation and causalgia. *In* Bonica, J.J. (ed.): Advances in Pain Research and treatment, pp. 305–329. New York, Raven Press, 1980.
24. Thomas, P.S., and Zauder, H.L.: Thermography. *In* Raj, P.P. (ed.): Practical Management of Pain, pp. Chicago, Year Book Medical Publishers, 1986.
25. Timmerman, G., and Sternbach, R.A.: Factors of human chronic pain: Analysis of personality and pain reaction variables. Science, *184*:806, 1974.
26. Winnie, A.P., and Collins, V.J.: Differential neural blockade in pain syndromes of questionable etiology. Med. Clin. North. Am., *52*:123, 1968.
27. Woodforde, J.M., and Merskey, H.: Personality traits of patients with chronic pain. J. Psychosom. Res., *16*:167, 1972.
28. Woolf, C., and Wiesenfeld–Hallin, Z.: The systemic administration of local anesthetics produces a selective depression of c-afferent fiber evoked activity in the spinal cord. Pain, *23*:361, 1985.
29. Wynn–Parry, C.B., and Withrington, R.: The management of painful peripheral nerve disorders. *In* Wall, P.D., and Melzack, R. (eds.): Textbook of Pain, pp. 395–401. Edinburgh, Churchill Livingstone, 1984.

27.2 PROGNOSTIC AND THERAPEUTIC LOCAL ANESTHETIC BLOCKADE

P. PRITHVI RAJ

Since the introduction of regional anesthesia in 1884 by Karl Koller, nerve blocks with local anesthetics or neurolytic agents have been used for the management of benign and malignant chronic pain (see Chap. 1, Appendices A and D). When skillfully administered, they are among the most effective methods of relieving pain. Despite their long use, some pain specialists are skeptical about their efficacy (see also Chap. 31). In this section the prognostic and therapeutic applications of local anesthetic block are discussed. The diagnostic applications and the role of neurolytic nerve blocks are described in Chapters 27.1 and 29, respectively.

RATIONALE

The rationale for the use of local anesthetic nerve blocks in chronic pain patients is the reliability with which they interrupt *sensory* and *nociceptive* pathways. Sensory nerve block thus obtained usually relieves pain and interrupts the afferent limbs of an abnormal reflex. With low concentrations of local anesthetic agents, one can block the A-delta, B, and unmyelinated C-delta fibers without clinically significant impairment of motor function.[16] Interestingly, in early phases of chronic pain, local anesthetic nerve blocks can produce prolonged pain relief that outlasts the pharmacological action of the drug by days or weeks. The mechanism for this is not yet understood, but one can speculate that this may be due to a reversal of physiologic changes, which accompany such chronic pain.[20]

INDICATIONS

Local anesthetic nerve blocks are useful for diagnosis, prognosis, and therapy of chronic pain.[16] The efficacy of diagnostic local anesthetic nerve blocks is discussed in Chapter 27.1.

Blocks For Prognosis

In certain painful states where surgical ablative procedures are being considered (*e.g.*, rhizotomy or sympathectomy), a single or prolonged local anesthetic nerve block can be used prognostically to allow the patient to experience and his surgeon to evaluate the effects of such a denervation.[10,12,13] Such an evaluation should help them to arrive at an appropriate decision whether or not to proceed with surgery. It is important to appreciate that although the immediate numbness experienced after a prognostic block may be a welcome relief, over time the prolonged numbness caused by surgical ablation may develop into a chronic deafferentation syndrome, followed by dysesthesia (see Chap. 30). The dysesthesia may be as distressing as the original nociception. Prognostic blocks may be helpful to arrive at decisions for surgery, but they certainly do not guarantee long-term pain relief (see Chap. 27.1 and Refs. 18 and 23 in that chapter).

Blocks for Pain Management

Therapeutically, the local anesthetic nerve blocks are effective in managing self-limiting diseases accompanied by severe pain and in breaking up the so-called vicious cycle in subacute and chronic pain, such as in patients with causalgia, reflex sympathetic dystrophy, or myofascial pain with reflex muscle spasm.[16] They have also been useful in treating ischemic and vasospastic pain syndromes of arterial embolus, Raynaud's disease, thromboangiitis obliterans, frostbite, acute herpes zoster, and phantom pain. Once the symptomatic pain relief is obtained by local anesthetic nerve blocks, other therapeutic measures, such as TENS (transcutaneous electrical nerve stimulation) and physical therapy, can be used for prolongation and maintenance of pain relief. However, therapeutic blocks for prolonged analgesia are usually attempted with neurolytic agents, especially for patients with pain resulting from cancer, chronic pancreatitis, and spastic paraplegia. Nerve blocks with local anesthetics and steroids, singly or in a series, have also been used therapeutically for pancreatitis and postherpetic neuralgia[73] and for back pain (see Chap. 27.3).

PAIN SYNDROMES

The subacute and chronic pain syndromes in which local anesthetic nerve blocks are indicated for prognostic and therapeutic effect can be classified into neurogenic pain, musculoskeletal pain, pain in somatic structures owing to abnormal sympathetic activity, and visceral pain. See Chapter 24.1 for classification and description of chronic pain syndromes.

NEUROGENIC PAIN

Neurogenic pain* syndromes in which local anesthetic nerve blocks may be useful are (a) neuralgias of the cranial and spinal nerves (trigeminal, occipital, glossopharyngeal, or intercostal nerves); (b) radiculopathies of cervical and lumbar nerve roots; (c) cervical, brachial, and lumbosacral plexalgias; (d) peripheral neuralgias and neuropathies (diabetic, nutritional); and (e) compression and entrapment syndromes.

Trigeminal Neuralgia

Trigeminal neuralgia is a manifestation of underlying disordered physiology. The syndrome is manifested by the classic features of unilateral painful paroxysms of lightning pains lasting for a few seconds to a couple of minutes; pain provoked by insignificant mechanical stimuli, such as touching the face or a breeze blowing across the face; pain confined to the zone of the trigeminal nerve, classically in V_2 or V_3; absent hypoesthesia; and prolonged pain-free intervals (see Chap. 24.1, Appendix B, Sect. II-1).

*See also Chap. 24.1, Appendix A.

The most common cause of the syndrome is the pressure exerted on the trigeminal nerve root entry zone in the posterior fossa by the loop of the superior cerebellar artery.[57] Multiple sclerosis is the second most common cause of the syndrome. Other possible causes are tumors, ectatic blood vessels, aneurysms, arteriovenous malformations, and arachnoidal scarring or cysts (see Chap. 24.1, Appendix B, Sect. II-2).[54]

Pain management of trigeminal neuralgia consists of medication, nerve blocks, percutaneous radiofrequency or thermocoagulation, and surgery. The rationale for the nerve block of trigeminal nerve or its branches with a local anesthetic or neurolytic agent is as follows: [a] it allows the patient to experience the facial numbness that would follow a surgical rhizotomy and decide whether or not he could tolerate it; [b] it allows the patient to recover from the debilitated state before surgery; [c] it helps to differentiate from "atypical" facial pain; and [d] it allows the patient to recover from severe pain immediately and thereby have a period of pain-free state before a permanent treatment is planned (see also Chaps. 29.2, 30).

Occipital Neuralgia

Occipital neuralgia is caused by compression of the anterior or posterior branch of the second cervical root. The patient complains of pain around the insertion of the trapezius and scalene muscles radiating along the course of the nerves. There is a persistent occipital scalp dysesthesia with tenderness over the exit of the nerve. Along with sore nuchal-occipital area, there may also be retro-ocular pain. If the occipital neuralgia is idiopathic, local anesthetic nerve block (plus steroids) can relieve the occipital headache. A series of three to six occipital nerve blocks is usually enough to provide prolonged relief.

Glossopharyngeal Neuralgia

Glossopharyngeal neuralgia has many of the characteristics of tic douloureux, but the pain occurs in the posterior third of the tongue and in the tonsillar and pharyngeal areas. The pain is usually described as stabbing, with periods of exacerbation and remission. Topical analgesia with local anesthetics (*e.g.*, cocaine in the oropharynx) relieves the pain and differentiates it from trigeminal neuralgia. Further therapeutic management consists of either repeated local anesthetic glossopharyngeal nerve blocks once a week for 6 weeks or use of neurolytic agents (alcohol) when repeat local anesthetic blocks have failed to prolong the relief (see Chap. 24.1, Appendix B, Sect. II-7).

Intercostal Neuralgia

Herpes zoster and postherpetic neuralgia are the most common causes of intercostal neuralgia. Metastatic and spreading tumors from the thoracic cavity, as well as post-thoracotomy scarring, can entrap intercostal nerves and produce intolerable radiating pain in the distribution of the intercostal nerves. Specific management of herpes zoster or nerve entrapment is described in the specific sections (see below).

Radiculopathy

Acute radicular pain results from irritation and inflammation of the nerve root by a herniated disk, usually in lower cervical and lumbar regions. Chemical radiculitis results from degenerating glycoprotein from the extruded herniated nucleus pulposus.[72] Neural swelling, ischemia, and, eventually, loss of neural elements and fibrosis occur, leading to chronic pain. Injection of corticosteroids into the epidural space adjacent to the irritated nerve root produces tolerable relief in the majority of the patients with early radicular pain.[2] Early treatment probably prevents some of the irreversible changes that occur with chronic inflammation. Further details of the efficacy of epidural steroid injection are given in Chapter 27.3.

Peripheral Neuralgia, Including Plexalgias

Severe pain and marked cutaneous hyperesthesia may result from many types of peripheral nerve pathology. Trauma, laceration, avulsion, and compression may cause degeneration of sensory axons. During and after regeneration, the cutaneous area supplied by the nerve remains hyperpathic. Toxic and metabolic neuropathies, such as those caused by diabetes, alcoholism, and certain drugs, may produce constant neuralgic pain and dysesthesias. Herpes zoster causes similar dysesthesias in addition to the cutaneous rash. In mixed nerves the larger fibers are susceptible to ischemia with preservation of small afferent fibers that subserve nociceptive functions.[49]

Multimodality treatment is helpful in controlling neuralgic pain. Diphenylhydantoin and carbamazepine are often effective in the episodic type of neuralgias. Sympathetic or peripheral nerve blocks with local anesthetic or anesthetic–steroid mixtures may be helpful for constant neuralgic pain and hyperpathia (see also Chap. 24.1, Appendix B, Sect. X-3).

Compression and Entrapment Syndromes

The peripheral nerve trunks of thorax and extremities are prone to compression and entrapment. The common entrapment neuropathies involve the intercostal, lateral femoral cutaneous nerve (meralgia paresthetica), carpal tunnel syndrome, delayed ulnar and common peroneal nerve palsy. A light touch on the scar produces intense radiating pain, sometimes accompanied by burning pain owing to associated reflex sympathetic dystrophy. Peripheral nerve or sympathetic blocks with a local anesthetic or a mixture of local anesthetic and steroid are useful to treat such entrapment syndromes. A series of three to six blocks are usually required for effective adequate pain relief in 60% of the patients. Single injections are usually short-lived and inadequate. Injection of the scar with a local anesthetic mixed with a steroid is likely to provide long-term relief.

Neuroma

A palpable neuroma in the scar, loss of pinprick sensation over the skin, and elicitation of pain on palpation are diagnostic. Repeated injection of a local anesthetic–steroid mixture may relieve the pain. Persistent pain from a well-localized neuroma may respond better to neurolytic injection of phenol or to cryolysis.

MUSCULOSKELETAL PAIN

Musculoskeletal pain[90] can be caused by inflammation, degeneration, or trauma to the skeletal or myofascial tissues. Myofascial pain[91] is the most common cause of chronic low back or cervical pain. Other conditions that produce soft tissue pain are bursitis, synovitis, and tendonitis (tennis elbow, golfer's elbow, leg compartment syndromes) (see Chap.

24.1). Skeletal pain can be due to osteoarthritis, degenerative arthritis, ankylosing spondylitis, inflammation of the facet joint, and spondylolisthesis.

Myofascial Pain

Skeletal muscle is the largest organ of the human body and accounts for 40% of body weight. Because the contractile muscle tissues are extremely subject to daily wear and tear, any muscle can develop myofascial trigger points that can cause pain and muscle spasm (see Chap. 24.1, Appendix B, Sect. I-9).

A major difficulty in understanding of myofascial pain has been the multiplicity of names given to this syndrome. Good used the term "muscular rheumatism" in 1938.[44] Later the same author used "non-articular rheumatism," "myalgic spots," "idiopathic myalgia," and "muscular sciatica" for the syndrome of myofascial pain.[13] Kelly used the term "fibrositis" and Travell used "idiopathic myalgia" and ended with "myofascial trigger points" in her later publications.[56,113,114] Many more names are given to this syndrome by other workers (*e.g.*, rheumatic myositis, myofasciitis, nodular fibromyositis, fibropathic syndromes).[81,102,109,124]

TABLE 27-3. PATHOPHYSIOLOGY OF A TRIGGER POINT: FIRST MECHANISM

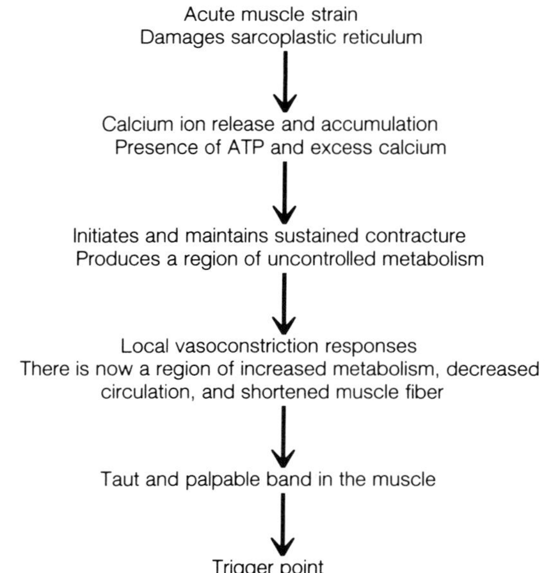

Acute muscle strain
Damages sarcoplastic reticulum
↓
Calcium ion release and accumulation
Presence of ATP and excess calcium
↓
Initiates and maintains sustained contracture
Produces a region of uncontrolled metabolism
↓
Local vasoconstriction responses
There is now a region of increased metabolism, decreased circulation, and shortened muscle fiber
↓
Taut and palpable band in the muscle
↓
Trigger point

(Raj, P.P. [ed.]: Practical Management of Pain. p. 694. Chicago, Year Book Medical Publishers, 1986).

It is believed that a myofascial trigger point starts as a neuromuscular dysfunction[87] and evolves into a histologically distinct lesion.[75] Miehlke and coworkers demonstrated biopsy findings that supported an initial dysfunction phase that developed into a dystrophic phase.[75]

Pathophysiology. An acute muscle strain may overload the muscle fibrils in one region of the muscle, causing tissue damage that includes damage to the sarcoplastic reticulum and release of stored calcium with loss of ability in that region to remove the calcium ions. The presence of normal adenosine triphosphate (ATP) and excess calcium will initiate and maintain a sustained contracture of the fibers exposed to the calcium. This produces a region of uncontrolled metabolism within the muscle, to which the body responds with local vasoconstriction. This could be a local response or a trigger point-mediated reflex response involving the central nervous system and the sympathetic nervous system. There is now a region of increased metabolism with decreased circulation with shortened muscle fibers. This group of taut fibers are palpable as a band in the muscle (Tables 27-3 and 27-4; see also Fig. 24-1).

A second mechanism may then take over. The total depletion of ATP could lead to conditions similar to others that are known to cause muscle contracture with electrical silence, as in McArdle's disease, carnatine deficiency, and rigor mortis. Without ATP, the myosin heads do not release actin filaments and the sarcomeres become rigid.

Nerve-sensitizing substances, such as histamine, serotonin, kinins, and prostaglandins, may be released in the trigger point zone by several mechanisms. With the tissue injury, some blood would extravasate, forming a large source for serotonin owing to increased platelets.[7] This could cause further local ischemia. Mast cells also increase in number at the site of muscle injury, causing a release of histamine.[7] The initial phase of increased metabolism with reduced circulation would accumulate local metabolic products that may result in the release of additional sensitizing agents, such as prostaglandins.[75,105]

Clinical Signs and Symptoms (see Chap. 24.1). The myofascial pain may appear acutely with muscle strain or begin insidiously as a sequel of chronic muscle fatigue. Pain may continue for months or years.[53] Regardless of the mode of onset, pain from a myofascial trigger point is steady, deep, and aching. Seldom is it burning. Myofascial trigger point pain can be augmented by strenuous use of the involved muscle, by passive stretch of the muscle, by pressure on the trigger point, during cold or damp weather, or by viral infections, stress, or fatigue. Even though pain may not be the main complaint, there is usually a limited range of motion as well as weakness. Limitation of motion and increased stiffness are worse in the morning and recur after periods of overactivity or immobilization during the day. Patients may report symptoms of autonomic dysfunction (*e.g.*, excessive lacrimation, pilomotor activity, changes in sweat patterns). The involved extremity may feel cold because of reflex vasoconstriction. Patients may have signs of depression, anxiety, and sleep disturbances, which in turn may lower the pain threshold.*

Clinically, a myofascial trigger point is a hyperirritable locus within the taut band of skeletal muscle, localized in the muscle or its associated fascia.[112] The trigger point is painful on compression and can evoke a characteristic referred pain and an autonomic response. A myofascial trigger point has to be distinguished from tender spots in skin, ligaments, and periosteum.

Trigger points can be either active or latent. An active trigger point causes pain whereas the latent trigger point may restrict movement and weaken the affected muscle. The latent trigger point persists for years after recovering from injury and predisposes to acute exacerbations of pain. The usual precipitating factors are jerky motion involving that muscle, fatigue, cold and damp surroundings, and emotional upset.

Examination. To palpate a taut band, the muscle is stretched until the fibers of the taut band are under tension. The stretch should evoke local discomfort but not referred pain. This usually occurs at two thirds of the muscle's normal range of stretch. The examiner palpates along the taut band to locate the point of maximum tenderness and then presses firmly on that spot to elicit the referred pain pattern. Flat palpation is used when the muscle can be pressed against underlying bony surface. Pincer palpation is used when the opposite sides of the muscle are accessible to grasping between the digits, for example, sternomastoid, lattisimus dorsi, biceps brachii, pectoralis major and minor (Figs. 27-6, 27-7).

There can be a local twitch response when the trigger point is rolled between fingers or touched by a needle.[56,60] Exploratory palpation for an active trigger point can elicit, simultaneously, a local twitch response, a jump sign, and a referred pain pattern. When a nerve passes through a muscle between taut bands or between a taut band and a bone, the patient may have two kinds of referred pain: aching pain from the trigger point or numbness, tingling, hyperesthesia, or hypoesthesia owing to nerve compression. Partial neuropraxia may be relieved within minutes after inactivation of responsible trigger points, and resulting muscle relaxation. Severe compression may require weeks for full recovery.

With an active trigger point, stretching of the involved muscle increases the pain[69] and the muscle spasm is initiated. This further increases the tension in the muscle and elevates the intensity of pain. The painful spasm does not allow further lengthening of the muscle unless therapeutic steps are taken to prevent the spasm.

Routine laboratory tests show no significant abnormalities with myofascial pain syndrome. The erythrocyte sedimentation rate, SMA, blood count, serum muscle enzymes are all normal. Radiograms and computed tomography scans are normal. Electromyography may show insertion potential, increased number of polyphasic potentials in muscles with trigger points. Thermograms of skin overlying active trigger points may show areas of increased skin temperature.[39] Sola and Williams observed low skin resistance over the trigger point.[104]

*Possibly by means of decreased central inhibitory noradrenergic (NA) mechanisms and increased peripheral NA sensitizing nociceptors.

TABLE 27-4. PATHOPHYSIOLOGY OF A TRIGGER POINT: SECOND MECHANISM

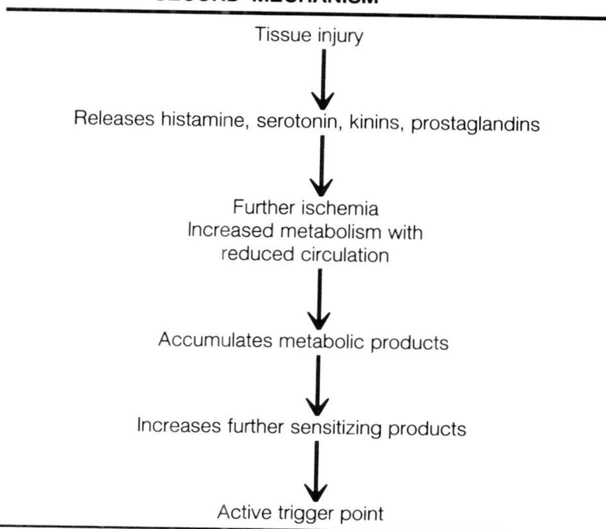

(Raj, P.P. [ed.]: Practical Management of Pain. p. 694. Chicago, Year Book Medical Publishers, 1986).

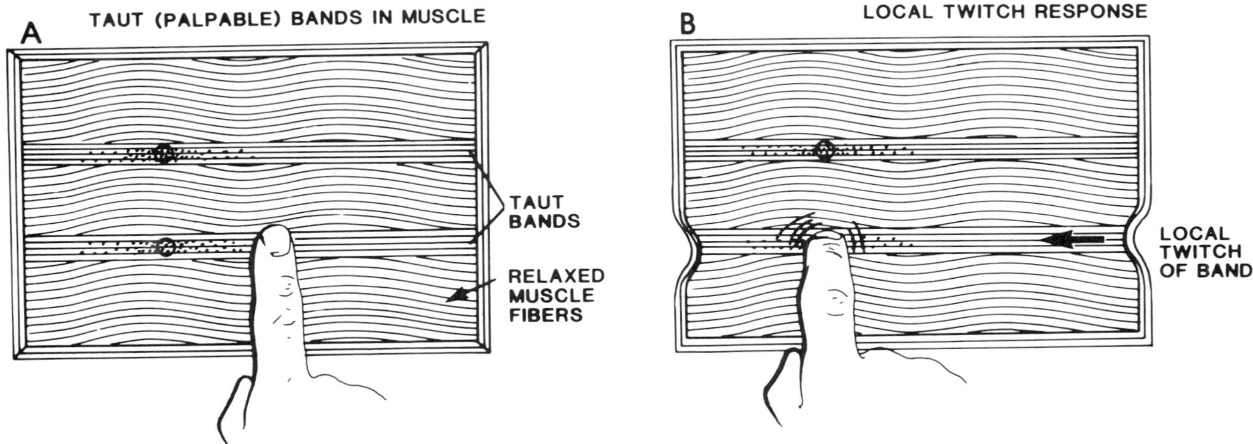

FIG. 27-6. Method of palpating a flat muscle to elicit a taut band in the muscle **(A)** of a local twitch **(B).** (Travell, J., and Simon, D.G.: Myofascial Pain and Dysfunction: The Trigger Point Manual. Baltimore, Williams & Wilkins, 1983.)

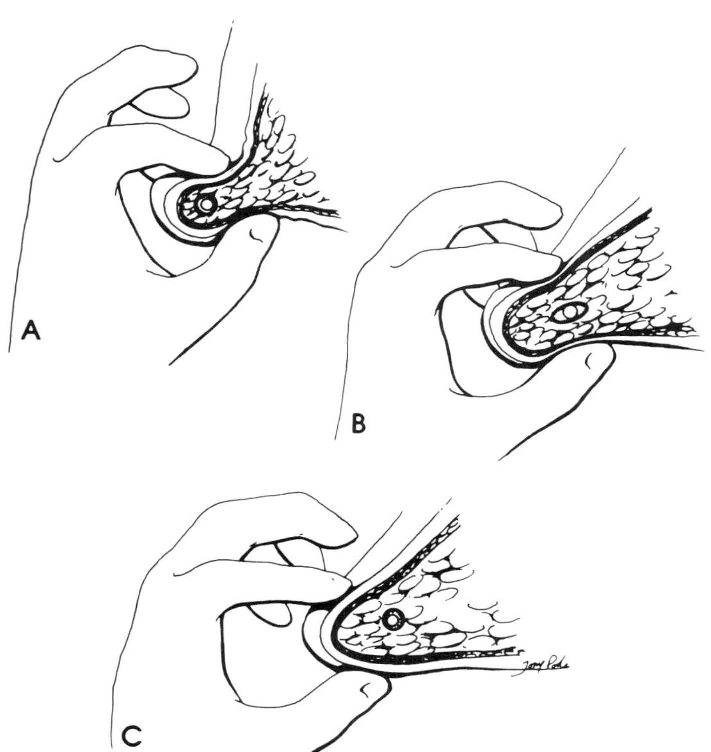

FIG. 27-7. Method of palpating the trigger point in a long thin muscle when the muscle can be grasped between the fingers and rolled through them. **A.** Muscle fibers surrounded by the thumb and fingers in a pincer grip; **B.** hardness of the taut band felt; **C.** edge of the taut band sharply defined with a local twitch response. (Travell, J., and Simon, D.G.: Myofascial Pain and Dysfunction: The Trigger Point Manual. Baltimore, Williams & Wilkins, 1983.)

Management of Myofascial Pain. The object of treating myofascial trigger point pain is to decrease pain to tolerable levels, improve function, and prevent permanent disability. This can be achieved by muscle relaxation, spray-and-stretch techniques or trigger point injection, exercise programs, and stimulation analgesia. The method of trigger point injection will be described in this chapter (see below).

Pain from Inflammation

In general, pain of soft tissues in the extremities is due to bursitis, tenosynovitis, and fibrositis.[90] Trauma is the most common cause of bursitis, but almost any illness characterized by joint synovitis may be associated with involvement of the lining of bursae. Tendon sheaths, like bursae, have synovial linings and can be involved by any process capable of inducing joint synovitis. Fibrositis is a poorly defined symptom complex characterized by pain and stiffness in varying areas, most often in the neck, shoulder girdle, and posterior aspect of the trunk.

Treatment. Generally, pain caused by these conditions is managed with physical measures (deep heat, massage, physical therapy, and TENS), nonsteroidal anti-inflammatory agents, and psychotherapy (relaxation technique, biofeedback, and so forth). If symptoms are acute, severe, or refractory to other treatments, local anesthetic nerve blocks (infiltration, trigger point injection, sympathetic and peripheral nerve blocks) with steroids are indicated. They are usually effective temporarily at the time of performing the nerve block, but for a more prolonged effect, a series of four to six blocks once a week may be required.

Pain from Sprains and Strains

Common examples of this syndrome are tennis elbow, groin strains, lumbosacral sprain, anterior and posterior compartment syndromes, and ankle sprains. Treatment consists of deep heat and rest in the acute stage and a series of local injections of local anesthetic and steroids (three to six) weekly with a graduated exercise program.

Torticollis

Torticollis is a severe state of contraction of the sternocleidomastoid muscle.[50] It may be either congenital or acquired. The congenital form may be muscular or postural, in which the striated muscle is replaced by fibrous tissue. Acquired torticollis may result from trauma or inflammatory disease of the cervical spine, or it may be a neuromuscular disorder of either neurologic or psychogenic origin (Fig. 27-8). Longstanding torticollis produces permanent contracture of the muscle, fibrotic changes in the tissues, and degenerative changes in the cervical spine. There may be variable degrees of pain. Psychological factors associated with this disorder may be responsible for either initiating or aggravating the problem.

Management. The lack of understanding of the cause of torticollis is exemplified by the diverse variety of therapeutic approaches that have been proposed: surgery (cervical rhizotomy, thalamotomy, dorsal column stimulation, sternocleidomastoid excision), psychotherapy (hypnosis, behavior modification, and biofeedback), drug therapy (amantidine, haloperidol, apomorphine),[41,42,110] and nerve blocks[94] (accessory nerve, cervical plexus, cervical epidural). Physical therapy is essential with all of the approaches in both acute and chronic stages.

Skeletal Pain

Skeletal pain may be due to pathology of the bone, periosteum, ligaments, or joints. Many systemic diseases cause skeletal pain (rheumatoid arthritis, osteoarthritis, degenerative arthritis, Paget's disease, osteoporosis). Metastatic tumors frequently involve bone at multiple sites and cause pain by periosteal pressure. Benign skeletal pain as part of low back or cervical pain may result from diffuse or focal spondylitic changes in the spine, inflammation of the facet joint, spondylolysis, spondylolisthesis, and pseudoarthroses (see also Chap. 27.3).

Management. In the management of skeletal pain, the following facts should be kept in mind: in most patients, the disease is chronic; spontaneous remissions occur in almost all patients; the majority of patients can lead active lives with varying degrees of restrictions; and complications of drug therapy (*e.g.*, steroids) can cause greater morbidity than the underlying disease.

A basic program that is applicable to all patients includes rest in the acute stage; maintenance of function by physical measures (deep heat, hydrotherapy, manipulation and mobilization, graduated exercise program, TENS); use of appropriate anti-inflammatory agents for maintenance of pain relief; and use of

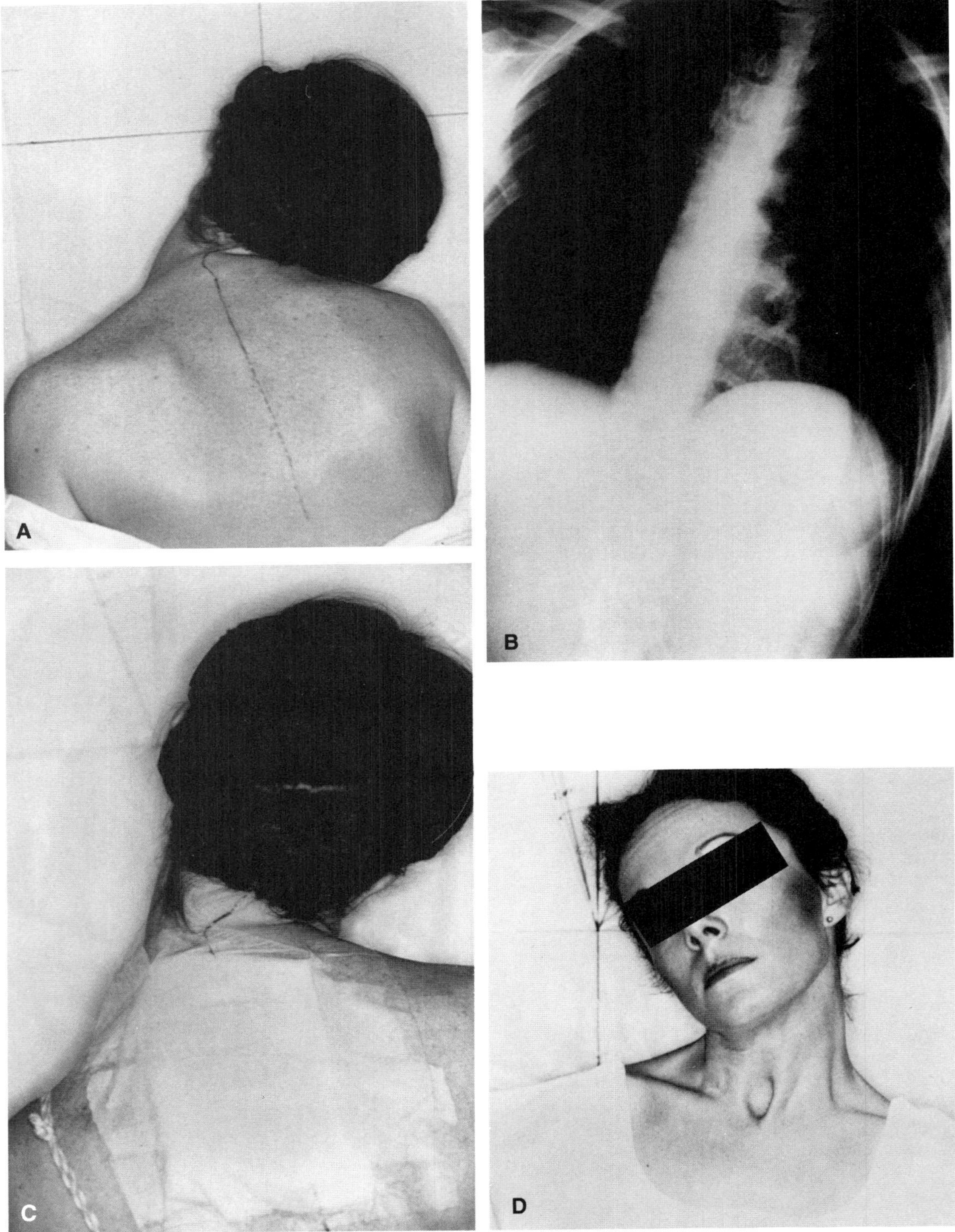

FIG. 27-8. Severe spasmodic torticollis in a 30-year-old woman. The torticollis developed acutely at 6 months of pregnancy after the administration of a phenothiazine. **A.** The condition 1 month after developing torticollis. (Raj, P.P. [ed.]: Practical Management of Pain, p. 426. Chicago, Year Book Medical Publishers, 1986.) **B.** X-ray of the patient showing thoracolumbar scoliosis as a compensation for torticollis. **C.** Patient with cervical epidural catheter. Note improvement of torticollis after a week of bupivacaine infusion. **D.** Patient condition 2 months after treatment.

local anesthetic nerve blocks for treatment of severe acute pain.

Local anesthetic nerve blocks could be as simple as trigger point injections if the pain is secondary to muscle spasms, or one may have to resort to joint or peripheral nerve injections of local anesthetics with or without steroids. Another technique that has recently been tried is prolonged infusion of the painful site with local anesthetic for 1 to 2 weeks if the pain is intractable. The technique of prolonged infusion is described later in this chapter.

PAIN IN SOMATIC STRUCTURES OWING TO ABNORMAL SYMPATHETIC ACTIVITY

The pain from this syndrome is due to the overactivity of the peripheral sympathetic nervous system involving the somatic structures. The two common syndromes that represent this pain are causalgia and reflex sympathetic dystrophy.[14,76] Peripheral vascular disease can also produce "sympathetic" pain.

Causalgia and Reflex Sympathetic Dystrophy

True causalgia follows partial injury to a major nerve trunk, such as the sciatic nerve, or its large branches. Reflex sympathetic dystrophy is much more common and may occur after the minor trauma to neural structures that accompanies fractures or soft tissue injuries. It is also not unusual as an iatrogenic complication of surgical or neurolytic therapy. Clinical characteristics include burning, poorly localized pain often with a stabbing component, hyperesthesia, and vasomotor and sudomotor alterations leading to trophic changes that themselves may provide noxious afferent stimuli to perpetuate the syndrome (Figs. 27-9 and 27-10).

The pathophysiology of these conditions may be based, at least partially, on reflex sympathetic hyperactivity with resultant hypoperfusion, release of algesic chemicals, such as prostaglandins or bradykinin, and increased sensitivity of nociceptors.[128] Increased spontaneous and evoked firing rates in afferent nerve fibers or in cells in the spinal cord may also play a role (see Chap. 24.1, Appendix B, Sects. I-4 and I-5).

During the early phases of the injury, the pain is due to the damage to A-delta and C fibers. These fibers promptly develop hypersensitivity to circulating norepinephrine, pressure, and movement. They then fire spontaneously, which produces the typical pain of sympathetic origin. Soon small neuromata are formed that sprout small myelinated and unmyelinated fibers.[117] These normally silent fibers can generate an ongoing barrage of impulses in the absence of stimulation that traverse in afferent fibers to the spinal cord. This barrage can initiate and sustain the burning pain of causalgia during its early phase (Fig. 27-11).

The peripheral pathophysiology further produces lesser inhibition or facilitation in dorsal horn and other regions of the central nervous system. Initially, this is reversible with effective therapy, but if the burning sympathetic pain does not improve sponta-

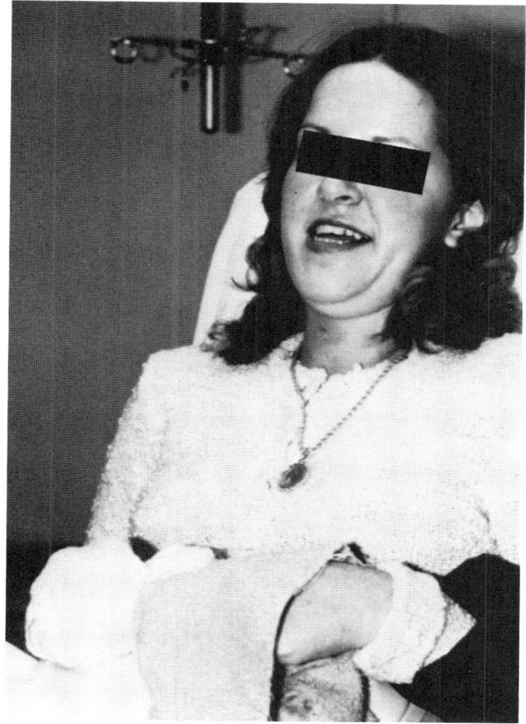

FIG. 27-9. Patient with gunshot wound of the right axilla with partial injury to the brachial plexus who developed causalgia within 48 hours with burning pain in right hand. This photograph was taken 2 months after the injury when the burning pain in right hand was extremely severe and would be precipitated by stroking left hand. The patient protected the left hand by covering it with a cloth. The photograph was taken after a stellate ganglion block had been done on the right side, which has relieved the causalgic pain as evidenced by her smile. (Raj, P.P. [ed.]: Practical Management of Pain, p. 454. Chicago, Year Book Medical Publishers, 1986.)

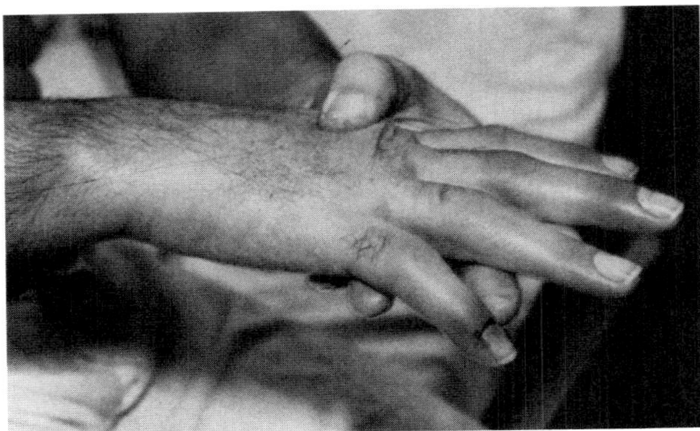

FIG. 27-10. Patient with reflex sympathetic dystrophy of the right hand. Note edema, stiffness, and loss of hair on the hand and digits.

neously, the abnormal function in the central nervous system becomes self-sustaining and independent of the abnormal peripheral input. The important clinical implication of this is that adequate therapy with chemical or surgical sympathectomy produces permanent relief in the early course of the disease and will fail to do so in the later stages.

Peripheral Vascular Disease

"Sympathetic pain" can be caused by peripheral vascular disease. This is based on the fact that in many of these conditions, there is an increased sympathetically induced vasoconstriction, ischemia, tissue damage, pain, and trophic changes that can be wholly or partially reversed by sympathetic interruption. The pain can be produced by the following conditions: [1] Acute vascular disorders with sudden severe circulatory insufficiency of the limb (*e.g.*, trauma, embolism, thrombosis, or chemical irritation). The local lesion initiates reflex spasm of the collateral vessels. If not relieved early by adequate therapy (*e.g.*, sympatholytic blocks), the reflex vasospasm leads to thrombosis and may terminate as gangrene; and [2] chronic vasospastic disorders. The common examples of these are Raynaud's phenomenon or disease, thromboan-

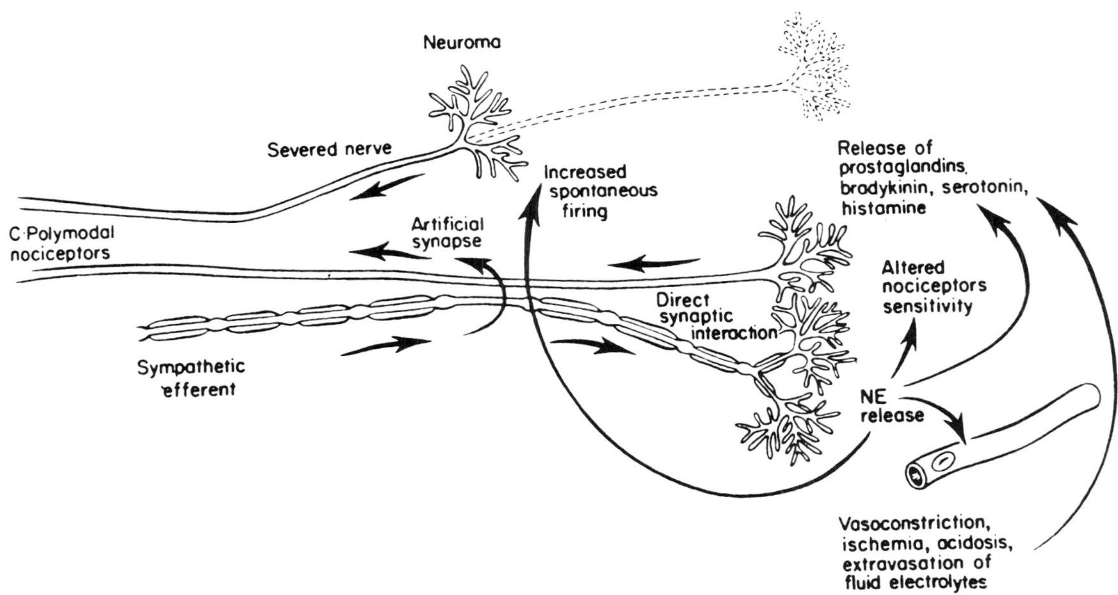

FIG. 27-11. Some proposed mechanisms of interaction between sympathetic efferent and nociceptive afferent fibers in causalgia. (Raj, P.P. [ed.]: Practical Management of Pain. p. 211. Chicago, Year Book Medical Publishers, 1986.)

giitis obliterans (Buerger's disease), and arteriosclerosis obliterans (Fig. 27-12) (see also Chap. 13).[17]

There are a number of less important disorders of the extremities in which sympathetic hyperactivity contributes to the pathophysiology and can produce sympathetic pain. These include hyperhydrosis, acute bursitis, tendinitis, tenosynovitis, and other traumatic and infectious disorders, including acute herpes zoster.

Repeated or prolonged anesthetic blocks of the sympathetic chain usually produce prompt permanent relief of symptoms in reflex sympathetic dystrophy. Such treatment benefits some patients with causalgia, but the majority require early sympathectomy to effect permanent relief. In both syndromes persistent pain and permanent disability are likely if appropriate therapy is not carried out early.

The conditions that may respond to interruption of sympathetic activity include atypical facial pain, certain neuropathies, Raynaud's disease, hyperhydrosis, and the chronic pain and vasoconstriction seen after frostbite (see Chap. 13).

VISCERAL PAIN

In general, the viscera have sensory receptors for no other modalities of sensation besides pain. Pain in the visceral tissues is usually diffuse, rather ill-defined, and frequently referred to distant points.[24] It is trans-

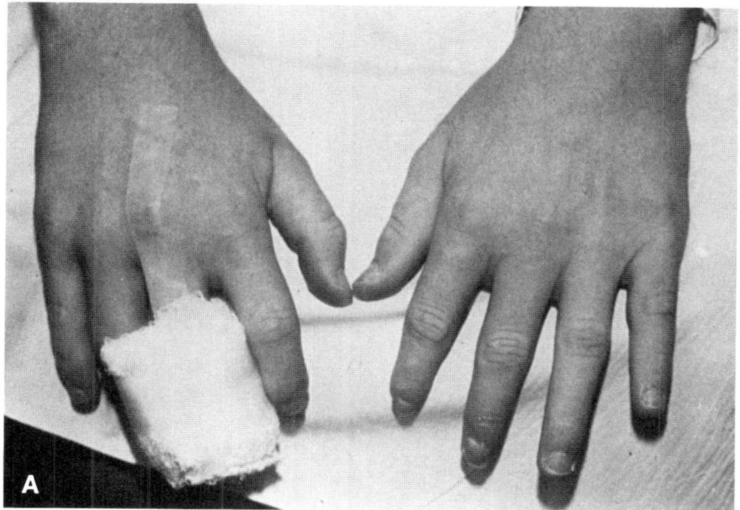

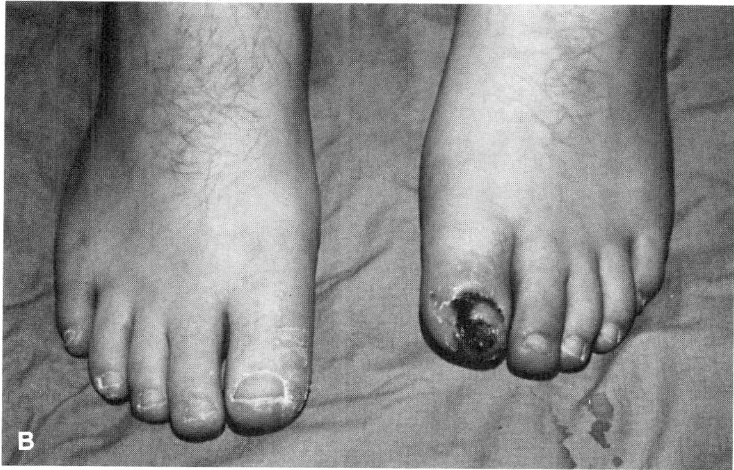

FIG. 27-12. Raynaud's disease in an 18-year-old boy. **A.** The disease first manifested in the hands with pain, synostosis, and ulceration. Treatment with stellate ganglion blocks brought relief. **B.** Later, ulceration and pain appeared in both great toes; treatment was with sympathetic blocks and hyperbaric oxygen.

mitted by visceral nociceptive afferent nerve fibers (see Fig. 13-1).

Any stimulus that excites nociceptive nerve endings in diffuse areas of the viscera causes visceral pain. Such stimuli include ischemia of visceral tissue, chemical damage to the surfaces of the viscera, spasm of the smooth muscle in a hollow viscus, distention of a hollow viscus, or stretching of the ligaments (see Chap. 24.2).

An important difference between somatic and visceral pain is that highly localized damage to the viscera seldom causes pain. For instance, a surgeon can cut the gut entirely in two in a patient who is awake without causing significant pain. On the other hand, any stimulus that causes diffuse stimulation of nociceptive nerve endings in the viscus causes extremely severe pain (*e.g.*, ischemia secondary to occlusion of the blood supply to a large area of gut).

Essentially all the true visceral pain originating in the thoracic and abdominal cavities is transmitted through afferent nerve fibers that run in the sympathetic nerves. These are small, unmyelinated type C fibers, and therefore can transmit only burning and aching types of pain (see also Fig. 13-1).

Pathophysiology

In addition to the following discussion, see Chapter 24.1 and Figure 24-2, and also Chapter 24.2.

Ischemia causes visceral pain similar to the way it causes somatic pain by the formation of acidic metabolic end products, such as bradykinin or proteolytic enzymes. These metabolites prime the nociceptors and stimulate them.

Chemical Stimuli. On occasion, damaging substances leak from the gastrointestinal tract into the peritoneal cavity. For instance, proteolytic acidic gastric juice often leaks through a ruptured gastric or duodenal ulcer. The juice causes widespread digestion of the visceral peritoneum, thus stimulating extremely large numbers of pain fibers. The pain intensity is usually severe.

Spasm of a Hollow Viscus. Spasm of the gut, the gallbladder, a bile duct, the ureter, or any other hollow viscus can cause pain in the same way that spasm of skeletal muscle causes pain. It may be due to mechanical stimulation of the nociceptors (*e.g.*, gut distention) or relative ischemia of the smooth muscle combined with increased metabolic demand for nutrients (see Figs. 24-1 and 24-2).

Often pain from a spastic viscus occurs in the form of cramps, the pain increasing to a high degree of severity and then subsiding, with this process continuing rhythmically once every few minutes. The rhythmic cycles result from rhythmic contraction of smooth muscle. For instance, each time a peristaltic wave travels along an overly excitable spastic gut, a cramp occurs. The cramping type of pain frequently occurs in gastroenteritis, constipation, menstruation, parturition, gallbladder disease, or ureteral obstruction.

Overdistension of a Hollow Viscus. Extreme overfilling of a hollow viscus results in pain, presumably because of overstretch of the tissues themselves. However, overdistension can also produce ischemic pain by collapse of the blood vessels that encircle the viscus or pass into its wall.

Visceral Pain Syndromes

Common examples of visceral pain for which local anesthetic nerve blocks are useful are acute myocardial infarction, angina pectoris, acute and chronic pancreatitis, ureteral and biliary colic, and visceral cancer.

Acute myocardial infarction often produces excruciating pain, and unless it is promptly relieved, reflex responses may exacerbate the myocardial pathophysiology.[15,124] The reflex responses may be composed of either the Bezold–Jarish effect of abnormal vagoreflex (bradycardia, arterial hypotension, and atrioventricular block) or, more frequently, segmental and suprasegmental sympathetic hyperactivity with a consequent increase in cardiac output and myocardial oxygen consumption.[126] Animal studies also suggest that segmentally induced sympathetic stimulation will produce reflex coronary vasoconstriction that further impairs oxygen delivery to the myocardium.[36,71,126] If this takes place in vessels perfusing myocardial tissue adjacent to the infarcted muscle, it can result in making previously healthy myocardial tissue ischemic and previously ischemic tissue necrotic. Suprasegmental reflexes stimulate autonomic centers and invariably increase general sympathetic tone and catecholamine release.[107,126] Moreover, the suprasegmental reflex responses are markedly enhanced by the severe anxiety that develops in patients with acute myocardial infarction.[126] In addition, emotional stress may cause cortically mediated increased blood viscosity and clotting,[31] fibrinolysis,[23] and platelet aggregation.[125]

The combined effects of segmental and suprasegmental reflexes, anxiety, and stress greatly increase the workload of the heart and its oxygen consumption and, by segmental vasoconstriction and alteration of blood clotting, may further decrease the already compromised arteriosclerotic coronary circulation. This may markedly increase the discrepancy between oxygen supply and demand and may cause extension of the infarction. It is therefore essential to promptly and effectively relieve the pain and anxiety and so inhibit adverse reflex responses.

Patients with excruciating pain who do not respond to narcotics will have effective analgesia for 8 to 10 hours if cervicothoracic sympathetic block is performed with a long-acting local anesthetic agent, such as 0.25% bupivacaine. The injection is made at the level of the stellate ganglion; however, a larger than usual amount of local anesthetic injected into the proper fascial plane (10–15 ml) will spread to involve the sympathetic chain from the middle cervical ganglion to the fourth or fifth thoracic ganglion (see Figs. 13-18 and 13-20). It thus blocks all sensory and sympathetic fibers to the heart. Alternatively, a thoracic sympathetic chain block can be performed to block T1–T4 sympathetic preganglionic fibers (see Fig. 13-21). In patients with pain predominant on one side, a unilateral block suffices. If the pain is bilateral, the block is done on the side with the severest pain first and, after an interval of 30 minutes, it is repeated on the opposite side. The value of sympathetic interruption in such cases is amply justified by animal studies. These demonstrate that sympathetic denervation of the heart significantly reduces both size of experimentally induced infarction and animal mortality.[27,70,98]

Angina pectoris, when severe and intractable to medical therapy, was formerly managed with block of the upper four or five thoracic sympathetic ganglia with local anesthetics and, subsequently, alcohol.[11,113] However, the advent of the coronary-aortic graft bypass operation has made chemical and surgical sympathectomy useless procedures. The indications for sympathetic block are patients with extensive coronary disease not amenable to the surgical procedure and in whom the anginal pain is disabling.[19] Acute angina pectoris can, however, be relieved by either a cervicothoracic sympathetic block or anterior chest wall (pectoralis major and minor) trigger point injections. Local anesthetic and neurolytic procedures may also be useful in relieving severe pain caused by aortic aneurysm.[10,119]

Acute pancreatitis frequently causes severe or excruciating continuous pain, severe abdominal muscle spasm and rigidity, marked abdominal tenderness, nausea and vomiting, and moderate ileus with consequent abdominal distention. In most patients the pain and associated reflex response impair pulmonary ventilation. Some patients develop progressive hypoxia and hypercapnia that may end in death. Although potent narcotics given intravenously partially relieve the pain, this condition is more effectively managed by regional block of the nociceptive afferents using splanchnic nerve block, celiac plexus block (see Fig. 14-6), or continuous segmental (T5–T10) epidural block. In one study it was suggested that in addition to relieving pain, interruption of nociceptive impulses decreases the severity and duration of the disease by combating reflex spasm of the duodenum, sphincter of Oddi, and the entire ductal system.[63] There is rapid release of extraductal pressure, and toxic fluid is emptied from the extrabiliary and pancreatic ductal systems. The procedure also relieves the visceral vasospasm and reflex ileus.

Ureteral and biliary colic are among the most excruciatingly painful conditions experienced by some patients.[12] Although potent narcotics administered intravenously produce adequate pain relief, they increase spasm of the smooth muscle. A block of nociceptive and efferent pathways with continuous segmental T5–T10 epidural block (see Chap. 8) is highly effective in providing pain relief and relieving the associated reflex muscle spasm caused by biliary colic. Segmental block of T10–L2 is equally effective for ureteral colic. In some patients the block also relaxes the ureter sufficiently to permit a stone to move down to a point where it can be removed through a cystoscope, thus obviating the need for an open operation.[10] An alternative method is paravertebral block of the splanchnic nerves and of the first and second lumbar sympathetic ganglia (see Figs. 14-8 and 13-25).

Visceral Intractable and Cancer Pain. Neurolytic block of the splanchnic nerves or celiac plexus performed with 50% alcohol or 5% to 7% phenol has been effective in relieving severe intractable pain caused by cancer of the pancreas, stomach, small intestine, gallbladder, or other abdominal viscera (see Figs. 14-6 and 14-8). Moore and associates used this procedure in 168 patients, and of these, 157 (94%) had good to excellent pain relief.[78] For such patients, prognostic block with a local anesthetic is indicated before the use of a neurolytic agent. At my institution, long-dwell Becton Dickinson catheters are placed for prolonged infusion of bupivacaine at the appropriate sites of the sympathetic block (Fig. 27-13). The catheters are then infused with 0.25% bupivacaine for 7 to 10 days and the pain relief and side-effects evaluated. If the sympathetic block is efficacious, then chemical sympathectomy is performed with a neurolytic agent. A similar technique may be indicated in patients with severe intractable pain of chronic pancreatitis, postcholecystectomy syndrome, or other chronic abdominal visceral diseases unrelieved by medical or surgical therapy.[15]

Rationale for the Use of Sympathetic Blocks for Visceral Pain

The technique of blocking the sympathetic nerves that innervate thoracic or abdominal viscera to relieve intolerable visceral pain not amenable to other therapies or as an important adjunct to these is well known. The rationale for this is as follows: The nociceptive pathways from the viscera accompany the efferent sympathetic nerves. When they are stimulated they produce segmental reflexes, which in turn produce skeletal muscle spasm and sympathetic hyperactivity. The condition is further aggravated by suprasegmental reflexes that stimulate hypothalamic autonomic centers and increase general sympathetic tone and catecholamine release. All of these responses increase cardiac output, blood pressure, the workload of the heart, metabolism, and oxygen consumption. Unless the severe pain and associated reflex responses are promptly eliminated, they become refractory and greatly aggravate the pathophysiology. Although narcotics administered by appropriate route in appropriate doses produce adequate pain relief, they do not eliminate abnormal reflex responses. Block with a local anesthetic or neurolytic agent not only relieves pain, but also interrupts the afferent and efferent limb and abnormal viscerovisceral and viscerosomatic reflexes that often develop and contribute to the pathogenesis (see Fig. 24-2).[15]

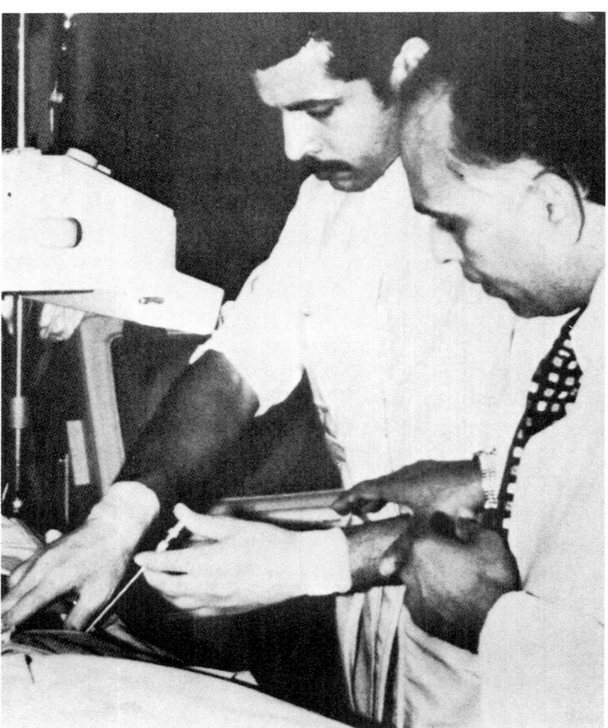

FIG. 27-13. A 20-gauge, 15-cm Longdwell Becton Dickinson nylon catheter is being placed in the region of the celiac plexus under fluoroscopy for prognostic block (48 hours) before neurolysis for carcinoma of the head of pancreas. (Raj, P.P. [ed.]: Practical Management of Pain, p. 676. Chicago, Year Book Medical Publishers, 1986.)

Chemical interruption of the peripheral sympathetic nervous system has produced prolonged and sometimes permanent relief of visceral pain. Pain in the visceral structures of the head, neck, and thoracic region can be relieved by stellate (see Fig. 13-9) or thoracic sympathetic chain interruption (see Fig. 13-21). Pain of the upper abdominal viscera can be relieved by the celiac plexus block, whereas the pain of the lower abdominal and pelvic viscera can be relieved by lumbar sympathetic blocks. Drugs like analgesics and antispasmodics for chronic visceral pain have not been efficacious. They may be useful as an adjunct and for short acute episodes of pain. Although physical methods like TENS have not been helpful, acupuncture may alleviate visceral pain in some patients. Biofeedback, hypnosis, and relaxation therapy also have advocates and may be successful in selected cases.

MISCELLANEOUS PAIN SYNDROMES AMENABLE TO LOCAL ANESTHETIC NEURAL BLOCKADE

Herpes Zoster and Postherpetic Neuralgia

Early lesions of herpes zoster are minute, unilocular vesicles in the epidermis. In addition, the dorsal root ganglion is hemorrhagic and swollen (Fig. 27-14). Maximum degeneration is seen in the posterior nerve root about 2 weeks after the dermal lesions first appear. Similar changes may be seen in the posterior column and sensory nerves and seldom in the anterior horn.[73]

Many theories have been proposed to explain the intractable nature of postherpetic neuralgia. Noxious impulses may become established in centrally located, self-perpetuating loops, and progressive facilitation develops in these synapses. Pain then occurs spontaneously. The possibility also exists that pain may be due to the involvement of higher pathways of spinal cord and brain. The gate control theory might explain some of the features involved in the production and persistence of postherpetic neuralgia. It is postulated that pain is carried by small unmyelinated and small myelinated nerve fibers to the central nervous system, where the input is modified by large myelinated nerve fibers. In acute herpes zoster, there is a tendency for proportionately more of the large fibers to be damaged than the small fibers. Hence there is an increase in the percentage of smaller fibers relative to large fibers.[49] In this state, without the modulation of large nerve fiber stimulation, a minimal small fiber stimulation may produce the sensation of pain. It is important to note that the older patient has fewer large fibers to begin with and loses more through the herpes zoster infection. The incidence of postherpetic neuralgia rises sharply after age 55 years (see Chap. 24.1, Appendix B, Sect. II-5).[64]

Management. The goals of treatment of herpes zoster are early resolution of the acute problem and prevention of postherpetic neuralgia. Aggressive management is imperative in the older patient, who is at greater risk of developing postherpetic neuralgia.

Usual methods of management of herpes zoster and postherpetic neuralgia include drug therapy (antiviral agents, analgesics, anti-inflammatory agents, antidepressants, vitamin B_{12}, B complex, and L-tryptophan), nerve blocks, psychosocial therapy, physical measures, and surgery. Only the efficacy of nerve block is discussed here.

Nerve blocks used for herpes zoster and postherpetic neuralgia are local infiltration, somatic nerve block, sympathetic nerve block, and epidural block.

Local Infiltration. In a large group of patients, Epstein injected 0.2% triamcinolone in normal saline subcutaneously in the areas of eruption and the sites of pain and itching. He obtained excellent results that approached 100%, and the development of postherpetic neuralgia was reduced to 2%. This study suggests that subcutaneous injection of steroid and local anesthetic is an effective therapy for acute herpes zoster. No significant complications were recorded, the technique is simple and inexpensive, and the response to treatment is fairly predictable.[33,34] My own experience with this technique corroborates these results (Fig. 27-15). It should be noted that no block technique prevents postherpetic neuralgia in a high percentage of older-age-group patients.[64]

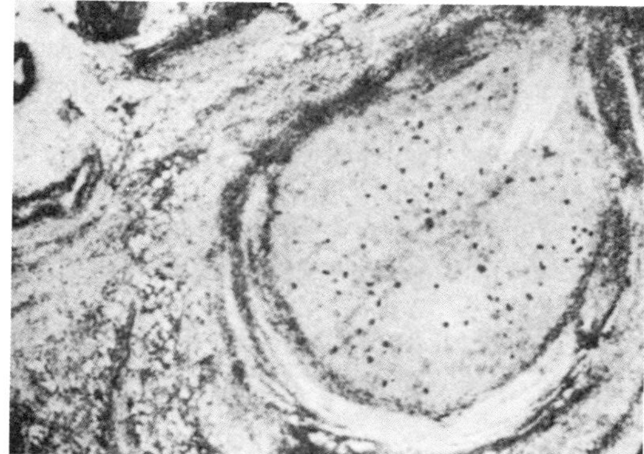

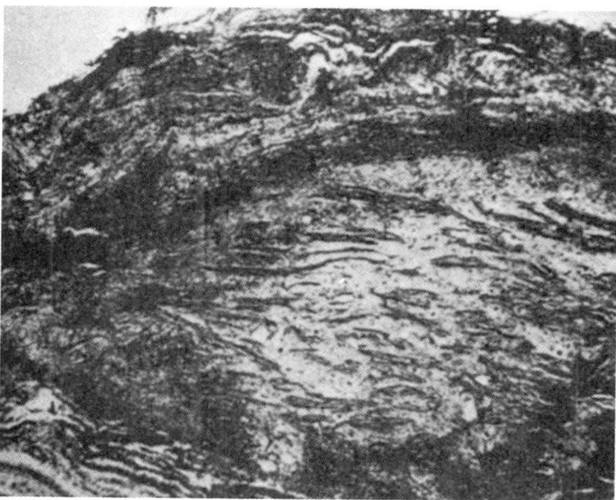

FIG. 27-14. Inflammatory reaction in the dorsal root ganglion owing to herpes zoster. **Top.** Ganglion and satellite cells show intranuclear inclusions. **Bottom.** The ganglion is swollen and hemorrhagic. (Raj, P.P. [ed.]: Practical Management of Pain, p. 347. Chicago, Year Book Medical Publishers, 1986.)

Somatic Nerve Blocks. Because nerve root involvement is suspected in acute herpes zoster, somatic nerve blocks have been used in its treatment. These blocks can include brachial plexus, paravertebral, intercostal, and sciatic blocks. Regrettably, they have been found to be of limited value in the acute phase and of no value in the postherpetic stage.

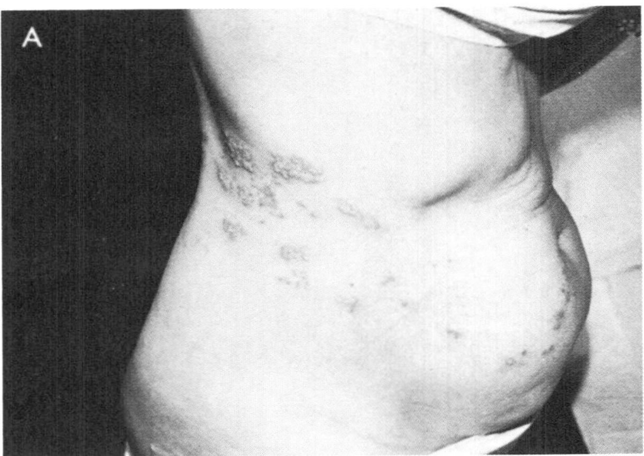

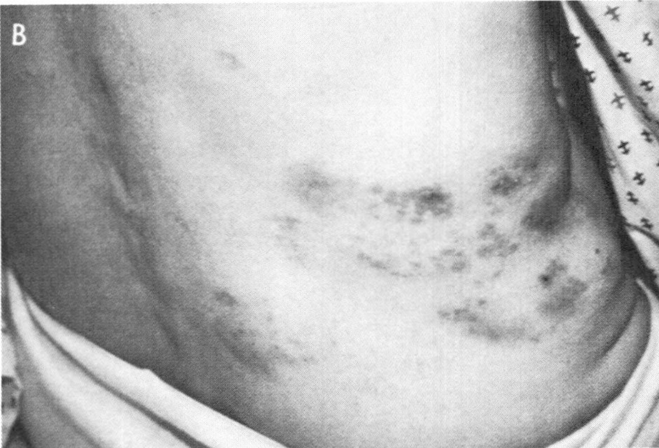

FIG. 27-15. **A.** Acute herpes zoster in the T10–T11 intercostal distribution before the intracutaneous injection of a steroid–local anesthetic mixture. **B.** Note healing of the vesicular lesions 3 days after the intracutaneous injection. Subcutaneous bruising is frequently seen for a few days after the injection. (Raj, P.P. [ed.]: Practical Management of Pain, plate 8. Chicago, Year Book Medical Publishers, 1986.)

Sympathetic Nerve Blocks. As understanding of the pathology of herpes zoster developed, attention was directed toward the sympathetic ganglia. Sympathetic blocks have been performed to relieve the vasospasm thought to cause the pain and nerve damage. Evidence suggests that sympathetic blockade performed during the acute phase of herpes zoster can help the immediate pain problem, often dramatically. Of greater value, however, is the possibility that it can prevent the development of postherpetic neuralgia. Although the evidence for this is less clear, it is probably a worthwhile prophylactic measure that should be used as early as possible.[79]

Trigeminal herpes zoster has been treated with a bupivacaine block of the ipsilateral stellate ganglion in a small study (Fig. 27-16). Dramatic and lasting relief of all dysesthesia was obtained in about 77% of patients. Some discomfort and paresthesia of the affected area persisted for several weeks in about 22%. Pain recurred after initial relief in about 22%. Vesicular skin lesions dried more quickly than in untreated patients. Transient side-effects included hoarseness, paresis of the ipsilateral arm, and paresis of the hemidiaphragm. The investigators were unable to draw any conclusions because of the informality of the study, but they believe that these preliminary results justify further investigation.[82]

In one large study more than 90% of patients with herpes zoster were treated successfully with one sympathetic block: the course of the disease showed definite improvement; pain disappeared or diminished within 15 minutes and lasted for 20 to 45 minutes initially, with spontaneous diminution of pain in 8 hours and complete relief in 24 hours; and blisters dried within 48 hours. Successfully blocked patients did not develop postherpetic neuralgia. Complete failure, in only a few patients, occurred when treatment was begun after the patient had been suffering for 10 days or longer and the disease had extended to a number of segments. A similar study reported complete recovery in 75% of patients after one block, while the rest responded to a second block 2 days later.[95]

Winnie has written that the incidence of success with sympathetic block depends on how soon after the onset of the disease the block is performed. If a sympathetic block is performed within the first 2 to 3 weeks, virtually 100% success is achieved. The success rate drops after that point. As postherpetic neuralgia supervenes, after 4 to 6 weeks, the success rate falls to about 20%. Thereafter, the incidence of success associated with sympathetic blocks decreases even more over the years.[121]

It is clear that if favorable results are to be obtained, it is absolutely necessary for patients to be treated in the first 2 to 3 weeks of the disease. This therapy also apparently prevents the disease from progressing to the postherpetic syndrome, at least in younger patients. However, few of these develop postherpetic neuralgia with no treatment. It is in the older age group that efficacy must be tested.

Epidural blocks using local anesthetic have been successful in acute herpes zoster. The duration of the infection is shorter, the lesions dry faster, and pain is relieved. In patients with herpes zoster of 7 weeks'

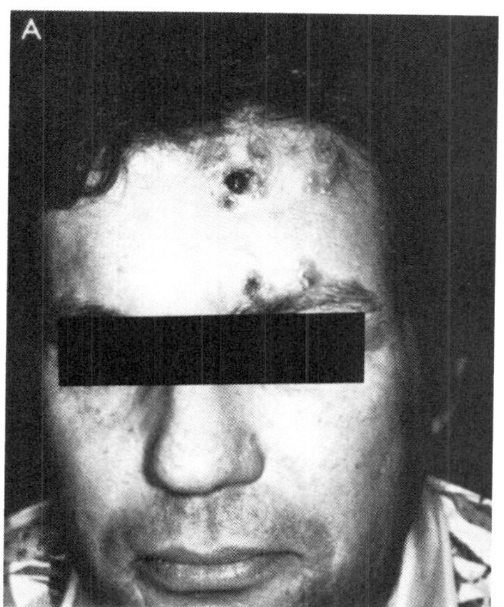

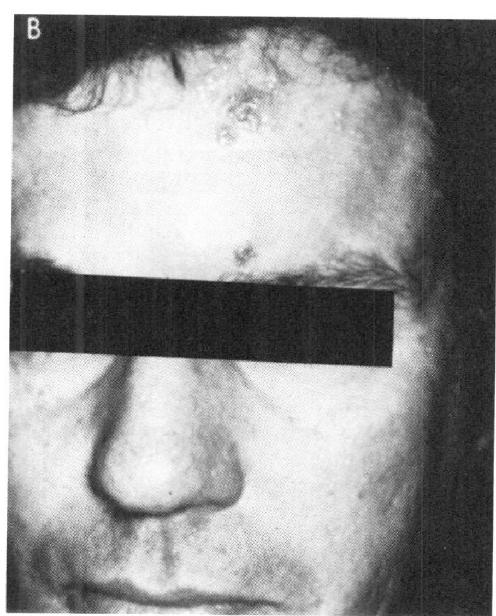

FIG. 27-16. **A.** Acute herpes zoster of the left eye and forehead before treatment with intralesional injection and left stellate ganglion block. **B.** Appearance 3 days after left stellate ganglion block. Note the clearing of the eye and the lesions of the forehead. (Raj, P.P. [ed.]: Practical Management of Pain, plate 7. Chicago, Year Book Medical Publishers, 1986.)

duration or less, Perkins and Hanlon, in a small series, achieved 70% to 100% relief 24 hours after treatment, and 100% relief in a 1- to 5-month follow-up. There was no subsequent report of postherpetic neuralgia. Their studies suggest that local anesthetic alone was effective and that the inclusion of corticosteroids did not increase benefits.[84] However, many patients were young. Currently no objective controlled studies confirm the efficacy of neural blockade in postherpetic neuralgia in older-age-group patients.[64]

Postamputation Pain Syndromes

Immediately after amputation of an extremity 80% to 90% of patients report feeling a phantom limb (or part). Of these, 10% to 15% have persistent severe pain in the phantom limb or the stump or both.[10,37] The characteristics of phantom limb pain vary, but two predominant types usually occur: [1] a burning, throbbing pain not unlike that of causalgia and the other reflex sympathetic dystrophies, which the patient describes as if the hand or foot were held too close to a fire; and [2] extremely abnormal position of the phantom limb with the hand or foot held in a painful, twisted, cramped, rigid, or flexed posture from which the patient is unable to release it. Pain in the stump is of three predominant types: [1] a constant, diffuse, burning, throbbing pain similar to that of reflex sympathetic dystrophies; [2] paroxysm of lancinating, shooting discomfort with a segmental or peripheral nerve distribution; or [3] a combination of these. Stump pain is usually associated with vasomotor and sudomotor disturbance manifested by coldness, cyanosis, edema, signs of vasoconstriction, and excessive sweating (see Chap. 24.1, Appendix B, Sects. I-2 and I-3).

In patients with predominantly burning, aching pain associated with vasomotor and sudomotor changes in the stump, sympathetic interruption with regional sympathetic block or Bier block are effective in relieving the symptoms temporarily and at times permanently.[10,12,74] Immediately after the block the patient feels partial or complete relief of pain and a warming of the stump. Sometimes the patient also feels the cramped or twisted extremity relax and assume a normal position. If the block affords complete or good relief of pain, it should be repeated several times to confirm the results and ascertain the duration of pain relief. If relief is of progressively longer duration and significantly outlasts duration of the block, surgical sympathectomy should be seriously considered.

Pain Secondary to Paraplegia or Quadriplegia

Among the most emotionally taxing people to deal with are those patients who have complaints of pain after fully realizing that they have paraplegia or quadriplegia. These patients are usually mentally alert, and yet they are so devastated from their spinal cord lesion. The physician wishes so much to be able to do something for their pain because he is unable to do anything for their spinal lesions. And yet these patients present with some of the most bizarre and unusual painful complaints, including pain in parts of the body that don't feel and spasms in parts of the body that don't move. In many of the interactions the unspoken theme is that if something is done for the pain, the patient "knows" that his function will improve. Fortunately, only about 15% to 20% of patients with severe spinal cord injury have such severe disabling pain.[55,80]

The etiology of spinal cord pain is not entirely clear. The primary lesion with interruption of the nervous continuity at the level of injury sets the stage for the subsequent pain. However, why do only 15% of the people have subsequent disabling pain when all cords at the site of lesion show hemorrhagic necrosis (see Central Pain in Chap. 24.1, Appendix B)?

The other causes of pain in paraplegics originate in the surrounding bony, ligamentous, and muscular structures. Bony instability at the site of injury can be painful.[67] Also, improper positioning and therapy of limbs and joints innervated above the level of a lesion can be the source of considerable pain.[48] Syrinx formation causes pain like syringomyelia syndrome (see Chap. 24.1, Appendix B, Sect. I-7).

The empirical fact does remain that the level of the cord just proximal to the lesion is the critical area in the genesis of the pain. This fact becomes apparent on review of all therapies involved in manipulating the nervous system distal to the level of the insult that show uniformly poor results.[66]

A number of hypotheses attempt to explain the physiologic basis for the anatomic location of the "spinal" pain in these debilitated patients. One hypothesis is that the pain from traumatized spinal cord is due to the hyperactivity of spinal neurons, which, having lost their inhibitory influences, fire abnormally and cause pain.

Another hypothesis brings up the possibility of collateral pathways that bypass the level of injury of the spinal cord in conducting the nociceptive impulses cephalad.

The third hypothesis believes that there is disruption of normal circuits, and when previously suppressed impulses become unsuppressed, they produce painful sensation. This may explain why partial conus lesions have the highest tendency to become painful afterward.[32]

Management. Any therapy for "spinal" pain must take into account the possible influence of outside factors in the management. Only in the context of the *total* patient can a rational approach be designed and a successful management scheme be executed.

With the exclusion of the extrinsic treatable inciting factors for spinal pain, one is left with three approaches to the problem: drug therapy, nerve blocks, or surgery. Sometimes a large syrinx may be "decompressed" surgically and give pain relief.

For those patients who have not responded to drug therapy, the next option appears to be nerve blocks. Sympathetic and epidural blocks with local anesthetics have been tried in the hope of predicting whether surgery or more permanent chemical blocks would be successful. This has not proved to be helpful.[67] A subarachnoid phenol block around and above the level of the injury and a segment or two higher has sometimes proved successful for varying periods.[67] The problem with the use of the nerve blocks for paraplegics is threefold: first, difficulty of the technique and nonspecificity of lesion; second, compromise of bowel and bladder function in incomplete lesions; and third, the inability to use the technique above the lower thoracic area because of potential compromise to respiratory control centers in cervical cord (see also Chap. 30).

NERVE BLOCKS USEFUL FOR SUBACUTE AND CHRONIC PAIN RELIEF

Local anesthetic nerve blocks useful for subacute and chronic pain include myofascial trigger point injections, subcutaneous infiltration, intravenous local anesthetic administrations, central and peripheral nerve blocks, and sympathetic blocks. It is important to keep in mind that when using such local anesthetic nerve blocks in chronic pain patients, the mechanisms of pain are frequently different from their acute counterpart, and nerve blocks seem to be less effective in chronic pain states.[106,127] In a recent study, Raj and colleagues found that with an identical objective level of lumbar epidural analgesia, chronic pain patients reported less pain relief and had more complaints of side-effects when compared with acute pain patients (Fig. 27-17).[93]

Prerequisites for Performing Local Anesthetic Nerve Blocks

To obtain good results, the anesthesiologist using these procedures must assume the responsibility of management of pain in such patients and not become a technical consultant at inserting needles.[16] He must have ample knowledge of various pain syndromes and of the advantages, disadvantages, limitations, and complications of the therapeutic modalities that may be available for each syndrome (see also Chaps. 24.1 and 31).

The anesthesiologist must be willing to devote the time and effort to obtain a detailed history, examine the patient thoroughly, and confirm the diagnosis. This is essential even if the patient has had a diagnosis made by the referring physician. The time spent in this exercise not only provides additional information, but affords an opportunity to develop rapport with the patient as well. A careful neurological examination also establishes a baseline to evaluate the effects of the block.

The anesthesiologist must be highly skilled in the indicated procedure and have a thorough knowledge of the expected immediate and long-term sequelae of the nerve block and the drugs used. Nerve blocks on chronic pain patients should not be done by unsupervised "learners."

It is important to inform the patient and family of the basic rationale of the procedure that is to be done and what will be accomplished by it. This information should be furnished during the initial visit and repeated just before the block. If the patient and family do not understand that the procedure is only to obtain information and may give only transient or no relief, they may be disappointed and the patient may not return for further care.

During and after the block it is essential to observe the patient's reaction to the procedure and evaluate the neurological changes that have occurred as a result of the administration of the local anesthetic. When the block is fully established, its effects on pain relief must be assessed and the implications for pathogenesis considered. This may require a few hours, several days, or perhaps weeks of evaluation. In addition to such observation by the physician, the results should be evaluated by the patient and the family (see also Chaps. 27.1 and 31).

It is essential that the patient and physicians realize that these procedures may produce side-effects with serious complications. Therefore, *no block should be done without an assistant present and resuscitative equipment ready for immediate use.* This should include an intravenous infusion set up before commencing the procedure for the prompt administration of drugs to combat systemic reactions, arterial hypotension, or high spinal anesthesia should it occur (see Chaps. 4 and 6).

MYOFASCIAL TRIGGER POINT INJECTION

Myofascial trigger point injection of local anesthetics is the simplest and most frequently used analgesic blocks in the treatment of pain. Simplicity and apparent innocuousness make this a method of choice among physicians treating chronic pain. By producing physicochemical interruption of reflex pathways almost at the source of the nociceptive process, it effectively relieves the pain (see Chap. 24.1, Appendix B, Sect. I-9).

Trigger point injection is helpful when a few trigger points are present and when the muscle cannot stretch because of excessive pain or because of its sequelae. An aseptic technique is required. The solutions, needles, and syringes should be properly sterilized before their use. Localization of a trigger point is mainly done by the sense of feel. It is the most sensitive spot in the palpable band. The muscle is placed on sufficient stretch to palpate the tight band and hold the trigger point in position.

With flat palpation, the trigger point can be localized by feeling the band roll back and forth between the fingers (Fig. 27-18). The trigger point is then fixed by keeping it between the fingers. The needle is inserted perpendicularly to the skin to the required depth of the trigger point by slowly advancing the needle toward the trigger point. The patient is asked to tell when he feels the worst pain. At that site the needle will usually impale the trigger point.

With pincer palpation, the trigger point is rolled between the digits. When located, the trigger point is held tightly between the thumb and fingertips for injection. This technique is useful for muscles like the pectoralis major and minor, latissimus dorsi, sternomastoid, and trapezius at the shoulder region (see Chap. 24.1, Appendix B, Sect. I-9).

Drugs Used for Injection

Dry needling of trigger points without injecting any solution may be effective but does not equal the therapeutic effectiveness of injecting a local anesthetic. Kraus noted that postinjection pain occurs after dry needling.[59] Sola and Kuitert treated a series of 100 patients with isotonic saline in their trigger points.[103] They found saline effective in relieving the pain. Hameroff and associates, on the other hand, found that long-acting local anesthetics, bupivacaine and etidocaine, provide better and longer pain relief for up to 7 days postinjection. Travell and Simons advocate the use of procaine for trigger point injections.[115] They

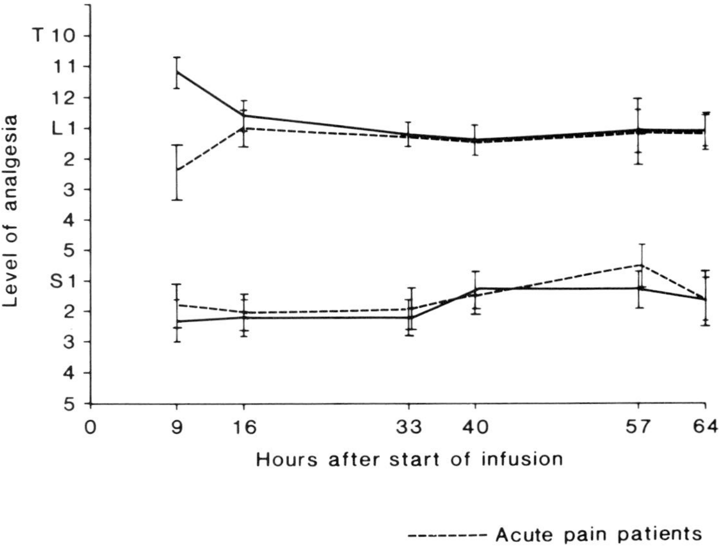

FIG. 27-17. **A.** Similar levels of analgesia as measured by pinprick in acute and chronic pain patients. **B.** (*Opposite page*) Acute pain patients rated the epidural analgesia as good or excellent higher (—92%) than chronic pain patients (—50%). **C.** (*Opposite page*) Acute pain patients show higher incidence of vomiting, pyrexia, and constipation, whereas complaint of backache is higher in chronic low back pain sufferers despite adequate sensory anesthesia above the pain segments. (Raj, P.P., *et al.*: Pain [submitted for consideration].)

argue that procaine has less systemic and local toxicity, in addition to its vasodilator effect and curarelike action at the myoneural junction. I have used a mixture of 0.5% etidocaine and 0.375% bupivacaine and found their effect long lasting without systemic toxicity or myotoxicity. In my experience this mixture has produced better relief than dry needling, saline, or lidocaine.

Travell and Simons advocate mixing a corticosteroid with a local anesthetic for trigger point injection[115] for only two groups of patients: patients with soft tissue inflammation (adhesive capsulitis) or those with postinjection soreness of muscles. They prefer oral steroids and believe that long-acting steroids are contraindicated because of their myotoxic properties[86] and delayed sequelae (Cushing's syndrome). I have used dexamethasone (4 mg/10 ml of local anesthetic solution), mixing it with bupivacaine and etidocaine, and have found no sequelae because of its use. It is true that steroid may be responsible for burning in the area of injection 24 to 48 hours postinjection. But this subsides and patients continue to have prolonged pain relief for 7 to 10 days afterward. If the patients are initially informed about the burning and its duration, it helps them to tolerate it.

Stretch after trigger point injections is important.[59,129] Vapocoolant spray or heat may also be applied after injection during stretching of the muscle to full length.

Alternative techniques to stretch-and-spray and trigger point injections have also been practiced for myofascial pain. They include ischemic compression techniques, massage, deep heat, TENS, biofeedback, and central modulation.[77,88,120] Combination of some or all may be required in chronic intractable trigger point pain. Commonly, however, the usual combination of techniques used are stretch-and-spray, trigger point injection, and TENS therapy. This is associated

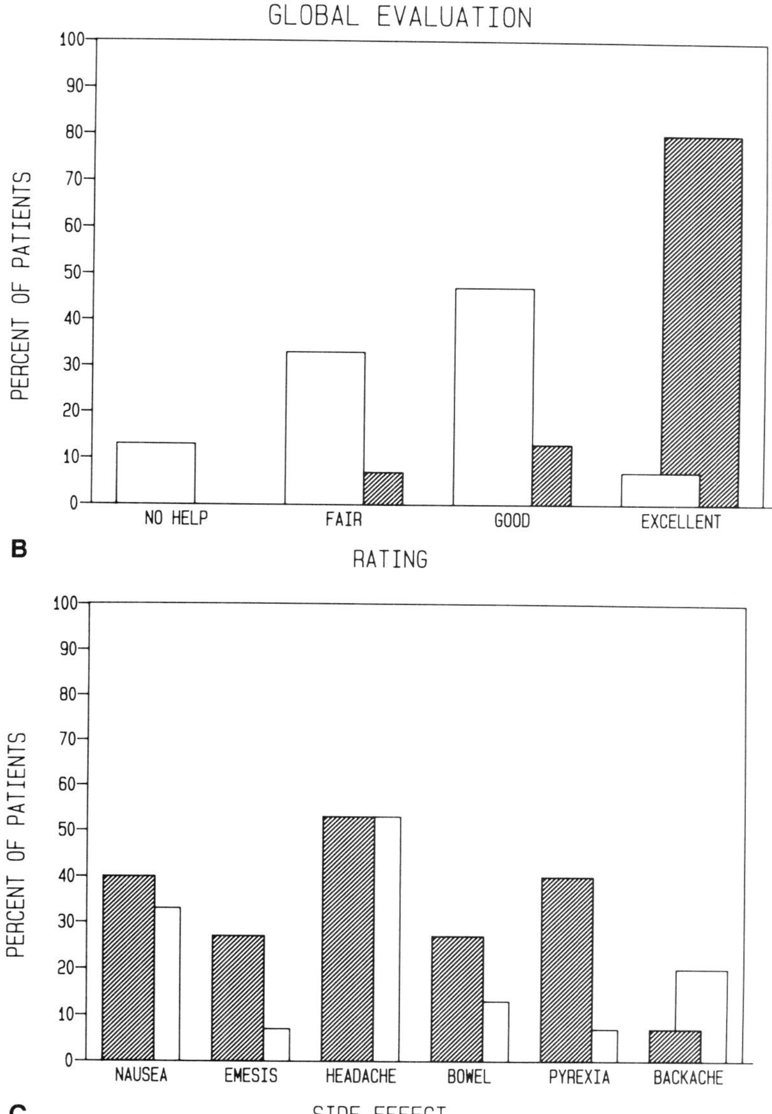

with muscle relaxants, nonsteroidal anti-inflammatory agents, and exercises. It is useful to know that the earlier the patient is treated, the more effective and longer lasting is the treatment. Generally, for a trigger point pain that is chronic (6–12 months), it takes a series of six injections at weekly intervals with other associated therapy to show improvement in pain relief. The management plan should be evaluated at such periodic intervals and a change made to other modalities if the one used is not effective.

SUBCUTANEOUS INFILTRATION

This technique is useful for acute herpes zoster and postherpetic neuralgia, neuroma, painful subcutaneous fibrotic nodules, and spermalgia or labial pain in the groin. For herpetic pain, a solution of 0.2% triamcinolone in 0.25% bupivacaine or dexamethasone (16 mg/50 ml) in 0.125% bupivacaine is prepared. The solution (10–50 ml) is injected subcutaneously throughout the area of intense pain or in the vesicular

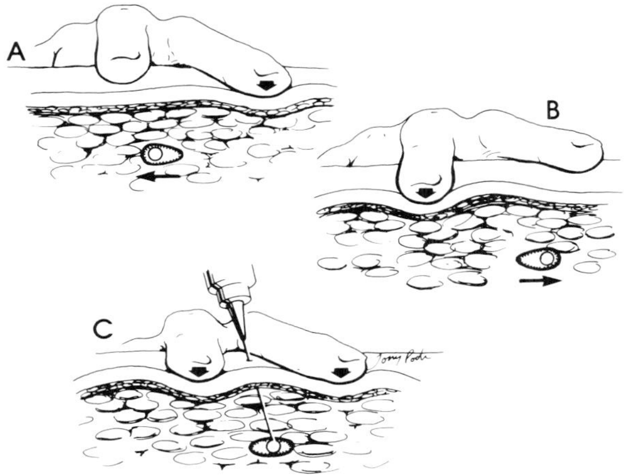

FIG. 27-18. Method of palpating and fixing the trigger point in the muscle with two fingers before inserting the needle tip in the trigger points for injection. **A.** Fixation of trigger point by the proximal finger. **B.** Fixation of trigger point by the distal finger. **C.** Needle on the trigger point. (Travell, J., and Simon, D.G.: Myofascial Pain and Dysfunction: The Trigger Point Manual. Baltimore, Williams & Wilkins, 1983.)

distribution. The total number of such treatments ranges from one to ten, with an average of four.[73] In acute herpes zoster the treatment is given two to three times weekly, whereas in postherpetic neuralgia it can be done weekly and may need as many as 12 treatments before the improvement in pain is seen.

For neuroma and other subcutaneous nodular or fibrotic pain, local anesthetic with steroid is injected four to six times on a weekly basis. The majority of patients obtain short-term pain relief with this regimen. Objective evidence of long-term pain relief is not available. Those with persistent pain after this may be candidates for neurolytic procedures; however, evidence for long-term efficacy is also lacking.

INTRAVENOUS LOCAL ANESTHETIC ADMINISTRATION

Since 1908 many reports describing the analgesic effect of intravenous (i.v.) local anesthetics have been published. This technique has been beneficial in managing such painful conditions as burns, postsurgical pain, central pain, deafferentation syndrome, Raynaud's disease, phantom limb pain, causalgia, neuritis, and myofascial pain.

Although the classic local anesthetic agent used has been procaine, the choice of drug has varied from chloroprocaine to tetracaine. When used for pain management, these local anesthetics have historically been administered in large, incremental dosages. However, techniques of administration have also used the flowmeter and the i.v. pump in an attempt to control the infusion rate of the local anesthetic agent.

Mechanism of Action

Various theories have been proposed to describe the pharmacodynamics of local anesthetics. In 1938 Leriche proposed that injury to tissue caused reflex vasoconstriction, resulting in anoxia, capillary dysfunction, and increased permeability.[61,62] This process would lead to the accumulation of nociceptive metabolites and to the irritation of peripheral nerve endings. Leriche believed that procaine, by acting directly on the arteriolar, meta-arteriolar, and capillary endothelia, produced widespread vasodilation, thereby anesthetizing the irritated endothelial nerve endings and breaking the reflex arc.

Lundy observed 4 hours of analgesia in several jaundiced patients with pruritus after the slow injection of 20 ml of 0.1% procaine solution.[68] His reported results supported Leriche's theory that peripheral irritation is accompanied by capillary hyperpermeability, allowing transudation of procaine into the tissues, anesthetizing the nerve endings.

Gordon, in 1943, produced analgesia in burn patients, but only in the burned area and tissues affected by edema.[45] One year later Bigelow and Harrison subcutaneously injected 5 to 40 ml of 2.0% procaine solution into the arms of normal subjects.[8] They noted a marked increase in the pain threshold in the forehead, and therefore asserted that the change resulted from a systemic action of procaine after circulatory absorption rather than from a direct action of the agent.

In 1946 Allen and coworkers discovered six to eight times more procaine in the transudate of the injured area than in normal tissue.[3] Using the work of Gordon, Bigelow, and Harrison, they postulated that analgesia resulted both from procaine's local anesthetic action in the inflamed and traumatized tissue and from central action in the nervous system, partially blocking the sympathetic nervous system and neutralizing the abnormal vasoconstriction resulting from the pain.

Graubard and Peterson combined these theories in 1950 and attributed the resulting relief of pain to the direct anesthetic action on irritated nerve fibers and to the indirect action of the procaine metabolite diethylaminoethanol on the vascular endothelium.[46]

Rowlinson and associates used i.v. lidocaine in normal volunteers and observed that blood levels below 3.0 μg/ml did not produce analgesia to ischemic pain caused by a tourniquet.[97]

Boas and colleagues used i.v. lidocaine (1.5 to 2.0 μg/ml, serum level) in patients with neuralgia and deafferentation syndrome to produce pain relief.[9] Anderson and co-workers[4] and Loeser and associates[65] hypothesized that pain associated with neurologic deafferentation may have a spinal electrogram pattern characterized by spontaneous high-frequency burst-discharge activity in the CNS; local anesthetics may relieve pain by reducing this activity.

Choice of Drug

Procaine has been the classic local anesthetic agent for i.v. administration because of its potency and low toxicity; however, its short action, even at maximum dosages, has been its major disadvantage. Since the mid-1940s other local anesthetics have been used in an attempt to increase analgesic effects without compromising potency and low toxicity; such anesthetic agents are tetracaine, lidocaine, and chloroprocaine.

Many authors have shown interest in the efficacy of i.v. lidocaine in managing painful conditions such as neuralgia, deafferentation syndrome, and paroxysmal attacks associated with postherpetic neuralgia. Hatangdi and colleagues used i.v. lidocaine, 1.0 to 1.5 mg/kg.[51] In general, there was complete relief of lancinating pain within seconds after injection. In addition, the degree of success with i.v. lidocaine often indicated patient response to oral antiepileptic drugs. Boas and associates used this local anesthetic agent in patients with deafferentation syndrome and noted significant pain relief within 15 to 20 minutes of starting the infusion.[9] In 1982 Atkinson advocated i.v. lidocaine for the management of intractable pain of adiposis dolorosa, administering a 0.1% solution of lidocaine i.v. until a total dose of 200 mg had been delivered over a 35-minute period.[6] Significant pain relief lasted for 2 to over 12 months.

Since 1952 focus has been placed on the i.v. administration of 2-chloroprocaine, the ortho-chloroderivative of procaine. Foldes and McNall found chloroprocaine to be two times more potent and to be hydrolyzed four times faster than procaine.[40] Because of its low toxicity and high potency, they recommended its use in poor-risk patients. In 1981 Parris and others successfully used a 60-ml bolus of i.v. 3% chloroprocaine solution to control pain associated with partial splenic embolization.[83]

Schnapp and colleagues used i.v. chloroprocaine to treat chronic intractable pain.[99] Forty-three percent of the patients reported more than 50% relief, lasting for longer than 30 days. Phero and associates considered i.v. chloroprocaine to be safe and efficacious in managing certain chronic intractable pain problems, particularly in patients with musculoskeletal pain.[85] Controlled studies of the efficacy of this technique in chronic pain syndromes are not currently available.

Technique of Administration

Two techniques have been used to administer i.v. local anesthetics in pain management, either as a single dose or with continuous infusion. Leriche was the first to use a single dose of 5 to 10 ml of 1% procaine infused over several hours for pruritus.[61] Graubard and Peterson devised the procaine unit, defined as 4 mg/kg of 0.1% procaine infused over 20 minutes by flowmeter.[46] Half of this dose was initially given as a bolus and then the rest of the dose was adjusted according to the incidence of side-effects. In 500 patients Bonica used one tenth of Graubard's procaine unit of pontocaine, delivering a total dose of 3.0 mg/kg (not exceeding 250 mg) over 2 to 3 hours.[10] The onset of analgesic effect was noted within one half hour and was reported to last longer than with procaine.

Boas and co-workers administered lidocaine at a rate of 4 mg/min using a Harvard pump for 1 hour in patients with deafferentation syndrome; these patients reported pain relief with serum lidocaine levels of 1.5 to 2.0 μg/ml.[9]

Foldes and McNall compared four local anesthetic agents (procaine, chloroprocaine, tetracaine, and lidocaine) in the conventional concentration ratios for toxicity in humans used in regional anesthesia.[40]

They observed no significant difference in the time of onset of signs and symptoms of toxicity among these agents. However, the signs and symptoms disappeared faster with 2-chloroprocaine, which was hydrolyzed four times faster than procaine. On the other hand, tetracaine hydrochloride was hydrolyzed 3.5 times slower than procaine (see Chap. 3). Investigators noted that the more rapidly an agent was hydrolyzed in the serum, the larger was the quantity of that agent required to maintain toxicity. Conversely, the slower an agent was hydrolyzed, the smaller was the dosage required to produce a toxic blood level.

In 1981 Schnapp and associates used 3% 2-chloroprocaine without preservatives delivered by a 30-ml syringe at a rate of 30 to 120 mg/min until either the pain had subsided or 900 mg had been injected.[99] In that study 44 patients were given a series of four i.v. 2-chloroprocaine injections 1 to 14 days apart. Forty-three percent of the patients had pain relief lasting for more than 30 days. Patients with allodynia or chronic pain responded favorably to this treatment.

Since 1981 the University of Cincinnati Pain Control Center has administered i.v. chloroprocaine by means of volumetric infusion pump to control the incidence of side-effects. The patients selected for i.v. local anesthetic therapy exhibited chronic pain problems refractory to conventional therapeutic modalities (surgery, nerve blocks, physical therapy, analgesics).

A 1% chloroprocaine solution is administered at a rate of 1.0 to 1.5 mg/kg/min until a total dose of 10 to 20 mg/kg is delivered. All infusions are conducted in a controlled environment where resuscitative equipment and drugs are immediately available. In addition, the patient's vital signs (ECG, blood pressure, heart rate, and mentation) are monitored. If evidence of CNS toxicity except for mild symptoms (tinnitus, metallic taste, light-headedness) occurred, the rate of infusion is decreased by one half, or if the symptoms persist or worsen, the infusion is discontinued. Patients are required to rest for 1 hour after conclusion of the treatment and then, if in satisfactory condition, are discharged home in the company of an escort.

Monitoring of the patient during i.v. infusion of a local anesthetic is essential. The patient's vital signs (ECG, blood pressure, heart rate, and mentation) are evaluated every 5 minutes. In more than 108 treatments, patients did not have any deleterious sequelae.

Evaluation. Patient's receive a series of four or five i.v. chloroprocaine infusions to evaluate efficacy of the modality. Pain relief scores are obtained before, during, and after the infusion. For the period between treatments in the diagnostic series, usually 1 to 3 weeks, patients are required to evaluate pain relief, function, and psychological scores on a visual analogue scale four times daily (morning, afternoon, evening, and night). In addition, the amount of oral medication consumed per day is documented.

Side-Effects. The side-effects of i.v. local anesthetics have long been documented and are associated with CNS toxicity.[25,26,28] Early signs and symptoms include metallic taste, tinnitus, light-headedness, agitation, and drowsiness. Moderate signs of CNS toxicity include difficulty with ocular focusing, nystagmus, slurred speech, dysarthria, numbness in the lips and tongue, and tingling or a heavy feeling in the extremities. Untoward effects of late CNS toxicity include hypotension or hypertension, bradycardia or tachycardia, seizure, and unconsciousness. Cardiac and respiratory failure, coma, and death may occur in the late stages of local anesthetic toxicity (see Chap. 4).

Prognosis. Patients with certain types of chronic intractable pain problems refractory to conservative modalities may respond well to this type of therapy. At my institution 38 patients received 178 i.v. chloroprocaine treatments over a 30-month period, an average of 4.7 treatments per patient. The time between treatments ranged from 3 days to 18 weeks, averaging 2.4 weeks per treatment. Of the 27 patients, 15 (56%) completed the diagnostic series of 4 to 5 i.v. chloroprocaine infusions; 12 of the 15 (80%) continued to receive additional treatments for continued pain relief. Fifty-eight percent of these patients (7 of 12) returned to usual conservative therapeutic modalities or were maintained on i.v. chloroprocaine infusions at a 3- to 6-month interval. Five of the seven patients (72%) with chronic intractable musculoskeletal pain had at least 30% pain relief for more than 11 months.*

BLOCK OF CRANIAL NERVES

Block of the cranial nerves is useful in the management of severe pain arising from the anterior two thirds of the head (see Fig. 15-2). Local anesthetic blocks are used to predict the effects of prolonged interruption with neurolytic agents or neurosurgical

*Administration of oral tocainide or mexilitine may be an option to maintain the beneficial effects of i.v. lidocaine. Tocainide may, however, depress bone marrow.

ablative procedures (Fig. 27-19). Alcohol block of one of the branches of the trigeminal nerve or Gasserian ganglion (see Figs. 15-3, 6) has long been used in patients with tic douloureux or severe cancer pain who are not suitable for neurosurgical operations.[12,18] More recently glycerol injection of the trigeminal ganglion has been used successfully (see Chap. 29.2). Although the advent of carbamazine and the recent reintroduction of thermocoagulation of Gasserian ganglion and percutaneous differential radiofrequency rhizotomy of the trigeminal sensory root have all decreased the use of alcohol block, there is still a definite place for such a neurolytic block in the management of cancer pain and, to a lesser extent, in the treatment of trigeminal neuralgia. Properly done, alcohol neurolytic block of Gasserian ganglion or its sensory root produces pain relief in 85% of patients with cancer pain of the anterior two thirds of the head.[12,18] Glycerol block is reported to be even more effective and less likely to produce side-effects (see Chap. 29.2). Block of the glossopharyngeal nerve alone or in combination with the vagus nerve below the jugular foramen (see Fig. 15-7) is also a useful prognostic procedure, in patients with glossopharyngeal neuralgia or cancer pain of the throat, before ablative section or percutaneous differential radiofrequency rhizotomy.[12,18]

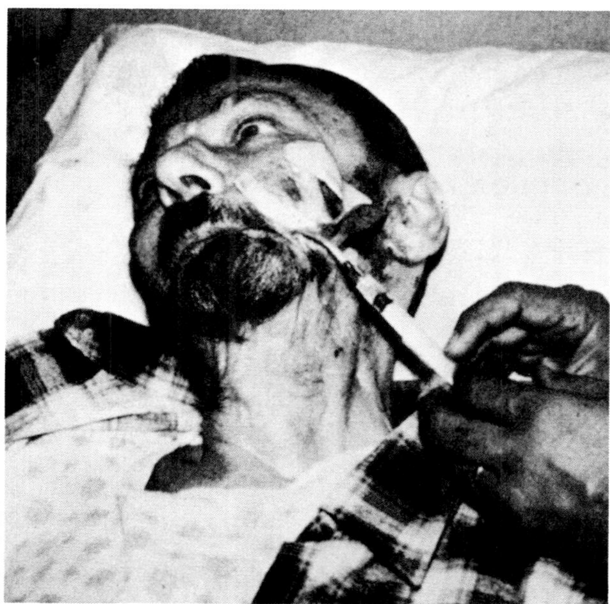

FIG. 27-19. The catheter has been inserted on the trigeminal ganglion under fluoroscopic control. A local anesthetic was injected through the catheter for initial pain relief, and alcohol was injected into the ganglion. (Raj, P.P. [ed.]: Practical Management of Pain, p. 588. Chicago, Year Book Medical Publishers, 1986.)

BLOCK OF THE SPINAL NERVES

Paravertebral Somatic Nerve Block

Paravertebral block of one or more of the spinal nerves is a useful procedure in the management of painful disorders of the back of the head, neck, trunk, and lower limbs (see Figs. 14-10, 15-11).[16] Because this procedure includes the recurrent meningeal nerve and posterior division and the branches that supply the vertebra, the facet joint, and the meninges, it is useful to help determine nociceptive pathways in patients with segmental neuralgia caused by vertebral pathology such as osteoporosis, scoliosis, or herniated intervertebral disk.[16]

Paravertebral somatic nerve block with local anesthetics usually produces only temporary pain relief and is therefore most useful in acute conditions, such as acute herpes zoster, when intercostal nerve or epidural block may not be possible.

Intercostal Block

Intercostal nerve block is one of the most useful procedures for relief of a severe acute post-traumatic, postoperative, or postinfectious pain in the thoracic or abdominal wall. It is highly effective in relieving severe pain resulting from fracture of one or more ribs or the sternum, dislocation of the costochondral junction, slipped rib cartilage, contusion chest pain, pleurisy, and acute herpes zoster. It is a useful therapeutic procedure in entrapment of the intercostal nerves in the rectal sheath, said to be a frequent cause of abdominal and chest pain (see Chap. 24.1, Appendix B, Sects. XVII-14, XX-3, XX-4, and XX- 5).[5]

Intercostal block produces analgesia two to four times the duration of that achieved with the same drug dose injected into the epidural space. Moore and others[78] reported that after intercostal block with 4 ml of 0.25% bupivacaine with adrenaline, analgesia lasted for 10 to 12 hours. This makes it practical to induce intercostal block in the morning and have the patient ambulate, cough, and be as active as possible during the analgesia that usually persists for the remainder of the day. If necessary, the block can be repeated in the evening, or at least each morning. Although intercostal block carries a risk of pneumothorax, when skillfully done the incidence of this complication is less than 1% (see Chap. 14 and Fig. 14-3).[16]

Peripheral Nerve Block

Block of the brachial (Chap. 10) or lumbosacral (Chap. 11) plexus or one or more of its major branches may be used as a prognostic measure. In the upper extremity, because all sympathetic fibers destined for the hand, forearm, and lower two thirds of the arm are carried with the nerves derived from the brachial plexus, block of the brachial plexus is an effective way to confirm the results of cervicothoracic sympathetic block in patients with reflex sympathetic dystrophy or those with painful peripheral vascular disorders (Fig. 27-20). It is also useful in providing temporary relief of severe acute pain after trauma or operation, or in patients with severe vasospasm caused by accidental intra-arterial injection of such agents as thiopental and in those with severe pain consequent to an embolus. Continuous brachial plexus block is especially useful in patients who have undergone reattachment of a severed limb or digits, and in those whose blood supply to the extremities is compromised.[96] In such circumstances prolonged sympathetic block and analgesia enhance survival of the limb and concomitantly provide pain relief.

The indications for block of the lumbosacral plexus or sciatic and femoral nerves are similar to those of the brachial plexus. These may be used to temporarily control acute pain and produce complete sympathetic interruption of the foot and leg. Block of the lateral femoral cutaneous nerve is indicated in the management of patients with meralgia paresthetica.[58,118] Obturator nerve block may be used in the management of adductor muscle spasm and differential diagnosis of patients with a painful hip.[12] A significant drawback to blocks of the somatic nerves to the extremities is the weakness or paralysis and loss of proprioception, touch, and sensation that produce a useless limb. Therefore, except in extreme cases of patients with terminal cancer pain, prolonged blocks with alcohol or other neurolytic agents are absolutely contraindicated.

EPIDURAL BLOCK

Continuous segmental epidural block is a practical technique to manage patients with subacute and chronic pain. By placing a catheter at different levels of the extradural space one can produce segmental analgesia involving two, three, or as many as ten spinal segments in virtually any part of the body (see Chap. 8). It reliably relieves severe pain of acute pancreatitis, biliary colic, renal and ureteral colic, multiple rib fractures, and other severe post-traumatic pain and controls postoperative pain in the thorax, abdomen, or lower limbs (see Chap. 26). It is indicated to provide immediate, albeit temporary, relief of severe pain owing to a herniated intervertebral

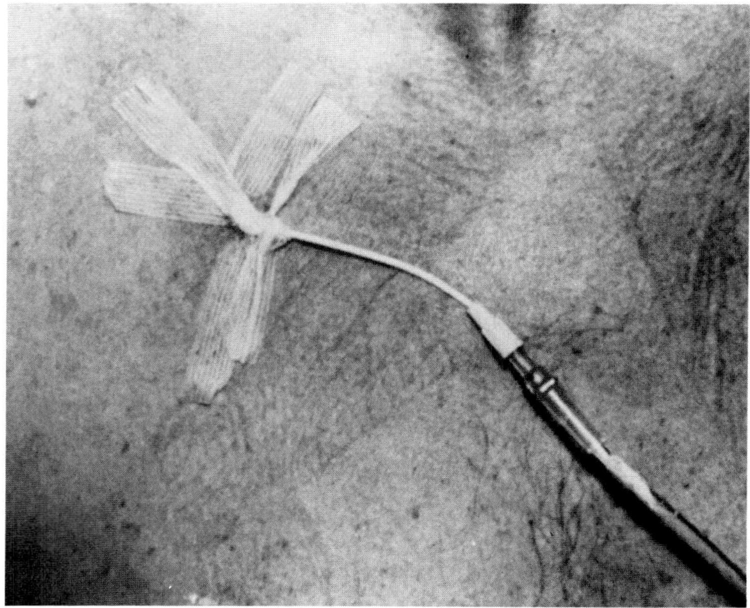

FIG. 27-20. For intractable pain secondary to reflex sympathetic dystrophy of the right upper extremity, an infraclavicular brachial plexus catheterization has been done for this patient. Bupivacaine 0.25% (10–15 ml/h) infusion is instituted after confirming with a bolus local anesthetic injection that brachial plexus block is effective. The object of the management plan is to provide adequate pain relief for a prolonged period (usually 1–2 weeks) to permit intensive physical therapy, withdraw addictive drugs, and maintain adequate vascularization of the extremity. (Raj, P.P. [ed.]: Practical Management of Pain, p. 694. Chicago, Year Book Medical Publishers, 1986.)

disk or a vertebral or pelvic fracture because it not only provides complete relief (in contrast to the partial relief achieved with narcotics), but also relieves the reflex muscle spasm and permits more definitive treatment.

Techniques of Prolonged Analgesia

The object of producing prolonged epidural analgesia for chronic pain is to have a prognostic and therapeutic effect. The volume and concentration of the local anesthetic agent is determined by how many segments need to be blocked. The bolus injections then maintain that quality of analgesia for a period of time, usually days, for the physician to evaluate the beneficial effect of pain relief and its side-effects. For the patient, this state of prolonged analgesia allows him to experience the feeling of numbness or weakness that accompanies the analgesia. The patient can then determine whether a proposed neurolytic block in that region could be tolerable. When prolonged analgesia is used for therapeutic regimen, one evaluates the benefits of prolonged sympathetic block, an exercise program during the pain-free period, and the benefits of reducing the nociceptive impulses on the reflex mechanisms.

Intermittent Bolus Technique. The bolus injection technique is similar to that used for postoperative or trauma patients. Because the need for prolonged analgesia is longest in patients with chronic pain, tachyphylaxis is common with this technique. Bromage and associates state that tachyphylaxis will appear if intervals between injections are long enough to allow analgesia to completely wear off (see Fig. 8-27 and its reference). On the other hand, augmentation of analgesia is seen when injections are given too closely.

Drugs. It is possible to administer any local anesthetic agent for bolus injection. Some agents, however, are more efficacious than others. The longer-acting local anesthetic agents are preferred to shorter-acting local anesthetic agents (see Chaps. 3 and 4). Bupivacaine is the drug of choice because of its prolonged analgesic effect and minimal motor effect.

Duration of analgesia with bolus injections in the epidural space is shorter than for surgical anesthesia. The addition of epinephrine does not appear to produce the prolongation of analgesia one sees during surgery. In most of patients 0.25% bupivacaine produces adequate analgesia. However, if the duration of the analgesia is short, it can be increased by using 0.375% or 0.5% bupivacaine. It should be cautioned that higher concentrations increase the chances of toxicity.

Volume of local anesthetic agent needed is determined by the region at which it is administered and how many segments need to be blocked. The largest volume is injected in the caudal region and the least, in the cervical region. The following are the maximum bolus injection volumes at various sites: caudal, 20 to 25 ml; lumbar, 15 to 20 ml; thoracic, 5 to 10 ml; and cervical, 2 to 5 ml.

With bolus injections, plasma concentrations of the drug will peak 15 to 20 minutes after each injection. Monitoring is mandatory for 45 minutes to prevent toxic reaction when the drug is peaking. If the injection is given at short intervals, it may produce a saw-toothed pattern, causing toxic concentration to be reached. This has been shown to occur rapidly with lidocaine and slowly with etidocaine (see Chap. 3).[116] Bupivacaine pharmacokinetics have not been studied in postoperative analgesia for bolus technique.

Infusion Technique. This method was developed to provide continuous analgesia between bolus injections. It provides continuous infusion of the drug into the epidural space that equals the rate at which it is removed from it.[30,47]

A bolus of 3% 2-chloroprocaine or 2% lidocaine is initially injected into a well-anchored epidural catheter to provide analgesia in the affected pain dermatomes. The volumes of the local anesthetic is determined by the site of catheter placement.[92] The maximum volume injected is similar to that used in the bolus technique (caudal, 25 ml; lumbar, 20 ml; thoracic, 10 ml; cervical, 5 ml). After confirming that the epidural is functioning, infusion of bupivacaine is started by means of a volumetric infusion pump (Fig. 27-21). Generally, 10 ml of 0.25% bupivacaine is needed for a 5′10″, 70-kg man when the catheter is placed in the lumbar space. Volume or concentration is changed by 12 hours if more than necessary segments are blocked (volume change) or motor and sensory block is intense (concentration change). In the thoracic space 5 to 10 ml is infused with similar concentrations. For the success of this technique, nursing monitoring is mandatory with ready availability of physician personnel when required (see also Chap. 26).

In a study by Raj and colleagues adequate pain relief was obtained in 75% of the patients with continuous infusion alone.[92] Twenty-five percent of the

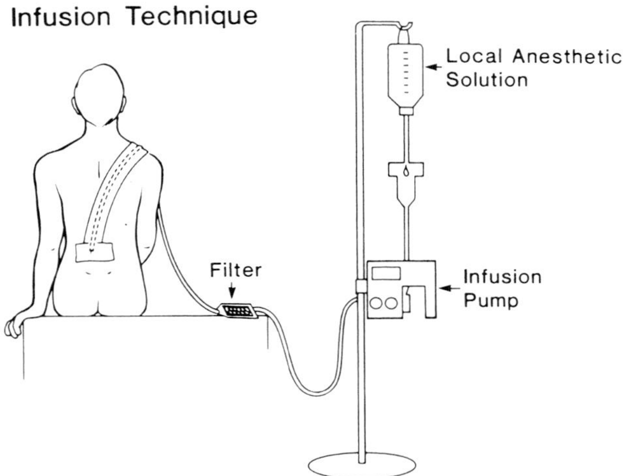

FIG. 27-21. Arrangement used for continuous epidural analgesia. Similar arrangement can be used at any other perineural site. (Pither, C., and Hartrick, C.: Postoperative pain. *In* Raj, P.P. [ed.]: Handbook of Regional Anesthesia. p. 104. New York, Churchill-Livingstone, 1985.)

remaining patients had less than 50% of pain relief and were administered bolus doses of 5 to 10 ml of 1% lidocaine once or twice a day. The initial concentration of infusion was 0.25% bupivacaine in patients with muscle spasm and pain (A-alpha and A-delta fibers) and 0.125% to 0.0625% bupivacaine in patients with C fiber pain. Most of the patients were infused for 7 days. Concentrations of bupivacaine were decreased if the patient had adequate relief but had motor paresis or numbness in other areas or urinary retention. Sixty-nine percent of patients with initial 0.25% concentration had their concentration changed, after 24 hours, to a lower concentration (0.125%). The volume of infusion per hour was determined by assessing the number of segments to be blocked. Usually 12 ml/h was infused for blocking of segments greater than six, 10 ml/h for segments between four and six, and 5 ml/h for segments less than four. Because the dose was reduced owing to increasing quality of block and adequate analgesia was seen in the majority of patients, the authors did not observe tachyphylaxis. With infusion up to 30 mg/h, a steady state was achieved in 18 hours in the plasma concentration, and accumulation was not observed up to 7 days. Steady-state plasma concentration was also achieved in one patient infused for 29 days.[30]

Pharmacokinetic Considerations. The pharmacokinetic parameters for 50 patients undergoing continuous extravascular perineural bupivacaine infusions for the treatment of their chronic pain were studied by Denson and associates.[30] The total plasma clearance, volume of distribution, and elimination rate were estimated from two blood samples. These parameters were compared with values obtained from the actual monoexponential decay curve at the termination of infusion. Estimated and actual pharmacokinetic parameters were found to be in excellent agreement (Table 27-5). No evidence of accumulation was seen, even after 5 days of continuous infusion. This study demonstrated a wide margin of safety during continuous perineural bupivacaine infusions at dosages up to 30 mg/h in normal patients. Such patients did not require determination of serum bupivacaine concentration to monitor the changes in dosages necessary for adequate clinical effect. On the other hand, in patients with renal or hepatic dysfunction, altered clearance rates were observed. In such patients monitoring of serum bupivacaine concentrations is necessary to determine the range of dosages available for adjustment to provide adequate clinical effect and to prevent systemic toxicity.

In one study on cancer and trauma patients, a significant decrease in bupivacaine total clearance with increasing alpha-1-acid glycoprotein concentrations was seen (Fig. 27-22).[92] Accumulation and concomitant increases in total serum bupivacaine concentration for a given infusion rate result from this decrease in total clearance. Increased plasma protein binding and corresponding decrease in the free fraction appear to prevent toxic reactions even at total serum bupivacaine concentrations above the apparent threshold level of 2.6 to 3.0 μg/ml (Fig. 27-23). Tinnitus occurred briefly in only one patient. The serum bupivacaine concentration for this patient was 7.1 μg/ml. The results of this study demonstrate the importance of measuring free fraction rather than the total serum bupivacaine concentration, since all five of the cancer patients exceeded the expected toxicity threshold (see also pp. 81–83).

Epidural Steroid Injection

Epidural steroid injection is performed after failure of conservative management of discogenic pain.[22] Even though some claim improved results with subarachnoid injection, most believe that epidural steroids are safer and produce equally good results. Because the nerve root compression is extradural in discogenic disease, it is rational to introduce the steroid epidurally at the site of compression rather than intradurally

TABLE 27.5. COMPARISON OF THE MEAN PHARMACOKINETIC VALUES FOR CONTINUOUS EPIDURAL, SYMPATHETIC, AND BRACHIAL PLEXUS INFUSIONS

		λz (l/h)	CL (l/h)	Vz (l)	Vz (ml/g) (BW)	Vz (ml/g) (LBM)
Brachial plexus	Estimated	±0.169	28.5	174.9	2.51	2.78
		±0.019	±4.2	±23.3	±0.40	±0.44
	Actual	0.165	26.0	155.3	2.58	2.80
		±0.018	±4.4	±14.6	±0.24	±0.38
Sympathetic	Estimated	0.181	30.4	177.9	3.02	2.80
		±0.021	±2.5	±14.5	±0.42	±0.31
	Actual	0.204	29.2	151.8	2.47	2.45
		±0.028	±2.8	±10.8	±0.25	±0.25
Epidural	Estimated	0.179	33.2	195.7	2.94	2.82
		±0.010	±2.4	±14.5	±.30	±.23
	Actual	0.176	29.6	173.7	2.36	2.61
		±0.010	±2.8	±18.2	±0.33	±0.28

(Denson, D.D., Raj, P.P, Saldahna, F., *et al.*: Int. J. Clin. Pharmacol. Ther. Toxicol., *21*:591, 1983).

Results shown are mean ± SEM.

λz = Elimination rate constant CL = Total clearance rate

Vz = Volume and distribution in the elimination phase

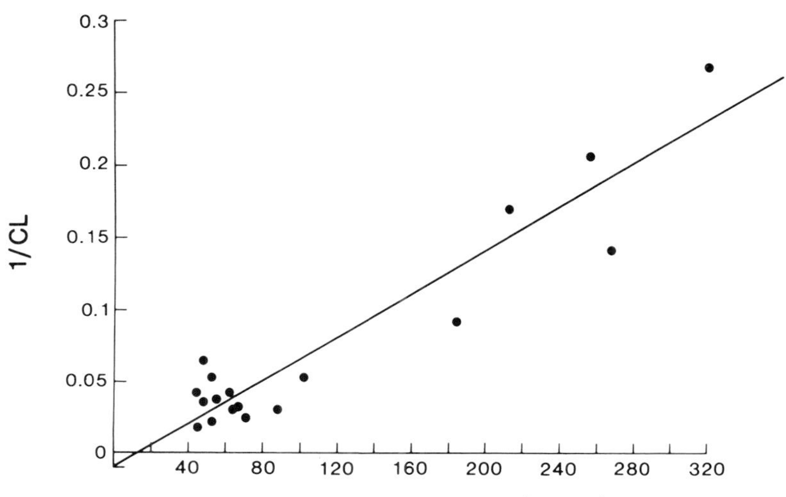

FIG. 27-22. Correlation between 1/CL on the *y*-axis and α_1-acid glycoprotein concentration on the *x*-axis. (Denson, D.D., *et al.*: Int. J. Clin. Pharmacol. Ther. Toxicol., *21*:591, 1983.)

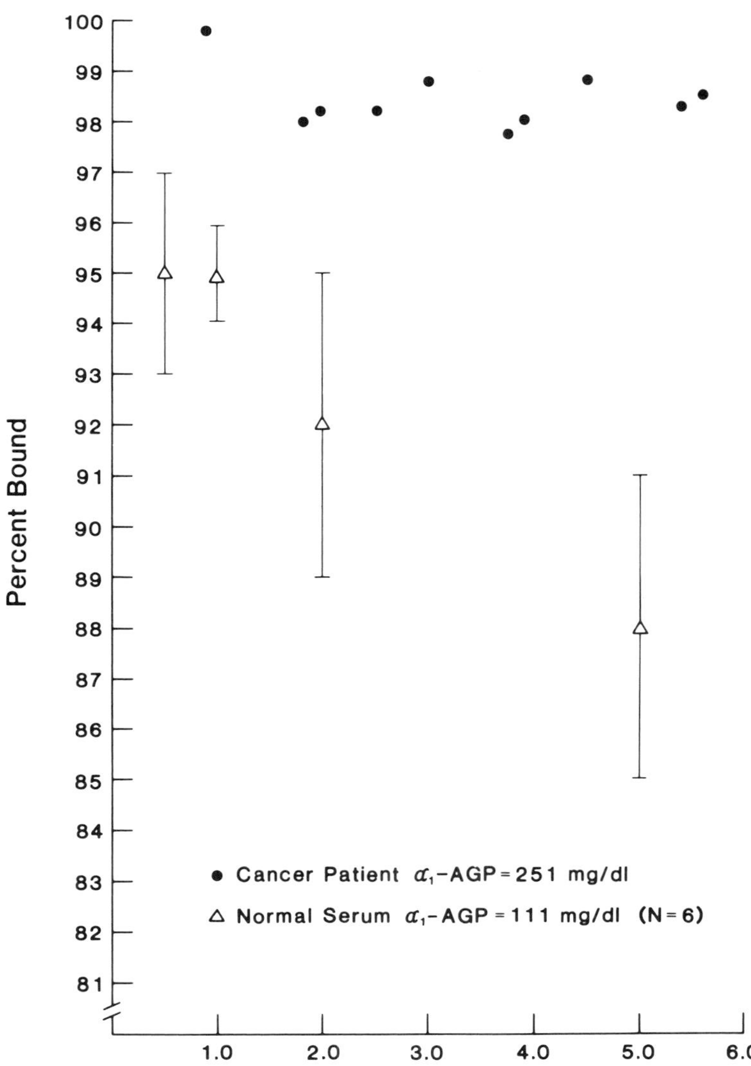

FIG. 27-23. Increased protein binding in cancer patients receiving continuous bupivacaine infusions is associated with a decrease in toxic reactions, despite high total serum concentrations of bupivacaine. (Raj, P.P. [ed.]: Handbook of Regional Anesthesia, p. 140. New York, Churchill-Livingstone, 1985.)

where it will be subject to dilution, dispersion, and precipitation (see also Chap. 27.3).

Technique. Epidural puncture should be done at the site of nerve root lesion, with the painful side down in the lateral decubitus position (see Chap. 8). When the epidural space has been identified by standard techniques, 80 mg of methylprednisolone acetate or 50 mg of triamcinolone diacetate is suspended in 10 ml of 0.25% or 0.125% bupivacaine and injected slowly into the epidural space. With previous back surgery, identification of the epidural space may be difficult. Initial local anesthetic administration will make identification of epidural space easier under these circumstances.

After epidural steroid injection a catheter can be introduced to inject another dose of steroid and local anesthetic, if needed, to reach the appropriate nerve root. This is determined by objectively measuring the improvement in straight leg-raising test and absence of radicular pain during the performance of the test.

The patient is kept in the lateral position for 10

minutes to keep the injected solution on the dependent side.

Two weeks after the epidural steroid injection, the patient is reevaluated. If there is significant improvement in function and subjective pain relief, no further epidural injection is administered. However, if after the first injection the initial improvement is not maintained, then epidural injection can be repeated up to a maximum of three. Similarly, if there is no change in the patient's condition after the first injection, then alternative measures are sought.

Many workers have reported impressive results with epidural steroid injections.[1,21,29,43,100,122] Winnie reported subjective total relief of symptoms in 80% of patients with either epidural or subarachnoid injections.[122] Brown reported "excellent to good" results in 100% of patients with acute discogenic disease of less than 3 months but in only 14% of those with pain that had lasted for more than 3 months.[21]

Arnhoff and co-workers reported a significant reduction in pain and improvement in function in their patients.[5a] Toomey and others extended their study to 5 years and found that gains noted at 1 to 2 years after epidural steroid injection were maintained at 5 to 6 years.[111]

Erdemir and associates studied 122 patients with postlaminectomy syndrome after treatment with intradural and extradural steroids. Fifty-three percent of patients reported satisfactory results (*i.e.*, 75%–100% of pain relief).[35]

When considering epidural steroid administration, the following points should be kept in mind:

- Histologic and biochemical evidence supports its use in the 30- to-50-year group; with low back or cervical pain with radiculopathy, the pain is primarily discogenic.
- Features of this pain are shooting pain in brachial plexus, sciatic or femoral distribution with sensory or motor deficits, reflex change, positive straight leg raising (SLR) above 30 degrees.
- Epidural versus subarachnoid injection has proponents on either side.
- Meningitis or arachnoiditis after intrathecal use and no appreciable advantage comparing with extradural route makes subarachnoid technique risky.
- Bupivacaine 0.125% or 0.25% with either Depo-medrol, 80 mg, or Aristocort, 50 mg, in 8 to 10 ml is commonly used.
- Three injections are recommended as maximum, 2 weeks apart in a 1-year period.
- Complications arise owing to excessive or frequent use.
- Two thirds of patients with acute discogenic disease will benefit by epidural steroids.
- Only one third will benefit after 6 months.
- Initial improvement is usually maintained; however, there seems to be no tendency for continued improvement.
- Epidural steroid injection is only one modality to treat low back pain.

See Chapter 27.3 for a critical appraisal of efficacy and safety of intrathecal and epidural steroids.

SUBARACHNOID BLOCK

There is usually no indication for local anesthetic subarachnoid block for chronic pain except for patients with spastic paraplegia, where it is used for diagnostic and prognostic purposes. For cancer patients, subarachnoid neurolysis is achieved by injection of small amounts of alcohol or phenol into the subarachnoid space, and it is one of the most effective methods for the relief of severe intractable pain below the neck (see Chap. 29.2).[38,52,108,123] Pain relief lasts for several days to several months, and sometimes longer, although frequently it is necessary to do several blocks to effect prolonged relief. Numerous reports suggest that neurolytic subarachnoid block produces complete relief in 50% to 60% of cancer patients, partial relief in 20% to 25%, and no relief in the rest.[12,52,108] This compares favorably with the results achieved with neurosurgical procedures. With subarachnoid block of the roots supplying the upper limb, there is a 15% to 20% incidence of muscle weakness. If the block is done to relieve pain in the pelvis or lower limbs, there is a 20% to 25% incidence of muscle weakness. If the block is done to relieve pain in the pelvis or lower limbs, there is a 20% to 25% incidence of bladder or rectal dysfunction and lower limb muscle weakness (see also Chap. 23).

SYMPATHETIC BLOCKS

Sympathetic blocks have been useful and commonly performed for pain in limbs and in viscera. The technique of sympathetic blocks has been described elsewhere in this book (see Chaps. 13 and 14). The mechanism of sympathetic efferent influence on pain perception is shown in Fig. 24-1. Nociceptive afferents from viscera travel to the spinal cord by way of sympathetic ganglia and can be blocked there.

However, they are not "sympathetic" (efferent) fibers (see Fig. 24-2). Sympathetic blocks represent one of the best risk-benefit ratios for neural blockade techniques. Even neurolytic sympathetic blocks of celiac plexus and lumbar sympathetic chain have a low incidence of complications if skillfully carried out. The many applications of sympathetic blocks in the limbs are described in Chapter 13. Treatment of thoracoabdominal visceral pain with sympathetic blocks is described in Chapter 14. There are also some conditions in the head and neck in which blockade of the cervicothoracic sympathetic chain may be of benefit; if there are symptoms or signs of abnormal sympathetic activity in this region, a diagnostic cervicothoracic sympathetic block is performed (see Chap. 13).

REFERENCES

1. Abram, S.E.: Subarachnoid corticosteroid injection following inadequate response to epidural steroids for sciatica. Anesth. Analg., *57*:313, 1978.
2. Abram, S.E., and Likavec, J.M.: Pain syndromes and rationale for management of neurogenic pain. *In* Raj, P.P. (ed.): Practical Management of Pain, pp. 182–191. Chicago, Year Book Medical Publishers, 1986.
3. Allen, F.M., Grossman, L.W., and Lyons, L.V.: Intravenous procaine analgesia. Anesth. Analg., *25*:1, 1946.
4. Anderson, L.S., Black, R.G., Abraham, J., and Ward, A.A.: Deafferentation neuronal hyperactivity: A possible etiology of paresthesias following retrogasserian rhizotomy. J. Neurosurg., *35*:444, 1971.
5. Applegate, W.V.: Abdominal cutaneous nerve entrapment syndrome. Surgery, *71*:118, 1972.

5a. Arnhoff, F.N., Triplett, H.B., and Pokorney, B.: Follow-up status of patients treated with nerve blocks for low back pain. Anesthesiology, *46*:170, 1977.

6. Atkinson, R.L.: Intravenous lidocaine for the treatment of intractable pain of adiposis dolorosa. Int. J. Obesity, *6*:351, 1982.
7. Awad, E.A.: Interstitial myofibrositis: Hypothesis of the mechanism. Arch. Phys. Med. Rehabil., *54*:440, 1973.
8. Bigelow, N., and Harrison, I.: General analgesic effects of procaine. J. Pharmacol. Exp. Ther., *81*:368, 1944.
9. Boas, R.A., Covino, B.G., and Shahnarian, A.: Analgesic responses to I.V. lignocaine. Br. J. Anesth., *54*:501, 1982.
10. Bonica, J.J.: Management of Pain. Philadelphia, Lea & Febiger, 1953.
11. Bonica, J.J.: Management of myofascial pain syndromes in general practice. J.A.M.A., *165*:732, 1957.
12. Bonica, J.J.: Clinical Applications of Diagnostic and Therapeutic Nerve Blocks. Springfield, Ill., Charles C. Thomas, 1959.
13. Bonica, J.J.: Current role of nerve blocks in the diagnosis and therapy of pain. *In* Bonica, J.J. (ed.): Advances in Neurology, Vol. 4, p. 445. New York, Raven Press, 1974.
14. Bonica, J.J.: Causalgia and other reflex sympathetic dystrophies. *In* Bonica, J.J., Liebeskind, J.C., and Albe-Fessard, D. (eds.): Advances in Pain Research and Therapy, Vol. 3, pp. 141–166. New York, Raven Press, 1979.
15. Bonica, J.J.: Blocks of the Sympathetic Nervous System. Vol. 2. Chicago, Frank J Corbett, 1981.
16. Bonica, J.J.: Management of pain with regional analgesia. Postgrad. Med., *60*:897, 1984.
17. Bonica, J.J.: Sympathetic Nerve Blocks. *In* Pain: Diagnosis and Therapy. Vol. 1: Fundamental Considerations and Clinical Applications. New York, Winthrop Breon Laboratories, 1984.
18. Bonica, J.J., and Madrid, J.L.: Cancer pain in the head and neck. Role of nerve blocks. *In* Bonica, J.J., Liebeskind, J.C., and Albe-Fessard, D. (eds.): Advances in Pain Research and Therapy. Vol. 3. New York, Raven Press, 1979.
19. Bonica, J.J., and Benedetti, C.: Postoperative pain. *In* Concon, R.E., deCosse, J.J., (eds.): Surgical Care: A Physiological Approach to Clinical Management, p. 394. Philadelphia, Lea & Febiger, 1980.
20. Brena, S.F.: Nerve blocks and chronic pain states: An update. Clinical Indications. Postgrad. Med., *78*:77, 1985.
21. Brown, F.W.: Management of diskogenic pain using epidural and intrathecal steroids. Clin. Orthop., *129*:72, 1977.
22. Carron, H., and Toomey, T.C.: Epidural steroid therapy for low back pain. *In* Stanton-Hicks, M., and Boas, R.A. (eds.): Chronic Low Back Pain, pp. 193–198. New York, Raven Press, 1982.
23. Cash, J.D., and Allan, A.G.E.: Effect of mental stress on the fibrinolytic reactivity to exercise. Br. Med. J., *2*:545, 1967.
24. Cervero, F.: Deep and visceral pain. *In* Kosterlitz, H.W., and Terenius, L.Y. (eds.): Pain and Society, pp. 263–282. Weinheim, Verlag Chemie, 1980.
25. Cousins, M.J., and Scott, D.B.: Clinical pharmacology of local anesthetic agents. *In* Cousins, M.J., Bridenbaugh, P.O. (eds.): Neural Blockade in Clinical Anesthesia and Management of Pain, pp. 86–121. Philadelphia, J.B. Lippincott Co., 1980.
26. Covino, B.G.., and Vassallo, H.G.: Local Anesthetics: Mechanism of Action and Clinical Use. Orlando, Fla., Grune & Stratton, 1976.
27. Cox, W.V., and Robertson, H.F.: The effect of stellate ganglionectomy on the cardiac function of intact dogs and its effect on the extent of myocardial infarction and on cardiac function following coronary artery occlusion. Am. Heart J., *12*:285, 1936.
28. deJong, R.H.: Local Anesthetics. 2nd ed. Springfield, Ill., Charles C Thomas, 1977.
29. DeLaney, T.J., *et al.*: The effects of steroids on nerves and meninges. Anesth. Analg., *59*:610, 1980.
30. Denson, D.D., *et al.*: Perineural infusions of bupivacaine for prolonged analgesia: Pharmacokinetic considerations. Int. J. Clin. Pharmacol. Ther. Toxicol., *21*:591, 1983.
31. Dreyfuss, F.: Coagulation time of the blood, level of blood eosinophils and thrombocytes under emotional stress. J. Psychosom. Res., *1*:252, 1956.

32. Druckman, R., and Lende, R.: Central pain of spinal cord origin. Neurology, *15*:518, 1965.
33. Epstein, E.: Triamcinolone-procaine in the treatment of zoster and postzoster neuralgia. Calif. Med., *115*:6, 1971.
34. Epstein, E.: Treatment of herpes zoster and postzoster neuralgia by subcutaneous injection of triamcinolone. Int. J. Dermatol., *20*:65, 1981.
35. Erdemir, H., Karamvir, M., and Gelman, S.: Intradural and extradural corticosteroids for postlaminectomy syndrome. Ala. J. Med. Sci., *19*:137, 1982.
36. Feigl, E.O.: Control of myocardial oxygen tension by sympathetic coronary vasoconstriction in the dog. Circ. Res., *37*:88, 1975.
37. Feinstein, D., Luce, J.C., and Langton, J.N.K.: The influence of phantom limbs. *In* Klopsteg, P.E., and Wilson, P.D. (eds.): Human Limbs and Their Substitutes, p. 79. New York, McGraw Hill, 1954.
38. Ferrer-Brechner, T.: Epidural and intrathecal phenol neurolysis for cancer pain. Anesthesiol. Rev., *8*:14, 1981.
39. Fischer, A.A.: Thermography and pain. Arch. Phys. Med. Rehabil., *62*:542, 1981.
40. Foldes, F.F., and McNall, P.G.: 2-Chloroprocaine: A new local anesthetic agent. Anesthesiology, *13*:287, 1981.
41. Gilbert, G.J.: Spasmodic torticollis treated effectively by medical means. N. Engl. J. Med., *285*:896, 1971.
42. Gilbert, G.J.: The medical treatment of spasmodic torticollis. Arch. Neurol., *27*:503, 1972.
43. Goebert, H.W., *et al.*: Sciatica: Treatment with epidural injections of procaine and hydrocortisone. Cleve. Clin. Q., *27*:191, 1960.
44. Good, M.G.: Objective diagnosis and curability of nonarticular rheumatism. Br. J. Phys. Med., *14*:1, 1951.
45. Gordon, R.A.: Intravenous novocaine for analgesia in burns. Can. Med. Assoc. J., *49*:478, 1943.
46. Graubard, D.J., and Peterson, M.C.: Clinical Uses of Intravenous Procaine. Springfield, Charles C. Thomas, 1950.
47. Green, R., and Dawkins, C.J.M.: Postoperative analgesia: The use of a continuous drip epidural block. Anaesthesia, *21*:372, 1967.
48. Guttman, L.: Spinal Cord Injuries: Comprehensive Management and Research. Oxford, England, Blackwell Scientific Publications, 1976.
49. Haas, L.F.: Postherpetic neuralgia: Treatment and prevention. Trans. Ophthalmol. Soc. N.Z., *29*:133, 1977.
50. Hansen, D.A.: Torticollis, S. Afr. Med. J., *40*:480, 1972.
51. Hatangdi, V.S., Boas, R.A., and Richards, E.G.: Post-herpetic neuralgia: Management with anti-epileptic and tricyclic drugs. *In* Bonica, J.J., Liebeskind, J.C., and Albe-Fessard, D. (eds.): Advances in Pain Research and Therapy, Vol. 1, pp. 583–587. New York, Raven Press, 1976.
52. Hay, R.C.: Subarachnoid alcohol block in the control of intractable pain. Anesth. Analg. Curr. Res., *41*:12, 1962.
53. Ingle, J.I., and Beveridge, E.E.: Endodontics. 2nd ed. Philadelphia, Lea & Febiger, 1976.
54. Janetta, P.J.: Trigeminal neuralgia and hemifacial spasm: Etiology and definitive treatment. Trans. Am. Neurol. Assoc., *100*:89, 1965.
55. Kahn,E.A., and Peet, M.M.: The technique of anterolateral cordotomy. J. Neurosurg., *5*:276, 1948.
56. Kelly, M.: The treatment of fibrositis and allied disorders by local anesthesia. Med. J. Aust., *1*:294, 1941.
57. Kerr, F.W.L.: Etiology of trigeminal neuralgia. Arch. Neurol., *89*:15, 1963.
58. Kopell, H.P., and Thompson, W.: Peripheral Entrapment Neuropathies, pp. 85–88. Melbourne, Florida, Krieger, 1976.
59. Kraus, H.: Clinical Treatment of Back and Neck Pain. New York, McGraw-Hill Book Co., 1970.
60. Lenman, J.A.R., and Ritchie, A.E.: Clinical Electromyography, 2nd ed, pp. 86–87. Philadelphia, J.B. Lippincott, Co., 1977.
61. Leriche, R.: Simple methods of easing pain in the extremities in arterial diseases and in certain vasomotor disorders. Presse Med., *49*:799, 1941.
62. Leriche, R.: Intra-arterial therapy of infections and other diseases. Mem. Acad. Chir., *64*:220, 1986.
63. Leung, J.W.C., *et al.*: Celiac plexus block for pain in pancreatic cancer and chronic pancreatitis. Br. J. Surg., *70*:730, 1983.
64. Loeser, J.D.: Herpes zoster and postherpetic neuralgia. Pain, *25*:149, 1986.
65. Loeser, J.D., Ward, A.A., and White, D.E.: Chronic deafferentation of human spinal cord neurons. J. Neurosurg., *29*:48, 1968.
66. Long, D.M.: Surgical therapy of chronic pain. Neurosurgery, *6*:317, 1980.
67. Long, D.M.: Neurological surgery. *In* Youmans, J.R. (ed.): Pain of Spinal Origin. Vol. 6. Philadelphia, W.B. Saunders Co., 1982.
68. Lundy, J.S.: Clinical Anaesthesia. Philadelphia, W.B. Saunders Co., 1941.
69. Macdonald, A.J.R.: Abnormally tender muscle regions and associated painful movements. Pain, *8*:197, 1980
70. McEachern, C.G., Manning, G.W., and Hall, G.E.: Sudden occlusion of coronary arteries following removal of cardiosensory pathways. Intern. Med., *65*:661, 1940.
71. Malliani, A., Schwartz, P.J., and Zanchetti, A.: A sympathetic reflex elicited by experimental coronary occlusion. Am. J. Physiol., *217*:703, 1969.
72. Marshall, L.L., Trethewice, E.R., and Curtain, C.C.: Chemical radiculitis. Clin. Orthop., *29*:61, 1977.
73. Mayne, G.E., Brown, M., Arnold, P., and Moya, F.: Pain of herpes zoster and postherpetic neuralgia. *In* Raj, P.P. (ed.): Practical Management of Pain, pp. 345–361. Chicago, Year Book Medical Publishers, 1986.
74. Melzack, R.W., and Wall, P.D.: Challenge of Pain. New York, Basic Books, 1980.
75. Miehlke, K., Schulze, G., and Eger, W.: Klinische und experimentelle Untersuchungen zum Fibrositis-syndrome. Z. Rheumaforsch., *19*:310, 1960.
76. Mitchell, S.W., Morehouse, G.R., and Keen, W.W.: Gunshot Wounds and Other Injuries of Nerves. Philadelphia, J.B. Lippincott Co., 1964.
77. Modell, W., *et al.*: Treatment of painful disorders of skeletal muscle. N.Y. State J. Med., *48*:2050, 1948.
78. Moore, D.C., Bridenbaugh, L.D., Thompson, C.E., Balfour,

R.I., and Horton, W.C.: Bupivacaine: A review of 11,080 cases. Anesth. Analg., *57*:42, 1978.

79. Murphy, T.: Herpes zoster. *In* Advances and Update in Pain Therapy, p. 40. ASA Annual Meeting, Oct. 25, 1982.

80. Nashold, B.S., and Bullit, E.: Dorsal root entry zone lesions to control center pain in paraplegics. Neurosurgery, *55*:414, 1981.

81. Neufeld, I.: Pathogenetic concepts of "fibrositis." Arch. Phys. Med. Rehabil., *33*:363, 1952.

82. Olson, E.R., and Ivy, H.B.: Stellate block for trigeminal herpes zoster (letter). Arch. Ophthalmol., *98*:1656, 1980.

83. Parris, W.C.V., Gerlock, A.J., and MacDonnell, R.C.: Intra-arterial chloroprocaine for the control of pain associated with partial splenic embolization. Anesth. Analg., *60*:112, 1981.

84. Perkins, H.M., and Hanlon, P.R.: Epidural injection of local anesthetic and steroids for relief of pain secondary to herpes zoster. Arch. Surg., *113*:253, 1978.

85. Phero, J.C., *et al.*: Controlled intravenous administration of chloroprocaine for intractable pain management. Reg. Anesth., *9*:50, 1984.

86. Pizzolata, P., and Mannheimer, W.: Histopathologic Effects of Local Anesthetic Drugs and Related Substances, pp. 40, 41, 60, 71. Springfield, Ill., Charles C. Thomas, 1961.

87. Popelianskii, I.I., Zaslavskii, E.S., and Veselouskii, V.P.: Medicosocial significance, etiology, pathogenesis, and diagnosis of nonarticular disease of soft tissues of the limbs and back (Russian). Vopr. Revm., *3*:38, 1976.

88. Prudden, B.: Pain Erasure: The Bonnie Prudden Way, pp. 18, 19. New York, M. Evans & Co., 1980.

89. Raj, P.P. (ed.): Handbook of Regional Anesthesia, pp. 104, 140. New York, Churchill-Livingstone, 1985.

90. Raj, P.P.: Pain of musculoskeletal origin. *In* Raj, P.P. (ed.): Practical Management of Pain, pp. 443–450. Chicago, Year Book Medical Publishers, 1986.

91. Raj, P.P.: Myofascial trigger point injection. *In* Raj, P.P. (ed.): Practical Management of Pain, pp. 569–577. Chicago, Year Book Medical Publishers, 1986.

92. Raj, P.P., and Denson, D.D.: Prolonged analgesia technique. *In* Raj, P.P. (ed.): Practical Management of Pain, pp. 687–703. Chicago, Year Book Medical Publishers, 1986.

93. Raj, P.P., Knarr, D., Vigdorth, E., Gregg, R.V., Denson, D.D., and Edström, H.H.: Difference in analgesia following epidural blockade in patients with postoperative or chronic low back pain. Pain (Submitted for consideration).

94. Ramamurthy, S.: Cervical Pain. *In* Raj, P.P. (ed.): Practical Management of Pain, pp. 418–430. Chicago, Year Book Medical Publishers, 1986.

95. Rosenak, S.S.: Paravertebral block for the treatment of herpes zoster. N.Y. State J. Med., *56*:2684, 1956.

96. Rosenblatt, R.M., Pepitone-Rockwell, F., and McKillop, C.: Continuous axillary analgesia for traumatic hand surgery. Anesthesiology, *51*:565, 1979.

97. Rowlingson, J.C., DiFazio, C.A., Foster, J., and Carron, H.: Lidocaine as an analgesic for experimental pain. Anesthesiology, *52*:20, 1980.

98. Schauer, G., Gross, L., and Blum, L.: Hemodynamic studies in experimental coronary occlusion. IV. Stellate ganglionectomy experiments. Am. Heart J., *14*:669, 1937.

99. Schnapp, M., Mays, K.S., and North, W.C.: Intravenous chloroprocaine in the treatment of pain. Anesth. Analg., *60*:844, 1981.

100. Sengal, A.D., and Gardner, W.J.: Place of intrathecal methylprednisolone acetate in neurological disorders. Trans. Am. Neurol. Assoc., *88*:275, 1963.

101. Slaff, J.I.: Management of pain in chronic pancreatitis. Hosp. Pract., *20*:53, 1985.

102. Sola, A.E., and Kuitert, J.H.: Quadratus lumborum myofascitis. Northwest Med., *53*:1003, 1954.

103. Sola, A.E., and Kuitert, J.H.: Myofascial trigger point pain in the neck and shoulder girdle. Northwest Med., *54*:980, 1955.

104. Sola, A.E., and Williams, R.L.: Myofascial pain syndromes. Neurology, *6*:91, 1956.

105. Stenger, R.J., *et al.*: Ultrastructural and physiologic alterations in ischemic skeletal muscle. Am. J. Pathol., *40*:1, 1962.

106. Sternbach, R.A.: Pain Patients, Traits and Treatment. New York, Academic Press, 1974.

107. Strange, R.C., Vetter, N., Rowe, M.J., and Oliver, M.F.: Plasma cyclic AMP and total catecholamines during acute myocardial infarction in man. Eur. J. Clin. Invest., *4*:115, 1974.

108. Swerdlow, M.: Subarachnoid and extradural neurolytic blocks. *In* Bonica, J.J., and Ventafridda, V. (eds.): Advances in Pain Research and Therapy, Vol. 2, p. 325. New York, Raven Press, 1979.

109. Telling, W.H.: "Nodular" fibromyositis, an everyday affliction, and its identity with so-called muscular rheumatism. Lancet, *1*:154, 1911.

110. Tolosa, E.S.: Modification of tardive dyskinesia and spasmodic torticollis by apomorphine. Arch. Neurol., *35*:459, 1978.

111. Toomey, T.C., Taylor, A.G., Skelton, M.A., and Carron, H.: Five-year follow-up status of chronic low back pain patients. Pain, *11*:272, 1982.

112. Travell, J.: Basis for the multiple uses of local block of somatic trigger areas (procaine infiltration and ethyl chloride spray). Miss. Valley Med. J., *71*:13, 1949.

113. Travell, J.: Myofascial trigger points: Clinical view. *In* Bonica, J.J., and Albe-Fessard, D. (eds.): Advances in Pain Research and Therapy, pp. 919–926. New York, Raven Press, 1976.

114. Travell, J., Rinzler, S., and Herman, M.: Pain and disability of the shoulder and arm: Treatment by intramuscular infiltration with procaine hydrochloride. J.A.M.A., *120*:417, 1942.

115. Travell, J., and Simons, D.G.: Myofascial Pain and Dysfunction: The Trigger Point Manual. Baltimore, Williams & Wilkins, 1983.

116. Tucker, G.T., *et al.*: Observed and predicted accumulation of local anaesthetic agents during continuous extradural analgesia. Br. J. Anaesth., *49*:237, 1977.

117. Wall, P.D., and Gutnick, M.: Ongoing activity in peripheral nerves: The physiology and pharmacology of impulses originating from a neuroma. Exp. Neurol., *43*:580, 1974.
118. Warfield, C.A.: Meralgia paresthetica: Causes and cures. Hosp. Pract., *21*:40A, 1986.
119. White, J.C.: Cardiac pain: Autonomic pathways and physiological mechanisms. Circulation, *16*:644, 1957.
120. Williams, H.L., and Elkins, E.C.: Myalgia of the head. Arch. Phys. Ther., *23*:14, 1942.
121. Winnie, A.P.: The patient with herpetic neuralgia. *In* Moya, F., and Gion, H. (eds.): Postgraduate Seminar in Anesthesiology (program syllabus), pp. 165–170. Miami Beach, 1983.
122. Winnie, A.P., *et al.*: Pain clinic. II. Intradural and extradural corticosteroids for sciatica. Anesth. Analg., *51*:990, 1972.
123. Wood, K.M.: Use of phenol as a neurolytic agent: A review. Pain, *5*:205, 1978.
124. Yawger, N.S.: Chronic "rheumatic" myositis (Muskelschwielen), with cases showing some common errors in diagnosis. Lancet, *2*:292, 1909.
125. Zahvadi, A., and Dreyfuss, F.: Second Congress of the International Society of Thrombosis and Hemostasis, Oslo, Norway, 1967.
126. Zanchetti, A., and Malliani, A.: Neural and psychological factors in coronary disease. Acta Cardiol., *20*:69, 1974.
127. Zarkowska, E., and Philips, H.C.: Recent onset vs. persistent pain: Evidence for a distinction. Pain, *25*:365, 1986.
128. Zimmerman, M.: Peripheral and central nervous mechanisms of nociception, pain and pain therapy: Facts and hypotheses. *In* Bonica, J.J., Liebeskind, J.C., and Albe-Fessard, D. (eds.): Advances in Pain Therapy, Vol. 3, pp. 3–32. New York, Raven Press, 1979.
129. Zohn, D.A., Mennell, J.McM.: Musculoskeletal Pain: Diagnosis and Physical Treatment, pp. 126–129, 190–193. Boston, Little, Brown, 1976.

27.3 BACK PAIN: ZYGAPOPHYSIAL BLOCKS AND EPIDURAL STEROIDS

NIKOLAI BOGDUK

The traditional approach to the diagnosis of spinal pain has been a morphologic one. The diagnostic process relies heavily on radiologic investigations designed to demonstrate the location and appearance of lesions that can be presumed to be the cause of pain (see Chap. 24.1, Appendix B, Sects. XXVI-1 to XXVII-15).

In this regard, plain radiographs can demonstrate fractures, dislocations, tumors, and infectious or inflammatory processes. Bone scans can supplement plain radiographs by revealing the metabolic activity associated with inflammation and tumor growth. Myelography shows the effect of space-occupying lesions on the spinal cord and spinal nerve roots, notably the effect of intervertebral disk herniation. Computed tomography (CT) allows soft tissues like bulging or herniated disk material to be visualized and permits the reconstruction of images of the vertebral column in any of three dimensions for the assessment of spinal and foraminal stenosis.

The morphologic approach, however, has suffered from several limitations. The lesions demonstrated by plain radiography and CT scanning are not the common causes of spinal pain. Fractures, tumors, and inflammatory diseases account for only a small minority of presentations of spinal pain. Even intervertebral disk herniation accounts for less than 30% of presentations of low back pain,[88] and even as few as 5% of total presentations.[59,64] In the cervical region, frank disk herniation is even less common than in the lumbar region.[123,166]

Although the changes of spondylosis are commonly reported in radiographs of the vertebral column, these cannot be regarded as the cause of pain, for their presence correlates poorly with the presence of symptoms. The incidence of spondylotic changes of the lumbar spine is virtually the same in patients with low back pain and in asymptomatic subjects.[113] Similarly, cervical spondylosis is essentially equally present in patients with and without neck pain.[66]

The lack of definitive, diagnostic radiologic criteria for spinal pain has prompted the development of alternative means of diagnosis, and these have been more of a physiologic nature. The principle of these investigations is that when pain-producing lesions cannot be demonstrated morphologically, their presence and location can nevertheless be demonstrated by provocation procedures or diagnostic blocks, or a combination of both.

Provocation is used principally in the diagnosis of pain arising from intervertebral disks. Symptomatic disks can be identified if and when an injection of contrast medium or normal saline into the nucleus pulposus reproduces the patient's pain. The rationale, technique, and clinical application of provocation discography, however, is beyond the scope of this text, but these issues are addressed extensively elsewhere.[17–19,44,45,47,97,127,138,148,165]

Diagnostic blocks are sometimes used to identify symptomatic nerve roots, and a few studies have reported the value of diagnostic spinal nerve

The spelling "zygapophysial" is accepted by the International Anatomical Nomenclature Committee and is used throughout this chapter. The alternative spelling "zygapophyseal" may be used in other chapters.

blocks.[100,155] However, diagnostic blocks are used more frequently in the diagnosis of pain stemming from zygapophysial joints, and this is the focus of the present chapter.

ZYGAPOPHYSIAL BLOCKS

HISTORICAL PERSPECTIVE

The lumbar zygapophysial joints were first incriminated in the pathogenesis of low back pain just after the turn of this century, when "arthritic" changes in these joints were highlighted as a radiologic feature of patients with low back pain.[3-5,96] However, "ligamentous strain" secondary to this arthritis was considered the actual cause of pain rather than the arthritis itself. It was not until 1933 that the joints themselves were considered the source of pain, and the term "facet syndrome" was introduced as a term of reference for this sort of pain.[70]

Initially, radiologic signs of degenerative joint diseases were considered the diagnostic criterion for zygapophysial joint pain, but epidemiologic studies later showed that such changes did not correlate with symptoms, having virtually an equal incidence in symptomatic and asymptomatic patients.[102,113] This lack of correlation led to doubts that the zygapophysial joints could be a significant source of pain,[122] and "facet syndrome" remained a disregarded diagnosis until the past 10 years.

PHYSIOLOGY

Interest in facet syndromes was resurrected in the 1970s, when clinicians began to treat low back pain by denervating the lumbar zygapophysial joints.[6,35,46,67,85,89,108,111,112,118,124,125,128,135,136,141,144-147,157] Prompted by these therapeutic reports, Mooney and Robertson provided the first physiologic evidence that the zygapophysial joints could cause back pain and referred pain in the lower limb.[119] They produced such pain in normal volunteers by experimentally stimulating lower lumbar zygapophysial joints, and these observations have since been corroborated by other workers.[110,160]

The striking feature of these experimental studies is that the pain produced in normal volunteers is remarkably similar in quality and distribution to the pain suffered clinically by many patients with low back syndromes. This similarity fostered the suspicion that the source of pain in these patients was one or other of the lumbar zygapophysial joints. Accordingly, several investigators developed and undertook diagnostic blocks of putatatively painful zygapophysial joints, and many studies have now reported the successful relief of low back pain syndromes after such blocks.[40-43,52,56,60,101,107,109,118,133,151]

Formal studies have not been performed to show that stimulation of the cervical zygapophysial joints can cause neck pain in normal volunteers, although Pawl[129] has reported the reproduction of pain in patients with neck pain and headache after injections of hypertonic saline into their cervical zygapophysial joints. Nevertheless, prompted by the results of lumbar diagnostic blocks, several authors ventured to perform diagnostic blocks of the cervical joints, and a growing number of studies have now reported the relief of neck pain and referred pain to both the head and the shoulder girdle after such blocks.[24-26,57,58,86,87,150,151,162]

CLINICAL FEATURES

Stimulation of the lumbar zygapophysial joints produces a dull, aching pain in the back associated with referred pain in the lower limb. The referred pain may be felt anywhere in the lower limb, but most commonly it occurs in the gluteal region or thigh.[110,119] However, there is considerable variation and overlap in the distribution of referred pain after stimulation of joints at different segmental levels,[60,110,119] and this distribution is in no way characteristic of the segment stimulated. The distribution of symptoms, therefore, cannot be used clinically to infer the location of a symptomatic joint.

Attempts have been made to identify some other clinical feature diagnostic of lumbar "facet syndrome." Features such as aggravation of pain on extension or on lateral flexion of the spine occur more frequently in patients with facet syndromes, but such features also occur in patients with other sources of pain and cannot be used to distinguish patients with facet syndromes from others.[60] Certain features have been noted to occur in CT scans of patients with facet syndromes, such as joint asymmetries, joint space narrowing, subchondral sclerosis, erosions, and facet hypertrophy,[42,43,82] but no studies have demonstrated that such changes are pathognomonic of symptomatic joints, and that they are not spurious findings. Radionuclide scanning has been evaluated as a putatative screening test for facet syndromes but has proved of no value.[134]

In the absence of diagnostic clinical features or

pathognomonic radiologic signs, the diagnosis of facet syndromes relies exclusively on the results of diagnostic blocks. A facet syndrome may be suspected in patients with dull, aching pain in the back and referred pain in the buttock, thigh, and even the leg, or a similar syndrome at cervical levels, but to make the diagnosis this suspicion must be confirmed by complete relief of symptoms after anesthetization of one or more zygapophysial joints.

DIAGNOSTIC BLOCKS

Two types of diagnostic blocks of the zygapophysial joints have been developed. One is essentially neurosurgical in origin and involves blocking the nerves that innervate the target joints.[21,108,128,132,151,159] The nerves supplying the zygapophysial joints are the medial branches of the dorsal rami of the spinal nerves, and blocks of these nerves are known as medial branch blocks. The other technique involves blocking the target joint intra-articularly and has been mainly propagated by orthopedic surgeons and radiologists.[40–43,52,56–58,60,101,109,110,119,131,133,151,162]

Preparation and Facilities

All of the blocks described below are performed under aseptic conditions under image-intensifier fluoroscopy. As well, resuscitation facilities should be available to deal with inadvertent complications, such as intravascular injection or spread of local anesthetic into the epidural space, although such complications should not occur with careful technique.

Lumbar Medial Branch Blocks

The medial branches of the lumbar dorsal rami emerge from their respective intertransverse spaces, and each nerve crosses the upper border of the lower transverse process and runs caudally along a groove formed by the junction of the transverse process with the root of the superior articular process.[16,20–22] Each nerve then hooks medially under the mamilloaccessory ligament[14] to cross the vertebral lamina (Fig. 27-24). Articular branches are given off to the zygapophysial joints above and below the nerve,[16,22,28,103,104,130] and eventually each medial branch enters the multifidus muscle.[22]

The anatomy differs at the L5 level in that the L5 dorsal ramus itself, rather than its medial branch,

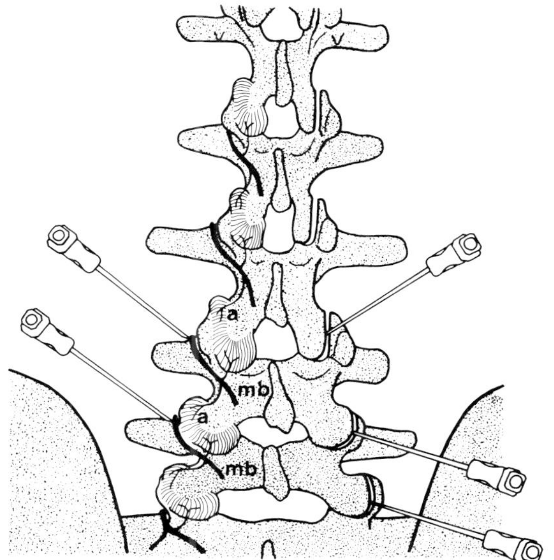

FIG. 27-24. Sketch of the needle placements used for lumbar medial branch blocks and lumbar intra-articular zygapophysial blocks. On the left, the courses of the medial branches of the lumbar dorsal rami *(mb)* and their articular branches *(a)* are shown. Needles have been introduced onto the L3 and L4 medial branches, which would be anesthetised to block the L4–L5 joint. On the right, the needle placement for intra-articular blocks of the L3–L4, L4–L5, and L5–S1 zygapophysial joints is depicted.

crosses the ala of the sacrum at its junction with the superior articular process of the sacrum (Fig. 27-24). Medial and intermediate branches are formed at the base of the lumbosacral zygapophysial joint,[22] and the medial branch hooks medially around the base of this joint, supplying it before entering the multifidus.[22,28]

As a result of this distribution of the lumbar medial branches, each lumbar zygapophysial joint is supplied by two nerves: the medial branch above its location and the one below. Small branches to the ventral aspect of each joint have been described by some investigators,[2,126] although denied by others,[22,109] but the bulk of the innervation seems to be derived from the two medial branches related to the joint. Therefore, a given joint can be substantially, if not completely, anesthetized by blocking these two nerves.

The constant location of the L1–L4 medial branches at the roots of the lumbar transverse processes, and the constant course of the L5 dorsal ramus over the ala of the sacrum allow the definition of suitable target points for diagnostic blocks of these nerves. The specific target point for the L1 – L4 nerves is the posterior surface of the most medial end of the transverse process just below its superior border (Fig. 27-24).[21] For the L5 dorsal ramus the homologous point is the medial end of the ala of the sacrum (Fig. 27-24). Needles introduced onto these target points will incur the respective nerves, which can be blocked with as little as 1.0 to 1.5 ml of local anesthetic.

With the patient lying prone on an x-ray table, the desired target point is visualized on posteroanterior screening and a puncture point through the skin of the back is selected about 5 cm lateral to the target point. The puncture point is anesthetized with a small volume of local anesthetic injected intradermally, and a 22-gauge, 90-mm spinal needle is then introduced through the skin. Using fluoroscopic guidance, the needle is directed ventrally and medially toward the target point. The oblique, lateral approach is recommended because enlarged superior articular processes may bulge laterally and overhang the target point, thereby preventing a direct posterior approach.[21]

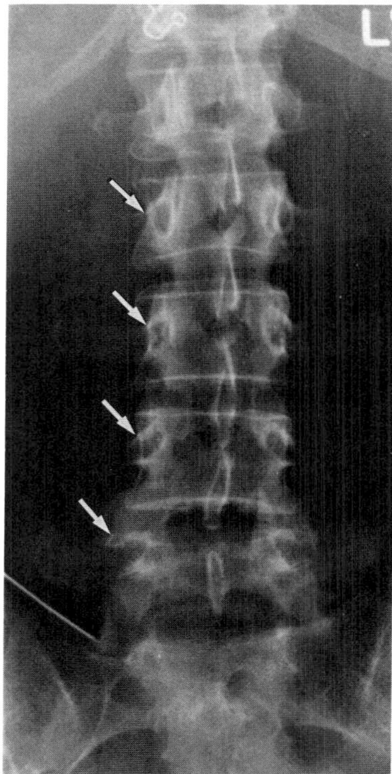

FIG. 27-25. Posteroanterior radiograph of the lumbar spine showing a needle in position for an L5 medial branch block. Target-points for the other lumbar medial branches are indicated by the arrows.

To facilitate accurate placement it is advisable to first introduce the needle onto the back of the transverse process. This familiarizes the operator with the depth of the target point and avoids inadvertent penetration into the intertransverse space and the risk of striking the ventral ramus, or spinal nerve or "dural cuff." Using fluoroscopic guidance, the point of the needle is readjusted until its image coincides with that of the target point.

Accurate positioning is indicated by the radiographic image and by the "feel" of the needle. If it is in correct position, the image of the tip of the needle should overlap that of the target point (Fig. 27-25). The needle should rest on bone (the back of the transverse process) and cannot be adjusted more medially (medial displacement being blocked by the superior articular process). To confirm that the needle rests at the upper border of the transverse process, it should be readjusted rostrally until it just slips over the superior border. It is then drawn back and repositioned behind and immediately below the superior border.

Once in position the needle can be used to inject 1.0 to 1.5 ml of local anesthetic. For the best diagnostic value, a long-acting agent, like 0.5% bupivacaine, is suggested. This will provide a maximum duration of possible relief that the patient can evaluate.

Provided the protocol as outlined is followed, there are no major structures that can be inadvertently punctured or injected during lumbar medial branch blocks, and the procedure should be free of any complications. However, intravascular injection may occur. Also, poor technique could result in injection into the spinal nerve, or dural cuff, and thus the subarachnoid space.

Lumbar Zygapophysial Blocks

Lumbar zygapophysial joint blocks are performed with the patient lying prone on the x-ray table, and the target joint is visualized on posteroanterior screening. If required, the x-ray beam is adjusted slightly obliquely so that the joint space is distinctly evident between the superior and inferior articular processes, and this space becomes the target for injection.[41]

A puncture point is selected overlying the target joint space and is anesthetized. A 20- to 22-gauge spinal needle is introduced through the puncture point and advanced toward the middle of the joint space until bony or cartilaginous resistance is felt. The needle is then randomly readjusted, probing for the joint space, until it is felt to slip into the joint (Fig. 27-24). The depth of penetration can then be checked by lateral screening of the joint.

Accurate location of the needle can be confirmed by injecting 0.5 ml or less of a contrast medium like iopamidol or methylglucamina diatrizoate.[41,43,60,109,133] If the needle is accurately placed, this injection will produce an arthrogram of the target joint. If the contrast medium remains within the joint, the perimeter of the arthrogram should be regular, but if too great a volume of contrast medium is injected, or if it is injected too forcefully, the medium may burst out of the joint capsule,[56] or it may leave the joint through naturally occurring apertures in the superior and inferior capsules to fill the superior and inferior (extracapsular) joint recesses.[104]

Once accurate location of the needle has been achieved, the contrast medium is aspirated, if possible, and replaced with local anesthetic. The volume of a typical lumbar zygapophysial joint is only about 1.0 ml,[127] so only this volume of local anesthetic should be used. Greater volumes are liable to leak or burst out of the joint, and thereby affect the specificity of the block.[56,133]

Cervical Medial Branch Blocks

The medial branches of the C4–C7 dorsal rami arise from their parent nerves in the cervical intertransverse spaces and then wrap around the waists of their respective articular pillars (Fig. 27-26).[15] Topographically, each medial branch is related to the articular pillar of the vertebra with the same segmental number as the nerve. Toward the posterior surface of the articular pillar, each medial branch furnishes articular branches to the zygapophysial joints above and below its course[15] before ramifying in the multifidus muscle (Fig. 27-26).

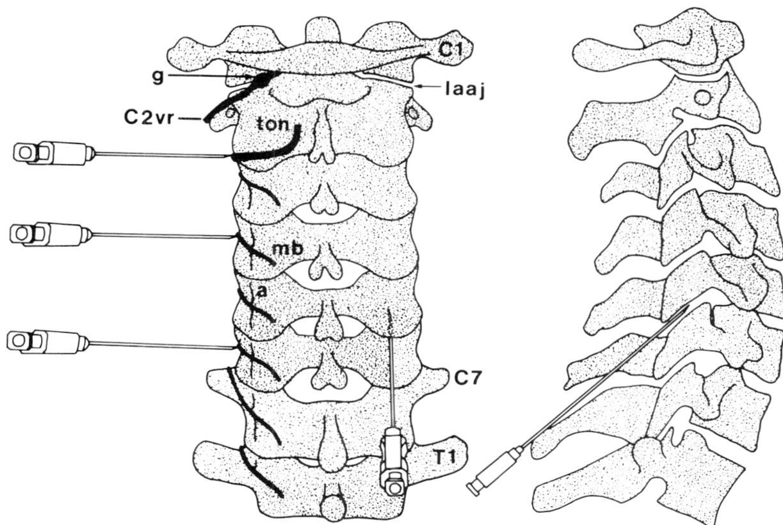

FIG. 27-26. Illustrations of the needle placement for cervical medial branch blocks and intra-articular zygapophysial blocks. **Left.** Posterior view of the cervical spine showing the location of the C2 ganglion *(g)* behind the lateral atlantoaxial joint *(laaj)*, the C2 ventral ramus *(C2vr)*, the courses of the medial branches of the cervical dorsal rami *(mb)*, their articular branches *(a)*, and the third occipital nerve *(ton)*. Needles are shown in position as they would be used for blocks of the C4 and C6 medial branches and the third occipital nerve. The articular pillar of C7 may be obscured by the shadow of the large C7 transverse process, in which case the C7 medial branch can be located midway between the lateral convexities of the C6–C7 and C7–T1 zygapophysial joints. **Right.** Lateral view of the cervical spine showing the course of a needle into the cavity of the right C5–C6 zygapophysial joint.

The constant location of the C4–C7 medial branches on the waists of the articular pillars permits accurate target points for blocks of these nerves to be defined.[15] In posteroanterior radiographs the cervical spine presents a scalloped lateral margin. The lateral convexities of this margin are formed by the zygapophysial joints, while the concavities are formed by the waists of the articular pillars. The medial branches of the cervical dorsal rami run in the depths of these concavities, and needles introduced onto these concavities will incur the respective medial branches (Fig. 27-26).

The medial branch of the C8 dorsal ramus crosses the root of the T1 transverse process, but instead of wrapping around an articular pillar, it hooks medially onto the lamina of T1, where it sends articular branches to the C7–T1 zygapophysial joint. The anatomy of the C8 medial branch is therefore similar to that of the lumbar medial branches, and the target point for the C8 medial branch is the concavity formed by the junction of the T1 transverse process and the T1 superior articular process (Fig. 27-26).

The second cervical nerve (anterior ramus) passes dorsal to the upper articular process of the axis and to the vertebral artery. The posterior primary ramus of the second cervical nerve is the largest of any of the cervical nerves. It divides into a small lateral branch and a large medial branch. The medial branch is the greater occipital nerve, which can be blocked superficially (see Fig. 15-10).

The C3 dorsal ramus forms two medial branches: a deep medial branch and a superficial medial branch known as the third occipital nerve.[15] The deep medial branch follows a course around the C3 articular pillar homologous to that of the lower cervical medial branches, and innervates the C3–C4 zygapophysial joint from above (Fig. 27-26). The target point for this nerve is the concavity of the C3 articular pillar.

The third occipital nerve wraps around the lateral and dorsal surfaces of the C2–C3 zygapophysial joint in its lower half, and the nerve is embedded in the connective tissue that invests the joint capsule (Fig. 27-26). Articular branches to the C2–C3 zygapophysial joint arise from the deep surface of the third occipital nerve or from the communicating loop between the third occipital nerve and the C2 dorsal ramus.[15] A suitable target point for the third occipital nerve is the lower half of the lateral margin of the C2–C3 zygapophysial joint as seen in posteroanterior radiograph of the neck (Fig. 27-26).[26]

Except at the C2–C3 level, each cervical zygapophysial joint is innervated by the medial branch above and below its location. Consequently, to anesthetize a typical cervical zygapophysial joint, two medial branches must be blocked. To anesthetize the C2–C3 joint, the third occipital nerve must be blocked.

Cervical medial branch blocks are performed with the patient resting prone on an x-ray table with the chest and head supported by pillows, leaving the mouth raised from the table and unobstructed and free to move. The target points for the C4 to C8 medial branches should be readily visible on posteroanterior screening.

Once the target point is identified, a puncture point is selected on the skin of the back of the neck 2 to 3 cm lateral to the target point. A 22-gauge spinal needle is introduced through the puncture point and directed ventrally and medially toward the target point. Repeated fluoroscopic screening is used to guide the course of the needle. To ensure that the needle is not introduced too deeply in the first instance, it is recommended that it first be directed onto the back of the articular pillar. From this location it can be readjusted laterally until its tip coincides with the lateral margin of the waist of the articular pillar (Figs. 27-26, 27-27). In the case of the C8 medial branch, the needle is introduced onto the T1 transverse process and then readjusted until its tip coincides with the target point for this nerve.[15] Once the needle is in position at the desired level, 1.0 to 1.5 ml of 0.5% bupivacaine may be injected onto the target nerve.

The target point for the third occipital nerve may be obscured by the mandible or the teeth. To visualize this target point, the patient may need to open the mouth and raise the forehead up or down the table, or even rotate the head slightly. These maneuvers displace the images of the mandible or teeth from over the C2–C3 joint. Once the joint is visualized, a needle is introduced onto the posterior aspect of the C2–C3 joint and is then readjusted laterally until its tip coincides with the lateral margin of the joint (Fig. 27-28).

Because the third occipital nerve is large, it is recommended that three injection sites be used.[26] All sites are located along the lateral margin of the joint, but one lies opposite the equator of the joint, the second lies at its lower margin, and the third lies between the first two (Fig. 27-28). This dispersion of injection sites ensures that the nerve is fully encompassed, and the injection of 0.5 ml of local anesthetic at each site is enough to infiltrate the nerve.[26] Adequate blockade of the nerve is indicated by the onset of a small patch of numbness over the suboccipital region, which is the cutaneous territory supplied by the third occipital nerve.

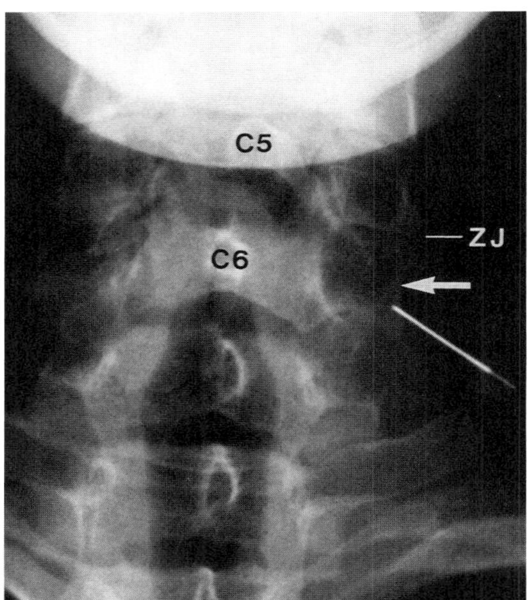

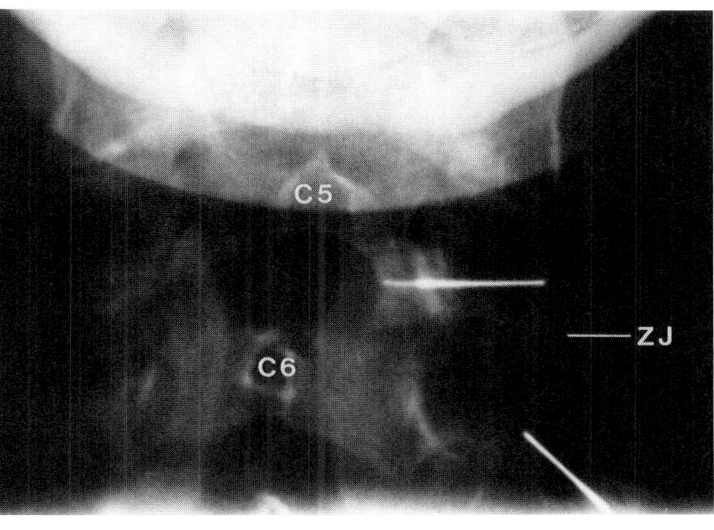

FIG. 27-27. **Left.** Posteroanterior radiograph showing a needle in position on the waist of the C6 articular pillar. The tip of the needle is slightly below the ideal location for a C6 medial branch block, which is indicated by the arrow. **Right.** Coned view of the same patient in which the upper needle has been correctly placed on the C5 articular pillar for a C5 medial branch block. The locations of the C5–C6 zygapophysial joint *(ZJ)* are indicated in each part of the figure.

If the protocols outlined are followed, there should be minimal risks of inadvertent puncture or injection of major structures. Using the posterolateral approach, the only structures penetrated are the posterior neck muscles. The vertebral artery lies in front of the zygapophysial joints and so is protected by bone from puncture. The epidural space could be entered, but only if the introduction of the needle onto the articular pillar is not carefully monitored fluoroscopically and the needle is allowed to pass too far medially.

A possible side-effect of upper cervical medial branch blocks is a sense of ataxia or dizziness. This is due to disturbances to the postural tonic-neck reflexes, and its mechanism is discussed elsewhere.[13,26] The effect is only temporary, frequently waning well before the offest of anesthesia. The patient should be warned of this possible effect. Its benign nature can be explained, and the patient can be shown how to accommodate for the apparent loss of balance by using visual cues rather than relying on subconscious mechanisms.

Cervical Zygapophysial Blocks

Intra-articular blocks of the cervical zygapophysial joints are performed using a posterior approach, with the patient lying prone on an x-ray table.[25,57,58,162] The target joint is identified and a puncture point is selected about two to three segments perpendicularly below the midpoint of the target joint. This is necessary because the cavity of the joint slopes posteroinferiorly. If required, the puncture point can be chosen by visualizing the target joint in a lateral view of the neck and plotting where the plane of the joint would intersect the skin of the back of the neck. Once the puncture point is anesthetized, a 3-inch (7.5-cm) 22-gauge needle is introduced through it and advanced upward and ventrally toward the target joint. The course of the needle should be carefully monitored using the fluoroscope to ensure that it *does not stray medially* toward the epidural space. Its course should stay strictly over the articular pillars.

The needle is advanced until it strikes the articular pillar immediately below the target joint. Its position

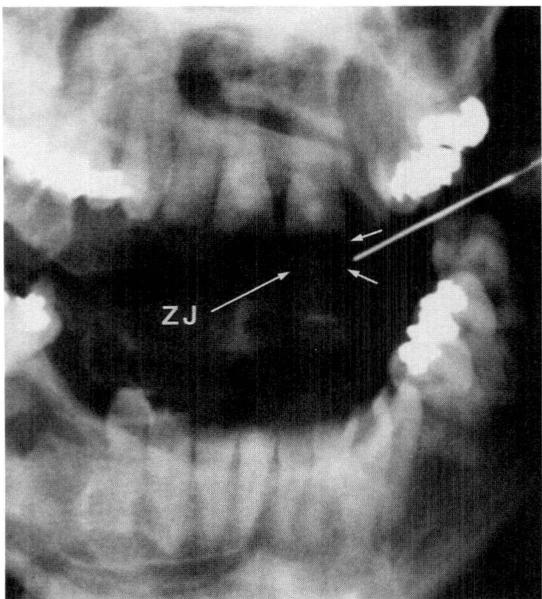

FIG. 27-28. Posterior radiograph of the upper cervical spine showing a needle in position at the target-point for a third occipital nerve block. The arrows indicate the other sites, which should be injected in order to fully block this relatively large nerve. The location of the C2–C3 zygapophysial joint is indicated *(ZJ)*.

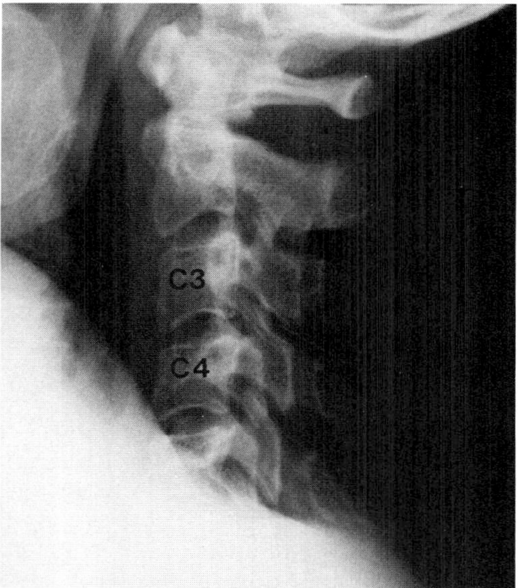

FIG. 27-29. Lateral radiograph of the cervical spine showing the appearance of a needle introduced into the C3–C4 zygapophysial joint.

can be checked at this stage by using lateral screening. The needle is then readjusted until its tip coincides with the lower margin of the target joint. During these maneuvers repeated lateral and posteroanterior screening are required to ensure correct location and to ensure that the needle does not deviate laterally or medially away from the middle of the joint. Minor readjustments are then performed until the tip of the needle is felt to slip into the joint cavity. Further penetration is then guided by a combination of posteroanterior and lateral screening, and the needle is advanced to the middle of the joint cavity (Fig. 27-29).

Once the needle has entered the joint space, its location within the joint can be confirmed by injecting 0.1 to 0.2 ml of contrast medium,[162] such as iothalamate meglumine, metrizamide, or methylglucamine diatrizoate.[57,162] The contrast medium should be aspirated, if possible, and about 1.0 ml of local anesthetic can be introduced to anesthetize the joint.

If the introduction of the needle is carefully monitored fluoroscopically, there should be no complications. However, because of the several major structures in the neck, the operator should be aware of potential risks.

With respect to penetration, the greatest risk is deflection of the needle medially into the epidural or subarachnoid space. A lesser risk is overpenetration superiorly and ventrally into the spinal nerve or vertebral artery or vein that lies in front of the joint. With respect to injection, there should be no problems, provided small volumes are injected slowly. If large volumes or forceful, rapid injections are used, the local anesthetic may rupture out of the joint capsule. This not only compromises the specificity of the block, but also risks the production of a cervical epidural block. As with any neural blockade procedure, resuscitation facilities should be on hand (see Chaps. 4, 6, and 8).

Lateral Atlantoaxial Joint Blocks

Diagnostic blocks of the lateral atlantoaxial joint (C1–C2) can be performed using a posterior approach in a manner analogous to that used for cervical zygapophysial joint blocks. A lateral approach is precluded at this level because the vertebral artery is a lateral relation of this joint.

With the patient in a prone position, the target joint is visualized on posteroanterior screening. Should the teeth or mandible interfere with a clear view, the patient's head can be maneuvered, as described for third occipital nerve blocks, until an unobstructed view of the joint is attained.

A puncture point is selected posterior to the joint and a 22- to 25-gauge needle is carefully introduced toward the back of the joint space. Penetration must be carefully monitored fluoroscopically because immediately medial to the joint the spinal cord and epidural space lie unprotected by bone at the C1–C2 space, and lateral to the joint run the vertebral artery and veins (see Figs. 10-3 and 15-11).

The needle is directed toward the lateral half of the joint space to avoid striking the C2 ganglion, which overlies the midpoint of the joint space (Fig. 27-26).[13] Contact with the ganglion will be indicated by an electrical shock sensation typical of striking a nerve. If this should occur, the needle should be directed more laterally or more medially, as appropriate.

Once the needle strikes the back of the joint, its location should be checked by lateral screening. It is then carefully readjusted until it enters the joint cavity. Its further penetration is monitored by posteroanterior and lateral screening until the tip of the needle reaches the middle of the joint cavity. Contrast medium can be used to control the location, and 1.0 ml of local anesthetic can be injected to anesthetize the joint (Fig. 27-30).

SELECTION OF TECHNIQUE

There are arguments for and against using either medial branch blocks or intra-articular blocks. However, while each technique has its particular technical and theoretical advantages and disadvantages, both reveal essentially the same diagnostic information: If anesthetization of a joint or its nerve supply relieves the patient's pain, that joint can be deemed the source of the pain. This conclusion is based on the patient's physiologic response to the block and can be made regardless of the presence or absence of any radiologically demonstrable morphologic changes in the joint.

A perceived disadvantage of medial branch blocks is that the joint responsible for the patient's pain is not directly anesthetized and the results have to be interpreted on the basis of a knowledge of the anatomy and distribution of the nerves. However, the advantages of medial branch blocks are that, technically, they are easier to perform and require less use of image-intensifier fluoroscopy. Needles are simply directed onto the target nerves using only posteroanterior fluoroscopy. In contrast, intra-articular blocks

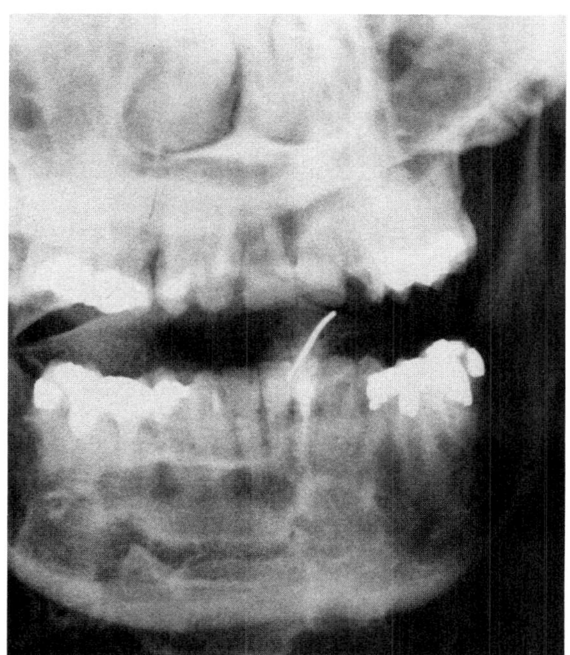

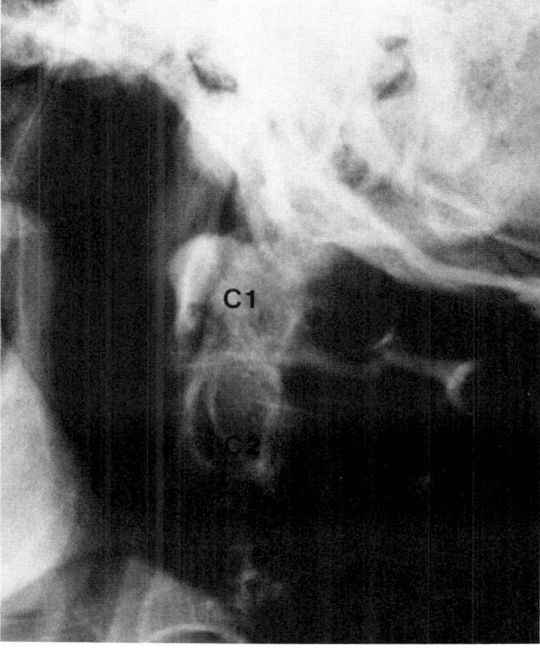

FIG. 27-30. Radiographs showing the appearance of a needle introduced into the right lateral atlantoaxial joint. **Left.** Posteroanterior view. **Right.** Lateral view.

require a certain dexterity to enter the joint and require facilities for repeated posteroanterior and lateral fluoroscopic screening, particularly at cervical levels.

Despite the associated technical difficulties, intra-articular blocks have been preferred by their proponents in the belief that they yield highly specific diagnostic information (*i.e.*, to prove that a joint is the source of pain, the joint itself must be blocked). However, there is good concordance between the results of intra-articular blocks and medial branch blocks, and it can be deduced that, for diagnostic purposes, medial branch blocks are just as specific as intra-articular blocks.[24,25] The choice between the two types of block is therefore mainly a reflection of the experience and personal preference of the operator.

It is suggested that, as a screening test, medial branch blocks are preferable because of their technical simplicity and because they do not require the penetration and injection of possibly normal, asymptomatic joints in the search for a symptomatic one. If required, intra-articular blocks can be used subsequently to corroborate the results of medial branch blocks.[25]

Notwithstanding these suggestions, there may be grounds to prefer one technique over the other, depending on the type of therapy to be used (see below). If intra-articular steroids are to be used, then intra-articular blocks are the appropriate diagnostic test, for the steroids may be injected simultaneously with the local anesthetic in order to minimize the total number of procedures undertaken.

On the other hand, if radiofrequency denervation of the joint is envisaged, then medial branch blocks are the appropriate diagnostic test. The operation performed to denervate zygapophysial joints is not a coagulation of specific articular nerves but is a medial branch neurotomy.[20,21] Therefore, by anesthetizing the nerves that are to be coagulated, these blocks not only provide diagnostic information, but also constitute a prognostic evaluation of the anticipated surgical procedure.

Although some authors base their use of denervation on the results of intra-articular blocks,[118,131,151] this is somewhat inferential. Because intra-articular blocks act on the joint capsule and not only the medial branches of the dorsal rami, they do not directly predict the effect of medial branch neurotomy. In contrast, medial branch blocks provide a direct evaluation of the putatative effects of medial branch neurotomy and should be an essential preoperative test.

APPLICATION AND INTERPRETATION

There are no clinical signs that constitute an indication for medial branch block or zygapophysial joint blocks. Facet syndromes can be suspected only on the basis of the type of pain of which the patient complains: deep, dull, aching pain in the back, with or without similar pain referred into the lower limb, or neck pain associated with referred pain in the head or the shoulder girdle. Blocks can then be used to test the hypothesis that the pain stems from one or other of the zygapophysial joints in the lumbar region or neck.

Although various clinical features have been used to determine which joint should be blocked first in a particular patient, no feature has been shown to be absolutely reliable. However, on the basis of published reports, most lumbar facet syndromes occur at the L4–5 or L5–S1 levels, and these should be the levels investigated in the first instance. Thoracolumbar pain syndromes have been described,[115–117] and sometimes it may be necessary to investigate upper lumbar levels.

In the cervical region, two main types of syndrome have been recognized: an upper cervical syndrome consisting of neck pain and headache and a lower cervical syndrome consisting of neck pain and shoulder pain.[25,150,151,162] The upper cervical syndrome most commonly stems from the C2–C3 level, whereas the lower syndrome stems from the C5–C6 level. In patients with one of these clinical presentations, the zygapophysial joints at the respective level should be investigated first. However, these guidelines are not absolute, and at either lumbar or cervical levels it may be necessary to block the joints one or two levels above or below the initially suspected level.

The clearest diagnostic information is obtained if single joints are blocked one at a time. If multiple joints are simultaneously blocked before pain relief is assessed, there is no way to determine exactly which of the anesthetized joints is the symptomatic one.

Once a joint is blocked, using either a medial branch block or an intra-articular block, the patient's immediate response should be assessed. In a clear-cut positive response, the patient will report complete relief of all pain within a few minutes of the block. Under these circumstances the patient should be discharged to undertake activities of daily living and assess the depth and duration of relief. If there is doubt about the degree of relief in the first few minutes, the patient may be asked to wait and the relief assessed over the next 10 to 20 minutes.

If no relief occurs immediately after the block, or if the relief is not clear-cut within 10 to 20 minutes, the opposite joint at the same level or the joint above or below may be blocked, depending on the distribution and laterality of the patient's pain. Once the second joint is blocked, pain relief is again assessed, and the process can be repeated at further levels, if required, until a clear-cut positive response is attained, or until all possible sources of pain among the zygapophysial joints is reasonably ruled out.

Pain relief may occur after anesthetization of one joint, both joints at a single level, or two consecutive joints. In any event complete relief of symptoms indicates that the anesthetized joint (or joints) is the source of pain. This information can then be used to direct specific therapy at the responsible joint(s). Conversely, if diagnostic blocks are negative, attention can be directed away from the zygapophysial joints to other possible sources of pain, like the intervertebral disks, dura mater, nerve roots, or paravertebral muscles.

CONTROLS

One of the major advantages of diagnostic blocks is that they can be made highly objective. At times, there may be doubt about the validity of the patient's response, particularly in medicolegal cases, but this can be tested using various types of control injections. Asymptomatic joints at adjacent levels can be anesthetized on a single-blind basis. Alternatively, different agents can be used during repeated or confirmatory blocks of the apparently symptomatic joint.

In this regard, a short-acting versus a long-acting local anaesthetic can be used, or even a placebo, on either a single-blind or a double-blind basis. If the patient's response is appropriate to the expected action of the drug used, then the reliability of his or her response can be endorsed. Conversely, an inappropriate response will deny a reliable positive diagnosis and invites an investigation of possible unrecognized psychological components of the patient's complaint.

INCIDENCE

The actual incidence of facet syndromes is difficult to determine from the literature because there have been no studies of zygapophysial blocks in a completely random selection of patients with spinal pain. In general, patients have been preselected on the basis of various clinical criteria or radiologic and CT findings, although typically the patients studied have been ones with deep, dull aching pain, without neurologic abnormalities.[42,43,52,57,60,101,108,109,119,128,133,162] Nevertheless, some estimate of the incidence of facet syndromes can be gained from the incidence of positive responses to diagnostic blocks among such patients.

In the lumbar region the incidence of positive responses after intra-articular blocks ranges from 48% to 67%,[42,43,52,101,119] and in one study that used a control injection at a randomly selected asymptomatic level in each patient the positive response rate at the putatatively symptomatic level was 56%.[60] However, some authors have reported a positive response rate of only 16%.[133] The reasons for this dramatic difference are not clear, but differences in the criteria used for patient selection may be a key factor.

There have been fewer studies of patients with cervical pain syndromes, but the positive response rate appears to be higher. Response rates of 86% and 69% have been reported after intra-articular blocks[57,162] and 70% after cervical medial branch blocks and third occipital nerve blocks.[25,26] In addition, 158 patients have been described as having responded to cervical dorsal ramus blocks, but the total population from which these patients were selected was not specified.[151]

Overall, the reasonably high positive response rates to zygapophysial blocks indicate that facet syndromes are fairly common causes of spinal pain in both the lumbar region and the neck. Because they cannot be diagnosed otherwise, diagnostic blocks are the only means of identifying these syndromes, and the use of diagnostic blocks will remain justified until less invasive diagnostic techniques are developed.

TREATMENT

The therapeutic armamentarium for zygapophysial joint pain is severely limited. The only techniques that have been used specifically for facet syndromes are intra-articular steroids and facet denervation.

Open trials indicate that appreciable numbers of patients with lumbar facet syndromes can get relief from intra-articular steroids. However, there have been no controlled trials of this procedure, and the duration of relief obtained is both limited and varied. In one study only 42% of patients maintained complete or good relief for more than 3 months,[107] and other studies have reported sustained relief for at least 6 months in proportions ranging from 25% to 63% of patients.[43,52,101,109,119] Similar variations occur with the use of steroids for cervical syndromes. The reported duration of relief has ranged from 2 weeks to 6 months in one study[162] and from 3 days to 13 months in another.[57]

These variations bring into question the suitability of steroids as a treatment for zygapophysial joint pain. In most studies, steroids have been injected along with local anesthetic during the performance of diagnostic blocks, on the presumption that they will exert a therapeutic effect that will outlast the duration of diagnostic, local anesthetic block. However, the therapeutic effect of steroids is only presumptive, and neither the rationale for their use nor their expected mechanism of action has ever been formally addressed.

There are no data that indicate that zygapophysial pain is caused by inflammatory processes, and it is not known whether the beneficial effect of steroids (when it does occur) is due to their anti-inflammatory properties or simply to some neurotoxic or neurolytic effect on the capsular nerve endings. Reciprocally, when steroids fail to have an effect, is it because the pain was not due to an inflammatory process or because the solution did not adequately infiltrate all inflammatory foci or all the nerve endings in the joint?

Clearly, there is a need for double-blind controlled trials not only to determine the true efficacy of intra-articular steroids, for both back and neck pain, but also to determine their mechanism of action. Only when the mechanism is determined can the indications for intra-articular steroids be properly defined, and only then can the reasons for their limited duration of action be addressed.

Percutaneous radiofrequency denervation of the zygapophysial joints was devised on the premise that pain from a target joint could be relieved by coagulating the nerves to that joint. In this respect the rationale for denervation is sound. By blocking conduction in the target nerve, coagulation simply reproduces the effect of a diagnostic medial branch block but for a more prolonged period of time. However, despite a valid rationale and despite an extensive literature,[6,35,61,63,86,87,108,111,112,118,124,125,128,131,132,141,144-147,159] percutaneous radiofrequency denervation of the zygapophysial joints has attracted a great deal of suspicion and controversy, and not without justification.

The early use of this procedure was compromised by the use of anatomically inaccurate target points,[20,21] and even though more accurate target points were later adopted, a recent study has shown the direction in which electrodes are applied to the target nerves greatly affects the reliability with which the nerves can be coagulated.[27] It is therefore likely that many of the reported failures of facet denervation have been due not to errors in diagnosis, but to technical errors. Therefore, the true benefit of this procedure cannot be assessed until trials have been performed with close attention to the anatomic accuracy and reliability of the technique used.

Notwithstanding these reservations, even using the best technique, denervation does not have the prospect of a long-term "cure." The coagulated nerves will eventually regenerate, and in my experience this occurs within about 12 months. Denervation, therefore, should not be misrepresented as a surgical cure. Rather, it is form of long-term block that can afford the patient satisfying but temporary analgesia which may permit other therapies to improve posture, activity, and so forth.

Denervation is potentially repeatable when pain recurs, but in many circles the need to repeat a procedure perhaps every 12 months is considered unacceptable. Therefore, unless the use of steroids or some alternative pharmacologic procedure is perfected, there will remain a need for the development of a more lasting, definitive surgical procedure for zygapophysial joint pain. In this regard, capsular excision has been reported for the treatment of thoracolumbar zygapophysial pain,[117] but it has yet to be evaluated at lower levels or cervical levels.

EPIDURAL STEROIDS

The epidural injection of corticosteroids is a widely used treatment for sciatica. It is practiced not only by orthopedic surgeons and anesthesiologists, but also by rheumatologists, specialists in physical medicine, and a large number of general practitioners. In all, about 5000 cases of its use has been reported in the literature and many more patients have been treated without report. Despite their widespread use, the administration of epidural steroids remains a controversial practice.

HISTORICAL PERSPECTIVE

The use of epidural steroids was first reported in the European literature in 1952.[137] There followed a large number of reports in foreign language journals[11,12,36–39,50,64,69,81,105,114,137,139,169,171]; the first English language reports appeared in 1961,[68,74] to be followed by an ever-increasing body of literature[7,8,10,23,30–33,48,49,54,55,73,76,78–80,83,84,91,92,95,106,120,121,140,143,152–154,161,164,167,168,170] and correspondence.[9,29,49,53,71,72,75,90,93,94,99,120,142,156,163] Controversies concerning the practice have related to its reputed efficacy and its side-effects.

RATIONALE

It is interesting that in much of the literature, the rationale for epidural steroids is not addressed.[32,36,39,50,64,73,83,95,121] It seems that the practice was introduced at a time when the intra-articular injection of steroids for rheumatic diseases was being explored,[105,137] and when used on a presumptive basis for sciatica, it appeared to be successful. For many authors the results of earlier uncontrolled trials appear to have justified the adoption of the technique without regard to its rationale.

When the rationale has been addressed, most authors have proposed an anti-inflammatory role for epidural steroids in lumbosacral root syndromes.[7,12,31,37,54,55,68,69,74,76,78,84,91,92,106,139,140,143,154,161,164,168,170] They consider the target to be neural or perineural inflammation, although some have used peridural steroids to prevent the development of periradicular fibrosis, or "adhesions," and couple the epidural injection of steroids and local anesthetic with manipulative procedures designed ostensibly to break down such adhesions.[33,68,74,120,121,161] However, the anti-inflammatory role for epidural steroids is essentially presumptive, and the little evidence in its support is only circumstantial or inferential.

Nevertheless, an emerging concept is that lumbosacral radiculopathy, at least in its early phase, involves a significant inflammatory component, evoked by chemical or mechanical irritation or an autoimmune response, and it is this phase that theoretically should be amenable to treatment with steroids (see Bogduk and Cherry[23] for review). Although parenteral steroids can be used,[77] the perceived advantage of epidural steroids is that the drug is delivered in full dose directly to the site of disease.

ROUTE OF ADMINISTRATION

Steroids have been injected into the epidural space either by the caudal (transsacral)[8,12,30,36–39,50,64,68,73,76,106,121,143,170] or lumbar[7,31–33,49,54,55,69,78–80,84,91,95,139,140,152,154,161,168,171] routes exclusively, or by either[74,83,92] or both concurrently.[164] The advantages of the caudal route are said to be the ease of the procedure and the avoidance of thecal puncture, but larger volumes have to be injected in order to reach the target level. The rationale for the lumbar route is that the injection is made at, or at least close to, the target pathology, thereby requiring a lesser volume to be injected. The imminent risk is that of thecal puncture, but in skilled hands this should be an uncommon complication.

AGENTS USED

A number of different agents and volumes have been reported in the literature. These have included steroid alone, or steroid mixed with or followed by local anesthetic or normal saline. Early studies used hydrocortisone or prednisolone as the steroid, each in various doses. Others have used dexamethasone, betamethasone, and triamcinolone, but most, and particularly the more recent studies, have used depot methylprednisolone usually is a dose of 80 mg.

The total volume injected has varied from 1 to 2 ml when steroid alone has been used[95,140,152,168] up to 20 or 40 ml when saline or local anesthetic has been added and when the caudal route has been used.[8,30,68,74,76,121] Large volumes have also been injected by the lumbar route,[7,33,79,84,161] but there is no evidence that large volumes are required when the lumbar route is used. Large volumes are associated with side-effects (see below), and there is no evidence that adding local anesthetic improves the efficacy.

NUMBER OF INJECTIONS

Some authors have used up to four or five injections,[12,36,39,50,64,73,79,139,168] and up to ten in one study,[91] but most have studied the efficacy of one[7,8,31–33,36,54,55,68,76,78,84,92,105,106,121,137,140,152,154,164,170] or one to three[37,38,74,80,83,91,95,143,161] injections at daily to weekly intervals. There is no clinical evidence to justify proceeding beyond three injections if these have not been of benefit.

SAFETY

Whereas it is established that steroids injected intrathecally can cause significant neural and meningeal damage,[10] there is no evidence that the same applies for epidural injections. The effects of epidural steroids on neural and perineural tissues have been studied in animals, and no deliterious changes have been found[51] (see Bogduk and Cherry[23] for review).

Few clinical complications have been reported in the literature on epidural steroids, and most complications have been of technical or enigmatic nature. Metabolic complications directly ascribable to steroids, have been exceedingly uncommon. The actual incidence of particular complications is difficult to calculate accurately, for many studies[12,30,36,38,39,50,64,69,83,84,92,143,168] do not mention the issue of complications. Some explicitly report no complications,[78,106,139,170] whereas others[7,54,74,76,80,91,95,152,154] mention complications and do not specify their incidence. However, a thorough review of the literature allows some measure of incidence to be determined from those studies that do provide actual figures.

Technical complications are those attributable to the act of epidural injection and are not directly caused by steroids. These include traumatic tap (one case[140]) and thecal puncture. In the literature that specifies an incidence,[8,33,55,95,161,170] dural puncture has a weighted mean incidence of 5%.[23] Enigmatic complications are those without a proven physiologic basis. They include headache (weighted mean incidence 2%[8,33,79,95]) and the temporary exacerbation of sciatic pain (weighted mean incidence 1.3%[33,73,79,95,121,161]). The former may well be due to unrecognized thecal puncture, and in this regard Jurmand,[95] in a study of 855 patients, found that the incidence of headache was 18% in patients who did suffer inadvertent dural puncture but was only 1% in those in whom there was no evidence of dural puncture. Abram and Cherwenka[1] suggest that headaches may be caused by the inadvertent injection of air into the subarachnoid space.

Analysis of the available data on transient exacerbation of pain suggests that this complication is due to the injection of large volumes into the epidural space, and it has been suggested[55] that this symptom can be avoided by injecting slowly. Other complications include those caused by the intercurrent injection of local anesthetic: procaine sensitivity (one case[74]), hypotension (1 case in 138[33]), and spinal anesthesia (two cases[74,121]).

Most recently there has appeared a report[142] of a patient who developed extensive severe spinal pains after an epidural injection of depot methylprednisolone. These symptoms remained unexplained for several months until, at laminectomy over the injection site, an adhesion of the dura mater to the roof of the vertebral canal was discovered. Resection of this adhesion resulted in prompt relief of the pain. To what extent this complication may be directly attributed to steroids is unclear. It may be that this adhesion was the result of an epidural hemorrhage rather than a reaction to the injected steroid, and for this reason it is mentioned in the context of technical complications.

Clinical studies have shown that epidural steroids do depress plasma cortisol levels for about 2 weeks,[34] but clinical manifestations of systemic side-effects have been uncommon. These include one case of congestive cardiac failure owing to fluid retention,[74] minor changes in serum glucose levels in susceptible patients,[95] and miscellaneous problems, each with an incidence of less than 1%, such as cramps, rash, malaise, fever, and digestive problems. Classic steroid side-effects have been reported only in four patients, all of whom received excessives doses of epidural steroids: between 200 and 400 mg of methylprednisolone over 1 to 3 days.[98]

EFFICACY

Although the principal indications for the use of epidural steroids have been the symptoms of either low back pain or sciatica, alone or in combination, the criteria used for the selection of patients for treatment have varied, and in the majority of studies the actual cause of symptoms was undetermined or only presumed. Because of these variations, few studies can be compared with one another in order to draw any concerted conclusions. Furthermore, follow-up periods have varied, and few controlled trials have been published. Most reports have been open trials of varying duration.

Without specifying any review period, some trials report an immediate success rate ranging from 25% to 89%.[12,36,38,39,50,54,68,73,76,79,80,83,95,121,140,154] Others report success rates of between 35% and 86% at review between 6 weeks and 5 years after treatment,[7,8,31,33,37,55,64,69,74,78,84,92,139,143,152,164,168] the average success rate being around 60% at 3 to 6 months review. There is, however, a decay in the success rate over time. Longitudinal studies have revealed a drop from 68% to 42% by 2 years,[37] and from 90% to 70% by 6 months.[106]

The most sobering longitudinal study has been that of White and others,[164] who carefully followed their patients hourly for 8 hours, daily for 2 weeks, and every 2 weeks for 6 months. They found a decay in overall success rate from 82% on the first day to 7% by 6 months. Only 4 of their 300 patients had no pain after 2 years.

Although overall success rates in the various open trials have been modest, retrospective analysis reveals that better results occurred in certain types of patients. Distinctly better results have been obtained in patients who had not previously undergone surgery,[78,83,84,95] and especially in patients with "acute" versus "chronic" complaints,[37,54,95,154] and more specifically, in those with histories shorter than 12 months,[33,91,161] 6 months,[84] 3 months,[31,78,79,91] and 2 months.[39]

This latter correlation was further borne out by Ryan and Taylor,[140] who found that complete relief was obtained in 77% of their patients who had symptoms for less than 2 weeks, but the response rates were 72%, 60%, and 43% for patients with histories of 4 weeks, 6 weeks, and more than 6 weeks, respectively. White and associates[164] found that patients with a history shorter than 2 weeks had a greater chance of sustaining relief, with 34% of such patients remaining pain-free at 6 months.

Apart from the open trials, epidural steroids have been assessed in several types of comparison and controlled trials. When compared with intrathecal steroids, epidural steroids have been shown to be equally[168] or slightly more effective.[80] When compared with epidural local anesthetic or saline, epidural steroids have been shown to be superior.[8,30,50,83,154,170] In a recent study[49] epidural steroids were compared with epidural local anesthetic and no significant differences in results were found. However, this study has been challenged on various technical grounds,[62,99] and it is noteworthy that most of the patients studied had long histories, in excess of the 2 to 4 weeks that the open trials have suggested is the optimal time for use of epidural steroids.

Although comparison with epidural saline[30] constitutes a controlled trial, two trials have compared epidural steroids with absolute placebo treatment. In both, the placebo was an injection of normal saline into an interspinous ligament and the active treatment was a lumbar epidural injection of methylprednisolone.

In the first study[152] the patients were highly selected. All had to have neurologic deficits and myelographic defects at the appropriate site. After treatment no significant differences were found between the treated and the control patients. This result demands agreement with the authors' conclusion[152] that epidural steroids are not worthwhile in patients with established neurologic signs and myelographic defects.

In contrast, the other controlled trial[55] studied an unselected population of 36 patients with various clinical features and revealed significant differences between the treated and the control groups. At 3 months after treatment fewer of the treated group had failed to return to work, more had decreased analgesic consumption, and fewer had persistent or severe pain. This trial, therefore, demonstrated that epidural steroids have a definite effect over strict placebo and validates the impression created by the open trials.

DISCUSSION

Open trials of the use of epidural steroids suggest that a certain proportion of patients can benefit, at least for short periods. Comparison trials have established a superiority of epidural steroids over epidural local anesthetic or normal saline, and controlled trials, while denying a value in patients with chronic, myelographically positive radiculopathy, have revealed an unequivocal value in less specific cases.

What remains unresolved are the indications for the optimal use of epidural steroids. Although the study of Dilke and colleagues[55] demonstrated a superiority over placebo, the overall success rate was only 45%, which compares poorly with the high success rates reported in other studies using patients with short histories. Indeed, there is a strong impression in the literature that the best results are obtained in early or acute cases, and this is in accord with the proposed anti-inflammatory rationale for the use of epidural steroids. Steroids would be expected to have a greater effect early in the course of an inflammatory radiculopathy, rather than later, when acute inflammation has changed to chronic inflammation and fibrosis. The impressive results obtained in early cases, however, are still compromised by three issues: longevity, reality, and indications.

In only one study[164] have patients with short histories been thoroughly followed after treatment, and then only a modest proportion remained pain-free after 6 months. This observation warns against enthusiasm based only on initial observations and against partisan viewpoints that epidural steroids may be anything more than perhaps an intermittent or temporizing form of therapy.

More significant, it must be realized that no studies of acute cases have been controlled. The possibility of spontaneous resolution looms strongly in patients with histories of less than 2 to 4 weeks. It is, therefore, imperative that to formalize the apparent efficacy of epidural steroids, appropriate controlled trials be undertaken, testing the hypothesis that treatment by epidural steroids early in the course of the illness offers benefits more desirable than those obtained from other conservative and less invasive therapy.

Even if it is acceptable that epidural steroids have a role to play in the early treatment of acute inflammatory radiculopathy, the problem remains as to how to identify such patients clinically. It has been shown that the best results are obtained in acute cases with raised cerebrospinal fluid protein levels.[140] Raised protein levels are consistent with the diagnosis of inflammatory radiculopathy[23] and provide an objective indication for epidural steroids. However, it is unattractive to suggest that all patients should be first screened by lumbar puncture and cerebrospinal fluid analysis before undergoing epidural steroid therapy.

"Irritative" Versus "Compressive" Neuropathy

To circumvent this requirement, there may be value in certain clinical features highlighted by Ryan and Taylor.[140] These authors distinguished between "irritative" and "compressive" neuropathies. Irritative lesions are ones in which sciatica is the predominant or only symptom, while compressive lesions are characterized by sensory, motor, or reflex disturbances.

In this regard, Ryan and Taylor[140] found that the response rate in patients with "irritative" lesions of 2, 4, and 6 weeks' duration were 100%, 100%, and 83%, respectively, whereas patients with compressive lesions of the same durations had response rates of only 70%, 69%, and 25%. These results suggest that "irritative" lesions can be used as a clinical indication for epidural steroids, but the partial, but nevertheless substantial, response rate in patients with compressive lesions indicates that responders cannot be perfectly distinguished on this basis alone. The concept of "irritative" lesions carries with it a high false-negative rate, which, therefore, compromises its suitability as an absolute indicator for therapy.[23]

REFERENCES

1. Abram, S.E., and Cherwenka, R.W.: Transient headache immediately following epidural steroid injection. Anesthesiology, *50*:461, 1979.
2. Auteroche, P.: Innervation of the zygapophyseal joints of the lumbar spine. Anat. Clin., *5*:17, 1983.
3. Ayers, C.E.: Lumbo-sacral backache. N. Engl. J. Med., *196*:9, 1927.
4. Ayers, C.E.: Lumbo-sacral backache. N. Engl. J. Med., *200*:592, 1929.
5. Ayers, C.E.: Further case studies of lumbo-sacral pathology with consideration of the involvement of the intervertebral discs and the articular facets. N. Engl. J. Med., *213*:716, 1935.
6. Banerjee, T., and Pittman, H.H.: Facet rhizotomy. Another armamentarium for treatment of low backache. N.C. Med. J., *37*:354, 1976.
7. Barry, P.J.C., and Kendall, P.H.: Corticosteroid infiltration of the extradural space. Ann. Phys. Med., *6*:267, 1962.
8. Beliveau, P.: A comparison between epidural anaesthesia with and without corticosteroid in the treatment of sciatica. Rheumatol. Phys. Med., *11*:40, 1971.
9. Bellhouse, C.P., Watson, J.R., Farrow, M.A., and Lyatt, D.B.: Spinal injections of corticosteroids (letter). Med. J. Aust., *1*:11, 1982.
10. Bernat, J.L.: Intraspinal steroid therapy. Neurology, *31*:168, 1981.
11. Beyer, W.: Das zervikale an lumbale Bandscheibensyndrom und seine Behandlung mit Novocain-Prednisolon-Injektionen and die Nervenwurzeln. Munch. Med. Wschr., *102*:1164, 1960.
12. Biella, A., and Cicognini, P.: L'acetato di idrocortisone nel trattemento della sindrome sciatalgica. Minerva Med., *1*:1863, 1954.
13. Bogduk, N.: Local anaesthetic blocks of the second cervical ganglion: A technique with an application in occipital headache. Cephalalgia, *1*:41, 1981.
14. Bogduk, N.: The lumbar mamillo-accessory ligament. Its anatomical and neurosurgical significance. Spine, *6*:162, 1981.
15. Bogduk, N.: The clinical anatomy of the cervical dorsal rami. Spine, *7*:319, 1982.
16. Bogduk, N.: The innervation of the lumbar spine. Spine, *8*:286, 1983.
17. Bogduk, N.: Neck pain. Aust. Fam. Physician, *13*:26, 1984.
18. Bogduk, N.: Low back pain. Aust. Fam. Physician, *14*:1168, 1985.
19. Bogduk, N.: The innervation of intervertebral discs. *In* Ghosh, P. (ed.): The Biology of the Intervertebral Disc. CRC Press. (In press).
20. Bogduk, N., and Long, D.M.: The anatomy of the so-called articular nerves and their relationship to facet denervation in the treatment of low back pain. J. Neurosurg., *51*:172, 1979.
21. Bogduk, N., and Long, D.M.: Percutaneous lumbar medial branch neurotomy. A modification of facet denervation. Spine, *5*:193, 1980.

22. Bogduk, N., Wilson, A.S., and Tynan, W.: The human lumbar dorsal rami. J. Anat., *134*:383, 1982.
23. Bogduk, N., and Cherry, D.: Epidural corticosteroid agents for sciatica. Med. J. Aust., *143*:402, 1985.
24. Bogduk, N., and Marsland, A.: Third occipital headache. Cephalalgia, *5* [*Suppl.*]:310, 1985.
25. Bogduk, N., and Marsland, A.: The cervical zygapophyseal joints as a cause of neck pain. Paper submitted for the First Cervical Spine Research Society Award, 1986.
26. Bogduk, N., and Marsland, A.: On the concept of third occipital headache. J. Neurol. Neurosurg. Psychiatry, *49*:775, 1986.
27. Bogduk, N., Macintosh, J.E., and Marsland, A.: A technical limitation to the efficacy of radiofrequency neurotomy for spinal pain. Neurosurgery. (In press).
28. Bradley, K.C.: The anatomy of backache. Aust. N.Z. J. Surg., *44*:227, 1974.
29. Bradley, K.C., Corrigan, A.B., and Ingpen, M.L.: Spinal injections of corticosteroids (letter). Med. J. Aust., *1*:11, 1982.
30. Breivik, H., Hesla, P.E., Molnar, I., and Lind, B.: Treatment of chronic low back pain and sciatica. Comparison of caudal epidural injections of bupivicaine and methylprednisolone with bupivicaine followed by saline. *In* Bonica, J.J., and Albe-Fessard, D. (eds.): Advances in Pain Research and Therapy. Vol. 1. Pp. 927–932. New York, Raven Press, 1976.
31. Brown, F.W.: Management of diskogenic pain using epidural and intrathecal steroids. Clin. Orthop., *129*:72, 1977.
32. Bullard, J.R., and Houghton, F.M.: Epidural steroid treatment of acute herniated nucleus pulposus. Anesth. Analg., *56*:862, 1977.
33. Burn, J.M.B., and Langdon, L.: Lumbar epidural injection for the treatment of chronic sciatica. Rheumatol. Phys. Med., *10*:368, 1970.
34. Burn, J.M.B., and Langdon, L.: Duration of action of epidural methyl prednisolone. A study in patients with the lumbosciatic syndrome. Am. J. Phys. Med., *53*:29, 1974.
35. Burton, C.V.: Percutaneous radiofrequency facet denervation. Appl. Neurophysiol., *39*:80, 1976/77.
36. Canale, L.: Il desametazone per via epidurale sacrale nelle lombosciatalgie. Gaz. Med. Ital., *122*:210, 1963.
37. Cappio, M.: Il trattemento idrocortisonico per via epidurale sacrale delle lombosciatalgie. Reumatismo, *9*:60, 1957.
38. Cappio, M., and Fragasso, V.: Osservazioni sull uso dell idrocortisone per via epidurale ed endorachidea nelle lombosciatalgie. Riforma Med., *22*:605, 1955.
39. Cappio, M., and Fragasso, V.: Il prednisolone per via epidurale sacrale nelle lombosciatalgie. Reumatismo, *5*:295, 1957.
40. Carrera, G.F.: Lumbar facet arthrography and injection in low back pain. Wis. Med. J., *78*:35, 1979.
41. Carrera, G.F.: Lumbar facet joint injection in low back pain and sciatica. Description of technique. Radiology, *137*:661, 1980.
42. Carrera, G.F.: Lumbar facet joint injection in low back pain and sciatica. Preliminary results. Radiology, *137*:665, 1980.
43. Carrera, G.F., and Williams, A.L.: Current concepts in evaluation of the lumbar facet joints. CRC Crit. Rev. Diagn. Imaging, *21*:85, 1984.
44. Cloward, R.B.: Cervical diskography. A contribution to the etiology and mechanism of neck, shoulder and arm pain. Ann. Surg., *150*:1052, 1959.
45. Cloward, R.B.: The clinical significance of the sinu-vertebral nerve of the cervical spine in relation to the cervical disk syndrome. J. Neurol. Neurosurg. Psychiatry, *23*:321, 1960.
46. Collier, B.B.: Treatment for lumbar sciatic pain in posterior articular lumbar joint syndrome. Anaesthesia, *34*:202, 1979.
47. Collis, J.S., and Gardner, W.J.: Lumbar discography—An analysis of 1,000 cases. J. Neurosurg., *19*:452, 1962.
48. Corrigan, A.B., Carr, G., and Tugwell, S.: Intraspinal corticosteroid injections. Med. J. Aust., *1*:224, 1982.
49. Cuckler, J.M., Bernini, P.A., Wiesel, S.W., Booth, R.E., Rothman, R.H., and Pickens, G.T.: The use of epidural steroids in the treatment of lumbar radicular pain. J. Bone Joint Surg., *67A*:63, 1985.
50. Czarski, Z.: Leczenie rwy kulszowej wstrzykiwaniem hydrokortyzonu i nowokainy do rozworu krzyzowego. Przegl. Lek., *21*:511, 1965.
51. Delaney, T.J., Rowlingson, J.C., Carron, H., and Butler, A.: Epidural steroid effects on nerves and meninges. Anesth. Analg., *58*:610, 1980.
52. Destouet, J.M., Gilula, L.A., Murphy, W.A., and Monsees, B.: Lumbar facet joint injection: Indication, technique, clinical correlation and preliminary results. Radiology, *145*:321, 1982.
53. Dewey, P.: Spinal injections of corticosteroids (letter). Med. J. Aust., *1*:9, 1982.
54. D'Hoogue, R., Compere, A., Gribmont, B., and Vincent, A.: Peridural injection of corticosteroids in the treatment of the low back pain/sciatica syndrome. Acta Orthop. Belg., *42*:157, 1976.
55. Dilke, T.F.W., Burry, H.C., and Grahame, R.: Extradural corticosteroid injection in management of lumbar nerve root compression. Br. Med. J., *2*:635, 1973.
56. Dory, M.A.: Arthrography of the lumbar facet joints. Radiology, *140*:23, 1981.
57. Dory, M.A.: Arthrography of the cervical facet joints. Radiology, *148*:379, 1983.
58. Dussault, R.G., and Nicolet, V.M.: Cervical facet joint arthrography. J. Can. Assoc. Radiol., *36*:79, 1985.
59. Eisenstein, S.M., Wood, P., O'Brien, J.P., Park, W.M., and McCall, I.W.: Pain patterns in low back syndromes: A preliminary report (abstract). J. Bone Joint Surg., *60B*:295, 1978.
60. Fairbank, J.C.T., Park, W.M., McCall, I.W., and O'Brien, J.P.: Apophyseal injection of local anesthetic as a diagnostic aid in primary low-back pain syndromes. Spine, *6*:598, 1981.
61. Fassio, B., Bouvier, J.P., and Ginestie, J.F.: Denervation articulaire posterieure per-cutanee et chirurgicale. Rev. Chir. Orthop., *67*[*Suppl.*]:131, 1981.
62. Fisher, R.H.: Letter. J. Bone Joint Surg., *68A*:789, 1986.
63. Florez, G., Eiras, J., and Ucar, S.: Percutaneous rhizotomy of

the articular nerve of Luschka for low back and sciatic pain. Acta Neurochir. [Suppl.] Wien, *24*:67, 1977.

64. Fragasso, V.: Il prednisolone idrosolubile per via epidurale sacrale nelle lombosciatalgie. Gaz. Med. Ital., *118*:358, 1959.
65. Friberg, S.: Lumbar disc degeneration in the problem of lumbago sciatica. Bull. Hosp. Joint Dis., *15*:1, 1954.
66. Friedenberg, Z.B., and Miller, W.T.: 1963 Degenerative disc disease of the cervical spine. A comparative study of asymptomatic and symptomatic patients. J. Bone Joint Surg., *45A*:1171, 1963.
67. Fuentes, E.: La neurotomia apofisiaria transcutanea en el tratamiento de la lumbalgia cronica. Rev. Med. Chile, *106*:440, 1978.
68. Gardner, W.J., Goebert, H.W., and Sehgal, A.D.: Intraspinal corticosteroids in the treatment of sciatica. Trans. Am. Neurol. Assoc., *86*:214, 1961.
69. Gerest, M.F.: Le traitement de la nevralgie sciatique par les injections epidurales d'hydrocortisone. J. Med. Lyon, *39*:261, 1958.
70. Ghormley, R.K.: Low back pain with special reference to the articular facets with presentation of an operative procedure. J.A.M.A., *10*:1773, 1963.
71. Gibb, D.: Spinal injection: Corticosteroids (letter) Med. J. Aust., *2*:302, 1981.
72. Giles, K.E., Finch, P.M., Gee, G., and Jacobs, S.: Spinal injections of corticosteroids (letter). Med. J. Aust., *1*:9, 1982.
73. Gilly,R.: Essai de traitement de 50 cas de sciatiques et de radiculalgies lombaires par le Celestene chronodose en infiltrations pararadiculaire. Marseille Med., *107*:341, 1970.
74. Goebert, H.W., Jallo, S.J., Gardner, W.J., and Asmuth, C.E.: Painful radiculopathy treated with epidural injections of procaine and hydrocortisone acetate: Results in 113 patients. Anesth. Analg., *140*:130, 1961.
75. Gonski, A.: Spinal injections of corticosteroids steroids (letter). Med. J. Aust., *1*:9, 1982.
76. Gordon, J.: Caudal extradural injection for the treatment of low back pain. Anaesthesia, *35*:515, 1980.
77. Green, L.N.: Dexamethasone in the management of symptoms due to herniated lumbar disc. J. Neurol. Neurosurg. Psychiatry, *38*:1211, 1975.
78. Green, P.W.B., Burke, A.J., Weiss, C.A., and Langan, P.: The role of epidural cortisone injection in the treatment of diskogenic low back pain. Clin. Orthop., *153*:121, 1980.
79. Harley, C.: Extradural corticosteroid infiltration. Ann. Phys. Med., *9*:22, 1967.
80. Hartman, J.T., Winnie, A.P., and Ramamurthy, S.: Intradural and extradural corticosteroids for sciatic pain. Orthop. Rev., *3*:21, 1974.
81. Hellens, A.: Lumbar nerve-root compression treated with epidural hydrocortisone (Finnish). Duodecim, *78*:28, 1962.
82. Hermanus, N., de Becker, D., Baleriaux, D., and Hauzer, J.P.: The use of CT scanning for the study of posterior lumbar intervertebral articulations. Neuroradiology, *24*:159, 1983.
83. Hesla, P.E., and Breivik, H.: Epidural bupivacaine and depot methylprednisolone for low back pain and sciatica compared with epidural bupivacaine and saline or epidural bupivacaine and intramuscular depot methylprednisolone (abstract). Proceedings of the Second World Congress on Pain, Montreal, 1978. Pain Abstr., *1*:25, 1978
84. Heyse-Moore, G.H.: A rational approach to the use of epidural medication in the treatment of sciatic pain. Acta Orthop. Scand., *49*:366, 1978.
85. Hickey, R.F.J., and Tregonning, G.D.: Denervation of spinal facet joints for treatment of chronic low back pain. N.Z. Med. J., *85*:96, 1977.
86. Hildebrandt, J., and Argyrakis, A.: Die perkutane zervikale Facettdenervation-ein neues Verfahren zur Behandlung chronischer Nacken-Kopfschmerzen. Man. Med., *21*:45, 1983.
87. Hildebrandt, J., and Argyrakis, A.: Percutaneous nerve block of the cervical facets — A relatively new method in the treatment of chronic headache and neck pain. Pathological-anatomical studies and clinical practice. Manual Med., *2*:48, 1986.
88. Horal, J.: The clinical appearance of low back disorders in the city of Gothenburg, Sweden. Acta Orthop. Scand. [Suppl.], *188*:1, 1969.
89. Houston, J.R.: A study of subcutaneous rhizolysis in the treatment of chronic backache. J. R. Coll. Gen. Pract., *25*:692, 1975.
90. Ireland, B.J.: Spinal injections of corticosteroids (letter). Med. J. Aust., *1*:10, 1982.
91. Ito, R.: The treatment of low back pain and sciatica with epidural corticosteroids injection and its pathophysiological basis. J. Jap. Orthop. Assoc., *45*:769, 1971.
92. Jackson, D.W., Rettig, A., and Wiltse, L.L.: Epidural cortisone injections in the young athletic adult. Am. J. Sports Med., *8*:239, 1980.
93. Jacobs, D.: Intrathecal and epidural/extradural injection of depo medrol (letter). Med. J. Aust., *2*:301, 1981.
94. Jacobs, D.: Intraspinal injection of depotcorticosteroids (letter) Med. J. Aust., *1*:49, 1984.
95. Jurmand, S.H.: Corticotherapie peridurale des lomblgies et des sciatiques d'origine discale. Le Concours Med., *94*:5061, 1972.
96. Key, J.A.: Low back pain as seen in an orthopedic clinic. Am. J. Med. Sci., *168*:526, 1924.
97. Kikuchi, S., Macnab, I., and Moreau, P.: Localisation of the level of symptomatic cervical disc degeneration. J. Bone Joint Surg., *63B*:272, 1981.
98. Knight, C.L., and Burnell, J.C.: Systemic side-effects of extradural steroids. Anaesthesia, *35*:593, 1980.
99. Korbon, G.A., Rowlingson, J.C., and Carron, H.: Letter. J. Bone Joint Surg., *68A*:788, 1986.
100. Krempen, J.F., Smith, B.S., and De Freest, L.J.: Selective nerve root infiltration for the evaluation of sciatica. Orthop. Clin. North Am., *6*:311, 1975.
101. Lau, L.S.W., Littlejohn, G.O., and Miller, M.: Clinical evaluation of intra-articular injections for lumbar facet joint pain. Med. J. Aust., *143*:563, 1985.
102. Lawrence, J.S., Bremner, J.M., and Bier, F.: Osteoarthrosis: Prevalence in the population and relationship between symptoms and X-ray changes. Ann. Rheum. Dis., *25*:1, 1966.
103. Lazorthes, G., and Gaubert, J.: L'innervation des articulations

inter-apophysaire vertebrales. Comptes Rendues de l'Association des Anatomistes, 43- Reunion. p 488–494. 1956.

104. Lewin, T., Moffet, B., and Viidik, A.: The morphology of the lumbar synovial intervertebral joints. Acta Morphol. Neerl. Scand., *4*:299, 1962.

105. Lievre, J.A., Bloch-Michel, H., Pean, G., and Uro, J.: L'hydrocortisone en injection locale. Rev. Rhum. *20*:310, 1953.

106. Lindholm, R., and Salenius, P.: Caudal, epidural administration of anaesthetics and corticoids in the treatment of low back pain. Acta Orthop. Scand., *1*:114, 1964.

107. Lippit, A.B.: The facet joint and its role in spine pain. Spine, *9*:746, 1984.

108. Lora, J., and Long, D.M.: So-called facet denervation in the management of intractable back pain. Spine, *1*:121, 1976.

109. Lynch, M.C., and Taylor, J.F.: Facet injection for low back pain. J. Bone Joint Surg., *68B*:138, 1986.

110. McCall, I.W., Park, W.M., and O'Brien, J.P.: Induced pain referral from posterior lumbar elements in normal subjects. Spine, *4*:441, 1979.

111. McCulloch, J.A.: Percutaneous radiofrequency lumbar rhizolysis (rhizotomy). Appl. Neurophysiol., *39*:87, 1976/77.

112. McCulloch, J.A., and Organ, L.W.: Percutaneous radiofrequency lumbar rhizolysis (rhizotomy). Can. Med. Assoc. J., *116*:30, 1977.

113. Magora, A., and Schwartz, A.: Relation between the low back pain syndrome and X-ray findings. I. Degenerative osteoarthritis. Scand. J. Rehab. Med., *8*:115, 1976.

114. Mahner, A.: Die peridurale Injektion von Novocain und Kortikosteroiden in der Therapie des lumbalen radikularen Syndrom. Zentralbl. Chir., *85*:625, 1960.

115. Maigne, R.: Low back pain of thoracolumbar origin. Arch. Phys. Med. Rehab., *61*:389, 1980.

116. Maigne, R.: Le syndrome de la charniere dorso-lombaire. Sem. Hop. Paris, *57*:545, 1981.

117. Maigne, R., Le Corre, F., and Judet, H.: Lombalgies basses d'origine dorso-lombaire: Traitement chrirurgical par excision des capsules articulaires posterieures. Nouv. Presse Med., *7*:565, 1978.

118. Mehta, M., and Sluijter, M.E.: The treatment of chronic back pain. A preliminary survey of the effect of radiofrequency denervation of the posterior vertebral articulations. Anaesthesia, *34*:768, 1979.

119. Mooney, V., and Robertson, J.: The facet syndrome. Clin. Orthop., *115*:149, 1976.

120. Mount, H.T.R.: Hydrocortisone in the treatment of intervertebral disc protrusion (letter). Can. Med. Assoc. J., *105*:1279, 1971.

121. Mount, H.T.R.: Epidural injection of hydrocortisone for the management of the acute lumbar disc protrusion. *In* Morley, T.P. (ed.): Current Controversies in Neurosurgery. Pp. 67–72. Philadelphia, W.B. Saunders, 1976.

122. Nachemson, A.L.: The lumbar spine. An orthopaedic challenge. Spine, *1*:59, 1976.

123. Naylor, A.: Brachial neuritis, with particular reference to lesions of the cervical intervertebral discs. Ann. R. Coll. Surg., *9*:155, 1951.

124. Ogsbury, J.S., Simons, H., and Lehman, R.A.W.: Facet "denervation" in the treatment of low back syndrome. Pain, *2*:257, 1977.

125. Oudenhoven, R.C.: Articular rhizotomy. Surg. Neurol., *2*:275, 1974.

126. Paris, S.V.: Anatomy as related to function and pain. Orthop. Clin. North Am., *14*:475, 1983.

127. Park, W.M.: The place of radiology in the investigation of low back pain. Clin. Rheum. Dis., *6*:93, 1980.

128. Pawl, R.P.: Results in the treatment of low back syndrome from sensory neurolysis of the lumbar facets (facet rhizotomy) by thermal coagulation. Proc. Inst. Med. Chicago, *30*:150, 1974.

129. Pawl, R.P.: Headache, cervical spondylosis, and anterior cervical fusion. Surg. Annu., *9*:391, 1977.

130. Pedersen, H.E., Blunck, C.F.J., and Gardner, E.: The anatomy of lumbosacral posterior rami and meningeal branches of spinal nerves (sinus-vertebral nerves): With an experimental study of their function. J. Bone Joint Surg., *38A*:377, 1956.

131. Rashbaum, R.F.: Radiofrequency facet denervation. Orthop. Clin. North Am., *14*:569, 1983.

132. Ray, C.D.: Percutaneous radiofrequency facet nerve blocks: Treatment of the mechanical low-back syndrome. Burlington, Radionics Procedure Technique Series, Radionics Inc, 1982.

133. Raymond, J.R., and Dumas, J.M.: Intraarticular facet block: Diagnostic test or therapeutic procedure? Radiology, *151*:333, 1984.

134. Raymond, J.R., Dumas, J.M., and Lisbona, R.: Nuclear imaging as a screening test for patients referred for intraarticular facet block. J. Can. Assoc. Radiol., *35*:291, 1984.

135. Rees, W.S.: Multiple bilateral subcutaneous rhizolysis of segmental nerves in the treatment of the intervertebral disc syndrome. Ann. Gen. Pract., *16*:126, 1971.

136. Rees, W.S.: Multiple bilateral percutaneous rhizolysis. Med. J. Aust., *1*:536, 1975.

137. Robecchi, A., and Capra, R.: L'idrocortisone (composto F). Prime esperienze cliniche in campo reumatologico. Minerva Med., *98*:1259, 1952.

138. Roth, D.A. Cervical analgesic discography. A new test for the definitive diagnosis of the painful-disk syndrome. J.A.M.A., *235*:1713, 1976.

139. Ruggieri, F., and Capello, A.: L'idrocortisone nel trattamento della lumbosciatalgica. Minerva Orthop., *7*:388, 1956.

140. Ryan, M.D., and Taylor, T.K.F.: Management of lumbar nerve-root pain. Med. J. Aust., *2*:532, 1981.

141. Schaerer, J.P.: Radiofrequency facet rhizotomy in the treatment of chronic neck and low back pain. Int. Surg., *63*:53, 1978.

142. Sekel, R.: Epidural depo-medrol revisited (letter). Med. J. Aust., *2*:688, 1984.

143. Sharma, R.K.: Indications, technique and results of caudal epidural injection for lumbar disc retropulsion. Postgrad. Med. J., *53*:1, 1977.

144. Shealy, C.N.: Facets in back and sciatic pain. Minn. Med., *57*:199, 1974.

145. Shealy, C.N.: The role of the spinal facets in back and sciatic pain. Headache, *14*:101, 1974.

146. Shealy, C.N.: Percutaneous radiofrequency denervation of spinal facets. J. Neurosurg., *43*:448, 1975.

147. Shealy, C.N.: Facet denervation in the management of back and sciatic pain. Clin. Orthop., *115*:157, 1976.

148. Simmons, E.H., and Segil, C.M.: An evaluation of discography in the localization of symptomatic levels in discogenic disease of the spine. Clin. Orthop., *108*:57, 1975.

149. Sluijter, M.E.: Percutaneous thermal lesions in the treatment of back and neck pain. Burlington, Radionics Procedure Technique Series. Radionics, 1981.

150. Sluijter, M.E., and Koetsveld-Baart, C.C.: Interruption of pain pathways in the treatment of the cervical syndrome. Anaesthesia, *35*:302, 1980.

151. Sluijter, M.E., and Mehta, M.: Treatment of chronic back and neck pain by percutaneous thermal lesions. *In* Lipton, S., and Miles, J. (eds.): Persistent Pain. Modern Methods of Treatment. Vol. 3. Pp. 141-179. London, Academic Press, 1981.

152. Snoek, W., Weber, H., and Jorgensen, B.: Double blind evaluation of extradural methyl prednisolone for herniated lumbar discs. Acta Orthop. Scand., *48*:635, 1977.

153. Stanton-Hicks, M.: Therapeutic caudal or epidural block for lower back or sciatic pain. J.A.M.A., *243*:369, 1980.

154. Swerdlow, M., and Sayle-Creer, W.: A study of extradural medication in the relief of the lumbosciatic syndrome. Anaesthesia, *25*:341, 1970.

155. Tajima, T., Furukawa, K., and Kuramachi, E.: Selective lumbosacral radiculopathy and block. Spine, *5*:68, 1980.

156. Tarlov, E.: Therapeutic caudal or epidural block for lower back or sciatic pain. J.A.M.A., *243*:369, 1980.

157. Toakley, J.G.: Subcutaneous lumbar "rhizolysis"—An assessment of 200 cases. Med. J. Aust., *2*:490, 1973.

158. Torgersen, W.R., and Dotter, W.E.: Comparative roentgenographic study of the asymptomatic and symptomatic lumbar spine. J. Bone Joint Surg., *58A*:850, 1976.

159. Uyttendaele, D., Verhamme, J., Vercauteren, M., and Verschraegen, R.: Local block of lumbar facet joints and percutaneous radiofrequency denervation. Preliminary results. Acta Orthop. Belg., *47*:135, 1981.

160. Vlok, G.J.: Comparative radiographic findings in anteroposterior radiographs in symptomatic and symptomatic backs. J. Bone Joint Surg., *62B*:279, 1980.

161. Warr, A.C., Wilkinson, J.A., Burn, J.M.B., and Langdon, L.: Chronic lumbosciatic syndrome treated by epidural injection and manipulation. Practitioner, *209*:53, 1977.

162. Wedel, D.J., and Wilson, P.R.: Cervical facet arthrography. Reg. Anaesth., *10*:7, 1985.

163. Weisz, G.M.: Spinal injections of corticosteroids. (Letter). Med. J. Aust., *1*:9, 1982.

164. White, A.H., Derby, R., and Wynne, G.: Epidural injections for diagnosis and treatment of low-back pain. Spine, *5*:78, 1980.

165. Wiley, J.J., MacNab, I., and Wortzman, G.: Lumbar discography and its clinical applications. Can. J. Surg., *11*:280, 1968.

166. Wilson, C.B., and Hoff, J.T.: Clinical features and surgical treatment of cervical discogenic radiculopathy and myelopathy. *In* Genant, H.K. (ed.): Spine Update 1984. Pp. 273-279. San Francisco, Radiology Research and Education Foundation, 1984.

167. Wiltse, L.L.: Therapeutic caudal or epidural block for lower back or sciatic pain. J.A.M.A., *243*:369, 1980.

168. Winnie, A.P., Hartmen, J.T., Meyers, H.L., Ramamurthy, S., and Barangan, V.: Pain clinic. II. Intradural and extradural corticosteroids for sciatica. Anesth. Analg., *51*:990, 1972.

169. Yamazaka, N.: Interspinal injection of hydrocotrisone or prednisolone in the treatment of intervertebral disc herniation. (Japanese). J. Jap. Orthop. Soc., *33*:689, 1959.

170. Yates, D.W.: A comparison of the types of epidural injection commonly used in the treatment of low back pain and sciatica. Rheumatol. Rehab., *17*:181, 1978.

171. Zappala, G.: Iniezione peridurale segmentaria di Hydrocortone nella sindrome dolorosa da ernia discale. Policlinico—Sez Prat., *62*:1229, 1955.

28 ACUTE AND CHRONIC PAIN: USE OF SPINAL OPIOIDS

MICHAEL J. COUSINS
DAVID A. CHERRY
AND GEOFFREY K. GOURLAY

HISTORICAL PERSPECTIVE

The centenary of regional anesthesia was commemorated in Vienna in 1984 by a scientific meeting devoted to regional anesthesia and the relief of pain. It was significant that the meeting discussed many methods for pain relief, including use of spinal opioids.[104] However, all methods were judged by the great moment in medical history in 1884 when Karl Koller demonstrated that pain relief could be obtained by local anesthetic blockade, so that effects on the brain and other parts of the body were minimal or absent. This was the first pharmacologic attempt to aim at a "relatively" specific target for pain control—axons of peripheral nerves.

It had been accepted for thousands of years that pain relief could be obtained only at the expense of substantial central nervous system depression, as exemplified by the use of Mandragora, wine, and opium in ancient China (2000 B.C.), Mandragora and "poppy" in ancient Egypt, Rome, and Greece, and use of atropine, opium, cocaine, and hallucinogens by the Incas and ancient Peruvians. Thus, until Koller's daring step in 1884, the major target for pain control was the brain. Axon and brain remained the major options until the mid-1970s, when spinal opioid receptors were convincingly shown to be associated with relatively selective spinal analgesia. Thus, spinal cord neurons became an exciting new option with the promise of avoiding effects on the brain. Also during the 1970s, pharmacokinetic studies refined the use of opioids by the intravenous route with the objective of minimizing brain effects such as sedation and respiratory depression, while maintaining analgesia.[18,251,317,347]

Brain, spinal cord, and *axon* were viewed as three major targets for pain control. It soon became clear, however, that the picture was more complex and that there was significant overlap in the target sites for analgesic actions of the contemporary methods of pain control (Table 28-1). Local anesthetics were found to block axons of sensory tracts (superficial) and motor tracts (deep) in the spinal cord (see reference 104). Intravenous opioids were shown to have a powerful antinociceptive effect at a spinal cord level in animal studies and in humans[208,223] (see Chap. 24.2). Epidural opioids were reported to be absorbed rapidly into the blood, producing early effects on the brain (see below). Particularly hydrophilic (*e.g.*, morphine) but also lipophilic opioids were shown to migrate in cerebrospinal fluid (CSF) to the brain, producing analgesic and other effects, such as sedation, dysphoria, nausea and vomiting, and respiratory depression. Very hydrophilic drugs, such as morphine, diffuse slowly out of the brain, and thus produce long-lasting effects, such as "delayed respiratory depression." Although blood concentrations of spinal opioids rapidly decline and then contribute only minimally to analgesia, it is possible that morphine in the brain may make a significant and continued contribution to the analgesic effects of spinal morphine.

Because brain effects with spinal opioids are dose

TABLE 28-1. TARGET SITES FOR ANALGESIC ACTIONS

	Brain	Spinal Cord	Axons of Spinal Roots
Intravenous opioids	+++	+ (cell)	−
Intraspinal opioids	+	+++ (cell)	−
Intraspinal meperidine	+	+++ (cell)	+
Intraspinal LAs	−	+ (axon)	+++
Intraspinal etidocaine	−	++ (axon)	+++
Intraspinal LA + opioid	+	+++ (cell and axon)	+++

Reproduced with permission from Cousins, M.J., and Phillips, G.D. (eds.): Acute Pain Management. In Ledingham, I.A., and Grenvik, A. (eds.): Clinics in Critical Care Medicine. Edinburgh, Churchill Livingstone, 1986.

related (see below), it seemed logical to attempt to achieve effective analgesia by combining small doses of spinal opioids with low-dose spinal (epidural) local anesthetic.[214] This technique clearly emphasizes a spinal action but acts both at the level of axons and of neurons. In addition, it aims to block axons in spinal nerve roots. Such an approach has appeal for acute pain because it minimizes the potential for toxicity owing to vascular absorption of local anesthetic and decreases the degree of motor blockade, thus preserving motor activity.

In chronic pain the use of intrathecal and epidural morphine rapidly gained acceptance, particularly in patients with some, but not too much, prior exposure to oral opiates. In such patients there was a minimal incidence of side-effects such as pruritus, sedation, respiratory depression, and urinary retention. However, tolerance to spinal morphine, not surprisingly, was reported (see reference 418). Also some forms of cancer pain either responded poorly or not at all.[13] Help in this case came not from local anesthetics, but from brilliant experiments showing several populations of opioid receptors and nonopioid antinociceptive systems. Fortunately, it seems that there is a lack of cross tolerance among at least some of these systems. (see reference 418). Also, different types of pain may be associated with different antinociceptive systems, raising the hope that pain unresponsive to spinal opioid may sometimes be responsive to spinal administration of agents acting on other spinal antinociceptive systems.

Another important historical perspective relates to the realization that there are inevitable sequelae of acute and chronic pain that require attention. In the case of acute pain, anxiety and sleeplessness have a powerful influence on pain and the need for analgesic agents; failure to use the appropriate nonpharmacologic and pharmacologic measures for these symptoms may result in inappropriate and excessive use of analgesic techniques (see reference 105).

In the case of chronic pain, sleeplessness, anxiety, depression, anger, social isolation, and other complex factors play a major part; this is also so in cancer pain. Proper attention to these issues reduces the need for pain relief. The use of oral opioids and "adjuvant drugs" reduces the need for other methods of pain control, such as neurolytic blocks and spinal opioids, to less than 10% of patients with cancer pain (see Chap. 24.1). Nevertheless, spinal opioids have gained a significant place in the treatment of cancer pain, partly at the expense of more invasive techniques, such as neurolytic procedures (see Chap. 29.2) and percutaneous neurosurgical techniques (see Chap. 30).

In a comprehensive review in 1984, Cousins and Mather outlined a substantial number of key questions that required answers, for the safe and effective use of spinal opioids.[102] In 1986 Cousins and Bridenbaugh reevaluated the literature and concluded that many important questions remained unanswered[98] (see p. 1016), so that knowledge of spinal opioids was far less than knowledge of spinal local anesthetics with respect to acute pain.[44,97,331,363] In cancer pain there is an even greater need for clinical data; for example, by 1986 not a single controlled study had shown an advantage of spinal opioids over simple methods, such as regular oral opioid, despite enthusiastic clinical anecdotal reports of greatly superior pain relief with spinal opioids.

Two thousand years of essentially unchanged methods of treatment of acute and chronic pain with opioids were associated with little fundamental information about actions and side-effects of opioids. Spectacular progress in the past 10 years has been based on several important lines of new information (see also Chap. 24.2):

1. Knowledge of neurologic mechanisms of pain increased markedly and, to a large extent, overturned previously held views. At a spinal level, a pivotal event in 1965 was the publication of Melzack and Wall's "gate theory of pain," suggesting that nociception could be modulated in spinal cord.[263]
2. In 1976 Martin and associates confirmed an earlier proposal of 1967 that distinct, complimentary opiate receptors in the brain may be activated or blocked by selected drugs.[248] From their work emerged evidence of mu_1 receptors (analgesia,

miosis, euphoria, hypothermia) and mu_2 receptors (bradycardia, sedation, and respiratory depression). This raised the possibility of analgesia without respiratory depression (see reference 251).

3. Animal models for pain were refined and used to develop new and potent analgesic agents. Fundamental to this work was the synthesis in 1961 of the opioid receptor antagonist naloxone and the later synthesis of antagonists selective for different opioid receptors.
4. In 1969 behavioral analgesia was produced by electrical stimulation of the periaqueductal gray matter of the medulla.[315] This analgesia was similar to that achieved with microinjections of morphine into the same area. Both analgesic effects were antagonized by naloxone. The analgesia was shown to be due to descending monoaminergic systems acting on the dorsal horn of spinal cord (see Chap. 24.2).
5. Calvillo and associates[60] and Duggan and associates[132,133] provided evidence of spinal analgesic effects of morphine with electrophysiologic studies after iontophoretic application of morphine to the dorsal horn region. Again the effect was antagonized by naloxone.
6. Identification of receptors for opioids and naloxone was reported in 1973 independently by Pert and Snyder,[296] by Terenius,[356] and by Simon and co-workers.[340] This was followed in 1975 by the isolation and characterization of the endogenous opioids, the enkephalins, by Hughes and others.[196]
7. The distribution of opiate receptors was mapped in 1977 by autoradiographic techniques. Major sites with high density of receptors were the substantia gelatinosa of spinal cord, medullary dorsal horn, periaqueductal gray matter, and other brain sites.[16]
8. In 1976 Yaksh and Rudy reported that intrathecal morphine in rats produced dose-dependent, stereospecific, and naloxone-reversible behavioral analgesia to noxious stimulation. It was postulated that this analgesia was mediated at a spinal level, since H^3-morphine showed only limited rostral spread to the brain.[423] Brilliant exploitation of chronic intrathecal and epidural catheter techniques in various animal models provided carefully controlled data concerning dose relationships, relative potency, receptor affinities, tolerance and cross tolerance, neurotoxicity, and other fundamental aspects of spinal opioids.[415] Evidence for multiple forms of spinal opioid receptors has been provided. Also, nonopioid systems have been reported to be associated with antinociceptive activity[399,402,415] (see Chap. 24.2).

Clinical reports of "selective" and long-duration analgesia after spinal administration of opioids were tempered by documentation of a number of side-effects, such as sedation, pruritus, nausea and vomiting, urinary retention, and both early and late respiratory depression.[32,100,101,120,121,160,241,314] Fortunately, the serious complication of delayed respiratory depression was reported soon after clinical use began in humans[160,241] and acted as a stimulus to promote appropriate further studies of this and other side-effects of intrathecal and epidural opioids in humans.[98] At the same time there has been a rapid increase in knowledge fundamental to spinal use of opioids through extensive animal studies.[401,418]

This chapter summarizes animal data that provide the basis of the physiology and pharmacology of intrathecal and epidural administration of opioids. The reader will find a detailed description of the physiology and pharmacology of spinal mechanisms of pain and analgesia in Chapter 24.2 and in Tables 24-10, 24-11, and Figs. 24-6 through 24-10. The clinical use of spinal opioids will be described in both acute pain and chronic pain. Emphasis will be placed on controlled studies of efficacy and safety and on comparative studies with other techniques of pain relief.

OPIOIDS AND RECEPTORS: TERMINOLOGY

The old term *narcotic* ("narco" in Greek is to deaden) is applicable to many drugs and is so vague that it is of little use. The term *opiate* refers to morphine and drugs of related structure; *opioid*, a much broader term, includes all drugs with morphinelike properties *(exogenous)* and the *endogenous* peptides (see reference 251). Unfortunately, there have been many interpretations of the use of these terms and they have often been used interchangeably. For example, "opioid receptor" is the correct term; however, many classic studies have described "opiate receptors." Opioid agonists are defined pharmacologically by their ability to activate opioid receptors and for this action to be antagonized by the pure opioid antagonist naloxone. The "receptors" are specialized macromolecules that are acted on by molecules with appropriate three-dimensional shape ("stereospecificity"); such molecules are called "ligands." The part of the receptor molecule where ligands attach is called a "binding site." In order to produce an effect (*e.g.*, analgesia), the receptor needs to link up with an "effector mechanism."

An *agonist* is a drug that produces an effect; an *antagonist* blocks that effect. A "partial agonist" produces only a percentage of the maximum effect obtained with a "pure agonist." An agonist/antagonist may produce agonist effects as well as antagonize the effect of other agonists.

The *affinity* of a drug for a receptor describes its attraction to the binding site, and the *efficacy* (or intrinsic activity) is the ability of the drug to activate the effector mechanism when bound to the receptor. Thus, naloxone, a pure opioid antagonist, has high affinity and zero efficacy. Duration of action of opioid agonists is partly influenced by their rate of dissociation from opioid receptors. For example, the partial agonist drug buprenorphine has a slow rate of dissociation from its receptor and a long duration of action. For other drugs with a rapid rate of receptor dissociation, the concentration of opioid in the bloodstream or CSF, and, in turn, redistribution and rate of clearance (*e.g.*, by liver), may determine duration of action (see reference 251).

TABLE 28-2. PHYSICOCHEMICAL PROPERTIES OF OPIOIDS AND LOCAL ANESTHETICS

	Molecular Weight*	pK_a (25°C)	Partition Coefficient†
Local anesthetics‡			
Procaine hydrochloride	236	8.9	0.02§
Lidocaine hydrochloride	234	7.9	2.9§
Bupivacaine hydrochloride	288	8.1	27.5§
Etidocaine hydrochloride	276	7.7	141§
Opioids‡			
Morphine sulfate	285	7.9¶	1.42**
Meperidine hydrochloride	247	8.5	38.8**
Methadone hydrochloride	309	9.3	116**
Fentanyl citrate	336	8.4	813**
Sufentanil citrate	386	8.0	1,778**
(−)Lofentanil cis-oxalate	408	7.8	1,450**
β-endorphin	3,300	—	—

*Base.
†*n*-Heptane and octanol partition coefficients are strongly correlated for similar compounds in a log–log relationship.
‡Commonly used forms (see Mather,[250] Tucker and Mather[363]).
§*n*-Heptane/*p*H 7.4 buffer, partition coefficient.
¶Tertiary amino group.
**Octanol/*p*H 7.4 buffer partition coefficient.

PHYSICOCHEMICAL PROPERTIES AND ACTIONS OF OPIOIDS AND LOCAL ANESTHETICS

There are similarities in molecular weight and pK_a between local anesthetics and opioids. Although partition coefficients listed in Table 28-2 were derived from two systems, there is considerable overlap. The phenylpiperidine derivatives (meperidine, fentanyl, lofentanil) are closest in structure to local anesthetics. The rate of absorption of meperidine from the epidural space is similar to that of lidocaine, and like lidocaine, it has a rapid onset of analgesia after epidural use that coincides with early peak meperidine concentrations in CSF.[103,159,354] Of note, high concentrations (2%–4%) of meperidine can produce profound peripheral nerve block[378]; however, such concentrations are unlikely to be used epidurally. Fentanyl sufentanil, and lofentanil are highly lipid soluble. This property should promote rapid onset of action with minimal residual CSF concentrations of drug that could be available to migrate to the brain. In contrast, morphine has a lower lipid solubility. It has a slow onset of action after epidural use that coincides with delayed peak concentrations of morphine in CSF,[281,354] and its relative hydrophilicity results in slower efflux from the spinal cord and CSF, resulting in greater migration to the brain.[161,257]

At *p*H 7.4, the tertiary amine group in each of the opioids is mostly ionized, making the molecule water soluble. In addition, in the case of morphine, hydroxyl groups on the molecule confer significant water solubility, so that is why morphine base is much more water soluble than any other opioid base in clinical use (Table 28-3).

Studies in animals and humans (*vide infra*) now point to presynaptic and postsynaptic receptors in the substantia gelatinosa of the dorsal horn of the spinal cord as a major site of action of spinally administered opioids.[418] In contrast, local anesthetics act by axonal membrane blockade, predominantly in the spinal nerve roots (Table 28-4 and Figs. 28-1 through 28-5). Of the opioids, only intrathecal meperidine, 1 mg/kg, has been shown effective as a sole agent for surgery.[267] Presumably, this reflects combined local anesthetic and opiate effects. Spinal opioids are gen-

TABLE 28-3. PHYSICOCHEMICAL PROPERTIES OF OPIOIDS

At *p*H 7.4 N^3 group mostly ionized ∴ all H_2O soluble
Morphine (M̲) OH groups → ↑H_2O soluble + ↓lipid soluble
Cord uptake of M̲ and onset of analgesia is slow
Cord "washout" of M̲ is slow and analgesia prolonged
High residual levels of CSF M̲ reach brain
Highly lipid-soluble opioids → rapid cord uptake, rapid onset (and offset) of analgesia, ? low brain stem CSF levels

TABLE 28-4. COMPARISON OF ACTIONS AND EFFICACY OF SPINALLY APPLIED OPIOIDS AND LOCAL ANESTHETICS

	Opioids	Local Anesthetics
Actions		
Site of action	Substantia gelatinosa of dorsal horn of spinal cord*	Nerve roots (and long tracts in spinal cord)
Type of blockade	Presynaptic and (postsynaptic) inhibition of neuron cell excitation (Fig. 28-2)	Blockade of nerve impulse conduction in axonal membrane
Modalities blocked	"Selective" block of pain conduction	Blockade of sympathetic and pain fibers, often also loss of sensation and motor function (Fig. 28-4)
Efficacy		
Type of pain and efficacy of blockade		
Surgical pain	Partial relief	Complete relief possible
Labor pain	Partial relief	Complete relief
Postoperative pain†		
Early first 24 h	Partial to complete relief (high dose)	Complete relief
24 h +	Complete relief (low dose)	Complete relief
Chronic pain	Complete relief	Impracticable (usually)

*And/or other sites where opioid receptors (binding sites) are present.

†Pain after major surgery requires higher doses (*e.g.*, thoracotomy, 6 mg morphine) than pain after more minor surgery (*e.g.*, lower abdominal, 4 mg morphine). Continuous infusion reduces dose in both situations.

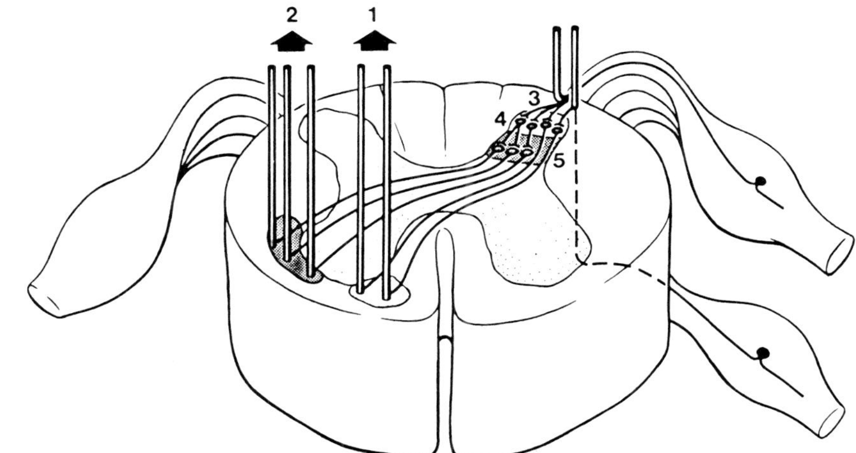

FIG. 28-1. Ascending pathways and dorsal horn region of spinal cord. Afferent fibers are shown entering the dorsal nerve root by way of dorsal root ganglion to reach Lissauer's tract *(3)*. Primary afferents have their cell body in the dorsal root ganglion. The second order neuron has its cell body in the substantia gelatinosa *(4)*. *(1)* and *(2)* = intermingled fibers of spinothalamic and spinoreticular tracts; *(5)* = Rexeds laminae IV, V, VI.

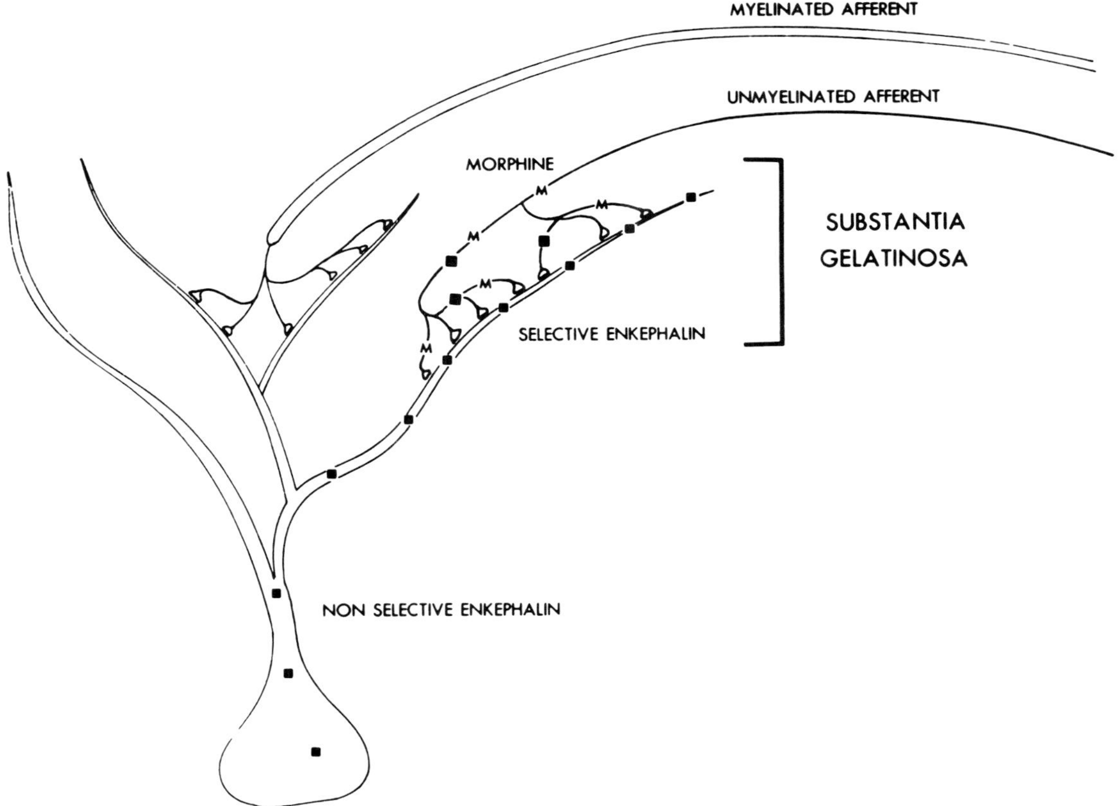

FIG. 28-2. Dorsal horn neuron. Proposed distribution of receptors for morphine (M) and enkephalin (■) in dorsal horn. The neuron is in laminae IV or V, with its dendrites projecting dorsally. In cats, morphine depressed nociceptive responses when administered by micropipette into the substantia gelatinosa (SG) but not at more ventral sites. Enkephalin depressed cell firing when ejected near cell body dendrites and at more dorsal sites, including SG. This suggested that receptors for morphine may be restricted to presynaptic terminals, whereas enkephalin also may act on postsynaptic dendrites. (Reprinted from Duggan, A.W., Johnson, S.M., and Morton, C.R.: Differing distribution of receptors for morphine and met ^{5}-enkephalinamide in the dorsal horn of the cat. Brain Res., *229*: 379, 1981, with permission of the publisher.)

erally ineffective, unless used with dilute local anesthetics, for second-stage labor pain. They are useful to provide the analgesic component of anesthetic techniques and provide an alternative technique for postoperative pain relief. A valuable application is in the management of chronic pain and, in particular, cancer pain (Table 28-5).

THERAPEUTIC ADVANTAGE

The term *selective spinal analgesia* was suggested by Cousins and associates[103] in 1979 to emphasize the difference between the analgesia obtained with relatively nonselective blockade of axonal conduction of local anesthetics and that of spinal opioids. Although subsequent clinical studies revealed effects of spinal morphine on systems other than antinociception, further animal studies have developed this concept of "selective spinal analgesia" by identifying opioid and nonopioid spinal systems and are progressively moving toward the goal of selective blockade of nociception with minimal or no effects on other systems. Even if this goal is reached, it is likely that the "selectivity" will still be relative, since high doses of any agonist are likely to progressively produce effects on systems other than the primary site of action. This may indicate the desirability of using two agonists acting on different antinociceptive systems, so that the dose of each can be kept at a level that eliminates side actions on systems other than antinociception (see Fig. 28-3).

The major advantages of "selective" blockade of pain by spinal opioids lies in the absence of sympathetic blockade and postural hypotension, potentially allowing easy ambulation of patients, and avoidance of cardiovascular collapse or convulsions — the major complications of local anesthetic blockade. However, early and late respiratory depression are major concerns with spinal opioids. The potential side-effects of intrathecal and epidural use of local anesthetics and opioids are summarized in Tables 28-6, 28-7. Decisions concerning the relative merits of spinal use of the two classes of drugs should be based on the therapeutic index for their respective life-threatening toxic effects compared with analgesic effects. Additional considerations should be based on any differences in rapidity of onset of toxic effects (Tables 28-6, 28-7). A large overdose of intrathecal opioid, or an inappropriate supplementary intravenous dose, may result in sudden apnea, necessitating rapid treatment. Usually onset of respiratory arrest is gradual, with more time available for diagnosis and implementation of treatment. However, in the case of morphine, prolonged and insidious depression of ventilatory response to carbon dioxide may occur and, if not diagnosed and treated, may be followed by sudden apnea, particularly if other risk factors, such as concomitant use of other central nervous system (CNS) depressants, are added. In contrast, local anesthetic-induced convulsions or circulatory depression is usually rapid in

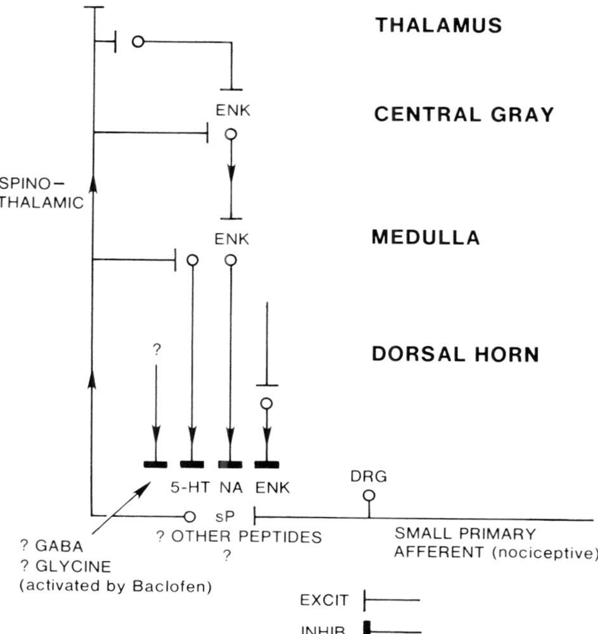

FIG. 28-3. Model of pain transmission. Proposed excitatory *(excit)* and inhibitory *(inhib)* pathways and transmitters are shown. DRG = dorsal root ganglion; SP = substance P; 5-HT = serotonin; NA = noradrenaline (norepinephrine); ENK = enkephalin; GABA = gamma-amino butyric acid. Primary afferent nociceptive impulses are conducted by way of DRG to spinothalamic and spinoreticular neurons in the dorsal horn with substance P as transmitter. Collaterals supply medulla and central gray matter. Enkephalin activates descending pathways (GABA, 5HT, NA), which inhibit primary afferent transmission. Within dorsal horn there are local enkephalin (opioid) inhibitory systems.

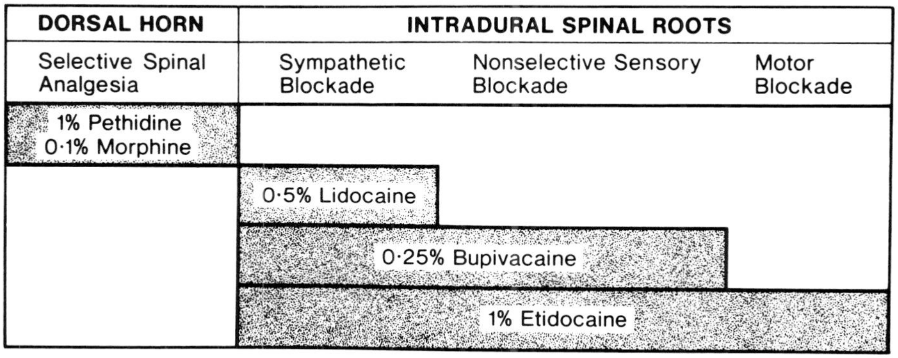

FIG. 28-4. "Selective spinal analgesia" by opioids, acting by means of selective action on presynaptic and postsynaptic opioid receptors (see Fig. 28-2). In comparison, local anesthetics nonselectively block axonal conduction with degree of sympathetic, sensory, and motor block, depending on local anesthetic used and its concentration.

DORSAL HORN	INTRADURAL SPINAL ROOTS		
Selective Spinal Analgesia	Sympathetic Blockade	Nonselective Sensory Blockade	Motor Blockade
1% Pethidine 0·1% Morphine			
	0·5% Lidocaine		
	0·25% Bupivacaine		
	1% Etidocaine		

TABLE 28-5. REPORTED CLINICAL APPLICATIONS OF INTRATHECAL AND EPIDURAL OPIOIDS

Reported Applications	Technique	References
Acute Pain		
During surgery (and postsurgery)		
Open heart	Intrathecal	17, 211, 255
Gynecologic	Epidural	80, 127
General surgery	Epidural	276, 349
	Intrathecal	156, 218, 327, 264
Orthopedic	Intrathecal	156
Postsurgery		
Thoracotomy	Epidural	73, 141, 159, 181, 281, 359, 382
Orthopedic	Epidural	6, 73, 138, 171, 247
	Epidural-intrathecal	26
	Intrathecal	218
Prostatectomy	Epidural	164, 348
Abdominal and general surgery	Epidural	14, 46, 112-114, 245, 300, 308, 309, 313, 359, 360, 379
	Epidural infusion	22, 86, 113
Anal and urogenital	Caudal epidural	40
	Epidural	157,164,359
Gynecologic	Epidural	56, 80, 107, 112, 127, 259
Posttrauma pain	Epidural	41, 209, 245, 359
Obstetrics		
Labor pain*	Intrathecal	3, 25, 289, 333, 345
	Epidural	37, 64, 152, 198-201, 245, 274, 283, 294, 295, 370
Postcesarean section	Epidural	28, 54, 55, 119, 227, 277, 391, 394
Second trimester abortion	Epidural	244
Complicated obstetrics (single ventricle) labor pain	Intrathecal	5
Acute medical conditions		
Myocardial infarction	Epidural	343
	Intrathecal	291
Thrombophlebitis	Epidural	245
Herpes zoster	Epidural	245, 359
Nephrolithiasis	Epidural	245
Chronic Pain		
Cancer pain	Intrathecal (single dose)	103, 290, 372, 375
	Intrathecal catheter with implanted pump	90, 288, 293
	Epidural top-up via percutaneous catheter	19, 103, 111, 159, 189, 349, 350, 393, 428
	Epidural via implanted "portal"	76
	Epidural infusion via implanted catheter and infusion pump	90, 92, 94
Chronic noncancer pain		
Bladder spasm	Epidural	286
Back pain	Epidural	19, 197, 245, 359
Ischemic rest pain	Epidural	234, 245, 359
Causalgia	Epidural	19, 245
Spasticity—muscle spasm	Epidural	148
Diagnosis of chronic pain	Epidural	77, 99

*Most studies reported unsatisfactory relief of labor pain with epidural morphine and satisfactory relief only after high-dose meperidine with added epinephrine. In comparison, intrathecal opioids were more effective. Combination of opioid and local anesthetic is effective.

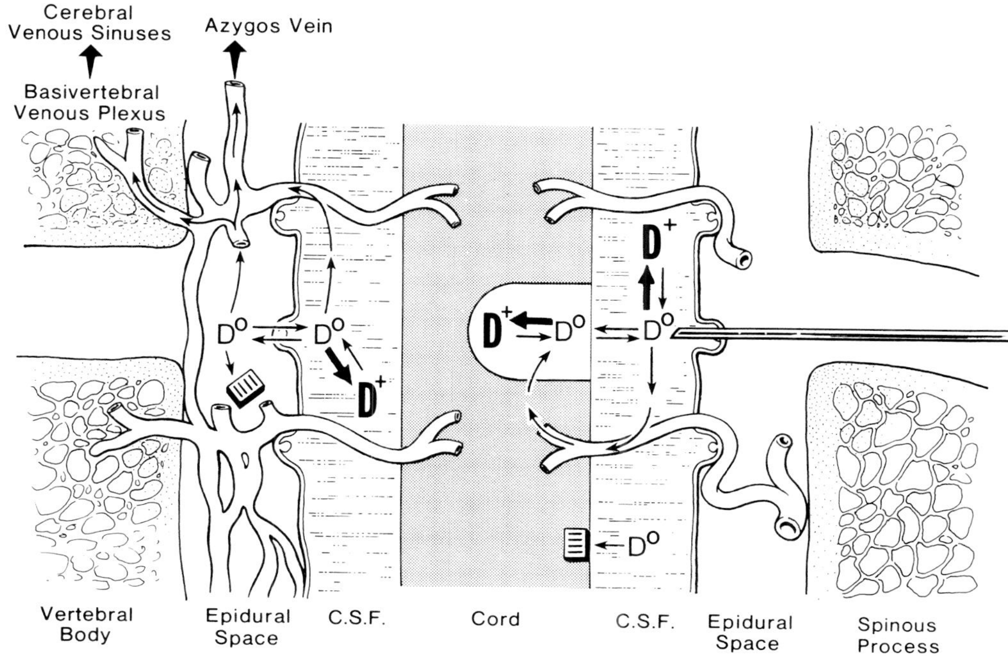

FIG. 28-5. Pharmacokinetic model: Subarachnoid injection of a hydrophilic opioid such as morphine. D^0 = un-ionized drug; D^+ = ionized hydrophilic drug. A spinal needle is shown delivering opioid directly to the CSF. Nearby spinal arteries are in proximity to arachnoid granulations (also see Fig. 28-11). In the spinal cord, equilibria of D^0 and D^+ on spinal receptors are shown, as well as nonspecific lipid binding sites *(shaded squares)*. Epidural veins, in proximity to arachnoid granulations, are depicted as the major spinal route of clearance of intrathecal opioid. The two alternative routes of venous drainage are shown.

onset and necessitates urgent treatment. The specific treatment of opioid-induced respiratory depression appears safer than that used to treat local anesthetic toxic effects (Table 28-7). Side-effects causing discomfort can result from both classes of drugs, with nausea and vomiting being more common from opioids and urinary retention similar from both classes of drugs, although tolerance to this effect develops with opioids and is antagonized by naloxone. Only spinal opioids appear to cause the strange phenomenon of pruritus (see Table 28-6).

NEUROTOXIC POTENTIAL

Another aspect concerning the safety of spinal opioids is their compatibility with CSF and neural tissue. Solutions of opioids of potential use in spinal injections (morphine, methadone, meperidine, fentanyl, alfentanil, lofentanil, and buprenorphine) and local anesthetics in normal saline had *p*H ranging from 4.52 to 6.85. When mixed with CSF, all lowered *p*H of the CSF by 0.3 or less, but etidocaine lowered *p*H by 0.82, with clouding of CSF.[39] Histologic examination of spinal cords of cancer patients who had epidural administration of bupivacaine–morphine mixture for 3 weeks[4] or morphine for up to 6 months[95] revealed no abnormality attributable to morphine. Two of seven patients had posterior column degeneration, which was suggested to be most likely caused by neuropathy associated with malignant disease.[91] Further studies of spinal cord pathology after prolonged spinal administration of opioids are required to resolve this question. A finding of technical significance was focal thickening of the dura in the vicinity of epidural catheters of four patients, with fibrous tissue cocoons surrounding the catheters (see pharmacokinetic section). Animal studies of the potential damage to the spinal cord of epidural catheters and repeated injection of opioids

TABLE 28-6. EFFECTS AND SIDE-EFFECTS

Effects and Side Effects	Spinal Opioids	Spinal Local Anesthetics
Cardiovascular	Minor heart rate changes	Low-block (below T10) sympathetic blockade: postural hypotension
	Usually not postural hypotension	High-block (above T4) sympathetic blockade: Postural hypotension
	Vasoconstrictor response intact	Cardio-accelerator block: ↓ HR, ↓ inotropic drive (see Chap. 8)
Respiratory	Early depression*† (0.1–1 h); systemically absorbed drug and ? CSF-borne drug Late depression*† (6–24 h); opioid in CSF migrating to brain (see Figs. 28-5, 28-7)	Usually unimpaired unless cardiovascular collapse
CNS		
Sedation	May be marked*	Mild or absent, depending on agent
Convulsions	Usually not seen with clinical doses; theoretical possibility at high doses	Expected toxicity from two times overdose or with rapid vascular absorption
Other neurologic abnormalities	Confusion, amnesia, catalepsy, hallucinations (reported with high doses intrathecally)	Not usually seen
Opioid withdrawal	If rapid discontinuation of systemic opioids	
Nausea	Yes*	Yes—low incidence
Vomiting	Yes*	Yes—low incidence
Pruritis	Yes*	No
Miosis	Yes	No (unless Horner's syndrome)
Urinary retention	Yes*†	Yes

*Antagonized by naloxone, but repeated doses may be required.
†Prevented by naloxone infusion 5–10 μg/kg/h without reversal of analgesic effects.[304,307]

TABLE 28-7. THERAPEUTIC RATIO AND SAFETY OF SPECIFIC TREATMENT OF TOXICITY

	Spinal Opioids	Spinal Local Anesthetics
Therapeutic ratio toxic effect versus analgesic effect*	Unknown ? Intrathecal >2, ? Epidural >2 (*Respiratory depression)	Approximately 2. (*Cardiovascular [CVS] depression or convulsions)
Time delay in onset of major toxic effect	May be hour(s). However, sometimes rapid if large intrathecal dose	May be seconds to minutes
Response time required for treatment	Minutes to hours unless marked respiratory depression or apnea	Seconds to minutes
Specific drug treatment	Naloxone—no other harmful effects (usually)	Atropine and α-, β-agonists, used to treat CVS depression, may themselves cause adverse CVS effects. CNS depressant drugs used to treat convulsions may themselves contribute to prolonged coma and may increase CVS depression.

Therapeutic ratio is the ratio of blood concentrations producing toxic effect to maximum blood concentrations attained during safe use of appropriate agents.
*See Table 28-6.

have not revealed significant histologic changes. Yaksh reported that 14 macaque monkeys with epidural catheters *in situ* for 4 to 16 months and receiving 15 to 122 injections of morphine had no abnormal neurologic signs. Three of the monkeys were sacrificed for autopsy after 6, 8, and 9 months and after 44, 68, and 72 intrathecal injections of a variety of opioids and peptides. No histologic evidence of cord pathology was found.[402,418] Abouleish and coworkers[4] found no immediate or chronic (42 days) changes in spinal cord histology attributable to a single intrathecal injection of a large dose of morphine (0.07 mg/kg).

In cats with *intrathecally* implanted catheters receiving only intrathecal saline and killed 19 to 21 days after implantation, an inflammatory response developed, with a thin fibrotic sleeve surrounding the catheter with no obstruction to the tip. Where the catheter lay in contact with the spinal cord, a mild deformation of the cord was present, with local demyelination at the point of contact. Animals that received the ED_{100} for alfentanil or sufentanil daily for 5 days showed spinal cord pathology indistinguishable from those receiving saline. Animals receiving ten times the ED_{100} of either drug showed results similar to controls.[419] Chronically implanted *epidural* catheters in rats resulted in the rapid development of a fibrotic reaction in 36 of 43 rats after only 1 day. After 10 days of catheterization, a thick fibrotic reaction obstructing the catheter tip was observed in 31 of 33 rats. Injection of methylene blue showed no spread into the epidural space; the dye filled the lumen of the catheter and then the sheath, making a blue spot on the skin if the injection was continued. A mild deformation of the dura was observed in all animals.[136]

Consideration of the well-controlled animal studies and the limited human data indicates that the opioid drugs are probably not neurotoxic at the doses and concentrations tested. However, fibrotic reactions were seen with intrathecal and epidural catheters made of polyethylene. In animal studies this may have contributed to mild indentation of dura (epidural catheters) and local demyelination (intrathecal catheters). This raises some concern about the posterior column degeneration reported in clinical cases. Clearly the use of more inert materials for chronically implanted intrathecal and epidural catheters should be investigated. Neuropathology of long-term administration of local anesthetics epidurally and intrathecally has only recently been investigated, as discussed in Chapter 29.1.

SITE OF ANALGESIC ACTION OF SPINAL OPIOIDS

The weight of evidence now points to the dorsal horn as the site of action of spinal opioids based on the following data:

1. Iontophoretic and microinjection data show a strong focus of activity in the substantia gelatinosa.
2. Autoradiographs after application of radiolabeled morphine or fentanyl to the surface of the spinal cord show that the front of radioactivity corresponds to the substantia gelatinosa at a time when the discharge of lamina V neurons to noxious stimuli was reduced significantly.
3. Latencies for inhibition of lamina V neurons after intrathecal administration of morphine are similar to those reported for the latency to block the skin twitch response after intrathecal morphine in the cat.[223,398] Also, it is likely that there is both presynaptic and postsynaptic inhibition of primary afferent transmission in the spinal cord (see Fig. 28-2).[134,154]
4. Release of the putative nociceptive neurotransmitter is inhibited by locally applied opioids.
5. Systemically administered low doses of opioids in decerebrate spinal animals selectively depresses A-delta and C fiber evoked activity in dorsal horn neurons and inhibits *in vivo* nociceptive reflexes.[12,398]
6. Intrathecal administration of opioid agonists produces powerful analgesia in all species examined (see Chap. 24.2).
7. Analgesic effects are antagonized by low doses of naloxone.
8. Order of time courses for onset of analgesia correspond closely with order of lipid partition coefficients of agents, which is known to correlate with rate of diffusion to CSF and presumably to the spinal cord.[418,419]

However, there may be differences in relative importance of sites of action for different opioid and nonopioid agonists. For example, intrathecal morphine probably acts predominantly at the spinal cord level, with a secondary analgesic effect owing to supraspinal migration of the drug.[161] Very lipid-soluble drugs with low affinity for spinal receptors (*e.g.*, fentanyl) may act only partly at a spinal level with significant brain effects, during the short time course of action.[419] Lipid-soluble drugs with high receptor affinity, such as lofentanil, may have predominant spinal action because of rapid delivery to spinal receptors and slow dissociation, as well as local deposition in spinal lipid[419] (see section on pharmacokinetics).

How do opioids produce their spinal analgesic effects? As discussed below, there is strong evidence of analgesic effects at mu, delta, and kappa receptors,[402,418] which constitute approximately 40%, 10%, and 50%, respectively, of the spinal opioid receptors.[115] Also, there is evidence of both presynaptic and postsynaptic sites of action of spinal opioids.[134,418]

The opioid effector mechanism at the neuronal level is probably inhibitory and likely to be mediated by means of ion channels.[431] Mechanisms have been most closely studied in peripheral nerve tissue, such as the myenteric plexus; however, it is thought that this may reflect the situation in the spinal cord.[431] *Mu and delta receptors* may be coupled to voltage- or calcium-dependent potassium channels; *kappa receptors* inhibit voltage-dependent calcium channels.[385] Mu and delta receptor activation could result in hyperpolarization of membranes and decreased neuronal responses to excitatory transmitters.[431] Kappa receptor activation could result in blockade of calcium ion influx in axonal terminals, and thus inhibition of transmitter release.[385] If the latter proves to be true, it could pose an exciting challenge for molecular engineering to design a drug with chemical and physical properties limiting its action to only *spinal* terminals of axons of A-delta C fibers.

Are there differences in spinal opioid efficacy for different types of pain? In *acute pain* states, sharp pain (A-delta fibers) seems to be blocked less readily than dull pain (C fibers). Thus, labor pain and surgical pain are not completely blocked. This may be due to the following factors:

1. The deeper location of A-delta fibers in the dorsal horn compared with C fibers.[411]
2. Opioids reduce the rate of the excitatory postsynaptic potential (EPSP) and thereby attenuate the temporal summating properties of the neuronal membrane. This effect is more likely to occur with the more slowly conducting C fibers compared with the more rapidly conducting A-delta fibers.[431]
3. Different opioid receptors may be associated with different types of pain: *Mu agonists* (*e.g.*, morphine, sufentanil) are active in cutaneous thermal tests (hot plate, tail flick), which may approximate somatic pain, and in tests using intraperitoneal administration of irritant chemicals (writhing test), which may approximate visceral pain. *Delta agonists* (*e.g.*, DADL) are active in cutaneous thermal tests but show no activity for visceral tests. *Kappa agonists* (*e.g.*, U-50488H) have no activity on cutaneous thermal tests but have activity on visceral tests.[418]
4. There may be pharmacokinetic factors determining how much drug reaches the three opioid receptor populations. For example, after epidural meperidine in pregnancy, rapid venous uptake from distended epidural venous plexuses results in much higher blood levels than in nonpregnant women. Thus, less drug is available to CSF and the spinal cord, resulting in less effective analgesia than in the nonpregnant state.

The relative importance of these factors in acute pain in humans is not clear. For example, in animal tests, intrathecal morphine is equally effective in both somatic-type and visceral-type testing.[423] Yet in humans, intrathecal morphine does not abolish sharp somatic pain associated with surgical incision.

In *cancer pain*, the situation is more complex. "Central" pain unresponsive to oral opioids is not likely to respond to spinal opioids. Also, it has been reported that *intermittent* sharp somatic pain from cutaneous structures and intermittent visceral pain respond poorly to spinal morphine.[13] Continuous dull somatic pain from deep structures and continuous visceral pain respond most predictably to spinal morphine. Other differences among opioids may relate to non-antinociceptive effects. For example, DADL does not produce the "scratching" phenomenon seen with high-dose morphine. Neither does it produce adverse motor effects, such as seizures and rigidity (see below).

It seems possible that the combined use of spinal opioids of different receptor affinities (see Table 24-11) may help to improve the situation. Also, the efficacy of nonopioid spinal analgesic drugs[404,406,420,424,425] needs evaluation for different types of human pain, in comparison with spinal opioids. At present there are no adequate animal models of all types of human cancer pain.

PROPOSED PATHWAYS AND TRANSMITTERS

Microiontophoretic studies previously suggested that GABA mediated presynaptic inhibition and glycine mediated postsynaptic inhibition.[154] However, enkephalin-containing neurons are present in substantia gelatinosa.[143] Evidence suggests that this intrinsic system is activated by segmental somatic input and is inhibitory.[132,407] In decerebrate rats, subarachnoid morphine selectively depressed activity in ascending axons of spinal cord evoked by electrical stimulation of primary nociceptive afferents.[129] There is also evidence for enkephalinergic systems located in medullary and brain stem regions, activated by input and producing descending inhibition of dorsal horn neurons. Such descending inhibition was shown to have a tonic component in experiments using reversible cold block of the cervical cord. It appeared that GABA and glycine were not involved in this process and that it was not mediated by way of a spinal opiate system. The most likely candidates as transmitters for these systems are serotonin and norepinephrine.[312,369,404,405] Subarachnoid injections of clonidine (α_2-adrenergic agonist) or ST-91 (α_1-adrenergic agonist) result in spinal analgesia,[420] which is antagonized by yohimbine and prazocin, respectively. Subarachnoid serotonin also produces spinal analgesia, which is antagonized by methysergide.[425]

Baclofen (which appears to act on a subpopulation of GABA receptors) also has been shown to produce behavioral analgesia when applied to the spinal cord and to be separate from the opioid system.[390,420] The benzodiazepine midazolam has been reported to produce selective spinal analgesia,[387] which is reversible by the specific benzodiazepine antagonist Ro 15-1788 (imidazobenzodiazepinone). It can be seen that there are complex transmission and modulation systems involved in the nociceptive process, considering the spinal cord only. Figure 28-3 is a model for some proposed mechanisms for inhibitory and excitatory pathways.

The neurotransmitter for nociception has not been identified clearly using the usual criteria.[261] Substance P (SP; 11 amino acids) is found in dorsal root ganglia type B cell bodies,[183-186] in peripheral nerve terminals,[204] and in central terminals of small myelinated and unmyelinated fibers. Substance P has been shown to be released into CSF *in vivo* by high-intensity electrical stimulation of all fiber types of peripheral nerves of rat and cat but not by electrical stimulation at low intensity of only myelinated fibers, and this release is inhibited by concurrent administration of morphine into the intrathecal space.[415] It also has been shown that depletion of dorsal horn SP in animals by intrathecal administration of capsaicin renders the animals insensitive to noxious thermal stimuli.[408] Other peptides have been demonstrated. These include vasoactive intestinal peptide (VIP; 28 amino acids), somatostatin (SOM; 13 amino acids), and cholecystokinin[406] (CCK; 33 amino acids) and may be candidates as neuromodulators or neurotransmitters of the nociceptive information (see Table 24-10). Prostaglandins and prostacyclins also have been implicated in central as well as peripheral mechanisms of nociception.[66,405] There is evidence that transmitters and peptides may be predominantly localized as follows:

Descending systems: Noradrenaline (NA; norepinephrine), serotonin (5-HT), and perhaps enkephalin, dopamine

Interneurons: Enkephalin, gamma-amino-butryic acid (GABA), acetylcholine, SP, neurotensin,[252] and SOM

Primary afferent terminals: VIP,[406] SOM, SP,[415] and CCK.[406] The "model" may be even more complex, since endogenous substances, such as calcitonin, also produce spinal analgesic effects, possibly at the level of the primary afferent terminal (see Chap. 24.2). Evidence for an analgesic effect of a number of these substances has been provided in animals (see Tables 24-2, 24-3) and in humans (see below).

Although this is an incomplete view of the mechanisms, a number of points can be made that have a bearing on clinical applications:

1. These multiple spinal inhibitory systems do not appear to act through a final common pathway, but appear to be independent.
2. These inhibitory systems do appear to be complementary and additive.
3. There has been good pharmacologic definition of the systems.
4. Tolerance (and tachyphylaxis) occurs.
5. Cross tolerance does not occur between the systems. (Also there are more than one population of opioid receptors involved in antinociception in the spinal cord.)
6. Physical properties of exogenous and endogenous drugs and modulators (such as lipophilicity) might be significant for intrathecal and epidural applications.
7. Pain appears to be blocked "selectively," leaving sensory, motor, and sympathetic function essentially intact (see Fig. 28-4).

Some further comment on points 1 through 5 is required, since each of these has clinical implications. Points 6 and 7 are discussed above.

Multiple Spinal Inhibitory Mechanisms. Local opioid inhibition, descending monoaminergic inhibition (activated by supraspinal opiate systems,[397–399] and baclofen (or GABA-type) inhibition have been shown not to act through a final common pathway.[399,404,420] This assertion must be qualified to state that there may be a final common pathway, but it is not opioid, monoaminergic, or GABA-ergic. There may be some overlap between noradrenergic and opioid systems, since intrathecal phentolamine attenuates the analgesia induced by 2.0 but not 7.5 mg/kg, subcutaneous morphine.[299] It has proved difficult to test (or identify) a specific SP antagonist, so the question of the role of SP in nociception is unclear. Capsaicin-treated rats, which are unresponsive to thermal stimuli, still appear to be capable of responding to certain noxious mechanical stimulation.[1,408] It is possible that one or more yet-unidentified transmitters may be responsible. However, it appears that morphine applied directly to the spinal cord is able to block all somatic nociception and at least some visceral nociception (writhing–peritoneal irritation). Spinal administration of the partial agonist nalbuphine had no effect on tail flick or hot plate latencies (thermal pain), but did modify writhing responses (?kappa receptors) to intraperitoneal acetic acid).[329] This implied that there are at least two populations of opioid receptors, some of which are associated with pain response evoked by thermal afferents and some with visceral afferents. Of interest, other partial agonists, pentazocine, cyclazocine, and nalorphine, have been reported to be devoid of any analgesic activity after spinal administration (quoted by Schmauss *et al.*[329]). Evidence has now been reported of at least three opioid receptors associated with antinociception (mu, delta, and kappa). Morphine is the prototype exogenous ligand at mu receptors, DADL at delta receptors and U 50 488H at kappa receptors (see Table 24-11).[402,403,409] Intrathecal administration of the kappa agonist U 50 488H produced analgesia to tail pressure, with a dose-response curve that was parallel to that of morphine. However, U 50 488H did not produce respiratory depression at any dose, whereas morphine was associated with dose-related respiratory depression.[65]

Synergism Occurs Without Cross Tolerance. These spinal inhibitory systems appear to be synergistic[401,402,405,420]; subanalgesic intrathecal doses of morphine, noradrenaline, and baclofen, administered together, produce significant analgesia. Similarly, there does not appear to be cross tolerance between the systems.[366] However, the roles of presynaptic actions (and transmitter depletion) need to be assessed further.

Pharmacologic Definition. The presence of separate opioid and monoaminergic analgesic systems in the spinal cord has been well defined.[401,404] Calvillo and associates administered opioids iontophoretically onto dorsal horn neurons and reported that morphine inhibition of these neurons was antagonized by naloxone.[60] Duggan and co-workers,[134] using micropipette electrophoretic administration, presented evidence for a predominantly presynaptic distribution of morphine-preferring receptors, while enkephalin-preferring receptors were located both presynaptically and postsynaptically (see Fig. 28-2) (see also Chap. 24.2, and Tables 24-10, 24-11).

Tolerance (or Tachyphylaxis) Develops in Each System. This phenomenon, presently unable to be prevented, may impose a time limit on the application of the spinal route to clinical pain management. However, the presence of at least four systems may allow this problem to be overcome by judicious alternation of administered drug. Modification of the synthesis, release, re-uptake, and metabolism of putative transmitters influences analgesic responses.[401] Substitution of drugs with similar structure activity may produce or mimic similar analgesic response, *e.g.*, ST-91, baclofen; opioids; ketamine. Enkephalinase inhibition within CSF also may influence analgesia. Co-administration of drugs acting on different systems, *e.g.*, ST-91 and morphine, seems to slow the development of tolerance.[401,420]

In the opioid system, tolerance to systemic administration of morphine can be demonstrated in dorsal horn neurons of the cat after 3 days' pretreatment with morphine.[207] In the primate, once-daily intrathecal administration of morphine, beta-endorphin, or metkephamid, in a dose producing a "just maximum effect," results in a daily reduction in the analgesic efficacy of the compound. The rate at which loss of responsiveness occurs is related inversely to the duration of analgesic effect produced by the fixed dose of the agonist. This indicates that the rate of onset of tolerance is linked to the time in which the receptor is exposed to the ligand. Primates made tolerant to intrathecal agents showed onset of recovery in 7 days and a near-maximum recovery during the first 1 to 2 weeks after the last intrathecal administration, indicating that the process was reversible.[420] It is possible that more effective pain relief, and slower development of tolerance, may be obtained by continuous administration of the opioid rather than intermittent exposure of the receptors to high concentrations from intermittent doses. Rats rendered tolerant to morphine by systemic administration show cross tolerance to spinal morphine administration, indicating that spinal morphine may not invariably solve the problem of loss of analgesic efficacy of oral morphine administration.[416] Withdrawal responses can follow a changeover from high oral morphine doses to much lower intrathecal doses.[416]

It should be noted in passing that the time course of development of tolerance is reported to be different in "normal" animals, compared with those under conditions of chronic pain. Colpaert found that animals exposed to acute pain (mechanical pinch) or chronic pain (arthritis model induced by *Mycobacterium butyricum*) failed to show tolerance to systemically administered opioids when compared with normal controls.[88] Similarly, Glynn and Mather[158] reported that tolerance was not an inevitable consequence of prolonged (1 year) treatment of chronic pain in patients receiving systemically administered meperidine. These observations would appear to be contrary to the experience of many practitioners and highlight the need for careful observations.

Cross Tolerance Apparently Does Not Develop Among Some of the Spinal Systems. Tolerance may develop in the opioid system throughout most of the range of opioid agonists, with the possible exception of DADL (D-ala^2, D-leu^5-enkephalin). However, recent studies in rat and primate suggest that there may be multiple spinal opioid receptor systems mediating analgesia.[366,403] Tung and Yaksh[366,367] demonstrated a range of potencies from dose–response curves, with lofentanil having high potency, DADL intermediate, and meperidine low potency. Dose–response curves for inhibiting the intrathecal analgesic effects of DADL, metkephamid, and morphine with systemically administered naloxone also were obtained. These data were analyzed in terms of the pA_2 (the negative log of the dose of naloxone that produces a doubling of the ED_{50} of the agonist). The pA_2 is thought to be proportional to the drug–receptor dissociation constant and reflects the interaction of that agonist with the particular antagonist (Table 28-8). The pA_2 value of 6.01 for DADL compared with 6.74 for morphine indicates that it takes approximately five times more naloxone to antagonize the antinociceptive effects of DADL than of morphine.

Animals rendered tolerant to morphine by daily intrathecal injections showed no loss of sensitivity to DADL or with only moderate tolerance to ethylketocyclazocine[366] (EKC) (Table 28-9). This indicates that there are at least two populations of spinal opioid receptors that are associated with antinociception (see Fig. 28-2). Other studies have reported spinal analgesic effects with the kappa agonist U 50 488H[62] (see above). These observations have potentially great clinical significance and suggest that it might be possible to maintain spinal opioid analgesia for prolonged periods by alternating opioid agonists of different receptor characteristic as tolerance develops.

TABLE 28-8. PARAMETERS OF THE DOSE-RATIO PLOT OF NALOXONE FOR INTRATHECALLY ADMINISTERED OPIOIDS IN THE PRIMATE ON THE SHOCK TITRATION THRESHOLD

		Dose-Ratio Parameters*†	
Drug	**N‡**	**Slope§**	**pA_2**
Morphine	4	-1.16 ± 0.21	6.74 ± 0.31
DADL	4	-1.04 ± 0.21	6.01 ± 0.13§
Metkephamid	4	-0.86 ± 0.17	6.25 ± 0.28

DADL = (D-ala^2, D-leu^5)-enkephalin.
(Reprinted from Yaksh, T.L.: In vivo studies on spinal opiate receptor systems mediating antinociception: I. Mu and delta receptor profiles in the primate. J. Pharmacol. Exp. Ther., *226*:303, 1983, with permission of the publisher)
*Details of calculation are as described in text.
†Mean ± SE.
‡N = number of animals.
§Slopes do not differ from −1; $p > 0.1$.
¶Differs from morphine; $p < 0.05$.

Relative loss of activity of various opioid ligands has been studied in rats and primates made tolerant to intrathecal morphine. Loss of analgesic efficacy is in the order: morphine ≥ β-endorphin >> metkephamid ≥ DADL = 0.[402,423,410] In animals made tolerant by intrathecal morphine or EKC, dynorphin β shows a significant loss of activity with the former but not the latter alkaloid.[175] Thus, animals made tolerant to spinal morphine (mu receptor) had little loss of effect of spinal DADL (delta receptor) or EKC (kappa receptor). On the other hand, dynorphin (kappa receptor) was ineffective in animals made tolerant to EKC. Yaksh has drawn attention to the fact that prediction of cross tolerance, or its absence, may be complex.[418] Factors may include dose of the agonists, time of exposure, selectivity of the various agonists, *e.g.*, in some tests metkephamid acts at both mu and delta receptors, yet it is resistant to loss of analgesic activity in morphine-tolerant animals.[418]

Nonopiate spinal analgesia is being intensely investigated in both animal and human studies. In particular, the α-agonists (*e.g.*, clonidine) have been shown

TABLE 28-9. ED$_{50}$ VALUES OF INTRATHECAL MORPHINE, EKC, DADL, AND THE POTENCY RATIOS IN NAIVE AND MORPHINE-TOLERANT ANIMALS

	Morphine	EKC	DADL
ED$_{50}$ before tolerance (μg)	3.9 (2.2–6.9)* (n = 12)	16.6 (11.8–23.4) (n = 25)	6.5 (5.5–7.7) (n = 15)
ED$_{50}$ after tolerance (μg)	27.54 (19.0–39.8) (n = 9)	47.7 (30.9–64.6) (n = 10)	5.9 (3.9–8.9) (n = 8)
ED$_{50}$ ratio (tolerant/naive)	7.1	2.7	0.9

(Reprinted from Tung, A.S., and Yaksh, T.L.: In vivo evidence for multiple opiate receptors mediating analgesia in the rat spinal cord. Brain Res., *247*:75, 1982, with permission of the publisher)
EKG = ethylketocyclazocine; DADL = (D-ala^2, D-leu^5)-enkephalin.
*95% confidence intervals.

to have powerful antinociceptive effects, which show no cross tolerance with opioid agonists.[404,405,420] Intrathecal and epidural clonidine have been successfully used in humans tolerant to spinal morphine[96] (see below). Alternative agonists from other spinal antinociceptive systems are summarized in Figure 28-2 and in Chapter 24.2, Table 24-11. Their use in humans is discussed below.

EFFECTS OF SPINAL OPIOIDS ON SYSTEMS OTHER THAN PAIN

Motor Function. At doses producing antinociceptive effects, spinal opioids have no measurable effects on motor power.[401,418] Monosynaptic stretch reflexes are unaffected, but spinal opioids do suppress polysynaptic flexion reflexes.[388,389] This is of significance, since in a paraplegic, spinal morphine blocks the polysynaptic flexion reflex elicited by sural nerve stimulation but has little effect on the monosynaptic "H" reflex.[165,388] Spinal morphine has now been successfully used for treatment of painful muscle spasms associated with spasticity[148] and multiple sclerosis.[352] This effect is naloxone reversible. At high doses intrathecal morphine in rats may produce two alarming syndromes: [1] convulsive seizures of the hind limbs and hyperreflexia in response to cutaneous stimuli, and [2] intense motor rigidity (the "banana rat" syndrome). Neither of these are antagonized by naloxone—implying an action on receptors other than those involved in antinociception. The mechanism is unknown but may result from high concentrations of morphine blocking the action of the inhibitory neurotransmitter glycine (see reference 418), since intrathecal strychnine or bicuculline produces a similar syndrome. There is a cautionary note here for the use of high doses of spinal opioids in humans.

Cardiovascular Function. Spinal morphine in antinociceptive doses does not change blood pressure and heart rate in animals and in humans, in the awake or the anesthetized state.[15,135] In dogs either anesthetized with halothane or unanesthetized, intrathecal morphine or DADL did not change cardiac output or peripheral resistance.[15,418] In humans, changes in skin temperature, blood pressure, and heart rate are absent with spinal opioids. Both sudomotor and vasomotor activity (*e.g.*, ice response, valsalva maneuver) remain intact.[47,50,103,159] The latter is important because of the retention of responses to posture and blood loss.

In the presence of noxious stimulation, in anesthetized animals and humans, sympathetic activity increases and is associated with increases in a number of neurohumoral markers[107,141,221] (see Chap. 5). Heart rate and blood pressure increase in this situation, and subsequent administration of spinal opioids results in a variable reduction in neurohumoral release and in cardiovascular responses in animals and humans (see reference 418). However, one study in dogs reported an increase in cardiac vagal activity after thoracic epidural morphine.[187]

Gastrointestinal Function. In humans, systemic opioids delay gastric emptying and decrease gastrointestinal motility. Intrathecal morphine in mice produce a dose dependent slowing of gastric transit time. Kappa and delta agonists produce similar effects (see reference 418). However, intrathecal morphine does not suppress the migrating motor complex associated with peristalsis (see reference 418). In humans, epidural morphine was reported to be associated with increased volume of gastric aspirate but with earlier recovery of intestinal motility after surgery in morbidly obese patients.[307] Systematic studies during both acute and chronic spinal opioid use in humans have not been reported.

Bladder Function. Spinal morphine in humans is associated with a naloxone-reversible inhibition of the volume-evoked micturition reflex.[314] A similar effect is reported in animals.[43,122] In humans, cystometrograms show increased bladder capacity owing to decreased detrusor muscle tone,[304] with a slight increase in the urethral sphincter tone (see reference 418). These effects are not dose-related in humans over the range of doses used epidurally.[304] However, they are reversed by naloxone.[304] Naloxone infusion of 5 μg/kg/hr in postoperative patients reversed urinary retention with only minimal effects on analgesia.[306]

Opioid ligands other than morphine also produce these effects; however, there is a clear structure–activity relationship when dose–response curves are carried out: β-endorphin ≥ DADL ≥ morphine > EKC >> SKF 10047 (see reference 418).

Anecdotal reports in humans suggest that incidence of bladder dysfunction may be less with spinal fentanyl[278], meperidine,[54,55] and methadone[149] compared with morphine; however, conclusive comparative studies are not available.

The precise mechanism of this effect of spinal opioids on bladder function has not been elucidated. However, it seems that a vesicosphincter dysynergia develops, and this points to inhibition of postganglionic nerves to the urinary bladder.[122] These effects are probably produced at a spinal level.

Unexpected benefits have become apparent from these new insights into spinal mechanisms of bladder function. Spinal morphine has been used as a treatment in patients with bladder spasm.[27] Naloxone augments the micturition reflex in spinal-transected animals (see reference 418). There are also anecdotal reports of short-term benefits of spinal morphine for enuresis.[62]

Respiratory Function. These effects are due to either bloodborne drug reaching the brain (early effects) or drug migrating cephalad in CSF (delayed effects). Such effects were not described in initial animal experiments and have been most clearly characterized in human studies (see section on side-effects below).

Premature ejaculation was described in subjects after a study of epidural morphine.[301] Further studies of effects of spinal opioids on sexual function are required.

Sedation, nausea and vomiting, pruritus, and other effects are described in the side-effects section below.

ONSET AND DURATION OF ANALGESIA

Onset of analgesia is directly related to lipid partition coefficient (see Table 28-2). The higher the lipid solubility, the more rapid the onset of analgesia. Other factors, such as molecular size and shape, may also contribute to some degree.[270] Morphine is an extreme example of low lipid solubility (and high water solubility), and thus has the slowest onset of action by a considerable amount. This relationship has been confirmed in rats,[401,419,423] cats,[400,401,419] primates,[402,410,417] and humans (see below).

For *intrathecal opioids,* in the primate, well-controlled comparative studies used the time to rise to half maximum shock titration threshold as an index of onset of analgesia: β-endorphin, 1.6 hours; morphine, 1.4 hours; DADL, 0.7 hour; metkephamid, 0.6 hour; meperidine, 0.5 hour; methadone, 0.4 hour; and lofentanil, 0.1 hour.

For *epidural opioids,* primate studies, as above, found similar onset times to those for intrathecal opioids: morphine, 2.9 hours; meperidine, 0.7 hour; and lofentanil, 0.2 hour.[402,418] Metkephamid and β-endorphin were inefficient epidurally in this primate preparation at doses several times those that were analgesic by intrathecal administration.[402,417,418] In other studies DADL also failed to completely block tail flick and hot plate responses in a rat epidural model.[136] This implies that these large molecules have difficulty establishing a concentration gradient from epidural space to spinal fluid. In rats the ED_{50} of epidural DADL is 30 to 50 times intrathecal values. Studies in humans confirm that analgesia can be obtained by epidural DADL administration (see below).

Duration of analgesia is inversely related to lipid solubility but is also influenced by rate of dissociation from receptors and perhaps by deposition in lipid of the epidural space. *For intrathecal opioids,* the primate shock titration model is used to determine time to fall to half maximum titration threshold, as indication of duration of analgesia[402,418]: β-endorphin, 22 hours; morphine, 16 hours; lofentanil, 7.6 hours; methadone, 6.8 hours; metkephamid, 6.1 hours; DADL, 5.2 hours; and meperidine, 5.1 hours. In rats, using hot plate and tail flick, the duration of analgesia for the fentanyl analogues, as well as morphine, was related to dose.[419] At doses producing an equal magnitude of inhibition, the duration of action was in the order: lofentanil > morphine > sufentanil > alfentanil ≥ fentanyl.

Intravenous naloxone resulted in dose-dependent antagonism of antinociceptive effects except that lofentanil was resistant to antagonism and required high doses of naloxone. This probably reflected lofentanil's high affinity and slow dissociation from receptors. Thus, lofentanil's long duration of action is partly due to lipid solubility but also to receptor binding.[419]

Interestingly, duration of analgesia for the fentanyl analogue sufentanil is reported to be increased by increasing *volume* of injectate (Janssen Pharmaceutica: Personal communication, 1986).

RELATIVE POTENCY OF SPINAL OPIOIDS IN ANIMALS

Based on studies in rat, cat, and primate models, the relative potency for intrathecal administration compared with morphine was estimated to be lofentanil, 250 : 1; sufentanil, 20 to 30 : 1; fentanyl, 3 : 1; alfentanil, 1 to 2 : 1.[419] Using Nordberg's estimate[281,282] in humans of minimum effective intrathecal analgesic dose of 250 μg of morphine, equivalent doses of fentanyl analogues were estimated to be lofentanil 1 to 2 μg, sufentanil, 10 to 20 μg; and alfentanil, 125 to 250 μg, respectively.[419]

PHARMACOKINETICS IN ANIMALS

Gustafsson and co-workers studied neuraxial distribution of [^{14}C]-morphine and [^{3}H]-meperidine after lumbar intrathecal injection in rats.[172] At 14 minutes after injection, spinal cord radioactivity was highest in the spinal cord close to the site of injection. For *morphine*, this was 215 times higher than would be observed if distribution in the body were homogeneous. The ratio of lower thoracic to upper cervical segment radioactivity was 0.2. For *meperidine*, spinal cord segments at a similar level to morphine contained maximal radioactivity, and this was 75 times higher than would be seen with even distribution in the body. The ratio of lower thoracic to upper cervical segment radioactivity was 0 : 1.[172] Morphine was much more evenly distributed over the lumbar and thoracic spinal cord than was meperidine.

The "distribution" of [^{14}C]-morphine throughout the neuraxis was studied in mice by whole-body autoradiography after lumbar intrathecal injections.[172] At 15 minutes after [^{14}C]-morphine injection, the entire spinal cord and ventral parts of the brain contained high levels of radioactivity. At 60 minutes, parts of the brain, that would include respiratory and vomiting centers and trigeminal nucleus, contained radioactivity; this was still present at 2 hours but not at 4 hours after injection. At 4 hours only the caudal part of the spinal cord contained radioactivity. Spinal cord radioactivity as a percentage of dose injected was 26% at 14 minutes, 20% at 44 minutes, 4.5% at 180 minutes. For meperidine, this figure was 7% at 14 minutes and 2% at 44 minutes.

These results indicate that the more lipophilic drug meperidine is rapidly taken up and eliminated from the spinal cord, whereas the hydrophilic drug morphine persists for much longer in the spinal cord. Also, morphine spreads rapidly into basal cisterns and then, after a delay, penetrates the brain.

Kinetics of [^{14}C]-labeled morphine and meperidine were studied after lumbar epidural and intrathecal administration in monkeys, using positron emission tomography at different levels of the spinal cord (C4, T4, T5, T6, L1, and L6).[170] This technique did not differentiate between epidural, intrathecal, or spinal cord sites, but could indicate spinal canal or whole body uptake. For meperidine, high activity was observed only in the lumbar region. For morphine, radioactivity was fairly constant along the spinal canal except at C4, where it was low. CSF taken from the cervical level showed peaks of radioactivity at about 60 minutes after injection of morphine and of meperidine. Injection in a large volume, as well as rapid injection, increased cephalad spread. Both drugs appeared rapidly in the blood, with peak concentration at 5 minutes after injection.[170] The terminal half-lives of disposition at the lumbar level were 47 and 60 minutes, respectively, for intrathecal and epidural administration. A pharmacokinetic "compartmental" model was proposed, based on these data.[170,172]

Strube and associates injected titrum-labeled morphine in the lumbar epidural region of anesthetized baboons and measured morphine in the CSF of cisterna magna for 22 hours. After a 1-hour delay, morphine was detected in the CSF and reached a peak at 3 hours. CSF concentration then declined with a half-life of 8 hours.[351]

Chrubasik and others measured CSF morphine in the cerebellomedullary cistern after epidural administration of either 2 mg in 10 ml saline or 2 mg in 1 ml saline, followed by an infusion of 0.16 mg per hour. Morphine was detectable near the brain stem after only 10 to 13 minutes. With the 1-ml volume, peak concentrations were reached later (2 – 3 hours) compared with the 10-ml volume (0.5 hour); peak concentrations were also much lower (1/40) for the low-volume (100 ng/ml) compared with the high-volume (4000 ng/ml) injection of morphine.[83] Both the time of initial detection and peak concentrations are similar to those obtained in cancer patients, using 10-ml volumes (see below).

After epidural injection of [^{3}H]-morphine and inulin in dogs, Durant and Yaksh studied distribution in lumbar CSF, azygos venous and femoral arterial

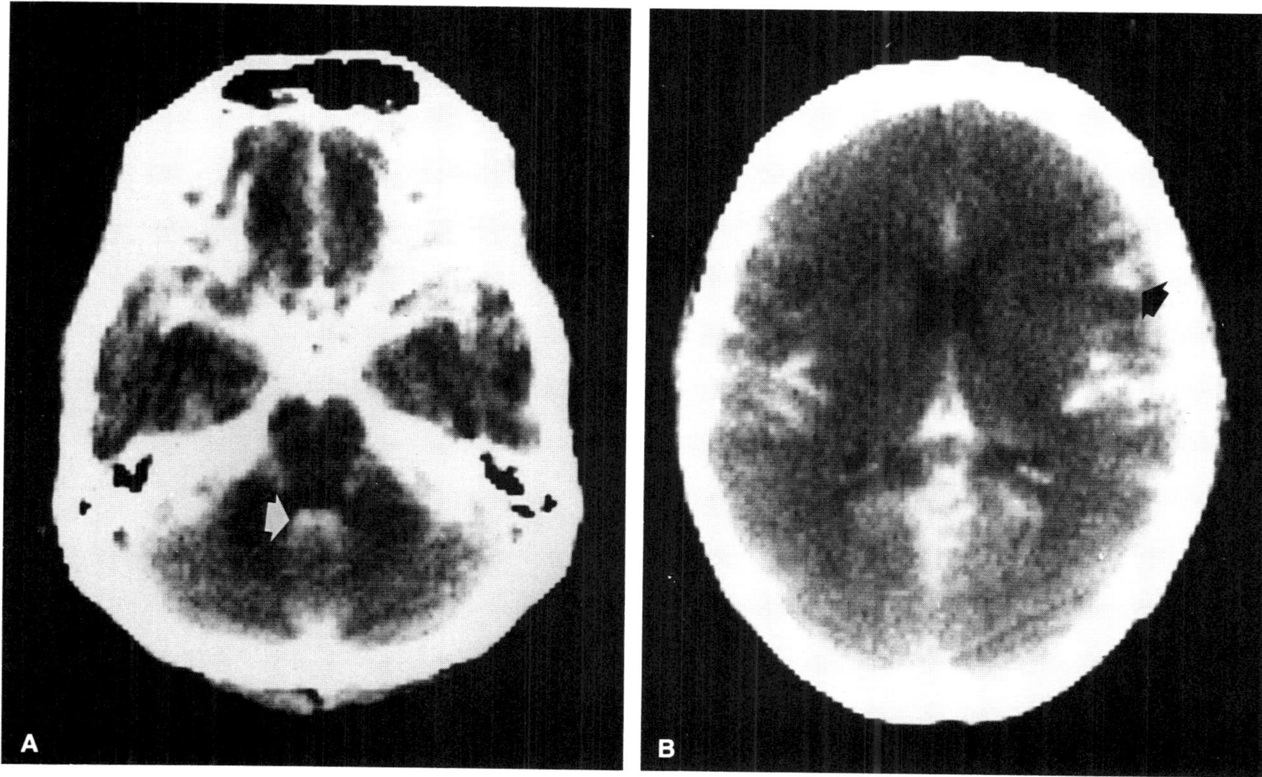

FIG. 28-6. CAT scans after injection of metrizamide into lumbar intrathecal space. **A.** Six hours after injection, contrast medium *(arrow)* is seen in fourth ventricle, indicating reflux through foramen of Luschka. **B.** Six hours after injection, significant penetration of central cortex is evident *(arrow)*. (Courtesy of Professor Michael Sage)

blood, and lymph.[137] During the first 20 minutes, morphine levels in the azygos blood were about three and ten times those in arterial blood and lymph, respectively. By 1 hour, approximately 50% of the morphine had passed into the azygos system. The elimination phase from CSF was about 106 minutes. Comparison of blood and lymph values indicated that morphine in lymph was derived from systemic distribution. Morphine appeared to be cleared from CSF by the azygos venous system at about the same rate as inulin. The fraction of morphine crossing the dura after epidural injection was about 0.3%. This was less than for inulin (0.6%). This indicates that *in vivo* molecular weight of the larger molecule inulin (MW 5175) compared with the smaller molecule morphine (MW 334) seems unimportant as a factor in dural penetration.[137]

Colpaert and co-workers studied opiate receptor binding and drug concentrations in plasma and brain after epidural and intravenous sufentanil in the rat.[89] Epidural sufentanil inhibited [^{3}H]-sufentanil binding in all areas of the brain and spinal cord, but particularly in the thalamus and lumbar spinal cord. Intravenous sufentanil inhibited [^{3}H]-sufentanil binding in brain areas at about the same dose at which it produced analgesia. The epidural dose inhibiting binding in the lumbar spinal cord was twofold lower than the intravenous dose. With intravenous sufentanil, more mu opiate binding occurred in the brain. However, the two routes differed by a factor of only about 2 in producing detectable levels of sufentanil in plasma and brain (intravenous > epidural). Analgesia with optimal epidural doses of sufentanil probably is due mostly to a spinal action, but a contribution from sufentanil in the brain is likely, at least during early stages of analgesia. High epidural doses of sufentanil are likely to progressively resemble intravenous administration, as the relative amount of drug in the brain increases.

The valveless internal vertebral venous plexus has connections with intracranial venous sinuses. Under conditions of increased epidural pressure, venous blood flow may be cephalad, with drug absorbed from epidural space potentially delivered direct to the brain. It has been reported that rapid epidural injection of a small dose of morphine in the cat sometimes resulted in retching, whereas the same dose given into the femoral vein produced no effect.[401] This suggested that, under certain conditions, opioids may reach the brain rapidly by way of a direct vascular channel, in addition to transport within spinal fluid. To test this hypothesis, [^{3}H]-naloxone or [^{14}C]-morphine was injected epidurally, and plasma concentrations of the label were measured in the azygos vein (representing epidural venous drainage to superior vena cava) and in the internal jugular vein (representing passage of the drug by way of the internal vertebral venous plexus to the intracranial venous sinuses and then to the brain). Compression of the vena cava lowered radioactivity in the azygos outflow but increased radioactivity in the jugular blood.[401] Changes in epidural venous blood flow may potentially influence clearance of opioids from the epidural space and influence their passage to the brain; however, this has not been proved in the clinical setting.

In a chronically catheterized maternal-fetal sheep model, Craft and associates[110] found that epidural morphine, 5 mg, caused no clinically significant changes in maternal or fetal hemodynamics or acid–base status. Maternal plasma concentrations of morphine peaked at 15 minutes (29 ng/ml), and fetal concentration levels peaked at 90 minutes (3–4 ng/ml).

An important potential interaction was suggested by studies of fentanyl infusion into the fourth ventricle with and without halothane anesthesia in the dog. Fentanyl combined with halothane 0.75%, but neither drug alone, caused a dose-related increase in arterial P_{CO_2}.[153]

SPINAL OPIOIDS IN HUMANS: AN OVERVIEW

It is clear from the studies in animals described above and from the incomplete data in humans that are described subsequently that the spinal administration of opioids is still in an investigational stage.[45,99,102,272] Some of the benefits and risks are now becoming known, but optimum patient selection still is not clear, and there may be risks that are yet to be defined. Despite this incomplete stage of knowledge, it can be stated that the discovery of "selective" mechanisms for pain inhibition at a spinal cord level has opened up a new era of options for acute[139] and chronic pain[316] management. Initially, investigational work in humans was largely restricted anatomically to the spinal cord and its inhibitory system, which operates by way of endogenous opioid substances and exogenous morphinelike and noradrenergic drugs. There are now reports that opioids (with or without alpha adrenoreceptor-blocking drugs) administered directly into the cerebral ventricles produce long-lasting analgesia in patients with inoperable cancer.[96,124,236,237,257]

Currently, none of the opioids used seems ideal for all applications. However, existing knowledge points to opportunity for improved clinical utility by manipulation of drug structure to achieve changes in physicochemical properties. This in turn may optimize such factors as transfer across dura, uptake into neural and perineural tissue, receptor binding, and efflux from CSF to minimize migration of the brain. It seems clear that lipid and water solubility are important, but other factors, such as molecular shape and receptor binding, also may be important.[271] Evidence of a selective spinal analgesic effect of opioids in humans is provided by two electrophysiologic studies of spinal cord function after intravenous morphine[249,389] and epidural morphine,[388] by pharmacokinetic studies, and by various indirect studies of changes of neurologic function after intrathecal and epidural opioids (see Table 28-10).

These studies in humans and in animals clearly refute claims that spinal opioids act predominantly on the brain.[109,110]

INTRATHECAL OPIOIDS IN HUMANS

In 1979, Wang and others[375] reported the first use of spinal intrathecal opioids in humans in the context of a double-blind placebo controlled cross-over study approved by a human studies committee. Wang and colleagues studied eight patients with intractable pain owing to malignancies of the genitourinary tract with invasion of the lumbosacral plexus. Patients received morphine 0.5 or 1.0 mg and physiologic saline at the second or third lumbar interspace to a total of 17 and 12 injections, respectively. Two patients reported pain relief after separate injections of morphine and saline, although the duration of pain relief after morphine was 15 hours, whereas that after saline injection was only 7 hours. This incidence (25%) of placebo effect and duration of effect is in keeping with many previous studies. Saline injections were ineffective in other patients, whereas morphine injection was followed by an onset of pain relief in 15 to 45 minutes, with a duration of 12 to 24 hours. The authors reported that there were no signs of sedation or respiratory depression, and all other neurologic functions remained intact.[375] However, it should be noted that all eight patients previously had been treated with opioids for prolonged periods. Also, in 1979, Cousins and colleagues reported that 1 to 2 mg of morphine injected in the thoracic region close to appropriate spinal cord segments relieved the pain of breast cancer and lung cancer for 24 to 48 hours.[103] These patients also had been taking opioids for long periods, and respiratory depression did not occur. Chauvin and associates reported that plasma morphine concentrations were low after 0.02 mg/kg of morphine intrathecally, and thus vascular absorption of morphine was unlikely to contribute to analgesia.[71] Use of intrathecal opioids for acute and chronic pain relief subsequently was reported in many clinical settings, including postoperative pain, cancer pain, chronic pain, obstetrics, postmyocardial infarction (see Table 28-4).

Postoperative pain consistently was relieved by intrathecal morphine; however, doses used have ranged from 0.25 and 0.5 mg[218,281] up to 20 mg.[326] Nordberg reported that the optimal intrathecal dose was 0.25 to 0.5 mg.[281] Katz and Nelson[218] reported excellent analgesia after herniorrhaphy when 0.5 mg of morphine was injected at the same time as spinal tetracaine. Seven patients receiving morphine had pain assessment scores recorded by the Visual Analogue Scale (VAS) of 11% to 20% for up to 24 hours postoperatively, while six control patients who received spinal tetracaine with only saline had scores of more than 69% from 1 to 2 hours postoperatively. However, five of the seven patients receiving morphine required bladder catheterization for urinary retention, while no control patient had this complication.

In another double-blind placebo controlled study, 0.3 mg of morphine given with intrathecal bupivacaine provided excellent pain relief in 17 of 23 patients after major hip surgery, with none of these patients requiring any other analgesia. In the placebo

TABLE 28-10. EVIDENCE OF SPINAL ACTION OF OPIOIDS IN HUMANS

Correlation of analgesic effects with CSF, but not blood, concentration of opioid
Antagonism of CNS side-effects, but not spinal analgesia, by naloxone intravenously
Analgesia without sedation with small doses spinally after sedation and poor analgesia owing to tolerance to high oral or intramuscular doses
Electrophysiologic studies after intravenous and after epidural morphine

group, all patients had severe pain and required additional analgesic medication[29] (see Table 28-11).

Mathews and Abrams[255] reported 40 patients who were given 1.5 to 4 mg of morphine by lumbar intrathecal injection under general anesthesia before open heart surgery. All awoke at the end of surgery free of pain and remained so for more than 17 hours postoperatively. Seventeen of the patients required no further opioid during their hospital stay. Other uncontrolled studies have reported good relief of postoperative pain.[156,211,216,326,327,364] Intrathecal heroin also is reported to be effective in humans[220] for postoperative pain.

Obstetric use of intrathecal opioids has been controversial. Initial clinical applications of the animal studies of Yaksh and others[426] were favorable.[8,53] One study reported that all of 31 patients had relief of labor pain with morphine 1 mg intrathecally.[53] Other clinical studies are in agreement that patients achieved adequate pain relief in the first stage of labor with 0.5 to 1.0 mg of morphine[3,118] (Table 28-11). However, more than 50% of patients had incomplete relief in the second stage and required local anesthetic blockade.[25,333,345] Baraka and coworkers[25] reported a high percentage of patients with nausea, vomiting, and skin itching. Two patients who received 2 mg of morphine had marked somnolence, skin itching, and nausea that persisted postpartum. Intravenous infusion of naloxone has been reported to decrease the incidence of side-effects without altering analgesia.[53,118] Oyama and colleagues reported that intrathecal beta-endorphin, 1 mg, relieved first- and second-stage labor pain in all of 14 parturients, and perineal discomfort was absent for 12 to 32 hours postdelivery.[289] Nausea and vomiting were noted in 4 of 14 patients studied; however, all patients were alert and there was no maternal respiratory depression. Apgar scores in infants were all in excess of 8, and umbilical blood gas values were normal. It was stated that the high molecular weight (3300 daltons)

TABLE 28-11. INTRATHECAL OPIOIDS: STUDIES OF EFFICACY

Type of Pain	Drug/Dose	Study Design	Outcome	Reference
Postoperative				
Postherniorrhaphy	Morphine 0.3 mg and tetracaine	DBPC	24 h pain relief in all given intrathecal morphine	218
Post major hip surgery	Morphine 0.3 mg and bupivacaine	DBPC	17/23 with intrathecal morphine; no other pain relief needed	29
Post cardiac surgery	Morphine 2 mg, 4 mg	DBPC, dose-response	Effective relief with 2 mg	17
Labor Pain	Morphine 0.5 mg versus 1 mg	Open, dose-response	0.5 mg and 1 mg—50% relief in 93% patients	3
	Morphine 1 mg	Open, 50% given i.v. naloxone or i.v. saline	50% relief in 82% given i.v. saline; 50% relief in 78% given i.v. naloxone; pruritus reduced by naloxone	118
	Morphine 1 mg	Open; objective tests [plasma β-endorphin]	Decreased β-endorphin ? due to pain relief	2
Cancer Pain	Morphine 0.5 to 1 mg single dose	DBPC	12-24 h pain relief in all given morphine; for 7 h in 25% given saline	375
	Morphine infusion	Open, long-term follow-up	Pain relief initially; invariable failure of relief at about 6 mo	92
	Morphine infusion	Open, comparison with other methods	Complete pain relief at 3 mo in 30% without other analgesics; 70% required other methods, mostly oral analgesics or neurolytic blocks	372

DBPC = double-blind placebo-controlled.

of beta-endorphin makes it necessary to administer the drug intrathecally; however, it does not pass the placenta and blood-brain barrier and cannot penetrate the fetal nervous system. In one report a patient with a single ventricle obtained good pain relief from intrathecal morphine during labor without cardiovascular compromise.[5]

Cancer pain management by repeated intrathecal injection is not practicable, not because the opioids are ineffective intrathecally, but because it is likely that the development of tolerance would occur and necessitate frequent lumbar puncture with increasing doses of opioid or peptide.[151] In an effort to overcome this problem, Onofrio and associates treated a patient with metastatic cancer pain by implanting a subarachnoid catheter and tunneling it to the pectoral region, where an infusion device (Infusaid, Metal Bellows Corp., Sharon, Massachusetts) was implanted.[288] The infusion reservoir gradually discharged its contents into the subarachnoid space at the rate of 0.62 mg per 24 hours. The reservoir could be refilled percutaneously by way of a septum. Their patient remained pain free for 10 days on the initial dose and then required 1.2 mg per 24 hours. After 28 days the dose was increased to 1.8 mg per 24 hours and remained at this level for a further 3 months. No sedation or respiratory depression was observed. The authors and an accompanying editorial commented that the slow development of tolerance may have been due to the maintenance of low concentrations of opioid at the spinal cord receptors.[288,316] Reference also was made to evidence that development of tolerance to opioids may be slower when they are used to treat chronic pain.[88] It was also pointed out that low-dose infusion limits the amount of drug in the CSF that is available at any one time for redistribution to supraspinal centers. Others have reported series of patients with cancer pain managed by implanted infusion devices and subarachnoid catheters.[92,236,374] A hazard of pain relief by intrathecal morphine is the possibility of opioid withdrawal syndrome if high doses of oral opioids suddenly are ceased.[264,365]

Tolerance to intrathecal morphine has been successfully treated with intrathecal DADL,[228] intrathecal clonidine,[96] and intraventricular morphine.[96] A sophisticated programmable pump is reported to be effective and to increase flexibility of dosing, since dose can be varied to suit patient needs.[293] Controlled studies of long-term intrathecal opioids compared with oral opioids and other methods of pain relief are not available. However, in a large comparative series of 3480 cancer patients, Ventrafridda and colleagues estimated that 29% of patients with spinal opioid infusions were pain free, without the need for other analgesic treatment, after 3 months.[372] In this series only 20% of patients required techniques other than oral opioid and adjuvant drugs; spinal opioids represented a small percentage of this group.[372] Use of implanted intrathecal and epidural systems for cancer pain is discussed in the section on epidural opioids and cancer pain.

MODEL OF INTRATHECAL OPIOIDS

Although clinical and animal data are incomplete, a working model of pharmacokinetics in relation to the actions of opioids after intrathecal injection can be proposed. For a highly ionized and hydrophilic drug such as morphine, intrathecal injection will produce extremely high CSF concentrations,[235,271,281] which will move slowly out of the CSF into spinal cord receptor sites[271] and into nonspecific binding sites and clearance sites (arachnoid granulations). Cephalad flow of CSF[328] will cause redistribution of the injected drug up the spinal subarachnoid space to the brain. Uptake into the systemic circulation competes for drug but results in plasma concentrations too low to produce any systemic analgesia.[72,281] For comparison, radiolabeled albumin (which is virtually membrane impermeable) passes cephalad so that 20% to 30% of an intrathecal dose reaches the endocranium within 12 hours and almost 100% within 24 hours.[125] It is possible that intermittent positive-pressure ventilation (or other respiratory maneuvers on the part of the patient) may enhance the spread of spinal CSF to the brain and results in the early onset of respiratory depression such as reported in elderly patients. Lazorthes and co-workers[235] measured morphine concentrations in lumbar spinal fluid after intrathecal administration of morphine 5 mg in a hyperbaric solution. They reported that the distribution half-life was 22 minutes, while elimination half-life was around 4 hours, the latter value being similar to values others have reported after intrathecal[281] and epidural[282] administration (see below), suggesting a common rate-limiting step. Interpretation of pharmacokinetic parameters in "models" such as these is extremely difficult, since compartment theory cannot be applied with confidence. The notion of a volume being cleared according to a particular rate constant applies only if the same is representative of a stirred pool contained within a volume. Neither representative sampling nor stirring of CSF would seem sufficient for rigorous compartment analysis. Nevertheless, the clinical relationship between the drug's properties and actions can be rationalized through pharmacokinetics. Loss of analgesia at 32 hours in a patient with cancer pain corresponded to a spinal fluid morphine concentration of 90 ng/ml.[235] Low lipid solubility and slow uptake into spinal cord receptors results in slow onset of action. Slow egress from the spinal cord results in a long duration of action (see Fig. 28-5; see also Ref. 341a).

In the case of a mostly ionized lipid-soluble drug such as fentanyl, there will be only a small amount of unionized lipid-soluble drug in CSF after subarachnoid injection. This will penetrate spinal cord receptors and nonspecific binding sites rapidly but will also have a rapid egress, unless it has particular affinity for lipid or high receptor binding. Thus,for fentanyl (which is less than 10% un-ionized at *p*H 7.4),[250] onset of analgesia is rapid but duration is not as long as for morphine. Lofentanil, which has similar lipid solubility but less ionization than fentanyl, has long duration, possibly because it tends to form a depot in lipid-binding sites in the spinal cord and because of high affinity for mu receptors.[250] Heroin disappears from CSF much more rapidly than does morphine because of its higher lipid solubility (minimal or no metabolism of heroin in the spinal cord was detected).[270] For drugs like these, systemic uptake occurs readily[159,198] and, presumably, concentration of residual ionized drug in CSF is low. Thus, analgesia tends to remain segmentalized, and a smaller amount of drug spreads to the brain. Concurrently, high lipid solubility gives easy access to the alternative arterial route into the spinal cord, as well as rapid passage across arachnoid granulations into venous and lymphatic clearance channels. The factors operating are identical to those depicted for epidural injection, apart from the initial equilibrium in the epidural space (see Fig. 28-14; see also Ref. 341a).

Respiratory Depression as Side-Effect of Intrathecal Opioids

Delayed respiratory depression after intrathecal morphine for postoperative pain was reported toward the end of 1979 independently by Glynn and associates[160] and by Liolios and Anderson.[241] Glynn and colleagues[160] reported two cases of prolonged respiratory depression persisting to 18 hours after a single dose of 3 mg and 5 mg of morphine, respectively. Repeated doses of naloxone were required, and the patients were managed with continuous surveillance of respiration in a critical care unit. It was noted that each naloxone dose did not alter the level of analgesia. High doses of morphine (20 mg) were injected in a hyperbaric solution of dextrose by Samii and co-workers[327] with a similar reported duration of analgesia to that reported by Wang and others.[375] Samii's patients were nursed semisitting, and side-effects were not noted. However, Liolios and Anderson,[241] using a hyperbaric solution of 15 mg of morphine, did observe respiratory depression. Early in 1980 Davies and colleagues reported delayed and prolonged respiratory depression in three patients who received 1 mg of morphine in an isobaric solution for postoperative analgesia.[120,121] It is worth noting that all three patients had premedication with a long half-life sedative, diazepam, and were nursed in the supine position postoperatively. In retrospect, it seems likely that the lack of respiratory depression in the patients reported by Cousins and others,[103,160] by Wang and others,[375] and by Sammi and others[327] was due to well-established tolerance, since all cases studied were patients with cancer pain who had been previously taking opioids for considerable periods. In contrast, the cases reported by Glynn and others[160] and Davies and others[120,121] were postoperative patients who had not had repeated treatment with opioids. Posture also may be important. No controlled study is available of the effect of posture in preventing delayed respiratory depression after intrathecal morphine injected in solutions of varying baricity. Only a small fraction of an intravenous dose of morphine is able to penetrate the central nervous system, perhaps as low as 0.1%.[346] Thus, with 100 mg of morphine intravenous, a dose that produces respiratory arrest in all subjects naive to opioids, only 0.1 mg distributed throughout the brain appears to be associated with this complication. Thus, the commonly used intrathecal dose of 1 mg is ten times the amount of morphine found in the brain at respiratory arrest and probably much higher than that found in respiratory center regions of the brain.[346] Wang and co-workers[375] found no difference between the analgesic effect of 0.5 mg and 1 mg of morphine. Gustafsson and associates found that [^{11}C]-morphine appeared at high cervical level after 60 to 170 minutes.[170] A patient who received 4 mg of morphine intrathecally was analgesic for 126 hours and had respiratory depression beginning 7 hours after the injection that did not respond to naloxone 0.4 mg intravenously.[339]

Critical information from animal studies (see above) is that regarding the dynamics of CSF flow and the pharmacokinetics of opioids after intrathecal administration, since there is strong evidence to connect respiratory depression to CSF concentrations of opioids. Lumbar intrathecal injection of radionuclides[125,126] or water-soluble contrast media[131] (metrizamide) is followed by a gradual movement of these substances rostrally to reach the fourth and lateral ventricles after 3 to 6 hours. Contrast media can be demonstrated in the fourth and lateral ventricles at 6 hours after injection, indicating major reflux into the ventricles by way of the foramina of Luschka. Contrast media also appear at 6 hours in the intrathecal space over the entire surface of the brain and show significant penetration of brain tissue (Fig. 28-6).[324,325] Studies in animals of cephalad migration of morphine after intrathecal administration indicate a more rapid time course, with drug reaching the ventral brain after only 15 to 30 minutes and the respiratory center regions by 60 minutes[170,172] (see above). Data in baboons and in humans after epidural administration indicate peak levels in CSF near the brain at about 3 hours[83,161,351] (see below). In animal studies, direct injection of opioids into the fourth ventricle or into CSF of the ventral brain stem region results in a rapid (3–5 minutes) onset of respiratory depression, which is similar for both sites of injection.[150] Thus, diffusion of the drug through the brain tissue to the respiratory centers in the brain stem appears to be rapid once the drug reaches this area in sufficient concentration.

In summary, if small volumes of opioid are injected slowly, it seems likely that they will follow the passive circulation of CSF in the spinal subarachnoid space to reach the cisterns of the brain and then reach the respiratory center by way of the ventral pons. Opioid traveling cephalad in CSF also may stream against the rapid and active intracranial CSF circulation to gain retrograde access to the fourth ventricle, with subsequent rapid access to respiratory centers (Fig. 28-7). An alternative site of respiratory depression is a group of cells in the ventrolateral medulla, the nucleus ambiguus, and retroambigualis. This area is involved in control of both inspiratory and expiratory motor pathways. However, the area is lacking in opioid receptors in comparison to the subependymal nuclei in the floor of the fourth ventricle. Once in the intracranial CSF, it seems likely that opioid removal may occur with great efficiency at the choroid plexus,[190] which appears to act as a "cerebral kidney" for these substances (Fig. 28-7).

Onset of respiratory depression after intrathecal administration seems to be quite vari-

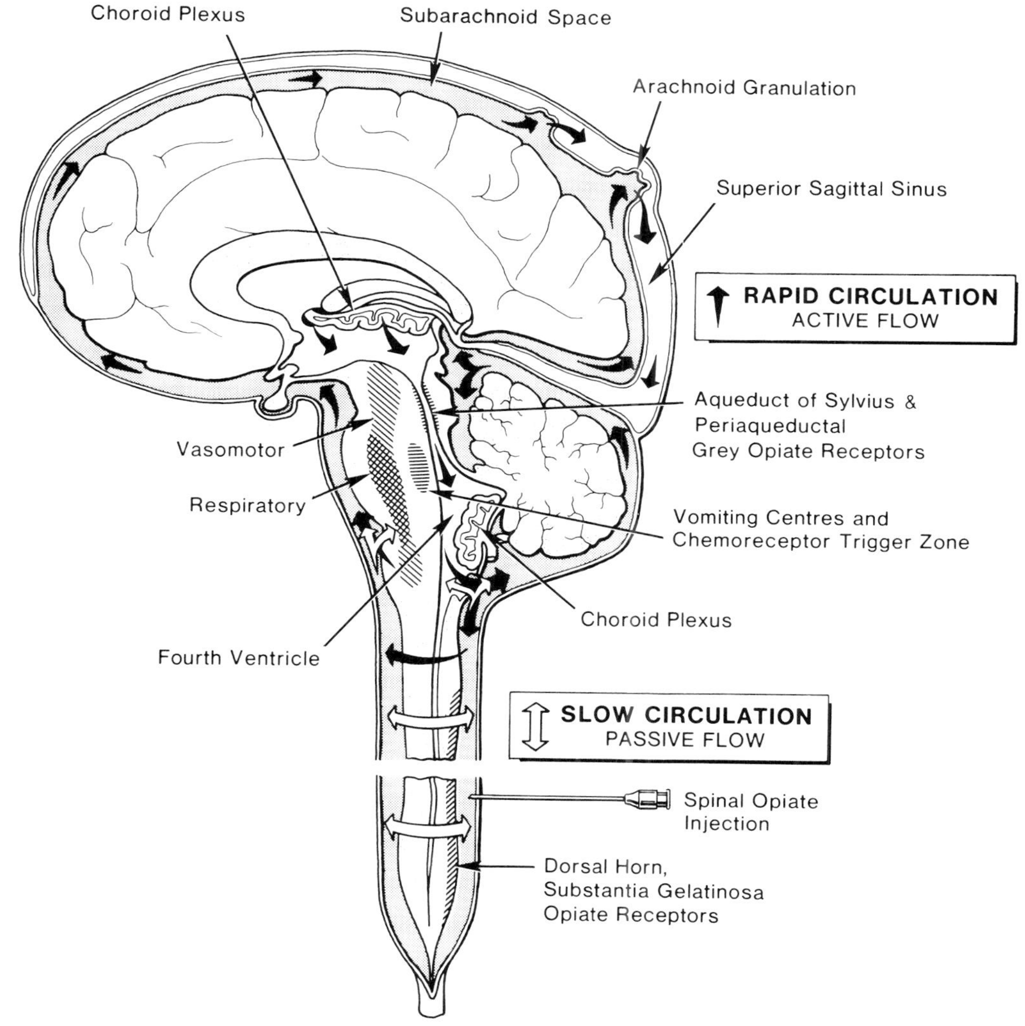

FIG. 28-7. Model of CSF-flow and spread of opioid in CSF. After lumbar intrathecal injection, opioid is carried in the passive flow of CSF to reach peak concentrations in brain after about 3 hours for morphine and 0.5 to 1 hour for meperidine (Demerol), as shown in Figure 28-15. Rapid spread ensues when the opioid mixes with the active flow of the rapid circulation of intracranial CSF. Spinal and brain stem opioid receptors are shown. The latter are seen to be in proximity to cardiorespiratory and vomiting control centers.

able.[120,121,156,160,210,241,284] In almost all cases intrathecal morphine has been used to provide postoperative analgesia.[120,121,156,160,173,284,292] In these patients, respiratory depression usually was evident within 6 to 10 hours after the opioid injection, although a delay of as long as 11 hours has been reported.[160] Return of normal respiration has required up to 23 hours after the injection. Case reports referring to further respiratory depression when opioids are injected in usual doses intramuscularly within 24 hours of intrathecal opioid,[284] therefore, are not unexpected. The timing of onset and offset of respiratory depression is in agreement with studies of time course of change in minute volume and carbon dioxide response after epidural morphine in volunteers (see below). In many of the case reports, antagonism of respiratory depression by naloxone has been reported, but often several doses of naloxone have been required.[120,160] Although respiratory depression was antagonized, analgesia was not[210] (see also Ref. 302a).

Factors predisposing to respiratory depression after intrathecal opioid administration appear to be advanced age[156]; poor general condition[302a]; use of water-soluble opioid, *i.e.*, morphine[173]; high doses[160]; marked changes in thoracoabdominal pressure, including artificial ventilation[156]; lack of tolerance to opioids[160]; concomitant administration, by other routes, of opioid or other CNS depressant drugs.[121,284] Patients with respiratory disease would be expected to be at risk, as they are with the use of opioids by any route. Age may influence spinal fluid volume and pressure, and the brain in elderly patients may be more susceptible to respiratory depression by opioids.[173] It has been claimed that the use of the sitting position and a hyperbaric solution of morphine protects against respiratory depression if higher doses of morphine are used.[327] However, these workers now have reported respiratory depression even when such maneuvers are used. As a general precaution it seems wiser to limit the dose of drug rather than to rely on the sitting position (see also Ref. 302a).

Other side-effects such as urinary retention, itching,[118] nausea, and vomiting are discussed under epidural opioids, since their etiology is the same, even though incidence is higher for intrathecal use.

EPIDURAL OPIOIDS IN HUMANS

Bahar and associates first reported the effective use of epidural opioids in humans in 1979.[19] A multitude of case reports followed (see Table 28-5). Systematic study of epidural opioids began with a brief report of pharmacokinetics of meperidine after epidural administration with simultaneous study of changes in neurologic function.[103] This initial study provided evidence that opioids reached the spinal fluid rapidly and that analgesia could be obtained in the absence

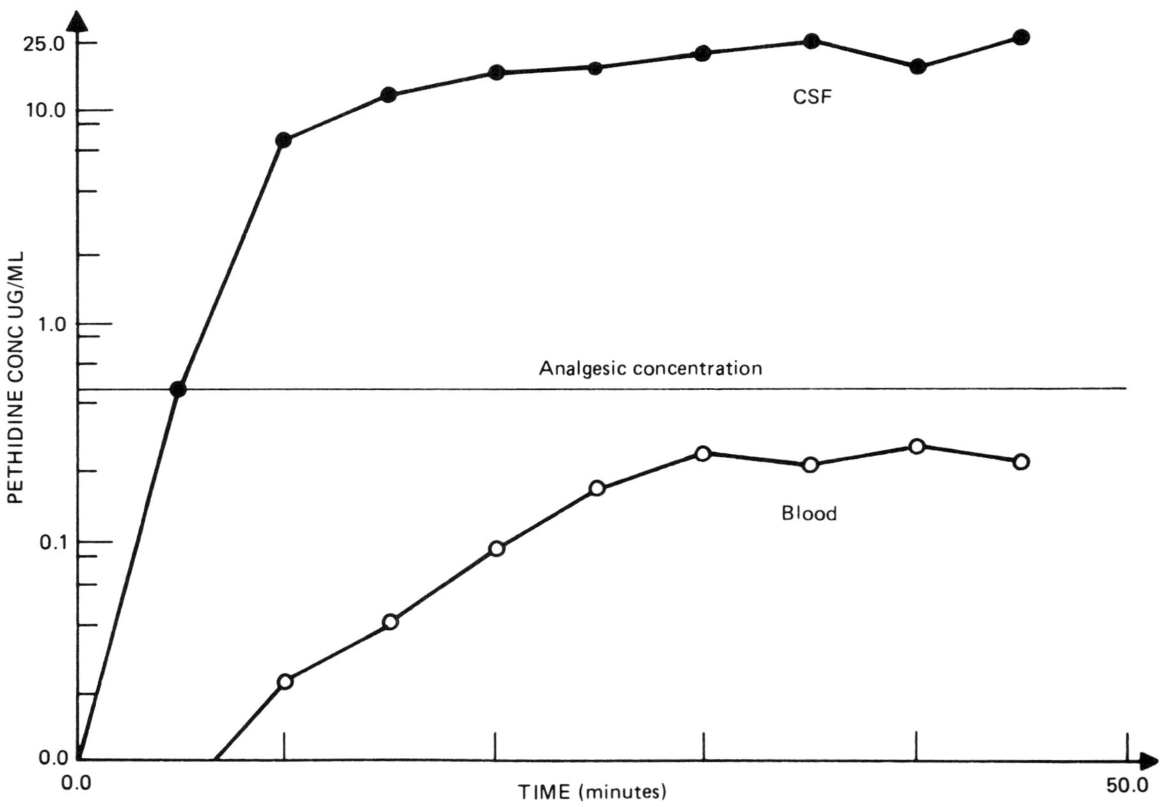

FIG. 28-8. CSF and blood concentrations after injection of epidural pethidine (meperidine) 100 mg. Onset of analgesia at 5 minutes after injection coincided with high CSF concentration of meperidine (Demerol). (Reprinted from Cousins, M.J., Mather, L.E., Glynn, C.J., *et al.*: Selective spinal analgesia. Lancet, *1*:1141, 1979, with permission of the publisher.)

of "analgesic" blood concentrations (Fig. 28-8). Because other neurologic functions, including sympathetic vasoconstrictor responses, were intact, the term "selective spinal analgesia" was suggested in comparing spinal opioids with spinal local anesthetics.[103]

PHARMACOKINETICS, PHARMACODYNAMICS, AND MODE OF ACTION

Compared with the intrathecal route, epidural administration is complicated by the pharmacokinetic aspects related to dural penetration, fat deposition, and systemic absorption. Pharmacodynamic aspects become complicated, since the larger doses of opioid used result in blood concentrations that cannot be ignored. More detailed study of epidural opioid pharmacokinetics has been made possible by studying blood concentration after separate injections of meperidine administered epidurally and intravenously in the same patients. This permitted calculation of the rate of absorption of meperidine from the epidural space into the systemic circulation[103,159] (Fig. 28-9). Absorption rate was exponential, with the log of fraction of dose unabsorbed at each time interval linearly related to time after injection. Absorption half-life ranged from 15 to 30 minutes. Analgesia appeared to be related to CSF concentrations in that patients having a high CSF-blood concentration ratio also had complete analgesia. There was considerable interpatient variability as reflected by a range of blood and CSF meperidine concentrations and of analgesic responses. A rapid increase in CSF meperidine concentrations in the first 5 minutes after injection coincided with onset of analgesia (see Fig. 28-8). The majority of patients who received 100 mg of meperidine epidurally had blood concentrations of 0.2 to 0.7 per liter within 20 minutes of epidural injection. These blood concentrations generally had been found to be associated with analgesia after a separate study in the same patient. However, two patients failed to achieve an "analgesic" blood concentration but still achieved rapid onset of analgesia. Also, analgesia lasted well beyond the time when blood concentrations had declined below analgesic levels (Fig. 28-9). These findings have been confirmed by others.[354] However, if similar doses of meperidine are given intramuscularly and epidurally, blood concentrations are similar and contribute to analgesia. Analgesia was significantly greater for epidural compared with intramuscular meperidine between 0.25 and 1 hour in one controlled study.[169,171] Also, some patients had evidence of hypalgesia, indicating a weak local anesthetic effect.[171] Thus, epidural meperidine dose (*e.g.*, 50 mg) should be lower than effective intramuscular doses (*e.g.*, 100 mg) if a predominantly spinal action is required (see Ref. 55 and 341b).

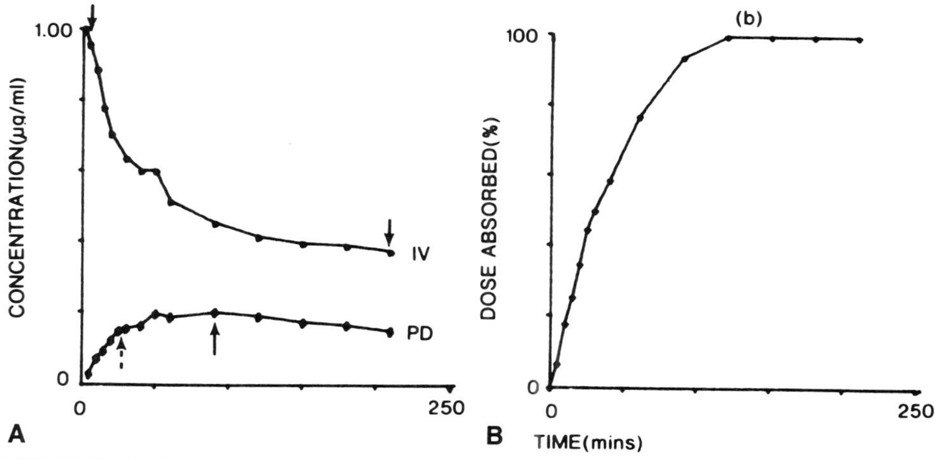

FIG. 28-9. **A.** Blood concentration after intravenous *(IV)* and epidural *(PD)* administration of 100 mg and 50 mg meperidine, respectively. Downward arrows (↓) indicate onset and regression of analgesia for IV meperidine. Upward arrows (⇡ ↑) indicate onset of partial and complete analgesia for PD meperidine. **B.** Meperidine absorption from epidural space. Calculated percentage of dose absorbed with time from data in **(A).** (Reprinted from Glynn, C.J., Mather, L.E., Cousins, M.J., *et al.*: Peridural meperidine in humans: Analgetic response, pharmacokinetics, and transmission into CSF. Anesthesiology, *55*:520, 1981, with permission of the publisher.) Pharmacokinetic data after epidural administration of meperidine are also available in Reference 341b.

With repeated dosing at short intervals, vascular absorption inevitably will lead to cumulation, since elimination half-life of meperidine is reported to be 5 to 7 hours.[169] As an aside, it should be noted that meperidine administered intravenously partitions from plasma into CSF according to the unbound fraction in plasma.[38,253] The clinical corollary of this is that meperidine administered epidurally will exert some central action from systemic absorption but that administered intravenously will not have its action enhanced by favorable partition into CSF.

Further support for a spinal analgesic effect of epidural opioids is provided by pharmacokinetic studies of epidural morphine.[48,72,168,270,281,282,308,354,357,379] Analogous to previous reports for meperidine *(vide supra),* mean peak serum morphine concentrations were similar for equivalent intramuscular and epidural doses[72] (Fig. 28-10); however, in one comparative study, vascular absorption was more rapid for epidural compared with intramuscular administration, with peak concentrations after only 10 minutes.[168] Compared with intravenous morphine, analgesic effect after epidural morphine correlated poorly with blood morphine concentration. After epidural morphine, some patients reported analgesia in the presence of extremely low serum morphine concentrations,[168,282,354] while others failed to achieve analgesia in the presence of typically analgesic concentrations.[72,118,308,379] In a cross-over study in volunteers, 1 hour after epidural or intravenous morphine, 10 mg, blood concentrations were similar; however, there was no analgesia in subjects who received intravenous morphine. Six hours after epidural injection, analgesia still was present despite low serum concentrations of morphine.[48,50] Concentration data from studies in which radioimmunoassays for morphine were used without steps to exclude metabolites are suspect, since some antisera used also cross-react with morphine metabolites. Because morphine metabolites can be detected in plasma shortly after administration, this particular analytic problem can lead to spurious conclusions regarding apparent "absorption" and persistence of morphine as well as concentration–analgesic effect relationships. Evidence of analgesia from epidural fentanyl and sufentanil has also been reported in patients in whom plasma concentrations were below analgesic levels.[355,391] Sufentanil peak blood concentrations are lower with epidural than with intravenous administration of equivalent doses.[355] Fentanyl blood con-

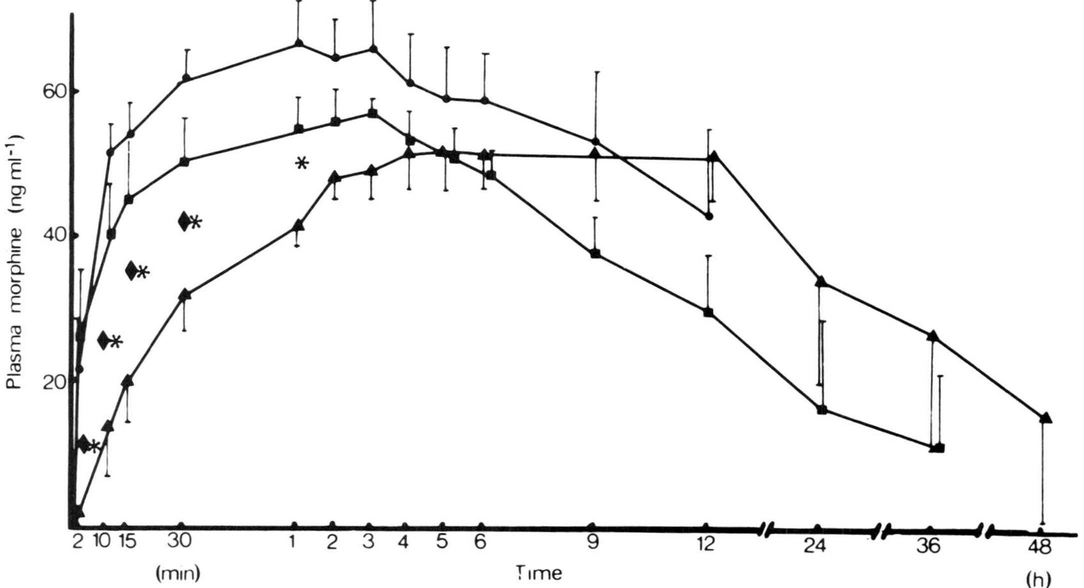

FIG. 28-10. Plasma concentration profiles after injection of morphine, 0.2 mg/kg (mean ± SEM). Intrathecal = ▲; epidural = ■; intramuscular = ● $p < 0.05$ intramuscular versus intrathecal; ◆ = $p < 0.05$ epidural versus intrathecal. (Reprinted from Chauvin, M., Samii, K., Schermann, J.M., *et al.*: Plasma concentration of morphine after im, extradural and intrathecal administration. Br. J. Anaesth., *53*:911, 1981, with permission of the publisher.) Note that the radioimmune assay used in this study co-determines morphine and its metabolites. Thus the apparent delay in reaching peak morphine concentrations may be a measurement artifact (see also pp. 283 and 284 and Refs. 341a and 341b).

centrations were reported to be lower for epidural than for intramuscular administration.[215,240] Also, analgesia was longer lasting and more profound when the same dose of fentanyl was given epidurally compared with intramuscularly.[215,240] Lower blood concentrations with epidural fentanyl may be partly due to deposition in epidural fat.[9]

Moore and co-workers[271] examined the permeability of isolated human dura to a variety of substances having different physicochemical properties. Their studies, which were based on correlation analysis, indicated that the molecular weight of the substance dominated the dural penetration rate. This finding was somewhat surprising and contrary to general expectation that lipid solubility would dominate. Close examination of their results, however, reveals that the lower-molecular-weight alcohols included in the test substances contributed heavily to the correlation. Extrapolation to clinical conclusions from widely differing substances is hazardous, since morphine and diamorphine, which have different lipid solubilities and molecular weight, demonstrated similar permeabilities. Fentanyl penetrated the dura several times faster than diamorphine, despite a similar lipid solubility. To account for this observation, the authors suggested that, for similar molecular weights, molecular shape ("long and thin" compared with "short and fat" morphine derivatives) also may influence membrane permeability. Their model developed for central neural transmission of epidurally applied opiates based on direct measurements of dural permeability is innovative and valuable as a starting point for future development. However, the conclusions reached by the authors are questionable and fail to consider that there are additional paths for drug entry to spinal cord receptors that only can be studied *in vivo. In vivo,* Durant and Yaksh found that the large molecule inulin diffused through dura at the same rate as the small molecule morphine.[137] Many studies in animals[170,401,402,404] and humans[79,171,256,257] indicate the important role of lipid solubility in dural transfer.[341a,341b]

The observation that meperidine reached the spinal fluid in high concentrations rapidly[159,354] suggests that lipid-soluble epidural opioids may gain rapid access to the spinal fluid by way of the arachnoid granulations in the dural cuff region (Fig. 28-11), in addition to dural membrane penetration.[271] This would permit facile access to the superficially located dorsal horn of the spinal cord. It is possible also that lipid-soluble drugs such as meperidine reach the spinal cord by rapid uptake into the posterior radicular branch of spinal segmental arteries, which run close to the dural cuff region. The posterior radicular ar-

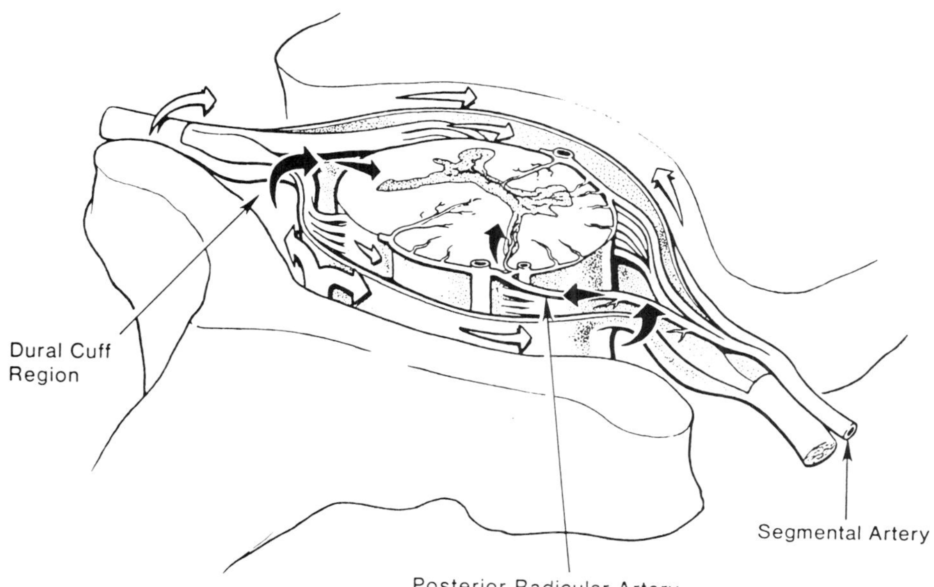

FIG. 28-11. Cross-section of spinal cord and epidural space. Opioid spread in epidural space is depicted by white arrows, and spread into CSF and spinal cord is depicted by black arrows. In dural cuff region, posterior radicular spinal artery is readily accessible to opioid, and this artery directly supplies the dorsal horn region of the spinal cord. Its role is currently speculative.

tery, in keeping with other segmental arteries, is known to reach the spinal cord at all levels but is quite small at most levels[97] and, thus, may be penetrated easily by lipid-soluble drugs. This artery gives branches that penetrate directly to the dorsal horn region (Fig. 28-11). Vascular transport of opioids to the spinal cord is indicated by the similarity in onset time for analgesia after intrathecal and epidural opioids (see above). The rapid concurrent absorption of meperidine into the systemic circulation (see Fig. 28-8) undoubtedly occurs by way of the extensive epidural venous plexus and then to the azygos vein. Obstruction of the inferior vena cava, as in pregnancy and other clinical situations, may cause distention of (epidural) veins as well as increased flow through the azygos vein (Fig. 28-12). This would result in an increased rate of systemic absorption of opioid from the epidural space, leaving less drug available for transfer across the dura to the spinal cord. Meperidine reaching the superior vena cava from the azygos vein will be distributed to the general circulation and then cleared rapidly at the liver. Studies in pregnant females during labor support the hypothesis of more rapid absorption of meperidine from the epidural space than occurs in nonpregnant women.[169,198,199] Also, in pregnancy, epidural absorption is even more rapid than after intramuscular injections[198] (Fig. 28-13). However, the analgesia obtained from meperidine 100 mg epidural in labor was of short duration (90 minutes) and appeared to correlate with plasma meperidine concentration. This brief and unsatisfactory analgesia from meperidine in pregnant patients was confirmed by Perriss.[294]

Although spinal fluid concentrations in pregnant patients have not been measured, it seems unlikely that sufficient meperidine reached the spinal cord to produce spinal analgesia. A lack of efficacy of low dose (2–5 mg) epidural morphine for labor pain also has been reported,[37,194,201,245] although in one study, assessment was made 30 minutes after injection, which is now known to be earlier than the peak analgesic effect of epidural morphine (60 minutes). Higher doses of epidural morphine (7.5 mg) were effective in 7 of 11 patients, supporting the hypothesis that less morphine reaches the spinal cord in pregnant patients.[194] In order to reduce epidural venous absorption of drug, Perriss used meperidine 50 mg with epinephrine 1 : 200,000 and injected the dose with the parturient in the lateral position, to minimize vena caval obstruction.[295] More than 80% of patients had a rapid onset (30 minutes) of complete pain relief, which lasted an average of 107 minutes. The brief duration probably reflected the transient effect of the epinephrine in decreasing epidural vascularity. However, the profound analgesia, without sedation, probably was indicative of effective concentrations of meperidine reaching spinal cord receptors, combined perhaps with some local anesthetic effect and some spinal analgesic effect of the epinephrine. Epidural fentanyl has been reported to relieve pain without sedation after cesarean section[277] at blood concentrations that are consistently less than those known to be analgesic.[70,391] Similar data have been reported during labor.[215] This indicates that epidural fentanyl may be transferred rapidly to the spinal cord by means of CSF and by way of

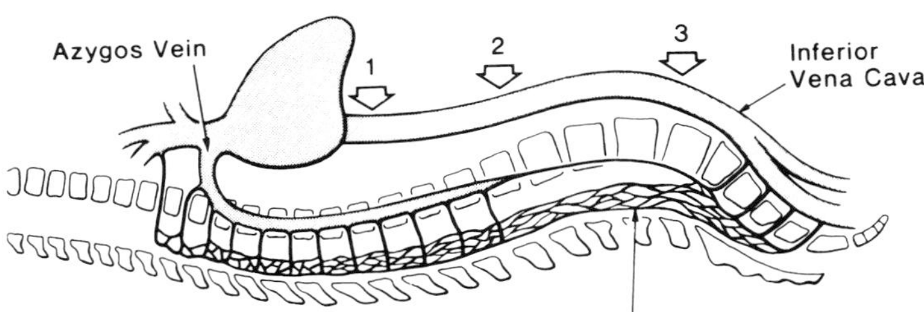

FIG. 28-12. Venous drainage of the epidural space into the inferior vena cava (IVC) by way of the azygos vein. Compression of IVC at 1, 2, or 3 results in rerouting of venous flow by internal vertebral plexus (epidural) veins to azygos vein. Increased intrathoracic pressure is transmitted to epidural veins and may result in increased flow up the portion of internal vertebral venous plexus that is protected within the vertebral body (also see Fig. 28-14). (Modified from Bromage, P.R.: Epidural Analgesia. Philadelphia, W.B. Saunders, 1978, with permission of the publisher.)

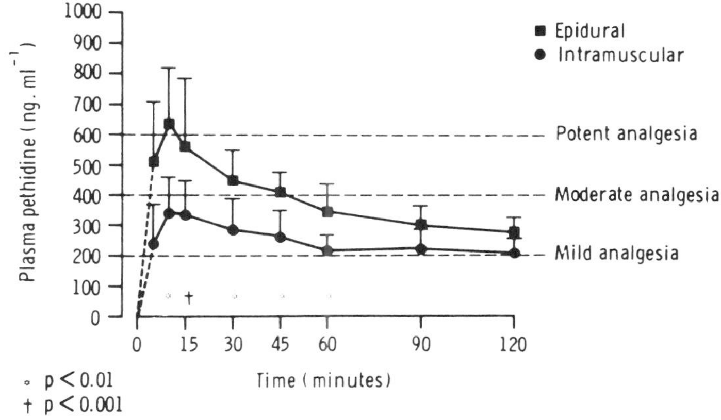

FIG. 28-13. Comparison of plasma meperidine (pethidine) concentrations after administration of 100 mg by epidural (■) or intramuscular (●) route during labor. Labeled broken lines refer to plasma meperidine concentrations associated with degrees of analgesia (Edwards and others[140]). (Reprinted from Husemeyer, R.P., Davenport, H.J., Cummings, A.J., *et al.*: Comparison of epidural and intramuscular pethidine for analgesia in labour. Br. J. Obstet. Gynaecol., *88*:711, 1981, with permission of the publisher.)

spinal radicular arteries, leaving only minimal amounts to be absorbed into epidural veins. "Buffering" of venous absorption also may occur as a result of uptake of fentanyl into epidural fat, analogous to the local anesthetic bupivacaine.[250]

Using sensitive electron-capture gas chromatography for plasma and CSF assay of morphine concentration, Nordberg and co-workers[282] reported that absorption of morphine into the vascular system was rapid, with peak arterial plasma concentrations occurring within 15 minutes owing to redistribution within the body. They reported that the ratio of morphine concentrations in CSF (lumbar) to plasma concentrations changed with the time after injection and ranged from 45 to 100 : 1 at 1 hour to 125 to 175 : 1 at 5 hours. However, this appeared to be caused by dysequilibrium between plasma and tissue concentrations, since the elimination half-lives of morphine in plasma and CSF were similar (approximately 4 hours). Gustafsson and colleagues[168] and other studies[354] have confirmed the rapid absorption of epidural morphine and reported that not only did peak plasma concentrations occur sooner, but were also higher (relative to dose) than morphine given intramuscularly. It is possible that the hydrophilic nature of morphine prevents significant buffering of venous absorption because of minimal uptake into epidural fat (see also Ref. 341b).

Bullingham and colleagues[59] reported that unexpectedly high plasma fentanyl concentrations could occur after epidural injection following aortic cross-clamping. There may be a number of reasons for these high plasma concentrations, including reduced clearance of fentanyl under general anesthesia, reduced distribution volume, and altered absorption from the epidural space.

A number of factors influence the analgesic effects of epidural opioids by way of pharmacokinetics. Factors now confirmed as having a significant pharmacokinetic effect are lipophilicity of drug, drug dose, mode of drug delivery (bolus vs. infusion), volume of injectate, use of epinephrine (with fentanyl analogues but not morphine). These factors and their effects are summarized in Table 28-12.

PHARMACOKINETIC MODEL OF EPIDURAL OPIOIDS

After *epidural injection of a highly ionized and hydrophilic drug* such as morphine (Fig. 28-14), only low concentrations of lipid-soluble un-ionized drug will be present in solution in the epidural space. Thus, transfer of morphine across arachnoid granulations will be slow, with a peak at 90 minutes,[354] and may rely partly on retrograde movements by way of the cyclic vacuolation in the epithelial cells of the arachnoid granulations. Similarly, direct access to spinal

TABLE 28-12. EPIDURAL OPIOIDS AND ANALGESIA: ANALYSIS OF FACTORS

Factor	Effect	References
Drug		
High hydrophilicity (*e.g.*, morphine)	Slow onset Long duration Cephalad spread Potential CNS effects are long lasting (slow in and out)	161, 281
High lipid solubility, moderate receptor affinity (*e.g.*, fentanyl, methadone)	Rapid onset Duration only slightly longer than i.m.	215 240 391
	Cephalad spread but smaller amounts of drug and effects short lived (rapid in and out)	
High lipid solubility, high receptor affinity (*e.g.*, sufentanil, lofentanil)	Rapid onset Medium to long duration Cephalad spread minor	355
Dose	Correlates with analgesia (efficacy and duration) up to plateau	6, 112, 247, 281
Major and extensive surgery (*e.g.*, thoracic, upper abdomen)	4-6 mg morphine or equivalent (young)* 2-3 mg " " " (old)	308, 348
More localized surgery (*e.g.*, hip, extremities, lower abdomen)	2-4 mg morphine or equivalent (young) 1-2 mg " " " (old)	247
Mode of Drug Delivery		
Bolus versus infusion	Infusion results in lower dose requirements, more effective analgesia, fewer side-effects	86, 91, 141
Volume of Injectate	? High volume (*e.g.*, 10 ml) increases cephalad spread compared with low volume (1 ml). Intensity of analgesia with 1 ml as good as with 10 ml but *duration* longer with 10 ml (? only for sufentanil)	83, 89
Epinephrine (EPI)		
EPI + meperidine	Increased analgesia (labor)	295
EPI (25 μg) + meperidine	No change in analgesia (postop)	171
EPI (1 : 200,000) + fentanyl	Below fentanyl concentration of 10 μg/ml, EPI increased analgesia	383
EPI + sufentanil	Increased duration of analgesia, decreased plasma sufentanil	355
EPI + morphine	No change in analgesia	46

*Refers to lumbar catheter. ? Dose may be reduced with a thoracic catheter to 2 to 4 mg (young) or 1 to 2 mg (old).

cord by way of spinal arteries may be limited (Fig. 28-11). Absorption into the venous system is rapid, and peak blood concentrations are reached in 10 minutes.[161] Blood concentrations are similar to those for an equivalent dose given intramuscularly.[72] Because most of the drug present in the spinal fluid will be ionized, only a small concentration gradient will pertain for transfer of un-ionized drug to spinal cord receptors. Egress from spinal cord to spinal fluid will be equally slow as the un-ionized species moves out along a small concentration gradient. The high concentrations of ionized drug in spinal fluid will be available to move upward with the spinal CSF flow, and thus extend the level of analgesia (also to migrate to supraspinal structures) (see Fig. 28-7). For morphine, the foregoing hypothesis is in keeping with the slow onset and long duration of analgesia as well as the significant incidence of delayed respiratory depression. These effects correlate well with delayed onset of peak morphine concentrations in CSF and prolonged elevation of CSF morphine.[161,281,341b,354]

In the presence of raised intrathoracic pressure, absorbed drug also could be redirected mainly up the internal vertebral venous system directly to the brain. This would account for rapid onset of nausea shortly after injection or transient periods of early respiratory depression. Consistent spread of opioid effects into the high cervical region has been reported after epidural injection in the lumbar region.[47,48,161,282] Also, lumbar epidural injection was as effective as thoracic

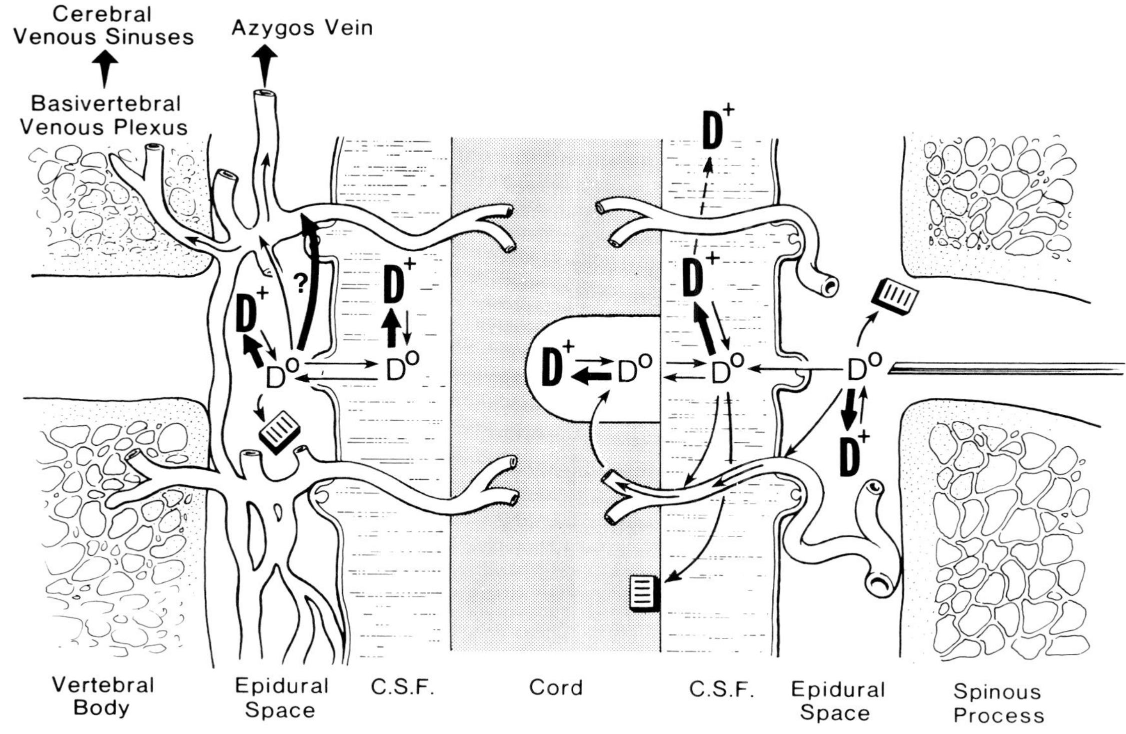

FIG. 28-14. Pharmacokinetic model: Epidural injection of a hydrophilic opioid such as morphine. D^0 = un-ionized lipophilic drug; D^+ = ionized hydrophilic drug. An epidural needle is shown delivering drug to epidural space. Model otherwise similar to Figure 28-5. The role of absorption by way of radicular arteries remains speculative. The shaded squares are nonspecific lipid binding sites.

injection for post-thoracotomy pain,[233,280] and caudal or lumbar epidural morphine seems equally effective for lower abdominal pain.[206] In cancer patients, epidural injection of morphine was followed by detection of morphine in cervical CSF 30 to 60 minutes after injection, with peak levels in this region at 3 hours (Fig. 28-15*A*). Pain in the cervical and thoracic regions was effectively managed with a lumbar catheter, confirming even distribution of morphine over the spinal cord.[161] All of these data, together with animal pharmacokinetic data, confirm that morphine reaches the spinal cord in the high cervical region after injection in the lumbar region. Also, quite high concentrations are achieved in the brain stem when a bolus of morphine is given in 10 ml of solution.[161] Some data indicate that reducing bolus volume to 1 ml and using an infusion may decrease brain stem morphine concentrations, but the effect is minimal.[341b]

After epidural injection of a *mostly ionized lipophilic drug* such as meperidine (Fig. 28-16), there will be low concentrations of lipid-soluble un-ionized drug in the epidural space, which rapidly will be transferred to CSF, into spinal radicular arteries, and into epidural veins. In the presence of brisk spinal artery blood flow and relatively slow epidural venous flow, transfer of the drug to the spinal cord will predominate while the concentration gradient is high. However, significant vascular absorption into epidural veins will reduce the concentration gradient relatively rapidly. Concurrently, there will be a potential for redirection up the basivertebral system to the brain if intrathoracic pressure is high. Egress from spinal cord receptors will be equally rapid and will be assisted by rapid uptake into epidural veins at the level of arachnoid granulations. Thus, analgesia will be rapid in onset and of only medium duration, and it will be reasonably independent of the specific lipid solubility of the agent. Therefore, the durations of meperidine, and fentanyl should not differ widely, and this is in keeping with clinical observations.[55,215] This contrasts with animal studies of the lipid-soluble

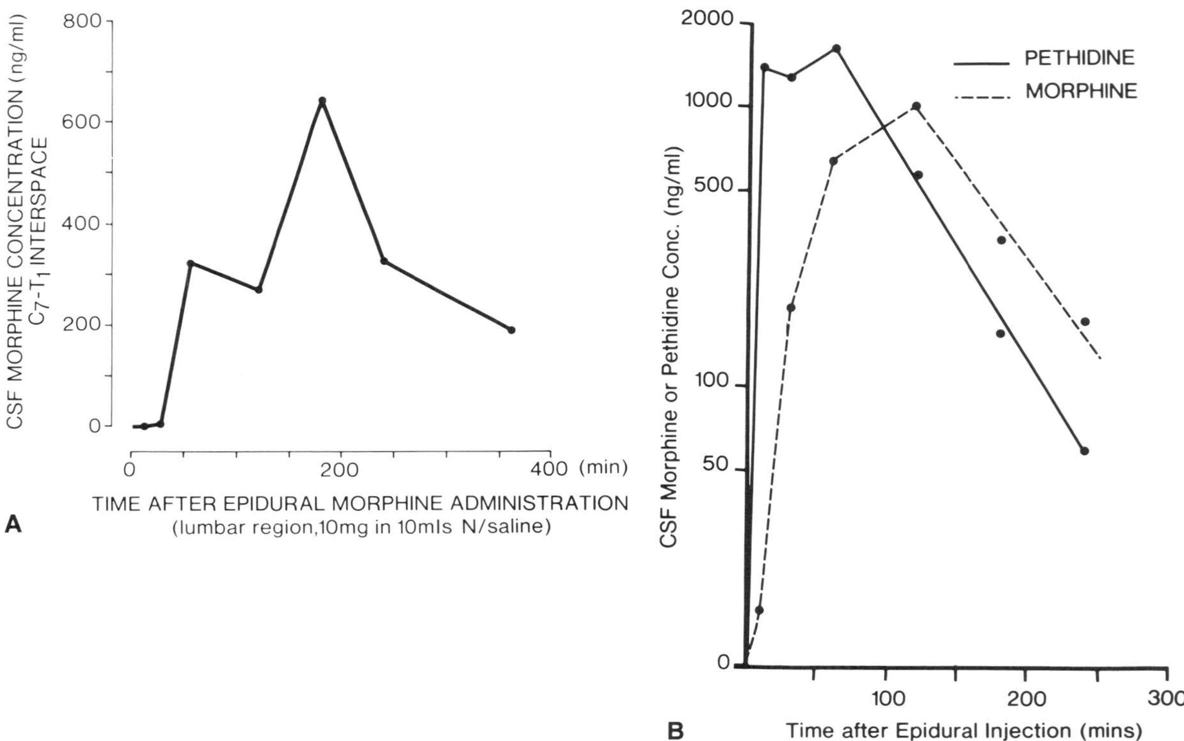

FIG. 28-15. **A.** Cervical cerebrospinal fluid (CSF) concentration of morphine. Cervical CSF samples were assayed for morphine at various times after lumbar epidural injection of morphine 10 mg in 10-ml saline. Note the early appearance of morphine in cervical CSF after 30 minutes and the peak concentration at about 3 hours. (Data from Gourlay, G.K., Cherry, D.A., Cousins, M.J.: Cephalad migration of morphine in CSF following lumbar epidural administration in patients with cancer pain. Pain, *23*:317–326, 1985.) **B.** Cervical CSF concentrations of morphine and pethidine (meperidine) as a function of time following lumbar epidural administration. Morphine (10 mg) and pethidine (50 mg) in 10 ml of normal saline were administered simultaneously by means of a lumbar epidural catheter at L2–L3 interspace, and CSF samples were collected from the C7–T1 interspace at the times shown on the graph. Peak cervical CSF concentrations of pethidine were achieved earlier and declined sooner in comparison to those of morphine. Also the peak concentrations of pethidine were lower than those of morphine, considering the doses of the two drugs injected. The rapid appearance of pethidine in CSF is in keeping with rapid diffusion through the dura. (Reproduced with permission from Gourlay, G.K., Cherry, D.A., Armstrong, P.A., Plummer, J.L., and Cousins, M.J.: Pain, 31:297–305, 1987.)

drugs lofentanil and sufentanil, which have long durations of action, possibly by nonspecific binding to spinal cord lipid combined with higher affinity for the mu receptor.[250,419]

Blood concentrations will be influenced greatly by the dynamics of vertebral venous and arterial blood flow. It seems probable that early respiratory depression will result from rapid early vascular absorption and transient increases in CSF concentrations at the base of the brain (cervical and cisternal CSF). However, for lipid-soluble opioids, such increases are much smaller and more transient than for morphine (see Fig. 28-15).[161,170,257] Late respiratory depression will be unlikely, unless there is a sudden redirection of blood flow through basivertebral veins to the brain as a result of increased intrathoracic pressure, or unless a large dose is accidentally injected into the subarachnoid space. It is of interest that to date, no reports of respiratory depression have followed the use of epidural fentanyl in the absence of other opioids.

This is supported by a study of the time course of the respiratory effects of intramuscular and epidural fentanyl in which resting ventilation, end-tidal P_{CO_2}, and CO_2 response remained normal throughout the 24-hour observation period after fentanyl 0.1 mg epidurally.[229] Studies in patients support these data.[6]

Redistribution, rather than systemic clearance, probably is more important in reducing risk of potential respiratory effects resulting from blood-borne drug, since dosing intervals for most epidural opioids will be greater than plasma half-lives. An exception is methadone, which has an epidural dosing interval of approximately 4 to 8 hours but may have a plasma half-life as long as 24 to 48 hours.[163] Thus, repeated doses of epidural methadone at 8 hour intervals could pose a risk of systemic cumulation in some patients with increased risk of delayed and prolonged respiratory depression owing to bloodborne drug.

MECHANISM OF RESPIRATORY EFFECTS

Early Respiratory Depression

Most reports of early respiratory depression after epidural meperidine have been in postoperative patients within 1 hour of injection,[173,332,405] and thus probably reflect vascular absorption by way of epidural veins or possibly rapid redirection to brain by way of the basivertebral system as discussed earlier. However, simultaneous lumbar epidural injection of morphine and meperidine in patients results in detectable levels of both drugs in cervical CSF at about 30 minutes after injection. Thereafter, CSF meperidine concentrations in the cervical region declined rapidly (unpublished observations; see Fig. 28-15B). Thus, it is possible that lipid-soluble drugs may cause early res-

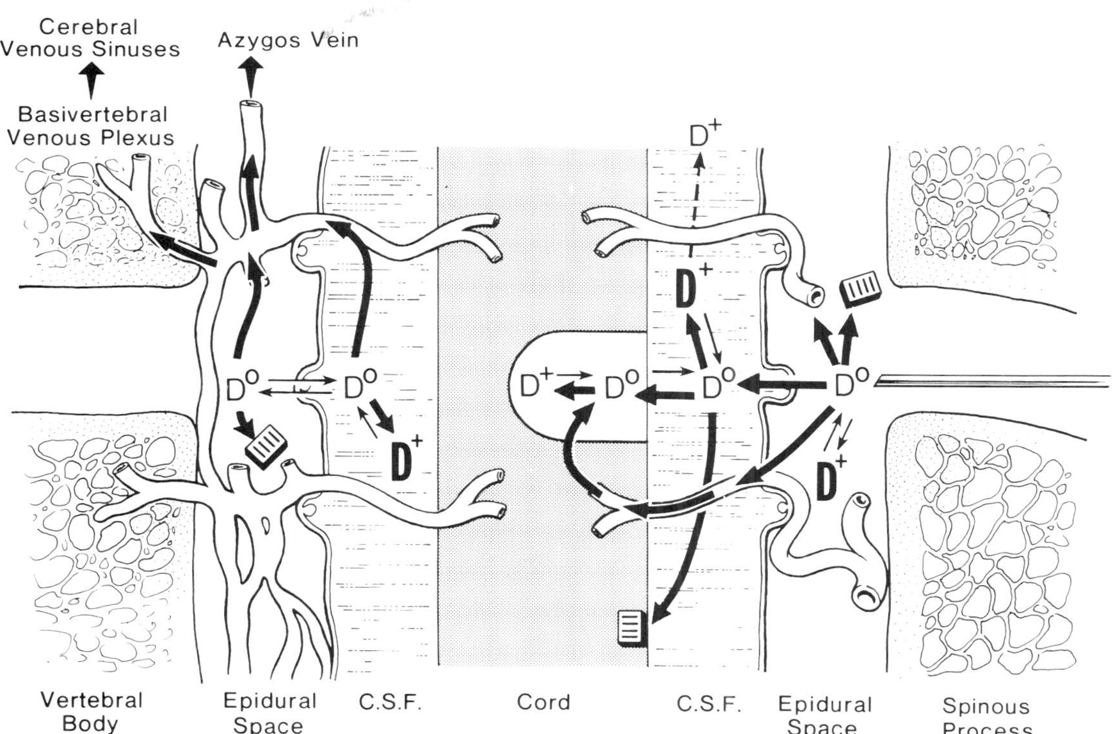

FIG. 28-16. Pharmacokinetic model: Epidural injection of a lipophilic opioid such as meperidine or fentanyl. Symbols as in Fig. 28-5. Note the rapid passage of unionized species (D^0) into CSF and thence to spinal opioid receptors. Thus the amount of ionized species (D^+), which remains to migrate to the brain, is less than that for morphine (see Fig. 28-14).

piratory depression at least partly as a result of rapid penetration of the brain after achievement of peak concentrations near the brain stem at about 30 minutes. This is supported by studies of plasma pharmacokinetics and respiratory effects of fentanyl: plasma fentanyl concentrations peak after 5 minutes and then decline rapidly, whereas respiratory depression is seen between 15 and 60 minutes.[6,240]

Late Respiratory Depression

Late respiratory depression has only been reported with epidural (and intrathecal) morphine. Postoperative patients may have the following factors potentially contributing to delayed respiratory depression:

1. Residual effects of parenteral opioids given before, during, or after surgery. In a number of cases, sizeable doses of intramuscular opioid were given either before epidural opioid[332] or after epidural opioid[32] at a time when it now is known that significant respiratory effects of epidural opioid are still present (see below).
2. Residual effects of other CNS-depressant drugs used in anesthesia.
3. Lack of tolerance to opioids, since most operative patients have not received opioids for prolonged periods before surgery. Thus, they are not tolerant to side-effects, such as respiratory depression.
4. Raised intrathoracic pressure, with "grunting" respiration associated with pain.
5. Raised intra-abdominal pressure and obstruction of inferior vena cava with increased blood flow through azygos system.
6. Inadvertent dural puncture[56,381] by needle or delayed catheter penetration.
7. Large doses (10 mg) of morphine sometimes required for pain relief after major surgery are associated with a higher incidence of respiratory depression that is persistent and prolonged, compared with lower doses of morphine (2–4 mg),[307] which pose a lesser risk of respiratory depression.[302a]

As in the case of intrathecal administration, old age, poor general condition, and respiratory disease probably predispose to respiratory depression.[32,81,224,302a] Patients subject to Stokes–Adams attacks also require caution.[79] From pharmacokinetic considerations, delayed respiratory depression would be expected to be most common with epidural morphine[31,81,276,313,379] and absent with epidural fentanyl.[6,229]

Studies in volunteers by Bromage and others[48,50,61] suggested a pattern for the rostral spread of morphine in the spinal fluid as judged by the upward progression of analgesia to ice and pin scratch, in parallel with observations of changes in CO_2 response curve (Fig. 28-17). Early and similar respiratory depression occurred after both intravenous and epidural morphine 10 mg, approximately 30 minutes after injection and associated with high-peak serum morphine concentrations. Between 3 and 6 hours, respiratory depression became maximal after epidural morphine and remained so until the 10th hour. Marked ventilatory depression remained at 16 and 22 hours postinjection (Fig. 28-17). The rostral spread of analgesia after epidural injection followed a similar time course: +3 hours, T9–11; +4.5 hours, above T5; +5 hours, loss of cold pressor response in hands (T1–C8-7); +6 to 9 hours, trigeminal analgesia. The onset of nausea and vomiting also occurred at +6 ±2 hours (Fig. 28-18). The coincidental onset of trigeminal an-

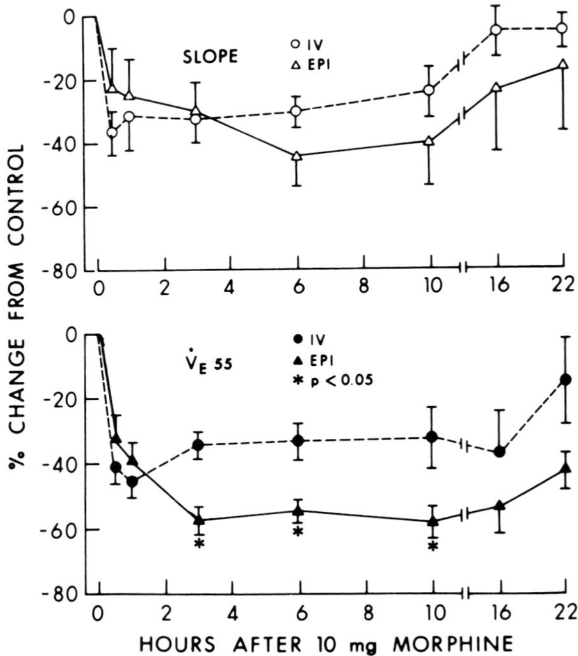

FIG. 28-17. Ventilatory response to endogenous CO_2 after epidural *(Epi)* and i.v. morphine 10 mg by separate injections 2 to 4 weeks apart in six subjects. Mean ± SEM percentage change in slope and ventilation at end-tidal P_{CO_2} of 55 mm Hg (V_E 55). (Reprinted from Neilsen, C.H., Camporesi, E.M., Bromage, P.R., *et al.*: CO_2 sensitivity after epidural and iv morphine. Anesthesiology, *55*:A372, 1981, with permission of the publisher.)

FIG. 28-18. Respiratory and other side-effects following epidural morphine.

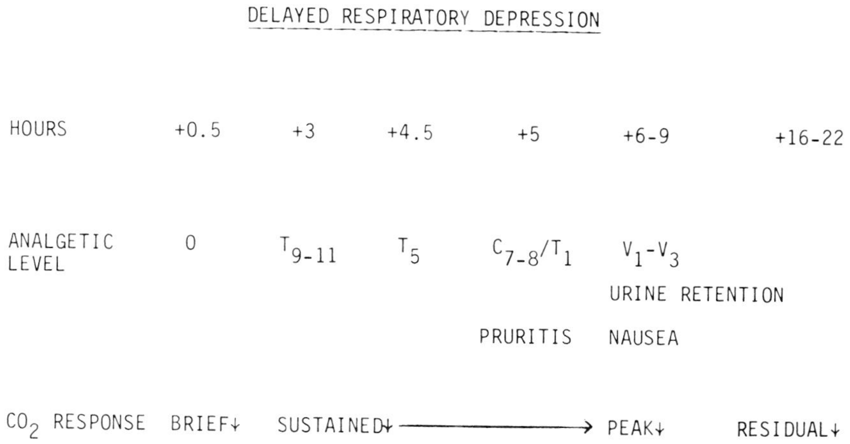

DELAYED RESPIRATORY DEPRESSION

HOURS	+0.5	+3	+4.5	+5	+6-9	+16-22
ANALGETIC LEVEL	0	T_{9-11}	T_5	C_{7-8}/T_1	V_1-V_3	
					URINE RETENTION	
				PRURITIS	NAUSEA	
CO_2 RESPONSE	BRIEF↓	SUSTAINED↓ ⟶			PEAK↓	RESIDUAL↓

algesia, nausea and vomiting, and peak respiratory depression at approximately 6 to 10 hours is strong evidence that this is the time at which significant concentrations of opioid are reached in the brain. There appears to be a relatively slow progression of analgesia as morphine is carried in the passive flow of the slow circulation of the spinal subarachnoid space and then comes into contact with the active intracerebral CSF circulation (see Fig. 28-7). This is in keeping with studies by Gourlay and associates[161] reporting peak morphine concentrations in cervical CSF after 3 hours (see Fig. 28-15*A*), with further time then required to penetrate neural tissue (? 1½ hours as in lumbar region). These data in humans are in broad agreement with animal pharmacokinetic data[170,172] (see above). The studies by Bromage and others[48,50,61] and Gourlay and others[161] help in understanding the time delay of approximately 3 to 12 hours in cases of delayed respiratory depression after epidural morphine.[173,276,313,379] It is significant that the time delay is similar after intrathecal morphine,[120,160,241,302a] confirming the role of rostral spread of morphine in CSF.

The interpretation of ventilation changes driven by exogenous CO_2 is difficult in the absence of data concerning resting ventilation. In a small number of volunteers, Knill and colleagues determined that epidural morphine 3.5 mg or 7 mg reduced resting minute volume and increased end-tidal carbon dioxide progressively with time. Six hours after injection, the ventilatory response to carbon dioxide was reduced considerably. These changes persisted for 24 hours.[225] From these studies it may be surmised that further systemic injection of "usual" doses of opioid would be dangerous at this stage. Indeed, the expected degree of depression can be gauged from the 40% reduction in slope and ventilation after 10 mg of morphine intravenously, which would be added to the residual 20% reduction in slope and 40% reduction in ventilation remaining at 22 hours after epidural morphine.[50] These results in volunteers are likely to be more exaggerated than those in postoperative patients, since the latter may have the counteracting effects of respiratory stimulation owing to postoperative pain. In patients receiving epidural morphine 10 mg for analgesia after lower abdominal or lower limb surgery under epidural local anesthetic, Doblar and co-workers[128] measured ventilatory responses to CO_2 in 10 patients before and after epidural morphine. Minute inspired ventilation (VI) and airway occlusion pressure (P 100) responses to CO_2 during rebreathing were determined. In the postoperative period, at 1 hour after epidural morphine, there was a 22% decrease in VI versus P_{CO_2} slope and a 33% decrease in average P 100 versus P_{CO_2} slope. At 6 hours after morphine, average decrease in VI versus P_{CO_2} slope was not significant; however, P 100 vs. P_{CO_2} slope was decreased by 27%. The authors concluded that epidural morphine caused decreased respiratory drive and that there was a high degree of individual variability in the time course and magnitude of this effect. *The moral is clear:* respiration must be carefully assessed if parenteral opioid is to be given within 24 hours of epidural morphine, and dosage must be reduced appropriately, preferably with the aid of cautious intravenous titration. In a "between-patient" study, the sitting position was reported to be associated with less respiratory depression than the supine position after epidural morphine.[258] However, a controlled study showed no effect of 45-degree elevated posture in protecting against respiratory depression.[269] Use of a minimal effective dose of morphine is important, since respiratory depression is dose-related.[6,310] Doses of 2 to 4 mg morphine result in a much less profound and briefer depression of respiration than do doses of 10 mg morphine,[6,310] which continue to depress respiration for more than 17 hours.[310] Fortunately, 2 to 4 mg of morphine is often adequate for "peripheral surgery," and 4 to 6 mg is adequate for more extensive surgery, provided sufficient time is allowed for onset.[6,231,348] An even better "therapeutic ratio" can be obtained between analgesia and respiratory depression by using low-dose epidural morphine infusion preceded by a bolus dose in a *low* volume (1 ml), so that peak concentrations of morphine in brain stem regions are decreased and incidence of respiratory depression is low.[83,86,141] Respiratory depression can be prevented, or antagonized when it occurs, by naloxone infusion at a dose of 5 μg/kg/h without antagonizing analgesia.[305] This indicates that the relative amount of morphine in the spinal cord is much greater than in the brain and/or that naloxone gains more facile access to mu receptors in the brain.

More lipophilic drugs may produce early respiratory depression, possibly by blood-borne drug (brief effects) but more likely by a transient peak concentration of drug in cisternal CSF[170,172] (see Fig. 28-15*B*). Because most of these drugs move rapidly into and out of neural tissue, it seems that delayed respiratory depression is unlikely. Also, drugs with high affinity for spinal receptors, such as sufentanil and lofentanil probably are associated with small amounts of drug reaching cisternal CSF (see above). In a small number of clinical studies, these theoretical considerations have been borne out, provided the dose of fentanyl analogue has been kept within the therapeutic margin of about 2, between safe epidural dose and "analgesic" intramuscular dose. Low-dose epidural fentanyl infusion (0.5 μg/kg/h) after a bolus of 1.5 μg/kg was not associated with changes in continuously monitored end-tidal CO_2 or respiratory rate, over an 18-hour monitoring period in 21 postoperative patients.[6] In volunteers, epidural fentanyl did not alter CO_2 response curves over a 24-hour period of study, apart from a brief early depression.[229] Other studies of epidural fentanyl in postoperative patients report no evidence of delayed respiratory depression.[240] Initial studies of epidural sufentanil also report no evidence of delayed respiratory depression.[130] However, all of the lipophilic opioids are reported to be associated with a brief period of *early* respiratory depression.[56,70,377] This has sometimes been confused with delayed respiratory depression. A question that remains is the importance of the relative resistance of sufentanil and lofentanil to antagonism by naloxone; much higher doses are needed, reflecting greater affinity of these opioids for mu receptors.[12,419] Presumably this would mean using a higher dose and continuing a naloxone infusion for a substantial period of time. If an inadvertently high dose of these drugs was given intrathecally, a large amount of drug would reach the brain and produce both early and *prolonged* respiratory depression, rather than delayed depression. However, it is theoretically possible for a small amount of residual lofentanil in the brain to produce delayed depression if a "usual analgesic dose" of parenteral opioid was given many hours after an epidural dose. This question has been answered for fentanyl, where morphine was given intravenously in addition to a fentanyl epidural infusion; no delayed respiratory depression was seen.[6] Such studies need to be extended to sufentanil and lofentanil.

SELECTIVITY OF EPIDURAL OPIOID BLOCKADE IN HUMANS

As discussed in the physiology section, epidural opioids may be associated with effects on other systems. Some of these may be regarded as effects of abuse of the technique (*e.g.*, respiratory depression owing to simultaneous epidural and intravenous opioid). However, it is now clear that epidural opioids, particularly morphine, produce effects other than analgesia. Despite this, use of minimally effective doses results in analgesia that is far more selective than that obtained with local anesthetics.

In one study, neurologic examination of patients after epidural meperidine (up to 1% solutions) failed to reveal evidence of sensory or motor blockade.[159] Specific tests of efferent sympathetic activity have included cobalt blue sweat test and skin blood flow response (measured by venous occlusion plethysmography) to the application of ice to skin outside the blocked area.[99,159] These indicated that sudomotor activity and vasoconstrictor sympathetic activity were unaffected by epidural meperidine (in contrast to the abolition of vasoconstrictor responses to ice when local anesthetic was injected epidurally[159]). In one patient there was a small increase in blood flow in the feet after epidural injection of meperidine, despite the retention of vasoconstrictor response to ice. This increase in resting blood flow was transient and probably reflected a direct effect of absorbed meperidine on the peripheral vasculature.[99,159] Zenz and colleagues found that plethysmograhic measurements were unchanged after epidural morphine.[430] Indirect evidence of normal efferent sympathetic activity was provided by Bromage and co-workers.[50] They found that the psychogalvanic response (PGR) and the arterial pressure response to Valsalva maneuver was abolished below the level of blockade when 2% chloroprocaine was injected epidurally. In contrast, both responses remained intact after epidural hydromorphone. Also, the blood pressure response to immersion of "nonblocked" hands in ice water was retained in contrast to "blocked" lower limbs, which elicited a smaller change in blood pressure when immersed in ice water. The latter finding implied that the afferent limb of the blood pressure reflex response to noxious stimuli had been obtunded. One subject in their study retained a normal PGR response when the ice was applied to the nonblocked area, but with thoracic epidural opioid, the blood pressure response to Valsalva was abolished. They interpreted this to mean that afferent signals from the thoracic area had been obtunded by the epidural opioid.[50] All of the above data indicate that efferent sympathetic vasoconstrictor fibers within the blocked area are unaffected by epidural opioid blockade. This is supported by an elegant study in dogs by Liao and others,[238] in which reflex vasoconstriction owing to hypotension (intravenous acetylcholine) and reflex vasodilatation owing to hypertension (intravenous norepinephrine) were not altered by epidural or cisternal administration of morphine (see also the physiology section).

In many studies, efferent motor activity has been reported to be unimpaired, so that patients ambulated normally.[50,159] Also, touch and proprioception are unimpaired, but bladder function may be impaired.[202,303] Urinary retention is common in volunteers,[50,303,304,357,358] less common after surgery,[54,308,359] and uncommon in patients with cancer[159,407] when epidural morphine is used for pain relief. Mechanisms are not clear; however, naloxone antagonism of urinary retention indicates involvement of opioid receptors, perhaps by means of inhibition of acetylcholine release from efferent postganglionic neurons innervating detrusor muscle.

It seems likely that generalized pruritus associated with spinal opioids is due to widespread alteration in sensory modulation, since it occurs when there is evidence of opioid migration over the entire spinal cord to the brain. Sensory modulatory mechanisms in the upper cervical spinal cord and trigeminal system may be involved, since the onset coincides with the spread of hypalgesia to this region.[47] The dominant feature of facial pruritus that often is reported may be explained by rapid penetration of opioid to the superficially placed caudal portions of the nucleus of the spinal tract of the trigeminal nerve.[170,172] Also, pruritus often subsides, like loss of bladder function, with subsequent doses of opioid, presumably because of adaptation to the change in sensation. It is not due to preservatives in opioids, since it occurs with non-preservative-containing agents. It is unlikely to be due to histamine release, since the time of onset is approximately 3 hours after epidural or spinal opioid administration[47,48,50] and occurs with fentanyl, which does not cause systemic histamine liberation as does morphine.[322] Intravenous naloxone antagonizes pruritus.[47,306]

SIDE-EFFECTS AND THEIR INCIDENCE

Respiratory Depression

Respiratory depression seems uncommon in patients previously made tolerant to opioids,[92,159,401] and thus there have been few reports in such patients with chronic pain. Even in patients who are naive to opioids, the incidence of life-threatening respiratory depression has been low when epidural opioids are used in the absence of opioid administration by other routes.[173] To date, only a handful of cases have been reported after many thousands of administrations of epidural opioid, for example, one case among 1200 patients receiving epidural morphine.[314] The predisposing factors noted earlier should be kept in mind. Also, it should be recognized that there is always some change in respiratory response, even if it is not detectable by usual clinical observations.[50] It is likely that epidural opioids have a much better safety margin in the patient whose respiratory and other intracranial structures already have become tolerant to opioid, which will be conveyed inevitably to the brain during epidural opioid administration (see Fig. 28-15). This is borne out by the failure to observe respiratory depression in many patients with cancer who are treated with long-term spinal opioids.[76,92,94,111,428]

In a nationwide retrospective study of epidural and intrathecal opioids, Gustafsson and colleagues[173] obtained data on approximately 6000 patients† who had received epidural morphine, 220 who received epidural meperidine, and 90 who received intrathe-

†A follow-up study of 14,000 patients given epidural morphine (4 mg) in 1986 revealed an incidence of delayed respiratory depression of 1 : 1000. In comparison the incidence for intrathecal morphine (0.2 – 0.8 mg) was 1 : 275.[302a]

cal morphine. Ventilatory depression requiring naloxone was reported in 22 patients receiving epidural morphine (approximately 0.33% of patients) and in 6 given intrathecal morphine (approximately 5.5% of patients.) Only two of the patients receiving epidural morphine had respiratory depression later than 6 hours after the last dose of opiates. Only 3 of the 22 patients did not receive opioids in addition to epidural morphine in the periods during or after operation. Ten of them were 70 or more years of age, and ten had thoracic injections. Brownridge[54] reported 9000 doses of meperidine 50 mg administered epidurally in 2000 women after cesarean section, with only one case of respiratory depression.[54] This was shown to result from migration of the epidural catheter into the subarachnoid space.[56] It has been reported that epidural fentanyl does not cause delayed respiratory depression in volunteers,[229] in accord with predictions. These results underscore the contributing factors to respiratory depression outlined in the pharmacokinetic section earlier and the importance of understanding physicochemical properties of the drug in addition to the pharmacologic properties. Comparative incidence data for early and delayed respiratory depression for the different opioids are not available from controlled studies.

Opioid Withdrawal Syndrome

In patients receiving epidural opioid after previous long-term treatment with parenteral opioids, the amount of opioid reaching the tolerant brain may not be sufficient to prevent a withdrawal response if opioid, by other routes, suddenly is ceased when pain relief is obtained. Withdrawal response has been observed in a patient with cancer who required epidural morphine 20 mg every 8 hours after failing to obtain pain relief from 1200 mg of morphine orally every 8 hours. Later in treatment, the same patient had withdrawal during a period of epidural local anesthetic treatment after long-term epidural morphine (Cousins, M.J.: Unpublished observations). Others also have reported patients whose pain was relieved by intrathecal morphine and who developed opioid withdrawal syndrome when parenteral opioid was abruptly ceased.[264,365] Withdrawal may occur also if epidural opioid treatment is antagonized by substitution of a pure agonist with a partial agonist or agonist–antagonist. This was demonstrated dramatically in a patient who developed a shocked state when the partial antagonist buprenorphine was injected epidurally after long-term epidural morphine treatment.[78] However, the two drugs were successfully alternated in one series.[63]

Nausea and Vomiting

In a cross-over study in volunteers, Bromage and colleagues[47] observed nausea and vomiting in 50% of subjects approximately 6 hours after epidural morphine, which coincided with other evidence of rostral spread of morphine in spinal fluid to intracerebral structures, including the vomiting center and the chemoreceptor trigger zone (see Fig. 28-18). In contrast, after intravenous morphine only one out of ten subjects had nausea lasting 2 hours. In a prospective study of 1085 postoperative patients, Stenseth and associates[348] reported that epidural morphine (dose 4–6 mg) was associated with nausea or vomiting in 34% of patients. In a series of 1200 postoperative patients, nausea and vomiting were present in 17% of the patients,[314] while in another series nausea was present in 12%, with vomiting in 24%.[232] In the latter series, the incidence of nausea and vomiting was similar whether morphine was used intramuscularly or epidurally, or saline was injected epidurally. Others, too, have reported a low incidence of nausea and vomiting after epidural morphine in the postoperative period.[359] In labor, the incidence of nausea and vomiting has been reported to be low with epidural opioid[54,295] in contrast to a high incidence with intrathecal opioid.[25,333] Epidural use of lipid-soluble opioids such as meperidine, fentanyl, and sufentanil[54,130,383] may be associated with the lowest incidence of nausea and vomiting. Fortunately, the incidence of nausea and vomiting seems to be much less with repeated epidural dosing and is low in patients with cancer who require long-term epidural opioid.[92,159,189,428] Perhaps the brain becomes tolerant to those side-effects as it does to respiratory depressant effects. It should be remembered that a 30% incidence of nausea and vomiting accompanies routine parenteral use of opioids in postoperative patients, while pain itself has been implicated, also, as a cause of nausea.[348] Nausea and vomiting are antagonized by intravenous naloxone, without diminishing analgesia, at doses of 5 $\mu g/kg/h$.[307]

Urinary Retention

As noted earlier, urinary retention is a more frequently reported complication[46,304,357,358,373] of spinal opioids administered to volunteer subjects than of spinal opioids administered to patients. Significantly, two subjects in Bromage's series[47] failed to respond to bethanecol 5 mg subcutaneously but then responded to naloxone 0.4 mg intravenously. All subjects in Rawal and others' study responded to naloxone 0.8 mg intravenously, indicating the involvement of some opioid receptors.[303,304] Thirty-nine per cent of postoperative patients required bladder catheterization in one series[133] after approximately 8 mg of morphine epidural. In a study of morphine, 6 mg, Torda and Pybus[359] found that only 1 patient out of 24 required bladder catheterization. Rawal and others reported an incidence of 22% urinary retention in 90 patients receiving epidural morphine.[308]

In a dose–response study of epidural morphine for postoperative pain relief, Martin and associates found that the incidence of urinary retention was the same for doses of morphine of 0.5, 1.0, 2.0, 4.0, and 8.0 mg.[247] This was in keeping with a urodynamic study in 30 volunteers in whom increased bladder capacity and relaxation of detrusor muscle was similar for epidural doses of morphine of 2, 4, and 10 mg.[304] Thus, current evidence indicates that urodynamic effects of epidural morphine are not dose related. It is not yet known if the incidence varies with the opioid used, the duration of treatment, or between males and females. That these factors may be important is suggested by a series of 40,000 injections of epidural meperidine 50 mg for pain after cesarean section in which catheterization of the bladder was not necessary.[54] In this large series, patients routinely had bladder catheterization intraoperatively and for the first 12 hours postoperatively and then did not require recatheterization. This is of interest, since another study reported a low incidence of urinary retention using this approach compared with a high incidence with "in, out" catheterization intraoperatively followed by epidural morphine.[222] In a study of postoperative patients using CO_2 cystometry, a great variation in bladder response to epidural morphine was found on the day after surgery. Intravenous naloxone reversed bladder effects in those patients who developed urinary retention.[202] Lipid-soluble opioids of the fentanyl type also cause urine retention, since they also act on spinal mu receptors. However, the incidence may be relatively low. In one study, incidence of urine retention was less with methadone than with morphine.[149] Also, there is evidence in animal studies that kappa agonists may be devoid of this urinary effect; studies of analgesic efficacy and side-effects in humans are not available. For patients with chronic pain, long-term epidural opioids would appear to be without a need to catheterize the bladder.[76,159,407]

Pruritus

In volunteer studies of epidural morphine, 10 mg, pruritus occurred in 100% of subjects in one study[46] and in three of four subjects in another study.[358] In postoperative patients, pruritus was present in 28% of patients receiving epidural morphine 10 mg in one study[232] but in only 1% of patients in studies of morphine 5 mg[46] and 2 mg, respectively.[313] Pruritus also has been reported with epidural meperidine, fentanyl, and diamorphine, but few comparative data are available. When meperidine 50 mg was used for post-cesarean section pain, Brownridge reported that 50% of 2000 patients admitted to pruritus (but only on direct questioning) and in only 1 patient was it troublesome.[54] In contrast, in some series, epidural morphine resulted in pruritus in up to 70% of patients, but there was no relationship between incidence of pruritus and dose.[247] However, the incidence of severe pruritus that troubles the patient appears to be close to 1%.[46] It has been reported that prior use of bupivacaine epidurally reduces the incidence of pruritus with epidural opioids.[334] An unexplained observation is that pruritus does not follow intrathecal administration of β-endorphin.[289,290]

Dysphoria, and Other CNS Effects

Dysphoria has been reported in volunteer studies,[47,225] and sedation has been observed in clinical studies.[27] These are familiar adverse effects of parenteral opioids. An uncommon complication of prolonged opioid administration epidurally for cancer pain was reported to be catatonia.[146,147]

Sedation has been reported to have a low incidence in cancer patients treated with epidural opioid after prior treatment with oral opioid.[76,92,396] Also, sedation is much less in opioid-naive patients if morphine dose is the minimum effective dose.[231,307] Sedation is reported to be minimal or absent with a bolus[240] or low-dose infusion of fentanyl[6] or with low-dose boli of meperidine.[55] The very lipophilic drug sufentanil has a high incidence of sedation shortly after its epidural administration; this is reduced (but not eliminated) by decreasing the dose from 75 μg to 50 μg.[130] *Hyperesthesia* has been reported after high doses of spinal morphine in patients with cancer pain.[413] It seems that this results from an action of morphine on receptors other than those involved in antinociception, since hyperesthesia is not antagonized by naloxone.[254] Fortunately, even high doses of sufentanil and alfentanil do not appear to be associated with this side-effect.[413]

An unusual hazard of CNS effects of epidural opioids is reported to be their use in patients with undiagnosed sleep apnea syndrome — where a small epidural dose of morphine resulted in severe sedation and respiratory depression.[230]

RELATIONSHIP BETWEEN DOSE AND PAIN RELIEF

Double-blind studies have confirmed a dose–response relationship between epidural morphine and the relief of postoperative pain,[6,112,247] labor pain,[193,194] or pain after cesarean section.[195,277] After lower abdominal and lower limb surgery, Martin and associates found morphine 2, 4, and 8 mg equipotent and more effective than morphine 0.5 and 1.0 mg.[247] Morphine 5 mg and 10 mg were equally effective for post-gynecologic surgery pain,[112] while morphine 5.0 mg and 7.5 mg were effective for post-cesarean section pain.[195] In both studies, morphine 2 mg provided unsatisfactory pain relief.[112,195] In a double-blind randomized study, Nordberg found a dose-related analgesic duration after epidural morphine, 2, 4, or 6 mg: 2 mg — 514 minutes; 4 mg — 718 minutes; 6 mg — 938 minutes.[281] In a within-patient double-blind study of pain relief after major thoracic and abdominal surgery, Pybus and Torda were not able to distinguish between 4, 6, and 8 mg of morphine in terms of efficacy. However, increasing the dose increased the mean duration of analgesia (4 mg — 593 minutes; 6 mg — 722 minutes; 8 mg — 885 minutes.[300] Rawal and others reported that morphine 4 mg was effective after upper abdominal surgery, but 2 mg was sufficient after lower abdominal surgery.[308] After peripheral vascular and total knee replacement surgery, Allen and associates found a dose–response relationship for epidural morphine with respect to efficacy and duration.[6] A dose–response relationship was reported for epidural met-enkephalin and postoperative pain relief.[10] In a double-blind study of morphine 5 and 2 mg and placebo, McClure and co-workers[258] found no significant difference in postoperative pain relief among the three at 20 minutes after epidural injection, but the frequency of successful analgesia was greater for the 5-mg dose. However, these results are difficult to interpret, since more than 35 minutes are required for complete onset of analgesic effect of morphine. Furthermore, some of these differences in results may be due to methodological problems in all current methods of pain assessment in humans, which are not present in experimental animal preparations. A plot of analgesic index (area under time–analgesic response curves) against log dose gives a clear dose–response relationship for epidural morphine, meperidine, methadone, and lofentanil in the cat.[367] The weight of evidence also points to a dose–response relationship for pain relief in humans. However, the relationship between dose and intensity of analgesic response would seem to plateau more quickly than that of the dose and duration of analgesia. Little clear therapeutic benefit would seem to accrue from increasing the dose further once effective intensities of analgesia have been reached.

Minimum effective analgesic doses have been determined for a number of opioids, for different types of acute pain. These studies have attempted to define an effective analgesic dose with minimal side-effects.

Morphine. The minimum effective dose for postoperative pain after major surgery is 6 to 8 mg[348]; after peripheral surgery and lower abdominal surgery, 2 to 5 mg.[6,231] Doses of morphine as high as 10 mg improved analgesia after major surgery but were associated with significant respiratory depression.[6,310] Infusion of morphine postoperatively at approximately 0.1 to 0.2 mg per hour[91,141] after a bolus of 2 mg is reported to be effective and to have a low incidence of side-effects. However, increments of morphine are needed on a demand basis.[91,141] For labor pain, a randomized study found that morphine 2 and 5 mg required supplementation with local anesthetic, but that morphine 7.5 mg gave satisfactory analgesia in 7 of 11 patients until delivery, when local anesthesia was needed in all 11 patients.[194] For cancer, doses vary greatly, depending on the patient and disease factors (see below).

Fentanyl. During surgery under epidural bupivacaine, fentanyl 50 μg decreased pain in all patients. Doses of 12.5 and 25 μg were less effective, while doses of 75 and 100 μg were no more effective but had a slightly more rapid onset. Postoperatively, 50 μg also was the optimum dose.[277] In a double-blind study of postoperative pain, fentanyl 100 μg was found to be optimal in patients who had received epidural lidocaine for their previous "top-up." Addition of 1 : 200,000 epinephrine to a 50-μg dose of fentanyl made it equieffective to the 100-μg dose.[383] When used by infusion for thoracic surgery, it was found that 60 μg per hour was the optimum rate of infusion.[384]

Meperidine. Systematic dose–response studies are not available. However, after cesarean section, meperidine 50 mg epidurally was as effective as bupivacaine 0.25% (10 ml).[55]

Sufentanil. Postoperatively, after orthopedic surgery, an open dose–response study found that 50 μg was the optimal dose[130] and gave excellent analgesia for 6 hours. Even at this dose, significant sedation was present.[130] After cesarean section, epidural sufentanil 50 μg provided effective analgesia for 219 ± 118 minutes.[355]

Other opioids such as methadone, hydromorphone, alfentanil, lofentanil, buprenorphine, nalbuphine, and pentazocine have been reported to be effective epidurally. Precise dose–response data are not available.

DIFFERENCES IN DURATION AND EFFICACY AMONG OPIOIDS

There are no data in humans indicating differences in *efficacy* among different opioids at equivalent doses. The exception to this may be morphine when used by a lumbar epidural catheter for thoracic pain,[282] since it spreads more evenly over the spinal cord than other opioids (see reference 170, 172).

Data from animals suggest that different types of pain may be more effectively relieved by opioids acting on different spinal opioid receptors, or on nonopioid receptors (see section on the site of action). This remains to be investigated in humans. Duration of analgesia does vary considerably for the different opioids.

Postoperative pain relief was assessed after epidural administration of three different opioids compared with intravenous morphine.[46] Methadone (5 mg) and hydromorphone (Dilaudid; 1 mg) effectively controlled pain for 7 and 11 hours, respectively, while morphine (5 mg) was longer acting (18 hours). In comparison, intravenous morphine (5–10 mg) lasted for only 3 hours. The onset of pain relief was more rapid with methadone and hydromorphone, compared with morphine[46] (Table 28-13). In another study of 24 postoperative patients, each patient received four different opioids epidurally in a double-blind "latin square" design, so that each of the 24 possible sequences of the four drugs was given to one patient.[360] Duration of pain relief was longest with morphine, intermediate with methadone and meperidine, and shortest with fentanyl (Table 28-13). These results were confirmed in another double-blind study.[323] Epidural diamorphine has been reported to be longer acting than epidural fentanyl,[188] possibly because of uptake into the spinal cord as diamorphine and then continued action through hydrolysis to its active metabolites, first to mono-acetyl morphine and then to morphine,[252] possibly in the spinal cord or CSF.[271] In one study, epidural diamorphine was only as effective as intramuscular diamorphine,[202] while in a further study, epidural diamorphine 5 mg was more effective than the same dose intramuscularly.[246] In a double-blind study, epidural

TABLE 28–13. EPIDURAL OPIOIDS: LATENCY AND DURATION OF POSTOPERATIVE ANALGESIA

Drug	Dose	Detectable Onset (min) (Mean ± SD or Range)	Complete Pain Relief (min) (Mean ± SD or Range)	Duration (h) (Mean ± SD or Range)	References
Meperidine	30–100 mg	5–10	12–30	6 (median)	159
				4–20	
				6.6 ± 3.3	360
Morphine*	5–10 mg	23.5 ± 6.0	60	20	112
	5 mg		37 ± 6	18.1 ± 6.8	46
				12.3 ± 7.7	360
	2–6 mg		60–90	8–15	281
Methadone	5 mg	12.5 ± 2.0	17 ± 3	7.2 ± 4.6	46
				8.7 ± 5.9	360
Hydromorphone	1 mg	13 ± 4	23 ± 8	11.4 ± 5.5	46
Fentanyl	0.1 mg			5.7 ± 3.7	360
	0.1 mg	4–10	20	2.6–4.0	391
Diamorphine	5 mg	15	30	8.4 ± 1	243a
	6 mg	5	15	12.4 ± 6.5	203
				2–21	
Phenoperidine	2 mg	15	30	6.0 ± 0.4	243a

*Increasing the dose from 2 mg to 6 mg of morphine increases the duration of pain relief from approximately 514 minutes to 938 minutes.[281]

methadone was reported to be more effective than morphine or bupivacaine.[28] However, the dosing interval for methadone was shorter than the plasma half-life, and it is possible that maintenance of significant concentrations of drug in the circulation added to analgesia.[163] In a double-blind study,[31] lofentanil 5 μg was more effective than buprenorphine 0.3 mg.

COMBINATION OF SPINAL OPIOIDS AND LOCAL ANESTHETICS

In **labor pain,** addition of 2 mg of morphine in 10 ml of saline to bupivacaine 0.25% 10 ml resulted in excellent pain relief for 131 minutes compared with 57 minutes for bupivacaine alone.[280] Morphine 2 mg given after bupivacaine 0.25% gave pain relief after episiotomy for up to 12 hours.[243] Addition of fentanyl 80 μg to 4 ml of 0.3% bupivacaine increased the rapidity of onset and the efficacy and duration of analgesia.[214] This approach has great appeal because it minimizes motor blockade (and perhaps increases spontaneous delivery rate) while providing effective analgesia. Case series in France and Belgium indicate that doses of fentanyl greater than 50 μg are effective when added to 10 ml of 0.25% bupivacaine. This is broadly supported by a dose–response study during cesarean section under epidural bupivacaine (see below).[278] Addition of meperidine 50 mg to 10 ml bupivacaine 0.25% results in similar effects to those noted earlier for fentanyl (Brownridge, P.: Unpublished observations, 1986).

During cesarean section, epidural fentanyl 50 μg relieved residual pain in all patients who were managed with epidural bupivacaine until the delivery of the baby.[277] This dose of fentanyl also provided significantly longer postoperative analgesia compared with 25, 12.5 or 0 μg of fentanyl.[277] In a controlled study, epidural morphine 3 mg enhanced the analgesia of epidural bupivacaine.[177] **After surgery,** the combination of morphine and bupivacaine epidurally (low-dose infusion) was superior to bupivacaine or morphine alone, in a randomized controlled study.[113]

EFFICACY OF EPIDURAL OPIOIDS IN COMPARISON WITH OTHER ACUTE PAIN RELIEF TECHNIQUES

Postoperative Pain Relief

In postoperative pain relief, epidural opioids are capable of relieving both visceral pain, such as after abdominal or thoracic surgery,[46,159,308,359] and somatic pain, such as after orthopedic surgery[26,138,168,247] (see Tables 28-5, 28-14). Using forced expiratory volume in 1 second (FEV_1), as an index of pain relief and improved respiration, Bromage and others found that epidural morphine 5 mg improved FEV_1 to 67% of control values compared with 45% with intravenous morphine 10 mg or 68% with epidural local anesthetic[46] (Fig. 28-19). Respiratory function was significantly better after epidural morphine compared with intravenous morphine in postthoracotomy patients.[337] In a controlled study, after arthrotomy, epidural morphine 0.05 mg/kg resulted in more pronounced and more prolonged analgesia than did morphine 0.05 mg/kg intramuscularly.[168] In patients after gallbladder surgery, 4 mg epidural morphine produced more effective and longer lasting analgesia than did intramuscular opioid (ketobemidone 5.0–7.5 mg) or intercostal nerve block with 0.5% bupivacaine. Also, the changes in blood gases and peak expiratory flow rate were more favorable with epidural morphine. Of the patients given epidural morphine, 40% did not require any further analgesia in the postoperative period, while the remainder were pain free for a mean duration of 19 hours.[309] In a double-blind, randomized, cross-over study, epidural morphine 4 to 8 mg was compared with 4 to 8 ml 0.5% bupivacaine after major abdominal or thoracic surgery.[361] Peak expiratory flow rate was improved equally, and pain relief was similar for each drug. However, three patients had significant hypotension after epidural bupivacaine. Patient preference seems to favor epidural opioid over intramuscular opioid for postoperative pain.[11,55,268] Another study compared epidural morphine 5 mg with 6 to 8 ml of 0.5% bupivacaine for postoperative pain relief. After total hip replacement, morphine provided pain relief for an average of 28 hours, compared with 4.3 hours with bupivacaine.[268] After upper abdominal operations, thoracic epidural morphine relieved pain for 9.8 hours, compared with 3.8 hours for 0.5% bupivacaine; however, one case of delayed respiratory depression occurred after the morphine.[268] In high-respiratory-risk patients, epidural morphine and lidocaine were equally effective in relieving pain after upper abdominal surgery and were superior to intravenous boli of morphine. Although vital capacity and FEV_1 were improved by epidural morphine, maximal inspiratory and expiratory pressures at the mouth remained markedly decreased after surgery and were not improved by epidural morphine or lidocaine.[27]

Pain relief by epidural morphine 2 mg after prostatectomy was judged by nursing staff to be superior to bupivacaine 0.5% (5–8 ml) and had a longer mean

TABLE 28-14. EPIDURAL OPIOIDS: STUDIES OF EFFICACY

Type of Pain	Drug/Regimen	Study Design	Outcome	References
Postoperative				
Hip replacement	Meperidine 1 mg/kg i.m. versus 20, 60 mg EPI	RPDB	Kinetics of i.m. and EPI the same. Pain (VAS) less after EPI only for 0.25–1 h. Hypalgesia to pinprick in some EPI patients for 2 h.	169 171
Knee arthrotomy	Morphine 0.05 mg/kg^{-1} EPI versus 0.1 mg kg^{-1} i.m.	RPDB	Time to C_{max} less for EPI (12 min) and C_{max}/dose greater for EPI. No correlation between plasma concentration and analgesia. Analgesia with EPI > i.m. between 2 and 11 h. Maximum analgesia after 2h.	168
Knee arthrotomy	EPI versus oral controlled-release morphine (CRM)	Controlled study	9/10 with EPI good relief. CRM not effective.	23
Total knee replacement	EPI bupivacaine versus EPI + meperidine versus i.m. opioid	RPDB	Both epidural regimens superior to i.m. for analgesia and hospital stay. Less sensory/motor block with combination.	302
Abdominal surgery	EPI versus i.m. morphine	Controlled	Pain relief superior with EPI.	35
Abdominal surgery	EPI morphine versus EPI bupivacaine versus EPI morphine + bupivacaine versus EPI saline versus no EPI [EPI by infusion]	RPDB	Morphine + bupivacaine infusion superior for pain relief, mobilization, and respiratory function.	113
Thoracic surgery	EPI bupivacaine boli versus EPI morphine bolus versus EPI morphine infusion	Controlled study	EPI morphine infusion as effective as other two methods, but fewer side-effects	141
Abdominal surgery for obesity	EPI morphine versus i.m. morphine	RPDB	Analgesia same for both, but dose of morphine less for EPI. EPI superior for mobilization, pulmonary complications, bowel function, hospital stay.	307
Upper abdominal	EPI morphine versus intercosal local anesthetic versus i.v. fentanyl infusion + "on-demand" boli	Controlled study	Pain at 2 and 24 h similar in all three groups. Efficacy rating similar. Time to supplemental analgesia longest in EPI morphine group. Pulmonary effects similar.	321
Thoracotomy	EPI versus i.v. boli of morphine	RPDB	EPI, less pain at 2 and 8 h. No differences in pulmonary function.	337
Abdominal surgery	EPI morphine versus EPI saline given intraoperatively	Double-blind multicenter	EPI morphine significantly longer analgesia, decreased requirements for i.m. morphine	394
Thoracotomy	EPI versus i.m. nicromorphine on patient demand	Controlled study	Both groups rapid and effective analgesia. Fewer pulmonary complications in epidural group.	180 181
Laminectomy	EPI versus i.m. morphine	Controlled study	Pain relief superior with EPI, but dose of morphine same.	311
Abdominal surgery	i.m. morphine versus EPI bupivacaine 1st 24 h then EPI morphine 72 h.	Controlled study	Pain better controlled with epidural. No difference in pulmonary, cardiac, wound, metabolic, thrombotic indices. Convalescence not improved by epidural.	182
Postcesarean Section	EPI morphine versus i.v. morphine	Controlled study	Excellent pain relief in 74% in epidural group, in 32% in i.m. group.	87
	EPI bupivacaine versus EPI meperidine versus i.m. meperidine	RPDB "within patient"	Epidural regimens superior to i.m. Significant patient preference for EPI meperidine.	55
During Labor	EPI fentanyl versus i.v. fentanyl in patients receiving EPI bupivacaine	RPDB	EPI fentanyl produced more rapid, intense, and long-lasting analgesia than i.v. fentanyl despite higher plasma concentrations with i.v.	371

RPDB = randomized prospective double-blind; i.m. = intramuscular; EPI = epidural; VAS = Visual Analogue Scale.

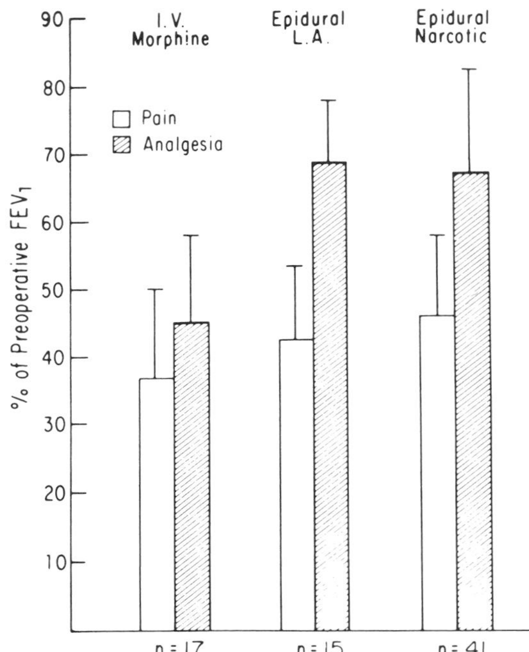

FIG. 28-19. Postoperative pain and respiratory effects of epidural opioids. FEV_1 values are shown as a percentage of preoperative values, after **upper abdominal surgery**. Results are given before and after relief of pain with intravenous morphine, epidural local anesthetic, and epidural opioid. Means ± SD. (Reprinted from Bromage, P.R., Camporesi, E., and Chestnut, D.: Epidural narcotics for postoperative analgesia. Anesth. Analg., *59*:473, 1980, with permission of the publisher.)

duration (12 hours) compared with bupivacaine (5.3 hours). Furthermore, 5% of patients receiving bupivacaine had a reduction of systolic blood pressure of more than 30 mm Hg.[164] In another study, after prostatectomy, single-dose epidural block with bupivacaine combined with morphine (4 mg) was compared with epidural bupivacaine alone. Patients receiving the morphine had an average of 27 hours of pain relief and requested no further analgesia. Those receiving bupivacaine alone had pain relief for an average of 6.2 hours, and all required opioids for in excess of 24 hours.[335] In a double-blind study of pain after orthopedic surgery, Lanz and associates compared morphine intramuscularly or epidurally (0.1 mg/kg) or epidural saline[232] and showed that patients receiving epidural morphine had pain less frequently and of less intense duration and required lower total doses of opioid. Chambers and co-workers[68] found that epidural morphine 10 mg, given at the time of epidural local anesthetic block for major gynecologic surgery, resulted in prolonged postoperative analgesia (707 minutes) compared with morphine 10 mg intramuscularly (371 minutes). However, when morphine was given epidurally after the onset of postoperative pain, it often "failed" to relieve pain. It is possible that the latter may have been related to the ward staff's response to the slow onset of epidural morphine.

Controlled studies of intravenous opioid infusion[347] compared with epidural opioid infusion[22] are not available. However, intravenous demand analgesia has been used to assess the success of epidurally applied opioids, while intramuscular and oral opioids have been reported to be as effective as "demand intravenous analgesia" if given regularly,[144] and continuous epidural infusion of local anaesthetics[155] and opioids[142] have been used successfully; precise definition of the relative merits of each of these methods of postoperative pain relief awaits further studies. Epidural bupivacaine has been reported to be superior to intravenous and intramuscular morphine, in a controlled study.[114] In another controlled study, epidural bupivacaine (0.25%) 6 to 15 ml per hour was compared with epidural bupivacaine (0.125%) plus meperidine (0.1%) 6 to 15 ml per hour and with standard intramuscular opioid on demand after total knee replacement. Both epidural regimens were equivalent in analgesic effect and superior in pain relief to intramuscular opioid. Motor and sensory loss were less in the bupivacaine plus meperidine epidural group. Hospitalization was shorter in the two epidural groups.[302] Intravenous fentanyl infusion plus "on-demand boli" of fentanyl was compared with epidural morphine boli and intercostal nerve blocks for upper abdominal surgery. Pain relief was similar in all three groups, as was pulmonary function. The time to first supplementary analgesia was longest in the epidural group.[321] In the meantime there is no doubt that the use of intravenous opioid infusion[321,347] or regular intramuscular injections of opioid[18] can provide analgesia less invasively and with a lower rate of complications than the use of epidural opioid. Thus, the potential advantage of superior analgesia with epidural opioid (see Table 28-14) has to be justified in individual cases against the "price" of greater invasiveness and currently recognized complications of epidural opioids[45] (see Tables 28-6, 28-7). For example, a study of the partial agonist buprenorphine reported a similar pattern of vascular absorption, similar efficacy and duration of analgesia for sublingual compared with epidural administration.[33] Studies in animals of other partial agonists have questioned the efficacy of these drugs administered by spinal route for some types of pain[329] (see above).

An additional choice for long-duration postoperative pain relief is intravenous methadone, which, because of its low systemic clearance, is a kind of "poor man's infusion." A single intravenous 20-mg dose of this drug administered soon after induction resulted in approximately 24-hour analgesia after major surgery of the spine.[163,251] As for epidural opioids, great care is required with administration of supplementary doses of opioid because methadone is cleared slowly from the blood,[252] with great individual variability both in terminal half-life and resultant pain relief. This then poses a potential for cumulation if doses are given at inappropriate intervals. Thus, intravenous methadone may be as dangerous as epidural opioids when supplementary doses of methadone are required. However, intravenous doses can be titrated more readily than epidural doses, and a method aimed at optimizing the safety of supplementary doses recently has been described.[162] Epidural methadone is effective[28] and brain stem CSF concentrations are low after epidural administration.[257] Respiratory depression is infrequent in anecdotal reports. One comparative study reported less urinary retention with epidural methadone than with epidural morphine.[149] In view of these potential attractions of this drug, a comparative study of efficacy and blood concentrations for epidural vs. intravenous methadone is required. It is likely that repeated doses of methadone epidurally would result in sustained blood concentrations that would add to analgesic effect and may pose potential hazards of the type described earlier.

Epidural use of fentanyl analogues has attraction for postoperative pain because of a potential to restrict these lipid-soluble drugs to the spinal cord. The short-acting drugs fentanyl and alfentanil have been used successfully epidurally.[70,384] They both have suitable properties for continuous infusion epidurally.[384] Alfentanil was effective epidurally at doses that were ineffective intramuscularly.[70] Longer-acting drugs lofentanil and sufentanil are better suited to repeated bolus administration until regimens for low-dose infusion have been investigated. Lofentanil is very long acting, resistant to naloxone reversal, and associated with considerable sedation; however, it is more effective than the partial agonist buprenorphine, which is another drug with high receptor affinity.[31] Sufentanil also causes short-term sedation, but not delayed respiratory depression, and provides long duration and intense pain relief after surgery.[130] Comparative studies for these new fentanyl analogues are not yet available.

A comparative study of buprenorphine (0.3 mg) and morphine (4 mg) epidurally found the two to be equieffective in orthopedic surgery.[392a] A comparative study of analgesia and pharmacokinetics found that epidural diamorphine (heroin) and morphine were equieffective. However, serum morphine concentrations were higher with diamorphine and slowing of respiration occurred only with diamorphine.[297,377] Thus, diamorphine seems to offer little over morphine.

Stress Response and Postoperative Pain

Epidural local anesthetic blockade used intraoperatively and postoperatively has been shown to be capable of obtunding the neuroendocrine and metabolic response to surgery.[221] Increases in plasma glucose concentrations are prevented, and only minimal changes in plasma cortisol occur. However, these results were obtained with epidural block for lower abdominal surgery, which may provide only a mild stimulus for the stress response. Epidural morphine and diamorphine are ineffective in preventing intraoperative changes in plasma cortisol or glucose concentrations and tend merely to delay or modify these changes postoperatively to a lesser extent than does epidural local anesthetic.[80,107,213] These results indicate that epidural opioid is unable to block all of the afferent noxious impulses resulting from surgical stimulation. In another study, epidural bupivacaine 0.25% failed to prevent alterations in plasma glucose and cortisol.[107] It seems possible that the level of blockade may have been inadequate; also, the block was allowed to wear off after surgery and was then reinstituted. Other studies are in agreement that high epidural local anesthetic blockade can prevent a predominant part of the neuroendocrine response during and after surgery in the region of the lower half of the body,[36,57,58,145,221] but there is a lesser modifying influence during and after upper abdominal surgery.[52,221,362] In general, epidural opioid is ineffective in modifying neurohumoral responses to surgery and has only a mild effect compared with local anesthetics[182] (see Chap. 5). Indeed, one study reported increases in antidiuretic hormone secretion because of morphine migrating in CSF to the brain.[226] When pain relief is effective with epidural opioids, the cortisol response is modified but not abolished[322a] (see Chap. 5). The role of pain stimuli versus other neurogenic stimuli in initiating the stress response remains to be elucidated. Of interest, high-dose opioid "anesthesia" suppresses the intraoperative endocrine–metabolic responses during surgery but without a persistent effect on postoperative responses.[42,362]

Postoperative Pediatric Pain

After pediatric surgery, caudal block with morphine was associated with pain relief that was longer (610–2,195 minutes) than with bupivacaine (245–515 minutes).[205] Epidural morphine in a dose of 1 to 2 mg has been used in children aged 3 to 11 years, and anecdotal reports indicate that it is effective.[336] Although intrathecal morphine is reported to be effective for pain relief after cardiac surgery,[211] controlled studies are not available. It appears that vigorous evaluation of the place of spinal opioids after pediatric surgery has not begun. There is an urgent need for controlled studies of different methods of pain relief after pediatric surgery.

Labor Pain

In labor pain the efficacy of epidural opioids has been controversial.[283] High doses of morphine (7.5 mg) have provided satisfactory analgesia for 6 hours in 66% of patients only for stage 1, whereas morphine 2 to 5 mg was unsatisfactory in more than 50% of patients.[37,193,201,283,395] In comparison, epidural bupivacaine 0.5% was effective in all patients in one study in stages 1 and 2,[193] and 0.25% bupivacaine was fully effective in a second study.[395] Epidural meperidine 25 mg provided inferior analgesia to 0.125% bupivacaine,[174] whereas increasing the dose to 50 mg provided good relief in only 50% of patients.[294] However, adding 1:200,000 epinephrine to meperidine 50 mg and injecting in the lateral position was reported to increase efficacy to 83%.[295] Baraka and associates reported excellent pain relief in 12 of 13 primipara given 100 mg epidural meperidine.[24] They also found that this large dose of meperidine prolonged the duration and increased the efficacy of subsequent doses of 0.25% bupivacaine.

As discussed in the section on pharmacokinetics, the greater efficacy of 50 mg meperidine with epinephrine probably is due to a greater amount of the (lipid-soluble) meperidine reaching the spinal cord. In a study of meperidine 25 mg with or without epinephrine, Skjolderbrand and colleagues reported that 14 of 19 women had good or excellent analgesia for 50 to 160 minutes, regardless of the presence of epinephrine.[342] Plasma meperidine concentrations were less than those known to be analgesic.[18] However, plasma meperidine concentrations were sustained for over 4 hours, and the need to repeat doses could pose a risk of cumulation of meperidine in mother and fetus.[342] In view of this problem and the success rate of only 75% compared with over 95% for epidural bupivacaine,[97] the authors concluded that epidural meperidine should not be used routinely in place of epidural bupivacaine in labor.[342] The potential efficacy of spinal opioids in labor pain is confirmed by a study in which a single dose of morphine 1.0 to 1.75 mg intrathecally relieved labor pain in all of 25 parturients with plasma concentrations in mother and fetus that were low.[34] Thus, it seems that intrathecal opioid has an acceptable risk-benefit ratio, but that epidural opioid, as a sole agent, is inferior to epidural bupivacaine. Small doses of epidural opioid may add to the efficacy and duration of epidural bupivacaine without increased risk[214,280] (see section on opioid, local anesthetic mixtures). This hypothesis was examined by a double-blind study of fentanyl 0.08 mg plus bupivacaine 0.5% 4 ml compared with bupivacaine 0.5% 4 ml.[214] Analgesia was more rapid in onset and more complete in the group receiving the fentanyl and had a duration of 2.36 hours compared with 1.66 hours in the other group. There was no evidence of respiratory depression, but moderate reductions in blood pressure were more common in the former group. Other studies have reported favorably on the use of epidural fentanyl in labor.[64] An opioid that remains in the spinal cord for a longer time may be more valuable in the future. Lofentanil (1.25–5 μg) combined with an extremely small dose of bupivacaine (12.5 mg) has been used in this context, but its favorable analgesic properties have been counteracted by a near 50% incidence of nausea and vomiting.[370] Sedation has also been a feature of use of epidural lofentanil.[31,370] It is possible that the other fentanyl analogues, sufentanil and alfentanil, will be of more interest for labor. In the meantime fentanyl has proved to be an effective and safe drug.

It has been proposed that labor pain is mainly mediated by A-delta fibers and that some of these bypass opioid receptors in the spinal cord (see above). However, this observation may be of theoretic rather than of practical interest, in view of the efficacy of intrathecal opioids for labor pain. Thus, it seems that the major explanations for lack of efficacy and brief duration of epidural opioids in labor are related more to pharmacokinetic factors as discussed earlier rather than to anatomic factors. A major influence of pharmacokinetic factors also is suggested by a comparison of postoperative pain relief with epidural morphine, in which duration of up to 24 hours is reported[46] in contrast to a maximum of 5 hours in labor pain.[37] Local anesthetics also have a shorter duration in labor pain compared with other types of pain. The final criterion of the safety of epidural opioids in labor awaits comparative neurobehavioral studies, and such data are only in early stages of collection.[117]

Postcesarean Pain

Treatment of post-cesarean section pain is an effective application of epidural opioids. In a double-blind trial, Hughes and associates reported that 7.5 or 5 mg morphine epidurally gave an average of 29 hours of excellent pain relief; in comparison, morphine 7.5 mg intramuscularly gave pain relief for only 2 hours.[195] The efficacy of epidural morphine doses (approximately 5 mg) has been reported in several studies.[87,119,195] Epidural morphine 5 mg was significantly more effective than intravenous morphine or placebo. Also, there were no significant differences between the two in terms of nausea and vomiting, drowsiness, or requirement for urinary catheterization.[87] Epidural fentanyl also produces highly effective analgesia of approximately 4 hours' duration.[188,392] The optimal dose has been reported to be 50 μg.[277,278] The only reported complication of epidural fentanyl is mild itching. Epidural meperidine is also effective for post-cesarean pain, has a duration of effect of 4 to 6 hours, and has a low incidence of side-effects.[54,55] Patient preference favors epidural opioid over intramuscular opioid. This was convincingly demonstrated in a double-blind within-patient study in which all patients received, in random order, intramuscular meperidine 100 mg (+ epidural saline), epidural meperidine 50 mg (+ intramuscular saline), and epidural bupivacaine 25 mg (+ intramuscular saline) for pain relief after a cesarean section or lower abdominal surgery. Analgesia with epidural meperidine was significantly superior to intramuscular meperidine but not statistically different from epidural bupivacaine. Duration of analgesia was the same for all three treatments. Epidural meperidine was the preferred treatment by patients, based on rank order and statistical analysis[55] (see Fig. 28-20).

The potential problems also should be considered. An accidental (perhaps unrecognized) massive subarachnoid dose of opioid may result in immediate problems[56]; however severe respiratory depression may occur much later, perhaps after surveillance has been relaxed. In contrast, a similar accident with local anesthetic usually results in a rapid onset of adverse effects, which obviously are associated with the drug administration, and occurs during the predicted time of maximum surveillance.

Post-trauma Pain

After trauma, epidural morphine and fentanyl[41] have been reported to be effective. In one study, in six patients with multiple fractured ribs, epidural morphine 2 mg gave more than 6 hours' analgesia with each dose, and analgesia was reported to be as good as with 0.5% bupivacaine. Other uncontrolled reports of the efficacy of epidural morphine have included patients after trauma.[245,359] On theoretic grounds, patients with overt or covert hypovolemia would be managed more safely with epidural opioid rather than with local anesthetic. However, comparative studies of efficacy and safety are not available. Because traumatized patients often are naive to opioids and may have received an intramuscular dose of opioid during transport, it would seem an advantage in the situation to use the more lipophilic opioids epidurally. Furthermore, the requirement to treat such patients in a critical care facility, staffed to inject "top-up" doses, negates any advantage of longer action of morphine over meperidine or fentanyl. Continuous epidural infusion of fentanyl (alone or with bupivacaine) would seem to have great appeal, provided appropriately controlled infusion apparatus is available. In critical care units, low-dose epidural infusions of local anesthetics are increasingly being used with considerable efficacy and safety (see Chap. 26). As is the case in labor, it is desirable to minimize motor block and prevent the development of tachyphylaxis. Interestingly, an intravenous dose of opioid given when sensory block regresses during epidural bupivacaine, restores the level of block,[242] indicating a synergistic effect. It is thought that this is mostly due to a spinal action of the opioid. Thus, it is logical to combine the opioid and local anesthetic epidurally. This has been tested after major surgery and was found to be superior to other techniques[113]; to date no controlled study has been reported in post-trauma patients. In some units it has been decided empirically to use local anesthetic epidural blockade for the first 24 hours and then change to epidural opioid from this time onward, with boli of local anesthetic for incident pain (see reference 106). However, it now seems more logical to use a low-

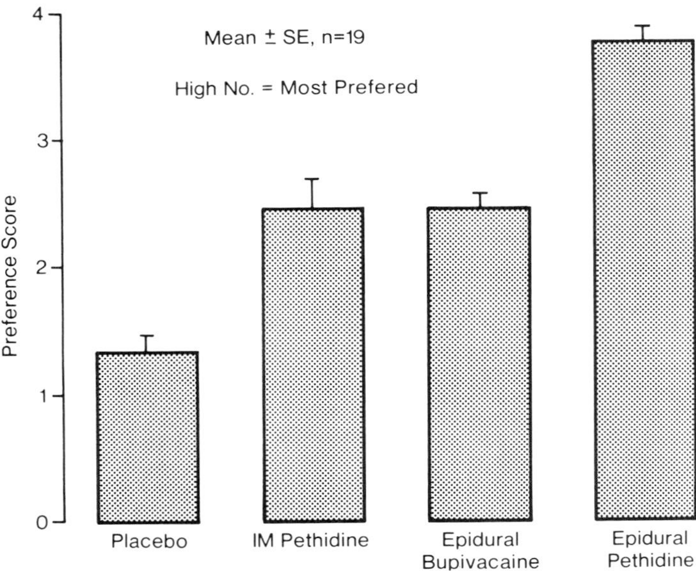

FIG. 28-20. Efficacy of epidural pethidine (meperidine) or postoperative pain relief. A double-blind within-patient comparison was made with each patient receiving four treatments in random order. Intramuscular saline (+ epidural saline); intramuscular pethidine 100 mg (+ epidural saline); epidural bupivacaine 0.25%, 10 ml (+ intramuscular saline); epidural pethidine 50 mg (+ intramuscular saline). Comparison of preference scores (maximum = 4). Epidural pethidine was superior to i.m. pethidine and epidural bupivacaine. (Reproduced with permission from Brownridge, P., Frewin, D.: A comparative study of techniques of postoperative analgesia following cesarean section and lower abdominal surgery. Anaesth. Intens. Care, *13*:123, 1985.)

dose infusion of epidural local anesthetic (0.25% bupivacaine) and opioid combined. This has been shown to be capable of relieving pain at rest as well as incident pain.[113] The choice of opioid agent in post-trauma pain may be important. Pharmacokinetic studies indicate that morphine spreads more evenly over the spinal cord, and that lumbar sites of injection are as effective as thoracic sites for post-thoracotomy pain.[233,280] Thus, for extensive pain after major trauma (*e.g.*, arms, legs, chest, abdomen), epidural morphine seems a logical choice. There is ample evidence from the treatment of cancer pain that a lumbar catheter will permit relief of pain even as high as cervical segments (see below). In more restricted areas of pain, it may theoretically be an advantage to place the catheter close to the segments involved and to use a lipid-soluble agent such as fentanyl (Table 28-15). The relative efficacy of thoracic versus lumbar injection of fentanyl (*e.g.*, for thoracic pain) has not been tested.

CANCER PAIN

Cancer pain management would seem to provide an excellent risk-benefit ratio for the epidural use of opioids. This is particularly so for patients who already are tolerant to parenteral opioids and, thus, are less liable to develop respiratory depression from the smaller doses that are required epidurally. By way of example, a patient with massive pelvic metastases required morphine 300 mg intravenously after careful intravenous titration to relieve her pain but with significant sedation and some respiratory depression. Oral bioavailability studies revealed that this was equivalent to 1200 mg morphine orally every 4 hours, and she received this for the next month until she became unhappy about the sedation. Epidural doses of morphine of 40 to 80 mg every 6 to 12 hours were sufficient to relieve her pain with no sedation or respiratory depression for the 3 months before her death. (Cousins, M.J.: Unpublished observations, 1979).

Indications

Indications for spinal opioids in cancer pain are as follows:

In patients treated with oral opioids who can achieve effective pain relief, but only with unacceptable side-effects, such as clouding of consciousness, nausea, and vomiting

In patients, whose pain cannot be adequately controlled with the use of oral opioids

In both indications it is assumed that appropriate adjuvant drugs have been combined with an adequate dosage regimen of an opioid agent, preferably with some form of pharmacokinetic monitoring. Ongoing chemotherapy or radiotherapy is not necessarily a contraindication to the implantation of a spinal catheter.

The site, nature, and degree of metastatic spread of the cancer, the character of the pain, and the predicted survival of the patient are important factors to be considered when making decisions about commencing spinal opioid therapy. Cancer pain of central origin (neuropathic, and "deafferentation" pain) is not amenable to epidural opioids (see Chap. 24.1). The best response is for deep, constant somatic pain. Some types of cancer pain respond variably: cutaneous pain, intermittent somatic pain (*e.g.*, pathologic fracture), intermittent visceral pain (*e.g.*, intestinal obstruction), coexistent malignant and nonmalignant pain.[13] Thus, it may be useful to carry out a trial of epidural opioid through a standard percutaneous catheter[77,396] before embarking on a more invasive implantation of an epidural or intrathecal system for long-term therapy.

In a series of 55 cancer patients whose pain was carefully evaluated, only 28 of the 55 became pain free. In 21 patients, pain relief was obtained only for one type of pain, leaving other pain unrelieved. In six patients, treatment was totally ineffective because of pain of the type discussed above.[13] It should be emphasized that less than 10% of patients with cancer pain will require techniques such as epidural opioids or neurolytic blocks (see Chap. 29.2) and other neurodestructive techniques (see Chap. 30). The majority should be effectively managed with oral opioids and adjuvant drugs.[372] Thus, such treatment should be optimized before considering intrathecal or epidural opioids (see Chap. 24.1). Despite the preceding qualifications, spinal opioids provide an attractive alternative to neurolytic and neurodestructive techniques. Spinal opioids are generally more suitable for patients with widespread pain, whereas neurolytic techniques may still be useful for patients with specific localized pain (*e.g.*, perineal pain when bladder function is absent) or with classic celiac plexus pain (*e.g.*, pancreatic cancer), as discussed in Chapters 29.2 and 30.

TABLE 28-15. SEVERE ACUTE PAIN MANAGEMENT: EPIDURAL OPIOIDS

Minor Lower Abdominal and Minor Lower Limb Surgery
Lumbar epidural catheter and fentanyl or meperidine (top-ups or infusion) + trained staff in medium care area ("open plan")
OR
Lumbar epidural catheter and low-dose morphine infusion (? preferable to top-ups) + trained staff + ? respiratory monitoring
NALOXONE AVAILABLE AND PROTOCOL FOR MANAGEMENT
Major and Extensive Surgery
Lumbar epidural catheter
Local anesthetic infusion (0.25% bupivacaine) for 24 h; then morphine infusion epidurally with local anesthetic epidural boli or small i.v. opioid boli for incident pain
OR
Lumbar epidural catheter
Local anesthetic and morphine infusion
OR
Thoracic epidural catheter (thoracic and abdominal pain)
Local anesthetic and/or fentanyl infusion
IN CRITICAL CARE UNIT (OR EQUIVALENT EXPERTISE)
NALOXONE AVAILABLE, RESPIRATORY MONITORING, AND PROTOCOL FOR MANAGEMENT

Contraindications

The same contraindications apply to the insertion of a spinal catheter for cancer pain control as they do for acute pain management (*e.g.*, in obstetrics and operative surgery; (see Chap. 8).

1. *Bleeding diathesis.* Hemorrhagic conditions that may result in long-term neurologic deficit secondary to the development of an epidural hematoma (see Chap. 8).
2. *Sepsis.* Local sepsis is unlikely to prevent the insertion of a spinal catheter because the segmental level chosen is not nearly as critical as when using local anesthetic, as explained earlier in this chapter. Septicemia is an absolute contraindication because the presence of a foreign body in the epidural space predisposes to the formation of an epidural abscess and its sequelae. If a patient with

an implanted epidural catheter subsequently becomes septicemic (*e.g.*, after chemotherapy), then prophylactic removal of the catheter, in most circumstances, is indicated.

3. Insulin-dependent diabetics have proved to be susceptible to infection at the portal site with potentially serious effects, resulting in the decision by some not to use spinal catheters in such patients.[76]
4. Immunologic suppression has, in clinical practice, been shown not to cause the problems that could be expected.
5. The known presence of *epidural metastases* is a relative contraindication, and unless the catheter can be positioned away from such lesions, it is probably wise to avoid spinal catheterization in such cases. The possibility of either the spinal needle or catheter penetrating a friable epidural mass, with the consequent development of paraplegia, is a risk that must always be assessed. The potential for eventual distal loculation of the CSF because of pressure on the subarachnoid space by an epidural mass should encourage the siting of catheters cephalad to metastases in patients with known or suspected spinal metastases.[75]

LONG-TERM INTRATHECAL VERSUS EPIDURAL SYSTEMS

Long-term access to enable the spinal administration of opioids in practice means the use of an intrathecal (see also intraventricular opioids below) or epidural catheter system connected to an injection system, with or without a reservoir.[76,90,92,94,95,178,298]

It is important to appreciate the reasons both for and against the epidural versus intrathecal administration of opioids on a long-term basis. The dura–arachnoid membrane offers a significant barrier to infection, and therefore the incidence of meningitis should be decreased with epidural access; also, the risk of severe dural puncture headache is less with this route of administration. However, the epidural space with its plentiful venous drainage, is known to absorb a large percentage of the drug deposited. This has the effect of adding a not insignificant systemic effect to any selective spinal action achieved. The total amount of drug required after intrathecal administration to achieve a similar effect as when given epidurally, has been estimated to be of the order of 1% to 10%. Pharmacokinetic studies confirm that substantial amounts of morphine reach the brain by way of CSF during both epidural and intrathecal administration.[161,257] The relative effects of drug absorbed into the circulation are likely to be much less after intrathecal use because of the significantly smaller dose required, compared with epidural administration. Thus, it is clear that long-term epidural or intrathecal opioids produce analgesic effects both by spinal and brain actions (see Table 28-1). It seems unlikely that intrathecal or epidural catheters would be more or less effective on the basis of these data.[92] However, a controlled study of efficacy is not available. Of practical significance is clear evidence in animal studies of rapid formation of a fibrous tissue sheath around epidural catheters, eventually preventing diffusion of drug into the epidural space.[95,136] This may partly explain the high failure rate in follow-up studies at about 3 months.[92] Whether such a reaction occurs in the subarachnoid space has not been determined, but the fluid environment may make it less likely; comparative neuropathology data are needed. Of some concern is the report of formation of a fibrous mass, in response to an epidural catheter, which compressed the spinal cord[320] (see also the neuropathology section above and Chap. 29.1). Although large molecules such as peptides have been shown to produce some analgesic effects with epidural administration in humans, they are ineffective when given epidurally in animals but are highly potent by the intrathecal route.[136,410,414,417,418,424] Thus, it remains to be seen if the intrathecal route will be more effective in humans for such molecules as DADL, metkephamid, somatostatin, and calcitonin. On the basis of physicochemical factors, it would seem that they may be best used intrathecally.

We prefer the epidural route for chronic morphine administration because of the avoidance of dural puncture headache and the protective barrier of the dura against infection. The latter seems important when using a "portal" system into which the patient or nurse makes frequent injections.[76] It is possible that the implanted reservoir pump may be more suited to an intrathecal catheter; however, it has been successfully used both epidurally and intrathecally.[92]

INSERTION TECHNIQUES: EXTERNALIZED CATHETER

When a percutaneous catheter is used, after a period of approximately 3 to 7 days, the exit site of the catheter through the skin can become erythematous, or even frankly infected. One means of attempting to prevent organisms from tracking along the catheter route into the epidural space is to tunnel the catheter away from the lumbar interspace and bring it out percutaneously onto the anterolateral chest wall (Fig. 28-21). A chronic inflammatory response occurs at the catheter exit site from the skin. However, so long as the exit site is not obstructed, seropurulent material has the opportunity for extrusion, creating a chronic sinus. A method of minimizing or preventing this problem is to place an adhesive air tight, water proof dressing over the catheter exit site, with the epidural catheter then running under the dressing to its edge.

There are now case reports documenting the relative safety of this technique in many hundreds of patients, with few documented cases of fistula formation[376] or an epidural abscess[90,279] occurring, despite the immunologically depressed state of many of these patients.[275,428,429] The catheter used in most cases was the relatively inexpensive and easy-to-insert polyethylene (nylon) catheter. These catheters do not require a stylet for insertion. Contrary to some opinion, these catheters do not become excessively brittle and break. Catheters have been left *in situ* in patients with pain related to cancer for periods in excess of 1 year without apparent undue sequelae. Some centers have advocated the use of the softer and more pliable polyurethane and Silastic catheters, as these catheters are believed to cause less tissue reaction within the epidural space. There are no published studies to show that epidural fibrosis, which is a significant problem with the long-term use of polyethylene catheters[320] can be significantly decreased by the long-term use of Silastic catheters. However, such catheters have been used very successfully long-term, with very infrequent need to replace them.* Comparative studies in animal models are required.

Catheter migration from the epidural space into the subdural or subarachnoid space, or even intravascularly, can occur[179]; however, this is a uncommon occurrence (see Chap. 8). Allowing for the pressure changes that do occur in response to cardiovascular and respiratory pulsation, combined with some movement of the catheter tip in response to vertebral column movement by the patient, one would still expect the dura–arachnoid membrane to prevent this inadvertent migration. Unrecognized migration into the subarachnoid space could lead to profound respiratory depression.[56] Bacterial filters (see Fig. 28-21) can be fitted to the end of the catheter to prevent bacteria from entering the lumen of the catheter. These need to be changed regularly, adding a cost factor to this form of therapy.

*Dupen, S.L.: Anesthesiology, *65*:A195, 1986. Also, note that Silastic is the material of choice for chronic venous cannulation.

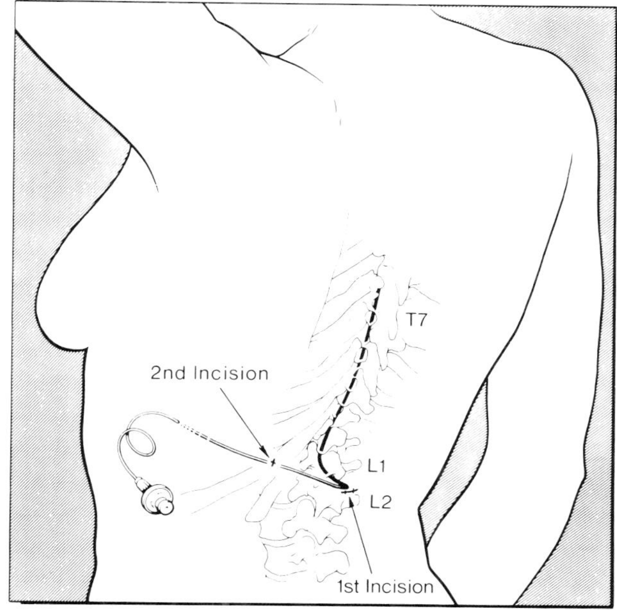

FIG. 28-21. Percutaneous epidural catheter tunneled to an exit on the lateral chest wall (see Fig. 28-23 for details of tunneling technique).

The entire system, which is efficacious, inexpensive, and potentially available worldwide, is somewhat inconvenient to wear and interferes, to some extent, with routine daily living activities such as washing, dressing, and sleeping. However, this system may be highly effective and quite acceptable.

TOTALLY IMPLANTED SYSTEMS

Systems that are implanted subcutaneously have obvious advantages in terms of sterility, comfort, and freedom of movement for the patient. This requires either a portal (bolus injection)-type of system for percutaneous access or an implanted, pump-driven, percutaneously refillable reservoir system. The portal or reservoir are connected to an epidural catheter and placed in a conveniently accessible position on the anterior chest or abdominal wall (Fig. 28-22).

Portal System

A portal system should have the following characteristics:

Easily palpable percutaneously

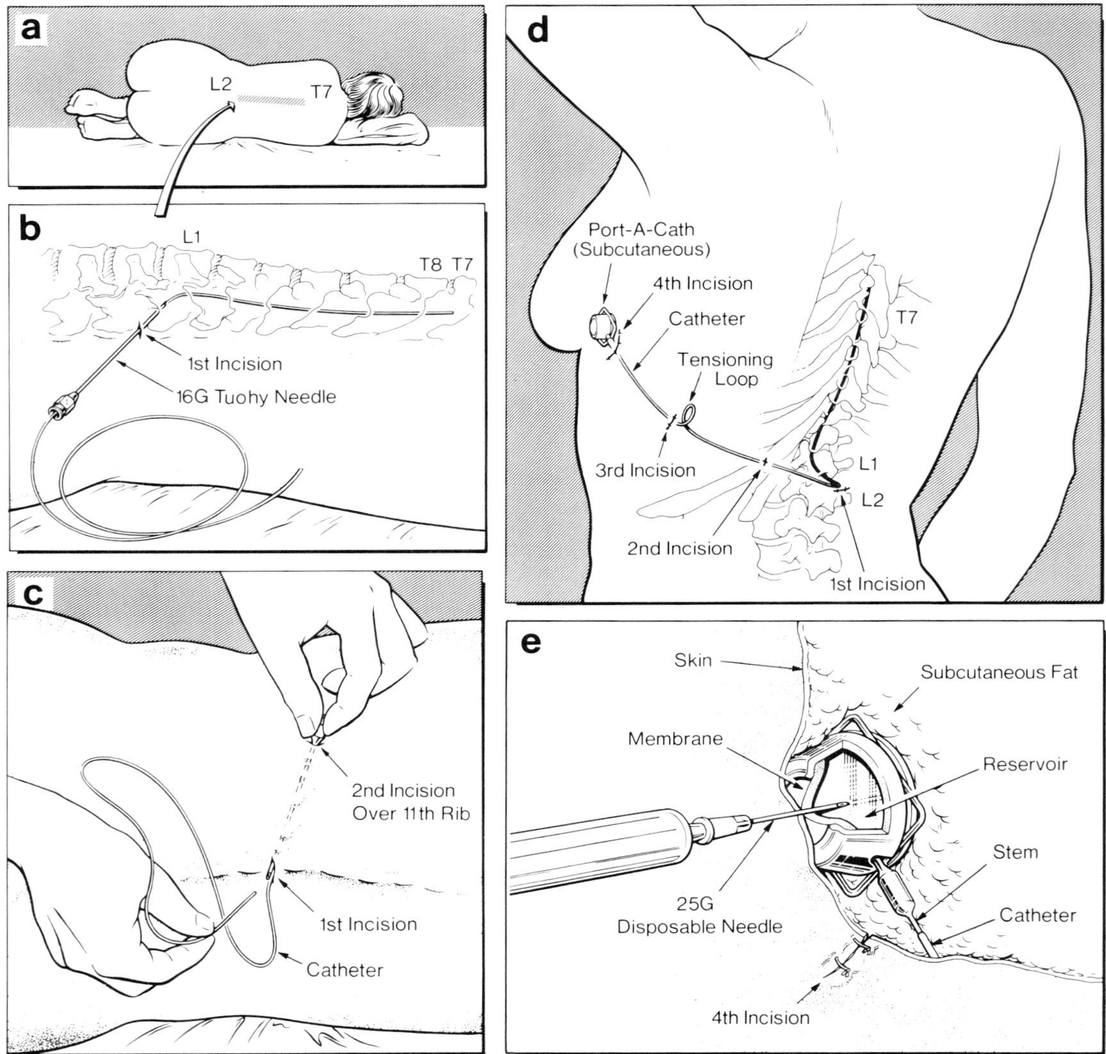

FIG. 28-22. Implantation of the epidural portal system. **a.** Position of patient before implantation. **b.** Insertion of 16-gauge epidural catheter through a Tuohy needle. **c.** Tunneling technique used to relocate the end of the epidural catheter to the anterior chest wall. **d.** Portal attached to the inserted epidural catheter. **e.** Injection technique and exposed view of the epidural portal.

Resealable membrane capable of withstanding 1000 injections under the pressure required to inject through a standard epidural catheter
Easily discernible end point to injection
Ability to remain patent
Injectable by non-medically trained people
Inexpensive
Simple to insert under local anesthesia
Filter system to prevent unwanted particulate matter from reaching the epidural or intrathecal space

The portal system introduced by Pharmacia (Porta-cath) is shown in Figure 28-23. In our series, these devices have been inserted for relief of cancer pain in more than 200 patients whose pain had previously been controlled by orally administered opioids.

Examples of other portal systems are shown in Figure 28-24. To date, we have found that the Pharmacia portal best meets the criteria outlined earlier. The portal itself has not been subject to leaking, the membrane has been robust, and staff and patients have found it easy to inject.

Blockage of Portal — Inability to Inject. Of our first 100 patients in whom a portal had been inserted for longer than 1 month, 14 patients needed exploration of the portal system because of blockage.[76]

Obstruction to the outlet of the portal by residue occurred in four patients. This residue, in most cases, consisted of silicone cores made by the repeated puncture of the membrane as well as plugs of dermal layers together with skin-swab material.[76] The latter problem has been practically overcome by placing the entrance to the outlet tube into the interior of the reservoir, thus avoiding the funneling effect that would otherwise occur.

Catheter blockage occurred in ten cases. This problem has been decreased by removing the end from the epidural catheter, so that the catheter is left with one terminal orifice. This decreases the tendency for fibrinous material to accumulate at the exit holes of the catheter and allows the catheter to be force-flushed, clearing any accumulation of fibrinous tissue.

Epidural Bolus Dosage. As mentioned earlier, morphine is the drug of choice for chronic use in patients suffering pain secondary to cancer. Morphine's relative hydrophilicity slows diffusion of morphine from the spinal cord (see Fig. 28-14), thus prolonging its therapeutic effect. Initially, morphine in appropriate dosage (2–10 mg) can be expected to provide pain relief for periods up to 12 hours. An initial dose of about one-tenth the dose that was effective by mouth is a general guide. However, considerable adjustment of dose may be needed if opioid therapy was ineffective before institution of epidural opioid therapy.

Infusion Techniques

On theoretical grounds, a continuous infusion of morphine epidurally or intrathecally would offer the potential for better pain control than bolus techniques. The peaks and troughs in CSF morphine concentration (which presumably reflect dorsal horn opioid concentration) that are associated with bolus-type injection would be avoided. One could also predict that less total drug would be required using an infusion, as compared with bolus administration, to achieve a similar state of pain relief, with less side-ef-

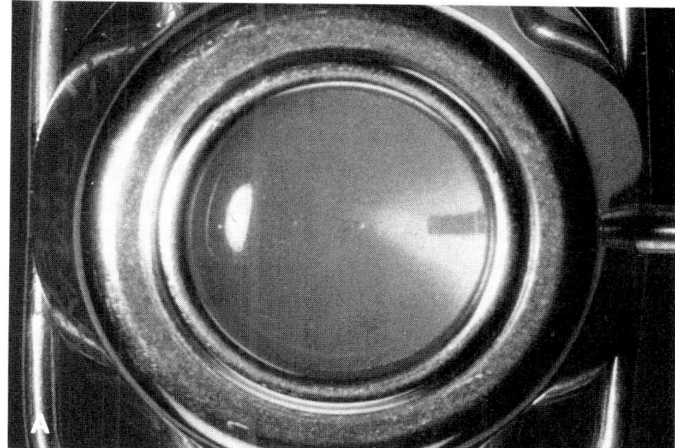

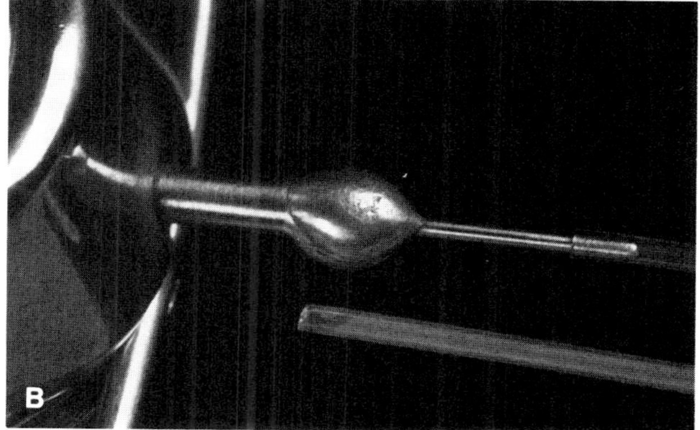

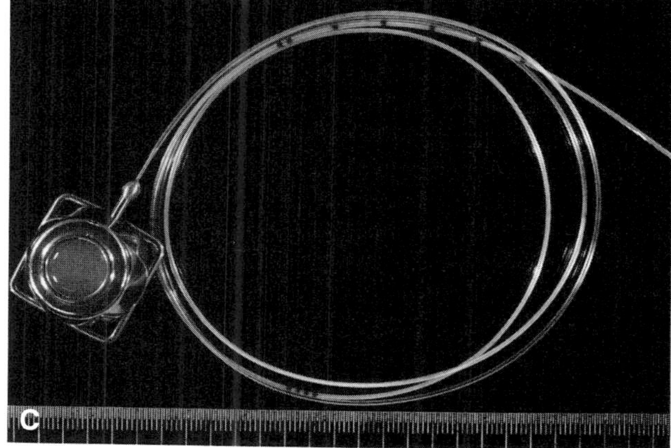

FIG. 28-23. Port-a-Cath epidural portal. **A.** Close-up of resealable injection membrane. **B.** Close-up of junction between portal and epidural catheter. Note that standard Port-a-Cath fitting for catheter attachment has been modified by soldering on a blunt length of 22-gauge needle. **C.** Entire assembly. Ruler shows size in centimeters.

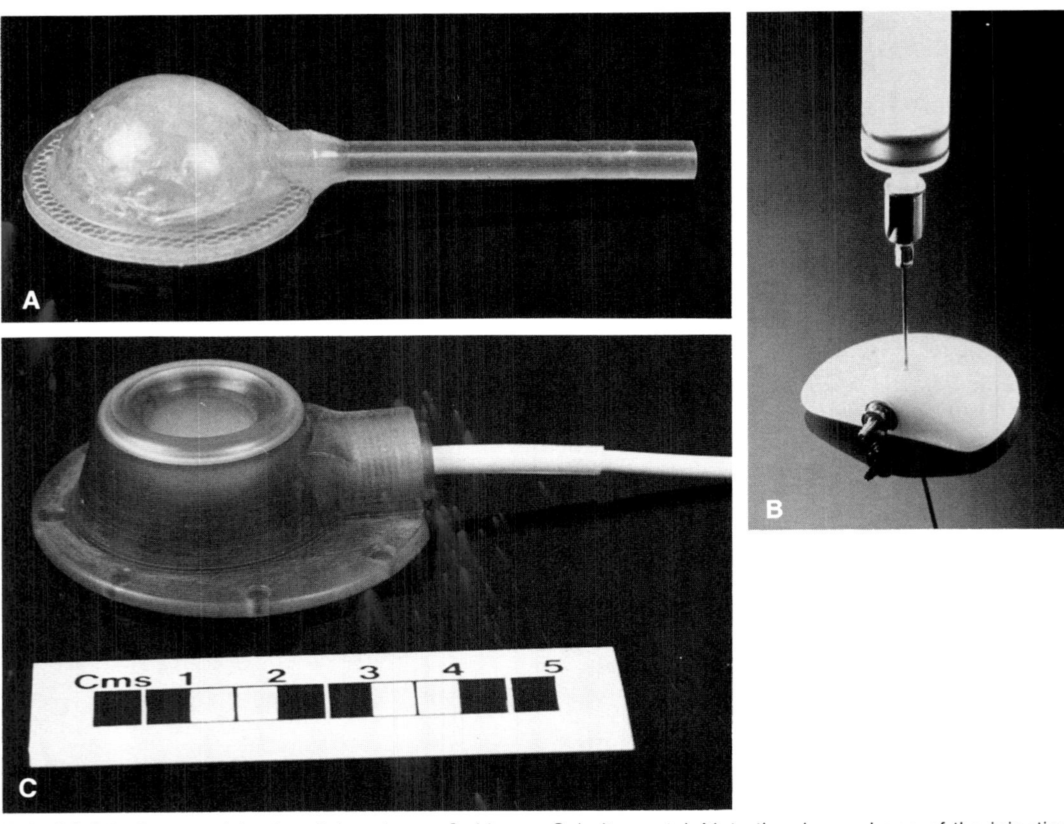

FIG. 28-24. Some epidural portal systems. **A.** Heyer–Schulte portal. Note the dome shape of the injection portion of the device and the somewhat "unprotected" side wall. Another similar device is the Holtner–Hausner system (Holtner–Hausner International, Inc., Bridgeport, PA.) **B.** Medtronic portal. The injection site in the center of the upper surface is quite small. The needle is shown penetrating this area. (Medtronic, Minneapolis, MN.) **C.** Infusaid portal. Similar to the Port-a-Cath with a readily palpable, well-defined injection septum. (Infusaid, Inc., Norwood, MA.)

fects and greater patient satisfaction. Data in animals[83] now indicate that peak brain stem concentrations of morphine are lower with low-volume injection, but effects in patients may be small.[341b] Comparative data in cancer patients are not available. Considering the relative costs of "portal" and pump systems, a comparative study is highly desirable.

External Pumps. Spinal opioid infusion can be provided through an externalized catheter connected to a small portable pump, such as the Fresenius (Injection MS26), Travenol Infusor and Patient Control Module, Graseby Dynamics Portable Infusion Pump (with self-administration option), Deltec Cadd-Pac, or an equivalent. This may be effective for bedridden terminal patients but is also an alternative for some ambulatory patients, since the pump can be worn in a shoulder holster and can be "loaded" for at least 24 hours of infusion.

Implanted Pumps. If the pump is to be implanted subcutaneously, then two prerequisites need to be satisfied: (1) a reservoir system needs to be incorporated and (2) a pump mechanism needs to be driven either internally or externally (by a transcutaneous induction device), or by a mechanical system operated by the patient.

Morphine can be commercially concentrated to 60 mg/ml or even greater. The patient requirement can vary from as little as 5 mg of morphine per day up to 60 to 100 mg per 24 hours. Assuming the larger dosage, the pump needs to deliver between 1 and 2 ml per 24 hours. To make the device a practical alternative to the portal/bolus devices, the reservoir capacity must be at least 20 ml. Epidural infusions of as little as 1.2 ml of a concentrated morphine solution in 24 hours have provided significant pain relief and effective morphine concentrations in CSF.[83]

Because of the reservoir, in addition to the pump mechanism, these devices are bulky, which, in a cachectic patient, can be a consideration regarding implantability. The most widely used system is the Infusaid (Fig. 28-25); however, other systems have been developed.[90] One such system is programmable, thus allowing flexibility in adjustment of delivered dose[293] (Fig. 28-26).

A detailed analysis of current and developing implanted spinal opioid systems has been made by Coombs (see reference 96). Broadly, there are three types of pump currently in use or under development[74,90]: [1] the Infusaid type, a continuous (constant rate) pump with a drug reservoir driven by a bellows-type vapor pressure outer chamber; [2] peristaltic pumps, driven by lithium batteries; [3] pumps with a pulsatile type of drug delivery, operated by solenoid valves driven by lithium batteries. Programmable pumps are available of the latter two types. However, they are currently expensive ($6–$10,000) compared with $2000 to $3500 for the Infusaid (or $300 for the Portacath portal system).

Pump-driven reservoir systems are currently

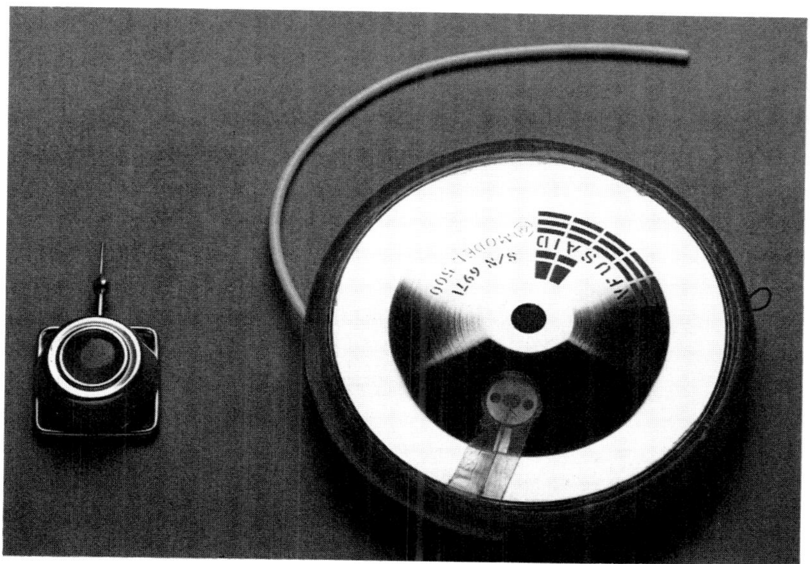

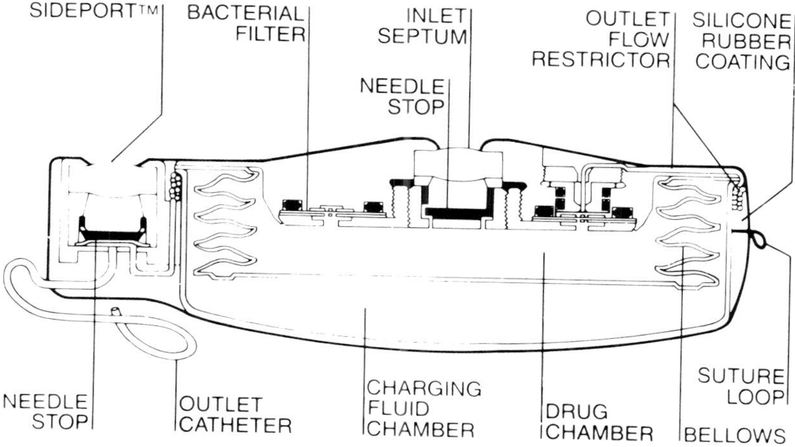

FIG. 28-25. Metal bellows constant infusion pump for totally implanted epidural or intrathecal opioid administration. **Top.** External view. Note size compared to Port-a-Cath portal. **Bottom.** Cross-section. Volatile hydrocarbon liquid in the "charging fluid chamber" expands and compresses the metal bellows, thus discharging fluid from the drug chamber into the outlet catheter and then into epidural space. The sideport permits the use of supplementary bolus doses.

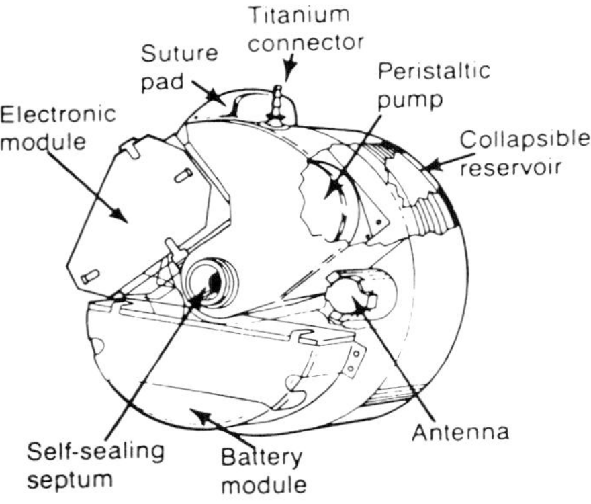

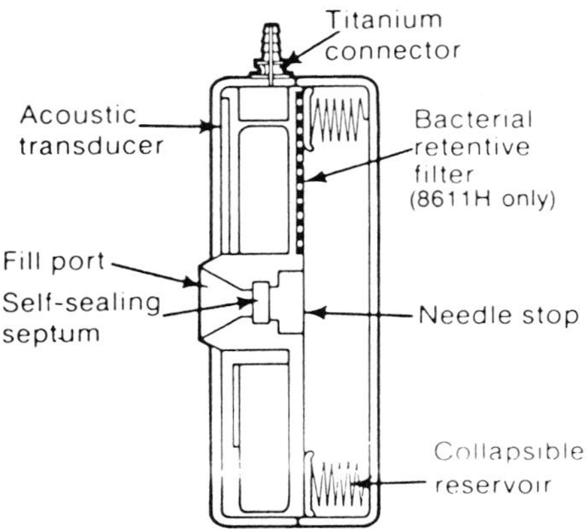

FIG. 28-26. Programmable implantable infusion system for epidural or intrathecal opioids. The Drug Administration Device (DAD) consists of an infusion pump with a collapsible drug reservoir, microprocessor-based circuitry, lithium battery-driven peristaltic pump, and an acoustic transducer attached to an antenna. An external programmer is used to control various parameters of drug delivery by means of coded radiofrequency signals from the "wand" of the programmer to the antenna of the DAD. The device shown is a Medtronic DAD. The Medtronic physicians' programmer is not shown. (Medtronic, Minneapolis, MN.)

nearly 2000% more expensive than the more readily available portal systems.

Ethical and Logistical Considerations

Certain ethical and logistical considerations must be addressed when such therapy is contemplated. If the patient is to be managed at home, when the portal system is being used, the patient or family must be allowed to keep a stock of sterile disposable needles and syringes, as well as up to 1 month's supply of morphine in the home setting. Care needs to be taken to ensure accurate accounting and safe housing of the morphine. The patient may have his portal injected by a district nurse, a member of the family, or self.

For the Pharmacia portal, the stainless steel plate onto which the needle is advanced has a distinct and reassuring feel to it, to which even nonmedically trained people readily adjust.

If the portal was to be injected by the district nurse, in today's climate of drug abuse, it would be an unnecessarily hazardous task to expect the district nurse to carry the drug with her. It is equally important for a responsible medically or nursing trained person to supervise and regularly check that the drugs are being properly administered by the patient or the patient's spouse or friends.

In the great percentage of cases, the patient's spouse has been only too pleased to inject the portal. This allows the spouse to actively take part in the caregiving process, rather than stand impotently to one side.

There has been resistance from some nursing administrations to allow nursing staff to inject an epidural opioid system. This is, in part, a reflection of their concern about nurses injecting local anesthetic into epidural catheters with the potential for serious autonomically induced side-effects. However, with the gradually evolving safety record of epidurally administered opioids in patients previously exposed to systemic opioids, these restrictions should gradually decrease. Use of spinal opioids in the context of a home-based palliative care program yields best results.

Ideally, a pain management unit should work in close harmony with a palliative care team. This forms a powerful hospital-based focus that can then act as a resource for the home care team of district nurse, volunteers, general practitioners, and other home care professionals. It is essential to conduct a training program for the district nurses and to have a well-organized system for regular liaison with them (see Chap. 32).

Reasons for Lack of Efficacy

Obstruction to CSF Flow. As mentioned previously in this chapter, epidural opioids act by passive diffusion from the epidural space through the dura and subarachnoid membranes into the CSF. Once in the CSF the opioids passively spread throughout the subarachnoid space and gain access to the dorsal horn of the spinal cord as well as the brain. In other words, the effect is nonsegmental as distinct from local anesthetic injected epidurally, which has a segmental effect. This has the practical implication that the site of the catheter is not critical when using epidural opioids. However, there have been four reported cases in which the epidural and subarachnoid spaces have been occluded by an extradural mass, effectively loculating the CSF distal to this mass and preventing the spread of opioid within the CSF to the appropriate dorsal horn cells, resulting in inadequate pain relief.[75,320]

Tolerance. It now seems that at least part of the problem of tolerance may be the formation of a fibrous sheath around epidural as well as intrathecal catheters (see above). However, there are also clear cases of pharmacologic tolerance to morphine, which were overcome by use of intrathecal DADL,[96,228] intrathecal clonidine,[96] and intraventricular morphine.[96] This is encouraging, since other drugs acting on systems besides the mu receptor are available, as indicated in the physiology section. Somatostatin has been reported to be effective in patients tolerant to morphine,[82] and calcitonin appears to add to the analgesic effects of morphine.[85] In one large series it was found to be beneficial to change from morphine to buprenorphine spinally and *vice versa.*[63] A rational regimen for avoiding tolerance needs to be developed first in carefully controlled animal experiments. Otherwise, undesirable side-effects may occur in humans, and at best, pain relief may only be partially successful. In a randomized, double-blind cross-over study of ten patients tolerant to morphine, DADL was more effective in six patients, equally effective in one patient, and less effective than morphine in three patients.[273]

Pain on Injection. The most common problem confronted is a burning pressure sensation, usually perceived in one or other hip, during injection of the morphine diluted in saline by way of the epidural catheter. This pain is postulated to be due to injection of the morphine solution onto a nerve root, but there are no data to prove or disprove this. The pain can be reduced by administering the injection over 5 to 10 minutes. Also, injection of a small dose of local anesthetic before injection of the opioid may help. Injection of steroid sometimes also helps. Neuropathology data now indicate that pain may be due to the fibrous sheath that forms around catheters.[136] Some patients still experience significant pain on injection, despite the measures taken above, and it is advised that the epidural catheter be repositioned. If, despite repositioning of the catheter, pain is still perceived on injection, then the catheter should be resited in the subarachnoid space. In our series of 200 cases, previously mentioned, with long-term epidural catheters, this has been found to be necessary on four occasions.[76]

INTRAVENTRICULAR OPIOIDS

Pharmacokinetic data indicate that epidural, intrathecal, and intraventricular opioids are likely to be equally efficacious.[257] Thus, it may be more appropriate or convenient in some patients to use the intraventricular route. It may prove to be less subject to fibrous sheath around catheter tips; however, this remains to be determined. A number of substantial series now report the efficacy of this technique for pain arising from all areas of the body.[96,237,257]

OUTCOME OF SPINAL OPIOID TREATMENT

Few follow-up series are reported.[90] Coombs and coworkers reported an almost invariable failure after about 3 months of treatment.[92] Ventafridda and colleagues reported that at 3 months, only 30% of patients were pain free; also, no patient had relief of incident pain.[372]

Follow-up of "Standard" Percutaneous Catheters with No Tunneling

Zenz has reported 139 patients treated for an average of just over 2 months, with 1 patient treated for more than a year.[428] Daily dosage ranged from 2 to 290 mg. In these 139 patients, catheters were *in situ* for a mean of 72 days. Twenty-six catheters were *in situ* for more than 100 days and 1 for 150 days. Patients not uncommonly required more than one catheter.[428] Complications included obstruction, breakage, kinking, cutting or removal of catheters (20%), local infection (11%),and nonfatal meningitis (1%; two cases). Both cases of meningitis resolved after removal of the catheter. Crawford and others reported 105 patients who required a total of 215 catheters.[111] It was common for patients to require more than one catheter. No cases of local infection became a clinical problem.

Subcutaneously Tunneled Catheters

In a series of 31 patients, technical problems were similar to those reported above, but no cases of clinical infection were reported (quoted in reference 90). In a large follow-up series of 810 patients from multiple anesthesia departments, an overall incidence of 40% side-effects of some type were reported (quoted in reference 90); however, this included any pain on injection, emesis, and urine retention.*

Implanted Portal Systems

Cherry and co-workers reported on 50 patients managed for up to 36 weeks with a Portacath portal system[76] (see Fig. 28-22). Seventy per cent of these patients were managed at home and the remainder in a hospice or hospital. Mean duration of use was 12 weeks. Five portals had to be removed: two infections occurred at the portal site (diabetes); one catheter became exposed through the skin; one because of local pain at the portal site; one because of reestablishment of effective treatment with oral opioids. Subsequently, more than 200 portals have been inserted (none in diabetics) with no spinal infections. District nurses and patients' relatives were quickly taught to inject through the skin into the portal (see Fig. 28-22).

Implanted Pump Systems

The Infusaid has been successfully used for both intrathecal and epidural infusion. In the United States alone, more than 8000 have been inserted in patients at more than 200 medical centers.[90] It has been found that flow delivery under clinical conditions does not vary by more than 15%.[90]

Follow-up of 14 patients (six intrathecal, eight epidural) treated with an Infusaid indicated good pain control for up to 6 months.[92] Initial starting dose was based on 0.5% to 1% of the oral morphine intake for intrathecal infusion, or 5% to 10% for epidural infusion. Comparison with preimplant narcotic requirements revealed equal or reduced narcotic use for up to 6 months of therapy but with a definite trend toward dose escalation.[92] This should be compared with well-controlled oral opioid treatment, in which opioid requirements often remain stable once pain control has been obtained. In Coomb's series, dose escalation was common after 2 months, and adjunctive measures such as supplementary oral analgesics and neurolytic procedures were used.[92] Failure of pain control occurred in most patients after 6 months. Side-effects were minimal: there was no respiratory depression and no infection. There appeared to be no clear difference between epidural and intrathecal infusion.[92]

It is surprising, in view of the widespread use and cost of spinal opioid systems, that controlled evaluation, compared with oral opioids and other treatments, is virtually nonexistent. There is an urgent need for these data.

*A tunneled Silastic catheter of the Broviac type has been used epidurally in more than 100 patients with excellent analgesia and minimal need to replace catheters. (Dupen, S.: Personal Communication). This catheter is made by Davol Co., Cranston, RI 02920.

CHRONIC NONCANCER PAIN

Epidural morphine has been used alone and in combination with steroids for back pain (see Chap. 27.2). The rationale for this is to permit mobilization and increase both physical and mental activity. It is theoretically possible that a vicious circle of spinal reflex activity may be modified or broken up. Controlled data for this approach are not available (see also Chap. 27.3). Other potential applications, such as pain caused by bladder spasm, are discussed in the physiology section.[286] One well-documented application is the treatment of muscle spasm and pain associated with spasticity.[148] In this study, patients who responded to an initial bolus dose of morphine then received an implanted epidural system, all with sustained relief of pain and muscle spasm.[148]

DIAGNOSTIC OPIOID BLOCK

The potential diagnostic application of spinal opioids was proposed in 1980 in the "New Horizons" chapter (Chap. 31) of the first edition of this text.[99] However, it was not until 1985 that Cherry and colleagues reported a series of cases, indicating that epidural opioid may be used to help differentiate pain of central origin (psychological as well as neurogenic, *e.g.*, "deafferentation") from pain arising peripheral to the dorsal horn of the spinal cord.[77] They used two injections of saline, one of fentanyl 1 μg/kg body weight, both epidurally, and then naloxone intravenously, followed by local anesthetic epidurally. The pattern of this response was used, together with physical and psychological evaluation, in a multidisciplinary setting. Relief of pain with opioid and reversal with naloxone pointed to a "peripheral" nociceptive focus. Failure to relieve pain, however, required further investigation of a number of more central causes.[77] The technique requires further pharmacokinetic and pharmacodynamic assessment: How much opioid is optimal? What dose of naloxone reliably antagonizes the opioid? How much effect is there on the brain by way of blood or CSF from the fentanyl dose used? Does this provide a cue to the patient? What categories of pain respond to opioid or to local anesthetic or to both? (See also Chap. 27.1) If these questions can be answered, this application may become a useful tool in the assessment of chronic pain in the multidisciplinary pain unit setting.

CONCLUSION

Spinal administration of opioids has proved beyond doubt to produce a powerful antinociceptive action that is substantially due to a spinal action. However, significant effects on the brain contribute to analgesia, and this is more marked with some agents under specific conditions of clinical use. Studies of physiologic effects of spinal opioids have revealed significant alteration of function of systems other than antinociception. Some of these effects are produced at only high spinal doses of opioids. However, others, such as modification of bladder spasm and skeletal muscle spasm, are present at clinical doses and have proved useful in treatment of clinical syndromes not previously thought to be amenable to spinal opioids.

Clinical evidence of differences among opioids in efficacy for different clinical pain states is lacking. However, evidence in animal studies of a possible association between different spinal opioid receptors (mu, delta, and kappa) with different nociceptive stimuli indicates that future research should examine whether some pain states are more amenable to opioids acting on one or other of these three systems. Also, the relative efficacy of nonopioid spinal antinociceptive agents, such as clonidine (noradrenergic), baclofen (GABA-ergic), somatostatin, and calcitonin, is unknown with respect to their indications compared with opioids.

In **acute pain,** randomized prospective studies have provided clear evidence of superiority of epidural opioids as well as of local anesthetics over opioids given intramuscularly. There seems to be a patient preference for epidural opioids. However, pain relief with spinal opioids is rather similar, in a small number of studies, to carefully tuned intravenous infusion of opioids or meticulously maintained somatic nerve blocks, such as intercostal block. Further data are needed to indicate whether controlled intravenous opioid infusion or epidural opioid–local anesthetic infusion is preferable in certain clinical settings and for certain patient categories. The combination of low doses of local anesthetic and opioid for epidural infusion has been shown to be highly effective and safe in well-controlled studies. Logistical and administrative hurdles need to be overcome to safely implement such treatment. Lumbar catheters are as effective as thoracic catheters when morphine is used. It is not known whether this applies to lipophilic drugs such as fentanyl. Delayed respiratory depression seems to be limited to morphine, although drugs with high receptor affinity, such as lofentanil, require further study. Epidural fentanyl has been shown not to produce delayed respiratory depression, and thus has appeal for the opioid-naive patient, either alone or in combination with local anesthetic. Intrathecal use of morphine in doses as low as 0.3 mg appears to be effective and safer than doses previously used (1–2 mg) for postoperative pain, when given at the time of a spinal local anesthetic.

In **cancer pain,** spinal opioids are highly effective but not for all types of pain. Failure of pain relief occurs after about 3 to 6 months in a number of patients probably because of a combination of fibrous tissue response to the epidural catheter, increased nociception, and pharmacologic tolerance. The former problem requires replacement of the catheter at another epidural site or intrathecally. Changing to an opioid acting on another spinal system or to a nonopioid drug helps to overcome tolerance.

Intrathecal, epidural, and intraventricular opioid administration are indistinguishable in their clinical effects and have considerable similarities pharmacokinetically. Comparative studies of efficacy and safety are not available. Intrathecal and epidural opioids have given clear benefit to individual patients with cancer pain. However, there is an urgent need for controlled studies comparing spinal opioids with optimized treatment with oral opioids and "adjuvant" drugs with respect to pain relief, side-effects, quality of life, and patient satisfaction. As with many new techniques, spinal opioids have suffered from too much enthusiasm and too little careful documentation of efficacy, safety, indications, and contraindications in the clinical setting. This is a pity, since the animal studies forming the basis of the technique have been meticulous and clear in their implications for the clinician. Further development of spinal opioids must continue to be based on the relevant pharmacologic and neuropathology studies in animals before use in humans. Widespread clinical applications of any further agents or techniques should be preceded by controlled clinical studies.

APPENDIX: FUTURE DIRECTIONS

In **acute pain,** development seems possible of spinal opioid and nonopioid drugs that optimize spinal antinociceptive action and minimize or eliminate effects on the respiratory center. It is of interest that animal studies are now beginning to realize Martin's proposal of an analgesic receptor (mu_1) without effect on respiration (mu_2). Spinal kappa agonists also need investigation in humans to determine what types of pain they relieve and what degree of selectivity there is for analgesic vs. other effects, including respiration. It seems likely that small doses of nonopioid drugs (*e.g.,* clonidine) may be useful in combination with opioid drugs in order to obtain effective (and ? potentiated) analgesia, while minimizing cardiovascular effects of clonidine and respiratory (and other) effects of opioids. This approach seems more attractive than using antagonists such as naloxone; however, it is likely that antagonism of respiratory depression, and not analgesia, may be developed further.

In **cancer pain,** the problems of fibrous reaction in the epidural space could be minimized or solved by investigating more inert catheter materials. Data on the relative efficacy of bolus compared with low-dose infusion techniques are vital. The problem of tolerance is important because of clear evidence of failure of analgesia after about 2 to 3 months. However, dose escalation also leads to [a] hyperesthesia, [b] muscle contraction—sometimes of a convulsive nature—and [c] other potential side-effects described in the physiology section. If tolerance could be overcome, there would also be a further reduction in the need to use neurolytic and neurodestructive techniques, all of which have an inevitable percentage of loss of function. Alternation from mu to delta to kappa receptors or to nonopioid systems in order to avoid tolerance needs to be pursued. As noted earlier, this may include combining agents at lower doses to avoid side-effects as well as delaying development of tolerance. Detailed studies in animals are required to determine which sequence(s) of agents (and which combinations of agents) is most effective. Also, information is needed about different types of pain and the most appropriate agonists, either alone or in combination. There is no doubt that the goal of "selective spinal analgesia" is worthwhile and potentially achievable. It is one that our patients would hope that we can reach.

UNANSWERED KEY ISSUES IN USE OF EPIDURAL, INTRATHECAL, AND INTRAVENTRICULAR OPIOIDS

Pharmacokinetics

?? Factors determining clearance of opioids from CSF and residual CSF concentrations in brain stem region, after injection at different neuraxial levels, of various opioids.[72,125,126,131,150,170,172,273,281,285]

?? Time course of CSF-borne drug migration[48,161] and penetration of neuraxis for the various opioid and nonopioid drugs.[51]

?? Comparative rates of systemic bioavailability of water-soluble (*e.g.,* morphine)[137] and lipid-soluble (*e.g.,* fentanyl) opioids and nonopioid drugs.

?? Effects of CSF and blood *p*H changes on CSF and blood concentrations of opioids.[219]

?? Relationships between endogenous opioids[353] and exogenous spinal opioid administration.

?? Ease of antagonism of various opioid drugs[419] after spinal use in humans.

Pharmacodynamics

?? Confirmation of predominant spinal site of action in humans after intrathecal and epidural administration of newly developed opioids.

?? Selection of opioid with best duration and efficacy/safety ratio for spinal administration.

?? Do subtherapeutic doses of nonopioid[238] and opioid drugs have synergistic effects?

?? Role of peptides in selective spinal analgesia.[287,290,406,410,412,414,417,424]

?? Role of nonopioid drugs in selective spinal analgesia.[399,404]

?? Method of alternation of spinal opioid and nonopioid drugs to avoid tolerance.[399,402,416]

?? Relationship between epidural–intrathecal opioid dose and oral–intramuscular dose after chronic treatment.

?? Rates of development of tolerance to opioids with chronic "top-ups" compared with continuous infusion of epidural–intrathecal opioids.[288,316]

?? Efficacy of lumbar compared with thoracic injection of lipid-soluble opioids for pain originating above the lumbar region.

?? Efficacy, safety, and neuropathology of chronic intrathecal versus epidural administration.[76,94,288,419]

?? Optimum volume and concentration of injectate.

?? Comparison of spinal opioids with current options, for example, with "on-demand" intravenous opioids,[67,319,386] "continuous" opioid infusion,[347] epidural local anesthetic infusion,[123] transdermal opioid and patient-controlled oral opioids in postoperative pain[23] and cancer pain[365] and subcutaneous opioid infusion in cancer pain.

?? Significance of multiplicative analgesic interaction between intraventricular and intrathecal morphine.[427]

Side-Effects

?? Long-term neurologic effects of chronic, intraventricular, intrathecal, and epidural opioid administration in humans.

?? Reliable premonitory signs before respiratory depression, for example, pupil size,[20,21] changes in respiratory rate,[56,225,260,280] carbon dioxide or oxygen partial pressure in blood, change in level of consciousness.

?? Comparative respiratory effects of spinal opioids and continuous intravenous opioid infusion[317] in patients with pain.

?? Role of opioid antagonists, such as naloxone and other specific receptor antagonists, and nonspecific antagonists of somnolence, such as physostigmine,[338,380] in the prevention and treatment of side-effects.

?? Method of avoidance of withdrawal syndrome after changeover from oral to spinal opioid,[264] or after neurolytic block subsequent to long-term opioids.[176]

?? Comparative incidence and treatment of itching, vomiting, and urinary retention with different opioids, as well as the potential for prophylaxis.[14]

?? Mechanism of lower incidence of side-effects of long-term spinal opioid administration compared with spinal opioids in acute pain.

?? Method of prevention of hyperalgesia[254] owing to high-dose spinal morphine.

A significant portion of this chapter was previously published as a review by Cousins and Mather[102] and is reproduced with permission of the publisher of Anesthesiology, J. B. Lippincott. Alan Bentley (Medical Illustration and Media, Flinders Medical Centre) provided excellent artistic design and drawing for the original illustrations.

REFERENCES

1. Abay, E.O., and Yaksh, T.L.: Effects of intrathecal capsaicin on thermal, mechanical and chemical nociceptive response in the cat. Pharmacologist, *22*:204, 1980.
2. Abbound, T.K., Goebelsmann, U., Raya, J., Hoffman, D.I., and DeSousa, B.: Effect of intrathecal morphine during labor on maternal plasma beta-endorphin levels. An. H. Obstet. Gynecol., *149*:709, 1984.
3. Abbound, T.K., Shnider, S.M., Dailey, P.A., Raya, J.A., and Sarkis, F.: Intrathecal administration of hyperbaric morphine for the relief of pain in labour. Br. J. Anaesth., *56*:1351, 1984.
4. Abouleish, E., Barmada, M.A., Nemoto, E.M., Tung, A., and Winter, P.: Acute and chronic effects of intrathecal morphine in monkeys. Br. J. Anaesth., *53*:1027, 1981.
5. Ahmad, S., Hawes, O., Dooley, S., Faure, E., and Brunner, E.A.: Intrathecal morphine in a parturient with a single ventricle. Anesthesiology, *54*:515, 1981.
6. Ahuja, B.R., and Strunin, L.: Respiratory effects of epidural fentanyl. Anaesthesia, *40*:949, 1985.
7. Allen, P.D., Walman, T., Concepcion, M., Sheskey, M., and Patterson, M.K.: Epidural morphine provides postoperative pain relief in peripheral vascular and orthopedic surgical patients: A dose-response study. Anesth. Analg., *65*:165, 1986.
8. Alper, M.H.: Intrathecal morphine: A new method of obstetric analgesia? Anesthesiology, *51*:378, 1979.
9. Andersen, H.B., Christensen, C.B., Findlay, J.W., and Jansen, J.A.: Pharmacokinetics of epidural morphine and fentanyl in the goat. Pain *19*[*Suppl.*]:A564, 1984.
10. Anderson, H.B., Jorgensen, B.C., and Engquist, A.: Epidural met-enkephalin (FK 33-824). A dose–effect study. Acta Anaesthesiol. Scand., *26*:69, 1982.
11. Anderson, I., Thompson, W.R., Varkey, G.P., and Knill, R.L.: Lumbar epidural morphine as an effective analgesic following cholecystectomy. Can. Anaesth. Soc. J., *28*:523, 1981.
12. Aoki, M., Senami, M., Kitahata, L., and Collins, J.: Spinal sufentanil effects on spinal pain transmission neurons in cats. Anesthesiology, *64*:225, 1986.
13. Arner, S., and Arner, B.: Differential effects of epidural morphine in the treatment of cancer-related pain. Acta Anaesthesiol. Scand., *29*:32, 1985.
14. Asari, H., Inove, K., Shibata, T., and Soga, T.: Segmental effect of morphine injected into the epidural space in man. Anesthesiology, *54*:75, 1981.
15. Atchison, S.R., Durant, P., and Yaksh, T.L.: Studies in the anesthetized dog on the effects of lumbar intrathecal injection of DADL and morphine on respiratory and cardiovascular parameters. Anesthesiology, *60*:1986.
16. Atweh, S.F., and Kuhar, M.J.: Autoradiographic localization of opiate receptors in rat brain. I. Spinal cord and lower medulla. Brain Res., *124*:53, 1977.
17. Aun, C., Thomas, D., St. John-Jones, L., Colvin, M.P., and Savage, T.M.: Intrathecal morphine in cardiac surgery. Eur. J. Anaesthesiol., *2*:419, 1985.
18. Austin, K.L., Stapleton, J.V., and Mather, L.E.: Relationship between blood meperidine concentrations and analgesic response: A preliminary report. Anesthesiology, *53*:460, 1980.
19. Bahar, M., Olshwang, D., Magora, F., and Davidson, J.T.: Epidural morphine in treatment of pain. Lancet, *1*:527, 1979.
20. Bahar, M., Orr, I.A., and Dundee, J.W.: Central action of spinal opiates. Anesthesiology,*55*:334, 1981.
21. Bahar, M., Orr, I.A., and Dundee, J.W.: Shrinking pupils s a warning of respiratory depression after spinal morphine. Lancet, *1*:893, 1981.
22. Bailey, P.W., and Smith, B.E.: Continuous epidural infusion of fentanyl for post-operative analgesia. Anaesthesia, *35*:1002, 1980.
23. Banning, A.M., Schmidt, J.F., Chraemmer, J., *et al.*: Comparison of oral controlled release morphine and epidural morphine in the management of postoperataive pain. Anesth. Analg., *65*:385, 1986.
24. Baraka, A., Maktabi, M., and Noueihid, R.: Epidural meperidine-bupivacaine for obstetric analgesia. Anesth. Analg., *61*:652, 1982.
25. Baraka, A., Noueihed, R., and Hajj, S.: Intrathecal injection

of morphine for obstetric analgesia. Anesthesiology, *54*:136, 1981.

26. Barron, D.W., and Strong, J.E.: Postoperative analgesia in major orthopedic surgery. Epidural and intrathecal opiates. Anaesthesia, *36*:937, 1981.
27. Baxter, A.D., and Kiruluta, G.: Detrusor tone after epidural morphine. Anesth. Analg., *63*:464, 1984.
28. Beeby, D., MacIntosh, K.C., Bailey, M., and Welch, D.B.: Postoperative analgesia for cesarean section using epidural methadone. Anaesthesia, *39*:61, 1984.
29. Bengtsson, M., Lofstrom, J.B., and Merits, H.: Postoperative pain relief with intrathecal morphine after major hip surgery. Reg. Anaesth., *8*:138, 1983.
30. Benhamou, D., Samii, K., and Noviant, Y.: Effect of analgesia on respiratory muscle function after upper abdominal surgery. Acta Anaesthesiol. Scand., *27*:22, 1983.
31. Bilsback, P., Rolly, G., and Tampubolon, O.: Efficacy of the extradural administration of lofentanil, buprenorphine or saline in the management of postoperative pain. A double-blind study. Br. J. Anaesth., *57*:943, 1985.
32. Boas, R.A.: Hazards of epidural morphine. Anaesth. Intens. Care, *8*:377, 1980.
33. Boas, R.A., and Cahill, V.S.: Epidural buprenorphine compared to other analgesic methods for postoperative pain relief. Anesth. Intenzivmed. [In press]
34. Bonnardot, J.P., Maillet, M., Calou, J.C., Millot, F., and Deligne, P.: Maternal and fetal concentrations of morphine after intrathecal administration during labor. Br. J. Anaesth., *54*:487, 1982.
35. Bonnet, F., Blery, C., Zatan, M., *et al.*: Effect of epidural morphine on post-operative pulmonary dysfunction. Acta Anaesthesiol. Scand., *28*:147, 1984.
36. Bonnet, F., Harari, A., and Thibonnier, M.: Suppression of antidiuretic hormone hypersecretion during surgery by extradural anaesthesia. Br. J. Anaesth., *54*:29, 1982.
37. Booker, P.D., Wilkes, R.G., Bryson, T.H.L., and Beddard, J.: Obstetric pain relief using epidural morphine. Anaesthesia, *35*:377, 1980.
38. Boreus, L.O., Skoldefors, E., and Ehrnebo, M.: Appearance of pethidine and nor-pethidine in cerebrospinal fluid of man following intramuscular injection of pethidine. Acta Anaesthesiol. Scand., *27*:222, 1983.
39. Borner, U., Muller, H., Stoyanov, M., and Hempelmann, G.: Epidural opiate analgesia. Compatibility of opiates with tissue and CSF. Anaesthesist, *29*:570, 1980.
40. Boskovski, N., Lewinski, A., Xuered, J., and Mercieca, V.: Caudal epidural morphine for post-operative pain relief. Anaesthesia, *36*:67, 1980.
41. Bowen-Wright, R.M., and Goroszeniuk, T.: Epidural fentanyl for pain of multiple fractures. Lancet, *2*:1033, 1980.
42. Brandt, M.R., Korshin, J., Hanson, A.P., Hummer, L., Madsen, S.N., Rygg, I., and Kehlet, H.: Influence of morphine on the endocrine metabolic response to open heart surgery. Acta Anaesthesiol. Scand., *22*:400, 1978.
43. Brent, C.R., Harty, G., and Yaksh, T.L.: The effects of spinal opiates on micturition in unanesthetized animals. Soc. Neurosci., *9*:743, 1983.
44. Bromage, P.R.: Epidural Analgesia. Philadelphia, W.B. Saunders, 1978.
45. Bromage, P.R.: The price of intraspinal narcotic analgesia: Basic constraints. (editorial) Anesth. Analg., *60*:461, 1981.
46. Bromage, P.R., Camporesi, E., and Chestnut, D.: Epidural narcotics for postoperative analgesia. Anesth. Analg., *59*:473, 1980.
47. Bromage, P.R., Camporesi, E.M., Durant, P.A.C., and Nielsen, C.H.: Nonrespiratory side effects of epidural morphine. Anesth. Analg., *61*:490, 1982.
48. Bromage, P.R., Camporesi, E.M., Durant, P.A.C., and Nielsen, C.H.: Rostral spread of epidural morphine. Anesthesiology, *56*:431, 1982.
49. Bromage, P.R., Camporesi, E.M., Durant, P.A., and Nielsen, C.H.: Influence of epinephrine as an adjuvant to epidural morphine. Anesthesiology, *58*:257, 1983.
50. Bromage, P.R., Camporesi, E., and Leslie, J.: Epidural narcotics in volunteers: Sensitivity to pain and to carbon dioxide. Pain, *9*:145, 1980.
51. Bromage, P.R., Joyal, A.C., and Binney, J.C.: Local anesthetic drugs: Penetration from the spinal extradural space into the neuroaxis. Science, *140*:392, 1963.
52. Bromage, P.R., Shibata,. H.R., and Willoughby, H.W.: Influence of prolonged epidural blockade on blood sugar and cortisol responses to operations on the upper part of the abdomen and the thorax. Surg. Gynecol. Obstet., *132*:1051, 1971.
53. Brookshire, G.L., Shnider, S.M., Abboud, T.K., Kotelko, D.M., Nouiehed, R., Thigpen, J.W., Khoo, S.S., Raya, J.A., Foutz, S.E., and Brizgys, R.V.: Effects of naloxone on the mother and neonate after intrathecal morphine for labor analgesia. Anesthesiology, *59*:A417, 1983.
54. Brownridge, P.: Epidural and intrathecal opiates for postoperative pain relief. Anaesthesia, *38*:74, 1983.
55. Brownridge, P., and Frewin, D.B.: A comparative study of techniques of postoperative analgesia following cesarean section and lower abdominal surgery. Anaesth. Intens. Care, *13*:123, 1985.
56. Brownridge, P., Wrobel, J., and Watt-Smith, J.: Respiratory depression following accidental subarachnoid pethidine. Anaesth. Intens. Care, *11*:237, 1983.
57. Buckley, F.P., Kehlet, H., Brown, N.S., and Scott, D.B.: Postoperative glucose tolerance during extradural analgesia. Br. J. Anaesth., *54*:325, 1982.
58. Buckley, F.P., and Simpson, B.R.: Acute traumatic and postoperative pain management. *In* Cousins, M.J., and Bridenbaugh, P.O. (eds.): Neural Blockade in Clinical Anesthesia and Management of Pain. pp. 586–615. Philadelphia, J.B. Lippincott, 1980.
59. Bullingham, R.E.S., McQuay, H.J., and Moore, R.A.: Unexpectedly high plasma fentanyl levels after epidural use. Lancet, *1*:1361, 1980.
60. Calvillo, O., Henry, J.L., and Neuman, R.S.: Effects of morphine and naloxone on dorsal horn neurones in the cat. Can. J. Physiol. Pharmacol., *52*:1207, 1974.
61. Camporesi, E.M., Nielsen, C.H., Bromage, P.R., and Durant, P.A.: Ventilatory CO_2 sensitivity after intravenous and epidural morphine in volunteers. Anesth. Analg., *62*:633, 1983.
62. Cardan, E.: Spinal morphine in enuresis. Br. J. Anaesth., *57*:354, 1985.
63. Carl, P., Crawford, M.E., Ravlo, O., and Bach, V.: Long term

treatment with epidural opioids. A retrospective study comprising 150 patients treated with morphine chloride and buprenorphine. Anaesthesia, *41*:32, 19886.

64. Carrie, L.E., O'Sullivan, G.M., and Seegobin, R.: Epidural fentanyl in labour. Anaesthesia, *36*:965, 1981.
65. Castillo, R., Kissin, I., and Bradley, E.L.: Selective kappa opioid agonist for spinal analgesia without the risk of respiratory depression. Anesth. analg., *65*:350, 1986.
66. Cahl, L.A.: Pain induced by inflammatory mediators. *In* Beers, R.F. Jr., and Bassett, E.G. (eds.): Mechanisms of Pain and Analgesic Compounds. New York, Raven Press, 1979.
67. Chakravarty, K., Tucker, W., Rosen, M., and Vickers, M.D.: Comparison of buprenorphine and pethidine given intravenously on demand to relieve post-operative pain. Br. Med. J., *2*:895, 1979.
68. Chambers, W.A., Sinclair, C.J., and Scott, D.B.: Extradural morphine for pain after surgery. Br. J. Anaesth., *53*:921, 1981.
69. Chang, K-J., and Cuatrecasas, P.: Heterogeneity and properties of opiate receptors. Fed. Proc., *40*:2729, 1981.
70. Chauvin, M., Salbaing, J., Perrin, D., *et al.*: Clinical assessment and plasma pharmacokinetics associated with intramuscular or extradural alfentanil. Br. J. Anaesth., *57*:886, 1985.
71. Chauvin, M., Samii, K., Schermann, J.M., Sandouk, P., Bourdon, R., and Viars, P.: Plasma morphine concentration after intrathecal administration of low doses of morphine. Br. J. Anaesth., *53*:1065, 1981.
72. Chauvin, M., Samii, K., Schermann, J.M., Sandouk, P., Bourdon, R., and Viars, P.: Plasma pharmacokinetics of morphine after I.M. extradural and intrathecal administration. Br. J. Anaesth., *54*:843, 1981.
73. Chayen, M.S., Rudick, V., and Borvine, A.: Pain control with epidural injection of morphine. Anesthesiology, *53*:338, 1981.
74. Cherry, D.A.: Drug delivery systems for epidural administration of opioids. Acta Anaesthesiol. Scand., (in press).
75. Cherry, D.A., Gourlay, G.K., and Cousins, M.J.: Extradural mass associated with lack of efficacy of epidural morphine, and undetectable CSF morphine concentrations. Pain, *25*:69, 1986.
76. Cherry, D.A., Gourlay, G.K., Cousins, M.J., and Gannon, B.J.: A technique for the insertion of an implantable portal system for the long term epidural administration of opioids in the treatment of cancer pain. Anaesth. Intens. Care, *13*:145, 1985.
77. Cherry, D.A., Gourlay, G.K., McLachlan, M., and Cousins, M.J.: Diagnostic epidural opioid blockade and chronic pain: Preliminary report. Pain, *21*:143, 1985.
78. Christensen, F.R., and Andersen, L.W.: Adverse reaction to extradural buprenorphine. Br. J. Anaesth., *54*:476, 1982.
79. Christensen, P., and Brandt, M.R.: Extradural morphine and Stokes-Adams attacks. Br. J. Anaesth., *54*:363, 1982.
80. Christensen, P., Brandt, M.R., Rem, J., and Kehlet, H.: Influence of extradural morphine on the adrenocortical and hyperglycaemic response to surgery. Br. J. Anaesth., *54*:23, 1980.
81. Christensen, V.: Respiratory depression after extradural morphine. Br. J. Anaesth., *52*:841, 1980.
82. Chrubasik, J. *et al.*: Somatostatin, a potent analgesic. Lancet, *2*:1208, 1984.
83. Chrubasik, J., Scholler, K., and Bammert, J.: Epidural morphine injection and cisternal cerebellomedullary CSF bioavailability of morphine in dogs. *In* Erdmann, W., Oyama, T., and Pernak, M. (eds.): The Pain Clinic. pp. 47–49. Utrecht, UNU Science Press, 1985.
84. Chrubasik, J., Meynadier, J., Scherperell, P., *et al.*: The effect of epidural somatostatin on postoperative pain. Anesth. Analg., *64*:1085, 1985.
85. Chrubasik, J., Volk, J., Meynadier, J., *et al.*: Observations in dogs receiving chronic spinal somatostatin and calcitonin. Schmerz. Pain Doleur, *1*:10, 1986.
86. Chrubasik, J., and Wiebers, K.: Continuous-plus-on-demand epidural infusions of morphine for postoperative pain relief by means of a small, externally worn infusion device. Anesthesiology, *62*:263, 1985.
87. Cohen, S.E., and Woods, W.A.: The role of epidural morphine in the post cesarean patient: Efficacy and effects of bonding. Anesthesiology, *58*:500, 1983.
88. Colpaert, F.C.: Can chronic pain be suppressed despite purported tolerance to narcotic analgesia? Life Sci., *24*:1201, 1979.
89. Colpaert, F.C., Leysen, L.E., Michiels, M., and Van den Hoogen, R.: Epidural and intravenous sufentanil in the rat: Analgesia, opiate receptor binding, and drug concentrations in plasma and brain. Anesthesiology. [In press]
90. Coombs, D.W.: Management of chronic pain by epidural and intrathecal opioids. Newer drugs and delivery systems. *In* Sjostrand, U.H., and Rawal, N. (eds.): Regional Opioids in Anesthesiology and Pain Management. Int. Anesthesiol. Clin., *24*:58, 1986.
91. Coombs, D.W., Fratkin, J.D., Meier, F.A., *et al.*: Neuropathologic lesions and CSF morphine concentrations during chronic continuous intraspinal morphine infusion. Pain, *22*:337, 1985.
92. Coombs, D.W., Maurer, L.H., Saunders, R.L., and Gaylor, M.: Outcomes and complications of continuous intraspinal narcotic analgesia for cancer pain control. J. Clin. Oncol., *2*:1414, 19884.
93. Coombs, D.W., Saunders, R.L., Gaylor, M., LaChance, D., and Jensen, L.: Clinical trial of intrathecal clonidine for cancer pain. Pain, *18*[*Suppl.*]:21, 1984.
94. Coombs, D.W., Sanders, R.L., Gaylor, M., and Pageau, M.G.: Epidural narcotic infusion: Implantation technique and efficacy. Anesthesiology, *55*:469, 1981.
95. Coombs, D.W., Saunders, R.L., Harbaugh, R., *et al.*: Relief of continuous chronic pain by intraspinal narcotics infusion via an implanted reservoir. J.A.M.A., *250*:2336, 1983.
96. Coombs, D.W., Saunders, R.L., LaChance, D., Savage, S., Ragnarson, T.S., and Jensen, L.: Intrathecal morphine tolerance: Use of intrathecal clonidine, DADLE, and intraventricular morphine. Anesthesiology, *62*:358, 1985.
97. Cousins, M.J.: Epidural neural blockade. *In* Cousins, M.J., and Bridenbaugh, P.O. (eds.): Neural Blockade in Clinical Anesthesia and Management of Pain. pp. 176–274. Philadelphia, J.B. Lippincott, 1980.

98. Cousins, M.J., and Bridenbaugh, P.O.: Spinal opioids and pain relief in acute care. *In* Cousins, M.J., and Phillips, G.D. (eds.): Acute Pain Management. pp.151–185. New York, Churchill Livingstone, 1986.
99. Cousins, M.J., and Glynn,C.J.: New horizons. *In* Cousins, M.J., and Bridenbaugh, P.O. (eds.): Neural Blockade in Clinical Anesthesia and Management of Pain. pp. 699–719. Philadelphia, J.B. Lippincott, 1980.
100. Cousins, M.J., Glynn, C.J., Wilson, P.R., Mather, L.E., and Graham, J.R.: Aspects of epidural morphine. Lancet, *2*:584, 1979.
101. Cousins, M.J., Glynn, C.J., Wilson, P.R., Mather, L.E., and Graham, J.R.: Epidural morphine. Anaesth. Intens. Care, *8*:217, 1980.
102. Cousins, M.J., and Mather, L.E.: Intrathecal and epidural administration of opioids. Anesthesiology, *61*:276, 1984.
103. Cousins, M.J., Mather, L.E., Glynn, C.J., Wilson, P.R., and Graham, J.R.: Selective spinal analgesia. Lancet, *1*:1141, 1979.
104. Cousins, M.J., Mather, L.E., and Gourlay, G.K.: Axon, spinal cord and brain: Targets for acute pain control. *In* Scott, D.B., McClure, J., and Wildsmith, J.A. (eds.): Regional Anaesthesia 1884–1984. Denmark, J.H. Schultz, 1984.
105. Cousins, M.J., and Phillips, G.D.: Sleep, pain and sedation. In Shoemaker, W.L., Thompson, W.L., and Holbrook, P.R. (eds.): Society for Critical Care Medicine. Textbook of Critical Care, pp. 787–800. Philadelphia, W.B. Saunders, 1984.
106. Cousins, M.J., and Phillips, G.D. (eds.): Acute Pain Management. New York, Churchill Livingstone, 1986.
107. Cowen, M.J., Bullingham, R.E.S., Paterson, G.M.C., McQuay, H.J., Turner, M., Allen, M.C., and Moore, A.: A controlled comparison of the effects of extradural diamorphine and bupivacaine on plasma glucose and plasma cortisol in postoperative patients. Anesth. Analg., *61*:15, 1982.
108. Craft, J.B. Jr., Bolan, J.C., Coaldrake, L.A., Mondino, M., Mazel, P., Gilman, R.M., Shokes, L.K., and Woolf, W.A.: The maternal and fetal cardiovascular effects of epidural morphine in the sheep model. Am. J. Obstet. Gynecol., *142*:835, 1982.
109. Crawford, J.S.: Site of action of intrathecal morphine. Br. Med. J., *281*:680, 1980.
110. Crawford, J.S.: Site of action of intrathecal morphine. Br. Med. J., *281*:1144, 1980.
111. Crawford, M.E., Andersen, H.B., *et al.*: Pain treatment on outpatient basis utilizing extradural opiates: A Danish multicentive study comprising 105 patients. Pain, *16*:41, 1983.
112. Crawford, R.D., Batra, M.S., and Fox, F.: Epidural morphine dose response for postoperative analgesia. Anesthesiology, *55*:A150, 1981.
113. Cullen, M.L., Staren, E.D., el-Ganzouri, A., Logas, W.G., Ivankovich, A.D., and Economou, S.G.: Continuous epidural infusion for analgesia after major abdominal operations: A randomized, prospective, double-blind study. Surgery, *98*:718, 1985.
114. Cuschieri, R.J., Morran, C.G., Howie, J.C., and McArdle, C.S.: Postoperative pain and pulmonary complications: Comparison of three analgesic regimens. Br. J. Surg., *72*:495, 1985.
115. Czlonkowski, A., Costa, T., *et al.*: Opiate receptor binding sites in human spinal cord. Brain Res., *267*:392, 1983.
116. Dahlstrom, B., Tamsen, A., Paalzow, L., and Hartvig, P.: Patient controlled analgesic therapy. IV. Pharmacokinetics and analgesic plasma concentrations of morphine. Clin. Pharmacokin., *7*:266, 1982.
117. Dailey, P.A., Baysinger, C.L., Levinson, G., and Shnider, S.M.: Neurobehavioral testing of the newborn infant. Effects of obstetric anesthesia. Clin. Perinatol., *1*:191, 1982.
118. Dailey, P.A., Brookshire, G.L., Shnider, S.M., Abboud, T.K., Kotelko, D.M., Noueihid, R., Thigpen, J.W., Khoo, S.S., Raya, J.A., Foutz, S.E., *et al.*: The effects of naloxone associated with the intrathecal use of morphine in labor. Anesth. Analg., *64*:658, 1985.
119. Danielson, D.R., Coombs, D.W., Pageau, M., and Rippe, E.: Epidural morphine for post-caesarian analgesia. Anesthesiology, *55*:A323, 1981.
120. Davies, G.K., Tolhurst-Cleaver, C.L., and James, T.L.: CNS depression from intrathecal morphine. Anesthesiology, *52*:280, 1980.
121. Davies, G.K., Tolhurst-Cleaver, C.L., James, T.L.: Respiratory depression after intrathecal narcotics. Anaesthesia, *35*:1080, 1980.
122. DeGroat, W.C., Kawatani, M., *et al.*: The role of neuropeptides in the sacral autonomic reflex pathways of the cat. J. Auton. Nerv. Sys., *7*:339, 1983.
123. Denson, D.D., Raj, P.P., Joyce, T.H., Saldanha, F.M., and Turner, J.L.: Kinetics of continuous epidural bupivacaine infusions. Anesthesiology, *55*:A159, 1981.
124. Devaux, C.B., Mangez, J.F., Tessier, C., Zickler, P., and Alibert F.: Potentiation of opiates administered by intra-ventricular route. Anesth. Intenzivmed. [In press]
125. DiChiro, G.: Movement of the cerebrospinal fluid in human beings. Nature, *204*:290, 1964.
126. DiChiro, G.: Observations on the circulation of the cerebrospinal fluid. Acta Radiol. [Diagn.] (Stockh.), *5*:988, 1966.
127. Dirkson, R., and Nijhuis, G.M.M.: Epidural opiate and perioperataive analgesia. Acta Anaesth. Scand., *24*:367, 1980.
128. Doblar, D.B., Muldoon, S.M., Abbrecht, P.H., Baskoff, J., and Watson, R.L.: Epidural morphine following epidural local anesthetic: Effect on ventilatory and airway occlusion pressure response to CO_2. Anesthesiology, *55*:423, 1981.
129. Doi, T., and Jurna, I.: Analgesic effect of intrathecal morphine demonstrated in ascending nociceptive activity in the rat spinal cord and effectiveness of caerulein and cholecystokinin octapeptide. Brain Res., *234*:399, 1982.
130. Donadoni, R., Rolly, G., Noorduin, H., and Vanden Bussche, G.: Epidural sufentanil for postoperative pain relief. Anaesthesia, *40*:634, 1985.
131. Drayer, B.P., and Rosenbaum, A.E.: Studies of the third circulation. Amipaque CT cisternography and ventriculography. J. Neurosurg., *48*:946, 1978.
132. Duggan, A.W., Hall, J.G., and Headley, P.M.: Morphine, enkephalin and the substantia gelatinosa. Nature, *264*:456, 1976.
133. Duggan, A.W.,, Hall, J.G., and Headley, P.M.: Suppression of transmission of nociceptive impulses by morphine selec-

tive effects of morphine administered in the region of the substantia gelatinosa. Br. J. Pharmacol., *61*:65, 1976.

134. Duggan, A.W., Johnson, S.M., and Morton, C.R.: Differing distributions of receptors for morphine and met[5]-enkephalinamide in the dorsal horn of the cat. Brain Res., *229*:379, 1981.

135. Duggan, A.W., Morton, C.R., Johnson, S.M., and Zhao, Z.Q.: Opioid antagonists and spinal reflexes in the anaesthestized cat. Brain Res., *297*:33, 1984.

136. Durant, P.A., and Yaksh, T.L.: Epidural injections of bupivacaine, morphine, fentanyl, lofentanil and DADL in chronically implanted rats: A pharmacologic and pathologic study. Anesthesiology, *64*:43, 1986.

137. Durant, P.A., and Yaksh, T.L.: Distribution in cerebrospinal fluid, blood and lymph of epidurally injected morphine and inulin in dogs. Anesth. Analg., *65*:583, 1986.

138. Ebert, J., and Varner, P.D.: The effective use of epidural morphine sulfate for postoperative orthopedic pain. Anesthesiology, *53*:257, 1980.

139. Editorial: Spinal opiates revisited. Lancet, *1*:655, 1986.

140. Edwards, D.J., Svensson, C.K., Visco, J.P., and Lalka, D.: Clinical pharmacokinetics of pethidine. Clin. Pharmacokin., *7*:421, 1982.

141. El-Baz, N.M., Faber, L.P., and Jensik, R.J.: Continuous epidural infusion of morphine for treatment of pain after thoracic surgery: A new technique. Anesth. Analg., *63*:757, 1984.

142. El-Baz, N., and Goldin, M.D.: Continuous epidural morphine infusion for pain relief after open heart surgery. Anesthesiology, *59*:A193, 1983.

143. Elde, R., Hokfelt, T., Johansson, O., and Terenius, L.: Immunohistochemical studies using antibodies to leucine-enkephalin: Initial observations on the nervous system of the rat. Neuroscience, *1*:349, 1976.

144. Ellis, R., Haines, D., Shah, R., Cotton, B.R., and Smith, G.: Pain relief after abdominal surgery: A comparison of IM morphine, sublingual buprenorphine and self administered I.V. pethidine. Br. J. Anaesth., *54*:421, 1982.

145. Engquist, A., Brandt, M.R., Fernandes, A., and Kehlet, H.: The blocking effect of epidural analgesia on the adrenocortical and hyperglycemic response to surgery. Acta Anaesthesiol. Scand., *21*:330, 1977.

146. Engquist, A., Chraemmer, J., and Orgensen, B.: Epidural morphine-induced catatonia. Lancet, *1*:984, 1980.

147. Engquist, A., Jorgensen, B.C., and Andersen, H.B.: Catatonia after epidural morphine. Acta Anaesthesiol. Scand., *25*:445, 1981.

148. Erickson, D.L., Blacklock, J.B., Michaelson, M., Sperling, K.B., and Lo, J.N.: Control of spasticity by implantable continuous flow morphine pump. Neurosurgery, *16*:215, 1985.

149. Evron, S., Samueloff, A., Simon, A., Drenger, B., and Magora, F.: Urinary function during epidural analgesia with methadone and morphine in post-cesareasn section patients. Pain, *23*:135, 1985.

150. Florez, J., McCarty, L.E., and Borison, H.L.: A comparative study in the cat of the respiratory effects of morphine injected intravenously and into the cerebrospinal fluid. J. Pharmacol. Exp. Ther., *163*:448, 1968.

151. Foley, K.M., and Inturrisi, C.E.: Intrathecal beta-endorphin. Lancet, *1*:317, 1980.

152. Francis, D.M., Justins, D., and Reynolds, F.J.M.: Obstetric pain relief using epidural narcotic agents. Anaesthesia, *35*:69, 1980.

153. Freye, E., and Hartung, E.: Fentanyl in the fourth cerebral ventricle causes respiratory depression in the anesthetized but not in the awake dog. Acta Anaesthesiol. Scand., *25*:171, 1981.

154. Game, C.J.A., and Lodge, D.: The pharmacology of the inhibition of dorsal horn neurones by impulses in myelinated cutaneous afferents in the cat. Exp. Brain Res., *23*:75, 1975.

155. Gjessing, J., and Tomlin, P.J.: Patterns of postoperative pain: A study of the use of continuous epidural analgesia in the postoperative period. Anaesthesia, *34*:624, 1979.

156. Gjessing, J., and Tomlin, P.J.: Postoperative pain control with intrathecal morphine. Anaesthesia, *36*:268, 1981.

157. Glurel, A., Unal, N., Elevli, M., and Eren, A.: Epidural morphine for postoperative pain relief in anorectal surgery. Anesth. Analg., *65*:499, 1986.

158. Glynn, C.J., and Mather, L.E.: Clinical pharmacokinetics applied to patients with intractable pain: Studies with pethidine. Pain, *13*:237, 1982.

159. Glynn, C.J., Mather, L.E., Cousins, M.J., Graham, J.R., and Wilson, P.R.: Peridural meperidine in humans: Analgetic response, pharmacokinetics and transmission into CSF. Anesthesiology, *55*:520, 1981.

160. Glynn, C.J., Mather, L.E., Cousins, M.J., Wilson, P.R., and Graham, J.R.: Spinal narcotics and respiratory depression. Lancet, *2*:356, 1979.

161. Gourlay, G.K., Cherry, D.A., and Cousins, M.J.: Cephalad migration of morphine in CSF following lumbar epidural administration in patients with cancer pain. Pain, *23*:317, 1985.

162. Gourlay, G.K., Willis, R.J., and Wilson, P.R.: Postoperative pain control with methadone: Influence of supplementary methadone doses and blood concentration-response relationships. Anesthesiology, *61*:19, 1984.

163. Gourlay, G.K., Wilson, P.R., and Glynn, C.J.: Pharmacodynamics and pharmacokinetics of methadone during the perioperative period. Anesthesiology, *57*:458, 1982.

164. Graham, J.L., King, R., and McCaughey, W.: Postoperative pain relief using epidural morphine. Anaesthesia, *35*:158, 1980.

165. Grossi, P., and Armer, S.: Effect of epidural morphine on the Hoffman reflex in man. Acta Anaesthesiol. Scand., *28*:152, 1984.

166. Gustafsson, L.L., Ackerman, S., Adamson, H., Garle, M., Rane, A., and Schildt, B.: Kinetics of morphine in cerebrospinal fluid after epidural administration. Acta Anaesthesiol. Scand., *28*:535, 1984.

167. Gustafsson, L.L., Feychting, B., and Klingstedt, C: Late respiratory depression after concomitant use of morphine epidurally and parenterally. Lancet, *1*:892, 1981.

168. Gustafsson, L.L., Friberg–Nielsen, S., and Garle, M.: Extradural and parenteral morphine: Kinetics and effects in postoperative pain. A controlled clinical study. Br. J. Anaesth., *54*:1167, 1982.

169. Gustafsson, L.L., Garle, M., Johannisson, J., Rane, A., Stenport, J., and Walson, P.: Regional epidural analgesia: Kinetics of pethidine. Acta Anaesthesiol. Scand., *74[Suppl.]*:165, 1982.
170. Gustafsson, L.L., Hartvig, P., *et al.*: Kinetics of ^{11}C-labelled morphine and meperidine after epidural and intrathecal administration to Rhesus monkey. Drug Metab. Dispos., (in press)
171. Gustafsson, L.L., Johannisson, J., and Garle, M.: Extradural and parenteral pethidine as analgesia after total hip replacement: Effects and kinetics. A controlled clinical study. Eur. J. Clin. Pharmacol., *29*:529, 1986.
172. Gustafsson, L.L., Post, C., Edvardsen, B., and Ramsay, C.H.: Distribution of morphine and meperidine after intrathecal administration in rat and mouse. Anesthesiology, *63*:483, 1985
173. Gustafsson, L.L., Schildt, B., and Jacobsen, K.J.: Adverse effects of extradural and intrathecal opiates: Report of a nationwide survey in Sweden. Br. J. Anaesth., *54*:479, 1982.
174. Hammonds, W., Bramwell, R.S., Hug, C.C., Najak, Z., and Critz, A.: A comparison of epidural meperidine and bupivacaine for relief of labor pain. Anesth. Analg., *61*:187, 1982.
175. Han, J.S., Xie, G.X., and Goldstein, A.: Analgesia induced by intrathecal injection of dynorphin B in the rat. Life Sci., *34*:1573, 1984.
176. Hanks, G.W., Twycross, R.G., and Lloyd, J.W.: Unexpected complication of successful nerve block. Morphine induced respiratory depression precipitated by removal of severe pain. Anaesthesia, *36*:37, 1981.
177. Hanson, A.L., Hanson, B., and Matousek, M.: Epidural anesthesia for cesarean section. The effect of morphine-bupivacaine administered epidurally for intra and postoperative pain relief. Acta Obstet. Gynecol. Scand., *63*:135, 1984.
178. Harbaugh, R.E., Coombs, D.W., Saunders, R.L., Gaylor, M., and Pageau, M.: Implanted continuous epidural morphine system. Preliminary Report. J. Neurosurg., *56*:803, 1982.
179. Hartrick, C.T., Pither, C.E., Paj, V., Raj, P., and Tomsick, T.A.: Subdural migration of an epidural catheter. Anesth. Analg., *64*:175, 1985.
180. Hasenbos, M., Van Egmond, J., Gielen, M., and Crul, J.F.: Post-operative analgesia by epidural versus intramuscular nicomorphine after thoracotomy. Pt. I. Acta Anaesthesiol. Scand., *29*:572, 1985.
181. Hasenbos, M., Van Egmond, J., Gielen, M., and Crul, J.F.: Post-operative analgesia by epidural versus intramuscular nicomorphine after thoracotomy. Pt. II. Acta Anaesthesiol. Scand., *29*:577, 1985.
182. Hjorts, N.C., Neumann, P., Frsig, F., Andersen, T., Lindhard, A., Rogon, E., and Kehlet, H.: A controlled study on the effect of epidural analgesia with local anaesthetics and morphine on morbidity after abdominal surgery. Acta Anaesthesiol. Scand., *29*:790, 1985.
183. Hokfelt, T., Elde, R., Johansson, O., Luft, R., Nilsson, G., and Arimura, A.: Immunohistochemical evidence for separate populations of somatostatain-containing and substance P-containing primary afferent neurons in the rat. Neuroscience, *1*:131, 1976.
184. Hokfelt, T., Kellerth, J.O., Nilsson, G., and Pernow, B.: Experimental immunohistochemical studies on the localization and distribution of substance P in cat primary sensory neurones. Brain Res., *100*:235, 1975.
185. Hokfelt, T., Kellerth, J.O., Nilsson, G., and Pernow, B.: Substance P: Localization in the central nervous system and in some primary sensory neurons. Science, *190*:889, 1975.
186. Hokfelt, T., Ljungdahl, A., Elde, R., Nilsson, G., and Terenius, L.: Immunohistochemical analysis of peptide pathways possibly related to pain and analgesia: Enkephalin and substance P. Proc. Natl. Acad. Sci., USA, *74*:3081, 1977.
187. Hotvedt, R., and Refsum, H.: Cardiac effects of thoracic epidural morphine caused by increased vagal activity in the dog. Acta Anaesthesiol. Scand., *30*:76, 1986.
188. Houlton, P., and Reynolds, F.: Epidural diamorphine and fentanyl for postoperative pain. Anaesthesia, *36*:1141, 1981.
189. Howard, R.P., Milne, L.A., and Williams, N.E.: Epidural morphine in terminal care. Anaesthesia, *36*:51, 1981.
190. Hug, C.C., Jr.: Transport of narcotic analgesics by the choroid plexus and kidney tissues *in vitro.* Biochem. Pharmacol., *16*:345, 1967.
191. Hug, C.C., Jr.: Improving analgesic therapy. Anesthesiology, *53*:441, 1980.
192. Hughes, S.C.: Intraspinal narcotics in obstetrics. Clin. Perinatol., *1*:167, 1982.
193. Hughes, S.C., Abboud, T.K., Shnider, S.M., Stefani, S.J., and Norton, M.: Maternal and neonatal effects of epidural morphine for labor. Anesth. Analg., *61*:190, 1982.
194. Hughes, S.C., Rosen, M.A., Shnider, S.M., Abboud, T.K., Stefani, S.J., and Norton, M.: Maternal and neonatal effects of epidural morphine for labor and delivery. Anesth. Analg., *63*:319, 1984.
195. Hughes, S.C., Rosen, M.A., Shnider, S.M., Norton, M., and Curtis, J.D.: Epidural morphine for the relief of postoperative pain after cesarean section. Anesth. Analg., *61*:190, 1982.
196. Hughes, J., Smith, T.W., Koslerlitz, H.W., *et al.*: Isolation of two related pentapeptides from brain with potent opiate activity. Nature, *258*:577, 1975.
197. Huntington, C.T., Cohn, M.L., and Byrd, S.E.: Combined use of epidural morphine and steroid in recurrent postsurgical low back pain syndrome. Anesth. Analg., *61*:191, 1982.
198. Husemeyer, R.P., Cummings, A.J., Rosankiewicz, J.R., and Davenport, H.T.: A study of pethidine kinetics and analgesia in women in labour following intravenous, intramuscular and epidural administration. Br. J. Clin. Pharmacol., *13*:171, 1982.
199. Husemeyer, R.P., Davenport, H.T., Cummings, A.J., and Rosankiewicz, J.R.: Comparison of epidural and intramuscular pethidine for analgesia in labour. Br. J. Obstet. Gynecol., *88*:711, 1981.
200. Husemeyer, R.P., O'Connor, M.C., and Davenport, H.T.: Aspects of epidural morphine. Lancet, 2:583, 1979.
201. Husemeyer, R.P., O'Connor, M.C., and Davenport, H.T.: Failure of epidural morphine to relieve pain in labour. Anaesthesia, *35*:161, 1980.
202. Husted, S., Djurhuus, J.C., Husegaard, H.C., Jepsen, J., and Mortensen, J.: Effect of postoperative extradural morphine

on lower urinary tract function. Acta Anaesthesiol. Scand., *29*:183, 1985.

203. Jacobsen, L., Phillips, P.D., Hull, C.J., and Conacher, I.D.: Extradural versus intramuscular diamorphine. A controlled study of analgesic and adverse effects in the postoperative period. Anaesthesia, *38*:10, 1983.

204. Jansco, N.: Desensitization with capsaicin as a tool for studying the function of pain receptors. *In* Pharmacology of Pain. Oxford, Pergamon Press, *9*:33, 1968.

205. Jensen, B.H.: Caudal block for post-operative pain relief in children after genital operations. A comparison between bupivacaine and morphine. Acta Anaesthesiol. Scand., *25*:373, 1981.

206. Jensen, P.J., Siem–Jorgensen, P., Nielsen, T.B.: Wichmand–Nielsen, H., and Wintherreich, E.: Epidural morphine by the caudal route for postoperative pain relief. Acta Anaesthesiol. Scand., *26*:511, 1982.

207. Johnson, S.M., and Duggan, A.W.: Tolerance and dependence of dorsal horn neurones of the cat: The role of the opiate receptors of the substantia gelatinosa. Neuropharmacology, *20*:1033, 1981.

208. Johnson, S.M., and Duggan, A.W.: Evidence that opiate receptors of the substantia gelatinosa contribute to the depression by intravenous morphine of the spinal transmission of impulses in the unmyelinated primary afferents. Brain Res., *207*:223, 1981.

209. Johnston, J.R., and McCaughey, W.: Epidural morphine: A method of management of multiple fractured ribs. Anaesthesia, *35*:155, 1980.

210. Jones, R.D.M., and Jones, J.G.: Intrathecal morphine: Naloxone reverses respiratory depression but not analgesia. Br. Med. J., *281*:645, 1980.

211. Jones, S.E., Beasley, J.M., Macfarlane, D.W., Davis, J.M., and Hall–Davies, G.: Intrathecal morphine for postoperative pain relief in children. Br. J. Anaesth., *56*:137, 1984.

212. Jorgensen, B.C., Andersen, H.B., and Engquist, A.: CSF and plasma morphine after epidural and intrathecal application. Anesthesiology, *55*:714, 1981.

213. Jorgensen, B.C., Andersen, H.B., and Engquist, A.: Influence of epidural morphine on postoperative pain, endocrine-metabolic, and renal responses to surgery. A controlled study. Acta Anaesthesiol. Scand., *26*:63, 1982.

214. Justins, D.M., Francis, D., Houlton, P.G., and Reynolds, F.: A controlled trial of extradural fentanyl in labor. Br. J. Anaesth., *54*:409, 1982.

215. Justins, D.M., Knott, C., Luthman, J., and Reynolds, F.: Epidural versus intramuscular fentanyl: Analgesia and pharmacokinetics in labor. Anaesthesia, *38*:937, 1983.

216. Kalso, E.: Effects of intrathecal morphine, injected with bupivacaine, on pain after orthopaedic surgery. Br. J. Anaesth., *55*:415, 1983.

217. Kanto, J., Erkkola, R., Aaltonen, L., and Aarimaa, L.: Epidural morphine as postoperative analgesic following cesarean section under epidural analgesia. Int. J. Clin. Pharmacol. Ther. Toxicol., *23*:43, 1985.

218. Katz, J., and Nelson, W.: Intrathecal morphine for postoperative pain relief. Reg. Anesth., *6*:1, 1981.

219. Kaufman, J.J., Semo, N.M., and Koski, W.S.: Microelectrometric titration measurements of the pka's and partition and drug distribution coefficients of narcotics and narcotic antagonists and their pH temperature dependence. J. Med. Chem., *18*:647, 1975.

220. Kaufman, L.: Intrathecal heroin. Lancet, *1*:1341, 1981.

221. Kehlet, H.: The modifying effect of general and regional anaesthesia on the endocrine metabolic response to surgery. Reg. Anaesth., *7[Suppl.]*:538, 1982.

222. Kerr–Wilson, R.H., and McNally, S.: Bladder drainage for caesarean section under epidural analgesia. Br. J. Obstet. Gynaecol., *93*:28, 1986.

223. Kitahata, L.M., and Collins, J.G.: Spinal action of narcotic analgesics. Anesthesiology, *54*:153, 1981.

224. Klinck, J.R., and Lindop, M.J.: Epidural morphine in the elderly. A controlled trial after upper abdominal surgery. Anaesthesia, *37*:907, 1982.

225. Knill, R.L., Clement, J.L., and Thompson, W.R.: Epidural morphine causes delayed and prolonged ventilatory depression. Can. Anaesth. Soc. J., *28*:537, 1981.

226. Korinek, A.M., Languille, M., and Bonnet, F., Thibonnier, M., Sasano, P., Lienhart, A., and Viars, P.: Effect of postoperative extradural morphine on ADH secretion. Br. J. Anaesth., *57*:407, 1985.

227. Kotelko, D.M., Dailey, P.A., Shnider, S.M., Rosen, M.A., Hughes, S.C., and Brizgys, R.V.: Epidural morphine analgesia after cesarean delivery. Obstet. Gynecol., *63*:409, 1984.

228. Krames, E.S., Wilkie, D.J., and Gershow, J.: Intrathecal d-Ala2-d-Leu5-enkephalin (DADL) restores analgesia in a patient analgetically tolerant to intrathecal morphine sulphate. Pain, *24*:205, 1986.

229. Lam, A.M., Knill, R.L., Thompson, W.R., Clement, J.L., Varkey, G.P., and Spoerel, W.E.: Epidural fentanyl does not cause delayed respiratory depression. Can. Anaesth. Soc. J., *30*:578, 1983.

230. Lamarche, Y., Martin, R., Reiher, Y., and Blaise, G.: The sleep apnoea syndrome and epidural morphine. Can. Anaesth. Soc. J., *33*:231, 1986.

231. Lanz, E., Kehrberger, E., and Theiss, D.: Epidural morphine: A clinical double-blind study of dosage. Anesth. Analg., *64*:786, 1985.

232. Lanz, E., Theiss, D., Riess, W., and Sommer, V.: Epidural morphine for postoperative analgesia: A double-blind study. Anesth. Analg., *61*:236, 1982.

233. Larsen, V.H., Iversen, A.D., Christensen, P., and Andersen, P.K.: Postoperative pain treatment after upper abdominal surgery with epidural morphine at thoracic or lumbar level. Acta Anaesthesiol. Scand., *29*:566, 1985.

234. Layfield, D.J., Lemberger, R.J., Hopkinson, B.R., and Makin, G.S.: Epidural morphine for ischaemic rest pain. Br. Med. J., *282*:697, 1981.

235. Lazorthes, Y., Gouarderes, C.H., Verdie, J.C., Monsarrat, B., Bastide, R., Campan, L., Alwan, A., and Cros, J.: Analgesie par injection intrathecale de morphine. Etude pharmacocinetique et application aux douleurs irreductibles. Neurochirurgie, *26*:159, 1980.

236. Leavens, M.E., Hill, C.S., Jr., Cech, D.A., Weyland, J.B., and Weston, J.S.: Intrathecal and intraventricular morphine for pain in cancer patients: Initial study. J. Neurosurg., *56*:241, 1982.

237. Lenzi, A., Gali, G., Gandolfini, M., and Marini, G.: Intraventricular morphine in paraneoplastic painful syndrome of the cervicofacial region: Experience in thirty-eight cases. Neurosurgery, *17*:6, 1985.

238. Liao, J., Harrison, P., Buckley, J.J., and Takemori, A.: Sympathetic reflexes in morphine vs lidocaine spinal block. Anesthesiology, *55*:A148, 1981.

239. Liolios, A., and Andersen, F.H.: Selective spinal analgesia. Lancet, *2*:357, 1979.

240. Lomessy, A., Magnin, C., Viale, J–P., Motin, J., and Cohen, R.: Clinical advantages of fentanyl given epidurally for postoperative analgesia. Anesthesiology, *61*:466, 1984.

241. Lord, J.A., Waterfield, A.A., Hughes, J., and Kosterlitz, H.: Endogenous opioid peptides: Multiple agonists and receptors. Nature, *267*:495, 1977.

242. Lund, C., Mogensen, T., Hjorts, N.C., and Kehlet, H.: Systemic morphine enhances spread of sensory analgesia during postoperative epidural bupivacaine infusion. Lancet, *2*:1156, 1985.

243. Macdonald, R., and Smith, P.J.: Epidural morphine and pain relief following episiotomy. Br. J. Anaesth., *56*:1201, 1984.

243a. Macrae, D.J., *et al.*: Double-blind comparison of the efficacy of extradural diamorphine, extradural phenoperidine and I.M. diamorphine following caesarean section. Br. J. Anaesth., *59*:354, 1987.

244. Magora, F., Donchin, Y., Olshwang, D., and Schenker, J.G.: Epidural morphine analgesia in second-trimester induced abortion. Am. J. Obstet. Gynecol., *138*:260, 1980.

245. Magora, F., Olshwang, D., Eimerl, D., Shorr, J., Katzenelson, R., Cotev, S., and Davidson, J.T.: Observations of extradural morphine analgesia in various pain conditions. Br. J. Anaesth., *52*:247, 1980.

246. Malins, A.F., Goodman, N.W., Cooper, G.M., Prys–Roberts, C., and Baird, R.N.: Ventilatory effects of pre- and post-operative diamorphine. A comparison of extradural with intramuscular administration. Anaesthesia, *39*:118, 1984.

247. Martin, R., Salbaing, J., Blaise, G., Tetrault, J.P., and Tetrault, L.: Epidural morphine for post-operataive pain relief. A dose–response curve. Anesthesiology, *56*:423, 1982.

248. Martin, W.R., Eades, C.G., Thompson, J.A., *et al.*: The effects of morphine and nalorphine-like drugs in the non-dependent and morphine dependent chronic spinal dog. J. Pharmacol. Exp. Ther., *197*:517, 1976.

249. Maruyama, Y., Shimoji, K., Shimizu, H., Sato, Y., Kuribayashi, H., and Kaieda, R.: Effects of morphine on human spinal cord and peripheral nervous activities. Pain, *8*:63, 1980.

250. Mather, L.E.: Clinical pharmacokinetics of fentanyl and its newer derivatives. Clin. Pharmacokinet., *8*:422, 1983.

251. Mather, L.E., and Cousins, M.J.: Pharamacology of opioids. Basic and clinical aspects. Med. J. Aust., *144*:424, 1986.

252. Mather, L.E., and Gourlay, G.K.: Biotransformation of opioids: Significance for pain therapy. *In* Nimmo, W., and Smith, G. (eds.): Opioid Agonists/Antagonist Drugs in Clinical Practice, pp. 31–46. Amsterdam, Excerpta Medica, 1984.

253. Mather, L.E., and Pavlin, E.G.: Transfer of pethidine to CSF following intravenous administration. Anaesth. Intens. Care, *9*:205, 1981.

254. Mathews, E.: Epidural morphine. Lancet, *1*:673, 1979.

255. Mathews, E.T., and Abrams, L.D.: Intrathecal morphine in open heart surgery. Lancet, *1*:543, 1980.

256. Max, M., Inturrisi, C.E., Grabrinski, P., Kaiko, R.F., and Foley, K.M.: Epidural opiates: Plasma and cerebrospinal fluid (CSF) pharmacokinetics of morphine, methadone and beta-endorphin. Pain, *1*[*Suppl.*]:S122, 1981.

257. Max, M.B., Inturrisi, C.E., Kaiko, R.F., Grabinski, P.Y., Li, C.H., and Foley, K.M.: Epidural and intrathecal opiates: Cerebrospinal fluid and plasma profiles in patients with chronic cancer pain. Clin. Pharmacol. Ther., *38*:631, 1985.

258. McCaughey, W., and Graham, J.L.: The respiratory depression of epidural morphine. Time course and effect of posture. Anaesthesia, *37*:990, 1982.

259. McClure, J.H.: Chambers, W.A., Moore, E., and Scott, D.B.: Epidural morphine for postoperative pain. Lancet, *1*:975, 1980.

260. McDonald, A.M.: Complication of epidural morphine. Anaesth. Intens. Care, *8*:490, 1980.

261. McLennan, H.: Synaptic Transmission. Philadelphia, W.B. Saunders, 1963.

262. McQuay, H.J., Bullingham, R.E.S., Evans, P.J.D., Lloyd, J.W., and Moore, R.A.: Demand analgesia to assess pain relief from epidural opiates. Lancet, *1*:768, 1980.

263. Melzack, R., and Wall, P.D.: Pain mechanisms: A new theory. Science, *150*:971, 1965.

264. Messahel, F.M., and Tomlin, P.J.: Narcotic withdrawal syndrome after intrathecal administration of morphine. Br. Med. J., *283*:471, 1981.

265. Meynadier, J., Chrubasik, J., Dubar, M., and Wunsch, E.: Intrathecal somatostatin in terminally ill patients. A report of two cases. Pain, *23*:9, 1985.

266. Miller, M.: Role of endogenous opioids in neurohypophysical function of man. J. Clin. Endocrinol. Metab., *50*:1016, 1980.

267. Mirceau, N., Constaninescu, C., Jianu, C., Busi, G., Ene, C., Nedelcu, A., Vrejau, G., Daschievici, S., Struja, D., Ungureanu, D., and Horvat, D.: Anesthesie sous-arachnoidienne par la pethidine. Ann. Fr. Anesth. Reanim., *1*:167, 1982.

268. Modig, J., and Paalzow, L.: A comparison of epidural morphine and epidural bupivacaine for postoperative pain relief. Acta Anaesthesiol. Scand., *25*:437, 1981.

269. Molke Jensen, F., Madsen, J.B., Guldager, H., Christensen, A.A., and Eriksen, H.O.: Respiratory depression after epidural morphine in the postoperative period. Influence of posture. Acta Anaesthesiol. Scand., *28*:600, 1984.

270. Moore, R.A., Bullingham, R.S.J., McQuay, H.J., Allen, M., Baldwin, D., and Cole, A.: Spinal fluid kinetics of morphine and heroin in man. Clin. Pharmacol. Ther., *35*:40, 1984.

271. Moore, R.A., Bullingham, R.S.J., McQuay, H.J., Hand, C.W., Aspel, J.B., Allen, M.C., and Thomas, D.: Dural permeability to narcotics: In vitro determination and application to extradural administration. Br. J. Anaesth., *54*:1117, 1982.

272. Morgan, M.M.: (Editorial). Quidquid Agas, Prudenter Agas, et respice finem. Anaesthesia, *37*:527, 1982.

273. Moulin, D.E., Max, M.B., Kaiko, R.F., Inturrisi, C.E., Maggard, J., Yaksh, T.L., and Foley, K.M.: The analgesic efficacy of intrathecal d-Ala2-d-Leu5-encephalin in cancer patients with chronic pain. Pain, *23*:213, 1985.
274. Muller, A., Laugner, B., Farcot, J.M., Singer, M., Gauthier–Lafaye, P., and Gandar, R.: Epidural morphine for obstetrical pain relief. Anesth. Analg. (Paris), *38*:35, 1981.
275. Muller, H., Borner, U., Stoyanov, M.,, Gleumes, L., and Hempelmann, G.: Peridurale opiatapplikation bie malignombedingten chronischen schmerzen. Anaesth. Intensivther. Notfallmed., *16*:251, 1981.
276. Muller, H., Borner, U., Stoyanov, M., and Hempelmann, G.: Intraoperative peridural opiate analgesia. Anaesthesist, *12*:656, 1980.
277. Naulty, J.S., Datta, S., Ostheimer, G.W., Johnson, M.D., and Burger, G.A.: Epidural fentanyl for postcesarean delivery pain management. Anesthesiology, *63*:694, 1985.
278. Naulty, J.S., Johnson, M., Burger, G.A., Datta, S., Weiss, J.B., Morrison, J., and Ostheimer, G.W.: Epidural fentanyl for post cesarean delivery pain management. Anesthesiology, *59*:A415, 1983.
279. Nielson, T.H., Husegaard, H.C., and Joensen, F.: Tunnelleret spiduralkateter og infektion. Ugeskr. Laeger, *147*:1548, 1985.
280. Niv, D., Rudick, V., Golan, A., and Chayen, M.S. Augmentation of bupivacaine analgesia in labor by epidural morphine. Obstet. Gynecol., *67*:206, 1986.
281. Nordberg, G.: Pharmacokinetic aspects of spinal morphine analgesia. Acta Anaesthesiol. Scand., *79*:1, 1984.
282. Nordberg, G., Hedner, T., Mellstrand, T., and Dahlstrom, B.: Pharmacokinetic aspects of epidural morphine analgesia. Anesthesiology, *58*:545, 1983.
283. Nybell–Lindahl, C., Carlsson, C., Ingemarsson, I., Westgren, M., and Paalzow, L.: Maternal and fetal concentrations of morphine after epidural administration during labour. Am. J. Obstet. Gynecol., *139*:20, 1981.
284. Odoom, J.A.: Respiratory depression after intrathecal morphine. Anesth. Analg., *61*:70, 1982.
285. Oldendorf, W.H., Hyman, S., Braun, L., and Oldendorf, S.Z.: Blood brain barrier: Penetrataion of morphine, codeine, heroin and methadone after carotid injection. Science, *178*:984, 1972.
286. Olshwang, D., Shapiro, A., Perlberg, S., and Magora, F.: The effect of epidural morphine on ureteral colic and spasm of the bladder. Pain, *18*:97, 1984.
287. Onofrio, B.M., and Yaksh, T.L.: Intrathecal delta-receptor ligand produces analgesia in man. Lancet, *1*:1386, 1983.
288. Onofrio, B.M., Yaksh, T.L., and Arnold, P.G.: Continuous low dose intrathecal morphine administration in the treatment of chronic pain of malignant origin. Mayo Clin. Proc., *56*:516, 1981.
289. Oyama, T., Matsuki, A., Taneichi, T., Ling, N., and Guillemin, R.: Beta-endorphin in obstetric analgesia. Am. J. Obstet. Gynecol., *137*:613, 1980.
290. Oyama, T., Toshiro, J.I.N., and Yamaya, R.: Profound analgesic effects of beta-endorphin in man. Lancet, *1*:122, 1980.
291. Pasqualucci, V., Moricca, G., and Solinas, P.: Intrathecal morphine for the control of the pain of myocardial infarction. Anaesthesia, 68, 1980.
292. Paulus, D.A., Paul, W., and Munson, E.S.: Neurologic depression after intrathecal morphine. Anesthesiology, *54*:517, 1981.
293. Penn, R.D., Paice, J.A., Gottschalk, W., and Ivankovich, A.D.: Cancer pain relief using chronic morphine infusion. Early experience with a programmable implanted drug pump. J. Neurosurg., *61*:302, 1984.
294. Perriss, B.W.: Epidural pethidine in labour. A study of dose requirements. Anaesthesia, *35*:380, 1980.
295. Perriss, B.W., and Malins, A.F.: Pain relief in labour using epidural pethidine with adrenaline. Anaesthesia, *36*:631, 1981.
296. Pert, C.B., and Snyder, S.: Opiate receptors demonstration in nervous tissue. Science, *179*:1011, 1973.
297. Phillips, D.M., Moore, R.A., Bullingham, R.E., Allen, M.C., Baldwin, D., Fisher, A., Lloyd, J.W., and McQuay, H.J.: Plasma morphine concentrations and clinical effects after thoracic extradural morphine or diamorphine. Br. J. Anaesth., *56*:829, 1984.
298. Poletti, C.E., Cohen, A.M., Todd, D.P., Ojemann, R.G., Sweet, W.H., and Zervas, N.T.: Cancer pain relieved by long-term epidural morphine with permanent indwelling systems for self-administration. J. Neurosurg., *55*:581, 1981.
299. Proudfit, H.K., and Hammond, D.L.: Alterations in nociceptive threshold and morphine-induced analgesia produced by intrathecally administered amine antagonists. Brain Res., 218:393, 1981.
300. Pybus, D.A., and Torda, T.A.: Dose–effect relationships of extradural morphine. Br. J. Anaesth., *54*:1259, 1982.
301. Pybus, D.A., and Torda, T.: Opiates and sexual function. Nature, *310*:636, 1984.
302. Raj, P.P., Knarr, D., Vigdorth, E., *et al.*: Comparative study of continuous epidural infusions versus systemic analgesics in postoperative pain relief. Anesthesiology, *63*:A238, 1985.
302a. Rawal, N., Arner, S., Gustaffson, L.L., and Allvin, R.: Present state of extradural and intrathecal opioid analgesia in Sweden. A nationwide follow-up survey. Br. J. Anaesth., 59:791–799, 1987.
303. Rawal, N., Mollefors, K., Axelsson, K., Lingardh, G., and Widman, B.: Naloxone reversal of urinary retention after epidural morphine. Lancet, 2:1411, 1981.
304. Rawal, N., Mollefors, K., Axelsson, K., Lingardh, G., and Widman, B.: An experimental study of urodynamic effects of epidural morphine and of naloxone reversal. Anesth. Analg., *62*:641, 1983.
305. Rawal, N., Schott, U., Dahlstrom, B., Inturrisi, C.E., Tandon, B., Sjostrand, U., and Wennhager, M.: Influence of naloxone on analgesia and respiratory depression following epidural morphine. Anesthesiology, *64*:194, 1986.
306. Rawal, N., Schott, U., Tandon, B., *et al.*: Influence of intravenous naloxone infusion on analgesia and untoward effects of epidural morphine. Anesth. Analg., *64*:270, 1985.
307. Rawal, N., Sjostrand, U., Christoffersson, E., Dahlstrom, B., Arvill, A., and Rydman, H.: Comparison of intramuscular and epidural morphine for postoperative analgesia in the

grossly obese: Influence on postoperataive ambulation and pulmonary function. Anesth. Analg., *63*:583, 1984.

308. Rawal, N., Sjostrand, U.H., and Dahlstrom, B.: Postoperative pain relief by epidural morphine. Anesth. Analg., *60*:726, 1981.

309. Rawal, N., Sjostrand, U.H., Dahlstrom, B., Nydahl, P.A., and Ostelius, J.: Epidural morphine for postoperative pain relief: A comparative study with intramuscular narcotic and intercostal nerve block. Anesth. Analg., *61*:93, 1982.

310. Rawal, N., and Wattwil, M.: Respiratory depression following epidural morphine. An experimental and clinical study. Anesth. Analg. *63*:8, 1984.

311. Rechtine, G.R., Reinert, C.M., and Bohlman, H.H.: The use of epidural morphine to decrease postoperative pain in patients undergoing lumbar laminectomy. J. Bone Joint. Surg. [Am.], *66*:113, 1984.

312. Reddy, S.V.R., and Yaksh, T.L.: Spinal noradrenergic terminal system mediates antinociception. Brain Res., *189*:391, 1980.

313. Reiz, S., Ahlin, J., Ahrenfeld, B., Andersson, M., and Andersson, S.: Epidural morphine for postoperative pain relief. Acta Anaesthesiol. Scand., *25*:111, 1981.

314. Reiz, S., Westberg, M.: Side effects of epidural morphine. Lancet, *2*:203, 1980.

315. Reynolds, D.V.: Surgery in the rat during electrical analgesia induced by focal brain stimulation. Science, *164*:444, 1969.

316. Richelson, E.: Spinal opiate administration for chronic pain: A major advance in therapy. Mayo Clin. Proc., *56*:523, 1981.

317. Rigg, J.R.A., Ilsley, A.H., and Vedig, A.E.: Relationship of ventilatory depression to steady state blood pethidine concentrations. Br. J. Anaesth., *56*:613, 1981.

318. Robertson, K., Douglas, M.J., and McMorland, G.H.: Epidural fentanyl, with and without epinephrine for post-Caesarean section analgesia. Can. Anaesth. Soc. J., *32*:502, 1985.

319. Robinson, J.O., Rosen, M., Evans, J.M., Revill, S.I., David, H., and Rees, G.A.: Self-administered intravenous and intramuscular pethidine. A controlled trial in labour. Anaesthesia, *35*:763, 1980.

320. Rodan, B.A., Cohen, F.L., Bean, W.J., and Martyar, S.N.: Fibrous mass complicating epidural morphine infusion. Neurosurgery, *16*:68, 1985.

321. Rosenberg, P.H., Heino, A., and Scheinin, B.: Comparison of intramuscular analgesia, intercostal block, epidural morphine and on-demand-i.v.-fentanyl in the control of pain after abdominal surgery. Acta Anaesthesiol. Scand., *28*:603, 1984.

322. Roscow, C.E., Moss, J., Philbin, D.M., Savarese, J.J.: Histamine release during morphine and fentanyl anesthesia. Anesthesiology, *56*:93, 1982.

322a. Rutberg, H., Hakanson, E., Anderberg, B., *et al.*: Effects of the extradural administration of morphine or bupivacaine, on the endocrine response to upper abdominal surgery. Br. J. Anaesth., *56*:233, 1984.

323. Rutter, D.V., Skewes, D.G., and Morgan, M.: Extradural opioids for postoperative analgesia: A double blind comparison of pethidine, fentanyl and morphine. Br. J. Anaesth., *53*:915, 1981.

324. Sage, M.: Kinetics of water-soluble contrast media in the central nervous system. Am. J. Neuro. Radiol., *4*:897, 1983.

325. Sage, M., *et al.*: Brain parenchyma penetration by metrizamide following lumbar myelography. Aust. Radiol., *28*:90, 1984.

326. Samii, J., Chauin, M., and Viars, P.: Postoperative spinal analgesia with morphine. Br. J. Anaesth., *53*:817, 1981.

327. Samii, K., Feret, J., Harari, A., and Viars, P.: Selective spinal analgesia. Lancet, *1*:1142, 1979.

328. Sato, O., Asai, T., Amaro, Y., Hara, M., Tsugane, R., and Yagi, M.: Formation of cerebrospinal fluid in spinal subarachnoid space. Nature, *233*:129, 1971.

329. Schmauss, C., Doherty, C., and Yaksh, T.L.: The analgetic effects of an intrathecally administered partial opiate agonist, nalbuphine hydrochloride. Eur. J. Pharmacol., *86*:1, 1983.

330. Schoeffler, P., Pichard, E., Ramboatiana, R., *et al.*: Bacterial meningitis due to infection of a lumbar drug release system in patients with cancer pain. Pain, *25*:75, 1986.

331. Scott, D.B., and Cousins,M.J.: Clinical pharmacology of local anesthetic agents. *In* Cousins, M.J., and Bridenbaugh, P.O. (eds.): Neural Blockade in Clinical Anesthesia and Management of Pain, pp. 86–121. Philadelphia, J.B. Lippincott, 1980.

332. Scott, D.B., and McClure, J.: Selective epidural analgesia. Lancet, *1*:1410, 1979.

333. Scott, P.V., Bowen, F.E., Cartwright, P., Mohan Rao, B.C., Deeley, D., Wotherspoon, H.G., and Sumrein, I.M.A.: Intrathecal morphine as sole analgesic during labour. Br. Med. J., *281*:351, 1980.

334. Scott, P.V., and Fisher, H.B.: Intraspinal opiates and itching: A new reflex? Br. Med. J., *284*:1015, 1982.

335. Shapiro, L.A., Hoffman, S., Jedeikin, R., and Kaplan, R.: Single-injection epidural anesthesia with bupivacaine and morphine for prostatectomy. Anesth. Analg. (Cleve.), *60*:818, 1981.

336. Shapiro, L.A., Jedeikin, R., Shalev, D., and Hoffman, S.: Epidural morphine analgesia in children. Anesthesiology, *61*:210, 1984.

337. Shulman, M., Sandler, A.N., Bradley, J.W., Young, P.S., and Brebner, J.: Post-thoracotomy pain and pulmonary function following epidural and systemic morphine. Anesthesiology, *61*:569, 1984.

338. Shulman, M.S., Sandler, A., and Brebner, J.: The reversal of epidural morphine induced somnolence with physostigmine. Can. Anaesth. Soc. J., *31*:678, 1984.

339. Sidi, A., Davidson, J.T., Behar, M., and Olshwang, D.: Spinal narcotics and central nervous system depression. Anaesthesia, *36*:1044, 1981.

340. Simon, E.J., Hiller, J.M., and Edelman, I.: Opiate receptors: Specific binding of the potent narcotic analgesic tritium labelled etorphine to rat brain homogenate. Natl. Acad. Sci. Proc. USA, *70*:1947, 1973.

341. Sjostrand, U.H., and Rawal, N. (eds.): Regional opioids in anesthesiology and pain management. Int. Anesthesiol. Clin., *24*:1. Boston, Little, Brown, 1986.

341a. Sjostrom, S., Tamsen, A., Persson, P., Hartvig, P.: Pharmacokinetics of intrathecal morphine and meperidine in man. Anesthesiology. (In press)

341b. Sjostrom, S., Hartvig, P., Persson, P., Tamsen, A.: Pharmacokinetics of epidural morphine and meperidine in man. Anesthesiology. (In press)

342. Skjolderbrand, A., Garle, M., Gustafsson, L.L., Johansson, H., Lunell, N-O., and Rane, A.: Extradural pethidine with and without adrenaline during labor: Wide variation in effect. Br. J. Anaesth., *54*:415, 1982.

343. Skoeld, M., Gillberg, L., and Ohlsson, O.: Pain relief in myocardial infarction after continuous epidural morphine analgesia (letter). N. Engl. J.Med., *312*:650, 1985.

344. Spence, A.A.: Relieving acute pain. Br. J. Anaesth., *52*:245, 1980.

345. Srinivasan, T.: Intrathecal morphine for obstetric analgesia. Anesthesiology, *55*:A298, 1981.

346. Stanley, T.H.: Intrathecal opiates a potent tool to be used with caution. Anesthesiology, *53*:523, 1980.

347. Stapleton, J.V., Austin, K.L., and Mather, L.E.: A pharmacokinetic approach to pain control: continuous infusion of pethidine. Anaesth. Intens. Care, *7*:25, 1979.

348. Stenseth, R., Sellevold, O., and Breivik, H.: Epidural morphine for postoperative pain: Experience with 1095 patients. Acta Anaesthesiol. Scand., *29*:148, 1985.

349. Stoyanov, M., Muller, H., Borner, U., and Hempelmann, G.: Value of morphine derivatives administered by the peridural route. Ann. Anesthesiol. Fr., *22*:311, 1981.

350. Stoyanov, M., Muller, H., and Hempelmann, G.: Epidural opiates for relief of chronic pain. Anesth. Analg. (Paris), *38*:375, 1981.

351. Strube, P.J., Downing, J.W., and Brock–Utne, J.G.: CSF pharmacokinetics of extradural morphine. Br. J. Anaesth., *56*:921, 1984.

352. Struppler, A., Burgmayer, B., Ochs, G., *et al.*: The effect of epidural application of opioids on spasticity of spinal origin. Life Sci., *33*:607, 1983.

353. Tamsen, A., Sakuroda, T., Wahlstrom, A., Terenius, L., and Hartvig, P.: Postoperative demand for analgesics in relation to individual levels of endorphins and substance P in cerebrospinal fluid. Pain, *13*:171, 1982.

354. Tamsen, A., Sjostrom, S., Hartvig, P., Persson, P., Gabrielsson, J., and Paalzow, L.: CSF and plasma kinetics of morphine and meperidine after epidural administration. Anesthesiology, *59*:A196, 1983.

355. Tan, S., Cohen, S.E., and White, P.F.: Sufentanil for analgesia after cesarean section: Intravenous versus epidural administration. Anesth. Analg., *65*[*Suppl.*]:1, 1986.

356. Terenius, L.: Stereospecific interaction between narcotic analgesics and a synaptic plasma membrane fraction of rat cerebral cortex. Acta Pharmacol. Toxicol., *32*:317, 1973.

357. Thompson, W.R., Smith, P.T., Hirst, M., Varkey, G.P., and Knill, R.L.: Regional analgesic effect of epidural morphine in volunteers. Can. Anaesth. Soc. J., *28*:530, 1981.

358. Torda, T.A., Pybus, D.A., Liberman, H., Clark, M., and Crawford, M.: Experimental comparison of extradural and I.M. morphine. Br. J. Anaesth., *52*:939, 1980

359. Torda, T.A., and Pybus, D.A.: Clinical experience with epidural morphine. Anaesth. Intens. Care, *9*:129, 1981.

360. Torda, T.A., and Pybus, D.A.: A comparison of four narcotic analgesics for epidural analgesia. Br. J. Anaesth., *54*:291, 1982.

361. Torda, T.A., and Pybus, D.A.: Extradural administration of morphine and bupivacaine. A controlled comparison. Br. J. Anaesth. *56*:141, 1984.

362. Traynor, C., Paterson, J.L., Ward, I.D., Morgan, M., and Hall, G.M.: Effects of extradural analgesia and vagal blockade on the metabolic and endocrine response to upper abdominal surgery. Br. J. Anaesth., *54*:319, 1982.

363. Tucker, G.T., and Mather, L.E.: Clinical pharmacokinetics of local anaesthetics. Clin. Pharmacokinet., *4*:241, 1979.

364. Tung, A., Maliniak, K., Tenicela, R., and Winter, P.M.: Intrathecal morphine for intraoperative and postoperative analgesia. J.A.M.A., *244*:2637, 1980.

365. Tung, A.S., Tenicela, R., and Winter, P.M.: Opiate withdrawal syndrome following intrathecal administration of morphine. Anesthesiology, *53*:340, 1980.

366. Tung, A.S., and Yaksh, T.L.: In vivo evidence for multiple opiate receptors mediating analgesia in the rat spinal cord. Brain Res., *247*:75, 1982.

367. Tung, A.S., and Yaksh, T.L.: The antinociceptive effects of epidural opiates in the cat: Studies on the pharmacology and the effects of lipophilicity in spinal analgesia. Pain, *12*:343, 1982.

368. Twycross, R.G.: Morphine and diamorphine in the terminally ill patient. Acta Anaesthesiol. Scand., *74*:128, 1982.

369. Tyce, G.M., and Yaksh, T.L.: Monoamine release from cat spinal cord by somatic stimuli: An intrinsic modulatory system. J. Physiol. (Lond.). *314*:513, 1981.

370. Van Steenberge, A.: Epidural lofentanil for pain relief in labor. Anesth. Intenzivmed. [In press]

371. Vella, L.M., Willatts, D.G., Knott, C., Lintin, D.J., Justins, D.M., and Reynolds, F.: Epidural fentanyl in labour. An evaluation of the systemic contribution to analgesia. Anaesthesia, *40*:741, 1985.

372. Ventafridda, V., Tamburini, M., and DeConno, F.: Comprehensive treatment in cancer pain. *In* Fields, H., *et al.* (eds.): Advances in Pain Research and Therapy, *9*:617–628. New York, Raven Press, 1985.

373. Walts, L.F., Kaufman, R.D., Moreland, J.R., and Weiskopf, M.: Total hip arthroplasty. An investigation of factors related to postoperative urinary retention. Clin. Orthop., *194*:280, 1985.

374. Wang, J.K.: Intrathecal morphine for intractable pain secondary to cancer of pelvic organs. Pain, *21*:99, 1985.

375. Wang, J.K., Nauss, L.E., and Thomas, J.E.: Pain relief by intrathecally applied morphine in man. Anesthesiology, *50*:149, 1979.

376. Wanscher, M., Riishede, L., and Krogh, B.: Fistula formation following epidural catheter: A case report. Acta Anaesthesiol. Scand., *29*:552, 1985.

377. Watson, J., Moore, A., McQuay, H., Teddy, P., Baldwin, D., Allen, M., and Bullingham, R.: Plasma morphine concentrations and analgesic effects of lumbar extradural morphine and heroin. Anesth. Analg., *63*:629, 1984.

378. Way, E.L.: Studies on the local anaesthetic properties of isonipecaine. J. Am. Pharm. Assoc., *35*:44, 1946.

379. Weddel, S.J., and Ritter, R.R.: Serum levels following epidural administration of morphine and correlation with relief of post surgical pain. Anesthesiology, *54*:210, 1981.

380. Weinstock, M., Davidson, J.T., Rosin, A.J., and Schnieden, H.: Effect of physostigmine on morphine induced postopertive pain and somnolence. Br. J. Anaesth., *54*:429, 1982.

381. Welch, D.B.: Epidural narcotics and dural puncture. Lancet, *1*:55, 1981.

382. Welch, D.B., and Hrynaszkiewicz, A.: Postoperative analgesia using epidural methadone. Administration by the lumbar route for thoracic pain relief. Anaesthesia, *36*:1051, 1981.

383. Welchew, E.A.: The optimum concentration for epidural fentanyl. Anaesthesia, *38*:1037, 1983.

384. Welchew, E.A., and Thornton, J.A.: Continuous thoracic epidural fentanyl. Anaesthesia, *37*:309, 1982.

385. Werz, M.A., and McDonald, R.L.: Dynorphin reduces calcium-dependent action potential duration by decreasing voltage-dependent calcium conductance. Neurosci. Lett., *46*:185, 1984.

386. White, W.D., Pearce, D.J., and Norman, J.: Postoperative analgesia: A comparison of intravenous on demand fentanyl with epidural bupivacaine. Br. Med. J., *2*:166, 1979.

387. Whitwam, J.G.: Benzodiazepine receptors. Anaesthesia, *38*:93, 1983.

388. Willer, J.C., Bergeret, S., and Gaudy, J.H.: Epidural morphine strongly depresses nociceptive flexion reflexes in patients with postoperative pain. Anesthesiology, *63*:675, 1985.

389. Willer, J.C., and Bussel, B.: Evidence for a direct spinal mechanism in morphine-induced inhibition of nociceptive reflexes in humans. Brain Res., *187*:212, 1980.

390. Wilson, P.R., and Yaksh, T.L.: Baclofen is antinociceptive in the spinal intrathecal space of animals. Eur. J. Pharmacol., *51*:323, 1978.

391. Wolfe, M.J., and Davies, G.K.: Analgesic action of extradural fentanyl. Br. J. Anaesth., *52*:357, 1980.

392. Wolfe, M.J., and Nicholas, A.D.G.: Selective epidural analgesia. Lancet, *1*:150, 1979.

392a. Wolff, J., Carl, P., and Crawford, M.E.: Epidural buprenorphine for postoperative analgesia. A controlled comparison with epidural morphine. Anaesthesia, *41*:76, 1986.

393. Woods, W.A., and Cohen, S.E.: High dose epidural morphine in a terminally ill patient. Anesthesiology, *56*:311, 1982.

394. Writer, W.D., Hurtig, J.B., Evans, D., Needs, R.E., Hope, C.E., and Forrest, J.B.: Epidural morphine prophylaxis of postoperative pain: Report of a double-blind multicentre study. Can. Anaesth. Soc. J., *32*:330, 1985.

395. Writer, W.D.R., James, F.M., and Wheeler, A.S.: Double blind comparison of morphine and bupivacaine for continuous epidural analgesia in labor. Anesthesiology, *54*:215, 1981.

396. Yablonski–Peretz, T., Klin, B., Beilin, Y., Warner, E., Baron, S., Olshwang, D., and Catane, R.: Continuous epidural narcotic analgesia for intractable pain due to malignancy. J. Surg. Oncol., *29*:8, 1985.

397. Yaksh, T.L.: Opiate receptors for behavioral analgesia resemble those related to the depression of spinal nociceptive neurons. Science, *199*:1231, 1978.

398. Yaksh, T.L.: Inhibition by etorphine of the discharage of dorsal horn neurons: Effects on the neuronal response to both high and low threshold sensory input in the decerebrate spinal cat. Exp. Neurol., *60*:23, 1978.

399. Yaksh, T.L.: Direct evidence that spinal serotonin and noradrenaline terminals mediate the spinal antinociceptive effects of morphine in the periaqueductal gray. Brain Res., *160*:180, 1978.

400. Yaksh, T.L.: Analgesic actions of intrathecal opiates in the cat and primate. Brain Res., *153*:205, 1978.

401. Yaksh, T.L.: Spinal opiate analgesia: Characteristics and principles of action. Pain, *11*:293, 1981.

402. Yaksh, T.L.: In vivo studies on spinal opiate receptor systems mediating antinociception. I. Mu and delta receptor profiles in the primate. J. Pharmacol. Exp. Ther., *226*:303, 1983.

403. Yaksh, T.L.: Multiple opioid receptor systems in brain and spinal cord. Pts. 1 and 2. Eur. J. Anaesthesiol., *1*:171, 1984.

404. Yaksh, T.L.: Pharmacology of spinal adrenergic systems which modulate spinal nociceptive processing. Pharmacol. Biochem. Behav., *22*:845, 1985.

405. Yaksh, T.L.: Spinal Afferent Processing. New York, Plenum Press, 1986.

406. Yaksh, T.L., Abay, E.O., and Go, V.L.: Studies on the location and release of cholecystokinin and vaso-active intestinal peptide in rat and cat spinal cord. Brain Res., *242*:279, 1982.

407. Yaksh, T.L., and Elde, P.R.: Factors governing the release of methionine enkephalin-like immunoreactivity from the mesencephalan and spinal cord of the cat in vivo. J. Neurophysiol., *46*:1056, 1981.

408. Yaksh, T.L., Farb, D., Leeman, S., and Jessel, T.: Intrathecal capsaicin depletes substance P in the rat spinal cord and produces prolonged thermal analgesia. Science, *206*:481, 1979.

409. Yaksh, T.L., Frederickson, R.C., Huang, S., and Rudy, T.: In vivo comparison of the receptor populations acted upon in the spinal cord by morphine and pentapeptides in the production of analgesia. Brain Res., *148*:516, 1978.

410. Yaksh, T.L., Gross, K.E., and Li, C.H.: Studies on the intrathecal effects of beta-endorphin in the primate. Brain Res., *241*:261, 1982.

411. Yaksh, T.L., and Hammond, D.L.: Peripheral and central substances involved in rostrad transmission of nociceptive information. Pain, *13*:1, 1982.

412. Yaksh, T.L., and Harty, G.J.: Effects of thiorphon on the antinociceptive actions of intrathecal (D-Ala^2, Met^5) enkephalin. Eur. J. Pharmacol., *79*:293, 1982.

413. Yaksh, T.L., Harty, G.J., and Oofrio, B.M.: High doses of spinal morphine produce a non-opiate receptor mediated hyperesthesia. Practical and theoretical implications. Anesthesiology. [In press]

414. Yaksh, T.L., Huang, S.P., Rudy, R.T., and Frederickson, R.C.: The direct and specific opiate-like effect of met^5-enkephalin and analogues on the spinal cord. Neuroscience, *2*:593, 1977.

415. Yaksh, T.L., Jessel, T.M., Gamse, R., Mudge, A.W., and Leeman, S.E.: Intrathecal morphine inhibits substance P release from mammalian spinal cord in vivo. Nature, *286*:155, 1980.
416. Yaksh, T.L., Kohl, R.L., and Rudy, T.A.: Induction of tolerance and withdrawal in rats receiving morphine in the spinal subarachnoid space. Eur. J. Pharmacol., *42*:275, 1977.
417. Yaksh, T.L., and Li, C.H.: Studies on the intrathecal effects of beta-endorphin in primate. Brain Res., *241*:261, 1982.
418. Yaksh, T.L., and Noueihed, R.: The physiology and pharmacology of spinal opiates. Ann. Rev. Pharmacol. Toxicol., *25*:443, 1985.
419. Yaksh, T.L., Noueihed, R.Y., and Durant, A.C.: Studies of the pharmacology and pathology of intrathecally administered 4-aminopiperidine analogues and morphine in the rat and cat. Anesthesiology, *64*:54, 1986.
420. Yaksh, T.L., and Reddy, S.V.: Studies on the primate on the analgetic effects associated with intrathecal actions of opiate alpha-adrenergic agonists and baclofen. Anesthesiology, *54*:451, 1981.
421. Yaksh, T.L., and Rudy, T.A.: Analgesia mediated by a direct spinal action of narcotics. Science, *192*:1357, 1976.
422. Yaksh, T.L., and Rudy, T.A.: Chronic catheterization of the spinal subarachnoid space. Physiol. Behav., *17*:1031, 1976.
423. Yaksh, T.L., and Rudy, T.A.: Studies on the direct spinal action of narcotics in the production of spinal analgesia in the rat. J. Pharmacol. Exp. Ther., *202*:411, 1977.
424. Yaksh, T.L., Schmauss, C., Micevych, P.E., Abay, E., and Go, V.L.: Pharmacological studies on the application, disposition and release of neurotensin in the spinal cord. Ann. N.Y. Acad. Sci., *400*:228, 1982.
425. Yaksh, T.L., and Wilson, P.R.: Spinal serotonin terminal system mediates antinociception. J. Pharmacol. Exp. Ther., *208*:446, 1979.
426. Yaksh, T.L., Wilson, P.R., Kaiko, R.F., and Inturissi, C.E.: Analgesia produced by a spinal action of morphine and effects on parturition in the rat. Anesthesiology, *51*:386, 1979.
427. Yeung, J.C., and Rudy, T.A.: Multiplicative interaction between narcotic agonism expressed at spinal and supraspinal sites of antinociceptive action as revealed by concurent intrathecal and intracerebro-ventricular injections of morphine. J. Pharmacol. Exp. Ther., *215*:633, 1980.
428. Zenz, M.: Epidural opiates long term experiences in cancer pain. Klin. Wochenschr., *63*:225, 1985.
429. Zenz, M., Schappler-Scheele, B., Neuhans, R., Piepenrock, S., and Hilfrich, J.: Long term peridural morphine analgesia in cancer pain. Lancet, *1*:91, 1981.
430. Zenz, M., van den Berg, B., and van den Berg, E.: Plethysmographic study on sympathetic block in peridural anaesthesia and peridural morphine analgesia. Anaesthesist, *30*:70, 1981.
431. Zieglgansberger, W.: Opioid actions on mammalian spinal neurons. Int. Rev. Neurobiol., *25*:243, 1984.
432. Zukin, R.S., and Zukin, S.R.: Multiple opiate receptors and emerging concepts. Life Sci., *29*:2681, 1981.

29.1 NEUROPATHOLOGY OF NEUROLYTIC AND SEMIDESTRUCTIVE AGENTS

ROBERT R. MYERS
JORDAN KATZ

The specialized structure of a peripheral nerve bundle is essential to its normal sensory and motor functions. Pathologic alterations in the structure of nerve fibers or changes in the biochemistry and biophysics of their environment are associated with abnormal function. Although these changes are usually caused by diseases or injuries to nerves, it may be therapeutically desirable to induce temporary nerve injury with neurolytic agents or mechanical devices for the clinical purpose of interrupting nerve sensory function. We review here the important neuropathologic features of peripheral nerves relevant to the neurolytic management of pain, highlighting the factors necessary for nerve regeneration. The role of edema and the biophysics of the nerve fiber environment, important factors in the functioning of peripheral nerves that have pathogenic significance in nerve injury, will also be presented. Last, the effect of specific neurolytic and semidestructive agents and techniques will be discussed with respect to their capacity to relieve pain by altering the structure and function of peripheral nerves.

NERVE STRUCTURE AND NORMAL FUNCTION

Peripheral nerve fibers are processes of cell bodies located in the spinal cord of the central nervous system or the dorsal roots of the peripheral nervous system (see Figs. 2-1 and 2-4). As such, they are conduits for the axonal transport of structural proteins and organelles necessary for the metabolic activity and growth of these fibers. Interruption or compression of the axon results in axonal swelling of the proximal portion caused by accumulation of transport particles and degeneration in the distal portion (discussed later in the chapter).

The axonal particles include mitochondria, endoplasmic reticula, neurofilaments, microtubules, and dense particles (Fig. 29-1).

The mitochondria are 0.1 to 0.3 μm in diameter, 0.5 to 0.8 μm in length, and are divided into outer and inner compartments. The outer compartment contains monoamine oxidase, which is responsible for degradation of catecholamines. The inner compartment, bounded by highly infolded membranes called cristae, contains the respiratory electron transport and energy transport enzymes and coenzymes involved in the Krebs cycle. The nucleotides ATP and ADP are also contained in the intracellular compartment. The concentration of mitochondria is greater in smaller axons. They are probably formed in the cell body and then slowly transported down the axon, where they are usually randomly located throughout the peripheral nerve; their movement seems to be dictated by the location of microtubules and neurofilaments.

The smooth endoplasmic reticulum (SER) is generally an agranular, irregular structure in the peripheral axon. With electron microscopy, SER may appear as vesicles, tubules, or cisternae generally arranged in rows parallel to the length of the axon. The wall of the endoplasmic reticulum has a trilaminar appearance,

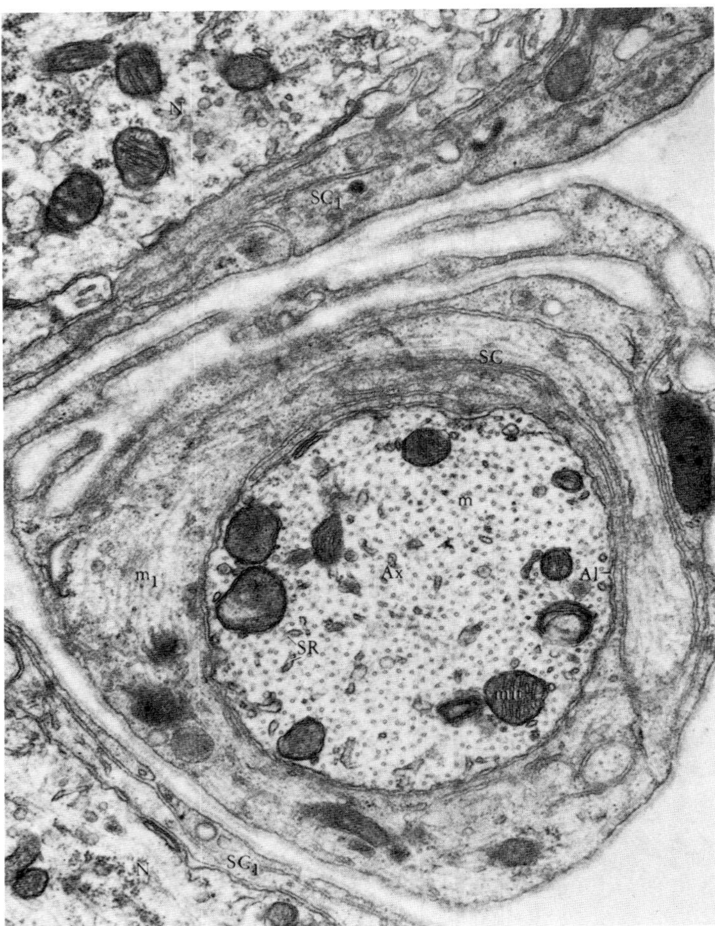

FIG. 29-1. Electron micrograph of transverse section from mouse ganglion cell axon. The axolemma *(A1)* is the boundary of the axoplasm and is surrounded by Schwann cell processes *(Sc)* containing microtubles *(m1)*. Within the axoplasm, microtubules *(m)* are homogeneously dispersed. Mitochondria *(mit)* and tubular profiles of smooth endoplasmic reticulum *(SR)* are also seen in this section. (Original magnification × 26,000) (Peters, A., Palay, S.L., and Webster, H.deF.: The Fine Structure of the Nervous System, p. 103. Philadelphia, W.B. Saunders, 1976.)

containing none of the ribosomes observed in the rough (granular) endoplasmic reticulum (RER). The RER takes part in protein synthesis, whereas the SER probably does not.

The neurofilament is a tubular structure 100 Å in diameter with a single wall approximately 30 Å thick. The wall seems to be a helically coiled thread composed of globular protein. The function of neurofilaments is thought to be related to the intracellular transport of ions and metabolites and to skeletal support of the cell.

The microtubules are composed of tubules that measure approximately 250 Å in diameter with walls 60 Å thick. The center may contain a thin central filament or row of granules. Microtubules seem to be most prevalent in unmyelinated axons, where neurofilaments are rare. The function of microtubules is thought to be similar to that of the neurofilaments.

Dense particles are often aligned in the cytoplasm next to the plasma membrane adjacent to the axolemma. Groups of dense particles are sometimes seen in the cytoplasm near the node of Ranvier. The function of dense particles is unknown; however, they may be lysomal in nature and indicate a normal turnover of axonal organelles.

These are the major particles in the axoplasm that, along with its cytoplasmic fluid, display a viscosity about five times that of water.[19] The basic properties of axoplasmic transport and the role of axonal transport in disease have recently been reviewed[3,46] and will not be discussed here. Rather, we shall consider the connective tissue components and support cells of peripheral nerves because they have an important pathogenic role that is less widely known.

CONNECTIVE TISSUE

Peripheral nerve fibers are maintained in a specialized environment created by the selective permeability of the connective tissue elements of nerve bundles and the blood–nerve barrier of the vasa nervorum.

The epineurium is the outermost covering of the nerve (see also Fig. 2-4) and has numerous blood vessels of arteriolar and venular size running longitudinally along its axis, as well as fat cells that help

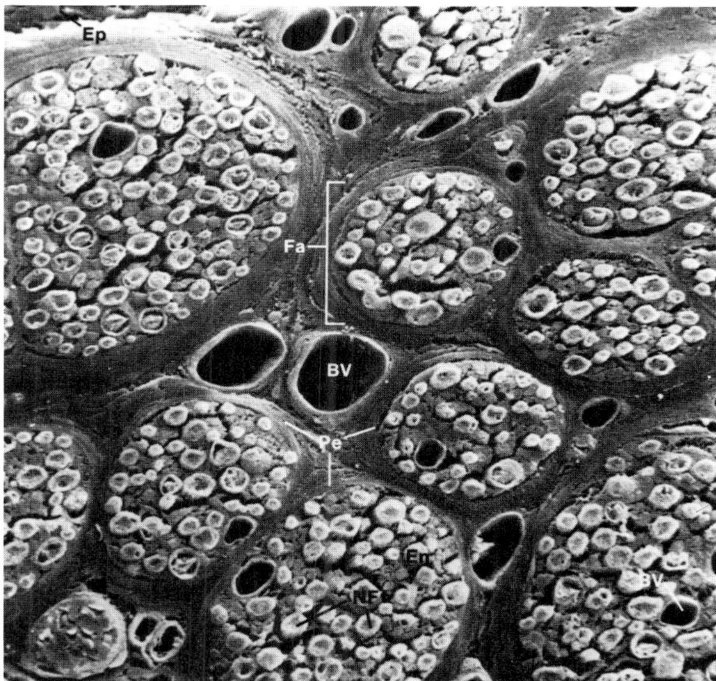

FIG. 29-2. Scanning electron micrograph of a peripheral nerve in cross-section. Nerve fibers *(NF)* are organized in bundles called fascicles *(Fa)*, each of which is surrounded by a collagen-rich sheath, the perineurium *(Pe)*. Loose connective tissue forms the epineurium *(Ep)*, which encircles groups of fascicles. The endoneurium *(En)* is a division of the perineurium that forms thin layers of connective tissue surrounding nerve fibers. In practice, the entire space bounded by the perineurium is referred to as endoneurial space. Blood vessels *(BV)* with fenestrated endothelial cells are numerous in the epineurial space. Somewhat smaller vessels within the endoneurium form the vasa nervorum with tight endothelial cell junctions. These two circulations communicate via vessels that pass obliquely through the perineurium. (Kessel, R.G., and Kardon, R.H.: Tissue and Organs, p. 79. W.H. Freeman, 1979.)

cushion the nerve against compression injury (Figs. 29-2, 29-3).[64] Additionally, the epineurium may contain fibroblasts and a variable number of mast cells. Epineurial vessels have a fenestrated endothelium that allows the extravasation of macromolecules such as Evans blue-albumin or horseradish peroxidase.[47] The epineurial tissue itself consists of areolar connective tissue that is loosely attached to the perineurium, which it surrounds. Collagen bundles are oriented primarily in the longitudinal axis, giving the epineurium high yield strength when pulled along this axis.[20] Lundborg reports that small segments of the epineurium can be removed without affecting peripheral nerve function because of an extensive anastomosis of the extrinsic epineurial circulation with the intrinsic vasa nervorum (Figs. 29-3, 29-4).[33] The radicular epineurial vessels pass through the epineurium and perineurium at an acute angle to anastomose with the intrinsic nerve circulation where capillary exchange occurs (Fig. 29-3).

The perineurium (see also Fig. 2-4) is an especially important tissue because of the vessels that pass through it and because of its functions as a semielastic, semipermeable membrane that organizes nerve fibers into fascicles and helps regulate their interstitial fluid environment. The perineurium consists of a laminated arrangement of flattened polygonal cells up to 15 layers thick bounded by a basal lamina.[64] The junctions between perineurial cells are tight and do not normally permit the free entry of macromolecules. Vesicular transport does occur, however, and is a route for macromolecular exchange between the epineurial and endoneurial spaces. Collagen fibrils are oriented primarily in the longitudinal axis; their relative lack in the circumferential axis contributes to the ballooning or stretching of the perineurium when edema occurs in the endoneurial space of the nerve.

Finally, the endoneurium (see also Fig. 2-4) comprises the intrafascicular connective tissue. Although the endoneurium is defined as a connective tissue element of nerve, the term is generally used to identify the space and tissue surrounded by the perineurium. Thus the endoneurium contains the individual myelinated and unmyelinated nerve fibers, their Schwann cells, the capillaries of the intrinsic vasa nervorum, collagen, and an interstitial fluid environment that promotes conduction of electrical nerve impulses.

MYELINATED FIBERS

Peripheral myelinated axons are surrounded by a tubular myelin sheath derived from Schwann cells (see Fig. 2-2). The axon is bounded by a surface membrane, the axolemma, which is about 8 nm thick. Internal to the axolemma is the axoplasm, which contains the neurofilaments,neurotubules, vesicles, and organelles previously discussed. The Schwann cell insulation allows increased conduction velocity that enhances the direct relationship between axonal diameter and the velocity of impulse conduction. The Schwann cell is trapezoidally shaped and wrapped spirally around the axon and axolemma. The number of concentric layers of wrapped myelin is directly proportional to the diameter of the axon. Myelin

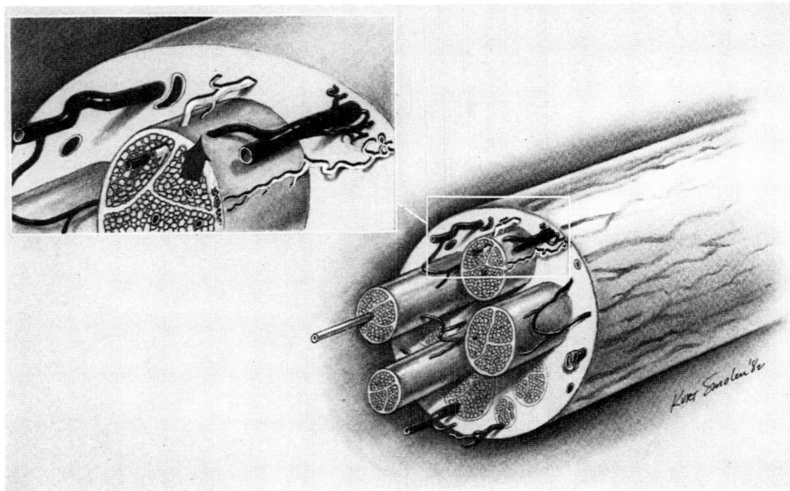

FIG. 29-3. Schematic diagram of multifascicled peripheral nerve illustrating the major connective tissue components of the nerve. The epineurial tissue contains the longitudinally oriented extrinsic vasculature consisting of the larger microvessels. The insert shows these vessels passing through the perineurium to anastomose with the intrinsic vasa nervorum where capillary exchange occurs. A pathologic valve mechanism is thought to exist in the extrinsic vasculature where it traverses the perineurium *(arrow)*. The endoneurial space contains the nerve fibers and is enclosed by the perineurium. The endoneurium has a specialized chemical environment appropriate for nerve conduction that is created by the selective permeability of the vasa nervorum and the perineurium.

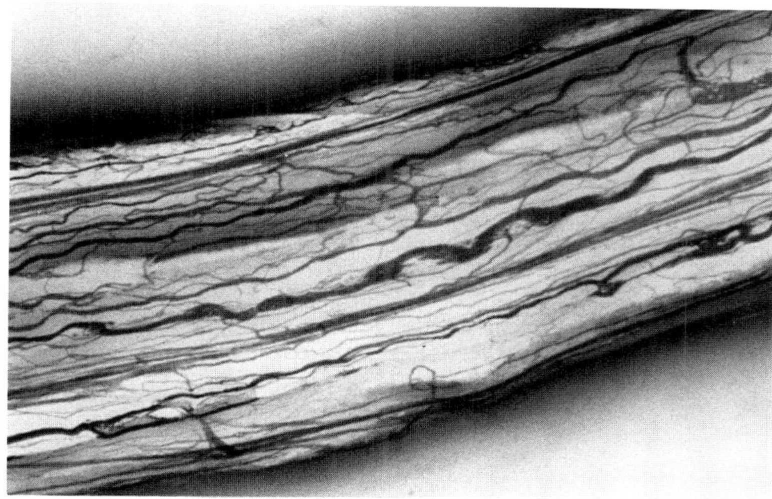

FIG. 29-4. Gelatin cast of rat sciatic nerve illustrating the extrinsic epineurial circulation. The cast was made by injecting a gelatin mass into the vasculature at systolic pressure. After the gelatin hardened, the tissue was cleared with methyl methacrylate. Note sinusoidal course of vessels to allow for stretching and the extensive anastomoses between vessels.

completely covers the axon except at the axon terminal, where there is usually a 1 to 2 μm gap, and at the nodes of Ranvier, the sites between adjacent Schwann cells. At a node of Ranvier, the axolemma is exposed for 1 to 1.5 μm (see Fig. 2-2). On either side of the gap, the total myelin thickness is somewhat less than average owing to a progressive reduction in the number of lamellae and their terminal myelin loops. The axoplasm is also reduced in volume and cross-sectional area in the nodal and paranodal spaces; however, the nodal region is critical to proper nerve function because it is the site of sodium channels between the axoplasm and endoneurial environment that are responsible for the saltatory conduction of nerve impulses. The paranodal region contains potassium channels[5] not normally observed except during fiber injury; paranodal demyelination is an early pathologic change. The Schwann cell is contained by a continuous basal lamina that extends across the node of Ranvier, forming a tubular scaffolding important in nerve regeneration.

UNMYELINATED FIBERS

The chief morphologic difference in myelinated and unmyelinated fibers is the lack of myelin lamellae in unmyelinated fibers. The axoplasms are qualitatively similar in their constituents. Myelinated and unmyelinated fibers are not randomly distributed, and groups of unmyelinated fibers cluster together (Fig. 29-5). The Schwann cell encompasses a variable number of unmyelinated axons in a common compartment, separating them by Schwann cell tongues. Thin septa also prevent axon–axon contact. Collagen pockets are included in the Schwann cell tubes and help separate axons. Finally, a basal lamina contains the packet of axons and Schwann cell. Some concern has existed about electrical cross-talk between unmyelinated axons, but the variable longitudinal course of axons within unmyelinated nerve fibers reduces the impact of this hypothesized artifact.

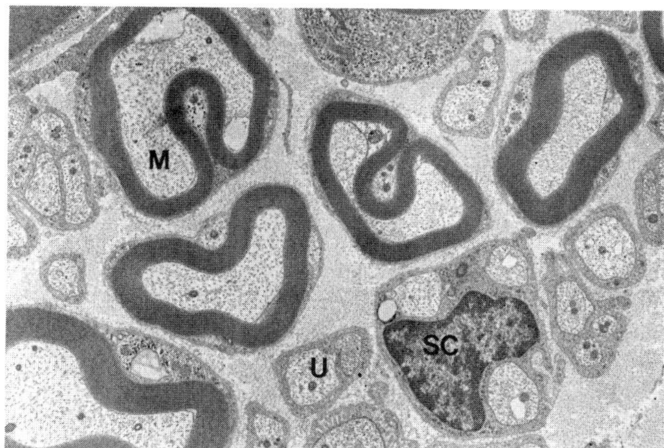

FIG. 29-5. Electron micrograph of normal human peripheral nerve illustrating coexistence of myelinated (with dark staining myelin sheaths) *(M)* and unmyelinated *(U)* fibers. A Schwann cell nucleus *(SC)* is seen in the lower right associated with a group of three unmyelinated fibers. Mitochondria and smaller organelles can be seen in the axoplasm of both myelinated and unmyelinated fibers. (Uranyl acetate and lead citrate) (Courtesy of Dr. Henry C. Powell, University of California, San Diego)

ENDONEURIAL ENVIRONMENT

The endoneurial environment is a delicately balanced fluid space that serves as a sink for electrolyte exchange with nerve fibers, making possible the propagation of action potentials. Although the unique characteristics of this space had been hypothesized for some time, it was not until the recent introduction of quantitative neuropathologic and bioengineering techniques that the pathogenic significance of the endoneurial environment became apparent. Using an indirect technique involving the drying and ashing of whole nerves, Krnjevic[27] predicted elevated concentrations of electrolytes in endoneurial (interstitial) fluids. Myers and colleagues[36] have been able to aspirate 100-pl volumes of endoneurial fluid directly from rat sciatic nerve and confirm that endoneurial fluid electrolyte concentrations are hypertonic with respect to serum.[36] The method used was energy-dispersive x-ray spectrometry. When the ions in the fluid samples are excited with an electron beam, the resultant x-ray fluorescence can be quantified for each ion and expressed as a concentration. It was observed that when the blood–nerve barrier was damaged by the ingestion of lead, the endoneurial fluid electrolyte concentrations asymptotically approached serum levels. This occurred early during the course of the neuropathy when there was electrophysiologic dysfunction but no demyelination.[36,53] Mizisin and associates[35] have recently shown that endoneurial sodium concentrations in galactosemic neuropathy are nearly double the control value of 152 mEq/liter. In this neuropathy the blood–nerve barrier is not damaged, but there is significant endoneurial edema. This finding may help explain the source of the osmotic force responsible for endoneurial hydration and the edema that is a nearly ubiquitous finding in neuropathy.

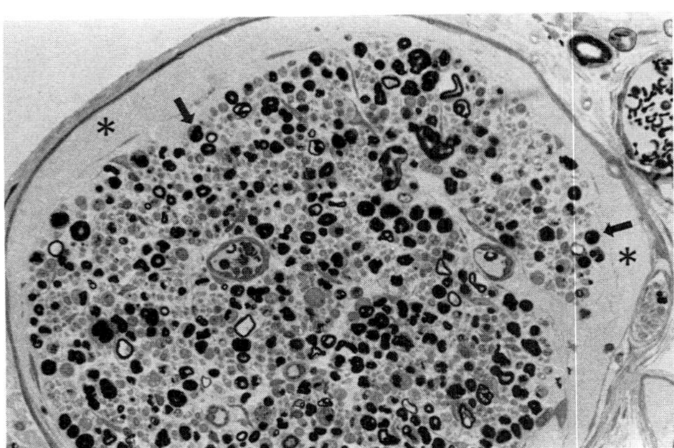

FIG. 29-6. Transverse section of rat sciatic nerve fascicle 6 days after crush injury. Note extensive endoneurial edema (*). Endoneurial fluid pressure was elevated about three times normal. Following axonal injury, wallerian degeneration is characterized by collapse of the myelin sheath and accumulation of osmiophilic debris into myelin ovoids, as is seen extensively here *(arrows)*. (paraphenylene diamine)

There are no lymphatic channels in peripheral nerve, and normal endoneurial hydration produces a slightly positive endoneurial fluid pressure of 2.0 ± 1.0 cm H_2O.[31,43] In galactosemic neuropathy and in many of the neuropathies caused by neurolytic agents, endoneurial fluid pressure can be significantly elevated.[31,41] The pathophysiologic significance of this is discussed below.

ABNORMAL STRUCTURE AND PATHOPHYSIOLOGIC FUNCTION

WALLERIAN DEGENERATION

Wallerian degeneration is the term used to describe the complex series of events associated with nerve fiber degeneration in the distal stump of a transected nerve. These events were originally described by Augustus Waller in 1850.[67] The term also applies to the pathologic events following crush injury and other injuries to nerve bundles that produce focal axonopathy,[51] including reduced nerve blood supply.[49] Initially, swelling occurs at the proximal stump mainly because of accumulation of mitochondria and lysosomes. The axolemma fragments and the axoplasm undergo granular dissolution. These primary events are followed by the collapse and digestion of the myelin sheath as a secondary change of wallerian degeneration; however, Schwann cells react within minutes of an injury to the nerve fiber. The myelin sheath retracts from the node of Ranvier and exposes the potassium channels. Eventually the myelin sheath collapses, forming darkly staining myelin ovoids (Fig. 29-6). Macrophages and Schwann cells, which also have a phagocytic role, are active during this time and assist in the removal of disintegrating material. Schwann cells proliferate within the confines of the old basal lamina vacated by degenerating nerve fibers, creating the bands of Büngner important to the successful regeneration of nerve fibers (Fig. 29-7). When nerves are transected, the basal lamina is interrupted, which makes it considerably more difficult for regenerating nerve fibers to find their appropriate end-organs.[61]

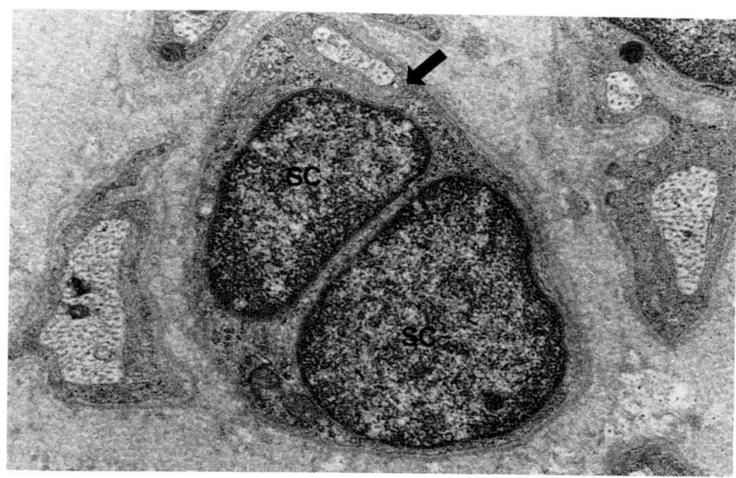

FIG. 29-7. Electron micrograph from human nerve showing the proliferation of Schwann cells *(SC)* within the existing basal lamina structure of a previous Schwann cell, creating a band of Büngner. Note two Schwann cell nuclei in the center and duplicate basal lamina surrounding them *(arrows).* (Uranyl acetate and lead citrate) (Courtesy of Dr. Henry C. Powell, University of California, San Diego)

REGENERATION PROCESS

The regeneration of the proximal portion of the axon is usually marked by the formation of an axoplasmic mass with filopodia at the end of the severed axon. Inside this growth cone can be seen increased mitochondria, dense bodies, vesicular elements, neurofilaments, and smooth endoplasmic reticulum (Fig. 29-8). Variation in mitochondrial shape and size may also be noted.

Accompanying the development of the growth cone, the Schwann cells undergo mitotic activity, forming a framework for developing fibers (Fig. 29-9). One axon may actually send out many growth cones. If all regenerating growth cones reach the end-organ, there may be more fibers distally than proximally. Many of these additional fibers degenerate over the course of 1 year. The growth of the regenerating axon is occasionally blocked by glial scars and cystic spaces that develop from lysis of neural debris. If a sensory fiber reaches a motor end-plate or a motor fiber reaches a sensory terminal, the fiber will eventually degenerate.[28]

Regeneration occurs at the rate of about 1 mm/day, so that reinnervation of a structure 5 cm away would take about 50 days; however, recovery of function may not always depend on regeneration, since alternative pathways may take over the impulse route. For example, after thoracic neurolytic subarachnoid block of posterior roots, pain conduction may "reroute" by way of the anterior roots that are known to possess about 10% to 12% afferent C fibers. Alternatively, overlapping innervation from adjacent dermatomes may compensate for denervated axons.

Clinically, after simple injuries, the ulnar nerve requires about 8 weeks until recovery begins; however, healing after a major injury, such as caused by gunshot, requires a minimum of 4 months. Return of voluntary muscle action after brachial plexus injury may be as early as 3 months, or it may be delayed for 2 or more years, depending on the severity of injury.[61]

ENDONEURIAL FLUID PRESSURE

Increased endoneurial fluid pressure is a frequent finding in neuropathies resulting from toxic, metabolic, or traumatic insult to nerve fibers, their supporting cells, or their environment.[41] Several different etiologic mechanisms are revealed in the process of wallerian degeneration after crush injury, where there is a complex series of changes in nerve hydration producing elevated EFP (Fig. 29-10). EFP is initially elevated due to damage of the blood–nerve

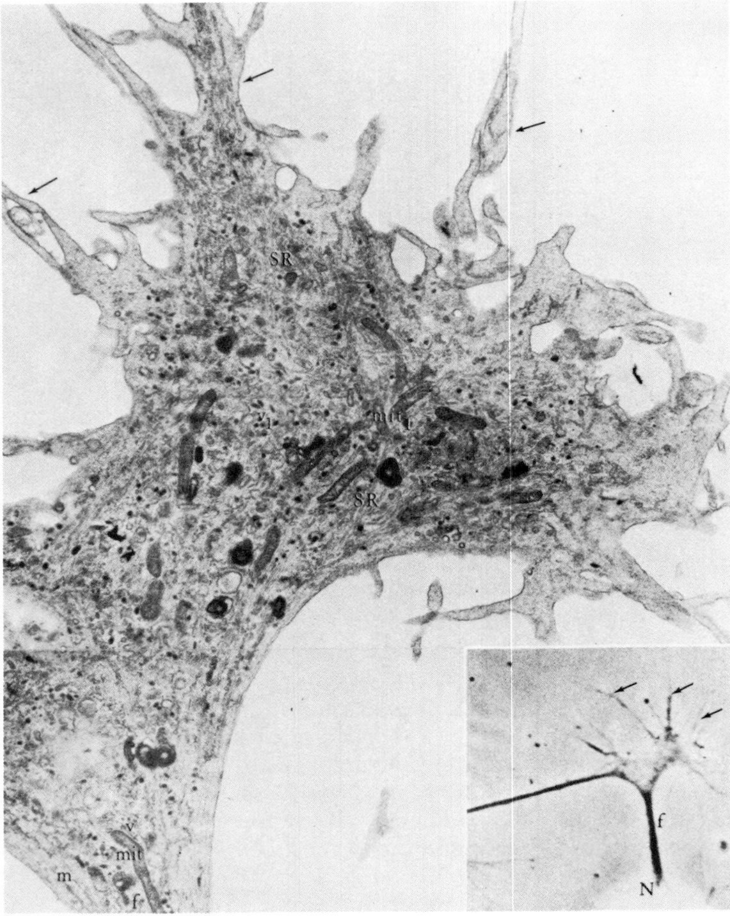

FIG. 29-8. Growth cone from sympathetic neuron in tissue culture. Insert is phase contrast micrograph showing fibers *(f)* extending from perikaryon *(N)* of a neuron. Filopodia *(arrows)* extend from growth cone. The electron micrograph from the same growth cone shows filopodia *(arrows)* and numerous cytoplasmic particles, including elongated mitochondria *(mit)*, smooth endoplasmic reticulum *(SR)*, vesicles *(v)*, vesicles with dense contents *(vl)*, and microtubules *(m)*. (Original magnification × 1400 for EM; × 1350 for phase contrast) (Peters, A., Parlay, S.L., and Webster, H.deF.: The Fine Structure of the Nervous System, p. 112. Philadelphia, W.B. Saunders, 1976.)

barrier but peaks about 6 to 7 days after the injury[52] and corresponds to the time of greatest discomfort in patients. The peak in EFP is due to a summation of events, each of which results in increased endoneurial volume. Mast cells degranulate, releasing vasoactive chemicals that increase the permeability of the blood–nerve barrier. Schwann cells proliferate, and phagocytic cells are active. EFP gradually declines and is normal 1 month after injury when regeneration is nearly complete.

ABNORMAL NERVE BLOOD FLOW

Nerve blood flow (NBF) has been measured recently with quantitative methods.[39,42,60,65] Normal NBF is about 16 ml/100 g tissue/min and is thus slightly less than the blood flow value for cerebral white matter. In edematous neuropathies with increased endoneurial fluid pressure, it has been shown that NBF is significantly decreased. Morphologic evidence supports ischemia as a pathogenic mechanism causing nerve fiber injury.[42,51] The pathogenic mechanism for reduced nerve blood flow in the presence of elevated EFP is actively being sought. Current hypotheses include separation of endoneurial capillaries by edema[65] and the apparent susceptibility of transperineurial vessels to occlusion when the perinerium is stretched by increased EFP—a pathologic valve mechanism in perineurial vessels.[32] The argument in support of the reduced capillary density hypothesis is based on blood flow per unit weight of tissue and an increased weight of edematous nerve; however, blood flow is still less than normal if the tissue weight is normalized by subtracting the excess water weight from the wet-weight of the nerve.[39] The existence of a

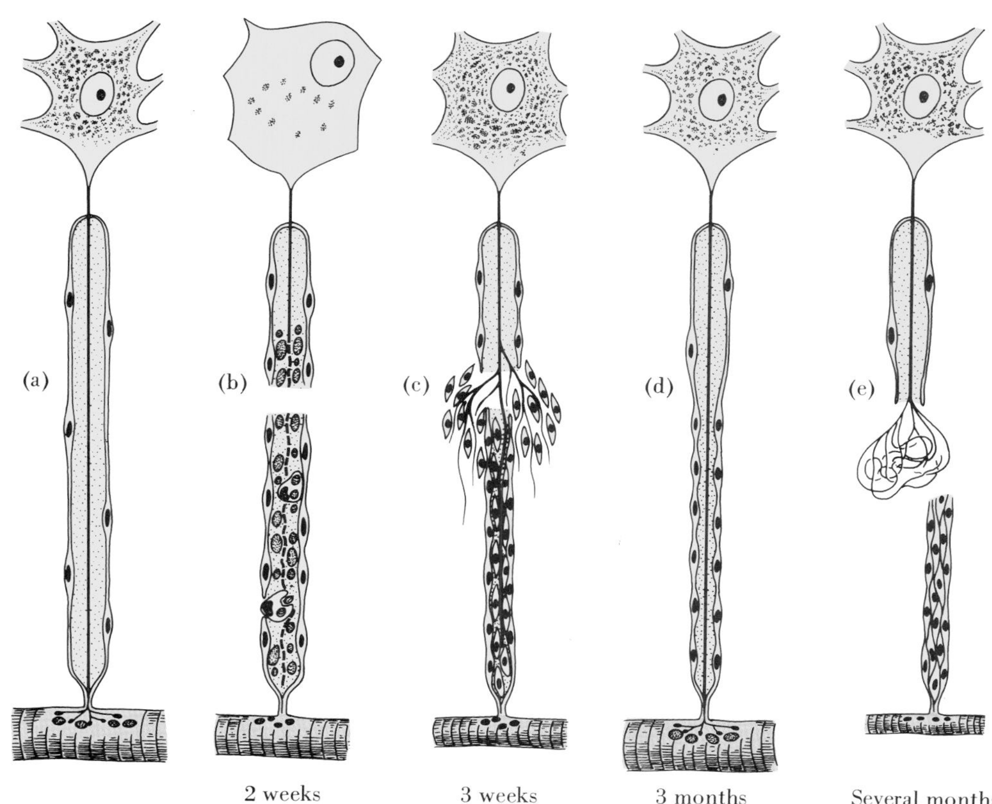

FIG. 29-9. Major changes associated with nerve fiber regeneration. *(a)* Normal nerve fiber with its perikaryon and its effector cell (striated skeletal muscle). The axon is surrounded by myelin generated by Schwann cells. *(b)* When the fiber is injured, the neuronal nucleus moves to the periphery and Nissel bodies in the perikaryon become greatly reduced in number. The nerve fiber distal to the injury degenerates along with its myelin sheath—wallerian degeneration. The blood–nerve barrier is damaged, and debris is phagocytized by macrophages. *(c)* By 3 weeks, the muscle fiber shows a pronounced disuse atrophy. Schwann cells proliferate, forming a compact cord through which an axon may grow. The axon grows at a rate of about 1 mm/day. *(d)* In this example, the nerve fiber has generated successfully 3 months after injury. *(e)* In other cases, however, the axon may not successfully find its original end-organ if growth is impeded by mechanical obstacles or is unorganized for other reasons. (Willis, R.A., and Willis, A.T.: The Principles of Pathology and Bacteriology. London, Butterworth, 1972; redrawn for Ross, M.H., and Reigh, E.J.: Histology. Philadelphia, J.B. Lippincott, 1985.)

pathologic valve mechanism in vessels traversing the perineurium is supported by both morphologic and theoretical evidence.[40] Morphologic evidence comes from serial sections of tissue that are reconstructed to follow the course of transperineurial vessels (Fig. 29-11). In the illustration, a sciatic nerve with increased EFP 48 hours after topical application of the clinical preparation of 2-chloroprocaine local anesthetic was fixed in phosphate-buffered gluteraldehyde and serially sectioned at 1-μm intervals. The reconstructed sections cover a distance of about 1.5 mm and show a venule traversing the perineurium. The segment surrounded by perineurium is greatly reduced in cross-sectional area, and stasis is seen in the epineurial segment. This can be explained by a biomechanical model studied by computer (Fig. 29-12). EFP is the force that stretches the perineurium and closes vessels, even though the EFP values

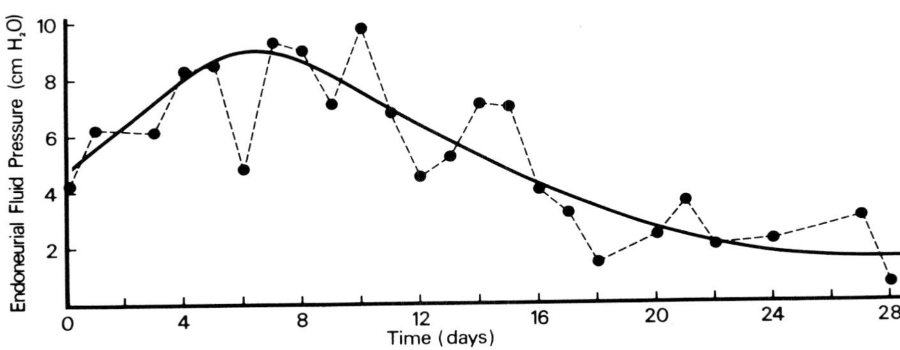

FIG. 29-10. Temporal changes in endoneurial fluid pressure (*EFP*) following proximal crush injury to rat sciatic nerve. Initially, EFP is elevated due to vascular damage associated with the crush. A peak in EFP is reached between the 6th and 7th days postcompression and represents a summation of events explained in the text. EFP gradually declines during the course of regeneration. (Myers, et al.: Ann. Neurol., *5*:550, 1979.)

are less than capillary closing pressures — the pathologic valve mechanism. This occurs because of the unequal stretching of the perineurium in the longitudinal and circumferential directions when subjected to a distending pressure in the endoneurial compartment.

AGENTS AND TECHNIQUES

HYPERTONIC AND HYPOTONIC SOLUTIONS

Subarachnoid injection of hypertonic and hypotonic solutions produces pathologic change in nervous system tissue[23,26,56] and has been used to treat pain.[22] The clinical impression that pain fibers are affected preferentially is not corroborated by histologic evidence.[45,56] Physiologically, it has been noted that osmotic swelling of the nerve bundle is associated with a deficit in nerve conduction.[10] Fink proposed a mechanism of hypo-osmotic conduction block based on the development of endoneurial edema in isolated peripheral nerves.[10] The presence of the perineurium was an essential factor in the conduction block, suggesting that the mechanism was a compression block caused by osmotic swelling of the fascicle, affecting nerve metabolism. Structural change to myelin and axon is not seen unless nerves are soaked for at least 1 hour in distilled water or solutions of osmolality of greater than 1000 mmol/liter. In this case, the myelin lamellae separate, and unmyelinated fibers may show total destruction. Thus the early functional change observed clinically is apparently not caused by acute structural damage, but rather by a change in the endoneurial environment that may later affect nerve structure and prolong the functional deficit.

HYPOTHERMIA AND FREEZE LESIONS

Hypothermia can produce either transient or long-lasting damage to peripheral nerves, depending on the degree to which temperature is lowered. In 1945, Denny-Brown and colleagues[6] reported on the pathology of nerves subjected to cold, noting the sensitivity of A-delta and C sensory fibers to damage. Subsequent studies have attempted to define the pathophysiologic changes of hypothermia and provide a theoretical rationale for its use on the spinal cord to relieve pain.[2,12,48] A physiologic effect, manifested as a prolonged axon potential, is seen in all fibers when cooled to 5°C. It is now generally agreed that unmyelinated axons are blocked at a lower temperature than myelinated axons[8] and that conduction is blocked in all myelinated fibers at approximately the same temperature.[48] Early cytopathology studies showed abnormalities of Schwann cells and endoneurial capillaries. This was thought to be due to accelerated enzyme production that affected Schwann cell metabolism. The pathogenic role of edema was not considered, however, even though Schwann cells are sensitive to ischemia and are easily damaged by elevated EFP.

Although the mechanisms of injury involving cooling are complex, it is clear that freezing results in formation of ice crystals, causing necrosis of all tissue elements.[63] Freezing produces a longer-lasting clinical deficit and has become an attractive method of neurolysis of intercostal nerves following thoracotomy that reduces the need for narcotic analgesia.[25] The technique is based on the freezing of a small nerve segment with a 2-mm diameter cryoprobe cooled to about −60°C by the rapid expansion of pressurized nitrous oxide from its tip. When left in contact with the nerve for 60 seconds, a 2- to 4-mm-

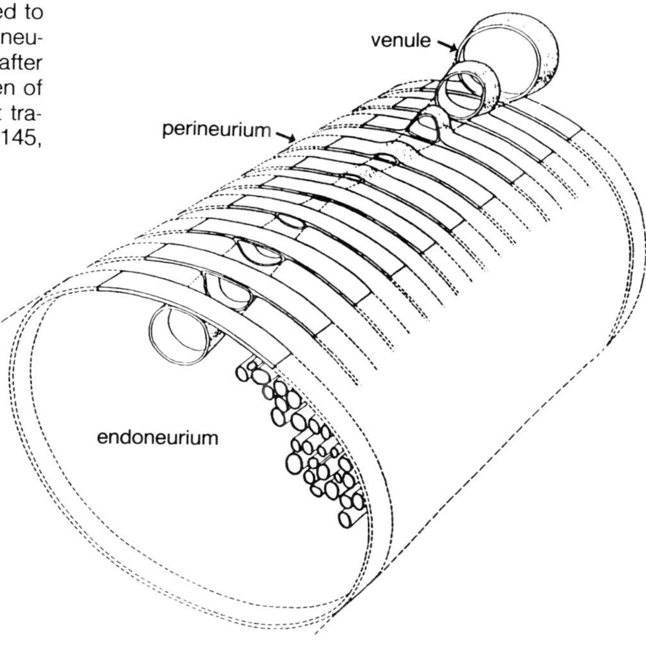

FIG. 29-11. Serial, transverse sections of nerve reconstructed to illustrate the passage of an epineurial vessel through the perineurium. In this actual example from an edematous nerve 48 hours after topical application of 3% 2-chloroprocaine, note that the lumen of the venous vessel is reduced in cross-sectional area when it traverses the perineurium. (Myers, et al.: Microvasc. Res., *32*:145, 1986.)

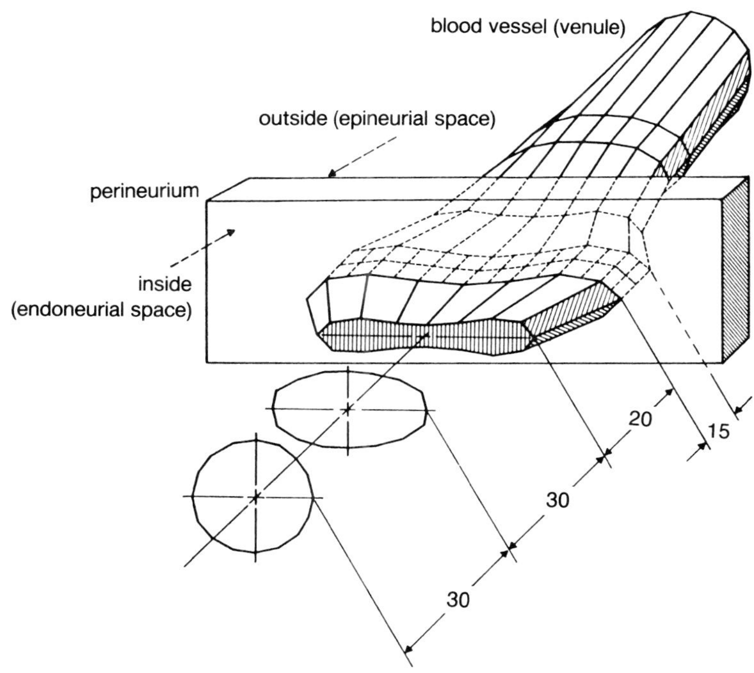

FIG. 29-12. Structural analysis of the transperineurial circulation modeling the pathologic valve mechanism. The three-dimensional computer analysis of the model produced deformation of the cylindrical blood vessel when EFP was elevated. The maximum compression of the vessel is seen inside the perineurium, even though the greatest elongation of the vessel occurs within the perineurium. Although many biomechanical factors affected the results of the analysis, EFP was a critical factor that directly led to significant reductions in luminal area. (Myers et al.: Microvasc. Res., *32*:145, 1986.)

diameter ice ball is formed that freezes the nerve and completely damages the nerve fibers.[44] This initially produces severe vascular injury and edema with diapedesis of polymorphonuclear cells through vessel walls (Fig. 29-13). Endoneurial fluid pressure is elevated within 90 minutes of the lesion, obtaining a level of approximately 20 cm H_2O, or twice that observed in edematous neuropathies developing more slowly. EFP is reduced, however, over the next 24 hours, presumably because of changes in the elastic characteristics of the perineurium. EFP then increases again to obtain a plateau at 6 days that is associated with wallerian degeneration of the distal fibers. Wallerian degeneration is the prominent pathologic feature in these nerves and affects the entire nerve (Fig. 29-14). Although freezing causes complete damage to nerve fibers, the basal lamina fortunately is spared and provides a conduit for nerve fiber regeneration. Thus freezing causes an acute, severe injury to all nerve fibers that will persist for about 1 month. Regeneration is aided by the presence of Schwann cell basal lamina, making possible the complete and appropriate reinnervation of distal structures.

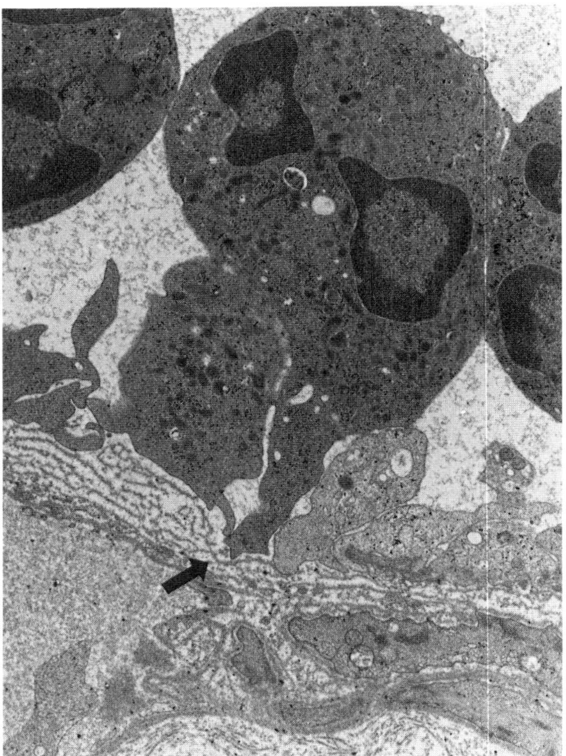

FIG. 29-13. Damage to the vasa nervorum 1 hour after cryoprobe freeze lesion to peripheral nerve. Electron micrograph shows polymorphonuclear cells with filopodia adjacent to exposed endothelial cell basement membrane *(arrow)*, which also appears fragmented and shows reduplication. (Uranyl acetate and lead citrate). (Myers, et al.: Ann. Neurol., *10*:478, 1981.)

HYPERTHERMIA AND LASER LESIONS

Heating of peripheral nerves with ultrasonic energy can produce three levels of nerve conduction effects: enhancement, reversible depression, and irreversible depression.[29] In Lele's study of nerves that were irreversibly damaged by heat, where irreversible implies a functional deficit lasting more than 18 hours, there was nodularity and fragmentation of axis cylinders with the perineurium apparently being unaffected. These nerves also showed poor staining in osmium tetroxide and vacuolation of myelin sheaths. Although these effects were largely dose dependent, there was wide variability in the results that could not be completely ascribed to biological variability in the subjects. Temperatures in the vicinity of the nerve never exceeded 42°C.

Heating of peripheral nerve can be better controlled with a laser because the energy output directly heats the nerve, not the surrounding tissue, and the output of the laser is controllable, both in magnitude and duration. Thus the severity of the lesion is influenced by the frequency, energy density, and duration of the irradiation, as well as by the absorption coefficients of the tissue. Laser irradiation of peripheral nerve produces localized lesions characterized histologically by a concentric zone of coagulation necrosis surrounded by persistent nerve edema. The perineurium is not damaged, and the resulting edema increases endoneurial fluid pressure.[37] In nerves irradiated for 0.5 seconds with 5 w of energy from a carbon dioxide laser, there was considerable damage to nerve fibers and endoneurial edema that affected adjacent fascicles (Fig. 29-15). Sections of laser-injured nerves showed discrete endoneurial lesions characterized by nerve fibers undergoing wallerian degeneration. Electron microscopy showed greatly swollen axons packed with organelles, changes characteristic of axonal dystrophy during acute wallerian degeneration. Because laser injury produces wallerian degeneration and can be finely controlled and focused, it could be a useful neurolytic technique provided that there is direct visual access to the nerve.

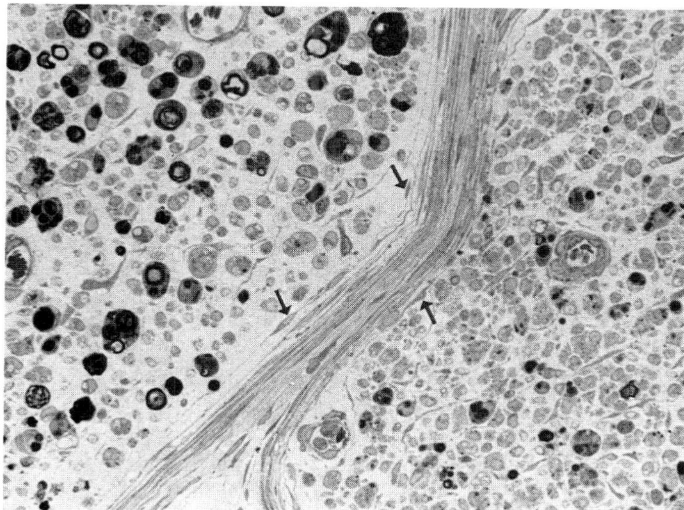

FIG. 29-14. Wallerian degeneration following cryoprobe freeze lesion to rat sciatic nerve. Light micrograph of two fascicles. Note complete degeneration of nerve fibers and fibroblast activity *(arrows)* in vicinity of perineurium. See also Figures 29-31 and 29-32. (Paraphenylene diamine)

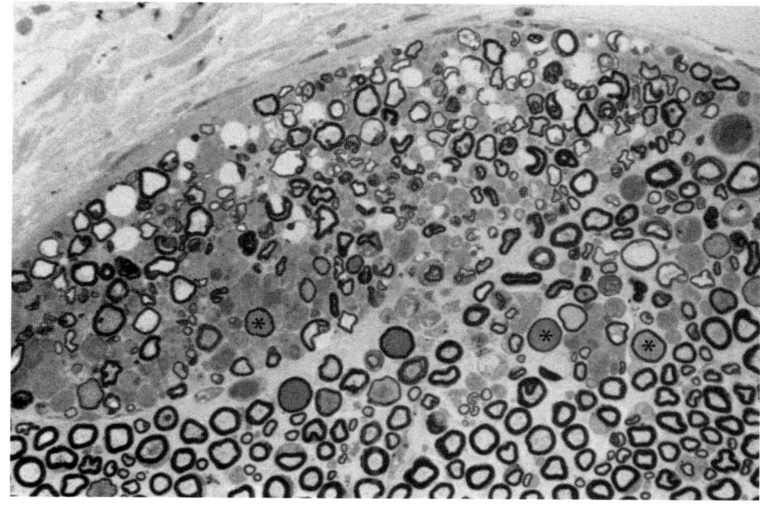

FIG. 29-15. Light micrograph of localized lesion caused by laser irradiation with a 5-watt carbon dioxide laser for 0.5 seconds. Note wallerian degeneration in this tissue 48 hours after irradiation. There is massive swelling of affected fibers with darkly stained axoplasm and attenuated myelin sheaths (*). (Paraphenylene diamine) (Myers, et al.: J. Neurol. Neurosurg. Psychiatry, *48*:1265, 1985.)

LOCAL ANESTHETIC SOLUTIONS

In an animal model, pure local anesthetic solutions alter the endoneurial environment and can produce nerve fiber injury when in prolonged contact with peripheral nerves.[24] The use of modern neuropathologic techniques has demonstrated that local anesthetic solutions administered to laboratory animals can cause nerve fiber injury and that the recently reported neurotoxic effects of antioxidants and *p*H[14] may be in addition to a direct effect of the local anesthetic *per se*.[24,38] In the late 1930s and early 1940s, anesthetic–oil mixtures were used for long-term nerve blockade; it was thought that oil suppressed absorption of the anesthetic and prolonged the effect. It was subsequently shown in 1943 that benzyl alcohol, a component common to all mixtures, was the likely cause of long-term neurologic dysfunction.[9]

In 1984 it was reported that bisulfite in "Nesacaine-Ce" chloroprocaine solutions could produce irreversible changes in neural function, which was dose and *p*H related.[14,66] Also, in epidural block it was postulated that large volume injection may increase CSF pressure. This may decrease spinal cord perfusion if combined with hypotension caused by a high level of blockade. This low level of spinal cord perfusion may increase susceptibility of the spinal cord to neurotoxicity.[14] In studies of neural function in which *p*H, bisulfite content, and volume of local anesthetic solution were controlled, the local anesthetic *per se* was not neurotoxic after short-term application.[14,54,66]

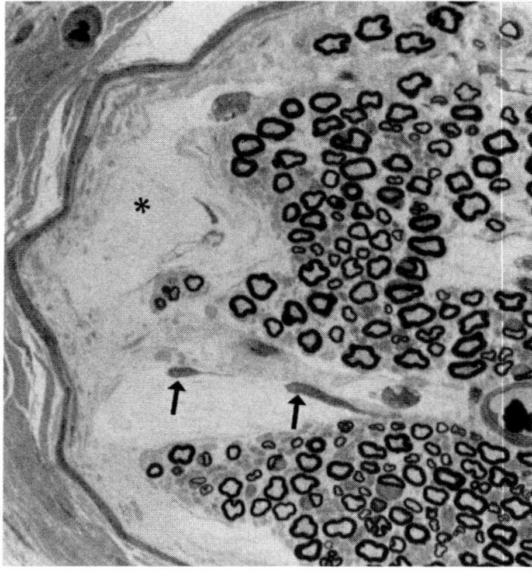

FIG. 29-16. Transverse section from rat sciatic nerve 48 hours after topical application of 2-chloroprocaine. Note extensive subperineurial edema (*) and fibroblasts *(arrows)*. Endoneurial fluid pressure was about three times the normal value. (Paraphenylene diamine)

Other work, however, indicates that local anesthetics may cause endoneurial edema and wallerian degeneration. It is important to assess the results of these animal studies with respect to mode of application, volume, concentration of local anesthetic, and presence of adjuvants.[14,54,66] For example, when local anesthetics are injected intrafascicularly, there are changes in the permeability of the blood–nerve barrier associated with edema and nerve fiber injury.[16,24,59] It has been reported that osmotic swelling, owing to application of hypo-osmotic solutions, results in a deficit of nerve conduction.[11] Injury can also occur even though the solutions are not injected into the endoneurial compartment. Recent unpublished results indicate that the endoneurial fluid in edematous nerves following exposure to local anesthetics is hypotonic to normal endoneurial fluid and may affect nerve conduction. When peripheral nerves are bathed in high concentrations of local anesthetics such as 3% 2-chloroprocaine, 1% tetracaine, or 10% procaine, the permeability of the perineurium is altered and endoneurial edema is striking 48 hours later (Fig. 29-16). Increased EFP is a consequence of this treatment, as is perineurial fibrosis.[38] Electron microscopy reveals abnormal mast cells and proliferation of endoneurial fibroblasts in addition to Schwann cell injury and axonal dystrophy. Schwann cell necrosis was characterized by cytoplasmic accumulation of myelin debris and lipid droplets (Fig. 29-17). Lipid droplets were also seen in the perineurium and in fibroblasts. At low concentration, local anesthetic-induced abnormalities were limited to changes in nerve hydration seen as subperineurial edema and mild structural damage to myelin and Schwann cells that rapidly resolved. These changes are dose dependent and are observed with local anesthetics not containing antitoxidants or preservatives.[24] More severe wallerian degeneration was observed at higher concentrations and was associated with abnormal function during the period of nerve regeneration.

Single lumbar subarachnoid injection in rabbits of a low volume of pure solutions of tetracaine, bupivacaine, lidocaine, and 2-chloroprocaine did not produce neural damage at usual clinical concentrations. Lidocaine and tetracaine could be prepared in high concentrations (16–32% and 4–8%, respectively), and these produced neurologic deficits at 48 hours that persisted until animals were killed at 5 to 7 days. This was also the case for bisulfite in concentrations

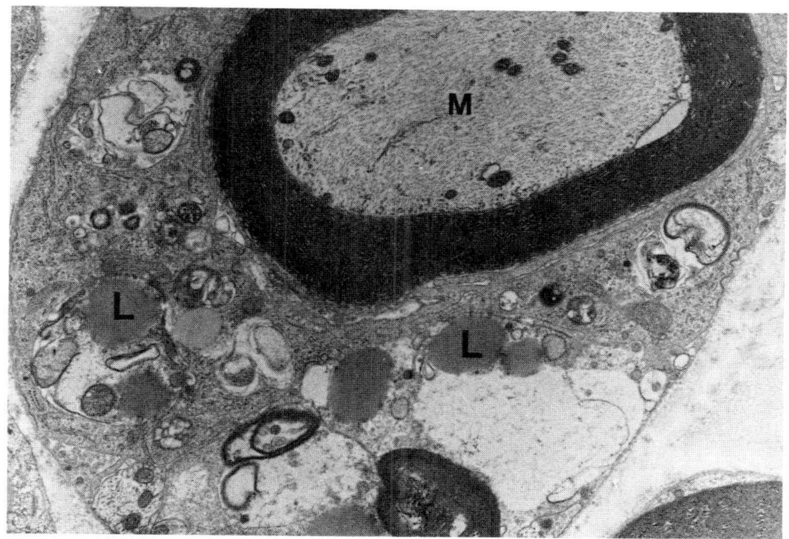

FIG. 29-17. Electron micrograph of lipid inclusions 48 hours after topical application of 2-chloroprocaine. Intact myelinated fiber *(M)* is surrounded by disintegrating Schwann cell and macrophage. Note numerous lipid inclusions *(L)*. (Uranyl acetate and lead citrate)

of 0.4% to 0.8% but not 0.2%. These effects were accompanied by histologic evidence of damage to spinal cord and nerve roots; however, there was not a good correlation between functional loss and histologic findings.[54]

Prolonged lumbar subarachnoid infusion of local anesthetic solutions in the rat resulted in spinal cord neurotoxicity and residual paralysis in more than half the rats studied. Bupivacaine 0.5% (*p*H 5.6), lidocaine 1.5% (*p*H 5.2), and chloroprocaine (*p*H 3.0 plus 0.2% bisulfite) all produced intraneuronal and perineuronal vacuolation in spinal cord gray matter. The neurotoxic effects were dose related: Thirteen of 15 receiving the infusion for 24 hours, 10 of 15 receiving it for 6 hours, and 4 of 15 receiving it for 3 hours had residual paralysis. No control animals receiving Hartman's solution were paralyzed. There was a poor correlation between neuropathologic and clinical findings. It was of interest that the damage with lidocaine and chloroprocaine was more severe than that with bupivacaine.[30] Since lidocaine and bupivacaine did not contain bisulfite, neurotoxicity with these solutions could be explained only by a neurotoxic effect of prolonged exposure to these drugs.

Clinical implications of these studies in animals are not certain; however, it seems that the following circumstances may pose a potential for neurotoxicity: excessive concentrations of bisulfite and low *p*H; high concentrations of local anesthetic on peripheral nerves; prolonged subarachnoid infusion of local anesthetics; and perhaps high CSF pressure and low spinal cord perfusion caused by hypotension in combination with local anesthetic effects. Many of these factors can be guarded against: Bisulfite can be kept at low concentrations or even eliminated from epinephrine-free local anesthetics; *p*H can be adjusted to above 5; high local anesthetic concentrations are unnecessary on peripheral nerves; large volumes should not be rapidly injected into the epidural space; and subarachnoid infusion is now unnecessary, and accidental subarachnoid placement can be detected clinically. The safety of long-term epidural infusion of local anesthetics remains to be examined by studies of neural function and neuropathology (Fig. 29-18). To understand fully local anesthetic neurotoxicity, it will be necessary to document further the sequence of pathologic events, since structural abnormalities are the basis of persistent functional deficit.

ALCOHOL

Alcohol is the classic neurolytic agent and has been used extensively as such in concentrations from 50% to 95%. Because of its hypobaric nature (specific gravity = 0.80) with respect to CSF (specific gravity = 1.1), special positioning of the intended lesion site is required, and it is not recommended for use by the unskilled.[68] When alcohol is injected in the CSF, it will rise and can diffuse quite rapidly from the injection site. After a slow injection, the highest concentration of alcohol will be at the top of the fluid space in contact with the injection site. Because of its non-

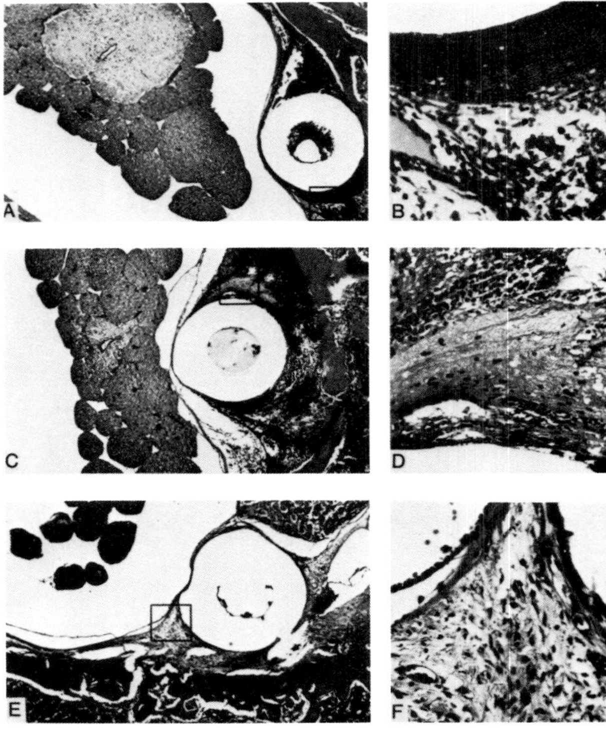

FIG. 29-18. Neuropathology of epidural catheter. Shown are histologic sections of vertebral columns of three epidurally implanted rats that did not receive any drug. After 1 day of catheterization, the epidural catheter is essentially surrounded by red blood cells (*A and B*, L3 section), after 2 days by edema (*C and D*, L4 section), and after 10 days by connective tissue (*E and F*, L4 section). The areas in the black squares on *A*, *C*, and *E* (original magnification, × 50) are shown on *B*, *D*, and *F* (original magnification, × 300). Granulomas, giant cells and fat are not present. (Durant, P.A.C., and Yaksh, T.L.: Epidural injections of bupivacaine, morphine, fentanyl, lofentanil, and DADL in chronically implanted rats: A pharmacologic and pathologic study. Anesthesiology, *64*:43, 1986.)

selective action, it can cause serious damage to neurologic tissue remote from the injection site if proper precautions are not exercised. Ethyl alcohol acts on nervous system tissue by extraction of cholesterol, phospholipid, and cerebroside and also causes precipitation of lipoproteins and mucoproteins.[57] Its widest application has been in the central nervous system, where it has been injected into the trigeminal ganglion, subarachnoid space, and the celiac plexus and lumbar sympathetic chain. The effective duration of intrathecal alcohol is about 4 months or less (see Chap. 30). A disadvantage of this technique is that fairly often only partial relief is seen or that relief lasts only briefly. Histologic sections of these tissues show spotty areas of demyelination and mild, focal inflammatory changes in the meninges.[13] With subarachnoid injection, the injury is often confined to the posterior portion of the cord and involves Lissauer's tract. Remote degeneration of the spinal cord can be seen and is probably due to wallerian degeneration of the distal fibers.

Alcohol applied topically to peripheral nerves produces damage to both the Schwann cell and axon. Schwann cell cytoplasm has swollen mitochondria, and the myelin sheath is disrupted. Dilated vesicles can be seen in the dystrophic axons, and wallerian degeneration is a prominent feature (Fig. 29-19).[70] *In vivo* electrophysiologic investigation of peripheral nerves of cats revealed significant depression of compound action potentials (CAP) when tested 8 weeks after injection of alcohol close to the nerve. There was a small increase in effect on CAP as alcohol concentration increased from 50% to 100%; however, the 100% solution caused marked skin slough.[17]

PHENOL

Phenol has been used extensively as a neurolytic agent.[69] Its primary effect is to coagulate proteins[50]; it is similar to alcohol in its potency and nonselective damage to nervous system tissue. Phenol is diffusely distributed throughout the endoneurium; autoradiography of labeled phenol gives no clear indication of its localization.[50] Subarachnoid injection of 5% to 8% phenol produces a mild meningeal reaction, although larger concentrations cause extensive fibrosis and thickening of the arachnoid. The histologic findings after phenol injection are similar to those for ethyl alcohol and include degeneration of fibers in the posterior columns and posterior nerve roots (Fig. 29-20). Both segmental demyelination and wallerian degeneration are characteristic of phenol injury. The specific neurotoxic reaction is related to the concentration of phenol, with wallerian degeneration resulting from exposure to a higher concentration; Schaumburg reports that the amount of wallerian degeneration increases in proportion to the strength and duration of application of phenol.[58] Axonal abnormalities are apparent only with high concentrations or long exposure to phenol. This finding is similar to that of Denny-Brown and Brenner, who found that mild trauma damages the myelin sheath, whereas more severe injury involves the axon as well, in experiments of ischemia of peripheral nerve.[7] Another

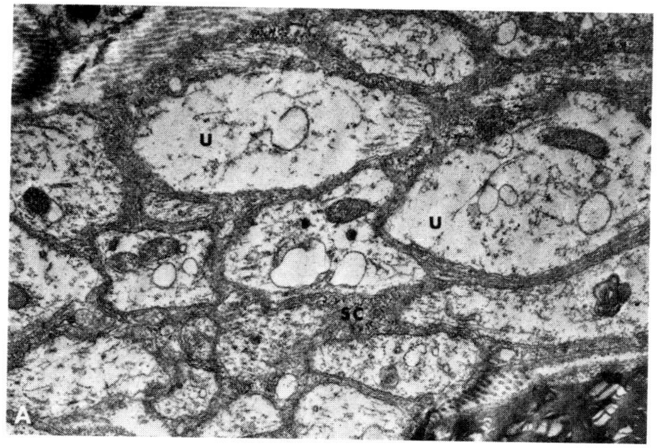

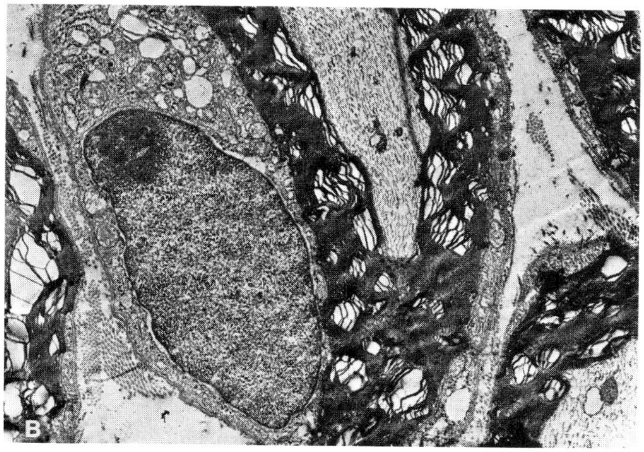

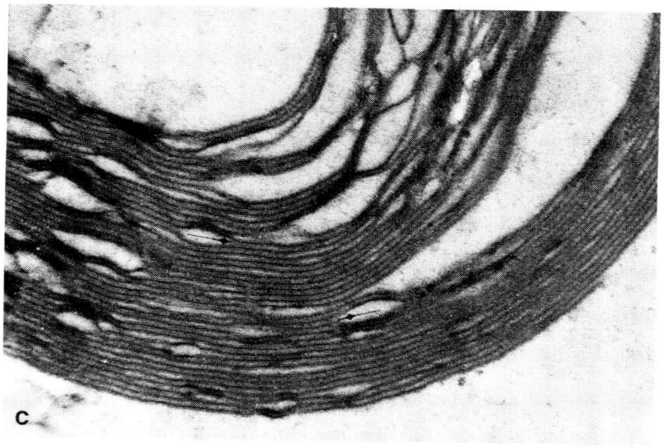

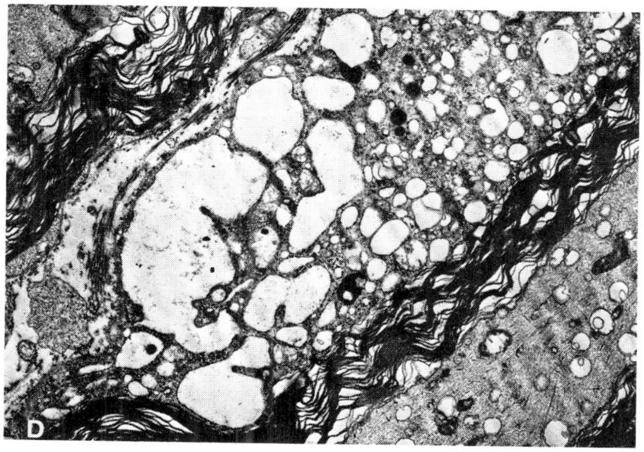

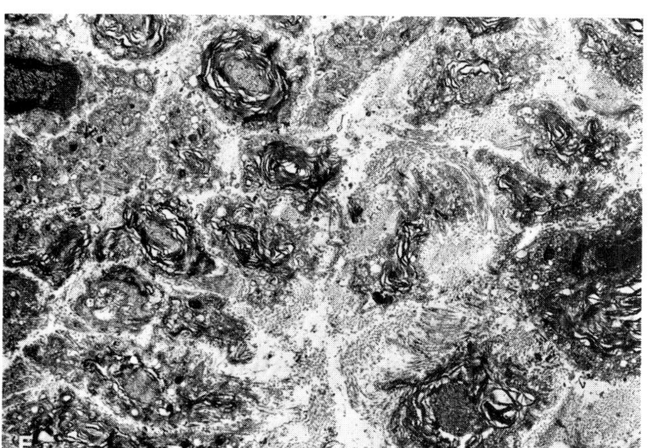

FIG. 29-19. **A.** Effect of alcohol on peripheral nerve, 15 seconds after topical application of 100% alcohol. Electron micrograph shows the sciatic nerve of a mouse after alcohol application. The arrows denote swelling of unmyelinated nerve fibers *(U)*; S denotes Schwann cell cytoplasm that is clumped and granular — Schwann cell destruction. (× 5000) **B.** Electron micrograph shows the Schwann cell after alcohol exposure. Note splitting of myelin sheath *(MS)* and dilated endoplasmic reticulum *(ER)*, indicating acute injury to Schwann cell and myelin sheath. (× 4300) **C.** Effect of alcohol on peripheral nerve, 1 minute after application. Electron micrograph shows splitting of myelin sheath after exposure to topical 100% alcohol. (× 9600) **D.** Effect of alcohol on peripheral nerve, 24 hours after a 15-second exposure to 100% alcohol. Note degenerating axons *(A)*, splitting myelin lamellae *(M)*, and beginning of connective tissue reaction. (× 2200) **E.** Effect of alcohol on peripheral nerve, 4 hours after a 15-second exposure. Electron micrograph shows vacuolization in Schwann cell after 100% alcohol exposure. (Woolsey, R.M., Taylor, J.J., and Nagel, J.H.: Acute effects of topical ethyl alcohol on the sciatic nerve of the mouse. Arch. Phys. Med. Rehabil., *53*:410, 1972.)

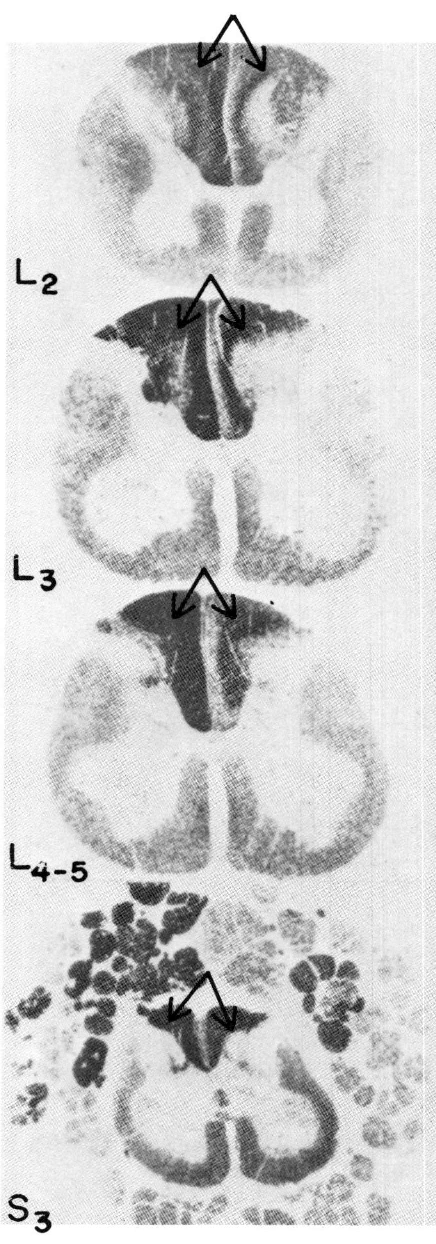

FIG. 29-20. Effect of phenol on spinal cord. Micrographs show transverse sections through a patient's spinal cord. Note posterior column degeneration *(arrows)* after subarachnoid injection of phenol. These sections were taken at the levels of spinal cord indicated adjacent to the section. Injection was made at bony spine level L3–L4. (Smith, M.C.: Histological findings following intrathecal injections of phenol solutions for relief of pain. Br. J. Anaesth., *36*:387, 1964.)

analogy can be made with nerve entrapment.[50] Low doses cause a transient conduction block, whereas higher doses cause an irreversible block by damaging axons. As in nerve crush injuries, the onset of wallerian degeneration occurs earlier in smaller diameter axons. Such findings contribute to the controversy regarding the capability of phenol to produce a differential block of nerve fibers; however, a combined electrophysiologic and histologic study of the effect of phenol on peripheral nerve by Schaumburg and associates concluded that phenol's neurotoxic effect is dose related and that there is no differential effect on nerve fibers.[58] Finally, in a series of experiments reviewed by Wood,[69] it was seen that the overall destructive effect of phenol contributed to its neurolytic effect. The affinity of phenol was greater for vascular tissue than for brain neurophospholipid, suggesting that injury to blood vessels may be an important pathogenic factor contributing to the observed neuropathology. Also, this raises a concern about the use of large amounts of phenol near major blood vessels. This is the basis for some specialists preferring alcohol over phenol for celiac plexus block. Electrophysiologic and histopathology investigation of phenol in Renografin injected close to peripheral nerves of cats *in vivo* revealed a highly significant, concentration-related depression of CAP at 1 and 2 weeks after injection. Maximum effect required 12% phenol. By 8 weeks, remyelination was clearly evident and CAPs had returned to normal.[18]

GLYCEROL

The neurolytic effect of glycerol was discovered accidentally[21] and rapidly led to the use of the agent in treating facial pain.[34,62] The technique of percutaneous retrogasserian glycerol rhizotomy for the treatment of tic douloureux is reported to be far superior to radiofrequency rhizotomy because no permanent injury to surrounding structures occurs and there is preservation of facial sensation in most patients.[34] The histologic study of experimental material shows that intraneural injection of glycerol is more damaging than topical application, although significant, localized, subperineurial damage is seen following topical application of a 50% glycerol solution.[55] The histologic changes include the presence of numerous inflammatory cells, extensive myelin swelling, and axonolysis. Myelin disintegration occurs weeks after the injury along with ongoing axonolysis during periods of myelin restitution,[55] indicating an ongoing nerve fiber injury possibly caused by secondary events such as compression of transperineurial vessels and ischemia. Electron microscopy shows evidence of wallerian degeneration; with intraneural injection, essentially all nerve fibers are destroyed. Lipid droplets are seen in Schwann cells and phagocytic cells (Fig. 29-21), and there is mast cell degranulation. The molecular basis of the toxic effects is unknown, but Rengachary suggests that it might be similar to that of ethanol, since both compounds are structurally related.[55] Despite evidence for the differential effect of glycerol on the electrophysiologic function of peripheral nerves,[4] histologic data are lacking.

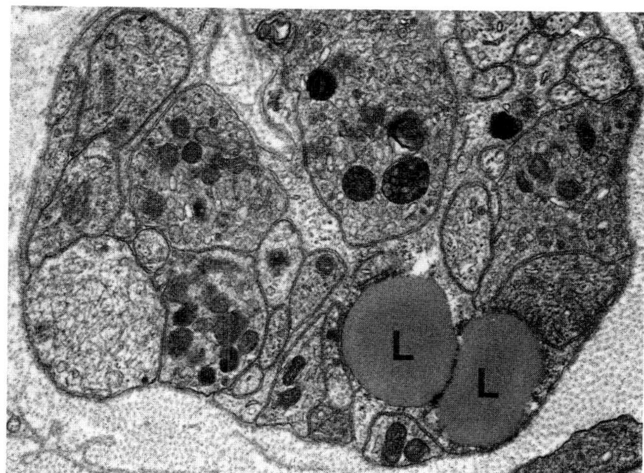

FIG. 29-21. Electron micrograph of glycerol-treated nerves. Lipid droplets *(L)* are seen in the cytoplasm of a Schwann cell in an unmyelinated nerve fiber. Increased numbers of organelles are present in some axons. They include mitochondria and electron-dense, membrane-enveloped structures resembling lysosomes and vesicular inclusions. These changes are consistent with axonal degeneration. (Uranyl acetate and lead citrate)

AMMONIUM SALTS

The first reported use of salts for long-term relief of pain was in 1935 when Judovich used pitcher plant distillate *(Sarracenia purpnea)* for certain forms of neuralgia. It was later reported that the ammonium ion in the form of ammonium chloride or ammonium hydroxide (depending on the *p*H of the distillate) was the active component.

In 1942, a report on the use of ammonium salts for nerve pain stated the following:[1]

> In no instance has there been any motor weakness, following injection of peripheral nerves nor loss of touch, pressure, pinprick, and temperature sensibility. In some instances, one infiltration of the distillate is sufficient to provide permanent relief of pain even in cases of long duration. . . ."

> In man, perineural infiltration of 0.5% to 1% solutions of ammonium chloride produces the same effects as does the infiltration of pitcher plant extract. The immediate effect of the injection is an increased intensity of the pain which then subsides during the first 30 minutes after injection. The neuralgic pain is relieved, the zone of hyperesthesia contracts and disappears, and when injected around the sciatic nerve there results no weakness and the sensations of touch, pressure, pinprick, and temperature on the outer aspect of the leg are unimpaired. . . .

The action of ammonium salts on nerve impulses produces obliteration of C fiber potentials with only a small effect on A fibers. Subsequent clinical information has shown that with concentrations of 10% of ammonium salts, motor function can be retained despite good analgesia. Limited pathologic studies suggest that injection of ammonium salts around a peripheral nerve causes an acute degenerative neuropathy affecting all fibers.

CONCLUSION

Neurotoxic agents can produce neurolysis of nerve fibers, depending on the concentration of agent in direct contact with the tissue. Agents applied topically can alter perineurial permeability to gain access to nerve fibers, but their effects may be diluted. Intraneural injection of neurotoxic agents produces the most severe damage, almost always resulting in significant axonal abnormalities and wallerian degeneration. Techniques that physically damage the nerve with heat or cold produce similar results. There appears to be no differential effect of these agents or techniques on electrophysiologic function; rather, variations in concentration produce different clinical findings, suggesting a dose-related response. When nerve fibers are damaged, wallerian degeneration is often the major finding and accounts for the desirable, long-lasting clinical effect. The persistence of the basal lamina around the Schwann cell tube (the bands of Büngner) allows the successful and appropriate regeneration of nerve fibers, eliminating the formation of painful neuromas and justifying the use of neurolytic agents over surgical interruption of nerve fibers in the treatment of chronic pain. There is often a poor correlation between findings at autopsy in humans and clinical effects produced by neurolytic block.

Changes in the endoneurial environment are thought to affect electrophysiologic function by altering the electrolyte concentration of endoneurial fluid. Local anesthetic-induced edema reduces endoneurial electrolyte concentration and increases endoneurial fluid pressure, which may lead to ischemia by compressing transperineurial blood vessels. These subtle pathogenic factors may exacerbate the principal neuropathologic effect of neurolytic agents—wallerian degeneration.

Supported by the Veterans Administration Research Service and USPHS Grant NS18715.

REFERENCES

1. Bates, W., and Judovich, B.D.: Intractable pain. Anesthesiology, *3*:663, 1942.
2. Basbaum, C.B.: Electrophysiological observations. J. Neurocytol., *2*:171, 1973.
3. Brimijoin, S.: The role of axonal transport in nerve disease. In Dyck, P.J., Thomas, P.K., Lambert, E.H., and Bunge, R. (eds.): Peripheral Neuropathy. pp. 477. Philadelphia, W.B. Saunders, 1984. (119 refs.)
4. Burchiel, K.J., and Russell, L.C.: Glycerol neurolysis: Neurophysiologic effects of topical glycerol application on rat saphenous nerve. J. Neurosurg., *63*:784, 1985.
5. Chiu, S.Y., and Richie, J.M.: Potassium channels in nodal and internodal axonal membrane of mammalian myelinated fibers. Nature, *284*:170, 1980.
6. Denny-Brown, D., Adams, R., Brenner, C., and Doherty, M.M.: The pathology of injury to nerve induced by cold. J. Neuropathol. Exp. Neurol., *4*:305, 1945.
7. Denny-Brown, D., and Brenner, C.: The effect of percussion of nerve. J. Neurol. Neurosurg. Psychiatry, *7*:76, 1944.
8. Douglas, W.W., and Malcolm, J.L.: Effect of localized cooling on conduction in cat nerves. J. Physiol. (Lond.), *130*:63, 1955.
9. Duncan, D., and Jarvis, W.H.: A comparison of the actions on nerve fibers of certain anesthetic mixtures and substances in oil. Anesthesiology, *4*:465, 1943.
10. Fink, B.R.: Mechanism of hypo-osmotic conduction block. Reg. Anaesth., *5*:7, 1980.
11. Fink, B.R., Barsa, J., and Calkins, D.F.: Osmotic swelling effects of neural conduction. Anesthesiology, *51*:418, 1979.
12. Franz, D.N., and Iggo, A.: Conduction failure in myelinated and non-myelinated axons at low temperatures. J. Physiol., *199*:319, 1968.
13. Gallager, H.S., Yonezawa, T., Hay, R.C., and Derrick, W.S.: Subarachnoid alcohol block II. Histologic changes in the central nervous system. Am. J. Pathol., *35*:679, 1961.
14. Gissen, A.J., Datta, S., and Lambert, D.: The chloroprocaine controversy. Reg. Anaesth., *9*:124, 1984.
15. Gasser, H.S.: Properties of dorsal root unmedullated fibers on the two sides of the ganglion. J. Gen. Physiol., *38*:709, 1955.
16. Gentilli, F., Hudson, A.R., Hunter, D., and Kline, D.G.: Nerve injection injury with local anesthetic agents: A light and electron microscopic, fluorescent microscopic, and horseradish peroxidase study. Neurosurgery, *6*:263, 1980.
17. Gregg, R.V., Constantini, C.H., Ford, D.J., and Raj, P.P.: Electrophysiologic investigation of alcohol as a neurolytic agent. Anesthesiology, *63*:A250, 1985.
18. Gregg, R.V., Costantini, C.H., Ford, D.J., and Raj, P.P.: Electrophysiologic and histopathologic investigtion of phenol in Renographin as a neurolytic agent. Anesthesiology, *63*:A239, 1985.
19. Haak, R.A., Kleinhauys, F.W., and Ochs, S.: The viscosity of mammalian nerve axoplasm measured by electron spin resonance. J. Physiol. (Lond.), *263*:115, 1976.
20. Haftek, J.: Stretch injury of peripheral nerve. Acute effects of stretching on rabbit peripheral nerve. J. Bone Joint Surg. [Br.], *52B*:354, 1970.
21. Hakanson, S.: Trigeminal neuralgia treated by the injection of glycerol into the trigeminal cistern. Neurosurgery, *9*:638, 1981.
22. Hitchcock, E.: Osmolytic neurolysis for intractable facial pain. Lancet, *1*:434, 1969.
23. Jewett, D.L., Kind, J.S.: Conduction block of monkey dorsal rootlets by water and hypertonic saline solutions. Exp. Neurol., *33*:225, 1971.
24. Kalichman, M.W., Powell, H.C., Reisner, L.S., and Myers, R.R.: The role of 2-chloroprocaine and sodium bisulfite in rat sciatic nerve edema. J. Neuropath. Exp. Neurol., *45*:566, 1986.
25. Katz, J., Nelson, W., Forest, R., and Bruce, D.L.: Cryoanalgesia for post-thoracotomy pain. Lancet, *1*:512, 1980.
26. King, J.S., Jewett, D.L., Phil, D., and Sundberg, H.R.: Differential blockade of cat dorsal root C fibers by various chloride solutions. J. Neurosurg., *36*:569, 1972.
27. Krnjevic, K.: The distribution of Na and K in cat nerves. J. Physiol. (Lond.), *128*:473, 1955.
28. Lampert, P.W.: A comparative electron microscopic study of reactive, degenerating, regenerating, and dystrophic axons. J. Neuropath. Exp. Neurol., *26*:345, 1967.
29. Lele, P.P.: Effects of focused ultrasound radiation on peripheral nerves, with observations on local heating. Exp. Neurol., *8*:47, 1963.
30. Li, D.F., Bahar, M., Cole, G., and Rosen, M.: Neurological toxicity of the subarachnoid infusion of bupivacaine, lignocaine, or 2-chloroprocaine in the rat. Br. J. Anaesth., *57*:424, 1985.
31. Low, P.A.: Endoneurial fluid pressure and microenvironment of nerve. In Dyck, P.J., Thomas, P.K., Lambert, E.H., Bunge, R., (eds.): Peripheral Neuropathy. p. 599. Philadelphia, W.B. Saunders, 1984.
32. Lundborg, G.: Structure and function of intraneural microvessels as related to trauma, edema formation, and nerve function. J. Bone Joint Surg., *57A*:938, 1975.
33. Lundborg, G., and Branemark, P.-L.: Microvascular structure and function of peripheral nerves. Vital microscopic studies of the tibial nerve in the rabbit. Adv. Microcirc., *1*:66, 1968.
34. Lunsford, L.D., and Bennett, M.H.: Percutaneous retrogasserian glycerol rhizotomy for tic douloureux: Part 1, Technique and results in 112 patients. Neurosurgery, *14*:424, 1984.
35. Mizisin, A.P., Myers, R.R., and Powell, H.C.: Endoneurial so-

dium accumulation in galactosemic rat nerves. Muscle and Nerve, *9*:440, 1986.

36. Myers, R.R., Heckman, H.M., and Powell, H.C.: Endoneurial fluid is hypertonic. Results of microanalysis and significance in neuropathy. J. Neuropath. Exp. Neurol., *42*:217, 1983.

37. Myers, R.R., James, H.E., and Powell, H.C.: Laser injury of peripheral nerve: A model for focal endoneurial damage. J. Neurol. Neurosurg. Psychiatry, *48*:1265, 1985.

38. Myers, R.R., Kalichman, M.W., Reisner, L.S., and Powell, H.C.: Neurotoxicity of local anesthesia: Altered perineurial permeability edema and nerve fiber injury. Anesthesiology, *64*:29, 1986.

39. Myers, R.R., Mizisin, A.P., Powell, H.C., and Lampert, P.W.: Reduced nerve blood flow in hexachlorophene neuropathy. J. Neuropath. Exp. Neurol., *41*:391, 1982.

40. Myers, R.R., Murakami, H., and Powell, H.C.: Reduced nerve blood flow in edematous neuropathies—A biomechanical mechanism. Microvasc. Res., *32*:145, 1986.

41. Myers, R.R., and Powell, H.C.: Endoneurial fluid pressure in peripheral neuropathies. In Hargens, A. (ed.): Interstitial Fluid Pressure and Composition, p. 193. Baltimore, Williams & Wilkins, 1981.

42. Myers, R.R., and Powell, H.C.: Galactose neuropathy: Impact of chronic endoneurial edema on nerve blood flow. Ann. Neurol., *16*:587, 1984.

43. Myers, R.R., Powell, H.C., Costello, M.L., Lampert, P.W., *et al.*: Endoneurial fluid pressure: Direct measurement with micropipettes. Brain Res. *148*:510, 1978.

44. Myers, R.R., Powell, H.C., Heckman, H.M., Costello, M.L., *et al.*: Biophysical and Pathological effects of cryogenic nerve lesions. Ann. Neurol., *10*:478, 1981.

45. Nicholson, M.F., and Roberts, F.W.: Relief of pain by intrathecal injection of hypothermic saline. Med. J. Aust., *1*:61, 1968.

46. Ochs, S.: Basic properties of axoplasmic transport. In Dyck, P.J., Thomas, P.K., Lambert, E.H., Bunge, R. (eds.): Peripheral Neuropathy. p. 453. Philadelphia, W.B. Saunders, 1984. (180 refs.)

47. Olsson, Y., and Kristensson, K.: Recent applications of tracer techniques to neuropathology, with particular reference to vascular permeability and axonal flow. In Smith, W.T., and Cavanagh, J.B. (eds.): Recent Advances in Neuropathology. pp. 1. Edinburgh, Churchill Livingstone, 1979.

48. Paintal, A.S.: Block of conduction in mammalian myelinated nerve fibers by low temperatures. J. Physiol., *180*:1, 1965.

49. Parry, G.J., and Brown, M.J.: Arachidonate-induced experimental nerve infarction. J. Neurol. Sci., *50*:123, 1981.

50. Politis, M.J., Schaumburg, H.H., and Spencer, P.S.: Neurotoxicity of selected chemicals. In Spencer, P.S., and Schaumburg, H.H. (eds.): Experimental and Chemical Neurotoxicity. p. 613. Baltimore. William & Wilkins, 1980.

51. Powell, H.C., and Myers, R.R.: Pathology of the peripheral myelinated axon. In Adachi, M. (ed.): Current Trends in the Neurosciences. vol. 3, p. 96. New York. Igaku-Shoin, 1985.

52. Powell, H.C., Myers, R.R., Costello, M.L., and Lampert, P.W.: Endoneurial fluid pressure in Wallerian degeneration. Ann. Neurol. *5*:550, 1979.

53. Powell, H.C., Myers, R.R., and Lampert, P.W.: Changes in Schwann cells and vessels in lead neuropathy. Am. J. Pathol., *109*:193, 1982.

54. Ready, B.L., Plumer, M.H., Haschke, R.H., Austin, E., *et al.*: Neurotoxicity of intrathecal local anesthetics in rabbits. Anesthesiology, *63*:364, 1985.

55. Rengachary, S.S., Watanabe, I.S., Singer, P., and Bopp, W.J.: Effect of glycerol on peripheral nerve: An experimental study. Neurosurgery, *13*:681, 1983.

56. Robertson, J.D.: Structural alterations in nerve fibers produced by hypotonic and hypertonic solutions. J. Biophysic. Biochem. Cytol., *4*:349, 1958.

57. Rumbsy, M.G., and Finean, J.B.: The action of organic solvents on the myelin sheath of peripheral nerve tissue-II (short-chain aliphatic alcohols). J. Neurochem., *13*:1509, 1966.

58. Schaumburg, H.H., Byck, R., and Weller, R.O.: The effect of phenol on peripheral nerve. A histological and electrophysiological study. J. Neuropath. Exp. Neurol., *29*:615, 1970.

59. Selander, D., Brattsand, R., Lundborg, G., Nordborg, C., *et al.*: Local anesthetics: Importance of mode of application, concentration and adrenaline for the appearance of nerve lesions. Acta Anaesthesiol. Scand., *23*:127, 1979.

60. Sladky, J.T., Greenberg, H.H., and Brown, M.J.: Regional perfusion in normal and ischemic rat sciatic nerves. Ann. Neurol., *17*:191, 1985.

61. Sunderland, S.: The anatomical basis of nerve repair. In Jewett, D.L., McCarroll, Jr., H.R., (eds.): Nerve Repair and Regeneration. p. 14. C.V. Mosby, St. Louis, 1980.

62. Sweet, W.H., Poletti, C.E., and Macon, J.B.: Treatment of trigeminal neuralgia and other facial pain by retrogasserian injection of glycerol. Neurosurgery, *9*:647, 1981.

63. Thomas, P.K., and Holdroff, B.: Neuropathy due to physical agents. In Dyck, P.J., Thomas, P.K., Lambert, E.H., and Bunge, R. (eds.): Peripheral Neuropathy. p. 1479. Philadelphia, W.B. Saunders, 1984.

64. Thomas, P.K., and Olsson, Y.: Microscopic anatomy and function of the connective tissue components of peripheral nerve. In Dyck, P.J., Thomas, P.K., Lambert, E.H., Bunge, R. (eds.): Peripheral Neuropathy. p. 97. Philadelphia, W.B. Saunders, 1984. (158 refs.).

65. Tuck, R.R., Schmelzer, J.D., and Low, P.A.: Endoneurial blood flow and oxygen tension in the sciatic nerves of rats with experimental diabetic neuropathy. Brain, *107*:935, 1984.

66. Wang, B.C., Hillman, D.E., Spielholz, N.I., and Turndorf, H.: Chronic neurologic deficits and Nesacaine-CE. Anesth. Analg., *63*:445, 1984.

67. Waller, A.: Experiments on the section of the glossopharyngeal and hypoglossal nerves of the frog and observations of the alterations produced thereby in the structure of their primitive fibers. Philos. Trans. R. Soc., Lond. [Biol.], *140*:423, 1850.

68. Wilson, F.: Neurolytic and other locally acting drugs in the management of pain. Pharmacol. Ther., *12*:599, 1981.

69. Wood, K.M.: The use of phenol as a neurolytic agent: A review. Pain, *5*:205, 1978. (124 refs.)

70. Woolsey, R.M., Taylor, J.J., and Nagel, H.H.: Acute effects of topical ethyl alcohol on the sciatic nerve of the mouse. Arch. Phys. Med., Rehabil., *53*:410, 1972.

29.2 CHRONIC PAIN AND NEUROLYTIC NEURAL BLOCKADE

MICHAEL J. COUSINS
With assistance from
BRIAN DWYER and
DAVID GIBB

GENERAL CONSIDERATIONS

Neurolytic blockade offers a great potential for pain relief in patients with severe pain, mostly caused by advanced cancer[21,31,32,40] but also owing to other non-curable conditions such as occlusive vascular disease. The techniques of subarachnoid, celiac plexus, and lumbar sympathetic block are capable of a high degree of success with an acceptable level of side-effects in the patient who has not obtained satisfactory pain relief by other methods. It should be stressed that neurolytic blockade is generally not suitable for young patients with undiagnosed medical problems or for patients (apart from occlusive vascular disease) who are likely to live for a long period of time.

Neurolytic block should be regarded as only one aspect of the overall management of patients with intractable pain.[3,4,13,21,31,32,39,40,106–108,110] The general care of these patients is best undertaken in a pain relief clinic in which a multidisciplinary approach helps to determine the cause of pain and to formulate a management plan; this approach improves the results of treatment.[14,35,74,102] Consultations among specialists in the fields of anesthesiology, neurology, neurosurgery,[13,71] psychiatry, clinical psychology, radiology,[52] radiotherapy, and social work within the structure of the Pain Relief Clinic have proved invaluable. Assistance from dentists[95] and orthopedic or general surgeons is essential in specific instances (see Chap. 31).

At the first interview, a detailed history should be taken with emphasis on the features of the pain; the preceding pathology and its treatment; and the personal, social, and domestic situation of the patient. A physical examination is then performed, concentrating primarily on the painful condition.

Psychological support by means of personal interest, reassurance, and encouragement is an integral part of the management. Depression is a common accompaniment of chronic pain and requires appropriate treatment, usually with a tricyclic antidepressant (*e.g.*, imipramine, amitriptyline, or nortriptyline). A suggested regimen is amitriptyline, 25 mg three times a day and 75 mg at night, gradually increased over a period of 2 weeks. Slow increase and adequate evening dosage reduce the unpleasant anticholinergic, hypotensive, and sedative effects of the drug. It is important to inform the patient that no subjective improvement in his mood will occur for 2 to 3 weeks. Analgesic effects may occur more rapidly. When anxiety, agitation, and muscle spasm are present, diazepam, 5 mg two to four times daily, should be added to the drug regimen. Barbiturates are avoided because they tend to be antanalgesic, and long-term therapy frequently induces depression. Combination analgesic-barbiturate drugs (*e.g.*, sodium pentobarbitone and codeine) are particularly unsuitable for these reasons. Phenothiazines are prescribed by some clinicians, but, again, they may aggravate depression and are best reserved for the treatment of insomnia or, in terminal cases, to keep the patient totally unaware of the environment.[83]

Patients with chronic pain have invariably been treated with analgesic drugs for a considerable time. It is usually failure of the powerful opioid analgesics to relieve pain, or the unfounded fear of producing addiction, that motivates the medical practitioner to seek advice on alternative forms of therapy. The best time to refer a patient for assessment is when the moderately strong, oral analgesics (*e.g.*, codeine phosphate) have ceased to be effective. This may be due to an increase in the intensity of the pain, the development of tolerance to the analgesic, or the appearance of such distressing side-effects as loss of appetite, gastric irritation, or constipation. Once a patient has become physically dependent on a powerful opioid analgesic, it may be exceedingly difficult to assess the efficacy of a nerve block or plan a satisfactory sequential analgesic regimen. It should be remembered that even when a neurolytic block has been a technical success, supplementary analgesics may be required because the disease has spread beyond the anatomic limits of the block or the patient has developed drug dependence. In malignant disease a primary objective of a neurolytic block is to keep the patient ambulant and on oral medication during the advanced stages of the illness. Regular injections of morphine or meperidine (pethidine) may be required, but the patient can usually be maintained on oral codeine, morphine, or methadone.

Techniques. Precise unilateral segmental blocks can be produced at any spinal level from the cervical region to the perineum by the *subarachnoid injection* of a neurolytic agent. *Epidural injection* can achieve similar results, but the anesthesia is bilateral and may not be as profound. Because the pain-carrying fibers of a spinal nerve cannot be selectively destroyed, neurologic complications are unavoidable in some patients; they are uncommon in the midthoracic region but are more common in the sacral area.

Celiac plexus block will denervate upper abdominal organs and relieve pain caused by disease in these viscera and in the abdominal aorta. The latter may occur with lower limb pain and necessitate lumbar sympathetic block as well. *Lumbar sympathetic block* alone will relieve lower limb pain when it has an autonomic component (see Table 24-3 and Figs. 24-4 and 24-5).

Peripheral nerves may effectively be blocked with a neurolytic agent by simple modification of the standard techniques used with local anesthetics. In the sensory branches of the cranial nerves, the effect of these blocks in relieving pain from head and neck cancer has been most encouraging. With peripheral sensory nerves, however, experience has been less rewarding, owing to the relatively high incidence of neuritis, tissue necrosis, and, more rarely, transverse myelitis and motor paresis. In some clinics, cryoprobe block has been an exception to these problems.

When a destructive procedure is contemplated, careful consideration should be given to the most effective method available. For example, evidence is now accumulating that balloon compression, *thermogangliolysis*, and *glycerol injection* are excellent alternatives to surgical section of the trigeminal ganglion.[100] These are the treatments of choice for trigeminal neuralgia, which is unresponsive to carbamazepine, since the results of these new approaches are more predictable than alcohol injection. Recently, *cryoanalgesia* has been used to control pain of both benign and malignant origin.[9,70] While the technique appears useful for postoperative pain, its role in the treatment of chronic pain requires further evaluation.

The results of neurolytic nerve block are disappointing in patients with widespread or poorly localized pain, when drug dependence dominates the clinical picture, in midline lower back pain, in the ambulant patient with minimal pain, and, in subarachnoid block, in the presence of vertebral metastases.[64]

Before any permanent nerve block is performed, the implications must be discussed with the patient or his relatives and the advantages and possible complications of the procedure fully understood by all. It is most unwise to attempt such procedures in unwilling or uncooperative patients. Workers at many pain clinics believe that it is essential to use an initial diagnostic block with reversible local anesthetic agent as part of the workup to assess the suitability of the patient for a permanent block. Sometimes the use of placebo agents is also favored in assessment (see Chap. 31).

Assessment of Results. Considerable objective improvement in drug requirements, sleep pattern, appetite, general activity, and mood can be observed after a technically successful nerve block. Subjectively, however, patients may deny any significant relief. This response may be due to the unmasking of other pains, preoccupation with side-effects of the block, depression, narcotic dependence, or other causes. Assessment of the results of a block is, therefore, difficult, and while it is not suggested that the patient's opinion be disregarded, other factors should also be considered.[53,64,74,102] In contrast, success may be obscured by withdrawal symptoms after too rapid cessation of analgesic therapy; it is thus extremely important to reduce analgesic therapy slowly. Finally, the opinions of relatives, friends, and nursing staff are invaluable in the assessment.

ROLE OF NEUROLYTIC BLOCKS COMPARED WITH ALTERNATIVES

The more effective use of oral opioid drugs and "coanalgesics" (see Table 24-1) has made it possible to treat more than 70% of patients with these measures alone. In one major study of 1229 cancer patients with pain, neurolytic blocks were required in less than 30% of patients, but a significant percentage of these patients still needed to continue with a reduced dose of oral opioid[108] (see Chap. 24.1). Neurolytic blocks are mainly indicated in localized unilateral pain, except for pituitary adenolysis, which is suitable for diffuse areas of pain. It should be noted that 60% of cancer patients have or develop multiple pain sources. Thus most neurolytic blocks can relieve cancer pain only temporarily. Because neurolytic blocks may result in long-lasting or permanent sequelae, there has been a definite trend toward the use of oral opioids, subcutaneous opioid infusion, or spinal opioids (see Chap. 28). Some authorities hold that percutaneous neurosurgical techniques, such as percutaneous cordotomy, are more controllable and longer lasting than neurolytic injection techniques (see Chap. 30). However, controlled studies of the relative efficacy and side-effects of the various options for treatment of cancer pain are not available. In particular, objective evaluation of results and side-effects of neurolytic blocks is reported in few studies (see below).

In general, neurolytic blocks are suitable for patients with short life expectancy and well-localized pain. Percutaneous cordotomy can be used to cover a wider area, but not diffuse pain, and with a longer duration of effect than neurolytic blocks. Pituitary adenolysis is still controversial, but recent results indicate an acceptable percentage of patients achieving relief of diffuse pain for in excess of 3 months. Spinal opioids may also be used for diffuse pain and for long periods; however, certain types of cancer pain respond poorly to spinal opioids, and tolerance to opioids may necessitate a change to other spinal antinociceptive drugs (see Chap. 28).

NEUROLYTIC AGENTS

The neuropathologic effects of neurolytic agents are discussed in Chapter 29.1. The agents in most frequent clinical use are ethyl alcohol and phenol. Glycerol is also now used for trigeminal ganglion block. Less commonly used agents include chlorocresol, ammonium sulfate, and cold saline. Lesions can also be made with radiofrequency "heating" (see Chap. 30) and with a cryoprobe (see below). Laser techniques are under development (Chap. 29.1). There are few data on which to base a rational choice of agent. However, glycerol appears to have unique properties for trigeminal block (see below).

Phenol has local anesthetic as well as neurolytic effects. This is an advantage because it is painless to inject and provides a clear indication of the area affected by neurolytic agent. Large systemic doses (8.5 g and above) cause convulsions and then central nervous system depression and cardiovascular collapse. Chronic poisoning results in skin eruptions, gastrointestinal symptoms, and renal toxicity. Clinical doses of phenol in the range of 1 to 10 ml of 1% to 10% solutions (up to 100 mg) are unlikely to cause serious toxicity; however, the foregoing possibilities should be kept in mind. There is some evidence that phenol has a more marked effect on blood vessels than does alcohol (see Chap. 29.1).

SUBARACHNOID BLOCK

The subarachnoid injection of a neurolytic agent is an effective method of pain control and is restricted, ideally, to patients with advanced malignancy in whom the pain is unilateral and limited in extent to a few spinal segments. It should be used with great caution when the pain is bilateral or widespread and when it is due to neurologic or undiagnosed disease.[55,72,102]

Particular care must be taken to avoid increasing the patient's disability through motor weakness, sphincteric incompetence, and loss of positional sense, unless it can be justified by the degree of pain relief that is achieved. The aim is to produce a chemical posterior rhizotomy and interrupt the pain pathways from the affected area. Alcohol, phenol, chlorocresol, cold saline, and ammonium salts have been used in the manner described below.

Subarachnoid Absolute Alcohol

The use of alcohol was first described by Dogliotti in 1931.[30] To produce a precise block of profound intensity and adequate duration, the patient must be carefully positioned so that the maximum concentration of the hypobaric alcohol solution reaches the posterior nerve roots. This means that the patient is placed in the lateral oblique position with the painful side uppermost. Alcohol may be injected where the affected nerve leaves the spinal cord or where it leaves the vertebral canal through the intervertebral foramen. Hay[53] and Swerdlow[102] state that the injection should be at cord level because alcohol exerts its maximal effect on the fine rootlets leaving the spinal cord. On the other hand, the alcohol concentration is probably greater where the posterior root enters the dura, and, for this reason, injection at the vertebral level may be preferred. The controversy relates only to the lumbosacral and lower thoracic spinal nerves because at higher levels the nerves pass horizontally from the cord to their point of exit at intervertebral foramina (Fig. 29-22). The principal pathologic effects produced by alcohol are demyelination and degeneration of the dorsal root with some chromatolysis and swelling of the dorsal root with secondary degeneration of the posterior columns (see Chap. 29.1).[53,54]

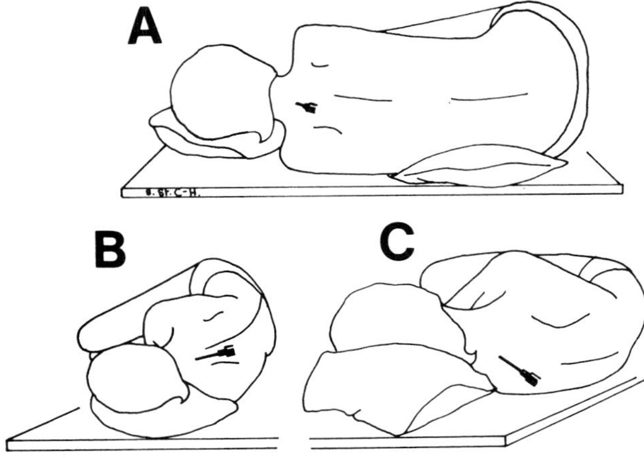

FIG. 29-23. Positioning of the patient for a cervical subarachnoid injection. **A.** Posterior view. **B.** Lateral-prone position used for the injection of absolute alcohol. **C.** Lateral-supine position used for the injection of hyperbaric solutions.

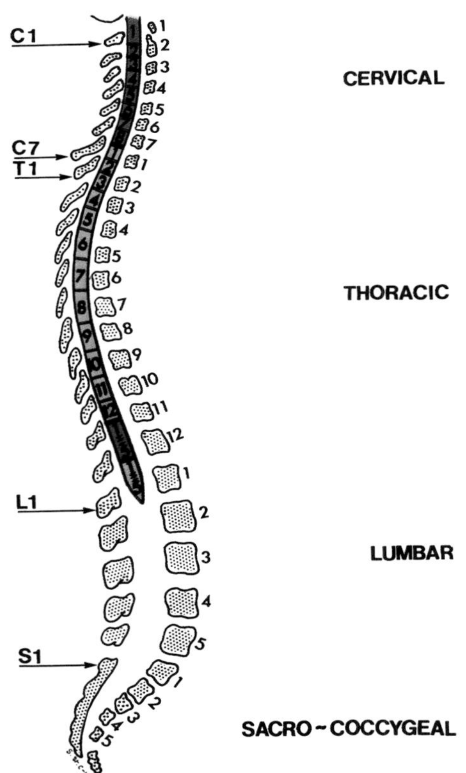

FIG. 29-22. This drawing of the vertebral column and spinal cord indicates their segmental relationships. Significant difference between the vertebral and cord levels occurs only in the lower thoracic and lumbosacral regions.

Technique has been well described.[15,53,54,72,102] The patient is placed on an operating table with the affected side upward, in the oblique lateral position with the body about 45° to the horizontal (Figs. 29-23 to 29-25). Breaking the table at the proposed injection site assists in maintaining the posterior roots in the uppermost position. The free-flow of cerebrospinal fluid (CSF) through a fine needle may be minimal, owing to low intrathecal pressure, but it may be improved through rotation of the spinal needle or aspiration with a 1-ml tuberculin syringe.

To limit the spread of alcohol in the subarachnoid space to the affected segments, the volume of solution injected should be small and the rate of injection slow. If the area involved is relatively extensive, multiple segmental injections of a small volume are preferable to a single larger injection. If the pain is confined to one or two spinal segments, a single injection of 0.5 to1.0 ml may be injected at each alternate interspace up to a total dose of 1.5 ml, and the injection time should be more than 2 minutes at each site. The patient may experience a burning pain or unpleasant paresthesia for a few seconds, but this rapidly subsides as complete analgesia supervenes. However, it can be a valuable guide that the correct segments are being blocked.

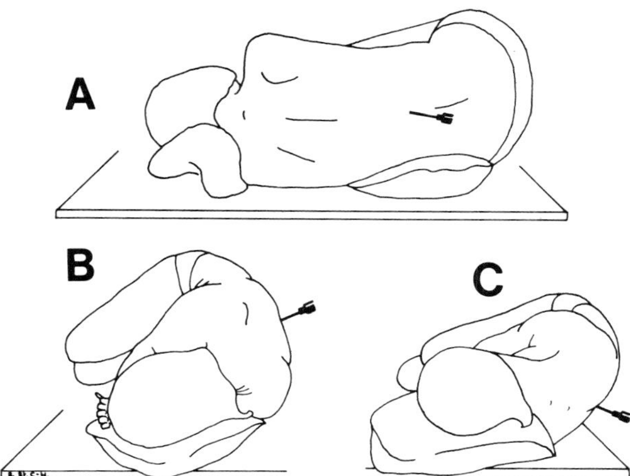

FIG. 29-24. Positioning for the patient for subarachnoid injection in the thoracolumbar region **A.** Posterior view. **B.** Lateral-prone position used for the injection of absolute alcohol. **C.** Lateral-supine position used for the injection of hyperbaric solutions.

Matsuki, Kato, and Ichiyanagi demonstrated that when the dose does not exceed 1 ml, the alcohol concentration in the CSF falls rapidly and allows the patient to be repositioned in the supine posture in 15 to 20 minutes without any fear of an unwanted extension of the block.[81] The supine position will reduce the incidence of spinal headache, particularly when a dural tap has been performed at several levels.

Bilateral Pain. Two techniques have been described to treat bilateral pain. The patient may be placed in the prone position with the affected segments uppermost over the break in the operating table. The injected alcohol will then spread to both posterior roots. Alternatively, each side may be blocked on separate occasions, 2 to 3 days apart, when the effect of the initial injection can be assessed before the second procedure is attempted.

Results. The difficulty of assessing results has already been mentioned, but within the limitations imposed by the subjective nature of the patient's response, various authors have claimed that approximately 50% of the results are good, 30% fair, and 20% poor (Table 29-1).[17]

A review of a large number of series of alcohol subarachnoid blocks reported an average of 60% good relief, 21% fair relief, and 18% poor relief.[32] It should be acknowledged that there were large differences in types and sites of tumor, sites and doses of alcohol injection, and methods of pain assessment. Thus it is possible that better results can be obtained for some cancer pain problems with specific neurolytic techniques; current data do not permit such an analysis. In most clinics, alcohol is injected close to the affected segments, and it is held that this increases efficacy and safety. The authors are aware of some clinics where injections are often made in the high lumbar region and then posture is used to attempt to direct the neurolytic solution to the affected segments of the spinal cord. This may account for the unacceptably high complication rates in some parts of the world, since large doses injected close to the lumbosacral enlargement of the spinal cord pose a considerable risk of spinal cord damage to segments involved in urinary bladder and lower limbs as well as other areas of the spinal cord. An important aspect of safe technique is precise placement of solution, correct use of posture, and use of minimal effective doses.

Duration of pain relief has seldom been documented with careful follow-up studies. In Table 29-1. "good" means complete relief of pain for more than 1 month; "fair" means complete pain relief for less than 1 month or reduction of pain for more than 1 month; "poor" means relief for several days or no relief. Some reports indicate a mean duration of pain relief of between 2 weeks and 3 months (see references 32 and 102). A few patients obtain pain relief for 4 to 12 months.

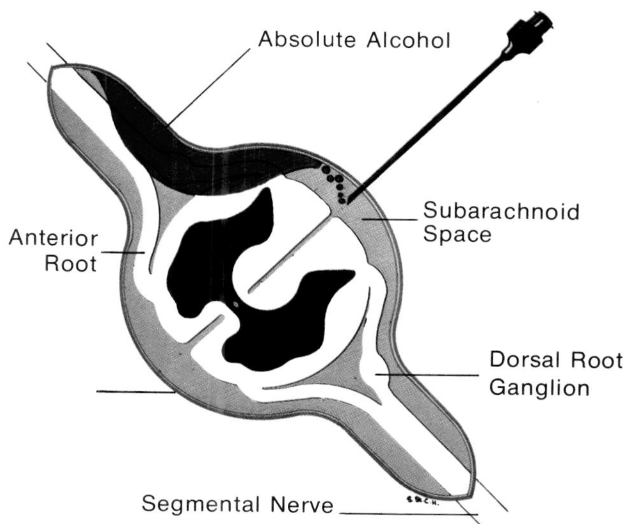

FIG. 29-25. The lateral-prone position used for the injection of absolute alcohol places the posterior nerve roots uppermost.

TABLE 29-1. RESULTS OF SUBARACHNOID BLOCK WITH ALCOHOL

Author	Number of Cases	Percentage Results		
		Good	Fair	Poor
Dogliotti (1931)[30]	150	59	25	16
Stern (1934)	50	63	27	10
Greenhill and Schmitz (1935)	25	80	12	8
Abbot (1936)	25	84	8	8
Adson (1937)	36	44	25	31
Peyton, Semansky, and Baker (1937)	33	34	27	39
Greenhill (1947)	>100	60	10	30
Bonica (1958)[17]	Unstated	50	30	20
Hay (1962)[53]	252	46	32	22
Tank, Dohn, and Gardner (1963)	13	54	15	31
Kuzucu, Derrick, and Wilber (1966)[64]	322	58.2	26.1	15.7
Combined series in review by Drechsel (1984)[32]	1908	60	21	19

(Data from Kuzucu, E.Y., Derrick, W.S., and Wilbur, S.A.: Control of intractable pain with subarachnoid alcohol block. J.A.M.A., *195*:541, 1966; and Swerdlow, M. [ed.]: Relief of Intractable Pain. 3rd ed. Amsterdam, Excerpta Medica, 1983)

Subarachnoid Phenol

Phenol has been recommended as a neurolytic agent on the basis that its action is differential, sparing the large myelinated fibers while destroying the small unmyelinated C fibers.[77,80,87] However, Bonica[15] and Lund[72] do not regard this differential effect as clinically significant, and there is now a wealth of experimental evidence to support this view (see Chap. 29.1). The block produced by phenol tends to be less profound and of shorter duration than that produced by alcohol (Tables 29-1 and 29-2). The incidence of bladder paresis is reported to be lower than with alcohol (see Table 29-4). However, Swerdlow[102] reported a series of 145 patients who received subarachnoid phenol and had complication rates similar to those reported for alcohol (see reference 18).

Phenol has been used as a 5% to 6% solution in glycerine (with or without silver nitrate, 0.6 mg/ml) or as a 7.5% to 10% solution in iophendylate.[6,72,77,80,87,102] Silver nitrate as an additive has largely been abandoned because of the meningeal irritation it can produce.[87] Phenol in glycerine is more effective than phenol in iophendylate because the glycerine diffuses more rapidly from the solvent to produce a higher neurolytic concentration.[80,87] Unlike absolute alcohol, all these phenol solutions are hyperbaric and viscous and deteriorate during storage, although this has been overemphasized, since deterioration takes at least 1 year.[79] Glycerine delays release of the active constituent phenol and thus facilitates the use of gravity to direct the neurolytic solution downward past structures not to be blocked and onto nerve roots delineated for blockade (Fig. 29-26).

Technique. Segmental subarachnoid blocking with phenol requires that the patient lie on the painful side in a semilateral/supine position so that the posterior nerve roots are dependent (see Figs. 29-23, 29-24, and 29-26). This may be quite distressing for some patients. In other respects, the technique similar to that previously described for alcohol. Swerdlow states that phenol acts on the nerve root just before it pierces the dura, and therefore the injection should be made at the vertebral level that corresponds to the spinal cord segments involved.[102]

The phenol solution should have been prepared within the past 6 to 12 months or within an expiration date determined by the pharmacy. It may be warmed to reduce viscosity, but a moderately wide-bore spinal needle is still required for the injection (although the use of a 1-ml tuberculin syringe obviates this). Swerdlow places emphasis on choosing the most favorable interspace in relation to the segments required to be blocked but injects up to 1 ml at this single site with subsequent posturing of the patient to assist with the spread of solution to adjacent segments.[101]

In addition to its neurolytic effect, phenol has an initial local anesthetic action, producing warmth and a tingling, or prickling sensation over the distribution of the affected nerve. Ichiyanagi and colleagues considered that if this local anesthetic effect does not

TABLE 29-2. RESULTS OF SUBARACHNOID BLOCK WITH PHENOL

<table>
<tr><th rowspan="2">Author</th><th rowspan="2">Number of Cases</th><th colspan="3">Percentage Results</th></tr>
<tr><th>Good</th><th>Fair</th><th>Poor</th></tr>
<tr><td>Mark and colleagues (1962)[38]</td><td>57
(phenol in iophendylate)</td><td>26</td><td>24</td><td>50</td></tr>
<tr><td></td><td>30
(phenol in glycerine)</td><td>30</td><td>40</td><td>30</td></tr>
<tr><td>Stovner and Endresen (1962)</td><td>151</td><td colspan="2">77</td><td>23</td></tr>
<tr><td>Tank, Dohn, and Gardner (1963)</td><td>23</td><td>48</td><td>18</td><td>34</td></tr>
<tr><td>Wilkinson, Mark, and White (1963)</td><td>30</td><td colspan="2">70</td><td>30</td></tr>
<tr><td>Ball, Pearce, and Davies (1964)[6]</td><td>51</td><td>41</td><td>33</td><td>26</td></tr>
<tr><td>Maher (1972)</td><td>433</td><td>62</td><td>6</td><td>32</td></tr>
<tr><td>Brown (1972)</td><td>114</td><td>68</td><td>5</td><td>27</td></tr>
<tr><td colspan="5">(Data from Swerdlow, M. [ed.]: Relief of Intractable Pain. 3rd ed. Amsterdam, Excerpta Medica, 1983)</td></tr>
<tr><td>Papo and Visca (1976)</td><td>282</td><td>40</td><td>35</td><td>25</td></tr>
<tr><td>Swerdlow (1983)[102]</td><td>200</td><td>56</td><td>19</td><td>25</td></tr>
</table>

develop within 2 to 3 minutes, the concentration of phenol is insufficient to produce an effective neurolytic block.[56] They state that rapid dilution and diffusion of the phenol in the CSF prevents extension of the block even if the patient is repositioned. Like alcohol, the concentration of phenol in the CSF falls below that required for neurolysis within 15 minutes, and the patient need be specially positioned only for that period.[56]

Because phenol is hyperbaric, it has a particular advantage when it is used to produce saddle block anesthesia in patients with midline pain owing to pelvic cancer.[58,91] With the patient in the sitting position, 1 to 2 ml of 6% phenol in glycerine injected at L4–5 or L5–S1 provides excellent pain relief with minimal or transient motor weakness or sphincteric disturbance (Fig. 29-27). Swerdlow, however, prefers unilateral blocks on both sides and reserves the saddle block for terminal or advanced cases and when unilateral block fails.[102]

Results. The results, as reported in Table 29-2, are generally slightly inferior to the figures for subarachnoid alcohol block and the effects are of shorter duration.

A series of 200 patients reported by Swerdlow had pain relief of similar efficacy and duration to that reported for alcohol (see Refs. 18 and 102).

Subarachnoid Chlorocresol

Maher[78] and Swerdlow[102] have reported the use of intrathecal chlorocresol and claimed that the agent

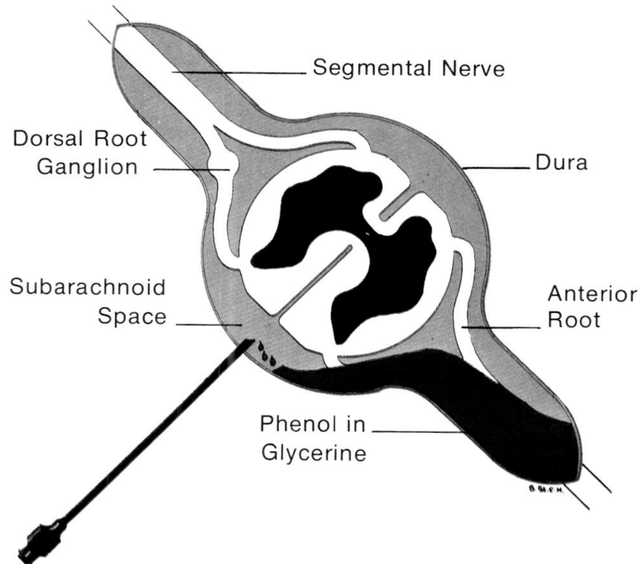

FIG. 29-26. The lateral-supine position used for the injection of phenol and other hyperbaric solutions ensures that the posterior nerve roots are dependent.

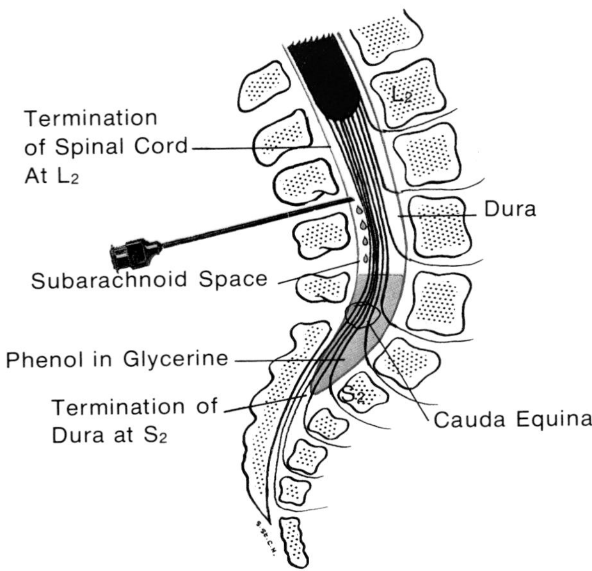

FIG. 29-27. Saddle block with phenol and other hyperbaric solutions is used in the treatment of midline perineal pain of malignant origin.

was more effective than phenol (Table 29-3), although Swerdlow recorded an increased incidence of complications (in particular, paresis and numbness; Table 29-4).[78,102] The solution used, 1:50 or 1:40 chlorocresol in glycerine, is hyperbaric. The technique was similar to that described for phenol. Chlorocresol does not produce any sensation on injection, and the anesthesiologist must wait for the disapperance of pain or onset of numbness to confirm the correct positioning of the needle. Swerdlow uses the repeated injection of 0.1-ml increments of chlorocresol at a single site and tilts the operating table to produce the desired effect. Five-tenths to 0.7 ml is recommended in the sacral region, 0.5 to 0.8 ml in the lumbar region, and 0.6 to 1.0 ml in the thoracic region.

Subarachnoid Cold Saline

The intrathecal injection of cold 0.9% saline (2°–4°C), is claimed to have a specific action on the pain-carrying C fibers, sparing the larger fibers that subserve other sensory, motor, and autonomic functions. Cerebrospinal fluid is withdrawn, and the cold saline is then injected rapidly. Ten milliliters is the recommended dose, although up to 60 ml has been given. The procedure is quite distressing to the patient, and heavy sedation or even general anesthesia is recommended. The incidence of complications with subarachnoid cold saline is low but significant, and the pain relief is usually only short-lived.[102]

Subarachnoid Ammonium Salts

In 1943, Bates described the intrathecal use of an extract of the insectivorous pitcher plant, *Sarracenia purpurea*, for the treatment of intractable pain.[10] The active ingredient was ammonium sulfate, which appeared to exert a specific action on the pain-carrying C fibers.

Prolonged pain relief was reported but Hand,[15] Bonica,[51] and Lund[72] were disappointed with the results. Complications such as nausea and vomiting, headache, paresthesia, and spinal cord damage have been documented.[49,51]

Overview of Results of Subarachnoid Neurolytic Blocks

In the hands of highly skilled experts, the results of phenol and alcohol are probably similar, with good results in about 50% of patients. Provided selection of patients is appropriate and technique is meticulous, complication rates in the range of 1% to 14% occur. These complications may be an acceptable "price" in some patients. For example, if a bladder catheter is *in situ*, bladder paresis is no price to pay. However, ambulatory patients will never choose to lose control of bladder function even if pain relief by alternative methods is slightly inferior. There are still too few data on efficacy of neurolytic blocks for specific tumor site and types, for different types of pain (somatic versus visceral) and for different pain characteristics (continuous, intermittent, and so forth). It is possible that some series include cancer pain that is unlikely to be responsive to neurolytic blocks (*e.g.*, "deafferentation" pain; see Chap. 24.1). Current re-

TABLE 29-3. COMPARISON OF NEUROLYTIC EFFECTS OF PHENOL AND CHLOROCRESOL

		Percentage Results		
Agent	**Number of Cases**	**Good**	**Fair**	**Poor**
Phenol	46	41	26	33
Chlorocresol	42	48	33	19

(Data from Swerdlow, M.: Intrathecal chlorocresol. A comparison with phenol in the treatment of intractable pain. Anaesthesia, *28*:297, 1973)

ports indicate that subarachnoid neurolytic blocks are best for relatively localized somatic pain of the trunk or in bilateral saddle pain in patients with colostomy and permanent bladder catheter.[32] More controversial uses are in neck and shoulder pain. In limb pain, the risk of producing a useless limb seldom justifies use of subarachnoid neurolytic blocks.

COMPLICATIONS

The complications encountered are usually of two kinds. First, there are those seen with any intrathecal injection — the self-limiting spinal headache — or the rare problems of mechanical neural damage, infection, and arachnoiditis.[72,102]

Second, there are complications that result from the action of neurolytic substances on nerve fibers not concerned in the mediation of pain. These include motor paresis, loss of sphincteric function, impairment of touch and proprioception, and troublesome dysesthesias[102,103] (see Chap. 23).

Complication rates reported by various authors are shown in Table 29-4 (see also Tables 23-1 through 23-4). Fortunately, complications are usually transient, although fatal meningitis, paraplegia, and permanent impairment of urinary function have been recorded.[53,64] The reported case of fatal meningitis was believed to have arisen as a result of meningeal irritation from silver nitrate incorporated in the neurolytic solution. The patients with postblock paraplegia were subsequently found to have vertebral metastases.

Complications should be analyzed with respect to the *site* of neurolytic injection and the *duration* of any resulting complications. Injections in the region of the brachial plexus or lumbar plexus have a high risk of motor paresis. This is less likely in the case of the brachial plexus, where posterior roots can be blocked with a reasonable chance of sparing anterior roots. In the lumbosacral enlargement of the cord, nerve roots are grouped closely between the levels of T11 and L1 spinous processes (see Fig. 29-22). Injection of even small volumes may affect anterior roots of a considerable number of segments. Below L1, injection will be made onto the *cauda equina,* where anterior and posterior roots are not separated; thus both motor and sensory effects must be expected.

Injection in the thoracic region has a low complication rate if the dose injected at any one level is minimal. However, patients with severe respiratory disease may be at risk of respiratory failure. Unintentional block of several ventral roots may (rarely) precipitate respiratory failure owing to loss of intercostal activity at those levels.

Techniques aimed at perineal pain in the S4–5 region hope to avoid the bladder segments (S2, S3, S4). However, injection at the L5–S1 level inevitably relies on solution moving by gravity past the important bladder segments to "pool" predominantly in the S4–S5 region. It is claimed that use of a lateral as well as a posterior tilt helps to expose S2–S3 segments minimally and only on one side. However, the risk of bladder paresis with all such techniques is at best 25% and at worst 60% or more.[18,32,58]

Duration of complications has seldom been re-

TABLE 29-4. COMPLICATIONS THAT RESULT FROM INTRATHECAL NEUROLYTIC BLOCK

			Percentage Recorded			
Author	**Agent**	**Paresis**	**Rectal and Urinary Dysfunction**	**Sensory Loss**	**Paresthesia Neuritis**	**Other**
Maher (1955)[77]	Phenol (± silver nitrate)	8	13			Headache, vomiting
Nathan and Scott (1958)[87]	Phenol (± silver nitrate)	14	12			Meningitis
Bonica (1958)[17]	Alcohol	25				
Hay (1962)[53]	Alcohol	1	0.7	1		
Mark and colleagues (1962)[80]	Phenol	8	2.3	3.0	3.4	
McEwen and colleagues (1965)[74]	Alcohol	5	10	10		
Kuzucu and colleagues (1966)[64]	Alcohol	4.6	3.4	3.7	0.3	Tremor, headache
Swerdlow (1973)[101]	Phenol		24	8.7	4	Headache
	Chlorocresol	12	26	21	2.4	Headache

ported. In one series of 2125 alcohol blocks in 1478 patients, the duration of 232 complications was as follows: 28% of the total complications resolved within 3 days, 23% resolved within 1 week, 21% within 1 month, 9% within 4 months, and only 18% lasted longer than 4 months (see Ref. 32). Bladder paresis lasting for more than 7 days was reported by Swerdlow in 7 of 145 patients receiving subarachnoid phenol. In this series, bowel paresis occurred in one patient, muscle paresis and numbness in four patients. A most serious complication is paraplegia owing to interference with the vascular supply to the spinal cord. Presumably, trauma, thrombosis, or direct neurotoxic effects (see Chap. 29.1) result in ischemia when injection is unintentionally made close to a major feeder artery (see Fig. 7-11). This complication is discussed further in Chapters 7 and 23.

Patients with complete obstruction of the subarachnoid space owing to cancer are at risk of neurological deterioration if a lumbar puncture is performed below the level of obstruction. It appears that removal of CSF below the level of spinal obstruction results in downward spinal coning after lumbar puncture.[55] A review was made of 100 patients with complete spinal block demonstrated by myelography. In 50 cases the myelography was done by C1–C2 puncture and in 50 cases by lumbar puncture. Seven patients (14%) had deterioration after lumbar puncture, whereas none deteriorated after C1–C2 puncture.[55]

As discussed later and in Chapter 23, the risk of medicolegal problems resulting from complications can be minimized by observing some practical measures on a routine basis (see Ref. 103).

FAILURE

Finally, the block may fail for reasons that are often difficult to explain anatomically or physiologically. However, it is reported that previous radiation therapy, inflammation in the region of the nerve roots, widespread disease, or opioid dependence will reduce the efficacy of the procedure.[64,102]

Deafferentation Pain and Neurolytic Blocks, and Neuralgic Pain

Neurolytic blocks are mainly effective in pain of "nociceptive" type (see Chap. 24.1). "Deafferentation" pain ("neurogenic") does occur in patients with cancer, for example, those with long-standing brachial plexopathies or well-established complete spinal cord lesions.[21,40] This type of pain responds poorly, if at all, to neurolytic procedures, despite misleading temporary relief with local anesthetic blocks (see Chap. 30). It should also be recognized that sometimes neurolytic blocks may result in sufficient denervation to produce a deafferentation type of pain. On the other hand, incomplete neural destruction by neurolytic blocks may produce a neuralgic type of pain. Both of these problems are most appropriately treated by transcutaneous electrical nerve stimulation, centrally acting drugs, or, less commonly, dorsal column stimulation[21] (see Chap. 30).

SUBDURAL BLOCK

Cancer pain involving the cervical segments is difficult to relieve with subarachnoid neurolytic block. This is because the neurolytic solution is rapidly diluted by the CSF from the nearby rapidly circulating intracranial CSF (see Fig. 28-7). Also, there is some difficulty restricting the neurolytic agents to the desired segments. Subdural extra-arachnoid neurolytic block has been used in an attempt to overcome these problems.[21,38,59] The subdural space is a potential space between the dura and the arachnoid mater, and the two membranes are separated by a thin fluid film (see Fig. 7-7). The subdural space is separated from the subarachnoid space by the arachnoid mater and extends laterally for a short distance, where it widens in the region of the nerve roots (see Fig. 7-7). It is apparent that injection of fluid into the space converts a potential space into an actual space that extends cranially to the foramen magnum and caudally to the level of the termination of the dura at S2. The subdural space is wider in the cervical region and is thus easier to enter there than at other levels of the spine. Throughout the subdural space there are trabeculae of connective tissue coursing between dura and arachnoid—similar to those shown in Figure 7-7 in the subarachnoid space. These trabeculae in the subdural space, and its narrow width, account for the "honeycomb" appearance in radiographs taken after injection of contrast media subdurally (see Fig. 7-6).

It may appear difficult, or even impossible, to place a needletip in the subdural space. However, radiologists performing myelograms report that they frequently enter this space. Subdural injection is probably the explanation for at least some failed or "patchy" attempted subarachnoid and epidural local anesthetic blocks.

Technique

Investigation of the pathology in the cervical region should precede any type of block (see below under "epidural"). A short-bevel needle is introduced into the epidural space using standard technique (see Chap. 8). It is desirable to keep the needle in the midline to aid subsequent bilateral spread of injected solution in the subdural space. The level of insertion of the needle may be chosen close to the affected segments; however, it may be convenient to use the C7–T1 interspace (see Chap. 8). The spread of solution is minimally affected by gravity and depends more on the volume injected and any local deformities in the spinal canal. An image intensifier is used to check that the needle is in the midline. In the anteroposterior view, the needletip should lie precisely in the line of the spinous processes. In the lateral view, the tip of the needle should be in line with the posterior wall of the cervical canal (see Fig. 29-28). A 0.5-ml syringe or a 1-ml tuberculin syringe filled with saline is connected to the needle in the epidural space. The needle is advanced while continuous pressure is exerted on the plunger of the syringe. As the needle enters the subdural space, an *increased* resistance is felt. Injection of 0.1 to 0.2 ml of contrast medium (*e.g.*, metrizamide) produces a classic "fine line" a few millimeters anterior to the plane of the posterior wall of the spinal canal. Injection of larger volumes does not increase this line. Also, a second line is produced anteriorly, where the contrast medium tends to arrange itself like a "rosary" in the dural root sleeves (Fig. 29-28). In contrast, epidural injection would produce only a blurred, patchy image. Subarachnoid injection produces a small, pulsating cylinder that moves gravitationally. The anteroposterior view is quite characteristic: bilateral images like a nail scratch shape are seen, confined to the spinal canal over four or more segments (Fig. 29-29). Injection of a large amount of contrast medium produces a trabecular honeycomb appearance outlining the dural space. Approximately 24 hours later an image of the nerve roots may appear if the patient is screened under radiography. Racz and associates have reported a soft-tip, wire spiral, fluoropolymer-coated catheter. It is claimed that the catheter is less likely to kink or migrate into the CSF. Also, the catheter is radiopaque and its position can be confirmed under image intensifier control.[93]

Phenol 5% to 10% in glycerin has been used in doses from 0.5 to 2.5 ml.[59] However, phenol 10% in metrizamide would have the advantage of direct visualization during injection. In a series of 25 patients with head/neck cancer, results were evaluated as follows: "good" if the patient was free of pain until death or until the end of follow-up at 3 months; "fair" if there was a decrease in use of analgesics or if pain disappeared completely for at least 20 days; lesser degrees of pain relief were classified as failures. Nine of the 25 patients (36%) had good results, 7 (28%) had fair results, and 9 (36%) were "failures."[59] The criteria used are quite demanding, and the results indicate that the technique may be useful for some patients. In particular, there is no need for the use of posture; the patient may be sitting or lying. Also, a catheter may be inserted and subsequent doses given to improve block. The results may be slightly inferior

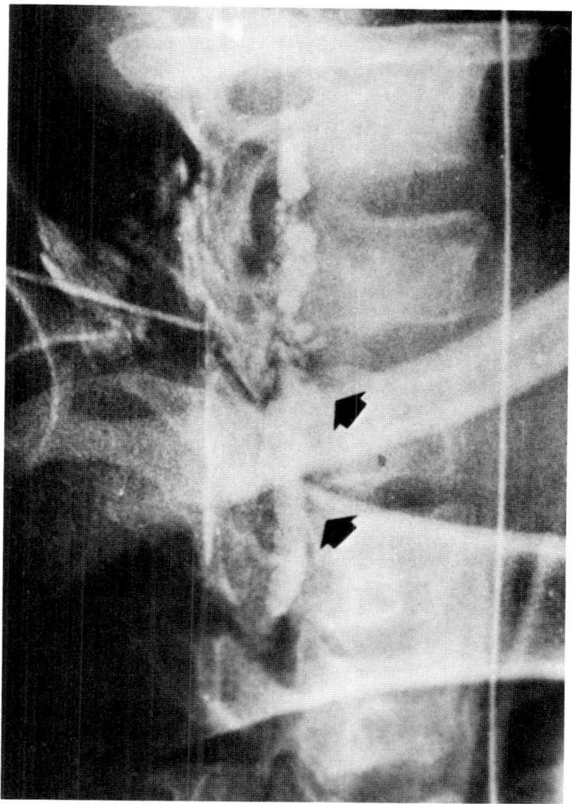

FIG. 29-28. Subdural block. Radiograph showing lateral view. Needletip has been placed in the subdural space and 0.5 ml of iophendylate (Myodil) has been injected. Note the fine line extending up and down from needletip. Also, there is a second broader line (arrows) in which contrast medium tends to arrange itself like a "rosary." (Ischia, S., Maffezzoli, G.F., Luzzani, A., and Pacini, L.: Subdural extra-arachnoid neurolytic block in cervical pain. Pain, *14*:347, 1982)

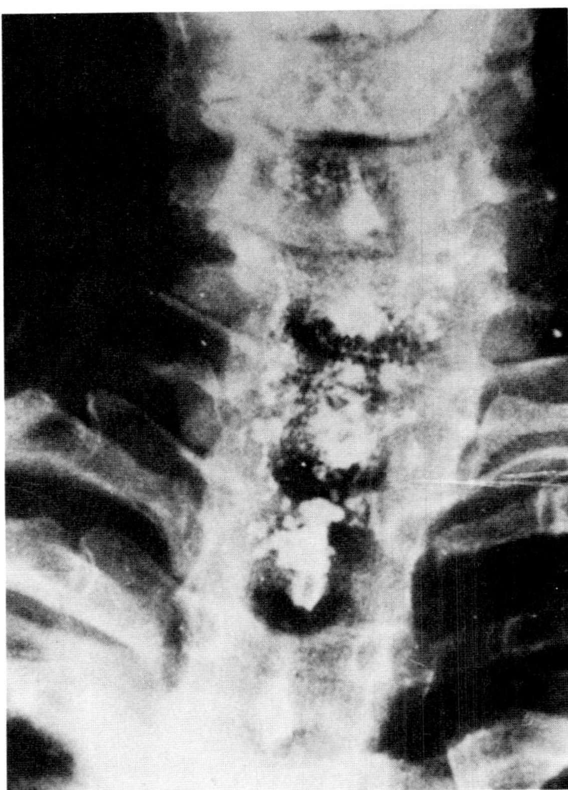

FIG. 29-29. Subdural block. Radiograph showing anteroposterior view after injection of 0.5 ml of Myodil. Note the bilateral spread confined to the interior of the canal, over several segments. The appearance of the contrast medium is like a "nail scratch" shape. (Ischia, S., Maffezzoli, G.F., Luzzani, A., and Pacini, L.: Subdural extra-arachnoid neurolytic block in cervical pain. Pain, *14*:347, 1982)

to subarachnoid block, although the evaluation criteria are different.

Cervical subdural block has been reported to be useful for pain caused by neoplastic disease of the ear, nose, and throat[59] as well as by other cancer encroaching on the cervical region, such as Pancoast syndrome and cervical vertebral metastases.[59] The place of this technique compared with subarachnoid neurolytic block and spinal opioids remains to be determined.

EPIDURAL NEUROLYTIC BLOCK

Some authorities use epidural neurolytic block above the T6 level because of the greater difficulty in obtaining consistent results with subarachnoid block, owing to the shape and capacity of the spinal canal at this level[21] (see above). Epidural neurolytic block is thus an alternative to the "subdural" approach for pain in the region of the neck, shoulder, and arm.[21,39] Myelography, computed tomography (CT) scan, or nuclear magnetic resonance (NMR) scan should be performed before making a decision to use epidural neurolytic block. This is because epidural or intrathecal invasion by tumor poses a risk of bleeding that may result in spinal cord compression and neurological deficit, including quadriplegia. Also, the distortion of the epidural space may lead to unpredictable spread of the neurolytic solution.

Technique

The C7–T1 interspace is the easiest space anatomically, since the spinous processes are almost horizontal at this level (see Table 8-3). An epidural catheter is inserted using standard technique, as presented in Chapter 8. The placement of the catheter may be checked by the injection of a small amount of contrast media (*e.g.*, metrizamide), which should produce a rather diffuse outline immediately anterior to the posterior wall of the vertebral canal. This is distinguished from subarachnoid and subdural injection as described earlier. Catheter placement can also be checked by injecting small doses of local anesthetic (*e.g.*, 2-ml doses of 1% lidocaine) at 15- to 20-minute intervals. Such doses should result in a narrow band of segmental sensory loss. In comparison, subdural block with such a dose is a diffuse and "patchy" type of block and subarachnoid block would result in a wide area of block accompanied by hypotension and perhaps bradycardia. Once the volume of local anesthetic required to block the affected dermatomes is determined, the block is allowed to wear off and at least 2 hours is allowed for recovery. This is important, since residual local anesthetic may cause the subsequent phenol injection to spread further and have a more profound effect, at least initially. In particular, the combination of the two drugs may produce an alarming degree of motor block. This may cause embarrassment of respiratory function in patients with respiratory disease but may also cause considerable anxiety to the patient and doctor. If bupivacaine is used for the diagnostic block, it is preferable to allow 24 hours between diagnostic and therapeutic blocks to avoid motor effects of the combination of bupivacaine and phenol.[93] The neurolytic solution most widely used is phenol in concentrations ranging from 5% to 10%. Swerdlow reports the use of 7% to 10% phenol, in glycerine (see

Ref. 18). Brown uses 7.5% phenol in glycerine,[21] Doyle uses 5% phenol in oil,[31] Ferrer–Brechner reports the use of 10% phenol in 10% glycerine,[39] and Racz and colleagues use 6% phenol in saline.[93] The ideal concentration and composition of solution of phenol has not been determined. It may be beneficial to inject the phenol as an emulsion in a water-soluble contrast medium, such as metrizamide; this would permit visualization of the spread of solution under image intensifier. However, no data on this approach are available.

Racz and co-workers report a technique of multiple epidural injections of 6% phenol in saline. Approximately 1 to 5 ml is injected on each occasion.[93] Other authorities prefer to limit the volume to only 1 ml at a time.[21] With phenol-in-saline solutions, onset of pain relief is rapid (1 to 2 minutes). With phenol-in-glycerine solutions, onset of pain relief takes 5 to 10 minutes. During the next 24 to 48 hours, sometimes attacks of lancinating pain may occur and this may require temporary treatment with opioid drugs.[21] After 2 or 3 days the pain is reassessed and, if necessary, a further dose is given. Sometimes pain relief is adequate for 2 to 3 weeks and then pain returns and the injection needs to be repeated.[93]

In a series of 18 patients with cancer pain treated by epidural phenol, 6 of 7 patients with metastatic cancer had pain relief on discharge from hospital. Pain relief lasted for 1 to 3 months in two of the patients with metastases and in three of the patients with primary cancer. A second series of injections increased the duration of relief in these patients experiencing pain relief of less than 1 month.[93] This is a small series and other reports are anecdotal.[21,31] This technique requires further objective evaluation of efficacy and incidence of side-effects.

It is claimed that satisfactory results can also be obtained at lumbar and caudal sites of catheter insertion.[21,93] However, data are not available.

TRANSSACRAL NEUROLYTIC NERVE BLOCK

Perineal pain caused by inoperable secondary cancer of the rectum or after abdominoperineal resection may be treated by transsacral neurolytic block. Perineal sensory innervation is predominantly derived from the S4 dermatome. The S4 nerve root is accessible on each side by way of the appropriate posterior sacral foramen (see Chap. 9). The S5 root is immediately adjacent to S4 and is likely to be blocked at the same time. However, the use of small volumes of solution prevents cephalad spread.

The detailed anatomy of the sacral nerve roots is shown in Figures 9-1 and 9-2, and block technique is shown in Figure 11-4. Briefly, the skin is infiltrated over the foramen, a needle is inserted to contact the posterior surface of the sacrum, and the depth is noted. The foramen is then located and the needle is inserted 1 cm into the foramen. Position may be checked with an image intensifier. After careful aspiration, 2 to 2.5 ml of 6% aqueous phenol is injected, followed by 0.25 ml of local anesthetic to clear the needle before removal. An initial diagnostic block, 24 hours previously, with the same volume of 0.5% bupivacaine may be helpful in deciding whether to use the neurolytic technique.[94] In a series of nine patients, pain relief with the first injection was less than 1 weeks' duration in six of the patients, 10 days in one, and 202 and 414 days in the other two. A second injection resulted in pain relief ranging from 18 days to 122 days.[94] However, treatment was repeated on an outpatient basis and there were no disturbances of bladder or motor function and sensory changes were limited to the perineum.[94] Another application is the treatment of bladder spasticity and pain. A prospective study evaluated the results of injection of 2 ml of 6% of aqueous phenol at S3 in 15 patients.[97] Patients initially received a diagnostic block with 0.5% bupivacaine. Then 2 ml of 6% aqueous phenol were injected through the right S3 sacral foramen using standard techniques (see Fig. 11-4). If pain relief was inadequate after 24 to 48 hours, another injection was made through the left S3 sacral foramen. Sometimes further injections were required 24 to 48 hours later through S2 or S4 foramina. Ten of the patients who received bupivacaine subsequently received phenol. Of these, seven reported significant long-lasting pain relief, one had pain relief for 1 week, and two received no benefit. The average follow-up period was 24 months and the duration of response in patients with persistent pain relief was at least this long. No patient suffered urinary or rectal incontinence. In the patients responding, 5 of 11 patients with interstitial cystitis had complete or significant sustained pain relief. Of three patients with postirradiation hemorrhagic cystitis, two had persistent pain relief, while the third had temporary relief. One patient with a neurogenic spastic bladder had no recurrence of pain after 22 months.[97]

TRIGEMINAL NERVE BLOCK

Neurolytic block of the trigeminal nerve and its branches has been used effectively in the management of chronic pain. Maxillary and mandibular nerve blocks are particularly useful in controlling pain of malignant origin that arises from structures that the nerves supply. In the past, injection of the gasserian ganglion with alcohol was widely used in the treatment of trigeminal neuralgia, but as indicated earlier, other methods, such as balloon compression, glycerol injection,[50,73] surgical rhizotomy, and thermogangliolysis[71,96,100] have largely superseded this technique. Gasserian ganglion blockade is a difficult procedure, and of the many methods described, Härtel's approach has proved most popular (see Fig. 15-5). This technique has been well described and illustrated in Chapters 15 and 30.

Hakanson reported that 86% of patients were initially free of pain after injection of 0.2 to 0.4 ml of glycerol.[50] However, subsequent follow-up has revealed a 31% recurrence rate over 1 to 6 years in 100 patients (see Chap. 30). The advantage of the glycerol technique is the minimal change in facial skin sensation. Histopathology and evoked potentials were studied in cats after glycerol injection into trigeminal ganglion. Glycerol increased the average latencies and reduced the average amplitude of brain stem-evoked potentials. Histopathology included focal demyelination and axonal swelling. It was proposed that glycerol injection results in further destruction of the abnormally myelinated fibers implicated in the etiology of trigeminal neuralgia.[73] This may be the basis of pain relief with only minimal interference in function of normal fibers.

Fluoroscopic control of needle placement in the trigeminal ganglion by way of the foramen ovale has been greatly refined.[46] A radiopaque marker is placed 3 cm lateral to the labial commissure. Then, under fluoroscopy, the patient's head is turned until the marker is projected vertically, over the foramen ovale. The needle is then advanced along the anatomically safe line determined by the foramen ovale and the lateral labial puncture site[46] (see Fig. 15-5).

Maxillary Nerve Block

The maxillary nerve supplies the maxilla, the maxillary antrum, the teeth of the upper jaw, the lower part of the nose, the nasopharynx, the roof of the mouth, part of the tonsillar fossa, and the skin over the middle third of the face (see Fig. 15-2). Maxillary nerve block is used to treat intractable pain in this area that commonly results from malignant disease as well as trigeminal neuralgia, or posttraumatic neuralgia. Because tumors, which initially arise in the structures supplied by the maxillary nerve, may spread locally to areas innervated by other cranial nerves or metastasize to glands in the neck, additional blockade of the appropriate nerves is often necessary.

Technique. Maxillary nerve block can be performed by lateral percutaneous, oral, or transorbital routes (see Chaps. 15 and 16). The lateral percutaneous method described by Macintosh and Ostlere is preferred because it is simple and predictable.[75] The skin landmark lies over the anterior border of the masseter where a vertical line from the lateral orbital margin crosses a horizontal line through the middle of the upper lip. With the patient supine, the needle is passed into the pterygopalatine fossa to a depth of 4 cm by following a line in the direction of the pupil, 30° to the horizontal and immediately posterior to the tuberosity of the maxilla (see Fig. 15-5). The injection should be free from any resistance, and there should be no distension of the lower eyelid, which indicates diffusion of the solution into the periorbital tissues through the inferior orbital fissure. Accurate positioning of the needle is essential because it is possible to advance the needle to too great a depth and thereby come into proximity to the optic nerve. A test dose of 2 ml of 2% lidocaine with epinephrine is desirable to confirm the siting of the needle and to reduce the pain of injection of the neurolytic agent. Larger volumes of local anesthetic should be avoided because they will dilute the neurolytic agent, which would reduce the effectiveness and duration of the neurolytic block and increase the risk of neuralgia when alcohol is used.

Because the injection is painful, heavy sedation or general anesthesia is recommended. Intravenous meperidine, 50 mg (or fentanyl, 50 μg), promethazine, 25 mg, and, when required, diazepam, 5 to 10 mg will generally produce adequate sedation. Once the patient is satisfactorily prepared, 1 to 2 ml of absolute alcohol is injected. The needle, cleared with 1 ml of air, is then repositioned, and the procedure is repeated, yielding a total volume of 2 to 4 ml of alcohol.

The technique for glycerol injection is more demanding. The needle must be placed in the CSF in the dural fold of Meckel's cavity (see Fig. 15-5). CSF is drained out of the cavity and then metrizamide is slowly injected, under image intensifier control, until the cistern of Meckel's cavity is filled. The head is then positioned to allow metrizamide to drain away from the maxillary parts of the trigeminal root, which are intended to be affected by glycerol. Then glycerol is slowly injected in a volume of 0.2 to 0.4 ml (see Chap. 30).

In maxillary carcinoma, preliminary tomography of the base of the skull is recommended to exclude direct spread of the disease because once the tumor has invaded the skull, the results of maxillary blockade are likely to be disappointing.

A diagnostic block with 2 ml of local anesthetic should be performed 1 to 2 days before the neurolytic injection to indicate the probable extent of the proposed neurolytic block. An alternative technique is described in Chapter 15 for both local anesthetic and neurolytic maxillary nerve block (see Fig. 15-6).

Results. The patient is reviewed on the next day when the effect of the heavy sedation has worn off. If the pain relief is incomplete, consideration is given to a further block after 2 to 3 weeks.

The results of alcohol injection have been similar to those described by McEwen and colleagues (70% of patients with good or fair relief and 30% with little or no relief).[74] Pain alleviation may last from a few weeks to more than a year. Glycerol injection relieves pain in about 86% of patients with fewer side-effects compared with alcohol[50] (see above). Nerve block can be repeated, but as the tumor spreads, producing a satisfactory result becomes increasingly difficult. Once the base of the skull has become infiltrated, the patient is best managed on potent oral analgesics, such as morphine, 20 to 60 mg, every 2 to 4 hours, or methadone, 10 mg, every 8 to 12 hours.*

Mandibular Nerve Block

The mandibular nerve carries sensory fibers from the lower jaw, the anterior two-thirds of the tongue, the external auditory meatus, the temporal region and anterior part of the ear, the temporomandibular joint, and the lower part of the face (see Fig. 15-2).

Intractable pain caused by malignancy and other lesions in this area may be effectively treated by mandibular nerve block.[15,17,28,36,74] The distribution of pain varies. It may be confined to the site of the lesion or may spread widely over the entire area supplied by the mandibular nerve. The pain may be aggravated by the associated trismus, difficulty in swallowing and speaking, facial swelling, foul breath, anorexia, and malnutrition. Occasionally pain limited to the distribution of the inferior dental nerve may be relieved by blocking that nerve alone. A technique has been described using radiographic control[69] (see Figs. 16-17 and 16-18).

*These are baseline starting doses in patients not previously treated with opioids. Adjustment of dose and dosing interval is necessary to suit individual patients.

Metastatic spread to the cervical glands or postoperative neuromas of the cervical plexus can produce a constant or a triggered pain into and behind the ear, around the angle of the jaw, and into the neck or shoulder. Local or metastatic spread can, therefore, involve branches of the facial, glossopharyngeal, and vagus nerves and the cervical plexus. Partial failure of a mandibular nerve block may be due to involvement of these other nerves.

Technique. Mandibular nerve block may be performed intraorally or extraorally. Two extraoral methods have been described; a lateral approach in which the needle is passed perpendicular to the skin through the mandibular notch and an anterolateral approach similar to that used to block the gasserian ganglion.[15,74] Radiographic localization has been recommended, but if the lateral extraoral method is used, the landmarks (mandibular notch, lateral pterygoid plate) are sufficient to allow accurate placement without radiography. A diagnostic block with 2 to 5 ml of 2% lidocaine with epinephrine may be used to indicate the probable extent of the proposed neurolytic block (see Figs. 15-5 and 15-6).

Absolute alcohol is used for the therapeutic block. Again, heavy sedation is necessary because the injection of absolute alcohol is extremely painful. The pain of the injection may also be modified by an injection of 2 ml of 2% lidocaine with epinephrine immediately before the alcohol block. One milliliter to 2 ml of absolute alcohol is injected initially, the needle is repositioned, and the procedure repeated, using a total of 2 to 4 ml of alcohol (see also Chaps. 15 and 16).

Results. When the patient is reviewed on the next day, if pain relief is incomplete, the area of anesthesia produced is determined, and a decision is made whether to repeat the mandibular block or to extend the area of anesthesia by performing a glossopharyngeal, vagus, or intrathecal cervical plexus block. Table 29-5 records the combination of blocks used by

TABLE 29-5. NERVE BLOCKS TO CONTROL PAIN OWING TO CARCINOMA OF TONGUE AND FLOOR OF MOUTH

Blocks Performed	Number of Patients	Number of Treatments
Mandibular nerve block	27	35
Intrathecal cervical plexus block	15	25
Mandibular nerve block and cervical plexus block	5	5
Mandibular glossopharyngeal, and vagus block	5	5
Total	52	70

Dwyer in 52 patients with carcinoma of the tongue and floor of the mouth.[36] Eighty percent of these patients received significant relief from the injection. The pain of the remaining 20% was unrelieved, and opioid oral analgesics were required.

The glycerol technique (see above) by way of the foramen ovale may be a useful alternative. In this case, the mandibular portion of the trigeminal root is exposed to the glycerol. Another approach is to use radiofrequency lesioning of the mandibular portion of trigeminal root by way of the foramen ovale (see Chap. 30).

As with the maxillary block, pain relief may last from a few weeks to more than a year, and the block may be repeated if necessary. In malignancy, failure may be due to faulty technique but usually indicates spread of the disease to the skull and middle cranial fossa.

Complications of alcohol injections of the mandibular nerve have been reported to be oculomotor palsy and total sensory loss in the distribution of the branches of the gasserian ganglion.[41]

Glossopharyngeal and Vagus Nerve Blocks

Glossopharyngeal and vagus nerve blocks are used in the treatment of intractable pain that arises from the pharynx, larynx, and related structures. They may be used singly when the lesion is discrete and confined to the area supplied by the nerves or, more frequently, in combination with other blocks (*e.g.*, mandibular or maxillary).[15,17,28,36]

The glossopharyngeal nerve supplies the pharyngeal wall, the palatine tonsils, and the posterior one-third of the tongue. The vagus, through the internal branch of its superior laryngeal division, supplies sensory fibers to the base of the tongue, the epiglottis, the larynx above the vocal cords, and the immediately adjacent pharynx. Both nerves leave the skull through the jugular foramen where they are anatomically related to the internal jugular vein, the internal carotid artery, the accessory nerve, the hypoglossal nerve, and the cervical sympathetic trunk (see Fig. 15-7).

The glossopharyngeal and vagus nerves are blocked at the base of the skull, at their exit through the jugular foramen (see Chap. 15). Invariably, the accessory and hypoglossal nerves are affected at the same time, causing weakness of the trapezius muscle and partial paralysis of the tongue. A Horner's syndrome owing to sympathetic block also occurs. For these reasons, together with the effects of the laryngeal paralysis and persistent tachycardia that occurs when both vagus nerves are blocked, bilateral injections should not be attempted. McEwen and associates recorded a death caused by respiratory obstruction after a vagal block in a patient with postcricoid carcinoma.[74]

Technique. The method used to block the glossopharyngeal and vagus nerves at the base of the skull has been described by Macintosh and Ostlere.[75] The patient lies flat on the operating table facing straight upward, and the needle is inserted just anterior to the tip of the mastoid process. It is directed forward at a right angle to the body axis and at an angle of 50° to the horizontal, to a depth of 4 cm, having passed just in front of and beyond the tip of the transverse process of C1. Two to 3 ml of absolute alcohol is then injected after careful aspiration to eliminate the greater than usual risk of an intravascular injection (see also Chap. 15).

In order to block the glossopharyngeal nerve and spare the vagus, Bonica recommends inserting the needle perpendicular to the skin, midway between the tip of the mastoid and the angle of the jaw, and injecting just anterior and medial to the styloid process.[15] Montgomery and Cousins report that accurate placement at the jugular foramen is aided by radiographic control.[84] Bonica further suggests, as an alternative to a complete vagal block with its attendant risks, that the internal laryngeal branch of the superior laryngeal nerve may be injected separately.[15] This is of particular advantage when the lesion extends across the midline, and the pain is bilateral. The nerve is approached as it enters the thyrohyoid membrane just anterior to the superior cornu of the thyroid cartilage deep to the posterior border of the thyrohyoid (see Fig.15-8). The block can be performed by a midline or a lateral approach. Accurate placement of 2 to 3 ml of absolute alcohol is necessary to produce an effective block. The patient is instructed not to speak, swallow, or cough during the procedure.

Careful premedication and follow-up, as previously described, are essential.

Results. Glossopharyngeal and vagal nerve blocks are used infrequently, and it is difficult to assess their success. However, the results appear comparable to those achieved with other neurolytic blocks.

improved to produce a more extensive block. Some pain relief is usually apparent immediately after the block, but relief may take some days to be complete. Results of this technique are shown in Table 29-6.

Spread of the alcohol over the upper roots of the lumbar plexus may result in numbness and paresthesias over the lower abdominal wall and upper thigh and is a source of temporary discomfort. Injection of a small volume of air or saline through the needle at the termination of the block may assist in preventing contamination of the lumbar plexus with alcohol as the needle is withdrawn through the psoas major. Complications of this technique are shown in Table 29-7.

Another technique for celiac plexus block is described in Chapter 14 and illustrated in Figures 14-6 and 14-7. Spread of neurolytic solution may result in serious complications, including paraplegia.[26] Thus various modifications to the classic technique have attempted to reduce posterior spread of solution toward the lumbar plexus and other structures and to increase spread over the celiac plexus, *anterior* to the great vessels. The use of CT scan and a modification of the "classic" technique has been described.[98] The celiac artery was located by CT scan and a straight line path to celiac plexus was determined by CT to avoid the kidney and major vessels. This invariably required the needle to pass *through the crura of the diaphragm.* Sometimes variations in the level of the celiac artery necessitated needle placement at levels other than L1 – usually higher. Mostly the left needle was inserted 4 cm from the midline and the tip was localized immediately adjacent to the anterolateral wall of the aorta. The point of insertion of the right needle was more variable: to place the needletip between the vena cava and the aorta, immediately anterior to diaphragm crus, it was necessary to insert the needle anywhere from 5 to 10 cm lateral to the midline, limited by the vertebral body medially and the kidney laterally. Spread of solution mixed with contrast media with the classic technique is markedly posterior, with surprisingly little spread over celiac plexus. With the technique described above, spread was much more concentrated over the celiac plexus, with little posterior spread[98] (see also Chap. 14 and Figs. 14-6 and 14-7).

Another variation is to intentionally insert a single needle through the aorta, on the left side, at the level of the midpoint of L1 vertebral body, the so-called *transaortic technique*[57]; after initial local anesthetic injection, 30 ml of 75% alcohol was injected. CT scanning revealed anterior spread of solution.

Results. A comparison of the results of the different methods of celiac plexus block is not possible because of different methods of assessment in the studies reported. No prospective controlled study is available. However, it seems that efficacy and safety may be improved by injection of neurolytic solution mixed with contrast medium using image intensifier control. Also, there appears to be some advantage in techniques that emphasize spread anterior to the aorta, except perhaps in patients with extensive cancer deposits close to the aorta. The availability of CT scans *before* celiac block should help in choosing appropriate technique. On occasion CT scan may be useful while carrying out the block.

With the "classic" technique, 56% to 85% of patients with upper abdominal cancer obtain pain relief (Table 29.2-6) lasting from 1 month up to 1 year.[12,20,21a,104a] In chronic pancreatitis, it is claimed that 60% to 70% of patients obtain pain relief. However, in the experience of the current authors, pain relief in pancreatitis is invariably of a temporary nature and declines with subsequent blocks. Thus the techniques should be viewed only as temporary measures to aid the initiation of other measures.

With the transaortic technique, immediate pain relief was obtained in 93% of 28 patients with pain caused by abdominal cancer.[57] Two patients had only

TABLE 29-6. RESULTS OF "CLASSIC" CELIAC PLEXUS BLOCK WITH ALCOHOL

Author	Indication	Number of Cases	Percentage Results		
			Good	Fair	Poor
Bridenbaugh and colleagues* (1964)[20]	Upper abdominal cancer	41	73	24.5	2.5
Gorbitz and Leavens† (1971)[47]	Upper abdominal cancer	11 (9)	56	17.5	26.5
Black and Dwyer (1973)[12]	Carcinoma of pancreas	20	70	30.0	0.0
	Other abdominal malignancy	37	70	17.0	13.0
	Chronic pancreatitis	21	62	5.0	33.0
Brown and colleagues* (1987)[21a]	Pancreatic cancer	136	85‡	—	15.0

*Used 50 ml of 50% alcohol.
†Represents results for 9 of 11 patients.
‡In 75% of patients, good pain relief lasted through remaining life. The success of repeat blocks was also 85%.[21a]

TABLE 29-7. COMPLICATIONS THAT OCCURRED IN 104 CELIAC PLEXUS BLOCKS

Complication	Incidence (%)
Weakness or numbness T10–L2 distribution	8
Lower chest pain	3
Failure of ejaculation	2
Postural hypotension	2
Warmth and fullness of leg	1
Urinary difficulty	1

(Data from Black, A., and Dwyer, B.: Coeliac plexus block. Anaesth. Intensive Care, *1*:315, 1973)

24 hours of relief and required subsequent splanchnic nerve block; both patients had extensive preaortic neoplastic infiltration.[57] In a further seven patients, pain returned in 1 to 3 weeks. In the remaining 14 patients, pain relief persisted during the follow-up period of 20 days (one patient) 1 month (four), 1.5 months (four), 2 months (two), and 4 months (three), respectively.[57] In other series of blocks using more anterior spread of solution, the numbers of patients are small and follow-up data are not available. *Failure* of initial blockade, with any of the techniques, is an indication for repeat blockade, perhaps with an alternative technique, since the success rate of repeat blockade remains high.[21a]

Complications. With all techniques, back pain may occur around the site of injection. With the "classic" technique, postural hypotension,[21a] owing to the block of both celiac plexus and lumbar sympathetic ganglia, is a common and sometimes troublesome complication. Also, posterior spread of solution not uncommonly leads to involvement of lower thoracic and lumbar somatic nerves.[12,20,47] This may result in severe neuralgias in the region of the lower rib cage or upper thigh. These may persist for 2 or more months. Table 29-7 summarizes the incidence of persistent complications recorded by Black and Dwyer in 104 patients treated over a 10-year period.[12] Paraplegia has been reported to occur despite performance of celiac block under image intensifier control. It was speculated that posterior spread of solution resulted in thrombosis of a major feeder artery to the spinal cord.[26] Pneumothorax may also occur.[21a]

The transaortic technique was used in 28 patients without any neurologic sequelae. Orthostatic hypotension occurred in only 20% of patients and in each case resolved in 48 to 72 hours.[57] Diarrhea lasting for 36 to 48 hours occurred in 60% of patients, presumably because of sympathetic blockade of gut smooth muscle.[57]

Complications with the "classic" technique have motivated those using celiac block to move toward the use of radiography, CT scan, and the newer approaches described earlier. Also, the more effective use of oral opioids and the availability of spinal opioid techniques has placed emphasis on a careful evaluation of the benefit-risk ratio before celiac block.

Splanchnic Nerve Block

Blockade of the splanchnic nerves above the diaphragm is a further alternative that is favored by some clinics.[14a] In this technique, 10% phenol in contrast medium is injected under image intensifier control as described in Chapter 14. As illustrated in Figure 14-8, the needle passes through the crura of the diaphragm.

Data on efficacy, duration of analgesia, and incidence of complications are currently lacking. In some clinics, splanchnic nerve block has replaced celiac block.

Lumbar Sympathetic Block

In patients with peripheral vascular disease, causalgia, and phantom limb pain in the lower limb, a lumbar sympathetic block may be indicated (see Chap. 13 and Table 13-1). The lumbar sympathetic ganglia also convey visceral nociceptive afferents from pelvic viscera in males and females such as urogenital organs, colon, rectum (see Fig. 13-2). In males and females, pain caused by cancer of the sigmoid colon or rectum may be relieved by bilateral lumbar sympathetic block, if the disease is confined to those viscera. In males, pain caused by cancer of the seminal vesicles or prostate may sometimes be relieved by bilateral lumbar sympathetic block. Gynecologic pain is still poorly understood; pain pathways are shown in Figure 24-5. It is apparent that pain caused by cancer of the uterus and cervix may sometimes be relieved by bilateral lumbar sympathetic block, if the disease is confined to those viscera. However, it may be necessary to extend the block to the T12 ganglion (see Fig. 24-5). In patients with abdominal pain, it can often be difficult to clearly define the area of referred pain (see Fig. 24-4). Diagnosis of source of pain may be helped by lumbar sympathetic block and subsequent celiac plexus block (see Table 24-3). If local anesthetic lumbar sympathetic block relieves the pain, subsequent neurolytic block may be used as longer-term tretament.[33] Treatment of cancer of the cervix usually relieves pain until the disease progresses to involve lumbosacral plexus; thus the role of lumbar sympathetic blocks is limited.

The use of lumbar sympathetic block for occlusive

vascular disease of the lower limb and other conditions is described in detail in Chapter 13. Technical details are shown in Figures 13-20 through 13-31.

Thoracic Sympathetic Block

The controversial question of cervicothoracic and thoracic neurolytic sympathetic blocks is considered in Chapter 13. Technical details are shown in Figures 13-18 through 21. The potential complications of either "stellate ganglion" (cervicothoracic) block or thoracic sympathetic block limit the use of those techniques. The thoracic approach described in Chapter 13 probably minimizes the risks, provided that pleural puncture is avoided. This involves the use of an image intensifier. Also, injection of a neurolytic agent mixed with contrast medium helps to minimize the dose and optimizes efficacy. Some series of neurolytic "stellate" block have been reported, using small volumes of phenol (1 ml) (see Chap. 13).

NEUROLYTIC SOMATIC NERVE BLOCKADE

Although considerable benefit can be obtained in various pain states with local anesthetic somatic nerve blockade, neurolytic blockade has not enjoyed great popularity. The primary reasons for this are that it is generally held that the incidence of neuralgia is high and that the often accompanying motor blockade poses the risk of a useless limb. The former problem may be partially related to technical difficulties, since somatic neurolytic block must be performed with a smaller dose than the equivalent local anesthetic block, and thus needle placement must be precise. It is possible that some cases of neuralgia are due to imprecise needle placement and incomplete neurolysis. If larger volumes of neurolytic solution are used, necrosis of surrounding tissues may occur.

Despite the dictum by some authors that, apart from cranial nerve block, somatic nerve block should never be performed with a neurolytic agent, there may be occasions when the appropriate agent and sufficient technical skill, sometimes aided by a peripheral nerve stimulator, can greatly benefit the patient. Examples are intercostal block, infraorbital block, obturator nerve block, brachial plexus block,[86] facial nerve block,[37,104] various peripheral nerve blocks in the arms and legs of patients with acquired spasticity,[22,109] motor point blocks for spasticity,[42,43] intralesion neurolytic injection for bone metastases.[31] Blockade of the medial branch of posterior primary ramus and facet joint blocks are described in Chapter 27.3. The use of the cryoprobe for somatic blocks is described below. Percutaneous radiofrequency lesions are advocated by some clinics as permitting more precise control for all peripheral neurolytic blocks (see Chap. 30).

Intercostal Block

In intercostal nerve block, a maximum of 1 ml of neurolytic solution should be used for each intercostal nerve (see Fig. 14-3). Because of dermatomal overlap, it is also necessary to block the adjacent segments. In view of the high incidence of neuralgia with absolute alcohol, 6% to 7% aqueous phenol or 10% ammonium sulfate has been used. Cryoanalgesia may be used, although its duration of effect is often as little as 10 days.[9,70] At most clinics the subarachnoid approach is preferred because of its greater predictability and avoidance of the problem of neuralgia, although of course it may pose more serious complications.

Infraorbital Nerve Block

A maximum dose of neurolytic agent of 1 ml is used in infraorbital nerve block and care must be taken to avoid direct periosteal injection (see Chap. 15 and Fig. 15-3).

Some patients with trigeminal neuralgia have pain localized to infraorbital distribution and obtain complete relief with infraorbital block rather than the more extensive maxillary block. The advent of carefully controlled thermogangliolysis has probably substantially reduced the indications for infraorbital block. However, cryoanalgesia has been used with considerable success.[9]

Obturator Block

Pain caused by osteoarthritis of the hip may be relieved by obturator block and blockade of the nerve to quadratus femoris (for technique, see Fig. 11-9). The use of 0.25% bupivacaine often yields weeks of pain relief so that the indications for the use of neurolytic solutions are minimal. It is essential to use radiographic control (and often a peripheral nerve stimulator) if a neurolytic agent is to be used, since needle placement is difficult.

On occasion the neurolytic technique can be used to assist nursing patients with paraplegia and adductor spasm, although percutaneous adductor tenotomy is simple and effective.

Cervical Plexus and Brachial Plexus

Individual cervical nerve blockade is performed by a technique that is identical to the description of interscalene blockade, except that each cervical nerve is injected separately (see Fig. 15-11). In general, chronic pain that involves the cervical and brachial plexus is best treated by the cervical subarachnoid, subdural, or epidural techniques previously described. Some patients for whom the use of the subarachnoid approach presents problems may benefit from blockade of one or more cervical nerves. Initial block with 1 to 2 ml 0.25% bupivacaine should be tried, since it will often yield several weeks of pain relief. More rarely 1 ml of 6% to 10% phenol in water or 10% phenol in Conray-420 dye (with radiographic control) may be injected at each level.

Some authors report the use of brachial plexus block, by way of the interscalene technique, to provide relief of the severe pain associated with Pancoast's syndrome (see Ref. 18). It is vital to use an image intensifier and to ensure needle placement well clear of vertebral artery and dural cuff (see Fig. 10-3). Mullin reports the use of 10 ml of 3% phenol in water with apparently good short-term pain relief and a low incidence of motor effects.[86] However, other authors report that pain on movement is not relieved.[21] For pain in the distribution of cervical plexus, less than 5 ml of 5% to 6% phenol is injected at the level of each cervical transverse process, and it is claimed that pain relief is good and motor effects are minimal.[21] The relative efficacy/safety of such techniques compared with subdural or epidural neurolytic techniques requires further assessment.

Neurolytic Blocks of Peripheral Nerves for Spasticity

Patients with acquired spasticity develop muscle contractures and spasms that may be painful, may prevent useful function, and may complicate nursing.[22,43,109] Diagnostic blocks with local anesthetic may aid therapists in rehabilitation and may indicate the value of further blocks with neurolytic agents to improve function, relieve pain, and aid nursing.[22,43,109] In one series, phenol nerve blocks were performed for adult acquired spasticity — mostly resulting from closed head injury. Excessive elbow flexion was treated with phenol block of the musculocutaneous nerve. Excessive plantar flexion was treated with phenol block of the posterior tibial nerve. The nerve blocks produced a high success rate in terms of restoration of normal functional position of the limb.[43] Duration of block was usually 6 months, but after this stage, normal function of the limb was not maintained. However, during the period of nerve block, rehabilitation made considerable progress and more definitive treatment (*e.g.*, lengthening of Achilles tendon) was planned. The use of such blocks in children is described in Chapter 21.

Another approach to spasticity in head-injured and other patients is to use phenol blocks of motor points in affected muscles.[42] Motor points are located by finding the points that elicit maximum muscle contraction in each muscle, using a peripheral nerve stimulator. Percutaneous injection is then performed with 3% to 5% aqueous phenol. Relaxation of muscle function lasts for approximately 2 months and allows control of spasticity and functional training of a limb (*e.g.*, hand) while neurologic recovery is occurring.[42]

Facial Nerve Block for Hemifacial Spasm

Hemifacial spasm of unknown cause can be debilitating to patients and is often resistant to any form of treatment. Blockade of the facial nerve with phenol has been described in some reports and has been successful in abolishing spasms. In one series of 20 patients, facial spasms were abolished for 6 to 12 months but then recurred.[37] In another report, a nerve stimulator was used to locate the facial nerve and decrease the dose of neurolytic agent required.[104]

Other Peripheral Neurolytic Techniques

Coccydynia. Neurolytic solutions have been used in the treatment of coccydynia. Either 10% phenol or 10% ammonium sulfate is injected onto the last sacral and coccygeal nerve. Superficial slough is a hazard, and at many clinics more conservative measures are preferred, since these patients usually have a long life expectancy and are otherwise healthy.

Nerve Entrapment. In general, diagnostic local anesthetic blocks are used for nerve entrapment, and if successful, the patient may be best managed by surgical lysis or sometimes by local anesthetic blocks with steroid included in the solution. The same applies to the syndrome in which a thoracic cutaneous nerve is trapped in the posterior wall of the rectus sheath. However, on occasion, if surgery is not feasible, injection of 5% to 7% aqueous phenol into the lateral part of the rectus compartment may be considered.

Trigger Point Injection. Some clinics inject "trigger points" in muscles with 5% to 6% aqueous phenol in patients who respond to local anesthetic block. Data on the efficacy and safety of this technique are lacking.

SOMATIC BLOCKADE BY CRYOANALGESIA

The term *cyroanalgesia* was coined by Lloyd, Barnard, and Glynn to describe the destruction of peripheral nerves by extreme cold to achieve pain relief.[70] The analgesic properties of extreme cold have been known for centuries. Indeed, the use of extreme cold constituted the earliest report of effective anesthesia, in an Anglo-Saxon manuscript from about 1050. Gratton and Singer translated this manuscript, which was attributed to a monk, Lacnunga. It says, in part, "Again, for eruptive rash, let him sit in cold water until it is deadened, then draw him up. Then cut four scarifications around the pocks and let them drip as long as he will."[48]

Refrigeration anesthesia was rediscovered over the succeeding centuries by such people as Bartholinus (1646) and Baron Larrey (1807). The latter, who was Napolean's surgeon general, noticed that amputation was painless for soldiers who had been in the snow for some time. Armstrong Davidson states that "the discovery that cold, especially ice, would relieve pain must have been made time and again in the long history of man; Hippocrates himself knew of it, but never recommended its use for surgery. It was not until man's feelings in regard to pain had altered that general use could be made of this simple method of analgesia."[2]

Thus Armstrong Davidson predicted the development of cryoanalgesia. It is a direct result of the increased interest in the assessment and treatment of patients with intractable pain and also the development of more powerful systems for the generation and maintenance of extreme cold.[1]

Cryoanalgesia was introduced to produce destruction of peripheral nerves for the relief of intractable pain that required somatic blockade. All other methods of peripheral nerve destruction, for example, cutting, crushing, or burning, are associated with an unacceptable incidence of neuralgia. Certainly, somatic blockade by the injection of chemical corrosives, such as phenol, has been shown, morphologically, to cause incomplete destruction of the nerve.[88] This may be the cause of the neuralgia that, not uncommonly, follows these injections or any other cause of incomplete destruction of a peripheral nerve. Cryolesions are associated with less fibrous tissue reaction than other forms of destruction.[7,113]

There is complete functional loss after a cryolesion in peripheral nerves of experimental animals; however, recovery can be expected over a period of weeks. This functional loss is associated with a second-degree nerve injury, according to Sunderland's (1968) classification; that is, there is wallerian degeneration with axonal disintegration and breakup of the myelin sheaths, but with minimal disruption of the endoneurium and other connective tissue elements[99] (see Chap. 29.1 and Figs. 29-1 and 29-14).

The application and maintenance of extreme cold is achieved by using a 15-gauge cryoneedle. Blockade is based on the Joule–Thompson effect with nitrous oxide as the refrigerant gas.[1] The Joule–Thompson effect occurs when gas at about 700 lb per square inch is ejected through a nozzle, and, as it expands, cooling to around −75°C occurs. The cold gas impinging on the inner surface of the needletip absorbs heat from the surrounding tissue, and the warm gas is exhausted back up the needle and vented through a scavenging system. The Spembley–Lloyd cryoneedle incorporates a thermocouple to confirm the temperature achieved at the tip. In addition, there is an electrical connection at the tip of the probe connected to a peripheral nerve stimulator for precise location of nerves (Figs. 29-31 and 29-32).

Clinical Applications

The use of cryoanalgesia has limitations in that the duration of analgesia is determined by the time taken for normal regeneration of the peripheral nerve. Thus duration of pain relief is a function of the completeness of destruction of the peripheral nerve. The positioning of the needle is of paramount importance because the ice ball is of limited size and must incorporate the nerve to achieve complete destruction. Positioning of the needle is a function of the expertise of the clinician and the characteristics of the peripheral nerve to be frozen. The median duration of pain relief varies from about 2 weeks to about 5 months.[9,70] Cryoanalgesia should not be used on mixed nerves unless there are extenuating circumstances because it will result in complete loss of function in the nerve, including paralysis of the muscles supplied by that nerve.

The most fruitful uses for cryoprobe blockade appear to be special situations of postoperative and posttraumatic pain and medium-duration relief of

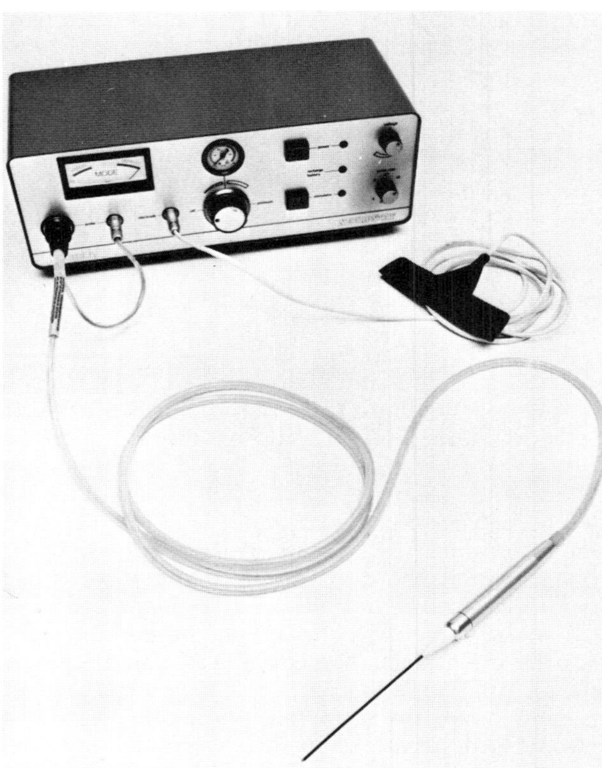

FIG. 29-31. Cryoanalgesia apparatus.

chronic pain. Analgesia by intercostal block has been provided for patients undergoing thoracotomy; there was a significant reduction in the number of narcotic injections and the number of days narcotic was required compared with a control group.[45] The intercostal nerves can conveniently be blocked under direct vision at the end of the operative procedure. However, if access from the chest is limited, an external approach can be used. This approach may also be used for analgesia for fractured ribs. Three important points should be noted.

First, the cryoprobe should not be withdrawn until it has fully thawed; otherwise, the surrounding tissue may adhere to the probe, and it is possible to tear blood vessels and neural structures.

Second, great care should be exercised with cryoprobe blockade in the dural-cuff region. It is possible for the cold lesion to extend to the spinal cord or for inadvertant thrombosis of a major "feeder artery" to result from the marked local reduction in temperature (see Fig. 7-11). Thus, in general, somatic blockade should be carried out lateral to the paravertebral muscles unless it is necessary to block the posterior primary ramus.

Third, a major disadvantage of percutaneous use is that the freezing that occurs along the needle may result in full thickness destruction of the skin. After healing there is usually a depigmented scar. This can be prevented by heating the skin with an ordinary infrared lamp. A large intravenous cannula can be used to provide a "sheath" for insertion of the cryoprobe, thus protecting the superficial tissues from cold lesions.

Applications in chronic pain management include some of the difficult problems that require somatic blockade, for example, occipital neuralgia (greater occipital nerve blocks), coccydynia (S5 and coccygeal nerve block), and atypical facial pain in the distribution of the infraorbital nerve (with an intraoral approach).[8,9] The cryoprobe has also been used for so-

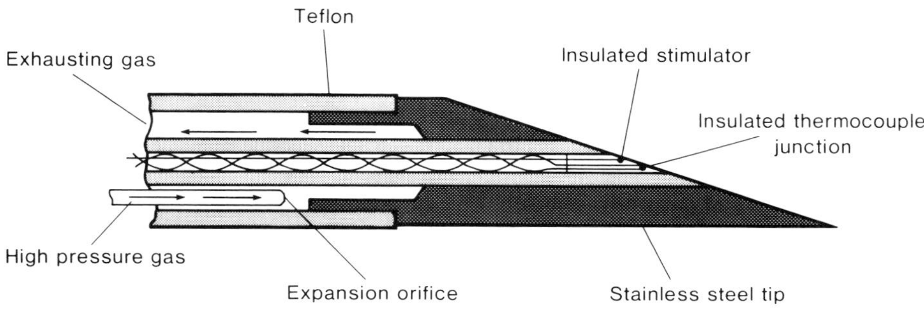

FIG. 29-32. Details of cryoprobe tip (Lloyd, J.W., Barnard, J.D., and Glynn, C.J.: Cryoanalgesia. A new approach to pain relief. Lancet, 2:933, 1976)

matic blockade in head/neck cancer. For example, mandibular and maxillary nerve blocks have been performed.[95] A cryoprobe technique for pituitary destruction has also been described[34] (see later).

CHEMICAL HYPOPHYSECTOMY

Injection of Alcohol into the Sella Turcica

One view of this technique is presented in Chapter 30. Because of the controversy that has surrounded the technique, it seems appropriate to present another somewhat more favorable view here. It should be stressed that a final evaluation cannot yet be made of the rationale and indications for use, results, complications, and mechanisms of action. However, the material presented below, and that of Chapter 30, should permit the reader to form a balanced view of the current status of this technique.

Injection of alcohol into the sella turcica was introduced in 1963 by Moricca of Rome, who called the procedure "neuroadenolysis of the pituitary" (see Ref. 44). The technique has also been called "pituitary ablation" and "chemical hypophysectomy" (CH). For simplicity, the latter term will be used in this discussion to refer to the injection of alcohol into the sella turcica.

Proposed Mechanism of Action. Hypophysectomy relieves pain in a similar percentage (60–90%) of cancer patients, regardless of whether it is carried out surgically by transcranial or open microsurgical technique, by transnasal cryoprobe, or by transnasal alcohol injection (see Refs. 67, 68). The *characteristics* of the pain relief are also similar, regardless of how the hypophysectomy is performed (see Refs. 44, 63, 65, 67, 68, 85).

1. Onset of relief is rapid and usually complete, in those who respond, within hours of the procedure. Sometimes pain relief is present at the end of the procedure.
2. Duration of relief is not related to tumor regression.
3. Degree of relief is not related to tumor regression. Some patients (50%) with no evidence of regression obtain long-lasting relief. Thus it appears that hormonal sensitivity of the tumor is not a factor in pain relief, and therefore not a consideration in deciding if the procedure will be helpful.
4. Pain relief is not related to degree of pituitary ablation or to any objective measurements of decreased pituitary function. Although a certain degree of pituitary damage is essential for pain relief, further damage does not appear to increase relief.
5. Level of relief varies from day to day, sometimes necessitating the addition of mild analgesics. In some patients (23%) there may be exacerbations of pain for 1 to 5 days, which then subside.
6. Acute episodes of pain, such as from acute injury or pathologic fracture, are not relieved.
7. There is no change in skin sensation, such as loss of pinprick sensation.

These clinical observations have been combined with other data to support a hypothesis that pain relief may be due to activation of a hypothalamic pain-suppressing response.

Evidence supporting stimulation of hypothalamic function is as follows:

1. Oophorectomy, adrenalectomy, and orchidectomy produce pain relief within hours of operation in patients with metastatic breast and prostate cancer, respectively. This pain relief occurs well before any evidence of tumor regression, and timing of its onset is similar to that for CH, suggesting a hypothalamic pain-suppressing response activated by the elimination of hormonal feedback.[68]
2. Neuropathology studies reveal no correlation between pain relief and degree of pituitary or hypothalamic damage. *Some* pituitary damage appears merely to indicate that sufficient alcohol was injected into the sella turcica. Regardless of the method of hypophysectomy, there is *retrograde* cell loss in the hypothalamus in the region of the paraventricular and supraoptic nuclei (PVN and SON). This appears to be quite adequate to initiate pain relief. The fact that it is seen even with meticulous microsurgical hypophysectomy indicates that it is a retrograde effect of hypophysectomy. Thus CH is unlikely to be a unique method of hypophysectomy, and this explains why pain relief is similar for all methods. The advantage of CH lies in its simplicity (see Refs. 65, 68).
3. Pituitary stalk section also produces retrograde cell loss in the hypothalamus and associated pain relief (see Ref. 68).
4. Measurements of pituitary and anterior hypothalamic function show no correlation between decreases in any hormone level and pain relief. For example, patients who develop diabetes insipidus after CH continue to have pain relief after the diabetes insipidus subsides (see Ref. 68).

5. A large body of animal data report on the efficacy of stress-induced analgesia. This involves exposing animals to a novel stress (*e.g.*, inescapable electrical foot shock). After this stress, animals exhibit long-lasting insensitivity to noxious stimulus. Stress-induced analgesia is well documented in humans in the situation of battle injuries and injuries in athletes where pain is absent after injuries that usually would be painful. Stress-induced analgesia and analgesia after hypophysectomy may both arise from activation of similar pain-suppressing hypothalamic mechanisms (see Ref. 68).

This evidence indicates that all methods of pituitary ablation may produce similar pain relief. Thus, for example, radiofrequency lesioning may become an alternative, as has cryoprobe ablation.[34]

Endogenous Opioid Involvement. The possible role of endogenous opioid involvement is controversial. In animal experiments using tooth pulp stimulation and electrical recording from pituitary and primary somatosensory cerebral cortex (PSC), CH resulted in increased electrical activity in pituitary and a decrease in PSC. Naloxone injection reversed these effects.[105] It was proposed that CH initiates a "wounding effect" in the pituitary associated with increased electrical activity, which may then decrease PSC activity by unknown mechanisms.[105] It is possible that the changes in hypothalamic activity discussed earlier may be the "link" in this chain. These data support a role for endorphins. However, the pain stimulus must be regarded as *acute* pain. In patients with chronic pain, naloxone failed to reverse the pain relief after CH for 29 cancer patients and 3 patients with thalamic pain.[67,68] However, in another series, 4 of 12 patients had pain relief after CH reversed when naloxone was injected (see Ref. 68). Assay of metenkephalin and beta-endorphin in lumbar CSF before and after CH showed no change (see Ref. 68).

In humans with cancer pain, the evidence seems weak for an involvement of endogenous opioids in pain relief resulting from CH.

Indications. CH has been used for pain that is widespread and due to multiple metastases. There is some evidence that pain relief occurs in a higher percentage of patients with breast or prostatic cancer. However, the results in other forms of cancer are little different.[68]

Less invasive methods should be used before considering CH. For example, oral nonopioid and opioid drugs and co-analgesic drugs should be carefully titrated (see Table 24-1, Chap. 24.1). The choice between CH and spinal opioids for diffuse pain seems to depend more on expertise available in each clinic. It is the view of the current authors that spinal opioid techniques are less invasive and have fewer complications than CH. However, CH undoubtedly provides highly effective and long-lasting relief in a substantial proportion of patients, with minimal need to take medication after CH. Refinements of CH technique using stereotaxic apparatus make it a more effective and safer alternative than it was initially.

The "freehand" technique of CH, with image intensifier control,[65] is described in Chapter 30. The stereotaxic technique was developed by Levin, Katz, and others[63,67,68] for the following reasons:

1. To permit precision in placement of needletip in sella turcica.
2. To permit the use of fine needles to prevent large holes in the floor of sella turcica, thus decreasing the chance of CSF leak, rhinorrhea, and subsequent possible meningitis. CSF leak is particularly likely in patients where a portion of the sella turcica is filled with a cystic extension of the subarachnoid space or in those in whom the diaphragma sella is incompetent.
3. To permit the use of a larger quantity of alcohol with only one needle placement. Such volumes of alcohol are unsafe with less precise needle placement.

Technique of Stereotaxic Chemical Hypophysectomy

1. Light general endotracheal anesthesia is used with any technique that preserves pupil responses as far as possible (*e.g.*, thiopental, N_2O/O_2, succinylcholine).
2. The patient is placed supine in a Todd–Wells stereotaxic head holder, using a transverse quadrant assembly (Fig. 29-33).
3. Under image intensifier control, the cross wires of the "target" are set on the posterosuperior aspect of the sella turcica, below the level of the posterior clinoid processes in the midline (Figs. 29-34 and 29-35).
4. Cocaine paste (4%) is applied to the nasal mucosa of one nostril to produce vasoconstriction. The nostril is chosen with least deviation of septum or obstruction by nasal turbinates.

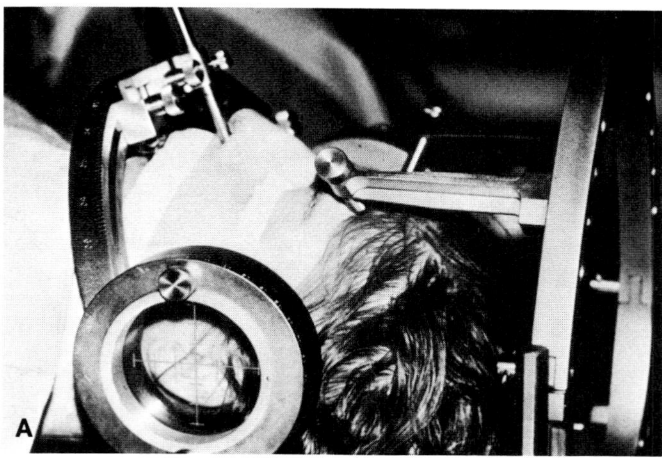

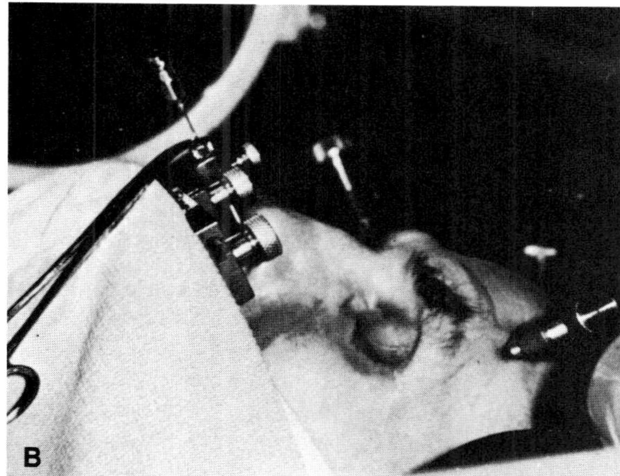

FIG. 29-33. Chemical hypophysectomy. **A.** Stereotaxic apparatus in place on patient's head. Note needle guide inserted into the nostril. **B.** Spinal needle (20-gauge) inserted into needle guide and then passed into sella turcica. (Levin, A.B., and Ramidel, L.L.: Treatment of cancer pain with hypophysectomy: Surgical and chemical. *In* Benedetti, C., *et al.* (eds.): Advances in Pain Research and Therapy, vol. 7, pp. 631–645. New York, Raven Press, 1984)

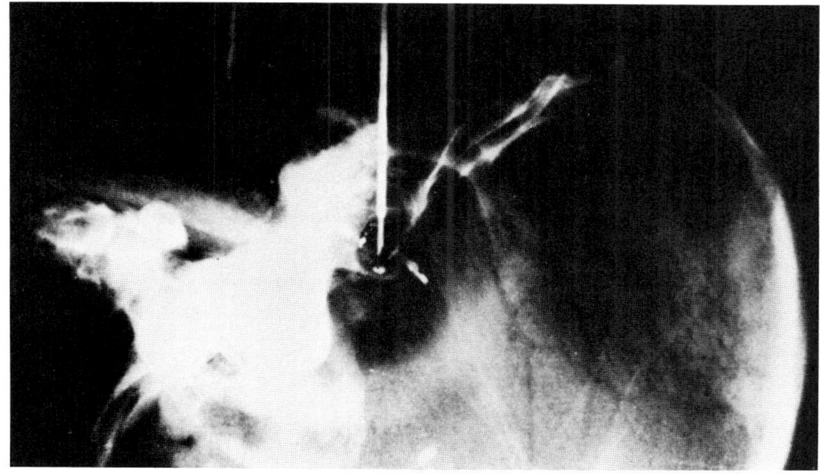

FIG. 29-34. Chemical hypophysectomy. Radiograph, lateral view, showing needle passing through sphenoid sinus and floor of sella turcica. Tip of needle is immediatey below level of posterior clinoid processes. Some injected Myodil can be seen moving up the pituitary stalk.

5. The nasal passage is swabbed with an organic iodine solution.
6. The needle guide of the stereotaxic apparatus is passed as far back as possible, toward the superior aspect of the nasal passage.
7. The angle of the transverse quadrant is adjusted so that the needle will have the greatest possible penetration of the pituitary gland on its way to the target.
8. The nasal mucosa at the tip of the guide is infiltrated with 1 ml of 1% lidocaine with 1 : 100,000 epinephrine.
9. An 18-gauge, 6-inch (15-cm) spinal needle is then passed through the guide and inserted through the floor of the sphenoid sinus. The sinus is then irrigated with bacitracin solution (5000 U/100 ml of saline).
10. The 18-gauge needle is removed from the guide and a 20-gauge, 6-inch (15-cm) spinal needle is passed through the guide and gently inserted through the floor of the sella turcica.
11. Anteroposterior (AP) and lateral views on the image intensifier are then examined to confirm that the needle has followed its intended path to the floor of the sella turcica. The AP view should confirm that the needle is following its line to the midline target.
12. The needle is now advanced to its target just below the posterior clinoid processes in the midline (see Fig. 29-34). AP and lateral views are again taken on the image intensifier to confirm correct placement (see Fig. 29-35).

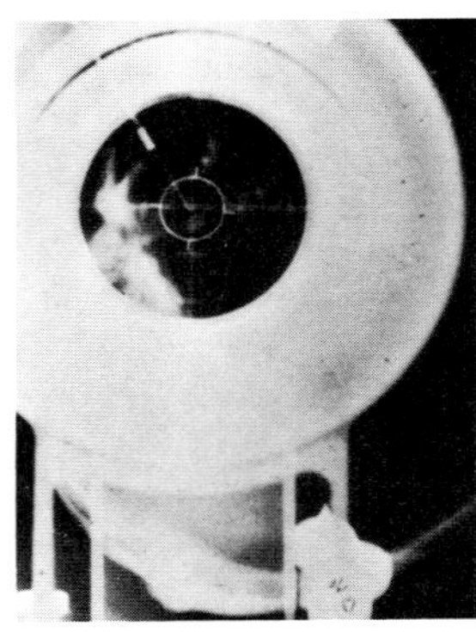

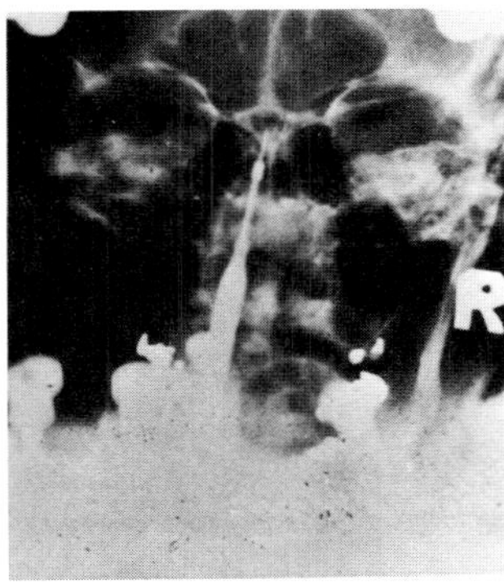

FIG. 29-35. Chemical hypophysectomy. **Left.** Lateral view radiograph showing needle at target of stereotaxic apparatus. **Right.** Anteroposterior view showing needle in midline at target. (Levin A.B., and Ramidel, L.L.: Treatment of cancer pain with hypophysectomy: Surgical and chemical. *In* Benedetti, C., *et al.* (eds.): Advances in Pain Research and Therapy, vol. 7, pp. 631–645. New York, Raven Press, 1984)

13. The needle stylet is removed and 1 to 2 ml of absolute alcohol is slowly injected, while the patient's pupils are monitored. Any sign of pupil enlargement is an indication to cease the injection.
14. If no pupil changes occur, the needle is withdrawn to a point halfway between the target and the floor of the sella turcica. A second injection of 1 to 2 ml is made, using the same precautions.
15. If the preceding injection is uneventful, the needle is withdrawn to a point halfway between the second injection and the floor of the sella turcica. A third dose of 1 to 2 ml of alcohol is injected as above.
16. The needle is withdrawn to just above the floor of the sella and 0.5 ml of "super glue" (alpha-ethyl cyano acrylate, slow polymerizing) is injected as the needle is being withdrawn through the floor of the sella. This seals the single hole and prevents CSF leak.
17. After the needle is withdrawn, the needle guide is withdrawn from the nostril. If there is evidence of bleeding from the nasal passage, it is packed with gauze impregnated with petroleum jelly. Otherwise, no packing is used.

    Some clinics routinely carry out a cisternal puncture, remove 10 ml of CSF, and then inject 50 to 100 mg of hydrocortisone succinate diluted with CSF.[65] Others carry out this step only if pupil dilatation has persisted despite ceasing alcohol injection.
18. After the procedure, all patients receive oral hydrocortisone supplement. Urine volume is monitored to detect the presence of diabetes insipidus; if necessary, vasopressin is given. Thyroid supplement is begun several days postoperatively.

Results. In an initial series of 13 patients, stereotaxic CH produced marked symptomatic relief in 11 patients, persisting in excess of 7 months.[63] In a later series, 82 patients with cancer pain and 3 patients with thalamic pain were treated with CH.[68] Good results were obtained in 84% of patients with cancer pain; this category represented patients reporting pain relief with no analgesics or with the need to use nonopioid analgesics or codeine. Six patients obtained good pain relief for about 1 month but later required cordotomy[5] or reinjection of alcohol, and these are not included in the "good result" category. Responses among breast, prostate, and other cancers were not different. Duration of pain relief was limited only by death. The mean postoperative survival was

5 months. As described above, there was some variation from day to day in the degree of pain relief.[68] Three patients with thalamic pain treated with CH all obtained pain relief.[68]

It is interesting to compare these results with those of Moricca and other groups using volumes of 3 to 5 ml of alcohol (see Ref. 44) and a "free hand" technique. Such groups have claimed "good" pain relief in more than 85% of patients. In contrast, careful documentation of results of "free hand" injection of volumes of 0.4 to 2 ml of alcohol revealed "good" pain relief in approximately 40% of patients.[65] This group found no correlation between pain relief and volume of alcohol injected in the range of 0.4 to 2 ml; however, this may not be the critical range of volume.

Complications. Since using the technique of sealing the hole in the sella turcica, there have been no CSF leaks in the series of Levin and colleagues.[68] In the 85 patients reported, there were five ocular nerve palsies, of which three cleared completely. Four patients had bilateral or unilateral temporal field loss and associated ocular nerve palsies; one cleared completely and two cleared partially.[68] All of these problems occurred in the first 40 patients with no complications in the subsequent 45 patients. There were no deaths in the series.

This compares favorably with complications using the freehand techniques.[65] In 100 patients who received CH for cancer pain, the complications were diabetes insipidus (39%), pupillary dilation (22%), severe postoperative headache (19%), blurring of vision (4%), diplopia (4%), focal sensory or motor neurologic deficit (4%), drowsiness or slow mentation (2%), rhinorrhea (2%), meningeal aseptic reaction (2%). These complications were reported to be "transient," except for one patient in whom diplopia and unilateral peripheral visual field deficit persisted for in excess of 2 months (see also Chap. 30).

Conclusion. Chemical hypophysectomy has proved to be capable of relieving severe pain owing to widely disseminated cancer in a high percentage of patients. The stereotaxic technique has much to offer in terms of its precision, efficacy, and minimal side-effects. However, other authors have reported large series using a "free hand" technique with radiographic control. In these series, often more than one needle was inserted with small volumes injected (1 ml) by way of each needle. Also, it was often necessary to repeat injection on a subsequent occasion to obtain lasting pain relief.[44,65] This approach may be safer if a stereotaxic apparatus is not used. It is of interest that Moricca originally advised that pain relief in a high percentage of patients required volumes of alcohol of 5 to 6 ml (see Ref. 44). In the view of the present authors, the stereotaxic technique would seem best suited to injecting such volumes "at one sitting." If this apparatus is unavailable, it may be best to limit the volume to 1 to 2 ml and be prepared to repeat the procedure.

REFERENCES

1. Amoils, S.P.: The Joule–Thompson cryoprobe. Arch. Ophthalmol., *78*:201, 1967.
2. Armstrong Davidson, M.H.: The history of anesthesia. *In* Gray, T.C., and Nunn, J.F. (eds.): General Anesthesia, p. 709. London, Butterworth, 1971.
3. Arner, S.: The role of nerve blocks in the treatment of cancer pain. Acta Anaesthesiol. Scand. [Suppl.], *74*:104, 1982.
4. Baines, M.J.: Cancer pain. Postgrad. Med. J., *60*:852, 1984.
5. Balamoutsos, N.G.: Infiltration block of the coeliac plexus using a plastic catheter. Reg. Anaesth., *5*:64, 1982.
6. Ball, H.C., Pearce, D.J., and Davies, J.A.: Experience with therapeutic nerve blocks. Anaesthesia, *19*:250, 1964.
7. Barnard, D.: The effects of extreme cold on sensory nerves. Ann. R. Coll. Surg. Engl., *62*:180, 1980.
8. Barnard, D., Lloyd, J., and Evans, J.: Cryoanalgesia in the management of chronic facial pain. J. Maxillofac. Surg., *9*:101, 1981.
9. Barnard, J.D.W., Lloyd, J.W., and Glynn, C.J.: Cryosurgery: In the management of intractable facial pain. Br. J. Oral Surg., *16*:135, 1978.
10. Bates, W.: Control of somatic pain. Am. J. Surg., *59*:83, 1943.
11. Bentley, F.H.: Observations of visceral pain. Visceral tenderness. Ann. Surg., *128*:881, 1948.
12. Black, A., and Dwyer, B.: Coeliac plexus block. Anaesth. Intensive Care, *1*:315, 1973.
13. Black, P.: Neurosurgical management of cancer pain. Semin. Oncol., *12*:438, 1985.
14. Bleasel, K.: The pain clinic at St. Vincent's Hospital, Sydney. Mod. Med. Aust., *17*:5, 1974.

14a. Boas, R.A.: Sympathetic blocks in clinical practice. Int. Anesthesiol. Clin., *16*:149, 1978.

15. Bonica, J.J.: The Management of Pain. Philadelphia, Lea and Febiger, 1953.
16. Bonica, J.J.: Management of pain with regional analgesia. Postgrad. Med. J., *60*:897, 1984.
17. Bonica, J.J.: Diagnostic and therapeutic blocks. A reappraisal based on 15 years' experience. Anesth. Analg. (Cleve)., *37*:58, 1958.
18. Bonica, J.J., and Ventafridda, V. (eds.): Pain of advanced cancer. *In* Advances in Pain Research and Therapy, vol. 2, pp. 325–403. New York, Raven Press, 1979.
19. Braun, H.: Ein Hilfsinstrument zur ausfeuhrung der Splanchnicusanasthesie. Zentralbl. Chir., *48*:1544, 1921.
20. Bridenbaugh, L.D., Moore, D.C., and Campbell, D.D.: Management of upper abdominal cancer pain. Treatment with celiac plexus block with alcohol. J.A.M.A., *190*:877, 1964.

21. Brown, A.S.: Current views on the use of nerve blocking in the relief of chronic pain. *In* Swerdlow, M. (ed.): The Therapy of Pain. Philadelphia, J.B. Lippincott, 1981.
21a. Brown, D.L., Bulley, C.K., Quiel, E.L.: Neurolytic celiac plexus block for pancreatic cancer pain. Anesth. Analg., 66:869–873, 1987.
22. Carpenter, E.B.: Role of nerve blocks in the foot and ankle in cerebral palsy: Therapeutic and diagnostic. Foot Ankle, *4*:164, 1983.
23. Carron, H.: Control of pain in the head and neck. Otolaryngol. Clin. North Am., *14*:631, 1981.
24. Challenger, J.H.: Sympathetic nervous system blocking and pain relief. *In* Swerdlow, M. (ed.): Relief of Intractable Pain. Amsterdam, Excerpta Medica, 1974.
25. Charlton, J.E.: Relief of the pain of unresectable carcinoma of pancreas by chemical splanchnicectomy during laparotomy. Ann. R. Coll. Surg. Engl., *67*:136, 1985.
26. Cherry, D.A., and Lamberty, J.: Paraplegia following coeliac plexus block. Anaesth. Intensive Care, *12*:59, 1984.
27. Dale, W.A.: Splanchnic block in the treatment of acute pancreatitis. Surgery, *32*:605, 1952.
28. Dam, W., and Larsen, J.J.V.: Peripheral nerve blocks in relief of intractable pain. *In* Swerdlow, M. (ed.): Relief of Intractable Pain. Amsterdam, Excerpta Medica, 1974.
29. De Takats, G.: Splanchnic anaesthesia: Critical review of theory and practice of this method. Surg. Gynecol. Obstet., *44*:501, 1927.
30. Dogliotti, A.M.: Traitement des syndromes douloureux de la peripherie par l'alcoolisation subarachnoidienne des racines posterieurs a leur emergencede la moelle epiniere. Presse Med., *39*:1249, 1931.
31. Doyle, D.: Nerve blocks in advanced cancer. Practitioner, *226*:539, 1982.
32. Drechsel, U.: Treatment of cancer pain with neurolytic agents. Recent Results Cancer Res., *89*:137, 1984.
33. Duthie, A.M., and Ingham, V.: Persistent abdominal pain. Treatment by lumbar sympathetic lysis. Anaesthesia, *36*:289, 1981.
34. Duthie, A.M., Ingham, V., Dell, A.E., and Dennett, J.E.: Pituitary cryoablation. The results of treatment using a transphenoidal cryoprobe. Anaesthesia, *38*:448, 1983.
35. Dwyer, B.: Le traitement de la douleur en australie. Cah. d'Anesthesiologie, *17*:633, 1969.
36. Dwyer, B.: Treatment of pain of carcinoma of the tongue and floor of the mouth. Anaesth. Intensive Care, *1*:59, 1972.
37. Elmqvist, D., Toremalm, N.G., Elner, A., and Mercke, U.: Hemifacial spasm: Electrophysiological findings and the therapeutic effect of facial nerve block. Muscle Nerve, *5*:S89, 1982.
38. Farcot, J.M., Laugner, B., Muller, A., Mercky, F., Thiebaut, J.B., and Foucher, G.: Subdural-arachnoid neurolytic block in cervical pain. Pain, *17*:316, 1983.
38a. Flanigan, D.P., and Kraft, R.O.: Continuing experience with palliative chemical splanchnicectomy. Arch. Surg., *113*:509, 1978.
39. Ferrer–Brechner, T.: Anesthetic management of cancer pain. Semin. Oncol., *12*:431, 1985.
40. Foley, K.M.: The treatment of cancer pain. N. Engl. J. Med., *313*:84, 1985.
41. Fujita, Y., and Nakazaki, K.: Complications of alcohol injection into the mandibular nerve. Gasserian palsy and oculomotor palsy. Reg. Anaesth., *5*:39, 1982.
42. Garland, D.E., Lilling, M., and Keenan, M.A.: Percutaneous phenol blocks to motor points of spastic forearm muscles in head-injured adults. Arch. Phys. Med. Rehabil., *65*:243, 1984.
43. Garland, D.E., Lucie, R.S., and Waters, R.L.: Current uses of open phenol nerve block for adult acquired spasticity. Clin. Orthop., *165*:217, 1982.
44. Gianasi, G.: Neuroadenolysis of the pituitary, of Moricca: An overview of development, mechanisms, technique and results. *In* Benedetti, C. *et al.* Advances in Pain Research and Therapy, vol. 7, pp. 647–678. New York, Raven Press, 1984.
45. Glynn, C.J., Lloyd, J.W., and Barnard, J.D.W.: Cryoanalgesia in the management of post-thoracotomy pain. Thorax, *35*:325, 1980.
46. Gomoro, J.M., and Rappaport, Z.H.: Transovale trigeminal cistern puncture: Modified fluoroscopically guided technique. A.J.N.R., *6*:93, 1985.
47. Gorbitz, C., and Leavens, M.E.: Alcohol block of the celiac plexus for control of the upper abdominal pain caused by cancer and pancreatitis. J. Neurosurg., *34*:575, 1971.
48. Gratton, J.H.G., and Singer, C.: Anglo-Saxon Magic and Medicine (Lacnunga), p. 165. Oxford, Oxford University Press, 1952.
49. Guttman, S.A., and Pardee, I.: Spinal cord level syndrome following intrathecal ammonium sulphate and procaine hydrochloride. A case report with autopsy findings. Anesthesiology, *5*:347, 1944.
50. Hakanson, S.: Trigeminal neuralgia treated by the injection of glycerol into the trigeminal cistern. Neurosurgery, *9*:638, 1981.
51. Hand, L.V.: Subarachnoid ammonium sulphate therapy for intractable pain. Anesthesiology, *5*:354, 1944.
52. Hartz, W.H., and Gatenby, R.A.: Interventional radiology in palliative care. Semin. Oncol., *12*:390, 1985.
53. Hay, R.C.: Subarachnoid alcohol block in the control of intractable pain. Report of results in 252 patients. Anesth. Analg. (Cleve.), *41*:12, 1962.
54. Hay, R.C., Yonezawa, T., and Derrick, W.S.: Control of intractable pain in advanced cancer by subarachnoid alcohol block. J.A.M.A., *169*:1315, 1959.
54a. Hegedus, V.: Relief of pancreatic pain by radiography-guided blocks. A.J.R., *133*:1101, 1979.
55. Hollis, P.H., Malis, L.I., and Zappulla, R.A.: Neurological deterioration after lumbar puncture below complete spinal subarachnoid block. J. Neurosurg., *64*:253, 1986.
56. Ichiyanagi, K., Matsuki, M., Kinefuchi, S., and Kato, Y.: Progressive changes in the concentrations of phenol and glycerine in the human subarachnoid space. Anesthesiology, *42*:622, 1975.
57. Ischia, S., Luzzani, A., Ischia, A., and Faggion, S.: A new approach to the neurolytic block of the coeliac plexus: The transaortic technique. Pain, *16*:333, 1983.
58. Ischia, S., Luzzani, A., Ischia, A., Magon, F., and Toscano, D.: Subarachnoid neurolytic block (L5–S1) and unilateral percutaneous cervical cordotomy in the treatment of pain

secondary to pelvic malignant disease. Pain, *20*:139, 1984.

59. Ischia, S., Maffezzoli, G.F., Luzzani, A., and Pacini, L.: Subdural extra-arachnoid neurolytic block in cervical pain. Pain, *14*:347, 1982.
60. Jackson, S.H., Jacobs, J.B., and Epstein, R.A.: A radiographic approach to celiac plexus block. Anesthesiology, *31*:373, 1969.
61. Jacobs, J., Jackson, S., and Doppman, J.: A radiographic approach to celiac ganglion block. Radiology, *92*:1372, 1969.
62. Kappis, M.: Erfahrungen mit localanasthesie bei Bauchoperationen. Verh. Dtsch. Ges. Chir., *43*:1, teil 87, 1914.
63. Katz, J., and Levin, A.B.: Treatment of diffuse metastatic cancer pain by installation of alcohol into the sella turcica. Anesthesiology, *46*:115, 1977.
64. Kuzucu, E.Y., Derrick, W.S., and Wilber, S.A.: Control of intractable pain with subarachnoid alcohol block. J.A.M.A., *195*:541, 1966.
65. Laheurta, J., Lipton, S., Miles, J. and Wells, C.B.: Update on percutaneous cervical cordotomy and pituitary alcohol neuro-adenolysis: An audit of our recent results and complications. *In* Persistent Pain, vol. 5, pp. 197–223. Orlando, Fla., Grune and Stratton, 1985.
66. Lassner, J.: L'Analgesie prolongee par l'alcoolisation du ganglion coeliaque. Traitement pallaitif des tumeurs abdominales hautes inoperables. Anesth. Anal. (Paris), *25*:335, 1968.
67. Levin, A.B., Katz, J., Benson, R.C., and Jones, A.G.: Treatment of pain of diffuse metastatic cancer by stereotactic chemical hypophysectomy: Long term results and observations on mechanism of action. Neurosurgery, *6*:258, 1980.
68. Levin, A.B., and Ramirez, L.L.: Treatment of cancer pain with hypophysectomy: Surgical and chemical. *In* Benedetti, C., *et al.* (eds.): Advances in Pain Research and Therapy, vol. 7, pp. 631–646. New York, Raven Press, 1984.
69. Littler, B.O.: Alcohol blockade of the inferior dental nerve under radiographic control in the management of trigeminal neuralgia. Oral Surg., *57*:132, 1984.
70. Lloyd, J.W., Barnard, J.D.W., and Glynn, C.J.: Cryoanalgesia: A new approach to pain relief. Lancet, *2*:932, 1976.
71. Long, D.M.: Surgical therapy of chronic pain. Neurosurgery, *6*:317, 1980.
72. Lund, P.C.: Principles and practice of spinal anesthesia. Springfield, Ill., Charles C. Thomas, 1971.
73. Lunsford, L.D., Bennett, M.H., and Martinez, A.J.: Experimental trigeminal glycerol injection. Electrophysiologic and morphologic effects. Arch. Neurol., *42*:146, 1985.
74. McEwen, B.W., *et al.*: The pain clinic: A clinic for the management of intractable pain. Med. J. Aust., *1*:676, 1965.
75. Macintosh, R., and Ostlere, M.: Local Analgesia: Head and Neck, ed. 2. Edinburgh, E & S Livingstone, 1967.
76. Macintosh, R.R., and Bryce-Smith, R.: Local Analgesia: Abdominal Surgery. Edinburgh, E & S Livingstone, 1953.
77. Maher, R.M.: Relief of pain in incurable cancer. Lancet, *1*:18, 1955.
78. Maher, R.M.: Intrathecal chlorocresol in the treatment of pain in cancer. Lancet, *1*:965, 1963.
79. Maher, R.M., and Mehta, M.: Spinal (intrathecal) and extradural analgesia. *In* Lipton, S. (ed.): Persistent Pain: Modern Methods of Treatment. New York, Grune and Stratton, 1977.
80. Mark, V.H., White, J.C., Zervas, N.T., Ervin, F.R., and Richardson, E.P.: Intrathecal use of phenol for the relief of chronic severe pain. N. Engl. J. Med., *267*:589, 1962.
81. Matsuki, M., Kato, Y., and Ichiyanagi, K.: Progressive changes in the concentration of ethyl alcohol in the human and canine subarachnoid spaces. Anesthesiology, *36*:617, 1972.
82. Melzack, R.: Phantom limb pain: Implications for treatment of pathologic pain. Anesthesiology, *35*:409, 1971.
83. Merskey, H.: Psychological aspects of pain relief: Hypnotherapy, psychotropic drugs. *In* Swerdlow, M. (ed.): Relief of Intractable Pain. Amsterdam, Excerpta Medica, 1974.
84. Montgomery, W., and Cousins, M.J.: Aspects of the management of chronic pain illustrated by ninth nerve block. Br. J. Anaesth., *44*:383, 1972.
85. Moricca, G.: Pituitary neuroadenolysis in the treatment of intractable pain from cancer. *In* Lipton, S. (ed.): Persistent Pain: Modern Methods of Treatment. New York, Grune and Stratton, 1977.
86. Mullin, V.: Brachial plexus block with phenol for painful arm associated with Pancoast's syndrome. Anesthesiology, *53*:431, 1980.
87. Nathan, P.W., and Scott, T.G.: Intrathecal phenol for intractable pain: Safety and dangers of the method. Lancet, *1*:76, 1958.
88. Nathan, P.W., Sears, T.A., and Smith, M.C.: Effects of phenol solutions on nerve roots of the cat: An electro-physiological and histological study. J. Neurol. Sci., *2*:7, 1965.
89. Ochsner, A.: Indications for sympathetic nervous system block. Anesth. Analg. (Cleve.), *30*:61, 1951.
90. Pereira, A., and de Sousa, A.: Blocking of the splanchnic nerves and the first lumbar sympathetic ganglion: Technic, accidents and clinical indications. Arch. Surg., *53*:37, 1946.
91. Porges, P., and Zdrahal, F.: Intrathecal alcohol neurolysis of the lower sacral roots in inoperable rectal cancer. Anaesthetist, *34*:627, 1985.
92. Quimby, C.W.: Intercostal-celiac block for abdominal surgery in the poor risk patient. J. Arkansas Med. Soc., *68*:266, 1972.
93. Racz, G.B., Heavner, J., and Haynsworth, P.: Repeat epidural phenol injections in chronic pain and spasticity. *In* Lipton, S. (ed.): Persistent Pain: Modern Methods of Treatment. New York: Grune and Stratton, 1977.
94. Robertson, D.H.: Transsacral neurolytic nerve block. An alternative approach to intractable perineal pain. Br. J. Anaesth., *55*:873, 1983.
95. Rowse, C.W.: Dental surgery's role in head and neck cancer management. Ear Nose Throat J., *62*:247, 1983.
96. Shapshay, S.M., Scott, R.M., McCann, C.F., and Stoelting, I.: Pain control in advanced and recurrent head and neck cancer. Otolaryngol. Clin. North Am., *13*:551, 1980.
97. Simon, D.L., Carron, H., and Rowlinson, J.C.: Treatment of bladder pain with transsacral nerve block. Anesth. Analg., *61*:46, 1982.
98. Singler, R.C.: An improved technique for alcohol neurolysis of the celiac plexus. Anesthesiology, *56*:137, 1982.
99. Sunderland, S.: Nerves and nerve injuries. 2nd ed., pp. 131, 180. Edinburgh, E & S Livingstone, 1978.
100. Sweet, W.H., and Wepsic, J.G.: Controlled thermocoagula-

tion of the trigeminal ganglion and rootlets for differential destruction of pain fibers. I. Trigeminal neuralgia. J. Neurosurg., *39*:143, 1974.

101. Swerdlow, M.: Intrathecal chlorocresol. A comparison with phenol in the treatment of intractable pain. Anaesthesia, *28*:297, 1973.

102. Swerdlow, M. (ed.): Relief of Intractable Pain. 3rd ed. Amsterdam, Excerpta Medica, 1983.

103. Swerdlow, M.: Medico-legal aspects of complications following pain relieving blocks. Pain, *13*:321, 1982.

104. Takahashi, T., and Dohi, S.: Hemifacial spasm: A new technique of facial nerve blockade. Br. J. Anaesth., *55*:333, 1983.

104a. Thompson, G.E., Moore, D.C., Bridenbaugh, L.D., and Artin, R.Y.: Abdominal pain and alcohol celiac plexus nerve block. Anesth. Analg., *56*:1, 1977.

105. Trouwborst, A., Yanagida, H., Erdmann, W., and Kok, A.: Mechanism of neuroadenolysis of the pituitary for cancer pain control. Appl. Neurophysiol., *47*:97, 1984.

106. Ventafridda, V., and De Conno, F.: The role of neurolytic therapy in blocking cancer pain. Minerva Med., *75*:1463, 1984.

107. Ventafridda, V., Tamburini, M., and De Conno, F.: Comprehensive treatment in cancer pain. *In* Fields, H.L., *et al.* (eds.): Advances in Pain Research and Therapy, vol. 9, pp. 617–627. New York, Raven Press, 1985.

108. Ventafridda, V., Tamburini, M., Carceni, A., Conno, F., and Naldi, F.: A validation study of the WHO method for cancer pain relief. Cancer (in press).

109. Wainapel, S.F., Haigney, D., and Labib, K.: Spastic hemiplegia in a quadriplegic patient: Treatment with phenol nerve block. Arch. Phys. Med. Rehabil., *65*:786, 1984.

110. Walsh, T.D., and Saunders, C.M.: Hospice care: The treatment of pain in advanced cancer. Recent Results Cancer Res., *89*:201, 1984.

111. Wendling, H.: Ausschaltung der nervi splanchnici durch leitungsanasthesie bei magenoperationen und andern eingriffen in der oberen bauchhohle ein beitrag zur kenntnis der sensibilitat der bauchhole. Beitr. Z. Klin. Chir., *110*:517, 1918.

112. White, T.T., *et al.*: Treatment of pancreatitis by left splanchnicectomy and celiac ganglionectomy. Am. J. Surg., *112*:195, 1966.

113. Whittaker, D.K.: An experimental study of the effects of cryosurgery on the oral mucous membrane. Ph.D. thesis, University of Wales, 1973.

114. Wilson, F.: Neurolytic and other locally-acting drugs in the management of pain. Pharmacol. Ther. *12*[Suppl.]:65, 1983.

30 NEUROSTIMULATION AND PERCUTANEOUS NEURAL DESTRUCTIVE TECHNIQUES

RONALD R. TASKER

Progress in pain relieving procedures consists of introducing new techniques and improving old ones, enhancing their effectiveness, precision, and safety, yet minimizing their invasiveness. Recent developments exemplify these features well, particularly through the elaboration of procedures that can be performed percutaneously.

BASIC CONSIDERATIONS

Before reviewing the spectrum of procedures available for treating pain, certain basic principles must be outlined. The normal pain-free state may be looked upon as a balance between noxious input to the nervous system and modulatory mechanisms generated by that input which tend to suppress that noxious input. Pain occurs with enhanced input or reduced modulation, or both. The procedures intended to relieve pain attempt to counteract these states.

In our present limited state of knowledge, noxious input to the nervous system may simply be considered as peripheral or central.

Peripheral Inputs. Peripheral input consists almost entirely of activation of nociceptors with resultant traffic in nociceptive pathways, usually resulting from actual or threatened tissue damage. Such pain will be referred to as "nociceptive pain," the treatment of which consists of direct interruption of nociceptive traffic or modulatory techniques that inhibit that traffic.

Possibly another type of peripheral input exists, but if so it is exceedingly rare and has never been clearly identified as a cause of chronic pain in humans: alteration of peripheral activity by neural damage so as to result in central transmission of a pathologic pattern of impulses, which upon arrival is interpreted as pain. Wall[153] has listed the consequences of peripheral nerve damage, any one of which could theoretically induce a peripheral type of what has come to be termed *deafferentation pain.*

Central Inputs. Central inputs that induce pain ("central pain") can be reduced to two gross types: *psychogenic* and the products of somatosensory *deafferentation* at various levels in the nervous system. The input of psychogenic pain, whether psychotic, hysterical, magnification, or due to other causes, is presumably cortical, whereas that of the various deafferentation syndromes, other than peripheral referred to above, could extend from dorsal horn to cortical levels.

DEAFFERENTATION PAIN

At present, it is sufficient to group deafferentation pain syndromes, including the pain that arises from nerve injury, the "causalgias," anesthesia dolorosa, post-traumatic syndromes, amputation and stump pain, the pain following brachial plexus avulsion, postherpetic neuralgia, spinal cord or cauda equina damage, cordotomy, stroke, and brain trauma. Although eventually it may turn out that various pathophysiologic processes are at work in these different conditions, their clinical features are similar:[132,134,138,140,141]

1. The pain is triggered by a lesion that interferes with somatosensory input, usually including spinothalamic fibers.
2. A series of apparently identical lesions does not result in pain every time. About 1 : 50,000 strokes, 20% of spinal cord injuries, 5% of cordotomies, 20% to 67% of brachial plexus avulsions, and 92% of preganglionic brachial plexus lesions are followed by pain.[138,159,162] In the case of strokes, there is some doubt about the incidence of pain because of the difficulty in communicating with some of the patients. Deafferentation pain of any kind is reported to be rare in children; however, precise data are not available.
   In the case of herpes zoster, postherpetic pain is more common the older that a victim is. Indeed, below the age of 45 years, only a small percentage of patients with zoster develop persistent postherpetic pain. Thus any form of treatment is likely to appear effective in this age group, whereas in the older age group no form of treatment has been clearly shown to be effective. Invasive procedures are thus not justified in the younger age group and are rarely helpful in older patients.
   Inbal and associates[45] and Levitt and Levitt[55] showed apparent genetically determined susceptibilities to what they deemed to be animal models of deafferentation pain.[58a]
3. The pain that results may have a delayed onset.
4. The pain is often dysesthetic or causalgic and is usually associated with areas of at least partial sensory loss to at least one modality and may be associated with allodynia, hyperpathia, or hyperesthesia.
5. The pain is usually relieved *temporarily* by proximal local anesthetic blockade but *permanently* in only 25% to 35% of cases after neural section at the same site.
6. The pain is more readily relieved temporarily by agents such as sodium thiopental than it is by opiates. Longer-term relief is sometimes possible with tricyclic drugs but rarely with opiates.
7. The pain can often be reproduced by electrically stimulating medial mesencephalic tegmentum, medial thalamus, somatosensory cortex, and sometimes the ventral basal complex.

The mechanism by which pain is produced is unknown although there are various central consequences of somatosensory deafferentation that theoretically could result in pain,[60,161] including activation of previously ineffective synapses; increased effect of surviving synapses; new aberrant connections; chemical hypersensitivity to neurotransmitters and neuromodulatory substrates; ephaptic connections; spontaneous activity generated at the injury site; altered somatotopic representation of one or more sensory modalities; loss of inhibitory connections; altered ascending or descending inhibitory paths; desensitization of pattern-generating systems; and spontaneous activity in denervated neurons. There is experimental and clinical evidence implicating denervation neuronal hypersensitivity as the substrate for deafferentation pain at the levels of dorsal horn and dorsal column nuclei and in the trigeminal system, whereas stimulation-induced reproduction of deafferentation pain in humans at the level of medial mesencephalon and thalamus is consistent with deafferentation neuronal hypersensitivity affecting the reticulospinal system.[132,134,138,140,141] Attempts to treat deafferentation pain must consider its peculiar pathophysiology.

DECISION TO USE A PAIN-RELIEVING PROCEDURE

Having categorized the patient's pain into an appropriate syndrome, the clinician must still decide whether it is appropriate to carry out a procedure and then must decide which procedure to use. Obviously it must be clear that the pain is intractable, that no treatable underlying causative disease exists, that the pain is not predominantly due to psychological factors, and that, even in pain with a clear physical component, the major disability is not derived from psychogenic magnification. Then the disability from the pain as distinct from that of the accompanying neurologic deficit must be weighed against the chance of success and the morbidity and mortality of the proposed procedure. This must be done by detailed physical and psychological assessment of the patient, including work, play, sleep, and use of medication. Following this, a program of treatment must be formulated starting with the simplest and progressing to more complex treatment as far as the disability warrants. For it must be remembered that there is a high failure rate in the treatment of chronic pain and that even successful treatment seldom achieves complete or permanent relief independent from other modalities of therapy.

Also there is a large element of placebo effect in the initial results of impressive procedures. The more impressive the procedure and the more convinced are the patient and surgeon that it will work, the more likely that initial result will be good. Initial success based on placebo effect has a rapid decline (see Chap. 25).

TECHNIQUES THAT INTERRUPT PAIN INPUT

Percutaneous techniques will be divided into interruptive and modulatory procedures, briefly mentioning the indications, highlights of technique, and results.

Destructive techniques are virtually confined to the treatment of nociceptive pain, and then almost entirely to *cancer pain* in patients with a short life expectancy. Changes induced by peripheral *deafferentation,* in patients with a medium to long life expectancy, may result in abnormal activity at the receptor or peripheral nerve levels as discussed above. Pain of this type that can be interrupted by neurectomy, rhizotomy, or other interruptive techniques, must be exceedingly rare to the point that it is virtually axiomatic that deafferentation pain is not only never relieved but also usually aggravated by destructive surgery, *even though local anesthetic blockade temporarily relieves that pain in 85% of cases.*

Destructive techniques have been accomplished by various means: injection of necrotizing substances such as alcohol and phenol, ionizing radiation, cold, heat, lasers, and physical cutting, among others; however, the use of such techniques is still sometimes beneficial in cancer pain (see Chap. 29). The precision of localization, the ease of physiologic corroboration of target size, the production of a controlled graded lesion, and the avoidance of injury to adjacent or intervening tissues make percutaneous thermocoagulation with radiofrequency current the contemporary method of choice for a number of situations in which neurodestructive techniques retain a limited but valuable place.

PERCUTANEOUS NEURECTOMY

Neurectomy of the trigeminal, glossopharnygeal, intercostal, occipital, and obturator nerves is readily performed percutaneously; however, neurectomy is rarely indicated in the treatment of pain for a variety of reasons. It is rarely successful in deafferentation syndromes. Only 25% of 44 patients with deafferentation pain caused by thoracotomy were relieved when the area of pain was rendered anesthetic by multiple intercostal neurectomy even though temporary pain relief was nearly always achieved by local anesthetic blockade of those same nerves. No controlled data to date support the use of neurectomy for post-thoracotomy pain. It is likely that the temporary response in 25% of patients is a placebo effect. In nociceptive syndromes such as those caused by cancer, pain is rarely subserved by one or a few peripheral nerves. Thus denervation of the pain area is seldom feasible by neurectomy. Finally the motor and sensory consequences of neurectomy are seldom acceptable. If such an approach appears desirable, it is better to use a subarachnoid neurolytic block (see Chap. 29).

On the other hand, even though the *spontaneous* pain of deafferentation is, naturally enough, not relieved by further surgical deafferentation, the hyperpathia or allodynia can be, for this unpleasant accompaniment of some deafferentation pain syndromes is dependent upon *partial* denervation and is relieved by completion of that denervation. By hyperpathia, or allodynia, is meant a painful experience elicited by a normally non-noxious stimulus or by one that is out of keeping with what would be expected from a noxious stimulus, delivered in an area of heightened threshold to at least one modality of somatosensory function. Sometimes there is accompanying temporal and spatial spread of that perceived sensation.

Procedures on the Trigeminal Nerve for Tic Douloureux

Trigeminal neurectomy is usually performed for tic douloureux. This is a condition without clinical signs or laboratory or imaging abnormalities, of controversial etiology, consisting of remitting attacks of lancinating pain affecting somatotopographically consistent areas in the trigeminal distribution, often associated with triggering during relapses, usually from within the pain territory. Progression of the pain to involve new areas of the face is somatotopic, and the disease affects both sides of the face in 3% of cases. In a minority of patients it is secondary to multiple sclerosis or trigeminal or acoustic neuroma, and occasionally it is associated with unexplained sensory loss.

Radiofrequency Coagulation of the Trigeminal Nerve

The treatment of choice for trigeminal tic douloureux after failure of medical treatment with carbamazepine is, in my opinion, percutaneous radiofrequency coagulation, preferably by the discrete selective technique (see below). In this manner pain relief can be achieved with minimal sensory loss at a risk a fraction of that faced with decompression of the trigeminal nerve root entry zone in the posterior fossa.

Conventional Procedure

The conventional technique will be discussed first. Based on the original work of Kirshner[49] and Härtel,[37] the technique required certain refinements, including radiofrequency lesion-making as described by Sweet and Wepsic,[124] before precision became great enough and risks low enough for general acceptance.

Technique. The patient is positioned supine, head precisely lateral, with lateral image intensification, under brief periods of thiopental anesthesia. A suitable varnish-insulated electrode with a 3-mm noninsulated tip fashioned from a No. 16 lumbar puncture needle* (Fig. 30-1) is introduced into the symptomatic side of the face a fingerbreadth lateral to the lateral angle of the mouth and advanced toward the intersection of the sagittal plane through the pupil of the eye and the coronal plane through the middle of the zygoma, avoiding the buccal cavity. The needle is advanced and followed radiographically, "walking" off the pterygoid plates or base of the skull into the foramen ovale. A sudden contraction of jaw muscles or an exacerbation of pain heralds its arrival in the foramen ovale. Although, theoretically, the needle can now be advanced until it impinges on the vault, the tip should not rise above the crest of the petrous ridge as its progress is followed on the image intensifier. For third division (V3) tic, the tip should lie relatively low on this trajectory, as shown in Figure 30-2; for first division tic (V1) relatively high, as shown in Figure 30-3. If cerebrospinal fluid return occurs, preferable in V1 tic, a more permanent and often more complete denervation is likely, since the electrode lies among preganglionic rootlets. In V3 tic this situation need not be sought, for the procedure is easily repeated in the event of recurrence when a postganglionic lesion is made. It may not be radiographically apparent when the electrode lies in alternate adjacent foramina except for the jugular, as shown in Figure 30-4—hence the dependence on physiologic localization. If arterial blood is encountered in foramen lacerum, the needle need only be withdrawn and reinserted. In proper position, stimulation at 1 to 5 Hz should elicit trigeminal motor contractions at thresholds under 2 to 3 V (Figs. 30-5, 30-6). There is no need to reposition to try to avoid motor denervation if motor contractions occur, for it will likely be transient. The patient is now awakened, and stimulation at 50 to 100 Hz is carried out. This should induce paresthesias in the area where the pain occurs, preferably at less than 0.5 V, certainly at no more than 1 V. Under brief thiopental anesthesia, a radiofrequency lesion is now made, progressively increasing current flow and needle tip temperature to 150 to 250 mA (average, 175–200) and 70° to 90°C, respectively, over 30 to 90 seconds. Too hurried a current and temperature rise, producing early fall-off of current, will prevent significant lesion-making owing to the insulation from heat produced by the gases that result from boiling of tissue at the needle tip. A visible flush will often appear in the denervated part of the

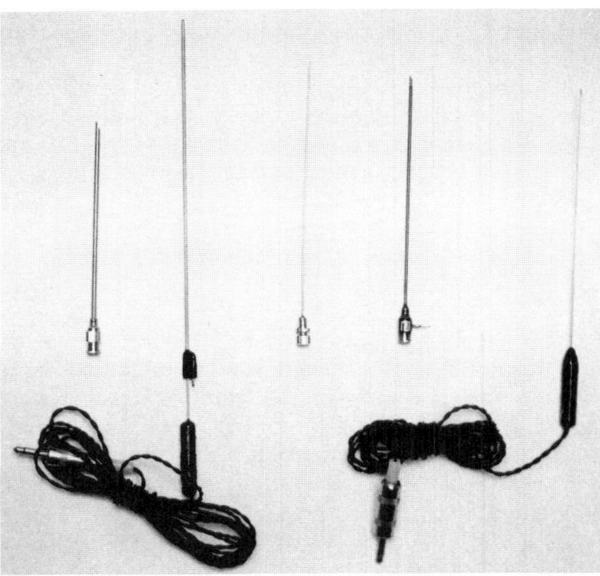

FIG. 30-1. Electrodes for percutaneous surgery. **Left.** Guide needle, and electrode with thermistor inserted, for "facet rhizotomy." **Right.** Stylet, electrode, and thermistor for conventional RF trigeminal coagulation. (Manufactured by Diros Technology)

*Manufactured by Diros Technology, 967 Pape Avenue, Toronto, Canada, M4K 3V6, or by Radionics Corporation, 76 Cambridge Street, Burlington, MA 01803, USA.

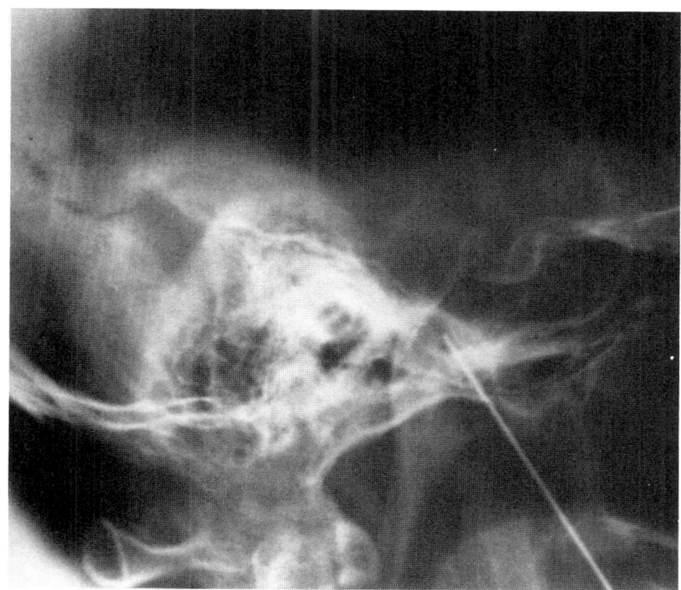

FIG. 30-2. Lateral x-ray showing electrode for conventional thermocoagulation of the trigeminal nerve inserted where stimulation and lesion-making produced effects in V3.

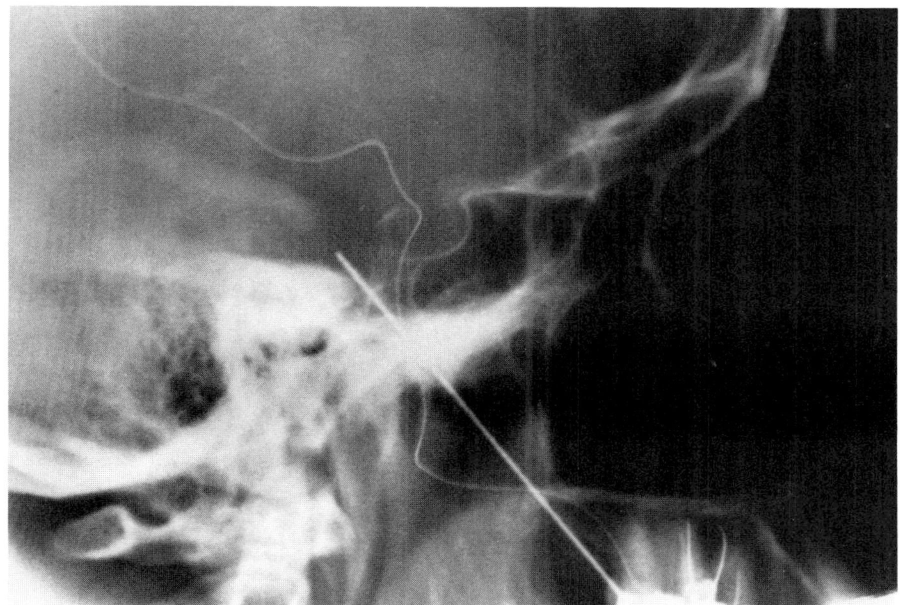

FIG. 30-3. Lateral x-ray, as in Figure 30-2, where stimulation produced paresthesias in the forehead.

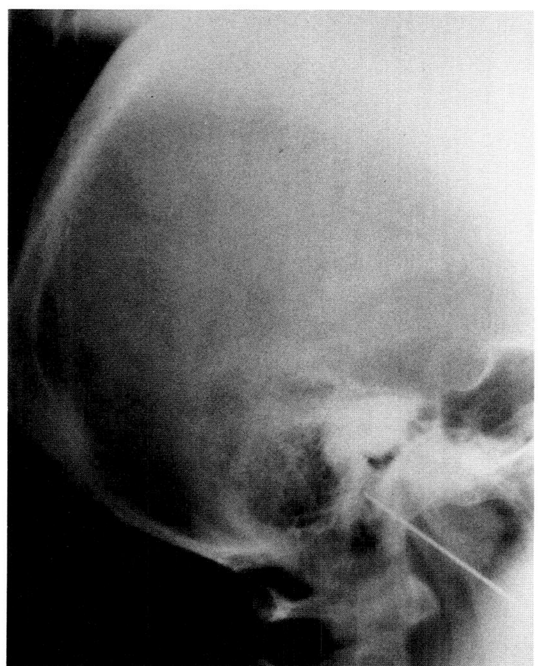

FIG. 30-4. Lateral x-ray, as in Figure 30-2, for thermocoagulation of glossopharyngeal nerve in jugular foramen.

face. The patient is reawakened and the sensory loss verified.

Discrete Selective Technique

A preferred variant of the procedure[87,144] consists of using an electrode similar to that for percutaneous cordotomy (Fig. 30-7) introduced through a No. 18 lumbar puncture needle. The tip of the cordotomy electrode is slightly bent so that by rotation a large number of sites in Meckel's cave can be stimulated using a single electrode introduction. A suitable electrode obtainable from Diros consists of a 0.4 mm electrolytically sharpened stainless steel wire projecting 2 mm beyond its shrunk-fit Teflon tubing, in turn projecting 2 mm beyond the tip of the lumbar puncture needle. The procedure is performed under local anesthesia or neuroleptanalgesia as described for the conventional technique. A site is sought at which paresthesias are produced exactly in the area of pain, then a graded lesion is made until selective analgesia is achieved in that area. Parameters of lesion-making are similar to those for percutaneous cordotomy described below, maximal lesions usually being achieved with 70 to 90 mA for 60 seconds.

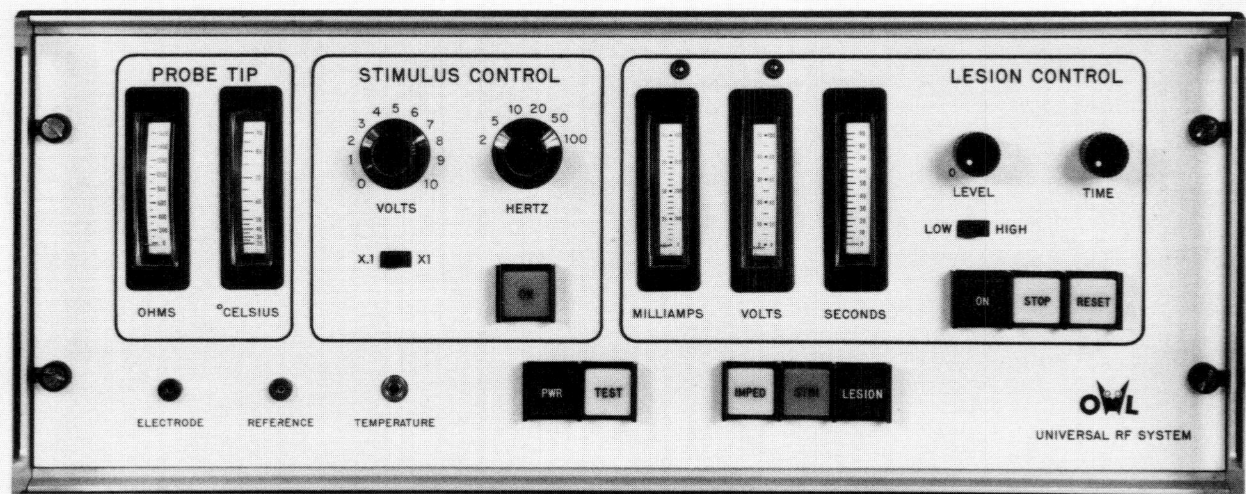

FIG. 30-5. Electronic backup for impedance monitoring, stimulation, and radiofrequency lesion-making with current, voltage, and temperature monitoring capabilities. (Manufactured by Diros Technology).

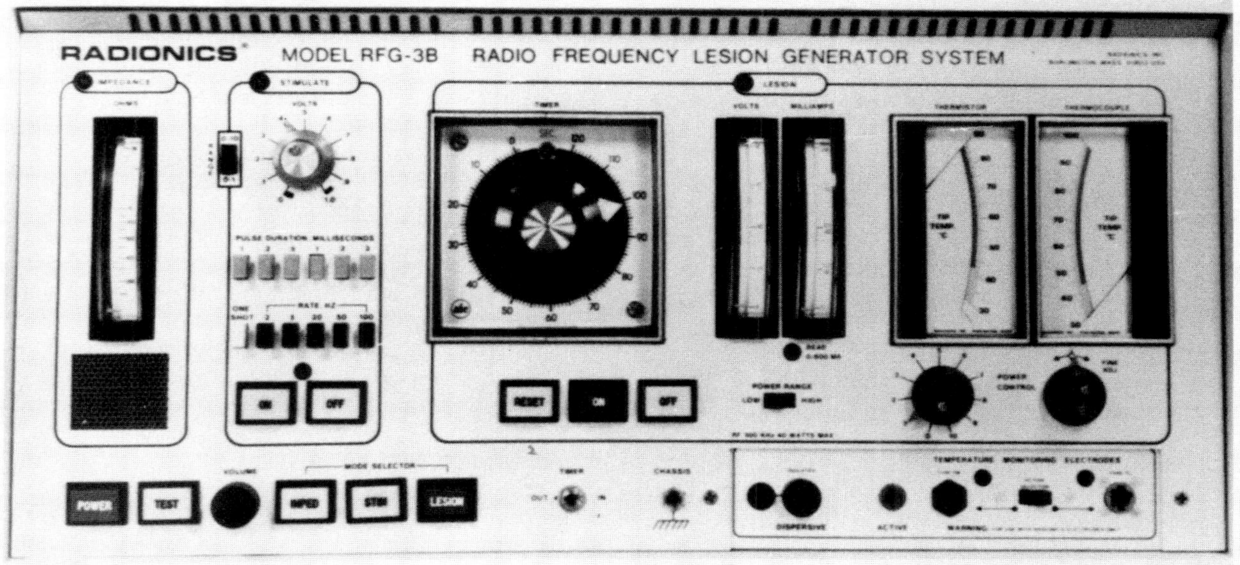

FIG. 30-6. Electronic backup, as in Figure 30-5. (Manufactured by Radionics Corporation).

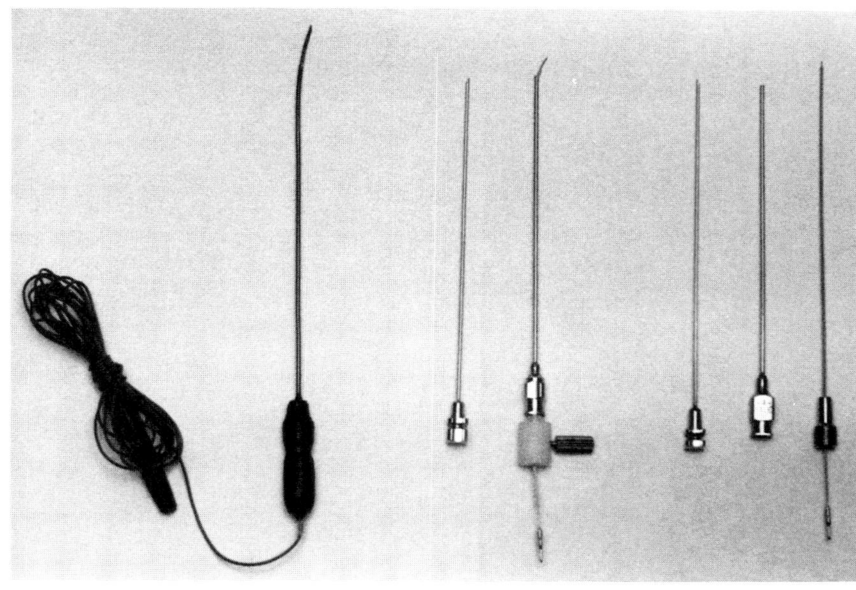

FIG. 30-7. Electrodes for percutaneous surgery. **Left.** Electrode for intercostal neurectomy. **Center.** Stylet, and curved electrode inserted in guide needle, for selective trigeminal thermocoagulation. **Right.** Stylet, guide needle, and electrode for percutaneous cordotomy. (Manufactured by Diros Technology)

Results. Tew and colleagues[143] reported 93% excellent to good results in 400 patients with tic using the conventional technique. Fourteen percent complained of unpleasant sensory effects, 1% so severe as to lead to excoriation of the face, nostril, or scalp. Only 2% developed keratitis, although 30% had corneal analgesia. Two percent exhibited transient diplopia and 22% paresis of the motor root, which also was usually transient. The latter was occasionally associated with complaints referred to the ear because of paralysis of the tensor veli palati or tensor tympani. Over 1 to 8 years, tic recurred in 14%, and 9% underwent a second operation. In a subsequent review,[144] Tew and associates reported 76% excellent, 17% good, 6% fair, and 1% poor results with 700 procedures also performed in the conventional way over a 10-year period. Of the 24% with recurrences, 9% were reoperated.

Using the selective technique and a curved electrode as described above, results in 200 patients were distinctly better, although the follow-up was only 12 months.

Complications in this larger series using the conventional method consisted of a 24% incidence of masseter weakness, 27% unpleasant paresthesias, 2% diplopia, and 4% keratitis. With the selective curved needle technique, there was a 9% incidence of masseter weakness, 11% unpleasant paresthesias, no diplopia, and 2% keratitis.

Latchaw and co-workers[51] reported 52% good results with the conventional method without recurrence in 96 patients with tic, particularly if the patient had not been previously exposed to open surgery and particularly if dense sensory loss was achieved. All patients without persistent sensory loss suffered recurrence. Twenty-six percent had depressed and 13% absent corneal reflexes, 2% keratitis, 5% masseter paresis, 42% unintended sensory loss, 26% unpleasant sensory effects, and 1% anesthesia dolorosa. The severity of the latter was related to the degree of sensory loss. Latchaw's useful literature review suggests a 7% to 22% incidence of corneal anesthesia, 0 to 5% keratitis, 1% to 19% dysesthesia, and 15% to 50% unintended sensory loss. Recurrences were reported in these series in 6% to 46% over 2 to 2½ years, 9% to 53% over 4 to 5 years, 18% to 22% over 7 to 8 years, and 80% in longer follow-ups.

Turnbull[147] reported his experience in 41 patients in a graphic and particularly interesting way. Anesthesia in at least part of the face occurred in 1 of 1 patient with V1 tic, 4 of 9 with V1-V2 tic, 6 of 14 with V2 tic, 3 of 9 with V2-V3 tic, and 2 of 11 with V3 tic. Pain was relieved in all, but recurred in 5 patients over 0 to 4 years. Motor weakness occurred in 9, keratitis in 2, and corneal areflexia in 8, 6 of whom did not have V1 tic to start with. Five developed dysesthesia and 1 anesthesia dolorosa. Anesthesia occurred in facial areas not afflicted with tic in 0 of 1, 1 of 9, 5 of 14, 1 of 9, and 0 of 11, and analgesia in 1 of 1, 2 of 9, 9 of 14, 2 of 9, and 2 of 11 of patients with V1, V1–V2, V2, V2–V3, and V3 tic, respectively.

Although percutaneous thermocoagulation of the trigeminal nerve is a procedure with low morbidity and mortality, I am aware of two incidences of fatal postoperative subarachnoid hemorrhage unrelated to the lesion, possibly caused by acute hypertension, one case of bacterial meningitis, one of temporal lobe abscess, and reported cases of stroke following carotid artery puncture and of carotid cavernous fistula.

Percutaneous Injection of Glycerol

Håkansson[35] has introduced the treatment of tic by the injection, through a 22-gauge needle, of 0.2 to 0.4 ml of glycerol into Meckel's cave cistern under local anesthesia using a technique similar to that employed for radiofrequency coagulation. CSF is drained and metrizamide slowly injected in 0.2- to 0.4-ml increments until the cistern is filled and dye starts to empty into the posterior fossa. Cisternal metrizamide is emptied by head positioning to remove the protective dye from parts of the root intended to be affected by glycerol. The calculated volume of the cistern is used to estimate the volume of glycerol needed. If the entire cistern is exposed to glycerol, all three divisions will be affected; leaving metrizamide in place to cover rootlets uninvolved with tic will protect them from the injection. In 15% of Håkansson's cases the first attempt failed, pain recurred in 18% over a period of 2 to 48 months, and 60% noted slight facial numbness for the first postoperative week. None suffered from dysesthesia, and alteration of facial sensation was barely detectable in "the majority." Eighty-six percent of 75 patients were totally free of their pain, half immediately and half within 4 to 6 days. One patient died of pulmonary embolism.

Sweet and Poletti[123] note that Håkansson's recurrence rate was 31% over 1 to 6 years in 100 patients. They themselves treated 31 patients, 27 suffering from tic, 3 from atypical facial pain, and 1 from posttraumatic pain. Pain was relieved in 24 of the 27 with tic. The only failures were in patients who did not develop analgesia during or after the injection, and 16 of their patients had persistent sensory loss, including 9 suffering from dysesthesia and 5 from reduced corneal reflexes.

Lunsford and Bennett[64] reported 67% complete and 23% partial control of tic in 112 patients followed over 4 to 28 months. Seventy-three percent of patients had no sensory loss, 3% developed aseptic meningitis, and 3.6% had severe postoperative dysesthesia. There was no motor weakness, oculomotor disturbance, or keratitis in their patients.

Percutaneous Compression of Trigeminal Nerve

Harking back to the technique of open compression or decompression of Meckel's cave advocated by Taarnhoj[126] and Sheldon and associates[109] for the treatment of tic, Mullan and Lichtor[80] have introduced a method for percutaneous compression of the nerve. Under general anesthesia with the patient intubated and using biplanar imaging, a No. 4 (0.75–1.0 ml capacity) Fogarty balloon catheter inserted to the tip of a liver biopsy needle is passed through the foramen ovale by the same method described above, after filling the air space with Conray. The catheter is now advanced 1 cm and slowly inflated with Conray diluted to a manageable viscosity until the balloon fills Meckel's cave and begins to assume a pear shape by slowly expanding into the posterior fossa. The balloon is held inflated 3 to 10 minutes with 0.5 to 1 ml Conray, then collapsed and withdrawn. Difficulties with a scarred cave may be encountered, including rupture of the balloon (not a dangerous occurrence). In 50 patients with tic, 49 obtained immediate relief, 6 experienced recurrence in 6 to 31 months, 3 suffered from dysesthesia, 4 from analgesia, and 1 from trochlear nerve palsy. All patients experienced subjective numbness and ipsilateral motor paralysis; some experienced sensory loss persisting 4 to 6 months.

Radiofrequency Coagulation of Trigeminal Nerve for Other Than Tic

The conventional percutaneous thermocoagulation technique can also be used to treat trigeminal pain caused by cancer and migrainous neuralgia consistently afflicting part of the trigeminal territory, although it should be avoided in atypical facial pain, deafferentation pain, and postherpetic neuralgia unless intended for the control of allodynia or hyperpathia alone.

In cancer, pain is rarely confined to the trigeminal territory so that trigeminal denervation alone is nearly always unsuccessful and cancerous destruction of the base of the skull may prevent needle positioning. In those few selected suitable candidates, denervation for the relief of cancer pain should be as complete as possible. Siegfried and Broggi[110] relieved pain in 10 of their 20 patients who had pain caused by cancer. Maxwell[67] relieved all 8 of his patients with migrainous neuralgia, although pain eventually recurred in 3. Watson and colleagues[155] reported pain relief in 8 of 13 patients with cluster headache treated by percutaneous thermocoagulation. One developed anesthesia dolorosa, and 5 suffered from recurrence, 1 of whom did not respond to repeated coagulation. Pain relief required sensory loss in the area of pain.

Percutaneous Thermocoagulation of the Glossopharyngeal Nerve

Essentially the same type of approach can be used to make lesions in the glossopharyngeal nerve in the jugular foramen.[11,12,46,52,102,144] The needle is passed 20° posterior and 5° to 10° medial to the course used to enter the foramen ovale, the x-ray (see Fig. 30-4) showing a more posterior position. Electrocardiogram and blood pressure should be monitored to avoid alterations in vagus nerve function, and correct positioning is indicated when 0.1 to 0.3 V stimulation produces paresthesias in the external auditory meatus or the ipsilateral side of the pharynx. Trapezius contractions, blood pressure, and cardiograph changes should be avoided. After a test lesion to ensure that untoward results do not occur, a 60-second 65° to 75°C lesion should be made, stopping short of producing alterations in blood pressure or pulse.

Isamat and associates[46] used this procedure on 4 patients with glossopharyngeal tic without complications, although pain recurred in 2. The procedure was successfully repeated in 1. Tew and co-workers[144] and Lazorthes and Verdie[52] relieved pain in 3 patients, but dysarthria and dysphasia were postoperative problems. Broggi[11] treated 6 patients with tic with 3 having good results and 1 fair results. Salar and colleagues[102] treated 3 patients with tic by a lateral approach, all of whom were relieved, although 75% showed transient vagal dysfunction. Tew and associates[144] treated 9 patients with cancer, 8 of whom were relieved. Broggi[11] used the procedure on 5 patients with cancer with 2 excellent results and 2 recurrences successfully managed by reoperation. Salar and co-workers[102] treated 5 patients with cancer in their series. Pagura and colleagues[91] relieved 11 of 15 patients with cancer pain at the expense of glossopharyngeal dysfunction in all.

Percutaneous Intercostal Neurectomy

Percutaneous intercostal neurectomy was first used by my colleagues and me in 1972 to treat pain in the chest wall, especially nociceptive pain caused by cancer of the sternum, ribs, or parietal pleura in patients in whom cordotomy was contraindicated. The procedure has limited usefulness in other types of nociceptive intercostal neuralgia but is of no help in managing deafferentation pain such as that of postherpetic neuralgia or post-thoracotomy pain unless hyperpathia alone is the problem.

Technique. The technique consists of using the basic radiofrequency lesion-making backup equipment (see Figs. 30-5, 30-6), with an electrode gently curved at its tip as shown in Figure 30-7. The latter is free of insulation over its 10-mm tip. With the patient anesthetized and positioned painful side up but not paralyzed, the electrode tip is slipped under the trailing edge of the appropriate rib at an appropriate distance along its length (see Fig. 14-3). Stimulation at 2 Hz and 10 V is continued as the needle tip is positioned while contractions in the appropriate intercostal muscles are watched for. Stimulation is reduced and repositioning carried out until intercostal contractions are obtained at the lowest possible threshold, preferably below 3 V when a graded radiofrequency lesion is made by gradually increasing current flow over 90 seconds from 75 mA until falloff occurs, usually at 175 to 250 mA. Stimulation is then repeated to identify a rise in threshold, preferably of 100%, or else a similar lesion is made at another site along the same nerve. The procedure is repeated at additional intercostal nerves as necessary. An upright chest x-ray film is done immediately postoperatively to identify pneumothorax.

Results. No published series have been seen, although the procedure is mentioned by Uematsu.[148] My colleagues and I have performed 52 intercostal neurectomies with a 25% incidence of relief of deafferentation syndromes, 100% in those caused by cancer. The only complication, pneumothorax, has occurred three times, twice resolving spontaneously. A third patient discharged by our thoracic surgery service without treatment underwent drainage at another hospital.

Percutaneous Occipital Neurectomy

A similar approach can be used to treat pain at the cervicocranial junction. Because the C1 root has no sensory input, pain in this region is largely mediated by C2 and particularly the greater occipital nerves. Blume[7] and Blume and Fromm[8] have reported 75% reduction in various syndromes with 1- to 4-year follow-up in 114 and 250 patients, respectively.

Percutaneous Obturator Neurectomy

Although strictly speaking not an operation for pain, percutaneous radiofrequency obturator neurectomy is sometimes helpful in the overall management of the patient with spinal cord injury with the combined problems of pain and spasticity. The patient is positioned supine with bladder emptied. Under local or neuroleptanalgesia, a conventional radiofrequency tic electrode is introduced under oblique image intensification, giving a "full face" view of the obturator foramen, from medial to lateral (see Chap. 11). The tip of the needle is slipped under the supralateral corner of the foramen where the obturator nerve enters it. Stimulation at 2 Hz should induce contractions in the adductor muscles at below 5 V when a radiofrequency lesion is made by maximizing current flow to falloff as described under intercostal neurectomy.

Nine such procedures have been performed successfully.

"FACET RHIZOTOMY"

In patients with spondylogenic back pain, Rees[98] introduced a procedure intended to sever facet nerves in the lower lumbar region using a knife as a treatment for spondylogenic back pain. Shealy[106] developed the means of performing the procedure percutaneously with radiofrequency current and physiologic localization. Fox and Rizzoli[32] and Pederson and associates[94] confirmed the anatomic course of the nerves taking off from the posterior ramus just distal to the ganglion and passing inferiorly and dorsally between facet joint and transverse process at interlumbar joints. At the lumbosacral space the facet nerve leaves the L5 root to enter the groove between the superior facet of the L5–S1 joint and the S1 transverse process (see Fig. 27-24).

Technique. The procedure is performed under local anesthesia or neuroleptanalgesia with brief periods of general anesthesia for lesion-making. The patient is postured prone. Some prefer the x-ray angle at 45°. Lateral views are used to check the depth of needle penetration. Usually bilateral rhizotomies at

L3 – L4, L4 – L5, and L5 – S1 are performed after diagnostic local anesthetic facet blocks have demonstrated satisfactory pain relief. Through a small stab wound a No. 14 needle is introduced at a 45° angle directed inferomedially so as to impinge on the base of the superior facet process distal to the corresponding foramen between the lower portion of the facet joint and the projection of the pedicle, as seen on end under image intensification. The equipment used is shown in Figure 30-1. The L5 – S1 joint is denervated by introducing the needle into the notch between the transverse process of L5 and the sacrum. An electrode with a 5-mm bare tip is now passed through the guide needle to the above-mentioned site and the needle withdrawn to avoid grounding out of current around the bare tip (see Fig. 30-1). Stimulation is now carried out at 2 and 100 Hz aimed at avoiding damage to anterior ramus and at precisely locating the facet nerve. A site is sought while the electrode tip is manipulated where paravertebral muscle contractions occur at 2 Hz, tetanization at 100 Hz at below 5 V affecting the paravertebral but not the pelvic or lower limb musculature. Stimulation at 100 Hz should produce paresthesias paravertebrally or in the pelvis but not below the knee, preferably at voltages below 0.5 V. The location of these paresthesias should be similar to that of the patient's pain. A graded lesion is now made until falloff occurs as described above (100 – 200 mA for 90 seconds sustaining a temperature of 70°C or more).

Results. Postoperative pain usually subsides within a few days, and the major risk of anterior ramus damage should be avoided by physiologic testing. Reported success in relieving pain varies from 50% to 70%. Oudenhoven described 74% excellent and 15% good results in 66 patients who had not had previous spinal surgery. Thirty-five percent excellent and 24% good results were achieved in 48 patients whose backs had been previously operated on.[89] Burton[13] found excellent results in 42% of 126 patients overall and in 67% of those not previously operated on. McCulloch[68] successfully relieved pain in 82% of patients not previously exposed to spinal surgery, whereas Dunsker and co-workers[24] reported 20% overall satisfactory results. Patients with previous spinal surgery never did well, but 40% of those whose pain was relieved by diagnostic local blockade of the facet nerve were helped (see also Chap. 27.3).

Shealy[106] reported 63% excellent results in 57 patients, including some with cervical and thoracic disease, none of whom had previously undergone spinal surgery. Only 25% excellent results occurred in 60 patients previously operated on without fusion, and 14% excellent results occurred among 90 with previous surgery, including fusion. Presumably, "facet rhizotomy" being a neurectomy, regeneration with pain recurrence should be expected in time. Thus the procedure does not provide a long-term solution but may be valuable as a means of pain relief to allow initiation of effective physical and psychologic, therapy during the pain-free interval.

SYMPATHECTOMY

Sympathetic ablation is valuable in ischemic pain (see Chap. 13) and in visceral pain caused by cancer (see Chap. 29).

In general, sympathectomy is less useful in controlling intractable "nonmalignant" pain, an exception being its *early* use in the occasional case of "major causalgia," affecting usually the sciatic nerve and selected cases of visceral pain. Nevertheless sympathectomy is frequently resorted to for the following reasons. Sympathetic dystrophic changes sometimes accompany deafferentation pain syndromes, just as hyperpathia does.[58] And just as denervation relieves hyperpathia but not the underlying spontaneous pain, sympathectomy, preferably performed percutaneously with phenol,[9] relieves the sympathetic dystrophy but without affecting the underlying pain.

The exceptions are rare cases of partial lesions of usually the sciatic nerve with reflex sympathetic dystrophy. Further, local sympathetic blockade may often temporarily relieve deafferentation pain just as local somatic blockade usually does, whereas sympathectomy, like permanent surgical denervation, does not. Presumably such relief is the result of inadvertent somatic blockade the salutary effect of which may be explained by Condouris' suggestion that local anesthetics induce some modulatory effect.[15]

In the case of visceral pain, pain fibers cross with the sympathetic system to reach the somatic afferents. Thus sympathetic denervation also produces nociceptive interruption. Sympathetic destruction may be useful in relieving intractable pain in such viscera as the pancreas. Originally achieved by open means, the pain caused by cancer of abdominal viscera may also be alleviated by the percutaneous injection of alcohol into the celiac plexus as in the experience of Moore,[76] who reported 94% excellent to good results in 168 patients undergoing 186 blocks (see Chap. 29). Complications included hypotension, iatrogenic pain, and inadvertent somatic nerve damage with the theoretical possibility of subarachnoid and intravisceral alcohol injection.

Wilkinson[157] has described a percutaneous radiofrequency technique for upper thoracic sympathectomy. With the patient prone under local anesthesia, a needle is introduced 6 to 7 cm from the midline and directed toward three sites. The most caudal site is lesioned first to best retain the pupillary response as a guide to lesion-making. An 18-gauge needle with a 10-mm bare tip is inserted within a 16-gauge needle between the third and fourth ribs medial to the scapular margin and aimed at a point 2 to 5 mm lateral and rostral to the midpoint of T3 vertebra. The electrode tip is positioned at the ventral edge of T3 in the lateral x-ray under the head of the third rib. The next lesion is made by passing the electrode between the second and third ribs to reach just lateral to the T2–T3 interspace. The third lesion is made through the same rib space, but the tip is directed to the midportion to rostral portion of T2 body beneath the head of the second rib. When each needle is properly positioned, stimulation is carried out and positioning effected so as to avoid a somatic motor or sensory response below 0.5 V. This avoids damage to the somatic roots. A test lesion at 60°C for 60 seconds is now made to guard against Horner's syndrome while plethysmography and hand temperature monitoring indicate whether sympathetic interruption is occurring. When all criteria have been satisfied, a 90°C 180-second lesion is made and enlarged by withdrawing the tip 8 to 10 mm. Twenty procedures on 27 sides produced 24 instances of sympathetic denervation. Two patients suffered from pneumothorax, three from brachial neuralgia, and one from unwanted Horner's syndrome.

USE OF PHENOL, ALCOHOL, AND OTHER SCLEROSING AGENTS AND SUBARACHNOID INJECTION OF COLD OR HYPERTONIC SALINE

I prefer, when feasible, to use percutaneous radiofrequency thermocoagulation rather than sclerosing agents for lesion-making in percutaneous techniques because it allows precise control of size and extent of lesion, avoids unpredictable spread, causes a uniform predictable degree of destruction of target tissue, and is more easily combined with physiologic localization, resulting in fewer complications and more accurate, effective, and enduring results.[47,77,93,125,150a,151] For a view in support of use of neurolytic techniques, see Chapter 29.

The use of cold and hypertonic saline injected into the subarachnoid space has the capacity to reduce intractable pain, but the uncertain results, the need for general anesthesia, and the incidence of side-effects leave little to recommend this technique.[125,152]

PERCUTANEOUS RADIOFREQUENCY DORSAL RHIZOTOMY

The same indications, limitations, and caveats apply to percutaneous radiofrequency dorsal rhizotomy as to neurectomy, although dorsal rhizotomy has the advantage over neurectomy of selective preservation of motor power with more widespread elimination of nociception. Nevertheless, dorsal rhizotomy in the limbs, particularly at more than one level, may result in significant disability. Formerly performed through open laminectomy, dorsal rhizotomy was described by Uematsu and associates using the percutaneous radiofrequency technique, which greatly diminishes the impact of the procedure in an often sick patient with major primary disease.[149] It is essential, however, to avoid inadvertent damage to vertebral or essential radicular arteries by avoiding lesions at C1, T1–T4, and T11–L1 levels.

Technique. The technique is similar to that of percutaneous radiofrequency neurectomy. With the patient under local anesthesia or neuroleptanalgesia, intermittent thiopental anesthesia, and image intensification, the latter so angled so as to view the appropriate intervertebral foramen "face on," an electrode such as that used for conventional-percutaneous-radiofrequency gasserian ganglion coagulation is introduced into the dorsal quadrant of the appropriate foramen. With 2 and 60 to 100 Hz stimulation using the appropriate electronic backup, the needle tip is positioned to avoid motor contractions but to produce paresthesias in the appropriate root with a low current flow (0.5 V or less). The radiofrequency lesion is then made progressively as described before. To block the C2 root the needle is introduced 1 cm below the mastoid in the midpoint of the foramen rostral caudally and in its dorsal one third. If CSF flow is obtained, the needle is withdrawn 1 mm. Stimulation at 2 Hz should produce motor contractions in trapezius at less than 1 V, and sensory stimulation should produce a response at less than 0.5 V.

Needles aimed at thoracic roots should be aligned from below upward into the foramen heading from the tip of the lower transverse process to the base of the one above. In the lumbar area the needle is introduced into the dorsal one third of the foramen from a point 4 cm from the midline with the patient's painful side up in the lateral recumbent position. At L5 the needle is introduced with the patient prone from laterally and inferiorly into the space between the transverse process of L5 and the ala of the sacrum aimed at the neck of the transverse process of L5. Progress is often impeded here by lumbarization or osteophytes. Sacral roots are reached through appropriate dorsal sacral foramina bringing the tip to the ventral foramina. Here one must be alert to the risks to bladder and sexual function.[148]

Results. Uematsu and colleagues[149] reported seven excellent and two good results among 17 patients with various pain syndromes. Pagura[90] relieved pain in 76% of 50 patients, 13 of whom suffered from cancer and 37 from lumbar disk disease. Two of these patients developed temporary postoperative paresis.

PERCUTANEOUS DESTRUCTIVE TECHNIQUES AIMED AT THE SPINAL CORD

Three percutaneous cord techniques have been proposed for the relief of chronic pain: percutaneous cervical cordotomy by the high lateral,[79] low anterior,[56] and posterior[38,39] techniques, percutaneous section of the descending tract of trigeminal nerve both at the medullary and upper cord level, and percutaneous high cervical commissurotomy. The first, percutaneous cordotomy, has enjoyed particularly wide acceptance.

Percutaneous Cordotomy

Cordotomy, long accepted as a major means of controlling pain, was first performed percutaneously by Mullan and co-workers using a radiostrontium source.[79] Rosomoff and associates[101] made the procedure practical by substituting radiofrequency lesion-making.

Indications. Percutaneous cordotomy is the neurodestructive treatment of choice for nociceptive intractable pain below the C4 level, largely restricted to pain caused by malignancy.

In my opinion, there is virtually no place for open cordotomy, and I have had no occasion to perform the procedure in 400 consecutive cordotomies. Percutaneous cordotomy has the advantage of low morbidity, high success rate, minimal impact on the patient, and, with physiologic localization, high precision. Not only is motor power not sacrificed as in neurectomy, but also somatosensory function other than spinothalamic is not lost as with rhizotomy. The result is that large areas of the body can be rendered pain-free without disabling neurologic consequences. Absolute contraindications other than deafferentation pain and pain at or rostral to the C4 dermatome include a solitary functioning lung ipsilateral to the proposed cord lesion when a high cervical level of analgesia is necessary. The latter will eliminate the strictly ipsilaterally distributed reticulospinal pathway responsible for unconscious respiration that lies sandwiched between the ventral horn and the spinothalamic tract. For similar reasons, if bilateral cordotomy is proposed, high levels of analgesia must not be produced bilaterally. Although most candidates suffer from cancer, there are exceptional patients with nociceptive pain not caused by cancer in whom cordotomy is indicated, particularly those with spinal cord injury and low or incomplete lesions with intermittent lancinating pain.[138,156] A relative contraindication to cordotomy is midline truncal, especially perineal, pain, better handled by the use of an epidural opiate reservoir or pump cannula system (see below), which avoids the 22% risk of impairment of bladder function occasioned by bilateral cordotomy.[71] The development of spinal opiate analgesia has greatly decreased the need for percutaneous cordotomy in some patients (see Chap. 28).

Technique. Three techniques are possible to achieve percutaneous cordotomy, of which the lateral high cervical technique is preferred because it allows a higher level of analgesia and more precise manipulation of electrode position in the cord. The low anterior approach[56] is useful when a high level of analgesia is not only unnecessary but also contraindicated to avoid respiratory complications. I have not had occasion to use the low anterior approach. A posterior approach has also been described.[18,38]

The lateral high cervical approach is performed with the patient positioned supine under neuroleptanalgesia with the dorsal spinal canal in the occipital C1 – C2 area positioned precisely horizontally to prevent loss of contrast medium. Lateral image intensification is necessary and anteroposterior x-ray film should be available. Uncooperative or extremely apprehensive patients may be operated on under general anesthesia without paralyzing agents, the only guiding parameter sacrificed being the reported sensory effects elicited by 60 to 100 Hz stimulation. A No. 18 lumbar puncture needle into which an electrolytically sharpened 0.4-mm stainless steel electrode with shrunk-fit Teflon insulation locks so that 2 mm of insulation and 2 mm of bare tip protrude in turn (see Fig. 30-7) is inserted in a rectilinearly lateral plane into the middle of the C1–C2 interspace or alternatively the occipital C1 interspace on the side opposite the pain. The lumbar puncture needle is advanced until the tip is felt to snap through first the ligamentum flavum and then dura, each inducing a twinge of ipsilateral neck pain. After the dura is entered, removal of the stylet results in cerebrospinal fluid drainage, verifying subarachnoid position as well.

Thereupon a one-to-one emulsion of CSF and ethiodan is injected to outline the dentate ligament, as shown in Figure 30-8. The dorsal dura and sometimes the dorsal or ventral root outlines and anterior cord margin may also be seen. The electrode is now introduced, aiming precisely at the image of the dentate ligament on the ipsilateral side while electrical impedance is monitored using the electronic back-up equipment (see Figs. 30-5, 30-6, 30-9). Impedance rises from 400 or 600 to 1000 or more ohms at the moment the cord is impaled. At this time a sense of gritty resistance is felt with the surgeon's fingers and the patient has a twinge of neck pain. X-ray film confirms the needle tip's position at the level of the dentate ligament in the lateral view and at about the middle of the dens in the anteroposterior view. Often the cord is displaced toward the contralateral side of the midline for several millimeters. Threshold stimulation is now carried out at 2 Hz and should result in contractions in some portion of the ipsilateral cervical musculature, usually the trapezius, below 5 V with the Owl equipment. Although such a response is also compatible with positioning in the anterior horn or rostral corticospinal tract, stimulation at 50 to 100 Hz induces no motor effect when the electrode is located in the spinothalamic tract, whereas tetanization occurs in the other two sites involving appropriate musculature. Fifty hertz to 100 Hz stimulation is now carried out. If the electrode lies in the spinothalamic tract, the patient should report a warm or cool, rarely paresthetic or burning effect referred to some portion of the contralateral body. If the effect is perceived in the hand, the electrode is somatotopographically centrally located, and a lesion at that level will likely induce widespread analgesia (Fig. 30-10). If the sensation is felt in the lower limb, the analgesia will likely affect lower trunk and lower limb. It is at such sites that paresis will occur, virtually always in the ipsilateral lower limb, but usually minor and temporary, so that one must carefully watch for tetanization in the ipsilateral limb during stimulation and reposition the needle tip slightly to avoid this.

Occasionally contralateral sensory effects are referred to chest, neck, or shoulder, in which case lesions are likely to induce suspended rostral levels of analgesia unsatisfactory for pain control. Occasionally ipsilateral paresthesias are felt, also indicating unsatisfactory positioning. To reposition the needle tip, one must withdraw the needle very carefully under impedance control, angle upward or downward as needs be and reinsert it under impedance

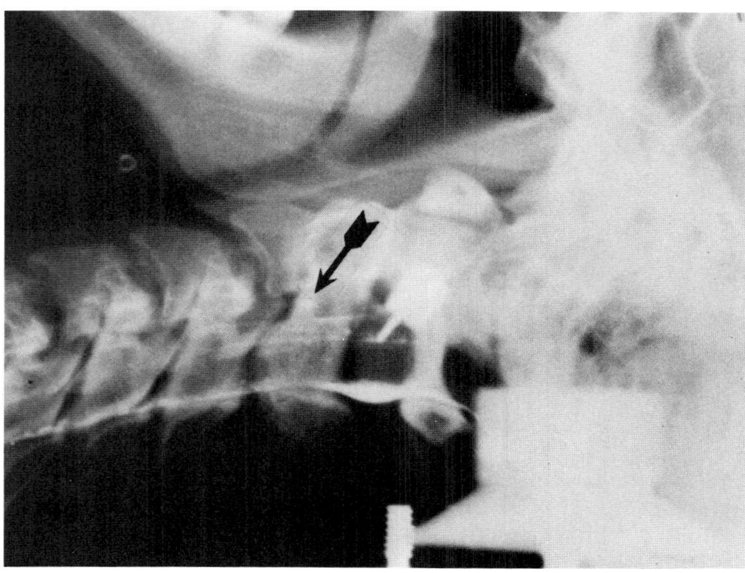

FIG. 30-8. Lateral x-ray of neck during percutaneous cordotomy. A drop of contrast medium *(arrow)* lies on the anterior cord margin. The ventral root line and dorsal dura are well outlined. The electrode tip is impaling the cord at the level of the dentate ligament, where a lesion produced analgesia up to T6 without complications.

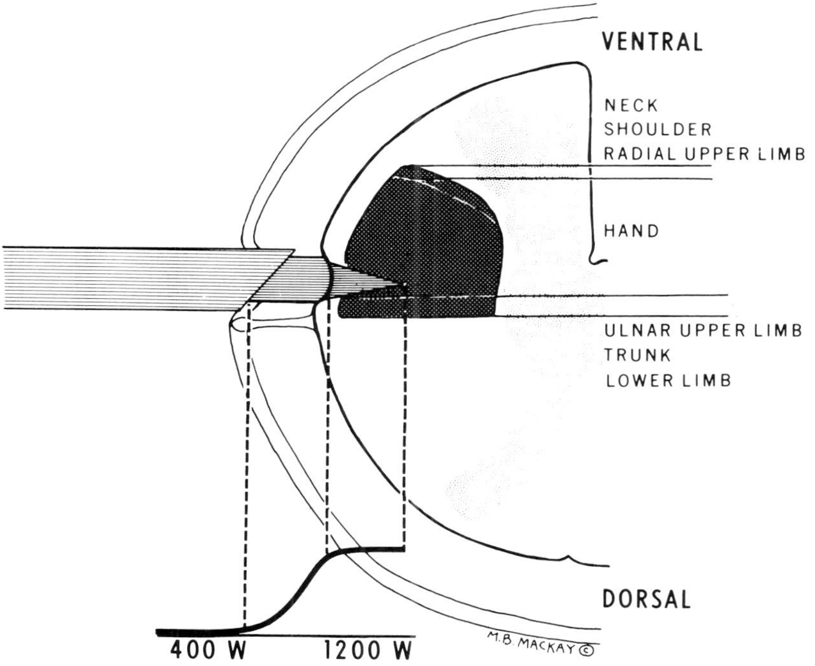

FIG. 30-9. Diagram illustrating technique of percutaneous cordotomy by the lateral high cervical approach, including impedance changes on cord impalation and anatomic organization of the region.

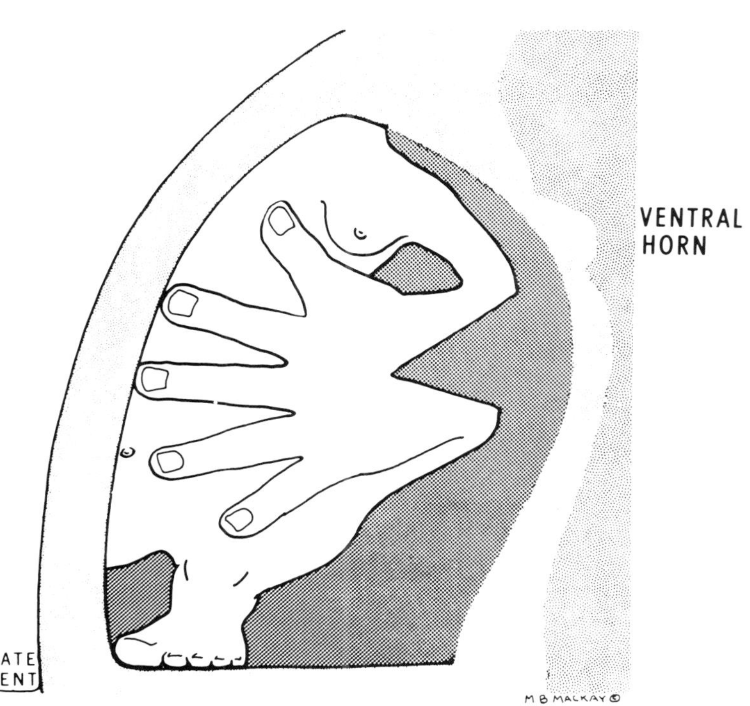

FIG. 30-10. Somatotopic organization of spinothalamic tract at C1.

control preparatory to repetition of stimulation. When radiologic and physiologic criteria of appropriate location have been met, a radiofrequency lesion is made with serial testing of the level of analgesia and ipsilateral leg strength under heightened levels of neuroleptanalgesia or brief thiopental anesthesia. Lesion-making is begun with 20 to 30 mA for 60 seconds and serially increased until falloff occurs, indicating that maximum lesion size has been achieved, or until adequate levels of analgesia occur. Maximum lesions are usually made at 50 to 70 mA for 60 seconds.

Second-side high cervical lateral cordotomy is performed after a 7- to 10-day interval. If the level on the second side must, to preserve respiratory function, be kept low, particular attention must be given to stimulation-induced sensory effects as mentioned above.

Results. In a personal series of 244 cases,[131] the procedure was completed in 99% of patients, achieving spinothalamic interruption in 92.4%. In unilateral cases, effective pain relief was obtained in 94.4% at the time of discharge from hospital and in 82.3% in longer-term follow-up. Incidence of pain relief after bilateral cordotomy obeys the P-squared rule and is therefore lower than for unilateral cordotomy. Recurrence of nociceptive pain for which the procedure was performed virtually never occurs in an area of persisting analgesia but rather in a region of fading or falling analgesia; however, ipsilateral pain appeared or intensified in 41% of our patients postoperatively, and 6% developed pain above the level of their previous pain contralateral to the lesion. Over years in those patients in whom cordotomy is performed for other than malignant disease,[138] analgesia levels tended to fade with recurrence of pain. In 5 of our 24 paraplegics undergoing cordotomy, this happened after 1, 1 1/12, 4, 5, 13, and 21 years. Pain relief was restored in 2 patients after 5 and 21 years, respectively, by repeating the cordotomy.[138]

Complications were as follows: 0.5% mortality from respiratory failure, 0.5% transient respiratory failure, 0.5% permanent significant paresis, 4% bladder dysfunction for unilateral cordotomy, 22% for bilateral cordotomy, 21% transient paresis, 24% Horner's syndrome, nearly always transient, and 4% postcordotomy dysesthesia.

Rosomoff[100] reported similar experience in 789 patients. Lipton[57] reported an 80% incidence of "complete" analgesia and thermanalgesia immediately postoperatively with 4% immediate fading of analgesic level. Eighty percent of his patients suffered from paresis, 40% to a noticeable degree, 20% enough to cause disability. Mortality was 6.2%, and the incidence of postcordotomy dysesthesia 2%, of ataxia 0.5%, of Horner's syndrome 100%, of bladder disturbance 0, amazingly, in unilateral, cordotomy and 100% in bilateral procedures.

In some clinics, the introduction of spinal opioid pumps or portals (see Chap. 28) has resulted in a sharp decline in use of percutaneous cordotomy, based on claims of fewer side-effects, less invasiveness, and ability to cover a wide area of pain stimulus. However, percutaneous cordotomy does not differ greatly in invasiveness to insertion of a spinal morphine pump, may cover a wide area of pain safely, and declines little in efficacy in patients with cancer who live an average of 3 months. A good case can be made for percutaneous cordotomy in such patients in view of emerging evidence of escalation of spinal morphine dose and loss of efficacy in some patients and other side-effects that occur at high morphine dose (see Chap. 28). Also the cost of spinal morphine pump devices is high.

Commissurotomy

Commissurotomy was originally introduced by Armour[4] with the intent of severing decussating spinothalamic and reticulothalamic fibers in the anterior commissure. It was widely used with an open technique, having the theoretical advantage of sparing respiratory pathways. The mechanism by which the procedure induces pain relief remains obscure, as lucidly reviewed by Cook and associates.[16] Pain relief is somewhat unpredictable and bears no relation to production of analgesia in the dermatomes corresponding to decussating fibers interrupted by the lesion or to section of anterior commissure itself. Moreover, Hitchcock,[41] who performed the procedure with the percutaneous radiofrequency technique at the occipital C1 interspace, was able to relieve pain at any level of the body without inducing cutaneous analgesia. Schvarcz[105] suggests that the procedure, in fact, interrupts some unknown extralemniscal pain pathway.

Indications. The procedure is an option in patients with pain caused by cancer, whereas its role in those with deafferentation pain needs further observation. It is particularly useful in patients with midline or bilateral trunk pain in the lower body; however, this pain is now mostly treated by epidural opiate instillation. I can see no role for commissurotomy by the open technique because of its morbidity, particularly in sick cancer patients, since similar problems can be managed by simpler and safer methods.

Technique. High cervical commissurotomy under local anesthesia is performed percutaneously through the occipital C1 interspace with the patient sitting, using a suitable frame. A cisternal Conray myelogram outlines the dorsal and ventral aspects of the medulla and cord. A sharpened 0.5-mm electrode is introduced under impedance control with stimulation for physiologic localization. It is passed toward a point 5 mm anterior to the dorsal cord margin in the midsagittal plane. As the electrode enters the cord, stimulation of dorsal columns produces paresthesias in both feet. More deeply near the central canal, stimulation effects are referred to more dorsal aspects of the lower limbs. At the central canal region paresthesias are encountered, starting in the soles and spreading to the dorsal aspects of the legs as the current is increased, sometimes also with paresthesias affecting the whole face, crossed limbs, or bilateral upper limbs, or else burning truncal sensations occur. Lesions are made as in cordotomy just anterior to or at the sites of distal lower limb responses. Lesions produce subjective analgesia without clinically demonstrable sensory loss unrelated in location to areas of pain relief.

Results. Hitchcock[41] reported 10 excellent and 2 good results in 14 patients with cancer pain and excellent results in 3 with deafferentation pain, producing unpredictable bilateral alterations in the appreciation of pinprick as painful. Eiras and co-workers[25] reported good results initially in patients with cancer pain with some degree of recurrence. Side-effects consisted of dysmetria and ataxia for up to 2 weeks in all patients. Schvarcz[105] reported 78% satisfactory pain relief in patients with midline and bilateral pelvic cancer pain. These patients experienced varying degrees of loss of appreciation of pinprick as painful postoperatively, although they retained the ability to realize it was sharp. Postoperative gait ataxia was reported as "common." Papo[92] found the pain relief short-lived in his patients.

This technique is now rarely, if ever, indicated because of the availability of the less invasive and more effective techniques.

Percutaneous Tractotomy of the Caudal Nucleus and Descending Tract of Trigeminal Nerve

Percutaneous tractotomy of the trigeminal nerve has been performed both at the lower medullary[19,20,31,145] and upper cervical[39–42,103,104] levels. Unlike the previously discussed destructive techniques aimed at interrupting nociception in the management of nociceptive pain, this procedure at the cord level has been directed toward the management of deafferentation pain in the face. The mechanism of relief for deafferentation pain by this method is unknown, one possibility being the destruction of deafferented hypersensitive neurons responsible for the pain, similar to the situation with lesions in the so-called dorsal root entry zone introduced by Hyndman,[44] elaborated by Sindou and co-workers[112] in the treatment of cancer pain, and popularized using a radiofrequency lesion-making technique at open laminectomy by Nashold and Ostdahl[83] for deafferentation pain. That procedure has recently been extended by Nashold[84] to include lesions in the upper cervical dorsal root entry zone affecting the trigeminal tract.

Crue and colleagues[19,20,145] first performed trigeminal medullary tractotomy primarily for the treatment of nociceptive pain; Fox[30,31] introduced radiographic localization.

Technique. *(Medullary).* The patient is positioned prone under local anesthesia. A No. 18 lumbar puncture needle is introduced between occiput and C1 into the midline of the cisterna magna and 1 ml of Pantopaque emulsified with 1 ml of CSF injected under lateral image intensification outlining the floor of the fourth ventricle, the dorsum of the brain stem, and the obex, the latter as a step in the shadow of the contrast medium. Four centimeters lateral to the midline, a second 18-gauge thin-wall lumbar puncture needle is passed over C1 lamina and aimed toward cisterna magna, terminating 12 mm from the midline as measured uncorrected on the posteroanterior film and 8 mm caudal to obex at the level of the dorsum of the brain stem on the lateral film (also uncorrected). These x-rays are achieved with a 30- inch tube to target and a 40-inch tube to film distance so as to afford reproducible measurements. A second electrode such as the stylet of a 22-gauge 4½-inch lumbar puncture needle insulated with vinyl tubing except for a 3-mm bare tip is passed through the laterally placed guide needle into the brain stem under impedance control at a site 0 to 10 mm from the midline of odontoid on the uncorrected posteroanterior film and at, or just caudal to, the obex and 4 mm anterior to the level of the floor of the fourth ventricle on the lateral film. Fifty hertz stimulation should cause ipsilateral facial sensation whereupon a graded radiofrequency lesion up to 50 mA for 10 to 60 seconds is made with serial sensory testing.

(Cervical). Hitchcock and Schvarcz[42] performed the procedure in the sitting position using a stereotactic frame under local anesthesia. A needle is passed through the occipital C1 interspace in the midsagittal plane and 50% Conray injected to outline the anterior/posterior aspects of the cord and the cisterna magna. The caudal dermatomes of the spinal tract of the fifth nerve at this location are said to lie 3 to 4 mm anterior to the posterior aspect of the cord and 6 mm lateral. Rostral dermatomes lie more laterally and anteriorly and intermedius, 9th, and 10th dermatomes more posteriorly and medially. A 0.5-mm sharpened varnish-insulated electrode with a 2-mm bare tip enclosed in a nylon tube is advanced under radiologic and impedance control using monopolar stimulation until stimulation induces sensation in the face, said to be paresthetic[103] or painful.[42] Stimulation of the dorsal columns or their nuclei may induce ipsilateral sensory effects, of the spinothalamic tract contralateral sensory effects, whereas the trigeminal effects are ipsilateral. At the level of C1 all of the trigeminal fibers, including circumoral dermatomes, are present. More distally circumoral dermatomes are not represented. As soon as satisfactory positioning is achieved, a graded radiofrequency lesion is made.

Figure 30-11 summarizes the physiologic anatomy in this area.

Results. Fox[31] operated on eight patients with neoplasms, two with postherpetic neuralgia, one with tic, and one with questionable iatrogenic deafferentation facial pain. Analgesia of the 5th, 7th, 9th, and 10th nerves occurred in seven, V2–V3 analgesia in the rest. Complications included transient ipsilateral ataxia (common), three instances of contralateral body analgesia, and "nearly all patients suffered from postoperative hyperpyrexia of 101 to 102°F."

Schvarcz[103,104] reported 53 procedures in 52 patients with 87.5% relief of postherpetic neuralgia, 56% of anesthesia dolorosa, and 74% of "dysethetic pain." He reported 83.8% relief of pain in 31 cancer patients. Complications consisted of contralateral hypalgesia and ipsilateral ataxia. Full evaluation of

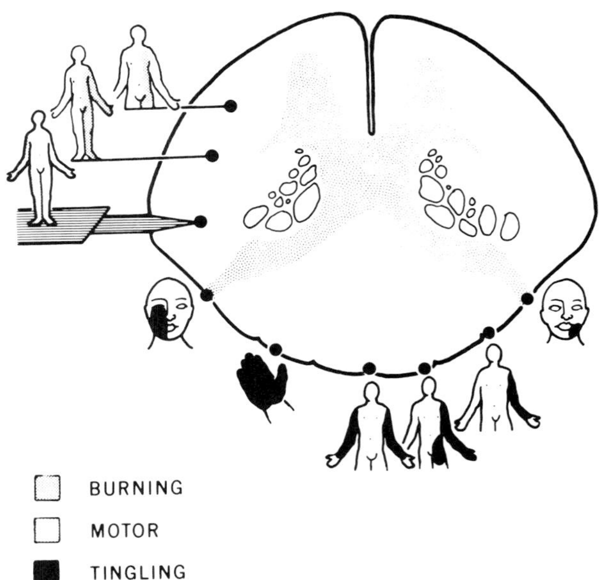

FIG. 30-11. Stimulation-induced effects at C1 in a single patient, at 100 Hz, using above cordotomy equipment. Ipsilateral tingling in face and upper limb arose in trigeminal tract and dorsal columns, respectively, ipsilateral tetanization in corticospinal tract, contralateral burning (usually hot or cold) in spinothalamic tract.

this interesting technique awaits wider experience. Epidural opiate techniques now offer a less invasive option in patients with cancer.

TECHNIQUES THAT MODULATE PAIN

Modulating procedures can be separated into those that appear to modulate nociceptive pain and those that affect deafferentation pain. The former include techniques for the epidural or intrathecal instillation of opiates as well as percutaneous hypophyseal alcohol injection. The latter include various techniques of chronic stimulation of which only spinal epidural and trigeminal can be considered as percutaneous techniques.

MODULATION OF NOCICEPTIVE PAIN: SPINAL OPIATE ADMINISTRATION

As soon as it was realized that opiates were taken up in spinal cord as well as in brain to block nociceptive access to the nervous system,[160] attempts were made to control acute transient pain, such as that seen postoperatively, by short-term intrathecal and epidural opiate infusions and then to control chronic pain. The latter was treated by the permanent implantation of epidural or intrathecal cannulae fed by a refillable reservoir or pumps of varying complexity.[21,71,88,95,97] Although the technique is still under investigation, it has a clear use in the treatment of nociceptive pain caused by cancer and is rapidly replacing techniques such as rhizotomy and cordotomy, particularly for midline or bilateral pain of the lower trunk, pelvis, and perineum (see also Chap. 28).

Techniques for spinal opiate administration are described in Chapter 28. I use a Silastic reservoir of suitable capacity with a reinforced dome and a hard backing, such as is shown in Figure 30-12. (Manufactured by Holter–Hausner Int., Bridgeport, PA 19405, USA).

Penn and co-workers[95] reported eight excellent and five good results with intrathecal and epidural opiate installation in patients with cancer pain treated with programmable pumps. Meyerson and associates[71] had 62% good results without complications. D'Annunzio and colleagues[21] reported 60% satisfactory results with 60% minor side-effects. A more detailed presentation of theoretical basis, effects, side-effects, technique, and indications is given in Chapter 28.

HYPOPHYSEAL ALCOHOL INJECTION

Hypophysectomy for intractable pain was originally directed toward treating hormone-dependent cancers of breast and prostate using open transfrontal and various percutaneous or stereotactic and transsphenoidal means. Morrica[78] popularized the use of percutaneous injection of alcohol into the pituitary by transsphenoidal approach for the treatment of pain caused by hormone and non-hormone-dependent cancer alike. The method by which this treatment affects cancer pain, although unknown, presumably is a modulatory one affecting the processing of noxious afferent input. It is not related to pituitary destruction, involvement of hypothalamus, and manipulation of levels in blood or CSF of any recognizable substance, including enkephalins and endorphins, and the effect is not reversed by naloxone.[14]

Technique. The technique is performed under neuroleptanalgesia. After preparing the nasal cavity with cocaine paste, a No. 16-gauge 12-cm needle is introduced through the right nostril under biplanar x-ray control through sphenoid sinus, which is sterilized, until it impinges on sella. A No. 19 needle of greater length is now introduced through the first needle and hammered through the sellar floor (see Chap. 29). Aspiration is applied to be sure that blood or CSF

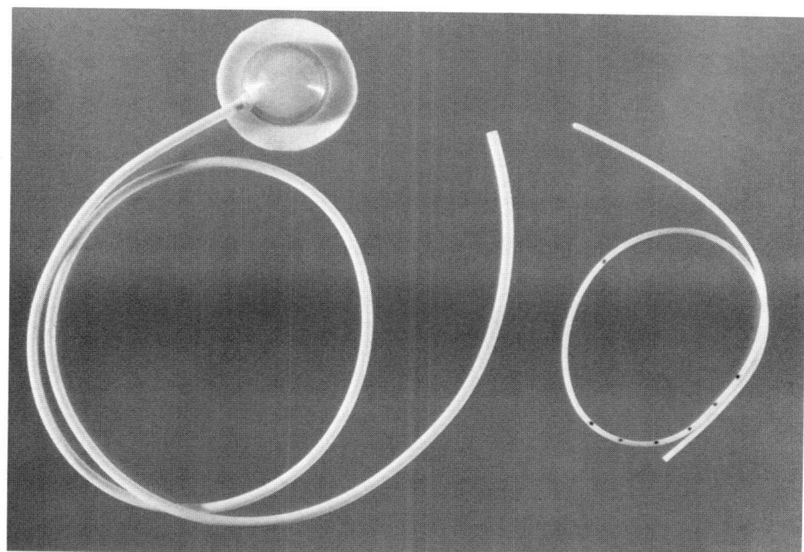

FIG. 30-12. Epidural cannula and subcutaneous metal-backed reservoir for continual epidural spinal morphine injection. (Manufactured by Holter–Hausner International)

return is not obtained. A total of 1.0 to 2.4 ml (average 2.0 ml) of pure ethanol is introduced by means of one to two such punctures with the radiologically localized needle tip lying in the midline almost against the posterior sellar wall. The needles are removed after 5 minutes and the nose packed. Pupillary responses and eye movements are monitored during the injection (see Figs. 29-33, 29-34, and 29-35).

Results. Miles[73,74] achieved 41% to 43% excellent and 30% partial pain relief in 122 patients, although relief persisted for 3 months or more in only 21% of patients. Eight of his patients died, and 5 suffered from visual or oculomotor disturbances, 2 from hypothalamic destruction, and 10% to 20% from CSF leakage and 1% from meningitis. There was a 60% incidence of diabetes insipidus, complications usually being transient. Madrid's patients[65] experienced 67% immediate relief of pain with 3% CSF rhinorrhea, 0.3% meningitis, and 3% visual-oculomotor disturbances. Takeda and colleagues[127,128] observed 80% immediate pain relief in 102 patients overall with 95% success in 43% of the patients with hormone-dependent cancer and 69% in the rest. Cancer in the hormone-dependent group sometimes regressed. Complications consisted of almost universal transient euphoria and polyphagia, 10% incidence of visual and 4% oculomotor disturbances, and 50% diabetes insipidus. A review of other publications on the subject[74] suggests that pain recurrence after 3 to 4 months, a 2% mortality, rhinorrhea, 2% visual complications, transient headache, diabetes insipidus, hyperthermia, and polyphagia are regular side-effects. Levin and co-workers[54] report relief of thalamic pain in 3 patients using this procedure. Again the use of this technique has decreased with the availability of epidural opiates for widespread cancer pain (see also Chap. 29.2).

MODIFICATION OF DEAFFERENTATION PAIN

Although the mechanism of deafferentation pain is unknown and may not be homogeneous, doubtless it is the result of some diffuse central neuronal functional aberration in cord or brain stem instituted by the deafferentation. Thus destructive lesions of conventional pain pathways seldom relieve deafferentation pain, apparent notable exceptions being lesions of the descending tract of the trigeminal nerve and of the spinal dorsal root entry zone, perhaps in patients in whom deafferentation-induced pathophysiology resides in the dorsal horns. In addition, destructive lesions of medial mesencephalon and medial thalamus afford some degree of success.[133,135,138] Possibly in both cases destruction of pathologically active cells outright is the mechanism of action.

The limited usefulness of these destructive procedures, however, as well as their complications, underscores the need for something better. On one count only — low risk — does chronic stimulation answer that need; incidence of success in treating deafferentation pain with chronic stimulation is still too low.

Chronic stimulation of the nervous system for pain relief was originally introduced for the treatment of nociceptive pain based on the prediction of the Melzack–Wall gate theory[69] by Wall and Sweet[154] at the peripheral nerve level. Extended to the spinal cord by Shealy and colleagues,[107] the technique became much more useful when percutaneous electrode introduction was introduced by Erickson,[26] Hoppenstein,[43] and Dooley.[23] Percutaneous testing allowed the exclusion of a large number of patients destined not to respond to chronic stimulation before commitment to an internalizing procedure with the use of expensive equipment. At the same time experience showed that chronic stimulation was a much more useful entity for the treatment of deafferentation pain than it was for that of nociceptive pain predicted by the Melzack–Wall theory. No other useful means exists other than percutaneous testing for the preselection of patients who will be relieved by stimulation at any level, just as it is impossible to predict which patients will develop deafferentation pain in the first place following a neurologic lesion.

Basically the technique of chronic stimulation consists of delivering artificial paresthesias over a test period of 1 week or more into the area of the patient's pain, either through peripheral nerve, cord, or brain stem. If the patient successfully "passes the test" of trial stimulation, implantation of a suitable receiver for radioactivation is carried out. The mechanism of action of chronic stimulation is unknown, possibly consisting of suppression of the deafferentation neuronal hypersensitivity through the dorsal-column lemniscal sensory input it induces. This is consistent with observations made in humans by Modesti and Wasak[75] and by Tsubokawa and associates[146] and with the evidence from various observations that dorsal cord stimulation suppresses the late events of the scalp-evoked potential[134] and with the suppression of deafferentation pain by sodium thiopental in those patients who will eventually respond to stimulation.[134] Of the various stimulation techniques, only those of trigeminal nerve and dorsal cord can be considered as percutaneous procedures, possibly also that of the descending tract of the fifth nerve.

The treatment technique of choice in deafferentation pain is a percutaneous trial of either peripheral nerve (practical only for trigeminal) or dorsal cord stimulation producing paresthesias in the area of pain. During this time the patient charts periods of stimulation and his level of pain on a 0 to 10 scale using a chart such as that shown in Figure 30-13. The risks of such treatment are very low; nonresponders are easily eliminated without further investment of time and equipment; successful treatment by chronic stimulation exposes the patient to far less risk than any of the alternatives such as brain stimulation, so-called DREZ lesions, or stereotactic brain lesions. As a rule dorsal cord stimulation is more useful than somatic nerve stimulation because of the larger field covered, the avoidance of damage to an already injured nerve, and the greater likelihood of satisfactory delivery of adequate paresthesias to the painful area.

CHRONIC TRIGEMINAL NERVE STIMULATION

Sheldon[108] originally conceived the idea of treating pain by trigeminal stimulation, but Meyerson and Håkansson[72] are responsible for introducing it as a treatment for deafferentation pain.

Technique. The technique consists of introducing a pliable electrode insulated except at its tip, such as the

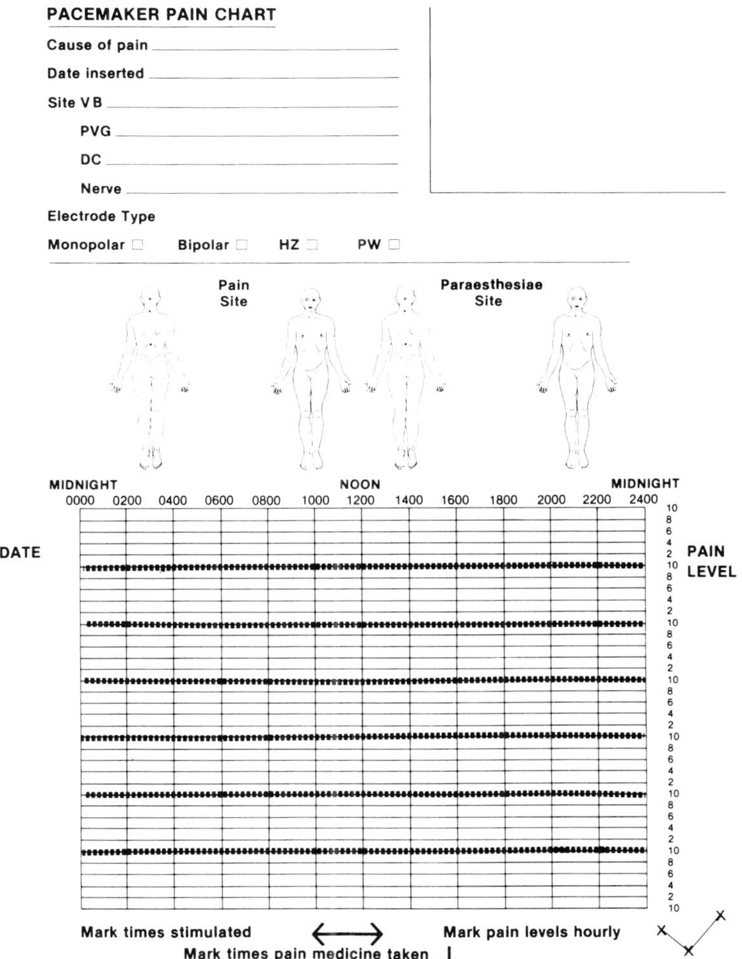
PACEMAKER PAIN CHART

Cause of pain

Date inserted

Site VB

PVG

DC

Nerve

Electrode Type

Monopolar ☐ Bipolar ☐ HZ ☐ PW ☐

Pain Site

Paraesthesiae Site

MIDNIGHT NOON MIDNIGHT

0000 0200 0400 0600 0800 1000 1200 1400 1600 1800 2000 2200 2400

DATE

PAIN LEVEL

10 8 6 4 2

Mark times stimulated ⟷

Mark pain levels hourly

Mark times pain medicine taken ↓

FIG. 30-13. Chart for percutaneous testing of trigeminal or spinal epidural stimulation upon which patient rates pain on a 0 to 10 scale against time, noting periods of stimulation and times of taking medications.

Medtronic Corporation's straight "Pisces" electrode, through a No. 16 thin-wall Tuohy needle into Meckel's cave using the same technique as for percutaneous thermocoagulation. It is preferable, but not essential, that CSF return be obtained and entry into the buccal cavity avoided. The electrode tip is positioned under lateral image intensification as shown in Figure 30-14 and trial stimulation performed so that paresthesias are induced in that part of the face where pain is located. The electrode is secured to the face with a stitch. The patient then undergoes a trial for up to 1 week using self-stimulation recording pain on a suitable chart (see Fig. 30-13). A decision is made as to whether the treatment is effective, and the electrode is then removed. For successful candidates either a straight "Pisces" electrode or a specially designed bipolar electrode, designed by the Medtronic Corporation to Meyerson's specifications, is sutured, at open operation, to the dura over Meckel's cave suitably positioned to produce appropriate paresthesias using the Frazier approach. The cable is tunneled subcutaneously to mate with a receiver such as that shown in Figure 30-15 (Manufactured by Medtronic Inc., Minneapolis, MN, USA) positioned below the ipsilateral collarbone. From then on, the patient controls the stimulator using an antenna and radio transmitter as shown in Figure 30-15. Steude[122] has internalized the test electrode itself, eliminating the need for a major operation.

Results. As yet little experience has been published concerning this technique. We have used the method in 11 patients, 4 with central pain caused by stroke, 4 with iatrogenic denervation of trigeminal nerve, 2 with postherpetic neuralgia, and 1 with traumatic trigeminal injury. Two patients with central pain, 2 with iatrogenic pain, and 1 patient with postherpetic neuralgia all derived relief, at least as followed thus far. One patient with anesthesia dolorosa caused by multiple sclerosis and prior radiofrequency coagulation failed to experience appropriate paresthesias. The only complication has been electrode migration in 2 patients that necessitated repositioning. Meyerson and Håkansson found that 56% of their 25 patients passed the stimulation test, of which 6 were implanted, all with satisfactory pain relief. The preferred stimulation rate was 50 to 100 Hz, producing paresthesias in the painful area. Steude[122] found that 3 of 10 patients were relieved of atypical facial pain. An alternative is to use high cervical epidural stimulation. This approach aims at the spinal tract of the trigeminal nerve.

DORSAL CORD STIMULATION

Most patients with deafferentation pain are candidates for a trial of percutaneous epidural cord stimulation, although success rate varies with type of causative lesion. Patients with pain caused by cord lesions, for example, may have such extensive damage that insufficient dorsal column fibers persist to allow stimulation-induced paresthesias in the painful area. Even so, patients with apparently clinically very complete cord lesions should still be tested by this simple and relatively innocuous method because they may still experience adequate paresthesias. Pa-

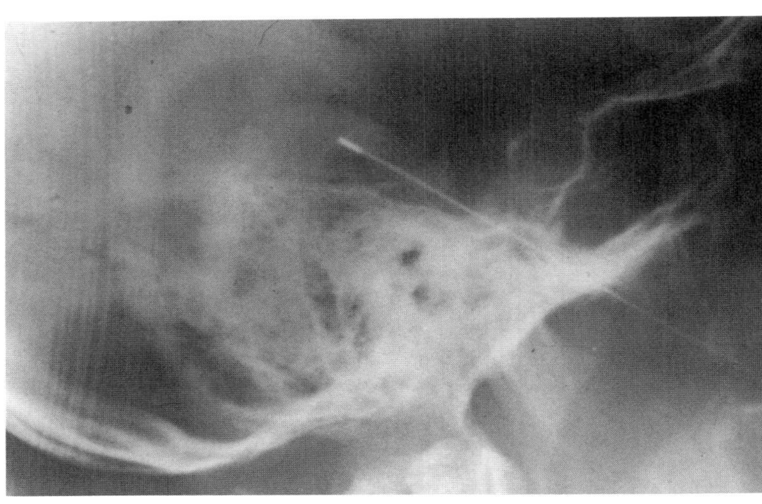

FIG. 30-14. Lateral x-ray showing Medtronic straight "PISCES"-type electrode introduced into Meckel's cave via foramen ovale and beginning to enter the posterior fossa.

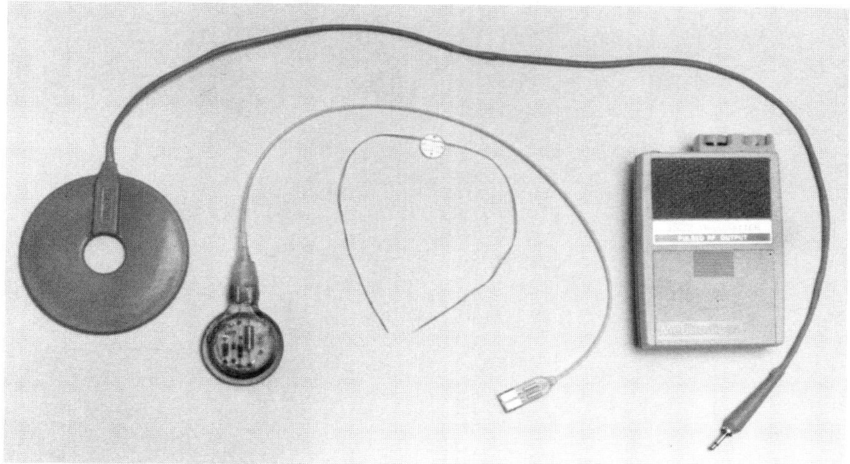

FIG. 30-15. Equipment for chronic epidural spinal stimulation. **Left to Right:** antenna, receiver, "sigma" "PISCES" electrode, transmitter. (Manufactured by Medtronic Corporation)

tients with cord injury may also be unsuccessful candidates because of obliteration of the appropriate epidural space by previous trauma or surgery. Those with prior surgery for disk disease, however, usually have an undamaged epidural space over the target area in the lower thoracic cord.

Technique. The technique consists of positioning the patient face down with vertebral flexion under anteroposterior image intensification. Under local anesthesia a No. 16 thin-wall Tuohy needle is introduced and angulated cephalad precisely in the midline between adjacent vertebral spines beginning 15 cm below the target dorsal horns. The needle is carefully advanced until the tip is felt to slip under the appropriate lamina, whereupon the epidural space is identified with the "loss of resistance" or "hanging drop" technique (see Chap. 8). A spring guide is now introduced and manipulated until it follows as precisely as possible a middorsal course to the desired level, taking care that it ends up either exactly in midline or, if off center, on the same side as the patient's pain. This is followed up with the introduction of a suitable epidural stimulating electrode. We most often use the Sigma "Pisces" electrode manufactured by Medtronic (shown in Figs. 30-15, 30-16). Once the electrode has been positioned so as to produce paresthesias in the area of pain, it is anchored in place to prevent rostral migration in the epidural space. It is then brought out through a paravertebral incision on the side opposite the patient's dominant hand to facilitate later control of the equipment. The patient tests the effect of the stimulator on his pain, charting the results on a pain chart as shown in Figure 30-13. Difficulties with the procedure consist of inability to enter the epidural space or to advance the electrode in the appropriate direction because of adhesions, inability to maintain a strictly dorsal midline position, and inability to achieve a position where appropriate or any paresthesias are produced, either because of damaged dorsal columns or problems in positioning. With extensive adhesions the subarachnoid space may be entered. In general this should be avoided because the risk of CSF leak and infection are increased and there is the tendency to produce unpleasant radicular effects. When these difficulties are encountered, introduction at a different space should be attempted. If subarachnoid introduction is inevitable, it should be accepted provided paresthesias are appropriate.

Although there is published evidence that anterior cord stimulation may also be effective in relieving pain,[137] most operators aim their electrodes over the dorsal cord, assuming that salutary results come from stimulating the dorsal columns. After an appropriate period of test stimulation, the electrode is removed if pain relief is not achieved; after successful test stimulation the electrode is internalized using a receiver transmitter antenna system such as that shown in Figure 30-15.

Results. In most series with an unspecified mix of pain syndromes, about 40% to 50% of patients pass the test of stimulation. Subsequently implanted devices usually yield 60% to 84% continuing pain relief, although there is a gradual attrition over the months and years despite continuing adequate technical performance of the device.[137] Complications consist of

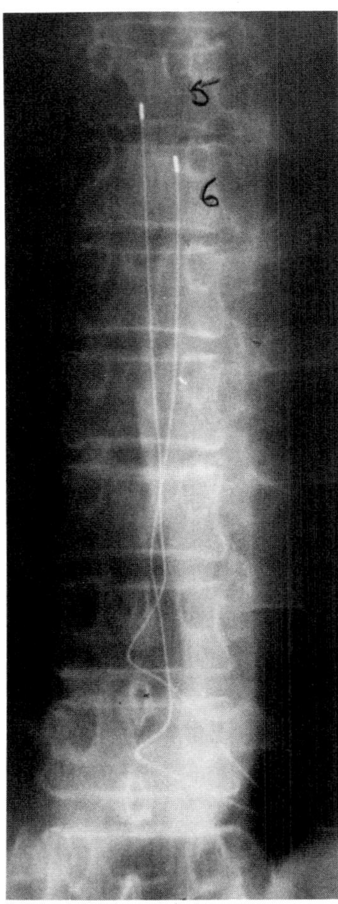

FIG. 30-16. Anteroposterior x-ray of thoracic spine showing two straight "PISCES"-type electrodes in epidural space.

electrode migration in up to 61% (average 25%), requiring repositioning or reintroduction, infection in 1% to 7%, incisional pain in up to 58%, electrode breakage in 4% to 23%, receiver failure in 0.5%, transmitter failure in 5%, and antenna failure in 100% within several years; skin irritation or breakdown at the antenna site occurs in 1% to 5% of patients.

My experience with dorsal cord stimulation in the treatment of deafferentation pain is shown in Table 30-1. Seven of the patients with cord lesions failed to experience paresthesias in their areas of pain, presumably because of degeneration of dorsal columns accounting in part for the high incidence of failure generally reported after cord lesions.[138] Relief was more likely when cord lesions were lower and incomplete. Published experience lists a 22% to 50% success rate with such patients.[138] My experience suggests that cauda equina and peripheral nerve lesions fare best with this form of treatment.

TRANSCUTANEOUS NERVE STIMULATION (TENS)

Use of TENS relates to acupuncture and traditional Western medicine through the ages. Although acupuncture analgesia is a modern concept, the traditional purpose being management of disease, the technique is the same, namely stimulation of designated body sites by manual rotation of a needle to produce a unique sensation known as "teh chi." This effect has been more recently reduplicated by slow (less than 5 Hz) electrical stimulation, which also produces powerful muscle contractions. The Western origins of TENS began with the Romans' use of electric fish and progressed to the modern use of stimulators

TABLE 30-1. TREATMENT OF DEAFFERENTATION PAIN WITH PERCUTANEOUS EPIDURAL DORSAL CORD STIMULATION: 1977-1984

Site of Lesion Causing Pain	Number of Patients	Percentage Relieved by Test Stimulation	Percentage of Continued Relief After Implantation
Brain	8	50	20
Cord	18	17	67
Cauda equina	8	88	86
Root	6	50	67
Nerve	25	60	80
Amputation	15	40	67
Disk	17	35	50
Unknown	8	25	100

employing rapid rates of stimulation inducing paresthesias. Interest in such treatment was rekindled after the publication of the Melzack–Wall gate theory of pain,[69] which suggested that the stimulation of large fibers would suppress pain transmission in small fibers, and hence suppression of nociceptive pain; however, experience taught that such rapid stimulation at the nerve, cord, or brain level was better suited to treat deafferentation pain.

The confusion over the appropriate roles of these various techniques for TENS has certainly not been resolved, but there is a suggestion that acupuncture or electrical acupuncture is most effective in managing nociceptive pain, whereas TENS at 30 to 100 Hz, applied so as to induce paresthesias in the area of pain, is more effective in treating deafferentation pain. The different patterns of TENS are illustrated in Figure 30-17.

Andersson[2] has thoughtfully compared and contrasted the two techniques, defining acupuncture as stimulation induced by manual manipulation of needles or else electrical stimulation below 10 Hz, and TENS as stimulation above 10 Hz. The former, a high-intensity stimulation, activates low and high threshold but mainly muscle afferents with a long induction time, producing both segmental and nonsegmental analgesia that long outlasts the stimulation, clearly indicating a neural-induced chemical modulatory effect. TENS, on the other hand, is a low-intensity stimulation and affects low threshold skin and muscle afferents, with a short induction and brief persistence producing only a segmental effect, relieving pain in the area in which it produces paresthesias. Acupuncture is best suited for the treatment of nociceptive syndromes such as pain resulting from acute injury in surgery, its effectiveness dependent on enhancing naloxone-reversible descending nociceptive inhibition through release of endorphins into the CSF. TENS, on the other hand, affects both nociceptive and deafferentation pain by a process not reversed by naloxone.[115]

This dichotomy between low- and high-frequency cutaneous stimulation has been explored further by Sjölund and his colleagues using "acupuncture-like TENS." The latter as contrasted with conventional TENS consists of trains of seven pulses at 100 Hz repeated at frequencies of 1.5 to 2 Hz,[27,118] resulting in powerful muscle contractions similar to the effects of acupuncture. Some patients who failed to obtain relief with conventional TENS obtained relief with "acupuncture-like TENS."[27,118] The Sjölund group showed that the action of acupuncture-like TENS in suppressing pain was blocked by naloxone[115] and resulted in the elevation of CSF levels of endorphins[116,120] at the same time profoundly inhibiting transmission from C fibers to spinal neurons.[117] The analgesia from conventional TENS, on the other hand, is not blocked by naloxone.[115] Most interestingly, Sjölund and Schouenborg[119] have shown in rats that nociceptive stimulation delivered in the form of heat or bradykinin injection elevated rate of glucose use in dorsal horn, especially in superficial layers of Rexed, an effect reduced with pretreatment with morphine and ipsilateral low-frequency sciatic nerve stimulation. On the other hand, the latter maneuver increased the use of glucose in substantia gelatinosa, suggesting a modulatory action there. These findings are in keeping with those of Takeshige and associates,[130] who showed parallel effects between acupuncture analgesia in rats and the action of morphine in periaqueductal gray stimulation, and of Takeda and co-workers,[129] who suggested that acupuncture analgesia implicated lower brain-stem nuclei such as the raphe group and locus ceruleus as well as neurochemical release.

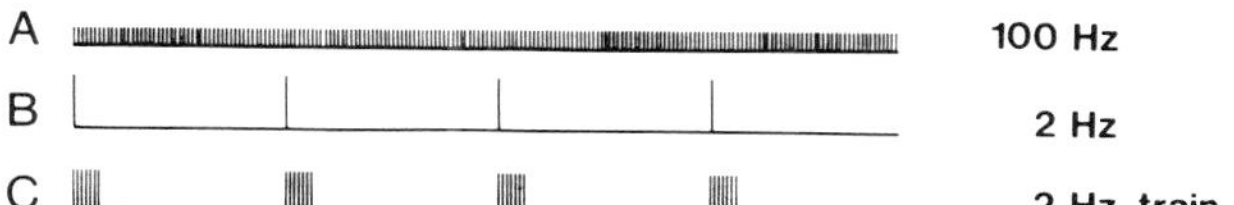

FIG. 30-17. Stimulation parameters of transcutaneous electrical nerve stimulation (TENS). **A.** *"High-frequency stimulation"* is usually at rates of 10 to 100 per second (10–100 Hz). A frequency of 80 Hz has been reported to be the most effective in inhibiting nociception in an animal model.[114] This type of stimulation (10–100 Hz) is also referred to as "conventional TENS." **B.** *"Low-frequency stimulation"* is usually at rates of less than 5 Hz (1–4 Hz). This produces local muscle contractions, which may stimulate afferents and play a role in the efficacy of the treatment. This is the type of stimulation used for *"electroacupuncture,"* where acupuncture needles are inserted into acupuncture points close to the painful area. Andersson and colleagues[2,3] found that similar pain-relieving effects can be obtained if large surface electrodes are used, provided adequate muscle contractions are obtained. **C.** *"Trains of impulses"* may be delivered at about 2 Hz. Sjolund and colleagues delivered trains of seven pulses at 100 Hz, repeated at frequencies of 2 Hz, and delivered by means of surface electrodes placed close to nerves to myotomes segmentally related to the painful area. This is termed *"acupuncture-like TENS."* It produces tolerable muscle contractions in the painful area and appears to be capable of obtaining pain relief when conventional TENS fails.[118] *Pulse configuration:* Current evidence[118] indicates that the most effective pulse configuration is a simple monophasic rectangular pulse, that is ⎍.

As for conventional TENS, its use has been summarized by Woolf[158] in Wall and Melzack's *Textbook of Pain.* In acute pain syndromes it was useful in posttraumatic states, especially the pain of fractured ribs,[81] the pain of labor,[5] and postoperative pain, especially on the first day. In postoperative pain it is best to use long skin electrodes placed on either side of the surgical wound. Sterile electrodes are now available. TENS is often not effective on its own but may achieve about 50% reduction in analgesic drug requirements (Table 30-2).[150] For chronic pain TENS was best in neurogenic syndromes not characterized by widespread or ill-localized pain. Nielzén and coworkers, in a blind screening procedure, reported on 66 patients with chronic pain. Patients without any relevant physical cause of their pain were generally treatment failures for TENS; these patients also had an excess of pathologic personality traits, mostly of a hysterical nature.[86] In practice it has been used most often for treating chronic pain of mixed etiologies employing unspecified stimulation parameters and strategies, especially deafferentation pain, with electrodes arranged over afferent nerves so as to produce paresthesias in the painful area (Table 30-3). This latter strategy is similar to that used with dorsal cord stimulation.

Meyerson,[70] in a review, has pointed out that TENS in the broad sense initially relieves pain in 60% of patients, with persistent success in only 30% after 5 months. Conventional TENS in a general way was more effective for nerve injury pain, whereas acupuncture and low-intensity stimulation were more effective for nociceptive pain. Sindou and Keravel[113] found TENS useful in 80% of cases of peripheral nerve injury. Gessler and Struppler[34] found 100 Hz TENS more effective than 2 Hz in the treatment of phantom pain. Keravel and Sindou[48] and Sindou[111] reviewed the use of TENS in 180 personal and 4200 published cases, finding more than 80% pain reduction after 3 weeks in 62% of patients with amputation pain and 61% with peripheral nerve injury. Relatively few patients with root lesions, postherpetic neuralgia, brachial plexus injury, and cord and brain lesions derived relief, and only 15% of patients with pain caused by cancer were helped. A world literature review[48] suggested that 62% of patients with amputation pain, 52% with nerve injury, 74% with radicular pain, 68% with postherpetic pain, 41% with cord injury, and 6% with thalamic pain derived relief. Frequency was not specified. In a series of 37 patients, 20 of whom suffered from nociceptive and 17 from deafferentation pain, treated with TENS at an unspecified rate, 50% of the former and 65% of the latter were still relieved after 30 days. Eriksson and co-workers[29] found 44% of patients with deafferentation facial pain were helped by conventional TENS and 33% by "acupuncture-like TENS." Twenty-nine percent of patients with tic douloureux

TABLE 30-2. EFFICACY OF TENS IN TREATING ACUTE PAIN

Type of Pain	Reference	Comment*
Acute trauma	81	Relief of rib fracture pain
Postoperative		
Abdominal thoracic surgery	150	47/61 with TENS had PR vs. 7/39 with "SHAM TENS." No change in respiratory complications
	17	77% with TENS had PR vs. 33% with placebo. No change in respiratory complications. Patients using preop opioids obtained no PR with TENS
	1	Reduced opioid requirements and PR. With TENS, less depressed PO_2, VC, and FRC than with "SHAM TENS"
Spine surgery	121	Reduced opioid requirements and PR. No PR if patients using opioid preoperatively
Total hip replacement	96	Reduced opioid requirements and PR
Abdominal hysterectomy	53	Implanted wire electrodes
Obstetric pain	5	PR may last up to 18 h after TENS. Need 1 pair electrodes at T10–L1 (1st stage) and 2nd pair at S2–S4 (2nd stage)
Acute orofacial pain	36	TENS more effective than "SHAM TENS" or aspirin

*PR = pain relief.

TABLE 30-3. EFFICACY OF TENS IN TREATMENT OF CHRONIC PAIN

Type of Pain	Reference	Comment*
Peripheral nerve injury	10	PR in 10/24 cases
	113	PR in 80% of cases
	48	PR in 52% of cases
Phantom limb pain	34	100 Hz more effective than 2 Hz
	82	PR in 8/11 cases
Amputation pain	48,111	4200 cases: PR in 62%
Deafferentation facial pain	29	PR in 44% of cases with TENS. PR in 33% of cases with "acupuncture-like TENS"
Tic douloureux	29	PR in 29% of cases with TENS. PR in 24% of cases with "acupuncture-like TENS"
Low back pain	61	Initial PR in 132/197 cases. Long-term PR in 71/104 cases followed up
	62	PR in 32% of 400 cases
	33	PR in about 30% of cases given 7-day trial of TENS: 84% of these continued to obtain PR
Deafferentation pain	59	PR in 6/33 cases
	22	PR in 2/11 cases
Radicular pain	22	PR in 3/9 cases
Spinal cord injury	22	PR in 8/11 cases. Electrodes close to pain
Brachial plexus avulsion	159	PR if electrodes placed over surviving afferents (*e.g.*, T2, C2–C4)
Postherpetic neuralgia	85	PR in 11/30 cases
Cancer (CA)	151	PR in 43% with CA in head and neck with "trigger areas." Used electroacupuncture. ?Pain of myofascial origin
Rheumatoid arthritis	50	PR in 55% with TENS, in 64% with acupuncture-like TENS, and in 37% with "SHAM TENS"
	66	PR in 5/20 cases with TENS at 3 Hz, PR in 18/20 cases at 70 Hz
Peripheral neuropathy	62	No PR
Central pain	62	No PR
Visceral pain	28	No PR
Ischemic pain	28	No PR
Psychogenic pain	86	No PR

*PR = pain relief.

were helped by conventional TENS and 24% by "acupuncture-like TENS." Long[61] reported initial excellent to good pain relief with conventional TENS in 132 of 197 patients, most of whom suffered from chronic low back pain. Seventy-one of 104 of these patients who responded to a questionnaire enjoyed longer-term relief, the only complication being dermatitis. It was necessary to avoid stimulation in patients with heart pacemakers. Long and Hagfors[62] estimated that TENS used in an unspecified 3000 patients in an unspecified way yielded 25% to 30% of patients "more or less completely relieved" of chronic pain, although up to 50% found it useful to some extent. Thirty-two percent of their 400 patients with low back pain had excellent results, and 56% of 45 suffering from deafferentation pain were helped. Patients with peripheral neuropathy or central pain did not benefit. Fried and associates[33] first eliminated nonresponders with a 7-day test of TENS with an overall 18.6% to 39.6% of 846 patients passing the test. Most of their patients suffered from low back pain. Once responders had been identified, 83.8% continued to gain relief. Loeser and associates[59] found long-term relief in 12.5% of 198 patients, 68% enjoying part-time short-term relief. TENS was used between 10 and 150 Hz. Of 33 patients with deafferentation pain, 6 were relieved.

Bohm[10] relieved pain in 10 of 24 patients with peripheral nerve injury and felt that relief occurred in most patients with sympathetic hyperactivity. Davis and Lentini[22] relieved pain localized around the injury site after spinal cord injury in 8 of 11 patients, placing electrodes adjacent to the pain. Radicular pain was relieved in 3 of 9 and deafferentation pain in 2 of 11. Naidu[82] found 8 of 11 amputees relieved of phantom pain. Wynn-Parry[159] found TENS most useful in treating pain from complete brachial plexus avulsion when the electrodes were placed over surviving afferent nerves such as in the inner upper arm, in the T2 distribution, and over the C2-C4 dermatomes in the neck. Nathan and Wall[85] found TENS useful in 11 of 30 cases of postherpetic neuralgia.

Ventafridda and colleagues[151] found electroacupuncture of unspecified rate helpful in 43% of patients with cancer pain, especially cancer of the head and neck, particularly in those with trigger points and hyperalgesic areas. They also note that it is especially effective in postherpetic neuralgia and early phantom pain, although efficiency declines with time. Andersson and associates[3] found that both low- and high-frequency infraorbital nerve stimulation increased the threshold for dental pain, as did Hoku acupuncture; however, high-threshold stimulation was less effective. Hansson and Ekblom[36] found that 100 Hz TENS decreased dental pain by more than half in 7 of 22 patients (32%); 2 Hz stimulation decreased the pain in 9 of 20 (45%). Augustinsson and colleagues[5] used TENS for the relief of labor pain at T10 to L1 during the first stage and S2 to S4 in the later stages. Forty-four percent reported good or very good relief. Andersson and co-workers[2] found 2 Hz TENS very useful in 48% of 27 patients in labor. Rosenberg and associates[99] found 50 to 100 Hz TENS useful in the first 2 days of management of postoperative pain. Langley and colleagues[50] found no difference between high-frequency, acupuncture-like, and placebo TENS in reducing rheumatoid arthritic hand pain by more than 50%. High-frequency TENS achieved 54.5%, low-frequency 63.6%, and placebo stimulation only 36.6% of pain reduction greater than 50%. Other factors such as drug intake and strength of grip showed little difference.

It would appear then that conventional high-frequency TENS has an important role in the treatment of deafferentation pain as long as afferent nerves can be stimulated so as to produce paresthesias in the area of pain. TENS is also useful in both acute and chronic nociceptive pain, particularly if lower-frequency or acupuncture-like TENS is applied, although patients are more likely to find the resulting strong muscular contractions unpleasant.

Problems that remain in the use of TENS include a clear definition of indications for its use, problems with skin irritation, and a progressive decline in efficacy with continued use. Initial responses of 50% to 70% of patients obtaining pain relief decline to 30% to 50% at 1 month, 20% to 30% at 1 year, and 10% to 20% after 1 year.[6,28,63,142] In comparison *placebo effect* accounts for pain relief initially in 30% of patients, declining very rapidly to 5% to 10% at 1 month and 1% to 2% at 1 year.

"FAILED BACK" PAIN

The pain associated with chronic degenerative lumbar disk disease consists of a variable mixture of psychogenic, nociceptive, spondylogenic, radicular, and deafferentation pain associated with root damage, whether produced by disease or previous surgery. Treatment strategies in these patients may include several different modalities tailored to the patients' needs after careful identification of the clinical problem. First, treatable conditions such as root compression, skeletal instability, and spinal stenosis must be recognized and dealt with. Then a decision must be made on the need for psychotherapy, supportive therapy, TENS, "facet rhizotomy," rarely, if ever, rhizotomy, and chronic spinal epidural stimulation (see Chap. 27.3).

CONCLUSION

The treatment of intractable pain consists of first dissecting the pain problem into the various categories such as psychogenic, deafferentation, and nociceptive problems. Then treatment techniques must be selected starting with the simplest, using percutaneous techniques whenever possible, and persisting to more complex techniques as far as disability caused by the pain, and not the underlying disease, warrants. The likelihood of success and justification of complications must be considered. Both interrupting and modulatory procedures are available for nociceptive and deafferentation pain syndromes. The treatments of choice for nociceptive pain are spinal opioids or percutaneous cordotomy. For deafferentation pain, chronic spinal epidural or trigeminal stimulation may be required if transcutaneous electrical stimulation is not effective. For tic douloureux the selective percutaneous radiofrequency thermocoagulation method, of the procedures that have been thoroughly explored, carries the highest chance of success with the lowest risk.

REFERENCES

1. Ali, J.A., Yaffee, C.S. and Serreti, C.: The effect of transcutaneous electric nerve stimulation on postoperative pain and pulmonary function. Surgery, *89*:507, 1981.
2. Andersson, S.A.: Pain control by sensory stimulation. *In* Bonica, J.J., Liebeskind, J.C., and Albe–Fessard, D.G. (eds.): Advances in Pain Research and Therapy. vol. 3, p. 569, New York, Raven, 1979.
3. Andersson, S.A., Ericson, T., Holmgren, T., and Lindquist, G.: Electroacupuncture. Effect on pain threshold measurement with electrical stimulation of the teeth. Brain Res., *63*:393, 1973.
4. Armour, D.: Surgery of the spinal cord and its membranes. Lancet, *2*:691, 1927.
5. Augustinsson, L.-E., Bohlin, P., Bundsen, P., and Carlsson, C.-A., Forsmann, L., Sjöberg, P., and Tyreman, N.O.: Pain relief during delivery by transcutaneous electrical nerve stimulation. Pain, *4*:59, 1977.
6. Bates, J.A.V., and Nathan, P.W.: Transcutaneous electrical nerve stimulation for thoracic pain. Anaesthesia, *35*:817, 1980.
7. Blume, H.G.: Radiofrequency denervation in occipital pain: a new approach in 114 cases. *In* Bonica, J.J., and Albe-Fessard, D.G. (eds.): Advances in Pain Research and Therapy. vol. 1, p. 691. New York, Raven, 1976.
8. Blume, H., and Fromm, S.: Radiofrequency denervation in occipital pain: A new approach. Sixth International Congress of Neurologic Surgeons. International Congress Series, *148*:221, 1977.
9. Boas, R.A., Hatangdi, V.S., and Richards, E.G.: Lumbar sympathectomy—a percutaneous chemical technique. *In* Bonica, J.J., and Albe–Fessard, D.G. (eds.): Advances in Pain Research and Therapy. vol. 1. p. 685. New York, Raven, 1976.
10. Bohm, E.: Transcutaneous electrical nerve stimulation in chronic pain after peripheral nerve injury. Acta Neurochir., *40*:277, 1978.
11. Broggi, G.C.: Surgical treatment of glossopharyngeal neuralgia and pain from cancer of the nasopharynx. J. Neurosurg.; *61*:952, 1984.
12. Broggi, G., and Siegfried, J.: Percutaneous differential radiofrequency rhizotomy of glossopharyngeal nerve in facial pain due to cancer. *In* Bonica, J.J., and Ventafridda, V. (eds.): Advances in Pain Research and Therapy. vol. 2, p. 469. New York, Raven, 1979.
13. Burton, C.V.: Percutaneous radiofrequency facet denervation. Appl. Neurophysiol., *39*:80, 1976.
14. Capper, S.J., Conlon, J.M., Lahuerta, J., Miles, J.B., and Lipton, S.: Peptide concentrations in the CSF following injection of alcohol into the pituitary gland. Pain, *2*[*Suppl.*]:S316, 1984.
15. Condouris, G.A.: Local anesthetics as modulators of neural information. *In* Bonica, J.J., and Albe–Fessard, D.G. (eds.): Advances in Pain Research and Therapy. vol. 1, p. 663. New York, Raven, 1976.
16. Cook, A.W., Nathan, P.W., and Smith, M.C.: Sensory consequences of commissural myelotomy. A challenge to traditional anatomical concepts. Brain, *107*:547, 1984.
17. Cooperman, A.M., Hall, B., Mikalacki, K., Hardy, R., *et al.*: Use of transcutaneous electrical stimulation in control of postoperative pain—results of prospective, randomized controlled study. Am. J. Surg., *133*:185, 1977.
18. Crue, B.L., and Todd, E.M., Carregal, E.J.A.: Posterior approach for high cervical percutaneous radiofrequency cordotomy. Confin. Neurol., *30*:41, 1968.
19. Crue, B.L., Todd, E.M., and Carregal, E.J.: Percutaneous radiofrequency stereotactic trigeminal tractotomy. *In* Crue, B.L. (ed.): Pain and Suffering. p. 69. Springfield, Illinois, Charles C. Thomas, 1970.
20. Crue, B.L., Jr., Todd, E.M., Carregal, E.J.A., and Kilham, O.: Percutaneous trigeminal tractotomy. Case report utilizing stereotactic radiofrequency lesion. Bull. Los Angeles Neurol. Soc., *32*:86, 1967.
21. D'Annunzio, V., Denaro, F., and Meglio, M.: Personal experience with intrathecal morphine in the management of pain from pelvic cancer. Acta. Neurochir. *33*[*Suppl.*]:421, 1984.
22. Davis, R., and Lentini, R.: Transcutaneous nerve stimulation for treatment of pain in spinal-cord-injured patients. Bull. Prosthet. Res., p. 298, Fall, 1974.
23. Dooley, D.M.: A technique for the epidural percutaneous stimulation of the spinal cord in man. Presented Annual Meeting AANS, Miami Beach, 1975.
24. Dunsker, S.B., Wood, M., Lotspeich, E.S., and Mayfield, F.H.: Percutaneous electrocoagulation of lumbar articular nerves. *In* Lee, J.F. (ed.): Pain Management. p. 123. Baltimore, Williams and Wilkins, 1977.
25. Eiras, J., Garcia, J., Gomez, J., Carcavalla, L.I., and Ucar, J.: First results with extralemniscal myelotomy. Acta Neurochir. Suppl., *30*:377, 1980.
26. Erickson, D.L.: Percutaneous trial of stimulation for patient selection for implantable stimulating electrodes. J. Neurosurg., *43*:440, 1975.
27. Eriksson, M.B.E., and Sjölund, B.H.: Acupuncture-like electroanalgesia in TNS-resistant chronic pain. *In* Zotterman, Y. (ed.): Sensory Functions of the Skin. p. 575. Oxford, Pergamon, 1976.
28. Eriksson, M.B.E. Sjölund, B.H., and Nielzén, S.: Long term results of peripheaarl conditioning stimulation as an analgesic measure in chronic pain. Pain, *6*:335, 1979.
29. Eriksson, M.B.E., Sjölund, B.H., and Sundbärg, G.: Pain relief from peripheral conditioning stimulation in patients with chronic facial pain. J. Neurosurg., *61*:149, 1984.
30. Fox, J.L.: Percutaneous trigeminal tractotomy. Variations in delineation of the obex using emulsified pantopaque. Confin. Neurol., *36*:97, 1974.
31. Fox, J.L.: Delineation of the obex by contrast radiography during percutaneous trigeminal tractotomy. Technical note. J. Neurosurg., *36*:107, 1972.
32. Fox, J.L., and Rizzoli, H.V.: Identification of radiological coordinates for the posterior articular nerve of Luschka in the lumbar spine. Surg. Neurol., *1*:343, 1973.
33. Fried, T., Johnson, R., and McCracken, W.: Transcutaneous electrical nerve stimulation: Its role in the control of chronic pain. Arch. Phys. Med. Rehabil., *65*:228, 1984.

34. Gessler, M., and Struppler, A.: Relief of phantom pain following modification of phantom sensation by TNS. *In* Bonica, J.J., Lindblom, U., Iggo, A. (eds.): Advances in Pain Research and Therapy. vol. 5. p. 591. New York, Raven, 1983.
35. Håkansson, S.: Trigeminal neuralgia treated by the injection of glycerol into the trigeminal cistern. Neurosurgery, *9*:638, 1981.
36. Hansson, P., and Ekblom, A.: Transcutaneous electrical nerve stimulation (TENS) as compared to placebo TENS for the relief of acute oro-facial pain. Pain, *15*:157, 1983.
37. Härtel, F.: Die Leitungsanästhesie und Injections—behandlung des Ganglion Gasseri und der Trigeminusstäme. Arch. Klin. Chir., *100*:193, 1912.
38. Hitchcock, E.R.: An apparatus for stereotactic spinal surgery. Lancet, *1*:705, 1960.
39. Hitchcock, E.R.: Stereotactic spinal surgery. A preliminary report. J. Neurosurg., *31*:386, 1969.
40. Hitchcock, E.R.: Stereotactic trigeminal tractotomy. Ann. Clin. Res., *2*:131, 1970.
41. Hitchcock, E.R.: Stereotactic cervical myelotomy. J. Neurol. Neurosurg. Psychiatry, *33*:224, 1970.
42. Hitchcock, E.R., and Schvarcz, J.R.: Stereotaxic trigeminal tractotomy for post-herpetic facial pain. J. Neurosurg., *37*:412, 1972.
43. Hoppenstein, R.: Percutaneous implantation of chronic spinal cord electrode for control of intractable pain. Preliminary report. Surg. Neurol., *4*:195, 1975.
44. Hyndman, O.R.: Lissauer's tract section. A contribution to chordotomy for the relief of pain. (Preliminary report). J. Int. Coll. Surgeons., *5*:394, 1942.
45. Inbal, R., Devor, M., Tuchendler, O., and Lieblich, I.: Autotomy following nerve injury: Genetic factors in the development of chronic pain. Pain, *9*:327, 1980.
46. Isamat, F., Ferrán, E., and Acebes, J.J.: Selective percutaneous thermocoagulation rhizotomy in essential glossopharyngeal neuralgia. J. Neurosurg., *55*:575, 1981.
47. Katz, J.: Current role of neurolytic agents. *In* Bonica, J.J. (ed.): Advances in Neurology, vol. 4. p. 471. New York, Raven, 1974.
48. Keravel, Y., and Sindou, M.: Anatomical conditions of efficiency of transcutaneous electrical neurostimulation in deafferentation pain. *In* Bonica, J.J., Lindblom, U., Iggo, A. (eds.): Advances in Pain Research and Therapy. vol. 5. p. 763. New York, Raven, 1983.
49. Kirschner, M.: Elektrokoagulation des Ganglion gasseri. Zentralbl. Chir., *47*:2841, 1932.
50. Langley, G.B., Sheppeard, M., Johnson, M., and Wigley, R.D.: The analgesic effect of transcutaneous electrical nerve stimulation and placebo in chronic pain patients. Rheumatol. Int., *4*:119, 1984.
51. Latchaw, J.P., Jr., Hardy, R.W., Jr., Forsythe, S.B., and Cook, A.F.: Trigeminal neuralgia treated by radiofrequency coagulation. Neurosurgery, *59*:479, 1983.
52. Lazorthes, Y., and Verdie, J.C.: Radiofrequency coagulation of the petrous ganglion in glossopharyngeal neuralgia. Neurosurgery, *4*:512, 1979.
53. Ledergerber, C.P.: Postoperative electroanalgesia. Obstet. and Gynecol., *151*:334, 1978.
54. Levin, A.B., Ramirez, L.F., and Katz, J.: The use of stereotaxic chemical hypophysectomy in the treatment of thalamic pain syndrome. J. Neurosurg., *59*:1002, 1983.
55. Levitt, M., and Levitt, J.H.: The deafferentation syndrome in monkeys: Dysesthesias of spinal origin. Pain, *10*:129, 1981.
56. Lin, P.M., Gildenberg, P.L., and Polakoff, P.P.: An anterior approach to percutaneous lower cervical cordotomy. J. Neurosurg., *25*:553, 1966.
57. Lipton, S.: Percutaneous cordotomy. *In* Wall, P.D., and Melzack, R. (eds.): Textbook of Pain. p. 632. Edinburgh, Scotland, Churchill Livingstone, 1984.
58. Livingston, W.K.: Pain Mechanisms: A physiologic interpretation of causalgia and its related causes. ed. 2. New York, Plenum, 1976.
58a. Loeser, J.D.: Herpes zoster and postherpetic neuralgia. Pain, *25*:149, 1986.
59. Loeser, J.D., Black, R.G., and Christman, A.: Relief of pain by transcutaneous stimulation. J. Neurosurg., *42*:308, 1975.
60. Loeser, J.D., Ward, A.A., and White, L.E.: Chronic deafferentation of human spinal cord neurons. J. Neurosurg., *29*:48, 1968.
61. Long, D.M.: Cutaneous afferent stimulation for relief of chronic pain. Clin. Neurosurg., *21*:257, 1974.
62. Long, D.M., and Hagfors, N.: Electrical stimulation in the nervous system: The current status of electrical stimulation of the nervous system for relief of pain. Pain, *1*:109, 1975.
63. Long, D.M., Campbell, J.N., and Gurer, G.: Transcutaneous electrical stimulation for the relief of chronic pain. *In* Bonica, J.J., Liebeskind, J.C., and Albe-Fessard, D.G. (eds.): Advances in Pain Research and Therapy. vol. 3. pp. 593–599. New York, Raven, 1979.
64. Lunsford, L.D., and Bennett, M.H.: Percutaneous retrogasserian glycerol rhizotomy for tic douloureux. Part 1. Technique and results in 112 patients. Neurosurgery, *14*:424, 1984.
65. Madrid, J.L.: Chemical hypophysectomy. *In* Bonica, J.J., Ventafridda, V. (eds.): Advances in Pain Research and Therapy. vol. 2. p. 381. New York, Raven, 1979.
66. Mannheimer, C., and Carlsson, C.A.: The analgesic effect of transcutaneous electrical nerve stimulation in patients with rheumatoid arthritis. A comparative study of different pulse patterns. Pain, *6*:329, 1979.
67. Maxwell, R.F.: Surgical control of chronic migrainous neuralgia by trigeminal ganglio-rhizolysis. J. Neurosurg., *57*:459, 1982.
68. McCulloch, J.A.: Percutaneous radiofrequency lumbar rhizolysis (rhizotomy). Appl. Neurophysiol., *39*:87, 1976.
69. Melzack, R., and Wall, P.D.: Pain mechanisms. A new theory. Science, *150*:971, 1965.
70. Meyerson, B.A.: Electrostimulation procedures: Effects, presumed rationale, and possible mechanisms. *In* Bonica, J.J., Lindblom, U., Iggo, A. (eds.): Advances in Pain Research and Therapy. vol. 5. p. 495. New York, Raven, 1983.
71. Meyerson, B.A., Arnér, S., and Linderoth, B.: Pros and cons of different approaches to the management of pelvic cancer pain. Acta Neurochir. Suppl., *33*:407, 1984.
72. Meyerson, B.A., and Håkansson, S.: Alleviation of atypical

trigeminal pain by stimulation of the gasserian ganglion via an implanted electrode. Acta Neurochir. Suppl., *30*:303, 1980.

73. Miles, J.: Chemical hypophysectomy. *In* Bonica, J.J., and Ventafridda, V. (eds.): Advances in Pain Research and Therapy. vol. 2. p. 373. New York, Raven, 1979.
74. Miles, J.: Pituitary destruction. *In* Wall, P.D., and Melzack, R. (eds.): Textbook of Pain. p. 656. Edinburgh, Scotland, Churchill Livingstone, 1984.
75. Modesti, L.M., and Waszak, M.: Firing pattern of cells in human thalamus during dorsal column stimulation. Appl. Neurophysiol., *38*:251, 1975.
76. Moore, D.C.: Celiac (splanchnic) plexus block with alcohol for cancer pain of the upper intra-abdominal viscera. *In* Bonica, J.J., and Ventafridda, V., (eds.): Advances in Pain Research and Therapy, vol. 2. p. 357. New York, Raven, 1979.
77. Moore, D.C.: Role of nerve block with neurolytic solutions for pelvic visceral cancer pain. *In* Bonica, J.J., and Ventafridda, V. (eds.): Advances in Pain Research and Therapy. vol. 2. p. 593. New York, Raven, 1979.
78. Morrica, G.: Chemical hypophysectomy for cancer pain. *In* Bonica, J.J., (ed.): Advances in Neurology. vol. 4. p. 707. New York, Raven, 1974.
79. Mullan, S., Harper, P.V., Hekmatpanah, J., Torres, H., *et al.*: Percutaneous interruption of spinal pain tracts by means of a strontium 90 needle. J. Neurosurg., *20*:931, 1963.
80. Mullan, S., and Lichtor, T.: Percutaneous microcompression of the trigeminal ganglion for trigeminal neuralgia. J. Neurosurg., *59*:1007, 1983.
81. Myers, R.A., Woolf, C.J., and Mitchell, D.: Management of acute traumatic pain by peripheral transcutaneous electrical stimulation South African Medical Journal, *52*:309–312, 1977.
82. Naidu, K.R.C.: Transcutaneous electrical stimulation in the management of phantom limb pain. J. Assoc. Physicians India, *30*:309, 1982.
83. Nashold, B.S., Ostdahl, R.H.: Dorsal root entry zone lesions for pain relief. J. Neurosurg., *51*:59, 1979.
84. Nashold, B.S., Lopes, H, and Chodakiewitz: Trigeminal DREZ; caudalis lesions for relief of facial pain. Presented at the International Symposium on surgery in and around the brain stem and third ventricle, Hannover, Feb 18–23, 1985. [In press].
85. Nathan, P.W., and Wall, P.D.: Treatment of post-herpetic neuralgia by prolonged electrical stimulation. Br. Med. J., *14*:645, 1974.
86. Nielzén, S., Sjölund, B.H., and Eriksson, M.B.E.: Psychiatric factors influencing the treatment of pain with peripheral conditioning stimulation. Pain, *13*:365, 1982.
87. Nugent, G.R., and Berry, B.: Trigeminal neuralgia treated by differential radiofrequency coagulation of the gasserian ganglion. J. Neurosurg., *40*:517, 1974.
88. Onofrio, B.M., Yaksh, T.L., and Arnold, P.G.: Continuous low-dose intrathecal morphine administration in the treatment of chronic pain of malignant origin. Mayo Clinic Proc., *56*:516, 1981.
89. Oudenhoven, R.C.: Articular rhizotomy. Surg. Neurol., *2*:275, 1975.
90. Pagura, J.R.: Percutaneous radiofrequency spinal rhizotomy. Appl. Neurophysiol., *46*:138, 1983.
91. Pagura, J.R., Schnapp, M., and Passarelli, P.: Percutaneous radiofrequency glossopharyngeal rhizolysis for cancer pain. Appl. Neurophysiol., *46*:154, 1983.
92. Papo, I.: Spinal posterior rhizotomy and commissural myelotomy in the treatment of pain. *In* Bonica, J.J., and Ventafridda, V. (eds.): Advances in Pain Research and Therapy. vol. 2. p. 439. New York, Raven, 1979.
93. Papo, I., and Visca, A.: Phenol subarachnoid rhizotomy for the treatment of cancer pain: a personal account on 290 cases. *In* Bonica, J.J., and Ventafridda, V. (eds.): Advances in Pain Research and Therapy. vol. 2. p. 339. New York, Raven, 1979.
94. Pedersen, H.E., Blunck, C.F.J., and Gardner, E.: The anatomy of lumbosacral posterior rami and meningeal branches of spinal nerves (sinu-vertebral nerves) with an experimental study of their functions. J. Bone Joint Surg., *38A*:377, 1956.
95. Penn, R.D., Paice, J.A., Gottschalk, W., and Ivankovich, A.D.: Cancer pain relief using chronic morphine infusion. J. Neurosurg., *61*:302, 1984.
96. Pike, P.M.: Transcutaneous electrical stimulation: Its use in management of postoperative pain. Anaesthesia, *33*:165, 1978.
97. Poletti, C.F., Cohen, A.M., Todd, D.P., Ojemann, R.G.: *et al.*: Cancer pain relieved by long-term epidural morphine with permanent indwelling systems for self-administration. J. Neurosurg., *55*:581, 1981.
98. Rees, W.E.S.: Multiple bilateral percutaneous rhizolysis in the treatment of the slipped disc syndrome. Presented at the Annual Meeting of the AANS, St. Louis, 1974.
99. Rosenberg, M., Curtis, L., and Bourke, D.L.: Transcutaneous electrical nerve stimulation for the relief of postoperative pain. Pain, *5*:129, 1978.
100. Rosomoff, H.L.: Percutaneous radiofrequency cervical cordotomy for intractable pain. Sixth International Congress of Neurologic Surgeons. International Congress Series, *148*:110, 1977. Amsterdam, Excerpta Medica.
101. Rosomoff, H.L., Carroll, F., Brown, J., *et al.*: Percutaneous radiofrequency cervical cordotomy: Technique. J. Neurosurg., *23*:639, 1965.
102. Salar, G., Ori, C., Baratto, V., Iob, I., *et al.*: Selective percutaneous thermolesions of the ninth cranial nerve by lateral cervical approach: Report of eight cases. Surg. Neurol., *20*:276, 1983.
103. Schvarcz, J.R.: Spinal cord stereotactic techniques re trigeminal nucleotomy and extralemniscal myelotomy. Appl. Neurophysiol., *41*:99, 1978.
104. Schvarcz, J.R.: Stereotactic spinal trigeminal nucleotomy for dysesthetic facial pain. *In* Bonica, J.J., Liebeskind, J.C., and Albe–Fessard, D.G. (eds.): Advances in Pain Research and Therapy. vol. 3. p. 331. New York, Raven, 1979.
105. Schvarcz, J.R.: Stereotactic high cervical extralemniscal myelotomy for pelvic cancer pain. Acta Neurochir. Suppl., *33*:431, 1984.
106. Shealy, C.N.: Percutaneous radiofrequency denervation of spinal facets. J. Neurosurg., *43*:448, 1975.
107. Shealy, C.N., Mortimer, J.T., and Hagfors, N.R.: Dorsal

column electroanalgesia. J. Neurosurg., *32*:560, 1970.

108. Sheldon, C.H.: Depolarization in the treatment of trigeminal neuralgia: Evaluation of compression and electrical methods; clinical concept of neurophysiological mechanisms. *In* Knighton, R.S., and Dumke, P.R., (eds.): Pain. p. 373. Boston, Little Brown, 1966.

109. Sheldon, C.H., Pudenz, R.H., Freshwater, D.B., *et al.*: Compression rather than decompression for trigeminal neuralgia. J. Neurosurg., *12*:123, 1955.

110. Siegfried, J., and Broggi, G.: Percutaneous thermocoagulation of the gasserian ganglion in the treatment of pain in advanced cancer. *In* Bonica, J.J., and Ventafridda, V. (eds.): Advances in Pain Research and Therapy. vol. 2. p. 463. New York, Raven, 1979.

111. Sindou, M.: Electro analgésies transcutanée dans les syndrome de déafférentation périphérique. Ann. Anesth. Franc., *19*:409, 1978.

112. Sindou, M., and Fischer, G., Goutelle, A., and Mansuy, L.: La radicellotomie postérieure sélective. Premiers résultats dans la chirurgie de la douleur. Neurochirurgie, Paris, *20*:391, 1974.

113. Sindou, M., and Keravel, Y.: Analgésie par la méthode d'électrostimulation transcutanée. Neurochirurgie Paris, *26*:153, 1980.

114. Sjölund, B.H.: Which are the most effective parameters for TENS? An experimental study. Pain. [In Press].

115. Sjölund, B.H., and Eriksson, M.B.E.: The influence of naloxone on analgesia produced by peripheral conditioning stimulation. Brain Res., *173*:295, 1979.

116. Sjölund, B.H., and Eriksson, M.B.E.: Endorphins and analgesia produced by peripheral conditioning stimulation. *In* Bonica, J.J., Liebeskind, J.C., and Albe–Fessard, D.G. (eds.): Advances in Pain Research and Therapy. vol. 3. p. 587. New York, Raven, 1979.

117. Sjölund, B.H., and Eriksson, M.: Naloxone reversible depression of C-fibre evoked flexion reflexes in low spinal cats after conditioning electrical stimulation of primary afferents. Neurosci. Lett., *3*[*Suppl.*]:264, 1979.

118. Sjölund, B.H., and Eriksson, M.: Stimulation techniques in the management of pain. *In* Kosterlitz, H.W. and Terenius, L.Y. (eds.): Pain and Society. pp. 415–43. Dahlem Workshop Report. Life Sciences Report 17. Verlag Chemie, GMBH, 1980.

119. Sjölund, B.H., and Schouenborg, J.: Site of action of anti-nociceptive acupuncture-like nerve stimulation in the spinal rat as visualized by the 14C-2-deoxyglucose method. *In* Bonica, J.J., Lindblom, U., and Iggo, A. (eds.): Advances in Pain Research and Therapy. vol. 5, p. 535. New York, Raven, 1983.

120. Sjölund, B.H., Terenius, L., and Eriksson, M.: Increased cerebrospinal fluid levels of endorphins after electro-acupuncture. Acta. Physiol. Scand., *100*:382, 1977.

121. Solomon, R.A., Viernstein, M.C., and Long, D.M.: Reduction of postoperative pain and narcotic use by transcutaneous electrical nerve stimulation. Surgery, *87*:142, 1980.

122. Steude, V.: Radiofrequency electrical stimulation of the gasserian ganglion in patients with atypical trigeminal pain. Acta Neurochir., *33*[*Suppl.*]:481, 1984.

123. Sweet, W.H., and Poletti, C.E.: Retrogasserian glycerol injection as treatment for trigeminal neuralgia. *In* Schmidek, H.H., and Sweet, W.H. (eds.): Operative Neurosurgical Techniques. Indications, Methods, and Results. p. 1107. New York, Grune and Stratton, 1982.

124. Sweet, W.H., and Wepsic, S.G.: Controlled thermocoagulation of trigeminal ganglion and results for differential destruction of pain fibres. J. Neurosurg., *29*:143, 1974.

125. Swerdlow, M.: Subarachnoid and extradural neurolytic blocks. *In* Bonica, J.J., and Ventafridda, V., (eds.): Advances in Pain Research and Therapy, vol. 2. p. 325. New York, Raven, 1979.

126. Taarnhøj, P.: Decompression of the trigeminal root and the posterior part of the ganglion as treatment in trigeminal neuralgia. Preliminary communication. J. Neurosurg., *9*:288, 1952.

127. Takeda, F., Fujii, T., Uki, J., Fuso, Y., *et al.*: Cancer pain relief and tumor regression by means of pituitary neuroadenolysis and surgical hypophysectomy. Neurol. Med. Chir., Tokyo, *23*:41, 1983.

128. Takeda, F., Uki, J., Fujii, T., Kitani, Y., *et al.*: Pituitary neuroadenolysis to relieve cancer pain: observations of spread of ethanol installed into the sella turcica and subsequent changes of the hypothalamopituitary axis at autopsy. Neurol. Med. Chir. (Tokyo), *23*:50, 1983.

129. Takeda, K., Taniguchi, N., Kuriyama, H., and Matsushita, A.: Experimental study on the mechanism of acupuncture anesthesia. *In* Bonica, J.J., Liebeskind, J.C., and Albe–Fessard, D.G. (eds.): Advances in Pain Research and Therapy. vol. 3. p. 623. New York, Raven, 1979.

130. Takeshige, C., Murai, M., Tanaka, M., and Hachisu,M.: Parallel individual variations in effectiveness of acupuncture, morphine analgesia, and dorsal PAG-SPA and their abolition by D-phenylalanine. *In* Bonica, J.J., Lindblom, U., and Iggo, A. (eds.): Advances in Pain Research and Therapy. vol. 5. p. 563. New York, Raven, 1983.

131. Tasker, R.R.: Percutaneous cordotomy—the lateral high cervical technique. *In* Schmidek, H.H., and Sweet, W.H. (eds.): Operative Neurosurgical Techniques. Indications, Methods, and Results. p. 1137. New York, Grune and Stratton, 1982.

132. Tasker, R.R.: Identification of pain processing systems by electrical stimulation of the brain. Human Neurobiology, *1*:261, 1982.

133. Tasker, R.R.: Thalamic stereotaxic procedures. *In* Schaltenbrand, G., Walker,, A.E. (eds.): Stereotaxy of the Human Brain. p. 484. Stuttgart, Thieme, 1982.

134. Tasker, R.R.: Deafferentation. *In* Wall, P.D., and Melzack, R. (eds.): Textbook of Pain, p. 119. Edinburgh, Scotland, Churchill Livingstone, 1984.

135. Tasker, R.R.: Stereotaxic surgery. *In* Wall, P.D., and Melzack, R. (eds.): Textbook of Pain. p. 639. Edinburgh, Scotland, Churchill Livingstone, 1984.

136. Tasker, R.R.: Surgical approaches to the primary afferent and the spinal cord. *In* Fields, H.L., Dubner, R., and Cervero, F. (eds.): Advances in Pain Research and Therapy. vol. 9. p. 799. New York, Raven Press, 1986.

137. Tasker, R.R.: Safety and efficacy of chronic neural stimula-

tors. Contract with Canada Dep't Health and Welfare, 1984. [In Press].

138. Tasker, R.R.: Pain due to central nervous system pathology. *In* Bonica, J.J. (ed.): Management of Pain in Clinical Practice. Philadelphia, Lea & Febiger (in press).

139. Tasker, R.R., Organ, L.W., and Smith, K.C.: Physiological guidelines for the localization of lesions by percutaneous cordotomy. Acta Neurochir., [*Suppl*] *21*:111, 1974.

140. Tasker, R.R., Organ, L.W., and Hawrylyshyn, P.: Deafferentation and causalgia. *In* Bonica, J.J. (ed.): Pain. p. 305, New York, Raven, 1980.

141. Tasker, R.R., Tsuda, T., and Hawrylyshyn, P.: Clinical neurophysiological investigation of deafferentation pain. *In* Bonica, J.J., Lindblom, U., and Iggo, A. (eds.): Advances in Pain Research and Therapy. vol. 5. p. 713. New York, Raven, 1983.

142. Taylor, P., Hallet, M., and Flaherty, L.: Treatment of osteoarthritis of the knee with transcutaneous electrical nerve stimulation. Pain, *11*:233, 1981.

143. Tew, J.M., Jr., Keller, J.T., and Williams, D.S.: Functional surgery of the trigeminal nerve: Treatment of trigeminal neuralgia. *In* Rasmussen T., and Marino R. (eds.): Functional Neurosurgery. p. 129. New York, Raven, 1979.

144. Tew, J.M., Jr., and Tobler, W.D.: Percutaneous rhizotomy in the treatment of intractable facial pain (trigeminal, glossopharyngeal, and vagal nerves). *In* Schmidek, H.H., and Sweet, W.H. (eds.): Operative Neurosurgical Techniques. Indications, Methods and Results. p. 1083. New York, Grune and Stratton, 1982.

145. Todd, E.M., Crue, B.L., and Carregal, E.J.A.: Posterior percutaneous tractotomy and cordotomy. Confin. Neurol., *31*:106, 1969.

146. Tsubokawa, T., and Moriyasu, N.: Follow-up results of centre median thalamotomy for relief of intractable pain. Confin. Neurol., *37*:280, 1975.

147. Turnbull, I.M.: Percutaneous rhizotomy for trigeminal neuralgia. Surg. Neurol., 2:385, 1974.

148. Uematsu, S.: Percutaneous electrothermocoagulation of spinal nerve trunk, ganglion, and rootlets. *In*: Schmidek, H.H., and Sweet, W.H. (eds.): Operative Neurosurgical Techniques, Indications, Methods, and Results. p. 1177. New York, Grune and Stratton, 1982.

149. Uematsu, S., Udbarhelyi, G.B., Benson, D.W., and Siebens, A.A.: Percutaneous radiofrequency rhizotomy. Surg. Neurol., 2:319, 1974.

150. Vanderark, G.D., and McGrath, K.A.: Transcutaneous electrical stimulation in treatment of postoperative pain. Am. J. Surg., *130*:338, 1975.

150a. Ventafridda, V., Fochi, C., Sganzerla, E.P., and Tamburami, M.: Neurolytic blocks in perineal pain. *In* Bonica, J.J., and Ventafridda, V. (eds.): Advances in Pain Research and Therapy. vol. 2. p. 597. New York, Raven, 1979.

151. Ventafridda, V., and Martino, G.: Clinical evaluation of subarachnoid neurolytic blocks in intractable cancer pain. *In* Bonica, J.J., and Albe–Fessard, D.G. (eds.): Advances in Pain Research and Therapy. vol. 1. p. 699. New York, Raven, 1976.

152. Ventafridda, V., and Spreafico, R.: Subarachnoid saline perfusion. *In* Bonica, J.J. (ed.): Advances in Neurology. vol. 4. p. 477. New York, Raven, 1974.

153. Wall, P.D.: Introduction. *In* Wall, P.D., and Melzack, R. (eds.): Textbook of Pain. p. 1. Edinburgh, Scotland, Churchill Livingstone, 1984.

154. Wall, P.D., and Sweet, W.H.: Temporary abolition of pain in man. Science, *155*:108, 1967.

155. Watson, C.P., Morley, T.P., Richardson, J.C., Schutz, H., *et al.*: The surgical treatment of chronic cluster headache. Headache, *23*:289, 1983.

156. White, J.C., and Sweet, W.H.: Pain and the Neurosurgeon. A forty year experience. p. 435. Springfield, Illinois, Charles C. Thomas, 1969.

157. Wilkinson, A.: Percutaneous radiofrequency upper thoracic sympathectomy: A new technique. Neurosurgery, *15*:811, 1984.

158. Woolf, C.J.: Transcutaneous and implanted nerve stimulation. *In* Wall, P.D., and Melzack, R. (eds.): Textbook of Pain. p. 679. Edinburgh, Scotland, Churchill Livingstone, 1984.

159. Wynn–Parry, C.B.: Brachial plexus injuries. Br. J. Hosp. Med., *32*:130, 1984.

160. Yaksh, T.L.: Spinal opiate analgesia: Characteristics and principles of action. Pain, *11*:293, 1981.

161. Zimmermann, M.: Peripheral and central nervous mechanisms of nociception, pain, and pain therapy: Facts and hypotheses. *In* Bonica, J.J., Liebeskind, J.C., and Albe–Fessard, D.G. (eds.): Advances in Pain Research and Therapy. vol. 3. p. 3. New York, Raven, 1979.

162. Zorub, D.S., Nashold, B.S., Jr., and Cook, W.A., Jr.: Avulsion of the brachial plexus: I. A review with implications on the therapy of intractable pain. Surg.Neurol. *2*:347, 1974.

31 NEURAL BLOCKADE IN THE MULTIDISCIPLINARY PAIN CLINIC

JOHN J. BONICA

For three-quarters of a century, neural blockade was used widely for the relief of acute and chronic pain syndromes. Its widespread use was related to the preeminent concepts of pain during the same period. An equally important fact was that besides systemic analgesics, neural blockade represented the only nonsurgical treatment modality for pain control. Before, during, and after World War II this trend was further engendered by the development of nerve block clinics in many parts of Australia, the United States, Britain, and continental Europe.

In recent years a marked increase in pain research has resulted in a great deal of new information on the physiologic, biochemical, and psychological substrates of acute pain, and the findings from research in behavioral sciences have added new dimensions to our view of chronic pain. These advances have markedly enhanced our knowledge of sensory coding and sensory modulation and have effected a significant change in our conceptualization of clinical pain and pain therapy, particularly with regard to chronic pain syndromes. For one thing, these advances have encouraged many physicians and other health professionals to become involved in managing patients with chronic pain within the context of multidisciplinary/interdisciplinary pain clinics/centers. For another, it has changed significantly the role of neural blockade in managing these patients. Indeed, some authorities[11,12] state that neural blockade currently has little or no role in managing patients with chronic pain. On the other end of the spectrum there are those who, because of their extensive experience with these techniques, firmly believe that neural blockade can be used to advantage, particularly within the setting of the multidisciplinary/interdisciplinary pain center.

In this chapter these issues are discussed in some detail. The material is presented in five parts: [1] the evolution of pain concepts and the use of neural blockade; [2] the organization of multidisciplinary pain clinics/centers; [3] basic principles for the use of neural blockade within the context of the multidisciplinary pain clinic; [4] a brief overview of pain clinics in various parts of the world; and [5] conclusions regarding the future use of neural blockade for pain control. Because of space limitations, only the most important "key" references containing extensive bibliographies are cited. A comprehensive review of the history of pain concepts can be found elsewhere.[8,9]

EVOLUTION OF PAIN CONCEPTS/ NEURAL BLOCKADE

Pain has always been a major concern of humankind and a subject of ubiquitous efforts to understand and control it. Ancient Egyptians, Babylonians, Chinese, and Hindus all recorded detailed descriptions of the concept of pain, its causes, and its treatment. Among these ancients it was widely believed that the heart and the blood vessels, not the brain, were responsible for pain (see Refs. 8 and 9). Among the ancient Greek thinkers and philosophers, Alcmaeon, without apparent precedent, produced the idea that the brain, not the heart, was the center of sensation and reason. Despite the support of Democritus, Plato, and others, this view did not gain widespread acceptance, in part because of the opposition of Empedocles and, above all, Aristotle, for whom the heart constituted the *sensorium commune.* Aristotle believed that pain resulted when an excess of vital heat caused an increase in the sensitivity of touch which arose from the flesh and was conveyed by the blood to the heart where it was experienced as pain. Like most other Greek philosophers, Aristotle believed that the pain experience was a negative passion, a quality of the soul and a state of feeling opposite to pleasure. Despite the repeated attempts by many anatomists and physiologists who followed, including Galen, Vaselius, da Vinci, and Descartes, to prove that pain was a sensation felt in the brain, the Aristotlean concept prevailed for two millenia.

EVOLUTION OF PAIN THEORIES AND THERAPIES

The scientific study of sensation in general and pain in particular in the modern sense really began in the first half of the 19th century when physiology emerged as an experimental science. This era was initiated in part by the publications of Bell and Magendie, who demonstrated with animal experiments that the function of the dorsal roots of the spinal nerves is sensory and that of the ventral roots is motor. The impetus to the scientific study of pain was further enhanced by Muller's proposal of "The Doctrine of Specific Nerve Energies"; published in 1840. This proposal stated that the brain received information about the external objects and body structures only by way of sensory nerves and that sensory nerves for each of the five senses carried a particular form of energy specific for each sensation. Muller's concept, then, was that of a straight-through system from the sensory organ to the brain center responsible for the sensation (Table 31-1) (see Ref. 8).

During the ensuing half a century numerous anatomic, physiologic, and histologic studies were done that prompted the formulation of two physiologic theories of pain: the specificity theory and the intensive theory. *The specificity theory* stated that pain was a specific sensation with its own apparatus, independent of touch and other senses. This theory, which had been suggested earlier by Avicenna and later by Descartes, was definitely formulated by Schiff in 1858 after his analgesic experiments in animals revealed that pain could be eliminated by section of the gray matter (see Ref. 8). This theory was supported by experiments carried out by many others but particularly by von Frey.[38] *The intensive theory,* first anticipated by Erasmus Darwin in 1790 and subsequently supported by Henle and Weber in the 1840s, was definitely formulated by Goldscheider,[20] who in 1894 stated that stimulus intensity of any sensation and central summation were the critical determinants of pain (Table 31-1).

Thus, by the end of the 19th century there existed three conflicting concepts on the nature of pain. The specificity theory and the intensive theory, which were in opposition to each other, were embraced by physiologists and a few psychologists. These two were opposed to the traditional Aristotlean concept that pain was an affective quality. During the first five decades of the present century, research on pain continued, and the published data acquired were used to support either the specificity theory or the intensive theory, or a modification of these. By mid-century, however, the theory of philosophers had been discarded and the specificity theory had prevailed and became taught universally.

TABLE 31-1. EVOLUTION OF PAIN CONCEPTS: EARLY HISTORY

320 B.C. Aristotle	Increased body heat in "flesh" conveyed by blood to heart (*sensorium commune*)
	Opposed unsuccessfully by Galen, Vaselius, da Vinci, Descartes—all favored brain as center where pain was felt
1810-20 Bell and Magendie	Dorsal roots sensory Ventral roots motor
1840 Muller	"Doctrine of specific nerve energies."
	Pain (and other senses) each had a specific *form of energy* carried from sensory organ to brain
1858 Schiff	"Specificity theory"—specific pain pathway to brain ("Private Line" Telephone Cable System)
1894 Von Frey	Specific pain receptors connected to pathways
1840 Henle and Weber	"Intensive theory" (originated by Erasmus Darwin in 1790)
1894 Goldscheider	Stimulus *intensity* and central summation are critical determinants of pain.

In the latter part of the 19th century the emerging preeminence of the concept of pain specificity provoked the development of two major methods of pain relief: neurosurgical operations and nerve blocking. Among the former procedures was the development of neurotomy, spinal rhizotomy, gasserian ganglionectomy, thoracic sympathectomy, and spinal cordotomy. These and other procedures subsequently developed and applied were based on the assumption that surgical interruption of pain pathways would produce permanent pain relief — a concept that prevailed and was widely applied until recent years (Table 31-2).

The concept of pain specificity also encouraged the use of nerve blocks for pain therapy. During the 1860s and 1870s numerous attempts were made to inject morphine, chloroform, osmic acid, and other agents near nerves to treat neuralgia. These efforts failed because these agents lacked specific local anesthetic action. The tongue numbing effects of cocaine observed by pharmacologists led Collins, Fauvel, Saglia, and others in France to apply the extract of cocaine leaves topically to the pharynx and larynx to control severe pain of tuberculosis and cancer (see ref. 20). This occurred 9 years before the demonstration of the efficacy of cocaine as a local anesthetic by Carl Koller in 1884. Promptly thereafter, Corning and others began to use cocaine to treat various pain problems in neurolgic disorders. Since the history of local and regional anesthesia is described in detail in Chapter 1, only a few comments relevant to their use for relief of nonsurgical pain will be made.

The first three decades of the 20th century can be considered the "golden age" of neural blockade because in this period, new and safer local anesthetics were developed, most of the techniques of regional anesthesia in current use were either developed or refined, and there appeared an unparalleled effort to apply all of these techniques for the control of nonsurgical pain and other medical disorders. One of the most brilliant chapters in the history of neural blockade was the application of paravertebral somatic and paravertebral sympathetic blocks in pain research and therapy. They were first used as research tools to confirm, in humans, the earlier findings from animal experiments of the specific spinal segments that provide sensory nerves, including those conveying pain to various viscera and somatic structures. Subsequently, paravertebral block was used widely as a diagnostic procedure and still later as a therapeutic measure to treat angina pectoris and various painful visceral diseases. The efficacy of these procedures led to the use of alcohol to produce a lasting interruption of sensory nerves to viscera and into the subarachnoid space to achieve chemical spinal rhizotomy for the treatment of cancer pain and other chronic painful conditions.

With few exceptions, all the contributions on the use of neural blockade for the diagnosis and therapy of nonsurgical pain made before World War II were achieved by surgeons, internists, and other physicians who were not anesthesiologists. The few exceptions were Woodbridge,[39] Ruth,[34] and Rovenstine and Wertheim,[32] who during this period wrote classic

TABLE 31-2. EVOLUTION OF PAIN CONCEPTS: RECENT HISTORY

1860s — ?1950s		Preeminence of "specificity" theory — thus surgical and neurolytic lesions in "Telephone Cable" to relieve pain (see Chap. 1, Tables 1-1 to 1-3)
1930s — 40s	Leriche, Livingstone, Ruth, Rovenstine	World War II, "Nerve Block" Clinics. Wrote of value of diagnostic and therapeutic nerve blocks
1946	Bonica	Concept of Multidisciplinary Pain Management Group
1946	Alexander	Concept of Multidisciplinary Pain Management Group
1953	Bonica	Publication of "Management of Pain" — Use of neural blockade described in broad context of multidisciplinary group
1960	Bonica	Multidisciplinary Pain Clinic (Seattle)
1960	Crue	Multidisciplinary Pain Clinic (California)
1966	Melzack and Wall	"Gate theory of pain." Spinal and central modulation — thus questioning the efficacy of lesions in a "straight through" pain system
1970s — present		Emphasis on multidimensional *sensory and emotional* aspects of pain
1974	Bonica and founding members of IASP	Founding of International Association for the Study of Pain (IASP)
1975	IASP	Publication of journal *Pain* — multidisciplinary basic science and clinical aspects of pain

review articles on the use of diagnostic and therapeutic nerve blocks. These writings encouraged a number of other American anesthesiologists to apply diagnostic and therapeutic blocks to the management of patients with pain. As a result of this trend, and other factors, anesthesiologists took over from internists, surgeons, and other physicians the primary responsibility of administering diagnostic and therapeutic nerve blocks. In the United States this trend was encouraged by some leaders of the then-new discipline of anesthesiology, who saw this as another area that would add breadth and depth to the scope of the new specialty. World War II gave a great impetus to both the development of anesthesiology as an important clinical discipline and the use of nerve blocks in the management of pain. Consequently, during and immediately after the war, many "nerve block clinics" for pain diagnosis, prognosis, and therapy within anesthesiology departments sprang up in the United States.

EVOLUTION OF PAIN CLINICS/CENTERS

It was this trend that was responsible for my assignment to the task of treating military personnel with intractable pain at Madigan Army Hospital, Tacoma, Washington, during World War II. The writings of Leriche[23] and Livingston[25] and the aforementioned reviews made surgeons, neurologists, and other physicians aware of the value of diagnostic and therapeutic nerve blocks. Consequently, I was referred many patients with major causalgia and reflex sympathetic dystrophy, painful phantom limb and other postamputation pain syndromes, myofascial pain syndromes, and obscure neurologic and musculoskeletal disorders. Not having had any experience with these procedures during my anesthesia training, I read the aforementioned reviews and all of the many articles cited in each of these.

In applying nerve blocks I noted that while patients with causalgia and other straightforward painful conditions responded to therapy, patients with complex chronic pain problems did not. This prompted me to search the literature to acquire the necessary knowledge about the broad field of pain, especially chronic pain problems. I found that [1] there was little information about the treatment of chronic pain, primarily because little research had been done; [2] other than the books by Leriche[23] and Livingston,[25] the available knowledge was scattered in numerous basic and clinical scientific journals and books, and thus accessible with difficulty to the average physician; and [3] that as a result of these factors, and because of lack of education in medical schools and postgraduate training for specialization, I, like most other clinicians, did not know the basic principles of managing patients with chronic pain.

Despite efforts to consult textbooks on medicine, neurology, and various other disciplines, I continued to experience great frustrations in trying to manage patients with many of the complex pain problems by myself. Consequently, I sought consultation of colleagues in neurology, neurosurgery, orthopedics, psychiatry, and other specialties in the usual manner inherent in traditional medical practice. Thus if I wished to have a patient with a complex pain problem seen in consultation by an orthopedist, neurologist, and psychiatrist, each of these individuals would evaluate the patient in his office or the patient's ward and then report his findings to me by telephone or by writing on the patient's chart, or both. After the patients had been seen by all consultants, I attempted to read the evaluation of each consultant, formulate a correct diagnosis, and develop the best therapy. It soon became apparent to me that these types of consultations in the isolation of each consultant's office were very slow and inefficient; this prompted me to have frequent face-to-face meetings with the various specialists with interest and expertise in dealing with complex problems.

These early experiences convinced me that complex pain problems could be treated more efficiently by a multidisciplinary/interdisciplinary team, each member of which would contribute his specialized knowledge and skills to the common goal of making a correct diagnosis and developing the most effective therapeutic strategy. These early experiences also led to the belief that much more research needed to be done on basic mechanisms of pain and that this similarly required a multidisciplinary/interdisciplinary effort by a team of scientists and clinicians who contributed their individualized expertise and skills to such studies.

By the end of my military duty in late 1946, I had developed deep convictions about the need for [1] widespread application of this multidisciplinary concept; [2] a better classification of pain syndromes; and [3] a textbook on the role and efficacy of diagnostic, prognostic, and therapeutic blocks. Promptly after the war, I put the concept of a multidisciplinary facility for the diagnosis and therapy of complex chronic pain problems into practice in Tacoma General Hospital, Tacoma, Washington. This group consisted of an anesthesiologist, neurosurgeon, orthopedist, psychiatrist, and radiation therapist, all of whom had special interest and some expertise in pain. Despite numerous problems inherent in individual private practice, for 13 years the group was successful in its objectives and goals, a fact that further strengthened my conviction on the value of the multidisciplinary approach. At about the same time F. A. D. Duncan Alexander had independently developed the same concept, and in 1947 he initiated a multidisciplinary pain diagnostic and therapeutic program at the Veterans Administration Hospital in McKinney, Texas.[1,2]

During this early postwar period, a number of other anesthesiologists organized and ran "pain clinics." Although some of these programs also involved other physicians as *ad hoc* consultants, the primary method of diagnosis and therapy consisted of various neural blockade procedures, including programs in the United States continued by Woodbridge,[39] Ruth,[34] Rovenstine and Wertheim,[32] Dittrick,[17] Stubbs,[36] Papper,[30] Ruben,[33] and Moore.[28] In the late 1940s and early 1950s similar facilities were developed by anesthetists in Britain,[22] Canada,[21] Italy,[10,14] Australia,[26] and a number of other European countries. The experience of these individuals as well as my own experience led me to develop basic principles and guidelines for proper application of neural blockade used for diagnostic, prognostic, prophylactic, and therapeutic measures; these will be discussed in a later section of this chapter. This experience led to the deep conviction that, properly applied (expertly done in properly selected patients), neural blockade was a highly valuable method of managing patients with acute and chronic pain and led me to the publication of the *Management of Pain.*[3]

During the early 1950s there were only three multidisciplinary pain facilities in the United States. In addition to the one directed by Alexander and the one in Tacoma, there was one at the University of Oregon, Portland, Oregon, directed by Dr. William K. Livingston, whose clinical research on pain and conceptualization of pain mechanisms made him one of the century's giants in this field. Working in collaboration with Haugen, chairman of anesthesiology, and others, that program not only managed patients with complex problems, but also was the first multidisciplinary pain research program supported by the National Institutes of Health of the United States.

The favorable experience with these programs prompted me, in the early 1950s, to begin espousing the multidisciplinary concept in numerous lectures and published papers, first in various parts of the United States, then, beginning in 1954, in other parts of the world (see Ref. 6). During this period, Alexander also promulgated the multidisciplinary concept, but because of personal illness he discontinued these efforts after the mid-1950s. Promptly after my appointment as chairman of anesthesiology at the University of Washington in 1960, I enlisted the help of Dr. Lowell White, a neurosurgeon, and Dr. D. Crowley, a member of the faculty of the School of Nursing, to develop a multidisciplinary pain clinic at that institution. Over the next few years we were joined by senior faculty of the Departments of Psychiatry, Orthopedics, Rehabilitation Medicine, Clinical Psychology, Oral Surgery, General Surgery, and Radiation Therapy. Despite a number of problems that have been discussed elsewhere,[6] during the ensuing decade the program evolved into a group of some 20 persons from 14 different medical specialists and clinical disciplines who participated in the activities of the program in varying degrees and devoted varying amounts of time and effort. In 1960 Crue[15,16] and associates also initiated a multidisciplinary pain clinic at the City of Hope Medical Center in California.

During the 1960s I continued my campaign to advocate the multidisciplinary pain center concept in various parts of the world. Despite several hundred lectures and the publication of numerous articles, the concept was ignored by the medical profession until the early 1970s, when a number of factors converged to cause others to put the concept into practice. These included the publication of the Melzack–Wall theory of pain[26] and the immense worldwide curiosity about the mechanisms and efficacy of acupuncture as a method of pain therapy and for surgical anesthesia. Another equally important development was the founding of the *International Association for the Study of Pain* in 1974, the publication of its journal *Pain* the following year, and a number of national chapters. These and other factors provoked an impressive surge of interest in research by neuroscientists and behavioral scientists in studying pain mechanisms and in collaborating with clinical investigators and practitioners to study clinical pain syndromes. The new knowledge has made it clear that pain is not a simple sensory phenomenon but the most complex multidimensional human experience that is often caused by a great variety of pathophysiologic, psychologic, and, in some patients, environmental factors. The new knowledge acquired in recent years has also prompted a revision to approaches to diagnosis and therapy of pain and has encouraged the development of an increasing number of multidisciplinary/interdisciplinary pain diagnostic and therapeutic programs in many countries throughout the world (Table 31-2).

These and other factors have caused an increasing number of physicians and other health professionals to become interested and actively involved in managing patients with chronic pain within the framework of pain clinics/centers. Moreover, in the United States and Britain and perhaps other countries there has merged a new breed of practitioners—algologists—as proposed in 1953 by Bonica.* The concept of the science and practice of algology is slowly gaining acceptance in the United States, as witnessed in 1983 by the founding of the American Association of Algology (AAA), whose primary purpose is to encourage the development of the specialty of algology with the long-range aim of applying for recognition as an American Board of Algology. Moreover, the agencies of some state governments have officially recognized the algologist as a physician, particularly qualified to render clinical opinions in cases of pain disabled patients.[12]

Marked increase in the number of pain clinic/centers throughout the world is most gratifying to me but is also a source of concern. The first source of concern by some clinical psychologists and other clinicians working in pain programs is the overemphasis of the operant mechanisms or the behavioral model of chronic pain. This has resulted from the relatively recent involvement of psychologists and some psychiatrists in the study of chronic pain, which has shown that the medical model is not sufficient to explain the normal illness behavior manifested by some patients and requires the inclusion of a behavioral model of pain.[18,35] This emphasis on chronic behavior resulting *primarily* from reinforcing environmental/psychologic influences or so-called operant mechanisms is long overdue and has had a favorable impact on the management of many patients with chronic pain. Because these investigators, particularly in the United States, have studied patients with intractable pain primarily due to behavioral/psychologic/sociologic factors, they have come to believe that in all patients with chronic pain, the pain results from operant mechanisms. Moreover, the numerous publications on this topic have misled American practitioners, who are not well informed on the makeup of the chronic pain population, into believing that such is actually the case. In view of the fact that in the United States only 3% to 4% of patients with pain are seen in pain clinics/centers[37] and since there are some 50 million Americans with pain caused by arthritis or other degenerative diseases, cancer, reflex sympathetic dystrophy, neuralgia, peripheral vascular diseases, and myofascial syndromes who are not seen in such facilities, the obvious conclusion is that patients with chronic pain caused by learning/environmental factors represent a relatively small percentage of the population with chronic pain in the United States.

A second and even more important concern is provoked by some of the facilities being staffed by physicians and other health professionals who have little or no training or experience in managing patients with chronic pain. Some of these are well-intentioned clinicians who have been attracted to the field because currently it is the fashionable "thing" to do or, in other words, pain is the "in thing" of modern medicine. Of even greater concern is that some facilities are being run by unscrupulous physicians and nonphysicians who are using the current surge of interest in pain to exploit patients, as occurred with acupuncture clinics during the height of the public's interest in acupuncture during the early 1970s. These facilities run by dilettantes will surely be detrimental to the general cause of pain research and therapy and to the current international movement in the field, and most importantly will do more harm than good to individual patients.

The recognition of the latter problem prompted Bonica in 1977 to recommend that the IASP encourage national chapters and to develop criteria, guidelines, and mechanisms for evaluating pain clinics/centers on a voluntary basis. Subsequently, the American Pain Society (APS) began to consider such an issue through a committee chaired by G. Aronoff (see Ref. 29). After considerable discussion by the committee and Board of Directors as well as by the membership of the APS, it was decided to approach the Commission on Accreditation of Rehabilitation Facilities (CARF) to undertake such a task. CARF, a nonprofit organization supported by the Joint Commission on Accreditation of Hospitals (JCAH) and a number of other national sponsoring organizations, has been surveying and accrediting rehabilitation facilities since the late 1960s. In 1981 the Board of Directors of CARF accepted the task of setting up criteria and surveying pain clinics/centers in the United States, and in 1982 convened 13 regionally distributed full-time pain center directors to form the National Advisory Committee on Chronic Pain Man-

*Initially Bonica[3] called such a professional a dolorologist, a hybrid word from Latin (dolor = pain) and Greek (logos = study), because at the time the term dolorimeter was widely used. Later Bonica proposed the term algologist as a more correct all-Greek-derived term.

agement Programs. This group developed criteria and guidelines that were subsequently approved by the APS and CARF, and surveying of pain management facilities was begun in July 1983. To date about 49 pain centers/clinics have been certified.*

ORGANIZATION AND FUNCTION OF THE MULTIDISCIPLINARY PAIN CLINIC/CENTER

Before discussing the organization and function of a multidisciplinary/interdisciplinary pain clinic/center, some definitions are in order. Review of the data contained in the *International Directory of Pain Clinic/Centers* published in 1979 by the American Society of Anesthesiologists suggests that there are various types of facilities which can be divided into either centers or clinics.

The term *center* should be used for units that are hospital based, have inpatient and outpatient facilities, have representatives from several disciplines, and have ample equipment to diagnose and treat most pain syndromes.

The term *clinic* should be used for facilities in which patients are managed in outpatient hospital clinics or in a nonhospital setting such as the physician's office. Moreover, each center can be arbitrarily classified according to the goals and objectives, personnel, equipment, and facilities as follows:

1. *Major comprehensive pain center* is a university-based unit, has both inpatient and outpatient facilities and personnel from various medical specialties and several disciplines, has equipment to diagnose and treat patients with various pain syndromes, has graduate and postgraduate teaching programs, and carries out research.
2. *Comprehensive pain center* is a hospital-based facility with the same characteristics of category 1 except it is not involved in teaching or research.
3. *Monodisciplinary pain center* is a facility that is directed and staffed by one or more persons in one discipline, has inpatient and outpatient facilities, has equipment to diagnose and treat a variety of pain syndromes, and has *ad hoc* consultants from other disciplines.
4. *Syndrome-oriented pain center* is a facility that has the characteristics of either category 1 or 2, but its diagnostic and therapeutic facilities and its teaching and research are oriented toward a specific pain syndrome such as headache center, low back pain center, orofacial pain center, and so forth.
5. *Modality-oriented pain program* is a facility with personnel from one or more disciplines and facilities that are focused primarily on the use of a specific modality, although other therapy may be used as an adjunct, such as the operant program for chronic pain, psychiatric pain program, rehabilitation pain programs, and neurosurgical pain program.

*The criteria for inpatient and outpatient programs may be obtained from CARF, 2500 North Pantano Road, Tucson, AZ 85715 USA.

Pain clinics can be categorized in a similar fashion, that is, major comprehensive (multidisciplinary/interdisciplinary) pain clinic, comprehensive pain clinic, monodisciplinary pain clinic, syndrome-oriented pain clinic, and modality-oriented pain clinic.

The characteristics of an "ideal" pain center/clinic depend on the environment and the personnel and resources available. In a university medical center, a facility should have the characteristics of a major comprehensive multidisciplinary/interdisciplinary pain center with a balanced program of patient care, education, training, and research. In a large nonuniversity medical center, it can be a multidisciplinary/interdisciplinary pain program with an appropriate number of medical specialists and health professionals from several disciplines capable of diagnosing and treating most of the important chronic pain syndromes. In smaller hospitals, a smaller facility that can manage the more common and simpler pain problems would be sufficient. Regardless of the size and scope of the facility, it is essential that it have sufficient personnel and ample physical facilities, equipment, and financial resources.

MAJOR COMPREHENSIVE MULTIDISCIPLINARY PAIN CENTER

To summarize the organization and function of the major comprehensive multidisciplinary pain center/clinic, I present the following description based on personal experience during the past four decades and especially that acquired at the University of Washington pain program. During the first decade, the collective efforts of this group were devoted primarily to patient care and education, with a modest amount of research being done by some members of the group who had individual projects. In 1970 we began to recruit basic scientists who would devote full-time to research. During the ensuing decade there evolved a progressively larger pain research program with about a dozen basic scientists and clinical scientists who had grants for individual and collaborative projects and "center grants" awarded by the National Institutes of Health of the United States. (A center grant is a large grant awarded to develop a research center.) As a result of the growth of the programs in patient care, education, and research, the program was designated by the Board of Regents of the University of Washington in 1980 as the U. W. Pain Center. Subsequently, the behavioral medicine division under the leadership of W. Fordyce of the Department of Rehabilitation Medicine, which existed parallel to the Pain Clinic, was made part of the Center.

Objectives and Missions

The primary objective of a major comprehensive pain center is to develop and maintain well-integrated, coordinated, and balanced multidisciplinary/interdisciplinary programs in patient care, education, training, and research. The specific mission should be as follows:

1. Provide high-quality care to patients with certain acute painful conditions and those with complex chronic pain syndromes.
2. Contribute to the education in algology of graduate and postgraduate students of medicine, dentistry, and other health professions.
3. Educate and train clinical algologists to pursue a career in pain management.
4. Enhance the transmission of new knowledge about the diagnosis and therapy of pain to all practitioners of the health professions.
5. Educate and train biomedical scientists who pursue a career of pain research.
6. Carry out studies on various aspects of acute and chronic pain through individual research projects, program projects, and demonstration projects.
7. Develop research teams composed of a critical mass of scientists and clinical algologists from the appropriate disciplines to study some of the most important clinical pain syndromes, to evaluate current therapeutic modalities, and to develop new and better modalities for the diagnosis and treatment of such syndromes.

The ultimate goal of these efforts should be to contribute to the improvement of the quality of life for millions of persons worldwide who currently suffer needlessly from acute and chronic pain.

To achieve these objectives, the U. W. Pain Center has been organized into two sections: a Clinical Pain Service (CPS) and a Pain Research Center (PRC). Currently the center includes a staff of about 40 basic and clinical scientists, physicians, and other health professionals from the following medical specialties and basic science disciplines (in alphabetic order): anatomy, anesthesiology, general dentistry, histology and morphology, neurosurgery, neurophysiology, nursing, oral medicine, maxillofacial surgery, orthodontics, orthopedics, clinical and experimental pharmacology, psychiatry and behavioral sciences, clinical and experimental psychology, rehabilitation medicine, sociology, social work, occupational therapy, physical therapy, and vocational counselors. Although some basic scientists have activities limited to research and teaching, most of the personnel are involved in all three aspects of academic pursuits of the center: research, education and training, and patient care. Their efforts are supported by about 30 technical and clinical personnel and administrative secretarial staff.

The key to such complex multidisciplinary efforts is an effective organization of personnel and ample physical facilities, equipment, and financial resources. One of the most important, and indeed essential, factors is to have a director who has the capabilities and time to provide vigorous medical, scientific, and administrative leadership to the group. Since the team comprises individuals who have appointments (and consequently allegiance) to their parent departments, it is essential that the director possess those qualities necessary to bring a heterogeneous group together and have it function as a single, efficient unit. The director is assisted by one or more associate directors. The organization of the U. W. Center is shown in Figure 31-1.

I shall now discuss the programs in patient care, education, training, and research.

CLINICAL PAIN SERVICE

The Clinical Pain Service (CPS) has outpatient and inpatient facilities for the diagnosis and treatment of complex pain problems and to carry out effective teaching and training programs for students of medicine, dentistry, and other health professions, physicians in specialty training, algology fellows, and practicing health professionals. This part of the

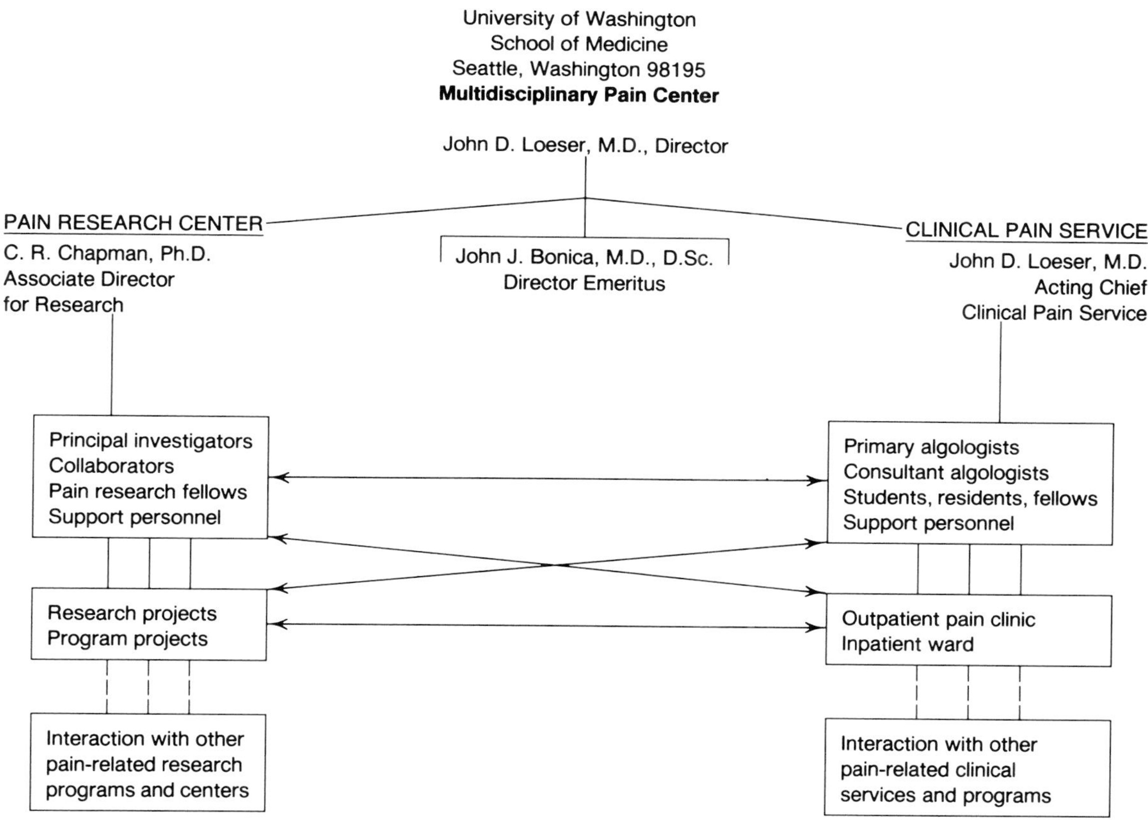

FIG. 31-1. Organization of the University of Washington Pain Center.

center is directed by the chief of the CPS who normally is an associate director of the center. The assistant director for inpatient services coordinates the day-to-day activity of the pain ward. The Chief of CPS has the responsibility of providing leadership in patient care, education, and training and for the overall administration and coordination of the service.

OTHER PERSONNEL

Patient Care Coordinator. The chief of the Service is assisted by a Patient Care Coordinator who is responsible for the initial review of referral letters, for making telephone contact with the referring physician, patient, and sponsoring agency coordinating and processing all inpatient and outpatient admissions and patient consultations, and for carrying out numerous other activities essential for the efficient function of the clinical facilities, including scheduling of case presentations at the conference.

Attending Physician/Psychologist. The other clinicians actively involved in patient care act either as the patient's attending physician/attending psychologist or as consultants. Each patient admitted to the Pain Service is assigned an attending physician who is an algologist and who has the responsibility for the initial work-up of the patient, including a detailed history and complete physical examination. The attending psychologist's task is to ascertain the role of affective and environmental factors in the genesis of the patient's pain, behavior, and disability. The physician and psychologist jointly determine the subsequent schedule of the patient's workup. Both of these individuals also act as liaison among the patient, his/her personal physician, and the rest of the Clinical Pain Service group, and also have the responsibility for writing progress reports and following up patients after discharge.

Professional Staff. The professional staff of the U.W. CPS includes medical specialists as follows: six from anesthesiology, one from Rehabilitation Medicine, two from Neurologic Surgery, one from Internal Medicine, and four clinical psychologists. In addition there are two physical therapists, two occupational therapists, three social workers/vocational counselors, and a total of six rotating nurses (three on duty at one time). To be a member of the CPS, each physician/health professional must have fulfilled the following requisites: [a] must have special interest in, and ample knowledge of, pain syndromes and the various therapeutic modalities currently available; [b] must possess specialized diagnostic or therapeutic skills, or both, in a particular field to contribute effectively to the care of patients and to the training of other health professionals; [c] must be willing and *able* to devote sufficient time and effort to the work of the group; and [d] most importantly, must have personal characteristics to be a member of the team and adhere to the five cardinal C's: *collaboration, coordination, cooperation, communication,* and *courtesy.* It deserves emphasis that each member of the team be *treated as an equal,* regardless of the professional title he/she has. Moreover, stability of the team members is an essential characteristic of a successful clinical pain service.

Trainees. Resident physicians (registrars) who rotate through the Pain Service, special Fellows in pain, and other health professionals assigned to the Service as part of their training constitute an important cadre of personnel who help with the workup and day-to-day care of these patients. The teaching program for these individuals is briefly described at the end of this section.

Secretary/Other Staff. The Pain Group must have ample secretarial support. Because of the secretary's interface with the public and the responsibilities of sharing details of clinic visits and admissions, the secretaries are among the most critical members of the group. Apart from typing correspondence and taking care of medical records and referrals, they must be available during regular office hours to handle phone calls and inquiries from physicians. Obviously, they also play an important role in maintaining optimal rapport among the Pain Group, the patient's physician, the family, and the public at large.

SPACE AND FACILITIES

To function optimally, the Multidisciplinary Pain Center requires space and equipment of several types: [a] space in the outpatient clinic; [b] inpatient hospital beds; [c] specialized space and equipment to meet the peculiar needs of a team actively engaged in patient care and teaching; and [d] facilities to carry out an active research program consisting of individual or collaborative projects, or both. The clinical facilities of our Clinical Pain Service include ample space in the outpatient clinic and ten inpatient hospital beds in a single ward.

Outpatient Clinic. The outpatient clinic facilities include [a] a comfortable waiting room; [b] four semiprivate carrels for the use of patients filling out the Minnesota Multiphasic Personality Inventory (MMPI) and other pain questionnaires; [c] five examining rooms equipped for general physical, neurologic, and orthopedic examinations; [d] a large room used to carry out nerve blocks and other nonsurgical procedures for diagnosis and therapy; [e] a recovery room (shared with Ambulatory Surgery) to monitor patients who have received nonsurgical diagnostic and therapeutic procedures; [f] three office rooms; [g] a conference room; and [h] a dictating room. The group also uses a common conference room that accommodates as many as 30 people to hold major conferences/lectures/seminars. The ten-bed inpatient ward is staffed by three nurses who rotate through the Pain Service for a 6-week period and an Assistant Head Nurse who concentrates exclusively on the patients in CPS.

Nerve Block Room. The nerve block room should include nerve block trays, resuscitative equipment, fluids, and drugs to promptly and effectively treat systemic reactions to local anesthetics or other possible complications. It should also include a regular operating table that allows for prompt change in position; an efficient operating room light; equipment to carry out various diagnostic and therapeutic nerve blocks; and complete facilities to permit prompt cardiovascular resuscitation in the event of toxic reaction. In addition, such a room usually has special equipment to measure sympathetic function, including sudomotor and vasomotor activity, and to carry out neurologic examinations before and after the block. Enough space must be provided for storing the necessary equipment and drugs and for moving the patient in and out of the room on a stretcher; also essential are sufficient space and electrical outlets for use of portable x-ray equipment, as well as x-ray viewing box. A portable x-ray machine, or preferably a C arm with image intensifier, is readily available but is stored in another space. The nurse(s) staffing the clinic should be permanent; she (they) must be thoroughly conversant with the procedures, methods, and equipment and with the care and positioning of the patients.

Inpatient Facilities. The U. W. CPS consists of ten beds in one ward, which is staffed with nurses who have special interest and knowledge of pain and which is under the direction and coordination of an assistant head nurse who concentrates exclusively on the pain service. Although familiar with all of the patients, each nurse selects three or four patients to follow through the specifics of their treatment program, from admission to discharge, and is called a "primary nurse." The primary nurse assures that the consults and diagnostic tests are done as prescribed and the rest of the program is optimized for each patient. Moreover, he/she presents his/her patient at weekly chart rounds and at nurse team conferences.

PATIENT CARE

The Multidisciplinary Pain Center of the University of Washington accepts only patients referred by physicians and other health professionals. The sources of referrals include [a] inpatients of the University Hospital system being cared for by faculty of other departments; and [b] patients referred by outside physicians from the community, Northwest region, and other parts of the United States and foreign countries.

Procedure for Admission of Patients

The first contact for referral of a patient will be either by letter sent by referring physician or a telephone call. One of our Pain Center physicians reviews each referral letter or speaks by telephone to the referring physician to ascertain the nature of the patient's problem and the type of assessment required. One of the six options is then elected: [1] The patient has a complex pain problem requiring multidisciplinary evaluation, and we label such a patient a "screener"; [2] the patient has a straightforward pain problem that one of our physicians or psychologists manages initially, and we label such a patient "a consultation"; [3] the patient has a severe chronic pain problem that represents an emergency, such as cancer or reflex sympathetic dystrophies, and requires direct admission to our inpatient service for both assessment and pain control; [4] further information is required before a decision can be made by our staff as to suitability of the patient for our Center, and this is requested of physicians or hospitals involved in prior management of the patient; [5] the patient clearly has unresolved medical issues that must be addressed before referral to our CPS, in which case we assist the referring physician to place the patient in the most appropriate treatment facility but continue to follow the patient in case our services may subsequently be required; [6] the patient is not suitable for further assessment or treatment at our facility, and we label such a patient a "reject." Included in the latter categories are patients who are "street addicts"; whereas we accept patients for detoxification of drugs prescribed by physicians, we reject the street addict because experience suggests that they resume drug abuse promptly after discharge. We also reject patients who have failed to benefit from other highly regarded pain treatment facilities, unless there has been a significant change in the patient's condition.

Once the decision has been made to accept the patient, the referring physician and the patient are notified and both are asked for additional information: The referring physician is requested to transmit all of the relevant records, x-ray, and laboratory findings, whereas the patient is asked to give the names and addresses of other physicians/health professionals who have treated the patient. Every effort is made by the staff to assemble the most complete documentation available. In addition the patient is sent [a] a *Pain Center brochure* that provides information about the procedures for admission and the comprehensive workup of the patient and emphasizes the importance of having the spouse accompany the patient during the initial visit and the probability of the patient's seeing several different specialists during the workup; [b] *daily diary forms* that the patient is requested to complete to maintain an accurate diary that records at hourly intervals during the day the frequency and intensity of the pain, the amount of medication taken, and the amount of time the patient spends lying down, walking, standing, and in social activities. Fourteen copies of the form are sent to keep a diary for each day of the 2-week period; [c] a questionnaire that the patient is expected to complete to provide the staff with demographic data and information on the history of the pain problem. The cover letter reemphasizes the importance of having the spouse accompany the patient and of completing the forms before the patient is admitted. Long experience has confirmed our deep conviction that evaluation of a patient's chronic pain requires assessment of the family/home situation and the information about the patient that only another person can provide.

Screening Evaluation

The screening evaluation occupies an entire morning for the patient and the spouse or significant other. The patient is seen usually by a physician in training or Pain Fellow and the person who will be the attending physician, and a complete history is elicited and comprehensive physical examination carried out. As previously mentioned, the patient and the patient's family member are interviewed separately by the psychologist. Following this the patient completes the Minnesota Multiphasic Personality Inventory (MMPI) and several other brief tests. Members of the CPS also use the McGill Pain Questionnaire as part of the diagnostic array, as well as a pain drawing and structured questionnaires to collect additional information. Once these have been completed, the physician and psychologist meet to review prior records, the diary and test data, and their own individual findings. These data allow the two individuals attending the patient to agree on assessment and the plans for either further diagnostic workup consultations or a treatment program. Usually two patients undergo a screening evaluation each working day.

A management conference is held following completion of the workup of the two patients and the interviews of the patient and spouse by the psychologist. About 30 to 45 minutes are devoted to review of the findings of each of the two patients. The physician, resident, or algology fellow presents the medical history and physical findings, and the psychologist or psychology trainee presents the psychologic and social history and MMPI interpretation. Other members of the CPS who have seen the patient make additional comments, whereas members who have not seen the patient are given an opportunity to ask questions and make comments. Often discussions are vigorous and continue until there is a consensus about the diagnosis and the therapeutic strategy. The patient and his significant other then go into the room for a feedback conference and are given an opportunity to ask questions. The process of evaluating the patient and meeting with the patient and significant other is very costly in terms of time and effort by CPS staff, but it seems necessary in order to come to the consensus for a correct diagnosis and the most appropriate therapeutic strategy.

In some patients, the screening evaluation does not provide sufficient information to make a diagnosis and to establish the appropriate treatment. The patient is then asked to undergo the appropriate additional diagnostic tests and is brought back for another conference after the necessary information becomes available. If the patient has litigation pending that is relevant to the pain problem, the staff asks the patient's permission to contact his attorney before embarking on a treatment program.

Long experience confirms our deep conviction that this face-to-face group discussion is much more effective and productive in making a correct diagnosis and formulating the appropriate therapeutic strategy than is communication by letter or telephone or through fragmented, independent efforts inherent in traditional medical practice. In addition to providing highly specialized consultant service to the referring physician and to the patient, these conferences serve as an excellent forum for the exchange of ideas and information and thus constitute a highly effective teaching mechanism.

TEACHING

The CPS carries teaching programs for medical students, residents (registrars) from the various medical specialties and disciplines with interest in pain, algology fellows, and practicing physicians who have special interest in pain.

Medical Students. The medical student teaching program includes a preceptorship for the first- and second-year students that gives them the opportunity to observe the patient care activities; a 4-week clerkship for fourth-year students who have completed their basic clerkships; and a variety of programs for students who work with the Pain Center faculty on research projects in the medical sciences. In addition, the faculty of the Pain Center participates in conjoint lectures related to the anatomic, physiologic, and psychologic substrates of nociception and pain.

Residents (Registrars). In the past, residents from the Departments of Anesthesiology and Rehabilitation Medicine, have regularly rotated through our service, as have, on occasion, residents from the Departments of Neurosurgery, Psychiatry, Medicine, and Orthopedics. The anesthesiology residents usually rotate for a 2-month period, and most of those who have rotated through the CPS have rated their experience among the best in the residency training program.

Psychology Intern. The University of Washington sponsors a psychology internship program that allows its trainees to elect a rotation on the pain service for a period of 4 months. In addition, psychology fellows from the geriatric training program spend 3 to 6 months in rotation. Special fellowships for psychologists funded by external sources have also been established at times.

Algology Fellows. The center has two algology fellowships of one-year's duration. During this time the physicians work in the capacity of house officers or junior instructors, depending on their qualification. In addition to the CPS preceptor basis, they receive formal courses and training by members of the CPS staff and are expected to carry out some of the pain-related research.

As previously mentioned, the algology fellows, psychology fellows, interns, and the residents who rotate through the service contribute significantly to the care of patients managed in both the inpatient and the outpatient service.

Short-term Visitors. During the past several years, an annual average of 20 to 25 health care providers have attended our pain service for periods ranging from a few days to a week. During this period they are given a formal presentation that describes the activities of the pain service as well as the Pain Center as a whole, and they are permitted to observe the management of patients who have a variety of chronic pain problems.

Long-term Visitors. Each year an average of seven to ten physicians visit the CPS for periods of 1 to 3 months. Most of these individuals are from countries in Western Europe, Latin America, and Asia. Some of these are not qualified to practice medicine in the state of Washington, so they spend their time observing, attending all of the conferences in the Pain Center, and are given advice as to sources of information about various aspects of pain. These long-term visitors who possess the appropriate licensure are treated as algology fellows. Although these long-term visitors make significant demands on the resources of the center, they represent a very worthwhile expenditure of the energies of the Pain Center staff.

RESEARCH

The research program and the U. W. Pain Research Center (PRC) have expanded impressively during the past decade or so. Despite continuing financial constraints on the budget of the National Institutes of Health and other federal agencies, the U. W. PRC has had impressive growth in support of its research programs. For example in the year 1985 – 1986, the total budget for research was $1.8 million. In recent years about 25% of the total research budget has come from sources other than the NIH. Growing reliance on nonfederal sources has provided the center with both flexibility and increased capability to endure the uncertainties and irregularities of federal spending for research. The research capability of PRC has grown in several ways: [1] There has been innovation on several hitherto neglected clinical areas related to acute pain; [2] efforts to foster research of medical school investigators have begun to reach fruition; and [3] the School of Dentistry has received unprecedented support for pain research. Moreover, three collaborative program projects have resulted in impressive interaction among the faculties of the School of Medicine, Dentistry, Nursing and Public Health, as well as those faculties at Harborview Medical Center on the Burn Trauma Unit and at the Fred Hutchinson Cancer Research Center. Although in the past the primary focus of pain research has been on *chronic pain,* in recent years *acute pain* has emerged as a major theme. In 1986 a satellite pain research program was initiated as a joint effort of the U. W. PRC and the Fred Hutchinson Cancer Research Center. This program, which addresses problems of pain associated with cancer treatment, has a 4-year research budget of $3.65 million. The U. W. PRC program involves 21 principal investigators who direct 30 individual projects. The satellite research program involves 3 principal investigators, 22 investigators, and 17 staff.

RESEARCH TRAINING

The PRC provides laboratory or clinical research training at the postdoctoral level for Ph.D. scientists and clinicians, physicians, dentists, and other health science professionals who have a long-range interest and commitment to the field of pain research. This effort is supported primarily by a research training grant awarded to the Pain Center. Since this program was initiated, eight research trainees have completed 1 to 3 years of training. Although most of these trainees have returned to their home universities, three have accepted faculty posts at the University of Washington and continue to remain as members of the PRC. Two Austrian psychologists have finished a 2-year research training fellowship that was sponsored by the NIH and Fogarty Center. In addition, foreign trainees from Japan, Australia, Germany, Brazil, and Italy have had research training with PRC investigators. The PRC has also a successful predoctorate training program that has accommodated a number of individuals who have obtained their Ph.D. degrees in the center.

PRINCIPLES OF USE OF NEURAL BLOCKADE IN PAIN CLINIC

Earlier in this chapter I emphasized that recently acquired scientific knowledge and the development of other therapeutic modalities have greatly altered the role of neural blockade in the management of pain. Thus the new knowledge about the deleterious effects of prolonged deafferentation suggests that neurolytic blocks (as well as ablative neurosurgery) not be used in patients with noncancer chronic pain who have a long life expectancy. The advent of intraspinal narcotics has markedly decreased the use of neural blockade with local anesthetics for the treatment of acute postoperative pain and post-traumatic pain, as well as in the management of patients with cancer pain. (In this regard I wish to mention that I consider intraspinal narcotics as a form of regional analgesia.) New knowledge on the preeminent role of psychological/environmental/sociologic factors in causing chronic pain in some patients (the so-called "chronic pain syndrome"), according to many behaviorists, contraindicates nerve blocking because this procedure may reinforce the conviction of a patient that he is ill, thereby fostering chronic illness behavior and consequent dependency and passivity. This has been emphasized by Brena.[10,11] As a result of his own clinical studies and experience, he has recently changed his views and has stated that most nerve blocks are obsolete as diagnostic or prognostic procedures and have little role in most patients with chronic pain. Similar opinions have been expressed by Fordyce[18] and other behaviorists, particularly those working in multidisciplinary/interdisciplinary pain clinics in the United States. As previously mentioned, this view results from the skewed perspective of those who have seen only patients with chronic pain due to operant mechanisms. This view is *not* shared by some psychiatrists and behavioral scientists and certainly not shared by many clinicians who have had a broad experience of patients with chronic pain associated with various pathologic and degenerative disorders.

Many algologists outside the United States, especially most of those working in Britain, Australia, Japan, and continental Europe, consider neural blockade as a therapeutic modality of major importance. Indeed, these procedures also constitute an important tool for physicians working in small or moderately sized pain clinics to which are referred patients with chronic pain that is amenable to this modality and that never reach the large multidisciplinary/interdisciplinary pain centers. Moreover, Brena[11] emphasizes an important point that may not be acceptable to the pure behaviorist: Sympathetic blockade, trigger point injection, and a number of other procedures are useful when they are part of the multimodal behavioral/rehabilitative programs. Brena and his colleagues have published several reports of studies that demonstrated the value of sympathetic blockade in patients with low back pain (see Refs. 11, 12).

From my own perspective that has evolved over more than four decades, I believe that while neural blockade no longer has the preeminent role of two decades ago, properly applied it remains a very useful tool to members of a multidisciplinary/interdisciplinary pain management program. Proper application requires skillful execution of the procedure and careful selection of patients taking into consideration the bases for the use of this modality and strict adherence of certain basic principles (Table 31-3).

TABLE 31-3. RATIONALE OF USE OF NEURAL BLOCKADE

- Neurolytic blocks not used if long life expectancy
- Neural blockade *one* tool in multidisciplinary pain clinic
- Interruption of nociception at or near its source
- Interruption of abnormal reflex mechanisms (*e.g.*, reflex muscle spasm)
- Sympathetic blockade to eliminate sympathetic hyperactivity contributing to pathophysiology of pain
- Sympathetic blockade to improve blood flow
- ? "Differential" block of sympathetic and visceral nociceptive fibers for pain diagnosis (see also Chaps. 4, 27, 28)
- Attention to a physical aspect of pain may gain patient cooperation in addressing psychological issues
- Neural blockade may enhance patient–doctor relationship and may be used in rehabilitation strategy

BASES FOR USE OF NEURAL BLOCKADE

The primary reason for the effectiveness and usefulness of neural blockade in patients with acute or chronic pain is the interruption of nociceptive input at its source or by blocking nociceptive fibers coursing in peripheral nerves. Blockade also interrupts the afferent limb of abnormal reflex mechanisms that may contribute to the pathogenesis of some chronic pain syndromes. Moreover, sympathetic blockade may be used to eliminate sympathetic hyperactivity that often contributes to the pathophysiology of postoperative and post-traumatic pain and plays an important role in chronic pain syndromes. In addition, through changes in peripheral blood flow, sympathetic blocks may decrease tissue damage and reestablish tissue homeostasis. By using low concentrations of the local anesthetic, blockade of the unmyelinated C and B preganglionic fibers and of the small myelinated A delta nociceptive fibers is achieved, with only minimal effect on somatic motor function. On the other hand, in certain conditions it may be useful to block somatomotor nerves to relieve severe skeletal muscle spasm.

By producing one or more of these effects, there is often prompt relief of pain that may last for varying periods of time depending on the characteristic of the local anesthetic used. Moreover, in certain conditions, the pain relief outlasts by hours and sometimes days and weeks the transient pharmacologic action of the local anesthetic. Melzack[27] has suggested that the block of sensory input for several hours stops the self-sustaining activity of the neuron pools in the neuraxis that may be responsible for some chronic pain states. Based on the concept of "hyperstimulation analgesia" first described by Fox and Melzack,[19] Brena[11] and Parris[31] suggest that neural blockade may alter or "jam" a pattern of central neural activities.

There are two other points with which Brena[11] and others[31] agree regarding the role of neural blockade in patients with multiple physical and emotional impairments: [a] because such patients usually have difficulty in accepting the idea that their discomfort is related to psychological/emotional factors, targeting of a medical intervention at the pain location may facilitate the patient's willingness to undertake psychophysiologic rehabilitation; and [b] when structured as part of the behavioral modification program, nerve blocking enhances the patient–physician relationship and strengthens the physician's role as an educator who reinforces the global roles of rehabilitation (Table 31-3).

INDICATIONS FOR CLINICAL APPLICATION

Neural blockade may be used as a diagnostic, prognostic, prophylactic, or therapeutic tool (see also Chaps. 27–29 and Table 31-4).[3]

Diagnostic Blocks. Certain nerve blocks are useful in ascertaining specific nociceptive pathways, differentiating referred from local pain, and determining the possible mechanisms of chronic pain states. Nerve block is also useful in the differential diagnosis of the site and cause of the pain and in determining the reaction if the pain is eliminated. Block of the appropriate nerves helps differentiate trigeminal neuralgia from atypical facial neuralgia, neuralgia involving the third division of trigeminal nerve from glossopharyngeal or vagal neuralgia; and pain due to visceral disease from pain of somatic origin. For example, complete relief of chest or epigastric pain following intercostal nerve block at the midaxillary line suggests that the pain is of somatic origin in the chest or abdominal wall, whereas lack of relief suggests it is a pain referred from viscera (see also Chap. 28).

Prognostic Blocks. Properly applied, certain nerve blocks may be used prior to prolonged interruption either by injection of neurolytic agents or by neurosurgical section. Interpretation of such blocks is discussed in Chapter 27.1. Moreover, prognostic blocks may give patients an opportunity to experience the numbness and other side-effects following surgery or neurolytic block and help them decide whether to have the procedure. Although clinical evidence suggests that this tool has certain limitations in predicting the long-term effects of spinal rhizotomy, it is still useful especially when prolonged interruption is to be carried out in patients with cancer pain (see also Chap. 30).

TABLE 31-4. INDICATIONS FOR NEURAL BLOCKADE IN THE PAIN CLINIC

Diagnostic
Dermatomal distribution
Somatic versus visceral etiology
Prognostic
Prophylactic
Acute pain
Chronic pain
Therapeutic
Interruption of "vicious cycles"
As adjunct to other therapies
Neurolytic sympathectomy for vascular disease
Neurolytic blocks for cancer (short life expectancy)

Prophylactic Blocks. A variety of nerve blocks are used to prevent pain and the delay of normal functional activity that follows trauma, infections, or operations. In some centers, nerve block procedures are considered some of the most efficient methods to control postoperative or post-traumatic pain, thus effecting earlier functional rehabilitation and prevention of complications (see Chap. 26). Moreover, there is evidence that analgesia achieved with regional block for several days decreases the incidence of reflex sympathetic dystrophy and other chronic pain syndromes.

Therapeutic Blocks. Local anesthesia and nerve blocks using local anesthetics are effective in treating self-limiting disease accompanied by severe pain and in breaking up the so-called "vicious circle" in patients with causalgia and other reflex sympathetic dystrophy, myofascial syndromes, and reflex muscle spasm. It provides symptomatic relief to permit other therapeutic measures or to use as an adjunct to other therapeutic modalities (see Chap. 27). Therapeutic blocks with neurolytic agents are usually limited to patients with cancer pain, although they may be indicated in selected patients with trigeminal neuralgia, causalgia, chronic pancreatitis, severe angina pectoris, or other chronic disorders in patients who cannot tolerate a neurosurgical operation (see Chap. 29.2). Neurolytic blocks are especially useful in patients with chronic peripheral vascular disease (see Chap. 13). These are discussed in detail in preceding chapters.

BASIC PRINCIPLES OF APPLICATION

For many years neural blockade was used in an empirical and often haphazard fashion, resulting not infrequently in failures and, at times, complications. These, in turn, resulted from deficiencies in applying this method by anesthesiologists or other physicians,[3,4] including [1] inadequate knowledge of pain syndromes; [2] inadequate evaluation of patients; [3] lack of knowledge of other therapeutic modalities that should be used in conjunction with nerve blocks as a multimodal form of therapy; [4] inadequate management of the patient before, during, and after carrying out the procedure; and [5] lack of appreciation of the specific indications, limitations, and possible complications of these procedures. The realization and full appreciation of these deficiencies prompted me soon after I began to use these tools to develop certain basic principles of application, first stated three decades ago in my book[3] and repeatedly reaffirmed with greater conviction as a result of increasing experience (Table 31-5).[4,5,7]

The first and one of the foremost principles is that the anesthesiologist or any other doctor using these procedures must assume the responsibility of the physician and not act as a mere technician, expert at inserting needles. Even when acting as a consultant skilled in neural blockade, it is important that the anesthesiologist have ample insight into the patient and his pain problem.

The second requisite is that the physician using this method must have ample knowledge of various pain syndromes, including the mechanisms and nociceptive pathways involved, the pathophysiology, and the symptoms. It is essential to know the advantages, disadvantages, limitations, and complications of the other therapeutic modalities that may be applicable for each syndrome. Only with this broad perspective can the best treatment or combination of treatments be chosen for each patient with a specific pain problem.

Third, the physician must be willing to devote the time and effort to examine the patient thoroughly and confirm the diagnosis. This is essential even if the patient is referred by a highly competent colleague who has already made the diagnosis. A detailed history and thorough physical examination not only provide additional information but also afford an op-

TABLE 31-5. PRINCIPLES OF USE OF NEURAL BLOCKADE

1. Avoidance of failures, complications, inappropriate use by
    - Knowledge of pain syndromes
    - Careful evaluation of patients
    - Knowledge of alternative treatments
    - Knowledge of adjunctive treatments
    - Careful management before, during, and after block
    - Appreciation of indications, limitations, complications
2. Assistant present and appropriate resuscitative equipment/drugs
3. High degree of skill and gentleness in neural blockade
4. Use of high-quality equipment
5. Clear explanation to patient of block, its rationale, and complications
6. Reassurance and appropriate supplementation before and during block
7. Precise localization, for example, with nerve stimulator, image intensifier
8. Use of minimal volumes (plus contrast media if needed)
9. Decisions based only on repeated blocks
10. Differing durations of local anesthetic and "placebo"
11. *Independent* assessment of success of nerve pathway block, degree of pain relief, change in blood flow, and so forth (see Chap. 13)
12. Use results of block in context of *all other information* from multidisciplinary group

portunity to become acquainted with the patient, to investigate his personality, and, most important, to establish rapport with, and win the confidence of, the patient. A careful neurologic examination not only provides useful information, but also constitutes a baseline in evaluating the effects of the block. These basic principles apply to all patients, particularly those with complex pain problems.

Once a tentative diagnosis has been made, it must be decided if the neural blockade is to be used at all and, if so, whether it is to be used to gain information to predict the effect of prolonged interruption or used for therapy. It is essential to avoid the haphazard use of this tool because it may cause more harm than good.

Another important requisite is that the individual be highly skilled in carrying out the appropriate neural blockade technique and thoroughly know the immediate and long-term effects of the agents used. Patients with chronic pain are not good subjects in whom to practice nerve blocks. The skill should be acquired by first observing experts doing the blocks and then performing them under their supervision. It deserves reemphasis that in patients with severe pain, especially complex chronic pain, neural blockade must be performed carefully with meticulous attention to anatomic detail, with utmost gentleness and by using high-quality equipment, including sharp needles, syringes that are in good working order and well-fitting, and a block tray adequately stocked with other necessary instruments (see Chap. 6).

It is important to inform the patient what procedure will be done, how it will be done, and what is to be accomplished by it. If the patient does not realize that the procedure is done only to gain information and that it may provide only temporary or no relief, he may be disappointed prematurely and may not return for further care. In addition to providing this information during the initial visit, it should be repeated just before the block. Moreover, the patient should be reassured that everything will be done to minimize discomfort, that he will be warned before each step of the procedure is carried out, and that he may ask for a brief rest any time he deems it necessary. In addition, if repeated therapeutic blocks are to be done, appropriate sedatives or narcotics may be used before and during the block.

If the procedure is to be done for diagnostic or prognostic purposes, depressant drugs should not be given because the patient must be alert to answer questions. It is essential to localize exactly the involved nerve or nerves. This can be accomplished by checking the position of the needle with an x-ray or image intensifier with or without prior injection of a contrast medium. Moreover, in using diagnostic or prognostic blocks, three essential principles must be adhered to: [1] Inject small (3–4 ml) amounts of solution to avoid diffusion to adjacent segments and to preclude misleading information; [2] no decision should be made until three or more blocks produce consistent responses; and [3] it is best to use local anesthetics of different duration and correlate the duration of the block with the duration of pain relief. Use of "placebo" block may be added to help determine the diagnosis.

During and after the block, it is essential to assess the results carefully. Observation of the patient's reaction to the insertion of a thin needle, the formation of intracutaneous analgesic wheals, and other parts of the procedure help in evaluating response to noxious stimuli. After the block, it is essential to ascertain whether the nerve pathways have been interrupted by repeating the neurologic examination, and, when that has been established, the effects on pain relief, the pathophysiology, or both must be carefully assessed. This may require a few hours or several days of observation. The amount, type, and duration of relief should be noted carefully and recorded on the patient's chart. In addition to observation by the physician, the results should be evaluated by the patient and his family, if they are available, and, most importantly, by the nursing staff.

All concerned must appreciate the fact that neural blockade is not a panacea and has limitations in helping to make a diagnosis or predict the effects of prolonged interruption. Although they are effective and have advantages in a significant percentage of properly selected patients, it is essential to use the results of blockade within the framework of all other information obtained. To make the final diagnosis solely on the results of one or even several blocks is hazardous and may subject the patient to a useless destructive operation.

The patient and physicians must realize that these procedures produce side-effects that may cause potentially serious complications. Therefore, all prophylactic measures against undesirable side-effects must be carried out. An absolute requisite is that *no block* (other than infiltration of 3–5 ml of local anesthetic into superficial parts of the body) be done *without an assistant present and resuscitative equipment ready for immediate use.* This should include an intravenous infusion started before the procedure is initiated so that it is available for prompt administration of drugs to combat systemic reactions, arterial hypotension, or high spinal anesthesia—the three complications of blocks that are most likely to be problematic (see Chaps. 4, 7, 8).

Finally, it is critical to use neural blockade, for the therapy of chronic pain in patients in whom environmental/sociologic/operant factors are the primary causes, as part of a multimodel rehabilitation program.

PAIN PROGRAMS IN OTHER COUNTRIES

Based on various sources of data, it can be crudely estimated that in 1986 there were between 1000 and 1200 pain programs in the United States and between 500 and 600 programs in other countries. According to data reported by Lipton and Wells[24] in 1983 and by Bullingham and associates[13] in 1985, it is estimated that between 200 and 225 programs exist in the United Kingdom. Moreover, assuming that the rate of growth of programs in other countries has followed the pattern suggested by the *International Pain Center/Clinics Directory* in 1979, there should be between 200 and 250 on the European continent, a similar number in Asia and Australasia, and between 60 and 75 in Canada.

It is likely that the organization and function of the programs in Canada are somewhat similar to those in the United States, whereas those in the United Kingdom and continental Europe (and to some extent in Asia and Australasia) are run mainly by anesthesiologists who have tended to rely heavily on neural blockade with local anesthetics for nonmalignant chronic pain syndromes and acute pain and neurolytic blocks, percutaneous cordotomy, and intraspinal narcotics for cancer pain control. There has been, however, a movement toward multidisciplinary clinics.

Based on the report by Bullingham and associates,[13] the degree of service offered in the United Kingdom varies from clinic to clinic. Although some clinics accept patients with any form of painful pathology referred by the hospital consultant or general practitioner, a minority will accept only patients with predetermined pathologic conditions such as cancer or arthritis. According to these authors, the services provided may be arbitrarily divided into three strata of complexity: minimal, limited service, and comprehensive service.

The minimal program involves only one consultant who sees patients outside the normal working hours. The facilities for both examining and treating patients will be available on an *ad hoc* basis, probably in a 1-day care unit or a recovery room in the operating theater. The secretary and other staff and the financial requirements for equipment are met from the parent department. Although this type of service is difficult and stressful to run, it usually constitutes the foundation of any further enlargement and evolution into the next stage.

Limited service programs are run by a consultant who has acquired a formal sessional commitment with which to provide his service that includes at least one session for consultation and one for treatment. Moreover, some of these programs eventually have one or more additional consultants to share the workload and gradually increase the referral area, accepting patients referred from both hospital colleagues and also from general practitioners. Such programs also eventually obtain a post for a secretary, which is deemed critical. A clinic providing limited service usually manages between 100 and 350 new patients per year. As the program increases, eventually it will require beds allocated for managing of inpatients. Once all of these resources have been acquired, the service can function adequately to provide a service to a district or population of 250,000.

A comprehensive service clinic seeks to provide a complete range of techniques and facilities for evaluation and treatment, along with structured training and research programs. The staffing for such service is based on a figure of two consultant sessions (one outpatient, one operating theater) for every 250,000 of population served and whether this service is regional or subregional, which would necessitate two or three consultants devoting half their sessional time to pain diagnosis and therapy. These authors believe that this is necessary not only to cope with the increased clinical administrative teaching and research programs, but also to provide continuity of service throughout the year. Apparently, a number of comprehensive pain centers have their own self-contained unit with outpatient and inpatient facilities and resources for administration, research, and training. These units have appropriate medical staff, nursing ancillary staff, and a formal allocation of junior medical staff that consists of anesthesia registrars who are required by the Faculty of Anaesthetists of the Royal College of Surgeons to have training in pain therapy.

In their report, Bullingham and colleagues[13] provided a concise description of these various programs and the different sources of funding currently available to support such programs. They emphasized the need for widespread publicity and other public relations programs to inform the lay public as well as their medical colleagues about the availability of such pain relief clinics. Lipton and Wells[24] also provide a general overview of the medical, nursing, and other staff personnel available, describe the referral system used and various procedures and agents employed by pain relief clinics, and give details about teaching programs for physicians and nurses, and seminars for members of the program.

CONCLUSION

The proper management of patients with pain remains one of the most important and pressing problems in the health care system of most medically advanced countries. This importance stems from the fact that acute and chronic pain requiring the care of physicians afflicts millions and millions of people worldwide and that many patients with acute pain, and most with chronic pain, are inadequately managed. Consequently, acute and chronic pain constitute the most frequent causes of suffering and disability. During the past 15 years, an increasing number of multidisciplinary/interdisciplinary pain clinics or centers have been developed to manage patients with a complex pain problem. Anesthesiologists have played an important role in this worldwide movement; indeed most of these programs are directed by anesthesiologists. Within the framework of multidisciplinary pain programs, neural blockade remains an important diagnostic and therapeutic tool in managing patients with various pain problems. Although as a result of new information the role of neural blockade in managing patients with nonmalignant chronic pain has diminished, this has been balanced by the advent and widespread use of intraspinal opioids and other spinal antinociceptive agents (see Chap. 28), which is an exacting development of neural blockade.

REFERENCES

1. Alexander, F.A.D.: Anesthesiology. In Hale, D. (ed.): Control of Pain, Chap. 28. Philadelphia, Davis, 1954.
2. McEwen, B.W., DeWilde, F.W., Dwyer, B., Woodforde, J.W., Bleasel, and Connelly, T.J.: The pain clinic: A clinic for the management of intractable pain. Med. J. Aust., *1*:676, 682, 1965.
3. Bonica, J.J.: The Management of Pain. Philadelphia, Lea & Febiger, 1953.
4. Bonica, J.J.: Diagnostic and therapeutic blocks. A reappraisal based on 15 years' experience. Anesth. Analg., *37*:58–68, 1958.
5. Bonica, J.J.: Clinical Applications of Diagnostic and Therapeutic Nerve Blocks. Springfield, Ill., Charles C Thomas, 1959.
6. Bonica, J.J., Benedetti, C., Murphy, T.M.: Functions of pain clinics and pain centres. In Swerdlow, M. (ed.): Relief of Intractable Pain, 3rd ed., pp. 65–84. Amsterdam, Elsevier, 1983.
7. Bonica, J.J.: Local anaesthesia and regional blocks. In Wall, P.D., Melzack, R. (eds.): Textbook of Pain, pp. 541–557. Edinburgh, Churchill Livingstone, 1984.
8. Bonica, J.J.: History of pain concepts and pain therapy. Semin. Anesth., *4*:189–208, 1985.
9. Bonica, J.J.: Evolution of pain concepts and pain clinics. In Brena, S.F., Chapman, S.L. (eds.): Chronic Pain: Management Principles. Clinics in Anaesthesiology, pp. 1–16. Philadelphia, W.B. Saunders, 1985.
10. Brena, S.F., Ferrero, B.: Die Sympaticus Blockade In der Behandlung einiger Schmerzsyndrome. Anesthetist., *7/11*:321–327, 1958.
11. Brena, S.F.: Nerve blocks and chronic pain states—an update. Postgrad. Med., *78*:62–90, 1985.
12. Brena, S.F.: Pain control facilities: Pattern of operation and problems of organization in the USA. In Brena, S.F., Chapman, S.L. (eds.): Chronic Pain: Management Principles. Clinics in Anaesthesiology, pp. 183–195. Philadelphia, W.B. Saunders, 1985.
13. Bullingham, R.E.S., McQuay, H.J., Budd, K.: Pain control centres: Problems of organization and operation in the U.K. In Brena, S.F., Chapman, S.L. (eds.): Chronic Pain: Management Principles. Clinics in Anaesthesiology, pp. 211–222. Philadelphia, W.B. Saunders, 1985.
14. Ciocatto, E., Bruzzone, P.L.: Terapie di blocco delle algie viscerali e periferiche. Gior. Ital. Anestesiol., *18*:241, 1952.
15. Crue, B.L.: What is a pain center? Bull. L.A. Neurol. Soc., *41*:160–167, 1976.
16. Crue, B.L.: Multidisciplinary pain treatment programs: Current status. Clin. J. Pain., *1*:31–38, 1985.
17. Dittrich, H.: The pain clinic. Curr. Res. Anesth. Analg., *29*:60, 1950.
18. Fordyce, W.E.: Behavioral Methods for Chronic Pain and Illness. St. Louis, C.V. Mosby, 1976.
19. Fox, A.J., Melzack, R.: Transcutaneous electrical stimulation in acupuncture: Comparison of treatment of low back pain. Pain, *2*:141–148, 1976.
20. Goldscheider, A.: Ueber den Schmerz in Physiologischer und Klinischer Hinsicht. Berlin, Hirschwald, 1894.
21. Gordon, R.A.: Application of nerve block in diagnosis and treatment. Can. Med. Assoc. J., *60*:251–257, 1949.
22. Lee, J.A.: Some therapeutic aspects of anaesthesia. Br. J. Anaesth., *27*:584–593, 1955.
23. Leriche, R.: Surgery of Pain. Baltimore, Williams & Wilkins, 1939.
24. Lipton, S., Wells, J.C.D.: Pain relief clinic: Starting an organization. In Lipton, S., Miles, J. (eds.): Persistent Pain, Vol. 4, pp. 159–172, New York, Grune & Stratton, 1983.
25. Livingston, W.K.: Pain Mechanisms: Physiologic Interpretation of Causalgia and Its Related States. New York, Macmillan, 1943.

26. Melzack, R., Wall, P.D.: Pain mechanisms: A new theory. Science, *150*:971–979, 1965.
27. Melzack, R.: The Puzzle of Pain. New York, Basic Books, 1973.
28. Moore, D.C.: Stellate Ganglion Block. Springfield, Ill., Charles C Thomas, 1954.
29. Morse, R.H.: Accreditation of USA chronic pain treatment facilities: Current status. In Brena, S.F., Chapman, S.L. (eds.): Chronic Pain: Management Principles. Clinics in Anaesthesiology, pp. 197–210. Philadelphia, W.B. Saunders, 1985.
30. Papper, E.M.: Some aspects of the therapy of painful states. Clin. Med. *58*:255–259, 1951.
31. Parris, W.C.V.: Nerve block therapy. In Brena, S.F., Chapman, S.L. (eds.): Chronic Pain: Management Principles. Clinics in Anaesthesiology, pp. 93–109. Philadelphia, W.B. Saunders, 1985.
32. Rovenstein, E.A., Wertheim, H.M.: Therapeutic nerve block. J.A.M.A., *117*:1599–1603, 1941.
33. Ruben, J.E.: Experiences with a pain clinic. Anesthesiology, *12*:601–603, 1951.
34. Ruth, H.: Diagnostic, prognostic and therapeutic block. J.A.M.A., *102*:419, 1934.
35. Sternbach, R.A.: Pain Patients: Traits and Treatment. New York, Academic Press, 1974.
36. Stubbs, D.: Cited by Dittrich, H. (Ref. 14).
37. Taylor, H.: The Nuprin Report: A survey of the prevalence of pain in the United States. Lou Harris and Associates, September 1985.
38. von Frey, M.: Ber. Verhandl. konig. Sachs. Ges. Wiss. Leipzig. Beitrage Physiol. Schmerzsinnes, *46*:185–196, 1894.
39. Woodbridge, P.D.: Therapeutic nerve block with procaine and alcohol. Am. J. Surg., *9*:278–288, 1930.

32 NEW HORIZONS

MICHAEL J. COUSINS

It is interesting to note that most of the "new horizons" discussed in the first edition of *Neural Blockade* have become significant areas in the second edition: *spinal opioids* (see Chap. 28); *cryoanalgesia* (see Chap. 29.2); *assessment of pain and its sequelae* (see Chaps. 13, 24.1, 25, 27.1, 31); and *pharmacokinetics* (see Chaps. 3, 6, 26, 27.2, 28). All of these areas continue to be vigorously investigated, and the new horizons are discussed in the appropriate chapters. *Education* has remained as an important horizon, perhaps the biggest challenge in all aspects of treatment of acute as well as chronic pain (see Chap. 24.1). Additional new horizons include

- pediatric pain relief;
- optimizing the use of neural blockade in a pain unit facility;
- optimizing local anesthetic action; and
- molecular engineering and a local anesthetic receptor.

EDUCATIONAL HORIZONS

In the treatment of most forms of acute pain, the knowledge and techniques are now available to achieve a high success rate.[1] One needs only to observe that the effective use of epidural blockade can relieve labor pain in more than 95% of patients (see Chap. 18). Yet in other areas of acute pain, the success rate in major hospitals in the developed world is less than 50% (see Chap. 24.1). The challenge lies in education: [1] of patients that better relief can and should be achieved; [2] of nursing staff that this aim is safe and desirable; [3] of nursing staff to develop protocols and expertise to manage the available techniques; [4] of house staff, surgeons, and others to help implement treatment; [5] of anesthesiologists; [6] of health authorities to provide the staff and funds. A critical step is the *collaboration* of anesthesiologists, nurses, and administrators to devise the practical steps required for implementation of effective treatment.[1] Ongoing education and review of results are vital. In some centers, pain is charted along with temperature, pulse, and other variables. Orders are written to respond to changes in pain score. The availability of such data and of a member of the nursing staff to provide quality control would achieve rapid results. The mere implementation of a method of charting pain and of an agreed-upon protocol for pain treatment is likely to effect improvement greatly. A small increment in the staff of a pain unit could add to the treatment of acute pain throughout a hospital, much as intensive care units have improved the overall quality of acute care in hospitals. I believe that it is desirable and cost effective for a pain unit in a hospital to act as an educational, treatment, and research focus for acute as well as chronic pain. This is offered as a challenge to those units that focus only on chronic pain.

Chronic cancer pain is able to be relieved in a large percentage of patients by simple measures.[6,13,14] Yet this is not occurring. All those involved in chronic pain treatment have an obligation to educate in the same areas as are indicated above under acute pain. Some pain clinics do not manage cancer pain at all, even when they are located in hospitals with a significant cancer service. This deprives patients of a full range of treatment options, narrows the educational base of those outside the pain clinic, and progressively distorts the view of pain clinic members. The syndromes of cancer pain[6] can act as a vital "reference point" for those involved in treating other types of chronic pain. The relief of cancer pain should be a top priority of pain clinics in hospitals, which should act as a treatment resource, and an educational resource with regard to the wider aspects of chronic pain. For example, some oncologists are unknowledgeable about "deafferentation" pain, yet some of their patients will develop this problem (see Chap. 30). On the other hand, only a percentage of patients with cancer pain need to be treated by pain clinic staff *provided* that palliative care/hospice resources are available and there is a good education program on the options for cancer pain treatment.

Chronic noncancer pain is undoubtedly the most difficult and most challenging educational horizon in both developed and developing countries. Education must include the general public, governments, undergraduates, and postgraduates in all of the health care professions. Substantial financial and physical resources are required. However, the costs in human suffering and financial terms *of not providing these resources* are even greater. Education programs are now being developed by the World Health Organization, by the International Association for the Study of Pain (IASP), and by other bodies. An encouraging development is the formation by the IASP of an International Pain Foundation that aims to support such educational programs. This could herald one of the most exciting and rewarding horizons in medicine.

Within the context of this upsurge of interest in treatment of cancer and noncancer pain, techniques of neural blockade will play a significant part. Before an education program can be mounted for neural blockade, important steps need to be taken:

1. For cancer pain, more definitive data are needed on the safety and efficacy of neurolytic and neurodestructive techniques as well as on spinal opioids for cancer pain (see Chaps. 28–30).
2. For cancer pain, data are needed on the role of (1) compared to less invasive options such as oral opioids, subcutaneous opioid infusion, and transdermal opioid and nonpharmacologic techniques.
3. For noncancer pain, data are required for the reliability of diagnostic and prognostic local anesthetic and "opioid" neural blockade, for the efficacy of therapeutic neural blockade, and for the safety, efficacy, and rationale of neurolytic blockade (see Chaps. 27.1, 27.2, 27.3, and 29).
4. For noncancer pain, data are required for the relative place of neural blockade compared to other options for diagnosis and treatment.
5. When available, the information from (1–4) needs to be developed into educational programs.
6. For all types of chronic pain, *protocols are needed* for nursing and other staff to manage patients safely during and after neural blockade.
7. Educational resources are needed to teach staff to use protocols in (6), for example, to teach "district nurses" (home care nurses) to manage patients at home with implanted epidural opioid systems and after other methods of neural blockade.

The need for more definitive data before formulating an educational program can be illustrated by the following examples of cancer pain treatment. Some experienced doctors involved in hospice/palliative care claim that almost all patients can have their pain effectively managed with oral medication, including opioids and "coanalgesics" (see Table 24-1). However, objective data in one study indicate that eventually about 30% of patients may require neural blockade of some type to obtain complete pain relief.[14] Some "pain specialists" are implanting spinal opioid systems in large numbers of patients and frequently are using neurolytic and neurodestructive techniques for cancer pain. There is an urgent need for comparative data to give perspective on efficacy, relative incidence of side-effects, and rational use of the various alternatives that now exist for cancer pain.

PEDIATRIC PAIN RELIEF

Relief of all forms of severe pain in children has received too little attention. Encouraging advances in intraoperative and postoperative use of neural blockade are described in Chapter 21. However, much remains to be done in critical care units, specialized medical units, accident and emergency departments, oncology units, and pain units that treat chronic noncancer pain in children. The myth that children feel less pain than adults has been exposed.[10] Unfortunately it was the ability of adults to assess and document pain in children that was lacking. A classic example is the chilling view that circumcision in young children is painless. Any anesthetist is familiar with the laryngeal spasm that is the result of too light a plane of general anesthesia for circumcision. Other evidence for this was recently obtained, in full-term infants, by the sharp decrease in oxygen saturation and increased heart rate and blood pressure in response to "cold" circumcision. In comparison, infants who received penile local anesthetic block showed no such changes. "Blind" observers could easily identify signs that all the unanesthetized infants were experiencing pain.[11]

Studies of the physiology and pharmacology of neural blockade are at last gaining impetus in children. It is significant to note that hemodynamic responses appear more favorable in children than in adults, particularly in those above 8 years of age.[3] The use of general anesthesia before "supplementary" neural blockade is sensible to avoid discomfort and establish baseline analgesia so that the block can provide postoperative pain relief (*e.g.*, epidural catheter technique). In the future another approach may be to use pretreatment with "transdermal" patches of local anesthetic (see below) before using any neural blockade technique. A further method of minimizing discomfort is the use of small doses of intravenous sedatives and opioids and of minimal electrical stimulus by means of a peripheral nerve stimulator to locate a nerve or plexus. Intraoperative nerve blocks, plexus blocks, epidural blocks, and other techniques are becoming more widely used in children. It is vital that their performance inflict no pain on the child—thus the need for an approach similar to that described above. It is to be hoped that successful techniques used in adults will be evaluated for their relative efficacy and safety in children, for example, continuous epidural infusion of local anesthetic or local anesthetic/opioid, intravenous opioid infusions, transdermal opioids, transdermal local anesthetics, and intrapleural local anesthetics.[12]

OPTIMIZING THE USE OF NEURAL BLOCKADE IN A PAIN UNIT FACILITY

To optimize the use of the neural blockade techniques described in *Neural Blockade,* I suggest an approach to develop funding, personnel resources, and facilities. *Funding* is likely to be more readily obtained from both government and private sources if a pain unit treats acute pain, cancer pain, and noncancer pain. *Personnel* can be much more economically employed in this situation. For example, acute pain would mainly involve anesthesiologists but also nurses, physical therapists, and clinical psychologists. In some hospitals, funding of these staff only for acute or chronic pain is not possible. As indicated above, the chronic noncancer pain expertise of this unit is invaluable for cancer pain. The type of outreach program that can be developed, and sometimes more easily funded, for cancer pain is very valuable for some forms of noncancer pain. Many pain clinics have little first-hand knowledge of the family, work, social, and other aspects of their patients that can be obtained only by staff working directly in these areas. In many countries there are social workers, "district" nurses, home care programs, work-associated nursing and medical staff and rehabilitation centers, clinics for sexual difficulties, and even home-care volunteer programs. Yet some pain clinics have minimal or no contact with these vital ingredients of effective cancer and chronic noncancer pain treatment. Minimal centralized liaison staff in a pain clinic may tap into these resources to ensure that patients gain access and that the clinic obtains feedback on these important areas.

LIAISON OF PAIN UNIT WITH HOSPITAL-BASED PALLIATIVE CARE SERVICE

The Flinders Medical Centre (FMC) Pain Management Unit (PMU) has a close liaison with a Palliative Care Service (PCS) based in FMC (Fig. 32-1). The PCS provides care either in FMC, in the patient's home (more than 70% of total treatment days) or in a small adjacent hospice unit. The PCS has close contact with oncologists and radiotherapists, among others. The PMU acts as a resource for symptom control of pain in all three sites where patients are treated. The PMU and PCS have centralized resources that allow them to arrange and coordinate the activities of general practitioners (GPs) and home-care professionals (domicillary care, district nurses) who visit patients in their homes and a team of volunteers who provide additional support and help. There is also a team of clergy who work with the unit, for those patients wishing to have such help. Nursing and medical staff from the PMU and the PCS also visit patients in the hospice and at home to supplement the above care as needed. Much interchange occurs through PMU and PCS liaison nursing staff who report back to PMU and PCS either in person at regular treatment discussions or by telephone. District nurses and GPs also regularly contact the units (PMU and PCS).

The availability of experienced nursing, administrative, and secretarial staff in the central facility is vital. Once peripheral staff are familiar with the work of the unit, they can carry out much of this care. Time invested in training programs and in "refresher courses" pays large dividends.

What has all of this infrastructure to do with neural blockade? It is likely that less invasive options will be used effectively in the setting described above. Also

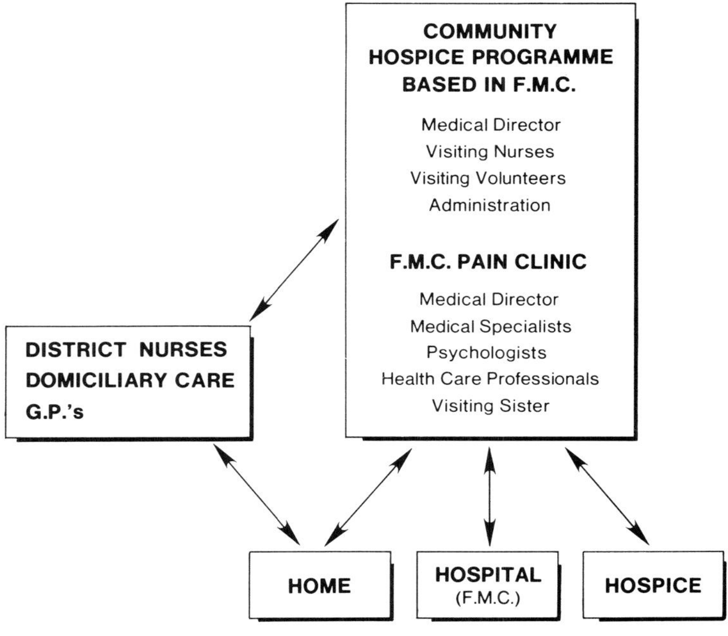

FIG. 32-1. FMC Pain Management Unit (PMU) and FMC "Community" Hospice Programme, Palliative Care Service (PCS) (see text). Staff in these two hospital-based units work closely together and coordinate with community-based staff such as general practitioners (GPs), district nurses, domiciliary care staff, and volunteers. Thus the two units can deliver pain relief as part of an integrated symptom-control program that cares for patients in the hospital (FMC), in a nearby hospice, or in the patient's home.

there is good access to ongoing review of the general medical condition of the patient, and thus the best possible review of the progress of the cancer and of the cause of the cancer pain. The safe and effective management of techniques such as spinal opioids depends heavily on this infrastructure. In the FMC PMU program, epidural portals and Infusaids were introduced by first running a training program for hospital, hospice, and district nurses. These staff and PMU staff now train patients and relatives to manage the epidural portals, with a high success rate (see Chap. 28). Patients can be maintained at home for most of their remaining lives because of the home support, the rapid liaison with expert help, and the knowledge that they can be readmitted to the hospice for readjustment of pain control. The latter is achieved speedily without having to go through the "system" of a large hospital. More minor problems are sorted out on a same-day basis in the PMU facility, which is designed for such treatment (see below). The unit has a policy of meeting cancer pain consultations within 24 hours or less.

DESIGN OF PAIN UNIT FACILITY

The FMC PMU advocated the foregoing rationale for the effective and economical treatment of severe pain for many years. In 1985, state government funding was provided for a purpose-designed facility and for appropriate staff. The principles of staffing are similar to those discussed in Chapter 31, except for the outreach component. The physical facility is self-contained but attached to the main hospital (Fig. 32-2). Both inpatients and outpatients are treated in the unit. Inpatient consultations are usually carried out in the inpatient wards; however, all inpatient treatments are performed in the unit. Some aspects of the design of the unit have a special bearing on the optimal use of neural blockade (Fig. 32-2):

1. "Day-care" patients have diagnostic and therapeutic local anesthetic blocks in a specially designed area. They then move to the adjacent holding area.
2. Patients who require pharmacokinetic studies for stabilization of oral opioid or other drug therapy are treated in an area within the unit. Thus this is an equally practicable option to neural blockade.
3. The design of the nurses station and the proximity of all areas allow considerable economy of nursing staff numbers.
4. A procedure room is equipped with operating table, translucent table top, and image intensifier. This room is used for neurolytic blocks, neurodestructive and neurostimulation procedures, and implantation of spinal opioid systems. All of these can be carried out under local anesthesia, on a day-care basis if required. For example, about five neurolytic sympathetic blocks are performed each week for pain caused by peripheral vascular disease.[2] This procedure takes 10 to 15 minutes, with an additional 30-minute rest before the patient returns home (see Chap. 13). Over the past 10 years the clinic has treated nearly 2500 patients with the technique with no direct mortality. The cost saving compared to inpatient treatment would be 15,000 to 25,000 inpatient bed days and surgical and other medical fees. Epidural opioid systems and other techniques can also be handled in this manner provided that a trained and capable team is available for home care or return to hospice or other venue. There is no doubt that many patients with cancer pain, and other forms of chronic

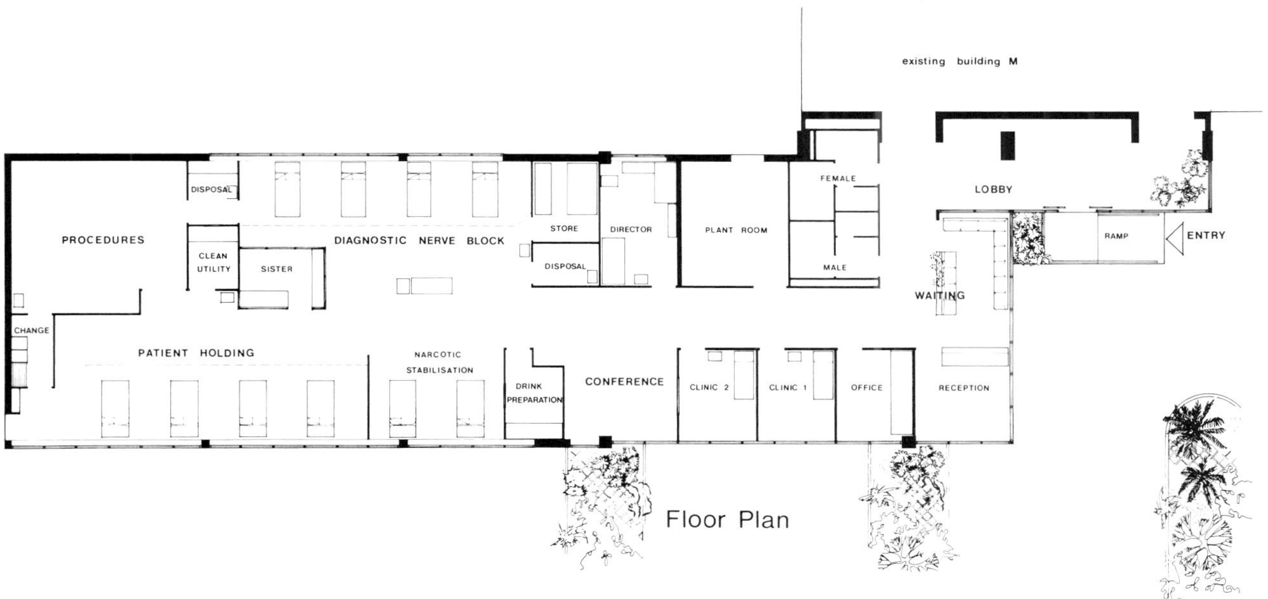

FIG. 32-2. FMC Pain Management Unit. The unit is purpose designed and self-contained; however, it is linked to the main hospital building (Building M) so that inpatients and outpatients can be transported to and from the unit and other areas if required. The ground level entrance allows easy access for patients delivered by car or ambulance. The outpatient clinic area adjoins a conference room and library. The *narcotic stabilization area* is used mostly for patients with cancer pain but also for some patients with refractory noncancer pain of nociceptive origin; opioid pharmacokinetic studies, pain evaluation, and side-effect monitoring are carried out. The *diagnostic nerve block area* is used also for adjunctive therapy, such as physical therapy after neural blockade. The *holding area* is used for outpatients and inpatients who are waiting for, or recovering from, procedures. The *nurses' station* has a clear view of all areas. The *procedure room* is used for all major neurolytic, neurodestructive, neurostimulation, and spinal opioid techniques.

pain, develop an aversion to hospitals, operating rooms, and similar environments. Direct "day-only" access to a pain unit, which has empathetic staff and a less-threatening environment than that of the major hospital, gives patients the courage to have the treatment they would otherwise often refuse. Some patients, of course, require inpatient assessment and treatment. However, the treatment aspect is much less of an ordeal when carried out in a familiar, reassuring environment.

The provision of specialized equipment, highly trained support staff, and a controlled environment allows much greater consistency in technique and greatly improves efficacy and safety of neural blockade. Any major region can and should afford such a facility.

OPTIMIZING LOCAL ANESTHETIC ACTION

DERMAL PREPARATIONS

A formulation of local anesthetic that was effective and safe for use on the skin would be highly desirable. Recently a cream comprising a eutectic mixture of 5% lidocaine and prilocaine has been reported to produce attenuation of pain associated with the insertion of a 16-gauge intravenous cannula; a minimum application time of 45 minutes is required.[5] Further development of dermal preparation would be invaluable as a prelude to all neural blockade, but particularly in children.

*p*H ADJUSTMENT

Adjustment of local anesthetic *p*H with the addition of bicarbonate solution before injection has been reported to shorten latency of onset of blockade, increase efficacy of block of certain segments, and increase duration of block.[7] These findings should be pursued with the aim of confirming efficacy and safety for the different methods of neural blockade. In the meantime *ad hoc* *p*H adjustment seems undesirable.

LONG-ACTING LOCAL ANESTHETIC FORMULATIONS

Rather than developing local anesthetic molecules with a longer duration of action, an innovative approach has been to develop novel formulations of local anesthetics that allow slow, sustained release of the drug. This is the same type of philosophy that resulted in slow-release formulations of oral morphine. One report describes the preparation of vesicles of L-a-phosphatidylcholine mixed with bupivacaine base to form a liposome-encapsulated bupivacaine suspension.[4] In this preparation, bupivacaine base was incorporated in the membrane and 0.75% bupivacaine hydrochloride was present in the lumen of the liposome and in the suspending watery medium. This formulation is about 38 times as viscous as bupivacaine hydrochloride solution. The liposome-encapsulated bupivacaine was compared with standard 0.75% bupivacaine hydrochloride by injecting it into the base of rat tail and testing withdrawal of tail from a heat stimulus. The liposome preparation produced analgesia of 34 hours duration compared to 5.7 hours for standard bupivacaine solution. There was no evidence of impaired function or tissue damage after the injection of either solution.[4] It was postulated that the high viscosity of the liposomes localized the blockade to the area of injection since the analgesia was present only distal to the injection site. The slow degradation of the liposomes is important in preventing the bupivacaine from reaching toxic local concentrations. The fast onset of action is due to the bupivacaine in the watery solution, and the prolonged duration is due to the multilayer phospholipid membrane acting as a storage for the lipophilic base form, which is in equilibration with the salt form in the watery phase (see p. 52).

Although not previously considered a local anesthetic, methoxyflurane has been prepared in a microdroplet formulation to produce long-lasting nerve block for chronic pain.[9] Methoxyflurane (6.7%) is encased in a monolayer of lecithin. This preparation was injected into the tail of rats and produced 25 hours of analgesia, compared to 3 hours for bupivacaine.[9]

Both of the above approaches may herald the use of conventional and nonconventional "local anesthetics" in different formulations and by different *methods of drug delivery.* This may allow greater flexibility and longer duration of analgesia for both acute and chronic pain treatment.

MOLECULAR ENGINEERING AND A LOCAL ANESTHETIC RECEPTOR

Molecular engineering has reached a high level of sophistication. Collaboration between molecular engineers, anesthesiologists, and pharmacologists resulted in spectacular improvements in molecules available for neuromuscular blockade. Drugs were "constructed" to do precisely what the clinicians requested. It is theoretically possible to apply the same approach to development of a "local anesthetic" that is much more specific than current agents. The spinal use of opioid and nonopioid drugs suggests that different molecules may be needed and that the site of action may be different from the traditional axonal blockade. One aim would be to develop a molecule that acts on a receptor capable of selective blockade of primary afferent nociceptive input to spinal cord without effects on sensory, motor, and sympathetic function. Such a molecule would be ideal for pain relief. Another aim would be a molecule with an action on receptors associated with sensory and motor fibers but without block of sympathetic fibers, so that surgery could be carried out without hypotensive side-effects. Recent studies have identified effects of local anesthetics on calcium and magnesium ATPase[8] and on other functions likely to be associated with receptors. The identification and the characterization of a "local anesthetic" receptor or receptors that fulfill the above clinical aims are important first steps before molecular engineering of ideal local anesthetic drugs.

REFERENCES

1. Cousins, M.J., and Phillips, G.D. (eds.): Acute pain management. *In* Clinics in Critical Care Medicine. Edinburgh, Churchill Livingstone, 1986.
2. Cousins, M.J., Reeve, T.S., Glynn, C.J., Walsh, J.A., *et al.*: Neurolytic lumbar sympathetic blockade: Duration of denervation and relief of rest pain. Anaesth. Intens. Care, *7*:121–135, 1979.
3. Delleur, M.M., Murat, I. and Saint-Maurice, C.: Hemodynamic changes during lumbar epidural anesthesia in children. Anesthesiology, *65*:A426, 1986.
4. Djordjevich, L., Ivankovich, A.D., Chigurupati, R., *et al.*: Efficacy of liposome-encapsulated bupivacaine. Anesthesiology, *65*:A185, 1986.
5. Evers, H., Von Dardel, O., Juhlin, L., *et al.*: Dermal effects of compositions based on the eutectic mixtures of lignocaine and prilocaine. A preliminary report (EM LA). Br. J. Anaesth., *57*:997–1005, 1985.
6. Foley, K.M.: The treatment of cancer pain. N Engl J Med., *313*:84–85, 1985.
7. Galindo, A.: pH-adjusted local anesthetics. Reg. Anesth., *8*:35–64, 1983.
8. Garcia–Martin, E., Gutijerrez–Merino, C.: Local anesthetics inhibit the Ca^{2+}, Mg^{2+} ATP-ase activity of rat brain synaptosomes. J. Neurochem., *47*:668–672, 1986.
9. Haynes, D.H., Kirkpatrick, A.F.: Ultra-long duration local anesthesia produced by injection of lecithin-coated methoxyflurane microdroplets. Anesthesiology, *63*:490–499, 1985.
10. Mather, L.E., Mackie, J.M.: The incidence of postoperative pain in children. Pain, *15*:271, 1983.
11. Maxwell, L.G., Yaster, M., and Wetzel, R.C.: Penile block reduces the physiologic stress of newborn circumcision. Anesthesiology, *65*:A432, 1986.
12. Reiestad, F., Stromskag, K.: Interpleural catheter in the management of postoperative pain: A preliminary report. Reg. Anesth., *11*:89–91, 1986.
13. Sternsward, J.: Cancer pain relief: An important global public health issue. *In* Fields, H.L., *et al.* (eds.): Advancees in Pain Research and Therapy, pp. 555–558. New York, Raven Press, 1985.
14. Ventrafridda, V., Tamburini, M., DeConno, F.: Comprehensive treatment in cancer pain. *In* Fields, H.L., *et al.* (eds.): Advances in Pain Research and Therapy, pp. 617–628. New York, Raven Press, 1985.

INDEX